Dietary Reference Intakes: Recommended Intakes for Individuals: Minerals

Life Stage Group	Calcium (mg/d)	Chromium (μg/d)	Copper (μg/d)	Fluoride (mg/d)	Iodine (μg/d)	Iron (mg/d)	Magnesium (mg/d)	Manganese (mg/d)	Molybdenum (μg/d)	Phosphorus (mg/d)	Selenium (μg/d)	Zinc (mg/d)
Infants												
0–6 mo	210*	0.2*	200*	0.01*	110*	0.27*	30*	0.003*	2*	100*	15*	2*
7–12 mo	270*	5.5*	220*	0.5*	130*	11	75*	0.6*	3*	275*	20*	3
Children												
1–3 y	500*	11*	340	0.7*	90	7	80	1.2*	17	460	20	3
4–8 y	800*	15*	440	1*	90	10	130	1.5*	22	500	30	5
Males												
9–13 y	1,300*	25*	700	2*	120	8	240	1.9*	34	1,250	40	8
14–18 y	1,300*	35*	890	3*	150	11	410	2.2*	43	1,250	55	11
19–30 y	1,000*	35*	900	4*	150	8	400	2.3*	45	700	55	11
31–50 y	1,000*	35*	900	4*	150	8	420	2.3*	45	700	55	11
51–70 y	1,200*	30*	900	4*	150	8	420	2.3*	45	700	55	11
> 70 y	1,200*	30*	900	4*	150	8	420	2.3*	45	700	55	11
Females												
9–13 y	1,300*	21*	700	2*	120	8	240	1.6*	34	1,250	40	8
14–18 y	1,300*	24*	890	3*	150	15	360	1.6*	43	1,250	55	9
19–30 y	1,000*	25*	900	3*	150	18	310	1.8*	45	700	55	8
31–50 y	1,000*	25*	900	3*	150	18	320	1.8*	45	700	55	8
51–70 y	1,200*	20*	900	3*	150	8	320	1.8*	45	700	55	8
> 70 y	1,200*	20*	900	3*	150	8	320	1.8*	45	700	55	8
Pregnancy												
≤ 18 y	1,300*	29*	1,000	3*	220	27	400	2.0*	50	1,250	60	13
19–30 y	1,000*	30*	1,000	3*	220	27	350	2.0*	50	700	60	11
31–50 y	1,000*	30*	1,000	3*	220	27	360	2.0*	50	700	60	11
Lactation												
≤ 18 y	1,300*	44*	1,300	3*	290	10	360	2.6*	50	1,250	70	14
19–30 y	1,000*	45*	1,300	3*	290	9	310	2.6*	50	700	70	12
31–50 y	1,000*	45*	1,300	3*	290	9	320	2.6*	50	700	70	12

NOTE: This table presents Recommended Dietary Allowances (RDAs) in **bold type** and Adequate Intakes (AIs) in ordinary type followed by an asterisk(*). RDAs and AIs may both be used as goals for individual intake. RDAs are set to meet the needs of almost all (97 to 98%) individuals in a group. For healthy breast-fed infants, the AI is the mean intake. The AI for other life stage and gender groups is believed to cover needs of all individuals in the group, but lack of data or uncertainty in the data prevent being able to specify with confidence the percentage of individuals covered by this intake.

Source: Trumbo, P., Schlicker, S., and Poos, M. *Dietary Reference Intakes: vitamin A, vitamin K, arsenic, boron, chromium, copper, iodine, manganese, molybdenum, nickel, silicon, vanadium, and zinc.* J. Am. Diet. Assoc. 101:294–301, 2001.

Recommended Energy and Protein Intakes

Category	Age (years) or Condition	Weight[a]		Height[a]		Average Energy Allowance (kcal)[b]		RDA for Protein
		(kg)	(lb)	(cm)	(in.)	Per kg	Per day[c]	(g/day)
Infants	0.0–0.5	6	13	60	24	108	650	13
	0.5–1.0	9	20	71	28	98	850	14
Children	1–3	13	29	90	35	102	1,300	16
	4–6	20	44	112	44	90	1,800	24
	7–10	28	62	132	52	70	2,000	28
Males	11–14	45	99	157	62	55	2,500	45
	15–18	66	145	176	69	45	3,000	59
	19–24	72	160	177	70	40	2,900	58
	25–50	79	174	176	70	37	2,900	63
	51+	77	170	173	68	30	2,300	63
Females	11–14	46	101	157	62	47	2,200	46
	15–18	55	120	163	64	40	2,200	44
	19–24	58	128	164	65	38	2,200	46
	25–50	63	138	163	64	36	2,200	50
	51+	65	143	160	63	30	1,900	50
Pregnant	1st trimester						+0	60
	2nd trimester						+300	60
	3rd trimester						+300	60
Lactating	1st 6 months						+500	65
	2nd 6 months						+500	62

[a]Weights and heights represent median values.

[b]In the range of light to moderate activity the coefficient of variations is ±20%.

[c]Figure is rounded.

Source: National Research Council, Food and Nutrition Board, *Recommended Dietary Allowance,* 10th ed. Washington, D.C.: National Academy Press, 1989.

NUTRITION

FROM SCIENCE TO LIFE

NUTRITION

FROM SCIENCE TO LIFE

MARY B. GROSVENOR, M.S., R.D.

LORI A. SMOLIN, PH.D.

University of Connecticut

HARCOURT COLLEGE PUBLISHERS
Fort Worth Philadelphia San Diego New York Orlando Austin San Antonio
Toronto Montreal London Sydney Tokyo

Publisher: Emily Barrosse
Acquisitions Editor: Nedah Rose
Marketing Strategist: Kathleen McLellan
Developmental Editor: Lee Marcott
Project Editor: Ellen Sklar
Production Manager: Alicia Jackson
Art Directors: Jacqui Lefranc, Caroline McGowan
Text Designer: Caroline McGowan

Cover Credit: Charles D. Winters

Nutrition: From Science to Life, 1/e
ISBN: 0-03-032159-X
Library of Congress Catalog Card Number: 2001090060

Address for domestic orders:
Harcourt College Publishers, 6277 Sea Harbor Drive, Orlando, FL 32887-6777
1-800-782-4479
e-mail collegesales@harcourt.com

Address for international orders:
International Customer Service, Harcourt, Inc.
6277 Sea Harbor Drive, Orlando FL 32887-6777
(407) 345-3800
Fax (407) 345-4060
e-mail hbintl@harcourt.com

Address for editorial correspondence:
Harcourt College Publishers, Public Ledger Building, Suite 1250, 150 S. Independence Mall West,
Philadelphia, PA 19106-3412

Web Site Address
http://www.harcourtcollege.com

Printed in the United States of America

0123456789 032 10987654321

Chapter Opener Photo Credits

Chapter 1 Opener: © Cohn

Cuthbert/Science Photo Library

Chapter 2 Opener: © Corbis

Chapter 3 Opener: © Department of Clinical Radiology, Salisbury District Hospital/Science Photo Library/Photo Researchers, Inc.

Chapter 4 Opener: © Charles D. Winters

Chapter 5 Opener: © Charles D. Winters

Chapter 6 Opener: © Brika Craddock/Science Photo Library/Photo Researchers, Inc.

Chapter 7 Opener: © D. Young-Wolff/Photo Edit

Chapter 8 Opener: © Carolyn A. McKeone/Photo Researchers, Inc.

Chapter 9 Opener: © Richard Hutchings/Photo Researchers, Inc.

Chapter 10 Opener: © Charles D. Winters

Chapter 11 Opener: © Bill Bachman/Photo Researchers, Inc.

Chapter 12 Opener: © Shaun Egan/Stone

Chapter 13 Opener: © John Eastcott/Photo Researchers, Inc.

Chapter 14 Opener: © Alain Jacquere, Agence Vandystadt/Photo Researchers, Inc.

Chapter 15 Opener: © Telegraph Colour Library/FPG International (baby); © David Parker/Science Photo Library/Photo Researchers, Inc. (silhouetted torso of pregnant woman)

Chapter 16 Opener: © Charles Thatcher/Stone

Chapter 17 Opener: © Reuters New Media Inc./Corbis

Chapter 18 Opener: © Bettmann/Corbis

Chapter 19 Opener: © Mitch Kezar/Stone

Chapter 20 Opener: © George Semple

Chapter Story Photo Credits

UNN1: © D. Young-Wolfi/PhotoEdit

UNN 2: © David Epperson/Stone

UNN 3: © Dick Luria/Photo Researchers, Inc.

UNN4: © Rodale Stock/Stone

UNN5: © Time Davis/Photo Researchers, Inc.

UNN 6: © Carl Purcell/Photo Researchers, Inc.

UNN 7: © Bob Thomas/Stone

UNN8: © Richard Hamilton Smith/Corbis

UNN 9: © Jerry Wachter/Photo Researchers, Inc.

UNN 10: © Amy C. Lira/PhotoEdit

UNN 11: © Gabriella Schiess

UNN 12: © Princess Margaret Rose Orthopaedic Hospital/Science Photo Library/Photo Researchers, Inc.

UNN13: © Eye Ubiquitons/Corbis

UNN 14: © AEP/Corbis

UNN15: © Richard Hutchinson/PhotoEdit

UNN 16: © Lori Adamski Peek/Stone

UNN17: © Lori Adamski Peek/Stone

UNN 18: © Bernd Wettich

UNN19: © Tom Uhlman/Visuals Unlimited

UNN 20: © Alan and Linda Detrick/Photo Researchers, Inc.

To our sons, Zachary and Max and David and John.
Their view of the world helps us to keep life in perspective.

To our husbands, David Knecht and Peter Ambrose,
who have given their support, patience, and understanding
over the years as well as their expertise as
computer and literary consultants.

About the Authors

Mary B. Grosvenor, M.S., R.D. Mary Grosvenor received her B.A. degree in English from Georgetown University and her M.S. in Nutrition Sciences from the University of California at Davis. She is a registered dietitian who worked for many years managing nutrition research studies at the General Clinical Research Center at Harbor–UCLA Medical Center. She has published in peer-reviewed journals in the areas of nutrition and cancer and methods of assessing dietary intake. She has taught introductory nutrition at the community college level and currently lives with her family in a small town in Colorado. She is continuing her teaching and writing career and is still involved in nutrition research via the electronic superhighway.

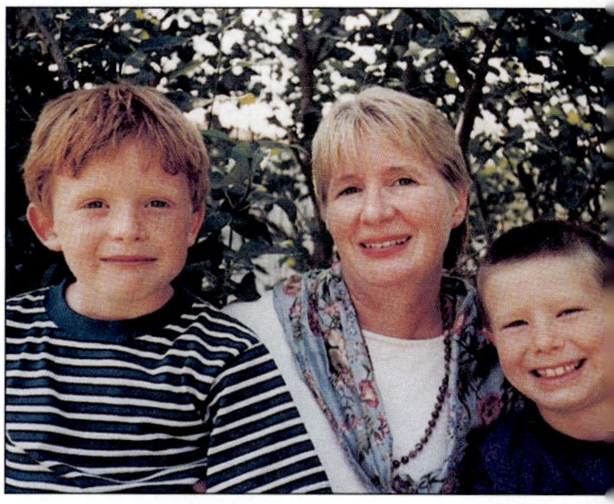

Lori A. Smolin, Ph.D. Lori Smolin received her B.S. degree from Cornell University, where she studied human nutrition and food science. She received her doctorate from the University of Wisconsin at Madison. Her doctoral research focused on B vitamins, homocysteine accumulation, and genetic defects in homocysteine metabolism. She completed postdoctoral training both at the Harbor–UCLA Medical Center, where she studied human obesity, and at the University of California at San Diego, where she studied genetic defects in amino acid metabolism. She has published in these areas in peer-reviewed journals. Dr. Smolin is currently at the University of Connecticut, where she has been involved in teaching, course development, and writing. She teaches both in the Department of Nutritional Science and in the Department of Molecular and Cell Biology. Courses she has taught include introductory nutrition, life cycle nutrition, food preparation, nutritional biochemistry, general biochemistry, and biology.

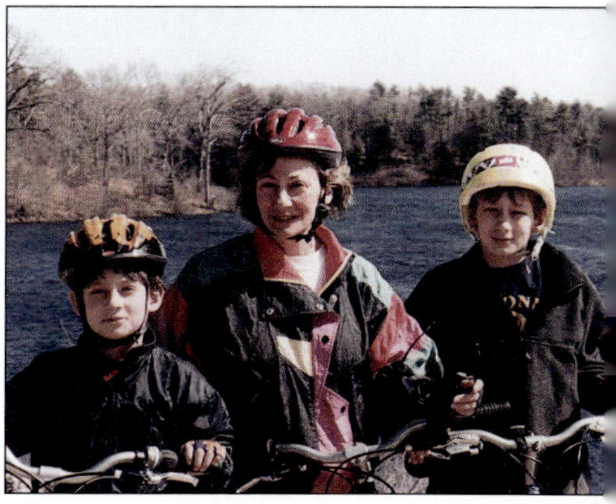

Preface

Nutrition: From Science to Life brings the science of nutrition off the pages of a book and into the lives of students. While all introductory nutrition courses offer students basic information about nutrients, their functions in the body, and their sources in the diet, this science-based text strengthens this foundation by providing students with the "how" and the "why" behind nutrition issues, allowing them to carry a broad-based knowledge out of the classroom and into their everyday lives both as consumers and as future scientists and health professionals.

This book is intended as an introductory text for a science-oriented nutrition course. A college student at any level, freshman to senior, will be comfortable with the material. Although there are no prerequisites for a course at this level, the strong biochemistry/metabolism coverage, clinical flavor, and in-depth approach to science and nutritional research make this a text that will prepare nutrition majors and other science majors for their future studies and careers. It is appropriate for either a one- or a two-semester course.

In designing a text to successfully lead students on the journey from science to life, we had several major objectives: First, to provide thorough discussions of nutrition science in a concise, consistent, engaging, and easy-to-read format; second, to introduce students to the logic needed to interpret nutrition information and make wise nutrition choices by providing examples of problem-solving and research methods; third, to be as up-to-date as possible; fourth, to intersperse nutrition science with applications that capture student interest; and finally, to provide illustrations and colorful and engaging photography along with graphics that are easy to follow and consistent from chapter to chapter. The features, themes, and learning aids used throughout the book support these objectives.

Approach and Features

Scientific Approach The study of nutrition should be alive and exciting. This book provides in-depth presentations of the methods of science while at the same time helping students understand how to make good nutrition a part their lives. In Chapter 1, we present the scientific method and discuss how it is used to evaluate the role of nutrition in health. This theme of scientific research is showcased throughout the text in *Research Discoveries,* a boxed feature that highlights recent research advances as well as classic nutrition studies. This material shows students how basic scientific research has led to discoveries that are key to our current understanding of nutrition. They also make students aware of the rich, colorful history of nutrition. For example, in Chapter 1, the Seven Countries Study is discussed. This classic study, begun in 1958, identified the relationship between saturated fat and heart disease. Other *Research Discoveries* topics include how weightlessness in space is used to study bone density, how obesity genes have been identified, how pellagra was determined to be a nutritional deficiency, and the discovery of LDL receptors, which help remove LDL cholesterol from the blood.

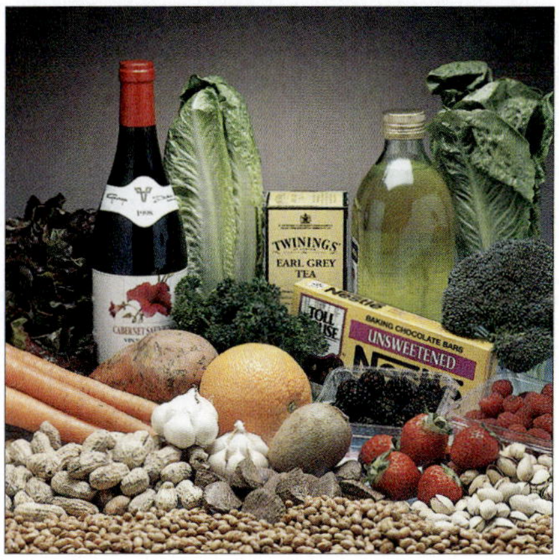

Critical Thinking and Decision-Making Skills Critical thinking skills are necessary both to understand how science works and to make decisions about nutrition and health. These skills allow students to apply their knowledge to situations that they have not previously encountered. Several features of this text promote critical thinking and the use of risk-benefit analyses in making decisions about dietary choices. *Making Decisions* is a feature that appears in each chapter to demonstrate the technique of thinking critically when making nutrition-related decisions. Each *Making Decisions* exercise demonstrates how to analyze the risks versus the potential benefits of such dietary choices as whether to use soy products, low-carbohydrate weight-loss diets, and dietary supplements. These discussions are a unique aspect of this text, briefly highlighting topics of special interest that deserve more explanation than the scope of a one-semester course allows. These can be read separately or in conjunction with the body of the text.

Each chapter also contains *Critical Thinking* exercises, which are designed to help students learn how to apply their nutrition knowledge to everyday situations. These case histories guide students through the logical thought processes involved in solving nutrition problems. Many of these support the theme of health promotion and disease prevention by focusing on optimizing diets to reduce disease risk and maintain health. Similar types of exercises are provided at the end of each chapter in a section called "Applying Critical Thinking Skills."

The theme of critical thinking through risk-benefit analysis is also applied to the text's extensive coverage of dietary supplements. Whether or not you support their use, dietary supplements are now a concern in the field of nutrition. Nutrition students should learn what supplements are, what they are marketed for, and what potential hazards they may pose. A text that does not address this topic leaves students seeking information from less reliable sources. The text's risk-benefit approach shows students how to make safe and valid decisions about the use of supplements.

Chapter Introductions Each chapter is introduced with a short case study. These health-oriented introductions help capture student interest and provide a taste of some of the critical thinking concepts that will be explored in the chapter. For example, the introduction to Chapter 6 discusses the experiences of a Peace Corps volunteer observing protein-energy malnutrition for the first time and wondering why a malnourished child would have a swollen abdomen. Chapter 10 examines the case of a toddler, adopted from China, who has rickets, and Chapter 11 recounts the story of an athlete who experienced dehydration during the 1984 Olympic marathon. Students are exposed to the critical thinking involved in understanding the issues associated with each case and are left with questions that are answered in the chapter that follows.

Integrated Metabolism Information Metabolism is one of the most challenging topics for nutrition students. This text integrates coverage of metabolism with discussions of the macronutrients, micronutrients, and exercise—rather than concentrating it into one long chapter. The information is then interspersed with applications that draw interest and highlight its importance. This approach also allows the student to build on and reinforce their understanding of metabolism gained in the previous chapter. For example, the information on fat metabolism in Chapter 5 builds on what is presented about carbohydrates in Chapter 4. Chapter 7 integrates all of the information on energy production, and Chapter 14 provides a review of it by applying its concepts to a discussion of fitness and the exercising body.

Health and Nutrition Relationships Discussions of the relationships among nutrition, good health, and disease are integrated throughout this text. Many students are drawn to the study of nutrition out of concern for personal or family health.

Integrating this information throughout the text engages students early on and continuously reinforces interest because it presents, for example, chronic diseases, such as cardiovascular disease and osteoporosis—topics of great interest—in association with those nutrients known to play a key role in increasing or decreasing the risk of such diseases. This approach keeps students motivated to learn the basics and prepares them to make decisions about their personal health and nutrition.

The Total Dietary Pattern Nutritional health depends on dietary patterns rather than on consumption of single foods or nutrients. The importance of the total dietary pattern is stressed throughout this text. While each chapter features individual nutrients, it also stresses the importance of the total diet. For example, while discussing recommendations for fat intake, the text incorporates a discussion of the importance of a varied diet based on grains, fruits, and vegetables. Several of the *Critical Thinking* exercises also help illustrate that each dietary change affects more than just one nutrient in the diet, thus helping students understand that one choice is not good or bad and does not make or break a diet.

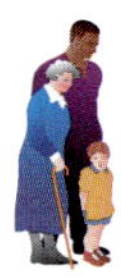

Life-Stage Integration Information about differences in nutrient requirements and nutrition concerns at various stages of life is integrated throughout the text. The completeness of the material contained in each chapter is thereby increased, offering information relevant to students in all phases of life. While there are separate chapters that cover nutrition for pregnancy, lactation, infancy, childhood, adolescence, and aging, often a one-semester course cannot encompass all this in-depth information. Thus, brief discussions—identified by **life-stage icons**—appear in each chapter to highlight issues and recommendations that apply to specific stages and circumstances of life.

Cultural Diversity College students today are a diverse cultural group. This text uses multicultural food and dietary examples to relate to all students and to expose students to the foods and eating patterns of other cultures. Differences in the disease risks of various ethnic groups in relation to their genetic makeups and their native diets are also addressed.

Environmental Issues Environmental issues can have an impact on the nutrient composition of foods as well as on consumer food choices. Advances in food production and technology that help provide a safe and adequate food supply are affecting the environment. In turn, concerns about depletion of natural resources, pollution of the air and water, and the risks of genetically modified plants and animals affect food production. These issues are addressed in a separate chapter on food technology as well as throughout the text as they relate to specific nutrients and topics.

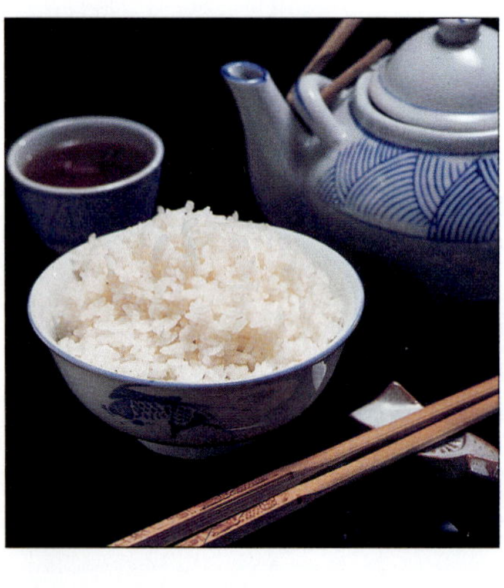

Learning Aids

Web-Enhanced Version This Harcourt textbook includes a dynamic new feature that directly links the user to additional relevant information on the Internet. Strategically placed :Cues from Digital:Convergence Inc., such as the one shown on the next page, enable students to instantly access complementary Web pages that amplify and further illustrate the principles and concepts described in the text. How does it work? Just download the free :CRQ software from www.crq.com, plug in a :CueCat reader, and start swiping the :Cues in a Web-enhanced Harcourt textbook. The software is available for both Windows and Macintosh users, and :CueCats can be obtained for free at any of the 7100 RadioShack stores nationwide. No more laborious typing of lengthy URLs! No more endless clicking to find nested information! If your computer already has a mouse, get a free :CueCat reader and take it out for an exciting and informative walk on the Web!

Each chapter of the text has a structure that reflects the authors' approach to learning. The features of this approach are:

Chapter Outline This brief outline of each chapter's content provides students and teachers with an overview of major topics presented in the chapter.

Learning Objectives Each chapter opens with a list of objectives that helps set distinct learning goals for students and instructors. These aid students in targeting important material and serve as a study check once the chapter is completed.

Margin Definitions Bold-faced type is used throughout the text to identify important terms and concepts. All such terms are defined in the margin for easy reference and as a study aid. These terms and many others are also included in the main glossary at the back of the book.

Web Menu Identified by a special marginal icon, this information guides students and instructors to sources of additional relevant nutrition information on the Internet.

Chapter Summary A summary at the end of each chapter provides quick access to the important concepts covered in the chapter.

Review Questions These brief questions direct students to the most important concepts covered in the chapter. They are designed to review in a simple manner the key points of each chapter and to serve as a study guide.

Applying Critical Thinking Skills These exercises, which appear at the end of each chapter, are divided into two parts: one that focuses on the student's personal diet and nutrition concerns and a second that relates to more general nutrition issues. Both require the student to think critically and apply key nutrition concepts. Some of these exercises feature clinical applications and therefore also support the health promotion and disease prevention themes of the book. Many can be done as collaborative learning exercises, in which students work together and learn from each other to solve a problem.

Ancillaries

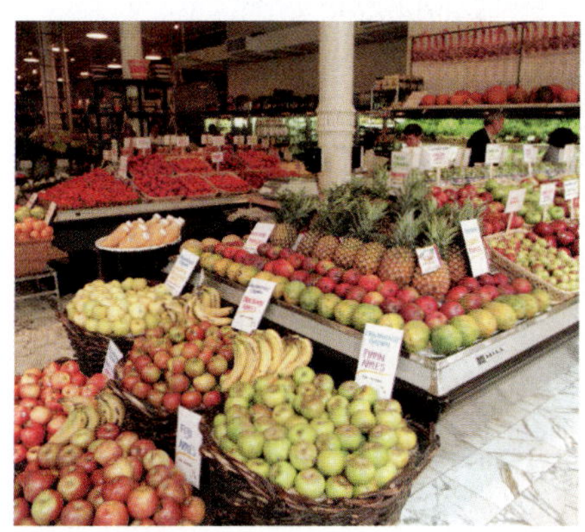

E-Book Available This Harcourt textbook is also available as a feature-packed Adobe Acrobat e-book that can be purchased and downloaded directly from the Internet. What's more, by buying online directly from Harcourt College Publishers, students can save up to 33% off the email price of a corresponding printed textbook. The Adobe Acrobat eBook Reader software is free and available for both Windows and Macintosh users. A Harcourt e-book on the Adobe platform offers a rich visual presentation in the Portable Document Format (PDF) that exactly matches the printed book, page for page. In addition, users can electronically annotate and highlight the text, look up definitions with a

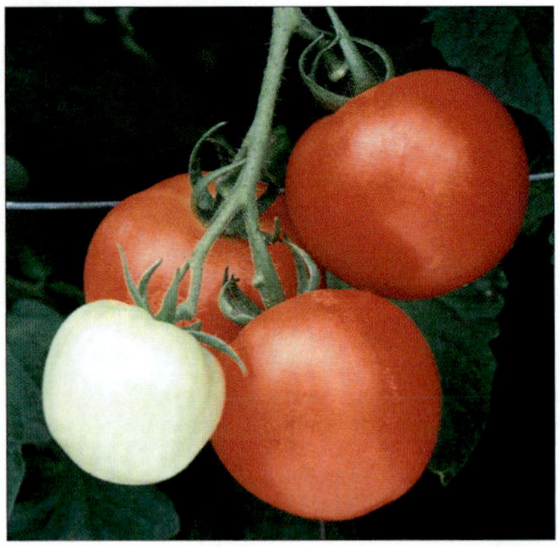

built-in dictionary, click instantly from section to section via internal hyperlinks, or, with a live Internet connection, link directly out to any URLs contained in the text. There's even a Read Aloud option! For more information about Harcourt e-books, or to download the free Adobe Acrobat eBook Reader, check out www.harcourtcollege.com/ebooks and get a glimpse of the future!

This title may also be available on other e-book platforms and devices. Consult your Harcourt sales representative for more details.

Nutrition: From Science to Life is accompanied by a supplementary set of teaching and learning materials. The materials available to students include:

Nutritionist Pro Student Version The nutrition software that accompanies this textbook provides powerful tools for analyzing diets, menus, and recipes. This comprehensive program allows for weight and exercise management and the customization of nutrient goals. When analyzing a recipe, cooking losses and gains are automatically accounted for and custom recipes can easily be stored in separate recipe books. Menus can be developed for individuals or groups and menu template can be used to simplify menu creation. The database contains over 80 nutrients and 13,000 foods including recipes and common brand-name foods, and an unlimited number of foods and recipes can be added to the database. Numerous reports are available including an analysis of a diet based on the number of servings recommended by the Food Guide Pyramid.

Nutrition Update This newsletter will be published in the summers of 2002 and 2003 to inform students and instructors of the ongoing updates of the DRIs and the Healthy People 2010 initiative, of changes in the Dietary Guidelines, and of other advances in nutrition science. The *Nutrition Update* is free and available with all new copies of the text.

Clinical Cases Supplement This supplement will expand on the *Critical Thinking* approach by including clinically oriented thinking problems that focus on health and disease, as well as some exercises that relate to institutional food production.

Study Guide This guide, written by Judy Driskell at the University of Nebraska, includes chapter outlines, multiple-choice questions, short-answer review questions, and a variety of learning activities designed for student use.

The teaching materials available to instructors include:

Instructor's Manual with Test Bank The *Instructor's Manual/Test Bank,* written by Nancy Kim Glaser of the University of Maryland, Baltimore County, includes key concepts, chapter outlines, new *Critical Thinking* exercises, key terms, student self-assessment forms, and sources for other teaching materials, including useful Web sites that are in addition to those listed in the text. The Test Bank includes multiple-choice questions as well as short case studies with questions that encourage students to apply what they have learned.

ExaMaster + This computerized version of the printed Test Bank makes preparing clear, concise tests quick and easy. It is available in both Windows and Macintosh formats.

Overhead Transparencies A set of 100 full-color overheads helps instructors show the book's concepts in the classroom. This set can be supplemented by using the image bank from the Instructor's Resource CD-ROM for Nutrition to create additional overheads for classroom use.

Instructor's Resource CD-ROM This dual-platform presentation CD-ROM (for Macintosh and Windows) features all of the line illustrations and selected photographs from the text. A variety of file formats include print- and screen-optimized PDFs and files for use in creating custom PowerPoint™ presentations and Web pages.

Frederick Essig of the University of South Florida has created **PowerPoint™ Lecture Presentations** to accompany each chapter of the text. These presentations are available on the IRCD-ROM as well as on the book companion Web site.

Companion Web Site The nutrition Web site is enriched with a number of unique features created by Nancy Berkoff, R.D., Ed.D., of Los Angeles Trade Technical College. A feature called "Food for Thought" offers a series of short articles on topics in food technology, food service, and general nutrition, with recommended further reading. Biographies of people who made various career choices in the nutrition field are featured. Also included is information on conducting research in the nutrition and food sciences. Student resources also include online "Quizzing & Testing," annotated Web links, a glossary, and a bulletin board. Instructors will find a syllabus generator, links to our "Class Act" course management system, an on-line image bank, and downloadable ancillaries, such as the *Instructor's Manual/Test Bank* and the PowerPoint slides.

Harcourt College Publishers may provide complimentary instructional aids and supplements or supplement packages to those adopters qualified under our adoption policy. Please contact your sales representative for more information.

Acknowledgments

Richard A. Ahrens
University of Maryland

S. Eugene Barnes
University of South Alabama

Nancy Berkoff
Los Angeles Trade Technical College

Donna Beshgetoor
San Diego State University

David Bissonnette
McGill University

George A. Bray
Pennington Biomedical Research Center
Louisiana State University

K. Shane Broughton
University of Wyoming

Alexander R. Doberenz
University of Delaware

Judy A. Driskell
University of Nebraska

Brenda Eissenstat
Pennsylvania State University

Frederick B. Essig
University of South Florida

Eugene J. Fenster
Longview Community College

Catherine J. Field
University of Alberta (Canada)

Betty Forbes
West Virginia University

Nancy Glaser
University of Maryland, Baltimore County

Shelley R. Hancock
University of Alabama

Sandra L. Hudak
University of Akron

Donna-Jean Hunt
Stephen F. Austin State University

Mary Ann Johnson
University of Georgia

Susan M. Krueger
University of Wisconsin, Eau Claire

Elaine M. Long
Boise State University

Mary S. Mead
University of California, Berkeley

Marilyn Mook
Michigan State University

Steven E. Nizielski
Texas A&M University

John C. Peters
Procter & Gamble Company

Melissa Shock
University of Central Arkansas

LuAnne Soliah
Baylor University

Susan S. Swadener
California Polytechnic State University

Michele L. Trankina
St. Mary's University
University of Texas Health Science Center at San Antonio

Susanne von Bodman
University of Connecticut

Yanyun Zhao
University of Connecticut

Contents Overview

Contents

1 Defining Nutrition

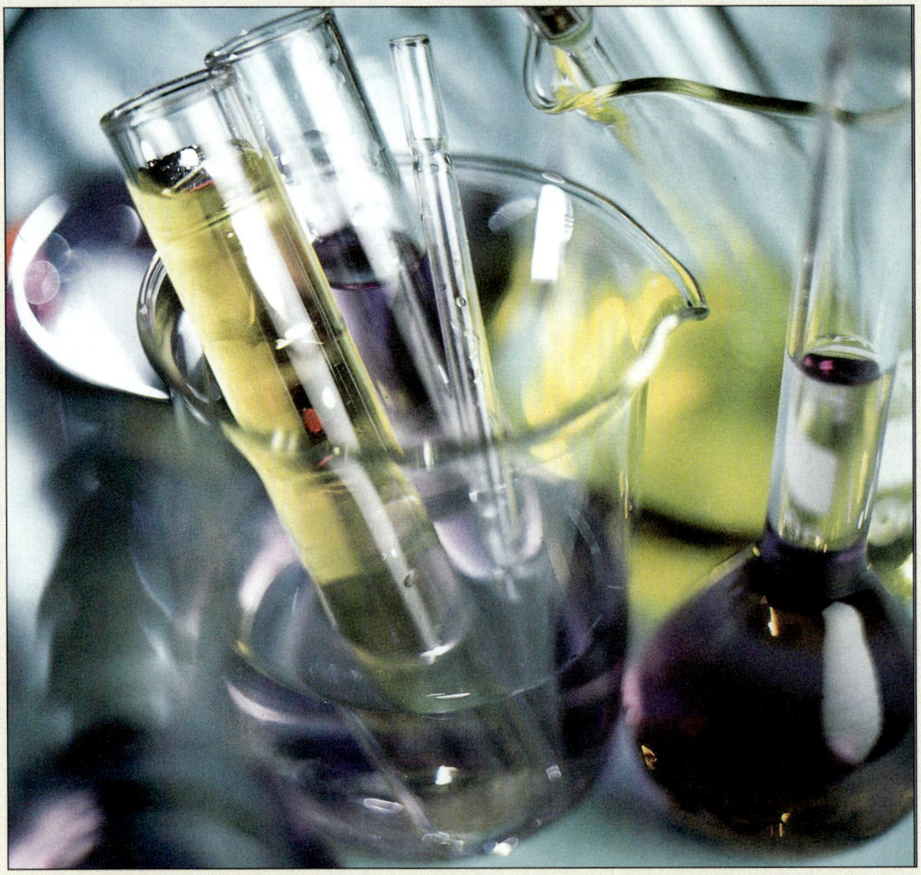

Learning Objectives

After reading this chapter, students should be able to:

1. Define the term "nutrition."
2. Discuss factors that affect food choices.
3. List the six classes of nutrients.
4. Explain the term "essential nutrient."
5. Describe the three general functions of nutrients.
6. Discuss how too little or too much of a nutrient can cause undernutrition or overnutrition.
7. List the steps of the scientific method.
8. Discuss experimental controls, including control groups, placebos, and blinded studies.
9. Explain the types of research studies used to investigate human nutrition.
10. Distinguish between reliable and unreliable nutrition information.

She knew the potato chips weren't a good choice—but they were the only thing in the vending machine that wasn't candy. Mary had had a busy day at school and work and now, studying late at night, she realized that she had missed dinner. She would need to eat something to keep her going until she finished that chapter in her nutrition book. Living in a dorm, she found that there are few food choices late at night for the unprepared. So, she opted for the chips and fruit punch—they seemed to be the healthiest choices available.

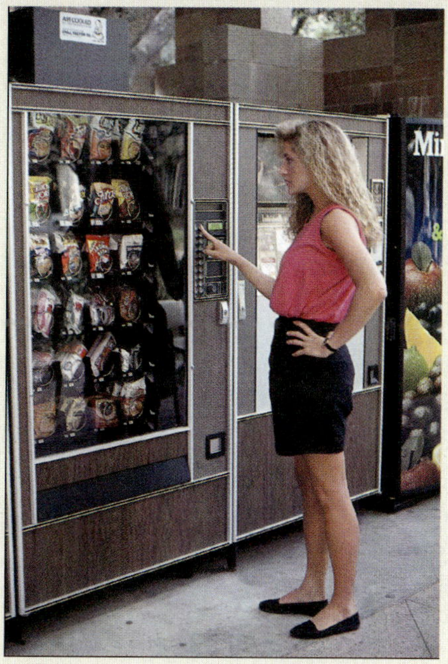

Mary is a college freshman away from home for the first time. She has gained a few pounds and is beginning to be concerned about her weight. Her father recently had cardiac bypass surgery and her mother is taking medication for high blood pressure. She knows from her family history that her diet is important for her future health. But she doesn't know how to change her diet. The dorm cafeteria offers a variety of foods, but because they aren't labeled with nutrition information, she doesn't know which are the best choices. She tries to keep some healthy snacks in her dorm room, but her options are limited because she doesn't have a refrigerator. Several of her friends have started taking dietary supplements like mega B to give them more energy and ginkgo biloba to improve their memories and mental function. She is tempted to start taking these but remembers her high school soccer coach saying that some supplements can be dangerous.

How can Mary figure out what is good for her, what she can eat without gaining weight, and what kind of diet will promote her nutritional health now and reduce her risk of chronic disease as she gets older? To meet these goals, she needs to understand the basics of nutrition science and the art of making nutritionally sound decisions and healthy food choices.

NUTRITION AND FOOD

Nutrition is a science that studies all the interactions that occur between living organisms and food. Food includes plant and animal products that, when consumed, can yield energy and provide **nutrients** needed to maintain life and allow growth and reproduction. The science of nutrition studies the physiologic functions of nutrients and their requirements from the diet, as well as the digestion, absorption, transport, and metabolism of food and the nutrients and other substances it contains. And, because there are numerous factors other than nutrient needs that affect our food choices, nutrition also considers the psychological, social, cultural, economic, and technological factors that influence which foods we choose to eat and the dietary patterns we adopt.

Nutrition A science that studies the interactions that occur between living organisms and food.

Nutrients Chemical substances in foods that provide energy, form body structures, and regulate body processes.

Determinants of Food Choice

Why do people choose the foods they choose? It may be that the food is available, or that it suits their personal or cultural preferences, or that it is thought to be a healthy choice (Table 1.1).

Availability The foods available to an individual or a population are affected by geography, socioeconomic factors, and health status. In many parts of the world,

TABLE 1.1 Factors That Can Affect Food Choices

Factor	Advantages and Limitations
Convenience	
Transport	Heavy or bulky items are difficult to transport from the store.
Storage	Some items require immediate cold storage or a large storage area.
Time	More time is needed to prepare or cook fresh or whole foods.
Geography	
Suburban	Large supermarkets offer year-round variety from around the world.
Rural	Stores may have less variety but better access to locally grown produce.
Inner city	Shopping may be limited to small local markets with less variety and higher prices.
Economics	
Income level	Finances affect which foods are purchased.
Living conditions	Food storage and cooking facilities may be limited.
Occupation and lifestyle	
Work location	Meals may be eaten outside or in an office, brought in a bag, purchased in a cafeteria, or heated in a microwave, if available.
Type of job	Frequency of travel, meals eaten in restaurants, and activity level during the day affect food choices.
Lifestyle	Time available for meal preparation and whether meals are eaten alone or with family members affect foods eaten.
Health status	
Chronic diseases	Many diseases, including cardiovascular disease, diabetes, hypertension, and obesity, require dietary modification.
Medications	Drugs may interact with certain foods or dietary components.
Allergies	Foods that cause allergic reaction must be eliminated from the diet.
Digestive problems	Certain types of foods, such as dairy products or wheat, may be restricted.
Dental disease	Texture and temperature of foods affect choices.
Personal and cultural background	
Personal preference	Taste, smell, appearance, and texture of food affect appeal; advertising and attractive packages affect choice.
Body image	Being uncomfortable about body size may limit what is eaten in public.
Religion and ethnicity	Some foods may be unacceptable.
Childhood experiences and habits	Foods people are used to eating they continue to consume; new foods are often intimidating.
Social interactions	Social events often involve food, and what is served affects consumption.
Peer pressure	Social acceptability dictates many food choices.
Body size	A person with higher energy needs can eat more.
Emotional comfort	Emotional stress may motivate food choices that make us feel good.
Past associations	A food that was eaten when you got sick may never be eaten again.
Health concerns	
Genetic background	People may modify food choices based on heredity in order to decrease personal disease risk factors.
Nutrition knowledge	An understanding of what foods make up a healthy diet affects choice.
Concern about specific deficiencies	Foods may be selected based on the amounts of specific nutrients, such as calcium or iron.
Body size	Concern about body weight may make energy and fat content a basis for food selection.
Environmental concerns	
Preservation of natural resources	Some foods use fewer natural resources.
Pesticides	Organically produced foods use fewer pesticides and other agricultural chemicals.

the diet is limited to foods produced locally. In other more developed areas, the ability to store, transport, and process food allows year-round access to seasonal foods as well as foods grown and produced at distant locations. However, even if foods are available in the store, they are not necessarily available to all individuals. Socioeconomic factors such as income and education level, living conditions, and lifestyle affect the types and amounts of foods that can be selected. Individuals living on limited incomes are restricted in their food choices. Those who don't own cars can purchase only what they can carry home on foot or on the bus or subway (Figure 1.1). Those without refrigerators and stoves are limited in what they can prepare at home. And, not knowing how to cook or not having time to cook or plan meals can limit food choices.

Health status also affects the availability of food. People who cannot carry heavy packages are limited in what they can bring home. People with food allergies, digestive disorders, and dental problems are limited in the foods they can consider for consumption. People consuming special diets for disease conditions are limited to foods that meet their dietary prescriptions.

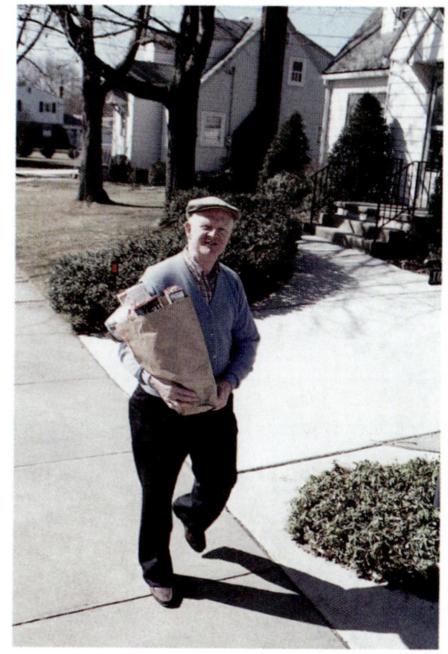

FIGURE 1.1 The availability of transportation can influence the amounts and types of food that one consumes. *(© Blair Seitz/Photo Researchers)*

Personal and Cultural Preferences Availability affects food choices, but individual palates and convictions also determine what is actually consumed, and tradition, religion, and social values may dictate what foods are considered appropriate. Personal preferences for taste, smell, appearance, and texture have a strong influence on which foods people select. Not wanting to give up the foods they like is the number one reason people give for not choosing a healthier diet.[1] Personal convictions also affect food choices; a vegetarian will not choose a meal that includes animal products and an environmentalist may not choose a food packaged in a nonrecyclable container.

Food preferences and eating habits are among the oldest and most entrenched features of every culture (Figure 1.2).[2] An individual of Asian descent may consider rice the focus of the meal, whereas Italians may include pasta with every meal. Almost every religion has dietary restrictions or special foods that are eaten in association with religious events or holidays. Seventh-Day Adventists are vegetarians; Jews and Muslims do not eat pork. Even for those who choose not to observe religious dietary rules, habit may dictate many mealtime decisions, since the foods people are exposed to as children influence what foods they buy and cook as adults. For example, Jewish kosher laws prohibit the consumption of meat and milk in the same meal. Even Jews who do not follow kosher law may choose not to serve milk at dinner because they never had it as children.

Food is a focus of social interaction, and food choices may determine social acceptance. For an adolescent, stopping for a cheeseburger or taco after school can be the basis for acceptance by one's peers. Food may also be an expression and moderator of moods and emotional states. Some people eat more when they are upset, while others eat less. And some people choose specific foods because to them these foods are associated with comfort, love, and security.

Web Menu: For more information on Americans' attitudes about health and nutrition issues, go to www.eatright.org/ and search for Trends 2000.

Health Concerns Individuals' perceptions of what makes a healthy diet affects their food and nutrition choices. For example, individuals may choose low-fat foods if they believe that these choices will help them lose weight. They may limit red meat intake to reduce their risk of heart disease, or they may purchase organically produced foods if they believe that reducing pesticide exposure will prevent illness. In a recent survey of attitudes about diet and nutrition, 85% of respondents said that diet and nutrition were important to them personally and more than 40% felt they were doing all they could to consume a healthy diet.[3]

Web Menu: For more information on food patterns and food availability in the United States today, go to the USDA Economic Research Service at www.ers.usda.gov/epubs/pdf/fanrr8/ and to the Interactive Healthy Eating Index at www.usda.gov/cnpp/.

Dietary Patterns in America

Each of the food choices individuals make contributes to their diet as a whole. This diet must provide enough energy to fuel the body and all the essential nutrients and other food components—in the right proportions—to prevent deficiencies, promote health, and protect against chronic disease. No single food choice is good or bad in and of itself, but all of our choices combined make up a dietary pattern that is either healthy or not so healthy.

In the beginning of the 20th century, the American diet was a meat and potatoes diet.[4] Food was plentiful, but seasonal availability and methods of

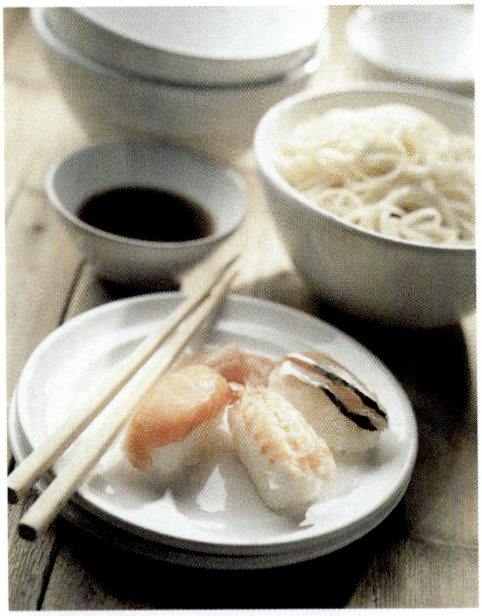

FIGURE 1.2 An individual's cultural background has a strong influence on the types of foods they eat. *(© Chris Everard/Tony Stone Images)*

food preservation limited variety. This was considered a healthy diet because, at the time, protein was known to be important but vitamins had not yet been discovered. Fresh fruits were seen as having little nutritional value, and eating greens was viewed as not worth the energy it took to chew them. Ethnic foods were scarce and unpopular because new immigrants wanted to blend in with American culture as fast as possible. To do so, they abandoned their traditional cuisine.

Over the last century, however, food production systems, tastes in food, and our understanding of nutrient needs have changed the American diet. The variety of foods available is enormous because of advances in transportation and storage. Ethnic foods are popular and are being incorporated into the American diet (Table 1.2). Health promotion campaigns recommend that Americans eat a diet

TABLE 1.2 Some Ethnic Foods That Are Common in the American Diet

Origin	Food	Nutritional Consideration
Mexico	Burritos, tacos, enchiladas, salsa	Based on beans, chili peppers, tomatoes, and rice that are good vegetable sources of protein and phytochemicals. Too much cheese and sour cream can make these high in fat.
China	Chow mein, stir fry, fried rice	Based on rice and vegetables with small amounts of meat—close to the recommendations of the Food Guide Pyramid. Choices that are breaded and fried can be high in fat.
Italy	Pasta, sauces, tomatoes and other vegetables, olive oil, wine	The Mediterranean diet is related to a lower incidence of heart disease than the U.S. diet. Cream sauces and sausages can make this high in saturated fat.
Greece	Moussaka, gyros (roasted seasoned meat served on pita bread with yogurt and cucumber sauce), eggplant, Greek salads, baklava	The Mediterranean diet is related to a lower incidence of heart disease than the U.S. diet. High in fat from olives and olive oil.
France	Rich sauces, pastries, wine	Often high in fat but served in small portions. The incidence of heart disease is lower in France than the United States.
India	Curried meat, lentils, rice, and vegetables with yogurt	Many of the traditional dishes are vegetarian using lentils and rice as the mainstay.
Japan	Vegetables, fish, noodles, and tofu and other soy products	Typically low in fat with lots of vegetables. Fish adds a low-fat protein source.
Middle East	Falafel, hummus (ground chick peas), tabuli (bulgur with vegetables), couscous, yogurt	Many vegetarian choices are based on lentils, chickpeas, and whole grains. Typically high in vegetable proteins.
Thailand	Varied cuisine that includes many vegetables and fruits as well as noodle dishes flavored with spicy sauces made with peanuts and coconut milk	Includes peanuts and many fruits and vegetables. Low in fat and very flavorful.
Vietnam	Pho (broth with noodles, vegetables, and meat) spring rolls, varied cuisine based on rice, wheat, and vegetables	Includes grains and vegetables that are streamed or grilled. Traditional food is low in fat.

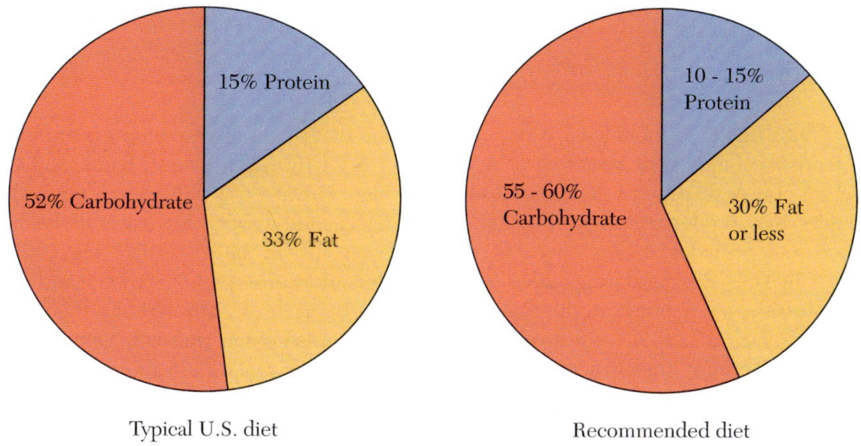

FIGURE 1.3 The typical American diet now contains amounts of carbohydrate, fat, and protein that are close to recommendations.

that is moderate in fat, adequate in protein, and based on high-carbohydrate foods such as grains, fruits, and vegetables.

The typical diet in the United States today comes close to the recommended proportions of protein, carbohydrate, and fat (Figure 1.3). However, the dietary pattern is not as healthy as it could be. The population doesn't meet recommendations for fruits, vegetables, dairy products, lean meats and meat substitutes or grains and exceeds the recommended intake of added fats and sugars (Figure 1.4).[5,6] This dietary pattern, along with a lack of physical activity, is a major contributor to the development of chronic diseases such as diabetes, obesity, heart disease, and cancer, which are the major causes of illness and death in our popu-

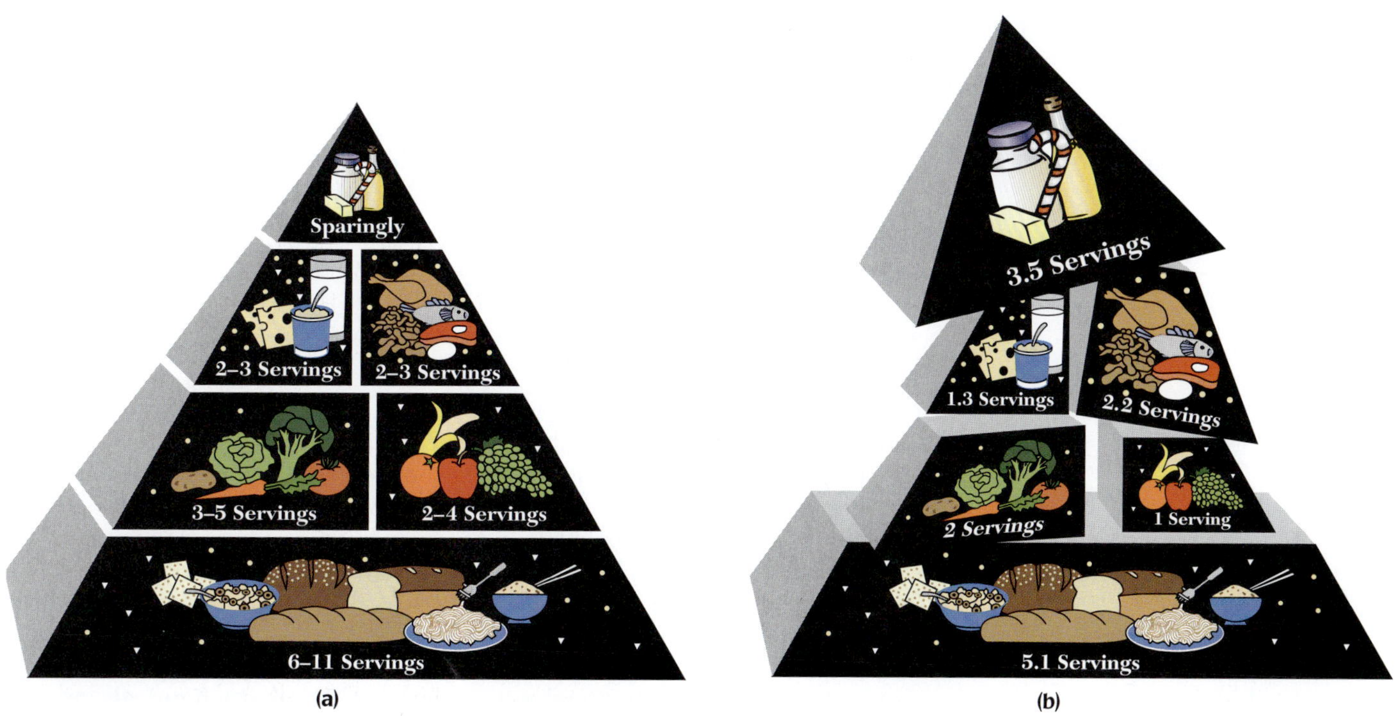

FIGURE 1.4 (a) The Food Guide Pyramid is a guide for planning diets that meet nutritional recommendations. (b) The typical American diet forms a top-heavy pyramid, with too many fats and sweets and too few fruits and vegetables, dairy products, and grains.

Making Decisions

Good Foods, Bad Foods?

Should you have that brownie with your milk? Should you skip breakfast to save kcalories? Should you be taking a calcium supplement? Should you be eating a vegetarian diet? Whether you are deciding to eat an extravagant dessert, skip a meal, or completely change your eating pattern, each decision has an effect on many other components of your diet and of your lifestyle. These dietary decisions have an impact now and may affect your health in future years. How can you decide?

The first step toward making healthy choices is understanding that there is no such thing as a good food or a bad food—any food can be part of a healthy diet. A healthy diet does not need to exclude the foods you love. Whether your cravings are for ice cream or potato chips, you can fit favorite foods into your diet. High-fat foods must be balanced with lower fat choices and sweet treats offset by foods naturally low in sugar. Choosing special foods like fat-free chips, sugar-free soda, or low-fat cookies doesn't guarantee a healthy diet. These foods are lower in fat and/or sugar, but they still add kcalories to the diet and contribute few other nutrients.

A healthy diet is based on grains, fruits, vegetables, dairy products, and meats or meat substitutes. It includes a wide variety of foods we enjoy. But selecting a healthy diet is not necessarily easy. The multitude of choices that modern food production and processing provides makes choosing difficult. Chicken, rice, and vegetables sounds like a healthy meal, but even purchasing the foods for such a simple meal involves hundreds of decisions that can impact on the overall healthiness and appeal of the diet. Should you purchase a whole raw chicken, boneless skinless chicken breasts, or frozen breaded nuggets of chicken? Should you use brown rice? Is it healthier than white rice because it adds more fiber to the diet? What about instant rice—it is convenient, but is it as nutritious and does it taste good? Is the packaged rice with added flavorings too high in fat and salt? Should you buy fresh, organically grown vegetables, or are canned as nutritious? And which vegetable is best? Carrots are a good choice, but what about adding variety to your diet? Choosing cherimoya, chayote, or bok choy would increase the variety of your vegetables, but how do you prepare them?

A healthy choice can be any choice that is part of an overall healthy diet. For example, fat-free ice cream sounds like a better choice than regular ice cream, but fat-free ice cream does not make a diet healthy if the diet's overall fat content is too high and it is low in whole grains, fruits, and vegetables. However, a diet rich in whole grains, fruits, and vegetables can still be healthy even if you have regular ice cream for dessert. Subsequent chapters and *Making Decisions* boxes throughout this text provide information that will help you understand what makes a healthy diet and how to make wise decisions about individual foods and supplements available to you.

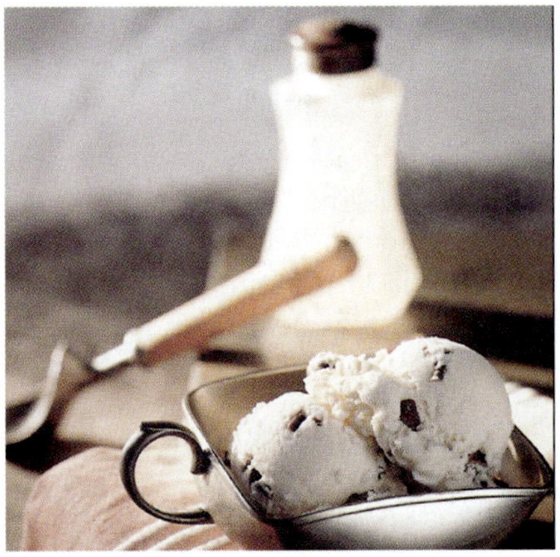

Ice cream and other favorite foods can be part of a healthy diet. *(© Angie Norwood Browne/Stone)*

lation.[7,8,9] Understanding nutrient needs and how to choose foods to meet these needs can help improve the American diet (see *Making Decisions*: "Good Foods, Bad Foods?").

NUTRIENTS

Essential nutrients Nutrients that must be provided in the diet because the body either cannot make them or cannot make them in sufficient quantities to satisfy its needs.

Phytochemical A substance found in plant foods ("phyto" means plant) that is not an essential nutrient but may have health-promoting properties.

To date, approximately 45 nutrients are considered essential to human life. **Essential nutrients** are those substances necessary to support life that must be supplied in the diet because they either cannot be made by the body or cannot be made in large enough quantities to meet needs. Vitamin A is an example of an essential nutrient; it cannot be made in the body but is needed for vision, growth, and reproduction. Food also contains substances that are required by the body but are not essential in the diet because they can be produced by the body in amounts sufficient to meet needs. For example, eggs contain lecithin, which is needed for nerve function; it is not an essential nutrient because it can be manufactured in the body. Other food components, such as **phytochemicals,** are not essential to sustain life but may have health-promoting properties. For example, broccoli contains sulforaphane, a phytochemical that is not a dietary essential but may reduce the risk of cancer (Figure 1.5).

Classes of Nutrients

Chemically, there are six classes of nutrients: carbohydrates, lipids, proteins, water, vitamins, and minerals. These classes can be grouped in a variety of ways—by whether they provide energy to the body, by how much is needed in the diet, and by whether their chemical structure contains carbon. Carbohydrates, lipids, and proteins provide energy to the body and thus are referred to as energy-yielding nutrients. Alcohol also provides energy but is not considered a nutrient because it is not needed to support life. The energy-yielding nutrients, along with water, constitute the major portion of most foods and are required in relatively large amounts in the diet. Therefore, they are referred to as **macronutrients** ("macro" means large). The amounts required are measured in kilograms (kg) or grams (g) (see Table 1.3 and Appendix N for metric conversions).

Vitamins and minerals are classified as **micronutrients** because they are needed in small amounts in the diet ("micro" means small). The amounts required are expressed in milligrams (1 mg = 1/1000 g) or micrograms (1 μg = 1/1,000,000 g). Structurally, carbohydrates, proteins, lipids, and vitamins are **organic molecules,** so they are referred to as organic nutrients. Minerals and water are **inorganic molecules** and so are referred to as inorganic nutrients.

Macronutrients Nutrients needed by the body in large amounts. These include water, carbohydrates, lipids, and proteins.

Micronutrients Nutrients needed by the body in small amounts. These include vitamins and minerals.

Organic molecules Molecules containing carbon atoms in their structure.

Inorganic molecules Molecules that do not contain carbon atoms in their structure, such as water and minerals.

Energy-Yielding Nutrients As already mentioned, carbohydrates, lipids, and proteins are the three classes of nutrients that can be broken down to provide energy. The energy provided by these nutrients is measured in units called **kilocalories** (abbreviated as kcalories or kcals) or in **kilojoules** (abbreviated as kjoules or kJs). The more common term, "calorie," is technically 1/1000 of a kilocalorie, but when it is spelled with a capital "C," it indicates kilocalories. For instance, the term "Calories" on food labels actually refers to kilocalories. However, in the popular press, the term "calorie" (small "c") is often used to express the kcalorie content of a food or diet. Throughout this book, the energy in food will be expressed in kcalories or kcals.

Kilocalorie A unit of heat that is used to express the amount of energy provided by foods.

Kilojoule A measure of work that can be used to express energy intake and energy output; 4.18 kjoules = 1 kcalorie.

Carbohydrates contain 4 kcalories per gram (Table 1.4) and provide a readily available source of energy to the body. Carbohydrates include sugars such as

TABLE 1.3 Measures Used in Nutrition

Metric Measure	English Conversion
Measures of weight	
1 kilogram (kg) = 1000 grams (g)	= 2.2 pounds (lb)
454 grams	= 1 pound = 16 ounces (oz)
28.4 grams	= 1 ounce
4 grams of sugar or salt	= about 1 teaspoon (tsp)
1 gram = 1000 milligrams (mg)	
1 milligram = 1000 micrograms (μg or mcg)	
Measures of volume	
1 liter = 1000 milliliters (ml)	= approximately 1 quart (qt) = 4 cups
240 milliliters	= 1 cup = 8 oz
5 milliliters	= 1 teaspoon
15 milliliters	= 1 tablespoon (Tbsp) = 3 teaspoons
30 milliliters	= approximately 1 fluid ounce
Measures of length	
1 meter (m) = 1000 centimeters (cm) = 1,000,000 millimeters (mm)	= 39.4 inches (in.) = 1.09 yards (yd)
2.54 centimeters	= 1 inch

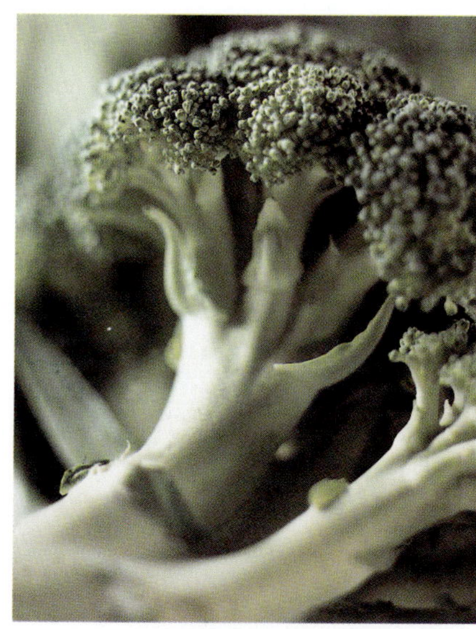

FIGURE 1.5 Food, such as this broccoli, contains essential nutrients as well as nonessential substances, many of which have health-promoting properties. *(© Alan Marsh/Tony Stone Images)*

TABLE 1.4 Energy Content of Carbohydrate, Protein, Lipid, and Alcohol

	Kcalories/gram	Kjoules/gram
Carbohydrate	4	16.7
Protein	4	16.7
Lipid	9	37.6
Alcohol	7	29.3

those in table sugar, fruit, and milk, and starches such as those in vegetables and grains. Sugars are the simplest form of carbohydrate, and starches are more complex carbohydrates made of many sugars linked together (Figure 1.6). Most fiber is also carbohydrate, but because it cannot be completely broken down by the body, it provides little energy. However, it is important for gastrointestinal health. Fiber is found in vegetables, fruits, **legumes,** and whole grains.

Legume The seed or pod of a plant that produces a pod (leguminous plant). Peas, beans, and peanuts are legumes.

Lipids, commonly referred to as fats and oils, provide a concentrated source of energy in foods and a storage form of energy in the body. They provide 9 kcalories per gram. Lipids in our diets come from foods that naturally contain fats, such as meat and whole milk, and from processed fats, such as

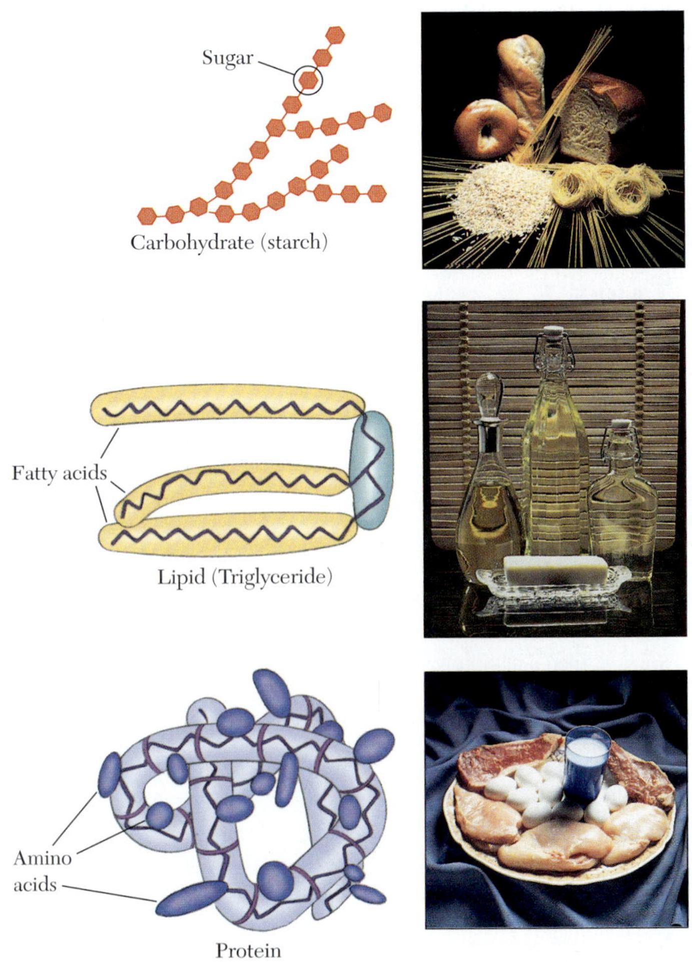

FIGURE 1.6 Starches are made of sugars linked together; most lipids, such as the triglyceride shown here, contain fatty acids; proteins are made of amino acids linked together. (*Photographs, Charles D. Winters*)

vegetable oils and butter, that are added to food in cooking and at the table. Most lipids in food and in our body are triglycerides (also called triacylgycerols). Triglycerides contain fatty acids, some of which are essential in the diet. The amount and type of lipid in the diet affect the risk of cardiovascular disease and certain types of cancer.

Protein is found in foods such as meat, fish, poultry, milk, legumes, nuts, and seeds. It provides energy—4 kcalories per gram—but is only used as an energy source when sufficient energy cannot be obtained from carbohydrate and fat or when the amount of protein in the diet exceeds the body's protein needs. Protein is made up of units called amino acids (see Figure 1.6). The body can make some amino acids, and others are essential in the diet. Protein consumed in the diet must provide all of the essential amino acids and is needed for growth and maintenance of body structures and regulation of body processes.

The amount of energy contained in a food can be calculated by multiplying the number of grams each of carbohydrate, protein, and fat by the energy each provides (4, 4, and 9 kcal/g respectively) and summing the answers (Table 1.5).

Water Water is a nutrient in a class by itself. It is a macronutrient that doesn't provide energy. Water makes up about 60% of the weight of the human body and is required in large amounts in the daily diet. It serves many functions in the body, including acting as a lubricant, a transport fluid, and a regulator of body temperature.

Micronutrients Vitamins are organic molecules that do not provide energy but are needed to regulate body processes. There are 13 essential vitamins. Some are soluble in water (the B vitamins and vitamin C) and others are soluble in lipid (vitamins A, D, E, and K). Each has a unique structure and function. Many are involved in the production of energy from carbohydrates, lipids, and proteins; others function in processes such as bone growth, blood clotting, vision, and tissue growth and development.

Minerals are inorganic elements. Like vitamins, they do not provide energy. Many have regulatory roles and some are important structurally. They are needed for bone strength, the transport of oxygen, the transmission of nerve impulses, and many other functions. Requirements have been established for many of the minerals, but some are required in such small amounts that their role in maintaining health is not fully understood.

Vitamins and minerals are found in most foods. Fresh foods are a good natural source of micronutrients, and many processed foods contain micronutrients

TABLE 1.5 Calculating the Energy in a Food

To calculate the energy in a food, multiply:

Grams of carbohydrate × 4 kcalories per gram
Grams of protein × 4 kcalories per gram
Grams of fat × 9 kcalories per gram

The sum of these is the energy in the food.
For example:

For a slice of bread that contains 17 grams of carbohydrate, 3 grams of protein, and 1 gram of fat:

Carbohydrate	17 g × 4 kcal/g = 68 kcal
Protein	3 g × 4 kcal/g = 12 kcal
Fat	1 g × 9 kcal/g = 9 kcal
Total energy	= 89 kcal

that are added to them during manufacture. For example, many breakfast cereals are good sources of iron and B vitamins because they are added during processing. Processing can also cause nutrient losses. Light, heat, and exposure to oxygen destroy some micronutrients, and others are lost in the water used for cooking and processing. Nevertheless, frozen, canned, and otherwise processed foods can still be good sources of vitamins and minerals. Vitamin and mineral supplements are also a common source of micronutrients in today's diet.

Nutrient Functions

By providing energy, contributing to structure, and regulating biological processes, nutrients allow the body to grow, maintain and repair itself, and reproduce.

Energy Inside the body, biochemical reactions release the energy contained in carbohydrates, lipids, and proteins. Some of this energy is used to synthesize new compounds and maintain basic body functions, some is used to fuel physical activity, and some is lost as heat. Energy-yielding nutrients that are not needed immediately can also be stored, primarily as fat. These stores can provide energy when dietary sources are unavailable. Over the long term, if more energy is consumed than is needed, body stores increase, causing weight gain. If less energy is consumed than is needed, the body will burn both its fat and carbohydrate stores, as well as body proteins, to meet its energy needs, and body weight will decrease.

Structure Water, proteins, lipids, and minerals are important structural nutrients. Muscle is made up primarily of protein and water, and bone is composed of a protein framework embedded with minerals. At the cellular level, lipids and proteins make up the membranes that surround cells. A lean adult male is approximately 62% water, less than 1% carbohydrate, 16% fat, 16% protein, and about 5% minerals and other substances.

TABLE 1.6 Examples of How Nutrients Function in the Body

Function	Nutrient	Example
Energy	Carbohydrate	Glucose is a carbohydrate that provides energy to body cells.
	Lipid	Fat is the most plentiful source of stored fuel in the body.
	Protein	Protein consumed in excess of protein needs will be used for energy.
Structure	Lipid	Lipids are the principal component of the membranes that surround each cell.
	Protein	Protein in connective tissue holds bones together and holds muscles to bones.
	Minerals	The minerals calcium and phosphorus make teeth and bones hard.
Regulation	Lipid	The lipid hormone, estrogen, helps regulate the female reproductive cycle.
	Protein	The protein, leptin, helps regulate the size of body fat stores.
	Carbohydrate	Sugar chains attached to proteins circulating in the blood signal whether the protein should remain in the blood or be removed by the liver.
	Water	Water lost as sweat helps cool the body to regulate body temperature.
	Vitamins	B vitamins regulate the use of macronutrients for energy.
	Minerals	The mineral sodium helps regulate blood volume.

Regulation Together, all of the reactions that occur in the body are referred to as **metabolism.** Metabolic processes must be regulated to maintain a constant environment inside the body, referred to as **homeostasis.** All six classes of nutrients have important regulatory roles. For example, water helps to regulate body temperature. When body temperature increases, water lost through sweat helps to cool the body by evaporation. Protein, vitamins, and minerals help to speed up or slow down the reactions of metabolism as needed to maintain homeostasis. Carbohydrate molecules on the surface of cells are important in regulating body processes by aiding cell communication (see Table 1.6 for further examples).

Metabolism The sum of all the chemical reactions that take place in a living organism.

Homeostasis A physiological state in which a stable internal body environment is maintained.

Nutrient Requirements

In order to support life, an adequate amount of each essential nutrient must be consumed in the diet. The optimal amount of a nutrient is an amount that will avoid deficiencies and excesses and optimize short-term and long-term health. The exact amount is different for each individual; it depends on body size, health status, and genetic makeup, as well as overall diet and lifestyle (Figure 1.7). A person with a genetic predisposition to heart disease may need to consume different amounts of certain nutrients to maintain long-term heart health than does a person with no genetic risk of heart disease. The amount of each nutrient required may also be dependent on the other nutrients in the diet. For example, adequate fat is essential for the absorption of vitamin A, and vitamin C increases the absorption of iron when they are consumed together. Lifestyle factors are also important. People who smoke require more

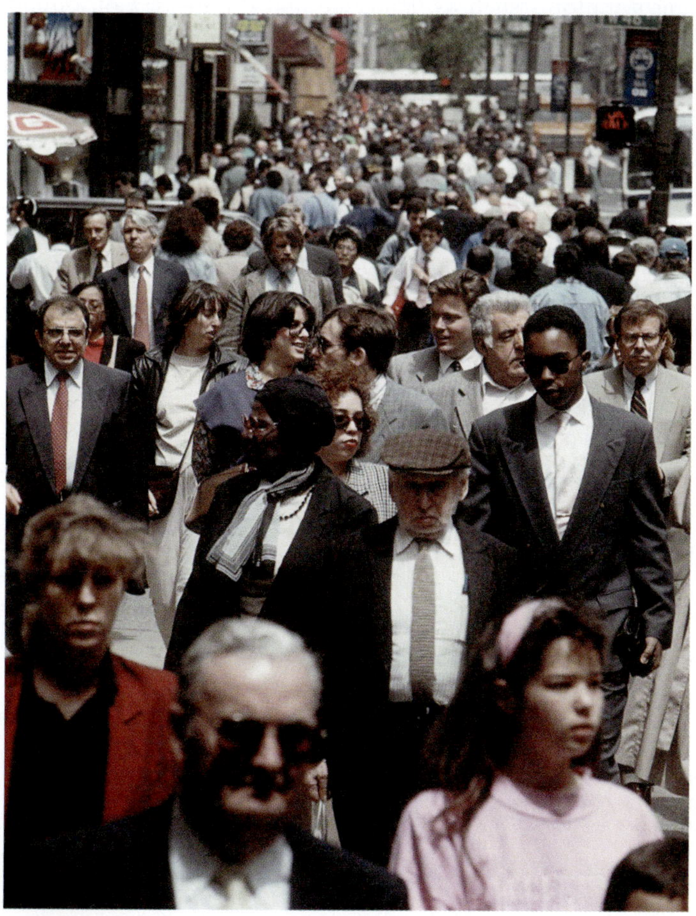

FIGURE 1.7 The specific nutrient requirements of individuals differ depending on their genetic makeup and lifestyle. *(© Veronika Burmeister/Visuals Unlimited)*

vitamin C, and active individuals have higher energy needs than their sedentary counterparts.

For more information on nutrition and health issues, go to the American Dietetic Association at www.eatright.org/.

Nutrients and Health

Consuming either too little or too much of one or more nutrients or energy can cause **malnutrition. Undernutrition,** a deficiency of energy or nutrients, is the form of malnutrition that usually comes to mind. Undernutrition may occur due to a deficient intake of energy or nutrients, increased requirements, or an inability to absorb or use nutrients. For example, iron deficiency is a form of undernutrition that is common in young children and adolescents because their diets are typically low in iron while their rapid growth increases iron needs. Vitamin B_{12} deficiency is a risk for older adults because changes in the stomach that often occur with age decrease vitamin B_{12} absorption. Starvation, the most severe form of undernutrition, is a deficiency of energy that causes weight loss, poor growth, the inability to reproduce, and, if severe enough, death.

Malnutrition Any condition resulting from an energy or nutrient intake either above or below that which is required.

Undernutrition Any condition resulting from an energy or nutrient intake below that which meets nutritional needs.

Overnutrition Poor nutritional status resulting from a dietary intake in excess of that which is needed to maintain health.

Toxic Possessing the capacity to produce injury at some level of intake.

Overnutrition is also a form of malnutrition, occurring when energy or nutrients are consumed in excess of needs. When energy is consumed in excess, the extra is stored as body fat. Some fat is necessary as insulation and energy storage, but an excess of body fat, called obesity, increases the risk for high blood pressure, heart disease, diabetes, and other chronic health problems (Figure 1.8). When excesses of specific nutrients are consumed, an adverse or **toxic** reaction may occur. Because foods generally do not contain high enough concentrations of nutrients to cause toxic reactions, most nutrient toxicities result from the overconsumption of vitamin and mineral supplements.

The symptoms of a nutritional deficiency or excess may appear rapidly or take a lifetime to develop. For example, a deficiency of water can occur quickly: An athlete exercising in hot weather may lose enough water in a few hours to become dehydrated, developing symptoms such as headache and dizziness. Consuming water will relieve these symptoms as rapidly as they appeared. Other nutritional imbalances, however, may take weeks or months to manifest themselves. For example, when excess energy is consumed, it may take months before a significant amount of weight is gained. Likewise, as anyone who has tried to lose weight knows, it can take months of reduced energy consumption to lose the excess fat.

The impact of nutritional imbalances over a much longer time frame is also an important health concern. An individual's nutrient intake today may affect the development of chronic diseases such as osteoporosis, cancer, or heart disease 20, 30, or 40 years from now. However, the effects of nutrition on the development of chronic disease are difficult to determine because other variables, or **risk factors,** such as age, genetics, and gender, are also often involved. These risk factors

Risk factor A characteristic or circumstance that Is associated with the occurrence of a particular disease. Risk factors include variables such as genetic background, dietary and lifestyle habits, and environmental conditions.

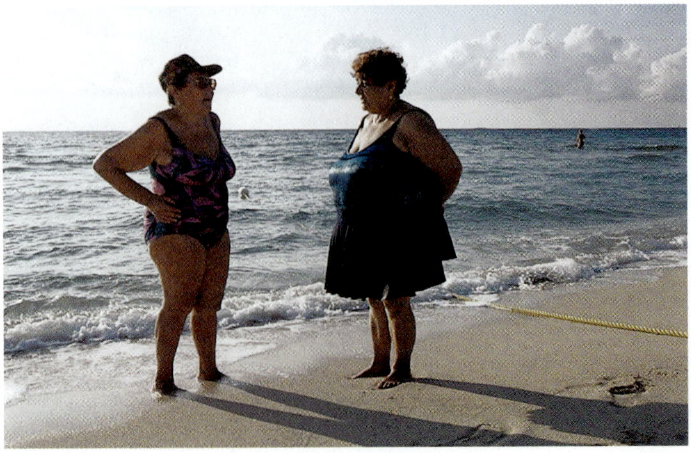

FIGURE 1.8 The incidence of obesity in the United States is on the rise. *(© Jeff Greenberg/Visuals Unlimited, Inc.)*

cannot be changed, but nutrition is a lifestyle variable that is determined by individual choices.

Nutrition Research

In order to understand nutrient needs and how to meet them, scientists use a variety of research tools to study nutrition. Advances are made by applying the **scientific method.** The results of well-designed and carefully-controlled experiments are used to make recommendations for nutrient requirements and food choices that will promote optimal nutritional health.

Scientific method The general approach of science that is used to explain observations about the world around us.

The Scientific Method

The scientific method offers a systematic, unbiased approach to evaluating the relationships among food, nutrients, and health. The first step of the scientific method is to make an observation and ask questions about the observation. The next step is to propose an explanation for the observation. This explanation is called a **hypothesis.** Once a hypothesis has been proposed, experiments can be designed to test it. The experiments must provide objective results that can be measured and repeated. If the experimental results do not prove the hypothesis to be wrong, a **theory,** or a scientific explanation based on experimentation, can be established (Figure 1.9). Scientific theories are accepted only as long as they cannot be disproved and continue to be supported by all new evidence that accumulates. Even a theory that has been accepted by the scientific community for years can be proved wrong. This flux allows the body of knowledge to increase, but it can be confusing as old theories give way to new ones.

Hypothesis An educated guess made to explain an observation or to answer a question.

Theory An explanation based on scientific study and reasoning.

The discovery of the relationship between nutrition and pellagra, a disease now known to be caused by a deficiency of the vitamin niacin, is an example of how the scientific method has been used in nutrition research. The events leading to this discovery began with the observation in 1914 that individuals in institutions such as hospitals, orphanages, and prisons suffered from pellagra—a disease marked by skin, digestive, and nervous disorders—but the staff did not. If pellagra was an infectious disease, as was believed by many at the time, both populations would be equally affected. Thus the hypothesis proposed was that pellagra was due to a lack of something in the diet. To test this hypothesis, nutritious foods such as fresh meats, milk, and eggs were added to the diet of children in orphanages. The symptoms of pellagra disappeared, supporting the hypothesis that pellagra was due to a lack of something in the diet. This experiment and others led to the theory that pellagra is caused by a dietary deficiency. This theory, further developed by the discovery of the vitamin niacin in 1937, still holds today (see Chapter 9, *Research Discoveries*: "Pellagra: Infectious Disease or Dietary Deficiency?").

Well-Designed Experiments

For the scientific method to generate reliable theories, the experiments done to test hypotheses must generate reliable results and be interpreted accurately. The first step is to understand what makes a good experiment. Well-designed, well-conducted experiments must use **objective measurements,** proper experimental controls, and the right experimental population.

Objective measurements Information that can be quantified and repeated by careful scientific methodology.

Objective Measurements Scientific experiments should be designed to provide measurable data that can be quantified and repeated. For example, the

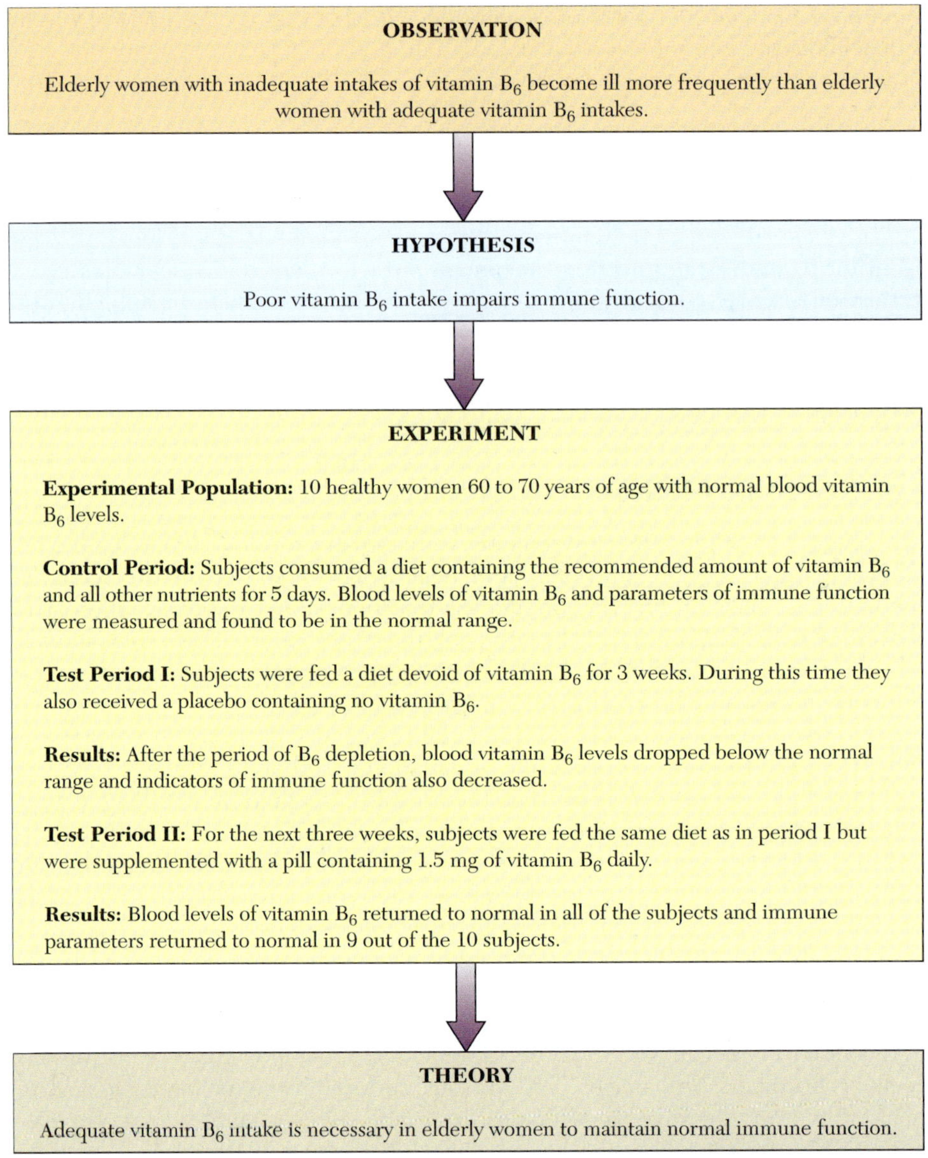

FIGURE 1.9 This example, which explores the relationship between vitamin B_6 and immune system function, illustrates how the scientific method can be used to formulate hypotheses based on observations, design experiments to test these hypotheses, and interpret the results to support or disprove the hypotheses, helping establish a theory.

concentration of a nutrient in the bloodstream, such as the level of vitamin B_6 discussed in Figure 1.9, is a parameter that can be quantified and repeated reliably. Individuals' opinions and feelings are referred to as subjective parameters. This type of information is often anecdotal and not sufficient to generate scientific theories. However, when subjective parameters such as how individuals feel about their energy level or general well-being need to be measured, standardized questionnaires can be administered before and after a treatment to objectively assess such parameters.

Experimental controls Factors included in an experimental design that limit the number of variables, allowing an investigator to examine the effect of only the parameters of interest.

Variable A factor or condition that is changed in an experimental setting.

Control groups Groups of participants in experiments to whom no experimental treatment is given. They are used as a basis of comparison.

Experimental groups Groups of participants in an experiment who are subjected to an experimental treatment.

Proper Controls **Experimental controls** ensure that each factor, or **variable,** studied can be compared with a known situation. A **control group** acts as a standard of comparison for the treatment being tested. This control group is treated in the same way as the **experimental groups** except that no experimental treatment is implemented. In some cases, the subjects participating in an experiment can serve as their own controls. For example, in the experiment described in Figure 1.9, the subjects are first fed an adequate control diet and control measurements are made. The values obtained from subsequent dietary changes are compared to this control value. The study could also have compared two groups of subjects matched for age, sex, and all other physiological parameters. The control group would then consume an adequate diet and the experimental group a deficient diet.

In some studies, a **placebo** is used to prevent participants or researchers from knowing who is receiving the experimental treatment. This placebo, often a sugar pill, is identical in appearance to the actual treatment but has no biological effect. In the studies described in Figure 1.9, the placebo is a pill that looks and tastes just like the vitamin B_6 supplement but doesn't contribute any vitamin B_6. In a **single-blind study,** experimental subjects do not know which treatment they are receiving, so their expectations cannot bias the results. For example, if the subjects believe that the pill they are taking will boost their immune response, the psychological well-being that results could have a physiological effect on the immune system. In a **double-blind study** neither the subjects nor the investigators know who is receiving the actual treatment until after the results have been analyzed. This prevents investigators' desire for a specific outcome from biasing the results.

Placebo A fake medicine or supplement that is indistinguishable in appearance from the real thing. It is used to disguise the control and experimental groups in an experiment.

Single-blind study An experiment in which either the study participants or the researchers are unaware of who is in a control or an experimental group.

Double-blind study An experiment in which neither the study participants nor the researchers know who is in a control or an experimental group.

Appropriate Experimental Population For an experiment to produce applicable results, it must be conducted in the right study population. For example, if a study is being conducted to test the hypothesis that vitamin B_6 supplements improve immune function in the elderly, then elderly subjects must be used as the study population. The number of subjects included in a study is also important. To be successful, an experiment must show that the treatment being tested causes a result to occur more frequently than it would occur by chance. A large number of subjects is needed to demonstrate an effect that occurs frequently by chance. Fewer subjects are needed when an effect rarely occurs by chance. **Statistical analysis** should be applied before a study is conducted to determine how many subjects are needed to show the effect of the experimental treatment. After the study is complete, statistics can be used to determine whether the experimental treatment had a significant effect.

Statistical analysis The process of collecting and analyzing numerical information to determine if an event is due to chance or to the effect of an experimental treatment.

Interpretation of Experimental Results In science, the interpretation of study results is as important as the way in which the study is done. For example, if the effects of vitamin B_6 intake are tested in elderly women, the study cannot conclude that the identical effect will occur in children. One way to ensure that experiments are correctly interpreted is to use a **peer-review** system. Most scientific journals require that reports of studies be reviewed by two or three experts in the field who did not take part in the research that is being evaluated. Before an article can be published in the journal, these scientists must agree that the experiments were well conducted and that the results were interpreted fairly. Nutrition articles can be found in peer-reviewed journals such as the *American Journal of Clinical Nutrition, Journal of Nutrition, Journal of the American Dietetic Association, New England Journal of Medicine,* and *International Journal of Sport Nutrition* (Figure 1.10).

Peer review Review of the design and validity of a research experiment by experts in the field of study who did not participate in the research.

Types of Nutrition Research Studies

Nutrition research studies are done to determine nutrient requirements, to learn more about the metabolism of nutrients, and to understand the role of nutrition in health and disease. Perfect tools do not exist for addressing all these questions. However, many types of research can be useful, including epidemiological observations and studies, human intervention studies, and a variety of types of laboratory studies.

Epidemiological Observations and Studies **Epidemiology** is the study of patterns that occur within populations. In nutrition, epidemiological studies are used

Epidemiology The study of the interrelationships between health and disease and other factors in the environment or lifestyle of different populations.

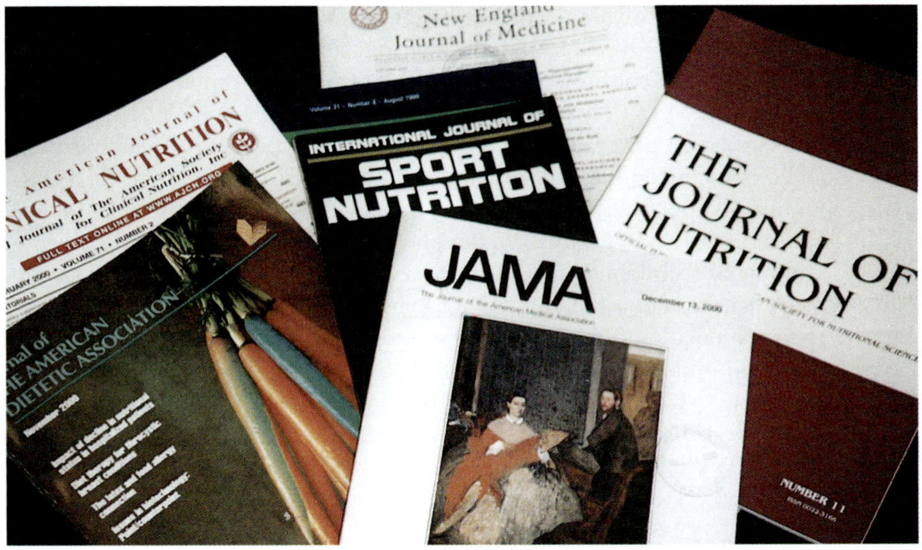

FIGURE 1.10 Nutrition articles published in journals such as these have been scrutinized by nutrition scientists to ensure the quality of the research and the accuracy of the interpretation. *(© Lori Smolin)*

to identify relationships between diet and health. Epidemiology does not determine cause and effect relationships—it just finds patterns. For instance, epidemiology was used to identify the association, or **correlation,** between diets high in fruits and vegetables and the incidence of cancer. This was done by looking at dietary patterns and the incidence of cancer in different countries. Some epidemiologic studies use **cross-sectional data,** which are collected from a cross section of the population at one point in time. The data could be used, for example, to identify associations between fat intake and blood cholesterol levels in a large population. **Longitudinal data** are collected from the same individuals over a period of time. Such data could be used, for example, to evaluate long-term relationships between dietary fat intake, blood cholesterol levels, and cardiovascular disease. However, this type of data is much more difficult, time consuming, and costly to collect because individuals have to be monitored for many years (see *Research Discoveries:* "From 'Seven Countries' to the Mediterranean Diet").

Correlation Two or more factors occurring together.

Cross-sectional data Information obtained by a single broad sampling of many different individuals in a population.

Longitudinal data Information obtained by repeatedly sampling the same individuals in a population over time.

Case-control studies are a type of epidemiological study that compares individuals with a particular condition to similar individuals without the condition. For example, a case-control study of colon cancer might compare the dietary intake of a 45-year-old African-American male with colon cancer to a man of the same age and background who is free of the disease. If a pattern were found in comparing cases to controls, further experimentation would then be needed to determine if a specific nutrient or dietary component that differed between the groups contributed to the colon cancer.

Case-control study A type of epidemiological study that compares individuals with a particular condition to those without the condition and then explores other variables that are different between the groups that might correlate with the presence of the condition being studied.

Human Intervention Studies The observations and hypotheses that come from epidemiology can be tested by human **intervention studies,** often referred to as **clinical trials.** This type of experiment actively intervenes in the lives of study participants and examines the effect of this intervention. Nutrition intervention studies generally explore the effects of altering people's diets. For example, if it is determined by epidemiology that populations that eat more broccoli have a lower incidence of various types of cancer, an intervention trial can be designed with an experimental group that consumes broccoli three to four days a week and a control group that consumes a typical diet, including broccoli once every other week. The groups would then be monitored to see if the dietary intervention affects the incidence of various types of cancer over the long term (see *Critical Thinking*: "The Scientific Method").

Intervention study or **clinical trial** A study of a population in which there is an experimental manipulation of some members of the population; observations and measurements are made to determine the effects of this manipulation.

Laboratory Studies Laboratory studies are conducted in the controlled environment of a laboratory or hospital. They include a variety of types of studies used to learn more about how nutrients function and to evaluate the relationships among nutrient intake, levels of nutrients in the body, and health. They may study nutrient requirements and functions in whole organisms—either humans or animals—or they may focus on nutrient functions at the cellular, biochemical, and molecular levels.

Studies Using Whole Organisms Many nutrition studies are done by feeding a specific diet to a person or animal and monitoring the physiological effects of that diet. **Depletion-repletion studies** are a classic method for studying the functions of nutrients and estimating the requirement of a particular nutrient. They involve depleting a nutrient by feeding a subject a diet lacking in that nutrient. After a period of time, if the nutrient is essential, symptoms of a deficiency will develop. The symptoms provide information on how the nutrient functions in the body. The nutrient is then added back to the diet, or repleted, until the symptoms are reversed. The requirement for that nutrient is the amount needed to reverse the deficiency symptoms. For example, depletion of magnesium from the diet causes a lack of muscle coordination. This tells scientists that magnesium is needed for muscle contraction. When enough magnesium is again added to the diet, muscle control returns; the requirement for magnesium is determined to be the amount of magnesium needed to return muscle control to normal. The experiment described in Figure 1.9 is an example of how a depletion-repletion study can be used to study the effect of vitamin B_6 on the immune system.

Depletion-repletion study A study that feeds a diet devoid of a nutrient until signs of deficiency appear, and then adds the nutrient back to the diet to a level at which symptoms disappear.

Another method for determining nutrient functions and requirements is to compare the intake of a nutrient with its excretion. This type of study is known as a **balance study.** If more of a nutrient is consumed than is excreted, it is assumed that the nutrient is being used or stored by the body. If more of the nutrient is excreted than is consumed, some is being lost from body stores. When the amount consumed equals the amount lost, the body is neither gaining nor losing that nutrient and is said to be in balance (Figure 1.11). By

Balance study A study that compares the total amount of a nutrient that enters the body with the total amount that leaves the body.

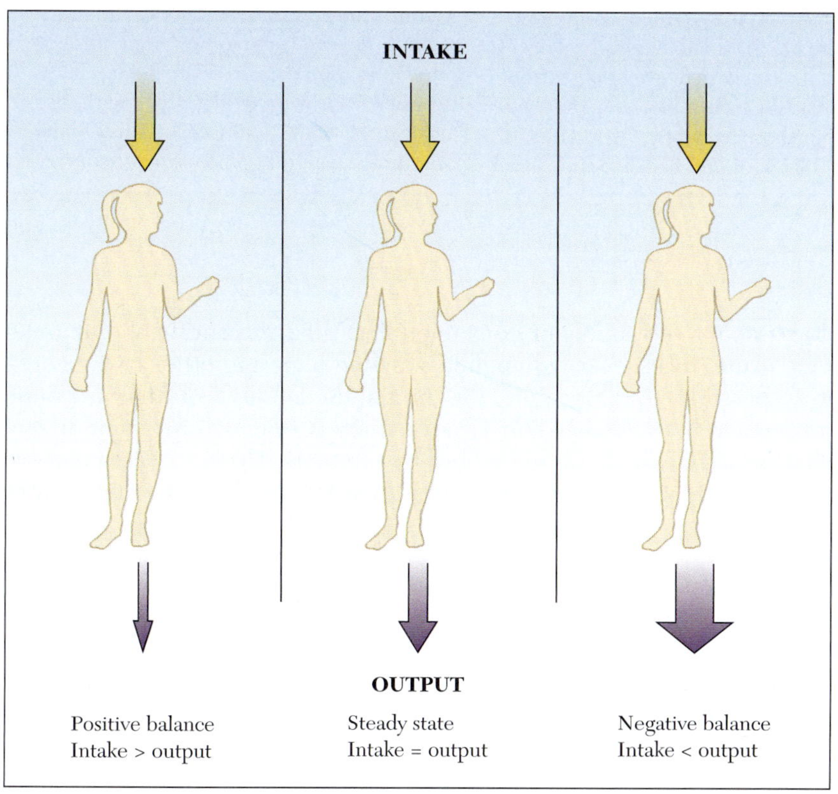

FIGURE 1.11 The concept of nutrient balance is illustrated here. If more of a nutrient is consumed than excreted, balance is positive. If the same amount is consumed and excreted, balance or a steady state exists. If less is consumed than excreted, balance is negative.

RESEARCH DISCOVERIES

From "Seven Countries" to the Mediterranean Diet

In 1916, Dutch internist C.D. de Langen hypothesized that a cholesterol-rich diet was associated with high blood cholesterol and the occurrence of coronary heart disease. But it was not until the 1950s that the associations among diet, blood cholesterol, and coronary heart disease were investigated. The question of whether the differences in the occurrence of heart disease between different populations could be explained by differences in diet and blood cholesterol was of interest to Professor Ancel Keys at the University of Minnesota. In 1958, he initiated one of the most extensive epidemiological studies in nutrition history. The Seven Countries Study was designed to test the hypothesis that atherosclerosis and coronary heart disease were nutritional problems related to fat intake. Between 1958 and 1964 the study enrolled 12,763 men from 40 to 59 years of age from 16 different regions within 7 countries on 3 continents.

Health status, dietary intake, body weight, blood pressure, blood cholesterol level, and other health-related parameters were evaluated at regular intervals over the duration of the study. As data were compiled, patterns began to emerge. In Northern European countries, the diet was high in dairy products; in the United States, it was high in meat; in Southern Europe, it was high in vegetables, legumes, fish, and wine; and in Japan, it was high in cereals, soy products, and fish.[a] After 10 years, 1512 of the study participants were dead—413 of them from coronary heart disease.[b] But, mortality from coronary heart disease differed strikingly with location. On the Isle of Crete there was only one coronary death out of 686 men studied. Yet in east Finland there were 78 coronary deaths among 817 participants.[c]

The coronary death rate was correlated with the average percentage of kcalories from saturated fat. In countries such as Japan, where the diet was low in total fat and saturated fat, blood cholesterol values were lower, and so was the risk of dying from heart disease. In countries such as Finland, where the diet was rich in saturated fat and cholesterol, blood cholesterol levels were higher, as was the incidence of heart disease. The results showed that blood cholesterol was strongly correlated with coronary heart disease deaths both for populations and for individuals. This meant that someone with a higher blood cholesterol level had a greater risk of dying from heart disease than someone with a lower cholesterol level.

A closer examination of the data revealed some paradoxes. In different populations, the same blood cholesterol level represented different degrees of cardiovascular risk. For example, someone living in Northern Europe who had a cholesterol level of 200 had five times the risk of dying of heart disease than someone with a cholesterol of 200 living in Mediterranean Southern Europe.[d] The data suggested that blood cholesterol was not the only risk factor involved in heart disease. When other dietary and lifestyle factors were examined, patterns emerged that were related to the risk of coronary heart disease. In the countries of Southern Europe around the Mediterranean Sea—countries where the incidence of coronary heart disease was low—the diet was plentiful in vegetables and whole grains, and, though not always low in total fat, relied on olive oil as the source of the fat. In addition, the lifestyle was not stressful and wine was routinely, but not excessively, consumed with meals. This pattern became known as the "Mediterranean diet."

Today, many of the features of the Mediterranean diet are included in population-wide recommendations that target a reduction in the risk of coronary heart disease (see Appendix H for the Mediterranean Food Guide Pyramid). The Seven Countries Study helped make diets low in saturated fat the standard prescription for reducing cardiovascular risk. The Mediterranean diet has taught us that including olive oil and other monounsaturated oils as the source of dietary fat is beneficial. Recommendations today also advocate other components of the Mediterranean diet, including plenty of

varying the amount of a nutrient consumed and then measuring the amount excreted (in urine, feces, sweat, sloughed skin and hair, and other body secretions), it is possible to determine the minimum amount of that nutrient needed to replace body losses. This type of study is effective for some nutrients, such as protein, which are not stored by the body. However, it cannot be used to study nutrients such as fat and iron, which are stored when excess is available.

Animals As Human Models in Nutrition Research Ideally, studies of human nutrition should be done in humans. However, because studying humans is costly, time consuming, inconvenient for subjects, and in some cases impossible for ethical reasons, many studies are done using experimental animals.

whole grains and fruits and vegetables. Exercise, smoking cessation, and stress reduction are also encouraged to reduce cardiovascular risk.

After over 40 years, survivors of the Seven Countries Study are still being studied and data are still being collected and analyzed. These epidemiological data have been the basis for countless laboratory studies and intervention trials. As more and more pieces of the coronary heart disease puzzle fall into place, scientists and government agencies will continue to modify their recommendations.

References

[a] Menotti, A., Kromhout, D., Blackburn, H., et al. Food intake patterns and 25-year mortality from coronary heart disease: cross-cultural correlations in the Seven Countries Study. The Seven Countries Research Group. Eur. J. Epidemiol. 15:507–515, 1999.

[b] The diet and all-causes death rate in the Seven Countries Study. Lancet 2(8237):58–61, 1999.

[c] Keys, A. *Seven Countries: A Multivariate Analysis of Death and Coronary Heart Disease.* A Commonwealth Fund book. Cambridge, Mass.: Harvard University Press, 1980.

[d] Kromhout, D. Serum cholesterol in cross-cultural perspective: the Seven Countries Study. Acta. Cardiol. 45:155–158, 1999.

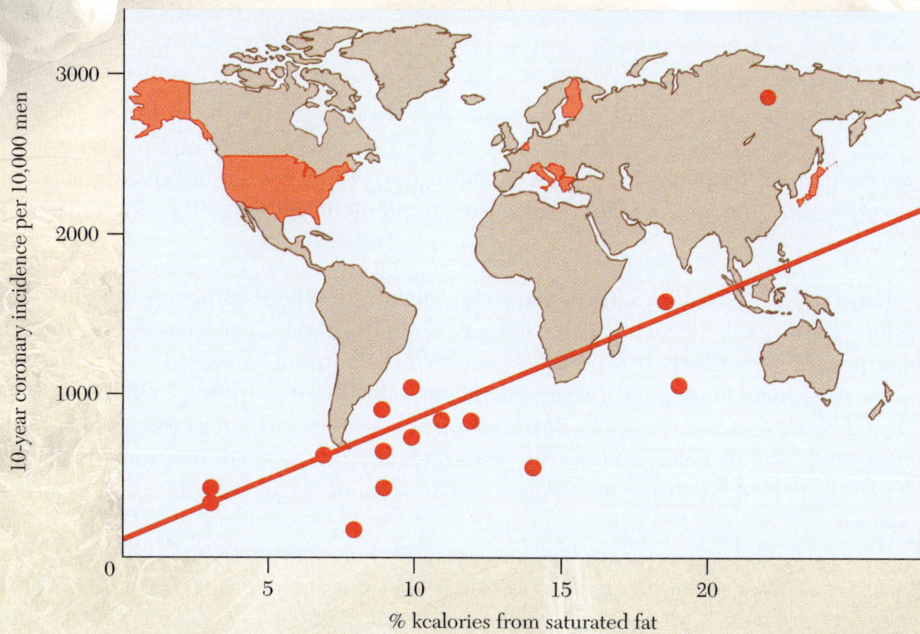

The data from the Seven Countries Study identified a relationship between the amount of saturated fat in the diet and the incidence of coronary heart disease. As the amount of saturated fat in the diet increases, so does the incidence of coronary heart disease. *(Keys, A.* **Seven Countries: A Multivariate Analysis of Deaths and Coronary Heart Disease.** *Cambridge, Mass.: Harvard University Press, 1980)*

An ideal animal model is one with metabolic and digestive processes similar to those in humans, such as a pig (Figure 1.12). However, in addition to digestion and metabolism, factors such as cost and time must be considered. Pigs and other large animals are expensive to use and take a long time to develop nutrient deficiencies. Smaller laboratory animals, such as rats and mice, are therefore the most common experimental animals. They are inexpensive, have short life spans, and reproduce quickly. Their food intake and excretions can be easily monitored, and the effects of nutritional changes develop rapidly. However, even when using small animals, a scientist must choose the species of animal carefully. For example, rats are more resistant to heart disease than are humans, so they are not a good model for studying the effect of diet on heart disease. Rabbits, on the other hand, do develop heart disease and can be used to study diet–heart disease relationships.

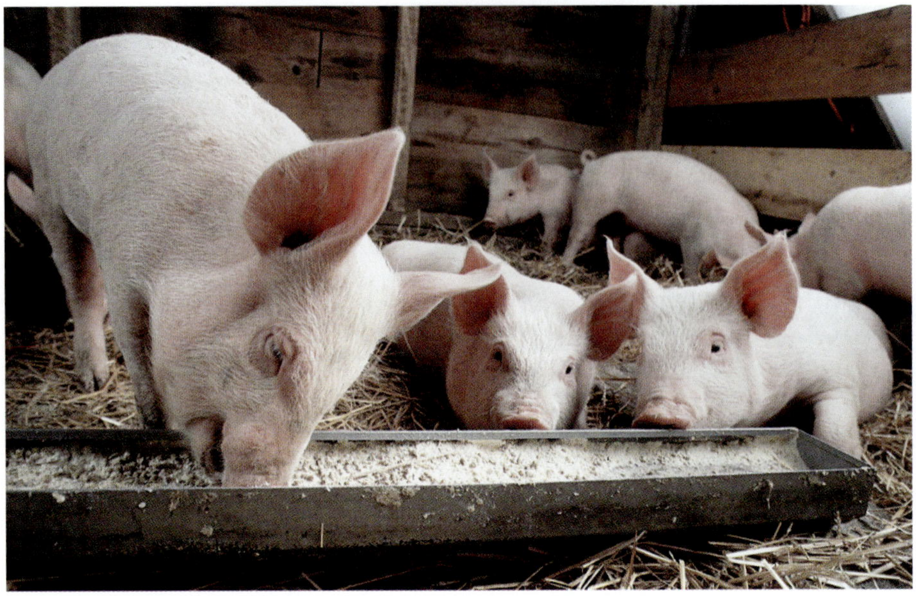

FIGURE 1.12 Pigs are a good animal model for human digestion and metabolism because they have similar digestive mechanisms and eat a similar type of diet. *(© Andrew Sacks/Tony Stone Images)*

Even the best animal model is not the same as a human, and care must be taken when extrapolating the results to the human population. For example, a study that uses rats to show that a calcium supplement increases bone density can hypothesize, but not conclude, that the supplement will have the same effect in humans.

Studying Cells Another alternative to conducting feeding studies in humans is to study either cells extracted from humans or cells grown in the laboratory for this purpose. Biochemistry can be used to study how nutrients are used for energy and how they regulate chemical reactions in cells. **Molecular biology** can be used to study how segments of **DNA (deoxyribonucleic acid),** called **genes,** regulate the functions of body cells and how the types and amounts of nutrients available to cells can affect the action of genes. For example, vitamin A can directly activate certain genes.

Knowledge gained from biochemical and molecular biological studies can be used to study nutrition-related conditions that affect the entire organism. These techniques may help to identify individuals at high risk of developing chronic diseases such as heart disease, diabetes, and cancer and to develop methods of prevention and treatment.

Molecular biology The study of cellular function at the molecular level.

DNA (deoxyribonucleic acid) The genetic material that codes for the synthesis of proteins.

Genes Lengths of DNA that provide instructions for heritable traits.

Ethical Considerations In addition to the issues of science, ethical issues are often raised in the process of conducting nutrition research. To avoid harm to study subjects or experimental animals, researchers use alternatives whenever possible: extracted fluids, cells grown in the laboratory, and, in some cases, computer models to predict how changes in nutrient intake affect body processes. Such alternatives cannot always be used; therefore, human and animal experimentation is still necessary to answer many questions.

To protect the rights of humans and animals used in experimental research, government guidelines and regulations have been developed. Before an experiment involving human subjects can be conducted, the study must be reviewed by a committee of scientists and nonscientists to ensure that the risks of physical, social, and psychological injury are balanced against the potential benefits of the research. This was not always the case. Much of what is known today about the effects of starvation in humans was determined during World War II by conducting depletion-repletion studies using conscientious objectors as experimental subjects. These subjects were monitored physically and psychologically while they

Web Menu For more information on government regulations regarding research involving human subjects, go to the NIH Office of Human Subjects Research at ohsr.od.nih.gov/.

were starved and then refed. Because starvation causes physical discomfort, these individuals experienced some level of suffering during the trials and risked longer-lasting physical and psychological harm.

As with experiments involving humans, the federal government mandates that panels of scientists review experiments that propose to use animals. These panels consider whether the need for animals is justified and whether all precautions will be taken to avoid pain and suffering. Animal housing and handling is strictly regulated, and a violation of these guidelines can close a research facility (Figure 1.13).

Finally, the development of the techniques of molecular biology created the need for guidelines and experimental review processes that assure that studies involving gene manipulation are safe and ethical. These guidelines and procedures are modified on an ongoing basis to stay abreast of advances in this area.

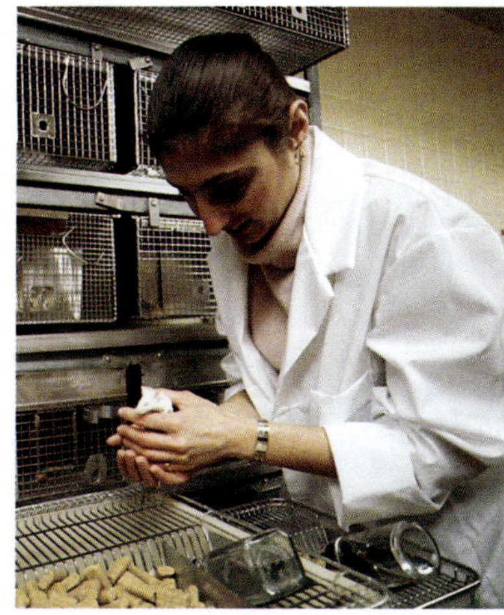

FIGURE 1.13 The care and housing of animals used in research are strictly regulated. *(Runk/Shoenberger/Grant Heilman Photography, Inc.)*

Critical Thinking

The Scientific Method

Observation

While examining epidemiological data, a scientist observes that the incidence of colon cancer is much greater in the United States than it is in Japan. He proposes a number of hypotheses to explain this observation.

Hypotheses

1. The difference may occur because the Japanese people inherit genetic factors that protect against colon cancer.
2. The difference may be due to differences between the diet in the United States and in Japan.
3. The difference may be due to some environmental factor that differs between Japan and the United States.

What other possible reasons could explain a difference in cancer incidence between these two populations?

Answer:

Experimentation

To explore the reasons for the difference in colon cancer incidence, the scientist reviews the medical records and dietary intakes of Japanese people living in the United States. These individuals are not different genetically from Japanese living in Japan but are now exposed to environmental factors in the United States rather than those in Japan. The results indicate that this group of people now consumes a typical American diet and that the incidence of colon cancer is similar to that of the rest of the U.S. population.

Which hypothesis has been disproved?

Answer:

Experimentation

To further explore this question, the scientist designs a human intervention trial. A group of Japanese Americans is instructed to consume a traditional Japanese diet. Those who adopt the traditional diet are monitored for many years. The results indicate that the incidence of colon cancer declines in this group when compared to Japanese Americans who continue to eat an American style diet.

What other experiments could you propose to obtain more information about the causes of colon cancer in the United States?

Answer:

Propose a theory based on the evidence presented here.

Answer:

Evaluating Nutrition Information

Web Menu: For a guide to health fraud, quackery, and evaluating information about food, nutrition, and health fads and fallacies, go to Quackwatch at www.quackwatch.com/index.html or the National Council for Reliable Health Information at www.ncahf.org/. For a site that reviews and rates nutrition information on the Web, go to Tufts Nutrition Navigator at www.navigator.tufts.edu/.

C 62 00 00 00 00 00 27 10

C 62 00 00 00 00 00 27 11

C 62 00 00 00 00 00 27 12

Nutrition, like all science, continues to evolve as new discoveries provide clues to the right combination of nutrients needed for optimal health. As knowledge advances, recommendations change. Sometimes established beliefs and concepts must give way to new ideas. For example, in the early part of the 20th century, exercise was considered dangerous for people at risk of cardiovascular disease; today, exercise is promoted to strengthen the heart and reduce the risk of heart attacks in individuals with cardiovascular disease. Consumers may find this evolution of nutrition knowledge frustrating because the experts seem to change their minds so often. In addition, consumers are bombarded with information from many sources. Some is accurate and some is incorrect or exaggerated to sell products or to make news headlines more enticing. How can a health-conscious consumer know what to believe?

Sources of Nutrition Information

The nutrition information that shapes our attitudes about what we should and should not eat comes to us in a variety of ways. Some comes from individual contact with physicians and dietitians; some is printed on food labels and in educational pamphlets. But much of it reaches us through television, radio, newspapers, magazines, and the Internet. Although dietitians and physicians are viewed as the most reliable source of nutrition information, Americans today get most of their food and nutrition information from the mass media, which are very powerful tools for promoting health and nutrition messages.[3] Information that would take individual health-care workers years to disseminate can reach millions of individuals in a matter of hours or days. Much of this information is reliable, but some can be misleading. At times, news stories are used to sell subscriptions or improve ratings, not to promote the nutritional health of the population. Advertisements paid for by food manufacturers are also a source of nutrition information. Because this information is designed primarily to sell products, it can be confusing to the consumer, who may not know how to interpret it. Knowing what information to believe and how to use it to choose a diet can be difficult but is essential to making appropriate food and nutrition decisions.

Judging Nutrition Claims

Just as scientists use the scientific method to expand their understanding of the world around us, consumers can use an understanding of the tools of science to judge the validity of nutrition headlines. The following sections and Table 1.7 list some steps to follow when judging a nutrition claim.

Does the Information Make Sense? The first question to ask when evaluating a nutrition claim is, Does the information make sense? Some claims are too outrageous to be true. For example, the hypothetical advertisement for ImmunoEnhance illustrated in Figure 1.14 states that this product will make illness a thing of the past. This is certainly appealing, but it is hard to believe, and common sense should tell you that it is too good to be true. The claim that ImmunoEnhance will reduce cold symptoms, however, is not so outrageous.

TABLE 1.7 Evaluating Nutrition Information

1. Does the information make sense?
   - Is it too outrageous to believe?
   - Is it based on a cultural or religious belief?
2. Where did the information come from?
   - Is it based on a government recommendation?
   - Is it based on a study in a peer-reviewed journal?
   - Have other studies confirmed the results?
   - Is it based on someone's personal experience?
   - Is it in a news story or an advertising promotion?
3. Were the experiments well designed?
   - Were proper controls used?
   - Were enough study subjects used to get reliable results?
   - Were the data objective?
4. Is the information interpreted accurately?
   - Were the results or importance of the study exaggerated?
   - If the study was done in animals, can it be applied to humans?
   - Was the level of food or nutrient used compatible with amounts in a human diet?
5. Who is making the recommendation and who stands to benefit?
   - Is it helping to sell a product?
   - Does the reporter stand to benefit from your believing the information?
   - Is it making a magazine cover or newspaper headline more appealing?
   - Is it designed to improve public health?

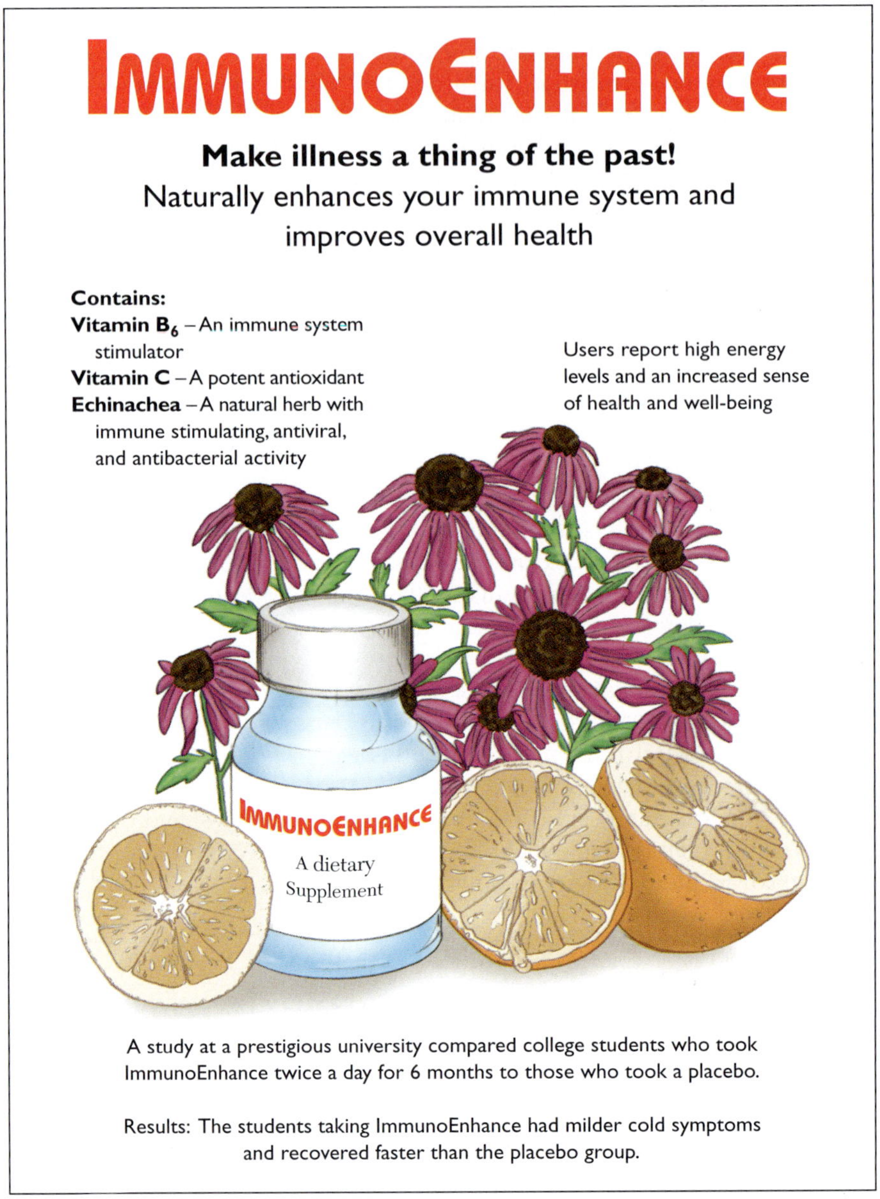
IMMUNOENHANCE
Make illness a thing of the past!
Naturally enhances your immune system and improves overall health
Contains:
Vitamin B_6 – An immune system stimulator
Vitamin C – A potent antioxidant
Echinachea – A natural herb with immune stimulating, antiviral, and antibacterial activity
Users report high energy levels and an increased sense of health and well-being
IMMUNOENHANCE
A dietary Supplement
A study at a prestigious university compared college students who took ImmunoEnhance twice a day for 6 months to those who took a placebo.
Results: The students taking ImmunoEnhance had milder cold symptoms and recovered faster than the placebo group.

FIGURE 1.14 This hypothetical advertisement illustrates some types of nutrition claims that consumers must be prepared to evaluate.

Where Did the Information Come From? If the claim seems reasonable, look to see where it came from. Was it based on a government recommendation or advice from a health professional? Was it the result of research studies, or one person's opinion? Is it in a news story or an advertising promotion?

Government guidelines regarding healthy dietary practices are developed by committees of scientists who interpret the latest well-conducted research studies and use their conclusions to develop recommendations for the population as a whole. The government provides recommendations about food safety, food choices, and specific nutrient needs. These recommendations are used to develop food-labeling regulations and are the basis for public health policies and programs. They are published in pamphlets and brochures designed for consumers.

Claims that come from individual testimonies have not been tested by objective experimentation. For example, the claim that ImmunoEnhance improves energy levels and overall sense of health and well-being is based on the comments of supplement users and is therefore anecdotal, and not based on measured parameters.

Research studies that are reported at conferences or published in popular magazines may be legitimate but have not been scrutinized by the scientific community to determine their quality and validity. The ImmunoEnhance ad does cite a university research study that demonstrated reduced cold symptoms. But, it does not indicate if the study was published, or if it was published in a peer-reviewed journal. Studies published in peer-reviewed journals are well scrutinized; however, even when published in a peer-reviewed journal, a single study is not necessarily enough on which to base a nutrition recommendation. Study results need to be verified and repeated if they are to be used to make dietary recommendations.

Was the Research Properly Designed? If the source of the information seems reliable, look to see if the research on which the claim is based was well designed. Did the study use the right population? Were enough subjects and the proper controls used? Were the data objective? For example, the university study described in the ImmunoEnhance ad compares the severity of cold symptoms and the cold recovery time (objective parameters) of college students who took the ImmunoEnhance supplement with the same parameters in a similar group of students who took a placebo. The results indicate that the experimental group had milder cold symptoms and quicker recovery times than the control or placebo group. This then supports the claim that the product can reduce cold symptoms.

Were the Data Accurately Interpreted? Even well-designed, carefully executed, peer-reviewed experiments can be a source of misinformation if the results are interpreted incorrectly or if the implications of the results are exaggerated. For example, the headline in Figure 1.14 states that ImmunoEnhance improves overall health. However, the study only shows that cold symptoms were reduced; overall health is not addressed.

Who Stands to Benefit? The final question in judging nutrition claims is, who is presenting the information, or who stands to benefit from the information? Is the claim making a magazine cover or newspaper headline more appealing? If a claim is part of a news headline, it may be true but exaggerated to sell the publication. Is the claim helping to sell a product? The claims for ImmunoEnhance are part of an advertisement to increase sales. The company stands to profit from your believing the claim.

Information presented in public health bulletins is designed to improve the nutritional health of the population. Information presented to individuals by nutritionists is designed to improve personal nutritional health. However, care must be taken even when obtaining information from a nutritionist or nutrition counselor. Although these individuals may provide accurate information, it is important to determine their credentials. The term "nutritionist" is not legally defined and is used by a wide range of individuals—from college professors with doctoral degrees from reputable universities to sales clerks in health-food stores with no formal nutrition education. One reliable source of nutrition information is registered dietitians (RDs), who have completed a four-year college degree in a nutrition-related field and who have met established criteria to certify them in providing nutrition counseling.

Summary

1. Nutrition is a science that encompasses all the interactions that occur between living organisms and food. Food provides energy and nutrients needed for growth, body maintenance and repair, and reproduction. Nutrition studies the physiological processes by which an organism ingests and uses food and nutrients, the biological actions and interactions of food with the body and their consequences for health and disease, and the psychological and sociocultural factors that influence food choices.
2. Food availability, personal tastes, sociocultural influences, and what is perceived to be healthy affect individual food choices.

No single food choice is good or bad, but together they make up a dietary pattern that is either healthy or not so healthy. The typical dietary pattern in the United States today is lower in fruits, vegetables, dairy products, lean meats, and whole grains, and higher in added sugars and fats, than recommended. This dietary pattern and lack of physical activity contribute to the increasing incidence of chronic diseases such as diabetes, obesity, and heart disease.

3. Nutrients are grouped into six classes: carbohydrates, lipids, proteins, water, vitamins, and minerals. Essential nutrients cannot be made by the body and therefore must be consumed in the diet. Nutrients provide energy, which is measured in kcalories or kjoules. They provide structure to the body and regulate the biochemical reactions of metabolism to maintain homeostasis.
4. When energy or one or more nutrients are deficient or excessive in the diet, malnutrition may result. Malnutrition includes both undernutrition and overnutrition. Too little or too much of a nutrient can cause effects that occur in the short term or over the course of many weeks, months, or even years.
5. The science of nutrition uses the scientific method to determine the nutrient needs of the body as well as the effects of nutrients and other dietary components on health promotion and disease prevention. The scientific method involves making observations of natural events, formulating hypotheses to explain these events, designing and performing experiments to test the hypotheses, and developing theories that explain the observed phenomenon based on the experimental results.
6. To be valid, a nutrition experiment must use objective measurements, appropriate controls, the right type and number of experimental subjects, and a careful interpretation of experimental results.
7. The science of nutrition uses many different types of experimental approaches to determine nutrient functions and requirements. Epidemiological observations identify relationships in populations. Intervention trials can test hypotheses developed from epidemiology. Laboratory studies, including those that study the whole organism (such as depletion-repletion and balance studies) and those that study cells (such as biochemical and molecular biological studies) are used to evaluate the relationships among nutrient intake, levels of nutrients in the body, and other parameters of metabolism or health.
8. When judging nutrition claims, consumers need to consider whether the information makes sense, whether it came from a reliable source, whether the studies were well done and accurately interpreted, and who stands to benefit from making the claim.

Review Questions

1. What is nutrition?
2. List three factors other than biological need that influence food choices.
3. What is an essential nutrient?
4. List the six classes of nutrients. Which nutrients provide energy?
5. List three functions of nutrients.
6. What is malnutrition? Overnutrition? Undernutrition?
7. What is toxicity?
8. List the steps of the scientific method.
9. What is a control group?
10. What is a placebo?
11. What is a double-blind study?
12. What type of information can be obtained using epidemiology?
13. Why are animal studies used to determine human nutrient requirements?
14. What factors should be considered when judging nutrition claims?

Applying Critical Thinking Skills

Personal nutrition:

1. What factors affect your food choices?
   a. List four food items you ate today or yesterday.
   b. For each food listed, indicate the factor or factors that influenced your selection of that particular food. For example, if you ate a candy bar before your noon class, did you choose it because the machine was available outside the lecture hall, because you didn't have enough money for anything else, because you just like candy bars, because you were depressed, because all of your friends were eating them, because it is good for you, or for some other reason?
   c. For each food, indicate what information you used in making the selection. For example, did you read the label on the product, or consider something you had read or heard recently in the news media?
   d. List three factors that commonly influence your food choices.
   e. List three types of information you regularly use to make your food choices.

General nutrition issues:

1. A large epidemiological study involving 40,000 middle-aged women has identified a relationship between magnesium intake and bone density. Women with the greatest intakes of magnesium—a nutrient plentiful in whole grains and green vegetables—had denser bones, which are associated with a decreased risk of osteoporosis.

a. Does this study show that magnesium deficiency causes osteoporosis? Why or why not?
b. Would you recommend that all women over age 45 take a magnesium supplement to increase their bone density? Why or why not?
c. Would it be accurate for an ad for a nutritional supplement containing magnesium to claim that taking the supplement twice a day prevents osteoporosis? Why or why not?

2. The Good Heart Study is evaluating the relationship between a new miracle drug and heart disease. Two hundred participants are divided into two equal groups. Pills identical in appearance are administered to all participants. Group 1 receives two tablets per day of the miracle drug and group 2 receives two placebo tablets per day. After one month, half of the subjects in group 1 have blood cholesterol levels at or below the recommended levels. In group 2, 49 of the subjects have blood cholesterol levels at or below the recommendations.
   a. Is the study blinded?
   b. Does the miracle drug lower cholesterol?
   c. What changes would you make to better control the study?
3. Examine a nutritional supplement ad provided by your instructor or select one from a health- or fitness-related magazine.
   a. Is the claim made about this product believable?
   b. Does the ad refer to any research studies? If so, do they seem well controlled? Were the results based on objective measurements? Were the conclusions consistent with the results obtained? Were they published in peer-reviewed journals?
   c. Were claims based on anecdotal reports of individual users?
   d. Who stands to benefit if you spend money on this product?
   e. Based on this ad alone, would you choose to take this supplement? Why or why not?

References

1. American Dietetic Association, 1997 Nutrition Trends Survey, Executive Summary. Chicago: American Dietetic Association, 1997.
2. Pratt, E. L. Historical perspectives: food, feeding, and fancies. J. Am. Coll. Nutr. 3:115–121, 1984.
3. American Dietetic Association. *Americans' Food and Nutrition Attitudes and Behaviors, Nutrition and You: Trends 2000.* Available online at **http://www.eatright.org/pr/2000/010300a.html.** Accessed 11 Nov 2000.
4. Dyson, L. K. American cuisine in the 20th century. Food Review 23:23–29, 2000. Available online at **http://www.ers.usda.gov/epubs/pdf/foodrevw/jan2000/.** Accessed 7 Nov 2000.
5. Bowman, S. A., Lino, M., Gerrior, S. A., and Bastiotis, P. P. *The Healthy Eating Index:* 1994–96. U.S. Department of Agriculture, Center for Nutrition Policy and Promotion, 1998. CNPP-5. Available online at **http://www.usda.gov/cnpp/usda_healthy_eating_index.htm.** Accessed 13 Nov 2000.
6. Kantor, L. S. A *Dietary Assessment of the U.S. Food Supply,* Food and Rural Economics Division, Economic Research Service, U.S. Department of Agriculture. Agricultural Economics Report 772, 1998. Available online at **http://www.ers.usda.gov/epubs/pdf/aer772/index.htm.** Accessed 7 Nov 2000.
7. Leontos, C., Wong, F., and Gallivan, J., for National Diabetes Education Program Planning Committee. National Diabetes Education Program: opportunities and challenges. J. Am. Diet. Assoc. 98:73–75, 1998.
8. National Institutes of Health, National Heart, Lung, and Blood Institute. *Clinical Guidelines on the Identification, Evaluation, and Treatment of Overweight and Obesity in Adults.* Executive Summary, June 1998. Available online at **http://www.nhlbi.nih.gov/guidelines/obesity/ob_xsum.htm.** Accessed 11 Nov 2000.
9. U.S. Department of Health and Human Services. Report from H Working Group on Sentinel Objectives, Leading Indicators for People 2010. U.S. DHHS Office of Disease Prevention and Promotion. Available online at **http://web.health.gov/healthypeople/.** Accessed 1

2 Applying the Science of Nutrition

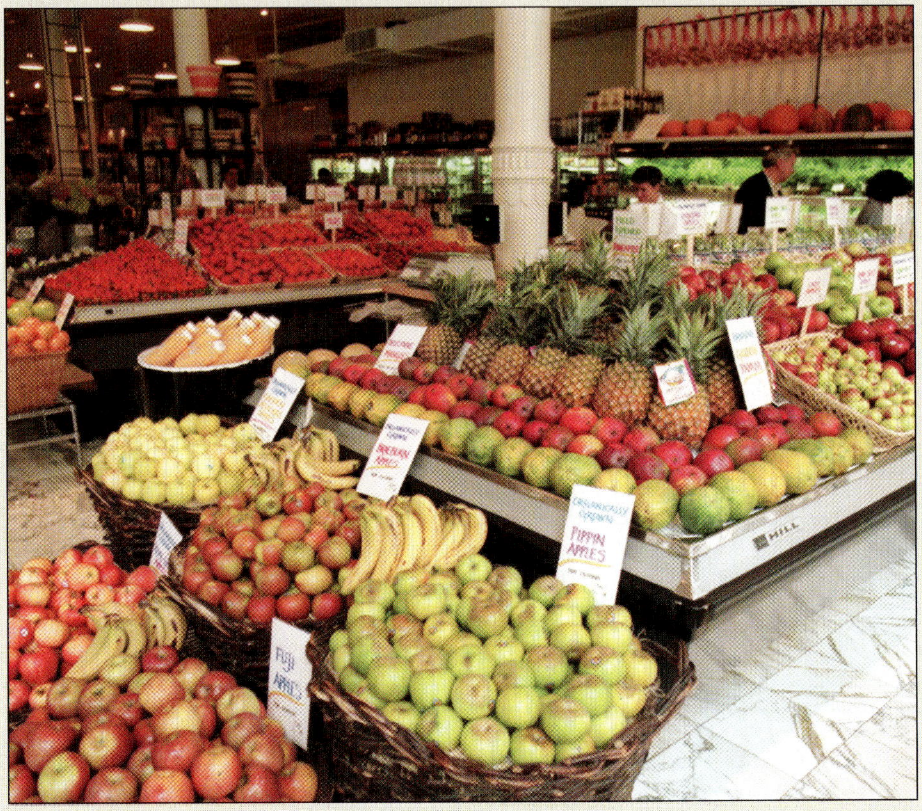

Learning Objectives

After reading this chapter, students should be able to:

1. Discuss how nutritional recommendations for populations are developed.
2. List the four types of standards that make up DRIs and explain the purpose of each.
3. Demonstrate to another student how to plan a diet using the Food Guide Pyramid.
4. Use the Nutrition Facts on a food label to select a food that contains less than 10% of the Daily Value for fat.
5. Identify from the ingredient list of a food label which ingredients are present in the greatest and least amounts.
6. Use a dietary supplement label to determine the amounts of each nutrient and other ingredients in the product.

…iscuss the three tiers of the Dietary Guidelines.

8. … a diet containing 1500 kcalories using the Exchange Lists.

9. Defi… …nutritional status" and explain the types of tools used to assess individua… …utritional health.

Hank had been the star of his high school track team. In college, Hank found the track competition to be much stiffer, and he began looking for ways to improve his times. He had heard that distance runners could benefit from extra protein, so he switched from eating cereal and toast at breakfast to eggs and sausage, and at lunch and dinner he skipped the starches that the cafeteria offered and increased his portions of meats. After a week on his new diet, Hank was feeling lousy. He was hungry and fatigued during workouts.

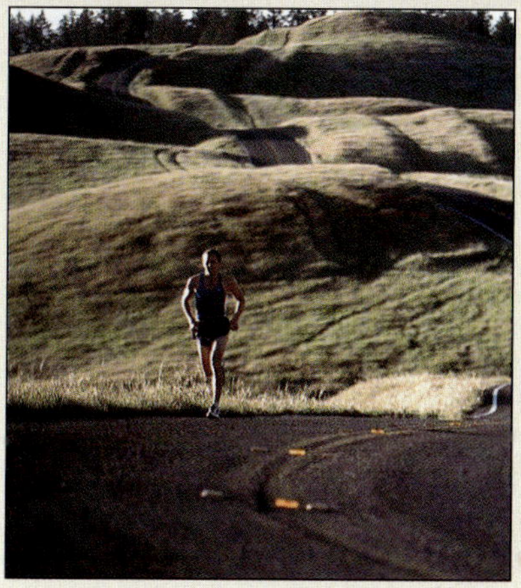

His coach sent him to the student health clinic to meet with the dietitian. After reviewing his diet and exercise schedule, she explained to him that he probably was not eating enough to meet his energy needs. In attempting to increase his protein intake, he had reduced his energy and carbohydrate intake. She explained that dietary carbohydrate is an important energy source for athletes. When he asked about the increased need for protein in distance runners, the dietitian explained that although the protein needs of a distance runner may be higher than the requirement set for the general population, a well-balanced diet can easily provide the extra protein. If Hank were to choose a balanced diet and eat enough to meet his energy needs, he would also be eating enough protein.

The dietitian helped Hank figure out how many servings of each group of the Food Guide Pyramid he would need to eat to meet his energy needs. By following the serving recommendations and choosing a variety of foods from each food group, he would get enough carbohydrates and protein and also meet his vitamin and mineral needs. She also gave him a copy of the Dietary Guidelines for Americans, which explains what components of the diet should be plentiful or limited and how to use food labels to choose foods to meet these goals. Knowing how to use these tools is key to consuming a healthy diet.

Nutritional Recommendations

Nutritional recommendations are standards for planning and evaluating healthy diets. They are developed by committees of scientists who interpret the latest well-conducted research studies and use their conclusions to establish recommendations for the population as a whole or for subsets of the population.

There are many types of nutritional recommendations. Some describe the amounts of individual nutrients that are needed and some recommend patterns of food intake to promote health and prevent disease. The nature of each set of recommendations depends on the population being targeted, who is developing the recommendations and why, and how they will be used. Is the recommendation for the general population? Is it for a particular gender, age, activity level, or ethnic group? Is it designed to promote health, prevent deficiencies, or prevent a specific disease? Is it designed for nutritionists to use when evaluating individual diets? Or is it intended to help the average consumer make individual food choices?

Because nutritional recommendations must satisfy a variety of needs, there are many different types available to the American public. These are updated periodically as new discoveries are made and our understanding of nutrition evolves.

Historical Perspective

Some of the first dietary recommendations were made in England in the 1860s, when the Industrial Revolution spurred a rise in urban populations, along with large numbers of homeless and hungry people. The government wanted to find the least expensive way to keep these underfed people alive and working. As a result, a dietary standard was established based on what the average working person ate in a typical day. This method of estimating nutrient needs was used until World War I, when the British Royal Society made specific recommendations about foods that not only would sustain life but also would be protective of health. The Society recommended that fruits and green vegetables be included in a healthy diet, and that milk be included in the diets of all children. Since then, the governments of many countries have established their own sets of dietary standards based on the nutritional problems and dietary patterns specific to their populations and the interpretations of their scientists. Most of the guidelines vary little from country to country. The World Health Organization and the Food and Agriculture Organization of the United Nations, organizations concerned with international health, also publish a set of dietary standards to apply worldwide[1] (see Appendix F).

Nutritional Recommendations in the United States

The U.S. government began considering recommendations for nutrient needs when food shipments were sent to its allies in Europe during World War I, but it was not until the early 1940s, when World War II created widespread food limitations at home, that the United States first set nutrition or dietary standards for its own population (Figure 2.1). The original dietary standards in the United States were the Recommended Dietary Allowances (RDAs). They were first published in 1943 and revised every few years until 1989 by the Food and Nutrition Board of the National Research Council.[2] The RDAs were set at levels that would prevent nutrient deficiencies. Recommendations were made for energy and nutrients likely to be deficient in the population's diet—protein, vitamins, and minerals.

Over the years since these first standards were developed, our knowledge of nutrient needs has increased and patterns of dietary intake and disease have changed. Overt nutrient deficiencies are now rare in the United States, but the incidence of chronic diseases that have a connection to diet quality, such as heart

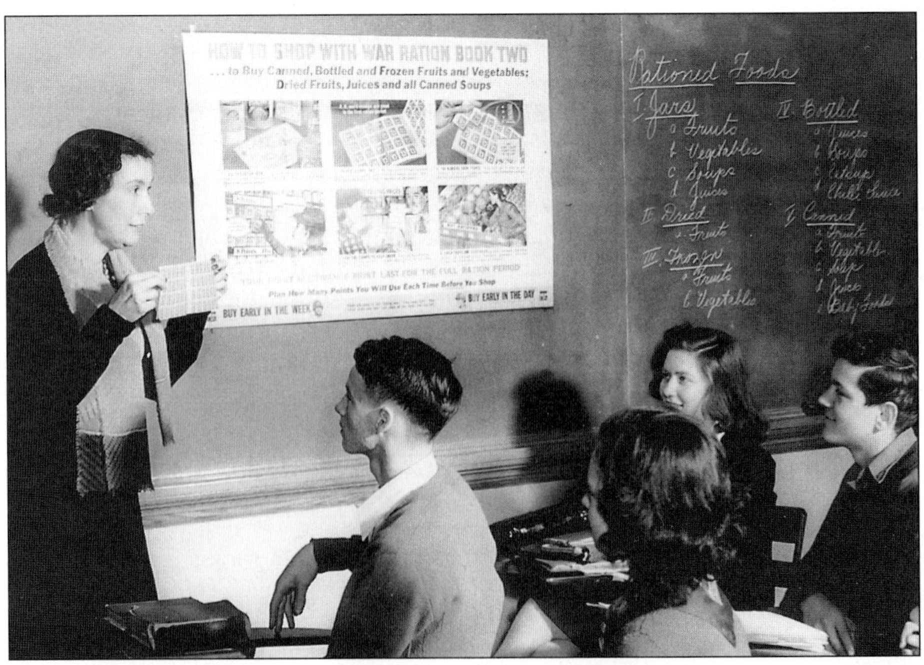
HOW TO SHOP WITH WAR RATION BOOK TWO
... to Buy Canned, Bottled and Frozen Fruits and Vegetables; Dried Fruits, Juices and all Canned Soups
BUY EARLY IN THE WEEK
BUY EARLY IN THE DAY
Rationed Foods

FIGURE 2.1 Food shortages during World War II led to food rationing and prompted the United States government to establish dietary standards. *(Office of War Information)*

disease, cancer, and obesity, has increased. Because of these changes in our diet and health, today's nutritional recommendations focus on health promotion as well as disease prevention. They come in many forms: Some define nutrient needs, others suggest healthy food and lifestyle choices. Some are designed to be used by health professionals and policy makers, and others are designed to provide accessible information to consumers.

DIETARY REFERENCE INTAKES: DEFINING NUTRIENT NEEDS

The current standard in the United States for recommended intakes of nutrients and other food components is a set of standards called **Dietary Reference Intakes (DRIs).** The DRIs are designed to be used for planning and assessing the diets of healthy people. They provide recommendations for the amounts of nutrients and other food components that should be consumed on an average daily basis—they are not requirements that must be consumed each day. The United States and Canada collaborated to develop the DRIs, which are replacing both the RDAs in the United States and the Recommended Nutrient Intakes (RNIs) in Canada (see Appendix E).[3] This joint United States–Canadian effort (with input expected from Mexico) will help to establish consistent recommendations for North America.

Web Menu

To view copies of the Dietary Reference Intake reports, go to the National Academy Press at www.nap.edu/ and search for Dietary Reference Intakes.

:C C 62 00 00 00 00 00 27 13

Dietary References Intakes (DRIs) A set of four reference values for the intake of nutrients and food components that can be used for planning and assessing the diets of healthy people in the United States and Canada.

The DRIs are an expansion of the concept developed in the original RDAs, which included recommended levels of energy, protein, and micronutrients that would prevent nutritional deficiencies in the healthy population. The DRIs differ from the original RDAs in a number of ways. First of all, the DRIs include values not only for energy, protein, and micronutrients, but also for macronutrients (carbohydrate, fat, and protein) and food components of nutritional importance, such as phytochemicals. Second, the recommendations of the DRIs aim to promote health and reduce the incidence of chronic disease, as well as prevent deficiencies. Third, unlike the original RDAs, which provided only a single set of values, the DRIs encompass four types of reference values.[4] Each type of DRI value includes recommendations that apply to different genders and life stages based on age and, when appropriate, pregnancy and lactation. The age divisions have been updated from those in the original RDAs and in some cases include additional categories.

The DRIs are being developed for seven nutrient groups: (1) calcium, phosphorus, magnesium, vitamin D, and fluoride; (2) B vitamins and choline; (3) antioxidants (vitamin C, vitamin E, selenium, and β-carotene); (4) vitamins A and K and the trace elements (e.g., iron, zinc, copper); (5) macronutrients (e.g., protein, fat, carbohydrate); (6) electrolytes and water; and (7) other food components, (e.g., fiber, phytochemicals). Values for some groups have been established and others are in the process of being finalized. At the time this book was published, values had been established for nutrients involved in bone formation (calcium, phosphorus, magnesium, vitamin D, and fluoride), for B vitamins and choline, for antioxidants, and for vitamins A and K and the trace elements (see inside covers).

DRI Values

As mentioned, the DRIs include four different sets of values. The **Estimated Average Requirement (EAR)** is the amount of a nutrient that is estimated to meet the needs of 50% of people in the same gender and life-stage group. The Estimated Average Requirement is a value that is useful for evaluating the adequacy of, and planning for, the nutrient intakes of population groups. The prevalence of inadequate nutrient intakes can be estimated by looking at the proportion of the population with intakes below the EAR.

Estimated Average Requirements (EARs) Intakes that meet the estimated nutrient needs (as defined by a specific indicator of adequacy) of 50% of individuals in a gender and life-stage group.

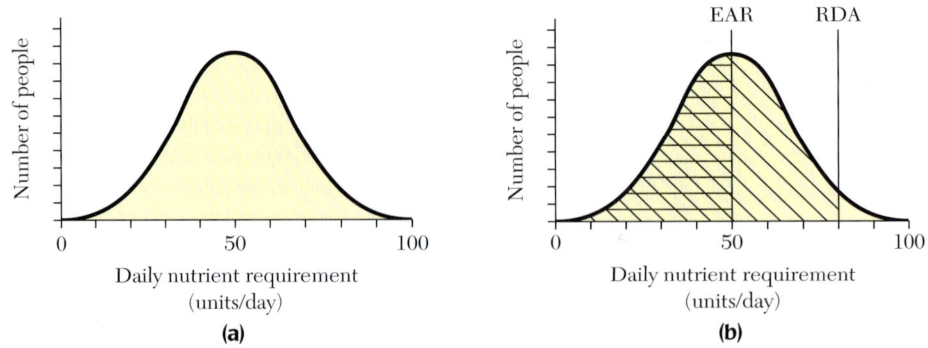

FIGURE 2.2 (a) When the amount of a particular nutrient required is determined for each person in a population and then the number of people requiring each amount is plotted, the result is theoretically a bell-shaped curve like the one shown here. In this example, the number of people who require 50 units of the nutrient is greater than the number who require only 10 units or who must have 80 units to maintain health. (b) This graph illustrates that the EAR is set as the average amount of a nutrient required. This amount will be enough to meet the needs of only half the population (shown as horizontal lines). When establishing the RDA, an amount is added to the EAR such that the RDA value is high enough to meet the needs of 97 to 98% of the population. The diagonal lines illustrate the proportion of the population whose needs will be met by the RDA.

Recommended Dietary Allowances (RDAs) Intakes that are sufficient to meet the nutrient needs of almost all healthy people in a specific life-stage and gender group.

The **Recommended Dietary Allowances (RDAs)** are calculated to meet the needs of nearly all healthy individuals in each gender and life-stage group. The RDAs are determined by starting with the EAR value and using the variability in the requirements among individuals to increase it to an amount that meets the needs of 97 to 98% of healthy individuals in a particular gender and life-stage group (Figure 2.2). The RDA is the value that can be used by individuals as a guide to achieving adequate nutrient intake. Because the RDA is only a target, an intake less than the RDA does not necessarily indicate that the needs of that particular individual have not been met.[5] Individual nutrient requirements are never known with certainty. However, the risk of a deficiency is low if intake meets the RDA and increases as intake falls below the RDA.

Adequate Intakes (AIs) Intakes that should be used as a goal when no RDA exists. These values are an approximation of the average nutrient intake that appears to sustain a desired indicator of health.

The **Adequate Intakes (AIs)** are estimates used when there is insufficient scientific evidence to set an EAR and calculate an RDA. The AIs are based on observed or experimentally determined approximations of the average nutrient intake by a healthy population. When an AI value rather than an RDA is set, it targets the need for more research on the requirement of that nutrient. The AI values, like the RDAs, can be used as a goal for individual intake. Even though they are derived from the mean intakes of groups, not individuals, it is assumed that if healthy individuals have an intake that is at or above the AI, there is a low risk that this intake is not adequate to maintain nutritional health.

Tolerable Upper Intake Level (UL) The maximum daily intake by an individual that is unlikely to pose risks of adverse health effects to almost all individuals in the specified life-stage and gender group.

The last set of values, the **Tolerable Upper Intake Levels (ULs),** represent the maximum level of daily intake of a nutrient that is unlikely to pose a risk of adverse health effects to almost all individuals in a specified group. It is not a recommended level but it is a level of intake that can probably be tolerated. Tolerable Upper Intake Levels are used as a guide for limiting intake when planning diets and evaluating the possibility of overconsumption. The exact level of intake that will cause an adverse effect cannot be known with certainty for each individual, but if an individual's intake is below the UL, there is good assurance that an adverse effect will not occur.

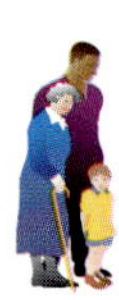

Life-Stage Groups

Life-stage groups Groupings of individuals based on stage of growth and development, pregnancy, and lactation that have similar nutrient needs.

The DRIs include values that apply to different **life-stage groups.** These have been established based on the physiological changes that occur in infants, children, adolescents, and older adults. The pregnancy and lactation life stages also include age categories to distinguish any unique nutritional needs of pregnancy and lactation in teenagers and older mothers (see inside front cover).

How the DRIs Are Determined

Designing standards to reduce the risk of chronic disease, developmental disorders, and other health problems—as well as to prevent deficiency diseases—is challenging. In order to meet this goal, appropriate criteria of adequate intake must be established for each life-stage and gender group for each nutrient. This **criterion of adequacy** is an indicator, such as the amount of a nutrient in the blood, that can be evaluated to determine the biological effect of a level of nutrient intake. One criterion may be used to determine the risk of deficiency, whereas another may help to assess the risk of chronic disease. Which criterion is used affects the recommendation made for a level of intake.

Criterion of adequacy An indicator such as the level of a nutrient in the blood or the appearance of a deficiency symptom that can be evaluated to determine the biological effect of a level of nutrient intake.

For each nutrient, an EAR and RDA, or an AI, is established to meet specific criteria for adequacy. The criteria may not be the same for different life-stage groups (Figure 2.3). For example, the AI for calcium for infants is based on the amount consumed in human milk. For children, the AI is based on the amount needed for maximal calcium accumulation to support bone growth. For older adults, the AI is set to support maximal calcium retention, which may decrease the risk of bone fractures. One or more criterion may be used to establish each EAR or AI. For all DRI values, the recommendations consider how much of a nutrient in the diet is available to the body for use.

To establish a UL, a specific adverse effect or indicator of excess is used. The lowest level of intake that causes the adverse effect is determined and the UL is set far enough below this level that even the most sensitive people in the population are unlikely to be affected. If adverse effects have been associated only with intake from supplements, the UL is based only on this source. Therefore, for some nutrients the UL represents intake from supplements alone; for some, it represents intake from supplements and fortified foods; and for others, it represents total intake from food, fortified food, water, nonfood sources, and supplements. For some nutrients, data are insufficient to establish a UL value.

Applications of the DRIs

The DRIs have many uses. They provide a set of standards that can be used to plan diets, to assess the adequacy of diets, and to make judgments about excessive intakes for individuals and populations.[4] For example, they are used as a standard for meals prepared for schools, hospitals, and other health-care facilities; for government feeding programs for the elderly; and even for meals for space-shuttle astronauts. They are used to determine standards for food labeling and to develop practical tools for diet planning, such as the Food Guide Pyramid.[6] They can also be used to interpret information gathered about the food consumed by a population to help identify potential nutritional inadequacies that may be of public health concern.

Despite their many uses, dietary standards cannot be used to identify with certainty whether a specific person has a nutritional deficiency or excess. To ascertain this, an evaluation of an individual's nutritional status using dietary, clinical, biochemical, and body-size measurements is needed, as discussed later in this chapter.

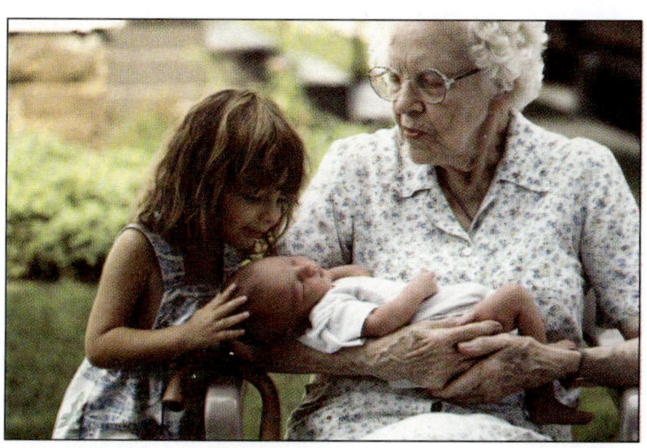

FIGURE 2.3 The nutrient requirements of infants and children differ from those of older adults. The criteria used to determine the DRI values for a particular nutrient, as well as the recommendations themselves, may be different for different life-stage groups. *(© Sue Ann Miller/Tony Stone Images)*

The Food Guide Pyramid: Planning Food Choices

The DRIs recommend amounts of specific nutrients and food components, but they do not recommend specific foods that should be consumed to meet these needs. To help individuals follow the recommendations for a healthy diet, a number of tools have been developed to translate the recommendations for nutrient intake into food choices. The most commonly used tools are food groups. These divide foods into groups based on the nutrients they supply most abundantly and then recommend the number of servings from each group needed to provide a healthy diet. The most recent version of a food group system used in the United States is the Food Guide Pyramid (Figure 2.4).

To learn more about the Food Guide Pyramid and pyramid modifications for different ethnic groups and types of diets, go to the USDA's Food and Nutrition Information Center at www.nal.usda.gov/fnic/Fpyr/pyramid.html.

What Is the Food Guide Pyramid?

The **Food Guide Pyramid** is a guide for planning diets that meet nutrient requirements and the recommendations for health promotion and disease prevention. It proposes a diet plan based on servings from five food groups: (1) Bread, Cereal, Rice, and Pasta Group; (2) Vegetable Group; (3) Fruit Group; (4) Milk, Yogurt, and Cheese Group; and (5) Meat, Poultry, Fish, Dry Beans, Eggs, and Nuts Group. The Pyramid also includes a recommendation to use Fats, Oils, and Sweets sparingly in the diet. The serving sizes within each group of the Pyramid are fairly constant. For instance, 1 serving from the grain group is equal to 1 slice of bread, 1 ounce of dry cereal, or 1/2 cup of cooked cereal, rice, or pasta (see Table 2.1). Foods within each food group supply similar nutrients. For example, foods in the milk group are good sources of protein, calcium, and riboflavin.

Food Guide Pyramid A guide for diet planning that is based on five major food groups. Following serving and selection recommendations helps individuals select diets that meet nutrient requirements and the recommendations for health promotion and disease prevention.

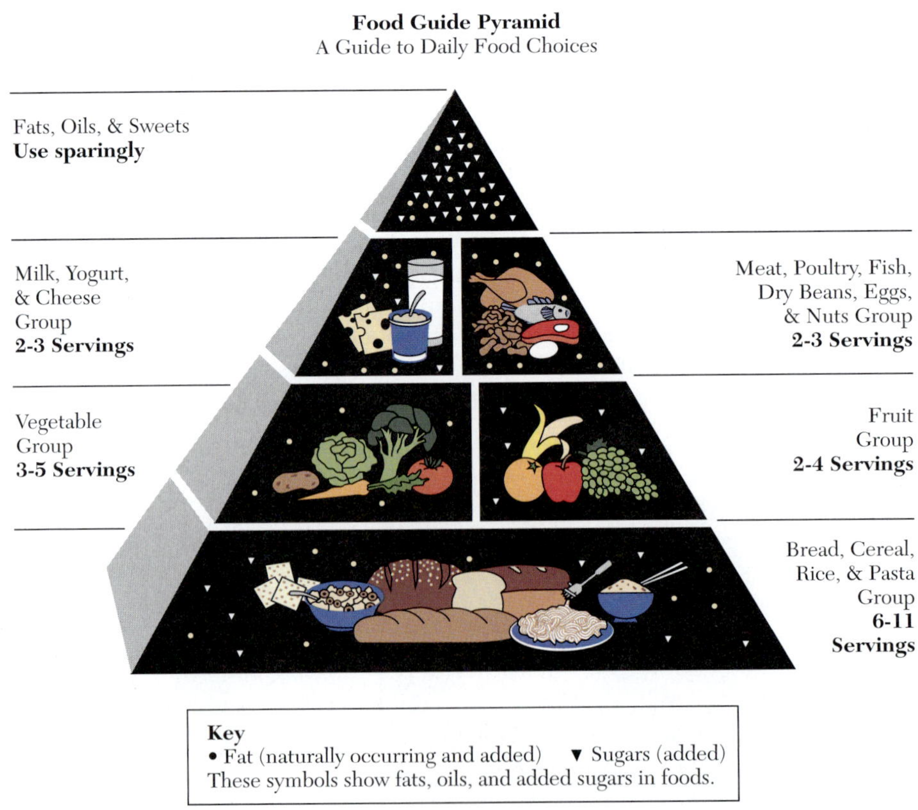

FIGURE 2.4 The Food Guide Pyramid. *(USDA, 1992)*

TABLE 2.1 Servings and Selections from the Food Guide Pyramid

Food Group/Serving Size	Nutrients Provided	Selection Tips
Bread, Cereal, Rice, & Pasta (6 to 11 servings) 1/2 cup cooked cereal, rice, or pasta 1 ounce dry cereal 1 slice bread, 1 tortilla 2 cookies 1/2 medium doughnut	B vitamins, fiber, iron, magnesium, zinc, complex carbohydrates	Choose whole-grain breads, cereals, and grains such as whole wheat or rye, oatmeal, and brown rice. Use high-fat, high-sugar baked goods such as cakes, cookies, and pastries in moderation. Limit fats and sugars added as spreads, sauces, or toppings.
Vegetable (3 to 5 servings) 1/2 cup cooked or raw chopped vegetables 1 cup raw leafy vegetables 3/4 cup vegetable juice 10 french fries	Vitamin A, vitamin C, folate, magnesium, iron, fiber	Eat a variety of vegetables, including dark-green leafy vegetables like spinach and broccoli, deep-yellow vegetables like carrots and sweet potatoes, starchy vegetables such as potatoes and corn, and other vegetables such as green beans and tomatoes. Cook by steaming or baking. Avoid frying, and limit high-fat spreads or dressings.
Fruit (2 to 4 servings) 1 medium apple, banana, or orange 1/2 cup chopped, cooked, or canned fruit 3/4 cup fruit juice 1/4 cup dried fruit	Vitamin A, vitamin C, potassium, fiber	Choose fresh fruit, frozen without sugar, dried, or fruit canned in water or juice. If canned in heavy syrup, rinse with water before eating. Eat whole fruits more often than juices; they are higher in fiber. Regularly eat citrus fruits, melons, or berries rich in vitamin C. Only 100% fruit juice should be counted as fruit.
Milk, Yogurt, & Cheese (2 to 3 servings) 1 cup milk or yogurt 1-1/2 ounces natural cheese 2 ounces process cheese 2 cups cottage cheese 1-1/2 cups ice cream 1 cup frozen yogurt	Protein, calcium, riboflavin, vitamin D	Use low-fat or skim milk for healthy people over 2 years of age. Choose low-fat and nonfat yogurt, "part skim" and low-fat cheeses, and lower-fat frozen desserts like ice milk and frozen yogurt. Limit high-fat cheeses and ice cream.
Meat, Poultry, Fish, Dry Beans, Eggs, & Nuts (2 to 3 servings) 2–3 ounces cooked lean meat, fish, or poultry 2–3 eggs 4–6 tablespoons peanut butter 1 to 1-1/2 cups cooked dry beans 2/3 to 1 cup nuts	Protein, niacin, vitamin B_6, vitamin B_{12}, other B vitamins, iron, zinc	Select lean meat, poultry without skin, and dry beans often. Trim fat, and cook by broiling, roasting, grilling, or boiling rather than frying. Limit egg yolks, which are high in cholesterol, and nuts and seeds, which are high in fat. Be aware of serving size; 3 ounces of meat is the size of an average hamburger.
Fats, Oils, & Sweets (use sparingly) Butter, mayonnaise, salad dressing, cream cheese, sour cream, jam, jelly		These are high in energy and low in micronutrients. Substitute low-fat dressings and spreads.

Human Nutrition Information Service. *The Food Guide Pyramid.* Home and Garden Bulletin No. 252. Hyattsville, Md: U.S. Department of Agriculture, 1992, 1996, revised.

The Pyramid Shape

The shape of the Pyramid helps emphasize the relative contribution each food group should make to the diet. The large base of the Pyramid is made up of foods that come from grains: bread, cereal, rice, and pasta. These high-carbohydrate foods are the foundation of a healthy diet; between 6 and 11 servings per day are recommended. In the next level of the Pyramid are two groups of foods that also come from plant sources: the Vegetable Group, of which 3 to 5 servings per day are recommended, and the Fruit Group, of which 2 to 4 servings per day are recommended. The next level, where the decreasing size of the Pyramid boxes reflects the smaller number of recommended servings, comprises two groups of foods that come primarily from animals: the Milk, Yogurt, and Cheese Group, of which 2 to 3 servings are recommended, and the Meat, Poultry, Fish, Dry Beans, Eggs, and Nuts Group, of which 2 to 3 servings a day are recommended. At the narrow tip of the Pyramid are Fats, Oils, and Sweets. These should be used sparingly after other nutrient needs have been met.

Planning Diets Using the Food Guide Pyramid

To plan a diet that satisfies the recommendations of the Food Guide Pyramid, several servings of breads and grains and fruits or vegetables should be included at each meal. From this base, servings from the milk and meat groups can be added. Mixed dishes can be planned with the Pyramid by considering the component parts. For example, a chicken taco consists of a tortilla (a bread), chicken (a meat), and lettuce and tomatoes (vegetables). A beef-with-broccoli stir-fry consists of beef (a meat) and broccoli (a vegetable), served over rice (a grain). However, just choosing the specified number of servings from each group of the Food Guide Pyramid will not assure an optimal diet. Wise choices must be made from each food group.

Nutrient density A measure of the nutrients provided by a food relative to the energy it contains.

Choosing for Balance and Variety Planning a diet to meet nutrient needs must consider the **nutrient density** of foods as well as the variety and balance of the foods chosen. Nutrient density refers to the amounts of essential nutrients in a food relative to the energy provided. For example, both skim milk and ice cream are in the Milk, Yogurt, and Cheese Group. However, a 1-cup serving of skim milk provides 300 mg of calcium in 90 kcalories, whereas a cup of ice cream provides 168 mg of calcium in 265 kcalories. The skim milk is considered to have a higher nutrient density because it provides more nutrients per kcalorie than the ice cream. The Food Guide Pyramid offers selection tips for choosing a nutrient-dense diet, which are listed in Table 2.1.

Choosing a variety of foods is also essential to meeting nutrient needs. There are similarities in the nutrients provided by different foods from within each food group, but there are also important differences in the amounts and types of nutrients. For example, white potatoes and carrots are both in the Vegetable Group of the Food Guide Pyramid. White potatoes are a good source of vitamin C but contain almost no vitamin A; carrots are high in beta-carotene (which can be converted to vitamin A in the body) but have little vitamin C. A diet that meets the recommended three servings of vegetables each day but includes three servings of potatoes will be missing out on vitamin A and other nutrients that would have been consumed in a more varied diet. Choosing a varied diet is also important because there are interactions between different foods and nutrients. These interactions may be positive, enhancing nutrient utilization, or negative, inhibiting nutrient use. For example, consuming iron with orange juice enhances the absorption of the iron, while consuming iron with milk may reduce its absorption. In a varied diet these interactions balance out. In addition, some foods may contain toxic substances such as pesticides, fertilizers, and natural toxins; choosing a variety of foods avoids an excess of any one of these substances.

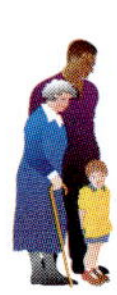

Meeting Individual Needs and Preferences The Food Guide Pyramid is designed to meet a variety of energy needs as well as to be flexible enough to suit the preferences of people from diverse cultures and lifestyles. By choosing within the range of recommended servings, individuals can satisfy a variety of energy needs. For example, someone who needs 1600 kcalories per day could meet their needs by using the low end of the range of servings—for instance, six bread servings per day. Someone who needs 2800 kcalories per day should choose from the high end of the range for each food group—for instance, 11 breads, 5 vegetables, 4 fruits,

TABLE 2.2 Number of Food Guide Pyramid Servings for Three Daily Energy Levels*

	1600 kcalories (sedentary women and some older adults)	2200 kcalories (children, teenage girls, active women, and many sedentary men)	2800 kcalories (teenage boys, many active men, and some very active women)
Bread, Cereal, Rice, & Pasta Group	6	9	11
Vegetable Group	3	4	5
Fruit Group	2	3	4
Milk, Yogurt, & Cheese Group	2–3†	2–3†	2–3†
Meat, Poultry, Fish, Dry Beans, Eggs, & Nuts Group	2 (5 oz total)	2 (6 oz total)	3 (7 oz total)

*Assumes that food choices are mostly low-fat and low kcalorie.

†Women who are pregnant or breastfeeding, teenagers, and young adults to age 24 need three servings.

U.S. Department of Agriculture. The Food Guide Pyramid. Home and Garden Bulletin 252, 1992, revised 1996.

and so on. See Table 2.2 and Appendix G for serving recommendations for various kcalorie levels.

The Pyramid can also be used for groups with special needs. For example, to consume adequate calcium, pregnant and lactating women, children, adolescents, and adults under 25 years of age need three servings from the milk group. Modified Food Guide Pyramids have been developed for young children, older adults, and vegetarians (see Chapters 6, 16, and 17). A number of pyramids have also been developed to provide food choices that meet the needs of various ethnic groups (see Appendix H).

LABELS: PROVIDING ACCESSIBLE INFORMATION

Food labels are designed to help consumers make healthy food choices. Unlike the Food Guide Pyramid, they do not provide the information needed to structure a whole diet. Rather, they provide information about the nutrient content of individual foods and how the amounts in a serving of the food compare to recommendations for health promotion and disease prevention. To make this information uniform and easy to use, food labeling standards are specified by the Nutrition Labeling and Education Act of 1990.[7] Dietary supplements must also bear standardized labels as specified by the Dietary Supplement Health and Education Act of 1994.[8]

Web Menu: For more information about the labeling of food and supplements, go to the FDA Center for Food Safety and Applied Nutrition at vm.cfsan.fda.gov/.

Food Labels

Food labels must follow standard formats. All labels contain basic product information such as the name of the product, the net contents or weight, the date by which the product should be sold, and the name and place of business of the manufacturer, packager, or distributor. In addition, most food labels contain a list of the food's ingredients and a "Nutrition Facts" panel that provides information about the nutrient content of the product and its contribution to a healthy diet.

Making Decisions
Restaurant Meals to Meet Your Goals

An occasional meal at a restaurant has little impact on the quality of an individual's diet. But, for many Americans eating out is more than an occasional treat. Today, more Americans than ever are eating away from home and the restaurant meals they consume are usually higher in fat and cholesterol than meals eaten at home.[a] The change in lifestyles to include more restaurant and fast-food meals has made choosing healthy foods from restaurant menus important in maintaining a healthy diet—but it can be a challenge.

Some healthy choices are easy, even at restaurants. If you are looking for a low-fat meal, skip the fried fish and have it broiled instead. Minimize sauces and spreads (like the honey butter on your corn bread) that add fat, sugar, and kcalories. Use less salad dressing by asking that it be served on the side so you can choose how much to use. Be conscious of portion sizes. Those served in restaurants are often much larger than what we prepare at home. You don't have to finish everything—take it home for tomorrow's lunch.

Other restaurant choices are more difficult to make. Items that sound like part of a healthy diet are not always what they seem. What's in that house special turkey tetrazzini, beef lo mein, or a fajita wrap? Without the chef's recipe it is impossible to know. The amounts of specific nutrients are usually not given on menus and the ingredients can be a mystery. Even when you know what ingredients are usually in a dish such as eggplant parmesan, you can never be sure how much oil or salt was used. Even an order of plain old green beans might come floating in butter.

Many restaurants and fast-food establishments have responded to consumer concern about healthy diets by offering healthier choices. Menus often highlight these items by making claims about their nutrient content, such as low-fat tostados, low-sodium lo mein, or reduced-kcalorie lasagna. The food labeling laws that regulate packaged foods also apply to menus so the definition of these terms must match those used on food labels. For example, if you order low-fat tostados, the term "low-fat" should mean the same as it does on labeled packaged foods—that it contains 3 g or less of fat per serving.

Menus may also include statements that give general dietary guidance or make specific claims about the relationship between a nutrient and a disease or health condition. For example, the salad section may start with the general statement that "eating five fruits and vegetables a day is an important part of a healthy diet."[b] A dish that is low in fat, saturated fat, and cholesterol might carry a claim that diets low in saturated fat and cholesterol may reduce the risk of heart disease. To carry a health claim, menu items must contain a significant amount of at least one of six key nutrients (vitamin A, vitamin C, iron, calcium, protein, or fiber) and cannot contain a food substance at a level that increases the risk of a disease or health condition.

Nutrient content claims and health claims referring to items on the menu must be backed up with appropriate nutrition information when requested. This information can be on the menu or in accompanying nutrition information available upon request. It can be presented in any format, such as printed in a notebook or recited by the staff, and only needs to provide information about the nutrient or nutrients to which the claim is referring. Restaurants do not have to provide nutrition information about items that do not carry nutrient content or health claims or that are referred to in general dietary messages.

When choosing from a menu, look for items that fit into a healthy diet—and are also things you enjoy. Choose foods you like and remember that a high-fat or high-kcalorie meal now and then doesn't make your overall diet unhealthy. If you eat out frequently, restaurant meals make up a greater part of your overall diet and should be chosen carefully.

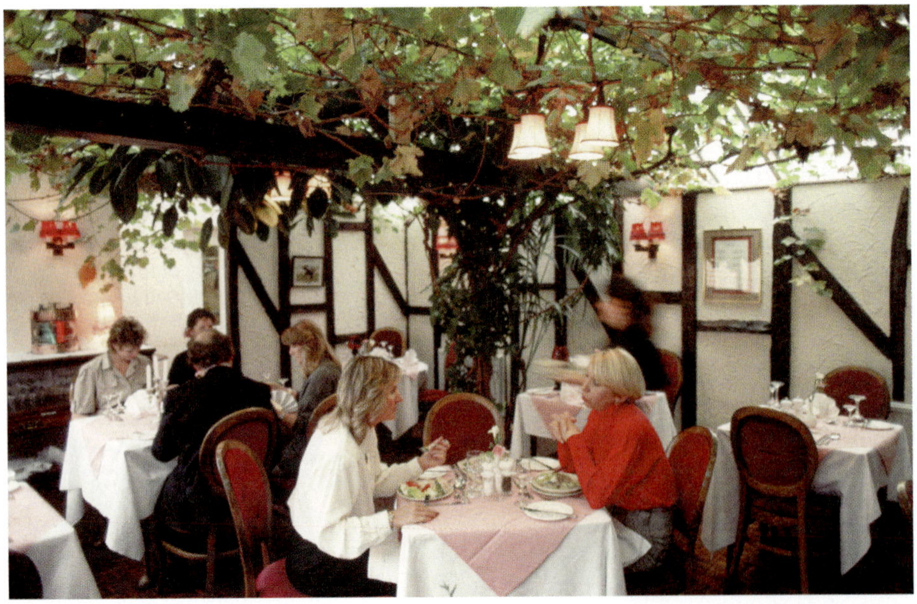
(© Bob Krist/Corbis)

References

[a] USDA, Agricultural Service, 1997. *Results from USDA's 1994–1996 Continuing Survey of Food Intakes by Individuals*, and *1994–1996 Health Knowledge Survey*. ARS Food Surveys Research Group. Available online at **http://www.barc.usda.gov/bhnrc/foodsurvey/home/htm** (Accessed 14 Nov 2000).

[b] Kurtzweil, P. Today's special nutrition information. FDA Consumer 31:21–25, May–June, 1997.

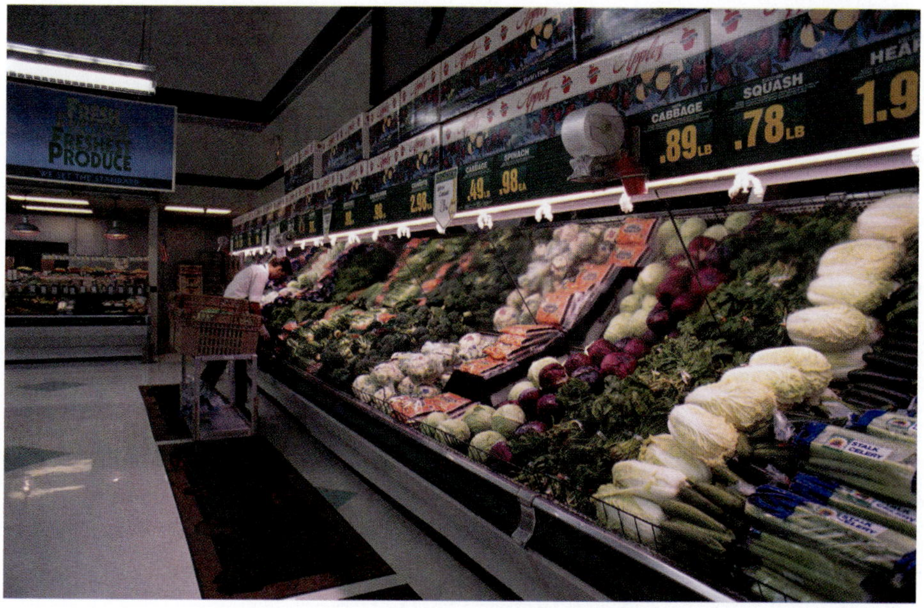

FIGURE 2.5 Fresh produce is not required to be labeled, but the information is usually displayed in the produce section of the store. *(© Bob Rowan; Progressive Image/Corbis)*

What Must Be Labeled Food labeling laws regulate about 75% of all food consumed in the United States.[9] The Food and Drug Administration (FDA) regulates the labeling of all foods except meat and poultry products, which are regulated by the U.S. Department of Agriculture (USDA). All packaged foods must be labeled except those produced by small businesses and those in packages too small to contain the labeling information. Some restaurant food and ready-to-eat food, such as that served in bakeries and delicatessens, is also exempt from labeling. However, if a claim about a food's nutritional content or health benefits—such as "low-fat" or "heart healthy"—is included on a menu, the eating establishment must provide nutritional information about this food when requested (see *Making Decisions:* "Restaurant Meals to Meet Your Goals"). Raw fruits, vegetables, fish, meat, and poultry are not required to carry individual labels. The FDA has asked grocery stores to voluntarily provide nutrition information for the raw fruits, vegetables, and fish most frequently eaten in the United States, and the USDA encourages voluntary nutrition labeling of raw meat and poultry. About 75% of stores comply with the request to provide nutrient information for raw produce and fish.[10] The information can appear on large placards or in consumer pamphlets or brochures (Figure 2.5).

Ingredient List The ingredients section of the label lists the contents of the product in order of their prominence by weight. An ingredient list is required on all products containing more than one ingredient. Food additives, including food colors and flavorings, must be listed among the ingredients.

Nutrition Facts The nutrition information section of the label is entitled "Nutrition Facts" (Figure 2.6). In this section, the size of a single serving is listed in common household and metric measures, and is based on a standard list of serving sizes. (These serving sizes are not always the same as the serving sizes in the Food Guide Pyramid.) The use of standard serving sizes allows comparisons to be made easily between products. For example, comparing the energy content of different types of crackers is simplified because all packages list energy values for a standard serving size of about 30 g.

The serving size on the label is followed by the number of servings per container. The label must then list the total kcalories and kcalories from fat. (On food

FIGURE 2.6 The Nutrition Labeling Act of 1990 required standardization of the information on food labels. (FDA Consumer *27:23, May 1993*)

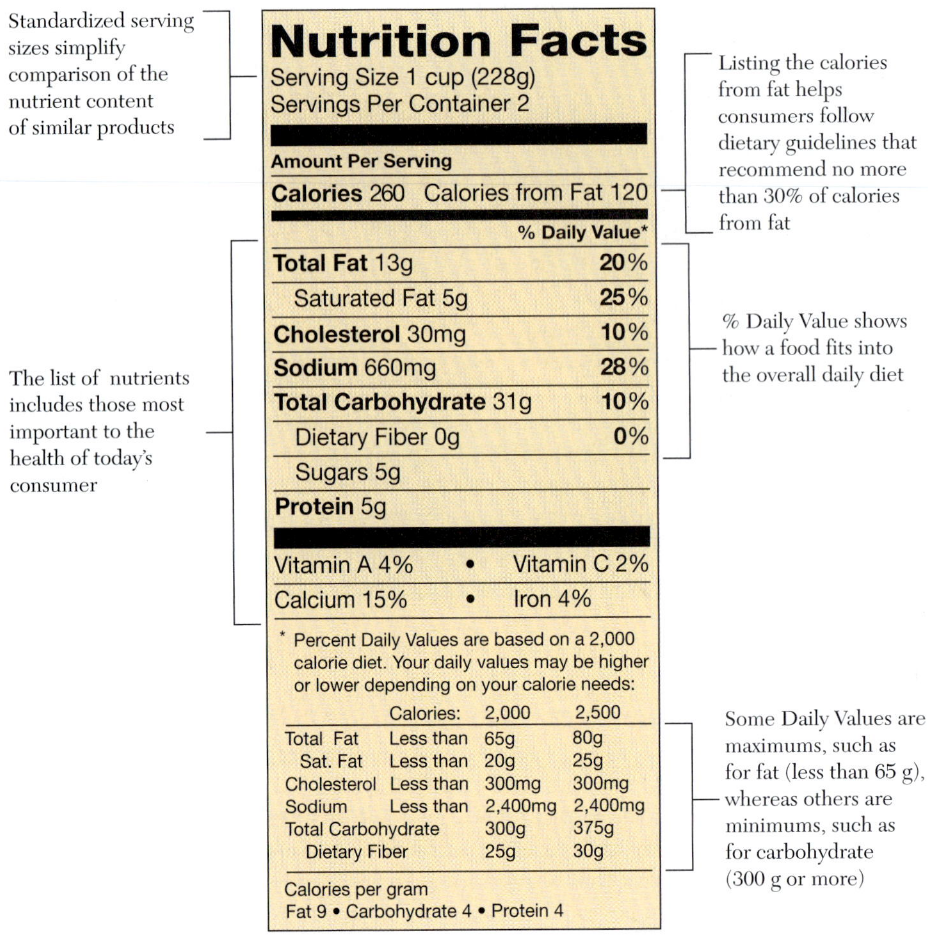

Daily Value A nutrient reference value used on food labels to help consumers see how foods fit into their overall diets.

labels, the term "Calorie" is used to refer to kcalories.) The amounts of total fat, saturated fat, cholesterol, sodium, total carbohydrate, dietary fiber, sugars, and protein per serving are listed next. The amounts of most of these nutrients are also listed as a percentage of a standard called the **Daily Value.** Daily Values are designed to help consumers determine how a food fits into their overall diet. The percent Daily Value is the amount of a nutrient in a food as a percentage of the recommendation for a 2000-kcalorie diet. For example, if a food provides 10% of

TABLE 2.3 Reference Daily Intakes*

Nutrient	Amount	Nutrient	Amount	Nutrient	Amount
Vitamin A	5000 IU†	Vitamin E	30 IU†	Biotin	300 μg
Vitamin C	60 mg	Vitamin B_6	2.0 mg	Pantothenic acid	10 mg
Thiamin	1.5 mg	Folic acid	400 μg	Vitamin K	80 μg
Riboflavin	1.7 mg	Vitamin B_{12}	6 μg	Chromium	120 μg
Niacin	20 mg	Phosphorus	1000 mg	Selenium	70 μg
Calcium	1000 mg	Iodine	150 μg	Molybdenum	75 μg
Iron	18 mg	Magnesium	400 mg	Manganese	2 mg
Vitamin D	400 IU†	Zinc	15 mg	Chloride	3400 mg
		Copper	2 mg		

*Based on National Academy of Sciences' 1968 Recommended Dietary Allowances.

†The RDIs for some fat-soluble vitamins are expressed in International Units (IU). The RDAs use a newer system of measurement.

the Daily Value for dietary fiber, then the food provides 10% of the recommended daily intake for dietary fiber in a 2000-kcalorie diet. Daily Values are based on two sets of standards, the **Reference Daily Intakes (RDIs)** and the **Daily Reference Values (DRVs)**. To avoid confusion, only the term "Daily Value" appears on food labels.

Reference Daily Intakes (RDIs) Reference values established for vitamins and minerals that are based on the highest amount of each nutrient recommended for any adult age group by the 1968 RDAs.

Daily Reference Values (DRVs) Reference values established for protein and seven nutrients for which no RDA has been established. The values are based on dietary recommendations for reducing the risk of chronic disease.

The Reference Daily Intakes are used to determine Daily Values for vitamins and minerals for which original RDAs were established (see Table 2.3). Although the name has changed, most of the current RDI values are the same as the old U.S. RDAs (U.S. Recommended Daily Allowances): They are based on the highest amount of each nutrient recommended for any adult age group by the 1968 RDAs. These may overestimate the amount of a nutrient needed for some groups, but they do not underestimate the requirement for any group (except pregnant and lactating women). Label regulations require that percent Daily Values, based on RDIs, be listed for vitamin A, vitamin C, calcium, and iron. In addition to these mandatory listings, a manufacturer may voluntarily include information about other vitamins and minerals.

Daily Reference Values are guidelines for the amounts of total fat, saturated fat, carbohydrate, fiber, cholesterol, sodium, potassium, and protein that should be included in a healthy diet (Table 2.4). The DRV for fat, for example, is based on the recommendation that dietary fat should account for less than 30% of energy, or less than 65 g for a 2000-kcalorie diet. The DRVs are used on food labels to calculate the percent Daily Values for nutrients based on a diet containing 2000 kcalories. To illustrate that the recommended intake of some nutrients depends on energy needs, Daily Values based on DRVs are listed on food labels for both a 2000- and a 2500-kcalorie diet.

TABLE 2.4
Daily Reference Values

Food Component	Daily Reference Value (2000 kcal)
Total fat	Less than 65 g (30% of energy)
Saturated fat	Less than 20 g (10% of energy)
Cholesterol	Less than 300 mg
Total carbohydrate	300 g (60% of energy)
Dietary fiber	25 g (11.5 g/1000 kcal)
Sodium	Less than 2400 mg
Potassium	3500 mg
Protein	50 g (10% of energy)

Nutrient Content Claims In addition to the required nutrition information, food labels often highlight specific characteristics of a product that might be of interest to the consumer, such as "low in Calories" or "high in fiber." Definitions for nutrient content descriptors such as "free," "low," and "light" have been established by the FDA and are based on how these terms relate to nutrient content. In selecting a product labeled with a descriptor such as "fat free," consumers can be assured that the food meets the defined criteria—in this case, that the product contains less than 0.5 g of fat per serving. The specific definition of each of these descriptors is given in Table 2.5, and their use in relation to specific nutrients is discussed in appropriate chapters throughout this text.

Health Claims Food labels are also permitted to include a number of health claims if they are relevant to the product. Health claims refer to a relationship between a nutrient or other substances in a food and the risk of a disease or health-related condition. They can be used on conventional foods or dietary supplements and can help consumers choose products that will meet their dietary needs or health goals. For example, low-fat milk, a good source of calcium, might include on the package label a statement indicating that a diet high in calcium will reduce the risk of developing osteoporosis. Health claims are permitted on food labels only after the scientific evidence is reviewed by the FDA and found to be factual and truthful. The claims listed in Table 2.6 are currently approved by the FDA for use on food labels.[11]

Despite the wealth of information available on food labels, today's consumer must be educated about the benefits and pitfalls of foods that are not labeled and about food and nutrition issues that are not addressed by food labels. Such issues include the advantages and disadvantages of fresh, frozen, and canned produce, and the safe selection, storage, and preparation of food. Food labels cannot tell you what you should eat, or how you should prepare it, but they are an important source of information about what you are eating.

TABLE 2.5 Nutrient Content Descriptors Commonly Used on Food Labels

Free	Product contains no amount of, or a trivial amount of, fat, saturated fat, cholesterol, sodium, sugars, or kcalories. For example, "sugar free" and "fat free" both mean less than 0.5 g per serving. Synonyms for "free" include "without," "no," and "zero."
Low	Used for foods that can be eaten frequently without exceeding the Daily Value for fat, saturated fat, cholesterol, sodium, or kcalories. Specific definitions have been established for each of these nutrients. For example, "low-fat" means that the food contains 3 g or less per serving, and "low cholesterol" means that the food contains less than 20 mg of cholesterol per serving. Synonyms for "low" include "little," "few," and "low source of."
Lean and extra lean	Used to describe the fat content of meat, poultry, seafood, and game meats. "Lean" means that the food contains less than 10 g fat, less than 4.5 g saturated fat, and less than 95 mg of cholesterol per serving and per 100 g. "Extra lean" means that the food contains less than 5 g fat, less than 2 g saturated fat, and less than 95 mg of cholesterol per serving and per 100 g.
High	Used for foods that contain 20% or more of the Daily Value for a particular nutrient. Synonyms for "high" include "rich in" and "excellent source of."
Good source	Food contains 10 to 19% of the Daily Value for a particular nutrient per serving.
Reduced	Nutritionally altered product contains 25% less of a nutrient or of energy than the regular or reference product.
Less	Food, whether altered or not, contains 25% less of a nutrient or of energy than the reference food. For example, pretzels may claim to have "less fat" than potato chips. "Fewer" may be used as a synonym for "less."
Light	Used in different ways. First, it can be used on a nutritionally altered product that contains one third fewer kcalories or half the fat of a reference food. Second, it can be used when the sodium content of a low-calorie, low-fat food has been reduced by 50%. The term "light" can be used to describe properties such as texture and color as long as the label explains the intent—for example, "light and fluffy."
More	Serving of food, whether altered or not, contains a nutrient that is at least 10% of the Daily Value more than the reference food. This definition also applies to foods using the terms "fortified," "enriched," or "added."
Healthy	Used to describe foods that are low in fat and saturated fat and contain no more than 360 mg of sodium and no more than 60 mg of cholesterol per serving and provide at least 10% of the Daily Value for vitamins A or C, or iron, calcium, protein, or fiber.
Fresh	Used on foods that are raw and have never been frozen or heated and contain no preservatives.

Federal Register 58, Jan. 6, 1993. U.S. Government Printing Office, Superintendent of Documents, Washington, D.C.

Dietary Supplement Labels

Dietary supplement Any product intended for ingestion as a supplement to the diet. These are classified as food and are regulated by the FDA.

Dietary supplements are currently a popular addition to the American diet. It is estimated that as many as 50% of adult Americans take some kind of supplement on a regular basis.[12] There are thousands of types of dietary supplements. Some contain essential nutrients, some are designed to alter the macronutrient content of the diet, and many are consumed for other purposes, such as to enhance athletic performance, promote weight loss, alleviate existing symptoms and conditions, or promote a longer life and prevent chronic disease. They take the form of pills, tablets, liquids, and powders.

TABLE 2.6 FDA-Approved Health Claims*

Calcium and osteoporosis	Adequate calcium intake throughout life helps maintain bone health and reduce the risk of osteoporosis.
Sodium and hypertension (high blood pressure)	Diets low in sodium may reduce the risk of high blood pressure in some people.
Dietary fat and cancer	Diets low in fat may reduce the risk of some types of cancer.
Saturated fat and cholesterol and risk of coronary heart disease	Diets low in saturated fat and cholesterol help reduce blood cholesterol and, thus, the risk of heart disease.
Fiber-containing grain products, fruits, and vegetables, and cancer risk	Diets low in fat and rich in fiber-containing grain products, fruits, and vegetables may reduce the risk of some types of cancer.
Fruits, vegetables, and grain products that contain fiber, particularly soluble fiber, and risk of coronary heart disease	Diets low in saturated fat and cholesterol and rich in fruits, vegetables, and grain products that contain fiber, particularly soluble fiber, may reduce the risk of coronary heart disease.
Fruits and vegetables and cancer	Diets low in fat and rich in fruits and vegetables may reduce the risk of some types of cancer.
Folic acid and neural tube birth defects	Adequate folic acid intake by the mother reduces the risk of birth defects of the brain or spinal cord in her baby.
Soluble fiber from certain foods and risk of coronary heart disease.	Diets low in fat, saturated fat, and cholesterol that include soluble fiber from whole oats or psyllium seed husk may reduce the risk of heart disease.
Dietary sugar alcohol and dental caries (cavities)	Sugar-free foods that are sweetened with sugar alcohols do not promote tooth decay and may reduce the risk of dental caries.
Soy protein and risk of coronary heart disease	Soy protein included in a diet that is low in saturated fat and cholesterol may reduce the risk of coronary heart disease by lowering blood cholesterol levels.
Plant sterol/stanol esters and risk of coronary heart disease	Plant sterols and plant stanols included in a diet that is low in saturated fat and cholesterol may reduce the risk of coronary heart disease by lowering blood cholesterol levels.

*A food carrying a health claim must be a naturally good source (10% or more of the Daily Value) for one of six nutrients (vitamin A, vitamin C, protein, calcium, iron, or fiber) and must not contain more than 20% of the Daily Value for fat, saturated fat, cholesterol, or sodium. These claims have been approved for use on food labels. The FDA continues to evaluate new claims, many of which are in various stages of approval.

What Must Be Labeled Any product intended for ingestion as a supplement to the diet must include the words "dietary supplement" on the label and carry a standardized label similar to a food label (Figure 2.7). According to the FDA definition, supplements may contain one or more of the following ingredients: vitamins; minerals; herbs, botanicals, or other plant-derived substances; amino acids; enzymes; concentrates; and extracts. The FDA also regulates nutrient and health claims made on supplement labels and in package inserts and accompanying literature. The Federal Trade Commission regulates dietary supplement advertising.

Supplement Facts and Ingredient List Dietary supplements must carry a "Supplement Facts" panel similar to the "Nutrition Facts" panel found on most processed foods. This panel lists the recommended serving size and the name and quantity of each ingredient per serving. The source of the ingredient may be given with its name in the "Supplement Facts" panel or in the ingredient list below the panel. The nutrients for which Daily Values have been established are listed first, followed by other dietary ingredients for which Daily Values have not been established.[13]

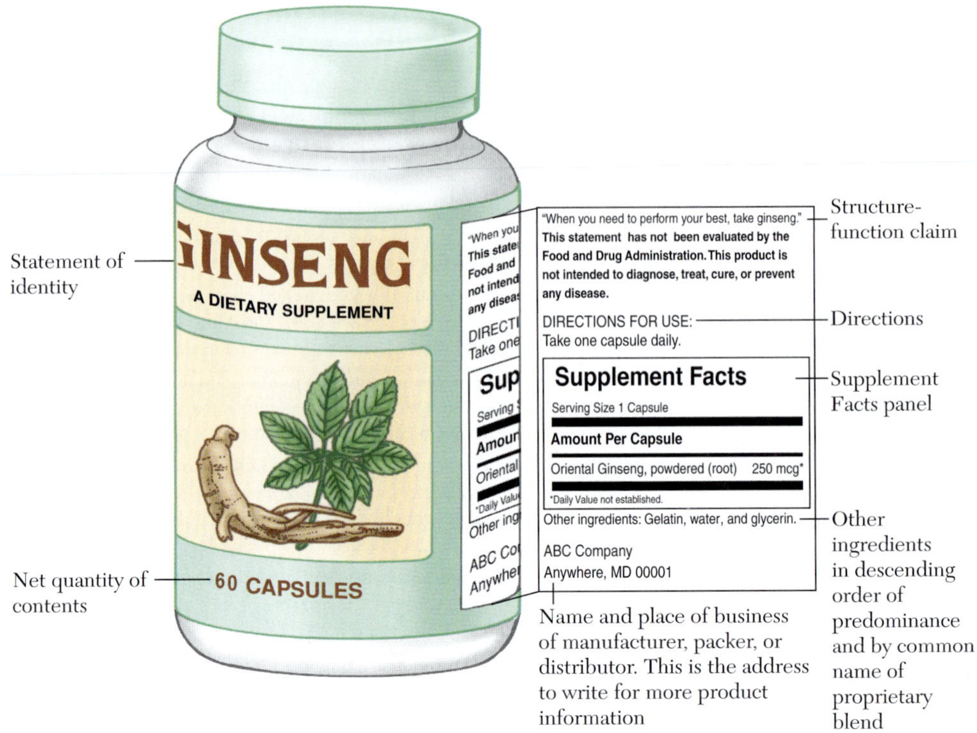

FIGURE 2.7 Products designed for use as dietary supplements must carry a standardized label.

Nutrient and Health Claims Three types of claims are allowed on the labels of dietary supplements: nutrient content claims, health claims, and nutrition support claims.[14] Nutrient content claims describe the level of a nutrient in a supplement. For example, a supplement containing at least 20% of the Daily Value of vitamin C per serving can state that it is an "excellent source of vitamin C." The terms "high potency" and "antioxidant" are also types of nutrient content claims that can only be used when the supplement meets certain criteria. When describing an individual vitamin or mineral, high potency means that one serving provides 100% or more of the Daily Value. For multinutrient products, it means that one serving provides more than 100% of the Daily Value for two thirds of the vitamins and minerals present. A supplement may use the term "antioxidant" if it is "a good source of" or "high in" a nutrient for which there is an established Daily Value and for which there is scientific evidence of its function as an antioxidant (see Chapter 10). For example, a supplement containing 60 mg of vitamin C could be labeled as an antioxidant supplement.

Health claims point out a link between a supplement and a disease or health-related condition. Only health claims approved by the FDA are permitted on the labels of dietary supplements, whereas nutrition support claims do not require FDA approval. This type of claim describes the relationship between a nutrient and a deficiency disease that can result if the nutrient is lacking in the diet. For example, a vitamin C supplement could state "vitamin C prevents scurvy." Nutrition support claims can also include structure-function claims. These refer to the effect of a supplement on maintaining the normal structure or function of the body. These may not directly or indirectly refer to a disease or health-related condition. For example, a calcium supplement might state "calcium builds strong bones." The ginseng supplement shown in Figure 2.7 claims that ginseng improves performance by stating that "when you need to perform your best, take ginseng." Structure-function claims are based on the manufacturer's review and interpretation of the scientific literature and must not be untrue or misleading. They must be accompanied by the disclaimer that "This statement has not been evaluated by the Food and Drug Administration. This product is not intended to diagnose, treat, cure, or prevent any disease."

Although the Dietary Supplement Health and Education Act limits the claims manufacturers can use on labels, products may still be promoted by using information in the form of articles, book chapters, and scientific abstracts that are displayed separately from the products. This information must not be false or misleading or promote a particular brand of supplement, and it must be presented in a balanced fashion.

What's Not on the Label Dietary supplements are classified as foods and not drugs, so they are not bound by the strict laws that regulate drug manufacturing. These products do not need to be approved by the FDA for safety and effectiveness before they are marketed. According to the Dietary Supplement Health and Education Act, the manufacturer is responsible for ensuring that a supplement is safe before it is sold. If a problem arises after the supplement is on the market, it is the responsibility of the FDA to prove that the supplement represents a risk and that it should be removed from the market.

In addition, there are no mandatory standards in supplement manufacturing, so the amount of an ingredient and how well it is absorbed by the body may vary from dose to dose. The U.S. Pharmacopoeial (USP) Convention, which sets the standards for drug manufacturing, is developing recommended standards for supplements. These standards will not be mandatory, but many companies will adopt them. While such standards will protect the consumer from inconsistencies in supplement composition, they may also increase the cost of dietary supplements.

The Dietary Guidelines for Americans: Tying It All Together

The **Dietary Guidelines for Americans** is a set of recommendations on diet and lifestyle designed to promote health, support active lives, and reduce chronic disease risks in the general population (Figure 2.8 and Appendix G).

Web Menu

For additional Information on the Dietary Guidelines, go to the USDA's Food and Nutrition Information Center at www.nal.usda.gov/fnic/dga/index.html.

Development of the Dietary Guidelines

The first broad-based recommendation for health promotion—rather than just deficiency prevention—was the Dietary Goals for the United States, established in 1977 by the Senate Select Committee on Human Needs.[15] The Dietary Goals were subsequently modified and published as the **Dietary Guidelines for Americans** in 1980 by the U.S. Department of Agriculture and the U.S. Department of Health and Human Services. Since then they have been revised every five years to reflect advances in scientific understanding of what constitutes a diet that promotes health. The most recent (fifth) edition was released in February 2000.[16]

The Dietary Guidelines for Americans 2000 take advantage of many of the other tools developed for selecting a healthy diet; for example, consumers are encouraged to use the Food Guide Pyramid and food labels to select a diet that meets the recommendations of the Dietary Guidelines. In this way, the Dietary Guidelines tie together other recommendations for a healthy diet to present a consumer-friendly package of information on choosing a healthy diet and lifestyle.

Dietary Guidelines for Americans A set of diet and lifestyle recommendations designed to encourage active lives and promote healthy and safe food choices for the purpose of improving health and reducing the incidence of nutrition-related chronic disease.

ABCs for Good Health

The Dietary Guidelines are organized using a three-tier system called the "ABCs for Good Health." The first tier, **Aim for Fitness,** contains two guidelines that focus on the importance of maintaining a healthy weight and being physically active. The second tier, **Build a Healthy Base,** contains four guidelines that focus on encouraging healthy food practices, and the third tier, **Choose Sensibly,** contains four guidelines that focus on dietary components that should be limited.

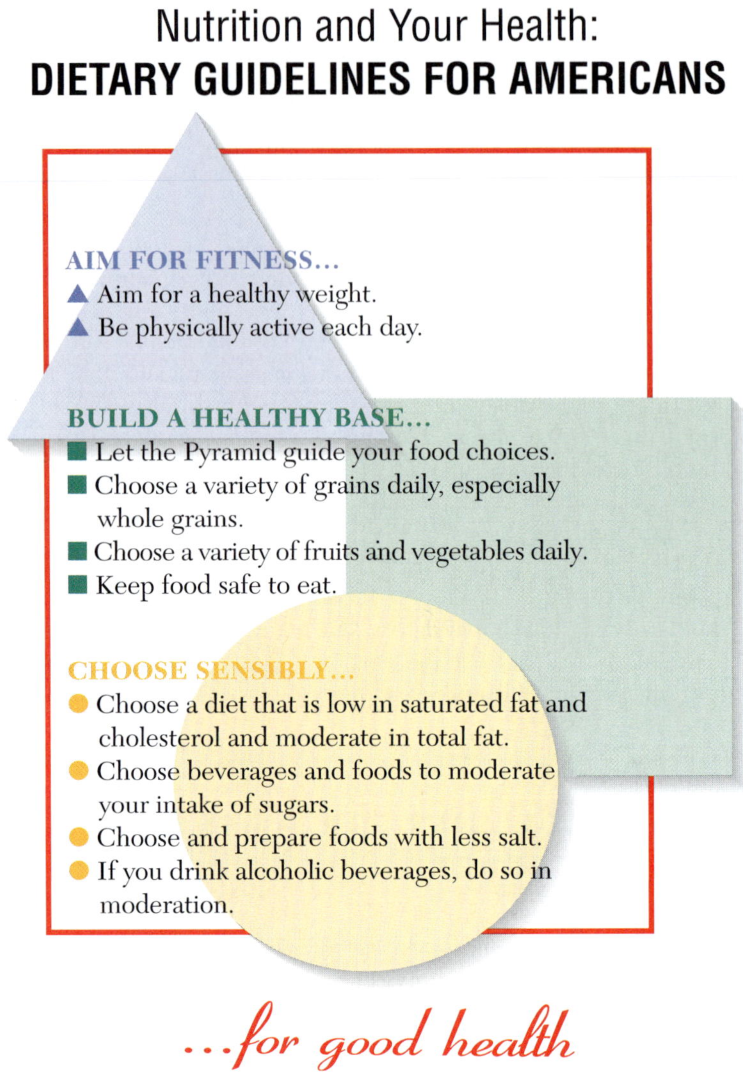

FIGURE 2.8 The Dietary Guidelines for Americans promote healthy diets. *(USDA, DHHS, 2000)*

Aim for Fitness Concerns about the rising incidence of obesity in the United States and the sedentary lifestyles of most Americans has prompted an emphasis in the Dietary Guidelines on a healthy body weight and active lifestyle. The tier called Aim for Fitness recommends that we "aim for a healthy weight." Specific guidelines for evaluating body weight are given (see Chapters 7 and 8). Emphasis is placed on encouraging healthy weight in children. This tier also encourages us to "be physically active each day." This guideline is backed up by specific recommendations about the intensity, amount, and variety of activity that will benefit health (see Chapter 14).

Build a Healthy Base This tier offers four guidelines on choosing a variety of foods and handling these foods safely. It emphasizes that no one food or food group provides all the nutrients and other healthful substances in the amounts needed. The first guideline recommends a diet based on the Food Guide Pyramid and emphasizes variety among food groups by advising "let the Pyramid guide your food choices." The next guideline emphasizes variety in the choices from the base of the Pyramid by stating "eat a variety of grains daily, especially whole grains." The emphasis on whole grains is based on increasing evidence that these foods may reduce the risk of coronary heart disease, bowel diseases, diabetes, and certain types of cancer (see Chapter 4). Variety is also encouraged in the guideline that suggests "eat a variety of fruits and vegetables daily." Fruits and vegetables are high in nutrients and health-promoting phytochemicals. Most Americans do not consume the recommended minimum of five servings of fruits and vegetables each day.

The fourth recommendation in this tier cautions Americans to "keep food safe to eat." This is the first edition of the Dietary Guidelines to include a food safety guideline. The topic has become a focus of public health education because most of the foodborne illness in the United States is caused by food prepared at home (Table 2.7).

TABLE 2.7
Steps to Keeping Food Safe

1. Clean—Wash hands and surfaces often.
2. Separate—Separate raw, cooked, and ready-to-eat foods while shopping, preparing, and storing.
3. Cook—Cook food to a safe temperature.
4. Chill—Refrigerate perishable foods promptly.
5. Follow the label.
6. Serve safely.
7. If in doubt, throw it out.

The Dietary Guidelines for Americans, 2000, USDA, DHHS, 2000.

Choose Sensibly The third tier focuses on choices designed to limit certain dietary components. The first guideline in this tier states that Americans should "choose a diet low in saturated fat and cholesterol and moderate in fat." This wording reflects the understanding that diets low in saturated fat and cholesterol can improve blood cholesterol levels, even if the diet is moderate rather than low in total fat. The guideline suggests that if one's total fat intake is more than 30% of kcalories it should be reduced by decreasing saturated and *trans* fats (see Chapter 5).

The guideline to "choose beverages and foods that limit your intake of sugars" is based on the fact that the intake of sugars in the United States has been on the rise and that the major source is soft drinks. The Dietary Guidelines points out that the Nutrition Facts label will indicate total grams of sugars in a food product, but to distinguish how much is from *added* sugars, consumers must be able to identify sources of added sugar listed in the ingredient list (see Chapter 4).

The guideline to "choose and prepare foods with less salt" is based on research that indicates that a diet high in salt increases blood pressure in some individuals. This recommendation is included because there is no way to identify who might benefit from reduced salt intake, and reducing salt intake is not harmful for healthy individuals. In addition, there is evidence that lower salt intake might reduce the loss of calcium from bone.

The final guideline states that "if you drink alcoholic beverages, do so in moderation." It emphasizes the dangers of excess alcohol consumption but includes the fact that in men over age 45 and women over age 55, moderate drinking can lower the risk of heart disease (see Chapter 17, *Making Decisions:* "The Risks and Benefits of Alcohol Use in Adults").

EXCHANGE LISTS: GROUPING BY ENERGY AND MACRONUTRIENT CONTENT

The **Exchange Lists** are a food group system that is useful in planning diets to meet specific energy and macronutrient goals. They were first developed in 1950 by the American Dietetic Association and the American Diabetes Association as a meal-planning tool for individuals with diabetes. Since then, their use has been expanded to planning weight-loss diets and diets in general. The latest revision of the Exchange Lists divides foods into three main groups based on their macronutrient content: the carbohydrate group, the meat and meat-substitute group, and the fat group (see Table 2.8 and Appendix I). The carbohydrate group includes exchange lists for groups of foods that are sources of carbohydrate: starches, fruits, milk, and vegetables. It also defines a list of other high-carbohydrate foods and indicates how to fit these foods into a diet based on exchanges. The meat and meat-substitute group includes an exchange list with four subgroups: very lean, lean, medium-fat, and high-fat meat. The fat group includes an exchange list with subgroups of monounsaturated, polyunsaturated, and saturated fats.[17]

Exchange Lists A system that groups foods according to energy and macronutrient content, often used in planning diabetic and weight-loss diets.

The serving sizes for foods within each exchange list are different from those in the Food Guide Pyramid. The exchanges are set so that a serving of each food within a list contains approximately the same amount of energy, carbohydrate,

TABLE 2.8 Energy and Macronutrient Values of the Exchange Lists

Exchange Group/Lists	Serving Size	Energy (kcals)	Carbohydrate (g)	Protein (g)	Fat (g)
Carbohydrate Group					
Starch	1/2 cup pasta, cereal, rice 1 slice bread	80	15	3	0–1
Fruit	1 small apple, peach or pear, 1/2 banana, 1/2 cup canned fruit (in juice)	60	15	0	0
Milk					
Non-fat	1 cup milk or yogurt	90	12	8	0
Low-fat		110	12	8	3
Reduced fat		120	12	8	5
Whole		150	12	8	8
Other carbohydrates	Serving sizes vary	Varies	15	Varies	Varies
Vegetables	1/2 cup cooked vegetables, 1 cup raw	25	5	2	0
Meat/Meat Substitute Group	1 oz meat or cheese, 1/2 cup legumes				
Very lean		35	0	7	0–1
Lean		55	0	7	3
Medium fat		75	0	7	5
High fat		100	0	7	8
Fat Group	1 tsp butter, margarine, or oil, 1 Tbsp salad dressing	45	0	0	5

protein, and fat. For instance, each fruit in the fruit exchange list provides about 60 kcalories, 15 g of carbohydrate, no protein, and no fat, whereas foods in the starch list provide about 80 kcalories, 15 g of carbohydrate, 3 g of protein, and 0 to 1 g of fat.

The Exchange Lists differ from the Food Guide Pyramid groups because the exchanges are designed to meet energy and macronutrient criteria whereas the foods in the Pyramid groups are selected based on the nutrients they provide regardless of their energy content. For example, a potato is included in the starch exchange list because it contains about the same amount of energy, carbohydrate, protein, and fat as breads and grains, but in the Food Guide Pyramid, a potato is in the Vegetable Group because it is a good source of vitamins, minerals, and fiber.

The Exchange Lists can be used to design diets to meet individual tastes and preferences at specific energy and macronutrient levels. For instance, a diet could be calculated to provide 1600 kcalories with 75 g of protein, 200 g of carbohydrate, and 50 g of fat. The consumer would meet these nutrient criteria by consuming a prescribed number of servings from each of the exchanges. For example, he would be asked to choose six starch exchanges, two milk exchanges, three vegetable exchanges, and so on.

OTHER GUIDELINES FOR HEALTH PROMOTION AND DISEASE PREVENTION

In addition to the recommendations and guidelines discussed earlier, there are a number of other types of recommendations that promote a healthy diet and lifestyle. The Healthy People Initiative is a general health promotion program that includes nutrition in its recommendations. Special-interest groups also make nutrition recommendations for reducing the risks of specific disease such as heart disease and cancer.

The Healthy People Initiative

The U.S. Public Health Service, along with 300 private and public organizations, has developed a set of public health objectives called **Healthy People.** The first set, Healthy People 2000, was developed in 1990 and was directed toward the year 2000. The most recent objectives, Healthy People 2010, target the current decade. Healthy People 2010 is committed to a single, overarching purpose: promoting health and preventing illness, disability, and premature death. From this broad view it defines goals and objectives for health promotion. The goals for the Healthy People initiative include increasing the span of healthy life for Americans and eliminating health disparities among Americans. These goals are to be met through the broad approaches to promoting healthy behaviors, protecting health, assuring access to quality health care, and strengthening community prevention.[18] Many of these objectives are directed toward improving the nutritional status of the population (see Appendix G). For instance, Healthy People is working toward reducing the number of cancer and heart disease deaths and the prevalence of obesity in adults by promoting active lifestyles and diets low in fat and sodium and high in fiber. It promotes a reduction in growth retardation in children by encouraging healthy feeding practices, including breast feeding for infants. Other nutrition-related objectives are designed to improve the delivery of nutrition information and services.

Web Menu: For more information on the Healthy People Initiative, go to web.health.gov/healthypeople/.

Healthy People A set of national health promotion and disease prevention objectives for the United States population.

Recommendations for Reducing Risks for Specific Diseases

In addition to guidelines for a healthy diet for the general population, recommendations to populations at risk for certain diseases have been published by groups such as the American Heart Association and the American Institute for Cancer Research (see Appendix G). These groups base their recommendations on sound scientific literature, but because of their special interest in preventing a specific disease, their recommendations may differ slightly from one another in emphasis and focus. For example, to reduce the risk of heart disease, the guidelines developed by the American Heart Association include a recommendation to restrict dietary cholesterol to less than 300 mg per day, whereas the recommendations of the American Institute for Cancer Research, which are designed to reduce the incidence of cancer, do not comment on cholesterol intake because a correlation has not been established between cholesterol intake and cancer incidence. On the other hand, the American Institute for Cancer Research recommends a reduction in the consumption of cured and smoked meats because of a correlation with cancer, but these foods are not mentioned in the American Heart Association guidelines.

Nutritional Status: Assessing Nutritional Health

To be healthy, people need to consume nutrients from the right combinations of foods in appropriate amounts. Scientists have developed standards for the amounts we need and tools for planning diets to meet these needs. An evaluation of the **nutritional status** of populations and individuals can identify nutritional needs and can be used to make public health recommendations and to plan diets to meet these needs.

Nutritional status State of health as it is influenced by the intake and utilization of nutrients.

Nutritional Health of the Population

We know that there is enough food available in the United States to meet the needs of the population. We also know that poor nutritional choices from this food supply result in diets high in some nutrients and low in others. This kind of information is obtained by monitoring what foods are available (the supply) and what is consumed. In the United States, the National Nutrition Monitoring and Related Research Program is responsible for providing an ongoing description of nutrition conditions in the population by collecting information about food availability and consumption, food composition, and the eating behaviors, health, and nutritional status of the population.[19] These epidemiological data are used for the purpose of planning nutrition-related policies and programs and predicting future trends of public health importance. The information gathered from population surveys is used to identify the need for nutrition education, food assistance programs, or addition of a specific nutrient to the food supply. These surveys are key in establishing relationships between diet, nutritional status, and the health of the U.S. population.

Food disappearance surveys A method that estimates the food use of a population by monitoring the amount of food that leaves the marketplace.

Monitoring the Food Supply The food available to a population is estimated using **food disappearance surveys.** The food supply includes all that is grown, manufactured, or imported for sale in the country. Food use or "disappearance" is estimated by measuring what food is sold. These types of surveys are used to estimate what is available to the population, to provide year-to-year comparisons, and to identify trends in the diet, but they tend to overestimate actual intake because they do not consider losses that occur during processing, marketing, and home use. Also, the surveys do not assess the distribution of food throughout the population. For example, Figure 2.9 illustrates the food disappearance data on milk consumption over the past 90 years. It shows that the consumption of whole milk, which is high in fat, has declined since the 1950s and the consumption of lower-fat milks has increased. From this it can be concluded that fat intake from milk has declined. But the graph also indicates that total milk consumption has been declining. This may alert the government that calcium intake from milk has decreased and that the population may be at risk for calcium deficiency. The numbers in this graph do not give any information about how much milk each person is drinking or who is at risk for inadequate calcium intake.

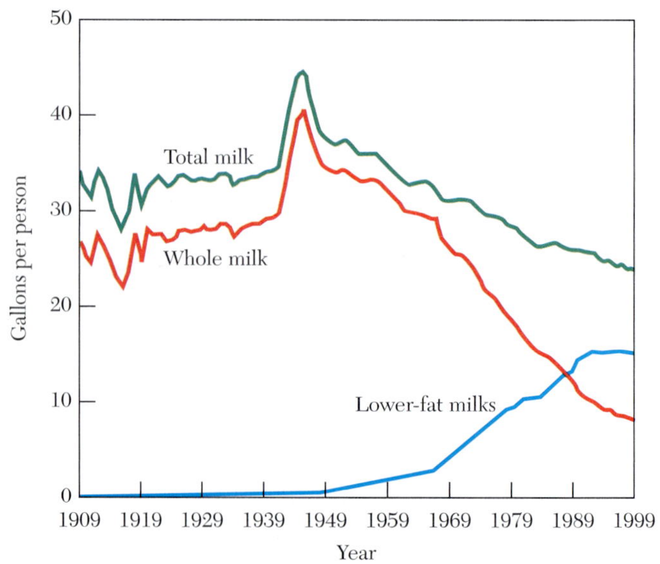

FIGURE 2.9 Food disappearance data can identify population trends in food intake such as the increase in the consumption of lower-fat milks and the decrease in whole milk consumption that has occurred over the last 50 years. *(USDA Economic Research Service, Major trends in the U.S. food supply, 1909–1999,* Food Review *23:12, 2000, Available online at http://www.ers.usda.gov/epubs/pdf/foodrevw/jan2000/)*

Monitoring Nutritional Status The nutritional status of the population is monitored by examining and comparing trends in food intake and health. This is done by interviewing individuals within the population to determine what food is actually consumed and by collecting information on health and nutritional status. The U.S. Department of Health and Human Services conducts the **National Health and Nutrition Examination Survey (NHANES),** which combines information on food consumption with medical histories, physical examinations, and laboratory measurements to monitor both nutritional and health information. Data on food, energy, and nutrient intake can be assessed by comparing population intakes with reference values such as the DRIs or with other guidelines such as the recommendations of the Dietary Guidelines or the Food Guide Pyramid. For example, these surveys show that few people eat the five or more servings of fruits and vegetables per day recommended by the Food Guide Pyramid, that there has been a slight drop in dietary fat intake, and that the number of people who are overweight has increased in all adult age groups in the past decade.

National Health and Nutrition Examination Survey (NHANES) A survey that collects information about the health and nutritional status of individuals in the population.

A system that has been developed to evaluate the adequacy of American diets is the Healthy Eating Index.[20] This summarizes the overall quality of a diet by scoring ten individual components, each representing different aspects of a healthy diet. Five of these components measure how well the diet complies with the serving recommendations for the food groups of the Food Guide Pyramid. The other five components score the diet based on how well it complies with the recommendations of the Dietary Guidelines for total fat, saturated fat, cholesterol, sodium, and variety. Each component has a maximum score of 10, so a diet that follows all of these guidelines would have a Healthy Eating Index score of 100 (10 points × 10 components). Since the index was first computerized in 1989, the typical American diet has improved slightly, from a score of 61.5 to 63.8 in 1996.[21]

Web Menu: To quickly evaluate your own diet with the Healthy Eating Index, go to the Interactive Healthy Eating Index at www.usda.gov/cnpp/.

C 62 00 00 00 00 00 06 28

Individual Nutritional Health

What is your nutritional status? Are you losing weight? Gaining weight? Do you have a family history of heart disease? Are you at risk for a nutrient deficiency because you can't get to the store, can't afford to buy healthy foods, or don't know what to eat or how to cook? An individual **nutritional assessment** requires a review of past and present dietary intake, assessment of body size, a medical history and physical exam, and laboratory measurements. Even with all these tools, diagnosing a nutritional deficiency or excess is not always clear-cut. Estimates of dietary intake are often inaccurate, and symptoms may be indistinguishable from other medical conditions.

Nutritional assessment The process of determining the nutritional status of individuals or groups for the purpose of identifying nutritional needs and planning personal health-care or community programs to meet these needs.

Dietary Intake A good place to start when evaluating an individual's nutritional status is to determine what they typically eat. This can be done by observing all the food and drink consumed by the individual for a specified period of time or by asking the individual to record or recall their intake. Neither system is ideal because being observed can affect an individual's intake. Similarly, recording and recalling food intake are imprecise measures because these methods rely on the memory and reliability of the consumer. For instance, a person who is attempting to lose weight may tend to report smaller portions than were actually eaten.[21] Despite this problem, the commonly used methods described here are the best tools available for evaluating dietary intake to predict nutrient deficiencies or excesses. Once this information has been collected, the nutrient content of the foods consumed can be estimated using food composition tables or computer software (see *Research Discoveries:* "The Art of Assessing Food Intake").

Twenty-Four-Hour Recall The most common method of assessing dietary intake is a **24-hour recall.** A trained interviewer asks the consumer to recall exactly what they ate during the preceding 24-hour period. A detailed

24-hour recall A method of assessing dietary intake in which trained interviewers ask individuals to recall what they ate the previous day.

RESEARCH DISCOVERIES

The Art of Assessing Food Intake

What did you have for dinner last night? Last week? Last year? It may be hard to remember, but information on dietary intake is critical for many aspects of nutrition research. To study nutrient requirements and functions, scientists need to know exactly how much of each nutrient their subjects are consuming. To identify possible nutrient deficiencies or excesses, a dietitian needs to know what a client's typical diet includes. To make nutrition recommendations for a population, public health officials need to know what the population is eating. Assessing how much of what foods people eat seems trivial, but in reality it is extremely difficult to do accurately. As a result, a great deal of research has gone into studying how to best determine the dietary intake of individuals and populations.

The most accurate way to know what a research subject is eating is to control what they are eating. To do this, subjects typically are housed in a research facility where all the food they consume is specially prepared and served specifically to them. The nutrient content of the diet is calculated to meet the study needs; the food is weighed before it is served, and everything that is served must be consumed. This method is ideal but is only practical for small numbers of subjects. Larger studies can be managed if a research facility prepares all food but subjects consume it in their home or workplace. This method is accurate only if the subjects are compliant with the diet, resist urges for a candy bar or bag of chips not included in the diet, and are honest about what they consume. Both of these techniques are useful for controlling the nutrient intake of a research study subject, but these methods do not provide information on what people typically eat. They are therefore not appropriate for assessing the usual dietary intake of either individuals or large groups of people.

Food frequencies, food records, and 24-hour recalls can be used to evaluate what individuals typically eat, to assess a population's nutritional health, or to study the relationships between nutrient intake and disease. Which tool is used depends on the type of information needed. But when collecting dietary information from large numbers of people, the time and cost involved must also be considered. The goal is to collect the most reliable data in the fastest and most cost-effective manner. For instance, a study that wants to look at fruit and vegetable consumption could use a food frequency questionnaire. This tool is easy for participants and relatively inexpensive to analyze. Food frequencies are often used in large epidemiological studies concerned with patterns of food intake. However, when more specific information on energy or nutrient intake is required, food frequencies may not be the best tool. A recent study that compared intakes determined by food frequency with weighed records of consumed foods found that food frequencies underestimated energy intake by about 20% and underestimated fat intake by as much as 36%.[a]

Food records and 24-hour recalls can provide more accurate information on nutrient intakes. Food records recorded by subjects as they consume their meals can be very reliable. However, the act of recording intake can affect intake. A subject may decide to skip that handful of chips they normally would have eaten rather than record that they ate it. In addition, food records are time-consuming for subjects and can be costly to collect and analyze. The 24-hour recall method has the advantage that large numbers of people can be surveyed in a short period of time. It is easy for the subjects and can provide information that is more comprehensive than a food frequency and more accurate than a food record because subjects are less likely to change their intake.[b] Currently, many large studies collect 24-hour recall data over the telephone from centralized study offices.

---

description of all food and drink, including descriptions of cooking and preparation methods, is recorded. Because food intake varies from day to day, repeated 24-hour recalls on the same individual provide a more accurate estimate of typical intake.

Food diary A method of assessing nutrient intake that involves an individual keeping a written record of all food and drink consumed during a defined period.

Food Diary or Food Intake Record Food intake information can also be gathered by having a consumer keep a **food diary,** or record, of all the food and drink consumed for a set period of time. The record should be as complete as possible, including all beverages, condiments, and the brand names and preparation methods. The individual may be asked to weigh and measure everything or simply to estimate the portions consumed. Typically, this is done for two to seven days, including at least one weekend day, because most people eat differently on weekends than during the school or work week. The tedious nature of this type of record can be a disadvantage; consumers may change their intake rather than record certain items.

Food frequency questionnaire A method of assessing nutrient intake that gathers information about how often certain categories of food are consumed.

Food Frequency A **food frequency questionnaire** lists a variety of foods and the consumer is asked to estimate the frequency with which each item or food group is consumed. This method cannot be used to itemize a specific day's intake,

With any of these methods, there is the possibility for error. Whether an individual's diet is being assessed to determine their saturated fat intake or a whole population is being surveyed to evaluate iron consumption, these methods depend on the memories and reliability of study subjects. The most common error in food intake data is underreporting of intake. This can occur because subjects do not remember all of the foods they have consumed or because they choose not to report them all. Even when a subject reports reliably, it can be difficult to accurately assess portion sizes. And when analyzing intake, it can be difficult to know ingredients in foods prepared away from home.

In order to recognize these biases, improve accuracy, and decrease or control for error in estimates of intake, researchers have studied methods of evaluating food intake and come up with some unique ways of validating their accuracy. Observation can be helpful in some situations. People can be placed in settings where they are allowed to choose the types and amounts of foods they wish to eat and their choices are secretly observed and recorded. This type of study can generate some general estimates on how well individuals report their intake. More recent methods to test the accuracy of food intake data rely on measuring energy balance (see Chapter 7). This principle of energy balance states that in someone who is not losing or gaining weight, the energy they eat will equal the energy they expend. A comparison of an individual's energy expenditure (either measured for a specific individual or estimated for an average individual) with their energy intake can be used to evaluate the reliability of their reported intake.[c,d] These types of investigations have found that underreporting of food intake is common. It occurs more often in women than in men and in persons who are older, overweight, or trying to lose weight.[d,e,f]

Public nutrition policies as well as individual dietary prescriptions are based on assessments of what people typically eat. This information is used to plan the food supply and to make and evaluate nutrition recommendations. Inaccurate dietary intake data can give an inaccurate view of the public's nutritional status or the effectiveness of nutritional guidelines. For example, current intake data indicate that Americans have not increased their energy intake over the last decade, yet body weight is increasing. Scientists have therefore concluded that the cause is a decrease in physical activity and have recommended that Americans increase their activity level. How might this conclusion and the recommendation change if it were determined that Americans were underreporting their food intake?

References

[a] Schaefer, E. J., Augustin, J. L., Schaefer, M. M., et al. Lack of efficacy of food frequency questionnaire in assessing dietary macronutrient intakes in subjects consuming diets of known composition. Am. J. Clin. Nutr. 71: 746–751, 2000.

[b] Fox, T. A., Heimendinger, J., Block, G. Telephone surveys as a method for obtaining dietary information: a review. J. Am. Diet. Assoc. 92:738–741, 1992.

[c] Martin, L. J., Su, W., Jones, P. J., et al. Comparison of energy intakes determined by food records and doubly labeled water in women partipating in a dietary-intervention trial. Am. J. Clin. Nutr. 63:483–490, 1996.

[d] Briefel, R. R., Sempos, C. T., McDowell, M. A., et al. Dietary methods research in the third National Health and Nutrition Examination Survey: underreporting of energy intake. Am. J. Clin. Nutr. 65(suppl): 1203S–1209S, 1997.

[e] Johansson, L., Solvoll, K., Bjørneboe, G- E. A., and Devron, C. A. Under- and overreporting of energy intake related to weight status and lifestyle in a nationwide sample. Am. J. Clin. Nutr. 68:266–274, 1998.

[f] Braam, L. A., Ocke, M. C., Bueno-de-Mesquita, H. B., and Seidel, J. C. Determinants of obesity-related underreporting of energy intake. Am. J. Epidemiol. 147:1081–1086, 1998.

but it can give a general picture of one's typical pattern of food intake (Figure 2.10).

Diet History A **diet history** is a general term for collecting overall information about dietary patterns. It may review eating habits: How many meals are consumed each day? Who cooks the meals? How much milk is consumed daily? It often includes a combination of methods to determine food intake, such as a 24-hour recall along with a food frequency questionnaire. The combination of two or more methods often provides more complete information than one method alone. For instance, if an individual's 24-hour recall does not include any milk, but a food frequency questionnaire suggests that the individual usually drinks milk once a day, information from the two tools can be combined to provide a more accurate picture of this individual's typical intake.

Diet history Information about dietary habits and patterns. It may include a 24-hour recall, a food record, or a food frequency questionnaire to provide information about current intake patterns.

Analyzing Nutrient Intake Once information on food intake has been obtained, the nutrient content of the diet can be compared to recommended intakes. This can be done in a number of ways. To get a general picture of dietary intake, an individual's food record can be compared with a guide for diet planning such as the

FIGURE 2.10 This section of a sample food frequency questionnaire is used to obtain information about dairy product consumption patterns.

Food Frequency Questionnaire

On the following pages, please check the appropriate column indicating how often you consume each food.

	Once a day	Twice or more a day	Once a week	Twice or more a week	Once a month	Twice or more a month
Milk						
Whole						
Reduced fat						✓
Nonfat	✓					
Yogurt						
Whole						
Reduced fat			✓			
Nonfat						
Cheese						
Hard					✓	
Soft						✓
Reduced fat						
Ice cream						
Regular						
Reduced fat	✓					

Food Guide Pyramid. For example, does the individual consume the recommended number of servings of milk per day? If an evaluation of the energy and macronutrient content of the diet is needed, it can be estimated using the Exchange Lists. A more precise diet analysis can be done by calculating the nutrient content of each food item in the diet.

To assess the nutrient content of foods in your diet, go to the USDA's Web site at www.nal.usda.gov/ and search for the Nurientdatabase for Standard Reference.

Information on the nutrient composition of foods is available on food labels, in published food composition tables, and in computer databases. Food labels provide information only for some nutrients and they are not available for all foods. Food composition tables generated by government and industry laboratories can provide more extensive information on food composition (see Appendix A for an abbreviated list). The major source of food composition data in the United States is the USDA Nutrient Database for Standard Reference, which is available online.[22] Computer programs with food composition databases are now readily available for professionals and for home use.

To analyze nutrient intake using a computer program, one must enter each food and the exact portion consumed into the program. If a food is not found in the computer database, an appropriate substitute can be used or the food can be broken down into its individual components. For example, homemade vegetable soup can be entered as generic vegetable soup, or as vegetable broth, carrots, green beans, rice, and so on, according to the recipe. If a new product has come on the market, the information from the food label can be added to the database. The advantage of computer diet analysis is that it is fast and accurate. A program can calculate the nutrients for each day or average them over several days. It can also compare nutrient intake to recommended amounts. However, the information generated by computer diet analysis is only useful if it is entered correctly and interpreted appropriately. Also, a nutrient intake that is below the recommended amount does not always indicate a deficiency, and intake that meets recommendations does not ensure adequate nutritional status. Figure 2.11 shows a typical printout for a computerized diet analysis.

Anthropometric measurements External measurements of the body, such as height, weight, limb circumference, and skin-fold thickness.

Anthropometric Measurements Evaluating nutritional health also involves an assessment of an individual's **anthropometric measurements**—that is, height, weight, and body size (Figure 2.12). These measurements can be compared with population standards (see Appendix B) or used to monitor changes

% comparison to: US Male (19 – 24 years)

Nutrient	Value	Goal %
Basic Components		
Calories	2917.80	102%
Protein	99.24 g	171%
Carbohydrates	407.81 g	98%
Dietary Fiber	17.04 g	60%
Soluble Fiber	1.18 g	
Sugar - Total	151.86 g	
Monosaccharides	64.19 g	
Disaccharides	79.36 g	
Other Carbs	182.01 g	
Fat - Total	100.34 g	105%
Saturated Fat	31.67 g	111%
Mono Fat	34.81 g	99%
Poly Fat	19.64 g	62%
Trans Fatty Acids	1.44 g	
Cholesterol	244.79 mg	82%
Water	1463.12 g	
Vitamins		
Vitamin A µg	631.63 µg	70%
Thiamin-B1	1.91 mg	134%
Riboflavin-B2	2.66 mg	155%
Niacin-B3	31.49 mg	167%
Niacin Equiv.	20.28 mg	107%
Vitamin-B6	2.27 mg	114%
Vitamin-B12	4.45 mcg	222%
Vitamin C	41.04 mg	68%
Vitamin D mcg	4.91 mcg	49%
Folate	278.46 mcg	139%
Pantothenic Acid	5.00 mg	71%
Minerals		
Calcium	1024.86 mg	85%
Copper	1.24 mg	138%
Iron	15.57 mg	195%
Magnesium	229.98 mg	66%
Manganese	58.66 mg	2550%
Phosphorus	1383.44 mg	115%
Potassium	3105.09 mg	83%
Selenium	67.61 mcg	97%
Sodium	3592.21 mg	150%
Zinc	11.75 mg	107%

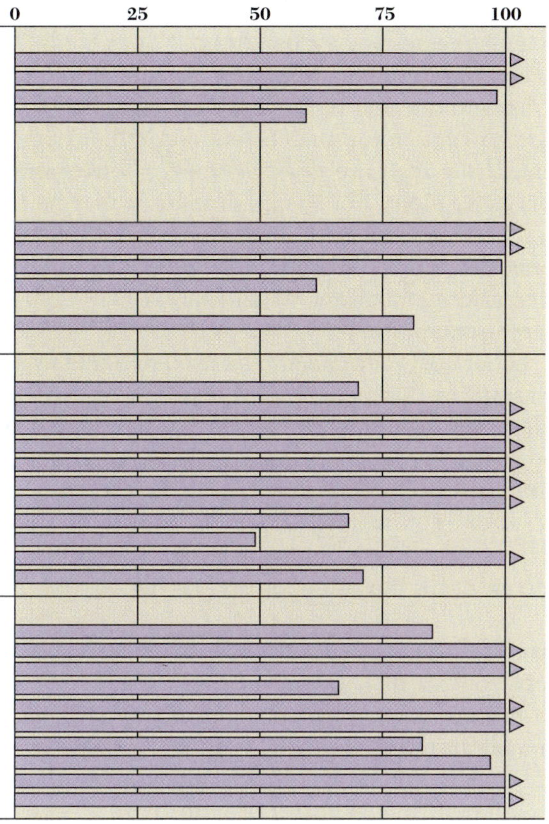

FIGURE 2.11 To be meaningful, the information on computer printouts from diet analysis must be accurately interpreted. This printout shows one day's intake for a 19- to 24-year-old male. The "Value" column gives the total amount of a nutrient consumed that day and the "Goal %" column compares this amount to dietary standards. For example, this individual's vitamin C intake on this day is only 68% of the recommended goal. For some nutrients, such as vitamin C, the goal is a target for average daily intake. A goal % that is consistently below 100% indicates an increased risk of inadequate intake. For others, such as fat, the goal is a maximum recommended amount, so a goal % below 100% is not a disadvantage.

in an individual over time. If an individual's measurements differ significantly from standards, it could indicate a nutritional deficiency or excess; however, this information should be evaluated only within the context of that person's personal and family history. For example, children who are small for their age may have a nutritional deficiency or may simply have inherited their small body size. Individuals whose weight is less than the standard may be adequately nourished if they have never weighed more than their current weight and are otherwise healthy.

Medical History and Physical Examination A medical history can be used to assess symptoms of, or risk factors for, nutrition-related diseases. This should include information about family medical history and individual health and socioeconomic status. For instance, a medical history could reveal that an individual's mother died of a heart attack at age 50. This individual thus has a higher than average risk of developing heart disease and therefore would want to select a diet that reduces the risk of developing this disease (see Chapter 5). Someone who has a family history of diabetes has an increased risk of developing this disease, especially if the individual carries excess body fat.

In a physical examination, all areas of the body, including the mouth, skin, hair, eyes, and fingernails, are examined for indications of poor nutritional status. Symptoms such as dry skin, cracked lips, or lethargy may indicate a nutritional deficiency, but these types of symptoms are nonspecific and may be due to factors unrelated to nutritional status. Determining whether symptoms noted in a physical exam are due to malnutrition or another disease requires that they be evaluated in conjunction with the results of laboratory measurements and within the context of each individual's medical history.

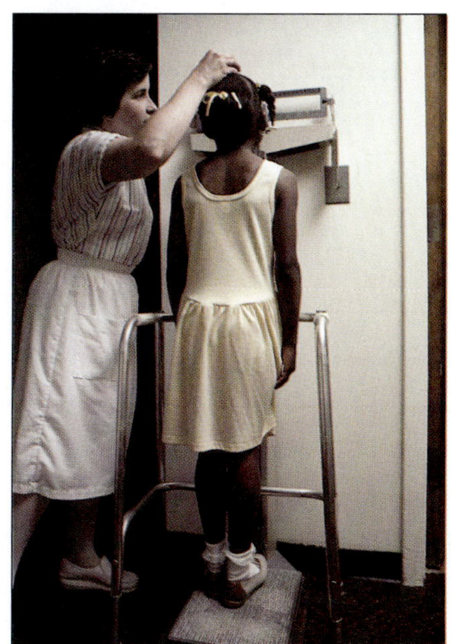

FIGURE 2.12 Measures of height, weight, and body circumference are examples of anthropometric measurements. *(© Blair Seitz/Photo Researchers, Inc.)*

Laboratory Measurements Measures of nutrients or their by-products in body cells or fluids such as the blood and urine can be used to detect nutrient deficiencies and excesses (see Appendix C). For example, levels of the blood protein albumin are often used to assess protein status. Because blood carries newly absorbed nutrients to the cells of the body, the amounts of some nutrients in the blood may reflect the amount in the current diet rather than the total body status of the nutrient. If the measure does not reflect body status, then it is not useful in nutritional assessment. For some nutrients, it may be better to analyze the cells in the blood or other tissues for indications of abnormal function such as altered rates of chemical reactions. For example, vitamin B_6 is needed for reactions involved in amino acid metabolism. When vitamin B_6 is deficient, the rate of these reactions is slower than normal.

Laboratory data can also be used to evaluate risk for nutrition-related chronic diseases. For instance, heart disease risk can be assessed by measuring levels of cholesterol in the blood. Measuring the amount of glucose in the blood can be used to diagnose diabetes. More sophisticated medical tests can be used to obtain additional information about the risk and progression of nutrition-related diseases. For example, procedures are available to determine the extent of coronary artery blockage in an individual with heart disease or to assess bone density in someone at risk for osteoporosis.

What Is Nutritional Deficiency? A nutritional deficiency usually takes time to develop. For example, an individual who is not meeting the requirement for protein may not suffer any physical signs of protein deficiency for months. Deficiencies generally progress through a number of stages. Appropriate nutritional assessment tools can identify deficiencies at any of these stages and allow intervention to restore nutritional health (Figure 2.13).

The earliest stage of nutrient deficiency is inadequate intake. Inadequate intake may occur due to a deficient diet, poor absorption, increased need, or increased losses from the body. Dietary intake data can help identify an insufficient intake and a physical exam and medical history can identify conditions that might increase need, increase losses, or reduce absorption. The next stage of deficiency is declining nutrient stores in the body. The most obvious measure of energy stores is body weight and body fat. Anthropometric measures can be used to estimate these and compare them with both an individual's weight history and population standards. Laboratory tests that measure levels of nutrients and their by-products in blood and tissues are also useful in determining nutrient deficiencies that have affected body stores. For instance, measuring the volume of red blood cells can be helpful in diagnosing iron deficiency anemia because red blood cells require iron for proper formation (see *Critical Thinking:* "Nutritional As-

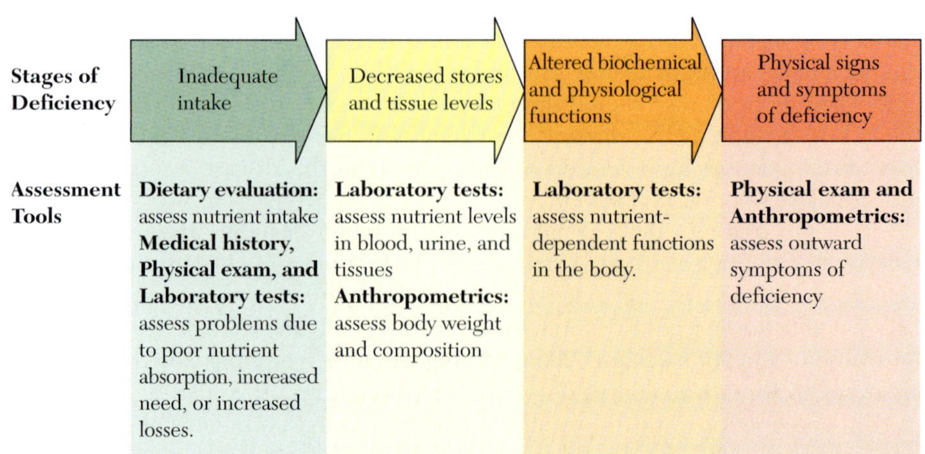

FIGURE 2.13 This figure illustrates the stages of nutrient deficiency and the assessment tools that are valuable for assessing each stage.

sessment" and Chapter 13). Finally, if a deficiency persists, function is disrupted enough that physical signs and symptoms referred to as clinical symptoms become apparent. For instance, a deficiency of the mineral iodine causes an enlargement of the thyroid gland in the neck (Figure 2.14)

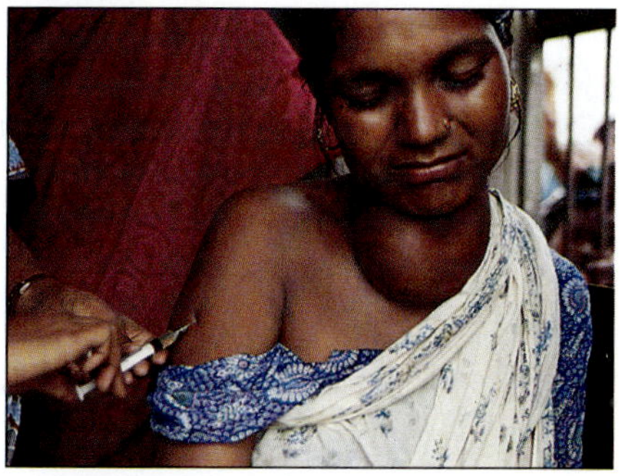

FIGURE 2.14 Iodine deficiency causes goiter, an enlargement of the thyroid gland. *(John Paul Kay/Peter Arnold, Inc.)*

Critical Thinking

Nutritional Assessment

Angelica is 19 years old and has just started college. Recently she has been feeling tired, is losing weight, and has had difficulty concentrating in class. She goes to the health clinic, where she is weighed and measured. A physician does a physical exam and asks about her medical history. Blood and urine samples are collected for laboratory analysis and she is referred to a dietitian to assess her dietary intake.

Anthropometric measures and physical exam

The physician notes that she appears thin and pale. Anthropometric measurements of height and weight indicate that she is 5 feet 4 inches tall and weighs 114 pounds. She recalls that a year ago she weighed 120 pounds and hasn't been trying to lose weight.

Using her height and weight, determine if her Body Mass Index (BMI) is in the healthy range (see Appendix B).

Although her BMI is in the healthy range, her unintentional weight loss is a concern.

Dietary intake

Angelica tells the dietitian that she stopped eating meat last year. Using information from a 24-hour recall, the dietitian enters her diet into a computer program. A portion of the analysis is shown here.

Nutrient	Value	Goal %
Kcalories	1400	64%
Protein	50 g	120%
Vitamin C	110 mg	147%
Vitamin A	1028 μg	147%
Iron	6 mg	33%
Calcium	900 mg	90%

Use the values given on this computer printout to identify nutrients that do not meet recommendations.

She consumes more than the recommended amounts of protein, vitamin A, and vitamin C. Her energy intake is less than the recommended amount and, since she is losing weight, is not enough to maintain her body weight. Her iron intake is well below the recommendation for young women.

Laboratory measurements

The results of her blood test indicate that blood hemoglobin level is 11.2 g per 100 ml of blood, and her hematocrit, which measures the total volume of blood cells, is 35 ml per 100 ml of blood.

Look up the normal values for hemoglobin and hematocrit in Appendix C. Are her values in the normal range?

Her values for both hemoglobin and hematocrit are below normal. This, along with her diet history, suggests that she hasn't been consuming enough iron to produce adequate hemoglobin, the oxygen-carrying protein in red blood cells. This reduces her ability to deliver oxygen to her cells, which could be the cause of her tiredness and difficulty in concentrating. The dietitian recommends that she take an iron supplement for a few months and improve her diet to include plant sources of iron such as leafy green vegetables.

What stage of nutrient deficiency is Angelica experiencing?

Answer:

Should she be concerned about the nutrients she is consuming in excess of her goal? Look up the UL for vitamin A to determine if her intake is likely to pose a risk (inside back cover).

Answer:

SUMMARY

1. Nutrition recommendations made to the public for health promotion and disease prevention are based on available scientific knowledge.
2. The Dietary Reference Intakes (DRIs) provide recommendations for intakes of nutrients and other food components that can be used to plan and assess the diets of individuals and populations. Intakes at these levels will avoid deficiencies and excesses and reduce the risk of chronic diseases in the majority of healthy persons.
3. The DRIs include four sets of standards. The Estimated Average Requirement (EAR) is the amount of a nutrient that is estimated to meet the needs of half of the people in a particular gender and life-stage group. The EARs can be used to evaluate and plan nutrient intakes for population groups and are the basis for the Recommended Dietary Allowances (RDAs). The RDAs are recommendations calculated to meet the needs of nearly all healthy individuals (97 to 98%) in a specific group and can be used by individuals as a guide to achieve an adequate intake. Adequate Intakes (AIs) serve the same purpose as the RDAs but are estimated from average intakes by healthy populations when there is insufficient scientific evidence to calculate an EAR and RDA. Tolerable Upper Intake Levels (ULs) provide a guide for a safe upper limit of intake.
4. The Food Guide Pyramid is a tool for planning diets. It recommends servings from each of five major food groups that can be used to plan diets that meet recommendations. The pyramid shape reflects the relative proportions of each food group that should be included in the diet. It includes a range of servings, so it can be used by individuals with a variety of energy needs.
5. Food labels follow a standard format and are designed to provide consumers with information they need to make wise food choices. The percent Daily Values show how foods fit into the recommendations for a healthy diet. Labels on dietary supplements are designed to help consumers make educated decisions about these products. Only FDA-approved health claims can appear on food and supplement labels. The manufacture of dietary supplements is not regulated, so the amounts of a specific ingredient may vary from dose to dose.

6. The Dietary Guidelines for Americans 2000 makes dietary and lifestyle recommendations that help Americans "Aim for Fitness" by targeting body weight and physical activity, "Build a Healthy Base" by encouraging healthy food choices and food safety, and "Choose Sensibly" by limiting certain dietary components. These recommendations promote good health and help reduce the risk of chronic diseases that are common in developed countries today. It instructs consumers on how to use the Food Guide Pyramid and food labels as tools to meet these guidelines.
7. The Exchange Lists are used to plan individual diets that provide specific amounts of energy, carbohydrate, protein, and fat.
8. The nutritional status of populations is monitored by measuring what foods are available, what foods are consumed, and how nutrient intake is related to overall health.
9. Individual nutritional status is assessed by evaluating dietary intake, examining clinical parameters such as body size, and interpreting laboratory values within the context of an individual's medical history.

Review Questions

1. Describe the four types of standards that make up the DRIs.
2. What is the basis for the shape of the Food Guide Pyramid?
3. List the food groups of the Food Guide Pyramid.
4. What is meant by nutrient density? Give an example.
5. Why is variety important to a healthy diet?
6. Why are the serving sizes standardized on food labels?
7. What determines the order in which food ingredients are listed on a label?
8. How do the Daily Values help consumers determine how foods fit into their diets?
9. What information must be included on dietary supplement labels?
10. How are the Exchange Lists used in planning diets?
11. What is nutritional status?
12. Explain the components of individual nutritional assessment.

Applying Critical Thinking Skills

Personal nutrition:

1. Keep a food diary of everything you eat for three days. Use a form similar to the sample shown here or one provided by your instructor. Because you may eat differently on weekends, record for two weekdays and one weekend day. To make sure you don't forget anything, carry your record with you and record food as it is consumed. This record will be used in exercises throughout this book to focus on particular nutrients. Make the record as complete as possible by using the following tips:
   a. Include all food and drink, and be as specific as possible. For example, did you eat a chicken breast or a thigh?
   b. Estimate as carefully as possible the portion size that you ate; for example, 1/2 cup of rice, 10 potato chips, 2 ounces of tofu, and 6 ounces of milk.
   c. Record the preparation or cooking method. For example, was your potato peeled? Was your chicken skinless? Was it baked or fried?
   d. Include anything added to your food—for instance, butter, ketchup, or salad dressing.
   e. Don't forget snacks, beverages, and desserts.
   f. If the food is from a fast-food chain, list the name.
   g. You may have to break down mixed dishes into their ingredients. For example, a tuna sandwich can be listed as 2 slices of whole-wheat bread, 1 tablespoon of mayonnaise, and 3 ounces of tuna packed in water.

   Food record

Food or Beverage	Kind/How Prepared	Amount

2. Make a form like the example shown here or use one provided by your instructor to list the foods and amounts from one day of your food record. Next to each food, list the Food Guide Pyramid food group to which it belongs. In the next column list the number of Food Guide Pyramid servings or fractions of servings it provides. For mixed foods, list all ingredients separately and identify the food groups and serving sizes that apply.

Food	Amount	Pyramid Group	Number of Servings

   a. How many servings from each food group did you consume?
   b. Does your diet meet the guidelines of the Food Guide Pyramid? If not, what types of food(s) do you need to add to or eliminate from your diet?
   c. Are your food choices consistent with the selection tips described in Table 2.1? How might you modify your food choices to more closely follow these suggestions?
3. From your kitchen cupboard or the grocery store, select three packaged foods with food labels.
   a. What is the percent of kcalories from fat in each of these foods?
   b. How much carbohydrate, fat, and fiber are in a serving of each?
   c. How does each of these foods fit into your overall daily diet with regard to total carbohydrate? Total fat? Dietary fiber?
   d. If you consumed a serving of each of these three foods, how much more fat could you consume that day without

exceeding the recommendations? How much more total carbohydrate and fiber should you consume that day to meet recommendations for a 2000-kcalorie diet?

General nutrition issues:

1. A college freshman has gained a few pounds and realizes she needs to pay more attention to the kinds of foods she eats. The foods and amounts she ate for one day are given below.
   a. Fill in the food groups from the Food Guide Pyramid and the number of servings each item provides.

Food	Serving Size	Food Group	Number of Servings
Breakfast			
Cornflakes	3/4 cup		
Whole milk	1/2 cup		
Orange juice	3/4 cup		
Coffee	1 cup		
with cream	1 Tbsp		
and sugar	1 tsp		
Snack			
Doughnut	1		
Lunch			
Tuna salad sandwich			
bread	2 slices		
tuna	2 oz		
celery	1 Tbsp		
onions	1 Tbsp		
mayonnaise	1 Tbsp		
Pretzels	1 oz		
Whole milk	1 cup		
Snack			
French fries	10 pieces		
Soda	1 can		
Dinner			
Frozen lasagna			
noodles	1/2 cup		
tomato sauce	1/4 cup		
ground beef	2 oz		
cheese	1 oz		
Soda	1 can		
Ice cream	1/2 cup		

   b. Does this student's diet meet the minimum number of servings recommended by the Food Guide Pyramid?
   c. How many foods did she have during the day that contribute primarily sugar and/or fat?
   d. Many of the foods this student chose were of low nutrient density. Suggest some more nutrient-dense alternatives.
2. To encourage healthy eating in her family, a nutrition student hangs a poster of the Food Guide Pyramid on the refrigerator. Her family is enthusiastic, but after one day, her mother and sister are complaining that they can't eat all that food. How could the serving recommendations from the Pyramid be individualized for:
   a. Her 45-year-old mother?
   b. Her 12-year-old sister?
   c. Her 16-year-old brother?
   d. Her 70-year-old grandmother?
3. Compare the label from a product such as cereal, crackers, or cookies purchased at the grocery store to the label from a comparable product from a "health" or "natural" food store.
   a. Which is higher in total fat? Saturated fat? Cholesterol?
   b. Which has more kcalories per serving?
   c. Which has more sugars?
   d. How do the ingredients differ?
   e. What other differences or similarities do you notice?

References

1. FAO/WHO/UNU. *Energy and Protein Requirements.* WHO Technical Report Series No. 724. Geneva: World Health Organization, 1985.
2. Natinal Research Council, Food and Nutrition Board. *Recommended Dietary Allowances,* 10th ed. Washington, D.C.: National Academy Press, 1989.
3. Health and Welfare Canada. *Nutrition Recommendations. Report of the Scientific Review Committee.* Ottawa: Minister of Supply and Services Canada, 1990.
4. Institute of Medicine, Food and Nutrition Board. *Dietary Reference Intakes for Calcium, Phosphorus, Magnesium, Vitamin D, and Fluoride.* Washington, D.C.: National Academy Press, 1997.
5. Institute of Medicine, Food and Nutrition Board. *Dietary Reference Intakes for Thiamin, Riboflavin, Niacin, Vitamin B-6, Folate, Vitamin B-12, Pantothenic Acid, Biotin, and Choline.* Washington, D.C.: National Academy Press, 1998.
6. U.S. Department of Agriculture. *The Food Guide Pyramid.* Home and Garden Bulletin No. 252. Hyattsville, Md.: Human Nutrition Information Service, 1992, revised, 1996.
7. Federal Register 58, Jan. 6, 1993. Washington, D.C.: U.S. Government Printing Office, Superintendent of Documents.
8. Dietary supplements: recent chronology and legislation. Nutr. Rev. 53:31–36, 1995.
9. United States Nutrition Labeling and Eduction Act of 1990. Nutr. Rev. 49:273–276, 1991.
10. Pennington, J. A. T., and Wilkening, V. L. Final regulations for the nutrition labeling of raw fruits, vegetables, and fish. J. Am. Diet. Assoc. 97:1299–1305, 1997.
11. Food and Drug Administration, Center for Food Safety and Applied Nutrition. *A Food Labeling Guide.* Appendix C, Health Claims, August 12, 1997. Available online at **http://vm.cfsan.fda.gov/label.html.** Accessed 13 Nov 2000.
12. American Dietetic Association. *Americans' Food and Nutrition Attitudes and Behavior: Nutrition and You: Trends 2000.* Available online at **http://www.eatright.org/pr/2000/010300a.html.** Accessed 11 Nov 2000.
13. New FDA labeling rules for dietary supplements. FDA Consumer 32:2, Jan./Feb., 1998.
14. Kurtzweil, P. An FDA guide to dietary supplements. FDA Consumer 32:28–35, Sept./Oct., 1998.
15. Report of the Select Committee on Nutrition and Human Needs, U.S. Senate. *Eating in America: Dietary Goals for the United States.* Cambridge, Mass.: MIT Press, 1977.

16. U.S. Department of Agriculture, U.S. Department of Health and Human Services. *Nutrition and Your Health: Dietary Guidelines for Americans,* 5th ed., 2000. Item Number 147-G. Hyattsville, Md.: U.S. Government Printing Office, 2000.
17. The American Diabetes Association, Inc., and the American Dietetic Association. Exchange Lists for Meal Planning, 1995.
18. Maiese, D. R., and Fox, C. E. *Laying the Foundation for Healthy People 2010—The First Year of Consultation.* Available online at **http://web.health.gov/healthypeople/** Accessed 13 Nov 2000.
19. Kuczmarski, M. F., Moshfegh, A., and Briefel, R. Update on nutrition monitoring activities in the United States. J. Am. Diet. Assoc. 94:753–760, 1994.
20. Bowman, S. A., Lino, M., Gerrior, S. A., and Bastiotis, P. P. *The Healthy Eating Index: 1994–96.* U.S. Department of Agriculture, Center for Nutrition Policy and Promotion, 1998. CNPP-5. Available online at **http://www.usda.gov/cnpp/usda_healthy_eating_index.htm** Accessed 13 Nov 2000.
21. Johansson, L., Solvoll, K., Bjørneboe, G-E. A., and Drevon, C. A. Under- and overreporting of energy intake related to weight status and lifestyle in a nationwide sample. Am. J. Clin. Nutr. 68:266–274, 1998.
22. USDA, USDA Nurientdatabase for Standard Reference. Available online at **http://www.nal.usda.gov/fnic/foodcomp/Data/SR13/sr13.html** Accessed 13 Nov, 2000.

3 Nutrient Digestion, Absorption, Transport, and Excretion

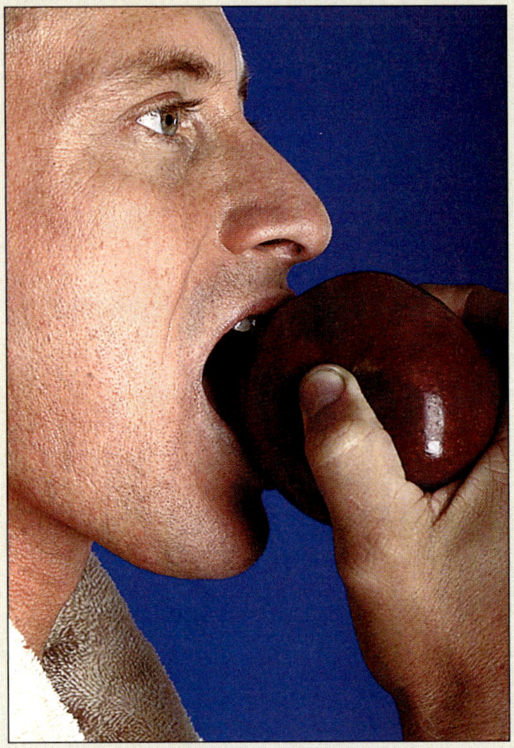

Learning Objectives

After reading this chapter, students should be able to:

1. Describe the organization of life from atoms to organisms.
2. Define "digestion" and "absorption" and list three organ systems involved in these processes.
3. Explain the roles of enzymes and hormones in the digestive tract.
4. Discuss the digestive processes that occur in the mouth, pharynx, esophagus, stomach, small intestine, and large intestine.
5. Define "peristalsis" and explain its function in digestion.
6. Describe how gastric secretion and motility are affected by the presence of food on the table, in the stomach, and in the small intestine.
7. Explain how the structure of the small intestine enhances its function.
8. Compare absorption via passive diffusion, facilitated diffusion, and active transport.
9. Contrast the transport of an absorbed water-soluble molecule from the intestine to the cells with that of a fat-soluble molecule.
10. Discuss the role of ATP in cellular metabolism.
11. List four ways that waste products are eliminated from the body.

Following an automobile accident, Gina had a 50-inch portion of her small intestine surgically removed. During the three months since the accident, she lost 15 pounds. She now feels gassy and bloated and has episodes of watery diarrhea after meals. How has the removal of part of her intestinal tract affected her ability to digest food and absorb nutrients?

The removal of part of Gina's ileum—the lower portion of her small intestine—made her intestine shorter, thereby reducing the absorptive surface area. The fact that the ileum is important for the absorption of water explains her watery stools. The lower ileum is also important for fat absorption, so the reduced ability to absorb fat would explain her gas and bloating, both of which are symptoms of fat malabsorption. This portion of the ileum is also important for the absorption of certain vitamins and minerals, suggesting a potential for micronutrient deficiencies.

An understanding of how and where foods are digested and nutrients are absorbed in a normal digestive tract is needed to determine what functions were lost when part of Gina's ileum was removed. This knowledge can be used to plan a diet that is modified to compensate for her digestive system deficiencies and minimize her symptoms. For example, frequent small meals will maximize the nutrients she can absorb without overloading her shorter gastrointestinal tract. Low-fat meals will reduce the symptoms that are due to fat malabsorption. Consuming extra fluid will help compensate for losses and prevent dehydration, and taking supplemental vitamins and minerals will reduce Gina's chances of micronutrient deficiencies.

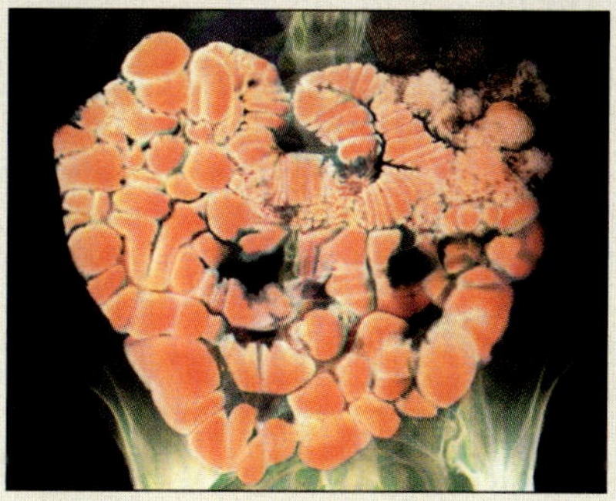

The Structural Organization of Life

The organization of life, as of all matter, begins with **atoms.** Atoms are units of matter that cannot be further broken down by chemical means. The atoms of different **elements** have different characteristics. Carbon, hydrogen, oxygen, and nitrogen are the most abundant elements in our bodies and in the foods we eat. These atoms can be linked by forces called **chemical bonds** to form **molecules**. The chemistry of all life on Earth is based on organic molecules—those that contain carbon. Carbohydrates, lipids, proteins, and vitamins are nutrient classes that are made up of organic molecules. Water and minerals are inorganic nutrients.

In any living system, whether a broccoli plant, a tadpole, or a human being, molecules are organized into structures that form **cells,** the smallest unit of life (Figure 3.1). Cells of similar structure and function are organized into **tissues.** The human body contains four types of tissues: muscle, nerve, epithelial, and connective. Muscle tissue allows movement, nervous tissue provides a means of internal communication, epithelial tissue covers surfaces and lines cavities, and connective tissue supports and protects the body. These tissues are organized in varying combinations into **organs,** which are discrete structures composed of two or more tissues that perform specialized functions in the body (Figure 3.2). The stomach, for example, is an organ; it contains all four types of tissues.

Most organs do not function alone but are part of a group of cooperative organs called an organ system. The organ systems in humans include the nervous system, respiratory system (lungs), urinary system (kidneys and bladder), reproductive system, cardiovascular system (heart and blood vessels), lymphatic/immune system, muscular system, skeletal system, endocrine system (hormones), integumentary system (skin and body linings), and digestive system (Table 3.1).

Atoms The smallest units of an element that still retain the properties of that element.

Elements Substances that cannot be broken down into products with different properties.

Chemical bonds Forces that hold atoms together.

Molecules Units of two or more atoms of the same or different elements bonded together.

Cells The basic structural and functional units of plant and animal life.

Tissues Groups of similar cells specialized to perform a specific function.

Organ A part of the body made up of more than one tissue type that act together to perform a specialized function.

Web Menu

For more information about the structure and function of the respiratory tract, the circulatory system, the urinary system, the lymphatic system, and other body systems, go to the BBC at www.bbc.co.uk/science/humanbody.

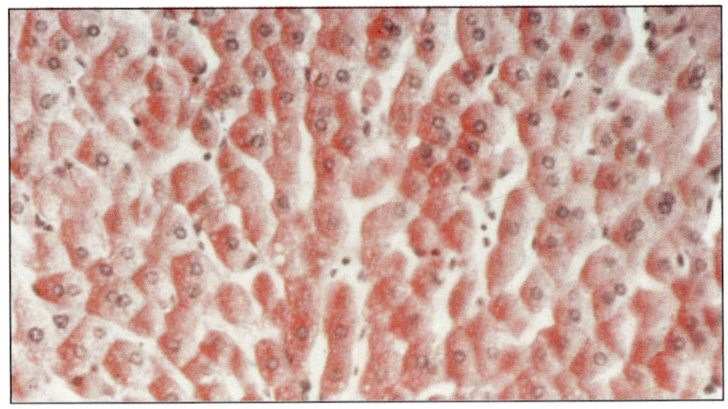

FIGURE 3.1 Living things are made up of cells such as these human liver cells. *(Dr. Roger Wagner)*

An organ may be part of more than one organ system. For example, the pancreas is part of the endocrine system as well as the digestive system. Organ systems work together to support the entire organism.

The digestive system is the organ system primarily responsible for the movement of nutrients into the body. Other organ systems that are important in processing nutrients for use in the body include the endocrine system, which secretes chemical messengers that help regulate food intake and absorption; the nervous system, which aids in digestion by sending nerve signals that help control the pas-

TABLE 3.1 The Roles of Body Organ Systems

Organ System	Components	Functions
Nervous	Nerves, sense organs, brain, and spinal cord	Responds to stimuli from the external and internal environments; conducts impulses to activate muscles and glands; integrates activities of other systems.
Respiratory	Lungs, trachea, and air passageways	Supplies the blood with oxygen and removes carbon dioxide.
Urinary	Kidneys and associated structures	Eliminates wastes and regulates the balance of water, electrolytes, and acid in the blood.
Reproductive	Testes, ovaries, and associated structures	Produces offspring.
Cardiovascular	Heart and blood vessels	Transports blood, which carries oxygen, nutrients, and wastes.
Lymphatic/ Immune	Lymph and lymph structures, leukocytes	Defends against foreign invaders; picks up fluid leaked from blood vessels; transports fat-soluble nutrients.
Muscular	Skeletal muscles	Provides movement and structure.
Skeletal	Bones and joints	Protects and supports the body, provides a framework for the muscles to use for movement.
Endocrine	Pituitary, adrenal, thyroid, and other ductless glands	Secretes hormones that regulate processes such as growth, reproduction, and nutrient use.
Integumentary	Skin, hair, nails, and sweat glands	Covers and protects the body; helps control body temperature.
Digestive	Mouth, esophagus, stomach, intestines, pancreas, liver, and gallbladder	Ingests and digests food; absorbs nutrients into the blood; eliminates nonabsorbed food residues.

Adapted from E. N. Marieb *Human Anatomy and Physiology*, 5th ed. Redwood City, Calif.: Benjamin/Cummings Publishing Co., 2000.

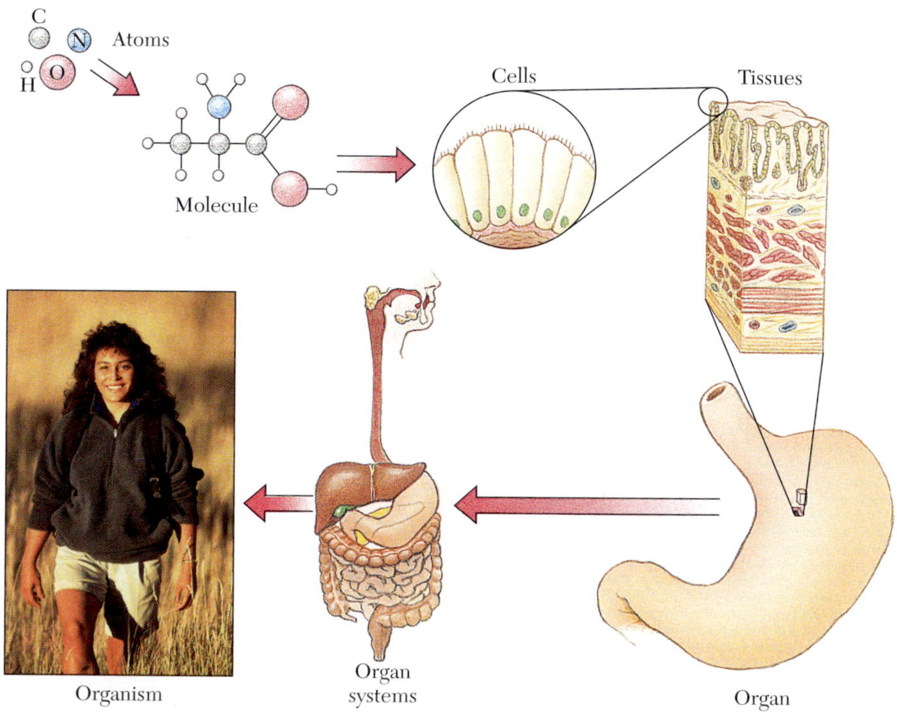

FIGURE 3.2 The organization of life begins with atoms that form molecules, which are then organized into cells to form tissues, organs, and organisms. *(Photo, © Brian Bailey/Tony Stone Images)*

sage of food through the digestive tract; the cardiovascular system, which transports absorbed nutrients to individual cells; and the urinary, respiratory, and integumentary systems, which allow for the elimination of metabolic waste products.

The Digestive System: An Overview

The digestive system provides two major functions: **digestion** and **absorption.** To be used by the body, food must be ingested and digested, and the nutrients must be absorbed and transported to the cells of the body. Carbohydrates, triglycerides, and proteins are digested and absorbed as sugars, fatty acids, and amino acids, respectively. Some substances, such as water, can be absorbed without digestion, and others, such as dietary fiber, cannot be digested by humans and therefore cannot be absorbed. Substances that cannot be absorbed pass through the digestive tract and are excreted in the **feces.**

Digestion The process of breaking food into components small enough to be absorbed into the body.

Absorption The process of taking substances into the interior of the body.

Feces Body waste, including unabsorbed food residue, bacteria, mucus, and dead cells, which is excreted from the gastrointestinal tract by passing through the anus.

Digestion and absorption occur as food is moved through the digestive system. The amount of time it takes for food to move through the digestive system—from the ingestion of food to the excretion of unabsorbed wastes—is referred to as **transit time.** In a healthy adult, transit time is about 24 to 72 hours. It is affected by the composition of the diet, physical activity, emotions, medications, and illnesses. To measure transit time, researchers add a nonabsorbable dye to a meal and measure the time between consumption of the dye and its appearance in the feces. The shorter the transit time, the more rapid the passage through the digestive tract.

Transit time The time between the ingestion of food and the elimination of the solid waste from that food.

Structure of the Gastrointestinal Tract

The main part of the digestive system is the **gastrointestinal tract.** It is also referred to as the GI tract, gut, digestive tract, intestinal tract, or alimentary canal. The organs of the gastrointestinal tract include the mouth, pharynx, esophagus, stomach, small intestine, large intestine, and anus (Figure 3.3). The GI tract can be thought of as a hollow tube that runs from the mouth to the anus. The inside

Gastrointestinal tract A hollow tube consisting of the mouth, pharynx, esophagus, stomach, small intestine, large intestine, and anus, in which digestion and absorption of nutrients occur.

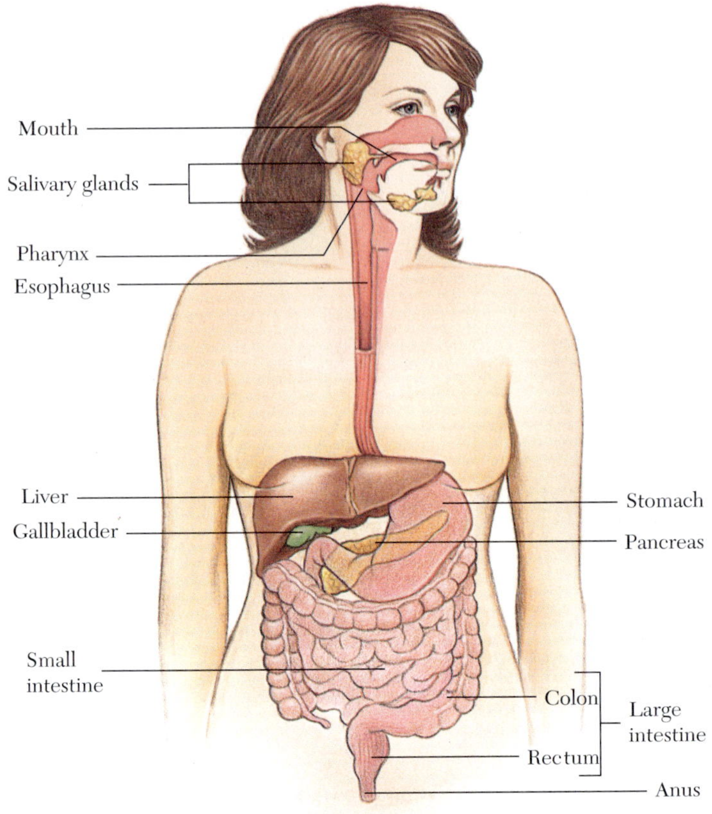

FIGURE 3.3 The digestive system consists of the organs of the gastrointestinal tract: the mouth, pharynx, esophagus, stomach, small intestine, large intestine, and anus, as well as a number of accessory organs: the salivary glands, liver, gallbladder, and pancreas.

of the tube that these organs form is called the lumen. Food within the lumen of the gastrointestinal tract has not been absorbed and is therefore technically still outside the body. Only after food is transferred into the cells of the intestine by the process of absorption is it actually "inside" the body.

Mucosa The layer of epithelial tissue lining the gastrointestinal tract and other body cavities.

The wall of the gastrointestinal tract contains four layers of tissue (Figure 3.4). Lining the lumen is a layer of moist epithelial tissue called the **mucosa.** The

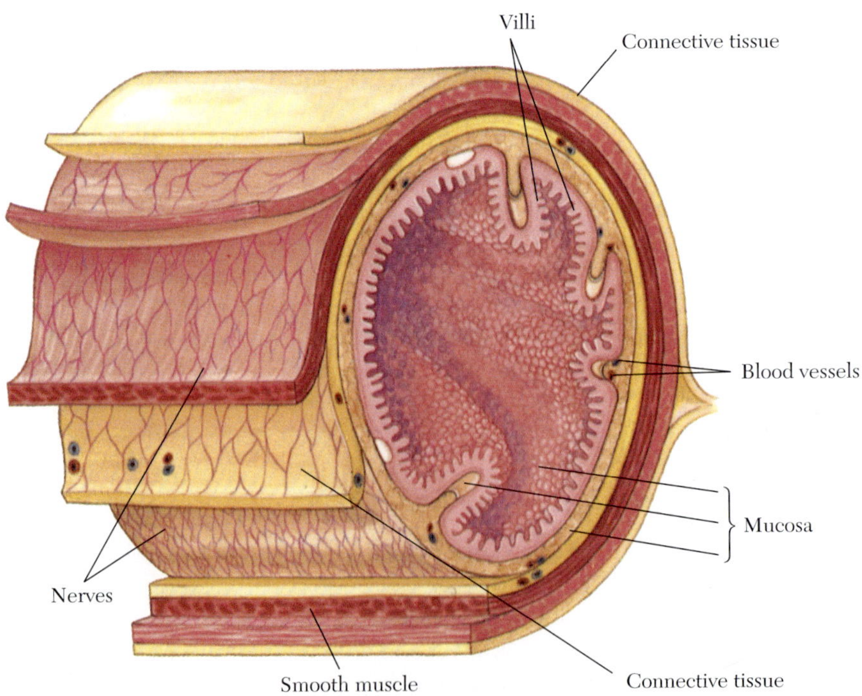

FIGURE 3.4 This cross section through the wall of the small intestine shows the four tissue layers: mucosa, connective tissue, smooth muscle layers, and outer connective tissue layer. *(Adapted from E. P. Solomon, R. R. Schmidt, and P. J. Adragna,* Human Anatomy and Physiology, *2nd ed. Philadelphia: Saunders College Publishing, 1990.)*

mucosa serves as a protective layer and is responsible for the absorption of the end products of digestion. The cells of the mucosa are in direct contact with churning food and harsh digestive secretions. Therefore, these cells have a short life span—only about two to five days. When these cells die, they are sloughed off into the lumen, where some components are digested and absorbed and what remains is excreted in the feces. Because its cells reproduce rapidly, the mucosa has high nutrient requirements and is therefore one of the first parts of the body to be affected by nutrient deficiencies.

Surrounding the mucosa is a layer of connective tissue containing nerves and blood and lymphatic vessels. This layer provides support, delivers nutrients to the mucosa, and provides the nerve signals that control secretions and muscle contractions. Layers of smooth muscle—the type over which we do not have voluntary control—surround this connective tissue layer. The contraction of smooth muscles mixes food, breaks it into smaller particles, and propels it through the digestive tract. The final, external layer is also made up of connective tissue and provides support and protection.

Regulators of Gastrointestinal Function

The digestion of food depends on secretions from the organs of the digestive system. The secretion of digestive substances as well as the movement of food through the gastrointestinal tract, is regulated by the nervous system and by the release of **hormones.**

Digestive Secretions Digestion inside the lumen of the gastrointestinal tract is aided by digestive secretions. One of the substances secreted into the digestive tract is **mucus,** a viscous material produced by **goblet cells** in the epithelial tissue that lines the gut. Mucus moistens, lubricates, and protects the digestive tract. **Enzymes,** another component of digestive system secretions, are protein molecules that speed up chemical reactions without themselves being consumed or changed by the reactions (Figure 3.5). In digestion, enzymes accelerate the breakdown of food. Different enzymes are needed for the breakdown of different food components. For example, an enzyme that digests carbohydrate would have no effect on fat, and one that digests fat would have no effect on carbohydrate. Digestive enzymes and their substrates are summarized in Table 3.2.

Hormones Chemical messengers that are produced in one location and released into the blood, and which elicit responses at other locations in the body.

Mucus A thick, viscous fluid secreted by glands in the gastrointestinal tract and other parts of the body. It acts to lubricate, moisten, and protect cells from harsh environments.

Goblet cells Cells that produce mucus.

Enzymes Protein molecules that accelerate the rate of specific chemical reactions without being changed themselves.

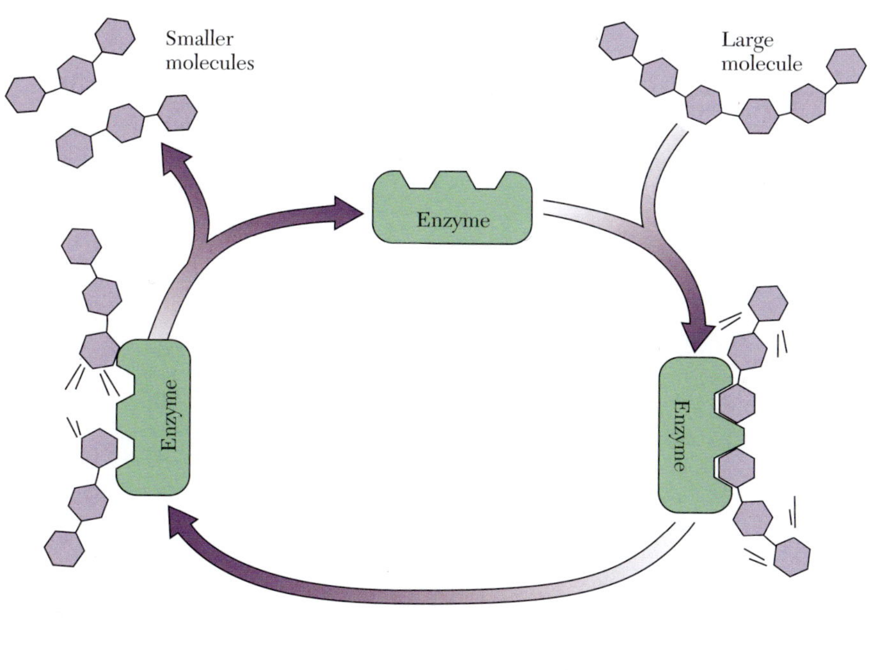

FIGURE 3.5 Enzymes speed up chemical reactions without themselves being altered by the reaction. In this example, an enzyme breaks a large molecule into two smaller ones.

TABLE 3.2 Functions of Some Important Gastrointestinal Enzymes

Site of Release	Enzyme	Activity
Salivary glands in the mouth	Salivary amylase	Breaks starch into shorter chains of glucose.
Gastric glands in the stomach	Rennin	Causes the milk protein casein to curdle.
	Pepsin	Breaks proteins into polypeptides and amino acids.
Secretions from the pancreas	Trypsin	Breaks proteins and polypeptides into shorter polypeptides.
	Chymotrypsin	Breaks proteins and polypeptides into shorter polypeptides.
	Carboxypeptidase	Breaks polypeptides into amino acids.
	Lipase	Breaks triglycerides into monoglycerides, fatty acids, and glycerol.
	Pancreatic amylase	Breaks starch into shorter glucose chains and maltose (2 glucose units).
Small intestine	Carboxypeptidase, aminopeptidase, and dipeptidase	Breaks polypeptides into amino acids.
	Lipase	Breaks monoglycerides into fatty acids and glycerol.
	Sucrase	Breaks sucrose into glucose and frutose.
	Lactase	Breaks lactose into glucose and galactose.
	Maltase	Breaks maltose into glucose.
	Dextrinase	Breaks short chains of glucose into individual glucose molecules.

TABLE 3.3 Functions of Some Important Gastrointestinal Hormones

Site of Release	Hormone	Stimulus	Activity
Stomach mucosa	Gastrin	Food in the stomach (particularly partially digested proteins); stretching of the stomach	Stimulates secretion of HCl and pepsinogen by gastric glands in the stomach and increases gastric motility and emptying.
Stomach and duodenal mucosa	Somatostatin	Food in the stomach; nerve stimulation	Inhibits the following: stomach secretion, motility, and emptying, pancreatic secretion, absorption in the small intestine, gallbladder contraction and bile release.
Duodenal mucosa	Secretin	Acidic chyme	Inhibits gastric secretion and motility; increases output of water and bicarbonate from the pancreas; increases bile output from the liver.
	Cholecystokinin (CCK)	Partially digested proteins; fatty chyme	Stimulates contraction of the gallbladder to expel bile; increases output of enzyme-rich pancreatic juice.
	Gastric Inhibitory Peptide	Fat and glucose in chyme	Inhibits gastric secretion and motility.

Nerves and Hormones The sight and smell of food, as well as the presence of food in the gut, stimulate nerves throughout the GI tract. Food in one part can trigger a nerve impulse that signals a later part of the gut to prepare for the food. These nerve signals cause muscle contractions that churn, mix, and propel food through the gut at a rate that allows for optimal absorption of nutrients. Nerve signals also stimulate or inhibit digestive secretions. For example, food in the mouth stimulates digestive secretions in the stomach. After food has passed through a section of the digestive tract, digestive secretions decrease and muscular activity slows to conserve energy and resources for other body processes. The nerves of the GI tract can also communicate with the central nervous system so that digestive activity can be coordinated with other body needs. For example, if the body is using muscles for physical activity, the digestive tract may receive signals that cause its muscular and secretive activity to decrease so energy can be used by skeletal muscles.

Activity in the digestive tract is also regulated by hormones released into the bloodstream. Hormones that affect gastrointestinal function are produced both by cells lining the digestive tract and by a number of accessory organs. Hormones send signals that help prepare different parts of the gut for the arrival of food and thus regulate the digestion of nutrients and the rate that food moves through the system. Some of the hormones released by the GI tract and their functions are summarized in Table 3.3.

Digestion and Absorption

Web Menu For more information on the anatomy and physiology of the digestive system, go to arbl.cvmbs.colostate.edu/hbooks/pathphys/digestion/.

The processes required for digestion and absorption begin even before food enters the mouth, and continue as food and waste products move through each organ of the GI tract (Figure 3.6). The unique structural characteristics and secretions of each organ provide for the digestion and absorption of almost all the nutrients in a meal.

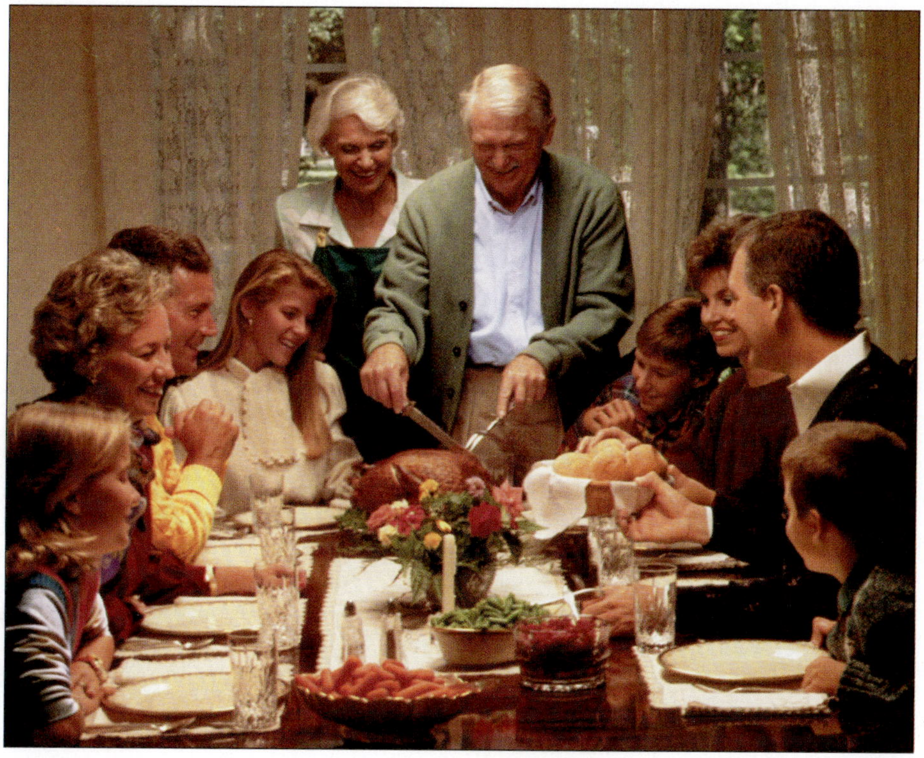

FIGURE 3.6 The sight and smell of food can initiate activity in the digestive tract even before any food is consumed. (© *Steve Chenn/Corbis*)

Eyes, Ears, and Nose

As a meal is being prepared, sensory input such as the clatter of a table being set, the sight of a fancy chocolate cake, or the smell of hot bread just out of the oven may make your mouth become moist and your stomach begin to secrete digestive substances. This response occurs when the central nervous system signals the digestive system to ready itself for a meal. This cephalic (pertaining to the head) response occurs as a result of external cues, such as the sight and smell of food, even when the body is not in need of nourishment.

Mouth

Go to the American Dental Association Oral Health Topics A–Z at www.ada.org/public/topics/ for information on oral health and hygiene.

Saliva A watery fluid produced and secreted into the mouth by the salivary glands. It contains lubricants, enzymes, and other substances.

Salivary amylase An enzyme secreted by the salivary glands that breaks down starch.

Lysozyme An enzyme in saliva, tears, and sweat that is capable of destroying certain types of bacteria

The mouth is the entry point for food into the digestive tract. Food is tasted here, and both the chemical digestion and mechanical breakdown of food begin. The presence of food in the mouth stimulates the flow of **saliva** from the salivary glands located internally at the sides of the face and immediately below and in front of the ears (see Figure 3.3). Saliva plays many roles: It moistens the food so that it can easily be tasted and swallowed; it begins the enzymatic digestion of starch; it cleanses the mouth and protects teeth from decay; and it lubricates the upper gastrointestinal tract. Saliva helps us taste because, as it moistens the food, molecules dissolve in the saliva and are carried to the taste buds, most of which are located on the tongue. This contact between food molecules and taste buds allows the flavors of the meal to be tasted and enjoyed. Saliva begins the chemical digestion of carbohydrate because it contains the enzyme **salivary amylase.** Salivary amylase can break the long sugar chains of starch in foods like bread and cereal into shorter chains of sugars. Saliva also protects against tooth decay because it helps wash away food particles and contains **lysozyme**—an enzyme that inhibits the growth of bacteria that may cause tooth decay.

Digestive enzymes can act only on the surface of food particles. Therefore, chewing is important because it mechanically breaks food into small pieces, increasing the surface area in contact with digestive enzymes. Adult humans have 32 teeth, specialized for biting, tearing, grinding, and crushing foods. The tongue aids chewing by constantly repositioning food between the teeth. Tongue movements also mix food with saliva and help form a bolus—a ball of chewed food mixed with saliva. Chewing also breaks apart fiber that traps nutrients in some foods. If the fiber is not broken, some nutrients cannot be absorbed. For example, unless it is thoroughly chewed, a raisin will travel intact through the digestive tract and the vitamins and minerals in the skin and the nutrients within the raisin will be unavailable.

Pharynx

Pharynx A funnel-shaped opening that connects the nasal passages and mouth to the respiratory passages and esophagus. It is a common passageway for food and air and is responsible for swallowing.

Epiglottis Elastic cartilage at the back of the throat that covers the opening of the larynx during swallowing.

The food that entered the mouth has now been formed into a bolus. In the mouth, the tongue initiates swallowing by moving the bolus back toward the **pharynx.** The pharynx is shared by the digestive tract and the respiratory tract: food and liquid pass through the pharynx on their way to the stomach, and air passes here on its way to and from the lungs. During swallowing, the air passages are blocked by a valvelike flap of tissue called the **epiglottis** so food passes to the stomach, not the lungs. Sometimes food can pass into an upper air passageway, where it is usually dislodged with a cough, but if it becomes stuck, it can block the flow of air and cause choking. A quick response is required to save the life of a person whose airway is completely blocked. The Heimlich maneuver, which forces air out of the lungs by using a sudden application of pressure to the upper abdomen, can blow an object out of the blocked airway (Figure 3.7).

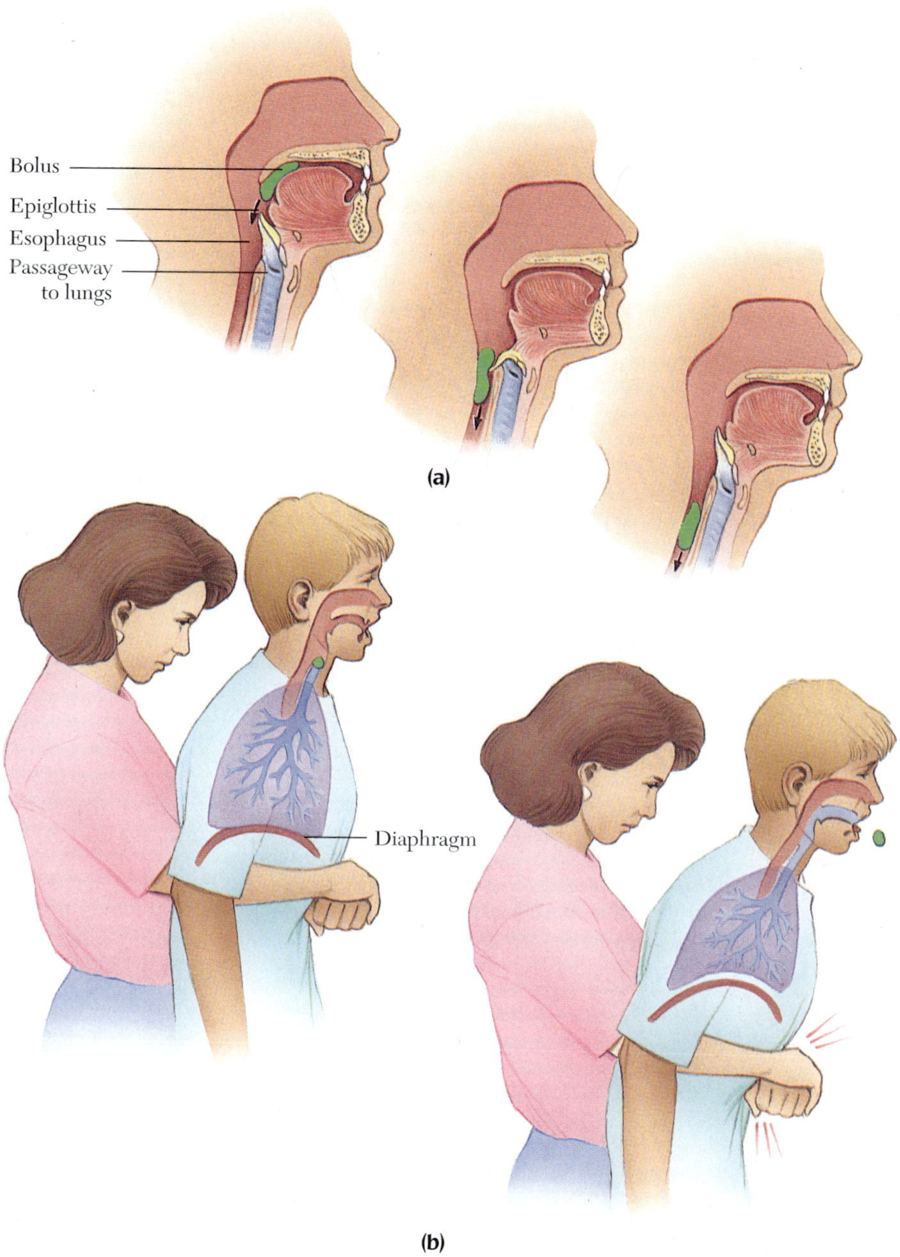

FIGURE 3.7 (a) When a bolus of food is swallowed, it pushes the epiglottis down over the opening to the air passageways. (b) If food does become lodged in the air passageways, it can be dislodged by the Heimlich maneuver, illustrated here.

Esophagus

The esophagus passes through the diaphragm, a muscular wall separating the abdomen from the cavity where the lungs are located, to connect the pharynx and stomach. In the esophagus, the bolus of food is moved along by rhythmic smooth-muscle contractions called **peristalsis.** It takes only about 4 to 8 seconds for solid food to move from the pharynx down the esophagus to the stomach and even less time for liquids to make the trip. The peristaltic waves in the esophagus are so powerful that food and fluids will reach your stomach even if you are upside down. Peristalsis is controlled automatically by the nervous system and occurs throughout the gastrointestinal tract, pushing the gastrointestinal contents along from the pharynx through the large intestine (Figure 3.8).

To move from the esophagus into the stomach, food must pass through the **gastroesophageal sphincter**—a muscle located between the esophagus and the stomach that encircles the tube of the digestive tract and acts as a valve (see Figure 3.8). When the muscle contracts, the valve is closed. Also called the cardiac or

Peristalsis Coordinated muscular contractions that move food through the gastrointestinal tract.

Gastroesophageal sphincter A muscular valve, also known as the cardiac or lower esophageal sphincter, that is located at the upper end of the stomach. It allows food to enter the stomach from the esophagus and prevents the acidic stomach contents from leaking up into the esophagus.

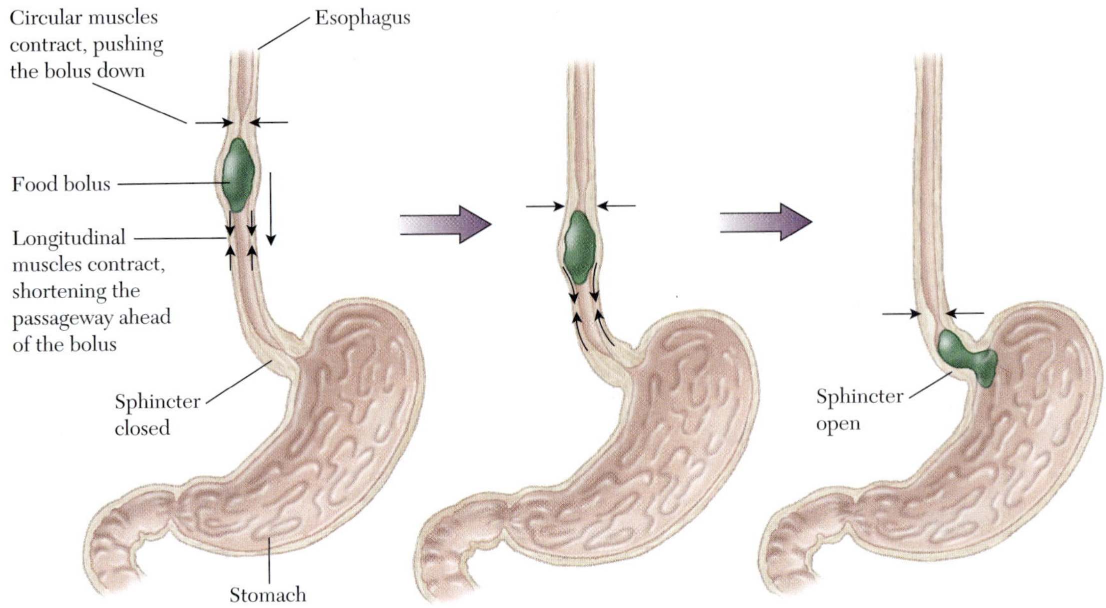

FIGURE 3.8 The rhythmic contractions of peristalsis propel food down the esophagus. Circular muscles contract to squeeze the bolus forward and longitudinal muscles contract to shorten the pathway in front of the bolus. When a peristaltic wave reaches the stomach, it causes the gastroesophogeal sphincter to relax allowing the food bolus to enter.

lower esophageal sphincter, it relaxes reflexively just before a peristaltic wave reaches it, allowing food to enter the stomach. This valve normally prevents foods from moving back out of the stomach. Occasionally, however, materials do pass out of the stomach through this valve. Heartburn occurs when acidic stomach contents leak up and out of the stomach into the esophagus, causing a burning sensation. Vomiting is the result of a reverse peristaltic wave that causes the sphincter to relax and allows the food to pass upward out of the stomach toward the mouth.

Stomach

The stomach is an expanded portion of the gastrointestinal tract that serves as a temporary storage place for food. The empty stomach has an internal volume of only about 50 milliliters (10 teaspoons), but when a meal enters, it can expand to hold as much as 4 liters (about 16 cups). While held in the stomach, the bolus is mixed with highly acidic stomach secretions to form a semiliquid food mass called **chyme.** Some digestion takes place in the stomach, but, with the exception of some water, alcohol, and a few drugs, including aspirin and acetaminophen (Tylenol), very little absorption occurs here.

Chyme A mixture of partially digested food and stomach secretions.

Stomach Structure The stomach walls are thicker and have stronger muscles than other segments of the GI tract, to promote the mixing of food. Two layers of muscle, one running longitudinally down the tract and one running around it, surround most of the gastrointestinal tract. The stomach contains a third layer that circles the stomach diagonally, allowing for powerful contractions that thoroughly churn and mix the stomach contents.

The surface of the stomach mucosa is composed of goblet cells that produce large amounts of protective mucus. This surface is interrupted by millions of tiny openings called gastric pits. These pits lead to gastric glands (Figure 3.9), which contain several different types of cells that secrete substances into the stomach. These stomach secretions are collectively referred to as gastric juice. Gastric glands also contain cells that secrete a variety of hormones and hormone-like compounds into the blood.

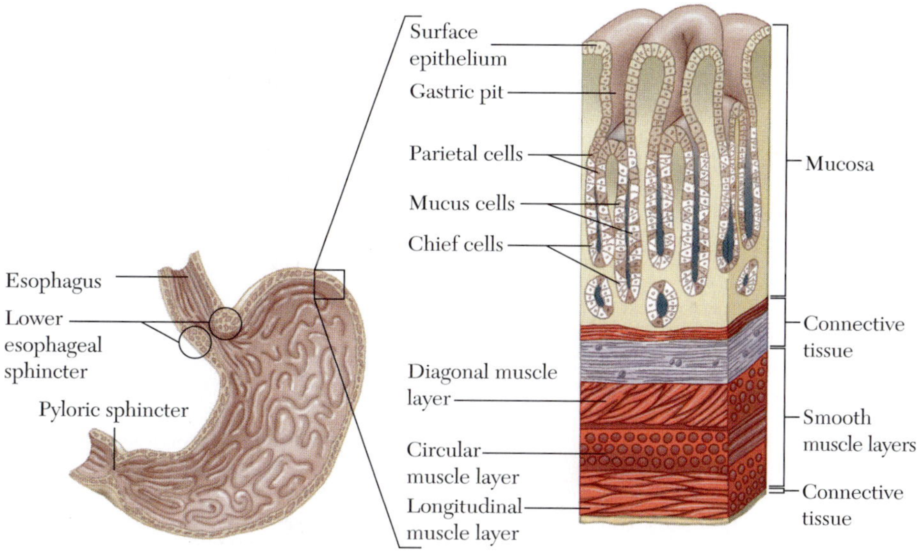

FIGURE 3.9 The stomach wall contains three layers of smooth muscle to produce powerful contractions to mix food. The stomach lining is covered with deep holes called gastric pits. Gastric pits contain a variety of cell types including mucus-producing cells, parietal cells, which produce hydrochloric acid and intrinsic factor, and chief cells, which produce pepsinogen. Together these secretions make up gastric juice.

Gastric Juice One of the components of gastric juice is hydrochloric acid, which is produced by **parietal cells.** Hydrochloric acid acidifies the stomach contents and also serves to kill most bacteria present in food. Parietal cells also produce intrinsic factor, a substance needed for the absorption of vitamin B_{12} (see Chapter 9). Another component of gastric juice is **pepsinogen,** produced by **chief cells.** Pepsinogen is an inactive form of the protein-digesting enzyme **pepsin.** Pepsin breaks proteins into short chains of amino acids called polypeptides. In children, the stomach glands also produce the enzyme rennin. Rennin acts on the milk protein casein to convert it into a curdy substance resembling sour milk.

Parietal cells Cells in the gastric mucosa that secrete hydrochloric acid and intrinsic factor.

Pepsinogen The inactive form of the protein-digesting enzyme pepsin.

Chief cells Cells in the gastric mucosa that produce pepsinogen.

Pepsin A protein-digesting enzyme produced by the stomach. It is secreted in the gastric juice in an inactive form (pepsinogen) and activated by acid in the stomach.

Pepsin and other protein-digesting enzymes, or proteases, are produced in inactive forms and activated in the gastrointestinal tract; otherwise, the active forms would digest the glands that produce them.

Pepsin functions best in the acidic environment of the stomach. This acidic environment stops the function of salivary amylase. Therefore, the digestion of starch from foods such as breads and potatoes stops in the stomach, and digestion of the protein from foods such as meat, milk, and legumes begins. The protein of the stomach wall is protected from the acid and proteases by a thick layer of mucus. If the mucus layer is penetrated, pepsin and acid can damage the underlying tissues and cause a **peptic ulcer,** an erosion of the stomach wall or some other region of the gastrointestinal tracts.

Peptic ulcer An open sore in the lining of the stomach, esophagus, or small intestine.

Regulation of Gastric Secretion Gastric secretions are regulated by both nervous and hormonal mechanisms. Signals from three different sites—the brain (central nervous system), stomach, and small intestine—stimulate or inhibit gastric secretion. The three phases of gastric secretion are therefore called cephalic, gastric, and intestinal (Figure 3.10). The **cephalic phase** occurs before food enters the stomach. During this phase, the thought, smell, sight, or taste of food causes the brain to send nerve signals that increase gastric secretion. This prepares the stomach to receive food.

Cephalic phase The phase of gastric secretion that is stimulated by the thought, sight, smell, and taste of food. It is characterized by an increase in the secretion of gastric juice.

The second phase, referred to as the **gastric phase,** begins when food enters the stomach. The presence of food in the stomach causes gastric secretion by stretching local nerves, by signaling the brain, and by stimulating the secretion of the hormone **gastrin** from the upper portion of the stomach. Gastrin triggers the release of gastric juice from gastric glands in the lining of the stomach.

Gastric phase The phase of gastric secretion triggered by the entry of food into the stomach. It is characterized by an increase in the secretion of gastric juice.

Gastrin A hormone secreted by the stomach mucosa that stimulates the secretion of gastric juice.

The third phase of gastric secretion, the **intestinal phase,** is begun by the passage of chyme into the small intestine. This triggers nervous and hormonal signals that decrease stomach motility and secretions and slow the release of food

Intestinal phase The phase of gastric secretion that is begun by the entry of food into the small intestine. It is characterized by a decrease in stomach motility and a decrease in the secretion of gastric juice.

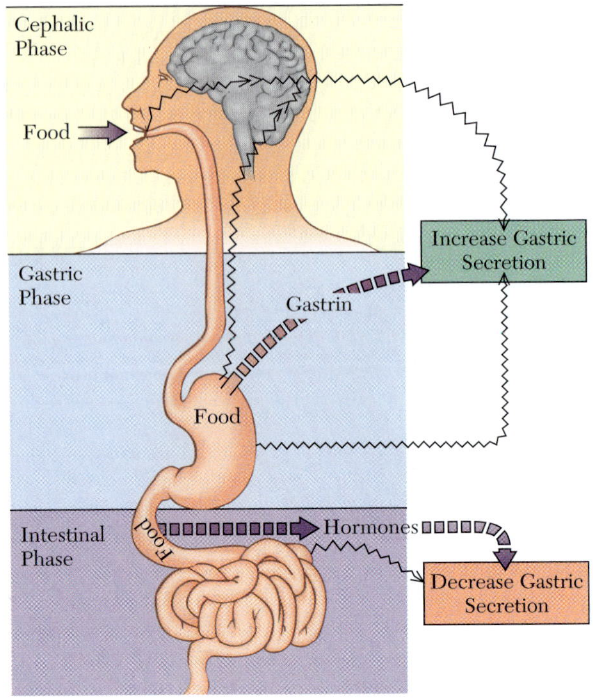

FIGURE 3.10 The regulation of gastric secretion is divided into three phases. In the cephalic phase, the sight, smell, and taste of food cause the brain to signal an increase in gastric secretions. In the gastric phase, food entering the stomach stimulates gastric secretions by stretching local nerves, signaling the brain, and causing gastrin release. In the intestinal phase, food entering the small intestine inhibits gastric secretions by triggering nervous and hormonal signals. In this diagram the zigzag arrows represent nerve signals and dashed arrows represent hormonal signals.

into the intestine. This ensures that the amount of chyme entering the small intestine does not exceed the ability of the intestine to process it.

Pyloric sphincter A muscular valve located at the lower end of the stomach that regulates the rate at which food leaves the stomach and enters the duodenum.

Regulation of Gastric Emptying Chyme normally leaves the stomach in 2 to 6 hours. The rate of stomach emptying is determined by the size and composition of the meal and by signals from the small intestine. Chyme moving out of the stomach must pass through the **pyloric sphincter** (see Figure 3.9). This sphincter helps regulate the rate at which food enters the small intestine. Each wave of peristaltic contraction that travels down the stomach causes the pyloric sphincter to relax and then tighten, allowing a few milliliters of chyme to squirt out into the small intestine. As chyme passes into the small intestine, the stretching of intestinal muscles and the increase in the concentration of acid, fat, and small particles are sensed. The small intestine then initiates nervous and hormonal signals that cause the pyloric sphincter to tighten and the contractions in the stomach to decrease, slowing stomach emptying. When the chyme has been neutralized, diluted, and moved further along the small intestine, stomach contractions increase again and the sphincter relaxes, allowing more chyme to enter the small intestine.

A large meal takes longer to completely leave the stomach than a small meal, and a solid meal will leave the stomach more slowly than a liquid meal. The nutritional composition of a meal also affects how long it stays in the stomach. A meal containing about 25% of energy as protein, 45% as carbohydrate, and 30% as fat that is partly solid and partly liquid, will be in the stomach for an average amount of time (about 4 hours). A high-fat meal will stay in the stomach the longest because fat entering the small intestine causes the release of hormones that slow GI motility, thus slowing stomach emptying. A meal that is primarily protein will leave more quickly, and a meal of mostly carbohydrate will leave the fastest. Thus, someone who consumes only dry toast and black coffee for breakfast is likely to feel hungry long before lunch time; someone who eats a larger meal with more protein and some fat, such as yogurt, cereal, and fruit will feel full longer and someone who has a high-fat breakfast of bacon and eggs will feel full even longer because the fat content slows stomach emptying.

Emotional factors can also affect gastric emptying. For example, sadness and fear tend to slow emptying, while aggression tends to increase gastric motility and speed emptying.

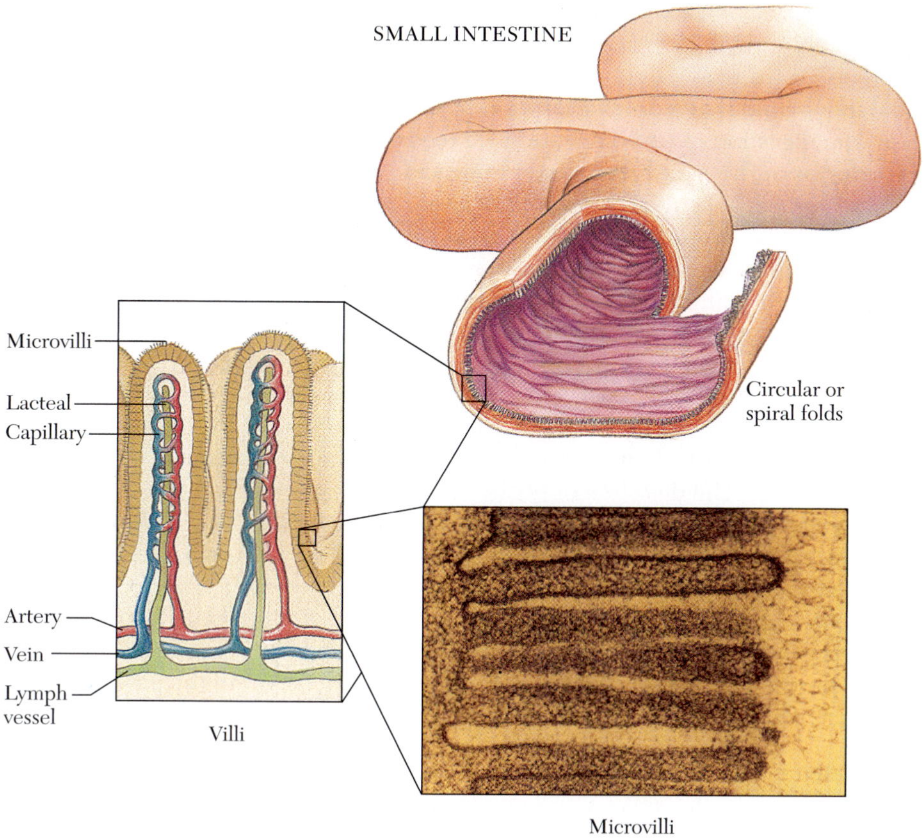

FIGURE 3.11 The small intestine contains folds, villi, and microvilli, which increase its absorptive surface area. *(Photo, © S. Ito, D. W. Fawcett/Visuals Unlimited)*

Villi (villus) Finger-like protrusions of the lining of the small intestine that participate in the digestion and absorption of foodstuffs.

Microvilli Minute brushlike projections on the mucosal cell membrane that contain digestive enzymes and increase the absorptive surface area in the small intestine.

Lacteal A lymph vessel in each villus of the small intestine that can transport large particles such as the products of fat digestion.

Bile A substance made in the liver and stored in the gallbladder. It is released into the small intestine to aid in fat digestion and absorption.

Small Intestine

The small intestine is a narrow tube about 20 feet in length. It is divided into three segments. The first 12 inches are the duodenum, the next 8 feet are the jejunum, and the last 11 feet are the ileum. The structure of the small intestine is specialized to allow maximal absorption of the nutrients. In addition to its length, the small intestine has three other features that increase the area of its absorptive surface (Figure 3.11). First, the intestinal walls are arranged in circular or spiral folds that increase the surface area in contact with nutrients. Second, its entire inner surface is covered with fingerlike projections called **villi** (singular, "villus"), which contain smooth-muscle cells that allow them to alternately shorten and elongate, increasing contact with nutrients in the lumen. And finally, each of these villi is covered with tiny **microvilli,** often referred to as the "brush border." Together, these features provide a surface area that is about the size of a tennis court (300 sq m or 3229 sq ft).

To facilitate nutrient absorption, each villus contains both a blood vessel and a lymph vessel called a **lacteal,** which are located only one cell layer away from the nutrients in the intestinal lumen.

Digestion in the Small Intestine About 95% of digestion and most absorption occurs in the small intestine. Chyme is propelled through the small intestine by peristalsis, and the mixing of chyme with digestive secretions is aided in the small intestine by rhythmic local constrictions called segmentation (Figure 3.12). Segmentation also enhances absorption by repeatedly moving chyme over the intestinal mucosa.

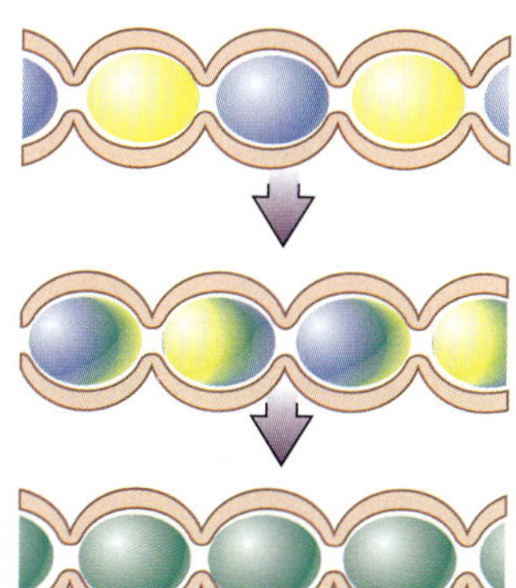

FIGURE 3.12 Segmentation refers to the alternating contraction and relaxation of segments of the intestine. Because the segments are separated by noncontracted regions, the food is moved forward and backward, mixing rather than propelling it.

Digestion in the small intestine is aided by secretions from the intestine itself and from two accessory organs, the gallbladder and pancreas. Although it is produced in the liver, **bile** is stored in and then secreted from the gallbladder. This yellow-green substance, consisting of bile salts, phospholipids, cholesterol, bile pigments, fats, and electrolytes, is important for lipid digestion and absorption. The pancreas secretes pancreatic juice containing bicarbonate ions and digestive enzymes. The bicarbonate neutralizes the hydrochloric acid in chyme. This reduction in acidity allows the enzymes present in pancreatic juice and those produced by the small intestine to continue the digestion of carbohydrates, fats, and proteins. Intestinal glands, or crypts, secrete intestinal juice, a watery mucus-containing fluid that aids in absorption.

The digestion of carbohydrate from foods such as grains and starchy vegetables begins in the mouth but stops in the acid environment of the stomach. Once the food reaches the neutral environment of the small intestine, the enzyme pancreatic amylase continues the job of breaking starch into sugars. The digestion of protein from meats, eggs, and legumes is begun by the acid and pepsin in the stomach. In the intestine pancreatic proteases such as trypsin, carboxypeptidase, and chymotrypsin, which are designed to work in the neutral environment of the small intestine, continue to break protein into shorter and shorter chains of amino acids. Like pepsin in the stomach, protein-digesting pancreatic enzymes are produced in an inactive form and are activated in the duodenum (see Chapter 6). Digestive enzymes attached to or inside the cells lining the small intestine are involved in both the digestion of sugars into single sugar units and the digestion of small polypeptides into amino acids.

Most of the digestion of fat, from foods such as whole milk, vegetable oils, and meats, occurs when the chyme reaches the small intestine. Here fat is mixed with bile, which emulsifies it (breaks it into small droplets). These smaller droplets allow pancreatic fat-digesting enzymes, called lipases, to more efficiently access the fat and digest it. Bile then forms small globules with the products of fat digestion and facilitates their absorption.

Regulation of Bile Release and Pancreatic Secretion The release of bile and pancreatic juice into the small intestine is controlled by two hormones secreted by the mucosal lining of the duodenum. **Secretin** is released in response to the presence of hydrochloric acid in the intestine. It signals the pancreas to secrete bicarbonate ions, which neutralize acid, and stimulates the liver to secrete bile into the gallbladder. **Cholecystokinin (CCK)** is released when fats and partially digested proteins enter the small intestine. CCK signals the pancreas to secrete digestive enzymes and causes the gallbladder to contract and release bile into the duodenum (Figure 3.13).

Secretin A hormone released by the duodenum that signals the pancreas to secrete bicarbonate ions and stimulates the liver to secrete bile into the gallbladder.

Cholecystokinin (CCK) A hormone released by the duodenum that signals the pancreas to secrete digestive enzymes and causes the gallbladder to contract and release bile into the duodenum.

Absorption in the Small Intestine The small intestine is the primary site of absorption for water, vitamins, minerals, and the products of carbohydrate, fat, and pro-

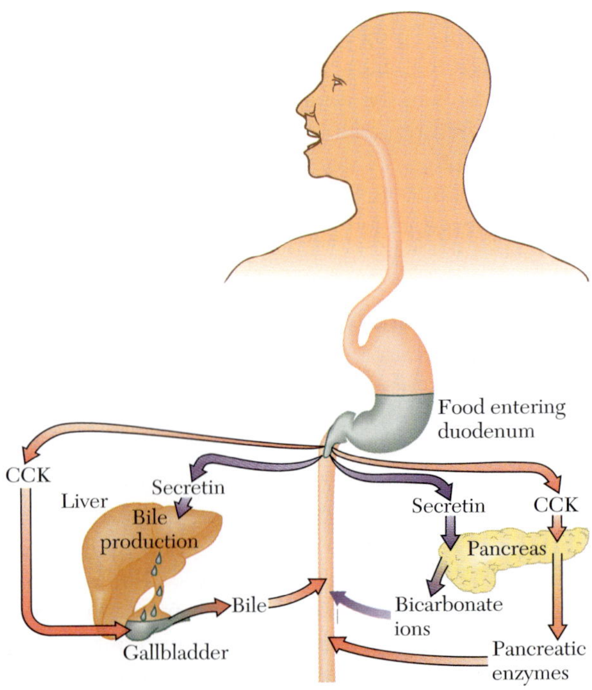

FIGURE 3.13 Food entering the duodenum triggers the release of the hormones secretin and cholecystokinin (CCK). Secretin increases the output of bile by the liver and the secretion of bicarbonate ions from the pancreas. CCK signals the release of bile by the gallbladder and the secretion of digestive enzymes from the pancreas.

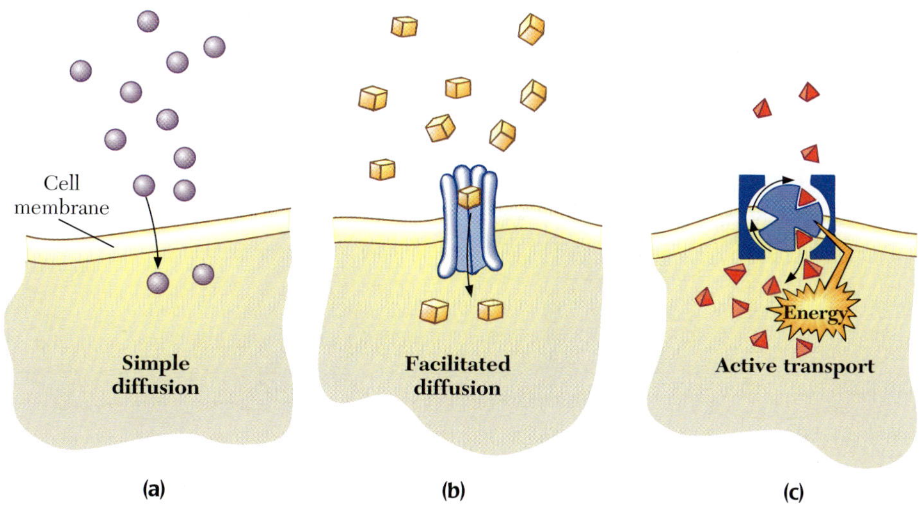

FIGURE 3.14 A number of mechanisms are used to transport nutrients from the lumen across the cell membrane into the mucosal cell during absorption. (a) Simple diffusion requires no energy and is shown here by the purple balls that move from an area of higher concentration to an area of lower concentration. (b) Facilitated diffusion requires no energy and is shown here by the yellow cubes that move from an area of higher concentration to an area of lower concentration with the help of a carrier. (c) Active transport requires energy and a carrier and is shown here by the red pyramids that move from an area of lower concentration to an area of higher concentration.

tein digestion. Several different mechanisms are involved (Figure 3.14). Some molecules are absorbed by diffusion—the process by which a substance moves from an area of higher concentration to an area of lower concentration. Substances that move from higher to lower concentrations are said to move down their concentration gradient. When a concentration gradient exists and the nutrient can pass freely from the lumen of the GI tract across the cell membrane into the mucosal cell, the process is called **simple diffusion.** This process requires no energy. Water, fatty acids, and fat-soluble vitamins are absorbed by simple diffusion.

Many nutrients cannot pass freely across cell membranes; they must be helped across by a molecule that acts as a carrier or forms a passageway in the cell membrane—a process called **facilitated diffusion.** Even though these nutrients are helped across the cell membrane by other molecules, they still move down a concentration gradient from an area of higher concentration to one of lower concentration without the expenditure of energy. The sugar fructose is absorbed by facilitated diffusion. Substances unable to be absorbed by diffusion must enter the body by **active transport,** a process that requires both a carrier molecule and energy. The use of energy allows substances to be transported against their concentration gradient from an area of lower concentration to an area of higher concentration. Glucose and amino acids are absorbed by active transport. These molecules, therefore, continue to be absorbed even when they are present in high concentrations inside the mucosal cells.

Simple diffusion The movement of substances from an area of higher concentration to an area of lower concentration. No energy is required.

Facilitated diffusion The movement of substances across a cell membrane from an area of higher concentration to an area of lower concentration with the aid of a carrier molecule. No energy is required.

Active transport The transport of substances across a cell membrane with the aid of a carrier molecule and the expenditure of energy. This may occur against a concentration gradient.

The digestion and absorption of carbohydrate, fat, and protein are summarized in Figure 3.15. More specific information about absorption of the products of carbohydrate, fat, and protein digestion will be discussed in Chapters 4, 5, and 6, respectively.

Large Intestine

Components of chyme that are not absorbed in the small intestine pass through the **ileocecal valve** to the large intestine, which includes the colon and rectum. Although most absorption occurs in the small intestine, water and some vitamins and minerals are also absorbed in the colon. Peristalsis here is slower than in the small intestine. Water, nutrients, and fecal matter may spend 24 hours in the large intestine, in contrast to the 3 to 5 hours it takes for chyme to move through the small intestine. This slow movement favors the growth of bacteria, referred to as **intestinal microflora.** These bacteria are permanent beneficial residents of this part of the gastrointestinal tract (see *Making Decisions:* "Probiotics and Prebiotics: Are They Beneficial?"). The microflora act on unabsorbed portions of food, such as fiber, producing nutrients that the bacteria can use or, in some cases, that can be absorbed into the body.[1] For example, the microflora synthesize small amounts of B vitamins and vitamin K, some of which can be absorbed.

Ileocecal valve A fold of mucous membrane that separates the ileum of the small intestine from the large intestine.

Intestinal microflora Microorganisms that inhabit the large intestine.

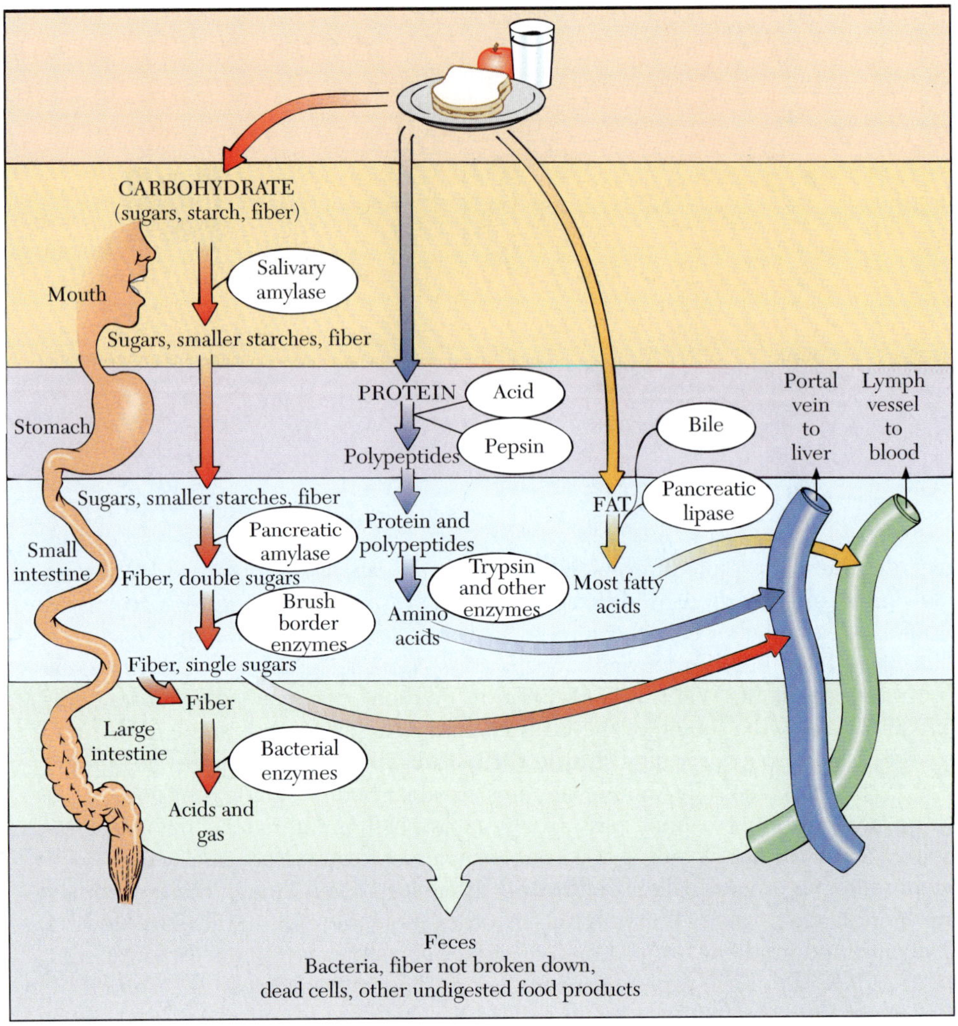

FIGURE 3.15 An overview of the digestion and absorption of a meal.

One additional by-product of bacterial metabolism is gas, which causes flatulence. About 500 ml of gas is produced each day and this amount is increased if the diet is rich in indigestible carbohydrates.

Materials not absorbed are excreted as waste products in the feces. Feces consist of material that is consumed but not digested and absorbed, dead intestinal bacteria (which make up about a third of the fecal solid matter), sloughed epithelial cells, and fluid. About 50 to 200 ml of water is typically excreted in the feces, but the amount varies depending on fiber and fluid intake. Fiber retains water, so when adequate fiber and fluid are consumed, feces have a high enough water content to be easily passed. When inadequate fiber or fluid is consumed, feces are hard and dry, and constipation can result.

The end of the colon leads to the rectum, where feces are stored prior to defecation. The rectum is connected to the anus, the external opening of the digestive tract. The rectum and anus work with the colon to prepare the feces for elimination. Defecation is regulated by a sphincter that is under voluntary control. It allows the feces to be eliminated at convenient and appropriate times.

Digestion and Health

The digestive system is adaptable and able to handle a wide variety of foods. However, minor problems related to the digestive tract are common and almost everyone experiences some type of GI distress at one time or another. The type of foods

Making Decisions

Probiotics and Prebiotics: Are They Beneficial?

The large intestine of a healthy adult is home to several hundred species of bacteria. The type and number of bacteria that make up this intestinal microflora are affected by the diet. The health of the consumer can in turn be affected by the microflora. Researchers are investigating how we can promote a healthy population of intestinal bacteria either by consuming products containing the bacteria, referred to as probiotics, or by consuming foods, called prebiotics, that nourish the right combination of bacteria.

The recognition that intestinal bacteria are important to human health is not new. In the early 1900s, Nobel Prize–winning Russian scientist Eli Metchnikoff observed that Bulgarian peasants who consumed large quantities of yogurt and other fermented milk products lived long, healthy lives. He proposed that the bacteria in these foods positively affected the microflora in the colon, "prevented intestinal putrification," and helped "maintain the forces of the body."[a] He isolated these bacteria and used them in human feeding trials. More recent research continues to support Metchnikoff's hypothesis that the bacteria in fermented dairy products, which include *Bifidobacterium* and *Lactobacillus*, provide health benefits.

When eaten live, these bacteria survive passage through the upper GI tract and live temporarily in the colon before being excreted in the feces. Consumption of probiotic bacteria has been hypothesized to reduce the risk of heart disease, stimulate immune function, prevent cancer, and improve the integrity of the gastrointestinal mucosa. Research has provided some support for these claims. Evidence from both human and animal studies suggests that the consumption of fermented dairy products has a moderate cholesterol-lowering effect.[b] This effect may occur because probiotic bacteria reduce the absorption of bile (made from cholesterol) from the intestine and produce metabolites that reduce cholesterol synthesis in the liver.[b] Probiotic bacteria have also been found to have beneficial effects on immune function in the intestine,[c] and studies in animal models have shown that they can prevent the formation and growth of cancerous cells in the colon.[d] Probiotics have been found to reduce the duration of diarrhea due to viral infections, and these bacteria may also be useful in treating other disorders in which the gut barrier is compromised, such as colitis.[e,f] A healthy bacterial population in the intestine may also help prevent constipation, flatulence, and gastric acidity.

One problem with probiotics is that when they are no longer consumed, the bacteria are rapidly washed out of the colon. In order to maintain the beneficial microflora, researchers are investigating ways to encourage the growth of particular types of bacteria. The principal food source for intestinal bacteria is dietary carbohydrates that have not been digested in the upper GI tract. Substances that pass undigested into the colon and serve as foods for bacteria are called prebiotics. Prebiotics can selectively stimulate the growth of certain types of bacteria. For example, nondigestible carbohydrates called fructooligosaccharides stimulate the growth of *Bifidobacteria*.[g] These bacteria break down the fructooligosaccharides, producing short-chain fatty acids that can inhibit the growth of harmful bacteria, serve as an energy source for the cells of the colon, and aid in the absorption of water and electrolytes. Fructooligosaccharides are found naturally in onions, bananas, garlic, and artichokes. They are currently sold as dietary supplements and are added to commercially prepared tube-feeding formulas to promote gastrointestinal health.

Our understanding of how probiotics and prebiotics can be used to treat disease and promote health is still growing. Today, healthy adults can eat yogurt or drink milk containing active cultures or take tablets containing them to get a dose of beneficial bacteria. To help friendly bacteria to flourish in the intestine, people can consume foods that are good sources of indigestible carbohydrates or take supplements containing fructooligosaccharides. The risks of using these products are negligible, but whether they provide benefits in a healthy adult is still being investigated. Research is focusing on the use of these products to treat disease and improve chronic conditions. Soon we may be able to take probiotics instead of antibiotics to kill hazardous bacteria in the gut. And, we may one day be paying attention to what we are feeding our microflora as well as ourselves.

References

[a] Metchnikoff, E. *The Prolongation of Life.* New York: G. P. Putnam's Sons, 1908.

[b] St-Onge, M. P., Farnworth, E. R., and Jones, P. J. H. Consumption of fermented and nonfermented dairy products: effects on cholesterol concentrations and metabolism. Am. J. Clin. Nutr. 71:674–681, 2000.

[c] Erickson, K. L., and Hubbard, N. E. Probiotic immunomodulation in health and disease. J. Nutr. 130:403S–409S, 2000.

[d] Brady, L. J., Gallaher, D. D., and Busta, F. F. The role of probiotic cultures in the prevention of colon cancer. J. Nutr. 130:410S–414S, 2000.

[e] De Roos, N. M., and Katan, M. B. Effects of probiotic bacteria on diarrhea, lipid metabolism, and carcinogenesis: a review of papers published between 1988 and 1998. Am. J. Clin. Nutr. 71:405–411, 2000.

[f] Rolfe, R. D. The role of probiotic cultures in the control of gastrointestinal health. J. Nutr. 130:396S–402S, 2000.

[g] Roberfroid, M. B. Functional effects of food components and the gastrointestinal system: chicory fructooligosaccharides. Nutr. Rev. 54 (part II):S38–S42, 1996.

that can be consumed and the function of the digestive tract are also affected by certain stages of life. Most gastrointestinal problems do not significantly affect health or nutritional status, but occasionally they can have serious implications, and alternative methods must be employed to provide the nutrients necessary for life.

Digestive Problems

Each of the organs and processes of the digestive system is necessary for the normal digestion and absorption of food. Problems at any step along the way can

For information on common gastrointestinal problems, go to the National Institute of Diabetes & Digestive & Kidney Diseases at www.niddk.nih.gov/, or the American College of Gastroenterology at www.acg.gi.org and click on patient information.

interfere with the ability to obtain nutrients from food and influence nutritional status. Many of these problems can be alleviated by simple dietary modifications or the use of over-the-counter medications such as antacids and laxatives.

Dry Mouth and Dental Problems The secretion of saliva and the ability to chew are important to nutritional health. A reduction in saliva can be caused by disease or by a host of different types of medications. A dry mouth can reduce the ability to taste foods, make chewing and swallowing difficult, and increase the likelihood of tooth decay and gum disease. Dental caries or loss of teeth can impair the ability to chew food and can limit the types of food consumed. When food is not properly chewed, digestive enzymes cannot access all parts of the food and nutrient digestion is incomplete. Changes in the consistency of food may be necessary to obtain adequate nutrition when dental problems are severe.

Heartburn Heartburn occurs when stomach acid backs up into the esophagus. Stomach acid is necessary for digestion, enhances the absorption of certain nutrients, and minimizes bacterial growth. The stomach has a thick mucus coating to protect it from stomach acid. However, when stomach acid comes in contact with other areas of the GI tract, such as the esophagus, it can cause pain and discomfort. Heartburn often results from overeating and tends to occur about an hour after a large meal. Anxiety and stress may also contribute to heartburn by stimulating stomach acid production. Heartburn is less likely to occur when the stomach is not overly full; therefore, reducing the size of meals, avoiding high-fat foods (which slow gastric emptying), and consuming liquids between, rather than with, meals can reduce heartburn. Also, because the stomach contents move with gravity, remaining upright for a few hours after eating can be helpful in reducing heartburn. The most common medications used to manage heartburn are antacids that neutralize stomach acid and drugs that block acid secretion.

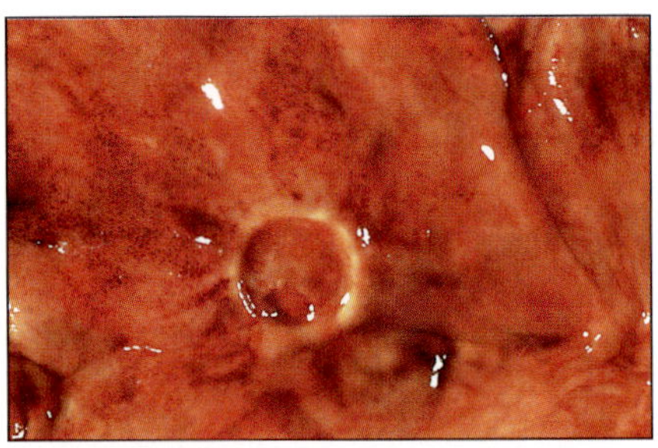

FIGURE 3.16 An ulcer in the lining of the stomach. *(© CNRI/Science Photo Library/Photo Researchers, Inc.)*

Ulcers Ulcers of the stomach and duodenum occur when the mucosa is eroded away, exposing the underlying tissues to the gastric juices (Figure 3.16). If the damage reaches the nerve layer, it causes pain, and if capillaries are damaged, gastrointestinal bleeding can occur, possibly leading to iron-deficiency anemia. If the ulcer perforates the wall of the GI tract, a serious abdominal infection can occur. The leading cause of ulcers is infection by the acid-resistant bacteria *Helicobacter pylori*, which penetrate the mucus layer and damage the epithelial lining of the gastrointestinal tract wall (see *Research Discoveries:* "Ulcers: A Bacterial Infection?").[2] This infection, which is also linked to stomach cancer, can be treated with antibiotics.[3] Ulcers are also caused by the chronic use of drugs such as aspirin and ibuprofen that erode the mucosa of the GI tract.

Vomiting Vomiting is a common GI complaint that can occur for many reasons—bacterial and viral infections, medications, and other illnesses. Vomiting can also be self-induced, as in eating disorders such as anorexia and bulimia nervosa (see Chapter 8).

Short episodes of vomiting, although uncomfortable, are unlikely to have long-term consequences in a healthy adult. But if vomiting is severe, continues for several days, or becomes chronic, it can lead to electrolyte imbalance and dehydration. Fluids, electrolytes, and glucose may need to be administered directly into the bloodstream to maintain homeostasis. Repeated vomiting as may occur with bulimia nervosa can also lead to irritation of the esophagus and mouth, tooth decay, and inflammation of salivary glands (see Chapter 8).

Pancreatic Disease Pancreatic disease can limit the availability of pancreatic enzymes needed to digest nutrients and bicarbonate needed to neutralize stomach acid. Lack of pancreatic lipase can lead to fat malabsorption and the inability to absorb fat-soluble vitamins. Lack of pancreatic proteases can impair vitamin B_{12}

RESEARCH DISCOVERIES

Ulcers: A Bacterial Infection?

Peptic ulcers are erosions or holes in the wall of the stomach or another portion of the GI tract. They cause pain and, sometimes, bleeding. For many years they were thought to be caused by the secretion of excess stomach acid. Over the years, many treatments have been used, including milk to coat the gastrointestinal lining, a bland diet devoid of spicy foods, stress reduction (because stress can increase stomach acid secretion), and drugs to neutralize acid (antacids) and, more recently, to reduce its secretion (histamine-2 blockers). These treatments usually reduced irritation and decreased symptoms, but the condition was considered chronic even with treatment. The observation, in 1982, that patients with ulcers frequently had a curvy-shaped bacteria, later named *Helicobacter pylori,* in their stomach mucosa has changed the way medical science approaches this condition.[a,b] A patient diagnosed with an ulcer today is given a different prescription for the same condition: antibiotics. This is now accepted treatment, but the hypothesis that ulcers could be caused by *H. pylori* was not immediately embraced by the scientific community. The accepted theory was that ulcers were caused by too much stomach acid. So how could bacteria survive in the strong acid of the stomach?

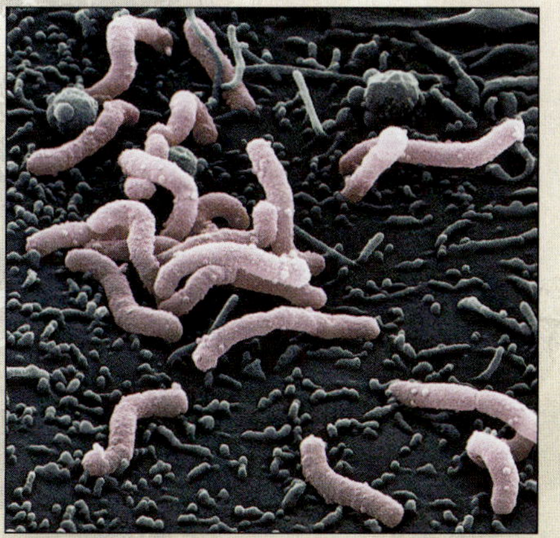

This magnification shows the helical shaped bacteria *Helicobacter pylori* attached to the gastric mucosa. *(© Juergen Berger, Max-Planck Institute/Science Photo Library/Photo Researchers, Inc.)*

Dr. B. J. Marshall was the first to identify *H. pylori* in the stomach mucosa and to hypothesize that it was the cause of peptic ulcers. However, to persuade other scientists that his hypothesis was correct, he needed more evidence. To provide proof that the bacteria caused the ulcer symptoms, he needed an animal model that could be infected with the bacteria and develop ulcer symptoms, such as gastric inflammation. However, a susceptible experimental animal model could not be found. Therefore, Marshall, in a bold move that would never have been approved by a human subjects ethics committee, decided to use himself as an experimental subject to gather evidence to support his theory.

Marshall's experiment involved first having a small sample of his gastric mucosa examined to confirm that it was normal and not infected with bacteria. He then drank a vial containing a culture of *H. pylori* that had been isolated from a patient with chronic gastric inflammation. Ten days later he developed symptoms that included vomiting, fatigue, irritability, and headaches. A follow-up sample of his gastric mucosa confirmed that his stomach lining was inflamed and that *H. pylori* bacteria could be seen attached to the mucosa (see figure).[c] Fortunately, his symptoms resolved quickly with antibiotic therapy.

As our understanding of how this organism survives in the acid environment of the stomach grew, the idea that bacteria caused ulcers became more universally accepted. When this organism enters the stomach, it produces substances that buffer the acid immediately around it. It is then able to swim through the thick gastric mucus and adhere to the mucosal cells. Once attached to the gastric mucosa, it is protected from stomach acid.[d] The bacteria damage mucosal cells and increase the release of gastrin, which subsequently increases stomach acid release.[e] The presence of bacteria causes inflammation and other immune responses that lead to additional tissue damage.

Today we know that about 50% of the world's population is infected with *H. pylori.*[f] Not everyone who is infected will have symptoms or go on to develop an ulcer, but *H. pylori* can be identified in about 90% of duodenal and 80% of gastric ulcers. Infection with this organism is now known to be associated not only with the development of stomach inflammation and duodenal and gastric ulcers, but also with cancers of the stomach. In the United States each year about 7 million people suffer *H. pylori*–related diseases, including ulcers and cancer.[g] Successful antibiotic therapy can allow the ulcer to heal, eliminate the bacteria that caused the disease, and cure the patient. Adding acid-suppression therapy speeds ulcer healing. A theory that was at first rejected by the scientific community is now supported and has helped to improve the lives and health of thousands of people.

References

[a] [No authors listed] Related Articles, OMIM Unidentified curved bacilli on gastric epithelium in active chronic gastritis. Lancet 1983 Jun 4; 1(8336): 1273–1275. No abstract available.

[b] Marshall, B. J., and Warren, J. R. Unidentified curved bacilli on gastric epithelium in active chronic gastritis. Lancet I:1311–1315, 1984.

[c] Marshall, B. J., Armstrong, J. A., McGechie, D. B., and Glancy, R. J. Attempt to fulfill Koch's postulates for pyloric *Campylobacter.* Med. J. Aust. 142:436–439, 1985.

[d] McGee, D. J., and Mobley, H. L. T. Mechanisms of *Helicobacter pylori* infection: bacterial factors. Curr. Top. Microbiol. Immunol. 241:156–180, 1999.

[e] Blanchard, T. G., Czinn, S. J., and Nedrud, J. G. Host response and vaccine development to *Helicobacter pylori* infection. Curr. Top. Microbiol. Immunol. 241:181–213, 1999.

[f] Mitchell, H. M. The epidemiology of *Helicobacter pylori.* Curr. Top. Microbiol. Immunol. 241:11–30, 1999.

[g] Christensen, D. Is your stomach bugging you? The rise and fall of the bacterium *H. pylori.* Science News 156:234–236, October 9, 1999.

absorption because this vitamin must be released from proteins before it can be absorbed. Cystic fibrosis is an inherited disease in which the pancreatic ducts become plugged with thick mucus, making pancreatic enzymes unavailable to the GI tract. Individuals with cystic fibrosis or other chronic pancreatic diseases must take oral enzymes to properly digest their food.

Gallstones A common problem related to the gallbladder is the formation of gallstones. Most gallstones are composed of cholesterol, bile pigments, and calcium salts. Gallstones often cause no symptoms, but if they become large enough or block the passage of bile into the duodenum, they can cause pain and interfere with fat absorption. Because dietary fat stimulates contraction of the gallbladder for the release of bile, a low-fat diet may reduce symptoms associated with gallstones. More severe cases are treated by surgically removing the gallbladder.

Diarrhea Diarrhea is characterized by frequent watery stools. It occurs when the intestinal contents move too quickly to allow normal fluid absorption or when fluid from the cells of the intestinal mucosa is drawn into the lumen. Occasional diarrhea may be caused by intestinal infections, medications, or food to which an individual is intolerant. Diarrhea can lead to significant fluid and electrolyte losses. In the short term, lost fluid must be replaced with water or electrolyte replacement solutions. Untreated diarrhea that leads to dehydration is a common cause of death among children in underdeveloped countries. A chronic syndrome of diarrhea may be due to a chronic bowel disorder such as irritable bowel syndrome, colitis, or Crohn's disease. For chronic conditions, long-term medical and nutritional therapy may be necessary to maintain fluid balance and nutritional health.

Constipation Alterations in the composition of the feces or a reduction in muscle tone in the large intestine can increase transit time and cause constipation. Constipation is uncomfortable and can damage the intestine, causing the formation of outpouches in the intestinal wall called diverticula (see Chapter 4). Dietary factors that contribute to constipation include a low fiber intake, a low fluid intake, or a high-fiber diet without adequate fluid intake. Also, lack of physical activity and muscular degeneration can reduce contractions in the intestine, contributing to constipation. To prevent constipation, physical activity and a diet high in fiber and fluid is recommended. A number of different types of over-the-counter laxative medications are available; some increase fecal bulk, others increase intestinal motility.

Digestive Concerns at Different Life Stages

The different stages of life affect the digestive system and can impact on its ability to digest food and absorb nutrients. Nutritional status can be maintained at all stages of life if the diet is properly managed.

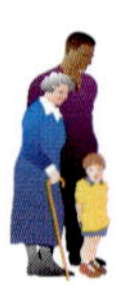

Infancy The digestive system is one of the last to fully mature in developing humans. At birth, the digestive tract is functional, but a newborn is not ready to consume an adult diet. The most obvious difference between the infant and adult digestive tracts is that newborns are not able to chew and swallow solid food. They are born with a suckling reflex that allows them to consume liquids from a nipple placed toward the back of the mouth. A protrusion reflex causes anything placed in the front of the mouth to be pushed out by the tongue. As head control increases, this reflex disappears, making spoon-feeding possible.

Digestion and absorption also differ between infants and adults. In infants, the digestion of milk protein is aided by rennin, an enzyme not produced in adults.[4] The stomachs of newborns also produce the enzyme gastric lipase, which begins the digestion of the fats in human milk. Low levels of pancreatic enzymes in infants limit starch digestion; however, enzymes at the brush border of the small intestine allow the milk-sugar lactose to be digested and absorbed.

The ability to absorb intact proteins is greater in infants than in adults. This can cause food allergies (see Chapters 6 and 16), but also allows infants to absorb immune factors from their mother's milk. These proteins provide temporary immunity to certain diseases.

The bacteria in the large intestine of infants are also different from those in adults because of the all-milk diet infants consume. This is the reason that the feces of breast-fed babies are almost odorless. Another feature of the infant digestive tract is the lack of voluntary control of elimination. Between the ages of two and three, this ability develops and toilet training is possible.

Pregnancy Physiological changes that occur during pregnancy often result in gastrointestinal problems. During the first three months, many women experience nausea, referred to as morning sickness. This term is a misnomer, because it can occur at any time of the day. Morning sickness is believed to be due to pregnancy-related hormonal changes. In most cases, it can be dealt with by eating frequent small meals and avoiding foods and smells that cause nausea. Eating dry foods such as crackers or cereal may also help. In severe cases where uncontrollable vomiting occurs, nutrients may need to be given intravenously to maintain nutritional status.

Later in pregnancy, the enlarged uterus puts pressure on the stomach and intestines, which can make it difficult to consume large meals. In addition, the placenta produces the hormone progesterone, which causes the smooth muscles of the digestive tract to relax. The muscle-relaxing effects of progesterone may relax the gastroesophageal sphincter enough to allow stomach contents to move back into the esophagus, causing heartburn. In the large intestine, relaxed muscles and the pressure of the uterus cause less efficient peristaltic movements and may result in constipation.

Advanced Age Although there are few dramatic changes in the nutrient requirements of humans as they age, changes in the digestive tract and other systems may affect the palatability of food and the ability to obtain proper nutrition. The senses of smell and taste are often diminished or even lost with age, reducing the appeal of food. A reduction in the amount of saliva can make swallowing difficult, decrease the taste of food, and also promote tooth decay. Loss of teeth and improperly fitting dentures may limit food choices to soft and liquid foods or cause solid foods to be poorly chewed. Intestinal secretions may also be reduced, but this rarely impairs absorption because the levels secreted in healthy elderly humans are still sufficient to break down food into forms that can be absorbed. A condition called **atrophic gastritis** that causes a reduction in the secretion of stomach acid is also common in the elderly. This may decrease the absorption of several vitamins and minerals and may allow bacterial growth to increase (see Chapter 17).

Atrophic gastritis An inflammation of the stomach lining that causes a reduction in stomach acid and allows bacterial overgrowth.

Constipation is a common complaint in the elderly and may be caused by decreased motility and elasticity in the colon, weakened abdominal and pelvic muscles, and a decrease in sensory perception. Although constipation occurs in about the same frequency in all age groups,[5] it is estimated that 20 to 30% of individuals over age 65 are dependent on laxatives[6] (see *Critical Thinking:* "Gastrointestinal Problems Can Affect Nutritional Status").

Alternative Feeding Methods

For individuals who are unable to consume food or digest and absorb the nutrients needed to meet their requirements, several alternative feeding methods have been developed. People who are unable to swallow can be fed a liquid diet through a tube inserted into the stomach or intestine. Carefully planned **enteral** or **tube feeding** can provide all the essential nutrients. Tube feeding can be used in patients who are unconscious or have suffered an injury to the upper gastrointestinal tract (Figure 3.17a). For individuals whose gastrointestinal tract is not functional, nutrients can be provided directly into the bloodstream (Figure

Enteral or tube feeding A method of providing nutrients to the gastrointestinal tract through a tube inserted through the nose or surgically placed through the abdominal wall.

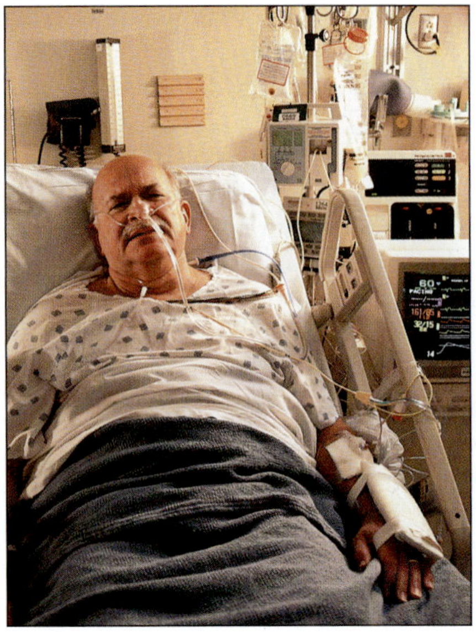

(a)

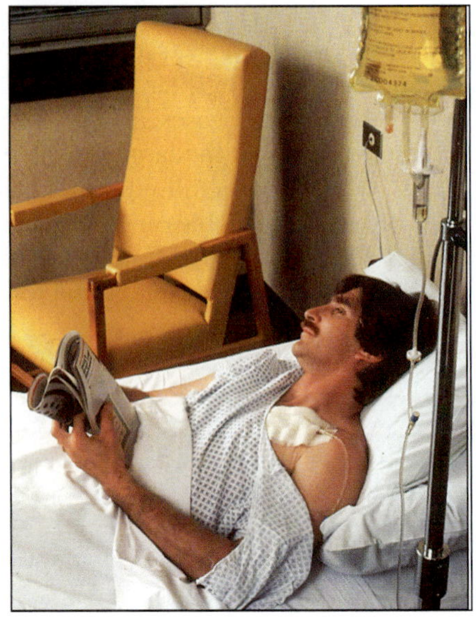

(b)

FIGURE 3.17 (a) Formulas providing complete nutrition can be delivered directly into the stomach or small intestine through a tube. (b) Individuals whose digestive tract is not functional can obtain all their energy and nutrients intravenously. *((a) © B. Seitz/Photo Researchers, Inc. (b) © W. L. Steinmark/Custom Medical Stock Photo)*

Total parenteral nutrition (TPN) A method of providing nutrients directly into the bloodstream.

3.17b). This is referred to as **total parenteral nutrition (TPN).** When all nutrients are not provided in a TPN solution, nutrient deficiencies develop quickly. Inadvertently feeding patients incomplete TPN solutions has demonstrated the essentiality of several trace minerals.

Critical Thinking

Gastrointestinal Problems Can Affect Nutritional Status

Many factors affect how well the processes of digestion and absorption work. For each situation described below, think about how digestion and absorption are affected and what the consequences are for nutritional status.

An individual is taking medication that reduces the amount of saliva produced.

What effect would this have on nutrition?

Answer:

A toddler with only four teeth gnaws on a carrot stick, swallowing the partially chewed pieces.

How will this affect the digestion and absorption of nutrients in the carrot?

Answer:

For breakfast, a man has cereal with skim milk and black coffee. His friend has scrambled eggs with sausage, biscuits with butter, and a glass of whole milk.

Which person's stomach will empty faster? Why?

Answer:

A 40-year-old woman weighing 350 lbs has undergone a procedure called stomach stapling to reduce the size of her stomach.

How will this affect the amount and types of foods that can be consumed at any one time?

Answer:

An individual has a disease of the pancreas that causes a deficiency of pancreatic enzymes.

What effect would this have on the digestion and absorption of protein?

Answer:

If the pancreas was not able to secrete bicarbonate into the duodenum, how would this affect digestion and absorption?

Answer:

An individual has gallstones, which cause pain when the gallbladder contracts.

What type of foods should be avoided and why?

Answer:

A 25-year-old woman is anorexic and is suffering from malnutrition. The malnutrition causes the intestinal villi to become flattened.

How will this affect absorption?

Answer:

An accident requires the removal of a large section of the small intestine.

How might this affect nutrient digestion and absorption?

Answer:

Treatment for colon cancer requires that most of the large intestine be surgically removed.

How would this affect fluid needs?

Answer:

After reading about the benefits of a high-fiber diet, an individual dramatically increases the amount of fiber consumed.

How might this affect the feces? The amount of intestinal gas?

Answer:

Nutrient Transport

Materials that are absorbed into the mucosal cells of the intestine must be transported and delivered to body cells. The primary nutrient transport and delivery system in the body is the cardiovascular system, which consists of the heart and blood vessels. The path by which nutrients enter the bloodstream varies with the nutrient. Amino acids from protein, simple sugars from carbohydrate, and the water-soluble products of fat digestion travel directly from the mucosal cells into the bloodstream. The products of fat digestion that are not water-soluble are taken into the lymphatic system before entering the blood.

Web Menu For more information on the heart, go to the Franklin Institute's online exploration of the heart at www.sln.fi.edu/biosci/heart.html.

Cardiovascular System

The cardiovascular system is a closed network of tubules through which blood is pumped. Blood carries nutrients and oxygen to the cells of all the organs and tissues of the body and removes waste products from these same cells. Blood also

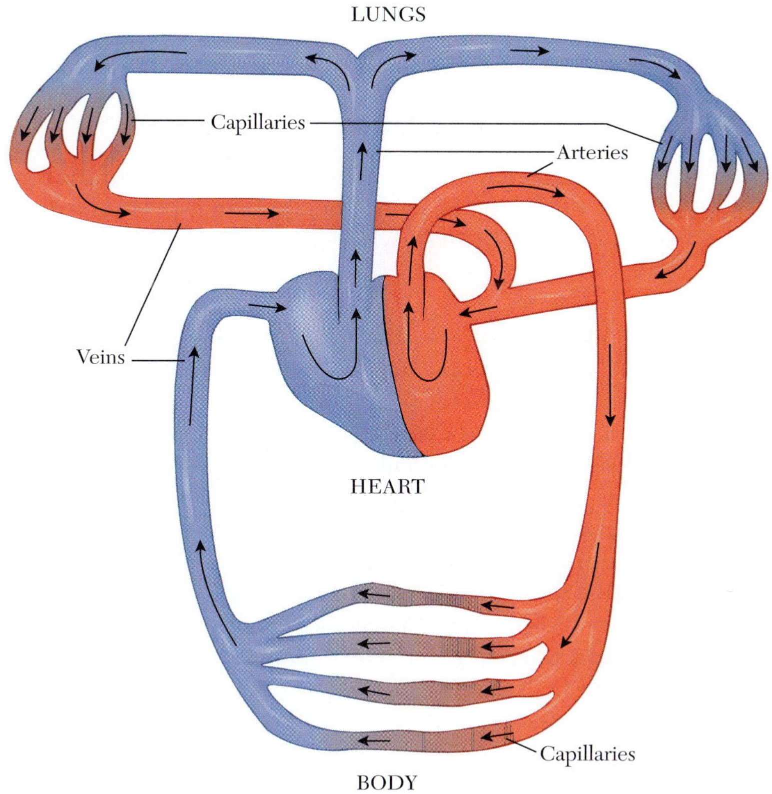

FIGURE 3.18 Blood is pumped from the heart through the arteries to the capillaries of the lungs, where it picks up oxygen. It then returns to the heart via the veins and is pumped out again into the arteries that lead to the rest of the body. In the capillaries of the body, blood delivers oxygen and nutrients and picks up wastes before returning to the heart via the veins. In this figure, red indicates blood that is rich in oxygen, and blue represents blood that is oxygen-poor and carrying more carbon dioxide.

carries other substances, such as hormones, from one part of the body to another (Figure 3.18).

The heart is the workhorse of the cardiovascular system. It is a muscular pump with two circulatory loops—one that delivers blood to the lungs and one that delivers blood to the rest of the body. The blood vessels that transport blood and dissolved substances toward the heart are called **veins,** and those that transport blood and dissolved substances away from the heart are called **arteries.** As arteries carry blood away from the heart, they branch many times to form smaller and smaller blood vessels. The smallest arteries are called arterioles. Arterioles then branch to form **capillaries,** which are thin-walled vessels that are just large enough to allow one red blood cell to pass at a time. From the capillaries, oxygen and nutrients carried by the blood pass into the cells, and waste products pass from the cells into the capillaries. In the capillaries of the lungs, blood releases carbon dioxide to be exhaled and picks up oxygen to be delivered to the cells. In the capillaries of the GI tract, blood picks up water-soluble nutrients absorbed from the diet. Blood from capillaries then flows into the smallest veins, the venules, which converge to form larger and larger veins for return to the heart. Therefore, blood starting in the heart is pumped through the arteries to the capillaries of the lungs where it picks up oxygen. It then returns to the heart via the veins and is pumped out again into the arteries that lead to the rest of the body. In the capillaries of the body, blood delivers oxygen and nutrients and removes wastes before returning to the heart via the veins.

Veins Vessels that carry blood toward the heart.

Arteries Vessels that carry blood away from the heart.

Capillaries Small, thin-walled blood vessels where the exchange of gases and nutrients between blood and cells occurs.

The volume of blood that flows to an organ or tissue, and hence the amounts of nutrients and oxygen that are delivered, depends on need. When a person is resting, about 24% of the blood goes to the digestive system, 21% to the skeletal muscles, and the rest to the heart, kidneys, brain, skin, and other organs.[7] After a large meal, a greater proportion of the blood supply will go to the intestines to support digestion and absorption and to transport nutrients. When a person engages in strenuous exercise, about 85% of blood flow will be directed to the skeletal muscles to deliver nutrients and oxygen and remove carbon dioxide and waste products. Attempting to exercise after a large meal creates a conflict. The body cannot direct blood to the intestines and the muscles at the same time. The muscles win, and food remains in the gastrointestinal tract, often resulting in cramps.

Hepatic Portal and Lymphatic Circulation

Hepatic portal circulation The system of blood vessels that collects nutrient-laden blood from the digestive organs and delivers it to the liver.

Lymphatic system The system of vessels, organs, and tissues that drains excess fluid from the spaces between cells, picks up fat-soluble substances absorbed from the digestive tract, and provides immune function.

Hepatic portal vein The vein that transports blood from the gastrointestinal tract to the liver.

Nutrients enter the blood circulation by either the **hepatic portal circulation** or the **lymphatic system.** The villi of the intestine contain both capillaries, which are part of the portal circulation, and lacteals, which are small vessels of the lymphatic system.

Hepatic Portal Circulation In the small intestine, water-soluble molecules—including amino acids, sugars, water-soluble vitamins, and water-soluble products of fat digestion—cross the mucosal cells of the villi and enter capillaries. These capillaries merge to form venules at the base of the villi. The venules then merge to form larger and larger veins, which eventually form the **hepatic portal vein.** The hepatic portal vein transports blood directly to the liver, where absorbed nutrients are processed before they enter the general circulation (Figure 3.19).

The liver acts as a gatekeeper between substances absorbed from the intestine and the rest of the body. Some nutrients are stored in the liver, some are changed into different forms, some are broken down to generate energy, and others are allowed to pass through unchanged. How an individual nutrient is handled depends on the immediate needs of the body. For example, the liver, with the help of hormones from the pancreas, keeps the concentration of glucose in the blood within a narrow range. The liver modulates blood glucose by removing absorbed glucose from the blood and storing it, by sending absorbed glucose on to the tissues of the body, or by releasing liver glucose (from stores or synthesis) into the blood. The liver also plays a key role in the synthesis and breakdown of amino acids, proteins, and lipids. It modifies the products of protein breakdown to form molecules that can be safely transported to the kidney for excretion. The liver also contains enzyme systems that protect the body from toxins absorbed by the gastrointestinal tract.

The Lymphatic System The lymphatic system consists of a network of tubules (lymph vessels) as well as structures and organs that contain infection-fighting cells. The lymphatic system carries fluid away from the tissues and filters it past its collec-

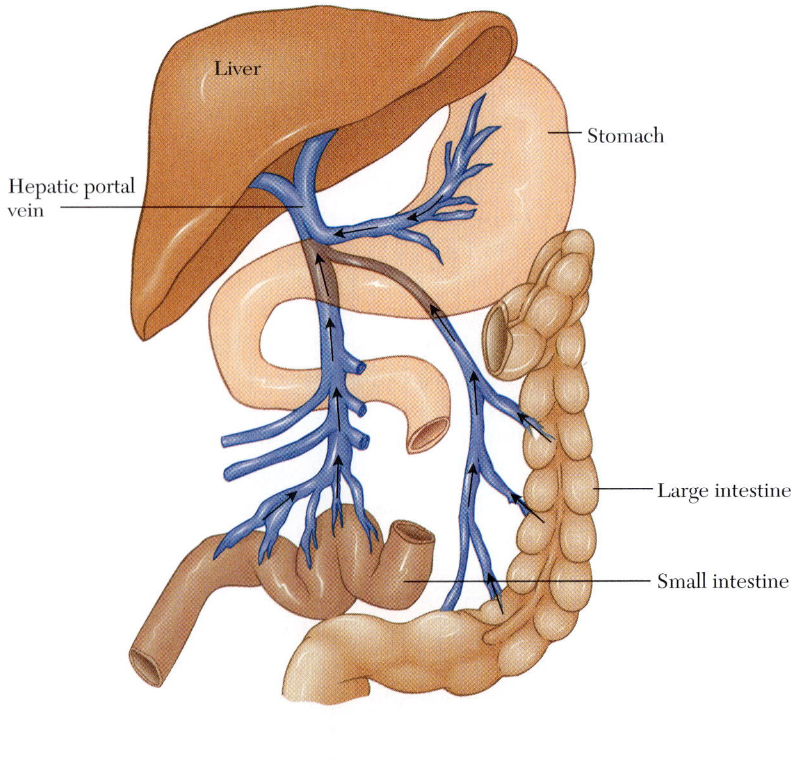

FIGURE 3.19 The hepatic portal circulation carries blood from the stomach and intestines to the hepatic portal vein and then to the liver.

tion of infection-fighting cells. The cleansed fluid is then returned to the bloodstream. By draining the excess fluid, and any disease-causing agents it contains, away from the spaces between cells, the lymphatic system provides immunity and prevents the accumulation of tissue fluid from causing swelling—a condition called edema. In the intestine, the lymphatic system transports absorbed materials too large to enter the intestinal capillaries such as fat-soluble substances. Fatty acids entering the mucosal cells of the intestine are assembled into triglycerides and combined with other fat-soluble molecules and protein to form particles that pass into the lacteals (see Chapter 5). Lacteals drain into larger lymph vessels. Lymph vessels from the intestine and most other organs of the body drain into the thoracic duct, which empties into the bloodstream near the neck. Substances that are absorbed into the lymph do not pass through the liver before entering the blood circulation.

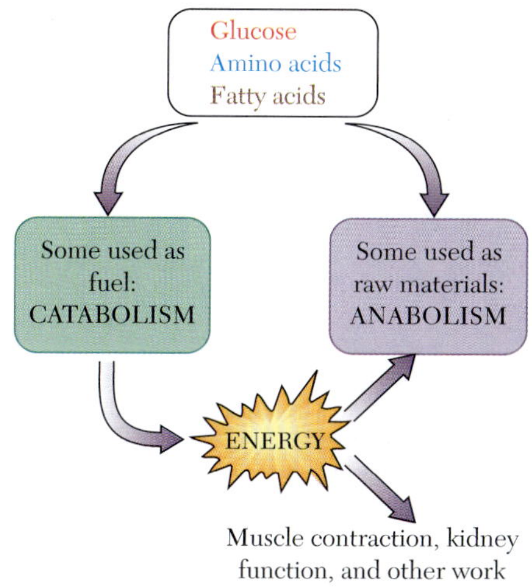

FIGURE 3.20 The products of digestion have now been absorbed, transported, and delivered to the cells. The carbohydrate has been broken down into glucose. The cells can use glucose to produce ATP or to synthesize other molecules for immediate use or storage. Protein has been broken down into amino acids that can be used by cells to synthesize needed protein, to make glucose if it is in short supply, or to produce ATP. Triglycerides have been broken down into fatty acids. These can be used to generate ATP or to produce lipids needed for body function, or they can be stored as body fat for later use.

Nutrient Utilization

By the mechanisms described thus far, foods are digested and the products of digestion absorbed, transported, and delivered to body cells. Once they have reached the cells, nutrients are used in chemical reactions. The sum of the chemical reactions that occur inside body cells is referred to as metabolism. Many of the reactions of metabolism occur in series known as metabolic pathways. Molecules that enter these pathways are modified at each step of the pathway with the help of enzymes. Some of the pathways are **anabolic,** using energy to build body structures, whereas others are **catabolic,** breaking large molecules into smaller ones and releasing energy (Figure 3.20).

Cell Structure

Cells are surrounded by a **cell membrane.** The cell membrane maintains homeostasis in the cell by controlling what enters and what exits. It is **selectively permeable** because some substances, such as water, can pass freely in and out of the cell, whereas the passage of others is regulated. Nutrients and other substances from the bloodstream are transported into cells by simple and facilitated diffusion and active transport.

Inside the cell membrane is the **cytoplasm,** or the cell fluid, that contains the cell **organelles** that perform functions necessary for cell survival. Organelles are also surrounded by membranes. The largest organelle is the nucleus, which contains the cell's genetic material (Figure 3.21).

Anabolic Energy-requiring processes in which simpler molecules are combined to form more complex substances.

Catabolic The processes by which substances are broken down into simpler molecules releasing energy.

Cell membrane The barrier that surrounds the cell contents.

Selectively permeable Describes a membrane or barrier that will allow some substances to pass freely but will restrict the passage of others.

Cytoplasm The cellular material outside the nucleus that is contained by the cell membrane.

Organelles Cellular organs that carry out specific metabolic functions.

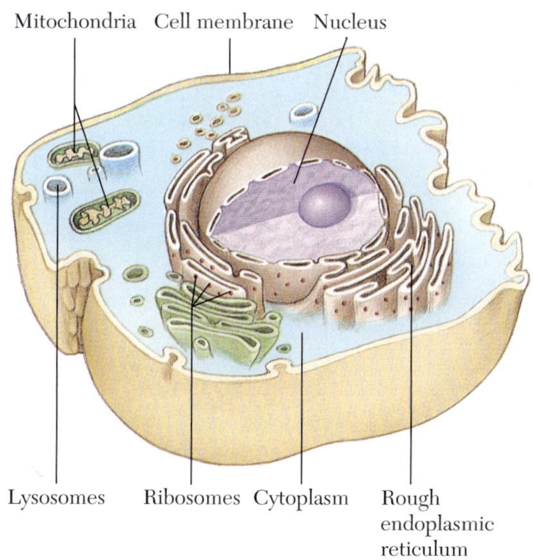

FIGURE 3.21 Structure of a general animal cell. Almost all human cells contain the organelles illustrated here.

Anabolic and catabolic processes occur in different cellular organelles. For example, the endoplasmic reticulum is an anabolic organelle. One type of endoplasmic reticulum specializes in the synthesis of lipid-based compounds such as the sex hormones estrogen and testosterone. Another type of endoplasmic reticulum is called "rough endoplasmic reticulum" because it is covered with small organelles called ribosomes, giving it a bumpy appearance. Ribosomes are the site of protein synthesis.

Lysosomes are catabolic organelles that act as a kind of digestive system for the cell. Lysosomes contain enzymes capable of breaking down carbohydrates, lipids, proteins, and other types of molecules that originate both inside and outside the cell. The **mitochondria** are catabolic organelles where the process of **cellular respiration** breaks down carbohydrates, lipids, and proteins to obtain energy.

Mitochondrion The organelle where cellular respiration occurs, generating energy in the form of ATP, that can be used for cellular activities.

Cellular respiration The reactions that break down carbohydrates, fats, and proteins in the presence of oxygen to produce carbon dioxide, water, and energy in the form of ATP.

ATP (adenosine triphosphate) The high-energy molecule used by the body to perform energy-requiring activities.

Cellular Respiration

Cellular respiration completely metabolizes carbohydrates, lipids, and proteins, in the presence of oxygen, to produce carbon dioxide, water, and **ATP (adenosine triphosphate).** The chemical bonds of ATP are very high in energy. When the bonds break, the energy is released and can be used to do cellular work. The energy contained in ATP can be used to pump blood, transport nutrients, and contract muscles—or it can be used to synthesize new molecules needed to maintain and repair body tissue (see Figure 3.20).

EXCRETION OF METABOLIC WASTES

As already discussed, substances that cannot be absorbed by the body are excreted from the GI tract in feces. The waste products generated by the metabolism of absorbed substances, such as carbon dioxide, nitrogen, and water, must also be removed from the body. The elimination of these waste products requires the respiratory, integumentary, and urinary systems (Figure 3.22).

Respiratory and Integumentary Systems

Carbon dioxide produced by cellular respiration leaves the cells and is transported to the lungs (respiratory system) by red blood cells. At the lungs, red blood cells release their load of carbon dioxide, which is then exhaled into the environment. In addition to carbon dioxide, a significant amount of water is lost from the lungs by evaporation. Water, along with protein breakdown products and minerals, is also lost through the skin (integumentary system) in perspiration or sweat and in the urine via the kidney (urinary system).

Urinary System

Nephrons Structural and functional units of the kidney consisting of the glomerulus and renal tubules.

Glomerulus A part of the nephron that consists of a cluster of capillaries where blood is filtered.

The kidney is the primary site for the excretion of water, metabolic waste products, and excess minerals. Each kidney consists of about 1 million **nephrons.** The nephrons consist of a **glomerulus** where the blood is filtered and a series of tubules where molecules that have been filtered out of the blood can be reabsorbed (Figure 3.23).

As blood flows through the kidney, it is filtered, removing most of the small dissolved molecules. Protein molecules and blood cells are too large to be filtered out by the glomerulus. Substances that are needed are then reabsorbed back into the blood. Much of the reabsorption that occurs in the kidney tubules takes place by active transport and requires energy in the form of ATP. Components that are

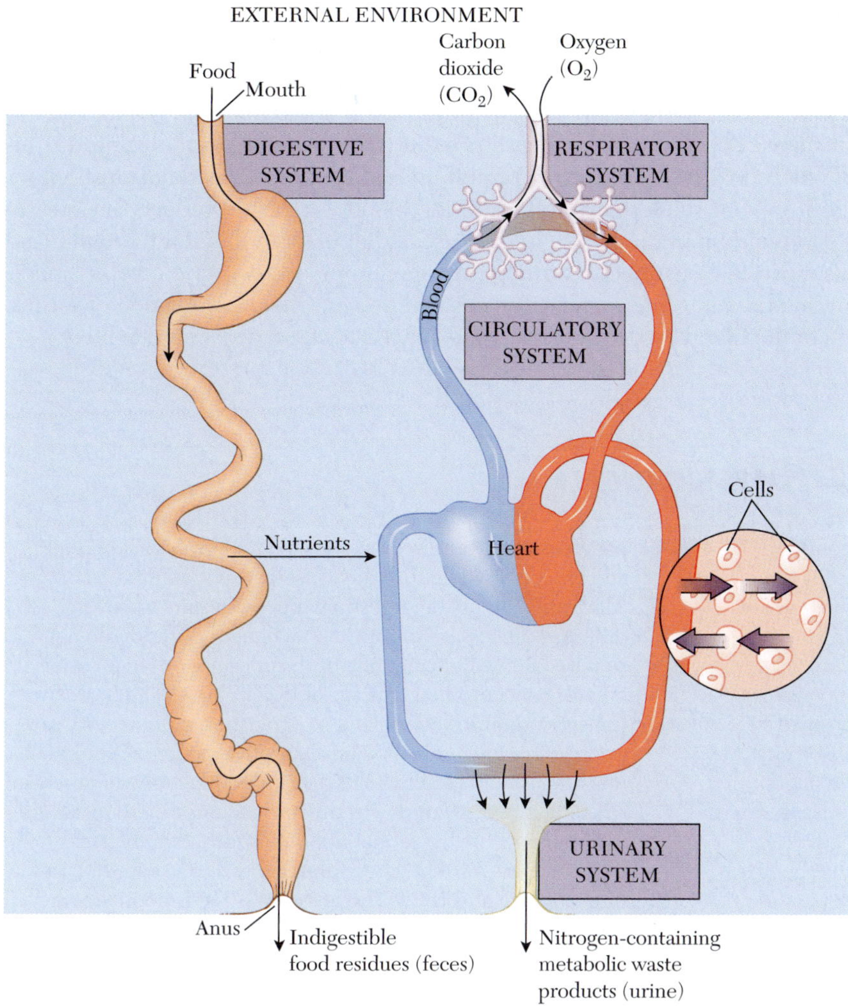

FIGURE 3.22 There are interrelationships among the body organ systems involved in the digestion, absorption, and transport of food and nutrients and the excretion of waste products. The digestive system takes in nutrients and the respiratory system takes in oxygen, which are then distributed to all the body cells by the circulatory system. The urinary and respiratory systems transfer metabolic wastes to the outside environment.

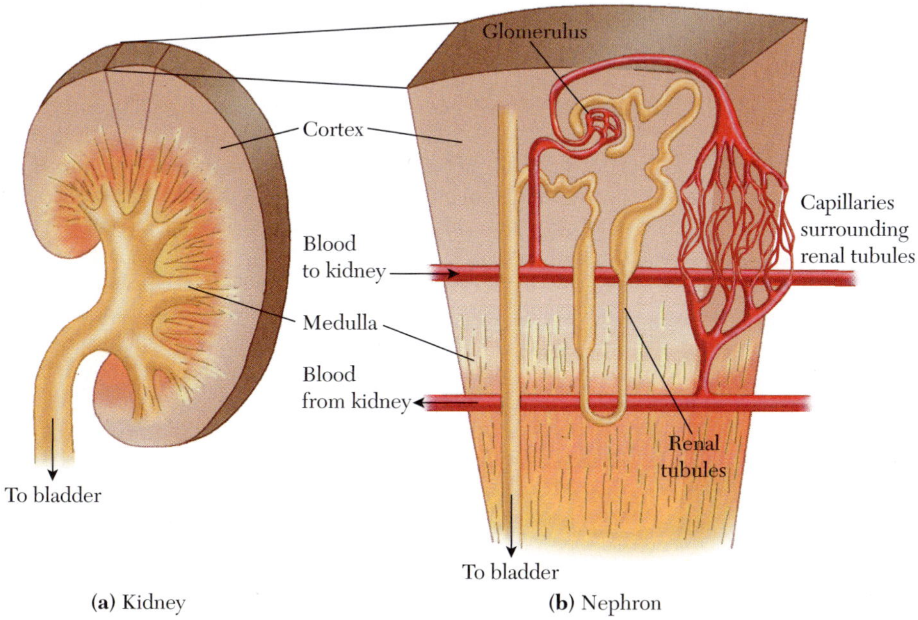

FIGURE 3.23 (a) The basic structure of a kidney. (b) In the nephron dissolved materials are filtered out of the blood by the glomerulus. The filtrate enters renal tubules where some materials are reabsorbed into the blood. Unabsorbed materials enter the collecting duct for delivery to the bladder and excretion in the urine.

not needed are not reabsorbed but are passed down the ureters to the bladder and excreted in the urine. The amounts of water and other substances excreted in the urine are regulated so that homeostasis is maintained (see Chapter 11).

Diseases of the kidney have a dramatic effect on homeostasis and can affect nutritional status. Some conditions cause protein to be excreted in the urine. In this case, the diet must provide enough protein to replace the excess that is lost. Other conditions prevent the kidneys from filtering blood, so waste products are not removed and build up in the blood. In this case, a diet restricted in fluid, protein, and minerals must be consumed in order to maintain homeostasis. When dietary modification can no longer meet nutrient needs and prevent the accumulation of wastes, filtration of the blood by a dialysis machine may be necessary to maintain life.

SUMMARY

1. The organization of all matter begins with atoms. Atoms are linked by chemical bonds to form molecules. The cell is the smallest unit of life. Cells of similar structure and function are organized into tissues, and tissues into organs and organ systems.
2. The digestive system is the organ system primarily responsible for the movement of nutrients into the body. The digestive system provides two major functions: digestion and absorption. Digestion is the process by which food is broken down into units that are small enough to be absorbed. Absorption is the process by which nutrients are transported into the body.
3. The gastrointestinal tract consists of a hollow tube that begins at the mouth and continues through the pharynx, esophagus, stomach, small intestine, large intestine, and anus. The passage, digestion, and absorption of food in the lumen of the gastrointestinal tract are aided by nerve signals and the secretion of mucus and digestive enzymes into the lumen and hormones into the blood.
4. The processes involved in digestion begin in response to the smell or sight of food and continue as food enters the digestive tract at the mouth. In the mouth, food is broken into smaller pieces by the teeth and mixed with saliva. Carbohydrate digestion is begun by the enzyme salivary amylase. From the mouth, food passes through the pharynx and into the esophagus. The rhythmic contractions of peristalsis propel it down the esophagus to the stomach.
5. The stomach acts as a temporary storage site for food. The muscles of the stomach mix the food into a semiliquid mass called chyme, and gastric juice containing hydrochloric acid and pepsin begins protein digestion. Gastric secretion is stimulated by the thought, sight, smell, or taste of food and by the entry of food into the stomach. Gastric secretion is inhibited by the passage of food into the small intestine. The rate of stomach emptying depends on the amount and composition of food consumed and is regulated by nervous and hormonal signals from the small intestine.
6. The small intestine is the primary site of digestion and absorption. In the small intestine, bicarbonate from the pancreas neutralizes stomach acid, and pancreatic and intestinal enzymes digest carbohydrate, fat, and protein. The digestion and absorption of fat in the small intestine is aided by bile from the gallbladder. Bile helps make fat accessible to fat-digesting enzymes by breaking fat into small droplets and helps to facilitate lipid absorption. Secretions from the pancreas and liver are regulated by the hormones secretin and cholecystokinin, produced by the duodenum.
7. Absorption across the intestinal mucosa occurs by several different processes. Simple and facilitated diffusion do not require energy but can only move substances from areas of greater concentration to areas of lower concentration. Active transport requires energy but can transport substances against a concentration gradient. The absorptive surface of the small intestine is increased by folds and finger-like projections called villi, which are covered with tiny projections called microvilli.
8. Components of chyme that are not absorbed in the small intestine pass into the large intestine, where some water and nutrients are absorbed. The large intestine is populated by bacteria that digest some of these unabsorbed materials, such as fiber, producing small amounts of nutrients and gas. The remaining unabsorbed materials, along with dead bacteria and sloughed mucosal cells, are excreted in feces.
9. Absorbed nutrients are delivered to the cells of the body by the cardiovascular system. The heart pumps blood to the lungs to pick up oxygen and eliminate carbon dioxide. From the lungs, blood returns to the heart and is pumped to the rest of the body to deliver oxygen and nutrients and remove carbon dioxide and other wastes before returning to the heart. Blood is pumped away from the heart in arteries and returned to the heart in veins. Exchange of nutrients and gases occurs at the smallest blood vessels, the capillaries.
10. The products of carbohydrate and protein digestion and the water-soluble products of fat digestion enter capillaries in the intestinal villi and are transported to the liver via the hepatic portal circulation. The liver serves as a processing center, removing some absorbed substances for storage, converting them into other forms, breaking them down for energy, or allowing them to pass unaltered. The liver also protects the body from toxic substances that may have been absorbed.
11. The fat-soluble products of digestion and other large materials enter the lymphatic system through lacteals in the intestinal villi. The nutrients absorbed via the lymphatic system enter the blood circulation without first passing through the liver.
12. Cells are the final destination of absorbed nutrients. To enter the cells, nutrients must be transported across cell membranes. Within the cells, some organelles are catabolic, specializing in the breakdown of nutrients to produce energy. Others are anabolic, specializing in the synthesis of molecules needed by the body. The sum of all the chemical reactions of

the body is called metabolism. The reactions that completely break down macronutrients in the presence of oxygen to produce water, carbon dioxide, and energy are referred to as cellular respiration.

13. Unabsorbed materials are excreted in the feces. The waste products generated by the metabolism of absorbed substances are excreted by the lungs, skin, and kidneys. The lungs eliminate carbon dioxide in exhaled air. The kidneys eliminate wastes by filtering small molecules out of the blood. Wastes are eliminated in the urine, but substances that are necessary to maintain homeostasis are reabsorbed.

Review Questions

1. What is the smallest unit of plant and animal life?
2. List three organ systems involved in the digestion and absorption of food.
3. How do teeth function in digestion?
4. What is the role of saliva?
5. What is peristalsis?
6. List three constituents of gastric secretions and their functions.
7. List some factors that regulate the rate at which materials move through the gastrointestinal tract.
8. List three mechanisms by which nutrients are absorbed.
9. Where does most of the digestion and absorption of food and nutrients occur?
10. How does the structure of the small intestine aid absorption?
11. What products of digestion are transported by the lymphatic system?
12. What path does an amino acid follow from absorption to delivery to the cell? What path does a large fatty acid follow from absorption to delivery to the cell?
13. What is the form of energy used by cells?
14. How are unabsorbed wastes excreted from the body?
15. How are metabolic waste products eliminated from the body?

Applying Critical Thinking Skills

Personal nutrition:

1. Select one meal from the food record you kept in Chapter 2 and review the protein, carbohydrate, and fat content of each food.
   a. List foods that might decrease your transit time if consumed with a meal.
   b. List foods that might require bile for digestion.
   c. List foods that might begin their digestion in your mouth.
2. Imagine you wake up on a Sunday morning and join some friends for a large breakfast consisting of: a cheese omelet and sausage (foods high in fat and protein), a croissant with butter (which contains carbohydrate but is also very high in fat), and a small glass of orange juice. After the meal, you remember that you have plans to play basketball with a friend in just an hour.
   a. If you keep your plans and play basketball, what problems might you experience while exercising?
   b. Had you remembered your plans for strenuous exercise before you had breakfast, what type of meal might you have selected to ensure that your stomach would empty more quickly?

General nutrition issues:

1. There are hundreds of products available to aid digestion. Go to the drug store, health food store, or search the Internet and select a product claiming to aid digestion.
   a. List the claims made for the product.
   b. Using the information in Chapter 1 on judging nutritional claims, analyze the information given.
   c. Does the product provide any nutrients?
   d. Does it carry any risk?
   e. Would you take it? Why or why not?
2. Plan a lunch menu for a senior center. It should provide one third of the recommended servings from the Food Guide Pyramid. Assume that many of the diners have difficulty chewing. Others are monitoring their sugar and salt intake, so these items should be limited on the menu.
   a. Evaluate whether your menu would be appropriate for someone with gallstones who needed to limit their intake of fat.
   b. Evaluate whether your menu would be appropriate for someone who is trying to increase their intake of fiber and fluid to prevent constipation.

References

1. Roberfroid, M. B., Bornet, F., Bouley, C., and Cummings, J. H. Colonic microflora: nutrition and health. Summary and conclusions of an International Life Sciences Institute (ILSI) [Europe] workshop held in Barcelona, Spain. Nutr. Rev. 53:127–130, 1995.
2. Damianos, A. J., and McGarrity, T. J. Treatment strategies for *Helicobacter pylori* infection. Am. Fam. Physician 55:2765–2774, 1997.
3. Mukhopadhyay, P. Gastric cancer and lymphoma. Curr. Top. Microbiol. Immunol. 241:57–69, 1999.
4. Marieb, E. N. *Human Anatomy and Physiology,* 5th ed. Redwood City, Calif.: Benjamin/Cummings Publishing Co., 2000.
5. Harari, D., Gurwitz, J. H., Avorn, J., et al. Bowel habit in relation to age and gender: findings from the National Health Interview Survey and clinical implications. Arch. Intern. Med. 156:315–320, 1996.
6. Brucker, M. C., and Faucher, M. A. Pharmacologic management of common gastrointestinal health problems in women. J. Nurse-Midwifery 42:145–162, 1997.
7. Rhoades, R., and Pflanzer, R. *Human Physiology,* 3rd ed. Philadelphia: Saunders College Publishing, 1996.

4 Carbohydrates

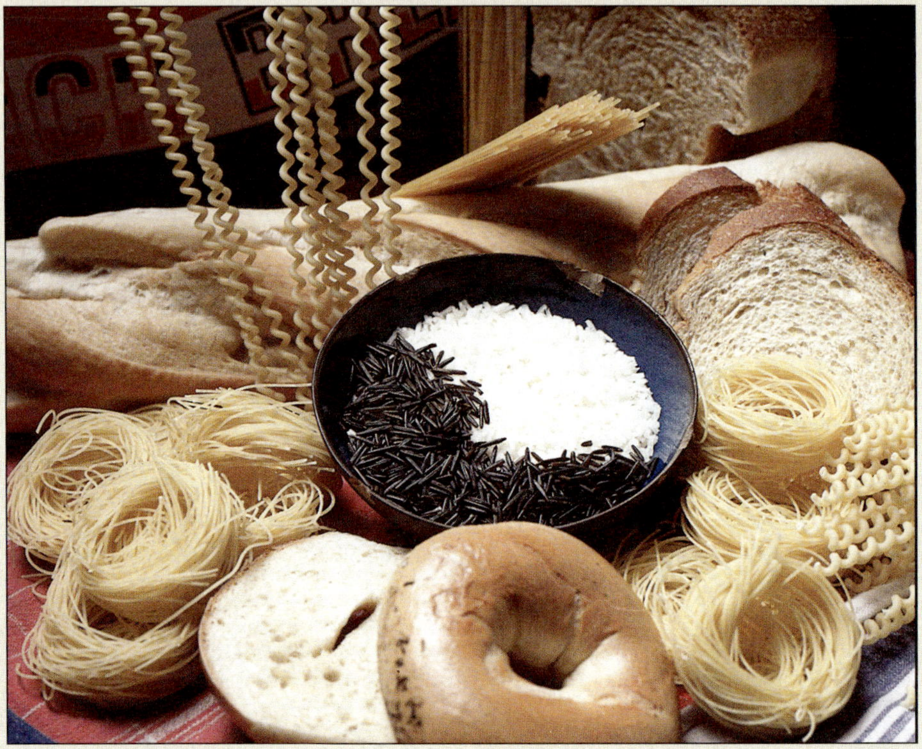

Learning Objectives

After reading this chapter, students should be able to:

1. Compare the structures of simple carbohydrates (monosaccharides and disaccharides) and complex carbohydrates (polysaccharides).
2. Distinguish between soluble and insoluble fiber and name food sources of each.
3. List sources of refined and unrefined simple and complex carbohydrates.
4. Discuss the effects of dietary fiber on gastrointestinal function.
5. Describe the steps involved in metabolizing glucose to produce energy in the form of ATP.
6. Explain how the hormones insulin and glucagon are involved in regulating blood glucose levels.
7. Discuss how diet can affect blood glucose levels, the risk of developing diabetes, and the management of existing diabetes.
8. Define "hypoglycemia" and discuss the dietary modifications recommended to reduce its symptoms.
9. Discuss the health risks and benefits associated with diets high in unrefined carbohydrates and those high in refined carbohydrates.
10. List some potential benefits and risks of sugar substitutes.

Elaine watched longingly as her coworker slid a cracker out of the sandwich bag, popped it in her mouth, and crunched it between her teeth. Elaine's lunch of baked chicken, string cheese, and celery sticks looked great to outside observers, but she longed for the sandwiches she used to bring. She missed not only sandwiches at lunch, but also spaghetti, rice, and potatoes at dinner, and cereal, muffins, and toast for breakfast. For the past three weeks Elaine had been on a low-carbohydrate weight-loss diet. She was allowed to consume only 20 g of carbohydrate a day. At first, the allowed foods made the diet appealing. She could eat bacon and scrambled eggs for breakfast, chicken nuggets for lunch, and steak and salad for dinner. But to keep her carbohydrate intake within the allowed limits, she had to eliminate all fruits and grain products and limit her vegetable intake.

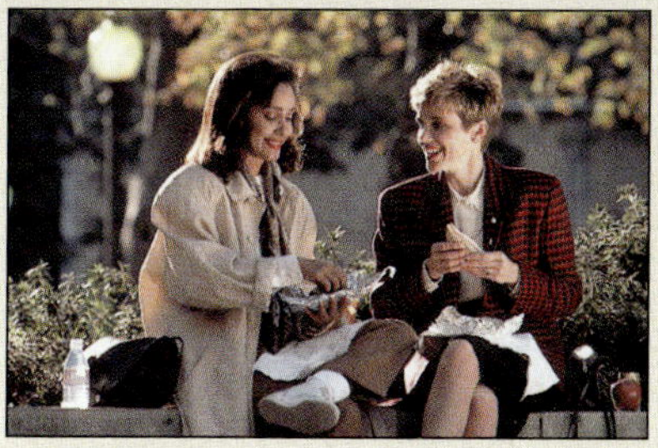

For the first few days Elaine was ecstatic. She seemed to be eating all she wanted of foods she enjoyed, and she lost 4 pounds. After a week she had lost an additional 2 pounds but was starting to miss the carbohydrate foods she loves. By the end of the second week she was bored with all her allowed food choices. Her weight loss continued at a slower rate and she began to feel light-headed and tired. She started having headaches and her husband noticed that her breath had a funny smell.

What was happening to cause these symptoms? An understanding of how carbohydrates function in the body will help to explain them. Elaine was eating only about 1100 kcalories a day. This was not enough to fuel all her body functions, so she began breaking down stored fat for energy. This helped promote weight loss, but, because not enough carbohydrate was available to completely metabolize fat, partial breakdown products, called ketones, began to accumulate, causing her headaches, light-headedness, and breath odor. In addition to these short-term symptoms, a diet this high in fat may increase the long-term risk of heart disease.

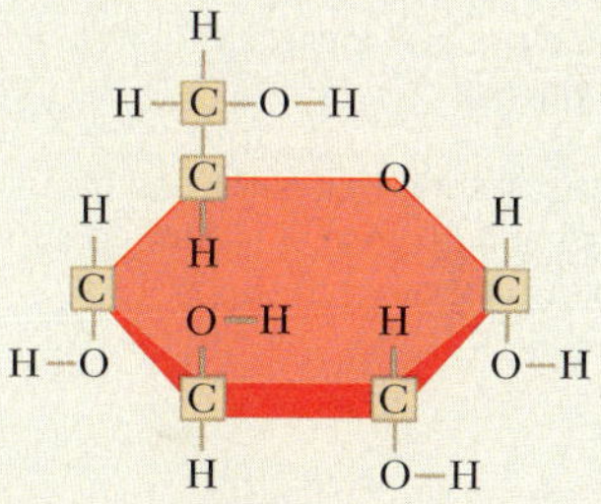

$C_6H_{12}O_6$

FIGURE 4.1 The general chemical formula for a sugar is $C_nH_{2n}O_n$ such that there are twice as many hydrogens as carbons or oxygens. The atoms of this glucose molecule are arranged in a cyclic or ring formation. Note that every carbon forms four chemical bonds, each oxygen forms two bonds, and each hydrogen one bond.

What Are Carbohydrates?

Chemically, **carbohydrates** are compounds that contain carbon ("carbo") as well as hydrogen and oxygen in the same proportion as in water ("hydrate"). In their simplest form, carbohydrates have two molecules of hydrogen for each molecule of carbon or oxygen, such that the general chemical formula is $C_nH_{2n}O_n$. A sugar with 6 carbons would therefore also contain 12 hydrogen atoms and 6 oxygen atoms (Figure 4.1). A sugar with 5 carbons would have 10 hydrogen atoms and 5 oxygen atoms. Carbohydrates range from single sugar units to complex branching chains of sugar molecules.

Carbohydrates Compounds containing carbon plus hydrogen and oxygen in the same proportions as in water. They include sugars, starches, and fibers.

Monosaccharide A single sugar molecule, such as glucose.

Disaccharide A sugar formed by linking two monosaccharides.

Simple carbohydrates Carbohydrates known as sugars that include monosaccharides and disaccharides.

Simple Carbohydrates

The basic unit of carbohydrate is a single sugar molecule, a **monosaccharide** ("mono" means one). When two sugar molecules combine, they form a **disaccharide** ("di" means two). Monosaccharides and disaccharides are known as simple sugars, or **simple carbohydrates**.

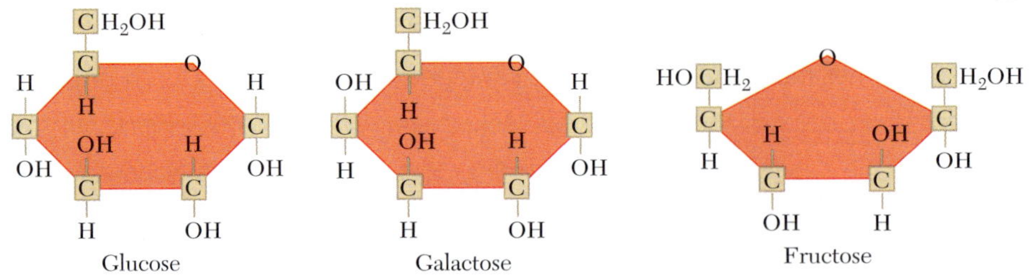

FIGURE 4.2 These common monosaccharides all contain six carbons. Glucose and galactose both form a 6-member ring but differ in the orientation of the hydroxyl groups (—OH) attached to the carbons. Fructose forms a 5-member ring so two of its carbon atoms extend from the ring. These structural differences affect the sweetness of these monosaccharides. Fructose is the sweetest followed by glucose and then galactose, which hardly has any sweet taste.

Glucose A monosaccharide that is the primary form of carbohydrate used to produce energy in the body. It is the sugar referred to as blood sugar.

Fructose A monosaccharide that is the primary form of carbohydrate found in fruit.

Galactose A monosaccharide that combines with glucose to form lactose or milk sugar.

Monosaccharides The three most common monosaccharides in the diet are glucose, fructose, and galactose. Each contains 6 carbon, 12 hydrogen, and 6 oxygen atoms but differs in the arrangement of these (Figure 4.2). **Glucose**, commonly referred to as blood sugar, is the most important carbohydrate fuel for the body. It is produced in plants by the process of photosynthesis, which uses energy from the sun to combine carbon dioxide and water (Figure 4.3). Glucose rarely occurs as a monosaccharide in food. It is most often found as part of a disaccharide or starch. **Fructose** is a monosaccharide that tastes sweeter than glucose. It is found in fruits and vegetables and makes up more than half the sugar in honey. **Galactose** occurs most often as a part of lactose, the disaccharide in milk, and is rarely present as a monosaccharide in the food supply.

Maltose A disaccharide consisting of two molecules of glucose.

Sucrose A disaccharide that is formed by linking fructose and glucose. It is commonly known as table sugar or white sugar.

Disaccharides Disaccharides are simple carbohydrates made up of two monosaccharides linked together (Figure 4.4). To form the link, a hydroxyl group (—OH) from one sugar and a hydrogen atom (H) from the other are lost as a molecule of water (H_2O). This type of reaction is called a condensation reaction. When the bond between two sugars is broken, a molecule of water is added to restore the hydroxyl group on one sugar and the hydrogen atom on the other. This type of reaction is called a hydrolysis reaction (Figure 4.5). **Maltose** is a disaccharide consisting of two molecules of glucose. This sugar is made whenever starch is broken down. For example, it is responsible for the slightly sweet taste experienced when bread is held in the mouth for a few minutes. As salivary amylase begins digesting the starch, some sweeter-tasting maltose is formed. **Sucrose,** or table sugar, is the

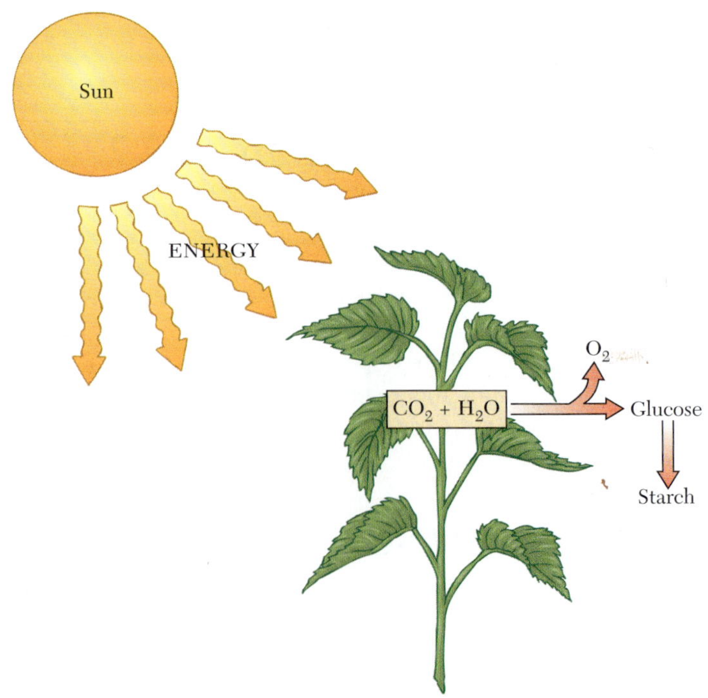

FIGURE 4.3 The process of photosynthesis uses energy from the sun to synthesize glucose from carbon dioxide and water. Glucose can then be stored as starch.

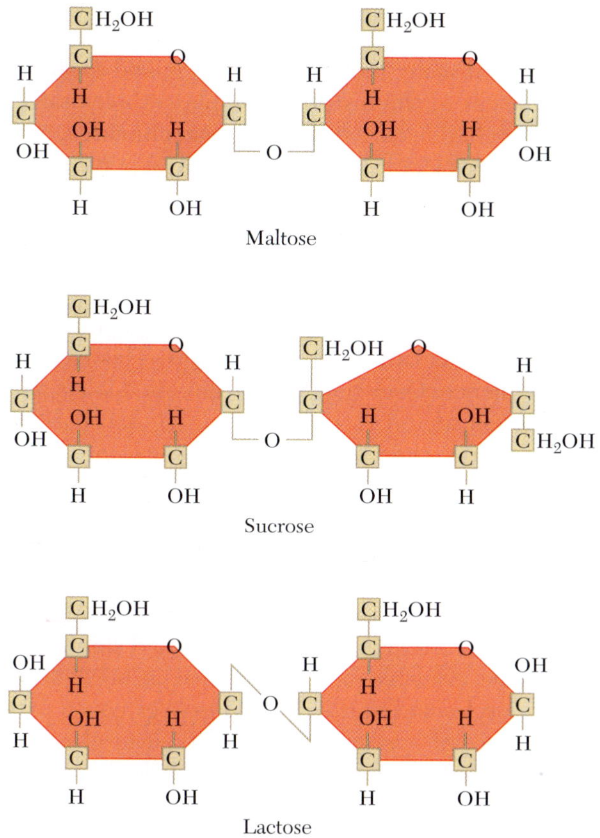

FIGURE 4.4 Structure of common disaccharides.

disaccharide formed by linking glucose to fructose. It is found in sugar cane, sugar beets, honey, and maple syrup. Sucrose is the only sweetener that can be called "sugar" in the ingredient list on food labels in the United States. **Lactose,** or milk sugar, is glucose linked to galactose. Lactose is the only sugar found in animal foods; it contributes about 30% of the energy in whole cow's milk and about 40% of the energy in human milk.

Lactose A disaccharide that is formed by linking galactose and glucose. It is commonly known as milk sugar.

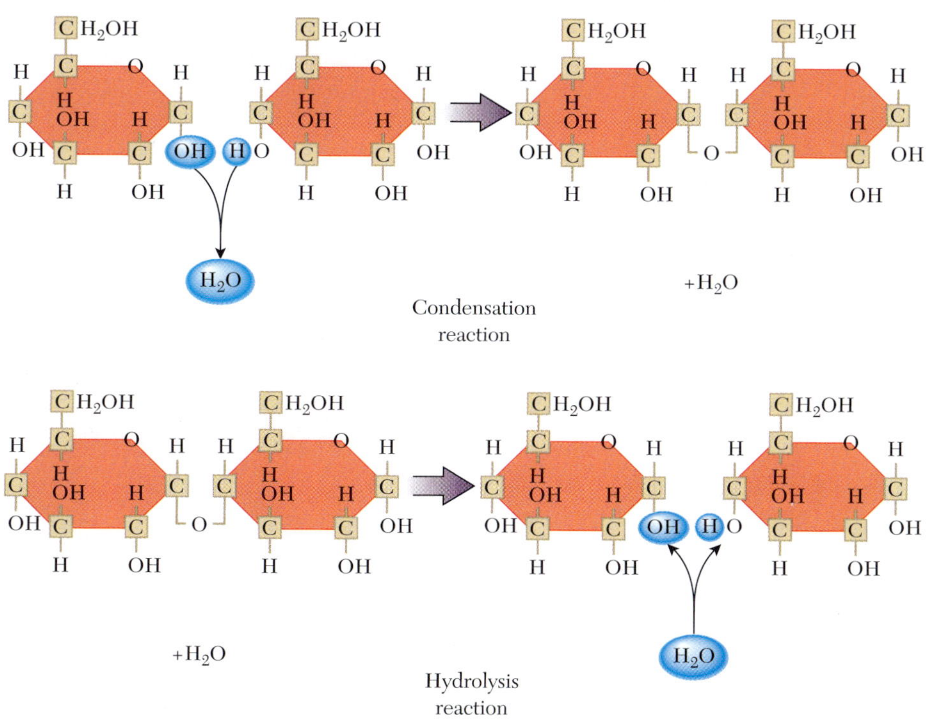

FIGURE 4.5 When two glucose molecules are joined in a condensation reaction, a molecule of water is lost and the disaccharide maltose is formed. A hydrolysis reaction breaks a bond by adding a molecule of water, as is shown here by the hydrolysis of maltose into its component monosaccharides.

Complex Carbohydrates

Complex carbohydrates are made up of many monosaccharides linked together in chains. They are generally not sweet to the taste like simple carbohydrates. Short chains of three to ten monosaccharides are called **oligosaccharides,** and longer chains are called **polysaccharides** ("poly" means many). The polysaccharides include glycogen in animals and starch and fiber in plants.

Oligosaccharides Short-chain carbohydrates containing three to ten sugar units.

Polysaccharides Carbohydrates containing many sugar units linked together.

Oligosaccharides Oligosaccharides such as raffinose and stachyose are found in beans and other legumes. These cannot be digested by enzymes in the human stomach and small intestine, so they pass undigested into the large intestine where bacteria digest them, producing gas and other by-products. This gas can cause abdominal discomfort and flatulence. Over-the-counter enzyme tablets and solutions (such as Bean-O) can be consumed to break down oligosaccharides before they reach the intestinal bacteria, thereby reducing the amount of gas produced.

Glycogen A carbohydrate made of many glucose molecules linked together in a highly branched structure. It is the storage form of carbohydrate in animals.

Glycogen **Glycogen** is the storage form of carbohydrate in animals. It is made up of highly branched chains of glucose molecules (Figure 4.6). The enzyme that breaks down glycogen removes one glucose at a time from the ends of the chains. The branched structure allows many glucose molecules to be released simultaneously. This allows glucose to become available quickly when it is needed. In humans, glycogen is stored in the muscles and in the liver. Muscle glycogen provides glucose to the muscles as a source of energy during activity; liver glycogen provides glucose that can be transported to cells throughout the body via the bloodstream.

The amount of glycogen in the body is relatively small—about 200 to 500 g.[1] The amount of glycogen stored in muscle can be temporarily increased by a diet and exercise regimen called "carbohydrate loading" or "glycogen supercompensation." This regimen is often used by endurance athletes to build up glycogen stores before an athletic event. Extra glycogen can mean the difference between

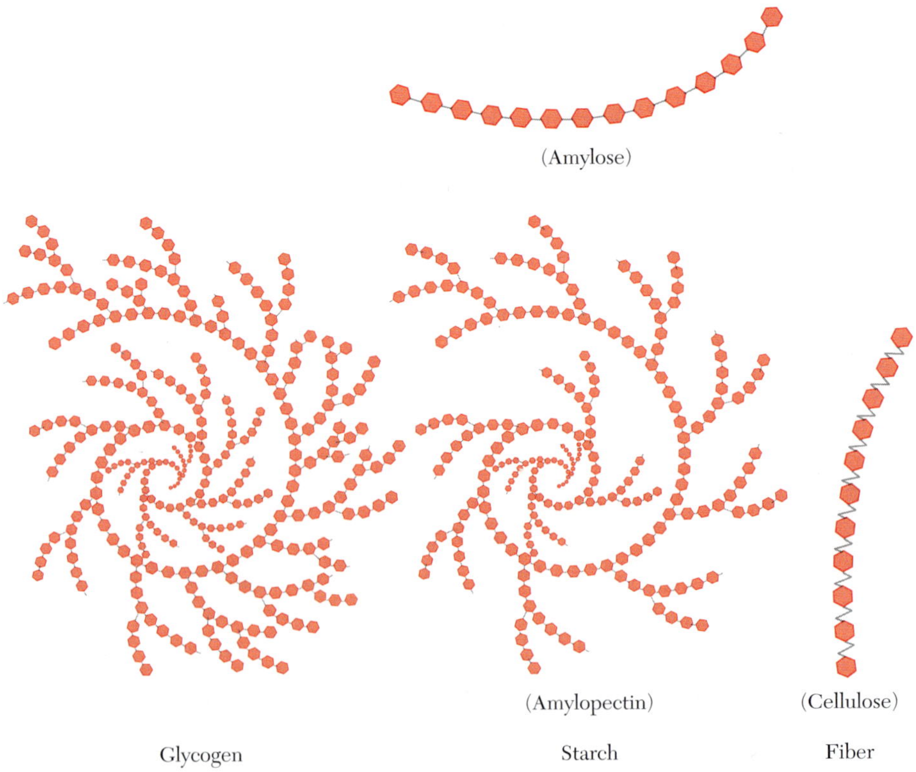

FIGURE 4.6 Complex carbohydrates are made up of straight or branching chains of monosaccharides. Glycogen contains hundreds of glucose molecules in highly branched chains. The starch amylopectin is similar in structure to glycogen but does not contain as many branches in the chain. The starch amylose consists of unbranched glucose chains. Fiber, such as this cellulose, is composed of unbranched chains of glucose, but the glucose molecules are linked by a type of bond that cannot be broken by human digestive enzymes.

TABLE 4.1 Dietary Sources of Soluble and Insoluble Fiber

Food/Serving	Total Fiber (g)	Insoluble Fiber (g)	Soluble Fiber (g)	Energy (kcal)
Wheat bran flakes, 1 cup	6.15	5.52	0.63	126
Broccoli, 1 cup	2.8	1.4	1.4	28
Celery, 1 stalk	0.29	0.19	0.10	3
Oatmeal, 1 cup	4.00	2.15	1.85	145
Apple, 1 medium	3.73	2.76	0.97	81
Carrot, 1 medium	1.84	0.92	0.92	26
Plum, 1 medium	0.99	0.46	0.53	36
Kidney beans, 1/2 cup	5.72	2.86	2.86	113
Green peas, 1/2 cup	4.40	3.12	1.28	62
Metamucil, 1 Tbsp	5.10	1.05	4.05	21

running only 20 miles or finishing a 26-mile marathon before exhaustion takes over. Glycogen supercompensation is discussed in more detail in Chapter 14.

Starches **Starch** is the storage form of carbohydrate in plants. It is found in two forms: amylose, which consists of long straight chains of glucose molecules, and amylopectin, which consists of branched chains of glucose molecules (see Figure 4.6). About 15 to 20% of the starch in the American diet is amylose and 80 to 85% is amylopectin. We consume starch in grain products and starchy vegetables, such as potatoes and squash.

Starch A carbohydrate made of many glucose molecules linked in straight or branching chains. The bonds that link the glucose molecules can be broken by human digestive enzymes.

Fiber Fiber or **dietary fiber** refers to plant materials that cannot be digested in the stomach and small intestine because humans lack the enzymes necessary to break the bonds that connect the monosaccharide units (see Figure 4.6). Because fiber cannot be digested, it cannot be absorbed into the body and used for energy. Some fiber is digested by microflora in the large intestine, producing gas and short-chain fatty acids, small quantities of which can be absorbed.

Dietary fiber Nonstarch polysaccharides in plant foods that are not broken down by human digestive enzymes.

Fibers are categorized by their ability to dissolve in water. **Insoluble fibers** are primarily those that are derived from the structural parts of plants, such as the cell walls. These substances include cellulose and some hemicelluloses, which are carbohydrates, and lignins, which technically are not carbohydrates but are classified as insoluble fiber. Food sources of insoluble fiber include wheat bran and rye bran, which contain hemicellulose and cellulose, and vegetables, such as broccoli and celery, that contain woody fibers composed partly of lignins. **Soluble fibers** are found around and inside plant cells. These carbohydrates either absorb water or dissolve in water, and most form viscous solutions. They include pectins, gums, mucilages, and some hemicelluloses. Food sources of soluble fibers include oats, apples, beans, and psyllium, the fiber used in bulk-forming laxatives such as Metamucil. Soluble fibers are also added in food processing to contribute texture to foods (see the next section). Most foods of plant origin contain mixtures of soluble and insoluble fibers (Table 4.1)

Insoluble fibers Fibers that, for the most part, do not dissolve in water. They include cellulose, hemicelluloses, and lignin.

Soluble fibers Fibers that either dissolve when placed in water or absorb water. They include pectins, gums, and some hemicelluloses.

CARBOHYDRATES IN THE DIET

Carbohydrates are found in grains, breads, legumes, fruits, vegetables, and milk, as well as in sweeteners such as honey and table sugar. Carbohydrates from all of these sources provide about 52% of the energy in the American diet.

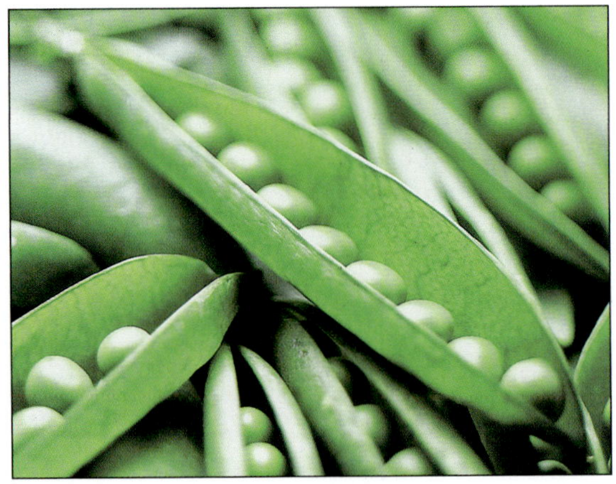

FIGURE 4.7 Legumes, like these peas, grow in a pod and are the seeds of leguminous plants. *(© Chris Everard/Stone)*

Complex Carbohydrates

Complex carbohydrates are found primarily in grains, legumes, and vegetables. Grains are the major source of complex carbohydrates in the North American diet. Grains are the seeds of plants such as rice, corn, oats, wheat, and barley. Legumes such as peas, lentils, soybeans, and kidney beans are starchy seeds from plants that produce seedpods (Figure 4.7). Starchy vegetables include roots (sweet potatoes, yams, cassava) and tubers (potatoes), which are an underground energy-storage organ produced by some plants. Grains, legumes, and starchy vegetables are good sources of vitamins, minerals, and fiber. Grains and legumes are also important sources of protein. Vegetables such as green beans and broccoli contain a relatively small amount of starch and are high in water, vitamins, minerals, and fiber.

Whole and Refined Grains Grain seeds or kernels are made up of three parts—the bran, the germ, and the endosperm (Figure 4.8a). The bran, which is the outermost layer, contains most of the fiber and is a good source of B vitamins. The germ, which lies at the base of the kernel, is the plant embryo where sprouting occurs. It is the source of vegetable oils such as corn and safflower oil, and is rich in vitamin E. The remainder of the kernel is the endosperm, which is the starchy food supply for the sprouting embryo. While primarily starch, the endosperm also contains protein and some vitamins and minerals. When we eat the entire kernel from a grain, such as brown rice or rolled oats, we are eating a whole-grain product (Figure 4.8b). Whole-grain flours such as whole-wheat flour include most of the bran, germ, and endosperm.

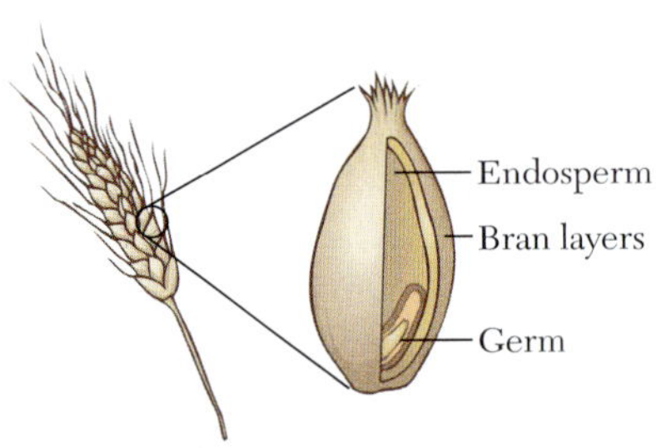

(a)

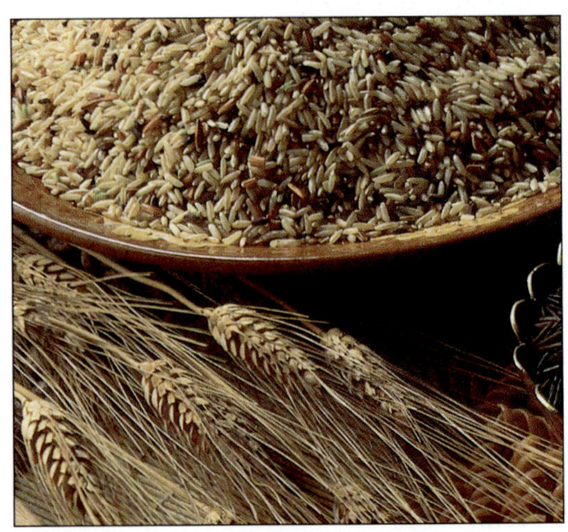

(b)

FIGURE 4.8 (a) A grain of wheat contains outer layers of bran, the plant embryo or germ, and a carbohydrate-rich endosperm. (b) Whole grains are good sources of dietary fiber. *((b) © Picture Perfect)*

Processing grains separates the parts of the kernel. For instance, during the milling of grain into flour, the grinding detaches the germ and bran from the endosperm. The term **refined** refers to the process whereby the coarse part of food products is separated and removed. White flour is a refined grain product because it is produced from just the endosperm; the bran and germ have been removed.

Refined Refers to foods that have been processed to remove the coarse parts, leaving behind a product of more uniform composition.

When the outer layers of the grain are lost in refining, fiber and some vitamins and minerals naturally found in the whole grain are also lost. In order to restore some of the lost nutrients, refined grains sold in the United States are enriched with some, but not all, of the nutrients lost in processing. For example, thiamin, riboflavin, niacin, and iron, which are removed by milling, are added back in the **enrichment** process (see Chapter 9). Vitamin E, magnesium, zinc, and vitamin B_6 are also removed by milling but are not added back.

Enrichment The addition of nutrients lost in processing to a level equal to or higher than that originally present.

Complex Carbohydrates Added to Foods Complex carbohydrates are often added to processed foods in order to change their texture. For example, starch is added to thicken foods such as sauces, puddings, and gravies. This works because starch, which is found as small granules in plants, swells when heated in water, causing the solution to become thicker (Figure 4.9). As a starch-thickened mixture cools, bonds form between the molecules, creating a gel. Cornstarch is frequently added to thicken or gel sauces and puddings. Food manufacturers also use a product called modified starch, or modified food starch. This is starch that has been treated to cause it to form a more stable gel.

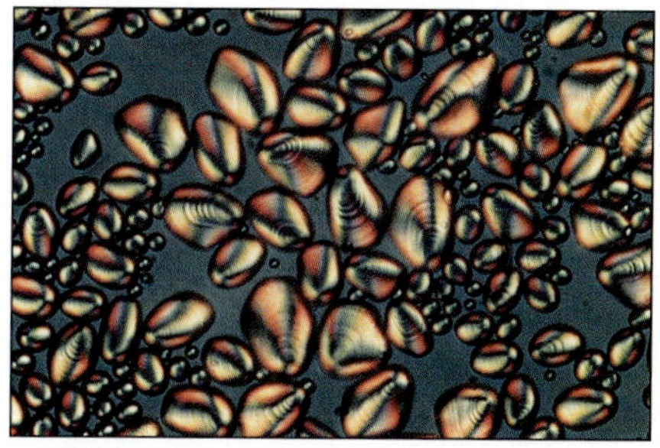

FIGURE 4.9 The starch molecules synthesized by plants are deposited in cells where they form starch grains or granules. Starch granules from different plants have different sizes and shapes. The organization of starch molecules within the granules accounts for some of the properties of various starches in food preparation. The granules shown here are from potato starch. *(© Eric V. Grave/Photo Researchers, Inc.)*

Pectin and carbohydrate gums are also used as thickeners and stabilizers. Pectin is a soluble fiber found in fruits and vegetables. It forms a gel when sugar and acid are added, such as in the preparation of jams and jellies. Gum arabic, gum karaya, guar gum, locust bean gum, xanthan gum, and gum tragacanth are carbohydrate gums extracted from shrubs, trees, and seedpods; agar, carrageenan, and alginates come from seaweeds. Carbohydrate gums combine with water to keep solutions from separating. Gravies, puddings, reduced-fat salad dressings, and frozen desserts are examples of products that contain carbohydrate gums. Pectins and gums are also used in reduced-fat products to mimic the texture of fat (see Chapter 5).

Simple Carbohydrates

Simple carbohydrates, or sugars, provide about 21% of the energy in the American diet. Half of this is from sugars naturally present in whole foods such as dairy products and fresh fruit.[2] The sugar in whole foods is consumed along with the other nutrients; therefore, these sources have a higher nutrient density—that is, they contain more nutrients per kcalorie than refined sugars. For example, kiwis contain sugars along with fiber, vitamins, and minerals (Figure 4.10).

Nutrient	Soda (12 fluid oz)	Kiwi (3 medium)
Vitamin A (μg)	0	7
Vitamin C (mg)	0	223
Folate (μg DFE)	0	87
Potassium (mg)	4	757
Calcium (mg)	7	60
Protein (g)	0	2
Fiber (g)	0	8
Carbohydrate (g)	37	34
Sugars (g)	37	26
Energy (kcals)	141	139

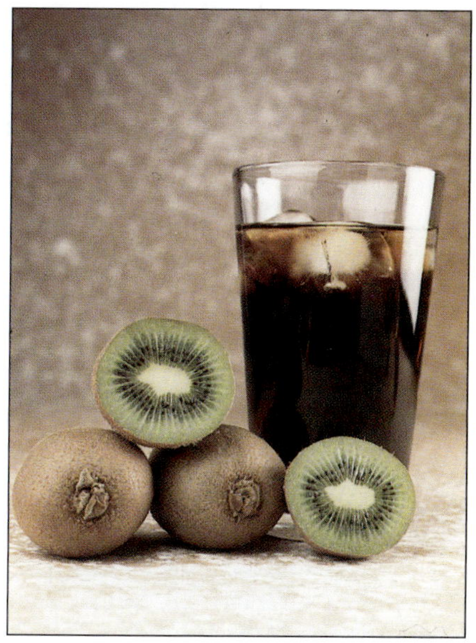

FIGURE 4.10 These two foods in the portions shown provide about the same amount of energy and carbohydrate, but the kiwis are also a good source of fiber and nutrients such as vitamin C and folate. *(© George Semple)*

The remaining half of the simple carbohydrate consumed in the American diet comes from refined sugars added to foods. Refined sugars are sugars that have been separated from the plants in which they are produced. They are not chemically different from sugars occurring naturally in foods, but they are no longer associated with most of the other nutrients present in the original plant source. Refined sugars are therefore low in nutrient density.

Simple Carbohydrates Added to Foods Simple carbohydrates are added to foods as sweeteners both by consumers and in the food manufacturing process. Americans consume about 150 pounds of sweeteners per person per year.[3] Simple carbohydrates are also added to provide texture and color and to serve as a preservative.

Sucrose, commonly called white sugar or table sugar, is the most common table sweetener. It is refined from sugar beets or sugar cane and contains few nutrients other than carbohydrate. Other sweeteners, such as honey, maple syrup, brown sugar, and molasses, are promoted as "natural" alternatives to white sugar. These products are actually all processed in some way, either by humans or, in the case of honey, by bees. Although these sweeteners contribute distinctive flavors to the foods to which they are added, the nutritional contributions of most are not significantly different from that of refined white sugar (Table 4.2). In addition, they may contain contaminants. For instance, honey may contain spores of the bacterium *Clostridium botulinum*, which can be dangerous if consumed by infants (see Chapter 19).

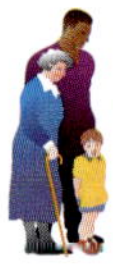

Sugars are also added in food manufacturing. Sucrose, fructose, high-fructose corn syrup, corn syrup, maltose, and others are added as sweeteners. In high concentrations, sugars are used as preservatives. For example, in jams and jellies sugars act as preservatives by drawing water away from microorganisms, preventing their growth. Sugars are also used to color foods, because they darken or caramelize when heated. Caramelized sugar is responsible for the brown color of caramel candy and the dark color of maple syrup.

One of the most popular sugars added in manufacturing is fructose. Fructose is a component of a number of sweeteners, including sucrose, honey, and high-fructose corn syrup. High-fructose corn syrup is produced by modifying starch extracted from corn to produce a syrup that is approximately half glucose and half fructose. Fructose dissolves more readily than sucrose, so it is preferred in soft drinks and canned fruits. It is also sweeter than sucrose. Because fructose does not cause as great a rise in blood glucose, it is sometimes used as an alternative to sucrose in products for diabetics. Fructose intake from sweeteners like high-fructose corn syrup, honey, and sucrose now makes up about 5% of the total energy

TABLE 4.2 Nutritional Contributions of Various Sweeteners

	Energy (kcal)	Protein (g)	Carbohydrate (g)	Calcium (mg)	Phosphorus (mg)	Sodium (mg)	Magnesium (mg)	Potassium (mg)	Iron (mg)
Daily Value*	–	*50*	*300*	*1000*	*1000*	*< 2400*	*400*	*3500*	*18*
Sweetener					***Nutrients per Tablespoon***				
Light molasses	40	0.4	10.0	25	7	2	31	138	0.6
Medium molasses	38	0.4	9.0	44	10	6	31	159	0.9
Blackstrap molasses	35	0.4	8.0	103	13	14	31	439	2.4
Honey	61	0.1	16.5	1	1	1	1	10	0.1
Brown sugar	52	0	13.4	11	5	3	9	32	0.4
White sugar	46	0	11.9	1	0	0	0	1	0

*Daily Value for a 2000-kcalorie diet.

intake in the United States.[2] Although current levels of fructose consumption are considered safe, fructose, like other simple sugars, can promote tooth decay and, in sensitive individuals, has been reported to cause an increase in insulin levels, blood lipids, and blood uric acid.[4] Fructose consumed in fruits or juices can also cause diarrhea in children.[5]

CARBOHYDRATES IN THE DIGESTIVE TRACT

Carbohydrates must be broken down into monosaccharides to be absorbed. Carbohydrates and other substances that are not digested and absorbed in the small intestine pass into the large intestine. Here, some additional digestion may occur due to the bacterial enzymes of the intestinal microflora.

Digestion and Absorption

The digestion of starch begins in the mouth, where the enzyme salivary amylase starts breaking the polysaccharides into shorter chains of glucose. This enzyme functions optimally at a pH of approximately 6.6 to 6.8. Its digestive activity therefore ceases when food moves into the acidic environment of the stomach (pH 1.5 to 3.5).

Carbohydrate digestion resumes in the small intestine, where pancreatic amylases complete the job of breaking starch into oligosaccharides and maltose. The final digestion of oligosaccharides and disaccharides is completed by enzymes attached to the brush border of the villi in the small intestine. Here, maltose is broken down into two glucose molecules by maltase, sucrose is broken down by the enzyme sucrase to glucose and fructose, and lactose is broken down by lactase to form glucose and galactose (Figure 4.11). The resulting monosaccharides—glucose, galactose, and fructose—are then absorbed into the mucosal cells and transported to the liver via the hepatic portal circulation. Glucose and galactose are absorbed by active transport, whereas fructose is absorbed by

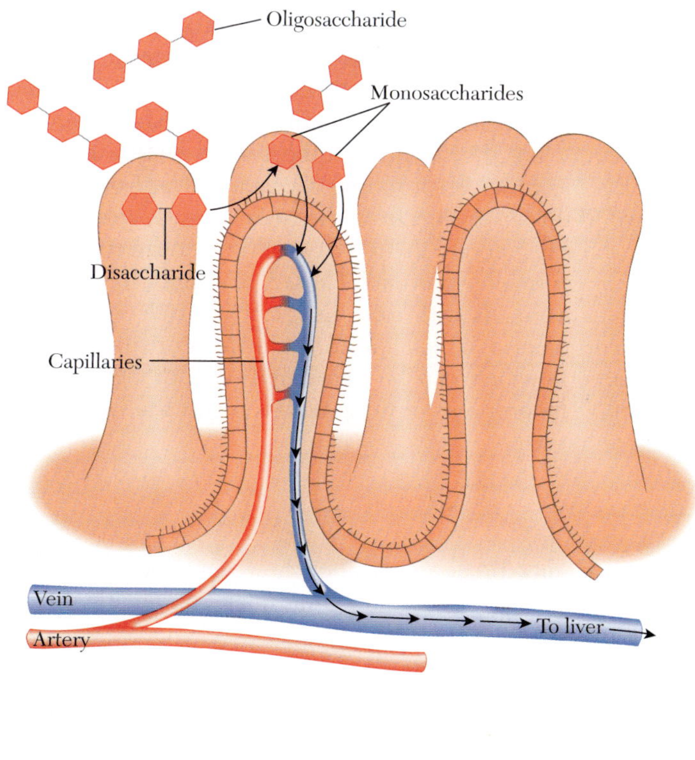

FIGURE 4.11 Oligosaccharides and disaccharides are hydrolyzed into monosaccharides by enzymes in the brush border of the small intestines. The end products of this hydrolysis enter the capillaries in the villi and are transported to the liver via the hepatic portal vein.

facilitated diffusion. Most monosaccharide absorption occurs in the upper portion of the small intestine.

Refined starches are digested efficiently, but the starch in grains and legumes is not completely digested, and from 1 to 10% may pass into the colon undigested.[6] This undigested starch is referred to as resistant starch. It is subject to bacterial degradation when it reaches the large intestine.

Lactose Intolerance

For more information about lactose intolerance, go to the National Institute of Diabetes & Digestive & Kidney Diseases at www.niddk.nih.gov/health/digest/digest.htm and click on lactose intolerance.

Lactose intolerance The inability to digest lactose because of a reduction in the levels of the enzyme lactase. It causes symptoms including intestinal gas and bloating after dairy products are consumed.

The disaccharide lactose, or milk sugar, is digested by the enzyme lactase. Lactase is synthesized by all humans during fetal life and is present at maximal activity at birth. Lactase levels decrease with age and in many individuals decline so much that lactose cannot be completely digested. **Lactose intolerance** is a reduced ability to digest lactose. In lactose-intolerant individuals, lactose consumed in the diet passes into the large intestine, where it is metabolized by bacteria. The undigested lactose and the acids and gas produced by the bacterial metabolism of lactose can draw water into the intestine and cause abdominal distension, flatulence, cramping, and diarrhea.

The percentage of adults with lactose intolerance ranges from a low of 5% or less in northwestern European populations to nearly 100% in some Asian and African populations.[7] In the United States, it is estimated that about 25% of the total adult population is lactose intolerant, but the incidence varies enormously depending on ethnic background. For instance, 80% of African Americans and 90% of Asian Americans experience symptoms after consuming lactose.[8] Lactose intolerance may also occur as a result of an intestinal infection or other disease. It is then referred to as secondary lactose intolerance and may disappear when the other condition resolves.

The degree of lactose intolerance varies. Some individuals cannot tolerate any lactose, whereas others can consume small amounts without symptoms. Because some of the lactose in yogurt and cheese is digested or lost in processing, many individuals with lactose intolerance can eat these products without developing symptoms. Although individuals with lactose intolerance must determine their own threshold for consuming dairy products without experiencing symptoms, research has shown that most individuals can consume one to two servings of dairy products daily if they are spread out over the course of the day.[8]

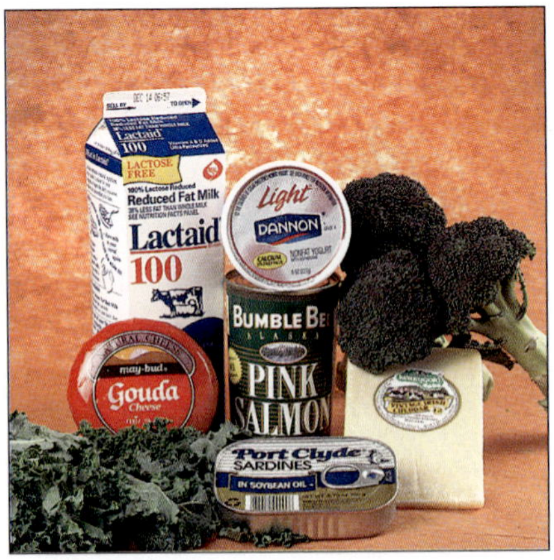

FIGURE 4.12 These foods are good sources of calcium and are low in lactose. *(© George Semple)*

Because dairy products are an important source of dietary calcium, individuals with lactose intolerance may need to consume other sources of calcium to meet their needs. In cultures where lactose intolerance is common, traditional diets provide sources of calcium other than milk. For example, in Asia, tofu and fish consumed with bones supply calcium, and in the Near East, fermented cheese and yogurt provide much of the calcium. In the United States, milk and other dairy products are the most important source of calcium. The Food Guide Pyramid recommends two to three servings from the Milk, Yogurt, and Cheese Group each day. Those who can tolerate lactose in small doses can divide the two to three servings into many smaller portions. Those who cannot tolerate any lactose can meet their calcium needs with tofu, fish, calcium-rich vegetables, milk treated with the enzyme lactase, or calcium-fortified foods or supplements (Figure 4.12). Lactase tablets, which can be consumed with or before milk products, are also available. The enzymes in these tablets digest the lactose before it passes into the large intestine.

Fiber

Human digestive enzymes cannot break down fiber; however, fiber does have important properties that affect the digestive tract and maintain healthy bowel function.

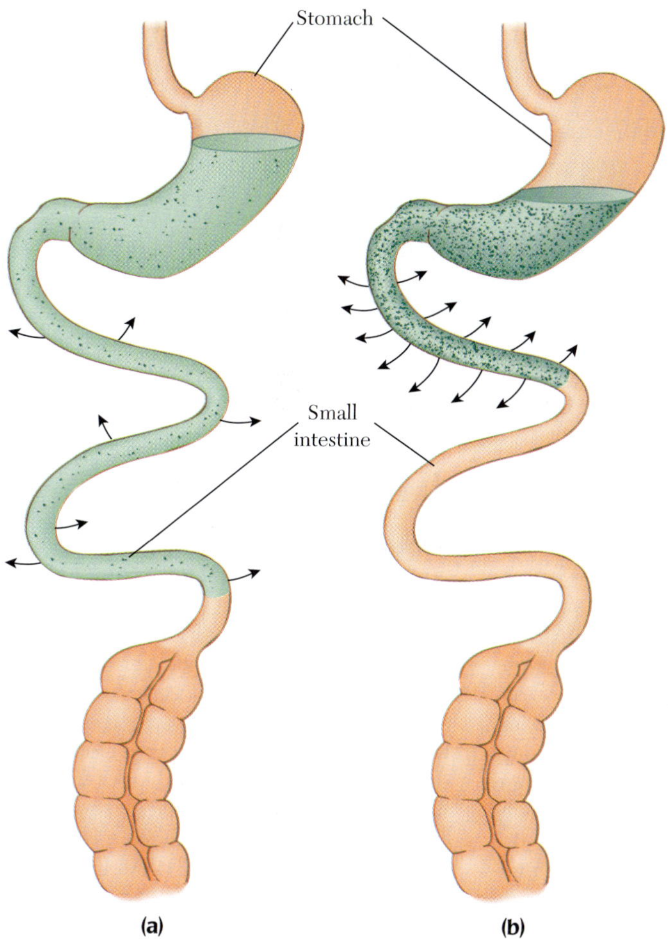

FIGURE 4.13 (a) This representation of the stomach and small intestine illustrates how a fiber-rich diet dilutes the intestinal contents and slows the digestion and absorption of nutrients (shown as green dots). (b) When a low-fiber diet is consumed, nutrients are more concentrated and digestion and absorption occur more rapidly.

Fiber is not a single substance. With the exception of lignin, fibers are complex carbohydrates, but they differ in the types of sugars that make up the polysaccharide chain. Fiber structure determines its physical properties and the effect it has on the gastrointestinal tract. Soluble fibers absorb water, forming viscous solutions in the gastrointestinal tract that slow the rate at which nutrients are absorbed. For example, in the stomach, soluble fiber causes distention and slows emptying. In the small intestine, it slows the absorption of sugars and other nutrients and decreases the absorption of bile (Figure 4.13). In the colon, soluble fibers are fermented by the bacterial microflora producing acids and gases. The by-products of this bacterial fermentation may affect cholesterol synthesis and the risks of heart disease and cancer. Insoluble fibers, such as wheat bran, also increase the amount of material in the intestine. They add bulk because they are not completely degraded by bacterial fermentation.

The combination of the increased bulk of insoluble fibers and the fluid drawn in by soluble fibers increases the volume of material in the intestine. This allows for easier evacuation of the stool. It also promotes healthy bowel function by stimulating peristalsis, which causes the muscles of the colon to work more and become stronger. The increase in peristalsis reduces transit time—the time it takes food and fecal matter to move through the GI tract. In African countries, where the diet contains 40 to 150 g of fiber per day, the transit time is 36 hours or less. In the United States, where the usual fiber intake is 14 to 15 g per day,[9] it is not uncommon for transit time to be as long as 96 hours (see *Research Discoveries:* "Cereal Fibers and Health").

RESEARCH DISCOVERIES

Cereal Fibers and Health

One hundred and fifty years ago, self-proclaimed health advocates Sylvester Graham, John Harvey Kellogg, and Charles W. Post promoted cereal foods as health tonics. These pioneers of what are now the breakfast cereal empires, Kellogg's and Post, were not scientists. Often the health information they promoted was outlandish. Graham preached that food should never be eaten hot, that water should not be consumed with a meal, and that lewdness, along with chicken pie, was the cause of cholera. Kellogg told his patients that coffee could cripple the liver and that bouillon was a solution of poisons. And Post advertised that his cereal, called Grape Nuts, tightened up loose teeth and cured tuberculosis and malaria.[a] However, the suggestion that the consumption of whole grains was a healthy approach to eating has held up over time. The Dietary Guidelines and the Food Guide Pyramid promote a diet that is based on cereals and other whole grains. This dietary pattern has been shown to promote gastrointestinal health and reduce the risks of the major chronic diseases of today—heart disease, cancer, and diabetes.

Scientific support for the role of cereal grain consumption in health began to accumulate in the 1940s, '50s, and '60s when scientists such as Denis Burkitt, Hugh Trowell, and A. R. P. Walker began observing and investigating the effects of high-fiber foods on health. Their hypotheses, which were based primarily on epidemiological observations, helped change the way we think about fiber. At the time they began their studies fiber was poorly defined, there was no consistent methodology to assess the amount of fiber in foods, and food composition tables did not include fiber values. Fiber was referred to as roughage and many regarded it as a gastrointestinal irritant rather than a dietary component important for health.

Walker and colleagues began to relate the dietary pattern in South African Blacks with their disease pattern—emphasizing the role of fiber.[b] They observed that in Western populations, where fiber intake was between 15 and 30 g per day, feces were smaller and harder than in African individuals consuming diets containing from 70 to more than 100 g of fiber per day. They hypothesized that fiber increased stool weight and decreased transit time. This hypothesis was supported by studies that compared intestinal transit time and stool weight in Ugandan villagers, who ate a high-fiber diet to British subjects, who ate a lower fiber diet (see figure).[c] To further test this hypothesis, they added unprocessed bran to the diet of British subjects. The added fiber reduced transit time and increased stool weight.[c]

In 1956, Denis Burkitt saw a patient in Uganda with a rare cancer involving his jaws (Burkitt's lymphoma). As he traveled in Africa to establish the geographical distribution of this type of cancer, he noticed that many diseases that were common among whites in Europe and whites in Africa were rare among African peasants. With these observations in mind, Burkitt studied a hypothesis that proposed that a variety of conditions common in industrialized society, including diabetes, obesity, coronary thrombosis, constipation, diverticular disease, hemorrhoids, and varicose veins, were caused by the overconsumption of refined carbohydrates. It postulated that three manufactured foods—refined sugar, white flour, and white rice—caused virtually all the diseases of civilization.[b] In response to his observations, Burkitt proposed that low fiber intake rather than high refined-carbohydrate consumption was the dietary connection. He suggested that the dietary fiber that had been removed during refinement created a deficiency of this substance that may underlie the development of these characteristically Western diseases.[c,d] This became known as the fiber hypothesis.

CARBOHYDRATES IN THE BODY

The main function of carbohydrate in the body is to provide energy. In order to provide this energy, a constant supply of glucose is delivered to cells via the bloodstream. There are a number of regulatory mechanisms in the body to ensure that glucose is available in the face of varying carbohydrate intakes.

Functions of Carbohydrate

Carbohydrates provide about 4 kcalories per g. The main source of this energy is glucose. Carbohydrates also have several other important roles. The sugar galactose is needed to form nerve tissue. It also combines with glucose to make lactose in women who are producing breast milk. Two other monosaccharides that are of great importance to the body are deoxyribose and ribose. These sugars have five carbon atoms and are components of DNA and RNA (ribonucleic acid), respectively, which contain the genetic information needed for the synthesis of proteins. Deoxyribose and ribose can be synthesized by the body and are not found in large amounts in the diet. Ribose is also a component of the vitamin riboflavin.

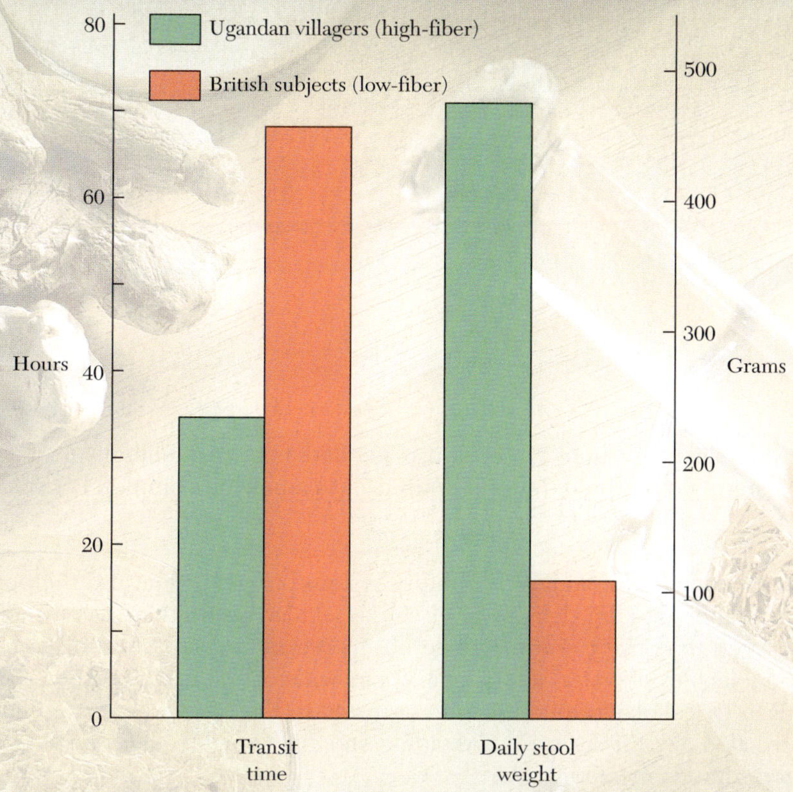

Ugandan villagers, who consume an unrefined diet high in fiber, have greater stool weights and shorter transit times than British citizens who consume a more refined lower fiber diet. *(Adapted from Burkitt, D. P., Walker, A. R. P., and Painter, N. S. Dietary fiber and disease. JAMA 229: 1068–1074, 1974.)*

Burkitt was often quoted as saying that the health of a country's people could be determined by the size of their stools and whether the stools floated or sank.[e]

The fiber hypothesis of Burkitt and others launched an era of fiber research in the United States and elsewhere. Their observations have been the stimulus for much of today's research on fiber and its importance in maintaining normal gastrointestinal function and reducing the incidence of chronic disease. Today the whole-grain cereals promoted by Graham, Kellogg, and Post are once again considered a sort of health tonic, but this time the concept is backed by scientific research.

References

[a] Deutsch, R. M. *The New Nuts Among the Berries.* Palo Alto, Calif.: Bull Publishing Company, 1977.

[b] Trowell, H. Dietary fibre: a paradigm. In *Dietary Fibre, Fibre-Depleted Foods and Disease.* Trowell, H., Burkitt, D., and Heaton, K., eds. London; Academic Press, 1985, 1–20.

[c] Burkitt, D. P., Walker, A. R. P., and Painter, N. S. Dietary fiber and disease. JAMA 229: 1068–1074, 1974.

[d] Burkitt, D. P., and Trowell, H. C. *Refined Carbohydrate and Disease: Some Implications of Dietary Fibre*. London; Academic Press, 1975.

[e] Story, J. A., and Kritchevsky, D. Denis Parsons Burkitt. J. Nutr. 124:1551–1554, 1994.

Oligosaccharides are also important in our bodies. They are found attached to proteins or lipids on the surface of cells, where they help to signal information about the cells. Another type of carbohydrate that is important in the body is the mucopolysaccharides. These are a class of polysaccharides that functions with proteins in body secretions and structures. Mucopolysaccharides give mucus its viscous consistency and provide cushioning and lubrication in connective tissue.

Carbohydrate Metabolism

After absorption, monosaccharides travel via the hepatic portal vein to the liver, where much of the fructose and galactose are metabolized for energy. The fate of the absorbed glucose depends on the energy needs of the body. If glucose is needed at the tissues, it is carried by the bloodstream and transported into cells. To generate energy, glucose is metabolized through **cellular respiration** to produce carbon dioxide, water, and energy in the form of ATP. If glucose is plentiful, the liver may store it as glycogen and, to a lesser extent, use it to synthesize fat. If glucose is in short supply, the liver can break down glycogen stores to maintain blood glucose. As glycogen stores are depleted, the liver must use other molecules, particularly amino acids from protein, to

Cellular respiration The reactions that break down carbohydrates, fats, and proteins in the presence of oxygen to produce carbon dioxide, water, and energy in the form of ATP.

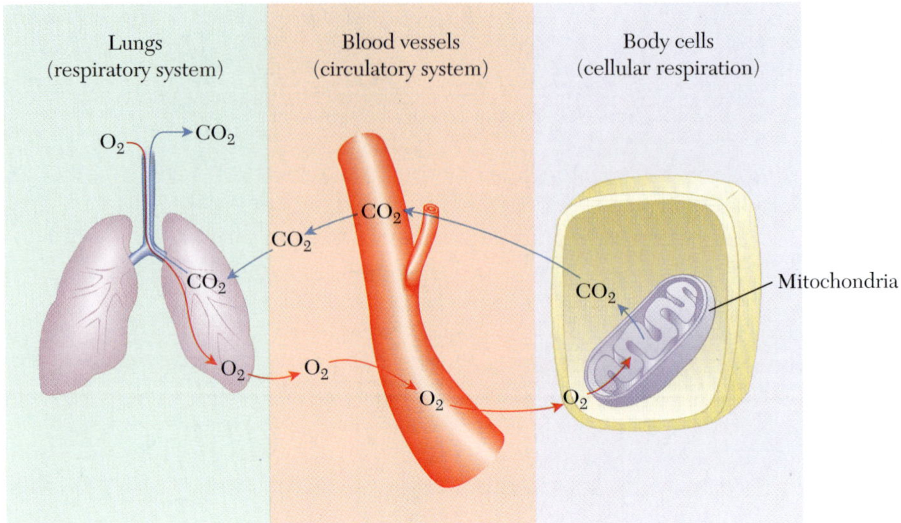

FIGURE 4.14 Oxygen enters the body via the lungs (respiratory system). It is transferred into the blood (circulatory system) and delivered to body cells where it is used to generate energy via cellular respiration. Cellular respiration produces carbon dioxide, which must be eliminated from the body. Carbon dioxide travels in the blood to the lungs where it is eliminated in exhaled air.

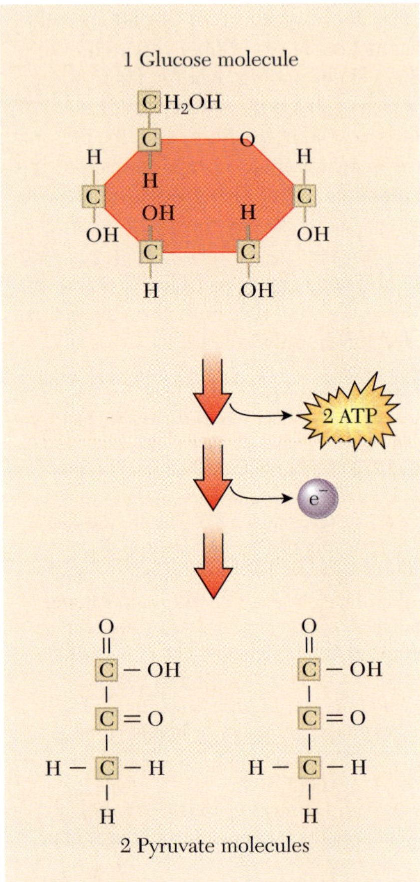

FIGURE 4.15 During glycolysis each molecule of glucose is broken into two molecules of pyruvate. Two ATP molecules are produced. These reactions occur in the cytoplasm of the cell and can proceed in the absence of oxygen.

Glycolysis A metabolic pathway in the cytoplasm of the cell that splits glucose into two 3-carbon pyruvate molecules. The energy released from one molecule of glucose is used to make two ATP molecules.

Citric acid cycle Also known as the Krebs cycle or the tricarboxylic acid cycle, this is the stage of respiration in which acetyl-CoA is broken down into two molecules of carbon dioxide.

Electron transport chain The final stage of cellular respiration in which electrons are passed down a chain of molecules to oxygen to form water and produce ATP.

make new glucose. Carbohydrate is also needed for the metabolism of fat. When the supply of carbohydrate is limited, fat cannot be completely broken down.

Cellular Respiration The body's respiratory system brings oxygen into the body and the circulatory system delivers it to cells. Cellular respiration uses 6 molecules of oxygen to convert one molecule of glucose into 6 molecules of carbon dioxide, 6 molecules of water, and about 38 molecules of ATP. The carbon dioxide produced by cellular respiration is transported to the lungs where it is eliminated in exhaled air (Figure 4.14). Providing energy through cellular respiration involves four interconnected stages.

Glycolysis The first stage of cellular respiration takes place in the cytoplasm of the cell and is called **glycolysis,** meaning glucose breakdown. In glycolysis, the 6-carbon sugar glucose is broken into two 3-carbon molecules called pyruvate (Figure 4.15). The reactions generate two molecules of ATP for each molecule of glucose and release high-energy electrons that are passed to shuttling molecules for transport to the last stage of cellular respiration.

Acetyl-CoA Formation In the second stage, which occurs in the mitochondria, one carbon, in the form of carbon dioxide, is removed from pyruvate and high-energy electrons are released. The remaining 2-carbon compound combines with a molecule of coenzyme A (CoA) to form acetyl-CoA (Figure 4.16). Acetyl-CoA then enters the third stage of breakdown, the **citric acid cycle.**

Citric Acid Cycle In the third stage, acetyl-CoA combines with oxaloacetate, a 4-carbon molecule derived from carbohydrate, to form a 6-carbon molecule and begin the citric acid cycle. The reactions of the citric acid cycle then remove one carbon at a time, to produce carbon dioxide. After two carbons have been removed in this manner, a 4-carbon oxaloacetate molecule is reformed and the cycle can begin again (Figure 4.17). These chemical reactions produce two ATP molecules per glucose molecule and also remove electrons, which are passed to shuttling molecules for transport to the fourth and last stage of cellular respiration, the **electron transport chain.**

The Electron Transport Chain The electron transport chain consists of a series of molecules, most of which are proteins, associated with the inner membrane of the mitochondria. These molecules accept electrons from the shuttling molecules and pass them from one to another down the chain until they are finally combined with oxygen to form water. As the electrons are passed along, their energy is used to pump hydrogen ions across the membrane. As these flow back through a special channel, the energy is used to make ATP (Figure 4.18). The reactions of cellular respiration are central to all energy-producing processes in the body. All four stages are shown together in Figure 4.19.

Sparing Protein When carbohydrate is adequate in the diet, amino acids from protein are not needed to synthesize glucose. Therefore, carbohydrate is said to spare protein. When carbohydrate intake is low, some glucose can be obtained from the breakdown of glycogen. This glucose is released into the blood to prevent blood glucose from dropping below the normal range. If carbohydrate intake remains low, glycogen stores are depleted. When glycogen breakdown can no longer provide glucose, it is synthesized from amino acids and other molecules by the process called **gluconeogenesis** (production of new glucose). Gluconeogenesis, which occurs in liver and kidney cells, is an energy-requiring process that forms glucose from 3-carbon molecules derived primarily from amino acids. Fatty acids cannot be used to make glucose because the reactions that break them down produce primarily 2-carbon molecules. Gluconeogenesis is essential for meeting the body's immediate need for glucose, particularly when carbohydrate intake is very low, but it uses amino acids from protein that could be used for other essential functions such as growth and maintenance of muscle tissue.

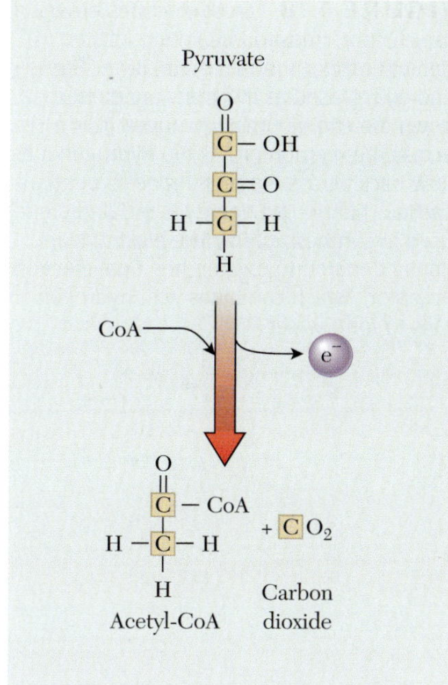

FIGURE 4.16 In the mitochondria, pyruvate loses a carbon as carbon dioxide and the remaining two carbons join with a molecule of coenzyme A (CoA) to form acetyl-CoA.

Gluconeogenesis The synthesis of glucose from simple noncarbohydrate molecules. Amino acids from protein are the primary source of carbons for glucose synthesis.

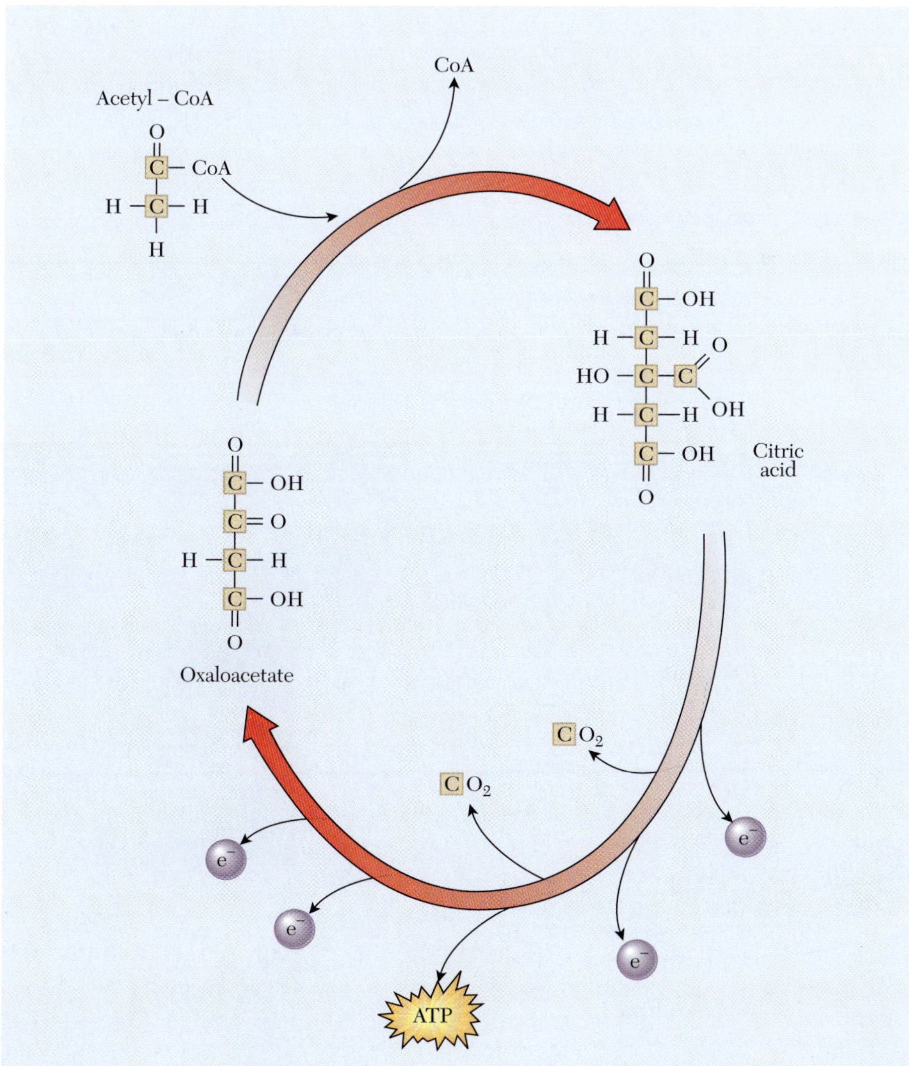

FIGURE 4.17 The reactions of the citric acid cycle take place in the mitochondria. Oxaloacetate combines with acetyl-CoA to form citric acid. The reactions then remove two carbons, one at a time, from citric acid as carbon dioxide to regenerate oxaloacetate. Two molecules of ATP can be produced here and high-energy electrons are released.

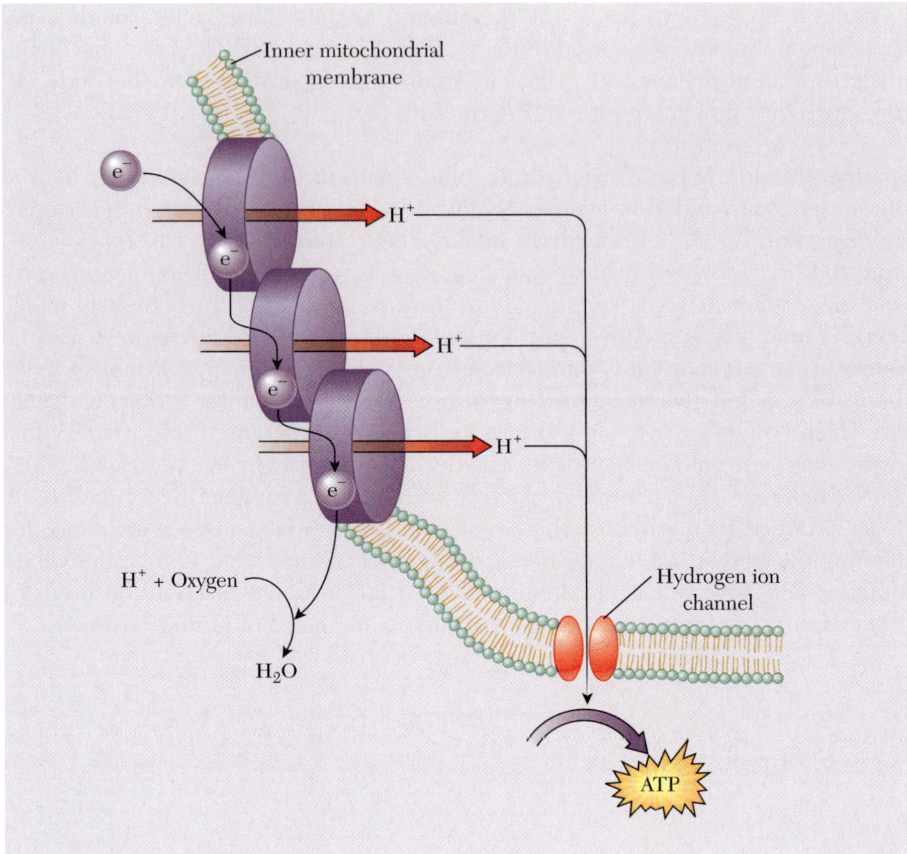

FIGURE 4.18 Most electron carriers of the electron transport chain are located in the inner mitochondrial membrane. The energy released as electrons are passed down the chain pumps hydrogen ions (H^+) across the membrane. As the hydrogen ions flow back across the membrane through a special channel the energy is reclaimed and used to synthesize ATP. The electrons are finally donated to oxygen (the final electron acceptor), which combines with hydrogen ions to form water.

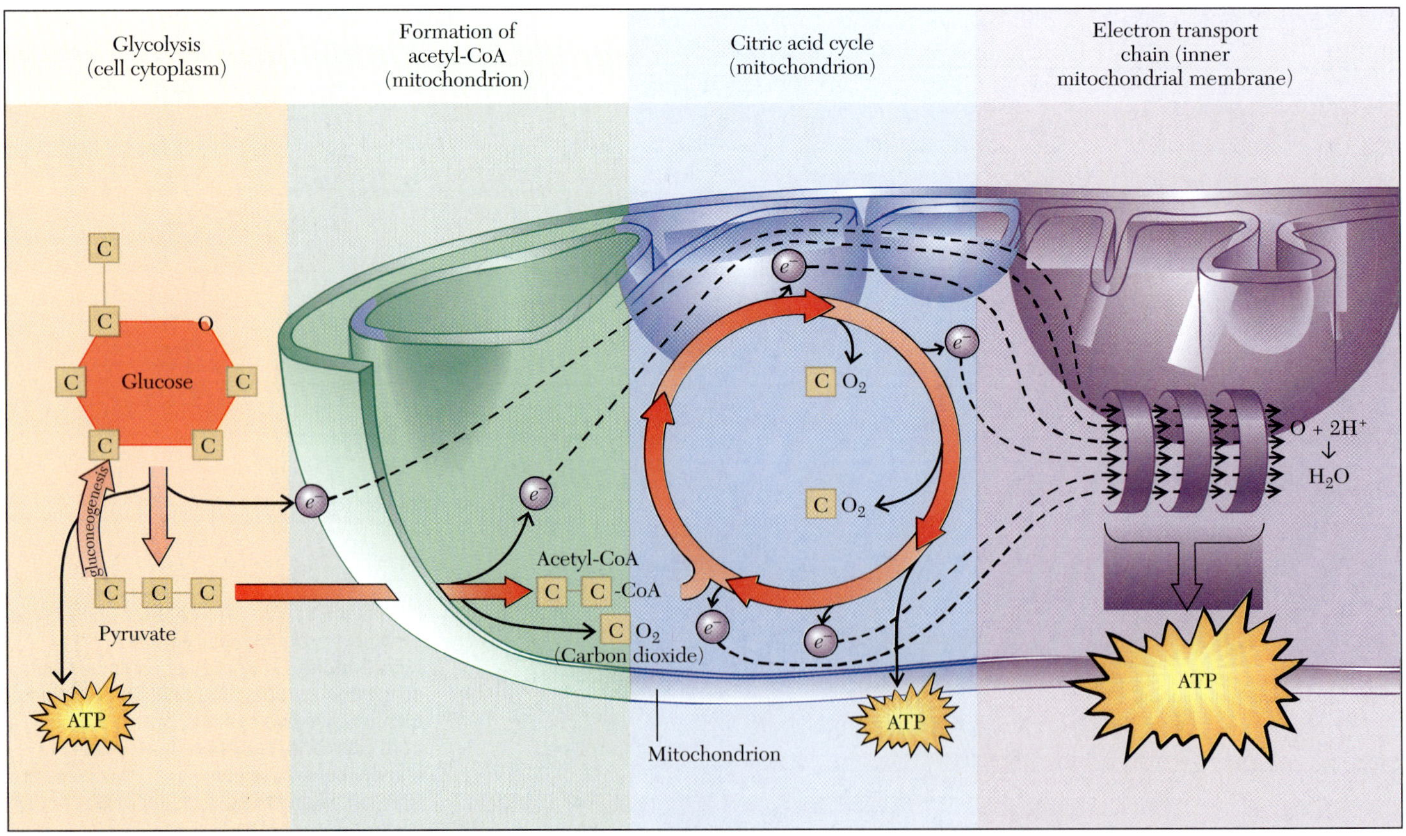

FIGURE 4.19 An overview of glucose metabolism. In the cytoplasm, glycolysis breaks glucose into two 3-carbon pyruvate molecules that enter the mitochondria, where they are converted into acetyl-CoA, which enters the citric acid cycle. High-energy electrons are released and transferred to the electron transport chain, where their energy is trapped to produce ATP.

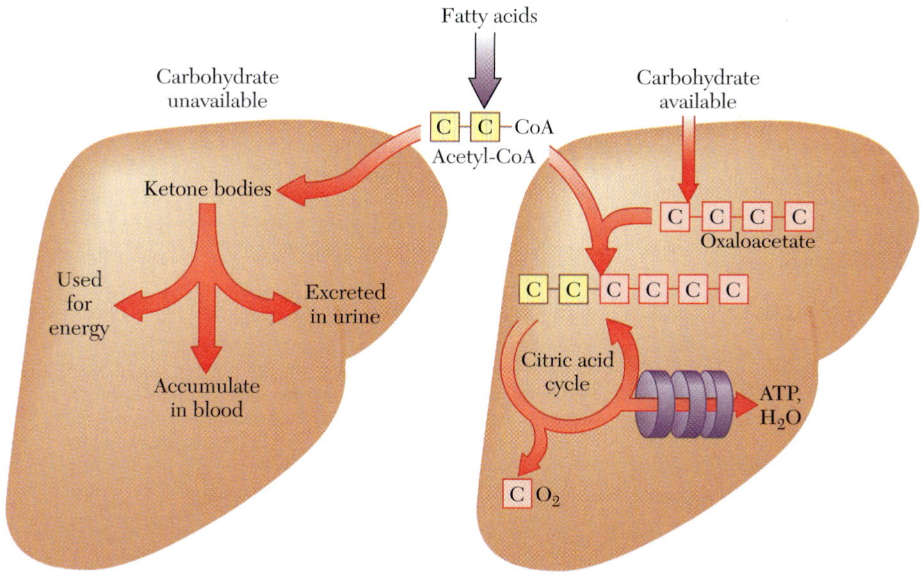

FIGURE 4.20 The availability of carbohydrate determines how fatty acids are metabolized. If carbohydrate is available, acetyl-CoA can combine with oxaloacetate to form glucose as is shown on the right of this figure. If carbohydrate is in short supply (as shown on the left), oxaloacetate will be limited. Acetyl-CoA from fatty acid breakdown will therefore not be able to enter the citric acid cycle. Instead, the liver uses it to make ketone bodies.

Fat Breakdown Carbohydrate is needed in order to completely break down fat to produce energy. Normally there is sufficient carbohydrate available to meet this need. When carbohydrate is available, acetyl-CoA (from fatty acid breakdown) can combine with oxaloacetate (derived from carbohydrate metabolism) and be metabolized via the citric acid cycle and electron transport chain to produce energy, carbon dioxide, and water. When carbohydrate intake is very low (generally less than 50 g per day) or when food intake in general is low, there is not sufficient oxaloacetate in the liver, so acetyl-CoA cannot be completely metabolized. Instead, the liver converts it into compounds known as **ketones** or **ketone bodies** (Figure 4.20).

Ketones or **ketone bodies** Molecules formed in the liver when there is not sufficient carbohydrate to completely metabolize the acetyl-CoA produced from fat breakdown.

The liver releases ketones into the blood. Ketones can be used as an energy source by tissues, such as those in the heart, muscle, and kidney. Ketone production is a normal response to starvation or to a diet very low in carbohydrate. Even the brain, which requires glucose, can adapt to obtain a portion of its energy from ketones.

Excess ketones are excreted by the kidney in urine. However, if fluid intake is too low to produce enough urine to excrete ketones, or if ketone production is high, ketones can build up in the blood, causing ketosis. Mild ketosis, which may occur during moderate energy restriction, such as might occur with a weight-loss diet, causes symptoms including headache, dry mouth, foul-smelling breath, and a reduction in appetite. High ketone levels, such as might occur with untreated diabetes (see following discussion), increase the acidity of the blood (ketoacidosis) and can result in coma and death.

Regulating Blood Glucose

In order to provide a steady supply of glucose to cells, the concentration of glucose in the blood is regulated by the liver and by hormones secreted from the pancreas. Normally, fasting blood glucose, which is measured after an 8- to 12-hour overnight fast, is maintained between about 60 to 100 mg per 100 ml of blood, or 70 to 110 mg per 100 ml of **plasma.** Maintaining this level ensures adequate glucose will be available to body cells. A steady supply of glucose is particularly important for nerve and red blood cells because these cells rely almost exclusively on glucose as an energy source.

Plasma The liquid portion of the blood that remains when the blood cells are removed.

Glycemic Response Blood glucose levels rise after carbohydrate is consumed. How quickly and how high blood glucose levels rise after a meal or a food is consumed and how quickly the body responds to bring levels back to normal is

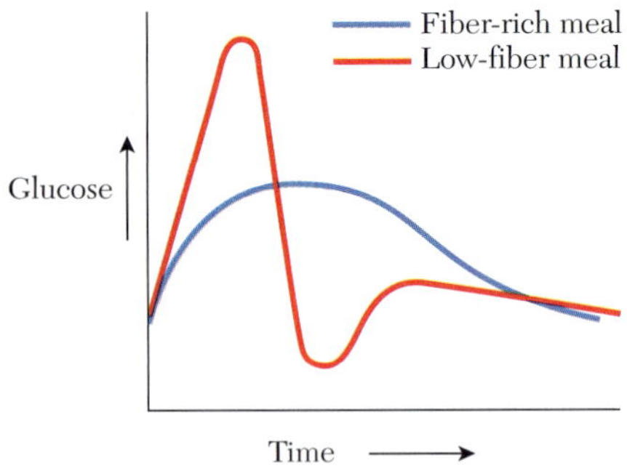

FIGURE 4.21 The fiber content of food affects the rise in blood glucose that occurs after a meal. After a high-carbohydrate, low-fiber meal, blood glucose rises rapidly. Consuming a fiber-rich meal slows the rise in blood glucose.

TABLE 4.3 Glycemic Index of Selected Foods

Food	Glycemic Index*	Food	Glycemic Index*
White bread	*100*	Rice, brown	79
White potatoes	121	Banana	76
Cornflakes	119	Green peas	68
Jelly beans	114	Spaghetti	59
Wheat bread	97	Milk, skim	46
Sugared soda	97	Kidney beans	42
Angel food cake	95	Milk, whole	39
Rice, white	83	Peanuts	21

*The glycemic index values are determined by comparing the rise in blood sugar following the consumption of a test food with the rise in blood sugar following consumption of a reference food (here, white bread; score = 100). The amount of the test food is chosen such that it contains the same amount of carbohydrate as the portion of the reference food.

Foster-Powell, K., and Miller, J. B. International tables of glycemic index. Am. J. Clin. Nutr. 62:871S–893S, 1995.

Glycemic response The rate, magnitude, and duration of the rise in blood glucose that occurs after a meal or a food is consumed.

Glycemic index A ranking of the effect on blood glucose of a food of a certain carbohydrate content relative to an equal amount of carbohydrate from a reference food such as white bread or glucose.

referred to as the **glycemic response.** This is affected by the composition of the foods that are consumed, the amount that is consumed, and the health of the consumer. Consuming sugar alone, such as in a sugar-sweetened soft drink, will cause blood glucose to increase rapidly. The more carbohydrate consumed at one time, the greater the glycemic response. And, consuming carbohydrate in a meal containing fat, protein, and/or fiber will slow the rise in blood glucose by slowing the rate at which the stomach empties and therefore the rate at which glucose enters the small intestine, where it is absorbed. Fiber also forms viscous solutions that slow glucose absorption from the intestine (Figure 4.21). The **glycemic index** is a ranking of how specific foods affect blood glucose compared with the response of a reference food of similar carbohydrate content. The glycemic index of a food, such as green peas, that contains fiber and protein as well as carbohydrate is about half that of carbohydrate alone. The glycemic index is also influenced by the type of starch (amylose or amylopectin) in the food, the way the food is processed, the physical structure of the food, and the other macronutrients in the food (Table 4.3).

Insulin A hormone made in the pancreas that allows the uptake and use of glucose by body cells and has other metabolic effects such as stimulating the synthesis of glycogen in liver and muscle.

Blood Glucose After Eating A rise in blood glucose triggers the pancreas to secrete the hormone **insulin,** which allows glucose to be taken into body cells to be metabolized for energy or stored. In muscle cells, insulin stimulates the uptake of glucose for energy production and the synthesis of muscle glycogen for energy storage. In lipid-storing cells, insulin increases glucose uptake from the blood and stimulates lipid synthesis. In liver cells, insulin allows glucose to be used and promotes the storage of glucose as glycogen, and, to a lesser extent, lipid. All of these actions remove glucose from the blood, decreasing levels to the normal range (Figure 4.22).

Glucagon A hormone made in the pancreas that stimulates the breakdown of liver glycogen and the synthesis of glucose to increase blood sugar.

Epinephrine The primary hormone produced by the adrenal medulla. It stimulates functions such as heart rate and respiratory rate that are important for conditions of stress, injury, emotional excitement, and strenuous physical activity. Also called adrenaline.

Blood Glucose Between Meals If no carbohydrate has been eaten for a few hours, the glucose level in the blood—and consequently the glucose available to the cells—begins to decrease. This triggers the pancreas to secrete the hormone **glucagon** (see Figure 4.22). Glucagon signals liver cells to break down glycogen into glucose, which is released into the bloodstream. Glucagon also stimulates the liver to synthesize new glucose molecules, via gluconeogenesis. Newly synthesized glucose is released into the blood to prevent blood glucose from dropping below the normal range. Gluconeogenesis can also be stimulated by the hormone **epinephrine,** also known as adrenaline. This hormone, which is released in response to dangerous or stressful situations, enables the body to respond to emergencies. It causes a rapid release of glucose into the blood to supply the energy needed for action.

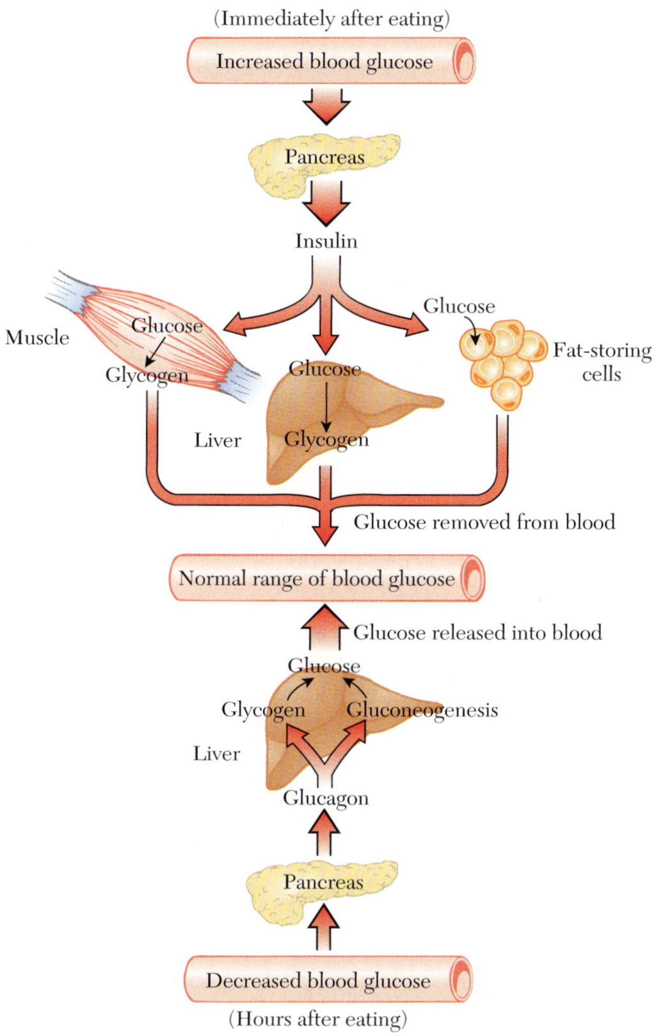

FIGURE 4.22 Blood glucose is regulated by hormones secreted by the pancreas. Immediately after eating, when blood glucose increases, insulin is released and stimulates the uptake and storage of glucose. Several hours after eating, when blood glucose levels begin to decrease, glucagon is released and stimulates the breakdown of glycogen into glucose and glucose production via gluconeogenesis.

Abnormal Blood Glucose Regulation

Insulin, glucagon, and other hormones normally regulate blood glucose levels. Abnormal blood glucose levels can result from either abnormal levels of these hormones or abnormal responses to these hormones. When glucose homeostasis is not maintained and blood glucose levels rise above the normal range, as occurs in diabetes, or drop below the normal range, as occurs in hypoglycemia, overall health is affected.

Diabetes

Diabetes mellitus is a disease in which blood glucose levels are elevated due to either a lack of insulin or an unresponsiveness of body cells to insulin. It is a major public health problem in the United States today, accounting for about $98 billion in direct medical costs and indirect costs due to disability, lost work, and premature death.[10] The elevated blood glucose causes damage to the large blood vessels, leading to an increased risk of heart disease and stroke.[11] It also causes changes in small blood vessels and nerves, leading to kidney failure, blindness, nerve dysfunction, and amputations. In the United States, diabetes is the leading cause of blindness in adults and accounts for 40% of all new cases of kidney failure and over half of all lower-limb amputations.[12]

Web Menu: For more information about diabetes and its diagnosis and management, go to the American Diabetes Association at www.diabetes.org/.

Diabetes mellitus A group of metabolic diseases characterized by high blood glucose levels resulting from defects in insulin secretion, insulin action, or both.

Type 1 diabetes A form of diabetes that is caused by the autoimmune destruction of insulin-producing cells in the pancreas, usually leading to absolute insulin deficiency; previously known as insulin-dependent diabetes mellitus or juvenile-onset diabetes.

Type 2 diabetes A form of diabetes that is characterized by insulin resistance and usually relative (rather than absolute) insulin deficiency; previously known as noninsulin-dependent diabetes mellitus or adult-onset diabetes.

Classification **Type 1 diabetes** is a form of diabetes that is usually diagnosed before the age of 30. It accounts for only about 5 to 10% of diagnosed cases.[13] What triggers this disease is unknown, but it is believed to be an autoimmune disease in which the immune system attacks the insulin-secreting cells of the pancreas. When these cells have been damaged or destroyed, insulin production is reduced or absent.

Type 2 diabetes is the more common form of diabetes.[13] It affects almost 16 million adults in the United States, and as many as 50% of these cases are undiagnosed.[12] The incidence is higher among minority groups, particularly African Americans, Hispanic Americans, and Native Americans.[12] Type 2 diabetes is believed to be due to a combination of genetic and lifestyle factors. Risk is increased in individuals who are overweight, in those who have a body type with more fat in the abdominal region, and in those with a family history of diabetes. This form of diabetes usually appears in persons over the age of 40, but lifestyle and dietary factors in the United States such as inactivity and excess body weight have contributed to an increasing incidence among younger individuals. In type 2 diabetes, insulin secretion may be low, normal, or even elevated, but blood glucose levels are high because body cells are insensitive to the effects of insulin.[13] Large amounts of insulin are therefore required to allow cells to take up enough glucose to meet their energy needs.

Gestational diabetes Any degree of glucose intolerance that begins or is first recognized during pregnancy.

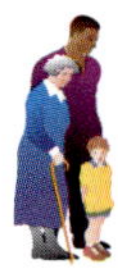

Gestational diabetes is a form of diabetes that occurs in women during pregnancy. It may be caused by the hormonal changes that occur during pregnancy and typically occurs between the 24th and 28th weeks of pregnancy, when the maternal demand for insulin is increased. The high levels of glucose in the mother's blood increase the risk of complications for the fetus (see Chapter 15). Gestational diabetes usually disappears once the pregnancy is complete and hormones return to nonpregnant levels. However, individuals who have had gestational diabetes have an increased risk for developing type 2 diabetes later in life.[14]

Diagnosis Diabetes is diagnosed by the presence of elevated blood glucose levels; greater than 126 mg of glucose per 100 ml of plasma after 8 hours without food (Figure 4.23). A fasting blood glucose level of 70 to 110 mg per 100 ml of plasma is considered normal. A blood glucose level that is higher than normal but not high enough to be classified as diabetes is referred to as impaired glucose tolerance or impaired fasting glucose. Impaired glucose tolerance affects more people than both type 1 and type 2 diabetes combined. It is an important public health concern because affected persons have an increased risk of developing diabetes and cardiovascular disease.

Effects Insulin is the hormone that is primarily responsible for the metabolism and storage of ingested body fuels. In diabetes, insulin is unavailable or ineffective, so glucose cannot be used normally. Cells that require insulin to take up glucose are starved for glucose. Cells that can use glucose without insulin are exposed to damaging levels of glucose.

Short-Term Effects The symptoms of diabetes may include excessive thirst, frequent urination, blurred vision, and weight loss. Excessive thirst and frequent urination occur because blood glucose levels rise so high that the kidneys excrete glucose, drawing fluid with it and increasing urinary output. Blurred vision occurs when excess glucose enters the lens of the eye, causing it to swell. Weight loss and impaired growth in children occur because glucose cannot be used for energy, so the body breaks down fat and protein to supply fuel.

Low levels of insulin or tissue insensitivity to insulin have short-term metabolic effects in the liver, muscles, and adipose tissue. The liver is unable to use glucose when insulin levels are inadequate. This leads to the production of glucose, via gluconeogenesis, that is released into the bloodstream and the use of fatty acids as an energy source. With limited carbohydrate for fatty acid metabolism, ketones are formed and released into the blood. Some ketones are used as fuel by muscle and adipose tissue, but in type 1 diabetes, they are produced more rapidly than they can be used and thus accumulate in the blood, possibly leading

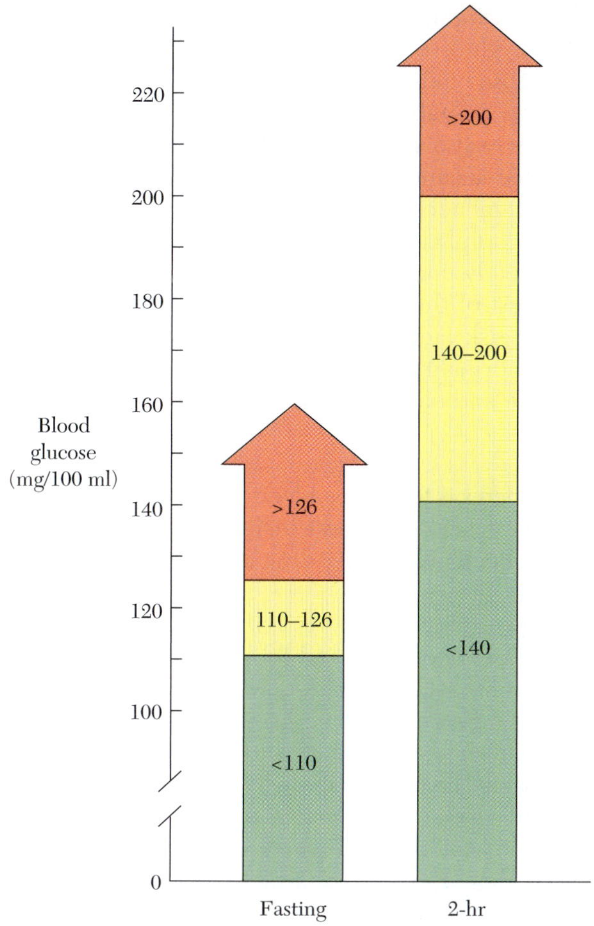

FIGURE 4.23 Blood glucose levels are used to diagnose diabetes. After an 8-hour fast, normal blood glucose is less than 110 mg/100 ml. Impaired fasting glucose is defined as a fasting blood glucose between 110 and 126 mg/100 ml and diabetes is defined as a fasting blood glucose greater than 126 mg/100 ml. Blood glucose measured two hours after consuming 75 g of glucose is normally less than 140 mg/100 ml. Impaired glucose tolerance is defined as a blood glucose level between 140 and 200 mg/100 ml two hours after a glucose load and diabetes is defined as a blood glucose greater than 200 mg/100 ml two hours after a glucose load. (*American Diabetes Association at* http://www.diabetes.org/diabetescare/supplement/98/s2.htm)

to diabetic ketoacidosis. In type 2 diabetes, ketoacidosis usually does not develop because there is enough insulin to allow some glucose to be used. Consequently, fewer ketones are produced.

Without adequate insulin, glucose cannot enter muscle or adipose tissue cells. As a result, glycogen is broken down in muscle to supply glucose. When the glycogen is depleted, muscle protein is broken down to provide amino acids for gluconeogenesis; the muscle uses fatty acids and ketones to meet energy needs. Adipose tissue responds to low insulin levels and the presence of glucagon by releasing fatty acids into the blood.

Long-Term Complications Long-term complications associated with elevated levels of blood glucose include damage to the nerves, blood vessels, and kidneys, and an increased risk of heart disease (Figure 4.24). The tissue damage is thought to

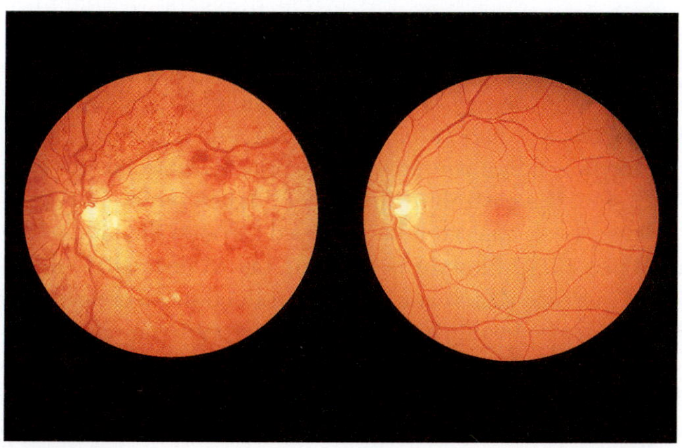

FIGURE 4.24 The retina of the eye is damaged by diabetes. (left) Damaged blood vessels in the retina caused by diabetes. (right) Normal blood vessels in the retina of the eye. (© *SBHA/Tony Stone Images, Inc.*)

be a result of exposure to high levels of glucose. Cells such as kidney and nerve cells that do not require insulin for glucose uptake, receive too much glucose when blood levels are elevated. Glucose binds to proteins and alters cell function, contributing to blood vessel damage and abnormalities in blood cell function. High levels of glucose in the cells may also cause damage because some is converted to polyols (sugar alcohols) that accumulate inside cells. Polyol accumulation can affect the function of peripheral nerves.

The most common long-term complication of diabetes is atherosclerosis. The reasons for this are not completely understood. Diabetics develop hypertension more frequently than the rest of the population and have an increased prevalence of other cardiovascular risk factors. High blood glucose and hormonal irregularities may cause abnormalities in the arterial wall, changes in white blood cells and blood clotting, and elevated blood lipids, all of which accelerate atherosclerosis.

Treatment The goal in treating diabetes is to reduce blood glucose to within the normal range and maintain it at that level. Treatment includes a modified diet, regular exercise, and, often, insulin injections or other drug therapy.

Diet To maintain normal blood glucose in either type 1 or type 2 diabetes, the amount of carbohydrate consumed at any one time and throughout the day must be controlled. Recommendations no longer restrict just sugar intake but rather suggest that total carbohydrate consumption be limited—whether the source is sucrose, fructose (which causes a smaller rise in blood glucose than sucrose), or starch. Carbohydrate consumption must be coordinated with medication and exercise schedules so that glucose and insulin are available in the proper proportions at the same time to maintain normal blood glucose levels. The diet can be planned based on either the Exchange Lists or on a system of carbohydrate counting (see Appendix I).[15] The diet must be adequate in energy and micronutrients, and protein should provide 10 to 20% of energy. To help maintain normal blood cholesterol and triglyceride levels and retard the development of atherosclerosis, the diet should meet the Dietary Guidelines recommendation of no more than 30% of energy from fat, with no more than 10% from saturated fat, and 300 mg or less of cholesterol each day. A high-fiber diet including 20 to 35 g of fiber per day is recommended because fiber reduces the glycemic response of a meal, may increase tissue insulin sensitivity, and can lower cardiovascular disease risk.[16] For overweight individuals, energy restriction can promote weight loss and be beneficial for maintaining blood glucose levels in the normal range.[15] Adherence to this type of dietary regimen, along with monitoring of blood glucose levels throughout the day, can reduce the incidence of elevated blood glucose levels and the complications it causes.

Exercise Exercise is an important component of diabetes management because it can improve glucose tolerance and increase the sensitivity of body cells to insulin. Because exercise can reduce blood glucose levels, individuals with diabetes are encouraged to maintain regular exercise patterns. A change in the amount of exercise an individual participates in may change the amount of insulin required.

Drug Therapy Drug therapy can involve insulin injections and oral medications to reduce blood glucose levels. In type 1 diabetes, insulin production is low or absent, so insulin must be provided. It is administered by injection because insulin is a protein that would be digested in the gastrointestinal tract if taken orally. In type 2 diabetes, normal blood glucose levels can often be achieved through diet and exercise without medication. When these lifestyle treatments fail to normalize blood sugar, oral medications that increase pancreatic insulin production, decrease glucose production in the liver, enhance insulin action, or slow carbohydrate digestion can be used. In about 40% of type 2 diabetes cases, insulin must be injected to achieve normal blood glucose levels.

Education Even careful adherence to diet, exercise, and drug therapy cannot prevent the long-term complications of diabetes, but the onset of these complications can be delayed and their progression slowed by good diabetic control—that is, keeping blood glucose levels within the normal range. The importance of good diabetic control was demonstrated by the Diabetes Control and Complications Trial. This study documented that improved diabetic control in type 1 diabetes decreased the development of diabetic eye complication, kidney disease, and nerve dysfunction.[17] Based on these findings, the National Institutes of Health and the Centers for Disease Control and Prevention have established the National Diabetes Education Program to reduce disability and death associated with diabetes.[18] This program is designed to increase public awareness of the seriousness of diabetes, promote better management among individuals with diabetes, and improve the quality of and access to health care.

Hypoglycemia

Hypoglycemia, or low blood glucose, is a common side effect of insulin therapy, but it may also result from abnormalities in the production of or response to insulin or other hormones involved in blood sugar regulation. The symptoms of hypoglycemia include low blood glucose, along with irritability, nervousness, sweating, shakiness, anxiety, rapid heartbeat, headache, hunger, weakness, and sometimes seizure and coma.

Hypoglycemia A low blood glucose level, usually below 40 to 50 mg of glucose per 100 ml of blood.

There are two forms of hypoglycemia. Reactive hypoglycemia occurs in response to the consumption of high-carbohydrate foods. In individuals with reactive hypoglycemia, the rise in blood glucose from the carbohydrate stimulates excess secretion of insulin and other hormones related to blood glucose regulation. Too much insulin is secreted or insulin levels remain elevated too long, resulting in a fall in blood glucose to an abnormally low level. The treatment for reactive hypoglycemia is a diet that prevents rapid changes in blood glucose. Small, frequent meals low in simple carbohydrates and high in protein and fiber are recommended. The second form of hypoglycemia, fasting hypoglycemia, is not related to food intake. In this disorder, abnormal insulin secretion results in episodes of low blood glucose levels. This condition is often caused by pancreatic tumors.

Carbohydrates and Health

Guidelines for a healthy diet recommend that Americans base their diet on foods rich in carbohydrates. Yet, it has been suggested that the consumption of carbohydrates is related to a host of chronic health problems from dental caries to heart disease, diabetes, obesity, and hyperactivity. This incongruity is due to differences in the health effects of different forms of dietary carbohydrates. Foods high in unrefined carbohydrates, particularly whole grains, vegetables, and fruits, are good sources of fiber, micronutrients, and phytochemicals. A dietary pattern that is high in these foods has been associated with a lower incidence of a variety of chronic diseases, including certain bowel disorders, colon cancer, heart disease, and diabetes.[19] On the other hand, diets high in refined carbohydrates may contribute to chronic disease risk.[20]

Web Menu

Go to the American Dental Association Oral Health Topics A–Z at www.ada.org/public/topics/ for information on oral health and hygiene.

Carbohydrates and Dental Caries

The most well-documented health problem directly associated with carbohydrate intake is dental caries, or tooth cavities. Dental caries are formed when bacteria that live in the mouth metabolize carbohydrate from the diet and produce acid. The acid can then dissolve the enamel and underlying structure of the teeth. Simple carbohydrates, particularly sucrose, are the most rapidly utilized food source for these microbes; however, any carbohydrate-containing foods that stick to the teeth can also cause cavities. The length of time that carbohydrate is in contact with the teeth determines the likelihood that a cavity will develop. Certain foods, such as sticky candies, cereals, crackers, and cookies, tend to remain on the teeth longer, providing a continuous supply of nutrients to decay-causing bacteria. Other foods, such as chocolate, ice cream, and bananas, are rapidly washed away from the teeth. Frequent snacking also increases contact time by providing a continuous food supply for the bacteria. Limiting sugar intake can help prevent dental caries, but because starch is eventually metabolized into acid, proper dental hygiene is important even if the diet is low in sugar.[21]

Carbohydrates and Heart Disease

Diets high in whole grains and fiber from cereals have been found to reduce the risk of heart disease.[9,22,23,24] There are a number of possible reasons for this beneficial effect. Diets high in fiber-rich foods are high in micronutrients and phytochemicals—some of which may reduce the risk of heart disease (see Chapters 5 and 10). And, this dietary pattern is relatively low in simple carbohydrates. Simple carbohydrates may increase fatty acid synthesis and lower levels of HDL cholesterol ("good" cholesterol) in the blood, and therefore increase the risk of cardiovascular disease.[25,26]

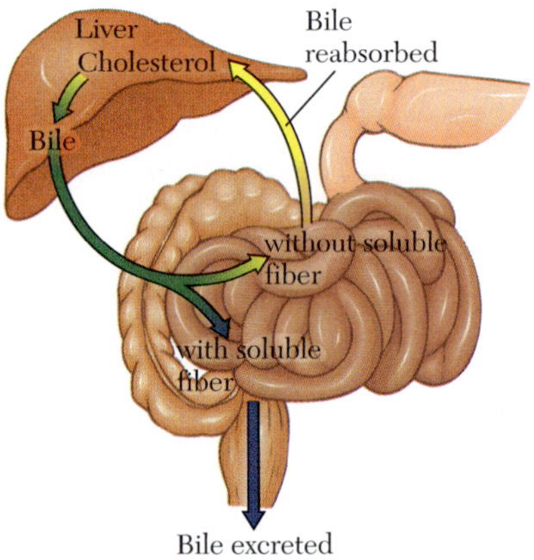

FIGURE 4.25 When the diet is low in soluble fiber, bile, which contains cholesterol and bile acids made from cholesterol, is absorbed and returned to the liver. When soluble fiber is present, it binds cholesterol and bile acids so they are excreted rather than absorbed.

Diets high in fiber-rich foods can reduce blood cholesterol levels, reducing the risk of heart disease.[9] Studies in humans indicate that soluble fiber such as that in legumes, rice and oat bran, guar gum, pectin, flax seed, and psyllium are more effective at lowering blood cholesterol levels than insoluble fibers such as wheat bran or cellulose.[9] Consumption of about 10 g of psyllium per day was found to lower total cholesterol by 4% and LDL cholesterol ("bad" cholesterol) by 7% and to have no effect on HDL cholesterol.[27] The reduction in blood cholesterol levels may be due to the ability of soluble fibers to bind cholesterol and bile acids, which are made from cholesterol, in the digestive tract. Normally, bile acids secreted into the GI tract are absorbed and reused. When bound to fiber, cholesterol and bile acids are excreted in the feces rather than being absorbed. The liver will then use cholesterol from the blood to synthesize new bile acids. This provides a mechanism for eliminating cholesterol from the body and reducing blood cholesterol levels (Figure 4.25). Soluble fiber may also lower cholesterol because the microbial degradation of soluble fiber produces short-chain fatty acids that can travel to the liver and inhibit cholesterol synthesis.[28] The FDA permits a health claim on food products containing either soluble fiber from psyllium seed husk or beta-glucan (found in whole oats) that states that these soluble fibers may reduce the risk of coronary heart disease.

Carbohydrate Intake and Diabetes

A dietary pattern that is high in refined starches and added sugars causes a greater glycemic response and therefore increases the amount of insulin needed to maintain normal blood glucose levels.[29] Evidence is emerging that long-term consumption of this dietary pattern may increase the risk of developing type 2 diabetes.[30,31] Epidemiological studies have shown that diabetes is rare in populations consuming a diet high in unrefined grains.[16] A correlation between low fiber intake and a higher prevalence of diabetes has also been identified among individuals within a population.[30] So although a diet high in simple carbohydrate does not cause diabetes, it does increase the demand for insulin required to maintain normal glucose levels, and may increase the risk of developing diabetes.

Carbohydrates and Obesity

Obesity is caused by consuming more energy than is expended. When energy (whether it is in the form of carbohydrate, protein, fat, or alcohol) is consumed in excess of needs, body weight will increase. Therefore, high intakes of carbohydrate do not directly cause obesity. And, because, gram for gram, carbohydrate (4 kcal/g) is lower in energy than fat (9 kcal/g), and because excess carbohydrate in the diet is less efficient at producing body fat than excess fat, carbohydrate is less "fattening" than fat (see Chapter 7).

One reason carbohydrates have been suggested to promote weight gain is that carbohydrates, eaten alone or in large quantities, increase secretion of the hormone insulin, which in turn has been hypothesized to stimulate food cravings, promote fat storage, and ultimately cause weight gain. Studies on the effect of sugar intake on food intake do not support this hypothesis. The effect of sugar consumption on overall food intake is consistent with what would be predicted by its energy content.[32] And, the sugar intakes of obese individuals are not different than normal-weight individuals.[33] Some research even supports the conclusion that obese individuals eat less sugar than normal-weight people and that sugar intake is inversely related to body weight.[32] Despite evidence to the contrary, a number of popular weight-loss diets recommend restricting carbohydrate intake based on this hypothesis (see *Making Decisions:* "Should You Be Eating a Low-Carbohydrate Diet?" and Chapter 8).

There is some evidence that an abnormal craving for carbohydrate-rich foods is a component of a variety of disorders including obesity, premenstrual syndrome, bulimia, depression, and seasonal affective disorder.[34,35] One theory proposed to explain carbohydrate craving is that these individuals have an abnormality in the regulation of brain levels of the neurotransmitter serotonin. This abnormality causes them to seek carbohydrate like a drug to increase serotonin levels and improve their mood.

Sugar and Hyperactivity

The consumption of sugary foods has been suggested as a cause of hyperactivity in children (see Chapter 16). The increase in blood glucose after a meal high in simple carbohydrates is hypothesized to provide the energy for the excessive activities of a hyperactive child. However, research on sugar intake and behavior has failed to support the hypothesis that sugar contributes to behavioral changes.[36] Hyperactive behavior that is observed after sugar consumption is likely the result of other circumstances in that child's life. For example, the excitement of a birthday party rather than the cake is more likely the cause of hyperactive behavior. Other situations that might cause hyperactivity include lack of sleep, overstimulation, caffeine consumption, the desire for more attention, or lack of physical activity.

Web Menu

For information on diverticulosis and diverticulitis, go to the National Institute of Diabetes & Digestive & Kidney Diseases at www.niddk.nih.gov/ and click on digestive or the American College of Gastroenterology at www.acg.gi.org/ and click on patient information.

Fiber and Chronic Bowel Disorders

High-fiber diets can relieve or prevent some chronic bowel disorders. Fiber adds bulk and absorbs water, making the feces larger and softer and reducing the amount of pressure needed for defecation. This helps to reduce the incidence of constipation and **hemorrhoids.** Too much fiber, however, can affect nutrient absorption and cause gastrointestinal discomfort.

Diverticulosis Reducing the pressure in the lumen of the colon can also reduce the possibility of developing **diverticulosis,** a condition in which the intestinal wall forms outpouches called diverticula (Figure 4.26). In the United States, about 50% of elderly people have diverticulosis. Fecal matter may occasionally accumulate in these outpouches, causing irritation, pain, inflammation, and infection. This condition is known as diverticulitis. Treatment of diverticulitis usually

C 62 00 00 00 00 00 27 22

C 62 00 00 00 00 00 27 23

Hemorrhoids Swollen veins in the anal or rectal area.

Diverticulosis The presence of sacs or pouches called diverticula (singular, "diverticulum") that protrude from the wall of the large intestine. When these become inflamed, the condition is called diverticulitis.

Making Decisions

Should You Be Eating a Low-Carbohydrate Diet?

Should you be eating a low-carbohydrate diet? The Dietary Guidelines, Daily Values, and the Food Guide Pyramid recommend a diet that provides about 55 to 60% of energy from carbohydrates. Yet, as Americans are attempting to incorporate these recommendations into their eating patterns, the incidence of obesity continues to rise and chronic disease remains a major public health problem. Are these recommendations healthy? Do they promote weight gain? There are those who believe that some of the health problems in the United States, including obesity, are due to our high carbohydrate intake. Their theories have made low-carbohydrate diets the current rage. The Atkins diet has been promoting low-carbohydrate diets for weight loss for 30 years and has recently gained renewed popularity along with a host of others programs promoting a reduction in carbohydrate intake for weight loss and improved health. Who should you believe?

The high-carbohydrate recommendations of the Dietary Guidelines, Daily Values, and the Food Guide Pyramid are based on the fact that diets high in complex carbohydrates from whole grains, fruits, and vegetables are high in micronutrients, phytochemicals, and fiber and low in fat and saturated fat. This dietary pattern has been correlated with a reduced incidence of gastrointestinal disease, heart disease, diabetes, and cancer.[a] And because carbohydrate has 4 kcalories per g, compared with fat at 9 kcalories per g, it would seem reasonable to recommend a high-carbohydrate, low-fat diet for weight loss. What then is the rationale for suggesting that a diet low in carbohydrate will improve your health and promote weight loss?

The premise of low-carbohydrate diets is that carbohydrate, eaten alone or in large quantities, triggers a rise in blood glucose, which in turn stimulates the release of insulin. Insulin is a hormone that is responsible for allowing glucose to enter cells and for stimulating the synthesis of fat. Therefore, proponents of these types of diets hypothesize that eating carbohydrate will stimulate hunger and overeating (because insulin causes blood glucose levels to drop) and promote an increase in body fat (because insulin stimulates fat storage). Consequently, restricting carbohydrate will prevent large rises in insulin levels, thereby reducing food cravings and fat storage.

Although some of the information upon which this hypothesis is based is correct, the physiology has been oversimplified. The effect of dietary carbohydrate on blood glucose and insulin and the role of insulin in the regulation of body weight are complicated. The rate and magnitude of the rise in blood glucose that occurs after the consumption of carbohydrate is affected by the structure of the carbohydrate, the food in which it is found, the way the food is cooked, what other foods are consumed in the meal, and the size and health status of the consumer. So simply assuming that carbohydrate causes high levels of insulin secretion is not necessarily accurate.

Some carbohydrates, particularly simple carbohydrates, do cause a rapid increase in blood glucose and insulin. But high-protein foods like eggs, cheese, and steak also cause insulin release. One study found that consuming a steak causes a greater rise in insulin than consuming the same number of kcalories as pasta.[b] There is research that supports the suggestion that a high-carbohydrate diet made up of high-glycemic-index foods will increase the amount of fat synthesized in adipose tissue.[c] However, these studies fed a diet that contained excess energy; total fat stores increase only when kcalories are consumed in excess of need. Scientific evidence also suggests that eating a diet of high-glycemic index foods increases the risk of chronic diseases, particularly heart disease and diabetes.[d] However, this research compares diets containing carbohydrate from high-glycemic-index foods to diets containing carbohydrate from whole grains and other fiber-rich foods. Diets low in total carbohydrate were not studied.

To assess the overall health effects of a low-carbohydrate diet, the total dietary pattern should be considered. Low-carbohydrate diets are based on a high intake of meat, meat products, and high-fat dairy products such as cheese—and limit the consumption of whole categories of foods such as whole grains, fruits, and most vegetables, because they are high in carbohydrate. This dietary pattern is high in protein, fat, saturated fat, and cholesterol. There is strong evidence that a diet high in saturated fat increases blood cholesterol and the risk of heart disease. There is also some evidence that a diet high in these foods may promote bone loss and damage the kidneys. The reduced consumption of whole grains, fruits, and vegetables is a dietary pattern associated with an increased risk of cancer, heart disease, and other chronic diseases.

The most common reason people try low-carbohydrate diets is to lose weight. These diets are perceived as more effective for weight loss for several reasons. First, they cause a rapid initial weight loss. This occurs because the lack of carbohydrate causes liver glycogen to be broken down, and the water stored with it to be released. Second, high-protein diets inhibit appetite. If you are not as hungry, you don't eat as much, and you lose weight. Finally, a diet based on meat is monotonous because the selection of allowed foods is quite small; intake decreases because the diet is boring, and weight loss follows.

So, will a low-carbohydrate diet promote weight loss? The answer is probably yes, but the weight loss is caused by the same thing that causes weight loss in other diets—it provides less energy than is expended. The overall rate of weight loss and the composition of weight loss are not different on low- versus high-carbohydrate diets.[e] But, is a low-carbohydrate diet a healthy diet? The answer is no, but a diet high in high-glycemic-index carbohydrates is also not healthy. A healthy dietary pattern should include whole grains, fruits, and vegetables.

References

[a] Slavin, J. L., Martini, M. C., Jacobs, D. R., Jr., et al. Plausible mechanism for protectiveness of whole grains Am. J. Clin, Nutr. 70(3 Suppl): 459S–463S, 1999.

[b] Holt, S. H., Miller, J. C., and Petocz, P. An insulin index of foods: the insulin demand generated by 100-kJ portions of common foods. Am. J. Clin. Nutr. 66:1264–1275, 1997.

[c] Aarsland, A., Chinkes, D., and Wolfe, R. R. Hepatic and whole body fat synthesis in humans during carbohydrate overfeeding. Am. J. Clin. Nutr. 65:1774–1782, 1997.

[d] Morris, K. L., and Zemel. M. B. Glycemic index, cardiovascular disease, and obesity. Nutr. Rev. 57:273–276, 1999.

[e] Galay, A., Allis, A. F., Morel, Y., et al. Similar weight loss with low- or high-carbohydrate diets. Am. J. Clin. Nutr. 63:174–178, 1996.

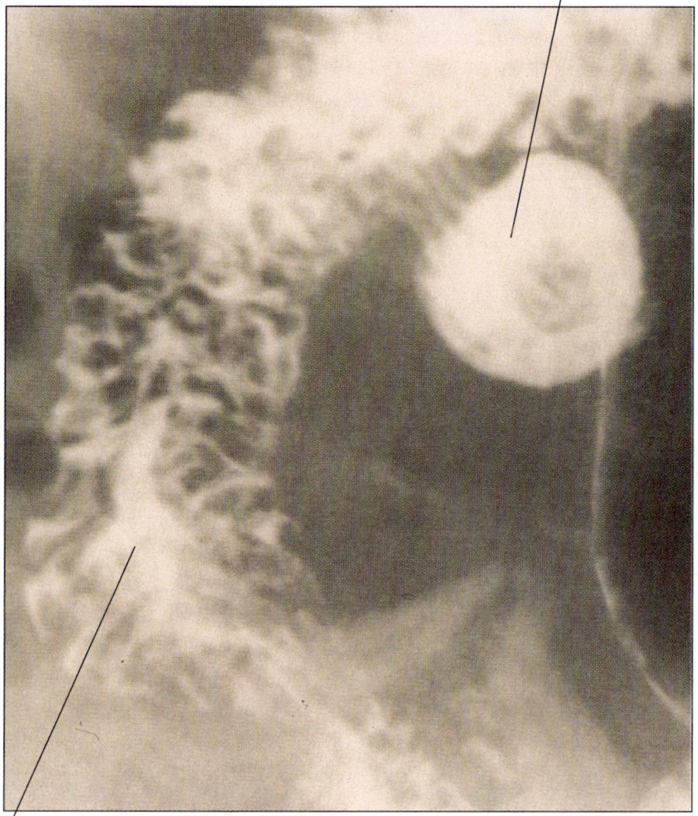

FIGURE 4.26 Diverticulum in the colon. (*L. V. Bergman/the Bergman Collection*)

includes antibiotics to reduce bacterial growth and a temporary decrease in fiber intake to prevent irritation of the inflamed tissues. Once the inflammation is resolved, however, a high-fiber diet is recommended to increase fecal bulk, decrease transit time, ease stool elimination, and reduce the possibility of future attacks.[9]

Problems with Excessive Fiber Intake Although a diet that meets the recommendation for fiber intake has many benefits, too much fiber can decrease the energy density of the diet, reduce nutrient absorption, and, if the diet is not adequate in fluid, cause constipation.

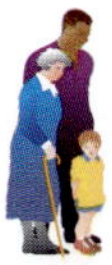

A high-fiber diet increases the volume of food needed to meet energy requirements. A person who has a small stomach capacity and consumes a diet that is very high in fiber may satisfy hunger before nutrient requirements are met. Generally this is only a problem when the diet is low in micronutrients or when young children, whose small stomachs limit the amount of food they can eat, consume high-fiber diets.

A high-fiber diet may decrease nutrient absorption for two reasons. First, the increase in the volume of intestinal contents caused by a high-fiber diet may prevent enzymes from coming in contact with food. If a food cannot be broken down, many of its components cannot be absorbed. Second, fiber may bind some micronutrients, preventing their absorption. For instance, wheat bran fiber binds the minerals zinc, calcium, magnesium, and iron, reducing their absorption. When mineral intake meets recommendations, a reasonable intake of high-fiber foods does not compromise mineral status.

A sudden increase in the fiber content of the diet can cause abdominal discomfort, gas, and diarrhea due to the bacterial breakdown of fiber. If fluid intake is too low, fiber can also cause constipation. The more fiber a diet includes, the more water is needed to keep the stool soft. When too little fluid is consumed, the stool becomes hard and difficult to eliminate. In severe cases when fiber intake is excessive and fluid intake is low, intestinal blockage can occur.[37] To avoid these problems, the fiber and fluid content of the diet should be increased gradually.

Fiber and Colon Cancer

Tumor initiator A substance that causes mutations and therefore may predispose a cell to becoming cancerous.

Tumor promoters Substances that stimulate a mutated cell to begin dividing.

Cells become cancerous as a result of mutations in their genetic material. The type of cancer depends on the type of cell that is originally affected—for example, lung, breast, or colon—and on how the genetic material is altered by the mutations. Most mutations are hypothesized to be caused by environmental factors, such as diet, tobacco use, or air pollution. In the case of the colon, mutations may be caused by substances consumed in the diet or produced in the gastrointestinal tract that come in contact with mucosal cells. Any substance that causes a potentially cancerous mutation is called a **tumor initiator.** For an affected cell to begin growing and dividing as a cancer cell, it must be exposed to **tumor promoters.** Although tumor promoters allow mutated cells to begin dividing, they do not cause mutations themselves.

Epidemiological studies have shown that the incidence of colon cancer is lower in populations consuming diets high in fiber.[9] Intervention trials have not been able to replicate these patterns by studying the effects of fiber supplements or of defined high-fiber, high-fruit and vegetable diets studied over the short term.[38,39] Nonetheless, the role of fiber in preventing the development of colon cancer is thought to be related to its ability to decrease contact between the mucosal cells of the large intestine and the fecal contents, which may contain tumor initiators or tumor promoters. Fiber increases fecal bulk, dilutes the colon contents, and speeds transit, thereby decreasing contact time between the mucosal cells and potentially cancer-causing substances. The presence of fiber in the colon also affects the intestinal microflora and the by-products of microbial metabolism, such as fatty acids, that accumulate there. These by-products may directly affect colon cells or may cause changes in the environment of the colon, such as pH, that may affect the development of colon cancer.[40] Some of the protective effect may also be due to the antioxidant vitamins and phytochemicals present in fiber-rich plant foods.

Meeting Carbohydrate Needs

Nutrition messages from the Dietary Guidelines, food labels, and the Food Guide Pyramid all recommend a diet high in unrefined carbohydrates and fiber and limited in refined carbohydrates. Planning a diet to meet these recommendations requires an understanding of the types and amounts of carbohydrate in our diets and in the food supply.

Recommendations for Carbohydrate Intake

There are currently no DRI values for carbohydrate or fiber; these are in the process of being developed. The 1989 RDAs suggest that a minimum of about 50 to 100 g of carbohydrate is needed to meet glucose needs and prevent ketosis. This amount is easily obtained. For example, two slices of toast and a cup of juice provide about 60 g. However, if only this small amount of carbohydrate is consumed, the total diet would be higher in fat and protein than is desirable.

The Daily Value used on food labels is based on the recommendation that the diet should provide 55 to 60% of energy as carbohydrate. This represents a slight increase from the typical intake in the United States of about 52% of energy. The Dietary Guidelines advise following the recommendations of the Food Guide Pyramid to plan a diet to meet this recommendation. They also encourage careful choices from the Pyramid food groups to increase consumption of whole grains while limiting the intake of beverages and foods that are high in refined sugars (Figure 4.27).

The recommended fiber intake in an adult diet is 10 to 13 g per 1000 kcalories or about 20 to 35 g per day. The Daily Value has been set at the midpoint—11.5 g per 1000 kcalories. This is greater than the amount typically consumed in the American diet of about 15 g per day.

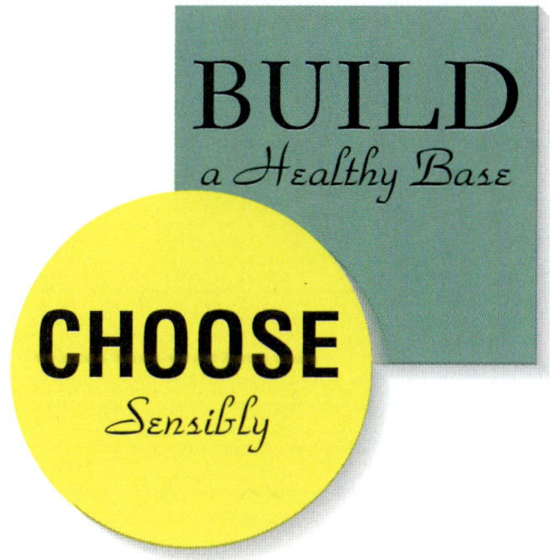

- Let the Pyramid guide your food choices.
- Choose a variety of grains daily, especially whole grains.
- Choose a variety of fruits and vegetables daily.
- Choose beverages and foods to moderate your intake of sugars.

FIGURE 4.27 The Dietary Guidelines for Americans make recommendations about the type and amount of carbohydrate in the diet. *(USDA, DHHS, 2000)*

Calculating Carbohydrate Intake

The recommendation for carbohydrate intake (55 to 60% of energy as carbohydrate) is based on energy intake. Table 4.4 illustrates how to calculate carbohydrate intake as a percent of energy. A similar calculation can be used to determine the percent of energy as carbohydrate in individual foods.

Computer databases and food composition tables (see Appendix A) provide information on the number of grams of carbohydrate and fiber contained in a wide variety of foods. Food labels provide a more accessible source of information on packaged foods. The Exchange Lists can be used to quickly estimate the total amount of carbohydrate in a food or in the diet (Table 4.5). The Exchange Lists cannot be used to calculate fiber, but Table 4.6 offers an exchange system for estimating fiber in foods.

TABLE 4.4 Calculating Percent Energy from Carbohydrate

Determine

- The total energy (kcalorie) intake for the day
- The grams of carbohydrate in the day's diet

Calculate Energy from Carbohydrate

- Carbohydrate provides 4 kcalories per g
- Multiply grams of carbohydrate by 4 kcalories per g

$$\text{Kcalories from carbohydrate} = \text{grams carbohydrate} \times 4 \text{ kcalories/gram carbohydrate}$$

Calculate % Energy from Carbohydrate

- Divide energy from carbohydrate by total energy and multiply by 100 to express as a percent

$$\text{Percent of energy from carbohydrate} = \frac{\text{kcalories from carbohydrate}}{\text{total kcalories}} \times 100$$

For example:

A diet contains 2500 kcalories and 350 g of carbohydrate

$$350 \text{ g of carbohydrate} \times 4 \text{ kcal/g} = 1400 \text{ kcal of carbohydrate}$$

$$\frac{1400 \text{ kcal of carbohydrate}}{2500 \text{ kcal}} \times 100 = 56\% \text{ of energy (kcal) from carbohydrate}$$

TABLE 4.5 Carbohydrate Content of the Exchange Lists

Exchange Groups/Lists	Serving Size	Carbohydrate (g)
Carbohydrate Group		
Starch	1/2 cup pasta, rice, cereal, potatoes; 1 slice bread	15
Fruit	1 small apple, peach, pear; 1/2 banana; 1/2 cup canned fruit (in juice)	15
Milk	1 cup milk or yogurt	
Nonfat		12
Low-fat		12
Reduced fat		12
Whole		12
Other carbohydrates	Serving sizes vary	15
Vegetables	1/2 cup cooked vegetables, 1 cup raw	5
Meat/Meat Substitute Group	1 oz meat or cheese, 1/2 cup legumes	
Very lean		0
Lean		0
Medium-fat		0
High-fat		0
Fat Group	1 tsp butter, margarine, or oil; 1 Tbsp salad dressing	0

A Diet to Meet Recommendations

Choosing a diet that provides 55 to 60% of energy as carbohydrate, that includes many whole foods, and that limits consumption of foods high in refined sugars seems complicated. But choosing carefully from the groups of the Food Guide Pyramid and using food labels to learn the composition of foods can provide a diet that meets these specifications (see *Critical Thinking:* "Meeting Carbohydrate Recommendations").

Carbohydrates in the Food Guide Pyramid A diet that follows the serving recommendations of the Food Guide Pyramid will be based on plant foods with smaller proportions of animal products. The shape of the Pyramid reflects these recommendations—the food groups made up of high carbohydrate plant foods are at the broad base of the Pyramid. A greater number of servings per day is recommended from these groups than those higher in the Pyramid. Six to eleven servings should be selected from the Bread, Cereal, Rice, and Pasta Group at the base of the Pyramid. Whole-grain products should be frequent choices from this group. The next level of the Pyramid contains the Vegetable Group and the Fruit Group, which are also good sources of complex carbohydrates and fiber as well as of naturally occurring simple carbohydrates. It is recommended that three to five servings from the Vegetable Group and two to four servings from the Fruit Group be consumed each day. The next level of the Pyramid, the Milk, Yogurt, and Cheese Group, provides unrefined simple carbohydrate in the form of lactose. Many of the choices in the Meat, Poultry, Fish, Dry Beans, Eggs, and Nuts Group contain no carbohydrate. Choosing dry beans from this group will provide a protein-rich food that is also a good source of complex carbohydrates and fiber.

Carbohydrate-based meals are also lower in fat and cost less than meat-based meals. For example, choosing a meal of chili with beans or spaghetti with tomato and meat sauce will cost less and provide the same energy with more carbohydrate and fiber than a meal of steak and french fries.

TABLE 4.6 Fiber Content of Food Groups Selections

Food Group/Serving	High Fiber	Medium Fiber	Low Fiber
Fiber per serving	***4–5 g***	***2 g***	***0.5–1 g***
Bread, Cereal, Rice, & Pasta Group			
Breads (1 slice)	—	Whole wheat Rye	White bread Bagel (1/2) Tortilla Roll (1/2) English muffin (1/2) Graham cracker
Cereals (1/2 cup)	All Bran Bran Buds 100% Bran Flakes	40% Bran Shredded Wheat	Cheerios Rice Krispies
Rice and pasta (1/2 cup)	—	Whole-wheat pasta Brown rice	Macaroni Pasta White rice
Fruit Group			
Fruits (1 medium or 1/2 cup)	Berries Prunes	Apple Apricot Banana Orange Raisins	Melon Canned fruit Juices
Vegetable Group			
Vegetables (1/2 cup)	Peas Broccoli Spinach	Green beans Carrots Eggplant Cabbage Potatoes with skin Corn	Asparagus Cauliflower Celery Lettuce Tomatoes Zucchini Peppers Potatoes without skin Onions
Dry Bean Group			
Beans (1/2 cup)	Pinto, red Kidney beans Blackeyed peas	—	—

[1]Adapted from Bright-See, E., Benda, C., Vartouhi, J., et al. Development and testing of a dietary fibre exchange system. Can. Diet. Assoc. J. 47:199–205, 1986; and Marlett, J. A. Content and composition of dietary fiber in 117 frequently consumed foods. J. Am. Diet. Assoc. 92:175–186, 1992.

Sugars in the Food Guide Pyramid To emphasize moderation in the consumption of refined sugar, the Food Guide Pyramid recommends that added sweeteners be used sparingly. The relative amounts of added sugar in each of the food groups are indicated by an upside-down triangle symbol (▽). The food groups that contain a higher proportion of foods with added sugar have more of these symbols. For example, the tip of the Pyramid, which includes sweets along with fats and oils, has the highest concentration of these symbols; the grain group, which includes sweetened bakery products like cakes and cookies, has a moderate concentration of symbols; and the Vegetable Group, which includes almost no foods with added sugar, has no symbols (Figure 4.28).

High-Fiber Choices To assure that a diet based on the Pyramid will meet the recommendations for carbohydrate and fiber intake, care must be used in choosing from the food groups. For example, switching from a breakfast of ham and eggs to one of whole grain cereal and toast will increase total carbohydrate and fiber intake. The choice of breakfast cereals however, can make a big difference in

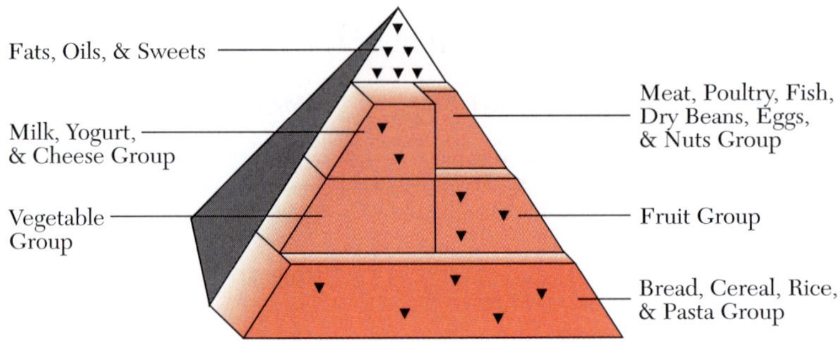

FIGURE 4.28 The Food Guide Pyramid groups that are sources of naturally occurring simple and complex carbohydrates are raised and colored red. The darker shades indicate groups with a greater proportion of high-carbohydrate foods. Note that the Meat, Poultry, Fish, Dry Beans, Eggs, and Nuts Group can provide complex carbohydrates if dry beans are chosen. Groups that provide good sources of fiber include the Bread, Cereal, Rice, and Pasta Group (if whole grains are chosen), the Vegetable Group, the Fruit Group, and the Meat, Poultry, Fish, Dry Beans, Eggs, and Nuts Group (if dry beans are chosen). The ▼ symbol indicates sources of added sugars.

fiber and sugar intake. A serving of Frosted Flakes has about 1 g of fiber and 13 g of sugars; a serving of bran flakes has about 5 g of fiber and only 6 g of sugars. Using fresh instead of canned fruit can also help increase fiber and decrease refined sugars. For example, half a cup of pear halves canned in heavy syrup provides 90 kcalories, 1 g of fiber, and almost 20 g of sugar, most of which is added in the syrup. One large fresh pear would provide 90 kcalories, 4 g of fiber, and no refined sugar. Choosing fresh fruit instead of juice also adds fiber (Table 4.7). An apple provides about 80 to 90 kcalories and 2.7 g of fiber, whereas 3/4 cup of apple juice provides the same amount of energy but almost no fiber (0.2 g).

Carbohydrates on Food Labels Food labels can be helpful in choosing foods high in carbohydrates and fiber and low in added refined sugar (Figure 4.29). Food labels list the amounts of carbohydrate, fiber, and sugars in a serving of food. To help determine how these amounts fit into the recommendations for an overall diet, total carbohydrate and fiber are also listed as a percent of the Daily Value. The Daily Value for total carbohydrate is calculated as 60% of the energy for a 2000-kcalorie diet. This represents 300 g of carbohydrate ([2000 kcal × 0.6]/4 kcal/g of carbohydrate = 300 g). The Daily Value for fiber is based on a recommended intake of about 11.5 g per 1000 kcalories, which is rounded to 25 g in a 2000-kcalorie diet. The amounts of soluble and insoluble fiber are not mandatory on food labels, but some manufacturers choose to include them.

Sugars on Food Labels No Daily Value has been established for sugars, but labels can help identify high-sugar products. The number of grams of sugars listed in the Nutrition Facts includes all monosaccharides and disaccharides but does not distinguish between refined and naturally occurring sugars. For example, the fructose found naturally in frozen strawberries, and that added as high-fructose corn syrup in soft drinks, are both listed as sugars. Nutrient claims provide some information about whether a food contains added refined sugar. The presence of

TABLE 4.7 Suggestions for Meeting Carbohydrate Recommendations

1. Increase intake of whole grains, fruits, and vegetables.
2. Use whole-grain products such as oatmeal, brown rice, and whole-wheat bread.
3. Increase consumption of legumes such as kidney, black, and pinto beans.
4. If fresh fruits are not available, choose frozen or canned fruits without added sugar.
5. Choose packaged foods that contain 10% or more of the Daily Value for fiber.
6. When baking at home, substitute whole-grain flour for one-fourth to one-half of the amount of flour specified in the recipe.
7. When cooking at home, use less sugar; try adding one-fourth less sugar than called for in the recipe.
8. Use less added sugar in beverages and on cereals and pancakes.
9. Eat fewer high-sugar prepared foods such as cookies and candies.
10. Read food labels to choose foods low in added sugars and high in fiber.

Whole Wheat Bread

Nutrition Facts
Serving Size 1 Slice (27g)
Servings Per Container 17
Calories 70
Calories from Fat 10

Amount/Serving	%DV*	Amount/Serving	%DV*
Total Fat 1g	**2%**	**Total Carb.** 12g	**4%**
Sat. Fat 0g	**0%**	Dietary Fiber 2g	**7%**
Cholesterol 0mg	**0%**	Sugars 2g	
Sodium 10mg	**0%**	**Protein** 2g	

Vitamin A 0% • Vitamin C 0% • Calcium 4% • Iron 4%
Thiamin 4% • Riboflavin 2% • Niacin 4%

*Percent Daily Values (DV) are based on a 2,000 calorie diet. Your daily values may be higher or lower depending on your calorie needs:

	Calories:	2,000	2,500
Total Fat	Less than	65g	80g
Sat Fat	Less than	20g	25g
Cholesterol	Less than	300mg	300mg
Sodium	Less than	2,400mg	2,400mg
Total Carbohydrate		300g	375g
Dietary Fiber		25g	30g

NOT A SODIUM FREE FOOD

INGREDIENTS: WHOLE WHEAT FLOUR, WATER, SWEETENERS (HIGH FRUCTOSE CORN SYRUP, MOLASSES), WHEAT GLUTEN, SOYBEAN OIL, CONTAINS 2% OR LESS OF THE FOLLOWING: YEAST, DOUGH CONDITIONERS (MONO & DIGLYCERIDES, ETHOXYLATED MONO & DI-GLYCERIDES, CALCIUM STEAROYL-2-LACTYLATE), YEAST NUTRIENTS (CALCIUM SULFATE, MONO- CALCIUM PHOSPHATE), CALCIUM PROPIONATE (A PRESERVATIVE).

FIGURE 4.29 Food labels provide a variety of information about the types and amounts of carbohydrates in foods.

a nutrient content claim such as "no added sugar" or "without added sugar" indicates that no sugars have been added in processing (Table 4.8). The ingredient list also provides information about the types of sweeteners added to a food. Only added sugars are listed here and the only type of sweetener that can be called "sugar" is sucrose. Because sucrose may represent only one of many added sweeteners, consumers need to increase their carbohydrate vocabulary to recognize all the sweeteners on the label. High-fructose corn syrups, invert sugar, dextrose, lactose, and honey are just a few (Table 4.9).

Fiber on Food Labels Nutrient content descriptors and health claims can be useful in identifying high-fiber foods. For example, foods that contain 20% or more of the Daily Value for fiber per serving can state on the label that they are "high in dietary fiber" (see Table 4.8). Food labels of products that are good sources of fiber may also include appropriate health claims related to fiber and the risk of certain chronic diseases (see Appendix J).

The ingredient list can also provide useful information about fiber and the degree of refinement if you understand the terminology. On breads, cereals, pastas, crackers, and other grain products, the term "whole" before the name of the grain indicates that the bran layer is still present in the food. Wheat flour, used to describe refined white flour made from wheat, is often confused with whole wheat flour. Only when whole wheat flour is the first ingredient is the product made with mostly wheat flour containing the bran layer. Fiber added to processed foods can also be identified from the list of ingredients. Insoluble fibers, such as wheat bran, are often added to wheat bread to decrease the energy content of the product or to meet consumer demands for a high-fiber product. The soluble fiber oat bran is also added for these reasons, but most added soluble fibers, such as pectins and gums, are used to thicken and stabilize foods and rarely contribute a significant amount of fiber.

TABLE 4.8 Sugar and Fiber Content Descriptors on Food Labels*

Sugar free	Product contains no amount, or a trivial amount, of sugars (less than 0.5 g per serving). Synonyms for "free" include "without," "no," and "zero."
Reduced sugar	Nutritionally altered product contains 25% less sugar than the regular or reference product.
Less sugar	Whether altered or not, a food contains 25% less sugar than the reference food. "Fewer" may be used as a synonym for "less."
No added sugars or without added sugars	No sugar or sugar-containing ingredient is added during processing.
High fiber	Food contains 20% or more of the Daily Value for fiber per serving. Synonyms for "high" include "rich in" and "excellent source of."
Good source of fiber	Food contains 10 to 19% of the Daily Value for fiber per serving. Synonyms for "good source of" include "contains" and "provides."
More fiber	Food contains 10% or more of the Daily Value for fiber per serving than an appropriate reference food. Synonyms for "more" include "added" (or "fortified" and enriched"), "extra," or "plus."

*If a food is not low in total fat, the label must state total fat in conjunction with any fiber claim such as "More Fiber."

Table 4.9 Sweeteners Used in Foods*

Brown sugar	Lactose
Confectioners' sugar (powdered sugar)	Levulose (same as fructose)
Corn syrup	Maltose
Dextrose (same as glucose)	Malt syrup
Fructose	Maple syrup
Fruit juice concentrate	Molasses
Glucose	Raw sugar
Granulated sugar	Sucrose
High-fructose corn syrup	Syrup
Honey	Table sugar
Invert sugar	Turbinado sugar (partially refined raw sugar)

*These ingredients often appear on food labels as added sweeteners.

Critical Thinking

Meeting Carbohydrate Recommendations

Maria knows that a healthy diet is important but is confused as to what makes a diet healthy. She meets with a dietitian to evaluate her diet.

Diet analysis

Maria's nutritional assessment indicates that her diet provides about 2100 kcalories, 20% of which come from protein, 36% from fat, and 44% from carbohydrate, and that she consumes about 8 g of fiber. Her diet is higher in fat and lower in carbohydrate and fiber than recommended.

How many more grams of carbohydrate would Maria need to meet the recommendation of 55 to 60% of energy from carbohydrate?

Her diet provides approximately 44% carbohydrate and 2100 kcal:

$$44\% \times 2100 \text{ kcal} = 924 \text{ kcal from carbohydrate}$$

Carbohydrate provides 4 kcal/g, so she consumes:

$$\frac{924 \text{ kcal}}{4 \text{ kcal/g}} = 231 \text{ g of carbohydrate}$$

A 2100-kcal diet with 55% of energy from carbohydrate would provide:

$$55\% \times 2100 \text{ kcal} = 1155 \text{ kcal from carbohydrate}$$

$$\frac{1155 \text{ kcal}}{4 \text{ kcal/g}} = 289 \text{ g of carbohydrate}$$

Maria's diet therefore needs to provide at least 58 additional g of carbohydrate:

$$289 \text{ g recommended} - 231 \text{ g consumed} = 58 \text{ g}$$

How does Maria's diet compare to the recommendations for fiber intake?

The recommendation is to consume 10 to 13 g of fiber per 1000 kcals. Because Maria's diet contains 2100 kcalories, she should consume between 21 and 27.3 g of fiber daily.

$$\frac{10 \text{ g fiber}}{1000 \text{ kcal}} \times 2100 \text{ kcal} = 21 \text{ g of fiber per day}$$

$$\frac{13 \text{ g fiber}}{1000 \text{ kcal}} \times 2100 \text{ kcal} = 27.3 \text{ g of fiber per day}$$

To improve her diet, the dietitian suggests some ways Maria could increase her intake of fruits, vegetables, legumes, and whole grains. These changes will increase the carbohydrate and fiber content of her diet and at the same time decrease her fat intake. The carbohydrate content of her original and modified diet is estimated using the Exchange Lists in Table 4.5 and the fiber is estimated using Table 4.6

Original Diet			**Modified Diet**		
Food	***Carbohydrate (g)***	***Fiber (g)***	***Food***	***Carbohydrate (g)***	***Fiber (g)***
Breakfast					
Coffee	0	0	Coffee	0	0
White toast (2)	30	1	Whole-wheat toast (2)	30	4
Margarine (1 tsp)	0	0	Margarine (1 tsp)	0	0
Jelly (1 tsp)	4	0	Jelly (1 tsp)	4	0
Chorizo (sausage) (2 oz)	0	0	Chorizo (sausage) (1 oz)	0	0
Apple juice (1 cup)	30	1	Apple juice (1 cup)	30	1
Lunch					
Burritos:			Burritos:		
Tortilla (2 large)	45	1	Tortilla (2 large)	45	1
Beef (3 oz)	0	0	Beef (3 oz)	0	0
			Kidney beans (1/2 cup)	15	4
Milk (1 cup)	12	0	Milk (1 cup)	12	0
Cookies (2 large)	30	0.5	Cookies (2 large)	30	0.5
			Orange	15	1
Snack					
Diet soda	0	0	Diet soda	0	0
Pretzels (1.5 oz)	22	0.5	Pretzels (1 oz)	15	0.3
Dinner					
Carne asada (beef) (4 oz) w/tomatoes	3	0.5	Carne asada (beef) (2 oz) w/tomatoes	3	0.5
Potatoes (1 cup)	30	4	Potatoes (1 cup)	30	4
			Green beans (1/2 cup)	5	2
			Salad (1/2 cup)	5	2
Milk (1 cup)	12	0	Milk (1 cup)	12	0
Ice cream (1/2 cup)	15	0	Nonfat frozen yogurt (1 cup)	19	0
			berries (1/2 cup)	15	4
Snack					
			Graham crackers (3 squares)	15	0.5
Total	**233**	**8.5**		**300**	**24.8**

Maria's diet now meets the recommendations for carbohydrate and fiber intake. How does her new diet compare to the recommendations of the Food Guide Pyramid?

Answer:

Web Menu

For more information on low-calorie sweeteners, go to the Calorie Control Council at www.caloriecontrol.org/ and click on low-calorie sweeteners.

Sugar Substitutes or Artificial Sweeteners

Americans' love of sweets and their desire to reduce their intake of sugar and energy have driven the technological development of an increasing number of artificial and nonnutritive sweeteners. These sugar substitutes, which provide little or no energy, are added to a host of low-kcalorie and "light" foods such as candies, cookies, yogurts, ice creams, and soft drinks. A 1998 survey by the Calorie Control Council found that 144 million adults in the United States regularly consume low-kalorie and sugar-free products such as diet sodas.[41] Artificial sweeteners are generally safe for healthy people. However, to assure that they are not misused, the FDA has set a level of intake, termed average daily intake (ADI), that should not be exceeded.

The Role of Sugar Substitutes in the Diet The average American eats about 20 teaspoons of refined sugar a day. Almost 60% of this comes from corn sweeteners used in sodas and sweetened drinks and another 40% is from sucrose used in products such as candy and sweetened baked goods.[42] Replacing some of these foods with sugar-free ones will decrease sugar and energy intake, but it will not increase the intake of whole grains or fresh fruits and vegetables—key components of a healthy diet. Because foods that are high in added sugar tend to be nutrient-poor choices, replacing them with artificially sweetened alternatives does not improve the nutritional quality of the diet. If, however, sugar substitutes and foods containing them are used in moderation as part of a diet that is based on whole grains, vegetables, and fruits, these products can be part of a healthy diet.

Artificial sweeteners have been shown to reduce the incidence of dental caries and can be helpful for managing blood sugar levels in diabetes, but their usefulness for weight loss is debatable. If individuals trying to lose weight replace sugar and high-sugar foods with artificially sweetened products, they will reduce their energy intake. When used as part of a weight-control program, artificial sweeteners may facilitate weight loss and long-term weight maintenance.[43] However, despite the variety of available artificial sweeteners, obesity has continued to increase in the American population. Clearly, artificial sweeteners are not a solution to the obesity epidemic.

Types of Artificial Sweeteners The main competitors in the artificial sweetener market in the United States today are saccharin and aspartame. Acesulfame K (acesulfame potassium), sucralose, and a variety of sugar alcohols or polyols such as sorbitol are also FDA-approved sugar substitutes. These are all used alone or in combination to sweeten a variety of foods sold in the United States. Stevia, used extensively in Japan, is a sweetener derived from a South American shrub. Though it can impart a sweet taste to foods, it cannot be sold as a sweetener in the United States because the FDA considers it an unapproved food additive. Stevia can be sold as a "dietary supplement," though it cannot be promoted as a sweetener.[42] Cyclamate, an artificial sweetener that was popular in the 1960s, was banned by the FDA in 1969. It is sold in Canada and some 50 other countries.

Saccharin Saccharin was inadvertently discovered in 1879 by a researcher trying to develop food preservatives. It was used in both World Wars to sweeten foods when sugar was in short supply. In 1977, after large doses of saccharin were found to increase the incidence of bladder cancer in rats, it was added to an FDA list of food carcinogens. The FDA proposed banning its use in the food supply, but because saccharin was the only artificial sweetener available at that time, the public and the food industry protested. In response, Congress decided to allow the use of saccharin in foods as long as a warning is included on the label stating that it had been shown to cause cancer. In May 2000, saccharin was dropped from the government's list of cancer-causing substances, although food labels still carry the saccharin warning.

Saccharin is 200 to 700 times sweeter than sugar. It has a long shelf life, can be made economically, and can be used in baked goods because it withstands high temperatures. Saccharin intake in the United States is estimated to be about 50 mg per person per day. The ADI is set at 5 mg per kg body weight per day. For a 145-pound (70 kg) individual, this would be about 350 mg/day, and for a 220-pound (100 kg) individual, about 500 mg per day.[44] A packet of sweetener sold under trade names such as Sweet 'n' Low contains 36 mg of saccharin. A 12-ounce diet beverage sweetened with saccharin alone contains about 120 mg. Because children weigh less than adults, they are more likely to exceed the ADI. A 6-year-old weighing 50 pounds (23 kg) would exceed the ADI of 115 mg/day by drinking a single 12-ounce saccharin-sweetened soft drink.

Aspartame In 1965, James Schlatter, at the pharmaceutical company G.D. Searle, was working with a chemical made up of two amino acids when he spilled some of the chemical on his fingers. Shortly afterward, he licked his finger to pick up a piece of paper and discovered an intensely sweet taste. This accidental discovery led to the development of the artificial sweetener aspartame. Because aspartame is made of two amino acids, the building blocks of protein, it is not a carbohydrate. It was approved for some uses in 1981 and for use in soft drinks in 1983. Because aspartame breaks down when heated, it works best in products that are not cooked, such as chewing gum, breakfast cereals, fruit spreads, yogurt, and beverages. Common trade names for this sweetener include NutraSweet, Equal, and NutriTaste. Each gram of aspartame contains 4 kcalories, but because it is about 200 times as sweet as sugar, only 1/200 as much of it needs to be used to achieve the same level of sweetness.

As with other artificial sweeteners, safety concerns have been raised about aspartame. It contains the amino acid phenylalanine and therefore can be dangerous to individuals with a genetic disorder called phenylketonuria (PKU). These individuals have an abnormality that affects the metabolism of phenylalanine. They must restrict their intake of this amino acid to prevent brain damage (see Chapter 6). There is also a concern that consuming aspartame might cause dangerously high blood phenylalanine levels in the general public. Phenylalanine occurs naturally in protein. A 4-ounce hamburger has 12 times more phenylalanine than a 12-ounce aspartame-sweetened soft drink. However, when phenylalanine is ingested without the other amino acids found in high-protein foods, blood or brain levels increase to a greater extent. There have been reports of headaches, dizziness, seizures, nausea, allergic reactions, and other side effects following ingestion of aspartame. There may be a small segment of the population that is sensitive to this sweetener or one of the by-products produced when it is metabolized. These individuals should restrict its use; however, double-blind placebo-controlled studies have not been able to reproduce these symptoms.[47] Concerns were also raised that an increase in the incidence of brain cancer in children might be associated with the use of aspartame. A review of the epidemiological data, however, found that cases of brain cancer began increasing in 1973—eight years before aspartame was approved. In addition, controlled studies have found no evidence that aspartame is a carcinogen.[45] Overall, the consensus of the scientific community is that aspartame is safe for most people.

Aspartame metabolism does cause the production of methanol, formaldehyde, and formate, substances that are considered toxic at high doses. The levels formed from aspartame metabolism in the body are well below that considered toxic.

The FDA has set an ADI of 50 mg of aspartame per kg of body weight. For a 70-kg individual, this would be 3500 mg/day of aspartame. A packet of sweetener contains about 37 mg of aspartame. A 12-ounce soft drink sweetened with aspartame contains about 200 mg. To exceed the ADI, a 70-kg adult would have to consume almost 16 aspartame-sweetened soft drinks a day, and a 23-kg child would have to consume almost six soft drinks.[44]

Acesulfame K (Acesulfame Potassium) Acesulfame potassium—or acesulfame K—was discovered in 1967. It is a noncarbohydrate, nonkcaloric sweetener that is approximately 200 times sweeter than sugar. Acesulfame K is not metabolized by the body and is excreted unchanged. It was approved for use as a tabletop sweetener in 1988, and is currently approved for use in chewing gum, powdered drink mixes, gelatins, puddings, baked goods, frozen desserts, candy, soft drinks, and nondairy creamers. It is heat stable, so it can be used in baking, and is sold under the brand names Sunett and Sweet One. More than 90 studies have demonstrated the safety of acesulfame K and it has been used in Europe since 1983 and in the United States since 1988 with no known documented adverse health effects. The ADI has been set at 15 mg per kg body weight. A packet of sweetener contains about 50 mg of acesulfame K.

Sucralose Sucralose was discovered in 1976 and is the only noncaloric sweetener made from sugar. Sucralose (trichlorogalactosucrose) is made by substituting three atoms of chlorine for three hydroxyl groups (—OH) on the sugar molecule. It is about 600 times sweeter than sucrose and contributes no kcalories because it cannot be digested so passes through the digestive tract unchanged. Sucralose has been used in Canada for many years and was approved for use in the United States in 1998. It is sold under the name Splenda and can be used as a general-purpose sweetener for all foods. Because it is heat stable, it can be used in baked goods.[44] Sucralose has been extensively tested for safety over a 20-year period and found to be safe even for children and pregnant and lactating women.[46]

Polyols Polyols, also called sugar alcohols, are chemical derivatives of sugar—part of their structure resembles sugar and part is similar to alcohols. The polyols currently being used in foods include erythritol, isomalt, lactitol, maltitol, mannitol, sorbitol, and xylitol.

Polyols provide energy, but because they are slowly and incompletely absorbed from the small intestine, they provide less than sugar. Maltitol provides 3 kcal per g, lactitol 2 kcal per g, and erythritol only 0.2 kcal per g. They also vary in sweetness from about half as sweet as the same amount of sugar to equally as sweet as sugar. Polyols are useful in diabetic diets because they cause less of an increase in blood glucose and insulin levels than sugars and other carbohydrates. They are useful for preventing dental caries because the bacteria in the mouth cannot metabolize polyols as rapidly as sucrose.[44]

Because polyols are not monosaccharides or disaccharides, they can be used in products labeled "sugar free." They are used to sweeten chewing gums, candies, ice cream, baked goods, and fruit spreads as well as toothpastes, mouthwashes, cough syrups, and throat lozenges. Sugar-free products sweetened with polyols may carry the health claim that states "does not promote tooth decay."

Polyols are safe for human consumption, but in some individuals large amounts can cause diarrhea. This is because polyols that are not absorbed pass into the large intestine where they are broken down into smaller segments, drawing water into the GI tract and causing diarrhea.[47] In children, even small amounts of the polyol sorbitol can cause diarrhea. This can be a problem for children consuming apple or pear juice, which contain sorbitol, or using sorbitol-containing gums or candies.

Summary

1. Carbohydrates are chemical compounds that contain carbon, hydrogen, and oxygen. In food, they include sugar, starch, and fiber. Simple carbohydrates include monosaccharides and disaccharides and are found in foods such as table sugar, honey, milk, and fruit. Complex carbohydrates are oligosaccharides and polysaccharides. Polysaccharides include glycogen in animals and starch and fiber in plants.
2. Fiber cannot be digested by enzymes in the human stomach or small intestine and therefore is not absorbed into the body. Insoluble fibers, such as those in wheat bran and the skins of fruits and vegetables, do not dissolve in water. Soluble fibers, such as those in oats and psyllium, can absorb or dissolve in water. Soluble fiber may reduce blood cholesterol levels. Fiber benefits gastrointestinal function by increasing the amount of water and bulk in the intestine, which increases the ease and rate at which material moves through the gastrointestinal tract.
3. In the body, carbohydrate, primarily as glucose, provides a source of energy. Glucose is metabolized through cellular respiration, involving glycolysis, which breaks glucose into pyruvate; acetyl-CoA formation; the citric acid cycle, which produces carbon dioxide and electrons; and the electron transport chain, which produces water and ATP. Several tissues, including the brain and red blood cells, require glucose as an energy source.
4. The bloodstream delivers glucose to body cells. Blood glucose levels are maintained by the hormones insulin and glucagon. When blood glucose rises, insulin is released from the pancreas to allow body cells to take up and use the glucose. When blood glucose falls, glucagon is released to increase blood glucose by stimulating glucose breakdown and gluconeogenesis.
5. Diabetes is a disease of glucose regulation that is a major public health problem. It occurs either because insufficient insulin is produced or because there is a decrease in the sensitivity of body cells to insulin. High blood glucose damages tissues and causes complications including heart disease, stroke, high blood pressure, kidney failure, blindness, and amputations. Treatment to maintain glucose in the normal range includes diet, exercise, and medication.
6. Hypoglycemia is a condition in which blood glucose falls to abnormally low levels, causing symptoms such as sweating, headaches, and rapid heartbeat.
7. Diets high in carbohydrates increase the risk of dental caries. Diets high in whole grains, vegetables, fruits, and legumes are good sources of fiber, vitamins, minerals, and phytochemicals. Diets high in fiber reduce the risk of chronic bowel disorders, heart disease, colon cancer, diabetes, and obesity.
8. Guidelines for healthy diets recommend 55 to 60% of energy from carbohydrates with a plentiful selection of whole food sources of complex carbohydrate. Whole grains, legumes, fruits, and vegetables should be increased in the American diet, and foods high in refined sugars should be consumed in moderation. Fiber intake should be increased to 10 to 13 g per 1000 kcalories per day.
9. Artificial sweeteners or sugar substitutes are used to replace energy-containing sweeteners. If used in moderation, they can be helpful in reducing the sugar and energy content of the diet.

Review Questions

1. What is the basic unit of carbohydrate?
2. List three common simple carbohydrates. In what foods are they found?
3. What is complex carbohydrate?
4. What foods are good sources of unrefined complex carbohydrates?
5. Why is refined sugar considered a source of empty kcalories?
6. How much energy is provided by a gram of carbohydrate?
7. Why doesn't fiber provide energy?
8. Why is carbohydrate said to spare protein?
9. What is the main function of glucose in the body?
10. What is diabetes? Why is ketosis less of a problem in type 2 than in type 1 diabetes?
11. What health benefits are associated with a diet high in unrefined carbohydrates?
12. How can the information on food labels be used to identify foods that are high in refined sugars? In fiber?
13. What are the risks and benefits of artificial sweeteners?

Applying Critical Thinking Skills

Personal nutrition:

1. Calculate your average carbohydrate and energy intake from the three-day diet record you kept in Chapter 2.
   a. What is the percent of energy from carbohydrate in your diet?
   b. How does this compare with the recommended 55 to 60% of energy from carbohydrate?
   c. If your diet does not meet the recommendations, suggest some modifications to increase your carbohydrate intake without changing your energy intake.
   d. Compare the fat content of your original diet with your modified diet. If it has changed, explain why.
   e. List sources of unrefined grains in your diet. Suggest whole-grain substitutes for refined grains.

2. Calculate the grams of fiber in your modified diet from question 1 above using a computer software program or the fiber exchanges in Table 4.6
   a. How many grams of fiber does your diet provide?
   b. How many grams of fiber per 1000 kcalories does your diet provide?
   c. If your diet does not meet recommendations, suggest modifications that would meet them.

General nutrition issues:

1. Bob weighs about 30 pounds more than he wants to weigh, so he decides to try to shed pounds quickly with a low-carbohydrate weight-loss diet. The diet allows an unlimited amount of beef, chicken, and fish as well as limited fruits and vegetables; breads, grains, and cereals are not allowed. Bob is overjoyed with his initial rapid weight loss, but after about a week his weight loss slows down and he begins to feel tired and light-headed. He is having headaches and notices a funny smell on his breath. A nutritional assessment suggests that Bob needs about 2500 kcalories a day to maintain his weight. His weight-loss diet provides about 1000 kcalories, 25 g of carbohydrate, 125 g of protein, and 44 g of fat per day. He consumes only about 3 cups of fluid daily.
   a. Explain why Bob is tired, light-headed, and has headaches and an unusual odor on his breath.
   b. What recommendations do you have to reduce these symptoms?
2. Go to a bookstore or the library and look up a sample one-day menu from a diet book that advocates a low carbohydrate intake. Enter these foods into the diet analysis computer program.
   a. How does this diet compare to the recommended intakes for saturated fat?
   b. For calcium?
   c. For fiber?

REFERENCES

1. Flatt, J. P. Use and storage of carbohydrates. Am. J. Clin. Nutr. 61(suppl):952S–959S, 1995.
2. Giboney, M., Sigmann-Grant, M., Stanton, J. L., and Keast, D. R. Consumption of sugars. Am. J. Clin. Nutr. 62(suppl):178S–194S, 1995.
3. USDA. *Food Consumption, Prices, and Expenditures.* 1997.
4. Glinsmann, W. H., and Bowman, B. A. The public health significance of dietary fructose. Am. J. Clin. Nutr. 58(suppl):820S–823S, 1993.
5. Dennison, B. A. Fruit juice consumption by infants and children: a review. J. Am. Coll. Nutr. 15:4S–11S, 1996.
6. Gray, G. M. Digestion and absorption of carbohydrate. In *Biochemical and Physiological Aspects of Human Nutrition.* Stipanuk, M., ed. Philadelphia: W. B. Saunders Company, 2000, 91–106.
7. Lee, M.-F., and Krasinski, S. D. Human adult-onset lactase decline: an update. Nutr. Rev. 56:1–8, 1998.
8. McBean, L. D., and Miller, G. D. Allaying fears and fallacies about lactose intolerance. J. Am Diet. Assoc. 98:671–676, 1998.
9. American Dietetic Association. Position of the American Dietetic Association: health implications of dietary fiber. J. Am. Diet. Assoc. 97:1157–1160, 1997.
10. American Diabetes Association. Economic consequence of diabetes mellitus in the United States in 1997. Diabetes Care 21:296–309, 1998.
11. Leontos, C., Wong, F., and Gallivan, J., for the National Diabetes Education Program Planning Committee. National Diabetes Education Program: opportunities and challenges. J. Am. Diet. Assoc. 98:73–75, 1998.
12. National Institutes of Diabetes and Digestive and Kidney Diseases, National Institutes of Health, National Diabetes Information Clearinghouse. *Fact Sheet on Diabetes Statistics.* NIH Publication No. 98-3926, Nov. 1997, updated Feb. 1998. Available online at **http://www.niddk.nih.gov/health/diabetes/pubs/dmstats/dmstats.htm**. Accessed 27 Nov 2000.
13. Report of the Expert Committee on the Diagnosis and Classification of Diabetes Mellitus. Diabetes Care 20:1183–1197, 1997.
14. Pasei, K., and McFarland, K. F. Management of diabetes in pregnancy. Am. Fam. Physician 55:731–738, 1997.
15. Schafer, R. G., Bohannon, B., Franz, M., et al. Translation of the diabetes nutrition recommendations for health care institutions: technical review. J. Am. Diet. Assoc. 97:43–51, 1997.
16. Anderson, J. W. Nutritional management of diabetes mellitus. In *Modern Nutrition in Health and Disease,* 9th ed. Shils, M. E., Olson, J. A., Shike, M., and Ross, A. C., eds. Baltimore: Williams & Wilkens, 1999. 1365–1394.
17. The Diabetes Control and Complications Trial Research Group. The Effect of Intensive Diabetes Therapy on the Development and Progression of Neuropathy. Ann. Intern. Med. 122:561–568, 1995.
18. National Institutes of Diabetes and Digestive and Kidney Diseases, National Institutes of Health. *National Diabetes Education Program.* Available online at **http://ndep.nih.gov/**. Accessed 27 Nov 2000.
19. Slavin, J. L., Martini, M. C., Jacobs, D. R., Jr., et al. Plausible mechanism for protectiveness of whole grains. Am. J. Clin. Nutr. 70(3 Suppl):459S–463S, 1999.
20. Willett, W. C. The dietary pyramid: does the foundation need repair? Am. J. Clin. Nutr. 68:218–219, 1998.
21. Konig, K. G., and Navia, J. M. Nutritional role of sugars in oral health. Am. J. Clin. Nutr. 62(suppl):275S–283S, 1995.
22. Jacobs, D. R., Meyer, K. A., Kushi, L. H., and Folsom, A. R. Whole-grain intake may reduce the risk of ischemic heart disease death in postmenopausal women: the Iowa Women's Health Study. Am. J. Clin. Nutr. 68:248–257, 1998.
23. Kushi, L. H., Meyer, K. A., Jacobs, D. R., Jr. Cereals, legumes, and chronic disease risk reduction: evidence from epidemiologic studies. Am. J. Clin. Nutr. 70(3 Suppl):451S–458S, 1999.
24. Wolk, A., Manson, J. E., Stampfer, M. J., et al. Long-term intake of dietary fiber and decreased risk of coronary heart disease among women. JAMA 281:1998–2003, 1999.
25. Starc, T. J., Shea, S., Cohn, L. C., et al. Greater dietary intake of simple carbohydrates is associated with lower concentrations of HDL cholesterol in hypercholesterolemic children. Am. J. Clin. Nutr. 67:1147–1154, 1998.
26. Hudgins, L. C., Seidman, C. E., Diakun, J., and Hirsch, J. Human fatty acid synthesis is reduced after substitution of dietary starch for sugar. Am. J. Clin. Nutr. 67:631–639, 1998.
27. Anderson, J. W., Allgood, L. D., Lawrence, A., et al. Cholesterol-lowering effects of psyllium intake adjunctive to diet therapy in men and women with hypercholesterolemia: meta-analysis of 8 controlled trials. Am. J. Clin. Nutr. 71:472–479, 2000.

28. Marlett, J. A. Sites and mechanisms for the hypocholesterolemic actions of soluble dietary fiber sources. In *Fiber in Human and Disease*. Kritevsky, D., and Bonfield, C., eds. New York: Plenum Press, 1997, 109–121.
29. Wolever, T. M. S., and Miller, J. B. Sugars and blood glucose control. Am. J. Clin. Nutr. 62(suppl):212S–227S, 1995.
30. Salmeron, J., Manson, J. E., Stampfer, M. J., et al. Dietary fiber, glycemic load, and the risk of noninsulin-dependent diabetes mellitus in women. JAMA 227:472–477, 1997.
31. Salmeron, J., Ascherio, A., Rimm, E. B., et al. Dietary fiber, glycemic load, and risk of NIDDM in men. Diabetes Care 20:545–550, 1997.
32. Anderson, G. H. Sugars, sweetness, and food intake. Am. J. Clin. Nutr. 62:195S–202S, 1995.
33. Hill, J. O., and Prentice, A. M. Sugar and body weight regulation. Am. J. Clin. Nutr. 62(supp):264S, 1995.
34. Wurtman, R. J., and Wurtman, J. J. Brain serotonin, Carbohydrate craving, obesity and depression. Obes. Res. 4:477S–480S, 1995.
35. Kurzer, M. S. Women, food, and mood. Nutrition Reviews 55:268–276, 1997.
36. Wolraich, M. L., Wilson, D. B., and White, J. W. The effect of sugar on behavior or cognition in children: a meta-analysis. JAMA 274: 1617–1618, 1995.
37. Miller, D. L., Miller, P. F., and Dekker, J. J. Small bowel obstruction from bran cereal. JAMA 263:813–815, 1990.
38. Alberts, D. S., Martinez, M. E., Roe, D. J., et al. Lack of effect of a high-fiber cereal supplement on the ocurrence of colorectal adenomas. N. Engl. J. Med. 342:1156–1162, 2000.
39. Schatzkin, A., Lanza, E., Corle, D., et al. Lack of effect of a low-fat, high-fiber diet on the recurrence of colorectal adenomias. N. Engl. J. Med. 342:1149–1155, 2000.
40. Gorbach, S. L., and Goldin, B. R. The intestinal microflora and the colon cancer connection. Rev. Infect. Dis. 12(Suppl.2):S252–S261, 1990.
41. Calorie Control Council National Consumer Surveys. Available online at **http://www.caloriecontrol.org/usfaves.html**. Accessed 27 Nov 2000.
42. Henkel, J. Sugar substitutes: Americans opt for sweetness and lite. FDA Consumer, November–December 1999. Available online at **http://vm.cfsan.fda.gov/~dms/fdsugar.html**. Accessed 4 Dec 2000.
43. Blackburn, G. L., Kanders, B. S., Lavin, P. T., et al. The effect of aspartame as part of a multidisciplinary weight-control program on short- and long-term control of body weight. Am. J. Clin. Nutr. 65:409–418, 1997.
44. American Dietetic Association. Position of the American Dietetic Association: use of nutritive and nonnutritive sweeteners. J. Am. Diet. Assoc. 98:580–587, 1998.
45. Gurney, J. G., Pogoda, J. M., Holly, E. A., et al. Aspartame consumption in relation to childhood brain tumor risk: results from a case-control study. J. Nat. Cancer Inst. 89:1072–1074, 1997.
46. Calorie Control Council. Low calorie sweeteners: sucralose. Available online at **http://www.caloriecontrol.org/sucralos.html**. Accessed 7 Mar 2000.
47. Payne, M. L. Craig, W. J., and Williams, A. C. Sorbitol is a possible risk factor for diarrhea in young children. J. Am. Diet. Assoc. 97: 532–534, 1997.

5 Lipids

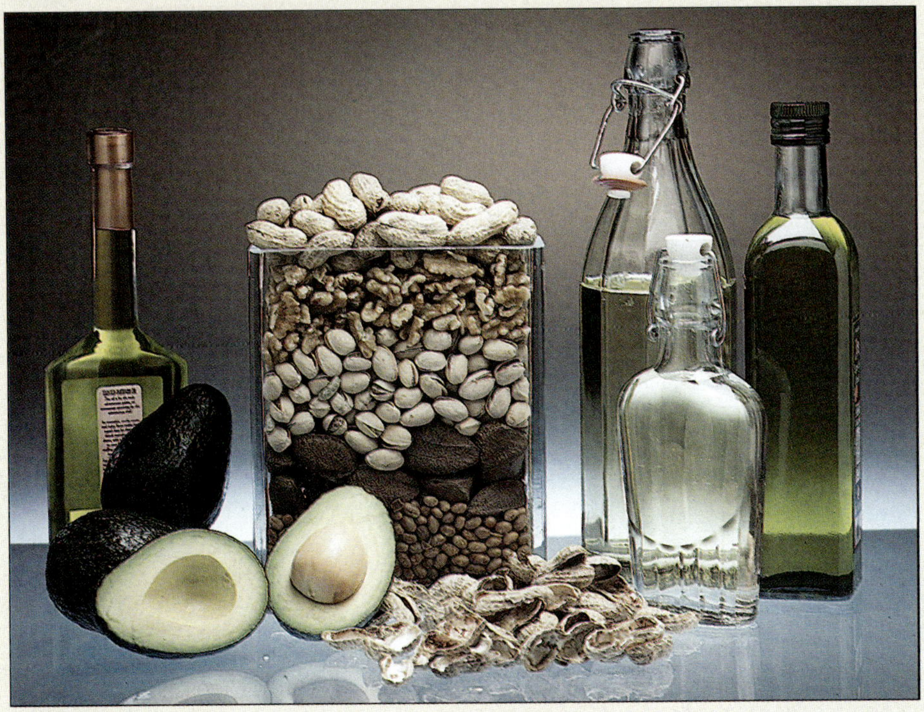

Learning Objectives

After completing this chapter, students should be able to:

1. Define the term "lipid" and describe the four classes of lipids.
2. Compare and contrast the chemical structures of a saturated fatty acid, a monounsaturated fatty acid, a polyunsaturated fatty acid, an omega-6 fatty acid, an omega-3 fatty acid, and a *trans* fatty acid.
3. List a food source of saturated fat, monounsaturated fat, polyunsaturated fat, omega-6 fatty acids, omega-3 fatty acids, and *trans* fatty acids.
4. Explain why hydrogenated fats are used to make margarine and vegetable shortening.
5. List and describe the events involved in fat digestion, absorption, transport, and delivery to cells.
6. Compare and contrast the functions of chylomicrons, VLDLs, LDLs, and HDLs.
7. List four functions of lipids in the body.
8. Discuss how fatty acids are used as an energy source to generate ATP.
9. List dietary factors that increase the risk of heart disease and those that decrease the risk.
10. Modify a diet to meet current recommendations for the types and amounts of fat.

Sam's grandfather died of a heart attack at the age of 50. That was 40 years ago. Sam is now a 20-year-old college student. At a recent health fair he took part in a risk assessment and found that he was about 25 pounds overweight, his percent body fat was higher than recommended, and his blood cholesterol was slightly elevated at 209 mg/100 ml. He was told that he should see a physician to evaluate his risk for a heart attack early in life. How could a 20-year-old be at risk for heart disease?

Sam began to think about changes he could make in his diet and lifestyle that would reduce his risk of developing heart disease. He currently eats a lot of red meat and drinks whole milk; he has only one or two servings of fruits and vegetables a day. He gets some exercise a couple of times each week playing Frisbee with his friends and lifting weights on Friday nights. When he tells his friends and family about his health concerns, everyone has some advice. His girlfriend is a vegetarian and she recommends that he eliminate meat from his diet. His lab partner in biology class tells him to eliminate all fat from his diet. His sister tells him about the Mediterranean diet and recommends he eat pasta with plenty of olive oil every night. His roommate tells him to eat more fish. His mother says he should stop using margarine because of all the *trans* fatty acids in it. Whose advice should he follow?

To know what Sam should do, you need to understand the role of fat in the body and the impact that the type and amount of dietary fat, as well as other dietary and lifestyle factors, have on the risk of heart disease and other disease processes. Sam may not be at risk of dying of a heart attack in the next few years, but his diet and lifestyle today affect his risk of heart disease in the future.

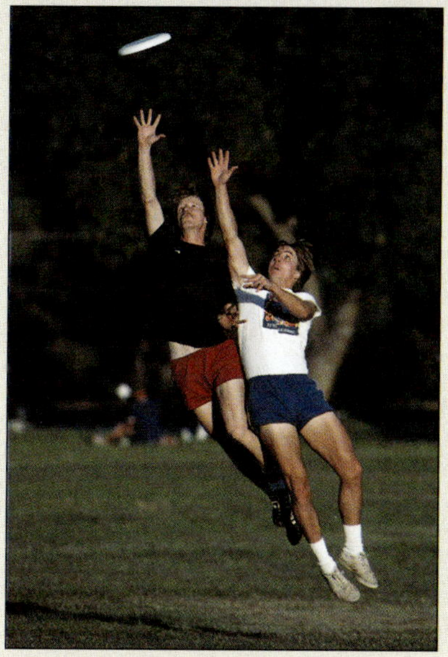

WHAT ARE LIPIDS?

Commonly known as fats or oils, **lipids** are a class of compounds that are soluble in organic solvents such as ether, chloroform, and acetone. They vary in size and the degree to which they are soluble in water. Lipids found in the body and in the diet include fatty acids, glycerides, phospholipids, and sterols. Each has a different structure and function.

Lipids A group of organic molecules, most of which do not dissolve in water. They include fatty acids, glycerides, phospholipids, and sterols.

Fatty Acids

Fatty acids consist of a chain of carbon atoms linked together by chemical bonds. The carbon chains of fatty acids vary in length from a few to 20 or more carbons. Each carbon atom forms four bonds linking it to four other atoms. If a carbon is not bound to four other atoms, double bonds are formed. At one end of the carbon chain, the carbon atom is attached to three hydrogen atoms (CH_3). This is referred to as the omega, or methyl, end of the carbon chain. At the opposite end of the chain is an acid group, formed by joining the carbon to an oxygen molecule by a double bond and to an OH group (COOH) by a single bond. Each of the carbons between the two ends is attached to two other carbons and up to two hydrogens (Figure 5.1). Fatty acids are typically found as components of larger molecules such as glycerides or phospholipids.

Fatty acids Organic molecules made up of a chain of carbons linked to hydrogens with an acid group at one end.

Categories of Fatty Acids Fatty acids are categorized based on the number of carbons in their carbon chain as well as on the types and locations of bonds between the carbons. These structural features affect their physical properties.

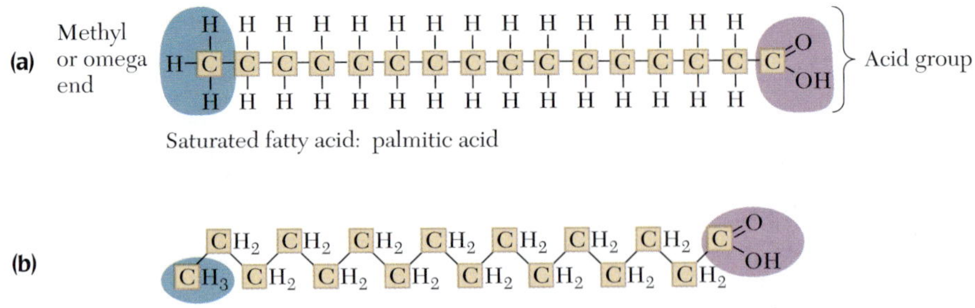

FIGURE 5.1 (a) In saturated fatty acids, such as the palmitic acid shown here, each carbon in the interior of the chain is bound to 2 hydrogen atoms. (b) The bonds between carbon atoms in the carbon chain of fatty acids are angled such that the chain takes on a zigzag configuration.

Carbon Chain Length Short-chain fatty acids range from four to seven carbons in length. They remain liquid at colder temperatures than do longer-chain fatty acids. For example, the short-chain fatty acids in whole milk remain liquid even at refrigerator temperatures. Medium-chain fatty acids, such as those in coconut oil, range from 8 to 12 carbons. They solidify in the refrigerator but remain liquid at room temperature. Long-chain fatty acids (greater than 12 carbons), such as those in beef fat, usually remain solid at room temperature. Most fatty acids in plants and animals, including humans, contain between 14 and 22 carbons.

Degree of Saturation Fatty acids are also categorized by the types of bonds between carbons in the chain. A fatty acid in which the chain is saturated with hydrogens so that each carbon has two hydrogens bound to it is called a **saturated fatty acid.** The most common saturated fatty acids are palmitic acid, which has 16 carbons, and stearic acid, which has 18 carbons. Saturated fatty acids are found in the greatest abundance in animal foods such as meat and dairy products, but there are some plant sources.

An **unsaturated fatty acid** contains some carbons that are not saturated with hydrogens. Double bonds form in the carbon chain between these carbons that are bound to only one hydrogen (Figure 5.2a). A fatty acid containing one double bond in its carbon chain is called a **monounsaturated fatty acid.** In our diets, the most common monounsaturated fatty acid is oleic acid, which is prevalent in olive and canola oils. A fatty acid with more than one double bond in its carbon chain is said to be a **polyunsaturated fatty acid.** The most common polyunsaturated fatty acid is linoleic acid, found in corn, safflower, and soybean

Saturated fatty acid A fatty acid in which the carbon atoms are bound to as many hydrogens as possible and which therefore contains no carbon-carbon double bonds.

Unsaturated fatty acid A fatty acid that contains one or more double bonds between carbons in the carbon chain.

Monounsaturated fatty acid A fatty acid that contains one double bond between carbons in the carbon chain.

Polyunsaturated fatty acid A fatty acid that contains two or more double bonds between carbons in the carbon chain.

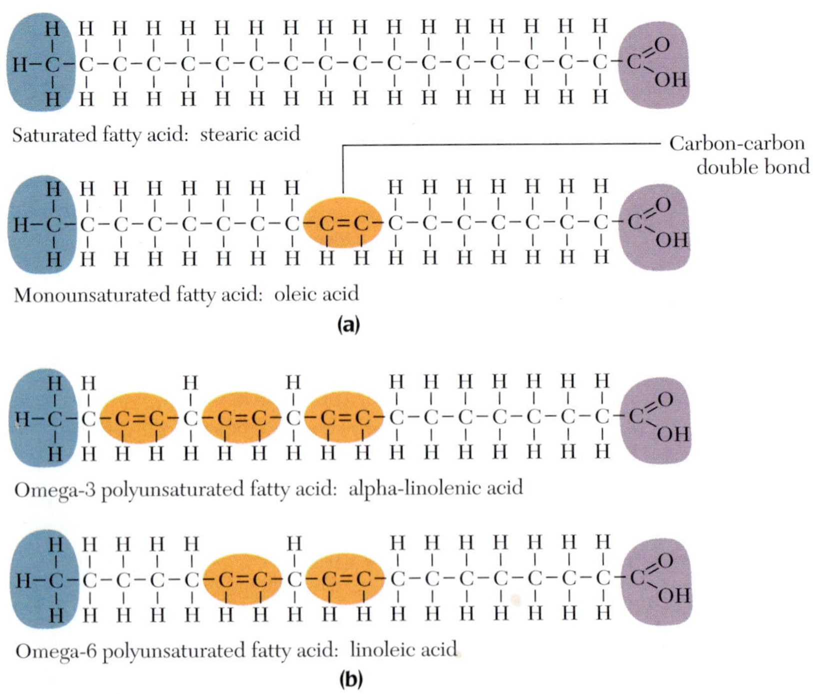

FIGURE 5.2 (a) Monounsaturated fatty acids contain a single double bond between carbons. The structure of the 18-carbon saturated fatty acid stearic acid and the 18-carbon monounsaturated fatty acid oleic acid are shown here. (b) The type of polyunsaturated fatty acid is determined by the position of the first double bond. In the omega numbering system, the bonds are counted beginning at the methyl (CH_3) end of the carbon chain. Shown here are the 18-carbon omega-3 polyunsaturated fatty acid alpha-linolenic acid and the 18-carbon omega-6 fatty acid linoleic acid.

oils. Unsaturated fatty acids melt at cooler temperatures than saturated fatty acids of the same chain length. Therefore, the more unsaturated bonds a fatty acid contains, the more likely it is to be liquid at room temperature. For example, margarine, which has more unsaturated bonds than butter, is more likely to melt at room temperature. The fat we consume in foods contains combinations of saturated, monounsaturated, and polyunsaturated fatty acids.

Location of the First Double Bond There are different categories of unsaturated fatty acids, depending on the location of the first double bond in the carbon chain. If the first double bond occurs between the third and fourth carbons, counting from the omega (CH_3) end of the chain (see Figure 5.2b), the fat is said to be an **omega-3 (ω-3) fatty acid.** Alpha-linolenic acid, found in vegetable oils, and eicosapentaenoic acid (EPA) and docosahexaenoic acid (DHA), found in fish oils, are omega-3 fatty acids. If the first double bond occurs between the sixth and seventh carbons from the omega end, the fatty acid is called an **omega-6 (ω-6) fatty acid.** Linoleic acid is the major omega-6 fatty acid in the North American diet. Both omega-3 and omega-6 fatty acids are precursors of compounds that help regulate blood clotting, blood pressure, and other body processes.[1] The correct ratio of the two is necessary to allow normal bodily functions.

Cis *versus* Trans *Double Bonds* The position of the hydrogen atoms around a double bond is another way of classifying unsaturated fatty acids. Most unsaturated fatty acids found in nature have both hydrogen atoms on the same side of the double bond, called the *cis* conformation. When the hydrogens are on opposite sides of the double bond—called the *trans* conformation—the fatty acid is a ***trans* fatty acid** (Figure 5.3). A *trans* fatty acid has a higher melting point than the same fatty acid in the *cis* conformation. *Trans* fatty acids are found naturally in some foods in small amounts and are formed during the **hydrogenation** of vegetable oils (see "Hydrogenated Fats" below).[2]

Essential Fatty Acids The body is capable of synthesizing most of the fatty acids it needs from glucose or other sources of carbon, hydrogen, and oxygen. However, humans are not able to synthesize double bonds in the omega-6 and omega-3 positions. Therefore, the fatty acids, linoleic acid (omega-6), and alpha-linolenic acid (omega-3), are **essential fatty acids.** They must be consumed in the diet to make other omega-6 and omega-3 fatty acids. Omega-6 fatty acids are important for growth, fertility, and maintaining skin and red blood cell structure. Omega-3 fatty acids are important for the structure and function of cell membranes, particularly in the retina of the eye and in the central nervous system. If the diet is low in linoleic acid or alpha-linolenic acid, the fatty acids synthesized from them become dietary essentials. Arachidonic acid is an omega-6 fatty acid synthesized from linoleic acid. Arachidonic acid is considered essential only when the diet is low in linoleic acid. It is found in both animal and vegetable fats. EPA and DHA are omega-3 fatty acids synthesized from alpha-linolenic acid. Arachidonic and DHA are necessary for normal brain development in infants and young children. They may be essential in the diets of infants, particularly in preterm infants, because the rate at which these are synthesized may not be sufficient to meet body needs.[3]

Glycerides

Most fatty acids in food and in the body are found attached to a three-carbon molecule called glycerol. When three fatty acids are attached, the molecule is called a **triacylglycerol,** commonly known as a triglyceride (Figure 5.4). When one fatty acid is attached, the molecule is called a monoacylglycerol, or monoglyceride, and when two fatty acids are attached, it is a diacylglycerol, or diglyceride. Triglycerides may contain any combination of fatty acids: long-, medium-, or

Omega-3 (ω-3) fatty acid A fatty acid containing a carbon-carbon double bond between the third and fourth carbons from the omega end.

Omega-6 (ω-6) fatty acid A fatty acid containing a carbon-carbon double bond between the sixth and seventh carbons from the omega end.

***Trans* fatty acid** An unsaturated fatty acid in which the hydrogens are on opposite sides of the double bond.

Hydrogenation The process whereby hydrogens are added to the carbon-carbon double bonds of unsaturated fatty acids, making them more saturated.

Essential fatty acids Fatty acids that must be consumed in the diet because they cannot be made by the body or cannot be made in sufficient quantities to meet needs.

Triacylglycerol (triglyceride) The major form of lipid in food and in the body. It consists of three fatty acids attached to a glycerol molecule. When only one fatty acid is attached, it is a monoacylglycerol or monoglyceride, and when two are attached, it is a diacylglycerol or diglyceride.

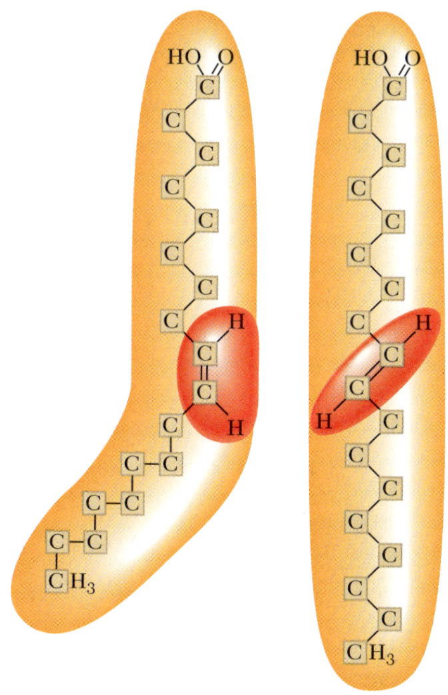

FIGURE 5.3 The orientation of hydrogen atoms around the double bond distinguishes *cis* and *trans* fatty acids. In *cis* fatty acids, the hydrogens are on the same side of the double bond and cause a bend in the carbon chain. In *trans* fatty acids the hydrogens are on opposite sides of the double bond and the carbon chain is straighter.

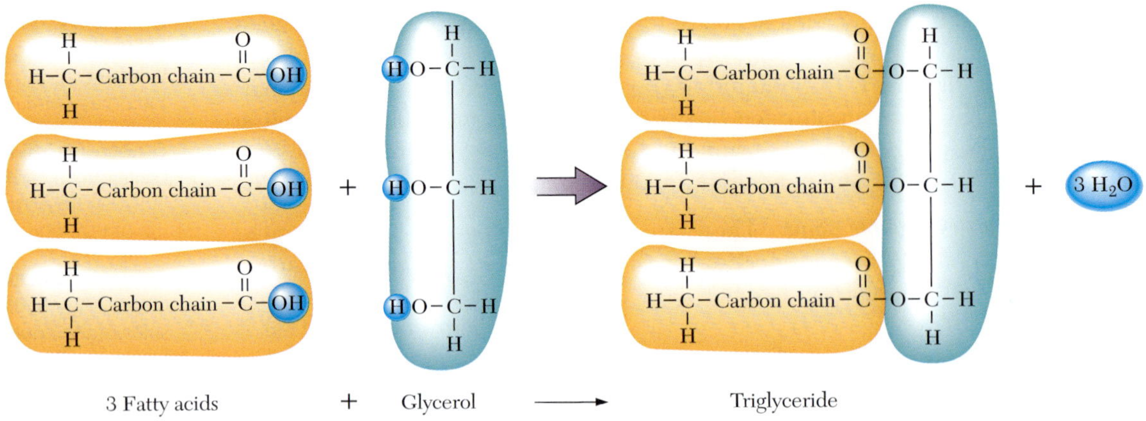

FIGURE 5.4 A triglyceride (triacylglycerol) is formed when three fatty acids are attached to a molecule of glycerol in a condensation reaction. A hydrogen atom (H) from the glycerol and a hydroxyl group (OH) from the acid end of the fatty acid combine to form water that is released when the bond is formed.

short-chain, saturated or unsaturated. Triglycerides make up most of the lipids in our food and in our bodies and are usually what are referred to when the term "fat" is used.

Phospholipids

Phosphoglycerides A type of phospholipid composed of a glycerol backbone with two fatty acids and a phosphate group attached.

Phospholipids are lipids attached to a chemical group containing phosphorus called a phosphate group. The **phosphoglycerides** are the major class of phospholipids. Like triglycerides, they have a backbone of glycerol. However, they have only two fatty acids attached to them. In place of the third fatty acid is a phosphate group, which is then attached to a variety of other molecules (Figure 5.5). The specific function of a phosphoglyceride depends on the molecule that is attached to the phosphate group. The fatty acid end of phosphoglycerides is soluble in fat, whereas the phosphate end is water-soluble. This allows phosphoglycerides to mix in both water and fat—a property that makes them important for many functions in the body and in foods. For example, lecithin, a phosphoglyceride that has a molecule of choline attached to its phosphate group, is a major constituent of cell membranes in the body. In cell membranes, lecithin and other phosphoglycerides form a lipid bilayer, in which the water-soluble phosphate groups orient toward the aqueous (water) environment both inside and outside the cell, while the water-insoluble fatty acids stay in the lipid environment sandwiched between them (Figure 5.6). This forms a barrier that helps regulate which substances can pass into

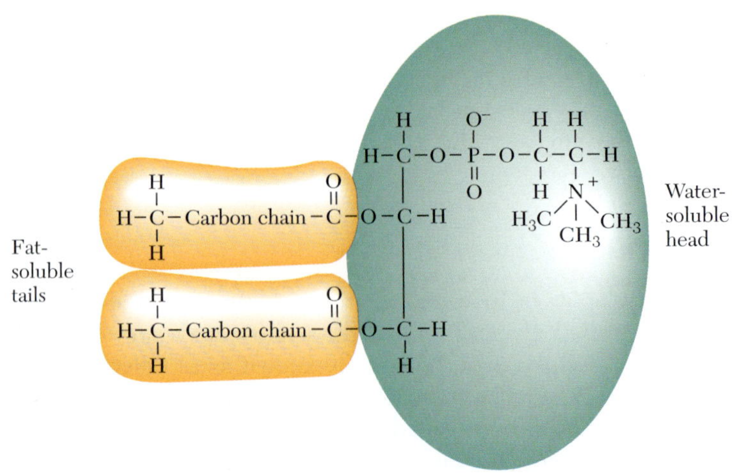

FIGURE 5.5 Phosphoglycerides, such as the lecithin shown here, consist of a water-soluble head containing a phosphate group and two lipid-soluble fatty acid tails.

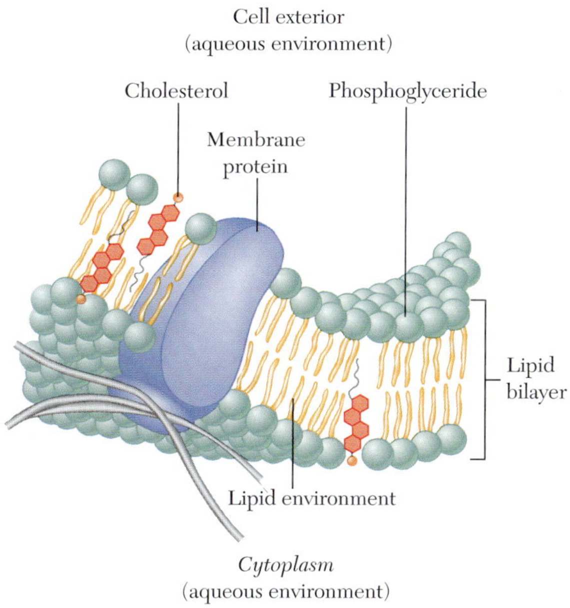

FIGURE 5.6 In cell membranes, phosphoglycerides form a lipid bilayer by orienting the water-soluble phosphate-containing head toward the watery environment inside and outside the cell and the fatty acid tails toward the interior of the membrane. Animal cell membranes also contain proteins and molecules of cholesterol.

Sterols Lipid compounds that contain atoms arranged in multiple ring structures with a variety of side chains attached.

Cholesterol A lipid made only by animal cells that consists of multiple chemical rings.

Anabolic steroids Synthetic fat-soluble hormones used by some athletes to increase muscle mass.

and out of the cell. In food, lecithin helps to keep the oil from separating from the water-soluble ingredients. It is used by the food industry as an additive to margarine, salad dressings, chocolate, frozen desserts, and baked goods.

Sterols

Structurally, **sterols** are composed of multiple rings, which makes them very different from triglycerides and phosphoglycerides (Figure 5.7). Like other lipids, they do not dissolve well in water. **Cholesterol** is a sterol necessary in the body, but because it is made in the liver, cholesterol is not essential in the diet. More than 90% of the cholesterol in the body is found in cell membranes (see Figure 5.6). Cholesterol is probably best known for its role in the development of cardiovascular disease. **Anabolic steroids** are also sterols. These drugs mimic the action of steroid hormones that stimulate muscle growth. Their use has been popular in athletes trying to increase muscle strength and muscle mass; however, they are illegal and can cause liver damage and other negative long-term health effects (see Chapter 14).

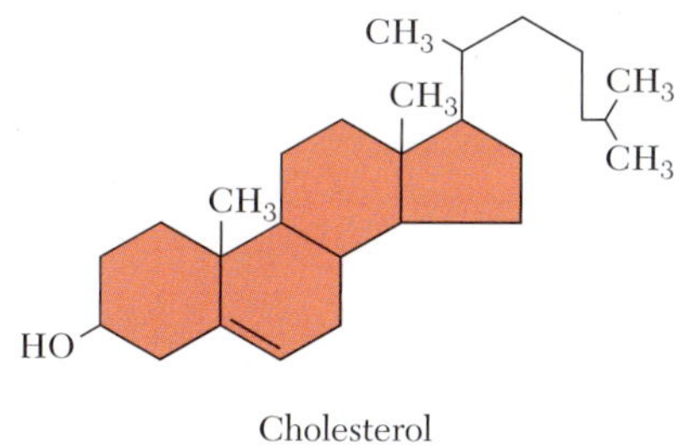

FIGURE 5.7 The four colored rings in this cholesterol molecule indicate the backbone structure common to all sterols.

Lipids in the Diet

Lipids (fats) occur naturally in foods and are added in processing and preparation. They contribute texture, flavor, and aroma to our food and can affect its stability and shelf life. The fat in ice cream gives it its smooth texture and rich taste. Olive oil imparts a unique taste to Italian food, and sesame oil gives Chinese food its distinctive aroma. Fats also provide a concentrated source of energy in food—9 kcalories per g.

Triglycerides and Fatty Acids

Triglycerides make up most of the fats we eat in food. Some of this fat occurs naturally, such as the fat on the outside of a cut of meat. And some is added to foods, such as dressing poured on a salad (Figure 5.8). These are visible examples of fat in food, but other sources, such as the fat used in processing, preparation, and cooking, are less obvious (Table 5.1).

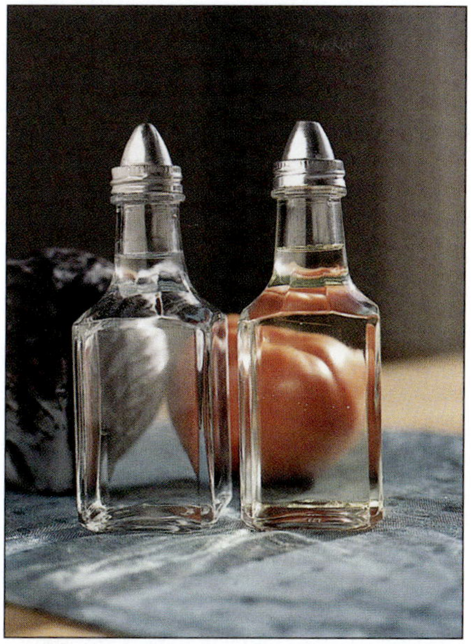

FIGURE 5.8 Oil added to salads is an obvious source of fat. *(© George Semple)*

TABLE 5.1 Comparison of Low-Fat and High-Fat Choices

Food	Serving	Fat (g)	Energy (kcal)
Steak, fat trimmed	3 oz	4.2	150
Steak, not trimmed	3 oz	8.0	186
Broiled chicken breast (no skin)	3 oz	3.0	140
Fried chicken breast (with skin)	3 oz	23.0	423
Salad without dressing	1 cup	0.2	14
Salad with dressing	1 cup	3.0	45
Potato, baked	1 medium	0.1	118
Potato, baked with sour cream	1 medium	5.6	174
French fries	1 small order	10.0	202
Bagel	1 large	1.0	236
Doughnut, glazed	1 large	22.0	436
Fresh broccoli	1 cup	0.2	24
Frozen broccoli with cheese sauce	1 cup	15.0	220
Egg noodles	1 cup	2.0	213
Ramen noodles	1 cup	12.0	275
Spaghetti with tomato sauce	1 cup	1.5	216
Spaghetti with cream sauce	1 cup	19.0	385

The types of fatty acids that make up the triglycerides in food determine the texture, taste, and physical characteristics that the fat gives to food. For example, the amounts and types of fatty acids in chocolate allow it to remain brittle at room temperature, snap when bitten into, and then melt quickly and smoothly in the mouth. The proportions of different types of fatty acids vary with the original food source. Typically, meats, dairy products, and other animal products are the main source of saturated fatty acids in the diet, but some plant oils, such as palm kernel and coconut oils, are also high in saturated fatty acids (see "Tropical Oils"). Unsaturated fats in our diet also come from both plant and animal sources. Olive, canola, and peanut oils are high in monounsaturated fatty acids (Figure 5.9). Other plant oils such as safflower, sunflower, and corn oils provide the omega-6

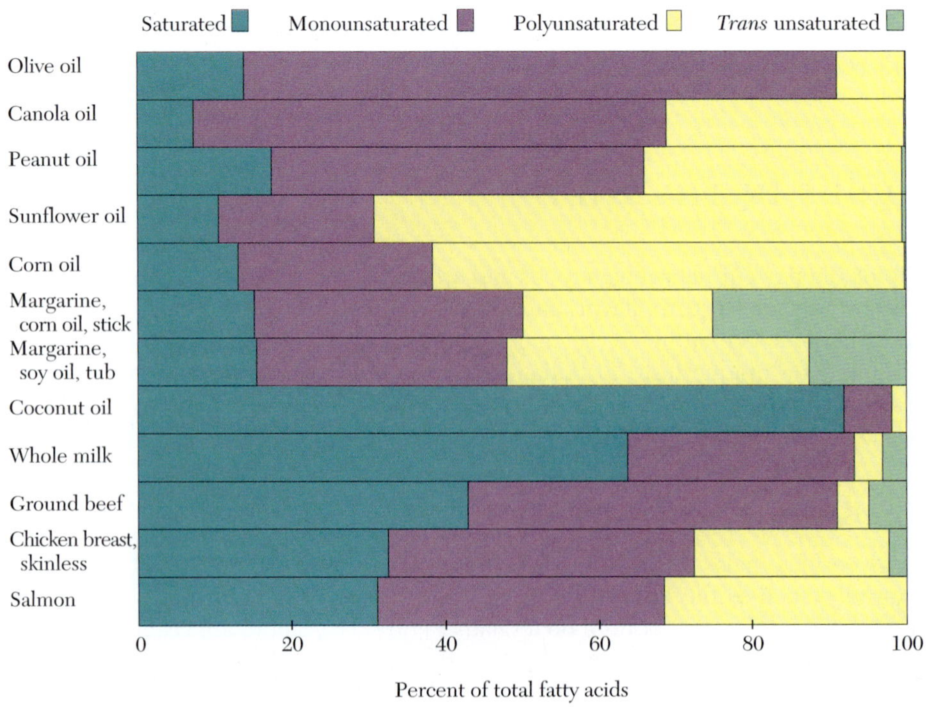

FIGURE 5.9 Foods contain varying amounts of saturated, monounsaturated, polyunsaturated, and *trans* unsaturated fatty acids. This graph shows the amounts of these types of fatty acids as a percentage of the total amount of fat in the product. *(From USDA, ARS, Beltsville Human Nutrition Research Center, Special Purpose Table No. 1. Fat and fatty acid content of selected foods containing* trans *fatty acids.)*

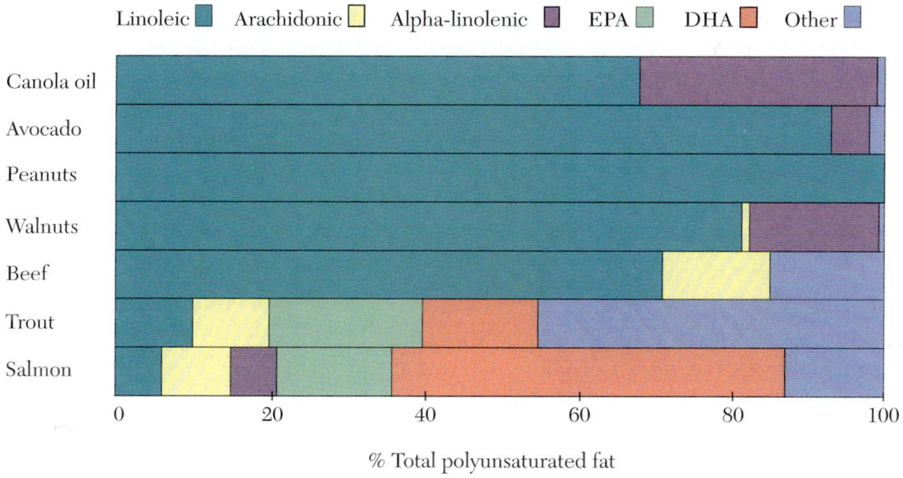

FIGURE 5.10 This bar graph shows the proportions of the omega-6 fatty acids linoleic and arachidonic acid and the omega-3 fatty acids alpha-linolenic acid, EPA, and DHA in selected foods as a percent of the amount of polyunsaturated fat in that food. Note that the amount of saturated fat found in these foods is not included in this graph.

polyunsaturated fatty acid linoleic acid. Meats are high in saturated fat but also supply linoleic and arachidonic acid. Fish and seafood provide the omega-3 polyunsaturated fatty acids EPA and DHA, and plant oils, nuts, seeds, and some vegetables provide alpha-linolenic acid (Figure 5.10).

Hydrogenated Fats Hydrogenated fats are made by bubbling hydrogen gas into an unsaturated liquid oil, causing some of the double bonds in the oil to accept hydrogen atoms and become saturated. The resulting fat is less susceptible to rancidity and has a higher melting point than the original oil. Hydrogenated or partially hydrogenated vegetable oils are a primary ingredient in margarine and vegetable shortening because they raise the melting point of the products, making them more solid at room temperature. In breakfast cereals and other processed foods such as cookies, crackers, and potato chips, they are used to lengthen shelf life (Figure 5.11).

Although beneficial in food manufacturing, the hydrogenation of vegetable oils creates some health concerns. During hydrogenation, some of the unsaturated bonds are converted from the *cis* to the *trans* conformation. The resulting product contains more *trans* fatty acids than the original oil. Consuming a diet high in *trans* fatty acids may increase the risk for both heart disease and cancer. *Trans* fatty acids are present naturally in small amounts in animal fats, but can account for as much as 20% of the total fat in hydrogenated products such as margarine and shortening (see Figure 5.9).

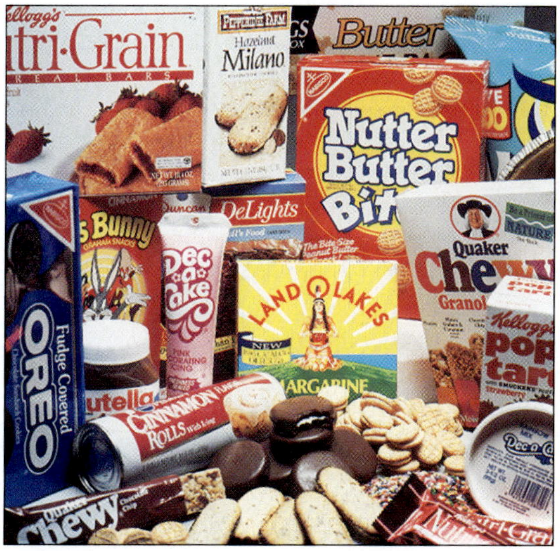

FIGURE 5.11 Products such as these are made with partially hydrogenated vegetable oil, which helps increase their shelf life. *(Charles D. Winters)*

Tropical Oils: Saturated Vegetable Oils Palm oil, palm kernel oil, and coconut oil are vegetable sources of saturated fatty acids. These are often called tropical oils because they are found in plants common in tropical climates. The tropical oils are rarely added to foods at home but are used by the food industry in cereals, crackers, salad dressings, and cookies. Products that contain these saturated fats are more resistant to spoilage and have longer shelf lives than those containing unsaturated fats.

Coconut, palm, and palm kernel oils provide only a small amount of the saturated fat in the American diet.[4] However, concern about the saturated-fat content of the diet has led many of the large food manufacturers to reformulate some of their products to use unsaturated vegetable oils. This reduces the saturated fat content of the foods but does not come without a cost to the consumer. Coconut oil, which comes primarily from the Philippines and Indonesia, and palm oil, which is imported from Malaysia, are usually cheaper than the soybean and corn oil produced in North America, so changing oils can increase the product price. Shorter shelf life and increased wastage of product can also increase consumer costs.

Cholesterol

Cholesterol is a lipid produced by animals, hence it is only found in foods of animal origin. Egg yolks and organ meats such as liver and kidney are high in cholesterol. One egg yolk contains about 213 mg of cholesterol. Organ meats contain about 300 mg per 3-ounce (85 g) serving. Lean red meats and skinless chicken contain about 90 mg in a 3-ounce serving, whereas fish contains 50 mg in 3 ounces. Plant foods do not contain cholesterol unless animal products are combined with them in cooking or processing.

Phospholipids

In foods, the ability of phospholipids to mix in water and fat makes them good emulsifiers, which are substances that allow water and fat to mix by breaking large fat globules into smaller ones. For example, egg yolks, which contain the phosphoglyceride lecithin, are added to cake batter to help the oil and water to mix.

Lipids in the Digestive Tract

Lipid digestion begins in the stomach due to the action of lipases produced in the mouth and stomach. These enzymes work best on triglycerides containing short- and medium-chain fatty acids such as those in milk, and so are particularly important in infants.[5] In healthy adults, most of the digestion of dietary fat takes place in the small intestine due to the action of lipases secreted by the pancreas.

Long-Chain Triglycerides

When the products of digestion enter the duodenum, the peristaltic movement of the small intestine and bile from the gallbladder help break large fat globules into smaller ones. The emulsifying action of bile keeps the fat droplets separate and allows water-soluble enzymes such as pancreatic lipase access to triglycerides, which are broken down to fatty acids and monoglycerides. These mix with bile to form smaller droplets called **micelles.** Micelles have a fat-soluble center surrounded by a coating of bile acids (Figure 5.12). Micelles facilitate the absorption of lipids into the mucosal cells of the small intestine. When the micelle comes close to the intestinal brush border, the monoglycerides and fatty acids diffuse into the mucosal cells. Because long-chain fatty acids are not soluble in water, further processing is necessary before they can be transported in the blood.

Micelles Small particles consisting of a core of fatty acids, monoglycerides, and other fat-soluble substances surrounded by bile acids that aid the absorption of lipids in the small intestine.

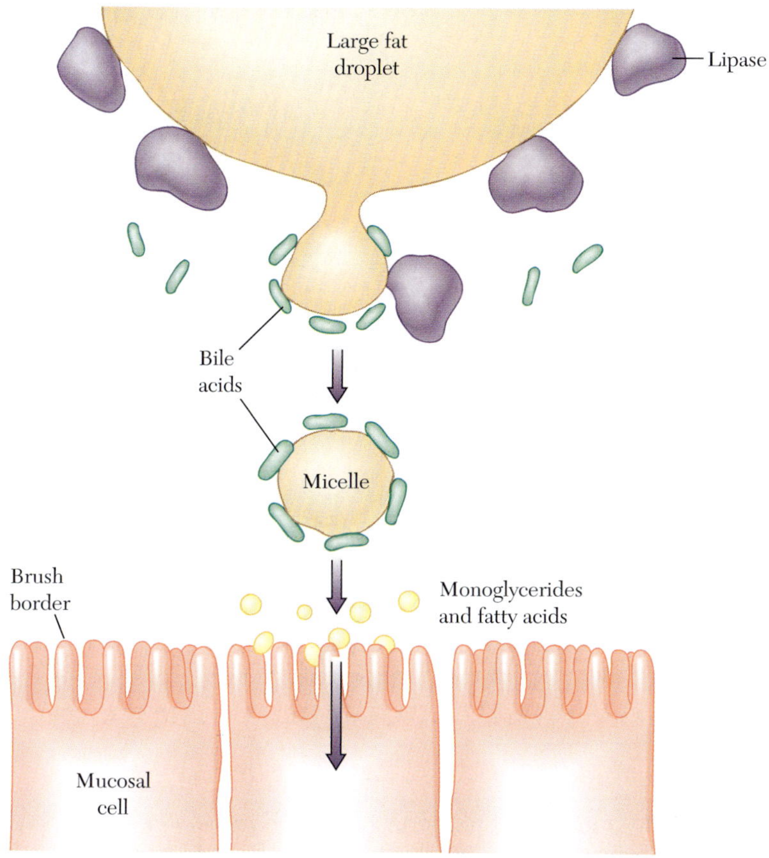

FIGURE 5.12 Bile acids help break fats into small droplets called micelles. The center of the micelle contains fatty acids, monoglycerides, cholesterol, and other fat-soluble substances. When the micelle moves close to the brush border, these fat-soluble substances are able to diffuse into the mucosal cells of the small intestine.

The processes necessary for the digestion and absorption of long-chain triglycerides are also necessary for the absorption of cholesterol, fat-soluble vitamins, and other fat-soluble molecules, such as beta-carotene. These lipid-soluble molecules must also be incorporated into micelles to be absorbed, and therefore their absorption depends on the presence of dietary fat. Most of the bile acids in micelles are also absorbed and returned to the liver to be reused.

Medium-Chain Triglycerides

Medium-chain triglycerides contain fatty acids that are 8 to 12 carbons in length and are water-soluble. They can be digested rapidly and do not require bile for digestion and absorption. Once these fatty acids enter the mucosal cell, they can be absorbed directly into the hepatic portal circulation along with the products of carbohydrate and protein digestion. Medium-chain triglycerides are found naturally in milk fat, palm kernel oil, and coconut oil. They are also sold commercially for use by individuals who cannot digest and absorb long-chain triglycerides due to diseases of or damage to the intestine.

Lipids in the Body

Just as water-insoluble lipids require special mechanisms to be absorbed into the body, they require special transport mechanisms to be circulated throughout the body. After lipids have been delivered to cells, they can be stored as an energy reserve, used to make structural and regulatory molecules, or be broken down via cellular respiration to produce carbon dioxide, water, and energy in the form of ATP.

FIGURE 5.13 Lipoproteins consist of a core of triglycerides and cholesterol with a shell of proteins, phospholipids, and cholesterol. Phospholipids orient with their fat-soluble tails toward the interior and their water-soluble heads toward the outside. This allows water-insoluble lipids to be transported in the aqueous environment of the blood.

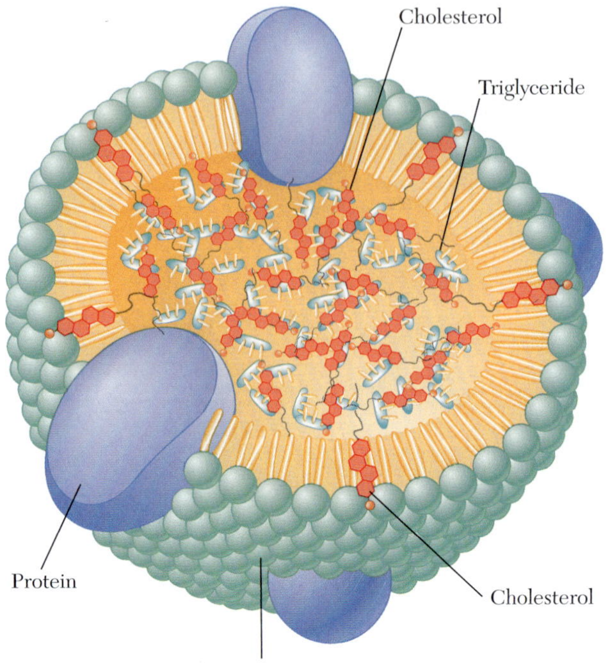

Lipid Transport

Lipoproteins Particles containing a core of triglycerides and cholesterol surrounded by a shell of proteins, phospholipids, and cholesterol. They transport lipids in blood and lymph.

Water-insoluble lipids are transported in the blood coated in a water-soluble envelope that is formed when the lipids combine with proteins to form particles called **lipoproteins** (Figure 5.13). Fat-soluble vitamins are also transported in lipoproteins.

Chylomicrons Lipoproteins that transport lipids from the mucosal cells of the intestine and deliver triglycerides to body cells.

Lipoprotein lipase An enzyme attached to cell membranes that breaks down triglycerides into fatty acids and glycerol.

Transport from the Small Intestine Lipids that are not soluble in water, such as long-chain fatty acids and cholesterol, cannot enter the bloodstream directly. After absorption into the intestinal mucosal cells, monoglycerides and long-chain fatty acids are assembled into triglycerides. These triglycerides are then combined with cholesterol, phospholipids, and a small amount of protein to form lipoproteins called **chylomicrons.** Chylomicrons enter lacteals in the intestinal villi. They are transported in the lymphatic system to the thoracic duct where they enter the bloodstream. By this route, they enter the blood circulation without first passing through the liver.

As chylomicrons circulate in the blood, the enzyme **lipoprotein lipase,** present on the surface of the cells lining the blood vessels, breaks the triglycerides down into fatty acids and glycerol, which enter the surrounding cells. The fatty acids can be either used as fuel or resynthesized into triglycerides for storage. What remains of the chylomicrons is chylomicron remnants composed mostly of cholesterol and protein. Chylomicron remnants travel to the liver where they are disassembled (Figure 5.14).

Very-low-density lipoproteins (VLDLs) Lipoproteins assembled by the liver that carry lipid from the liver and deliver triglycerides to body cells.

Transport from the Liver The liver is the major lipid-producing organ in the body. Here, excess protein, carbohydrate, or alcohol can be broken down and used to make triglycerides or cholesterol. Triglycerides made in the liver are incorporated into lipoprotein particles called **very-low-density lipoproteins (VLDLs).** Cholesterol synthesized in the liver or delivered in chylomicron remnants can also be incorporated into VLDLs or be used to make bile. VLDLs transport lipids out of the liver and deliver triglycerides to body cells. As with chylomicrons, the enzyme lipoprotein lipase breaks down the triglycerides in VLDLs so that the fatty acids can be taken up by surrounding cells.

Once the triglycerides are removed from the VLDLs, a denser, smaller, intermediate-density lipoprotein (IDL) remains. About two thirds of the IDLs are

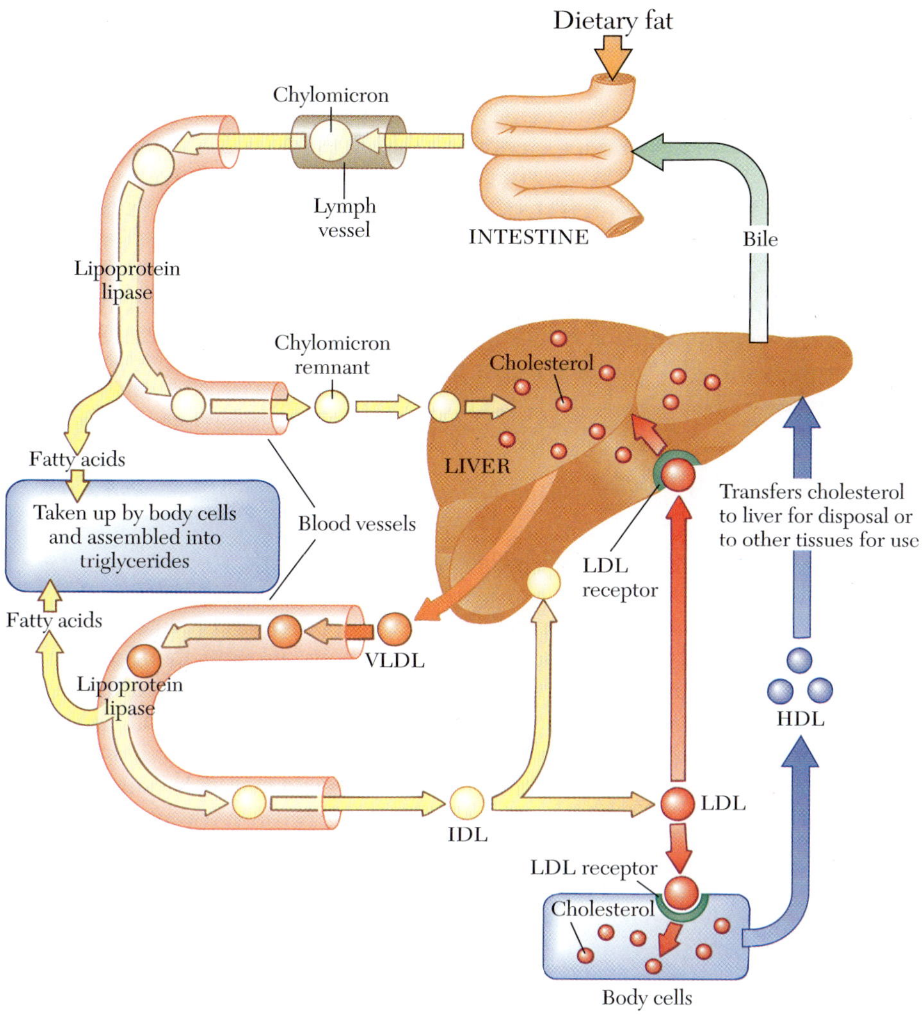

FIGURE 5.14 Chylomicrons carry lipids from the intestines into the lymph and then the bloodstream. With the help of lipoprotein lipase, they deliver fatty acids to body cells. The remainder of the chylomicron, called a chylomicron remnant, is delivered to the liver. VLDLs formed in the liver carry lipids from the liver to body cells. The activity of the enzyme lipoprotein lipase is needed for VLDLs to deliver fatty acids to body cells. After the triglycerides in VLDLs have been broken down to fatty acids and removed, IDLs remain. Some IDLs are transformed into LDLs, which are the primary cholesterol delivery system for body cells. LDLs are taken into cells after first binding to the LDL receptor. HDLs carry cholesterol away from cells and return it to the liver.

returned to the liver, and the rest are transformed in the blood into **low-density lipoproteins (LDLs).** LDLs contain an even higher proportion of cholesterol than VLDLs and are the primary cholesterol delivery system for cells (Figure 5.15). For LDLs to be taken up by cells, a protein on the surface of the LDL particle must bind to a receptor protein on the cell membrane, called an **LDL receptor.** This binding allows LDLs to be removed from circulation and enter cells

Low-density lipoproteins (LDLs) Lipoproteins that transport cholesterol to cells. Elevated LDL cholesterol increases the risk of cardiovascular disease.

LDL receptor A protein on the surface of cells that binds to LDL particles and allows them to be taken into the cells making their contents available for use by the cell.

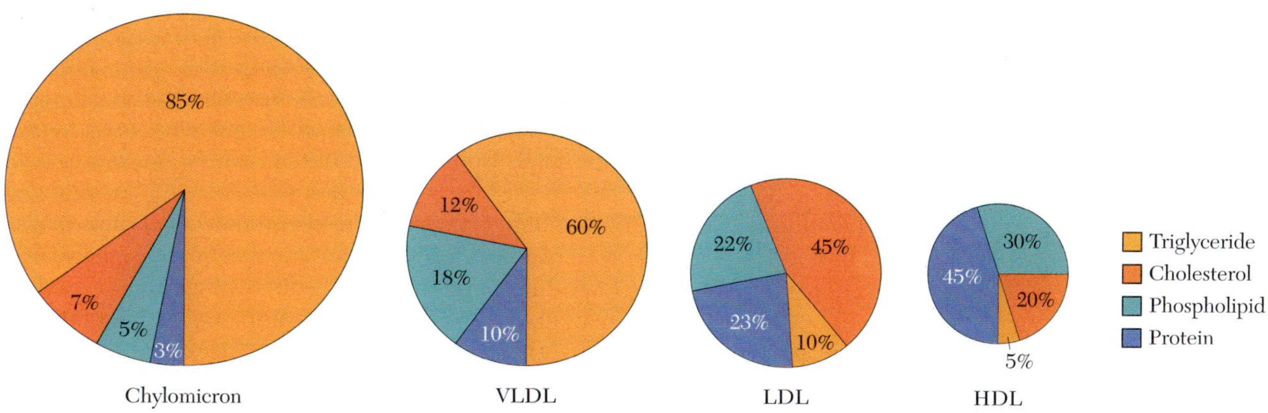

FIGURE 5.15 All lipoproteins consist of a shell of phospholipid, protein, and cholesterol and a center of triglycerides and cholesterol, but they vary in size and density. The proportions of these in the different lipoproteins are shown here. Chylomicrons are the largest, least-dense particles and contain the most triglyceride, whereas HDLs are the smallest, densest particles and have the greatest percentage of protein.

where their cholesterol and other components can be used (see Figure 5.14). High levels of LDLs in the blood have been associated with an increased risk of heart disease.

Because most body cells have no system for breaking cholesterol down, it must be returned to the liver to be eliminated from the body. This reverse cholesterol transport is accomplished by the densest of the lipoprotein particles, called **high-density lipoproteins (HDLs).** These particles originate from the intestinal tract and liver and circulate in the blood, picking up cholesterol from other lipoproteins and body cells. Some of the cholesterol in HDLs is taken directly to the liver for disposal, and some is transferred to other lipoproteins or organs that have a high requirement for cholesterol, such as those involved in steroid hormone synthesis. High levels of HDL in the blood are associated with a reduction in heart disease risk.

High-density lipoproteins (HDLs) Lipoproteins that pick up cholesterol from cells and transport it to the liver so that it can be eliminated from the body. A low level of HDL increases the risk of cardiovascular disease.

Functions of Lipids

In the body, lipids are a concentrated source of energy. They also provide a number of protective, structural, and regulatory roles.

Energy Lipids can be used as an immediate source of energy or stored for future use. Triglycerides, the most abundant lipid in the body, provide about 85% of the stored energy in a normal weight adult. Most triglyceride is stored in **adipose tissue,** which lies under the skin and around internal organs. Each gram of triglyceride provides 9 kcalories, compared with only 4 kcalories per g from carbohydrate or protein. Because triglycerides are a concentrated energy source, a large amount of energy can be stored without a great increase in body size or weight.

Adipose tissue Tissue found under the skin and around body organs that is composed of fat-storing cells.

Protection and Lubrication In addition to providing an energy storage site, adipose tissue protects the body from changes in temperature. It forms an insulating layer and cushions the internal organs to protect them against shock. Lipids are also important for lubricating body surfaces. Glands in the skin and mucous membranes release lipids that lubricate these tissues.

Structure Phospholipids and cholesterol are also important structural components of the membranes that surround cells and the internal membranes surrounding organelles (see Figure 5.6). Lipids are particularly important structural components of the brain and nervous system, where the cholesterol-rich membranes of specialized cells surround nerve cells to form the myelin coating that is essential for nerve transmission.

Regulation Lipids also have important regulatory roles. A number of signaling molecules both inside and outside the cell are made of lipid. Inside the cell, lipid molecules help relay signals from the cell membrane to enzymes in the cell cytoplasm or to proteins that regulate the activity of genes in the nucleus (see Chapter 6). Outside the cell they send signals from one part of the body to another to help regulate body functions.

Lecithin, which is a phospholipid important in membrane structure, is also used to synthesize the neurotransmitter acetylcholine. Acetylcholine signals muscle cells to contract and is important in the memory center of the brain. Based on these functions, lecithin is marketed to consumers as a supplement that improves memory and maintains proper cell function. Lecithin is not essential in the diet and is made in ample amounts by the body.

Cholesterol is used to synthesize bile salts, needed for digestion and absorption. It is also the precursor for a number of steroid molecules that travel through the blood and affect cell functions. For example, the following are all synthesized from cholesterol: vitamin D, a vitamin needed for calcium absorption; cortisol, a hormone that promotes glucose synthesis in the liver; and the sex hormones, which promote growth and the development of sex characteristics.

Both omega-3 and omega-6 fatty acids are precursors of a group of compounds called **eicosanoids** or **prostaglandins.** Eicosanoids are hormone-like molecules that help regulate blood clotting, blood pressure, immune function, and other body processes.[1] The particular eicosanoid synthesized and its effect depends on the fatty acid precursor. For example, when the omega-6 fatty acid arachidonic acid is the starting material, the eicosanoid that is synthesized enhances blood clotting; when the eicosanoid is made from the omega-3 fatty acid EPA, it inhibits blood clotting. The correct ratio of the two is necessary to allow appropriate blood clotting.

Eicosanoids or **prostaglandins** A group of hormone-like regulatory molecules that can be synthesized from omega-3 and omega-6 fatty acids.

Lipid Metabolism

Fatty acids delivered to cells can be used directly for energy or reassembled into triglycerides and stored for future use. In muscle cells, fatty acids and glycerol are used primarily to produce energy in the form of ATP. During this process, the carbon chain of fatty acids is broken into two-carbon units that form acetyl-CoA and release high-energy electrons (Figure 5.16). Acetyl-CoA can then enter the citric acid cycle, which generates more high-energy electrons. The high-energy electrons released in both steps are shuttled to the electron transport chain to generate ATP (Figure 5.17). Glycerol is a 3-carbon molecule, so it can be used to make glucose or to produce ATP. Glycerol makes up only a small proportion of the carbon in a triglyceride molecule, so the amount of glucose that can result from triglyceride breakdown is small.

Fatty acids delivered to adipose tissue cells are usually reassembled into triglycerides for storage. Throughout the day, some stored triglycerides are broken down and new triglycerides are formed as the energy needs of the body change. For example, after a meal, some triglyceride will be immediately stored; then, between meals, some of the stored triglyceride will be broken down to provide energy. When the energy in the diet equals the body's energy requirements, the net amount of stored triglyceride in the body does not change.

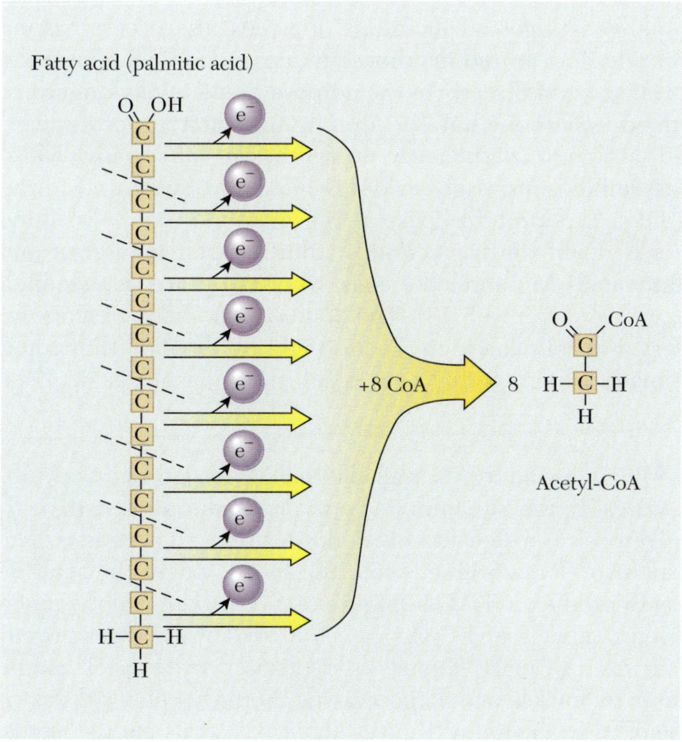

FIGURE 5.16 Fatty acids can be broken down to yield two-carbon fragments that combine with CoA to form acetyl-CoA. Electrons released at each step of this process are passed to the electron transport chain. This molecule of palmitic acid, which contains 16 carbons, can generate eight molecules of acetyl-CoA.

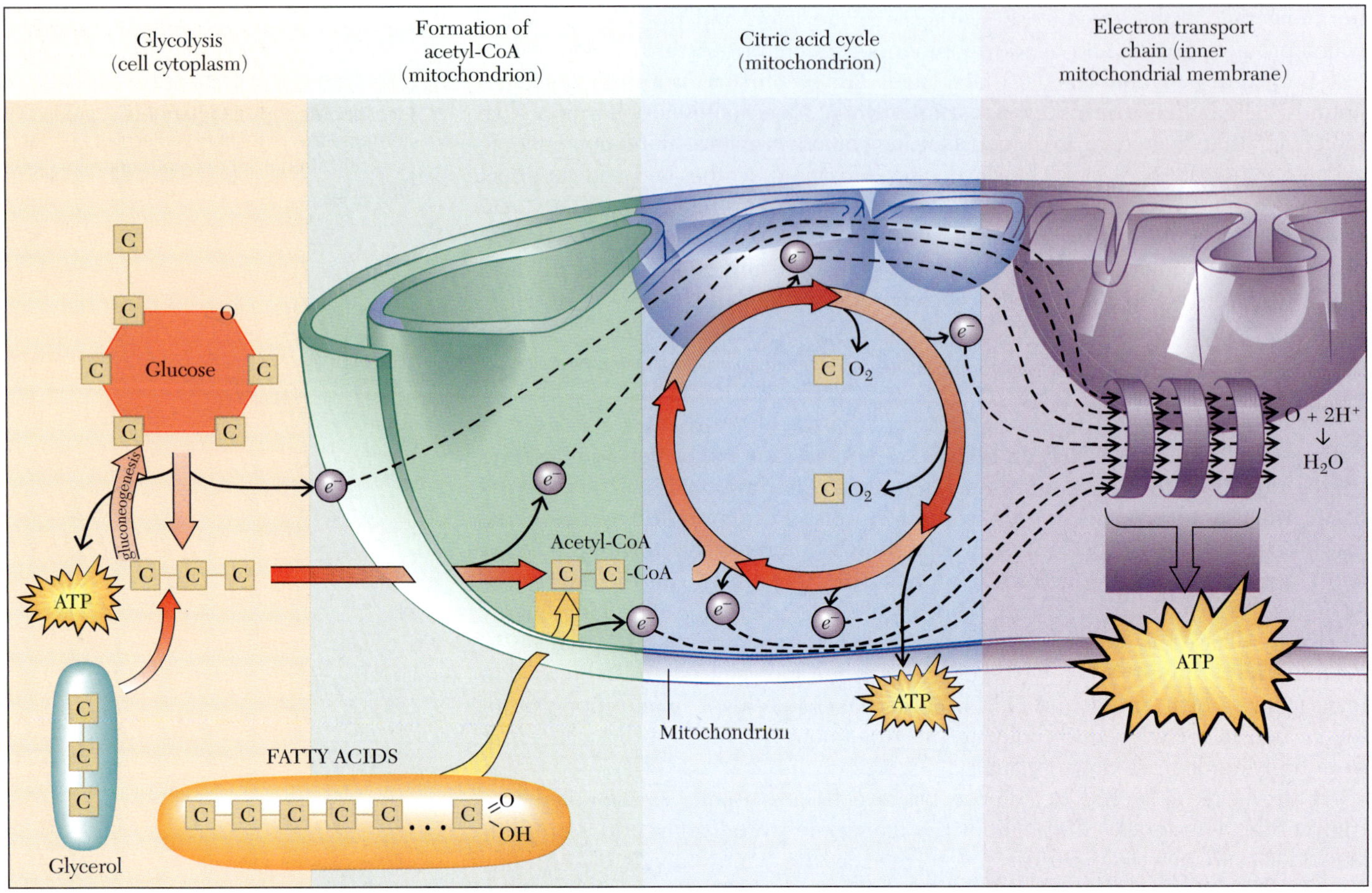

FIGURE 5.17 Triglycerides are broken down to fatty acids and glycerol to produce energy. Fatty acid breakdown yields high-energy electrons that are shuttled to the electron transport chain and two-carbon units that enter the citric acid cycle as acetyl-CoA. Glycerol is a three-carbon molecule that can be converted into pyruvate.

Storing Fat When energy is ingested in excess of needs, the excess can be converted into triglycerides and stored in adipose tissue. Dietary fat consumed in excess of needs is transported directly to the adipose tissue in chylomicrons. Excess energy consumed as carbohydrate or protein must first go to the liver, where it can be used, although inefficiently, to synthesize fatty acids. These fatty acids are then assembled into triglycerides, which are transported to the adipose tissue in VLDLs. Lipoprotein lipase at the membrane of cells lining the blood vessels breaks down the triglycerides from both chylomicrons and VLDLs so that the fatty acids can enter the cells, where they are reassembled into triglycerides for storage (Figure 5.18). The ability of the body to store fat is theoretically limitless. Fat cells can increase in weight by about 50 times, and new fat cells can be made when existing cells reach their maximum size (see Chapter 7).

Releasing Stored Fat When less energy is available than is needed, the body obtains energy from fat stores. In this situation, the enzyme **hormone-sensitive lipase** inside the fat cells receives a signal to break down stored triglycerides. The fatty acids and glycerol are released directly into the blood, where they can be taken up by body cells to produce ATP (see Figure 5.18). If there is not enough carbohydrate in the liver to allow acetyl-CoA from fat breakdown to enter the citric acid cycle, it will be used to make ketones (see Chapter 4). Ketones can be used as an energy source by muscle and adipose tissue. During prolonged starvation, the brain can adapt to use ketones to meet about half of its energy needs.

Hormone-sensitive lipase An enzyme present in adipose cells that responds to chemical signals by breaking stored triglycerides into fatty acids and glycerol for release into the bloodstream.

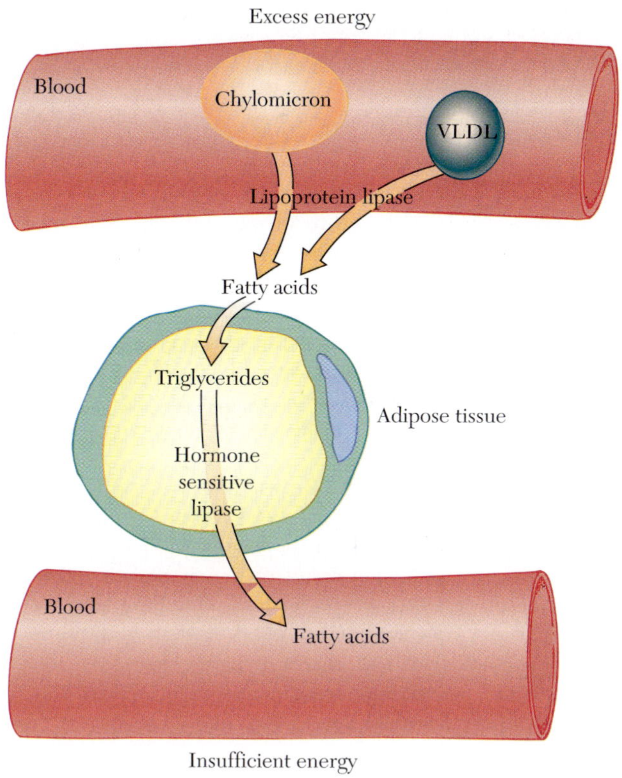

FIGURE 5.18 When excess dietary energy is available, lipoprotein lipase helps remove triglyceride from chylomicrons and VLDLs so it can be stored in adipose tissue. When dietary energy is insufficient, the enzyme hormone sensitive lipase helps break down stored triglycerides to make fatty acids available as an energy source.

The other half of the brain's energy needs must be supplied as glucose. Fatty acids cannot be used to make glucose, and only a small amount of glucose can be made from glycerol.

Lipids and Health

Adequate amounts of essential fatty acids are required to maintain normal body function. However, too much fat, and in particular the wrong types of fats in the diet, increases the risk of chronic disease. Diets high in total fat are associated with obesity because high-fat diets are usually high in energy and promote body fat storage. Excess body fat in turn is associated with an increased risk of diabetes, cardiovascular disease, and high blood pressure. Diets high in saturated fat increase the risk of heart disease, and polyunsaturated fat intake may be related to cancer incidence. In addition to the type and amount of fat consumed, other dietary and lifestyle factors are also important in reducing disease risk and maintaining health.

Essential Fatty Acid Deficiency

People often think of fat as unhealthy; however, if adequate amounts of linoleic and alpha-linolenic acid are not consumed, an **essential fatty acid deficiency** will result. Symptoms include scaly, dry skin, liver abnormalities, poor healing of wounds, impaired vision and hearing, and growth failure in infants. Essential fatty acid deficiency is rare because the requirement for essential fatty acids is well below the typical intake. Deficiencies have been seen, however, in infants and young children fed low-fat diets, in individuals who are unable to absorb lipids, and in adults consuming a weight-loss diet consisting of only nonfat milk.

Essential fatty acid deficiency A condition characterized by dry scaly skin and poor growth that results when the diet does not supply sufficient amounts of the essential fatty acids.

RESEARCH DISCOVERIES

A Genetic Disease Helps Us Understand How Blood Cholesterol Is Regulated

Children with a rare form of the inherited disease familial hypercholesterolemia have blood cholesterol levels that range from 650 to 1000 mg/100 ml—six times the normal level. Cholesterol is so high in their blood that it deposits in the tissues, forming soft, yellow, raised bumps on the skin called xanthomas (see figure). The elevated cholesterol damages blood vessels, leading to premature atherosclerosis. Chest pain, heart attacks, and death are common before the age of 15.[a] One patient had a heart attack at 18 months of age.[b] It is rare for individuals with this disease to survive past the age of 30. Research into the causes of this disease led doctors Michael Brown and Joseph Goldstein to a discovery that is key to our understanding of how blood cholesterol is regulated.

There are two forms of familial hypercholesterolemia. The children described above inherited two genes for this disease, causing them to have a rare and more severe form that affects only about one in a million people. About 1 in 500 persons inherits only one gene and has a less severe form of the disease. These individuals have moderately elevated blood cholesterol levels from birth and do not usually develop clinical symptoms of heart disease until after age 30. Adults with this disease have blood cholesterol levels ranging from 300 to 550 mg/100 ml. About 75% of men with this condition will have a heart attack before the age of 60, compared to only 15% of unaffected men.[c]

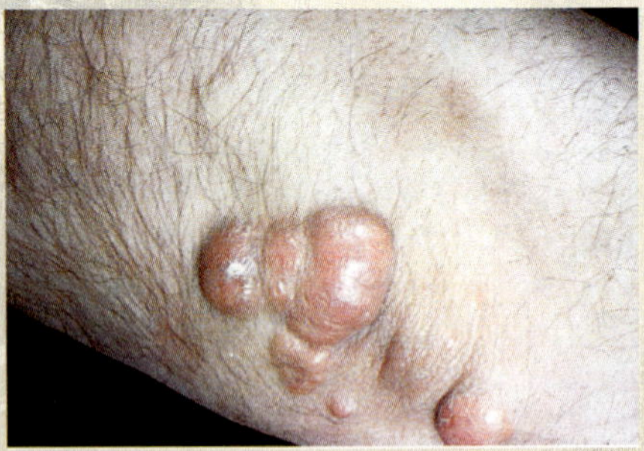

In familial hypercholesterolemia, cholesterol deposits called xanthomas form in the skin.

To study this disease, Brown and Goldstein grew cells in culture. They observed that when LDL cholesterol was added to the culture medium, the rate of cholesterol synthesis in cells from normal subjects decreased. But, in cells from individuals with familial hypercholesterolemia, the presence of LDL in the medium did not cause a decrease in cholesterol synthesis.[d] By using radioactively labeled LDL particles, Brown and Goldstein were able to demonstrate that in cells from normal individuals, LDL particles bind to the cells and are removed from the surrounding media. In cells from individuals with familial hypercholesterolemia, the LDL particles are unable to bind to the cells and therefore cholesterol could not be removed from the surrounding media.[e] The binding of LDL to the cell was found to be due to a protein on the surface of the cell membrane that was named the LDL receptor.

The discovery of the LDL receptor led to an understanding of how the body controls the concentration of LDL cholesterol in the blood. The LDL receptor is a cell surface receptor; it is synthesized by the cell and inserted into the cell membrane. The binding of an LDL particle to the receptor results in the movement of the LDL particle into the cell. Cholesterol entering the cell suppresses the synthesis of new cholesterol. An individual who inherits one gene for familial hypercholesterolemia has about half the number of LDL receptors as someone without the disease. Someone who inherits two genes has no LDL receptors. This means that LDL cholesterol is not removed from the blood and the liver continues to synthesize large amounts of cholesterol, causing LDL particles to accumulate in the blood. The elevated cholesterol leads to atherosclerosis and eventually heart attacks.

In 1985 Brown and Goldstein were awarded the Nobel Prize in Medicine for their work on cholesterol and LDL receptors. As a result of their research, scientists now understand the basis for the development of heart disease. And, physicians and pharmacologists have been able to develop treatments to reduce blood cholesterol levels.

References

[a] Fredrickson, D. S., Goldstein, J. L., and Brown, M. S. The familial hypercholesterolemias. In *The Metabolic Basis of Inherited Disease,* 4th ed., eds. Stanbury, J. B., Wyngaarden, J. B., and Fredrickson, D. S. New York: McGraw-Hill, 1974, 604–655.

[b] Goldstein, J. L., and Brown, M. S. The LDL receptor locus and the genetics of familial hypercholesterolemia. Ann. Rev. Genet. 13:259–289, 1979.

[c] Stone, N. J., Levy, R. I., Fredrickson, D. S., and Verter, J. Coronary artery disease in 116 kindred with familial type II hyperlipoproteinemia. Circulation 49:476–478, 1974.

[d] Goldstein, J. L., and Brown, M. S. The low-density lipoprotein pathway and its relation to atherosclerosis. Ann. Rev. Biochem. 46:897–930, 1977.

[e] Brown, M. S., and Goldstein, J. L. Familial hypercholesterolemia: defective binding of lipoproteins to cultured fibroblasts associated with impaired regulation of 3-hydroxy-3-methylglutaryl coenzyme A reductase activity. Proc. Nat. Acad. Sci. 71:788–792, 1974.

Diet and Heart Disease

Cardiovascular disease Any disease affecting the heart and blood vessels.

Over 58 million people in the United States suffer from one or more forms of heart or **cardiovascular disease.** The relationship between diet and heart disease is one of the most extensively studied of all diet and health relationships. Since 1916, when Dutch internist C. D. de Langen first hypothesized that a cholesterol-rich diet was associated with high blood cholesterol and the occurrence of coronary heart disease, millions of hours and research dollars have been spent studying the relationships between diet and heart disease. Laboratory studies using cells and animal models have helped demonstrate the mechanisms by which blood lipids affect the heart and blood vessels. Feeding studies have examined the effect of different types of fat on blood lipid levels, and epidemiological studies, including the famous Seven Countries Study of Dr. Ancel Keys, have demonstrated a number of relationships between the amount and type of dietary fat and heart disease risk (see Chapter 1, *Research Discoveries:* "From Seven Countries to the Mediterranean Diet"). A high incidence of heart disease has been reported in populations consuming a diet high in saturated fat,[6,7] whereas a low incidence of heart disease is seen in populations, such as the Inuits in Greenland, that consume a diet high in omega-3 fatty acids.[8] In Mediterranean countries, where the diet is high in monounsaturated fat as well as grains and vegetables, deaths from heart disease are less frequent.[9,10]

The Development of Heart Disease **Atherosclerosis** is a type of cardiovascular disease in which lipids are deposited in the artery walls, reducing elasticity and eventually reducing or completely blocking the flow of blood. When cells do not receive blood, they are deprived of oxygen and die very quickly. If blood flow to the heart muscle is interrupted, heart cells die, resulting in a heart attack, or myocardial infarction. If the blood flow to the brain is interrupted, brain cells die and a stroke results. It was originally hypothesized that this was caused by dietary cholesterol transported into the bloodstream and deposited in the arteries.[11] We now know the mechanisms are more complicated and are affected by other dietary and lifestyle factors as well as individual genetic makeup.

Atherosclerosis A type of cardiovascular disease that involves the buildup of fatty material in the artery walls.

LDL Receptors Our current understanding of how atherosclerosis develops is based on the work of Michael Brown and Joseph Goldstein (see *Research Discoveries:* "A Genetic Disease Helps Us Understand How Blood Cholesterol Is Regulated"). They identified LDL receptors on cell membranes and demonstrated how the receptors bind LDL particles in the blood, allowing the LDL to be taken up by the cells and shutting off cholesterol synthesis in the body.[12] Excess LDL cholesterol in the blood can lead to the deposition of cholesterol in the artery walls, causing plaque formation and eventually atherosclerosis.

Plaque Formation The exact events that lead to the buildup of cholesterol in arterial walls are still not fully understood. One theory is that an injury to the arterial wall—possibly caused by high blood pressure, high cholesterol levels, microorganisms, chemicals, or some other factor—begins the process. The injury may be caused by LDL particles that become stuck to molecules in the blood vessel wall while they are passing through to reach nearby cells.[13] After the injury occurs, white blood cells, blood platelets (cell fragments involved in blood clotting), and more LDL particles enter the artery wall. Inside the artery wall, LDL that comes in contact with highly reactive oxygen molecules is transformed into **oxidized LDL cholesterol.** Oxidized LDL cholesterol binds to receptors, called scavenger receptors, on the surface of white blood cells and is transported into these cells.[14] As white blood cells fill with more and more oxidized LDL cholesterol, the white blood cells are transformed into cholesterol-filled foam cells. Foam cells accumulate in the artery wall and then burst, depositing cholesterol to form a fatty streak (Figure 5.19). Platelets signal muscle cells to invade the fatty streak and secrete fibrous proteins. The result is a mass of cholesterol, muscle cells, and fibrous tissue called a **plaque.** Eventually, calcium collects in the plaque and causes it to harden. Blood clots form around the plaque and it continues to enlarge, causing the artery to narrow and lose its elasticity. The buildup of material can become so large that it completely blocks the artery, or a blood clot can break loose from the plaque and block an artery elsewhere. When an artery is blocked, blood can no longer move through it to supply oxygen and nutrients to the cells, and they die quickly.

Oxidized LDL cholesterol A modified cholesterol formed when the cholesterol in LDL particles is oxidized by reactive oxygen molecules. It is key in the development of atherosclerosis because it is taken up by scavenger receptors on white blood cells.

Plaque The cholesterol-rich material that is deposited in the blood vessels of individuals with atherosclerosis. It consists of cholesterol, smooth muscle cells, fibrous tissue, and calcium.

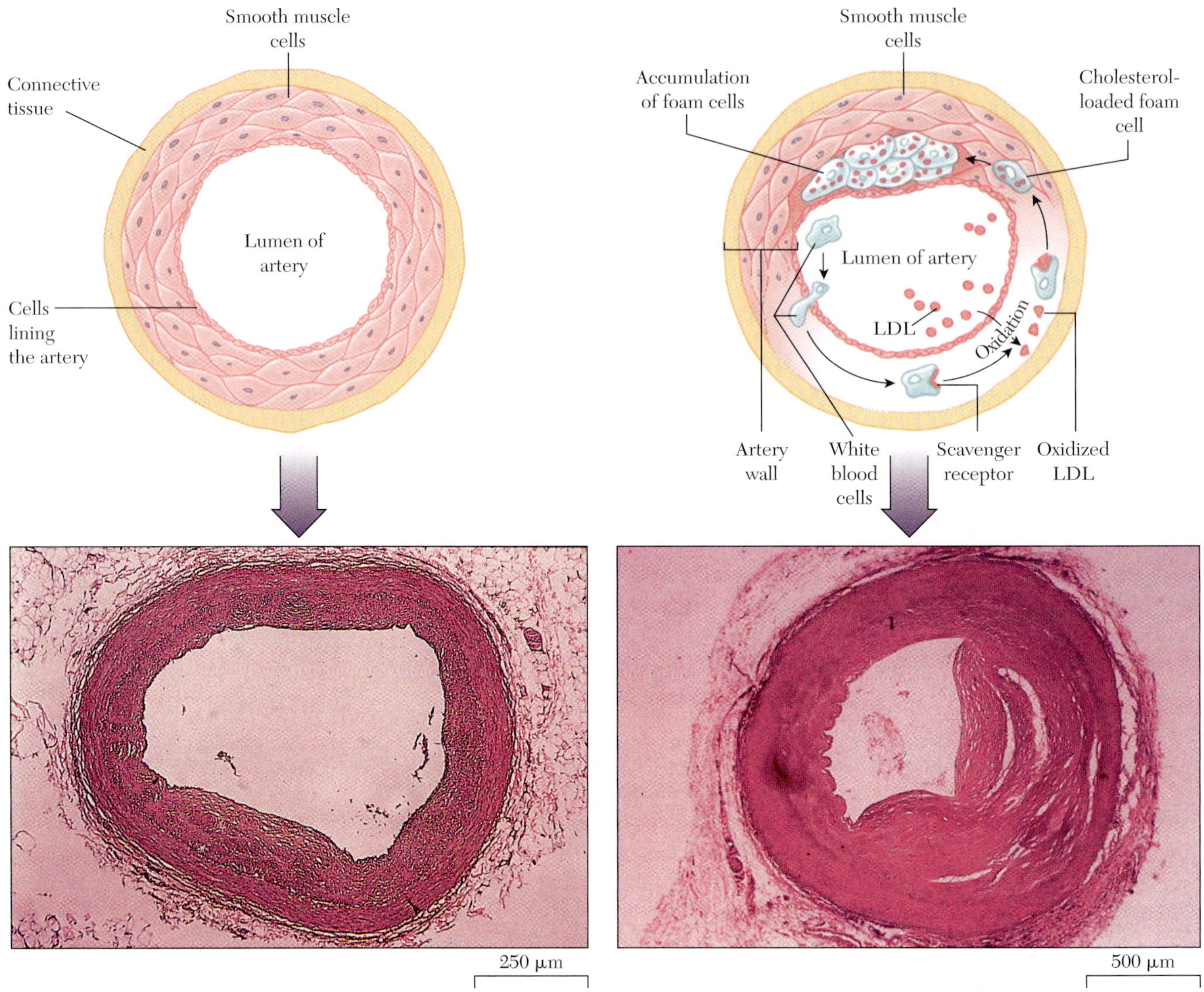

FIGURE 5.19 On the left are a drawing and photograph of a normal artery. On the right are a diagram showing the development of an atherosclerotic plaque and a photograph of a cross section of an artery partially blocked by atherosclerotic deposits. Plaque develops when white blood cells and LDL particles penetrate the artery wall. LDLs become oxidized and enter the white blood cells by binding to scavenger receptors. The cholesterol-filled white blood cells are transformed into foam cells that burst, depositing cholesterol in the artery wall. *(left, © Cabisco/Visuals Unlimited; right, © Ober/Visuals Unlimited)*

Web Menu

The American Heart Association at www.americanheart.org/ provides information on heart disease, its risk factors, incidence, prevention, and treatment.

Risk Factors for Heart Disease Factors that directly increase the risk of developing heart disease include diabetes, high blood pressure, obesity, and high blood cholesterol levels. Other factors that affect risk include age, gender, genetics, and lifestyle factors such as smoking, exercise, and diet. These may directly change risk or act indirectly by altering the risk of diabetes or affecting blood pressure, body weight, or blood cholesterol levels (Table 5.2).

Primary Risk Factors Diabetes increases the risk of heart disease. The high levels of blood glucose that can occur with this disease cause damage to blood vessels. Elevated blood pressure can also increase risk by damaging blood vessels. In addition, high blood pressure forces the heart to work harder, causing it to enlarge and weaken over time. Obesity increases the amount of work required by the heart and the risk of heart disease by affecting blood pressure, blood cholesterol levels, and the risk of diabetes. High blood cholesterol levels, and, in particular,

TABLE 5.2 Factors That Affect Heart Disease Risk

Age: Risk increases with increasing age.

Sex: Males have a higher risk until age 65, then risks do not differ between the sexes.

Disease factors:

Diabetes: fasting blood sugar greater than 126 mg/100 ml
High blood pressure: greater than 140/90
Obesity: body mass index greater than 27*
High blood lipid levels:

	Low Risk	Moderate Risk	High Risk
Total cholesterol (mg/100 ml)	< 200	200–239	≥ 240
LDL cholesterol (mg/100 ml)	< 130	130–159	≥ 160
HDL (mg/100 ml)	≥ 40	< 40	< 40

Lifestyle:

Risk is increased by:
- Cigarette smoking
- Stress
- A sedentary lifestyle

Risk is decreased by: regular exercise

Diet:

Risk is increased by:
- High total fat intake
- High saturated fat intake
- High cholesterol intake
- High intake of *trans* fatty acids

Risk is decreased by:
- A high intake of omega-3 fatty acids
- A high fiber intake
- A diet high in fruits and vegetables
- A diet high in antioxidant nutrients such as vitamin E

*See Chapter 7 for information about body mass index and how it can be calculated.

high levels of LDL cholesterol, may injure artery walls as well as promote plaque formation.

The desirable level of total **blood cholesterol** in adults is below 200 mg per 100 ml. LDL cholesterol levels should be below 130 mg per 100 ml and HDL cholesterol levels should be 40 mg per 100 ml or greater. Currently, 51% of American adults have blood cholesterol levels of 200 or more, and 20% have values of 240 mg per 100 ml or greater.[15]

Blood cholesterol level A term generally used to describe the concentration of cholesterol in the blood, plasma, or serum. Plasma is the clear portion of blood that remains when the cells are removed. Serum is plasma with clotting factor proteins removed. Blood, plasma, and serum cholesterol values are similar and the term "blood cholesterol" will be used throughout regardless of which specific measurements were made.

Other Risk Factors Many other risk factors have been identified for heart disease. Some of these are unavoidable. For instance, the risk of heart disease increases with age; four out of five people who die of heart disease are 65 or older.[16] Men and women are both at risk, but men are generally affected a decade earlier than women.[17] This is due in part to the protective effect of the hormone estrogen in women. As women age, the effects of menopause—including the decline in estrogen level and gain in weight—increase heart disease risk. Although it is unclear why, the incidence of heart disease among men has been declining since the 1950s, whereas the incidence among women has increased.[18] Heart disease is currently the single largest killer of American women. Genetics, including ethnic background, also affect risk. Individuals with a male family member who exhibited heart disease before the age of 55 or a female family member who exhibited heart disease before the age of 65 are considered to be at greater risk. African-Americans are at greater risk than other ethnic groups; the death rate from cardiovascular disease is 49% higher in African-American men and 67% higher in African-American women than among Caucasian men and women respectively.[15]

Age, gender, and genetics are risks that cannot be changed, but lifestyle and diet can be modified to reduce risk. Lifestyle factors that affect risk include activity, smoking, and stress. An inactive lifestyle increases the risk of heart disease, as do cigarette smoking and stress. On the other hand, regular exercise decreases risk by promoting the maintenance of a healthy body weight, reducing the risk of diabetes, increasing HDL cholesterol, and reducing blood pressure.[19] A number of dietary components, including the amount and type of fat, affect heart disease risk.[20] Some dietary factors increase risk while others offer a protective effect (see *Critical Thinking:* "Heart Disease Risk").

Dietary Factors That Promote Heart Disease Excessive intake of cholesterol, saturated fat, *trans* fatty acids, and energy can increase the risk of cardiovascular disease. Some or all of their effect is due to their influence on blood cholesterol levels.

Dietary Cholesterol The extent to which cholesterol intake affects blood levels depends on an individual's genetic makeup. Cholesterol in the blood comes from cholesterol both consumed in the diet and synthesized by the liver. Generally, the liver makes about three to four times more cholesterol than is consumed in the diet. In some individuals, as dietary cholesterol increases, liver cholesterol synthesis decreases, so that blood levels do not change.[21] In others, however, liver synthesis does not decrease in response to an increase in dietary cholesterol, so blood cholesterol levels rise.

Dietary Saturated Fat Diets high in saturated fat increase LDL cholesterol in the blood. Increased LDL then increases the risk of atherosclerosis. When the diet is high in saturated fatty acids, liver production of cholesterol-carrying lipoproteins increases and the activity of LDL receptors in the liver is reduced, so that LDL cholesterol cannot be removed from the blood.[13] When the diet is low in saturated fats, the number of LDL receptors increases, allowing more cholesterol to be removed from the bloodstream.[22] There are some saturated fats, such as the stearic acid found in chocolate and beef, that do not increase blood cholesterol levels.[23] Despite this, stearic acid, like other long-chain saturated fatty acids, has been found to increase the risk of heart disease.[24] This may occur because stearic acid depresses HDL cholesterol and because it accelerates the progression of heart disease by affecting blood platelets and blood clotting, both of which are involved in plaque formation.[25]

Trans *Fatty Acids* Both clinical and epidemiological studies provide evidence that *trans* fatty acid intake increases the risk of heart disease.[26] Some of this increase in risk is due to the effect of *trans* fatty acids on cholesterol levels. *Trans* fatty acid intake increases blood cholesterol levels more than does the same amount of polyunsaturated fatty acids but less than does an equivalent amount of saturated fatty acids. Therefore, when partially hydrogenated vegetable oils high in *trans* fatty acids replace unhydrogenated vegetable oils in the diet, the total and LDL cholesterol concentrations in the blood increase and HDL concentrations decrease.[26] When partially hydrogenated vegetable oils, such as those in margarine, replace fats rich in saturated fatty acids, such as those in butter, total as well as LDL and HDL cholesterol concentrations in the blood decrease.[27,28] Epidemiological studies indicate that an increase in the amount of *trans* fatty acids in the diet increases the risk of heart disease even more than an equivalent increase in saturated fat.[20] This suggests that *trans* fatty acids may have effects on heart disease risk that are independent of its effect on blood cholesterol.

Excess Energy Excess energy intake increases the risk of heart disease because it increases body fat, which is a separate risk factor for elevated blood cholesterol levels, high blood pressure, diabetes, and heart disease in general. A reduction in body weight has been shown to reduce blood cholesterol levels, blood pressure, and heart disease risk, and to help control diabetes.[29]

Dietary Factors That Protect Against Heart Disease Diets high in polyunsaturated fats, monounsaturated fats, and plant foods all tend to decrease the risk of heart disease. Moderate amounts of alcohol may also decrease risk. Some of these dietary factors reduce risk by reducing LDL cholesterol and increasing HDL cholesterol. Some protect against heart disease in other ways.

Dietary Polyunsaturated Fat: Omega-6 and Omega-3 When saturated fat in the diet is replaced by any type of polyunsaturated fat, there is a beneficial decrease in LDL cholesterol.[22] However, a high intake of omega-6 polyunsaturated fatty acids may also decrease HDL cholesterol, which is undesirable in terms of heart disease risk. Omega-3 fatty acids have a similar effect on LDL levels but do not lower HDL cholesterol.[30] In addition to these effects on blood lipids, omega-3 fatty acids may reduce heart disease risk by preventing the development of atherosclerotic plaque and by altering the types of eicosanoids synthesized, which in turn affects blood clotting, blood pressure, and immune function.[31,32] The beneficial effects are greater when the omega-3 fatty acids are consumed in fish, such as salmon and albacore tuna, rather than in supplements (Table 5.3).[33]

TABLE 5.3 Omega-3 Fatty Acid Content of Fish and Seafood

Food*	Omega-3 Fatty Acids (g)
Swordfish	1.16
Salmon	1.16
Trout	1.16
Sole	0.44
Cod	0.44
Shrimp	0.27
Mussels	0.26
Clams	0.26
Tuna, canned	0.23
Lobster	0.07

*All values represent amounts in a 3-oz cooked portion.

Monounsaturated Fat Populations consuming diets high in monounsaturated fats, such as those in Mediterranean countries where olive oil is commonly used, have a mortality rate from heart disease that is half of that in the United States. This is true even when total fat intake provides 40% or more of energy intake.[34] Substituting monounsaturated fat for saturated fat reduces LDL cholesterol without decreasing HDL cholesterol and makes LDL cholesterol less susceptible to oxidation.[30] Diets high in monounsaturated fat have also been found to lower triglyceride concentrations in the blood.[35] However, monounsaturated fat in the diet is unlikely to be the only factor involved in the differences in the incidence of heart disease between the Mediterranean countries and the United States.

Plant Foods: Fiber and Antioxidants Epidemiology has shown that diets high in plant foods are associated with a lower risk of heart disease. Plant foods such as fruits, vegetables, whole grains, and legumes are a good source of fiber, vitamins, minerals, and phytochemicals. As discussed in Chapter 4, soluble fibers, such as those in oat bran, legumes, psyllium, pectin, and gums, have been shown to reduce blood cholesterol levels. In addition, many of the vitamins, minerals, and phytochemicals in plant foods have antioxidant properties. Antioxidants are postulated to protect against plaque formation by decreasing the formation of oxidized LDL cholesterol (see *Making Decisions:* "Dietary Supplements to Reduce Blood Cholesterol").

Moderate Alcohol Consumption Moderate alcohol consumption has been shown to reduce stress, to raise levels of HDL cholesterol, and to reduce blood clotting. This has a protective effect against heart disease. Red wine may provide the greatest effect because it contains compounds known as phenols, which are antioxidants that may protect against lipoprotein oxidation, thereby preventing the development of atherosclerotic plaques.[36] Similar effects have been seen with grape juice.[37] The Dietary Guidelines recognize that in men over age 45 and women over age 55, moderate drinking can lower the risk of heart disease. Moderate drinking is defined as no more than one drink per day for women and two drinks per day for men (a drink is 12 ounces of beer, 5 ounces of wine, or 1.5 ounces of 80-proof distilled spirits). Greater intakes of alcohol increase the risk of accidental deaths, heart disease, cancer, birth defects, and drug interactions and should be avoided. Alcohol consumption is not recommended for children or adolescents, pregnant women, individuals who cannot restrict their drinking to a moderate

Making Decisions

Dietary Supplements to Reduce Blood Cholesterol

High levels of blood cholesterol increase the risk of developing heart disease. In turn, diet, lifestyle, and medications can all affect blood cholesterol levels. The standard therapy for reducing blood cholesterol involves a diet low in fat, particularly saturated fat, and high in grains, fruits, and vegetables, along with an active lifestyle. When these measures fail, cholesterol-lowering drugs are available.

In addition, to these standard therapies, there is a variety of dietary supplements, ranging from fibers and vitamins to garlic and phytochemicals, that are marketed for lowering blood cholesterol. Are these safe and reasonable alternatives to diet modification or prescription medication?

Fiber Supplements

The safest supplements for lowering cholesterol are probably soluble fibers such as psyllium, pectin, guar gum, or locust bean gum. Many studies have shown that fiber supplements lower total and LDL cholesterol in those with elevated levels. One study found that consumption of about 10 g of psyllium per day lowered total cholesterol by 4% and LDL cholesterol by 7% without affecting HDL cholesterol.[a] The effectiveness of a fiber supplement depends on how the fiber is processed and thus varies with the brand. An alternative to fiber supplements is to increase intake of high-fiber foods such as beans, whole oats, and fruit. These add not only soluble fiber to the diet but also the other nutrients and phytochemicals present in these foods.

Niacin

Niacin is a vitamin that can lower blood cholesterol. Doses of 2 to 3 g per day of a form of the vitamin called nicotinic acid have been shown to lower LDL cholesterol and raise HDL cholesterol.[b,c] But at doses this high, niacin is not really a vitamin—it is a drug. The amount used to treat high blood cholesterol is more than 50 times higher than the Tolerable Upper Intake Level (UL) of 35 mg per day that has been set for adults.[d] High doses can cause liver damage, ulcers, impaired glucose tolerance, headaches, flushing, nausea, heartburn, and diarrhea. Although readily available over the counter, niacin should not be taken at these high doses without a doctor's supervision.

Garlic

Garlic has been used medicinally for centuries. Many health-promoting phytochemicals have now been identified in garlic, and today one of the promises used to market garlic supplements is that they will lower blood cholesterol. The results of studies on the effectiveness of garlic have not been consistent—some reports have found that garlic supplements are effective at reducing blood cholesterol,[e,f] whereas others have found no effect.[g,h] The doses used in these studies are equivalent to consuming one or more cloves of raw garlic daily. The primary side effect of this is a strong garlic body odor. Garlic supplements are available as capsules containing garlic extract or garlic oil and as garlic powder or garlic powder tablets. Some of these preparations are odorless.

Phytochemicals

Phytosterols are phytochemicals that are marketed for their cholesterol-lowering effects. Phytosterols are plant sterols that resemble cholesterol chemically, making it difficult for the digestive tract to distinguish them from cholesterol. They are believed to lower blood cholesterol by inhibiting cholesterol absorption.[i] A Western diet provides about 200 to 400 mg of phytosterols a day from foods such as soybeans, wheat, and rice.[j] Intakes of 1500 to 3000 mg a day have been shown to reduce total cholesterol and LDL cholesterol levels in the blood and to have no effect on HDL cholesterol. A tablet of the phytosterol supplement Cholestatin contains 380 mg, so it would take four to eight tablets a day to supply the amounts that have been shown to reduce cholesterol in these studies. Phytosterols have been incorporated into several brands of margarine, including Take Control and Benecol. When sufficient quantities are consumed, these spreads lower blood cholesterol.[k] No side effects have been reported with phytosterol consumption.[i]

amount, or individuals who plan to drive or perform other activities that require concentration.

Dietary and Lifestyle Patterns and Heart Disease Individual dietary components affect the risk of heart disease, but each of these components is only part of an overall pattern of intake. Risk is affected not just by individual components but by patterns that are followed over the course of a day, a week, and a lifetime. For example, reducing saturated fat intake by limiting red meat consumption to three times a week can help to reduce blood cholesterol levels. However, if this same diet is high in energy and *trans* fats and low in fiber and antioxidant nutrients, the impact of reducing saturated fat intake on the overall risk of heart disease may be small. Combining changes in individual dietary components to create a pattern of intake that is not only low in saturated fat and *trans* fat, but also high in fruits, vegetables, and whole grains, will more significantly affect overall heart disease risk.

Phytochemicals called tocotrienols, which are related to vitamin E, have also been sold to lower cholesterol. They are found in rice, oat bran, and barley. They are believed to lower cholesterol by interfering with the liver's ability to make it. One study found that a dose of 200 mg a day for a month lowered LDL cholesterol by 13% in subjects with high cholesterol.[l] Tocotrienols have the potential to lower blood cholesterol, but to obtain these effects would require taking four to eight times the dosage recommended on supplement packages.

If You Choose to Use Supplements

To assess your risk of heart disease, you should have your blood cholesterol measured. If it is higher than recommended, you should be under a doctor's care. The best treatment can only be determined by a physician who assesses the levels of all types of lipid fractions in your blood. The use of any type of dietary supplement should be discussed with your doctor, since these products may impact the effectiveness of other treatments. With the exception of niacin, these supplements have few side effects, but dietary supplements are not tested as extensively as drugs, so less is known about their safety and effectiveness. For example, Cholestin, a supplement made from Chinese red yeast rice, contains the chemical lovastatin. Lovastatin is the active ingredient in some prescription cholesterol-lowering medications. Unlike prescription lovastatin, the amount of this drug in each dose of Cholestin is not regulated and may vary. Lovastatin can cause serious side effects and should not be used by people with infections or organ transplants and those who consume more than two alcoholic beverages a day.

Cholesterol-lowering supplements should not take the place of adequate exercise and a diet low in total fat, saturated fat, and cholesterol and high in fiber, fruits, vegetables, and whole grains. Most of the active ingredients contained in these supplements can be obtained from a healthy diet. This type of diet benefits not only blood cholesterol levels but blood pressure, body weight, and cancer risk as well.

References

[a] Anderson, J. W., Allgood, L. D., Lawrence, A., et al. Cholesterol-lowering effects of psyllium intake adjunctive to diet therapy in men and women with hypercholesterolemia: meta-analysis of 8 controlled trials. Am. J. Clin. Nutr. 71:472–479, 2000.

[b] O'Connor, P. J., Rush, W. A., and Trence, D. L. Relative effectiveness of niacin and lovastatin for treatment of dyslipidemias in a health maintenance organization. J. Fam. Pract. 44:462–467, 1997.

[c] McKenney, J. M., McCormick, L. S., Weiss, S., et al. A randomized trial of the effects of atorvastatin and niacin in patients with combined hyperlipidemia or isolated hypertriglyceridemia. Collaborative Atorvastin Study Group. Am. J. Med. 104:137–143, 1998.

[d] Institute of Medicine, Food and Nutrition Board. *Dietary Reference Intakes for Thiamin, Riboflavin, Niacin, Vitamin B-6, Folate, Vitamin B-12, Pantothenic Acid, Biotin, and Choline.* Washington, D.C.: National Academy Press. 1998.

[e] Adler, A. J., and Holub, B. J. Effect of garlic and fish oil supplementation on serum lipid and lipoprotein concentrations in hypercholesterolemic men. Am. J. Clin. Nutr. 65:445–450, 1997.

[f] Bordia, A., Verma, S. K., and Srivastava, K. C. Effect of garlic (*Allium sativum*) on blood lipids, blood sugar, fibrinogen and fibrinolytic activity in patients with coronary artery disease. Prostaglandins Leukot. Essent. Fatty Acids 58:257–263, 1998.

[g] Berthold, H. K., Sudhop, T., and von Bergmann, K. Effect of garlic oil preparation on serum lipoproteins and cholesterol metabolism: a randomized controlled trial. JAMA 279: 1900–1902, 1998.

[h] Isaacsohn, J. L., Moser, M., Stein, E. A., et al. Garlic powder and plasma lipids and lipoproteins: a multicenter, randomized, placebo-controlled trial. Arch. Intern. Med. 158:1189–1194, 1998.

[i] Ling, W. W., and Jones, P. J. Dietary phytosterols: a review of metabolism, benefits and side effects. Life Sci. 57:195–206, 1995.

[j] Jones, P. J., MacDougall, D. E., Ntanios, F., and Vanstone, C. A. Dietary phytosterols as cholesterol-lowering agents in humans. Can. J. Physiol. Pharmacol. 75:217–227, 1997.

[k] Weststrate, J. A., and Meijer, G. W. Plant sterol–enriched margarines and reduction of plasma total- and LDL-cholesterol concentrations in normocholesterolemic and mildly hypercholesterolemic subjects. Eur. J. Clin. Nutr. 52:334–343, 1998.

[l] Qureshi, A. A., Bradlow, B. A., Brace, L., et al. Response of hypercholesterolemic subjects to administration of tocotrienols. Lipids 30:1171–1177, 1995.

Analysis of heart disease incidence around the world demonstrates the benefits of a healthy dietary pattern. The incidence of heart disease is low in Asian and Mediterranean countries. The Asian diet is low in total fat and based on rice and vegetables; the Mediterranean diet is rich in monounsaturated fat and is high in grains, vegetables, and fruit. The diets in both of these regions contain relatively small amounts of animal products such as fish, poultry, eggs, and red meat (see Appendix H: The Asian and Mediterranean Food Guide Pyramids). Changing one's diet to mimic only one component of these diets does not impart the benefits of the total pattern. For example, switching to olive oil will not make your diet a Mediterranean diet. And, even when a complete dietary pattern is duplicated, heart disease risk may not be the same because dietary factors interact with genetics and lifestyle factors, such as stress and activity, to determine risk. It is the sum of an individual's dietary pattern, lifestyle, and genetic makeup that determines their overall risk.

Critical Thinking

Heart Disease Risk

Selma is 45 years old and generally healthy, but when she read that heart disease is the leading killer of women in the United States, she became concerned. She has high blood pressure for which she takes medication, and her father had coronary bypass surgery at age 52. She knows she should be consuming a diet low in fat but isn't sure how to do this. Her son is taking a nutrition class and decides to analyze his mother's heart disease risk for his class project. He makes the following list of Selma's potential risk factors:

Sex	Female
Age	45
Family history	Father had heart disease before the age of 55
Height/weight	66 inches/140 lb
Blood pressure (with medication)	120/70
Stress level	Moderate
Smoker	No
Activity level	Sedentary
Blood values	
Total cholesterol	210 mg/100 ml
LDL cholesterol	160 mg/100 ml
HDL cholesterol	34 mg/100 ml

What risk factors does she have for developing cardiovascular disease?

Answer:

He asks her to record everything she eats for three days. A sample day is shown below.

Food	Serving	Food	Serving
Breakfast		*Snack*	
Bran muffin	1 medium	Cola	1 can
Butter	1 tsp	*Dinner*	
Coffee	1 cup	Fish sticks	5
Apple juice	1 cup	Tater Tots	10
Lunch		Ketchup	2 Tbsp
Bologna sandwich		Cookies	2 large
Bologna	2 slices	Tea	1 cup
White bread	2 slices	*Snack*	
Mayonnaise	1 Tbsp	Ice cream	1 cup
Potato chips	1 ounce		
Soda	1 can		
Apple	1 medium		

How does her diet compare to the serving recommendations of the Food Guide Pyramid? Do her choices follow the selection tips of the Food Guide Pyramid?

Answer:

Her son analyzes Selma's diet on the computer and shows her the following information.

Nutrient	Amount
Energy	2210 (kcals)
Fat	102 g
Saturated fat	37 g
Cholesterol	199 mg
Trans fat	8.7 g
Total fiber	13 g
Soluble fiber	5 g

How does Selma's diet compare to the recommendations for fat intake—30% of energy as fat, 10% as saturated fat, and less than 300 mg of cholesterol per day?

Answer:

What other dietary factors contribute to her risk of heart disease (see Table 5.2)?

Answer:

If Selma were to replace all of the added fat in her diet with olive oil, would she reduce her risk of cardiovascular disease to the level found in Mediterranean countries?

Answer:

Diet and Cancer

Cancer is the second leading cause of death in the United States, and it is estimated that 30 to 40% of cancers are directly linked to diet.[38] As with cardiovascular disease, there is a body of epidemiological evidence correlating diet and lifestyle with the incidence of cancer. Diets high in fat and low in fiber and plant foods are correlated with an increased risk of certain types of cancer, including breast and colon cancers.[39,40] The mechanism whereby a high fat intake increases the incidence of various cancers is less well understood than the relationship between dietary fat and cardiovascular disease; however, dietary fat has been suggested to be both a tumor promoter and a tumor initiator.

Web Menu

For information on nutrition and cancer prevention, go to the American Cancer Society at www2.cancer.org/prevention/ and click on nutrition and prevention, and the American Institute for Cancer Research at www.aicr.org/.

Dietary Fat and Breast Cancer Breast cancer is the leading form of cancer in women worldwide. In the United States it affects 182,000 women annually. The incidence is similar among all ethnic groups, but the mortality is higher among minority women. Breast cancer is more common in postmenopausal women, in women who have had no children or who had children late in life, and in women with a family history of the disease. In populations where the diet is high in fat and low in fiber, the incidence of breast cancer is high. In populations where the typical fat intake is low, the incidence is lower and the survival rate is better in people with the disease. Currently, several major studies are under way to determine if reducing fat intake to less than 15% of energy will reduce breast cancer risk or mortality.[41]

As is the case with heart disease, the type of fat is as important as the total amount of fat in determining risk. The incidence of breast cancer in Mediterranean women who rely on olive oil, which is high in monounsaturated fat, as a source of dietary fat is low despite a total fat intake similar to that in the United States.[42] Epidemiology also supports a protective effect from an increased intake of omega-3 fatty acids from fish, such as in the native Eskimos of Alaska and Greenland.[42] A higher intake of *trans* fatty acids found in foods such as stick margarines, however, may increase the risk of breast cancer.[43]

The tumor-promoting effects of diet on breast cancer cells has been studied in laboratory animals. Because most laboratory animals do not get breast cancer tumors, studies are conducted by implanting breast tumors and examining how diet affects their growth. The tumors are more likely to grow in mice fed a high-fat diet than in those fed a low-fat diet. The type of fat also affects growth; diets high in linoleic acid, which is found in polyunsaturated vegetable oils, are stronger tumor promoters than diets high in saturated fatty acids or omega-3 fatty acids.[11] So, unlike heart disease, where polyunsaturated fats reduce risk, a high polyunsaturated fat intake may be detrimental in terms of cancer risk.

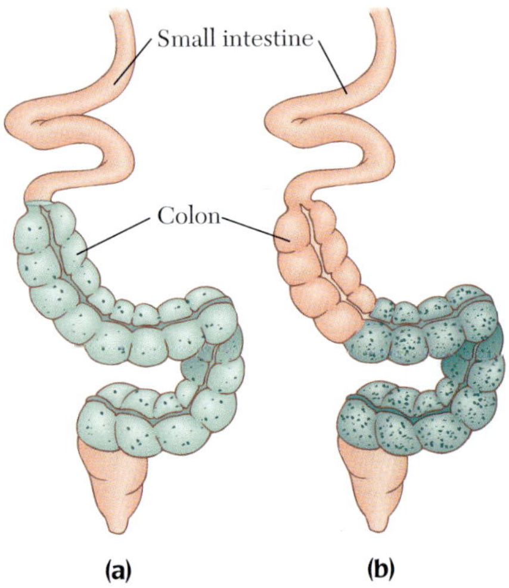

FIGURE 5.20 (a) When the diet is high in fiber, the volume of material entering the colon is greater and any mutagens present (shown as green dots) will be diluted. (b) When the diet is low in fiber, the volume of material in the colon is smaller, so any mutagens present will be more concentrated and therefore more likely to come in contact with the cells lining the colon.

Diet and Colon Cancer Epidemiology has correlated the incidence of colon cancer with high-fat, low-fiber diets.[45] The correlation is stronger for diets high in animal fats, in particular those from red meats.[46] The connection between dietary fat and colon cancer may be related to the breakdown products of fat in the large intestine. Here, bacteria metabolize dietary fat and bile, producing substances that may cause mutations. These mutation-producing substances, or mutagens, may act as tumor initiators. A high intake of fiber tends to dilute these mutagens by increasing the volume of colon contents (Figure 5.20). High-fiber diets also decrease transit time. Both of these effects reduce the exposure of the intestinal mucosa to the hazardous substances (see Chapter 4).

Meeting Lipid Needs

About 33% of the energy in the typical North American diet comes from lipids.[47] Guidelines for a healthy diet recommend a diet low in saturated fat and cholesterol and moderate in total fat intake.

Recommendations for Fat Intake

Recommendations for fat intake are based on meeting needs for essential fatty acids while limiting fat intake to reduce the risks of chronic disease. Although there is no 1989 RDA for fatty acids, the recommendation for a minimally adequate adult intake is 1 to 2% of energy, or 3 to 6 g per day, from the omega-6 fatty acid, linoleic acid. This is well below the approximately 7% of energy from linoleic acid in a typical adult diet in the United States. There is no 1989 RDA for omega-3 fatty acids, but DRIs are being considered. The World Health Organization recommends a ratio of linoleic to alpha-linolenic acid in the diet of between 5 : 1 and 10 : 1, a ratio much lower than currently provided by a typical Western diet.[48,49]

The amounts of essential fatty acids needed are minuscule compared with the total amount of fat most Americans consume. Public health guidelines recommend a diet low in saturated fat and cholesterol and moderate in total fat (Figure 5.21). Total dietary fat intake should be no more than 30% of energy, divided approximately equally between saturated fat, polyunsaturated fat, and monounsaturated fat. Cholesterol intake should be no more than 300 mg per day, and *trans* fatty acid intake should not increase above the current level of intake—about 2.6% of total energy or 7.4% of fat energy.[2]

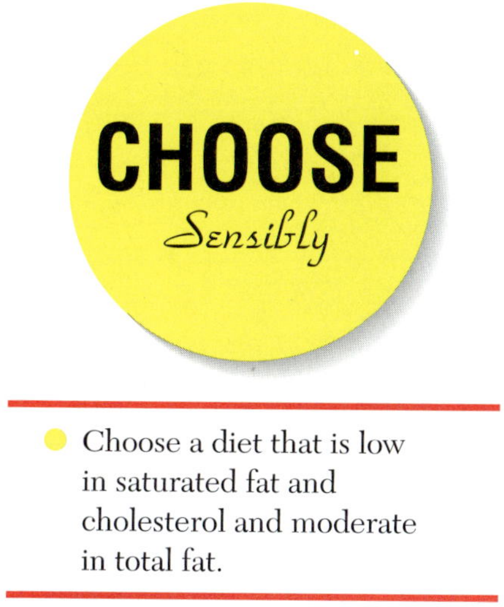

FIGURE 5.21 The Dietary Guidelines for Americans recommend a diet low in saturated fat and cholesterol and moderate in total fat *(USDA, DHHS, 2000)*

For more information about coronary heart disease and how to lower your blood cholesterol, go to the National Heart, Lung, and Blood Institute and the National Cholesterol Education Program's interactive site at www.nhlbi.nih.gov/chd/.

Recommendations for Reducing Disease Risk In addition to these general recommendations for fat intake, some dietary recommendations are made to target specific diseases such as heart disease and cancer (see Appendix G). For example, the goals of Healthy People 2010 include reducing the prevalence of heart disease and elevated blood cholesterol levels in the American population. Both the American Heart Association (a private organization) and the National Cholesterol Education Program (NCEP) (a federally sponsored program) have developed dietary recommendations to promote heart health.

Recommendations designed to reduce the risks of specific diseases may not always be appropriate for the general population. For example, the NCEP recommends that all adults have their blood lipids measured every five years (Figure 5.22).[50] Individuals with blood cholesterol levels in the moderate risk category (see Table 5.2) and who have heart disease or two other risk factors for heart disease, should begin the Step I dietary program shown in Table 5.4. If, after six months of consuming this diet, blood cholesterol levels have not decreased, the Step II diet is recommended. The NCEP also recommends drug therapy for individuals with extremely high cholesterol levels or for those for whom diet therapy fails. The most prominent drugs used to treat elevated cholesterol are those in the statin family, such as lovastatin (Mevacor), atorvastatin (Lipitor), and pravastatin (Pravachol). These work by blocking cholesterol synthesis in the liver and by increasing the capacity of the liver to remove cholesterol from the blood. Drugs such as cholestyramine (Questran) and colestipol (Colestid) act in the gastrointestinal tract by preventing cholesterol and bile absorption. Nictotinic acid, a form of the B vitamin niacin, can also be used to lower cholesterol (see *Making Decisions:* "Dietary Supplements to Reduce Blood Cholesterol" and Chapter 10).

Guidelines for Children, Pregnant Women, and the Elderly Recommendations to reduce fat intake to 30% or less of energy intake and cholesterol to less than 300 mg per day apply to all individuals over two years of age. Children under the age of two should not consume diets restricted in fat and cholesterol because lipids

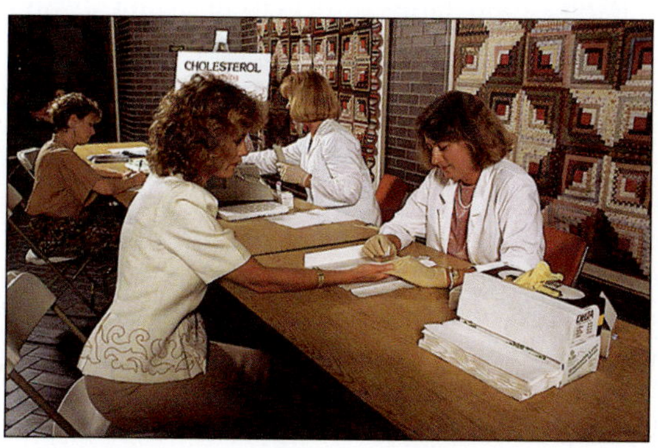

FIGURE 5.22 The National Cholesterol Education Program recommends that all adults have their blood cholesterol levels checked at least every five years. *(© Blair Seitz/Photo Researchers, Inc.)*

TABLE 5.4 National Cholesterol Education Program Step I and Step II Diets*

	Recommended Intake	
Nutrient	***Step I***	***Step II***
Total Fat†	30% or less	30% or less
Saturated fatty acids†	8–10%	Less than 7%
Cholesterol	Less than 300 mg/day	Less than 200 mg/day
Sodium	Up to 2400 mg	Up to 2400 mg
Total energy	To achieve and maintain desired weight	To achieve and maintain desired weight

*Adapted from National Cholesterol Education Program. Available online at http://www.nhlbisupport.com/cgi-bin/chd1/step1intro.cgi.

†Values are % of total energy intake.

are needed to support their rapid brain development and high energy needs. Beginning at two years of age, fat intake should be decreased to 30% or less of energy, and children should get most of their energy from whole-grain products, fruits, vegetables, low-fat dairy products, legumes, and lean meats. The American Academy of Pediatrics specifies a lower limit of 20% of energy from total fat for children and adolescents.[51]

During pregnancy, there is an increase in blood cholesterol. This increase appears to be independent of diet, and levels return to normal about eight weeks after the baby is born. Consuming a diet containing 30% of energy as fat has not been shown to be detrimental during pregnancy as long as energy, protein, and micronutrient needs are met.

In the elderly, the value of dietary fat reduction must be balanced with the risk of undernutrition. Reducing fat intake to 30% of energy causes little risk, though further reduction may increase the risk for protein or micronutrient malnutrition in this group.

Calculating Fat Intake

The amount of fat that is recommended in a diet is based on energy intake. Table 5.5 illustrates how to calculate fat intake as a percent of energy. This same equation can be used to calculate the percent of energy from monounsaturated, polyunsaturated, or saturated fat in the diet or to determine the percent of energy from fat in individual foods. Databases and food composition tables provide information on the number of grams of fat contained in a wide variety of foods. Food labels provide a more accessible source of information on packaged foods. Unfortunately, food label information is not always available on fresh meats, which are one of the main contributors of fat in the American diet.

The Exchange Lists can be used to estimate the total amount of fat in a food or in the diet (Table 5.6; see also Appendix I). An exchange of fruits, vegetables, or breads contains 1 g or less. The amount of fat in an exchange of dairy products varies. A serving of nonfat milk provides less than a gram of fat, but a serving of whole milk contains 8 g. Likewise, the amount of fat in a meat exchange depends on your choice; very lean meat such as turkey breast contains 1 g of fat or less, whereas a serving of bologna contains 8 g. An exchange from the fat list contains 5 g of fat.

TABLE 5.5 Calculating Percent of Energy from Fat

Determine

- The total energy (kcalorie) intake for the day
- The grams of fat in the day's diet

Calculate Energy from Fat

- Fat provides 9 kcalories per g
- Multiply grams of fat by 9 kcalories per g

$$\text{Kcalories from fat} = \text{grams fat} \times 9 \text{ kcalories/gram fat}$$

Calculate % Energy from Fat

- Divide energy from fat by total energy and multiply by 100 to express as a percent

$$\text{Percent of energy from fat} = \frac{\text{kcalories from fat}}{\text{total kcalories}} \times 100$$

For example:

A diet contains 2000 kcalories and 75 g of fat

$$75 \text{ g of fat} \times 9 \text{ kcal/g} = 675 \text{ kcalories from fat}$$

$$\frac{675 \text{ kcal from fat}}{2000 \text{ kcal}} \times 100 = 34\% \text{ of energy (kcal) from fat}$$

A Diet to Meet Recommendations

Choosing a diet that limits cholesterol and total fat, that divides fats equally among saturated, monounsaturated, and polyunsaturated fat, and that meets needs for essential fatty acids as well as all other nutrients seems like an overwhelming task. In reality, diet planning does not need to be that difficult. Choosing carefully from the groups of the Food Guide Pyramid and using food labels to learn the composition of foods can provide a diet that meets all of these specifications. There is also a multitude of fat-modified products on the market that may be helpful in meeting recommendations for fat intake.

TABLE 5.6 Fat Content of the Exchange Lists

Exchange Groups/Lists	Serving Size	Fat (g)
Carbohydrate Group		
Starch	1/2 cup pasta, rice, cereal, potatoes; 1 slice bread	0–1
Fruit	1 small apple, peach, pear; 1/2 banana; 1/2 cup canned fruit (in juice)	0
Milk	1 cup milk or yogurt	
Nonfat		0
Low-fat		2–3
Reduced-fat		5
Whole		8
Other carbohydrates	Serving sizes vary	Varies
Vegetables	1/2 cup cooked vegetables, 1 cup raw	0
Meat/Meat Substitute Group	1 oz meat or cheese, 1/2 cup legumes	
Very lean		0–1
Lean		3
Medium fat		5
High fat		8
Fat Group	1 tsp butter, margarine, or oil; 1 Tbsp salad dressing	5

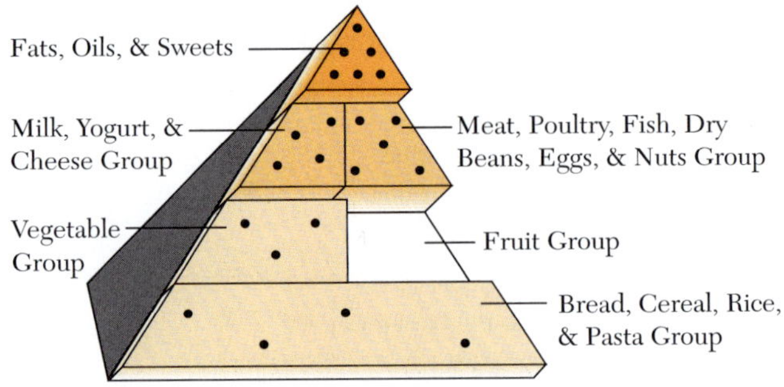

FIGURE 5.23 The groups that are sources of naturally occurring and added fat contain circles and are raised and colored orange. The darker the shade and the more circles, the more high-fat foods the group contains.

Fat in the Food Guide Pyramid The recommendations for fat intake are reflected in the shape of the Food Guide Pyramid. In Figure 5.23, the circle (•) symbol indicates the concentration of high-fat choices. The large food groups in the lower half of the Pyramid—grains, vegetables, and fruits—contains few high-fat items and therefore few of these symbols. The food groups in the next higher level of the Food Guide Pyramid—the Milk, Yogurt, and Cheese Group and the Meat, Poultry, Fish, Dried Beans, Eggs, and Nuts Group—contain more high-fat choices. The animal foods in these upper groups contain saturated fat and are the only sources of cholesterol in the diet. The most concentrated sources of fat—oils, butter, margarine, and salad dressings—are separated into the narrow tip of the Pyramid.

Meeting the recommendations for fat intake requires careful choices from each of the Food Guide Pyramid groups. Simply consuming the recommended number of servings from each group will not assure that nutrient recommendations are met because choices from within each group differ greatly in fat content and nutrient density. Grain products, vegetables, and fruits are naturally low in fat as long as fat is not added in processing or preparation. For example, within the grain group, choosing high-fat baked goods such as doughnuts, cookies, and muffins adds more fat and energy and fewer nutrients than whole-grain breads, rice, and pasta. Within the Fruit Group, fresh fruits are a nonfat choice while fruits that are baked into pies and tarts add fat and refined sugar. Most fresh vegetables have little or no fat, but fried vegetables such as french fries and fried onion rings are high in fat and energy. The fat content of choices from the meat and dairy groups varies widely. Choosing reduced-fat dairy products and lean meats, such as chicken, turkey, flank and round steak, and vegetable sources of

TABLE 5.7 Suggestions for Reducing Fat Intake

1. Instead of frying, bake, broil, barbecue, roast, steam, or microwave.
2. Skip added fats such as butter, margarine, mayonnaise, and salad dressing—or use low-fat or fat-free spreads and dressings.
3. Use egg whites or egg substitutes in baking.
4. Use cocoa instead of chocolate in baking.
5. Use reduced-fat milk instead of coffee creamer.
6. Use reduced-fat cheeses or limit the amounts consumed.
7. Reduce the emphasis on meat as the centerpiece of meals:
   - Base meals on whole-grain products.
   - Reduce the portion size of meats served.
8. Trim visible fat from meats before cooking, and skin poultry before eating if not before cooking.
9. Choose meats with little marbling:
   - "Prime grade" contains an abundant amount of marbled fat.
   - "Choice grade" contains a modest amount of marbling.
   - "Select grade" contains a comparatively slight amount of marbling.

protein, such as legumes, will reduce fat intake from these groups. Choices from the tip of the Pyramid are the most concentrated sources of dietary fat intake. These should be added sparingly to the diet.

Limiting total fat intake requires limiting the amount of fat added to food at the table and in cooking (Table 5.7). Many low-fat and nonfat salad dressings and spreads are available that offer the taste and texture of the original products with much less fat. Careful choices in added fats can help meet the recommendations to limit total fat as well as saturated and *trans* fats. Choosing vegetable oils that are high in monounsaturated fat (such as canola and olive oils), and high in polyunsaturated fat (such as corn and soybean oils) instead of butter and lard will reduce saturated fat intake. Limiting the used of hard margarines and shortening will reduce *trans* fatty acid intake. Following these recommendations will provide a dietary pattern that is low in saturated fat and cholesterol, moderate in total fat, and plentiful in grains, vegetables, and fruits.

Fat on Food Labels The information about fat on food labels is designed to make it easier to identify the sources and types of fat in foods. Understanding how to use this information can help consumers make more informed choices about the fats they include in their diet.

The ingredient list includes the source of fat, such as corn oil, soybean oil, or partially hydrogenated vegetable oil. The Nutrition Facts section provides the number of kcalories from fat, the number of grams of fat, the number of grams of saturated fat, and the number of milligrams of cholesterol in a serving (Figure 5.24). These are also presented as a percent of the Daily Value. Daily Values help determine how much fat, saturated fat, and cholesterol are in a food relative to the daily amount recommended for a 2000-kcalorie diet. The Daily Value for total fat is calculated as 30% of energy. For a 2000-kcalorie diet this represents about 65 g of fat ([2000 kcal × 0.3]/9 kcal/g of fat = 67 g, which is rounded to 65 g). The Daily Value for saturated fat is based on 10% of energy, and the Daily

Web Menu

For more information on lipids on the food label, go to the Food and Drug Administration's Center for Food Safety and Applied Nutrition, Food Labeling and Nutrition page at vm.cfsan. fda.gov/label.html.

C 62 00 00 00 00 00 27 33

Cheese Sandwich Crackers

Nutrition Facts

Serving Size 1 Package (43g)
Servings Per Container 12

Amount/Serving	
Calories 230	Calories from Fat 120
	% Daily Value*
Total Fat 14g	**22%**
Saturated Fat 3.5g	**18%**
Cholesterol 5mg	**2%**
Sodium 410mg	**17%**
Total Carbohydrate 23g	**8%**
Dietary Fiber Less than 1g	**2%**
Sugars 6g	
Protein 3g	
Vitamin A 0% •	Vitamin C 0%
Calcium 6% •	Iron 6%

*Percent Daily Values are based on a 2,000 calorie diet. Your daily values may be higher or lower depending on your calorie needs:

	Calories:	2,000	2,500
Total Fat	Less than	65g	80g
Sat Fat	Less than	20g	25g
Cholesterol	Less than	300mg	300mg
Sodium	Less than	2,400mg	2,400mg
Total Carbohydrate		300g	375g
Dietary Fiber		25g	30g

INGREDIENTS: ENRICHED FLOUR (WHEAT FLOUR, NIACIN, REDUCED IRON, THIAMINE MONONITRATE {VITAMIN B1}, RIBOFLAVIN {VITAMIN B2}, FOLIC ACID), PARTIALLY HYDROGENATED SOYBEAN OIL, WHEY (FROM MILK), SUGAR, HIGH FRUCTOSE CORN SYRUP, BUTTER (PASTEURIZED CREAM, SALT, ANNATTO COLOR), CHEDDAR CHEESE (CULTURED MILK, SALT, ENZYMES, AND ANNATTO EXTRACT COLOR), BUTTERMILK SOLIDS, SALT, LEAVENING (BAKING SODA, CALCIUM PHOSPHATE), DISODIUM PHOSPHATE (STABILIZER), NATURAL FLAVOR, SOY LECITHIN (EMULSIFIER), COLOR ADDED (INCLUDES YELLOW 6), MALTED BARLEY FLOUR, PEANUTS.

FIGURE 5.24 Food labels provide information about the types and amounts of lipids in foods.

Value for cholesterol is set at 300 mg per day regardless of the amount of energy in the diet. The percent Daily Value on labels allows consumers to tell at a glance how one food will fit into the recommendations for fat intake for the day. For example, if a serving provides 50% of the Daily Value for fat—that is, half the recommended maximum daily intake for a 2000-kcalorie diet—the rest of the day's intake will have to be carefully selected to not exceed the recommended maximum.

There are no Daily Values for polyunsaturated and monounsaturated fat, but the amounts of these may be included voluntarily on the labels of some products. For example, in addition to listing the 2 g of saturated fat, the label on a bottle of olive oil may indicate that it contains 2 g of polyunsaturated fat and 10 g of monounsaturated fat per tablespoon. The amount of *trans* fat in a product is not listed in the Nutrition Facts section of the food label. However, if a food's ingredient list includes hydrogenated or partially hydrogenated oils, the food is a source of *trans* fatty acids. Some products may state that the food does not contain *trans* fat.

Food labels may also include standard descriptors such as "fat free," "low cholesterol," or "lean." As shown in Table 5.8, a product labeled "low-fat," for example, cannot contain more than 3 g of fat in a serving.[52] These terms can be used only in ways that do not confuse consumers. For instance, because saturated fat in the diet raises blood cholesterol, a food that is low in cholesterol but high in saturated fat, such as crackers containing coconut oil, cannot be labeled "low cholesterol," because it may actually raise blood cholesterol.

Some products may claim to be a certain percent fat free. These may be confusing to consumers because it refers to a percent of the product's weight,

TABLE 5.8 Nutrient Content Descriptors Related to Fat and Cholesterol

Descriptor	Definition
Fat-free	Contains less than 0.5 g of fat per serving.
Low-fat	Contains 3 g or less of fat per serving.
Percent fat-free	May be used only to describe foods that meet the definition of fat-free or low-fat.
Reduced- or less fat	Contains at least 25% less fat per serving than the regular or reference product.
Saturated fat-free	Contains less than 0.5 g of saturated fat per serving and less than 0.5 g *trans* fat per serving.
Low saturated fat	Contains 1 g or less of saturated fat and not more than 15% of kcalories from saturated fat per serving.
Reduced- or less-saturated fat	Contains at least 25% less saturated fat per serving than the regular or reference product.
Cholesterol-free	Contains less than 2 mg of cholesterol and 2 g or less of saturated fat per serving.
Low cholesterol	Contains 20 mg or less of cholesterol and 2 g or less of saturated fat per serving.
Reduced- or less cholesterol	Contains at least 25% less cholesterol than the regular or reference product and 2 g or less of saturated fat per serving.
Lean	Contains less than 10 g of fat, 4.5 g or less of saturated fat, and less than 95 mg of cholesterol per serving and per 100 g.
Extra lean	Contains less than 5 g of fat, less than 2 g of saturated fat, and less than 95 mg of cholesterol per serving and per 100 g.

not of energy. To avoid deception, labeling laws require that a product can claim to be a certain percent fat free only if it is also a fat-free or low-fat food. For example, low-fat hot dogs that are labeled 97% fat free contain 1.5 g of fat per serving and therefore meet the definition of a low-fat food. Although packaged meats must be labeled, fresh raw meats such as steak, which are one of the greatest contributors of fat, are not required to carry standard labels. Labels on ground beef can be particularly misleading because they may mention a certain "% lean." In this case "% lean" refers to the weight of the meat that is lean. So when the label says it is 78% lean, it means that 22% of the weight of the meat is fat, or that there are 22 g of fat in 100 g (3.5 ounces) of raw hamburger. This works out to about 55% of energy as fat. Only ground beef that is 90% lean or greater meets the government's definition of lean: less than 10 g of fat per serving.

Reduced-Fat Foods and Artificial Fats

Web Menu: For more information on fat substitutes, go to the Calorie Control Council at www.caloriecontrol.org/ and click on fat replacers.

In response to recommendations that Americans decrease their fat intake, a wide variety of reduced-fat and fat-free foods have become available. These products are designed to mimic the taste, texture, and cooking properties of fat without adding fat to the diet. Some of these are made by simply reducing the amount of fat added to a product during manufacturing. Others rely on artificial fats. These products help reduce fat intake when used in place of high-fat choices and can be part of a healthy diet.

Do Fat-Modified Foods Help Reduce Energy Intake? High-fat snack foods such as potato chips and corn chips are a major contributor to the fat in the American diet.[53] If these foods are replaced with reduced-fat versions, the fat and energy in the diet will decrease. Studies examining the use of products containing the artificial fat Olestra have shown that substituting these foods can reduce total fat and energy intake.[53] About 75% of adult Americans and 93% of dieters consume reduced-fat snack products so they can enjoy these snacks without adding excess fat and energy to their diets.[54] Used in moderation, they can be part of a weight reduction or maintenance program.

However, despite the multitude of reduced-fat products that are on the market today, more Americans are overweight than ever before. One reason for this is that consumers do not always reduce energy intake when they reduce fat consumption. The Dietary Guidelines reminds us that low-fat foods are not always low in kcalories. In many products, fats are replaced with other energy-containing nutrients, so the energy content of fat-free foods may not be significantly reduced. For instance, a regular brownie contains about 6.5 g of fat and 112 kcalories. A reduced-fat brownie contains 2 g of fat and 89 kcalories. Replacing one regular brownie with a reduced-fat one will reduce energy intake by only 23 kcalories. If consumers use reduced-fat products too generously, total energy intake will increase.

Americans have reduced their fat intake as a percent of energy intake—from about 40% of kcalories in the late 1950s to 33% of kcalories today. But, because we now consume more energy, our total fat intake has not really changed.[55] Fat-free products can help reduce the amount of fat in the diet—but they cannot be eaten liberally without affecting energy intake.

Are Reduced-Fat Foods a Healthy Choice? A healthy low-fat diet does not need to include fat-modified foods. Likewise, using fat-modified products does not transform a poor diet into a healthy one or improve overall diet quality. If reduced-fat desserts and snack foods replace whole grains, fruits, and vegetables, the resulting diet could be low in fat but also low in fiber, vitamins, minerals, and phytochemicals. This dietary pattern may actually increase the risk of some chronic diseases. A diet low in fat and high in simple sugars increases blood triglyceride levels and may increase the risk of heart disease.[56] Likewise, this diet affects insulin metabolism and may increase the risk of developing diabetes.[57] For a low-fat diet to be a healthy diet, it must include a variety of foods that are low in fat and high in fiber and micronutrients.

If used appropriately, fat-modified foods can be part of a healthy diet. Reduced-fat dairy products, for example, have a higher nutrient density than their full-fat counterparts. The majority of fat-modified foods, however, are sweets and snack foods, which are low in nutrient density to begin with. These foods, whether full- or reduced-fat, should make up only a small portion of the diet. If consumed in small amounts to replace full-fat treats, fat-modified foods can reduce dietary fat and energy without reducing the intake of fruits, vegetables, and whole grains. So, replacing a high-fat brownie with a low-fat one is not a bad choice, but replacing the brownie with an orange or a banana is an even healthier one.

Types of Artificial Fats Some artificial fats are made from carbohydrates or proteins, and thus contribute less energy than fat. Others are engineered by modifying the fat. These reduce fat and energy intake because the new fats are not well absorbed from the gastrointestinal tract.[58]

Carbohydrate-Based Fat Substitutes Carbohydrate-based fat replacers such as various pectins and gums have a slippery feel that mimics the texture of fat. These reduce the amount of fat contained in a product while adding soluble fiber. The USDA Agricultural Research Service has developed two carbohydrate-based products that provide the texture of fat: Oatrim, made from oats, and Nutrim, made from oats and barley. These can be used in baked goods, salad dressings, sauces, and ice cream and are a good source of a soluble fiber, which has been shown to reduce blood cholesterol levels.

Protein-Based Fat Substitutes The protein-based fat replacer Simplesse is a fat substitute made from egg-white and milk proteins that are modified by heating, filtering, and high-speed mixing. The resulting protein consists of millions of microscopic balls that slip and slide over each other to give it the creamy texture of fat. Because it is made from protein, Simplesse contains energy, but because the protein is mixed with water, it contains only 1.3 kcalories per g, which is much lower than the 9 kcalories per g provided by fat. It is used in frozen desserts, cheese foods, and other products, but it cannot be used for cooking, because heat causes it to break down.[55]

Web Menu

For more information on Olestra go to Procter & Gamble at www.pg.com/main.jhtml/ and search for Olestra.

Poorly Absorbed Fats As Fat Substitutes Some fat substitutes are made from fats that have been modified to reduce how well they are digested or absorbed. Caprenin, for example, consists of a glycerol backbone with three poorly absorbed fatty acids attached. It is digested like fat, but the fatty acids are only partially absorbed, so it provides only 5 kcalories per g.[55] The artificial fat Olestra is made from sucrose with fatty acids attached (sucrose polyester). Olestra cannot be digested by either the human enzymes or the bacterial enzymes in the gastrointestinal tract. It is therefore excreted in the feces without being absorbed. One of the problems with Olestra is that it reduces the absorption of other fat-soluble substances, including the fat-soluble vitamins A, D, E, and K. To avoid depleting these vitamins, Olestra has been fortified with them. However, it is not fortified with beta-carotene and other fat-soluble substances that may be important for health. Research done by Procter & Gamble, the company that manufactures Olestra, has not found an association between Olestra intake and a reduction in blood carotenoid concentrations,[59] but the extent to which Olestra impacts the absorption of other fat-soluble phytochemicals over the course of days or weeks

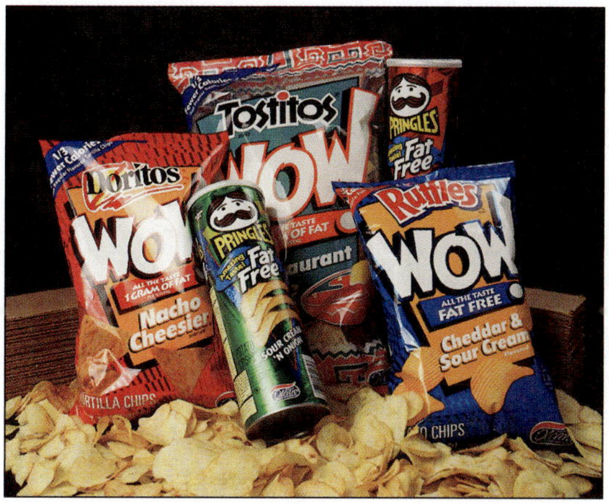

FIGURE 5.25 Products that contain Olestra (Olean), such as these snack chips, must carry the following health warning: "This product contains Olestra. Olestra may cause abdominal cramping and loose stools. Olestra inhibits the absorption of some vitamins and other nutrients. Vitamins A, D, E, and K have been added." *(George Semple)*

has not been determined. Another potential problem with Olestra is that it can cause gastrointestinal irritation, bloating, and diarrhea in some individuals because it passes into the colon without being digested.[57] Products containing Olestra must carry a warning label about these potential side effects (Figure 5.25).

SUMMARY

1. Lipids are a diverse group of organic compounds, most of which do not dissolve in water. In the body, they provide a concentrated source of energy, insulate against shock and temperature changes, act as a structural component of cell membranes, and are used to synthesize hormones and other regulatory molecules. In the diet, they provide energy and contribute to the texture and flavor of food.
2. Fatty acids consist of a carbon chain with an acid group at one end. The length of the carbon chain and the number and position of double bonds determine the characteristics of the fat. Linoleic acid (omega-6) and alpha-linolenic acid (omega-3) are considered essential fatty acids because they cannot be synthesized by the body. Other omega-6 and omega-3 fatty acids may become essential if they cannot be synthesized in amounts adequate for proper physiological function. In the body and in the diet, most fatty acids are found as part of triglycerides.
3. Triacylglycerols or triglycerides, commonly referred to as fat, are the storage form of fat. They consist of a backbone of glycerol with three fatty acids attached.
4. Phosphoglycerides are a type of phospholipid that consists of a backbone of glycerol, two fatty acids, and a phosphate group. Phosphoglycerides are an important component of cell membranes and lipoproteins because one end is water-soluble and one end is lipid-soluble.
5. Sterols, of which cholesterol is the best known, are made up of multiple chemical rings. Cholesterol is made by the liver and consumed in animal foods in the diet. In the body, it is a component of cell membranes and is used to synthesize vitamin D, bile acids, and a number of steroid hormones.
6. Most of the fat in food is triglycerides. These provide taste, texture, and aroma as well as energy (9 kcal/g). The types of lipids in foods depend on the source. Most saturated fats come from animal products; vegetable oils provide more unsaturated fats. Cholesterol is only found in animal products. The types of fats used in processing depend on the desired characteristic. Partially hydrogenated vegetable oils and tropical oils are used to improve shelf life and increase the melting point. The *trans* and saturated fatty acids in these products may increase health risks.
7. In the small intestine, churning and bile from the gallbladder help break fats from the diet into small droplets. This allows pancreatic lipase to access these fats for digestion. The products of fat digestion, primarily fatty acids and monoglycerides, combine with bile to form micelles, which facilitate the absorption of these materials into the cells of the small intestine. Medium-chain triglycerides do not require bile for digestion and absorption. Medium-chain-length fatty acids are water-soluble and so can be absorbed and transported via the bloodstream.
8. In body fluids, water-insoluble lipids are transported as lipoproteins. Long-chain-length triglycerides, cholesterol, and phospholipids absorbed from the intestine are packaged with protein to form chylomicrons, which enter the lymphatic system before entering the blood. The triglycerides in chylomicrons are broken down by lipoprotein lipase, an enzyme on the surface of cells lining the blood vessels. The fatty acids released are taken up by surrounding cells. The chylomicron remnants that remain are returned to the liver.

9. Very-low-density lipoproteins (VLDLs) are lipoproteins synthesized by the liver. With the help of lipoprotein lipase, they deliver triglycerides to body cells. Once the triglycerides have been removed, intermediate-density lipoproteins (IDLs) are transformed into low-density lipoproteins (LDLs). LDLs deliver cholesterol to tissues by binding to LDL receptors on the cell surface. High levels of LDL are associated with an increased risk of cardiovascular disease. High-density lipoproteins (HDLs) are made by the liver and small intestine. They help remove cholesterol from cells for disposal and protect against cardiovascular disease. High blood HDL cholesterol protects against heart disease.
10. After eating, chylomicrons and VLDLs deliver triglycerides to cells for energy or storage. During fasting, triglycerides stored in adipose cells are broken down by the enzyme hormone sensitive lipase and the fatty acids and glycerol are released into the blood.
11. The risk of heart disease is increased by diabetes, high blood pressure, obesity, and high blood cholesterol levels. Risk is also affected by age, gender, genetics, and lifestyle factors such as diet. Diets high in saturated fat, *trans* fatty acids, and cholesterol increase the risk of heart disease primarily by increasing blood cholesterol levels. Diets high in energy promote obesity. Diets high in omega-6 or omega-3 polyunsaturated fatty acids, monounsaturated fatty acids, and plant foods containing fiber, antioxidants, and phytochemicals reduce the risk of heart disease by affecting cholesterol levels and other risk factors. Total dietary and lifestyle pattern is more important than any individual dietary factor in reducing heart disease risk.
12. Diets high in fat correlate with an increased incidence of certain types of cancer. In general, diets very low in fat are associated with a lower risk of breast cancer. High intakes of linoleic acid may promote tumor growth. Diets high in fat and low in fiber increase colon cancer risk. As with heart disease, the overall diet is probably more important in cancer prevention than fat intake alone.
13. A minimum of 3 to 6 g of linoleic acid is recommended to prevent essential fatty acid deficiency. To reduce chronic disease risk it is recommended that the diet contain a moderate amount of total fat (30% of energy) that is divided equally among saturated fat, polyunsaturated fat, and monounsaturated fat; and that dietary cholesterol be no more than 300 mg per day.
14. Reducing fat intake requires decreasing intake of obvious sources of fat such as butter and oils, as well as baked goods, fast foods, and processed convenience foods that contain hidden fats. Saturated fat and *trans* fat intake can be reduced by limiting animal fats, margarine, and partially hydrogenated shortenings. To reduce health risks, the total dietary pattern, including consumption of grains, fruits, and vegetables, is as important as a moderate fat intake.
15. Artificial fats are used to create reduced-fat products with taste and texture similar to the original. Some low-fat products are made by using mixtures of carbohydrates or proteins to simulate the properties of fat, and some use modified lipids that are not well absorbed.

Review Questions

1. What is a lipid?
2. Name four types of lipids found in the body.
3. What distinguishes a saturated fat from a monounsaturated fat? From a polyunsaturated fat?
4. Name two functions of fat in foods.
5. What types of foods contain cholesterol?
6. What is hydrogenation and how is it related to *trans* fatty acids?
7. Is essential fatty acid deficiency common in developed countries? Why or why not?
8. List three functions of fat in the body.
9. In the body, what is the advantage of storing energy as fat rather than as carbohydrate?
10. What is the function of bile in fat digestion and absorption?
11. How do chylomicrons and VLDLs differ?
12. How do HDLs differ from LDLs?
13. How are blood levels of LDLs and HDLs related to the risk of cardiovascular disease?
14. What are the recommendations for dietary fat intake?
15. How do recommendations for fat intake compare to the typical intake in the United States?

Applying Critical Thinking Skills

Personal nutrition:

1. Using the food record you kept in Chapter 2, calculate your average fat, saturated fat, and cholesterol intake.
   a. How many grams of total fat and saturated fat do you consume?
   b. What percent of your energy intake is from fat? Saturated fat?
   c. How does your fat intake compare with the recommendation of no more than 30% of energy from total fat and no more than 10% from saturated fat?
   d. If your diet contains more than 30% of energy from fat, suggest substitutions that would decrease your fat intake to 30% or less of energy without changing your energy intake. If your diet already contains less than 30% of energy from fat, list foods you typically consume that are high in fat and some lower-fat alternatives.
   e. If your diet contains more than 10% of energy from saturated fat, suggest food substitutions that would decrease the amount of saturated fat in your diet.

f. How does your cholesterol intake compare with the recommendation of 300 mg or less per day?
g. Does your diet meet the recommendations of the Food Guide Pyramid?

2. Review all three days of the food record you kept in Chapter 2. Identify foods from your diet that are sources of each of the following lipids. If your diet does not contain any foods that are sources of these, name foods that do contain them.
   a. Cholesterol
   b. Saturated fat
   c. Polyunsaturated fat
   d. Monounsaturated fat
   e. Omega-3 fatty acids
   f. *Trans* fatty acids
3. Using the information in Table 5.2, assess your own risk of cardiovascular disease. Unless you have had a recent physical examination, you may not know your blood cholesterol values.
4. Select four packaged foods that you routinely consume. Examine the food labels. If you consumed only this food for an entire day, how many servings could you eat before exceeding the Daily Value for:
   a. Total fat?
   b. Saturated fat?
   c. Cholesterol?

General nutrition issues:

1. The typical fat intake in the United States has decreased over the last few years. There are thousands of reduced-fat products on the market and millions of dollars have been spent teaching Americans about the benefits of a low-fat diet. Nevertheless, there has been an increase in the incidence of obesity in the United States over this same period. How is it possible that people are cutting down on the percent fat in their diet and still gaining weight?
2. Many Americans are so confused about what type of fat to eat that they have given up paying any attention at all to recommendations. How would you explain the recommendations concerning the type of fat they should consume? If they were preparing a stir-fry, what type of fat would you suggest they use: Margarine? Butter? Olive oil? Why?
3. Ka Ming is 54 years old and has lived in the United States since 1964. An annual physical reveals that his total blood cholesterol is 280 mg/100 ml and his HDL cholesterol is 25 mg/100 ml. He is of normal weight and does not smoke. He works as a laboratory technician and so spends part of the day on his feet but gets little other exercise. A medical history reveals that none of Ka Ming's relatives in China have had cardiovascular disease.
   a. Assess Ka Ming's risk for developing cardiovascular disease.
   b. Why might the lack of cardiovascular disease in his family history not be a true indication of Ka Ming's risk?
   c. A diet analysis reveals that Ka Ming consumes a mixture of American foods and traditional Chinese foods. He likes a big breakfast but must bring a bag lunch to work. Dinner is often Chinese-style food that he cooks himself at home or buys from a family-owned Chinese-American restaurant near his home. His diet contains approximately 40% of its energy from fat, and 15% of this is from saturated fat. It contains about 350 mg of cholesterol a day. Below is a list of foods that Ka Ming routinely consumes. Which choices are low in fat and what modifications, selection suggestions, or cooking tips would decrease his intake of total fat, saturated fat, and cholesterol?

Breakfast foods

Scrambled eggs
Pancakes
Cheese omelet
Sausages

Lunch foods

Ham and cheese sandwich
Peanut butter and jelly sandwich
Tuna salad sandwich
Potato chips

Dinner foods

Crispy fried beef over white rice
Sweet and sour pork over white rice
Chicken and broccoli stir-fry over white rice
Pork fried rice
Egg rolls

References

1. Gerster, H. The use of n-3 PUFAs (fish oil) in enteral nutrition. Int. J. Vitam. Nutr. Res. 65:3–20, 1995.
2. Allison, D. B., Egan, S. K., Barrah, L. M., et al. Estimates of trans fatty and other fatty acids in the U.S. population. J. Am. Diet. Assoc. 99:166–174, 1999.
3. Crawford, M. A., Costeloe, K., Ghebremeskel, K., et al. Are deficits of arachidonic and docosahexaenoic acids responsible for the neural and vascular complications of preterm babies? Am. J. Clin. Nutr. 66(supp): 1032S–1041S, 1997.
4. Elson, C. E. Tropical oils: nutritional and scientific issues. Crit. Rev. Food Sci. Nutr. 31:79–102, 1992.
5. Hamosh, M., Iverson, S. J., Kirk, C. L., and Hamosh, P. Milk lipids and neonatal fat digestion: relationship between fatty acid composition, endogenous and exogenous digestive enzymes and digestion of milk fat. World Rev. Nutr. Diet. 75:86–91, 1994.
6. Krauss, R. M., Deckelbaum, R. J., Ernst, N., et al. Dietary guidelines for healthy American adults: a statement for health professionals from

the Nutrition Committee, American Heart Association. Circulation 94:1795–1800, 1996.

7. Keys, A. *Seven Countries: A Multivariate Analysis of Diet and Coronary Heart Disease.* Cambridge, Mass.: Harvard University Press, 1980.
8. Ascherio, A., Rimm, E. B., Stampfer, M. J., et al. Marine n-3 fatty acids, fish intake, and the risk of coronary disease among men. N. Engl. J. Med. 332:977–982, 1995.
9. Nestle, M. Mediterranean diets: historical and research overview. Am. J. Clin. Nutr. 61(suppl):1313S–1320S, 1995.
10. Keys, A. Mediterranean diet and public health: personal reflections. Am. J. Clin. Nutr. 61(suppl):1321S–1323S, 1995.
11. Gordon, T. The diet-heart idea. Am. J. Epidemiol. 127:220–223, 1988.
12. Brown, M. S., and Goldstein, J. L. How LDL receptors influence cholesterol and atherosclerosis. Sci. Am. 251:58–66, 1984.
13. Ginsberg, H. N., and Karmally, W. Nutrition, lipids, and cardiovascular disease. In *Biochemical and Physiological Aspects of Human Nutrition.* M. H. Stipanuk, ed. Philadelphia: W. B. Saunders Company, 2000, 917–944.
14. Brown, M. S., and Goldstein, J. L. Scavenging for receptors. Nature 343:508–509, 1990.
15. American Heart Association, Cardiovascular Disease Statistics. Available online at **http://www.amhrt.org/Heart_and_Stroke_A_Z_Guide/cvds.htm.** Accessed 2 Dec 2000.
16. Schaefer, E. J., Lichtenstein, A. H., Lamon-Fava, S., et al. Lipoproteins, nutrition, aging, and atherosclerosis. Am. J. Clin. Nutr. 61(suppl):726S–740S, 1995.
17. American and Canadian Dietetics Association. Position of the American Dietetic Association and the Canadian Dietetic Association: women's health and nutrition. J. Am. Diet. Assoc. 95:362–366, 1995.
18. Geil, P. B., Anderson, J. W., and Gustafson, N. J. Women and men with hypercholesterolemia respond similarly to an American Heart Association Step 1 Diet. J. Am. Diet. Assoc. 95:436–441, 1995.
19. Sagiv, M., and Goldbourt, U. Influence of physical work on high density lipoprotein cholesterol: implications for the risk of coronary heart disease. Int. J. Sports Med. 15:261–266, 1994.
20. Hu, F. B., Stampfer, M. J., Manson, J. E., et al. Dietary fat intake and the risk of coronary heart disease in women, N. Engl. J. Med. 337:1491–1499, 1997.
21. Denke, M. A. Review of human studies evaluating individual dietary responsiveness in patients with hypercholesterolemia. Am. J. Clin. Nutr. 62(suppl):471S–477S, 1995.
22. Dietschy, J. M. Dietary fatty acids and the regulation of plasma low density lipoprotein cholesterol concentrations. J. Nutr. 128:444S–448S, 1998.
23. Aro, A., Jauhiainen, M., Partanen, R., et al. Stearic acid, trans fatty acids and dairy fat: effects on serum and lipoprotein lipids, apolipoproteins, lipoprotein (a) and lipid transfer proteins in healthy subjects. Am. J. Clin. Nutr. 65:1419–1426, 1997.
24. Hu, F. B., Stampfer, M. J., Manson, J. E., et al. Dietary saturated fats and their food sources in relation to the risk of coronary heart disease in women. Am. J. Clin. Nutr. 70:1001–1008, 1999.
25. Watts, G. F., Jackson, P., Burke, V., and Lewis, B. Dietary fatty acids and progression of coronary artery disease in men. Am. J. Clin. Nutr. 64:202–209, 1996.
26. Asherio, A., and Willett, W. C. Health effects of trans fatty acids. Am. J. Clin. Nutr. 66(suppl):1006S–1010S, 1997.
27. Zock, P. L., and Katan, M. B. Butter, margarine and serum lipoproteins. Atherosclerosis 131:7–16, 1997.
28. Lichtenstein, A. H., Ausman, L. M., Jalbert, S. M., et al. Effects of different forms of dietary hydrogenated fats on serum lipoprotein cholesterol levels. N. Engl. J. Med. 340:1933–1940, 1999.
29. Eckel, R. H., and Krauss, R. M. American Heart Association call to action: obesity is a major risk factor for coronary heart disease. AHA Nutrition Committee. Circulation 97:2099–2100, 1998.
30. Katan, M. B., Zock, P. L., and Mensink, R. P. Dietary oils, serum lipoproteins, and coronary heart disease. Am. J. Clin. Nutr. 61(suppl): 1368S–1373S, 1995.
31. Stone, N. J. Fish consumption, fish oil, lipids, and coronary heart disease. Am. J. Clin. Nutr. 65:1083–1086, 1997.
32. Connor, S. L., and Connor, W. E. Are fish oils beneficial in the prevention and treatment of coronary artery disease? Am. J. Clin. Nutr. 66(suppl):1020S–1031S, 1997.
33. Schoene, N. W., and Fitzgerald, G. A. Thrombogenic potential of dietary long-chain polyunsaturated fatty acids: session summary. Am. J. Clin. Nutr. 56(suppl):825S-826S, 1992.
34. Willett, W. C., Sacks, F., Trichopoulou, A., et al. Mediterranean diet pyramid: a cultural model for healthy eating. Am. J. Clin. Nutr. 61(suppl):1402S–1406S, 1995.
35. Kris-Etherton, P. M., Pearson, T. A., Wan, Y., et al. High-monounsaturated fatty acid diets lower both plasma cholesterol and triacylglyceride concentrations. Am. J. Clin. Nutr. 70:1009–1015, 1999.
36. Waterhouse, A. L., German, B. L., Walzem, R. L., et al. Is it time for a wine trial? Am. J. Clin. Nutr. 68:220–221, 1998.
37. Stein, J. H., Keevil, J. G., Wiebe, D. A., et al. Purple grape juice improves endothelial function and reduces the susceptibility of LDL cholesterol to oxidation in patients with coronary artery disease. Circulation 100:1050–1055, 1999.
38. American Institute for Cancer Research, World Cancer Research Fund. Food, Nutrition and the Prevention of Cancer: A Global Perspective. Presented at the American Institute of Cancer Research Conference, Oct. 8–10, 1997.
39. Lichtenstein, A. H., Kennedy, E., Barrier, P., et al. Dietary fat consumption and health. Nutr. Rev. 56(II):S3–S28, 1998.
40. Kuller, L. H. Dietary fat and chronic diseases: epidemiologic overview. J. Am. Diet. Assoc. 97(suppl):S9–S15, 1997.
41. Wynder, E. L., Cohen, L. A., Muscat, J. E., et al. Breast cancer: weighing the evidence for a promoting role of dietary fat. J. Natl. Cancer Inst. 89:766-775, 1997.
42. Rose, D. P. Dietary fatty acids and cancer. Am. J. Clin. Nutr. 66(suppl):998S–1003S, 1997.
43. Greenwald, P., Sherwood, K., and McDonald, S. Fat, caloric intake and obesity: lifestyle risk factors for breast cancer. J. Am. Diet. Assoc. (suppl):S24–S30, 1997.
44. Noguchi, M., Rose, D. P., Earashi, M., and Miyazaki, I. The role of fatty acids and eicosanoid synthesis inhibitors in breast carcinoma. Oncology 52:265–271, 1995.
45. Reddy, B. S. Nutritional factors and colon cancer. Crit. Rev. Food Sci. Nutr. 35:175–190, 1995.
46. LeMarchand, L., Wilkens, L. P., Hankin, J. H., et al. A case control study of diet and colorectal cancer in a multiethnic population in Hawaii: lipids and foods of animal origin. Cancer Causes Control 8:637–648, 1997.
47. USDA, Agricultural Service. Results from USDA's 1994–1996 Continuing Survey of Food Intakes by Individuals and 1994–1996 Health Knowledge Survey. ARS Food Surveys Research Group, 1997. Available online at **http://www.barc.usda.gov/bhnrc/foodsurvey/home/htm.** Accessed 4 Dec 2000.
48. WHO and FAO Joint Consultation. Fats and oils in human nutrition. Nutr. Rev. 53:202–205, 1995.
49. Simopoulos, A. P. Essential fatty acids in health and chronic disease. Am. J. Clin. Nutr. 70(suppl):560S–569S, 1999.
50. National Heart, Lung, and Blood Institute, National Institutes of Health, National Cholesterol Education Program. Live Healthier, Live Longer. Available online at **http://rover.nhlbi.nih.gov/chd.** Accessed 4 Dec 2000.
51. American Academy of Pediatrics Committee on Nutrition. Statement on cholesterol. Pediatrics 101:141–147, 1998.
52. Kurtzweil, P. Skimming the milk label. FDA Consumer 32:22–25, Jan./Feb. 1998.

53. Miller, D. L., Castellanos, V. H., Shide, D. J., et al. Effect of fat-free potato chips with and without nutrition labels on fat and energy intake. Am. J. Clin. Nutr. 68:282–290, 1998.
54. Calorie Control Council. Light foods and beverages soar to new levels of popularity. Calorie Control Commentary 18:1–3, 1996.
55. American Dietetic Association. Position of the American Dietetic Association: fat replacers. J. Am. Diet. Assoc. 98:463–468, 1998.
56. Roche, H. M. Dietary carbohydrates and triacylglycerol metabolism. Proc. Nutr. Soc. 58: 201–207, 1999.
57. Salmeron, J., Manson, J. E., Stampfer, M. J., et al. Dietary fiber, glycemic load, and the risk of noninsulin-dependent diabetes mellitus in women. JAMA 277:472–477, 1997.
58. Sigman-Grant, M. Can you have your low-fat cake and eat it too? The role of fat-modified products. J. Am. Diet. Assoc. 97(suppl):S76–S81, 1997.
59. Procter & Gamble Co., Carotenoids and Olestra: Understanding the "Big Picture." June 1999.

6 Protein

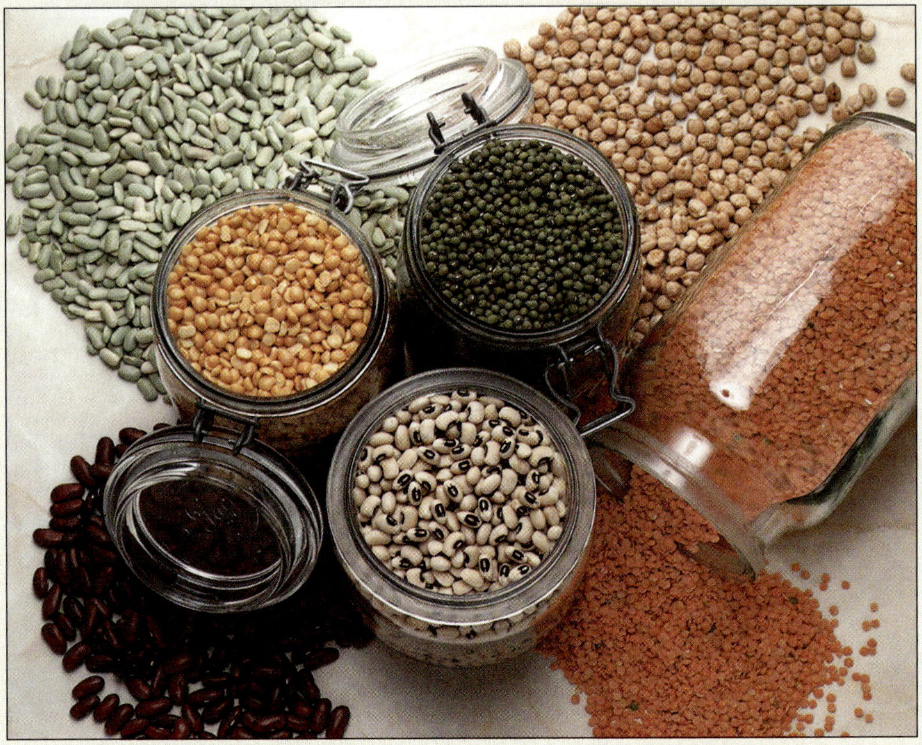

Learning Objectives

After reading this chapter, students should be able to:

1. Describe the general structure of an amino acid and a protein.
2. Explain why some amino acids are essential and others are not.
3. Give examples of dietary sources of plant and animal proteins.
4. List the sources of amino acids entering the "amino acid pool" and the uses for amino acids drawn out of the pool.
5. Explain what is meant by gene expression and describe the role of genes in protein synthesis.
6. List and describe functions of proteins in the body.
7. Define "protein-energy malnutrition" and explain why it develops more rapidly in small children than in adults.
8. Discuss how protein needs are determined and how protein quality affects needs.
9. Explain why protein complementation is important in vegetarian diets and give an example of complementary protein sources.
10. Discuss the benefits and risks associated with vegetarian diets.

Teresa has recently begun her year in the Peace Corps in Somalia. She has been assigned to assist with children in a refugee camp. She can't help noticing Songe's winning smile. He is a small boy about two years old. His hair is an odd color, his legs are scrawny, and his belly is so large he looks pregnant. Songe and his new baby brother live with their mother and three other siblings in the camp. His mother says that his symptoms began shortly after his younger brother was born. His gaunt look suggests that he isn't getting enough to eat, but why is his belly so large?

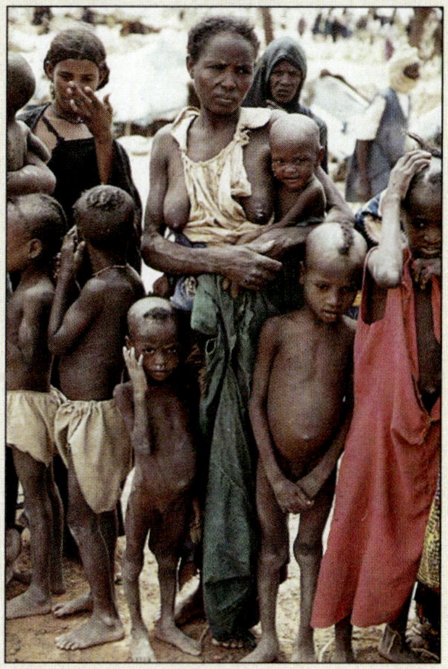

The clinic nurse explains to Teresa that Songe is suffering from protein-energy malnutrition. When his brother was born, Songe stopped nursing at his mother's breast. Instead, he was fed the camp diet, which is high in carbohydrate and fiber. As a result, his protein intake decreased drastically. He was no longer consuming enough protein to support the needs of his growing body. His belly is bloated because his abdomen is filling with fluid and his liver is filling with fat. There is not enough protein in his blood to hold the fluid there, so it seeps into his abdomen. Nor is there enough protein to transport fat, so it is trapped in his liver. Less visible changes are also occurring. Without adequate protein, Songe's immune system cannot function normally, making him more susceptible to illness. The immunizations provided in the camp are less likely to be effective.

Why don't his older siblings, who consume the same high-carbohydrate diet, look like this? Because his siblings are older, they have larger stomachs, and their protein needs per kcalorie are less than Songe's, so they are able to eat enough of the camp diet to meet their protein needs.

To treat his malnutrition, the clinic provides Songe with a special high-protein drink to consume along with his regular diet, and in a few weeks his belly begins to shrink.

Songe's case is a dramatic illustration of the importance of protein in the body. Severe protein deficiency is rare in the United States where the food supply is plentiful and varied. Most Americans have access to meats, eggs, and dairy products, which are very concentrated sources of animal protein, and to legumes, grains, and vegetables, which provide plant sources of protein. Even adults who choose a vegetarian diet can easily meet their protein needs. Nonetheless, protein drinks, pills, and powders fill the shelves of health-food stores. Consumers often choose high-protein foods and supplements because protein is associated with good health. How much protein do we need to stay healthy? Do we need to worry about eating too much protein or about which protein sources we choose? An understanding of the chemistry of protein and how the body metabolizes it is necessary to answer these questions.

What Are Proteins?

Proteins are a group of compounds that are made up of one or more chainlike strands of **amino acids.** The amino acid chains of each type of protein molecule contain a characteristic number of amino acids in specific proportions and are

Amino acids The building blocks of proteins. Each contains a carbon atom bound to a hydrogen atom, an amino group, an acid group, and a side chain.

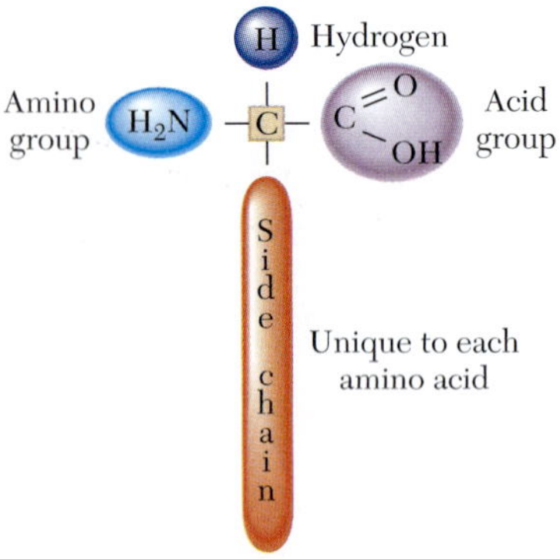

FIGURE 6.1 All amino acids have a similar structure, consisting of a central carbon bound to an amino group (NH_2), an acid group (COOH), a hydrogen (H), and a side chain that differs for each amino acid.

bound together in a precise order. The amino acid chain folds into different orientations, giving each protein a unique three-dimensional shape that is essential to its specific function. Variations in the number, proportion, and order of amino acids in the chain determine the three-dimensional shape and allow for an infinite number of different protein structures.

Like carbohydrates and lipids, proteins contain the elements carbon, hydrogen, and oxygen, but proteins are distinguished from the other energy-yielding nutrients by the presence of the element nitrogen in their structure.

Amino Acids

There are approximately 20 amino acids commonly found in proteins. Each amino acid consists of a carbon atom bound to four chemical groups: a hydrogen atom (H); an amino group (NH_2), which contains nitrogen; an acid group (COOH); and a fourth group referred to as a side chain that varies in length and structure (Figure 6.1). Different side chains give specific properties to individual amino acids. Some amino acids are acidic, some are basic, some are attracted to water, others repel water. Some are large and others are small enough to fit in tight spaces. (See Appendix L for amino acid structures.)

Of the 20 amino acids commonly found in protein, 9 cannot be made by the adult human body. These amino acids, called **essential,** or **indispensable, amino acids,** must be consumed in the diet (Table 6.1). If the diet is deficient in one or more of these amino acids, new proteins containing them cannot be made without the breaking down of other body proteins to provide them. The 11 **nonessential,** or **dispensable, amino acids** can be made by the human body and are not required in the diet. Most of the nonessential amino acids can be made by the process of **transamination,** in which an amino group from one amino acid is transferred to a carbon-containing molecule to form a different amino acid (Figure 6.2).

Some amino acids are **semiessential,** or **conditionally essential.** These are essential only under certain conditions. For example, the conditionally essential amino acid tyrosine can be made in the body from the essential amino acid phenylalanine. However, if phenylalanine is in short supply, tyrosine cannot be made and thus becomes essential in the diet. Likewise, the amino acid cysteine is only essential when the essential amino acid methionine is in short supply. Amino acids may also be essential under certain metabolic conditions. For example, in premature infants, cysteine and tyrosine are essential because the metabolic pathways to synthesize them in adequate amounts are not fully developed. These

Essential or **indispensable amino acids** Amino acids that cannot be synthesized by the human body in sufficient amounts to meet dietary needs and therefore must be included in the diet.

Nonessential or **dispensable amino acids** Amino acids that can be synthesized by the human body in sufficient amounts to meets needs.

Transamination The process by which an amino group from one amino acid is transferred to a carbon compound to form a new amino acid.

Semiessential or **conditionally essential amino acids** Amino acids that are essential in the diet only under certain conditions or at certain times of life.

TABLE 6.1 Classification of Amino Acids

Essential Amino Acids	Nonessential Amino Acids
Histidine	Alanine
Isoleucine	Arginine
Leucine	Asparagine
Lysine	Aspartic acid (aspartate)
Methionine	Cysteine (cystine)[a]
Phenylalanine	Tyrosine[a]
Threonine	Glutamic acid (glutamate)
Tryptophan	Glutamine
Valine	Glycine
	Proline
	Serine

[a]These amino acids are also classified as semi-essential. If not enough is supplied in the diet, they must be made in the body from essential amino acids. If those essential amino acids are in short supply, the semi-essential amino acids can become essential.

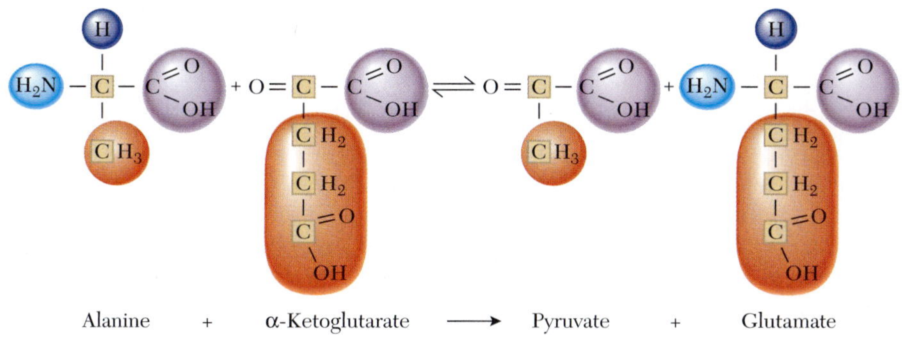

FIGURE 6.2 In this example, the process of transamination transfers the amino group from the nonessential amino acid alanine to the carbon compound alpha-ketoglutarate to form the three-carbon compound pyruvate and the amino acid glutamate.

amino acids are also essential in individuals with inherited disorders of the metabolic pathways that synthesize them.

Protein Structure

To form proteins, amino acids are linked together by a unique type of chemical bond called a **peptide bond.** This bond is formed between the nitrogen atom in the amino group of one amino acid and the carbon atom in the acid group of the next amino acid (Figure 6.3). Two amino acids linked with a peptide bond are called a **dipeptide;** three similarly linked amino acids form a **tripeptide.** Many amino acids bonded together constitute a **polypeptide.**

Peptide bond The linkage formed between the nitrogen in the amino group of one amino acid and the carbon in the acid group of another by a condensation reaction in which water is eliminated.

Dipeptide Two amino acids linked by a peptide bond. A **tripeptide** is three amino acids linked by peptide bonds, and a **polypeptide** is a chain of three or more amino acids linked by peptide bonds.

A protein is made of one or more polypeptide chains folded into a complex three-dimensional shape. The order and chemical properties of the amino acids in a polypeptide chain determine the three-dimensional shape of the protein. Folds and bends in the chain occur when some of the amino acids attract each other and other amino acids repel each other. For example, amino acids at various places along the chain that are attracted to each other may cause segments of the chain to coil like a telephone cord. Amino acids that are attracted to water will orient to the outside of the structure to be in contact with body fluids, whereas amino acids that repel water will fold to the inside to be away from body fluids. After polypeptide chains have folded, several may bind together to form the final protein, whose function may also depend on the addition of a metal ion or a vitamin molecule (Figure 6.4).

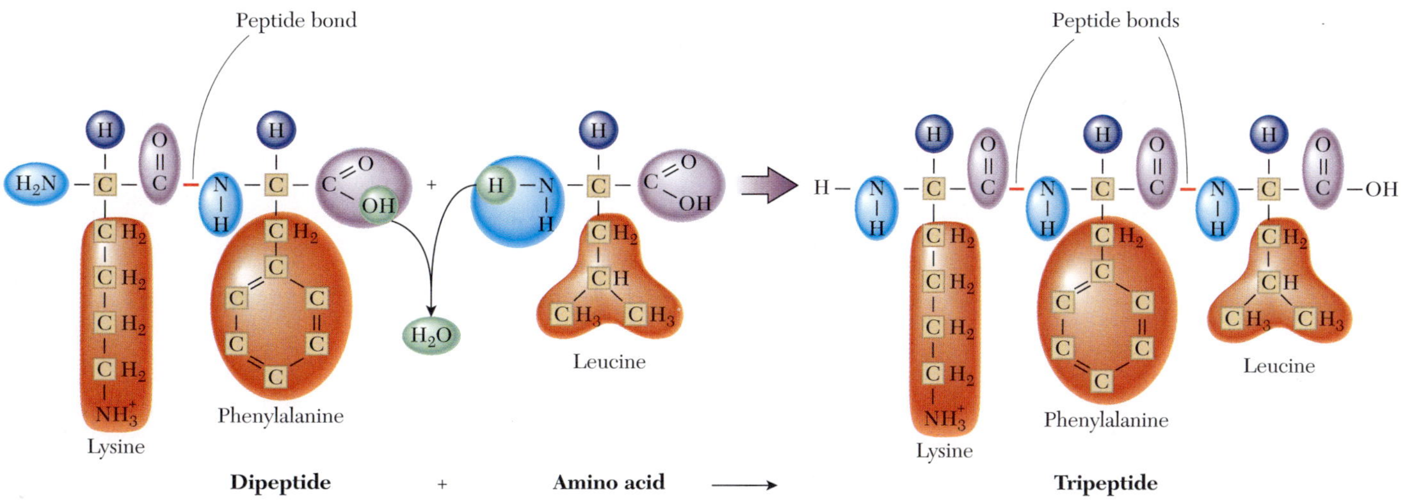

FIGURE 6.3 Amino acids in proteins are linked by peptide bonds that join the amino group of one amino acid to the acid group of the next. This example shows a dipeptide of lysine and phenylalanine joining with the amino acid leucine to form a tripeptide via a condensation reaction. A molecule of water is lost when the peptide bond is formed.

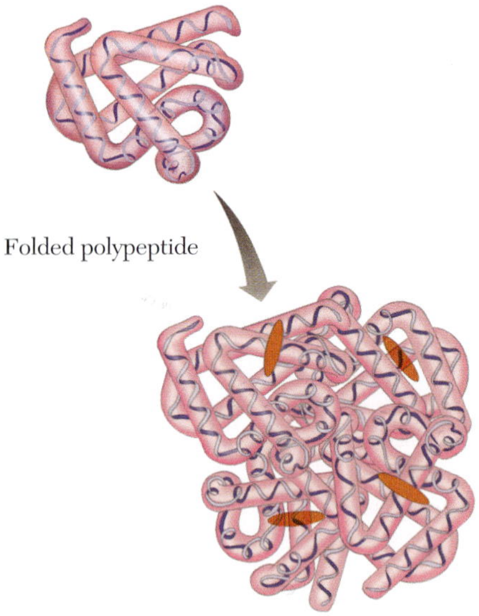

FIGURE 6.4 A polypeptide chain will often curl into a helical configuration that may then fold over itself to form a more complex three-dimensional shape. In the case of the protein hemoglobin, four folded polypeptides join to form the final protein. The rust-colored rings contain the element iron, which is needed for hemoglobin function.

Denaturation The alteration of a protein's three-dimensional structure.

It is the shape of this final protein that determines its function. For example, the connective tissue proteins, collagen and alpha-keratin, are in the shape of elongated helices. This structure allows these proteins to give strength to fingernails and ligaments, respectively. The oxygen-carrying protein hemoglobin has a spherical shape, which allows proper functioning of the red blood cells. If the shape of a protein is altered, its function may be disrupted. In the genetic disease sickle-cell anemia, a single amino acid in the hemoglobin molecule is altered, causing the protein molecules to bind together in long chains (Figure 6.5). Thus, a red blood cell containing these ropelike strands of sickle-cell hemoglobin has a distorted shape that resembles a crescent or sickle. (Normal hemoglobin molecules do not bind together and the red blood cells containing them are disc-shaped.) Sickle-shaped red blood cells can block capillaries, causing inflammation and pain. They also rupture easily, leading to anemia from a shortage of red blood cells.

Changes in protein structure can also be caused by changes in temperature and acidity. This change in structure is called **denaturation,** a change from the natural. During digestion, stomach acid denatures proteins, opening up their structure to allow digestive enzymes better access to the peptide bonds. In food, cooking denatures protein, thereby changing its shape and physical properties. For example, a raw egg white is clear and liquid, but once it has been denatured by cooking, it becomes white and firm (Figure 6.6).

PROTEIN IN THE DIET

Protein consumed in the diet provides the raw material to make all the various types of proteins that the body needs. Animal foods provide concentrated sources of dietary protein. Plant foods also contribute protein but are less concentrated sources. Despite this, plant foods provide most of the protein consumed by the Earth's population (Figure 6.7).

Protein also contributes to the texture, shape, and color of food. It is the protein in grains that provides the structure of breads and baked goods. Egg protein gives custard stability. The protein in cream allows it to stiffen when whipped,

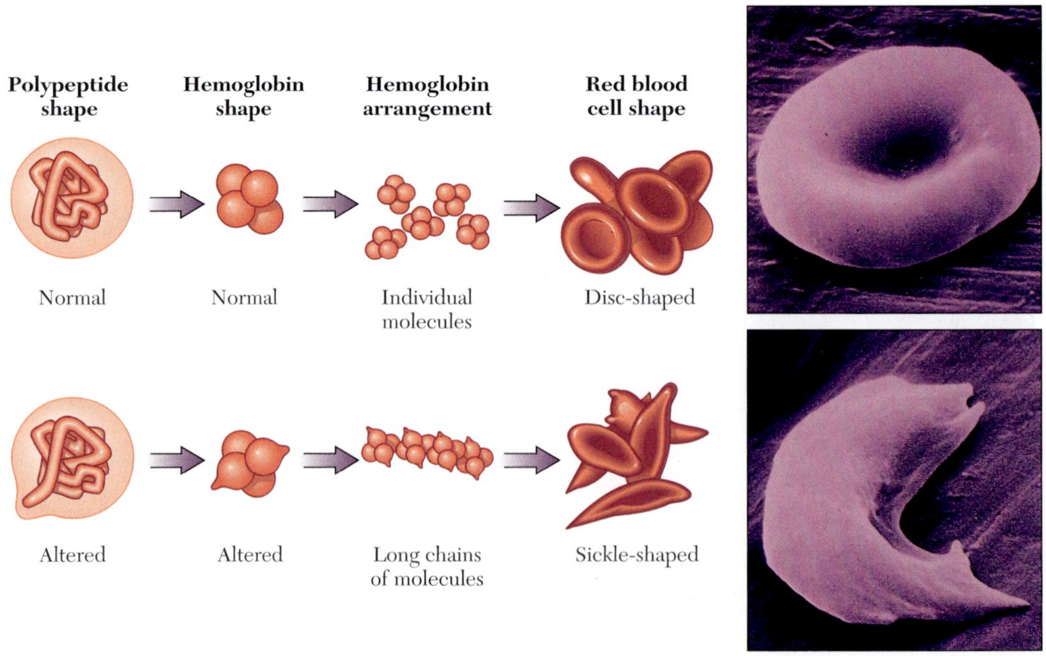

FIGURE 6.5 In sickle-cell anemia, a change in the sequence of amino acids in hemoglobin causes a change in the shape and function of the protein molecule. Sickle-cell hemoglobin forms long chains that distort the shape of red blood cells. *(© Stan Flegler/Visuals Unlimited)*

and myoglobin, the iron-carrying protein in muscle, gives meat its red color. The chemical and physical properties of proteins and amino acids have made them important additives in processed foods.

Sources of Protein

Animal foods are high in protein. A three-ounce portion of meat provides about 21 g of protein. Plants also provide good sources of protein but usually contain less protein per serving. Legumes such as lentils, soybeans, peanuts, black-eyed peas, chickpeas, red beans, pinto beans, kidney beans, and black beans provide 6 to 10 g of protein per half-cup serving. Nuts and seeds are also good sources of protein, providing about 5 to 10 g per quarter cup. A serving of grains or vegetables provides 2 to 3 g (Figure 6.8).

In addition to the amount of protein, the quality of protein must be considered in meeting dietary needs. **Protein quality** is a measure of how useful a dietary protein is for building body protein. Animal proteins usually contain a pattern of amino acids closer to that needed by the body than do plant proteins. Therefore, they are said to be of high quality or **complete protein.** Plant proteins are usually low in one or more amino acids in relation to body proteins. This amino acid is said to be the **limiting amino acid** of that protein source. It is the amino acid that limits the usefulness of the protein for meeting body needs. Proteins limited in one or more amino acids are said to be of low quality. Body needs can be met with low-quality proteins if a variety of proteins containing different limiting amino acids are consumed (see Protein Complementation later in this chapter).

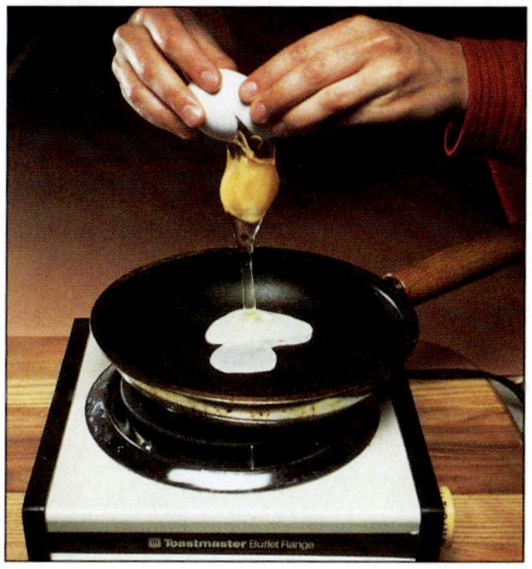

FIGURE 6.6 The protein in egg white is denatured by heat when the egg is cooked. *(Charles D. Winters)*

Protein quality A measure of how efficiently a protein in the diet can be used to synthesize body proteins.

Complete protein Protein that provides essential amino acids in the proportions needed to support protein synthesis.

Limiting amino acid The essential amino acid that is available in the lowest amount relative to the body's needs.

Proteins and Amino Acids Added to Foods

Proteins and amino acids are added to foods to modify taste and texture and to change their nutrient composition. The milk protein casein is often added to coffee whiteners and frozen dessert toppings to simulate the taste and texture of cream. Soy protein concentrate is used to aid in emulsification and provide texture in products such as canned gravies and candy bars. These additives also increase the protein content of the foods in which they are used. Gelatin, a protein derived from animal connective tissue, is used to gel yogurt; to whip foams such as cupcake fillings; to clarify fruit juices, wines, and beer; to increase viscosity (thicken); and to prevent the growth of ice crystals in frozen desserts. Although it is derived from an animal protein, gelatin is completely deficient in the essential amino acid tryptophan and low in other essential amino acids. So, though it is a useful additive for the food industry, gelatin is not a good source of high-quality

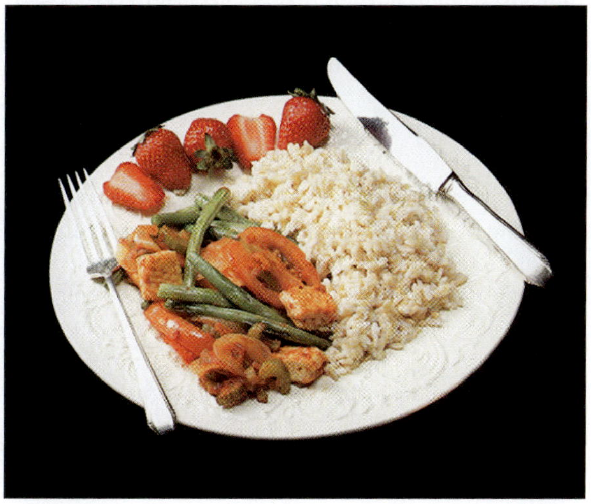

FIGURE 6.7 Foods of plant origin can supply plenty of protein *(ASAP/Photo Researchers, Inc.)*

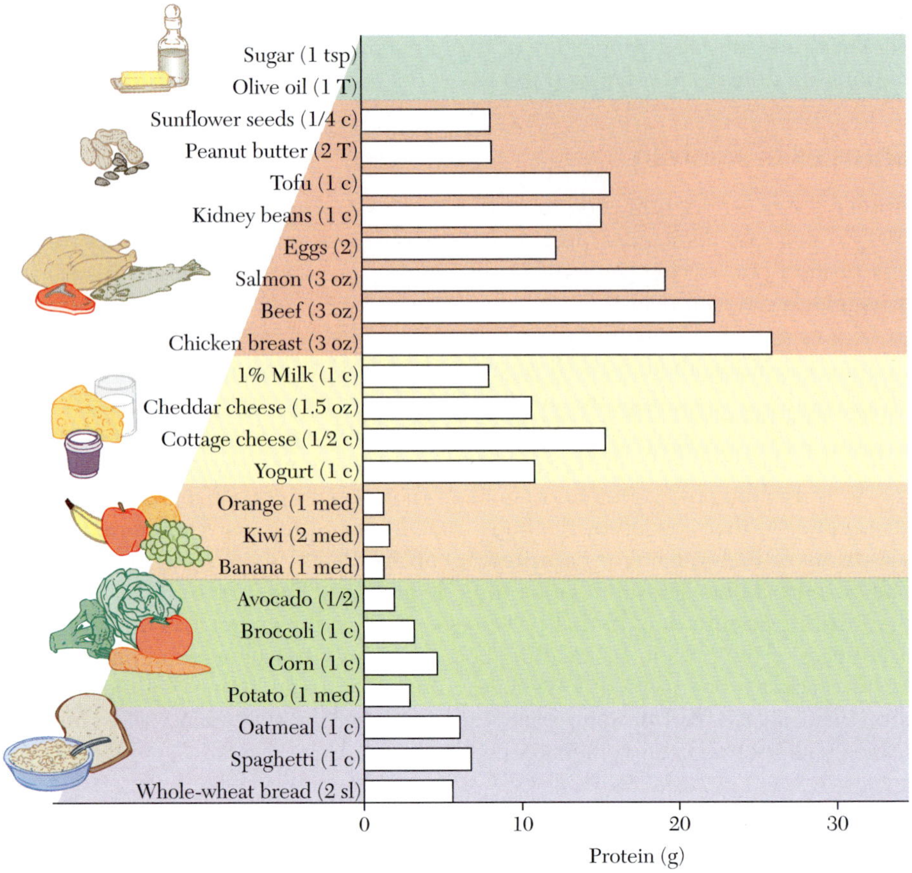

FIGURE 6.8 Protein content of selections from each food group of the Food Guide Pyramid. Foods in the Meat, Poultry, Fish, Eggs, Dry Beans and Nuts Group and the Milk, Yogurt, and Cheese Group contain the most protein per serving.

Protein hydrolysates or **hydrolyzed proteins** Mixtures of amino acids or amino acids and polypeptides produced when a protein is completely or partially broken down by treatment with acid or enzymes.

dietary protein. **Protein hydrolysates,** or **hydrolyzed proteins,** are also frequently added to food. These are proteins that have been treated with acid or enzymes to break them down into amino acids and small peptides. They are used as flavorings, flavor enhancers, stabilizers, or thickening agents in products such as packaged rice pilaf and potatoes au gratin.

Meat Substitutes Meat substitutes are processed vegetable products used to replace meat in the diet; most are soy based. Soy protein isolates and texturized soy protein are soy protein that can be formed into chunks, woven or spun into fibers, or otherwise shaped and flavored to form meat substitutes. They are used to make imitation hot dogs, meatballs, chicken, and veal, or they can be added to animal protein as an extender or filler. Although soybeans are limited in the sulfur amino acids methionine and cysteine, they are so high in total protein and the protein is so digestible that soy protein is considered to be equivalent to animal protein in quality.[1] (See *Making Decisions:* "Should You Increase Your Intake of Soy Protein?")

Fat Substitutes Protein can also be used in processed foods to simulate the texture of fat. The fat substitute Simplesse is made from egg-white and milk proteins that are modified by heating, filtering, and high-speed mixing. The resulting protein consists of millions of microscopic balls that slip and slide over one another, providing the slippery texture of fat.[2] Despite its "fatty" texture, Simplesse contains only a little more than 1 kcalorie per g, compared with 9 kcalories per g of fat.

Aspartame The amino acids aspartic acid and phenylalanine combine to form the artificial sweetener aspartame. Aspartame is used in a wide variety of foods, including carbonated beverages, gelatin desserts, and chewing gum (Figure 6.9). It cannot be used in cooked products because it breaks down

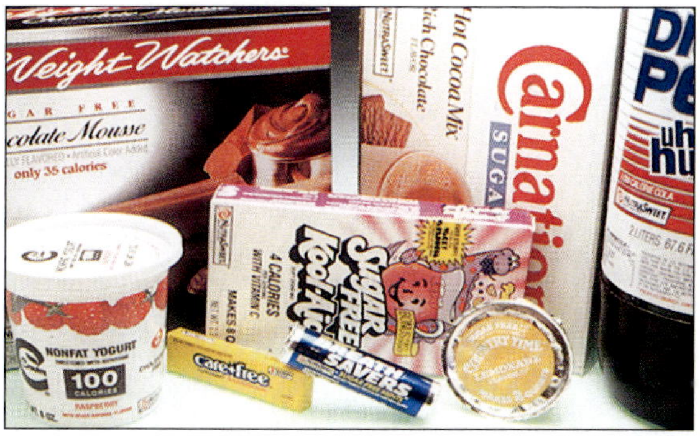

FIGURE 6.9 Although used to replace sugar in a variety of products, aspartame is made from the amino acids aspartic acid and phenylalanine. *(Charles D. Winters)*

when heated, losing its sweet taste. It became popular when it was suggested that both saccharin and cyclamates could cause cancer in laboratory animals (see Chapter 4).

Because aspartame contains the amino acid phenylalanine, it can be harmful to individuals with a genetic disorder called **phenylketonuria (PKU).** In individuals with PKU, the gene coding for an enzyme needed to metabolize the essential amino acid phenylalanine is abnormal. As a result, the enzyme does not function properly and these individuals are unable to convert phenylalanine to the semiessential amino acid tyrosine. Instead, phenylalanine is converted to compounds called phenylketones, which build up in the blood. High phenylketone levels can interfere with brain development, causing mental retardation. To prevent mental retardation, infants and children with PKU must consume a diet with just enough phenylalanine to meet the body's need for protein synthesis but not so much that the buildup of phenylketones occurs. The diet must also provide sufficient tyrosine since the enzyme deficit prevents conversion of phenylalanine to tyrosine.

Phenylketonuria (PKU) An inherited disease in which the body cannot metabolize the amino acid phenylalanine. If the disease is untreated, toxic byproducts accumulate in the blood and cause mental retardation.

Web Menu For more information about PKU, from special diets to the latest research, go to www.pkunews.org.

Monosodium Glutamate Monosodium glutamate (MSG) is a flavor enhancer that consists of the amino acid glutamic acid (or glutamate) bound to sodium. MSG is best known for its use in Chinese cooking. It is also added to canned soups, meats, and fish; packaged meals such as frozen seafood, chicken, and other entrees; cured meats and lunch meats; and potato chips and other snack foods. Seasonings that contain MSG include Accent, Ajinomoto, Zest, Vestin, Gourmet Powder, Subu, Chinese seasonings, Glutavene, Glutacyl, RL-50 Kombu extract, and Meijing or Wei-jing.

Consumption of MSG has been reported to cause adverse reactions in some individuals. MSG symptom complex, commonly called Chinese restaurant syndrome, is a set of symptoms including facial pressure or tightness, tingling sensations, headache, rapid heartbeat, chest pain, nausea, weakness, and drowsiness.[3] These symptoms are most likely to occur within an hour after consumption of a large quantity of MSG (about 3 g or more) on an empty stomach.[4] However, a typical serving of an MSG-containing food includes only about 0.5 g of MSG. In a placebo-controlled double blind study, reactions to MSG were infrequent, inconsistent, and not observed when MSG was given with food.[5] MSG has also been suspected of inducing asthma attacks in individuals with asthma; however, research studies have not conclusively established the existence of MSG-induced asthma.[6] In addition, some brain researchers are concerned that very high dietary intakes of glutamate could be toxic to nerves in humans because glutamate is a neurotransmitter. However, a review of scientific data has found no evidence that dietary MSG causes brain lesions or damages nerve cells in humans.[3,4] The FDA has therefore maintained glutamate on the list of substances generally recognized as safe (see Chapter 19). When MSG is added to a packaged food, it must appear in the label's ingredient list but the amount present is not included.

Making Decisions

Should You Increase Your Intake of Soy Protein?

Soy products have long been a major protein source in Asian diets. Recently the consumption of soy has been increasing in the United States. Sales exceeded $1 billion in 1997—a jump from $300 million in 1980. Why has soy increased in popularity? Soy is a high-quality plant protein that is low in fat and high in phytochemicals. Its popularity, however, is more likely due to evidence that it can reduce the risk of heart disease, cancer, and osteoporosis and lessen the symptoms of menopause. Can soy consumption really deliver on these promises? Should you be eating more?

Research indicates that the consumption of soybeans and products made from soybeans can reduce the risk of heart disease. Compared to animal protein, soy is low in fat and saturated fat and contains no cholesterol. When soy protein is substituted for animal protein in the diet, it lowers blood levels of LDL cholesterol and either increases or causes no change in HDL levels.[a] Some of this effect on blood lipids is believed to be due to the phytochemicals in soy. One class of phytochemical, isoflavones, which are also known as plant estrogens, or phytoestrogens, may also reduce the formation of plaque in artery walls and protect cholesterol from oxidation. The antioxidant effect of isoflavones is similar in magnitude to that of vitamin E.[b] Taking supplements of isoflavones, however, does not have the same effect as consuming them in soy foods.[c] It is hypothesized that there is something else in soy protein that allows the phytoestrogens to act. The evidence that soy reduces the risk of heart disease is viewed as strong enough that a health claim is now allowed on the labels of foods that are low in saturated fat and cholesterol and provide at least 6.25 g of soy protein per serving. Such a food might state that "25 g of soy protein a day, as part of a diet low in saturated fat and cholesterol, may reduce the risk of heart disease."

The isoflavones in soy may play a role in reducing the risks of certain types of cancer. These phytoestrogens are chemically similar to the hormone estrogen and may protect against hormone-related cancers, such as breast, prostate, and endometrial cancers.[d,e] It has been hypothesized that the high intake of soy in traditional Asian

Products Made from Soybeans

Food	Amount	Energy (kcal)	Protein (g)	Fat (g)
Soy milk, regular	1 cup	150	4	8
Soy milk, fat-free	1 cup	89	4	0
Tofu, regular	1 oz	22	2.3	1.4
Tofu, lowfat	1 oz	10	1.7	0.3
Miso	1 Tbsp	35	2	1
Tempeh	1 Tbsp	21	2	1
Roasted soybeans	1/4 cup	203	15	11
Soybean sprouts	1 cup	85	9	4
Texturized soy protein	1 oz	42	9	0.4
Veggie dogs	1 serving	112	10	6
Soy veggie burger	3 oz	120	15	5
Tofutti frozen dessert, regular	1/2 cup	120	2	2
Tofutti frozen dessert, low-fat	1/2 cup	87	2	0.2
Soy flour, regular	1 Tbsp	23	2	1
Soy flour, fat-free	1 Tbsp	21	3	0

Protein in the Digestive Tract

The protein digested in the gastrointestinal tract comes from the diet and from protein contained in digestive secretions and sloughed gastrointestinal cells. No matter what the source, the protein must be broken down to amino acids before entering the bloodstream.

Digestion

Protein digestion begins in the stomach, where hydrochloric acid denatures proteins, opening up their folded structure to make them more accessible to enzyme attack. Stomach acid also activates the protein-digesting enzyme pepsin, which breaks proteins into polypeptides and amino acids. When the polypeptides enter the small intestine, they are broken into smaller peptides, tripeptides, dipeptides, and amino acids by a host of pancreatic protein-digesting enzymes such as trypsin, chymotrypsin, and carboxypeptidases. As in the stomach, these enzymes are released in inactive forms and activated in the small intestine. The small peptides are further broken down by intestinal peptidases in the brush border of the in-

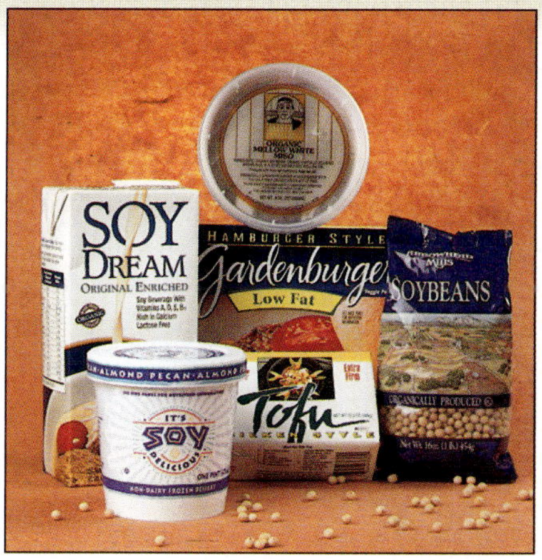

(George Semple)

diets is one reason that Asian women have a relatively low breast cancer incidence.[f] In cultured cells, soy protein preparations containing isoflavones prevent breast cancer cell growth. In animals, they reduce breast cancer initiation.

In addition to reducing the risks of heart disease and cancer, soy may reduce the risk of osteoporosis and alleviate some of the symptoms of menopause. Epidemiologic evidence suggests that populations who consume a large amount of soy have a lower incidence of osteoporosis.[g] Some soy products are a good source of calcium, but the effects on osteoporosis extend beyond this. When compared to women consuming a soy-free diet, women consuming a soy-containing diet show an increase in bone mineral density. A synthetic isoflavone, called ipriflavone, is currently used to treat women with osteoporosis.[h] Soy isoflavones may also be an alternative for hormone replacement therapy in postmenopausal women.

The health-promoting effects of soy are well documented—but how much do you need to eat to achieve these benefits? An analysis of the studies done on soy suggests that an intake of about 25 grams of soy protein per day is necessary to reduce cholesterol levels.[i] This is about half of a woman's daily protein requirement. How can you increase your intake of soy protein? Soy-based foods are available in many forms (see table). Soybeans can be eaten boiled or roasted. Soybean sprouts can be added to salads. Tofu, also known as bean curd, is a soft cheeselike product made by curdling fresh hot soy milk. It can be consumed cooked or raw. Miso and tempeh are fermented soybean products that are used in soups and mixed dishes. Soy flour can be incorporated into baked goods. Soy flour is also used to make texturized soy protein, which is a main ingredient in vegetarian burgers and hot dogs.

Although the evidence supporting the health-promoting effects of soy is strong, simply including soy-based foods, or any single food, in the diet is not the answer to good health. Replacing some of the animal sources of protein with soy protein may help, but other dietary and lifestyle factors also influence chronic disease risk.

References

[a] Anthony, M. S. Soy and cardiovascular disease: cholesterol lowering and beyond. J. Nutr. 130:662S–663S; 2000.

[b] Tikkanen, M. J., Wahala, K., Ojala, S., et al. Effect of soybean phytoestrogen intake on low-density lipoprotein oxidation resistance. Proc. Natl. Acad. Sci. USA 95:3106–3110; 1998.

[c] Nestel, P. J., Yamashita, T., Sasahara, T., et al. Soy isoflavones improve systemic arterial compliance but not plasma lipids in menopausal and perimenopausal women. Atheroscler. Thromb. Vasc. Biol. 17:3392–3398; 1997.

[d] Adlercreutz, H., Mazur, W., Bartels, P., et al. Phytoestrogens and prostate disease. J. Nutr. 130:658S–659S; 2000.

[e] Goodman, M. T., Wilkens, L. R., Hankin, J. H., et al. Association of soy and fiber consumption with the risk of endometrial cancer. Am. J. Epidemiol. 146:294–306; 1997.

[f] Stoll, B. A. Eating to beat breast cancer: potential role for soy supplements. Ann. Oncol. 8:223–225; 1997.

[g] Adlercreutz, H., and Mazur, W. Phytoestrogens and Western diseases. Ann. Med. 29:95–120; 1997.

[h] Potter, S. M., Baum, J. M., Teng, H., et al. Soy protein and isoflavones: their effects on blood lipids and bone density in postmenopausal women. Am. J. Clin. Nutr. 68(suppl):1375S–1379S; 1999.

[i] Anderson, J. W., Johnstone, B. M., and Cook-Newell, M. E. Meta-analysis of the effects of soy protein intake on serum lipids. N. Engl. J. Med. 333:276–282; 1995.

testinal mucosa. Single amino acids, dipeptides, and tripeptides can be transported into the mucosal cells of the small intestine. Once inside, enzymes in the cytosol complete the digestion of dipeptides and tripeptides into single amino acids.

Absorption

Amino acids and di- and tripeptides enter the mucosal cells of the small intestine using one of several transport systems. Amino acids with similar structures share the same transport system and therefore compete for absorption. For instance, the amino acids leucine, isoleucine, and valine, referred to as branched chain amino acids because their carbon side chains have a branching structure (see Appendix L), share the same transport system. If there is an excess of one of these, the transport of the other two will be slowed. The proportions of different amino acids in foods are generally not different enough to cause a problem with absorption of any one amino acid. However, taking an amino acid supplement can dramatically increase the amounts of one or a few amino acids in the intestine. The absorption of other amino acids that share the same transport system as the supplemented amino acids may be impaired. (Figure 6.10).

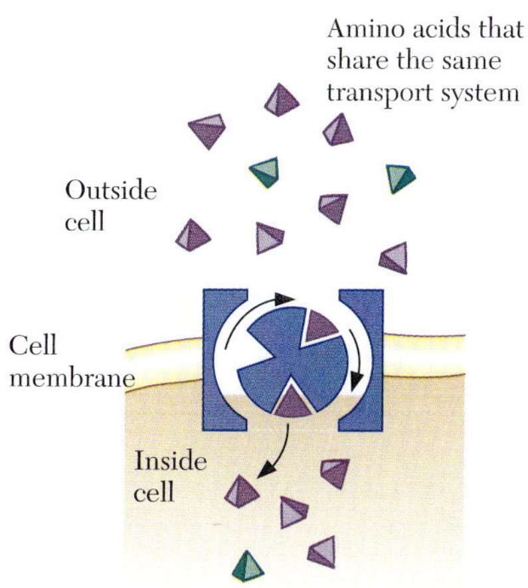

FIGURE 6.10 The amino acids (represented by pyramids) in this figure share the same transport system, and since there are more of the purple ones than the green ones, more of the purple amino acids are able to cross the membrane into the cell.

Food Allergies

For more information on peanut and other food allergies, go to Allergy, Asthma, and Immunology Online at allergy.mcg.edu/home.html, or to the Food Allergy and Anaphylaxis Network at www.foodallergy.org/.

If a protein from the diet is absorbed without being completely digested, the immune system may be activated, causing an allergic reaction (see Chapter 16). The absorbed protein is recognized as a foreign substance by the immune system, which mounts an attack resulting in the symptoms of a **food allergy.** Symptoms of food allergies can include reactions of the respiratory tract (sneezing and asthma), skin (rashes or hives), nervous system (headache and dizziness), cardiovascular system (rapid heart rate or change in blood pressure), urinary tract (blood in the urine), or digestive system (vomiting and diarrhea). Symptoms can be so mild that they are barely noticed or so severe that they are life threatening. For instance, a peanut allergy can be so severe that microscopic amounts of peanut protein that are eaten, touched, or even inhaled can cause a life-threatening reaction called anaphylaxis. Because of this, food products that contain peanuts—and even those that have a potential for cross-contamination from equipment or from foods made in the same facility—include peanuts in the ingredient list or provide a separate statement indicating that the food may contain peanuts.

Food allergy An adverse reaction involving the immune system that results from the exposure, generally through consumption, to a specific food.

Food allergies are most common in people with gastrointestinal disease, because their damaged intestine allows the absorption of whole proteins, and in infants, because their immature gastrointestinal tracts are more likely to allow larger polypeptides to be absorbed. Once an infant's intestinal mucosa matures, absorption of whole proteins is less likely and some food allergies disappear. The absorption of whole proteins by very young infants, however, can also be of benefit because antibody proteins present in breast milk can be absorbed and provide temporary protection against certain diseases (see Chapter15).

Protein in the Body

Once dietary proteins have been digested and absorbed, the amino acids travel to the liver via the hepatic portal vein. The liver plays an important role in determining how amino acids will be used by the rest of the body. The liver can release amino acids into the general circulation for use by other tissues, it can use amino acids to synthesize proteins or nonprotein molecules, or it can degrade amino acids for energy.

The proteins that make up our bodies serve a variety of functions. They provide structure to cells, tissues, and organs and are therefore essential for growth and repair. Proteins also regulate the body's ability to use other nutrients and aid in the transport of substances in the bloodstream and the movement of molecules into and out of cells.

Protein and Amino Acid Metabolism

Amino acid pool A term used to describe all of the amino acids in body tissues and fluids that are available to protein synthesis.

All of the available amino acids in the body are referred to collectively as the body **amino acid pool.** Of the approximately 300 g of protein synthesized by the body each day, only about 100 g is made from amino acids from the diet. The other 200 g is made from amino acids recycled from protein broken down in the body (Figure 6.11). When dietary intake of protein and energy are adequate but not excessive, most of the amino acids leaving the amino acid pool are used to synthesize body proteins and other nitrogen-containing compounds. Some amino acids are broken down and used for energy; the amount depends on the adequacy of the diet.

Protein turnover The continuous synthesis and breakdown of body proteins.

Protein Turnover Body proteins are not static but rather are continuously synthesized and broken down. This process is referred to as **protein turnover,** which is necessary for normal growth and maintenance of body tissues and for adaptation to changing situations. The rate at which proteins are made and de-

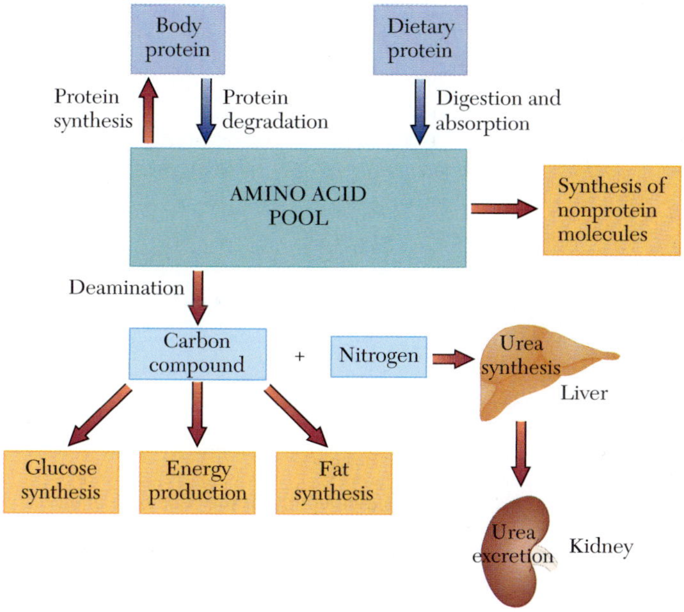

FIGURE 6.11 Amino acids enter the available amino acid pool from the diet and from the breakdown of body proteins. They are used to synthesize body proteins and nonprotein molecules. When the amino group is removed, they can be used to generate ATP or synthesize glucose or fat.

graded varies with the protein and is related to its function. Proteins whose concentration must be regulated and proteins that act as chemical signals in the body tend to have high rates of turnover—that is, synthesis and degradation. For example, the level of insulin in the blood can be increased by increasing its synthesis and decreasing the rate at which it is degraded. To decrease insulin levels, breakdown can be increased and synthesis slowed. Altering levels of synthesis and degradation allows protein levels to quickly change to maintain homeostasis as body conditions change. Structural proteins, such as collagen in connective tissue, have slower rates of synthesis and breakdown.

Protein Synthesis Which proteins are made and when they are synthesized are carefully regulated. When a protein is needed, the process of protein synthesis is begun. If all the amino acids in that protein are not available, the protein cannot be made. Just as on an assembly line, if one part is missing, the line stops—a different part cannot be substituted. If the missing amino acid is a nonessential amino acid, it can be synthesized in the body and protein synthesis can continue. If the missing amino acid is an essential amino acid, the body can break down its own proteins to obtain this amino acid. If an amino acid cannot be supplied, protein synthesis will stop. If all amino acids are present in adequate amounts at the time of synthesis, protein synthesis will proceed.

Transcription The structure of a protein is determined from a code or blueprint that is contained in DNA in the nucleus of each cell. A stretch of DNA that provides the blueprint for the structure of a polypeptide is called a **gene.** For a protein to be made, the information in the gene must first be transferred or transcribed into a molecule of RNA known as **messenger RNA (mRNA).** This process is called **transcription** (Figure 6.12). Messenger RNA takes this information from the nucleus to ribosomes in the cytoplasm of the cell where proteins are made. The mRNA attaches to the ribosome and specifies the sequence of amino acids that must bind together to form a particular polypeptide.

Translation The process of **translation** takes the information coded in mRNA and translates it into a sequence of amino acids. The mRNA message or code dictates which amino acids are used and in what order they will be bonded together. Another type of RNA, called **transfer RNA,** reads the code and delivers the needed amino acids. There is a different type of transfer RNA for each amino acid. Each transfer RNA binds to its amino acid and brings it to the ribosome.

Gene A section of DNA that codes for a polypeptide chain.

Messenger RNA (mRNA) A class of RNA molecules that carries the genetic message from DNA in the nucleus to ribosomes in the cytoplasm of the cell.

Transcription The process of copying the information in DNA to a molecule of mRNA.

Translation The process of translating the mRNA code into the amino acid sequence of a polypeptide chain.

Transfer RNA A class of RNA molecules that interprets the mRNA code by delivering specific amino acids to the ribosome and pairing with the mRNA code for those amino acids.

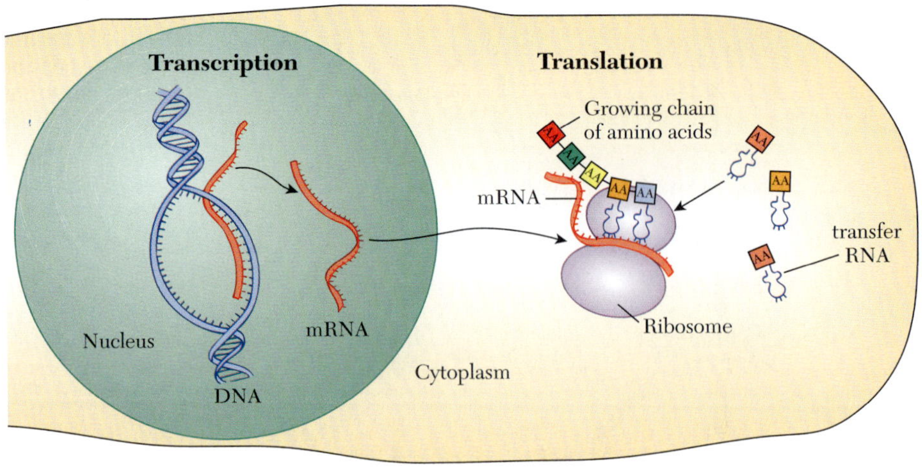

FIGURE 6.12 DNA in the nucleus of cells provides a blueprint for the sequence of amino acids in proteins. In the process of transcription the information in DNA is copied into a strand of mRNA. The mRNA leaves the nucleus and travels to the cytoplasm where it binds to a ribosome. Transfer RNA molecules in the cytoplasm collect amino acids and deliver them to the mRNA strand. The sequence in the mRNA dictates which transfer RNA, and its corresponding amino acid, will be added to the growing amino acid strand. As each amino acid is added, its transfer RNA is released to collect another amino acid. As the strand grows, the ribosome moves along the mRNA to read the next part of the code.

When the mRNA presents the code for that amino acid, it is set in place and enzymes add it to the growing polypeptide chain. When all the amino acids have been attached, the completed polypeptide chain is released for further processing by the cell. (See *Research Discoveries:* "Manipulating Genes.")

Gene expression The events of protein synthesis in which the information coded in a gene is used to synthesize a protein.

Gene Expression When the information in a gene is used to make a protein, the gene is being "expressed." Genes are not expressed in all cells or at all times. For example, the hormone insulin is a protein that is made in the beta cells of the pancreas. Insulin is not made by other body cells because the gene is not expressed in cells other than those in the pancreas. The expression of some genes changes depending on the need for the protein for which they code. For example, when iron intake is high, the expression of a gene that codes for the iron storage protein ferritin is turned on. This allows more of this protein to be synthesized so the capacity to store iron is increased.[7]

Nutrients can affect how and when genes are expressed. As discussed above, the amount of iron in the diet determines the amount of ferritin made. A rise in blood glucose causes an increase in the production of insulin. Vitamin A affects the expression of many genes involved in the maturation of cells, and vitamin D affects genes that code for calcium transport proteins (see Chapter 10). In this way, levels of nutrients can determine which proteins are made and can therefore regulate body functions. Who we are and how healthy we are depends not only on which genes we have but on which genes are expressed.

Synthesis of Nonprotein Molecules Some amino acids are also used to synthesize nonprotein molecules that contain nitrogen. For example, the amino acid tryptophan is used to synthesize the neurotransmitter serotonin, which acts in the relaxation center of the brain. Tyrosine is needed to synthesize the hormones epinephrine and norepinephrine. The nitrogen-containing units that make up DNA and RNA are derived partially from amino acids. Other molecules synthesized from amino acids include the skin pigment melanin; the vitamin niacin; creatine phosphate, which provides energy for muscle contraction; glutathione, needed to regulate oxidation reactions in the body; and histamine, which causes blood vessels to dilate.

RESEARCH DISCOVERIES

Manipulating Genes

Genetic engineering is the process of manipulating the genetic make-up of plants, animals, and microorganisms. By modifying DNA, scientists can change the proteins that a cell or organism can make. This technology, developed over the last 30 years, has allowed researchers to create bacteria that make medicines for humans, plants that are disease resistant, and foods that provide a healthier mix of nutrients.

To alter the genetic composition of a cell, a specific piece of DNA, or gene, from one type of cell must be clipped out and pasted into the DNA in another cell. The new DNA, called recombinant DNA, can then provide the blueprint for new proteins. For example, if scientists take a piece of human DNA containing the gene for the hormone insulin and paste it into the DNA of a bacterium, the bacterium can then make human insulin. Diabetics today are often treated with insulin that is produced by genetically engineered bacteria. Before 1970, however, none of this was possible because there was no way to cut DNA. The ability to cut DNA emerged from basic laboratory research that studied bacteria. In the 1950s it was recognized that some strains of bacteria were able to slice viral DNA into pieces.[a] This ability was found to be due to bacterial enzymes, called restriction enzymes, which cut DNA in specific places. By the late 1960s and early 1970s, restriction enzymes were being isolated and characterized.[b,c] At the same time, bacterial enzymes that repair breaks in DNA, called DNA ligases, were also being studied. DNA ligases had the ability to paste together two strands of DNA. At the time of their discovery restriction enzymes and DNA ligases were recognized as interesting in the field of microbiology but it was impossible to predict the impact they would have on the fields of biology and medicine. These seemingly obscure bacterial enzymes changed the course of technology and will impact many fields of science for years to come.

Restriction enzymes are present in bacteria as a form of protection. If a virus invades the bacterium it can defend itself by cutting the viral DNA into little pieces before the virus can cause harm. In the laboratory these enzymes act like precision scissors that can clip out a gene that produces a specific protein. Because DNA in all forms of life is made of the same building blocks, an enzyme from a bacterium can cut the DNA from a cow, a soybean plant, and a human cell with equal efficiency. When DNA from one cell is combined with that of another, the resulting cells can produce new proteins and provide new functions to the host. For example, a corn plant could be given a gene that makes a protein that is toxic to the corn borer, an insect that attacks corn plants. The corn plant would then be resistant to that insect pest.

The discovery of restriction enzymes and DNA ligase provided the raw materials for the techniques of molecular biology. Today scientists don't need to isolate these enzymes themselves but can purchase them from scientific suppliers. Scientists have the techniques to locate, isolate, prepare, and study small segments of DNA. Obscure experiments done 30 years ago with oddball enzymes have created an endless supply of human insulin for diabetics and clotting factors for hemophiliacs. They have led to new, more powerful cancer therapies and vaccines to prevent disease. Genetic engineering is also changing the foods we eat. It has created crops with greater yields and enhanced disease resistance, and tomatoes that ripen faster and squash less easily. However, despite the potential and realized benefits, this technology has raised new questions and concerns, both ethical and scientific. A reflection of this concern is the moratorium on importing genetically modified foods that was put in place by the European Union in 1999 (see Chapter 19).

References

[a] Old, R. W., and Primrose, S. B. *Principles of Gene Manipulation: An Introduction to Genetic Engineering*, 5th ed. London: Blackwell Science, Ltd., 1994.

[b] Meselson, M., and Yuan, R. DNA restriction enzyme from *E. coli*. Nature 217:1110–1114, 1968.

[c] Smith, H. O., and Wilcox, K. W. A restriction enzyme from *Hemophilus influenzae*. I. Purification and general properties. J. Mol. Biol. 51:379–391, 1970.

Energy Production Amino acids from dietary and body proteins can be used to produce energy. Although amino acids are continually used as an energy source, the amount increases both when the diet does not provide enough total energy to meet needs, as in starvation, and when protein is consumed in excess of needs.

During starvation, body protein provides the second largest store of energy after adipose tissue. Carbohydrate stored as glycogen is sufficient only in the short term and cannot meet energy needs for more than a few hours. After glycogen stores are gone, amino acids from protein breakdown are used to make glucose via gluconeogenesis. Unlike fat and carbohydrate, the protein that is broken down is not from a body store, but from functional body proteins. The most dispensable proteins are broken down first, conserving others for the numerous critical roles they play, but if the energy deficit continues, more critical proteins, such as those that make up the heart and other internal organs, will also be degraded. A loss of more than 30% of the body's protein reduces the strength of the muscles required for breathing and heart function, depresses immune function, and causes a general loss of organ function that is great enough to cause death.[8]

Amino acids are also used for energy when protein intake exceeds protein needs. If the diet is adequate in energy and high in protein, extra amino acids are not needed to make body proteins, so they are degraded and used to produce ATP—providing about 4 kcalories per g. If both energy and protein intake exceed needs, the extra amino acids are not stored as protein; rather, they are converted into either glucose or fatty acids, depending on their structure, and can contribute to weight gain.

Deamination The removal of the amino group from an amino acid.

Deamination Before amino acids can be used for energy, the nitrogen-containing amino group must be removed in a process called **deamination.** The remaining carbon structure can then be used to produce energy or be converted to glucose or fat. The amino group produces ammonia, which is toxic and must be excreted or converted to a less toxic molecule.

The Carbon Side Chain The carbon compounds remaining after nitrogen is removed from the amino acids can be used in a number of ways, depending on the needs of the body. Amino acids that break down to form three-carbon compounds can be used to make glucose via gluconeogenesis. Amino acids can also be converted into acetyl-CoA and, if energy is plentiful, can be used to synthesize fat for storage. If energy is needed, the carbon structure of the amino acids can be further broken down by the citric acid cycle and electron transport chain to produce ATP (Figure 6.13).

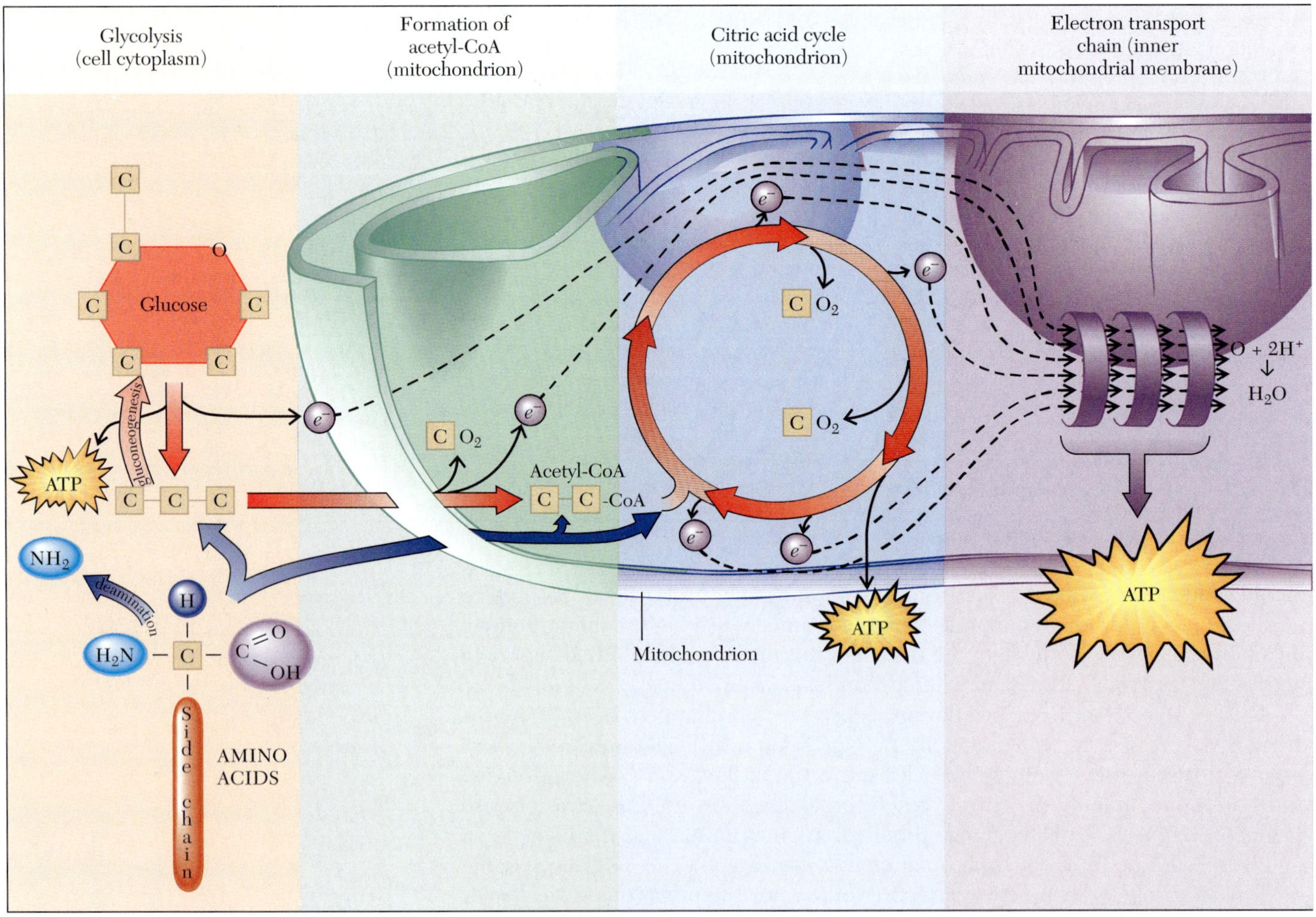

FIGURE 6.13 How the carbon structure of an amino acid that remains after deamination is metabolized varies depending on the structure of the original amino acid. Some can form three-carbon molecules and be used for gluconeogenesis. Some form molecules that are intermediates in the citric acid cycle. Some form acetyl-CoA and can be used to synthesize fatty acids. All can be broken down completely to generate ATP.

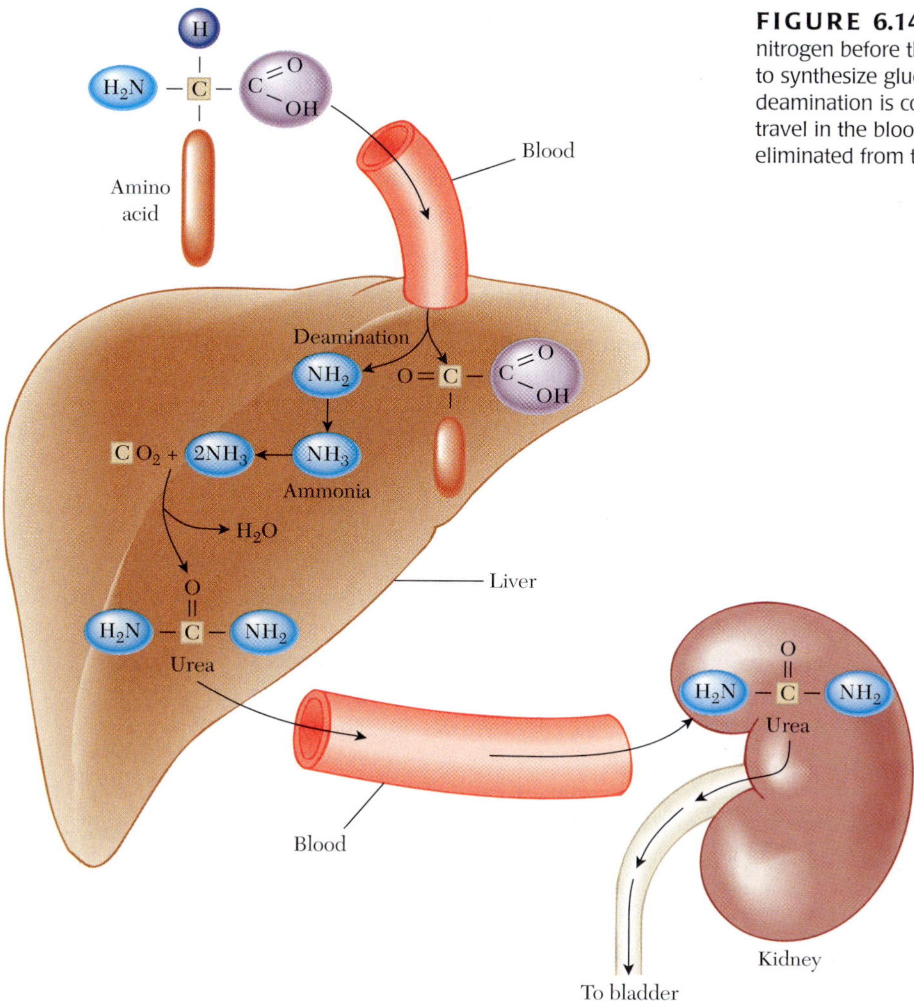

FIGURE 6.14 Amino acids must be deaminated to remove the nitrogen before they can be metabolized to produce energy or used to synthesize glucose or fat. The toxic ammonia produced by deamination is converted into urea by the liver. Urea can safely travel in the blood and is filtered out of the blood by the kidney and eliminated from the body in the urine.

Urea Formation To protect cells from ammonia, the liver combines it with carbon dioxide to produce the less toxic waste product **urea.** Urea is released into the blood and then travels to the kidney and is excreted in the urine (Figure 6.14). If the liver is damaged, the levels of ammonia in the blood may increase. If the kidney is unable to excrete waste products from the blood, the level of urea will increase. A high-protein diet increases the work of the liver because more ammonia must be converted into urea; it increases the work of the kidney because more urea must be eliminated in the urine. A high-protein diet also increases the amount of water lost from the body because more water is lost in the urine when extra urea is excreted.

Urea A nitrogen-containing waste product that is excreted in the urine.

Functions of Body Proteins

About 15% of our body weight is protein. Adequate protein must be consumed in the diet to supply amino acids in order to replace protein losses that occur during protein turnover, to repair damaged tissues, and to synthesize new body proteins for growth. Each protein molecule that is synthesized by the body has a specific function; some provide structure and others help regulate body processes.

Structural Proteins Proteins provide structure to individual cells and to the body as a whole. In cells, proteins are an integral part of the cell membrane, the cytoplasm, and the organelles. Skin, hair, and muscle are composed largely of protein. Bones and teeth are made up of minerals embedded in a protein framework.

When the diet is deficient in protein, these structures break down. The muscles become smaller, the skin loses its elasticity, and the hair becomes thin and can easily be pulled out by the roots. These outward signs of dietary protein deficiency have become the subject of marketing strategies for cosmetic companies. Shampoo and hand lotion manufacturers add protein to their products, suggesting that protein applied to the hair or skin will improve its structure. However, the proteins that make up hair and skin can only be made inside the body, so a healthy diet will do more for hair and skin quality than expensive protein shampoos or lotions.

Regulatory Proteins Proteins help regulate the body's many integrated processes to maintain homeostasis. Regulatory proteins include enzymes, transport proteins in the blood and in cells, immune system proteins, contractile or motile proteins, protein hormones, and proteins that aid in fluid, mineral, and acid–base balance.

Enzymes Enzymes are protein molecules that speed up metabolic reactions but are not used up or destroyed in these reactions. All the reactions involved in the production of energy and the synthesis and breakdown of carbohydrates, lipids, proteins, and other molecules are expedited by enzymes. Each reaction requires a specific enzyme protein with a specific structure. If the structure of the enzyme molecule is abnormal, it cannot function in the reaction it is intended to accelerate.

Enzymes that function in the body are synthesized by cells in the body, and therefore do not need to be consumed in the diet. In cooked foods, enzymes are denatured by the cooking process and are no longer functional when eaten. When raw foods are eaten, the enzymes present—such as papain in papaya—are broken down during digestion and are absorbed from the gastrointestinal tract as amino acids. Purified enzymes sold as dietary supplements are also broken down in the gut. If these are digestive enzymes they may provide some function in the gut before they are digested. For example, lactase, taken by individuals with lactose intolerance, breaks down lactose that is consumed while the lactase is in the gut. Pancreatic enzymes are available for individuals who do not produce sufficient amounts to digest nutrients. Eventually, these enzymes are digested and absorbed as amino acids. If enzymes that function inside the body in cells, in the blood, or in other body fluids are consumed in the diet they will not reach these locations as enzymes, but rather as the component amino acids. Oral supplements of these types of enzymes therefore do not provide enzyme function in the body.

Transport Proteins Proteins transport substances throughout the body and into and out of individual cells. Transport proteins in the blood carry substances from one organ to another. For example, hemoglobin, the protein in red blood cells, picks up oxygen in the lungs and transports it to other organs of the body. The proteins in lipoproteins are needed to transport lipids from the intestines and liver to body cells. Some vitamins, such as vitamin A, must be bound to a specific protein to be transported in the blood. When protein is deficient, the nutrients that require proteins for transport cannot travel to the cells. For this reason, a protein deficiency can cause a vitamin A deficiency even if vitamin A is consumed in the diet, because the vitamin A cannot be transported to the cells.

At the cellular level, transport proteins present in cell membranes help move substances such as glucose and amino acids across the cell membrane. For example, transport proteins in the intestinal mucosa are necessary to allow the body to absorb amino acids from the intestinal lumen into the mucosal cells. Cellular transport or binding proteins in the cytoplasm can help direct substances toward specific enzymes or functions in the cell. For example, in the nucleus, vitamin A must be bound to a protein before it can regulate gene expression (see Chapter 10).

Immune System Proteins Proteins play an important role in protecting the body from injury and invasion by foreign substances. Skin, which is made up primarily of protein, is the first barrier against infection and injury. Foreign particles, such as dirt or bacteria, that are on the skin cannot enter the body and can be washed away. If the skin is broken and blood vessels are injured, fibrinogen, thrombin, and other blood-clotting proteins help prevent too much blood from being lost. If a foreign particle such as a virus or bacterium enters the body, the immune system fights it by synthesizing proteins called **antibodies.** Each antibody has a unique structure that allows it to attach to a specific invader. When an antibody binds to an invading substance, the production of more antibodies is stimulated, and other parts of the immune system are signaled to help destroy the invader. The next time the same type of invading bacterium or virus enters the body, the immune system is already primed to produce specific antibodies to help destroy the invader. When you are immunized against diseases such as measles, mumps, and chicken pox, a small amount of dead or inactivated virus is injected into the body. The injected material does not cause disease, but it does stimulate the immune system to produce antibodies to the virus. The next time the body comes in contact with the same virus, a large-scale immune attack is mounted and the infection is prevented (Figure 6.15). When the immune system malfunctions as a result of protein deficiency or other causes, such as HIV infection, the ability to protect the body from infection is compromised.

Antibodies Proteins produced by cells of the immune system that destroy or inactivate foreign substances in the body.

Contractile or Motile Proteins Some proteins give cells and organisms the ability to move, contract, and change shape. Actin and myosin function in the contraction of muscle cells. These two proteins slide past each other to shorten the muscle and cause contraction. For example, when you do a pull-up or a biceps curl, the muscles in your arms shorten as the alternating actin and myosin proteins slide past one another (Figure 6.16). A similar process causes contraction in the heart muscle to pump blood throughout the body, and in the muscles that cause constriction in the digestive tract, blood vessels, and body glands. Actin and myosin can also cause contraction in nonmuscle cells. This contraction may help individual cells, such as white blood cells, change shape and move. The energy for contraction comes from ATP, which is derived primarily from the metabolism of carbohydrate and fat.

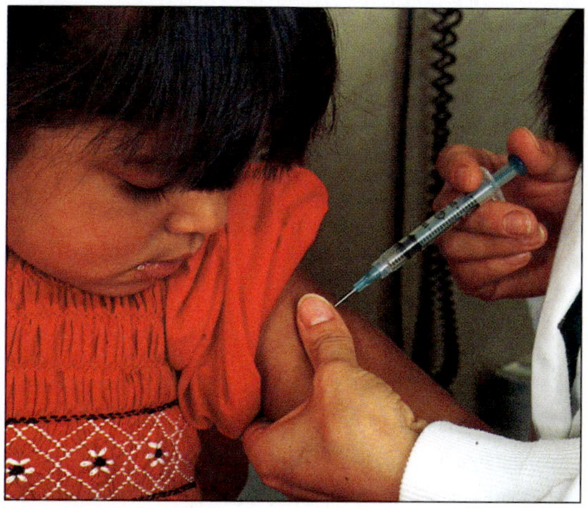

FIGURE 6.15 Immunizations stimulate the production of immune system proteins called antibodies. Antibodies bind to disease-causing organisms and participate in their inactivation. *(© Matt Meadows/Peter Arnold, Inc.)*

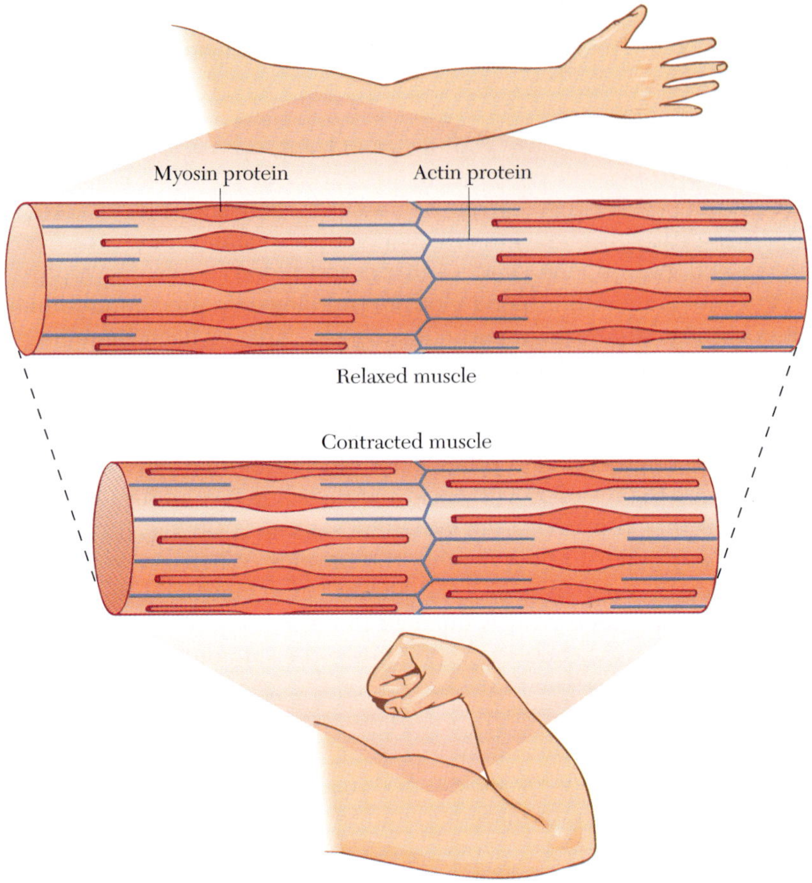

FIGURE 6.16 During muscle contraction the proteins actin and myosin slide past each other, causing the muscle fiber to shorten.

Protein Hormones Hormones are chemical messengers that are secreted into the blood by one tissue or organ, acting on target cells in other parts of the body. Some hormones are made of lipid; others are made of amino acids and are classified as peptide, or protein, hormones. For instance, insulin and glucagon are protein hormones. Some diabetics are treated by injections of the hormone insulin. Other hormones derived from protein or amino acids include thyroid hormones, which regulate metabolic rate; calcitonin and parathyroid hormone, which help regulate blood calcium levels; and oxytocin, which causes milk let-down during lactation.

Proteins in Fluid and Mineral Balance The distribution of fluid between the intracellular and extracellular spaces is important for health. Fluid moves back and forth across membranes to maintain appropriate concentrations of minerals and fluids inside and outside cells and tissues (see Chapter 11). Proteins help regulate this fluid balance in two ways. First, protein pumps located in cell membranes transport minerals from one side of a membrane to another. This not only helps keep fluids in the right places but maintains the correct proportions of minerals, such as sodium and potassium, needed for nerve conduction and muscle contraction. Second, large protein molecules present in the blood keep fluid in the blood both by preventing it from being forced into tissues and by drawing tissue fluids back into blood vessels. In cases of protein malnutrition, the concentration of these large proteins in the blood decreases and fluid is no longer held in the blood; it therefore accumulates in the tissues—a condition called **edema.**

Edema An abnormal accumulation of fluids in the spaces between cells or in body cavities.

pH A measure of acidity.

Proteins in Acid–Base Balance The chemical reactions of metabolism require a specific level of acidity, or **pH,** to function properly. An acid solution, which has a low pH, is one that has a high concentration of hydrogen ions (H^+). In the gastrointestinal tract, pH varies widely. The stomach contents are acidic; the small intestine is more neutral (Table 6.2). The digestive enzyme pepsin, which is secreted in gastric juices, works best in the acid environment of the stomach, whereas the pancreatic enzymes operate best in the neutral environment of the small intestine. Inside the body, metabolic reactions continuously produce both acids and bases. These must be neutralized in order to prevent changes in pH, which in turn can prevent metabolic reactions from proceeding normally. The lungs and kidneys help maintain a normal pH by eliminating some of these waste products. Proteins both in the blood and within the cells help prevent or buffer changes in pH by attracting or releasing hydrogen ions. For instance, the protein hemoglobin in red blood cells helps neutralize acid produced when carbon dioxide, a waste product of cellular respiration, reacts with water. Untreated diabetes is an example of what happens when the amount of acid produced exceeds the ability of the body proteins and other systems to neutralize it (see Chapter 4). When the production of ketones exceeds the ability of the body to excrete them, they accumulate, causing a drop in pH. The acid pH damages proteins and they are unable to perform their functions, resulting in coma and eventually death.

TABLE 6.2
Normal pH Values for Various Body Fluids[a]

Fluid	pH
Gastric juice	1.0–3.0
Pancreatic juice	8.0
Blood	7.35–7.45
Urine	4.8–8.4
Tears	7.35–7.45
Saliva	6.5–7.5
Human milk	6.3–7.5

[a]pH values range from 1 to 14, 1 being most acidic and 14 being most basic. Most chemical reactions in the body take place near pH 7.

PROTEIN AND HEALTH

A diet adequate in protein is essential to health. Dietary protein is needed to replace protein that is broken down and lost each day as a result of normal protein turnover. It is also needed for growth and healing. If too little protein is consumed, the consequences can be dramatic and devastating. Too much protein, particularly if it is derived primarily from animal sources, may also have negative health effects.

Protein-Energy Malnutrition

Protein-energy malnutrition (PEM) occurs when the body's need for protein, energy, or both is not met with diet. Because of the availability and variety of foods in developed countries, protein deficiency there is uncommon. However, in developing nations, concerns about inadequate protein are very real. Diets deficient in protein are most often deficient in energy as well, but protein deficiency can predominate when food choices are extremely limited and the staple food of a population is very low in protein. Protein-energy malnutrition is a continuum of conditions ranging from predominantly protein deficiency, called **kwashiorkor,** to overall energy deficiency, called **marasmus.**

Web Menu: For more information about protein-energy malnutrition and other world nutrition health issues, go to the World Health Organization Web page at www.who.int.

C 62 00 00 00 00 00 27 38

Kwashiorkor Kwashiorkor is typically a disease of children. The word "kwashiorkor" comes from the Ga tribe of the African Gold Coast (now Ghana). It means the disease that the first child gets when a second child is born.[9] When the new baby is born, the older child is no longer breast-fed. Rather than receiving protein-rich breast milk, the young child is fed a watered-down version of the diet eaten by the rest of the family. This diet is low in protein and is often high in fiber and difficult to digest. The child, even if able to get adequate energy, is not able to eat a large enough quantity to get adequate protein. Because children are growing, their protein needs per unit of body weight are higher than those of adults, and the effects of a deficiency become evident much more quickly.

The symptoms of kwashiorkor can be explained by examining the roles that proteins play in the body. People with kwashiorkor do not appear excessively thin because they are consuming enough energy to maintain some body fat. Their abdomens are swollen as a result of both fat accumulating in the liver because there is not enough protein to transport it and fluid accumulating in the abdomen because there is not enough protein to keep fluid in the blood (Figure 6.17a). Those

Protein-energy malnutrition (PEM) A condition characterized by wasting and an increased susceptibility to infection that results from the long-term consumption of insufficient energy and protein to meet needs.

Kwashiorkor A form of protein-energy malnutrition in which only protein is deficient. It is most common in young children who are unable to meet their high protein needs with the available diet.

Marasmus A form of protein-energy malnutrition in which a deficiency of energy in the diet causes severe body wasting.

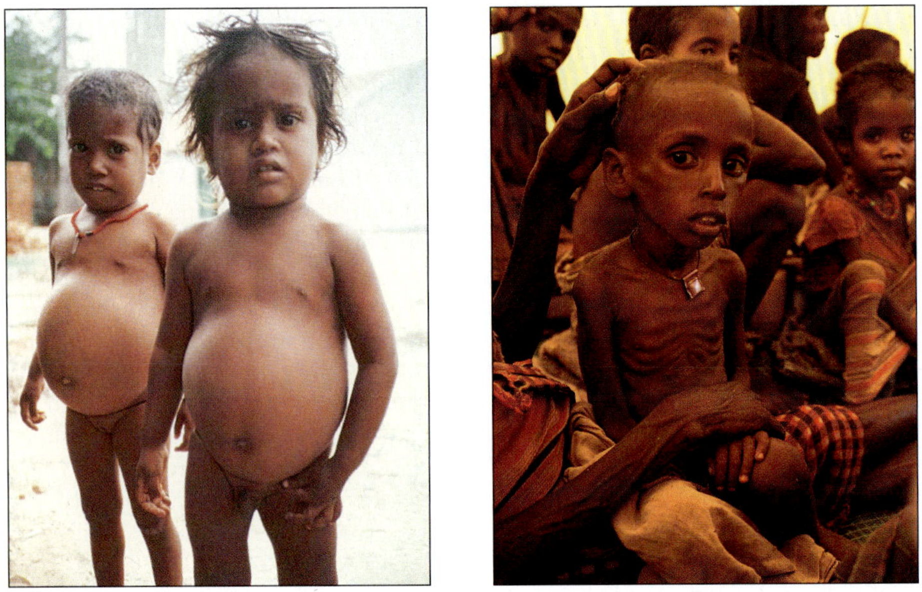

(a) (b)

FIGURE 6.17 Kwashiorkor (a) is characterized by a bloated belly, whereas marasmus (b) presents as severe wasting. Most protein-energy malnutrition is a combination of the two. *(a, Food and Agriculture Organization of the United Nations; b, Scott Dani Peterson/Gamma Liaison, Inc.)*

afflicted have a puffy appearance because fluid also accumulates in the tissues. Their hair is brittle, can be pulled out easily, and is of abnormal color because the pigment melanin is not made. Their skin flakes because structural proteins are not available to provide elasticity and support. There is an increased susceptibility to infection because immune system proteins are in short supply. Growth in height and weight is hampered because protein is needed for the synthesis of new tissue, and nutrient absorption is impaired because cells lining the digestive tract die and cannot be replaced.

Kwashiorkor occurs most commonly in Africa, South and Central America, the Near East, and the Far East. It has also been reported in poverty-stricken areas in the United States. Although more common in children, it is also seen in hospitalized adults who have high-protein needs due to infection or trauma and a low-protein intake because they are unable to eat.

Marasmus At the other end of the continuum of protein-energy malnutrition is marasmus, meaning to waste away. Marasmus is due to a deficiency of energy, but protein and other nutrients are usually also insufficient to meet needs. Marasmus may have some of the same symptoms as kwashiorkor, but there are also differences. In kwashiorkor, some fat stores are retained, because energy intake is adequate. Marasmic individuals appear emaciated because their body-fat stores have been used to provide energy (Figure 6.17b). Muscles waste away as proteins are broken down to provide amino acids for gluconeogenesis. Adaptations in metabolism occur to preserve body protein, but if energy continues to be inadequate, body protein continues to be lost to supply the body with glucose. Because fat is a major energy source and carbohydrate is limited, ketosis may occur in marasmus. This is not so in kwashiorkor because carbohydrate intake is adequate—only protein is deficient.

Marasmus occurs in individuals of all ages and is the form of malnutrition that occurs with eating disorders (see Chapter 8). It has devastating effects in infants and children because adequate energy is essential for growth. Because most brain growth takes place in the first year of life, malnutrition early in life impairs intelligence and learning ability. The effects persist throughout life. Marasmus often occurs in infants who are fed diluted formula prepared by caregivers trying to stretch limited supplies. Marasmus is less common in breast-fed infants.

Protein Excess: Can Too Much Be Harmful?

Adequate protein intake is absolutely essential to life. But is there such a thing as too much protein? Some research suggests that a high-protein diet has negative effects, while other studies find no ill effects. Still others suggest that the problem with high-protein diets is that in most cases they are also high in fat and low in fruits and vegetables. Despite these concerns about protein excess, protein and amino acid supplements remain popular among some segments of the population.

A Diet High in Protein The consumption of too much protein increases both the production of protein breakdown products and the need to eliminate them from the body. When protein is degraded, the amino groups from its amino acids form ammonia, which is converted into urea. The kidneys must then excrete the urea. To excrete more waste products requires more water. So unless sufficient fluid is consumed when protein intake is high, dehydration can result. Although not a problem for most people, this can be a problem if the kidneys are not able to concentrate urine, as is the case with the immature kidneys of newborns. Feeding a newborn infant formula that is mixed improperly can provide excess protein, which can increase fluid losses and lead to dehydration.

Another concern with high-protein diets is that they may be related to kidney and bone health. The long-term consumption of a high-protein diet may speed the progression of renal failure in individuals with kidney disease.[10] However, there is only weak evidence that a high-protein diet is associated with kidney disease within the healthy population.[11] Protein intake may also affect calcium balance and bone health. Protein is an important structural component of bone, but increasing protein intake increases calcium losses in the urine. Some studies have found that a diet high in animal protein may increase the risk of bone fractures (see Chapter 12).[12] Other studies have not found this to be true and diets higher in animal protein were found to reduce the risk of hip fractures in postmenopausal women.[13] High levels of protein are believed to negatively affect bone mass only if calcium intake is inadequate.[14]

The only concern about high-protein diets that is not disputed is that they are usually high in foods of animal origin. Diets high in animal products are generally low in grains, vegetables, and fruits. Low intakes of these plant foods are associated with a greater risk of cancer.[15,16] Diets high in animal protein are also typically high in saturated fat and cholesterol and therefore increase the risk of heart disease (see Chapter 5). Such diets are also usually high in energy and total fat, which may promote obesity (see Chapters 7 and 8).

The body is very efficient at disposing of excess nitrogen; therefore, it is believed that protein intakes moderately above recommendations are safe. The National Research Council recommends that protein intake not exceed twice the 1989 RDA.[17]

Protein Supplements Although protein is needed for proper immune function, healthy hair, and muscle growth, a supplement will affect these only if the diet is deficient in protein in the first place. Increasing protein intake above the requirement does not protect you from disease, make your hair shine, or stimulate muscle growth. Muscle growth occurs in response to exercise in the presence of adequate protein. Although protein supplements are not harmful for most people, they are an expensive and unnecessary way to increase protein intake. A typical protein drink provides 10 to 20 g of protein per serving, or 20 to 40% of the Daily Value. It can add about 100 to 200 kcalories to the diet, and thus can contribute to weight gain. If consumed consistently, a high intake of protein from supplements or from foods may also contribute to dehydration.

Amino Acid Supplements Amino acid supplements are also an unnecessary and expensive addition to a healthy diet. Many of these are marketed for specific reasons; for example, ornithine, arginine, and lysine are offered to increase lean body mass. Because amino acids share transport systems, a supplement of one may impair the absorption of others that share the same transport system (see Figure 6.10). For example, if a weight lifter takes large amounts of supplemental arginine in the hopes that it will enhance muscle mass, the absorption of lysine will be reduced because lysine and arginine share the same transport system.

Because amino acids are dietary supplements and not drugs, they are often not carefully tested for safety and purity. In 1989 supplements of L-tryptophan were found to contain a contaminant that was associated with an outbreak of a rare blood disorder. L-Tryptophan supplements can no longer be sold, but a metabolite of the amino acid tryptophan (5-hydroxy-L-tryptophan) is being promoted for the treatment of insomnia. In 1998 similar impurities were also found in 5-hydroxy-L-tryptophan.

PROTEIN REQUIREMENTS

How much protein the body needs depends on the individual's genetic makeup, age, body size, and whether they are pregnant, growing, injured, or healing. The amount of dietary protein required to meet these needs depends on the digestibility and amino acid composition of the diet consumed.

Determining Protein Requirements

Protein requirements are estimated using balance studies. Because protein is the only nutrient that contains nitrogen, the amount of protein used by the body can be determined by comparing nitrogen intake with nitrogen loss. Nitrogen intake is calculated from dietary protein intake. Nitrogen loss or output is measured by totaling the amounts of nitrogen excreted in urine and feces and that lost from skin, sweat, hair, and nails. The majority of the nitrogen lost is excreted in the urine as urea and other nitrogen-containing waste products. Comparing the amount of nitrogen consumed with the amount lost provides information about the amount of protein being synthesized and broken down within the body. An individual who is consuming enough protein to meet body needs is in **protein** or **nitrogen balance.** This means the amount of nitrogen or protein the individual consumes in the diet is enough to replace the amount that is lost from the body. If more nitrogen is lost than ingested, a negative nitrogen balance is said to exist. This indicates that more body protein is being broken down than is being consumed. This can occur when intake is too low or when the amount of protein broken down has been increased by a stress such as injury, illness, or surgery. Positive nitrogen balance occurs when less nitrogen is lost than is ingested, indicating that the body is using dietary protein for synthesis of new body proteins. This occurs when new tissue is synthesized, such as during growth, pregnancy, wound healing, or muscle building (Figure 6.18). (See *Critical Thinking:* "What Does Nitrogen Balance Tell Us?")

Protein or **nitrogen balance** A state in which the amount of protein nitrogen consumed in the diet is equal to the nitrogen excreted by the body, indicating that the amount of body protein is constant and there is no net protein synthesis or degradation.

The protein requirement of a specific individual can be determined by doing a balance study for that individual. Because this procedure cannot be done for everyone, the protein needs of populations must be estimated from balance study data. Recommendations for protein intake for the general public are actually higher than the requirements determined by balance studies for individuals. This is to allow a margin of safety that will ensure the needs of the majority of the population are met.

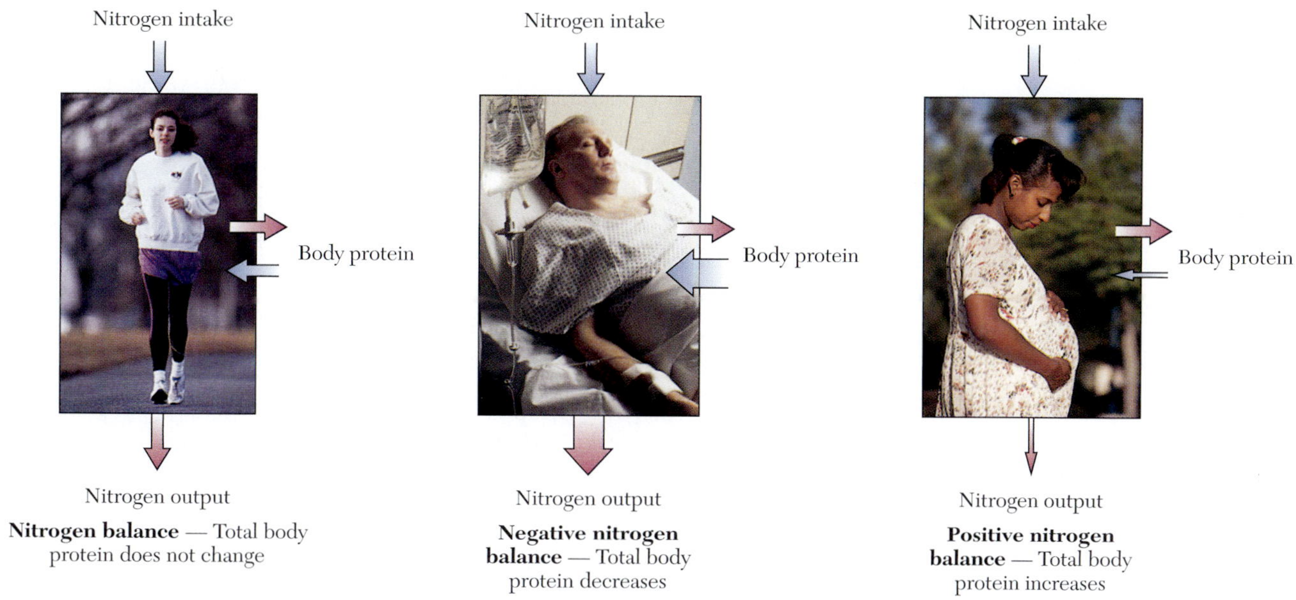

FIGURE 6.18 In nitrogen balance, nitrogen intake is equal to the nitrogen output; in negative balance, output exceeds intake because more body proteins are broken down than synthesized and the nitrogen is excreted; in positive balance, intake exceeds output because more protein is used to synthesize body proteins than is lost from protein breakdown. *(Photos: left, Dennis Drenner; center, © Brian Yarvin/Photo Researchers, Inc.; right, © Myrleen Cate/Tony Stone Images, Inc.)*

Critical Thinking

What Does Nitrogen Balance Tell Us?

The Groslin Company wants to include nitrogen balance studies in the assays it performs in its clinical laboratory. To test their methodology, they analyze nitrogen balance in three individuals. The technicians are given information about the daily nitrogen intake of these people and analyze samples of urine and feces to determine daily nitrogen losses.

Nitrogen Balance = Nitrogen In − Nitrogen Out

Subject A consumed 6.4 grams of nitrogen. The laboratory determines that she lost 8.0 grams of nitrogen in her urine and feces. The nitrogen balance equation for subject A is

$$6.4\text{ g} - 8.0\text{ g} = -1.6\text{ g}$$

This result of a balance of −1.6 grams per day suggests that the individual is breaking down body protein to meet her needs.

Does this make sense metabolically?

Subject A is a 35-year-old woman who weighs 120 kg but is on a weight-loss diet. She is consuming only 500 kcalories and 30 grams of protein per day. To meet energy needs, her body is breaking down body protein, resulting in an increased excretion of nitrogen in the urine. A negative nitrogen balance would be expected for someone consuming such a low-energy, low-protein diet.

Subject B is a healthy 29-year-old male who weighs 82 kg and consumes an adequate diet of 2700 kcalories and 70 g of protein a day. His nitrogen values are:

	Nitrogen In	Nitrogen Out
Subject A	11.2 g	11.2 g

What is his nitrogen balance?

Answer:

Does his nitrogen balance make sense metabolically?

Yes. He is in nitrogen balance. This means his protein intake meets his needs, and he is neither retaining protein for growth or repair of tissues nor breaking down body protein for energy.

Subject C is a 31-year-old pregnant woman of average prepregnancy weight who is consuming 2500 kcalories and 80 g of protein a day. Her nitrogen values are:

	Nitrogen In	Nitrogen Out
Subject C	12.8 g	10.4 g

What is her nitrogen balance?

Answer:

Does her nitrogen balance make sense metabolically?

Answer:

Recommendations for Protein Intake

The 1989 RDA for dietary protein is 0.8 g of protein per kilogram of body weight for adults. This value is calculated assuming that the diet contains both plant and animal sources of protein and is therefore of mixed quality. It is set to meet the needs of the majority of healthy people in the population. For a person weighing 70 kg (154 lb), the recommended intake would be 56 g of protein per day. Protein needs vary with life stage (Table 6.3). Growth during childhood, adolescence, and

TABLE 6.3 Calculating Protein Needs

To determine protein requirement:

- Determine body weight. If weight is measured in pounds, convert it to kilograms by dividing by 2.2:

$$\frac{\text{weight in pounds}}{2.2\ \text{pounds/kg}} = \text{weight in kg}$$

For example:

$$\frac{150\ \text{pounds}}{2.2\ \text{pounds/kg}} = 68\ \text{kg}$$

- Determine the grams of protein required per day. Multiply weight in kg by the grams of protein per kilogram recommended for the specific gender and life-stage group.
- For example, a 23-year-old female weighing 68 kg would require 0.8 g/kg × 68 kg = 54.4 grams of protein.

Gender or Condition	***Age (yrs)***	***1989 RDA (g/kg)***
Both sexes	0–0.5	2.2
	0.5–1	1.6
	1–3	1.2
	4–6	1.1
	7–10	1.0
Males	11–14	1.0
	15–18	0.9
	19 and older	0.8
Females	11–14	1.0
	15 and older	0.8
Pregnancy		Nonpregnant RDA + 10 g/day
Lactation	First 6 months	Nonlactating RDA + 15 g/day
	Second 6 months	Nonlactating RDA + 12 g/day

pregnancy increase protein requirements. Lactation increases the body's protein demand because the milk that is secreted is high in protein. Illness, injury, and recovery as well as the demands of some types of strenuous exercise can also increase protein needs.

Growth During the first year of life, a large amount of protein is required to support the rapid growth rate. Thus, the 1989 RDA for the first six months of life is 2.2 g per kilogram of body weight. For the second six months, 1.6 g per kilogram is recommended. As the growth rate slows, requirements per unit of body weight decrease but continue to be greater than adult requirements until about 18 years of age (see Table 6.3 and Figure 6.19).

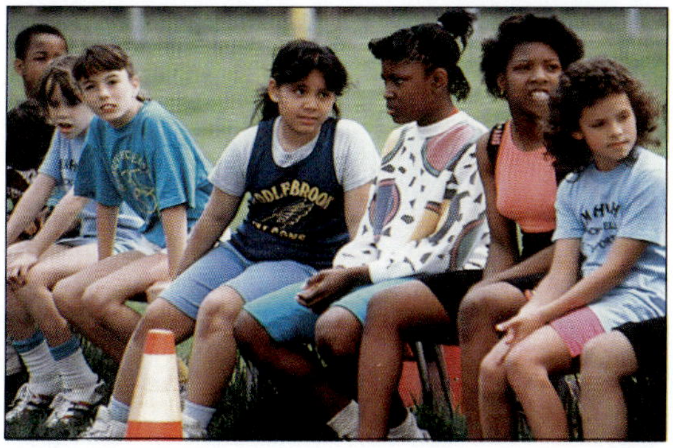

FIGURE 6.19 Protein needs are greater during periods of growth. *(© Jeff Greenberg/Visuals Unlimited)*

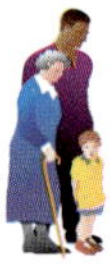

Pregnancy and Lactation Protein is needed in the pregnant woman's diet for the expansion of her blood volume, enlargement of her uterus and breasts, development of the placenta, and growth and development of the fetus. The 1989 RDA for pregnant women suggests an additional 10 g per day above the nonpregnant recommendation. Most women in North America already consume this much protein in their typical diets. The quantity of milk produced and the protein content of the milk determine the additional protein needs during lactation. The 1989 RDA recommends an additional 12 to 15 g per day of dietary protein during lactation.

Illness and Injury Extreme stresses on the body such as infections, fevers, burns, or surgery increase protein breakdown, causing negative nitrogen balance and muscle wasting. In a burn patient, protein losses are even greater because protein is lost in fluids lost through the burn. Dietary protein must be increased to support the needs of protein synthesis and minimize the amount of body protein that is broken down. Requirements for these types of stresses must be assessed on an individual basis, depending on the extent of protein breakdown. For example, a severe infection increases requirements by one third or more. Burns can increase requirements to two to four times the normal level.

Athletics The marketing of protein powders and amino acid supplements to athletes might lead people to believe that athletes need extra protein. In fact, most athletes can meet their protein needs by consuming the 1989 RDA of 0.8 g per kg of body weight. Endurance athletes such as distance runners and cyclers, and strength athletes, such as weight lifters and body builders, may require more protein. Endurance athletes metabolize protein for energy and to maintain blood glucose, so they need a total of 1.2 to 1.4 g of protein per kilogram per day. Strength athletes require extra protein to supply amino acids to build new muscle, so they need about 1.4 to 1.8 g of protein per kilogram per day[18] (Figure 6.20).

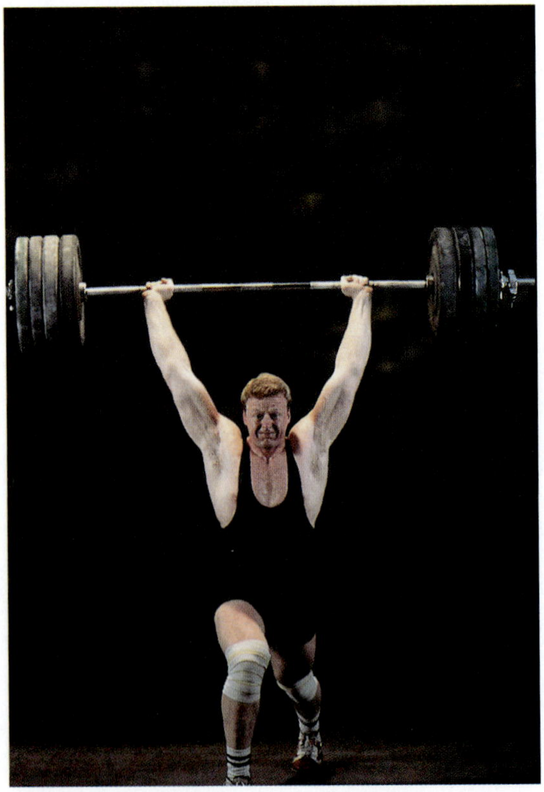

FIGURE 6.20 The protein needs of athletes who are building muscle can be met with a well-balanced diet. *(Amwell/Tony Stone Images)*

Because muscle growth occurs in response to exercise, which is fueled primarily by glycogen stored in the muscles, dietary protein in excess of this does not increase muscle growth. Even those athletes who require extra protein are likely to meet their needs by consuming a balanced diet. The typical American diet contains about 15% protein or about 100 to 150 g of protein per day. This can meet the requirements even for strength and endurance athletes. For example, if a 200-pound (91-kg) man consumes 3600 kcal per day, 15% of which is from protein (approximately the amount contained in a typical North American diet), he will consume 135 g of protein or 1.5 g per kilogram. The protein needs of athletes are also discussed in Chapter 14.

Assessing Protein Quality

Recommendations for protein intake assume that the protein consumed is of mixed quality (some high-quality, some low-quality). Protein quality is a measure of how useful a protein in the diet is for building body protein. Generally foods of animal origin, such as meat, eggs, and milk, are sources of high-quality protein. However, more specific measures of protein quality are available. These measures consider both the amino acid composition and the digestibility of the protein. These measures are useful for determining the quality of dietary protein available to populations. For example, the quality of protein in a dietary staple such as corn or cassava is extremely important in a country where both food and protein are scarce. Each of the measures discussed below has scientific advantages and drawbacks.

Web Menu

For more information on assessing protein quality, go to the Food and Agriculture Organization Web page at www.fao.org/ and search for protein quality.

Amino Acid Composition One way to evaluate protein quality is to compare the amino acid pattern of the food being evaluated with the amino acid composition of an ideal or reference amino acid pattern. A **chemical** or **amino acid score** is calculated by expressing each amino acid as a proportion of the amount found in the reference pattern. The lowest proportion of an amino acid as a percentage of that amino acid in the reference identifies the limiting amino acid and is used as the score for that protein. For example, 100 g of wheat protein has 1.7 g of lysine. The reference pattern contains 5.8 g of lysine per 100 g of protein. So the wheat protein contains only 29% of the amount of lysine in the reference. Because this is the smallest percentage of any of the essential amino acids in wheat protein, lysine is the limiting amino acid and the chemical score for wheat protein is 29. Proteins with the most desirable proportions of amino acids will have the highest chemical scores. For example, if a protein has a limiting amino acid that is present at 75% of the level found in the reference pattern, it will be assigned a chemical score of 75[19,20] (Table 6.4).

Chemical or **amino acid score** A measure of protein quality determined by comparing the amount of the limiting amino acid in a food with that in a reference protein.

TABLE 6.4 Measures of Protein Quality

Measure	Formula
Chemical or Amino Acid Score =	$\frac{\text{mg of limiting amino acid per g of test protein}}{\text{mg of amino acid per g of reference protein}} \times 100$
Protein Digestibility–Corrected Amino Acid Score (PDCAAS) =	Amino Acid score × digestibility factor
Protein Efficiency Ratio (PER) =	$\frac{\text{wt gain when fed test protein}}{\text{wt gain when fed reference protein}}$
Net Protein Utilization (NPU) =	$\frac{\text{nitrogen retained}}{\text{nitrogen intake}} \times 100$
Biological Value (BV) =	$\frac{\text{nitrogen retained}}{\text{nitrogen absorbed}} \times 100$

Digestibility Amino acid score is an easy way to estimate protein quality in theory, but it does not take into account how well the body can use the protein that is being evaluated. Some proteins are more digestible than others. Digestibility is important because only protein that is digested can contribute amino acids to meet requirements. The digestibility of most animal proteins such as milk, meat, and eggs is high, between 90 and 99%. Plant sources of protein are less digestible particularly when eaten raw, and digestibility ranges from 70 to 90%.[21]

Protein digestibility-corrected amino acid score A measure of protein quality that is calculated by adjusting the amino acid score with a correction factor for digestibility.

To account for digestibility, the amino acid score is multiplied by the percent digestibility of the protein. The value obtained is called the **protein digestibility-corrected amino acid score** (see Table 6.4). For example, if a protein has an amino acid score of 75, but only 80% of it is digested, it will have a protein digestibility-corrected amino acid score of 60% ($0.75 \times 0.8 = 0.6$). Despite some shortcomings, the protein digestibility-corrected amino acid score is currently used to assess the protein quality of foods for humans.[22] This is the method required by the FDA to assess the protein quality for food labels on products intended for people over one year of age (Figure 6.21).

Growth The most accurate way to assess protein quality would be to use human clinical studies that measure growth and other metabolic indicators. But, for both ethical and economic reasons, this is not always feasible. Therefore, techniques that measure the effectiveness of protein in promoting animal growth have been used. The **protein efficiency ratio** is calculated by comparing the weight gain of growing rats fed a test protein with the weight gain of those fed a reference protein such as egg protein. The PER method with casein as a standard is used to measure the protein quality of infant formulas and baby foods. The growth of rats is not a perfect indicator of human protein needs, and it is now recognized that PER overestimates the value of some animal proteins for human use and underestimates the value of some plant proteins.[20]

Protein Efficiency Ratio A measure of protein quality determined by comparing the weight gain of a laboratory animal fed a test protein with the weight gain of an animal fed a reference protein.

Protein Retention Several methods use human or animal balance studies to measure how well a protein is used for growth and maintenance. These include **net protein utilization** and **biological value**. Net protein utilization measures how much of the protein in the diet is retained for use by the body. With this method it is not possible to determine if a low value is due to the poor amino acid composition of the protein or to its poor digestibility. To avoid this problem, biological value compares the amount of nitrogen retained in the body for maintenance and

Net protein utilization A measure of protein quality determined by comparing the amount of nitrogen retained in the body with the amount eaten in the diet.

Biological value A measure of protein quality determined by comparing the amount of nitrogen retained in the body with the amount absorbed from the diet.

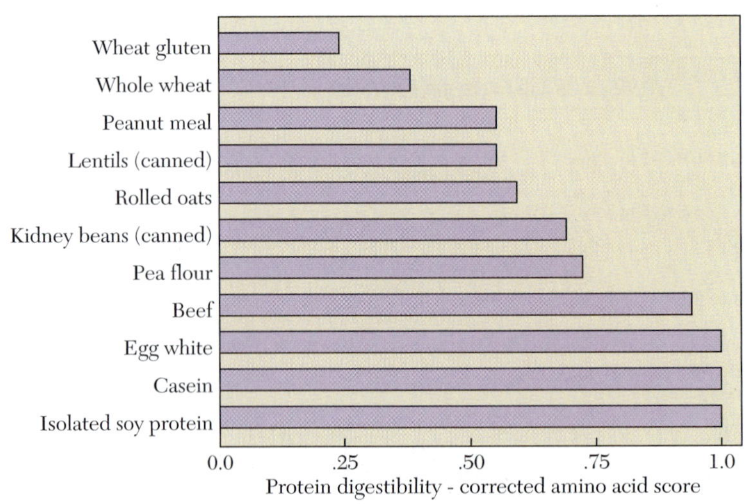

FIGURE 6.21 The protein digestibility-corrected amino acid score of plant foods is generally lower than that of animal foods. An exception is soy protein. The high digestibility of protein from most soy products such as tofu and soy protein isolate contributes to the overall high protein quality and protein digestibility–corrected amino acid score. *(Source: Protein Quality Evaluation, Report of the Joint FAO/WHO Expert Consultation, FAO/WHO, 1989)*

growth with the amount absorbed from the diet. The high-quality protein in egg has a biological value of 100, meaning that 100% of the egg protein that is absorbed is retained by the body. The protein in corn has a biological value of only 60, meaning that only 60% of that which is absorbed is retained for use by the body.

Meeting Protein Needs

In a typical North American diet, protein provides about 15% of the energy consumed, or 100 g of protein, an amount that is well above the 1989 RDA. The Food Guide Pyramid and the Dietary Guidelines both recommend an increase in the consumption of plant foods such as grains and vegetables. Following this recommendation will increase the proportion of protein from plant sources. The following sections discuss how to calculate the amount of protein in a diet, the benefits and risks of consuming a vegetarian diet, and how to plan a diet to meet needs.

Calculating Protein Intake

To maintain health, protein intake must meet needs. Table 6.3 illustrates how to calculate protein needs from the 1989 RDA. To calculate protein intake, the protein content of a diet or a food can be obtained using food composition tables or databases, the information on food labels, or Exchange Lists. Food composition tables and databases contain information on a wide range of foods and supplements. Food labels provide a more readily available source of information; however, because the labeling of raw meats and fish is voluntary, many of the greatest sources of protein in the diet do not carry food labels. The protein content of these and other foods can be estimated using the Exchange Lists shown in Table 6.5. According to the Exchange Lists, a 1-ounce serving of meat (28 g) provides 7

TABLE 6.5 Protein Content of the Exchange Lists

Exchange Groups/Lists	Serving Size	Protein (g)
Carbohydrate Group		
Starch	1/2 cup pasta, rice, cereal, potatoes; 1 slice bread	3
Fruit	1 small apple, peach, pear; 1/2 banana; 1/2 cup canned fruit (in juice)	0
Milk	1 cup milk or yogurt	
Nonfat		8
Low-fat		8
Reduced fat		8
Whole		8
Other carbohydrates	Serving sizes vary	Varies
Vegetables	1/2 cup cooked vegetables, 1 cup raw	2
Meat/Meat Substitute Group	1 oz meat or cheese, 1/2 cup legumes	
Very lean		7
Lean		7
Medium fat		7
High fat		7
Fat Group	1 tsp butter, margarine, or oil; 1 Tbsp salad dressing	0

g of protein. One cup of milk provides 8 g, and grains and vegetables provide 2 to 3 g per serving. For diets based primarily on plant proteins, protein quality must also be considered.

Vegetarian Diets

For more information on vegetarian diets, go to the Vegetarian Resource Group at www.vrg.org or the American Heart Association at www.americanheart.org, click on Heart and Stroke A to Z Guide, and select vegetarian diets.

In the United States and other affluent countries, the majority of dietary protein comes from animal sources—meat, poultry, fish, eggs, and dairy products. However, in many cultures animal protein is unavailable or unaffordable. These cultures rely on a dietary pattern that combines plant proteins with small amounts of animal proteins or with other plant proteins containing different limiting amino acids. Plant protein–based or **vegetarian diets** have evolved in most parts of the world out of necessity. In affluent societies, vegetarian diets are followed for a variety of reasons other than economics, such as health, religion, personal ethics, or environmental awareness. (See Chapter 18 *Making Decisions:* "Are Vegetarian Diets Better for the Environment?")

Traditionally, vegetarianism is defined as abstinence from meat, fish, and fowl. The current interpretation of vegetarianism includes a wide variety of eating patterns depending on the degree of abstinence from animal products. Semivegetarians are those who avoid only certain types of red meat, fish, or poultry—for example, individuals who avoid all red meat but continue to consume poultry and fish. Lacto-ovo vegetarians are those who eat no animal flesh but do eat eggs and dairy products such as milk and cheese. Lacto vegetarians are those who avoid animal flesh and eggs but do consume dairy products. **Vegans** are those who avoid all food of animal origin. Providing all the essential amino acids with a vegetarian diet requires that combinations of foods with complementary amino acids be consumed.

Vegetarian diets Patterns of food intake that eliminate some or all animal products.

Vegans Individuals who have a pattern of food intake that eliminates all animal products.

Protein Complementation Even though most plant proteins are limited in one or more amino acids, vegetarian diets meet protein needs by using **protein complementation,** a technique for combining foods containing different limiting amino acids in order to improve the protein quality of the diet as a whole. By eating plant proteins with complementary amino acid patterns, essential amino acid requirements can be met without consuming any animal proteins. The amino acids that are most often limited in plant proteins are lysine, methionine, cysteine, and tryptophan. As a general rule, legumes are deficient in methionine and cysteine but high in lysine. Grains, nuts, and seeds are deficient in lysine but high in methionine and cysteine. Corn is deficient in lysine and tryptophan but is a good source of methionine. Thus, consuming a diet containing foods from various categories provides an amino acid pattern similar to that of animal foods. For example, when rice, which is limited in the amino acid lysine but high in methionine, is eaten with beans, which are high in lysine but limited in methionine, the combination will provide a much higher quality protein than if either is eaten alone.

Protein complementation A method for combining proteins from different sources so that they collectively provide the proportions of amino acids required to meet needs.

Common combinations of grains and legumes that have become cultural staples include beans and rice or beans and wheat or corn tortillas in Central and South America; rice and soybean products such as miso and tofu in China and Japan; rice and lentils in India; rice and black-eyed peas in the southern United States; and peanut butter (peanuts are legumes) and bread throughout the United States (Figure 6.22). Plant proteins can also be complemented with animal protein in order to meet the need for essential amino acids. For example, in Asia rice is often flavored with a small amount of spiced beef, chicken, or fish. Although it is not necessary to consume complementary proteins at each meal, the entire day's diet should include proteins from complementary sources in order to satisfy the daily need for amino acids.[23]

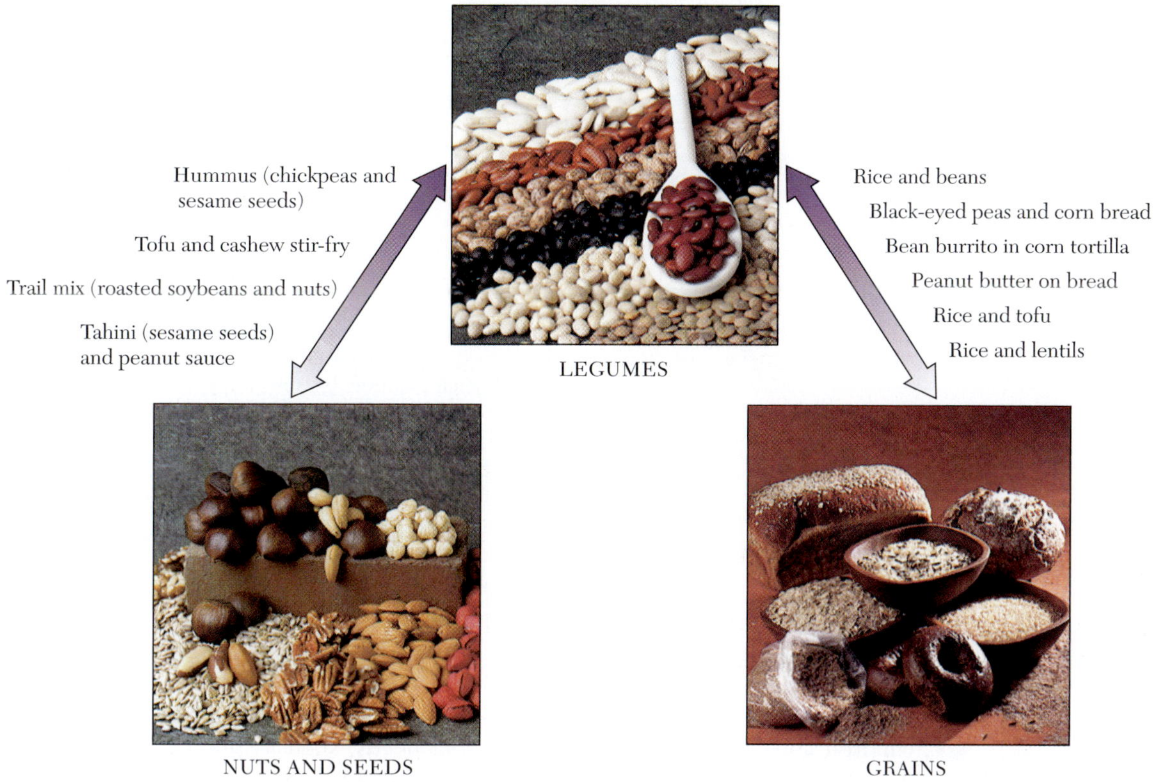

FIGURE 6.22 Combining complementary sources of incomplete plant proteins can provide a diet containing enough of all of the essential amino acids. *(George Semple)*

Benefits of Vegetarian Diets The health benefits of vegetarian diets have made them increasingly popular in affluent societies as people strive to adopt healthy lifestyles. Vegetarians have been shown to have lower risks for obesity, diabetes, cardiovascular disease, high blood pressure, and some types of cancer.[23,24] Studies of Seventh-Day Adventists, a religious group that espouses a diet containing no animal products as well as abstention from alcohol consumption and cigarette smoking, found that the incidence of heart disease is about half that of non–Seventh-Day Adventists living in the same area.[25] Even when lifestyle factors other than diet, such as abstinence from alcohol use and cigarette smoking, were kept constant by comparing Seventh-Day Adventists who do not consume vegetarian diets with their vegetarian counterparts, eating meat was associated with a higher incidence of heart disease and certain types of cancer.[26] Because vegetarian diets eliminate or limit the intake of animal foods, they are lower in saturated fat, cholesterol, and animal protein. The increased intakes of grains, legumes, vegetables, and fruits add fiber, vitamins (including antioxidant vitamins and folate), minerals, and phytochemicals to the diet.[27,28] It is not known whether the reduction in chronic disease is due to the amount and type of fat in the diet, the source of the protein, or the increase in fiber, micronutrients, and phytochemicals. It is likely that the total dietary pattern rather than a single factor alone is responsible.

In addition to reducing disease risks, diets that rely more heavily on plant proteins are more economical. A meal based on rice, pasta, or beans—even with a small serving of meat—costs less and can provide plenty of protein with less fat than a meal based on a large serving of meat. For example, a dinner of stir-fried vegetables and rice with a small amount of meat costs about half as much as a meal of steak and potatoes; a meal containing no meat, such as stir-fried vegetables and rice with tofu, costs even less. Yet both meals provide a significant portion of the day's protein requirement.

TABLE 6.6 Sources for Essential Nutrients Potentially Lacking in Vegan Diets

Nutrient	Sources in Vegan Diets
Protein	Soy-based products, legumes, seeds, nuts, grains, and vegetables.
Vitamin B_{12}	Products fortified with B_{12} such as soy beverages and cereals, vitamin supplements
Calcium	Tofu processed with calcium, broccoli, kale, bok choy, seeds, nuts, legumes, and products fortified with calcium such as soy beverages, grain products, and orange juice
Vitamin D	Sunshine, products fortified with vitamin D such as soy beverages and margarine
Iron	Legumes, tofu, green leafy vegetables, dried fruit, whole grains, iron-fortified cereals and breads (absorption is improved by vitamin C found in citrus fruit, tomatoes, strawberries, and dark green vegetables)
Zinc	Whole grains, legumes, nuts, tofu, and fortified cereals

Risks Associated with Vegetarian Diets Most people can easily meet their protein needs with lacto and lacto-ovo vegetarian diets. These diets contain high-quality animal proteins from eggs or milk, which complement the limiting amino acids in plant proteins. However, nutrient deficiencies can be a problem for people consuming unsupplemented vegetarian diets, particularly vegan diets.

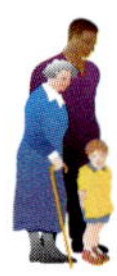

Protein deficiency is a potential risk when vegan diets are consumed by small children and adults with increased protein needs, such as pregnant women and those recovering from illness or injury. These individuals must plan carefully to consume a diet that provides enough of the essential amino acids to meet their needs.

Deficiencies of certain vitamins and minerals are a greater risk for vegetarians than protein deficiency.[12] Vitamin B_{12} is found almost exclusively in animal products; therefore, those consuming vegan diets must use supplements or fortified foods to meet needs. The major source of calcium in the North American diet is dairy products, so again, vegan diets must be carefully planned to meet calcium needs. Likewise, most dietary vitamin D comes from fortified dairy products, so vegans must get their vitamin D from sunshine or consume other sources of this vitamin, such as fortified soy milk. Iron and zinc may be deficient in vegetarian diets because the best sources of these minerals are red meats. They are also poorly absorbed from plant sources. Because amounts of iron and zinc are low in dairy products, lacto-ovo and lacto vegetarians as well as vegans are at risk for deficiencies. A special RDA for iron has been set for vegetarians. Vegetarian sources of nutrients are listed in Table 6.6 and discussed in Chapters 9 to 13. (See *Critical Thinking:* "Choosing a Vegetarian Diet.")

Critical Thinking

Choosing a Vegetarian Diet

A year ago Angela decided to stop eating meat. While studying protein in her nutrition class, she became concerned that her diet did not correctly complement protein sources. Angela is 19 years old and weighs 130 pounds. She wanted to know if her diet met her protein needs.

What is the 1989 RDA for protein for someone of her age and weight?

$$\frac{130 \text{ pounds}}{2.2 \text{ pounds/kg}} = 59 \text{ kg}$$

1989 RDA for adults = 0.8 g protein per kg body weight
Angela's 1989 RDA = 59 kg × 0.8 g/kg = 47.2 g of protein

She records her food intake for one day and then uses diet analysis software to calculate her protein intake.

Food	Serving	Protein (g)
Breakfast		
Grape Nuts	3 Tbsp	2.4
Milk, lowfat	1/2 cup	4
Orange juice	1/2 cup	0.8
Toast, wheat	2 slices	5
Peanut butter	1 Tbsp	4
Coffee	1 cup	0
Lunch		
Lentil soup	1 cup	9
Rice	1 cup	6
Banana	1	1
Apple juice	1 cup	0
Dinner		
Green salad	1 cup	1
with dressing	1 Tbsp	0
Rice	1 cup	6
Curried potatoes	1/2 cup	1.5
and chickpeas	1/3 cup	5
Dinner rolls	2 medium	6
Ice cream	1/2 cup	2
Total		*53.7*

Her diet provides 53.7 g of protein, which exceeds her calculated 1989 RDA of 47.2 g.

Do Angela's food choices include complementary proteins?

At breakfast, she has milk, which is a high-quality protein, and bread and peanut butter, which contain proteins that complement each other (see Figure 6.22). At lunch, the protein in the lentil soup complements the protein in the rice. At dinner, she has chickpeas, which complement both the rice and the wheat protein in the rolls. She also has ice cream, which provides high-quality protein.

How much protein would her diet provide if she decided to eliminate dairy products?

Answer:

How would eliminating dairy products affect her calcium and vitamin D intake?

The major source of calcium in her diet is dairy products, so she would have to carefully plan her diet to include other calcium sources. Likewise, most of her dietary vitamin D comes from fortified dairy products, so she would need to be sure to get her vitamin D from sunshine or other fortified foods. Vegetarian sources of these nutrients are listed in Table 6.6 and discussed in Chapters 10 and 12.

Does her diet meet the Food Guide Pyramid recommendations for vegetarians?

Answer:

A Diet to Meet Recommendations

Populations around the world meet their protein requirements with different types and amounts of protein. It is generally not difficult to meet protein needs when consuming an adequate diet that contains animal foods and/or a variety of plant foods. The Food Guide Pyramid provides information on meeting protein needs and can be modified to plan vegetarian diets. Food labels also provide information on the amounts and sources of proteins in food.

Protein in the Food Guide Pyramid A simple way to ensure an adequate protein intake from a combination of plant and animal proteins is to follow the recommendations of the Food Guide Pyramid. The groups in the Food Guide Pyramid that are highest in protein are the Milk, Yogurt, and Cheese Group and the Meat, Poultry, Fish, Dry Beans, Eggs, and Nuts Group (Figure 6.23). These two food groups are in the upper sections of the Pyramid, indicating that these foods should make up a relatively small proportion of the day's intake. Two to three servings per day are recommended from each. Two 8-ounce glasses of milk and two 2-ounce servings of meat provide about 44 g of protein. Consuming the minimum recommended servings from the Bread, Cereal, Rice, and Pasta Group and the Vegetable Group, six and three servings respectively, would bring the total to 71 g of protein—more than enough to meet most people's needs.

Vegetarians can meet their needs by making a few modifications to the traditional Food Guide Pyramid (see Table 6.7 and Appendix G). The food choices and recommended number of servings from the groups containing grains, vegetables, and fruits are the same as in the traditional Food Guide Pyramid. The groups in

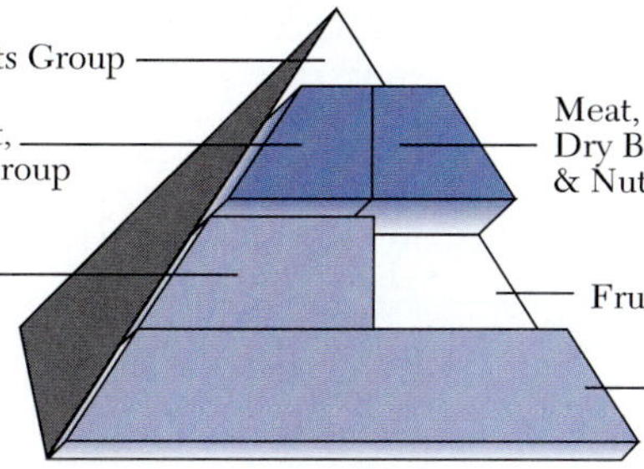

FIGURE 6.23 The Food Guide Pyramid groups that are raised and colored blue are good sources of protein. The groups shown in the darker shade contain a greater proportion of high-protein foods and are the only groups that include animal proteins.

the next level of the traditional Pyramid (meat and milk) include foods of animal origin. To modify this for vegetarian diets, two to three servings from a group containing dry beans, nuts, seeds, eggs, and meat substitutes are recommended. Lacto-vegetarians (those who consume dairy products) should also consume two to

TABLE 6.7 Selecting a Vegetarian Diet Using the Food Guide Pyramid[a]

Food Group	Suggested Number of Servings	Serving Sizes
Bread, Cereal, Rice, & Pasta Group	6 to 11	1 slice bread 1 oz cold cereal 1/2 cup rice, pasta, or cooked cereal
Vegetable Group[b]	3 to 5	1/2 cup cooked 1 cup raw leafy
Fruit Group	2 to 4	1 medium apple, orange, or banana 1/2 cup chopped or canned 3/4 cup juice 1/4 cup dried
Dry Beans, Nuts, Seeds, Eggs, & Meat Substitutes Group	2 to 3	1-1/2 cups cooked dry beans 4–6 Tbsp nuts, seeds, or peanut butter 1 cup soy milk 1/2 cup tofu 2–3 eggs[c]
Milk, Yogurt, & Cheese Group[d]	0–3	1 cup milk 1.5 oz cheese 1 cup yogurt
Fats, Oils, and Sweets Group	Use sparingly	Candy Butter Oil Salad dressing

[a]For vegan diets vitamin B_{12} supplements or vitamin B_{12}-fortified foods are necessary to meet needs.

[b]Include 1 cup of dark green leafy vegetables daily to help meet iron and calcium needs.

[c]Lacto vegetarians and vegans may eliminate this choice.

[d]Vegetarians who choose not to use milk need to select milk substitutes fortified with calcium and vitamin D, such as fortified soy milk, and other foods rich in calcium such as dark green leafy vegetables. At least two servings of calcium-rich foods should be consumed daily.

Modified from the National Center for Nutrition and Dietetics, the American Dietetic Association; based on the USDA Food Guide Pyramid, © ADAF, 1997.

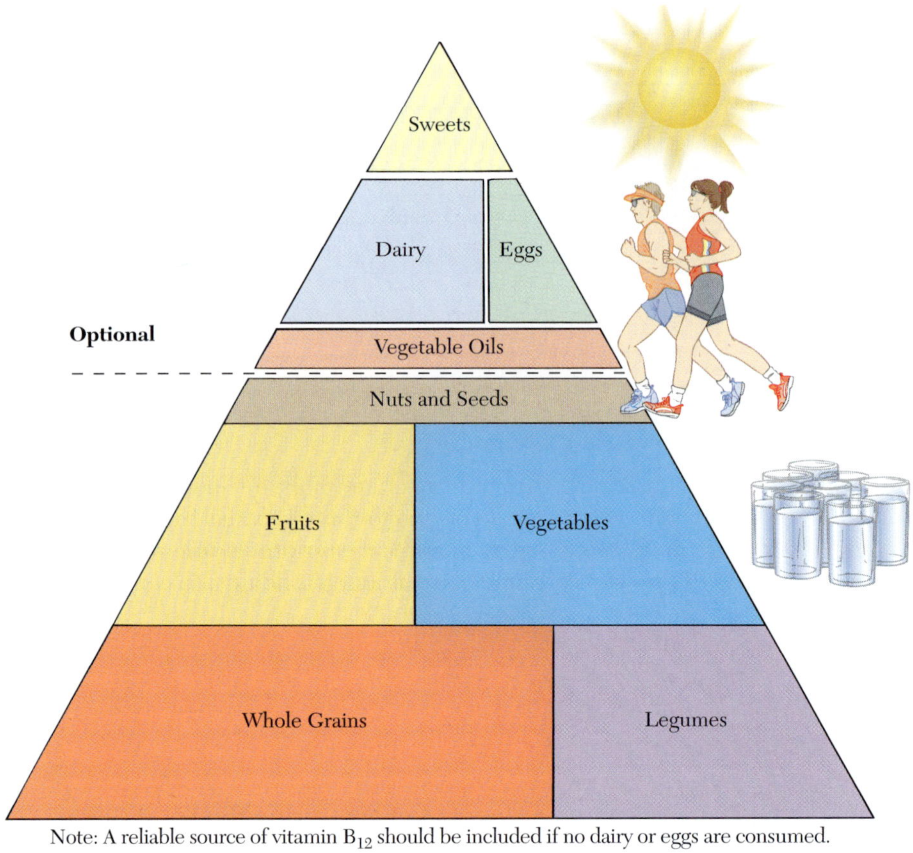

FIGURE 6.24 This Vegetarian Food Guide Pyramid can be used to select a diet that meets nutrient needs without including animal foods. All vegetarians should make selections from the five plant-based groups in the lower trapezoid-shaped portion of the pyramid. Depending on the type of vegetarian diet, additional selections can be made from one or more of the four groups in the upper portion of the pyramid. For example, a lacto-vegetarian would include selections from the dairy group. This pyramid also emphasizes the importance of moderate exposure to sunlight to ensure adequate vitamin D, and physical activity, and adequate water consumption for health. *(Source: Haddad, E. H., Sabaté, J., and Whitten, C. G. Vegetarian food guide pyramid: a conceptual framework. Am. J. Clin. Nutr. 70 (suppl):615S–619S; 1999. Or, online at http://www.llu.edu/llu/nutrition/vegguide.html.)*

three servings from the milk group. Vegans (those who do not consume any animal foods) should consume milk substitutes fortified with calcium and vitamin D, or other foods high in these nutrients. To obtain adequate vitamin B_{12}, vegans must take B_{12} supplements or use products fortified with vitamin B_{12}.[23]

A Food Guide Pyramid designed specifically for vegetarian diets is shown in Figure 6.24.[29] It includes five major plant-based food groups in the bottom portion of the pyramid. All vegetarians should consume selections from these groups, which include whole grains, legumes, fruits, vegetables, and nuts and seeds. The four food groups in the smaller upper portion of the pyramid are optional. These include dairy, eggs, vegetable oils, and sweets. One or more of these optional foods groups can be included in the diet depending on the philosophical values and health beliefs of the individual vegetarian. Although the dairy group is optional, the nutrients provided by this group are not, and adequate calcium and vitamin D must be obtained from other sources if no selections are made from this group. If no animal products are consumed, a reliable source of vitamin B_{12} must be included. In addition to providing for the dietary needs of vegetarians with diverse eating patterns, this Vegetarian Food Guide Pyramid also considers lifestyle factors. Moderate exposure to sunlight is important to ensure adequate vitamin D. Adequate physical activity and water intake are also important for health.

Using Food Labels to Pick Your Proteins Food labels provide information about the composition of foods and the contribution they make toward meeting daily nutrient intake recommendations. Because protein is a nutrient that is adequate in the diet of most Americans, the protein content of foods is listed but not emphasized on most food labels. For some individuals, however, such as those with allergies to certain proteins and those who wish to avoid specific foods for religious, ethical, or other reasons, food labels are an important source of information that can help identify foods appropriate for their diets.

Nutrition Facts Like other nutrients, information on protein is listed in the Nutrition Facts section of the food label as well as in the ingredient list. The Nutrition Facts section lists the number of grams of protein per serving. However, the percent Daily Value is required only on foods that contain protein of very low quality. When listed, the percent Daily Value is adjusted for protein quality using the protein digestibility-corrected amino acid score of the protein. For example, a food that contains 10 g of high-quality protein supplies 20% of the Daily Value for protein, whereas, for a food that contains 10 g of a protein with a protein digestibility-corrected amino acid score of 50%, the Nutrition Facts may indicate that it provides only 10% of the Daily Value for protein. Only foods with low-quality protein must list the percent Daily Value on the label.

Ingredient List The ingredient list can be used to determine the source of protein in packaged foods. This information is helpful to individuals who restrict their intake of certain proteins. For instance, if an individual's religion prohibits the consumption of pork, the ingredient list is needed to determine if a packaged food, such as frozen egg rolls, contains pork. This information is also helpful to vegetarians who restrict animal proteins.

Even foods that contain little or no protein may have small amounts of individual proteins, protein hydrolysates, or amino acids added to them. The sources of these must be listed in the ingredient list and be explicit enough to

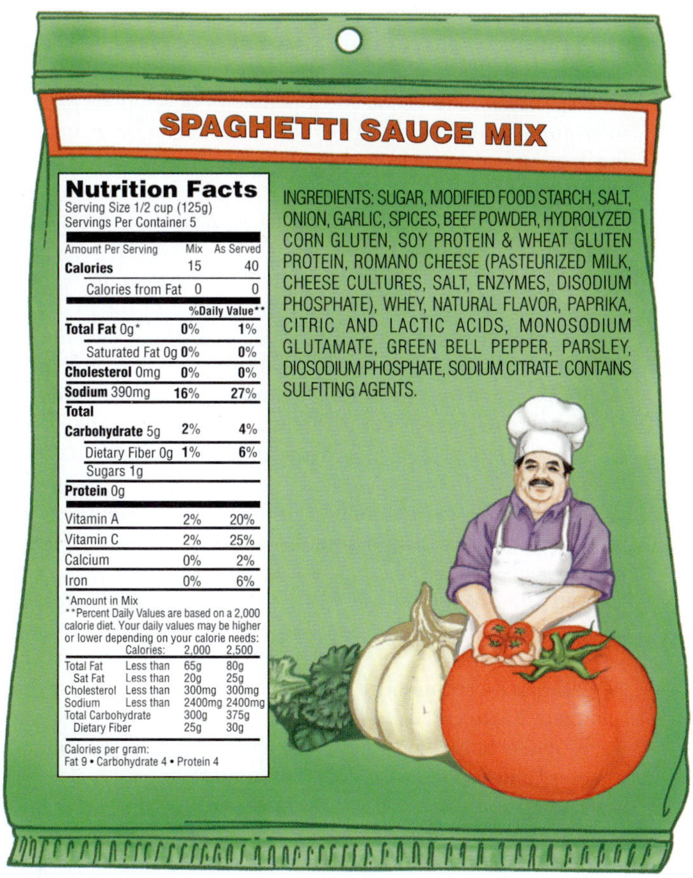
SPAGHETTI SAUCE MIX
Nutrition Facts
Serving Size 1/2 cup (125g)
Servings Per Container 5
Amount Per Serving Mix As Served
Calories 15 40
Calories from Fat 0 0
%Daily Value**
Total Fat 0g* 0% 1%
Saturated Fat 0g 0% 0%
Cholesterol 0mg 0% 0%
Sodium 390mg 16% 27%
Total Carbohydrate 5g 2% 4%
Dietary Fiber 0g 1% 6%
Sugars 1g
Protein 0g
Vitamin A 2% 20%
Vitamin C 2% 25%
Calcium 0% 2%
Iron 0% 6%
*Amount in Mix
**Percent Daily Values are based on a 2,000 calorie diet. Your daily values may be higher or lower depending on your calorie needs:
Calories: 2,000 2,500
Total Fat Less than 65g 80g
Sat Fat Less than 20g 25g
Cholesterol Less than 300mg 300mg
Sodium Less than 2400mg 2400mg
Total Carbohydrate 300g 375g
Dietary Fiber 25g 30g
Calories per gram:
Fat 9 • Carbohydrate 4 • Protein 4
INGREDIENTS: SUGAR, MODIFIED FOOD STARCH, SALT, ONION, GARLIC, SPICES, BEEF POWDER, HYDROLYZED CORN GLUTEN, SOY PROTEIN & WHEAT GLUTEN PROTEIN, ROMANO CHEESE (PASTEURIZED MILK, CHEESE CULTURES, SALT, ENZYMES, DISODIUM PHOSPHATE), WHEY, NATURAL FLAVOR, PAPRIKA, CITRIC AND LACTIC ACIDS, MONOSODIUM GLUTAMATE, GREEN BELL PEPPER, PARSLEY, DIOSODIUM PHOSPHATE, SODIUM CITRATE. CONTAINS SULFITING AGENTS.

FIGURE 6.25 Although the Nutrition Facts label on this spaghetti sauce mix lists 0 g of protein, the ingredient list indicates that it contains small amounts of a number of proteins and amino acids including beef powder, hydrolyzed corn gluten, soy protein, wheat gluten protein, romano cheese, whey, and monosodium glutamate.

minimize confusion about the contents of a food. This information is particularly helpful to individuals who have food allergies or intolerances. For example, a meatless spaghetti sauce mix may contain hydrolyzed soy protein (Figure 6.25). An individual with an allergy to soy should avoid this product and all products listing soy or hydrolyzed soy protein as an ingredient. Individual amino acids added to foods are also included in the ingredient list. For instance, some people try to avoid consuming the amino acid glutamate (glutamic acid) because they experience MSG symptom complex. When added, it must appear on the label in the ingredient list as monosodium glutamate or potassium glutamate, as shown in Figure 6.25. Glutamate may also be added to food as a component of a protein hydrolysate. Foods containing ingredients that are sources of glutamate, such as hydrolyzed protein, may not state "no MSG" or "no added MSG" on the label.[4]

Summary

1. Proteins are made of chainlike strands of amino acids linked together by peptide bonds. These strands fold over on themselves to create proteins with unique three-dimensional structures. The shape of a protein determines its function.
2. Amino acids consist of a central carbon atom with a hydrogen atom, a nitrogen-containing group, an acid group, and a unique side chain attached. Essential or indispensable amino acids are those that cannot be made in the body in sufficient quantities to meet needs and must therefore be consumed in the diet. Nonessential or dispensable amino acids can be made in the body, usually by the process of transamination.
3. Dietary protein comes from both animal and plant sources. Animal proteins contain a pattern of amino acids that matches the needs of the human body more closely than the pattern of amino acids in plant proteins. Therefore, they are said to be higher quality or more complete proteins than most plant proteins.
4. Digestion breaks protein into small peptides and amino acids, which can be absorbed. Amino acids can be used for the synthesis of protein and other nitrogen-containing molecules and can be deaminated and used for energy or to synthesize glucose or fatty acids.
5. Protein turnover refers to the continuous synthesis and breakdown of body proteins. The amino acids available to cells for protein synthesis, referred to as the amino acid pool, come from both the degradation of body proteins and dietary protein. Protein is made by the body in amounts necessary to maintain homeostasis.
6. The specific proteins that are made are determined by which genes are expressed. Genes are segments of DNA that code for the synthesis of proteins. The information in a gene is transferred to mRNA in the process of transcription. Messenger RNA carries the coded message from the nucleus to ribosomes in the cytoplasm where the process of translation interprets the mRNA code to form a polypeptide.
7. Body proteins provide structure and regulate body functions. Enzymes and some hormones are proteins. Proteins help transport molecules in the blood and into and out of cells. Antibody proteins are essential for immune system function and contractile proteins are needed for muscle contraction. Proteins help regulate fluid balance and acid balance. Proteins can also be used to generate ATP or to synthesize glucose or fat.
8. Protein-energy malnutrition is a public health concern, primarily in developing countries. Kwashiorkor occurs when the protein content of the diet is insufficient to meet needs. It is most common in children. Marasmus occurs when total energy intake is deficient. Most people in developed countries consume more than enough protein, although unnecessary protein and amino acid supplements remain popular. Excess amounts of individual amino acids can interfere with the absorption of other amino acids that share the same transport systems.
9. Protein requirements are determined by studying nitrogen balance. For healthy adults, the 1989 RDA for protein is 0.8 g per kilogram of body weight. Growth, pregnancy, lactation, and physical stress can increase requirements. Certain types of physical activity can also slightly increase protein needs.
10. The quality of protein in the diet is as important as the amount of total protein. There are numerous ways of assessing protein quality in the laboratory. In diet planning, animal proteins are generally considered to be complete proteins—that is, they provide the right combination of amino acids to meet needs. Diets that include little or no animal protein can provide adequate protein if the sources of protein are complemented to supply enough of all the essential amino acids.
11. Vegetarian diets can meet all amino acid needs if carefully planned. Lacto and lacto-ovo vegetarian diets provide high-quality animal proteins. Vegan diets must be carefully planned and supplemented with vitamin B_{12} to meet needs.

Review Questions

1. What are amino acids?
2. What is an essential amino acid?
3. What is the "amino acid pool"?
4. List some plant sources of protein.
5. How are gene expression and protein synthesis related?
6. List six functions of proteins in the body.
7. Why is protein deficiency most common in infants and children?
8. What does nitrogen balance suggest about the balance between protein synthesis and protein breakdown in the body?
9. How does the typical protein intake in North America compare to recommendations?
10. What effect does moderate exercise have on protein needs?
11. What is protein quality and how does it affect protein needs?
12. What are the health benefits of a vegetarian diet? The risks?
13. What is protein complementation? List three pairs of complementary protein sources.

Applying Critical Thinking Skills

Personal nutrition:

1. Calculate your average protein intake using the three-day food record you kept in Chapter 2.
   a. What is your average daily protein intake in grams?
   b. Is your intake higher or lower than the 1989 RDA for protein for someone of your weight, age, and life stage?
   c. If you consumed more than the 1989 RDA for protein, do you think you should decrease your protein intake? Why or why not?
   d. If you consumed less than the 1989 RDA for protein, modify one day of your diet to meet your protein needs.
2. Using the three-day record you kept in Chapter 2, record your total protein and fat intake for each day in the table below.

	Protein (g)	Fat (g)
Day 1		
Day 2		
Day 3		

   a. What is the relationship between the fat and protein in your diet?
   b. Look at the three foods that contribute the most protein to your diet each day. Are they animal or plant foods? How much fat does each of these provide?
3. Imagine that you have decided to become a lacto-vegetarian. Make a list of the nondairy animal foods in your diet and then list plant foods you could substitute. Use protein complementation (see Figure 6.22) to be sure that you meet your need for essential amino acids.
   a. Does your modified diet meet the vegetarian serving recommendations in Table 6.7? If not, what changes would you suggest?
   b. How much protein is in your lacto-vegetarian diet? Does it meet the 1989 RDA for protein for someone in your age and gender group?
   c. If you already consume a lacto-vegetarian diet, design a vegan diet by substituting plant sources of protein for dairy products. Make sure the diet includes at least two servings of calcium-rich foods.

General nutrition issues:

1. A friend of yours is a weight lifter. He has read that if he eats a high-protein diet he will build muscle more quickly. He is 5′8″ tall and weighs 160 pounds. He drinks two or three protein shakes daily and includes two eggs, a 4-ounce hamburger, and a 6-ounce steak in his daily intake.
   a. How much protein do the eggs, hamburger, and steak provide?
   b. Go to a health food store and read labels to determine how much protein a typical "protein shake" contains.
   c. How does his protein intake compare to his requirement (remember that protein needs may be slightly higher for weight lifters)?
   d. Does he need the protein shake to meet his protein needs?
2. Epidemiology suggests that individuals who consume a vegetarian diet have a reduced risk of heart disease. Examine the original and lacto-ovo vegetarian diets shown below.
   a. Which diet contains less total fat? Saturated fat?
   b. Compare the fiber content of the two diets.
   c. Compare the number of servings of fruits and vegetables in the two diets.

Original Diet	Lacto-Ovo Vegetarian Diet
Breakfast	
Fried eggs with ham	Banana
Toast with butter	Toast with peanut butter
Orange juice	Orange juice
Coffee with milk and sugar	Coffee with milk and sugar
Lunch	
Turkey sandwich on whole wheat bread with mayo	Swiss cheese sandwich on whole wheat bread with mayo
Whole milk	Whole milk
Pear	Pear
Potato chips	Potato chips
Dinner	
Spaghetti with meat sauce	Spaghetti with tomato sauce
Garlic bread with butter	Garlic bread with butter
Vegetable salad with bacon bits	Vegetable salad with garbanzo beans
Ice cream	Ice cream

3. For each food in column A, select one or more in column B that could be combined with it to provide a meal of high-quality protein.

Column A	Column B
Rice	Tofu
Wheat bread	Peanut butter
Corn tortilla	Cheese
Pasta	Kidney beans
Tofu	Cashews
Peanut butter	Corn tortilla
Corn bread	Wheat bread
Soybeans	Chickpeas
Black-eyed peas	Chicken

4. One of the most common examples of protein complementation is a peanut butter sandwich. The table here gives the essential amino acid composition of 100 grams of peanut butter protein and 100 grams of wheat bread protein and a reference amino acid pattern.

Amino acid	Peanut Butter	Wheat Bread	Reference Amino Acid Pattern
Isoleucine	4.0	3.4	5.9
Leucine	7.7	6.2	9.0
Lysine	3.9	1.7	7.2
Methionine + Cysteine	2.4	3.6	6.3
Phenylalanine + Tyrosine	10.8	6.4	10.3
Threonine	3.0	2.4	5.0
Tryptophan	1.2	1.0	1.3
Valine	4.6	3.8	6.7

a. Calculate the percentage of each amino acid in peanut butter and wheat bread relative to the amino acid reference pattern.

b. Which is the limiting amino acid in peanut butter? Which is the limiting amino acid in wheat bread? Which of the two food proteins has the higher amino acid score?

References

1. Young, V. R. Soy protein in relation to human amino acid nutrition. J. Am. Diet. Assoc. 91:820–827, 1991.
2. American Dietetic Association. Position paper of the American Dietetic Association: fat replacers. J. Am. Diet. Assoc. 98:463–468, 1998.
3. Walker, R., and Lupien, J. R. The safety evaluation of monosodium glutamate. J. Nutr. 130:1049S–1052S, 2000.
4. U.S. Food and Drug Administration. FDA and monosodium glutamate (MSG). FDA backgrounder, August 31, 1995. Available online at **http://vm.cfsan.fda.gov/~lrd/msg.html**. Accessed 1 Aug 2000.
5. Geha, R. S., Beiser, A., Ren, C., et al. Review of alleged reaction to monosodium glutamate and outcome of a multicenter double-blind placebo-controlled study. J. Nutr. 130:1058S–1062S, 2000.
6. Stevenson, D. D. Monosodium glutamate and asthma. J. Nutr. 130:1067S–1073S, 2000.
7. Kuhn, L. D. Iron and gene expression: molecular mechanisms regulating cellular iron homeostasis. Nutr. Rev. 56(II):S11–S19, 1998.
8. Matthews, D. E. Proteins and amino acids. In *Modern Nutrition in Health and Disease,* 9th ed. Shils, M. E., Olson, J. A., Shike, M., and Ross, A. C., eds. Baltimore: Williams & Wilkins, 1999; 11–48.
9. Williams, C. D. Kwashiorkor: nutritional disease of children associated with maize diet. Lancet 2:1151–1154, 1935.
10. Maroni, B. J., and Mitch, W. E. Role of nutrition in prevention of the progression of renal disease. Annu. Rev. Nutr. 17:435–455, 1997.
11. Millward, D. J. Optimal intakes of protein in the human diet. Proc. Nutr. Soc. 58:403–413, 1999.
12. Feskanich, D., Willet, W. C., Stampfer, M. J., and Colditz, G. A. Protein consumption and bone fractures in women. Am. J. Epidemiol. 143:472–479, 1996.
13. Munger, R. G., Cerhan, J. R., and Chiu, B. G-H. Prospective study of dietary protein intake and risk of hip fracture in postmenopausal women. Am. J. Clin. Nutr. 69:147–152, 1999.
14. Heaney, R. P. Excess dietary protein may not adversely affect bone. J. Nutr. 128:1054–1057, 1998.

15. van't Veer, P., Jansen, M. C., Klerk, M., and Kok, F. J. Fruits and vegetables in the prevention of cancer and cardiovascular disease. Public Health Nutr. 3:103–107, 2000.
16. Steinmetz, K. A., and Potter, J. D. Vegetables, fruit, and cancer prevention: a review. J. Am. Diet. Assoc. 96:1027–1039, 1996.
17. National Research Council. *Diet and Health: Implications for Reducing Chronic Disease Risk.* Washington, D.C.: National Academy Press, 1989.
18. Paul, G. L., Gautsch, T. A., and Layman, D. K. Amino acid and protein metabolism during exercise and recovery. In *Nutrition in Exercise and Sport,* 3rd ed. I. Wolinski, ed. Boca Raton, Fla.: CRC Press, 1998; 125–158.
19. FAO/WHO/UNU, Energy and protein requirements. Report of a joint FAO/WHO/UNU expert consultation. WHO Tech. Rep. Ser. No. 724. Geneva, WHO; 1985.
20. Boutrif, E. Recent developments in protein evaluation. Available online at **http://www.fao.org/docrep/u5900t/u5900t07.htm**. Accessed 19 Jan 2000.
21. Fuller, M. F. Protein and amino acid requirements. In *Biochemical and Physiological Aspects of Human Nutrition.* Stipanik, M. H., ed. Philadelphia: W. B. Saunders Company, 2000; 287–304.
22. Sarwar, G. The protein digestibility-corrected amino acid score method overestimates quality of proteins containing antinutritional factors and of poorly digestible proteins supplemented with limiting amino acids in rats. J. Nutr. 127:758–764, 1997.
23. Messina, V. K., and Burke, K. I. Position of the American Dietetic Association: vegetarian diets. J. Am. Diet. Assoc. 97:1317–1321, 1997.
24. Walter, P. Effects of vegetarian diets on aging and longevity. Nutr. Rev. 55(II):S61–S68, 1997.
25. Fonnebo, V. The healthy Seventh-Day Adventist. Am. J. Clin. Nutr. 59(suppl):1124S–1129S, 1994.
26. Fraser, G. Associations between diet and cancer, ischemic heart disease, and all-cause mortality in non-Hispanic white California Seventh-Day Adventists. Am. J. Clin. Nutr. 70(suppl):532S–538S, 1999.
27. Janelle, K. C., and Barr, S. I. Nutrient intakes and eating behavior scores of vegetarian and nonvegetarian women. J. Am. Diet. Assoc. 95:180–189, 1995.
28. Jacob, R. A., and Burri, B. J. Oxidative damage and defense. Am. J. Clin. Nutr. 63(suppl):985S–990S, 1996.
29. Haddad, E. H., Sabaté, J., and Whitten, C. G. Vegetarian food guide pyramid: a conceptual framework. Am. J. Clin. Nutr. 70(suppl): 615S–619S, 1999.

7 Energy Balance and Regulation of Body Weight

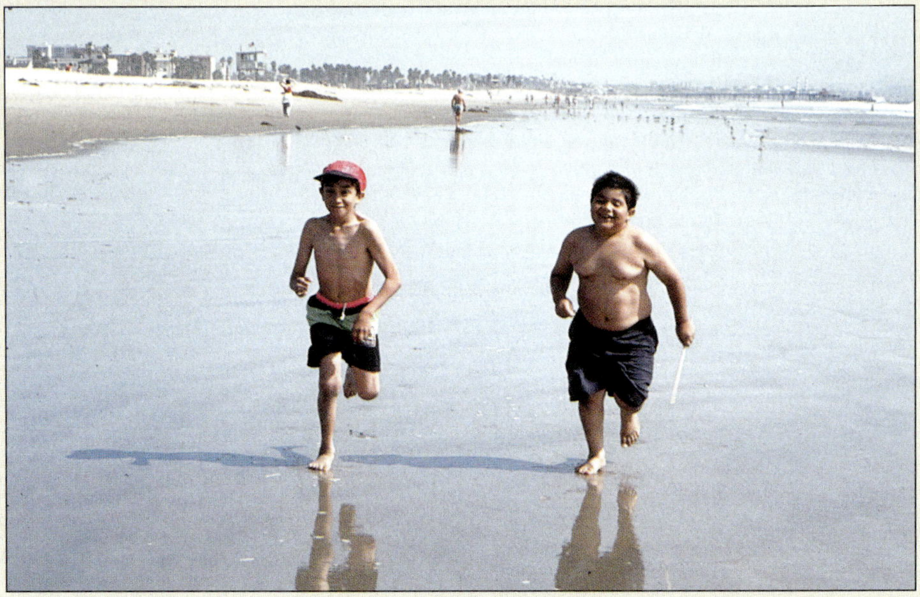

Learning Objectives

After reading this chapter, students should be able to:

1. Define the term energy and discuss how it is measured in terms of human needs.
2. Describe the relationships between energy, catabolism, and anabolism.
3. Explain the principle of energy balance.
4. List the sources of energy in the diet and those that are available from body stores.
5. Define "BMR," "physical activity," and "TEF" and discuss the contribution each makes to total energy expenditure.
6. Explain why the recommendations for energy intake may be too high for some and too low for others.
7. Compare three methods of evaluating body weight and fat.
8. Discuss external and internal factors that affect hunger and satiety.
9. Explain how leptin is involved in the long-term regulation of energy balance.
10. Give an example of how genetic and environmental factors interact to determine energy balance and body fat.

She had always been "the fat one." She and her sister had the same parents, were only three years apart in age, and yet were very different. Sara had brown hair, long legs, and a slender build. Why had Erin ended up with freckles, red hair, and chunky thighs? Erin was always the one who could stand to lose a few pounds. She would rather read than ride her bike and often spent the afternoon munching chips while she studied. Then one day when she was a college freshman she decided she didn't want to be "the fat one" any more. She changed her diet and started an exercise program. At first it was just a walk after dinner, but soon exercise became part of her daily routine. She covered a few miles every day whether at the gym, on her bike, or jogging. The extra pounds disappeared. On the other hand, Sara, the slender one, had spent the fall finishing law school and studying for the bar exam. She passed the bar 30 pounds heavier than she had ever been. At a recent family reunion, she heard a distant relative say to her sister, "Didn't you used to be the fat one?" What happened? How could two women with the same parents have such different builds? And how could they change so much?

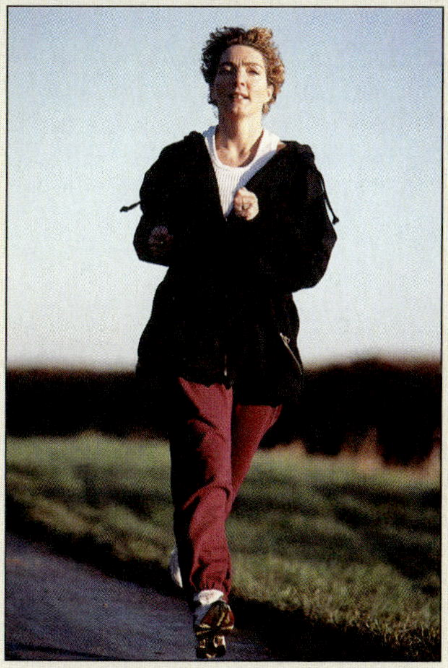

Although the two sisters have the same parents, they inherited different combinations of genes from them. These genes determined their body builds. However, lifestyle factors such as how much and what kind of food they eat and how much they exercise also affect body size. Sara inherited her slender build, but eating too much and exercising too little while she studied for the bar exam added pounds to her thin frame. Erin, on the other hand, may never have thin thighs, but when she exercises regularly and watches what she eats, she can maintain her weight in a healthy range. The principle of energy balance is simple: When energy consumption equals energy expenditure, weight remains constant. But, the mechanisms that regulate how much energy we consume and how much energy we expend are complex.

Energy Balance

In most people, body weight remains constant over long periods of time. This steady state is referred to as **energy balance.** It means that the total amount of energy in the body is neither increasing nor decreasing.

Energy Balance A state in which the amount of energy consumed is equal to the amount burned.

Energy

In the human body, **energy** is obtained from the energy-containing nutrients (carbohydrate, lipid, and protein) and alcohol in the diet and from energy stored in body tissues. Defined as the ability to do work, energy exists in many forms that can be converted from one to another. For example, the energy in flowing water can be converted into electrical energy, which can then be converted into the light energy emitted by a lightbulb (Figure 7.1). The transformations that occur in the human body are similar. For example, some of the chemical energy stored in a molecule of glucose can be converted into the energy in **adenosine triphosphate (ATP)**. In muscle, the process of muscle contraction converts the chemical

Energy The capacity to do work.

ATP (adenosine triphosphate) A high-energy molecule used by the body to perform energy-requiring activities.

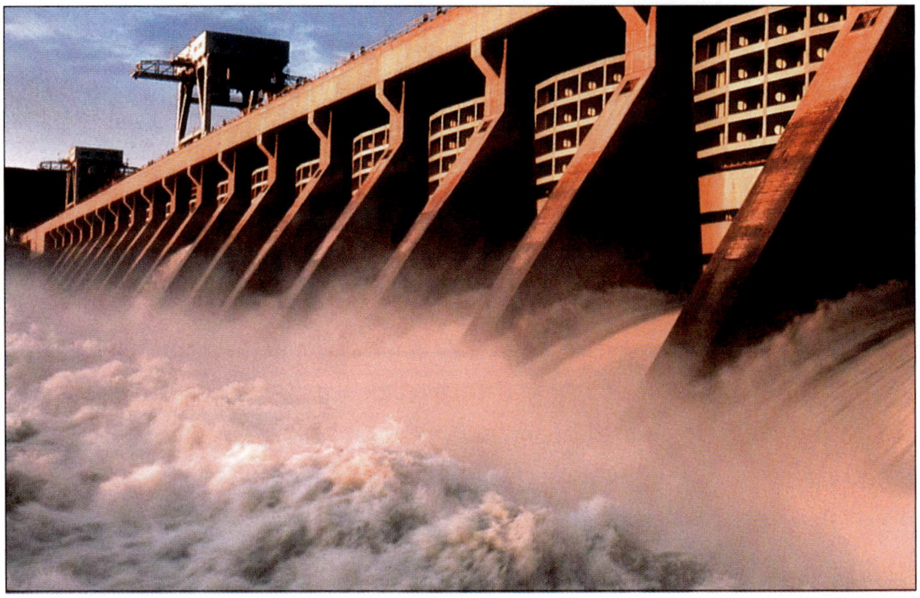

FIGURE 7.1 The energy in flowing water can be harnessed to produce electricity. *(USDOE)*

energy in the bonds of ATP to mechanical energy. Much of the energy consumed in food is converted to and lost from the body as heat.

Kilojoule (kjoule or kJ) The amount of work required to move an object weighing 1 kilogram a distance of 1 meter under the force of gravity.

Kilocalorie (kcalorie or kcal) The amount of heat required to raise the temperature of 1 kilogram of water 1 degree Celsius.

Energy is measured in **kilojoules (kjoules, kJ),** which are units of work, and in **kilocalories (kcalories, kcal),** which are units of heat. A kjoule is the amount of work required to move an object weighing 1 kilogram a distance of 1 meter under the force of gravity. In Europe, the kjoule is the standard measure of energy in food and the body. In the United States, kcalories are the measure most commonly used. Technically, a kcalorie is the amount of heat required to raise the temperature of 1 kilogram of water 1 degree Celsius. In practical terms, a kcalorie is a measure of the amount of energy that can be supplied to the body. We don't eat kcalories; we eat food, which provides energy measured in kcalories. Individuals who struggle with weight loss often think of kcalories as an enemy—something to be avoided. However, food and the energy it provides are essential to maintaining life. Just as gasoline is necessary to run an engine, kcalories are necessary to run the body.

Metabolism

Whether they involve the heart pumping blood through the vessels, the legs carrying the body weight up a flight of stairs, or the intestines contracting to move food through the gastrointestinal tract, body processes do work and therefore require energy. To obtain this energy, metabolic reactions break down carbohydrate, protein, and fat from the diet and the body (Figure 7.2 and Chapters 4–6). The released energy then fuels metabolic reactions that build and maintain body components and do work. The processes of metabolism that break down molecules to produce energy and those that use energy to build body structures occur continually and simultaneously in the body.

Catabolic reactions Energy-releasing reactions in which substances are broken down into simpler molecules.

Anabolic reactions Energy-requiring reactions in which simpler molecules are combined to form more complex substances.

Catabolism is the sum of all reactions that break down body compounds, releasing energy. **Catabolic reactions** take larger molecules and break them into smaller units. The reactions of cellular respiration are catabolic, breaking glucose, fatty acids, and amino acids into carbon dioxide and water and producing energy in the form of ATP. ATP contains three phosphate groups, two of which are linked by chemical bonds that are very high in energy (Figure 7.3). When these bonds are broken, the energy released can be used to fuel **anabolic reactions,** to

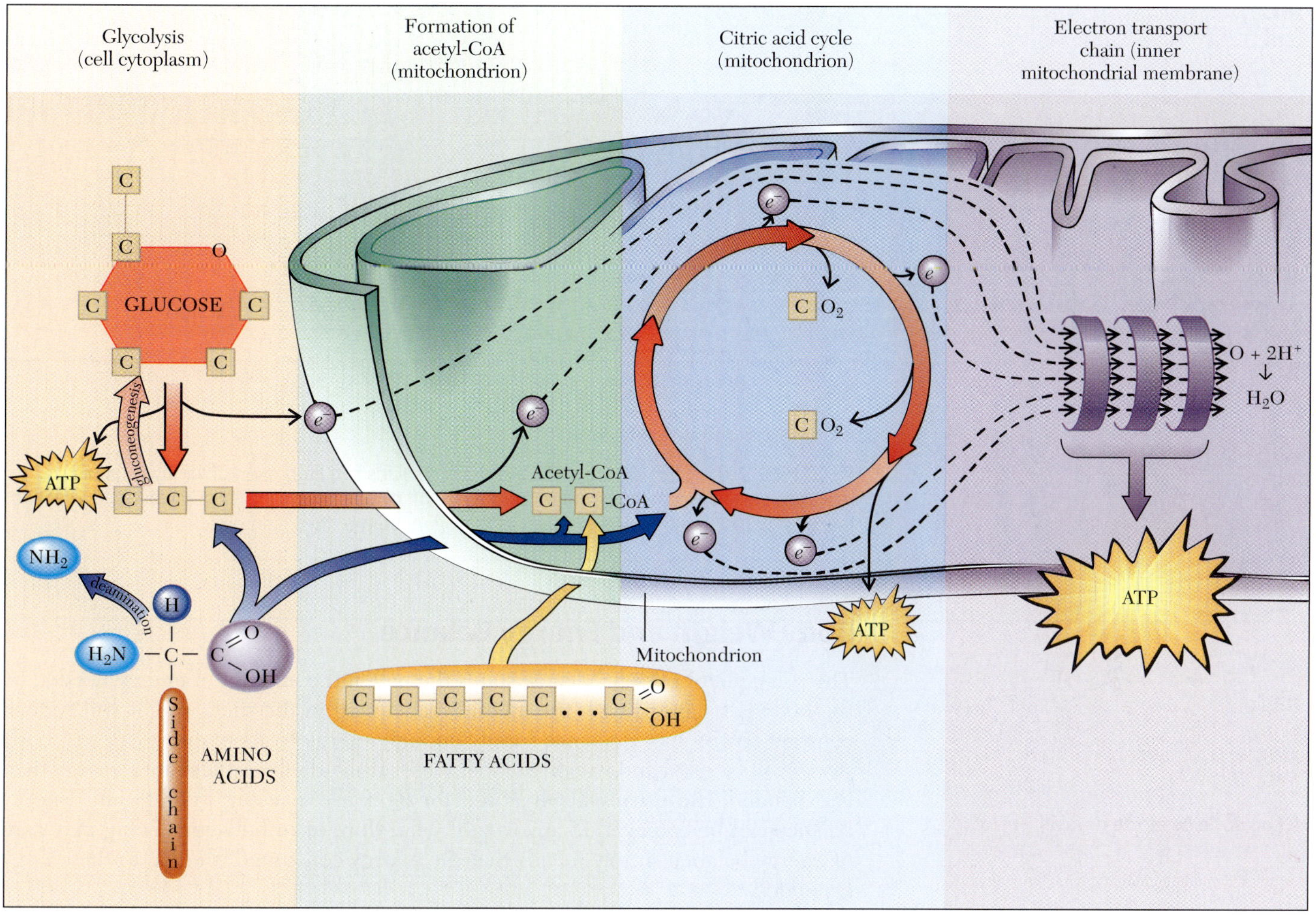

FIGURE 7.2 Energy is consumed in the diet as carbohydrates, triglycerides, and proteins. Glucose, fatty acids, and amino acids from these macromolecules can be broken down by the reactions of cellular respiration to yield carbon dioxide, water, and energy in the form of ATP.

maintain the internal environment of the body, to power activity, or do other body work.

The sum of reactions that build body compounds is referred to as anabolism. Anabolic reactions use molecules such as glucose, amino acids, or acetyl-CoA to form larger, more complex molecules such as glycogen, proteins, or fatty acids. Anabolic processes synthesize the carbohydrate, lipid, protein, and other molecules that are needed for structural and regulatory functions in the body. These reactions require energy (Figure 7.4).

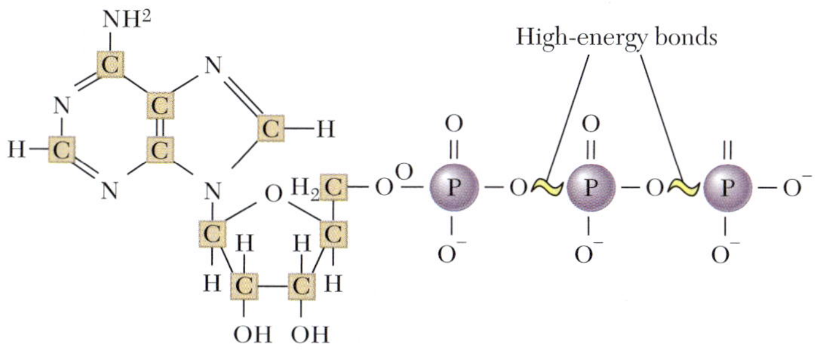

FIGURE 7.3 ATP contains two high-energy phosphate bonds shown here as wavy lines. When these bonds are broken, energy is released.

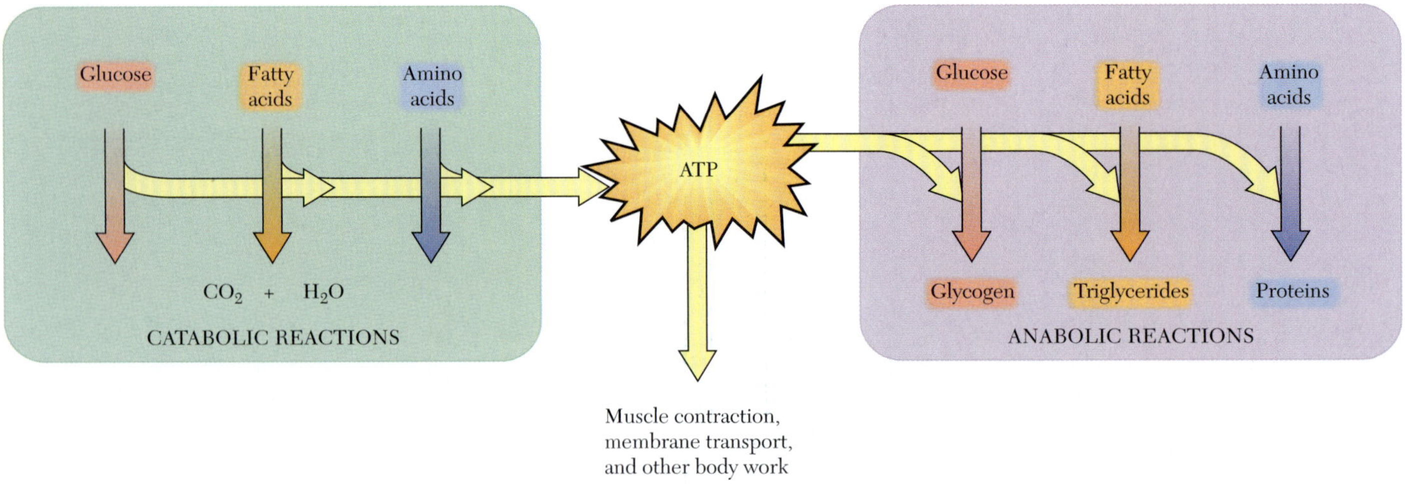

FIGURE 7.4 Glucose, fatty acids, and amino acids can be broken down by catabolic reactions, releasing energy in the form of ATP. ATP can be used to fuel body work and anabolic reactions, which build molecules such as glycogen, triglycerides, and proteins.

Body Weight and Energy Balance

The principle of energy balance states that when the amount of energy needed by the body is balanced with the amount consumed in the diet, weight will remain constant. If the diet does not supply enough energy to meet energy needs, body stores will be used and weight will decrease. If the diet supplies more energy than is expended, the extra will be stored for later use, causing weight gain. Energy balance can be achieved at any weight—fat, thin, or in between. Being in a state of energy balance simply means that the energy consumed is equal to the energy expended.

Energy Sources

Energy is supplied to the body by food. The amount of energy depends on the volume of food consumed and its nutrient composition.

Energy in Food

The energy content of the food we eat can be estimated from its nutrient composition or measured precisely in the laboratory. Protein and carbohydrate provide 4 kcalories per gram, alcohol provides 7 kcalories per gram, and fat provides 9 kcalories per gram.

Determining the Energy Content of a Diet The energy content of a diet can be calculated by summing the energy content of each food in the diet. When the nutrient composition of a food is known, the energy content can be approximated by totaling the energy from the carbohydrate, fat, protein, and alcohol in the food. For example, 5 g of sugar, which is almost pure carbohydrate, contains about 20 kcalories (5 g × 4 kcal/g of carbohydrate). Five grams of corn oil, which is almost pure fat, contains about 45 kcalories (5 g × 9 kcal/g of fat). The energy content of a mixed food can be calculated by multiplying the weight of each nutrient by the energy it provides (see Table 7.1). Vitamins, minerals, and water, though essential nutrients necessary for energy production, do not provide energy to the body.

TABLE 7.1 Estimating the Energy Content of Food

Determine:

- The number of grams of carbohydrate, protein, fat, and alcohol in a food or meal

Calculate the Energy Provided by Each:

grams of carbohydrate	× 4 kcal/g = kcal from carbohydrate
grams of protein	× 4 kcal/g = kcal from protein
grams of fat	× 9 kcal/g = kcal from fat
grams of alcohol	× 7 kcal/g = kcal from alcohol

Calculate the Total Energy:

- Total kcal = (kcal from carbohydrate) + (kcal from protein) + (kcal from fat) + (kcal from alcohol)

Example:

- A half-cup (100 g) serving of macaroni and cheese contains 8 grams of protein, 20 grams of carbohydrate, and 11 grams of fat:

20 grams of carbohydrate	× 4 kcal/g = 80 kcal
8 grams of protein	× 4 kcal/g = 32 kcal
11 grams of fat	× 9 kcal/g = 99 kcal

Total = 80 kcal + 32 kcal + 99 kcal = 211 kcal

Values for the energy content of foods are published in food composition databases and tables. Food labels are also a source of this information; the Nutrition Facts portion lists the total kcalories in a serving of food. The energy content of foods in a diet can also be estimated from the Exchange Lists (Table 7.2). The serving size of each food within an exchange is chosen to provide the same amount of energy. For example, one starch exchange, whether a slice of bread, one-half cup (100 g) of cereal, or six saltines, provides about 80 kcalories.

TABLE 7.2 Energy Content of Exchange Lists

Exchange Groups/Lists	Serving Size	Energy (kcal)
Carbohydrate Group		
Starch	1/2 cup pasta, rice, cereal, potatoes; 1 slice bread	80
Fruit	1 small apple, peach, pear; 1/2 banana; 1/2 cup canned fruit (in juice)	60
Milk	1 cup milk or yogurt	
Nonfat		90
Low-fat		110
Reduced-fat		120
Whole		150
Other carbohydrates	Serving sizes vary	Varies
Vegetables	1/2 cup cooked vegetables, 1 cup raw	25
Meat/Meat Substitute Group	1 oz meat or cheese; 1/2 cup legumes	
Very lean		35
Lean		55
Medium fat		75
High fat		100
Fat Group	1 tsp butter, margarine, or oil; 1 Tbsp salad dressing	45

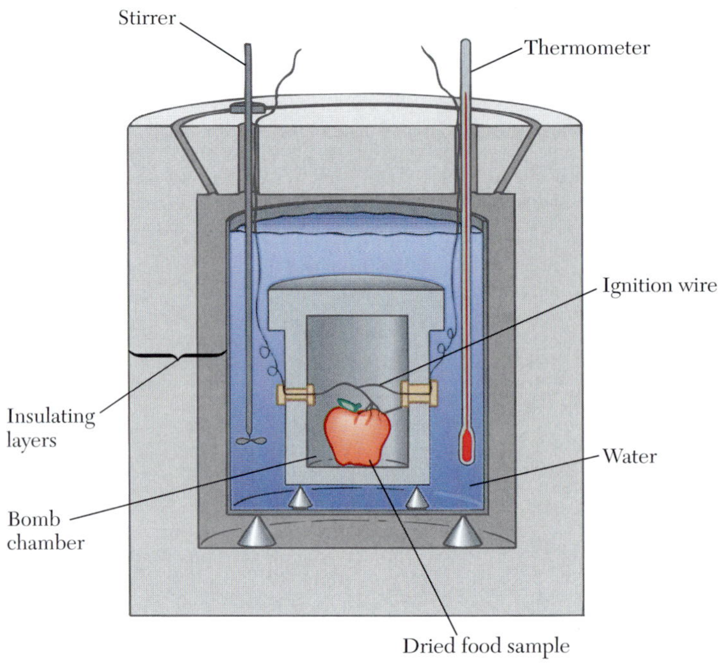

FIGURE 7.5 The energy content of a food can be determined by combusting a dried sample in the chamber of a bomb calorimeter and measuring the rise in temperature of the water surrounding the chamber.

Bomb calorimeter An instrument used to determine the energy content of food. It measures the heat energy released when a food is combusted.

Measuring the Energy Content of Food in the Laboratory The amount of energy in a food or a mixture of foods can be determined in the laboratory using a **bomb calorimeter.** A bomb calorimeter consists of a chamber surrounded by a jacket of water (Figure 7.5). Food is dried, placed in the chamber, and burned. As the food combusts, heat is released, raising the temperature of the water. The increase in water temperature can be used to calculate the amount of energy in the food based on the fact that 1 kcalorie is the amount of heat needed to increase the temperature of 1 kilogram of water by 1 degree Celsius.

Combusting a food in a bomb calorimeter determines the total amount of energy contained in that food. However, because the body cannot completely digest, absorb, and utilize all of the substances in a food, bomb calorimeter values are slightly higher than the amount of energy the body can obtain from that food. To correct for this difference, feeding experiments have been done to measure the energy not available to the body, such as that lost in urine and feces. Subtracting this unavailable energy from the values determined by the bomb calorimeter gives a more accurate estimate of the energy available to the body. These types of experiments determined the amount of energy in a mixed diet contributed by carbohydrate, fat, protein, and alcohol (4, 9, 4, 7 kcal/g respectively). As discussed earlier, these values are then used to calculate the amount of energy the body obtains from a food based on its macronutrient composition.

Energy Stores in the Body

Energy is stored in the body as glycogen and triglycerides. These stores come from nutrients consumed in the diet that are not used to meet immediate energy needs. This stored energy can be used when intake is less than needs, whether this occurs between meals or over the long term.

Using Body Stores The body must have a steady supply of energy, and some of it must come from glucose, which is needed to fuel cells in the brain and several other types of body cells. As we eat, energy is supplied by the diet. Between meals body stores are used to meet energy needs. Typically, these stores are then replaced by energy consumed in the next meal so that there is no net change in the amount of stored energy. However, if energy stores are not replenished, the amount of stored energy—and hence, body weight—will decrease.

TABLE 7.3 Sources of Stored Energy in the Body

Energy Source	Primary Location	Energy (kcalories)*
Glycogen	Liver and muscle	1400
Glucose or lipid	Body fluids	100
Triglyceride	Adipose tissue	115,000
Protein	Muscle	25,000

*Values represent the approximate amounts in a 70-kg male.

Cahill, G. F. Starvation in man. N. Engl. J. Med. 282:668–675, 1970; and Frayn, K. *Metabolic Regulation: A Human Perspective*. London: Portland Press, 1996, 78–102.

Energy needs are met between meals by the breakdown of glycogen to provide glucose, and of fat, to meet other energy needs. But, because glycogen stores are limited, over the long term the body must shift the way it uses energy to ensure that glucose continues to be available. The body generally stores only about 200 to 500 g of glycogen—enough to provide glucose for about 24 hours (see Table 7.3). Once these stores have been depleted, glucose is then supplied by the breakdown of small amounts of body protein, primarily muscle protein, to yield amino acids. Amino acids can then be used to make glucose via gluconeogenesis (see Chapters 4 and 6). Because protein is not stored in the body, protein breakdown to provide energy and glucose results in the loss of functional body proteins.

Energy for tissues that don't require glucose is provided by the breakdown of stored fat. If the supply of glucose is limited, such as during starvation, fatty acids delivered to the liver cannot be completely oxidized, so ketones are produced (see Chapter 4). Ketones can be used as an energy source by many tissues. After about three days of starvation, even the brain adapts to meet some of its energy needs from ketones (see Chapter 5). This reduces the amount of glucose needed and so slows the rate of protein breakdown.

During prolonged restriction of energy intake, substantial amounts of fat are used to provide energy and protein is degraded to provide glucose. This results in weight loss. The magnitude of the change in body weight depends on the degree of energy deficit and the length of time over which it occurs (see Chapter 8). It is estimated that an energy deficit of about 3500 kcalories results in the loss of a pound of fat.

Building Body Stores People typically eat three to six times during the day. The sum of the intake for all of these meals and snacks must meet energy needs for weight to remain stable, but at each occasion more energy is likely to be consumed than is needed at that moment in time. When excess energy is consumed, we generally say this excess is stored as fat. This is an oversimplification of a complex situation. After eating, the body prioritizes how nutrients are used based on body needs, which nutrients can be stored, and how efficiently they can be stored. Excess energy consumed over the long term will be stored as fat regardless of the composition of the diet.

Excess Energy Intake Increases Storage of Dietary Fat There is a metabolic hierarchy as to how nutrients are used. Because alcohol is toxic and cannot be stored in the body, it is rapidly **oxidized** for fuel. Amino acids from dietary protein are used to meet needs for the synthesis of body proteins and nonprotein molecules; any excess is then oxidized because there is no mechanism for storing them as amino acids or proteins. Carbohydrate is used to maintain blood glucose and to build glycogen stores. Once glycogen stores are full, the remaining carbohydrate is oxidized for energy. The body is capable of converting carbohydrate and amino acids into fat for storage. However, under normal dietary circumstances, this rarely occurs.[1] Most of the fat that is stored in

Oxidize To breakdown a molecule in the presence of oxygen to yield energy.

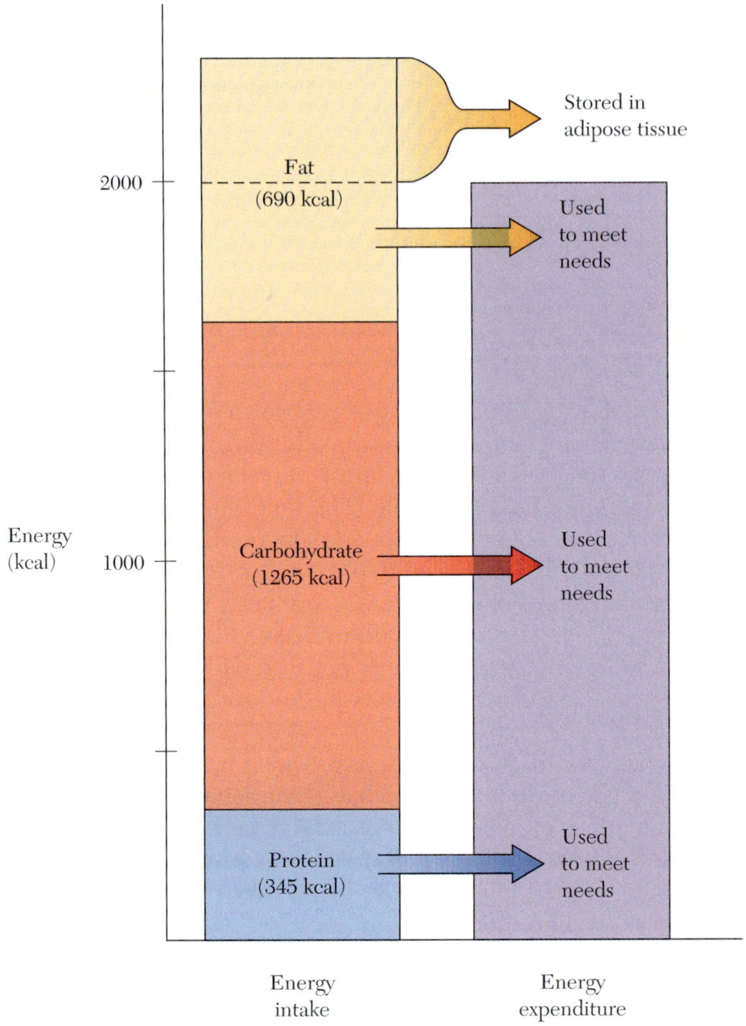

FIGURE 7.6 Although the body is capable of synthesizing fat from carbohydrate or protein, this generally does not occur to a great extent. Dietary carbohydrate and protein are preferentially oxidized to meet energy needs. Fat is then oxidized also, but if intake exceeds expenditure, the excess fat is stored. An example of a 2300-kcalorie mixed diet, consisting of 55% of energy from carbohydrate, 30% from fat, and 15% from protein, is shown here. It would provide 1265 kcalories from carbohydrate, 690 kcalories from fat, and 345 kcalories from protein. If energy expenditure was 2000 kcalories per day, the energy supplied by carbohydrate and protein together (1265 kcal + 345 kcal = 1610 kcal) would be insufficient to meet needs. Some of the fat would be oxidized to meet the remaining energy needs (2000 − 1610 = 390 kcal), but the remaining 300 kcalories from fat would not be needed and would be stored in adipose tissue.

Adipocytes Fat-storing cells.

the body comes from dietary fat. Fat, unlike the other energy-containing nutrients, is not needed as fuel or to build tissues and can be stored in the body in virtually unlimited amounts. Therefore, dietary fat is preferentially stored unless carbohydrate and protein do not meet immediate energy needs. In this situation, enough fat is oxidized to meet immediate energy needs and any remaining dietary fat is stored as triglycerides, primarily in adipose tissue (Figure 7.6).

Adipose tissue is made up of fat cells, or **adipocytes.** Adipocytes store triglycerides that they pick up from the blood with the help of the enzyme lipoprotein lipase (LPL). These cells grow in size as they accumulate more fat (Figure 7.7). The greater the number of adipocytes an individual has, the greater the ability to store fat. Most adipocytes are formed between infancy and adolescence. In adulthood, only excessive weight gain can cause the production of new fat cells.

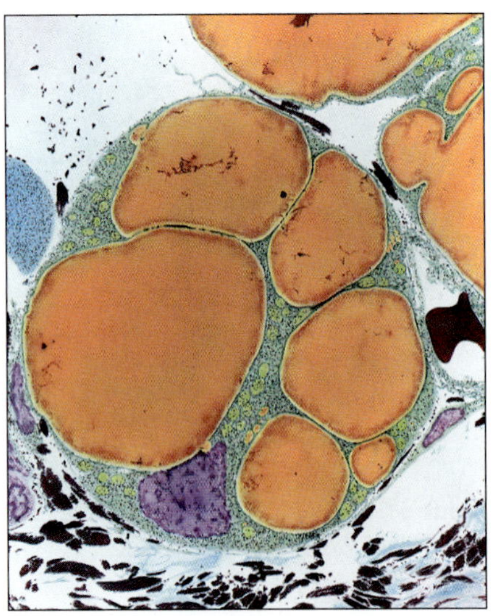

FIGURE 7.7 Adipocytes contain droplets of fat surrounded by other cell components. As body fat is gained, the size of the fat droplets increases. *(© Ed Reschke/ Peter Arnold, Inc.)*

Making Fat from Carbohydrate and Protein The body is capable of converting carbohydrate and amino acids into triglycerides for storage. However, these conversions are energetically costly. Making fat from glucose involves converting glucose to acetyl Co-A and then assembling fatty acids from the 2-carbon acetyl-CoA units. The fatty acids must then be joined to a molecule of glycerol to make triglycerides for storage. These conversions cost the cell about 20% of the energy originally present in the carbohydrate. The costs of converting amino acids into fat are even greater. The amino group must first be removed from each amino acid and then the carbon skeleton must be broken down to yield acetyl-CoA that

Making Decisions

Fat Burners: The Hot and the Cold

Do you have an extra ten pounds that you'd rather not carry around with you? You start an exercise program and lose a few pounds, but as weight loss slows, so does your motivation and soon the weight is back? Wouldn't it be nice if there were a pill that you could take to increase your metabolism without breaking a sweat? There are many dietary supplements that claim to do just this—but do they work and are they safe?

Weight loss supplements that claim to increase metabolism are called fat burners or thermogenic stimulators. They promise to boost metabolism, prevent loss of lean muscle tissue, suppress appetite, and increase the burning of stored fat. Most of these products contain some vitamins, minerals, and amino acids along with central nervous system stimulants such as ephedrine (ephedra) and methylxanthines (compounds such as caffeine found in coffee and theophylline found in tea). Many also contain aspirin.

Do they really boost metabolism? Ephedrine is a decongestant and a central nervous system stimulant that increases heart rate and blood pressure. It stimulates nerves called adrenergic neurons that (among other effects) inhibit hunger and stimulate energy expenditure, fat breakdown, and fat oxidation. There are different types of adrenergic neurons with different effects. Stimulation of a combination of adrenergic neurons can increase energy expenditure by 5 to 10% and increase the relative proportion of fat that is burned. This may be the mechanism responsible for the weight loss caused by agents such as ephedrine plus caffeine.[a] Research supports the claim that the combination of ephedrine and caffeine increases thermogenesis, depresses appetite, and enhances fat loss when compared to a placebo.[b] The addition of aspirin to this combination does not appear to further increase the thermic effect.[c] A mixture of ephedrine, caffeine, and theophylline was also shown to increase energy expenditure, particularly in individuals predisposed to obesity.[d] The results of this study suggested that dietary methylxanthines may work mainly by increasing the thermogenic response to food in individuals predisposed to obesity.[d]

Are fat burners the magic bullet that will help keep Americans slim? Despite evidence that they do increase energy expenditure, the cost to overall health may be higher than that of the extra pounds. Ephedrine is a powerful drug with dangerous side effects. Between 1993 and 1995 the Texas Department of Health received 500 reports of adverse effects, including eight deaths, in people who consumed dietary supplements containing ephedrine and substances related to ephedrine.[e] Side effects range from nervousness, dizziness, headache, gastrointestinal distress, and changes in blood pressure and heart rate to chest pain, heart attack, hepatitis, stroke, seizures, psychosis, and death. Combinations of caffeine and ephedrine cause side effects that are more severe than those caused by either compound alone. These symptoms have occurred in young, otherwise healthy individuals as well as those with other confounding conditions such as hypertension.

What if the supplement is "all natural"? Aspirin, ephedrine, and caffeine sound more like drugs than natural ingredients, and they are. But, supplements can contain these compounds and still claim to be "all natural" by using herbal sources. For example, *Citrus aurantium* is an herb that contains a chemical derivative of ephedrine called synephrine; Ma Huang is a Chinese herb that contains ephedrine; gaurana extract is an herbal source of caffeine; and white willow bark extract contains salicin, a compound similar to aspirin. Just because these compounds are added as components of herbs does not mean they are any less biologically active or cause fewer side effects than when they are present in over-the-counter or prescription medications.

So, should you take a fat burner or keep up your routine at the gym? The risks of ephedrine-containing supplements are very real and there is no evidence of long-term benefits. Boosting metabolism may cause short-term weight loss, but eventually intake is likely to catch up with expenditure, causing weight loss to slow or stop. The weight may be regained even with the supplement. To lose weight and keep it off requires changes in lifestyle and the behaviors that led to the accumulation of extra pounds in the first place.

References

[a] Astrup, A., and Lundsgaard, C. What do pharmacological approaches to obesity management offer? Linking pharmacological mechanisms of obesity management agents to clinical practice. Exp. Clin. Endocrinol. Diabetes 106 (Suppl 2): 29–34, 1998.

[b] Astrup, A., Toubro, S., Christensen, N. J., and Quaade, F. Pharmacology of thermogenic drugs. Am. J. Clin. Nutr. 55(1 suppl):246S–248S, 1992.

[c] Horton, T. J., and Geissler, C. A. Postprandial thermogenesis with ephedrine, caffeine and aspirin in lean, and predisposed obese and obese women. Int. J. Obes. Relat. Metab. Disord. 20:91–97, 1996.

[d] Dulloo, A. G., and Miller, D. S. The thermogenic properties of ephedrine/methylxanthine mixtures: human studies. Int. J. Obes. 10:467–481, 1986

[e] MMWR August 16, 1996: Adverse events associated with ephedrine-containing products—Texas, December 1993–September 1995. Available online at **http://vm.cfsan.fda.gov/~dms/ephedrin.html**. Accessed 25 Apr 2000.

can be used for fatty acid synthesis. In contrast, the conversion of dietary fat to body fat requires only the removal and reattachment of fatty acids to the glycerol backbone (see Chapter 5); the metabolic cost of converting dietary fat to stored body fat is 2 to 3% of the energy present. It is therefore more efficient for the body to oxidize carbohydrate and protein to meet immediate energy needs than to convert it to fat. The conversion of carbohydrate to fat becomes important only when the diet is composed primarily of carbohydrate and energy intake exceeds expenditure.[1] (See *Making Decisions*: "Fat Burners: The Hot and the Cold.")

Energy Expenditure

The energy expended by the body is the sum of all the energy needed for body functions. Some of this energy is used in anabolic reactions and processes such as muscle contraction. This energy utilization can be categorized based on whether it is needed to maintain basic body functions, to fuel physical activity, or to process the nutrients consumed in food.

Basal Metabolic Rate (BMR)

Basal metabolic rate (BMR) The minimum amount of energy that an awake resting body needs to maintain itself. BMR measurements are performed in a warm room in the morning before the subject rises, and at least 12 hours after the last food or activity.

For most people, the energy needed for the maintenance of basic body functions such as breathing, circulating blood, and maintaining a constant body temperature makes up 60 to 75% of the body's total energy requirement. This portion of the energy requirement is called the **basal metabolic rate (BMR),** which is the minimum amount of energy needed to keep an awake, resting body alive. BMR includes the energy necessary for all essential metabolic reactions and life-sustaining functions, but it does not include the energy needed for physical activity or for the digestion and absorption of food. To eliminate any residual energy expenditure from activity or digestion and absorption, BMR measurements must be performed in the morning in a warm room before the subject rises and at least 12 hours after food intake or activity. Because of the difficulty of achieving these conditions, measures of basal needs are usually made after only five to six hours without food or exercise. These measures yield values referred to as **resting energy expenditure (REE)** or **resting metabolic rate (RMR).** The difference between BMR and RMR values is less than 10% in most cases.[2]

Resting metabolic rate (RMR) or **resting energy expenditure (REE)** An estimate of basal metabolic rate that is determined by measuring energy utilization after 5 to 6 hours without food or exercise.

Lean body mass Body mass attributed to nonfat body components such as bone, muscle, and internal organs. It is also called fat-free mass.

RMR is affected by factors such as body weight, **lean body mass,** gender, growth rate, and age. It increases with increasing body weight, so is higher in heavier individuals. It also rises with increasing lean body mass; thus, RMR is generally higher in men than in women because men have greater lean body mass. RMR increases during periods of rapid growth because energy is required to produce new body tissue. It decreases with age, partly due to a decrease in lean body mass that usually occurs in older adults.

RMR can be altered by certain abnormal conditions. An elevation in body temperature, such as that due to a fever, increases RMR. It is estimated that for every 1 degree Fahrenheit above normal body temperature, there is a 7% increase in RMR. This extra energy use explains why weight loss can occur with fever. Abnormal levels of thyroid hormones can also affect RMR. Individuals who overproduce these hormones burn more energy; in fact, a symptom used to diagnose thyroid hormone excess is unexplained weight loss. Individuals with an underproduction of thyroid hormones require less energy. The fact that hormones produced by the thyroid gland affect energy expenditure is the reason that obesity was once explained as a glandular problem. It is now known that obesity due to a thyroid hormone deficiency is rare.

RMR may also be affected by low-energy diets. Energy intake below needs may depress RMR by 10 to 20%, or the equivalent of 100 to 400 kcalories per day.[3] This drop in RMR decreases the amount of energy needed to maintain weight. It is a beneficial adaptation in starvation, but it makes intentional weight loss more difficult. (Table 7.4)

Web Menu For information on fitness and the energy requirements of various activities, go to the Fitness Jumpsite at www.primusweb.com/fitnesspartner/.

Physical Activity

Physical activity is the second major component of energy expenditure. It represents the metabolic cost of external work, which includes the energy needed for exercise as well as for the functions of daily life, such as sitting, standing, and

TABLE 7.4 Factors Affecting Energy Expenditure

Factor	Effect
Resting Metabolic Rate (RMR)	
Age	As one grows older, RMR decreases.
Growth	Growing children and adolescents have a higher RMR.
Weight	An increase in body size increases RMR.
Body composition	Lean body mass requires more energy, so RMR is greater in individuals with more muscle mass. Men therefore have higher RMRs than women.
Body shape	Tall, thin people have higher RMRs than short, stout people of the same weight because they have more surface area per unit of body weight for heat loss.
Body temperature	A rise in body temperature such as a fever increases RMR.
Stress	Stress increases RMR through hormones and the nervous system.
Hormones	An increase in thyroid hormones or growth hormone increases RMR.
Nutritional state	Fasting and starvation decrease RMR and overeating increases RMR.
Pregnancy	Pregnancy involves tissue growth and so increases RMR.
Lactation	Milk synthesis increases RMR.
Physical Activity	
Duration	Energy expenditure increases as the duration of activity increases.
Intensity	More intense activities require more energy.
Body weight	Heavier people expend more energy to move their bodies.
Thermic Effect of Food (TEF)	
Meal size	Large meals increase TEF because energy is needed to store nutrients.
Meal composition	High-fat meals require less energy to store than high-carbohydrate or high-protein meals.

walking. For most people, physical activity accounts for 15 to 30% of energy requirements, but this varies greatly. The energy required to perform an activity, such as walking, increases with increasing body weight because it takes more energy to move a heavier body. Energy requirements also depend on how strenuous the activity is and the length of time it is performed. A professional athlete who spends many hours a day training at a strenuous activity level uses a great deal more energy in daily activities than does an office worker who spends most of his day sitting at a desk. Because technological advances have reduced the amount of physical activity needed for daily tasks, people today need to make a conscious effort to increase their exercise. This does not necessarily mean running marathons; choosing to take the stairs rather than the elevator, walking rather than taking the bus, and riding a bike rather than driving to the store all increase activity (Figure 7.8). The energy costs of specific activities are listed in Appendix K.

Thermic Effect of Food (TEF)

The **thermic effect of food (TEF),** also called **diet-induced thermogenesis,** is the increase in energy expenditure above BMR that occurs during the several hours after the ingestion of food. This effect is due to the metabolic cost of digesting food and absorbing, metabolizing, and storing nutrients from the meal. These processes cause body temperature to rise slightly for several hours after eating. The energy required for TEF is estimated to be about 5 to 10% of energy intake but can vary depending on the amounts and types of nutrients consumed.

Thermic effect of food (TEF) or **diet-induced thermogenesis** The energy required for the digestion of food and the absorption, metabolism, and storage of nutrients. It is equal to approximately 10% of daily energy intake.

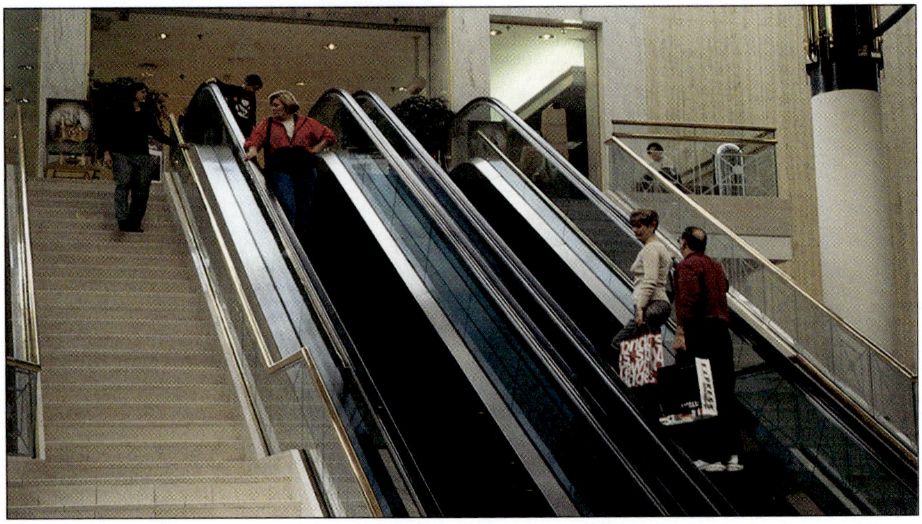

FIGURE 7.8 Even small increases or decreases in daily activity can affect energy balance. Walking up a flight of stairs burns three times as much energy as riding an escalator or an elevator. *(George Semple)*

Because it takes energy to store nutrients, TEF increases with the size of the meal. A meal that is high in fat has a lower TEF than a meal high in carbohydrate or protein, because dietary fat can be efficiently stored as body fat. The metabolic cost of either oxidizing or storing dietary fat is only 2 to 3% of the energy consumed, whereas the cost of using amino acids by either oxidizing them or incorporating them into proteins is 15 to 30% of the energy consumed, and the cost of oxidizing carbohydrate or storing it as glycogen is 6 to 8%.[4] The difference in the cost of storing energy means that a diet high in fat may produce more body fat than a diet high in carbohydrate.[5]

Energy Requirements

The amount of energy needed to maintain body weight is the sum of the needs for RMR, physical activity, and TEF (Figure 7.9). The energy expended by the body can be measured in a number of ways—some more precise than others. These estimations are then used to develop recommendations for energy intakes that will meet the needs of the general population for maintenance and growth.

Measuring Energy Expenditure

The most direct method for determining energy expenditure is to measure the heat produced by the body. Other methods make estimations based on measurements of the amount of oxygen used and carbon dioxide produced. Because of the equipment involved, these methods are not often used to determine individual requirements; rather, they are used experimentally to make estimates for the energy requirements of the general population.

Direct calorimetry A method of determining energy use that measures the amount of heat produced.

Direct Calorimetry The combustion of food in a bomb calorimeter is a type of **direct calorimetry.** Direct calorimetry can be used to measure energy expenditure in people by measuring the amount of heat given off by the body; the heat produced is proportional to the amount of energy used by the individual. This heat is generated by metabolic reactions that both convert food energy into ATP and use ATP for body processes.

Direct calorimetry is an accurate method for measuring energy expenditure, but it is expensive and impractical because it requires that the individual being assessed remain in an insulated chamber throughout the evaluation.

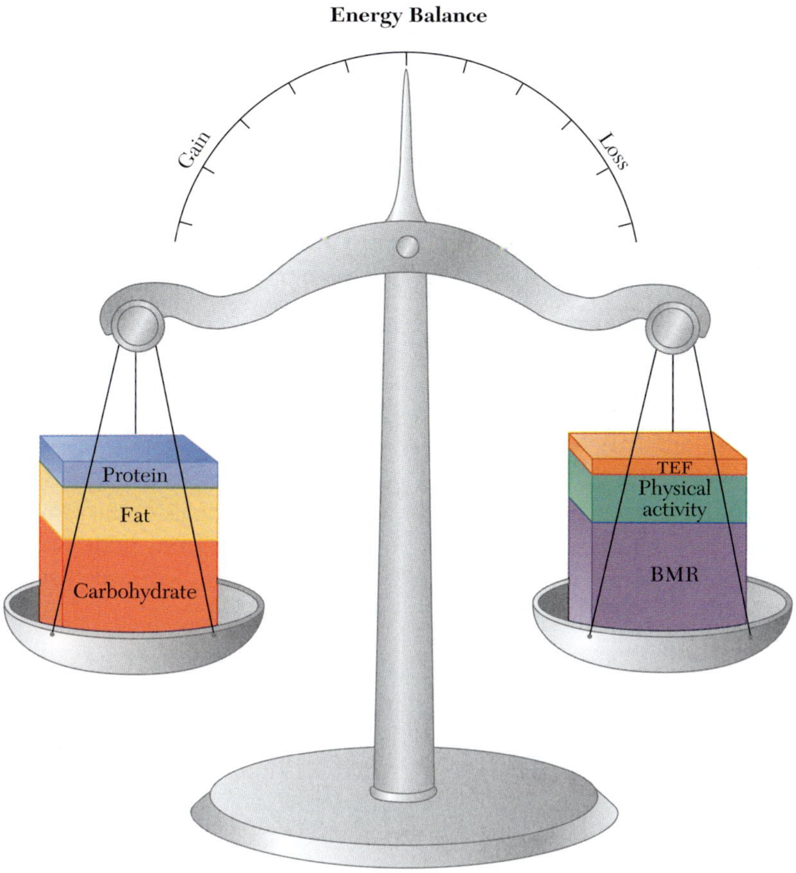

FIGURE 7.9 When the amount of energy expended by the body is balanced with the amount consumed, weight will remain stable.

Indirect Calorimetry The more commonly used method of estimating energy expenditure is **indirect calorimetry,** which estimates energy use by assessing nutrient utilization. One method of indirect calorimetry measures the amounts of oxygen consumed and carbon dioxide expired by the body. The body's energy use can be calculated from these values because the burning of fuels by the body in cellular respiration uses oxygen and produces carbon dioxide. Oxygen use and carbon dioxide production can be measured by analyzing the difference between inhaled and exhaled air.

Indirect calorimetry A method of estimating energy use that compares the amount of oxygen consumed to the amount of carbon dioxide expired.

Measuring respired gases requires that one breathe into a mask or ventilated hood so that the expired air can be measured. Some of these devices are large and designed for use in a hospital or research setting, but others are small and easily transported. Indirect calorimetry can be used to measure the energy used for individual components of expenditure, such as physical activity or RMR. It can also be used to estimate total energy needs, but it is not practical for measuring energy expenditure in free-living individuals because the equipment is uncomfortable and inappropriate for long-term use.

Total Daily Energy Expenditure Another type of indirect calorimetry involves having the individual ingest (or be injected with) water labeled with **isotopes** of oxygen and hydrogen. This is called the **doubly-labeled water method.** The labeled oxygen and hydrogen are used by the body in metabolism. By measuring the rate at which labeled oxygen and labeled hydrogen disappear from body fluids, the amount of carbon dioxide produced by the energy-requiring reactions in the body can be estimated.

Isotope An alternative form of an element that has a different atomic mass, which may or may not be radioactive.

Doubly-labeled water method An indirect calorimetry technique for measuring energy expenditure based on measuring the distribution of isotopes of hydrogen and oxygen in body fluids after consumption of a defined amount of water labeled with both isotopes.

The doubly-labeled water method does not require the individual to carry any equipment and can be used to measure expenditure in free-living subjects for periods up to two weeks. It has been used to estimate energy needs in some unusual situations. For example, one study measured the energy expenditure of mountain climbers during an ascent above 6000 meters and found it to be 4700 kcal/day.[6] Measurement of energy expenditure during short-term space flight revealed that it is similar to expenditure on Earth despite the lack of gravity.[7] Doubly-labeled water has also been used to validate dietary intake data obtained from diet records and histories. It is now the preferred method for determining the total daily energy expenditures of both healthy and clinical populations.[8] However, it is not helpful in determining the proportion of energy used for RMR, physical activity, or TEF.

Estimating Energy Needs

Energy needs can be estimated by totaling the approximate amount of energy expended for RMR, activity, and TEF.

Energy for RMR Resting metabolic rates for individuals of the same age, sex, and weight are fairly consistent and can be calculated from body weight using the equations given in Appendix N. Some of these have been calculated and are included in Table 7.5.

Energy for Physical Activity The energy required for various activities has been estimated using both direct and indirect calorimetry. These are available in tables and databases and can be expressed in a number of ways. Appendix K lists the energy costs of specific activities per hour; these energy costs can be multiplied by the time spent exercising to estimate energy use for that activity. Table 7.6 gives estimates of energy requirements for categories of activity based on RMR. The energy needed for RMR plus physical activity can be calculated by multiplying RMR per hour by the activity factor.

Total Energy Needs The energy needed for the thermic effect of food can be approximated as 10% of total energy intake. The sum of BMR or RMR, activity, and TEF equals the total daily energy requirement to maintain weight. See Table 7.7 for an example of how to calculate energy expenditure.

TABLE 7.5 Resting Metabolic Rate Based on Body Weight

Body Weight (kg)	40	50	57	64	70	77	84	91	100
(lb)	88	110	125	140	155	170	185	200	220
Kcalories per 24 hours									
Male									
Age (yr)									
10–18	1351	1526	1648	1771	1876	1998	2121	2243	2401
18–30	1291	1444	1551	1658	1750	1857	1964	2071	2209
30–60	1343	1459	1540	1621	1691	1772	1853	1935	2039
> 60	1027	1162	1256	1351	1423	1526	1621	1716	1837
Female									
Age (yr)									
10–18	1234	1356	1441	1527	1660	1685	1771	1856	1966
18–30	1084	1231	1334	1437	1525	1628	1731	1833	1966
30–60	1177	1264	1325	1386	1438	1499	1560	1621	1699
> 60	1016	1121	1195	1268	1331	1404	1478	1552	1646

Adapted from National Research Council, Food and Nutrition Board. *Recommended Dietary Allowances*, 10th ed. Washington, D.C.: National Academy of Sciences, 1989.

TABLE 7.6 Energy Requirements of Activities in Relation to Resting Metabolic Rate

Level of Activity	Activity Factor per Unit Time of Activity
Resting Sleeping, reclining	RMR × 1.0
Very light Seated and standing activities, painting, driving, laboratory work, typing, sewing, ironing, cooking, playing cards, playing musical instrument	RMR × 1.5
Light Walking on a level surface (2.5–3 mph), garage work, carpentry, house cleaning, child care, golf, sailing, table tennis	RMR × 2.5
Moderate Walking 3.5–4 mph, weeding and hoeing, carrying a load, cycling, skiing, tennis, dancing	RMR × 5
Heavy Walking with load uphill, tree felling, heavy manual digging, basketball, climbing, football, soccer	RMR × 7

National Research Council, Food and Nutrition Board. *Recommended Dietary Allowances*, 10th ed. Washington, D.C.: National Academy of Sciences, 1989.

TABLE 7.7 Calculating Total Energy Expenditure

Determine Energy for RMR

- Use Table 7.5 or Appendix B to determine daily energy needs for RMR based on age, weight, and sex.
- Calculate RMR per hour: RMR per day ÷ 24 hours per day = RMR per hour

  Example: A 23-year-old female who weighs 125 lb has an RMR of 1334 kcal/day 1334 kcal/day ÷ 24 hr = 55.6 kcal/hr.

Estimate Activity Level

- Estimate the number of hours per day spent in each activity category listed in Table 7.6

Calculate Energy for RMR Plus Physical Activity

- Multiply the number of hours spent at each level by the activity factor and RMR per hour

  Example: A 23-year-old female who spends 8 hours resting, 12 hours engaged in very light activity, and 4 hours engaged in light activity, would expend:

8 hours of resting requires 8 hr × (1 × RMR in kcal/hr)
= 8 hr × 1 × 55.6 kcal/hr = 445 kcalories

12 hours of very light activity requires 12 hr × (1.5 × RMR in kcal/hr)
= 12 hr × 1.5 × 55.6 kcal/hr = 1001 kcalories

4 hours of light activity requires 4 hr × (2.5 × RMR in kcal/hr)
= 4 hr × 2.5 × 55.6 kcal/hr) = 556 kcalories

Total energy required for RMR and activity = 2002 kcalories

Calculate Energy for the Thermic Effect of Food (TEF)

- TEF is about 10% of daily energy intake.

Example: A person consumes 2200 kcalories per day.
2200 kcalories × 10% = 220 kcalories.

Total Energy Expenditure

- Sum energy for RMR + physical activity and energy for TEF

  In this example, Total Energy Expenditure = 2002 + 220 = 2222 kcalories.

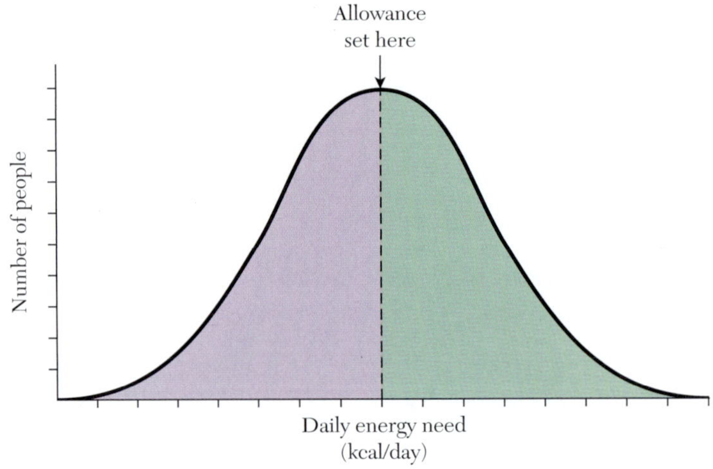

FIGURE 7.10 The recommended energy allowance is the average daily amount of energy needed by a specific gender and life-stage group. Individuals whose needs are below this average would gain weight if they consumed the recommended amount (purple), and those who require more energy than average would lose weight if they consumed the recommended amount (green).

Recommended Energy Intakes

The current standard for energy intake in the United States is the 1989 recommended energy allowances (the DRIs will replace these when they are completed). These values assume that individuals engage in light to moderate activity. For adults, values range from 30 to 40 kcalories per kilogram, depending on age and gender For example, the average energy allowance for a 51-year-old woman is about 30 kcalories per kilogram. The average energy allowance for a 23-year-old man is about 40 kcalories per kilogram (see inside front cover).

The 1989 energy allowances were calculated as the average amount of energy needed for weight maintenance by individuals in the same age and gender category. Because these values are expressed as an average, about half of individuals will have an actual requirement that is above the allowance, and the other half will have a requirement that is below the allowance (Figure 7.10).

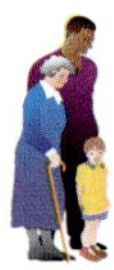

Energy needs per kilogram are higher during periods of rapid growth, such as infancy, adolescence, and pregnancy. The energy requirements for infants and children up to the age of ten are based on the amount needed for normal growth. From birth to six months of age, an intake of about 108 kcalories per kilogram of body weight is recommended. From one to three years, this decreases to about 102 kcalories per kilogram. Requirements per kilogram then drop off steadily until one reaches the age included in the adult recommendations—about age 25. With aging, requirements continue to decrease slowly because lean body mass and physical activity generally decrease.

Beginning with the onset of puberty, gender also affects energy requirements. The changes that occur with puberty cause an increase in muscle mass in males and in body fat in females. Because of these changes, males require more energy per kilogram than females.

Energy needs are increased during pregnancy. An additional 300 kcalories per day is recommended after the first three months of pregnancy. This is to allow for the growth of the fetus, placenta, and added maternal tissues. Additional energy is also needed to support lactation. An individual's energy needs during lactation increase with the volume of milk produced.

Web Menu For more information on the causes, consequences, diagnosis, and treatment of obesity, go to the National Institute of Diabetes & Digestive Kidney Diseases Weight Control Information Network at www.niddk.nih.gov/health/nutrit/win.htm.

Assessing Body Composition and Fat Stores

Body fat provides an energy store as well as insulation and protection, but too much body fat can increase the risk of chronic disease (see Chapter 8). There are many ways to measure body fat stores. The most common techniques measure body weight and make assumptions about body composition. Others make measurements that more directly assess body composition.

Body Composition

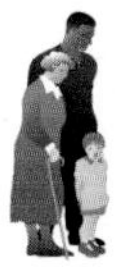

The body is composed of lean body mass and body fat. Lean body mass or fat-free mass includes bone, muscles, and all tissue except fat tissue. Body fat, or adipose tissue, lies under the skin and around internal organs. The amount of fat an individual carries and where that fat is deposited are affected by age and genetics as well as by energy balance.[9]

At birth, body fat is about 12% of body weight and increases in the first year of life. During childhood, as muscle mass increases, body fat decreases. During adolescence, females gain proportionately more fat and males gain more muscle mass. As adults, women have more stored body fat than men. A healthy level of body fat for a young adult female is between 20 and 30% of total weight; for young adult males, it is between 12 and 20%.[10] There is an increase in body fat during pregnancy to provide energy stores for the mother and fetus. With aging, lean body mass decreases; between the ages of 20 and 60, body fat typically doubles even if body weight remains the same.[11] This occurs regardless of energy intake. Some of this loss of lean body mass can be prevented by increasing physical activity.

Fat located under the skin is called **subcutaneous fat,** and that deposited around the organs is called **visceral fat.** Generally, fat in the hips and lower body is subcutaneous, whereas fat deposited around the waist in the abdominal region is primarily visceral fat. Where an individual deposits body fat is determined primarily by their genes.[12] For example, African-American women, who have an incidence of obesity that is 50% higher than that of Caucasian women, store less visceral fat.[13] Gender, age, and environment also influence where fat is stored. Visceral fat storage is more prevalent in men than in women. But after menopause, visceral fat increases in women. Stress, tobacco use, and alcohol consumption predispose people to visceral fat deposition, whereas activity reduces it.[14] The distribution of body fat affects the risks associated with carrying excess body fat. Excess visceral fat is associated with a higher incidence of heart disease, high blood pressure, stroke, diabetes, and breast cancer.

Subcutaneous fat Adipose tissue that is located under the skin.

Visceral fat Adipose tissue that is located around the body's internal organs.

Assessing Body Weight

Body fat stores can be estimated by evaluating weight for height. Tables of weight for height have historically been used as the standard for assessing body weight. Currently, **body mass index (BMI)**, which is calculated from a ratio of weight to height, is the standard for evaluating body weight. Although they do not directly assess percent body fat, BMI values correlate well with body fat in most people. An exception is athletes such as weight lifters or football players, who have an increased body weight due to a high level of muscle mass.

Body mass index (BMI) An index of weight in relation to height that is used to compare body size with a standard.

Body Mass Index Body mass index is calculated from the ratio of weight to height according to the following equation:

$$\text{BMI} = \frac{\text{weight in kg}}{(\text{height in m})^2}$$

$$\text{Or, BMI} = \frac{\text{weight in pounds}}{(\text{height in inches})^2} \times 704.5$$

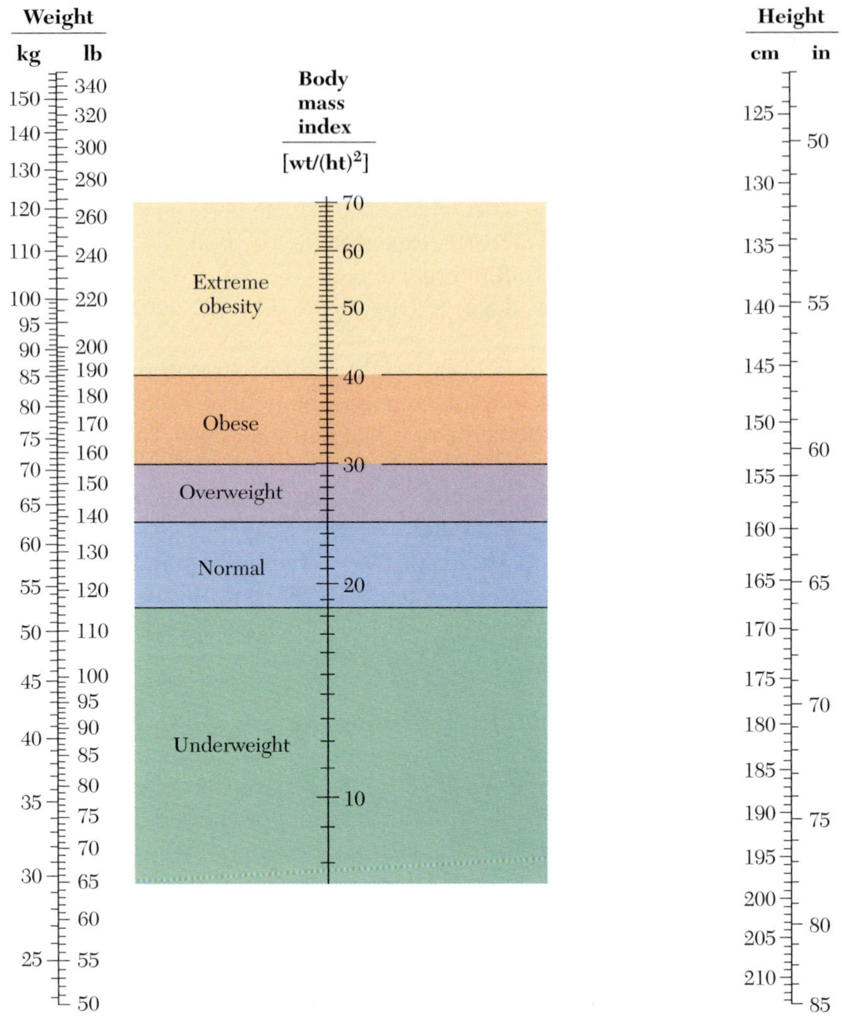

FIGURE 7.11 To determine body mass index using a nomogram, place a straightedge between your body weight in the left column and your height on the right. The point at which your line crosses the middle line is your body mass index. *(Copyright © 1978, George A. Bray. Used with permission.)*

For example, someone who is 6 feet (72 inches or 1.83 meters) tall and weighs 180 pounds (81.8 kg) has a body mass index of 24.5 kg/m^2. BMI can also be determined using the nomogram shown in Figure 7.11.

A healthy body weight is defined as a BMI between 18.5 to 24.9 kg/m^2. In general, people with a BMI within this range have the lowest health risks.[10] Underweight is defined as a body mass index of less than 18.5 kg/m^2, overweight is identified as 25 to 29.9 kg/m^2, and obese as 30 kg/m^2 or greater.[15] The increased health risks of being underweight or overweight are discussed in Chapter 8.

Weight Tables Weight tables that list ranges of healthy weight for height are still used in some settings to evaluate body weights.[15] The most commonly used weight tables are the Metropolitan Life Insurance Company tables. These present healthy weight ranges based on height, sex, and frame size, which is an approximation of weight due to bone mass (see Appendix B). The Metropolitan Life Insurance tables were developed by determining the weight at which individuals of a given age, sex, and height live the longest. Unfortunately, these tables were developed using weights recorded at the time individuals purchased insurance; because there was no follow-up to determine if individuals' weights had changed by the time of death, the weights in the table may not represent the healthiest weights. In addition, because they are based only on people who bought insurance, the values may underrepresent lower socioeconomic and minority groups who could not afford insurance.

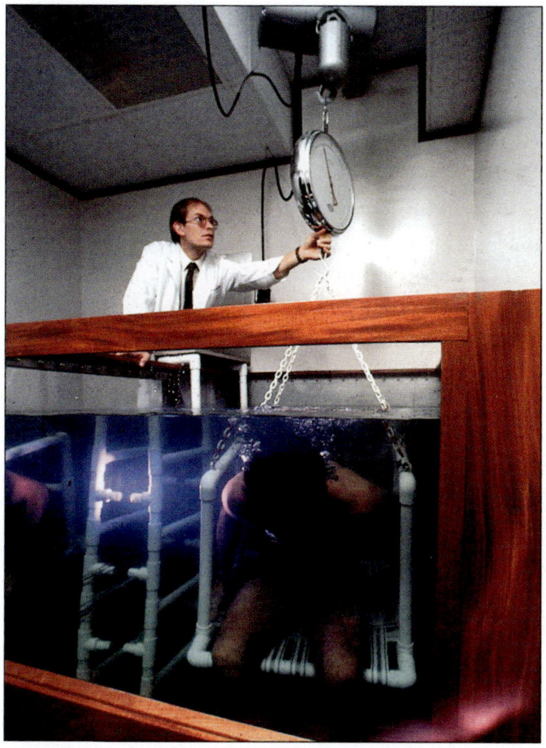

FIGURE 7.12 Underwater weighing can be used to determine body composition by measuring body weight on land and underwater. To measure weight underwater, the individual must expel air from their lungs and be lowered into a tank of water. *(© Jim Olive/Peter Arnold, Inc.)*

Body Weight and Body Fat

Assessing body composition is more cumbersome than simply measuring height and weight. Many of these techniques require expensive equipment and must be performed in a research setting by trained technicians. Others are more portable, so they are more appropriate for use in a clinic, office, or health club.

Underwater Weighing An accurate noninvasive technique for assessing body composition is **underwater weighing,** which involves weighing an individual both on land and in the water. These measures are used to determine body density, which is proportional to fat-free mass. The percentage of body fat can then be determined using standardized equations. To measure underwater weight, one must sit on a scale, expel the air from the lungs, and be lowered into a tank of water (Figure 7.12). Although this method is accurate, it requires special equipment and cannot be used for some groups such as small children or frail adults. A newer method for estimating body composition measures air displacement rather than water displacement to calculate body fat. The individual is placed in an air-filled chamber (known as the BOD POD) rather than water. It is accurate and more convenient than underwater weighing.[16]

Underwater weighing A technique that uses the difference between body weight underwater and body weight on land to estimate body composition.

Skinfold thickness A measurement of subcutaneous fat used to estimate total body fat.

Circumferences and Skinfold Thickness Measurements of circumference and **skinfold thickness** at various locations on the body can also be used to assess body composition. Measurements of waist and/or hip circumferences can be used to assess the location of body fat stores (see Chapter 8). Skinfold thicknesses measured at one or more locations using a caliper are used to assess subcutaneous fat. The most common sites for skinfold measurements are the triceps (the area over the muscles on the back of the upper arm) and the subscapular area (just below the shoulder blade) (Figure 7.13). Either a nomogram or mathematical equations are then used to estimate percent body fat from these measurements.

These measurements are noninvasive and, when performed by a trained observer, can accurately predict body fat in normal-weight individuals. They are more difficult to perform and less accurate in obese and elderly subjects.

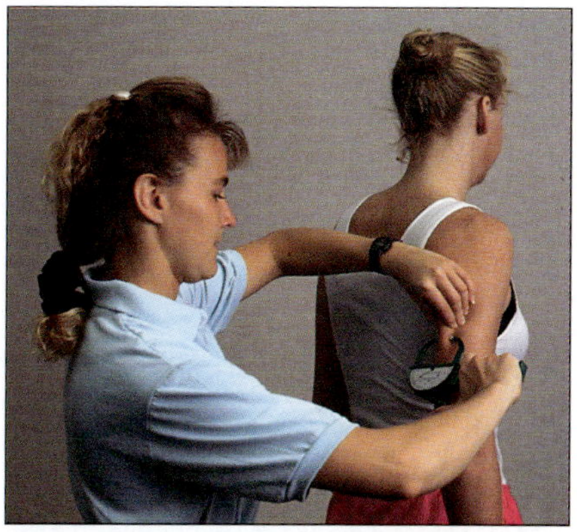

FIGURE 7.13 The triceps skinfold is measured at the midpoint of the back of the arm. This measure of the thickness of the fat layer under the skin can be used to estimate body fat. *(David Young-Wolff/PhotoEdit)*

Bioelectric impedance analysis A technique for estimating body composition that measures body fat by directing a low-energy electric current through the body and calculating resistance to flow.

Bioelectric Impedance Analysis **Bioelectric impedance analysis** estimates body fat by measuring the rate of electrical current flow through the body. A painless, low-energy electrical current is directed through the body by electrodes placed on the hands and/or feet. The rate of current flow through the body is then measured. Because fat is a poor conductor of electricity, it offers resistance to the current. Thus, the amount of resistance to current flow is proportional to the amount of body fat. The equipment needed for impedance measurements is inexpensive and the process is quick and painless. However, because impedance techniques assume the presence of a standard amount of water in the body, measurements must be performed when the GI tract and bladder are empty and body hydration is normal. Measurements performed within 24 hours of strenuous exercise are not accurate because body water has been lost in sweat.

Dilution Methods Body fat can also be assessed based on the principle of dilution. Because water is present primarily in lean tissue and not in fat, a water-soluble isotope can be ingested or injected into the bloodstream and allowed to mix with the water throughout the body. The concentration of the isotope in a sample of body fluid, such as blood, can then be measured. The extent to which the isotope has been diluted can be used to calculate the amount of lean tissue in the body, and body fat can then be calculated by subtracting lean weight from total body weight. Another technique measures a naturally occurring isotope of potassium. Because potassium is found primarily in lean tissue, a measure of the amount of this isotope in the body can be used to determine the total amount of body potassium, which can then be used to estimate the amount of lean tissue. Dilution techniques are expensive and invasive, usually requiring injections. They are used primarily for research purposes.

Radiologic Methods A variety of radiologic technologies have been used to assess body composition. These are less invasive but more expensive than dilution methods. Computerized tomography (CT), generally used as a diagnostic technique, can be used to visualize fat and lean tissue. CT is more accurate than underwater

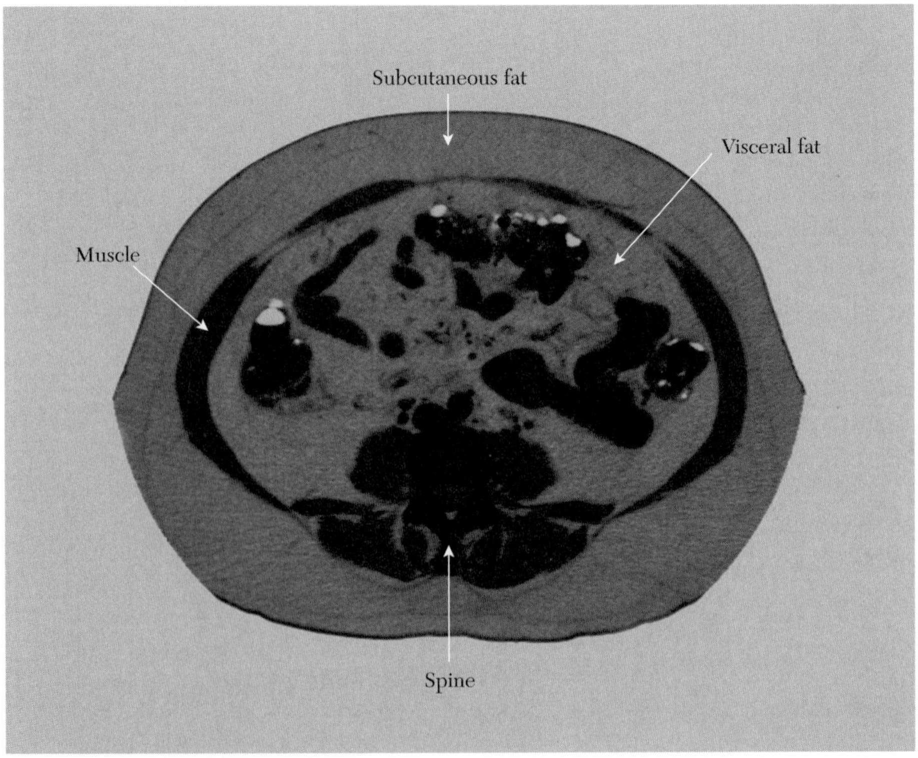

FIGURE 7.14 As shown in this CT scan taken at waist level in an overweight female, fat in the abdominal region is located both under the skin (subcutaneous) and around the internal organs (visceral). *(Courtesy of Michael S. Smolin M.D.)*

weighing, skinfold measures, and total body potassium for evaluation of body composition, and is particularly useful for measuring the amount of visceral adipose tissue (Figure 7.14).[17] Dual-energy X-ray absorptometry (DEXA) is another method that uses low-energy X-rays for assessing body composition. A single investigation can accurately determine total body mass, bone mineral mass, and percent body fat, but it does not distinguish between visceral and subcutaneous fat. Another method, magnetic resonance imaging (MRI), uses magnetic fields to create an internal body image. MRI can be used to accurately estimate the amount of abdominal fat, which is associated with the risk of heart disease and other chronic diseases. (See *Critical Thinking:* "Balancing Energy: Genetics and Lifestyle.")

Critical Thinking

Balancing Energy: Genetics and Lifestyle

Aysha was a chubby child. As an adolescent she continued to be heavy. No one was surprised because her parents are both obese. At home her mother served healthy meals, but the family never missed dessert and the house was always stocked with plenty of high-kcalorie snack foods. Her mother spent her spare time sewing or knitting and her dad was more inclined to watch sports on TV than to participate in them. During her freshman year at college, Aysha gained 10 pounds and became resigned to the inevitability that she would be fat like her parents. Then she noticed that many of her thin friends made different dietary choices than she did and spent more of their free time playing sports. Since she was now in charge of all her lifestyle choices, she decided to make some changes. She is 5 feet 4 inches tall, 23 years old, and weighs 155 pounds.

What is her BMI? Is it in the healthy range?

Answer:

By analyzing her lifestyle, Aysha realizes that she gets almost no exercise and often snacks from the vending machine while studying late at night. By recording and analyzing her food intake for three days, she determines that she eats about 2650 kcalories per day. By keeping an activity log, she estimates that a typical day includes 8 hours of sleep, 14 hours of very light activity such as studying, and 2 hours of light activity such as walking. To determine her expenditure, she estimates the energy she needs for RMR, activity, and the thermic effect of the food.

Is she in energy balance?

Answer:

By examining her food intake record, she estimates that by replacing desserts and trips to the vending machine with fruit, she can reduce her energy intake by about 150 kcalories. Her diet also contains a number of high-kcalorie, high-fat foods such as cheese Danish at breakfast, french fries at lunch, and extra gravy on her dinner entree. She can further decrease her energy intake by making substitutions for these high-energy choices. For instance, having a bagel instead of a cheese Danish would save 190 kcalories.

The biggest change she wants to make is in her activity level. She decides to devote one hour a day to doing something active, whether it is a game of tennis, a swim, a night out dancing, or just a brisk walk with a friend. She also tries to increase her daily activity by riding her bike or walking to class rather than taking the bus, and by using the stairs instead of the elevator in the dorm.

If she replaces one hour of her very light activity with one hour of moderate activity, how much additional energy will this burn?

Answer:

Is she destined to be obese?

If these small dietary changes decrease Aysha's daily intake by about 250 kcalories a day, and the changes in her activity increase her expenditure by about 200 kcalories a day, she will lose weight. If she can maintain these changes, making them a part of her lifestyle, her weight may settle at a new lower level that is healthier than her parents' weights.

Regulation of Body Fatness and Energy Balance

Most young adults maintain a relatively constant body weight over periods of weeks, months, or years despite fluctuations in intake and exercise. How does this happen? And, why are some of us fat and some of us lean? Energy balance appears to be regulated at different levels for different individuals.

Defending Body Weight and Fat

Body weight resists change. In some, body weight and the amount of fat are higher than in others. This can be explained by the set point theory, which suggests that body weight is genetically determined and that there are internal mechanisms that defend against weight change. A set point for body weight has been demonstrated experimentally by under- or overfeeding study subjects. The subjects lose or gain weight, but when they are allowed to return to their normal intake, their weight returns to its original "set" level.[18] Likewise, as anyone who has dieted can attest, it is difficult to decrease body weight, and most people who lose weight eventually regain all they have lost.

However, the mechanisms that defend body weight are not absolute. Changes in physiological, psychological, and environmental circumstances do cause the level at which body weight is regulated to change, usually increasing it over time. For example, body weight increases in most adults between the ages of 30 and 60 years, and after childbearing, most women return to a weight that is one to two pounds higher than their prepregnancy weight. This suggests that the mechanisms that defend against weight loss are stronger than those that prevent weight gain.[19]

Regulating Energy Balance

In order for weight to remain constant, the mechanisms that regulate body weight and fatness must respond to changes in both energy intake and output. The central controller of body fatness is the brain, which receives input from inside the body and from the external environment. It responds by sending signals that affect food intake and energy expenditure. Signals related to meal-to-meal food intake affect **hunger** and **satiety** and hence the size and timing of individual meals. Signals that trigger the brain to adjust food intake and energy expenditure for the long-term regulation of body weight come from adipose tissue and other body tissues.

Hunger Internal signals that stimulate one to acquire and consume food.

Satiety The feeling of fullness and satisfaction, caused by food consumption, that eliminates the desire to eat.

Short-Term: Meal-to-Meal Food Intake The short-term regulation of energy balance involves the control of food intake from meal to meal. We eat in response to hunger, which is the physiological drive to consume food. We stop eating when we experience satiety, the feeling of fullness and satisfaction that follows food intake. But, what, when, and how much we eat are also affected by **appetite,** the drive to eat that is not necessarily related to hunger. Signals to eat or stop eating can be external, originating from the environment, or they can be internal, originating from the gastrointestinal tract, circulating nutrients, or from higher centers in the brain[20] (Figure 7.15).

Appetite The desire to consume specific foods that is independent of hunger.

External Signals External factors such as the sight, taste, and smell of food, the time of day, cultural and social conventions, the appeal of the available foods, and ethnic and religious rituals can affect eating behavior.[21, 22] Some people eat lunch at noon out of social convention, not because they are hungry. Americans eat turkey on Thanksgiving because it is a tradition. Shoppers may eat cookies or cinnamon rolls while walking through the mall because the smell entices them. Likewise, external factors can signal us to stop eating. These signals can be anything from fasting in accordance with religious tradition to avoiding certain foods because they remind us of a negative experience. Many of these external stimuli are learned from prior experiences.

Internal Biological Signals Internal signals can also promote hunger and satiety. These internal signals originate both before and after food is absorbed. The simplest type of signal about food intake comes from local nerves in the walls of the stomach and small intestine that sense the volume or pressure of food and send a message to the brain to either start or stop food intake. The presence of glucose, fat, and amino acids in the gastrointestinal tract also sends information directly to

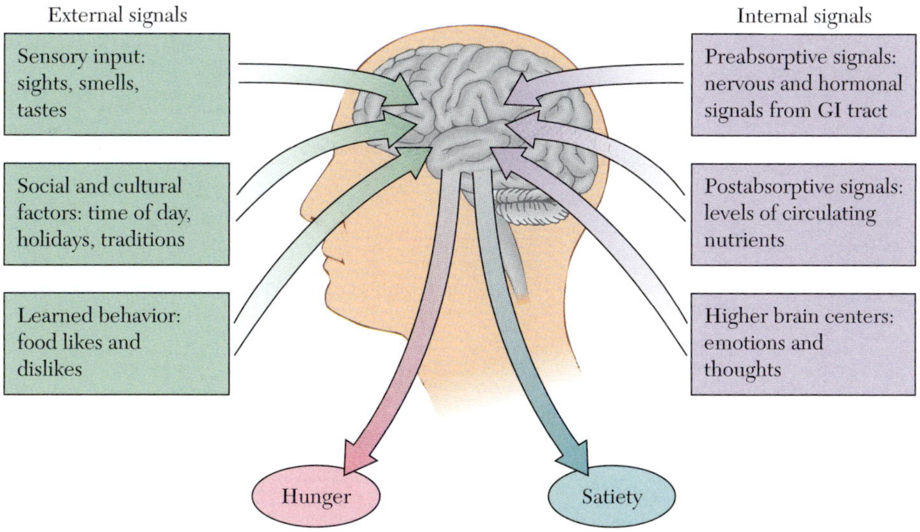

FIGURE 7.15 Signals that regulate the short-term intake of food (from meal to meal) come from both the external environment and inside the body. The brain integrates this information and responds by sending signals that trigger the sensations of hunger or satiety.

the brain. In addition, the presence of nutrients triggers the release of gastrointestinal hormones such as cholecystokinin that cause satiety. These hormones act by signaling the brain through peripheral nerves and by directly signaling control centers in the brain.[23]

Absorbed nutrients may also send information to the brain to modulate food intake. Circulating levels of nutrients, including glucose, amino acids, ketones, and fatty acids, are monitored by the brain and may trigger signals to eat or not to eat.[24] Nutrients that are taken up by the brain may affect neurotransmitter concentrations, which then affect the amount and type of nutrients consumed. For example, some studies suggest that when brain serotonin is low, carbohydrate is craved, but when it is high, protein is preferred.[24]

Other organs, such as the liver and pancreas, may also be involved in signaling hunger and satiety. The liver is in a unique position to monitor changes in fuel metabolism because absorbed water-soluble nutrients go there directly. Changes in liver metabolism, in particular the amount of ATP, are believed to modulate food intake.[21] The pancreas is also involved in food intake regulation because it releases insulin, which may affect hunger and satiety by lowering the levels of circulating nutrients. Insulin may also be involved in long-term regulation of body fat.

Psychological factors can also affect eating behavior. Psychological distress may come from events in the external environment, but the processing of these events occurs in the higher centers of the brain. The effect that emotions have on appetite depends on the individual. Some people eat for comfort and to relieve stress. Others may lose their appetite when these same emotions are felt.

Leptin: Long-Term Signals About Body Fat Short-term regulators of energy balance affect the size and timing of individual meals, but if a change in input is sustained over a long period it can affect long-term energy balance and hence body weight and fatness. To regulate the amount of fat at a set level, the body must be able to monitor how much fat is present. This information is believed to come

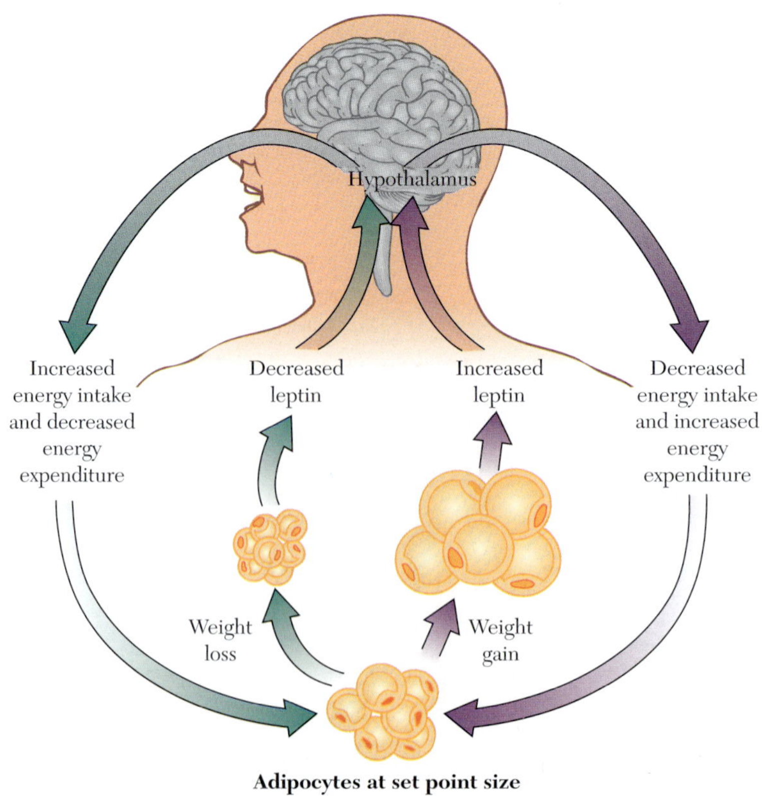

FIGURE 7.16 Leptin helps maintain body fat at a stable level. When an individual gains weight, adipocytes accumulate more fat and leptin levels are increased, triggering events that decrease food intake and increase energy expenditure. When an individual loses weight, fat is lost from adipocytes and less leptin is released, causing an increase in food intake and a decrease in energy expenditure.

from hormones, such as insulin and **leptin,** which are secreted in proportion to the amount of body fat.[23] Insulin is secreted from the pancreas when blood glucose levels rise; its circulating concentration is proportional to the amount of body fat. Insulin interacts with the hypothalamus to reduce food intake and body weight, and insulin levels are believed to affect the amount of leptin produced and secreted.[20] Leptin is a hormone produced by the adipocytes; the amount of leptin produced is proportional to the size of adipocytes, so more leptin is released as fat stores increase. Leptin exerts its effect on food intake and energy expenditure by binding to leptin receptors present in the brain and other tissues. This triggers mechanisms that affect intake and expenditure. When leptin levels are high, mechanisms that cause an increase in energy expenditure and a decrease in food intake are stimulated, and pathways that promote food intake and hence weight gain are inhibited. When fat stores shrink, less leptin is released. Low leptin levels in the brain allow pathways that decrease energy expenditure and increase food intake to become active.[25] Thus, leptin acts like a thermostat or lipostat to keep body fatness from changing (Figure 7.16). (See *Research Discoveries*: "Leptin: Discovery of an Obesity Gene.")

Leptin A protein hormone produced by adipocytes that signals information about the amount of body fat.

Hormonal signals involved in the long-term regulation of body weight act in the brain not only to favor shifts in energy balance, but also to affect the sensitivity of the brain to short-term signals of energy balance. For example, during weight loss, low levels of these hormones are hypothesized to decrease the efficacy of satiety signals, suppress pathways that cause weight loss, and activate pathways that contribute to weight gain.[20]

Genetic and Environmental Determinants of Body Fatness

Heredity plays a role in how much body fat we accumulate and where it is deposited. Hereditary factors account for many of the differences in the body weights of individuals in a population. But, body fat is not determined purely by genetics; environmental and behavioral factors are also involved. The influence of environmental factors on body weight accounts for changes in the average body weight of a population that occur over time.

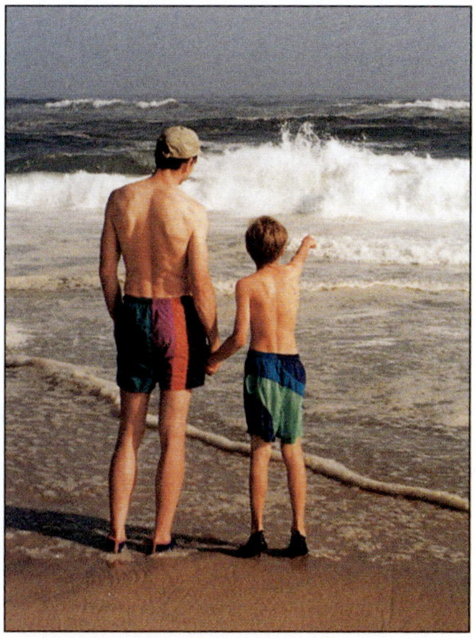

FIGURE 7.17 The genes we inherit from our parents are important determinants of our body size and shape. *(Lori Smolin)*

Heredity and Body Weight

Traditionally, it was assumed that fat people were fat because of the choices they made. They either ate too much or exercised too little or both. However, this theory does not explain why children have body shapes, sizes, and compositions similar to those of their parents (Figure 7.17). Some of us inherit tall, slender bodies with long, thin bones. Others inherit stocky bodies with short bones, wide hips, and stubby fingers. And some of us inherit a tendency to store excess body fat. If one or both of a child's parents is obese, his or her risk of being obese is increased. Individuals with a family history of obesity are two to three times more likely to be obese, and the risk increases with the magnitude of the obesity. In a study that overfed pairs of identical twins to the same extent, some individuals in the study gained only 9 pounds, whereas others gained as much as 29 pounds, indicating that different people utilize excess energy differently.[12] When the sets of identical twins were compared, it was found that each set of twins tended to gain the same amount of weight and that the fat was deposited in the same parts of their bodies. Because identical twins have the same genetic makeup, these results suggest that heredity affects the way humans use energy and gain weight (Figure 7.18).

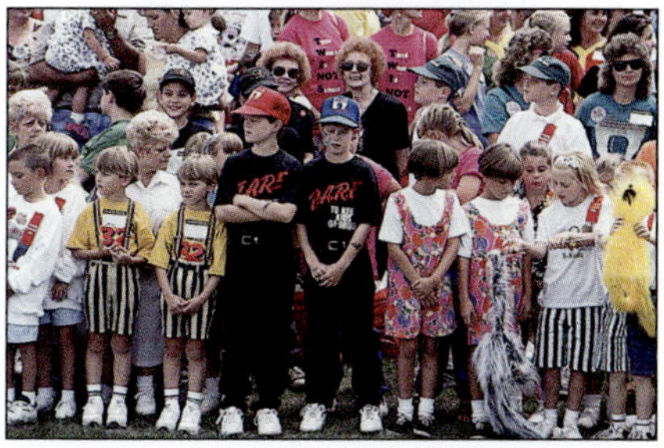

FIGURE 7.18 Identical twins inherit the same genes and thus tend to gain the same amount of weight and deposit fat in the same locations. *(© Mark C. Burnett/Stock Boston)*

RESEARCH DISCOVERIES

Leptin: Discovery of an Obesity Gene

A discovery made by Jeffrey Friedman and colleagues in 1994 brought hope to millions. Perhaps the cause of obesity had been found and a cure might be close behind. Was relief in sight for the millions of people who suffer from the physical and social consequences of obesity?

Dr. Friedman's work began with a strain of mice called *ob* for obese. *Ob* mice become grossly obese, gaining up to three times the normal body weight. The *ob* strain arose spontaneously in 1950 in the mouse colony at the Jackson Laboratory in Bar Harbor, Maine. Friedman and colleagues unraveled the cause for the obesity in this strain of mice when they identified and cloned the gene that was responsible.[a]

Researchers used a series of breeding experiments to localize the gene to a particular stretch of DNA. They then looked to see if any of the genes in this stretch of DNA were expressed in adipose tissue. The search yielded a single gene. Evidence that this gene was involved in the regulation of body weight was obtained by examining the gene and the protein it codes for in the *ob* mice. Researchers found that this protein, which they named leptin, was either not produced or produced in an inactive form in the obese mice. Soon afterward a similar gene was identified in humans.

Optimism about the role of the protein hormone leptin in human obesity was so great that a biotechnology firm (Amgen) paid $25 million for the commercial rights to leptin in the hope that it could be used to treat human obesity. Those hopes grew even higher when Friedman and colleagues were able to demonstrate that injections of the hormone could restore the genetically obese mice to normal weight.[b,c] Leptin's role appeared to be that of a lipostat: Fat stores rise and leptin rises and signals the brain to reduce energy intake and increase expenditure. Unfortunately, the role of leptin in human obesity has not lived up to expectations. A few cases of obesity have been linked directly to a defective leptin gene;[d] but mutations in this gene are not responsible for most human obesity. In fact, obese humans generally have high blood leptin levels.[e] A clinical trial with humans showed that high doses of leptin administered to obese humans produced only modest weight loss in some of the subjects.[f]

The leptin receptor—a protein in the brain to which leptin must bind to produce weight reduction—was identified soon after the leptin gene was.[g] The fact that obese humans have high levels of leptin suggested that the cause of human obesity might involve an abnormality in leptin receptors. If leptin receptors were defective, the leptin produced would have no place to bind and would not be able to signal mechanisms to promote weight reduction. Thus far, however, defective leptin receptors have not been found to be an important cause of human obesity.[h]

Continued study of the role of leptin in obesity has confirmed that it is an important signal involved in the long-term regulation of body fat, but it does not act alone. There are many steps, involving many genes, that occur between the production of leptin and alterations in food intake and energy expenditure. Researchers have discovered about a dozen molecules that interact with leptin in the brain to control appetite.[i] For example, neuropeptide Y and melanin-concentrating hormone boost appetite, whereas alpha-melanocyte stimulating hormone blunts appetite, and a protein called SOCS3 reduces the sensitivity of leptin receptors. Many of these compounds are now targets for the development of new obesity drugs.

Despite the fact that the identification of leptin has not produced a cure for human obesity, its discovery lit up the field. This research was an important advance in our understanding of the genetics of body weight regulation. Continued work will someday answer the questions that remain about why some of us are obese and some of us are lean.

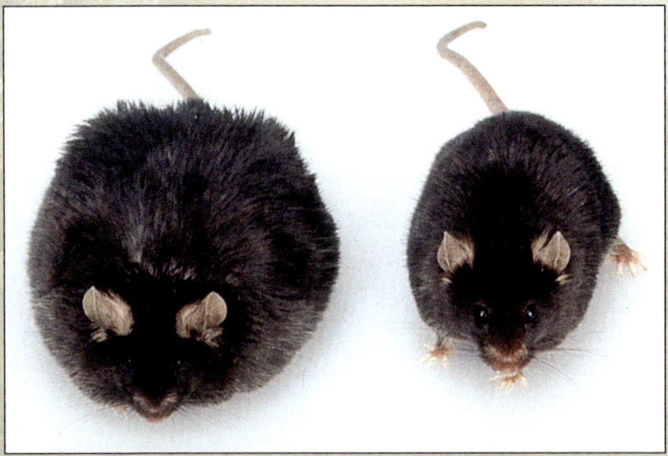

A mouse with a defect in the leptin gene *(ob)* may weigh three times as much as a normal mouse. Both of these mice have defective *(ob)* genes but the one on the right was treated with leptin injections. *(John Sholtis, Rockefeller University, New York/© 1995 Amgen, Inc.)*

References

[a] Zhang, Y., Proenca, R., Maffei, M., et al. Positional cloning of the mouse obese gene and its human homologue. Nature 372:425–432, 1994.

[b] Halaas, J. L., Gajiwala, K. S., Maffei, M., et al. Weight-reducing effects of the plasma protein encoded by the obese gene. Science 269: 543–546, 1995.

[c] Pelleymounter, M. A., Cullen, M. J., Baker, M. B., et al. Effects of the obese gene product on body weight regulation in *ob/ob* mice. Science 269:540–543, 1995.

[d] Montague, C. T., Farooqi, I. S., Whitehead, J. P., et al. Congenital leptin deficiency is associated with severe early onset obesity in children. Nature 387:903–908, 1997.

[e] Considine, R. V., Sinha, M. K., Heiman, M. L., et al. Serum immunoreactive-leptin concentrations in normal weight and obese humans. New Engl. J. Med. 334:292–295, 1996.

[f] Gura, T. Obesity research: leptin not impressive in clinical trial. Science 286:881–882, 1999.

[g] Tartaglia, L. A., Dembski, M., Weng X., et al. Identification and expression cloning of a leptin receptor, OB-R. Cell 83:1263–1271, 1995.

[h] Considine, R. V., Considine, E. L., Williams, C. J., et al. The hypothalamic leptin receptor in humans. Diabetes 19:992–994, 1996.

[i] Gura, T. Tracing leptin's partners in regulating body weight. Science 287:1738–1741, 2000.

Obesity Genes The information that regulates energy balance, body size, and body shape is contained in genes. A gene is a segment of DNA that provides the code or blueprint for the synthesis of a protein (see Chapter 6). A host of genes that code for proteins involved in the regulation of body weight have been identified in rodents, and similar genes have been found in humans.[25, 26, 27] Some of the proteins coded for by "obesity genes," such as leptin, are involved in signaling the brain about the amount of body fat present; some are receptors that bind signaling molecules in the brain, and others are involved in transmitting messages from the brain to other parts of the body to increase or decrease food intake or energy expenditure. A defect in one of the obesity genes could interfere with the regulation of body weight. When a gene is defective, the protein it codes for is not made, or is made incorrectly so that the signals that tell the brain about the amount of body fat or to change food intake or energy expenditure are not received correctly.

For more information on leptin and obesity genes, go to www.accessexcellence.org/ and search for leptin or to the "Understanding Obesity" Web site at www.understanding-obesity.com.

C 62 00 00 00 00 00 31 40

C 62 00 00 00 00 00 27 28

Although a number of genes involved in the regulation of body weight have been identified in humans, very few cases of human obesity have been traced to a specific defective gene. It is believed that most human obesity is due to variations in a number of genes that together create a situation that promotes the accumulation and storage of excess energy. For example, variations in levels of hormones, such as insulin and leptin, may play a role in determining the level at which body fat is maintained. Other proteins may affect an individual's response to external cues. For example, studies have shown that obese individuals may be more influenced by cravings for specific foods, such as sweet or salty items,[28] and tend to choose high-fat foods.[29] The impact on human energy balance of the proteins made by many of the obesity genes is still under investigation, and many genes involved in body weight regulation remain to be elucidated.

Do Genetics Affect Energy Expenditure? Many overweight people contend that they eat very few kcalories and yet continue to gain weight. This would imply that their energy expenditure is less than in normal-weight individuals. One possible explanation for this is that overweight individuals inherit a thrifty metabolism. An individual with a thrifty metabolism theoretically uses energy very efficiently so that more of the energy they consume is converted into ATP or deposited in energy stores than in someone with a less efficient metabolism. They would therefore need to eat less to maintain body weight. But actual studies of energy intake in overweight individuals have been inconclusive, in part because determining energy intake is difficult; there is evidence that overweight individuals are more likely to underreport their energy intake than their lean counterparts (see Chapter 2: *Research Discoveries*: "The Art of Assessing Food Intake").[8] Studies using doubly-labeled water have shown that energy expenditure increases with increasing body weight, suggesting that obese individuals need to eat *more* than lean controls to maintain their higher body weight.[8] Although some individuals may need fewer kcalories than others, there is little evidence that a thrifty metabolism is a factor in the majority of human obesity.

Adaptive Thermogenesis The regulation of energy expenditure in response to changes in circumstance, such as over- or underfeeding, changes in temperature, or trauma is referred to as **adaptive thermogenesis.** Increased energy expenditure through adaptive thermogenesis may prevent some of the weight gain that accompanies an increase in energy intake.[30, 31, 32] When body weight is increased above normal by overconsumption, energy expenditure increases in both lean and obese subjects to compensate for the increase and to return weight to normal. And, when body weight is reduced by restricting food intake, energy expenditure decreases in both groups.[18, 32] Some studies found the drop in RMR seen with weight reduction was greater in obese than in lean subjects, and the increase in RMR seen with weight gain was less in obese than in lean subjects.[18] These differences in the adaptive responses of lean versus obese subjects may help explain why it is difficult to maintain weight loss.

Adaptive thermogenesis The change in energy expenditure induced by factors such as changes in ambient temperature and food intake.

Several biochemical mechanisms have been proposed to explain adaptive thermogenesis. The first is substrate cycling or futile cycling, which wastes energy by allowing opposing biochemical reactions to occur simultaneously. For example, a molecule is formed, consuming ATP, and then is quickly broken down again. Energy is consumed but there is no net change in the number of molecules in the body.

A second way that excess energy might be dissipated is by separating or uncoupling the electron transport chain from the production of ATP so oxygen is consumed but no ATP is produced. Instead, the energy is lost as heat. For example, the increase in energy expenditure that occurs when mice are injected with leptin is believed to be due to the stimulation of receptors on a specialized type of adipose tissue called **brown adipose tissue.** Brown adipose tissue can waste energy as heat. This tissue contains many more mitochondria than other adipose tissue, and these mitochondria can be uncoupled from the electron transport chain by uncoupling proteins to release the energy in food as heat. In rats, brown adipose tissue generates heat to prevent weight gain during overfeeding and to provide warmth when the ambient temperature is low. With the exception of newborns, humans have only a very small amount of brown adipose tissue, but humans may be able to dissipate energy in other tissues. Several proteins that uncouple the electron transport chain from the production of ATP have been identified in human muscle, white adipose tissue, lungs, spleen, white blood cells, bone marrow, and stomach.[33] It is hypothesized that these uncoupling proteins may be involved in increasing energy output to regulate body weight in humans.

Brown adipose tissue A type of fat tissue that has a greater number of mitochondria than the more common white adipose tissue. It can waste energy by producing heat and is believed to be responsible for some of the change in energy expenditure due to adaptive thermogenesis in rodents.

Thermogenesis of Fidgeting Humans vary considerably in their susceptibility to weight gain when excess energy is consumed. Differences in basal metabolic rate and the thermic effect of food do not account for all this variability, but physical activity, the other component of energy expenditure, may play a role. We tend to think of physical activity as the amount of planned exercise we engage in, but energy is also expended in involuntary exercise, such as fidgeting, maintenance of posture, and the other small movements that occur during daily living. A study that overfed nonobese individuals found there was a tenfold variation in the amount of fat gained. Some subjects were able to increase energy expenditure to a greater extent and so gained less fat. About two thirds of the increase in energy expenditure that occurred with overfeeding was found to be due to an increase in involuntary exercise.[34] Individuals who gained little weight had a greater level of involuntary exercise than those who gained more weight. It is still not known what mechanisms control why some people respond to excess energy by becoming restless and fidgeting more while others remain lethargic in their daily activities.

Web Menu For more information on the American food supply, go to www.ers.usda.gov/publications/foodreview/jan2000/.

Environment and Body Weight

Influences from our environment and our personal choices are also important determinants of body weight. An individual with a genetic predisposition to obesity who has a limited supply of food or who engages in strenuous physical labor may never be obese, while someone with no genetic tendency toward obesity who consumes a high-energy diet and gets little exercise may become obese.

American Lifestyles The typical lifestyle in the United States today fosters increased food intake and discourages physical activity. This has been proposed as a major reason for the increasing prevalence of obesity in the United States.[35]

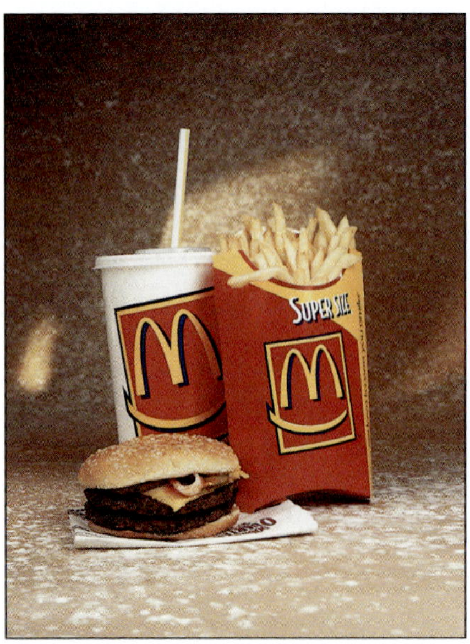

FIGURE 7.19 A supersized fast-food meal can contribute as much as 1500 kcalories and 55 grams of fat to daily intake. *(© George Semple)*

Food Availability Palatable, affordable food is available in abundance to the majority of the population. Supermarkets, fast-food restaurants, and all-night convenience marts provide ready access to food throughout the day and night. Snack foods, baked goods, and candy entice us at the checkout counter of the supermarket. Bigger is marketed as better in terms of portion sizes. Super-sized beverages often offer a liter of your favorite soft drink, which can contain over 600 kcalories (Figure 7.19). Also, living in a household where high-kcalorie foods are always

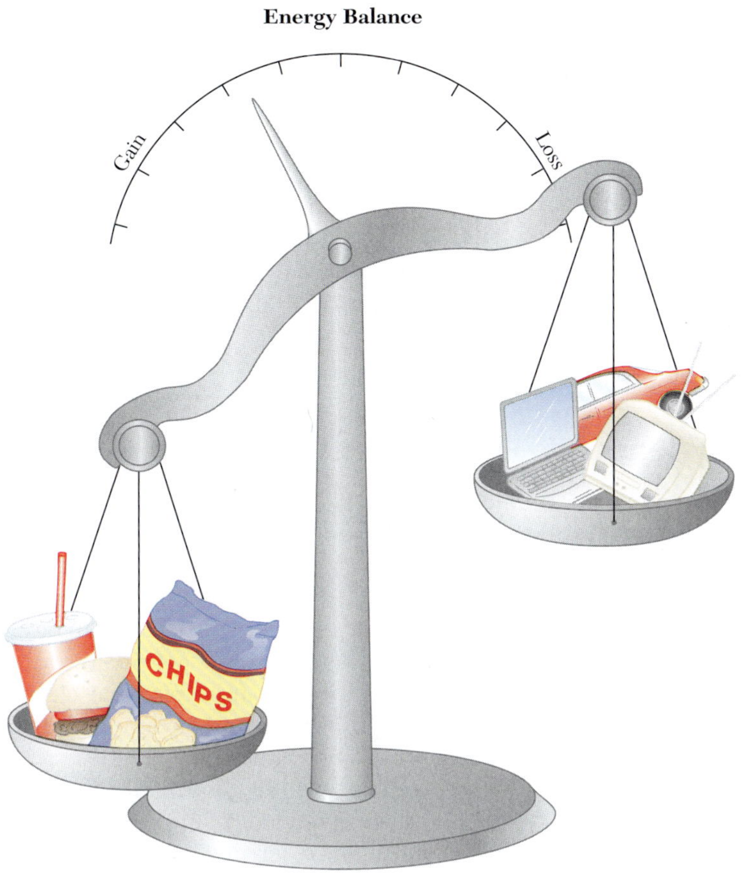

FIGURE 7.20 The constant accessibility of high kcalorie foods and the availability of labor-saving devices and low-activity entertainment have combined to tip the American population's energy balance scale in the direction of weight gain.

available and exercise is infrequent increases the likelihood of becoming overweight. Studies have shown that one of the reasons having obese parents increases one's risk of obesity is that obese families consume more high-energy foods than lean families.[36]

Modern Conveniences Along with the increase in food availability and portion sizes, there has been a decrease in the amount of energy needed for the activities of daily life. In 1900, a farmer who worked his field by hand did not have to plan an exercise program—his day-to-day life was active enough. Today, advances in technology have brought tractors, automobiles, elevators, and vacuum cleaners, which allow us to work without being as physically active. In addition, television, electronic games, and computers have given us sedentary ways to spend our leisure time (Figure 7.20).

Personal Choices Although genetics affect our predisposition both for body size and food choice,[8] and we live in an environment that encourages eating and makes exercising unnecessary, these factors do not have the final say in what we eat and how much exercise we get.

Dietary Choices The types and amounts of food one chooses affect body weight. Personal decisions to snack on fruit versus chips, to have a second helping of salad rather than french fries, or to have a bowl of ice cream every night determine how much energy we consume, and this, in turn, determines how much we weigh.

Physical Activity Choices The amount of energy an individual expends depends primarily on metabolic rate and physical activity. Genetics affect metabolic rate, but activity level is affected by both genetics and individual choices. When the energy expended for physical activity is compared with the amount of body fat, it is found that individuals with the most body fat have the lowest levels of physical activity, supporting the hypothesis that obesity is associated with inactivity.[37] This does not mean that reduced physical activity necessarily causes obesity. The reduction in activity may occur as a result of the obesity. Excess weight makes it more difficult to exercise or even to perform simple daily activities. Obese individuals carry extra weight with every action. A 230-pound man walking a mile is carrying the same weight as a 200-pound man walking a mile carrying a 30-pound suitcase. This extra burden reduces the inclination to increase activity. In addition to the physical stress, obese individuals often shy away from exercise because they don't want to be compared with their leaner counterparts. Obese children may avoid athletic activities because they are teased about their weight. Inactivity reduces energy expenditure regardless of whether it is a cause of obesity or not.

Web Menu For more information on the Pima Indians, go to www.niddk.nih.gov/health/diabetes/pima/.

C 62 00 00 00 00 00 31 41

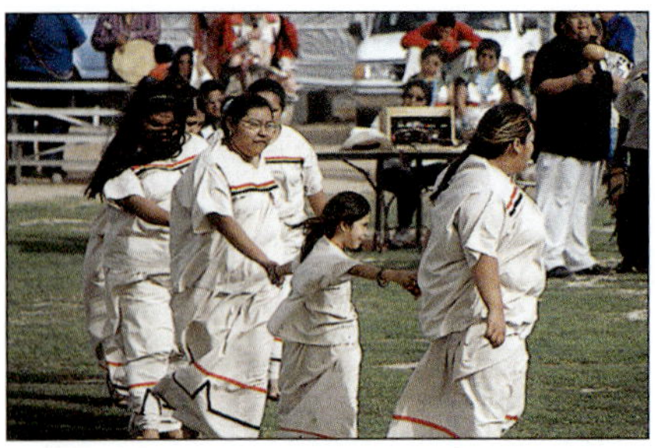

FIGURE 7.21 A genetic predisposition as well as environmental factors have led to the high incidence of obesity among the Pima Indians in the southwestern United States. *(© Marilyn "Angel" Wynn/nativestock.com)*

Interactions of Genes and Environment

The incidence of obesity in the United States has increased significantly over the last two decades.[38] The genes present in a population take many generations to change, supporting the view that nongenetic factors such as increased energy intake and decreased physical activity are major contributors to this increase in body weight. When genetically susceptible individuals find themselves in an environment where food is appealing and plentiful and physical activity is easily avoided, obesity is a likely outcome. An example of human obesity that clearly demonstrates the interaction of a genetic predisposition and an environment that is conducive to obesity is the Pima Indian tribe living in Arizona (Figure 7.21). More than 75% of this population is obese. Genetic analysis has identified a number of genes that may be responsible for this group's tendency to store more body fat.[39] Typically, Pimas have low energy requirements per unit of fat-free mass, which, coupled with a low level of physical activity and a high intake of an energy-dense diet, has caused body fat to be maintained at a high level. A group of Pima Indians living in Mexico is genetically the same as those in the United States, but they are farmers who consume the food they grow and have a high level of physical activity.[40] They still have higher rates of obesity than would be predicted from their diet and exercise patterns, suggesting genes that favor high body weight. However, they are significantly less obese than Arizona Pima Indians. These two Pima populations demonstrate the interactions between heredity and environment in determining body weight.

Summary

1. Energy is the ability to do work. It is measured in kcalories or kjoules. A kcalorie is the amount of heat needed to raise the temperature of 1 kilogram of water 1 degree Celsius.
2. Catabolic reactions are those that break down or oxidize molecules releasing energy as ATP. Anabolic reactions use ATP to synthesize molecules needed by the body. ATP is also used to provide energy for other body work.
3. The principle of energy balance states that if energy intake equals energy needs, body weight will remain constant.
4. Energy is provided to the body by carbohydrate (4 kcalories per gram), fat (9 kcalories per gram), protein (4 kcalories per gram), and alcohol (7 kcalories per gram).
5. When energy in the diet does not meet needs, body energy stores are used. When excess energy is consumed, it is stored for later use. Fat is preferentially stored while carbohydrate is used for energy and amino acids are used to meet protein needs.
6. In the adult body energy is required for basal metabolism, physical activity, and the thermic effect of food. Basal metabolic rate (BMR), usually measured as resting metabolic rate (RMR), is the largest component of energy expenditure. It differs with body size, body composition, age, and gender. The energy needed for physical activity typically accounts for 15 to 30% of energy expenditure but varies greatly depending on the individual. The thermic effect of food (TEF) is the energy required for the digestion of food and the absorption, metabolism, and storage of nutrients. It is equal to about 10% of energy consumed.
7. Energy expenditure can be determined by direct calorimetry, which measures the heat produced by the body, or indirect calorimetry, which measures nutrient utilization. Doubly-labeled water is a type of indirect calorimetry.
8. Because the 1989 recommended energy allowances are averages, they are too high for some and too low for others.

9. Body weight and fat can be measured in many ways. Body Mass Index (BMI) is the currently accepted standard for assessing body fatness. It correlates better with body fat than does comparing weight for height. Techniques that measure body composition, including underwater weighing, skinfold thicknesses, isotope dilution techniques, and imaging, can be used to assess the amount and distribution of body fat.
10. Body fat and body weight are regulated by internal mechanisms. Signals from the external environment, such as the sight and smell of food, and internal signals, such as nervous and hormonal signals from the GI tract and levels of circulating nutrients, regulate short-term hunger and satiety. Signals that relay information about the size of body fat stores, such as the release of leptin from adipocytes, regulate long-term energy intake and expenditure.
11. The amount of body weight or body fat an individual carries is the result of genetics, environmental influences, and personal choice. Genes have been identified that regulate body fatness in animals, and similar genes have been located in humans. It has been determined that much of the tendency to be obese is genetic. However, the availability of high-energy foods and labor-saving devices, as well as individual choices about food consumption and physical activity, also affect energy balance and body weight.

Review Questions

1. What is a kcalorie?
2. What is anabolism? Catabolism?
3. Define energy balance.
4. Which nutrients provide energy?
5. List the three components of energy expenditure.
6. What is BMR? RMR?
7. What is the thermic effect of food?
8. Describe three methods for measuring energy expenditure.
9. Why are the 1989 recommended energy allowances too high for some people and too low for others?
10. What is the accepted standard for assessing body weight?
11. List some methods for determining body fat?
12. Discuss the role of leptin in regulating body weight.
13. List some environmental factors that affect energy balance and discuss how these might interact with an individual's genetic predisposition to a particular body weight.

Applying Critical Thinking Skills

Personal nutrition:

1. Using the three-day food record you kept in Chapter 2, calculate your average energy intake.
   a. Estimate your average energy expenditure using your RMR (see Table 7.5), physical activity factors (see Table 7.6), and the thermic effect of food based on the energy intake you just calculated (see Table 7.7).
   b. How does your energy expenditure compare with your energy intake?
   c. If you consumed and expended these amounts of energy every day, would your weight increase, decrease, or stay the same?
   d. If intake does not equal output, how much would you gain or lose in a month? (Assume that a pound of fat is equal to 3500 kcal.)
   e. If your energy intake does not equal your energy expenditure, list some specific changes you could make in your diet or the amount of activity you get to make the two balance.
2. Record the following information to determine factors that may affect your body weight:

Your current BMI	
Your BMI a year ago	
Your mother's current BMI	
Your mother's BMI at age 21	
Your father's current BMI	
Your father's BMI at age 21	
Number of minutes of moderate exercise you currently get each day	
Number of minutes of moderate exercise you got a year ago	
Number of servings of snack foods, such as chips and candy bars, you eat each day	
Number of servings of fruits and vegetables you eat each day	
Number of servings of snack foods (chips, candy) you ate per day a year ago	
Number of servings of fruits and vegetables you ate per day day a a year ago	

   a. How has your weight changed over the last year?
   b. How much did your parents' weights change since they were 21?
   c. Do you eat more servings of snack foods such as chips and candy bars, or of fruits and vegetables daily? Has this changed over the last year?

   d. How has your activity changed over the last year?
   e. What patterns do you see emerging that can predict if your weight will change over the next year? The next 10 years? The next 20 years? What are your predictions?
   f. Are genetic factors or environmental factors a larger influence on your energy balance?

General nutrition issues:

1. Do a class survey by collecting everyone's answers to question 2 above. Tabulate the patterns that you see.
   a. Is weight generally increasing or decreasing?
   b. Is exercise increasing or decreasing?
   c. Which are the more popular snacks—prepackaged snack foods or fruits and vegetables?
   d. What percentage of your classmates has one parent whose BMI increased by 4 BMI units or more since they were 21?
   e. What percentage of your classmates has two parents whose BMI increased by 4 BMI units or more since they were 21?
2. Several strains of mice with mutations in genes that regulate body weight have been identified. For each of the following, predict whether the mouse will be over- or underweight and explain why.
   a. A mouse that makes excess leptin.
   b. A mouse that makes leptin normally, but the leptin receptor in the brain is defective, so it always acts as if large amounts of leptin are bound to it.
   c. A mouse that makes more leptin than normal, but the leptin molecule made is defective and cannot bind to receptors in the brain.
   d. A mouse that makes normal leptin and normal leptin receptors, but a compound released by the brain that stimulates appetite is inactive.

References

1. Hellerstein, M. K., De novo lipogenesis in humans: metabolic and regulatory aspects. Eur. J. Clin. Nutr. 53 (suppl 1):S53–S65, 2000.
2. National Research Council, Food and Nutrition Board. *Recommended Dietary Allowances*, 10th ed. Washington, D.C.: National Academy Press, 1989.
3. Wadden, T. A., Foster, G. D., Letizia, K. A., and Muller, J. L. Long-term effects of dieting on resting metabolic rate in obese patients. JAMA 264:707–711, 1990.
4. Kriketos, A. D., Peters, J. C., and Hill, J. O. Cellular and whole-animal energetics. In *Physiological and Physiological Aspects of Human Nutrition*, Stipanuk, M.H., ed. Philadelphia: W.B. Saunders Company, 2000, 411–424.
5. Horton, T. S., Drougas, H., Brachey, A., et al. Fat and carbohydrate overfeeding in humans: different effects on energy storage. Am. J. Clin. Nutr. 62:19–29, 1995.
6. Pulfrey, S. M., and Jones, P. J. Energy expenditure and requirement while climbing above 6,000 m. J. Appl. Physiol. 81:1306–1311, 1996.
7. Stein, T. P. Leskiw, M. J., Schluter, M. D., et al. Energy expenditure and balance during space flight on the space shuttle. Am. J. Physiol. 276:R1739–R1748, 1999.
8. Schoeller, D. A. Recent advances from application of doubly-labeled water to measurement of human energy expenditure. J. Nutr. 129: 1765–1768, 1999.
9. Albu, J., Allison, D., Boozer, C. N., et al. Obesity solutions: report of a meeting. Nutr. Rev. 55:150–156, 1997.
10. Abernathy, R. P., and Black, D. R. Healthy body weights: an alternative perspective. Am. J. Clin. Nutr. 63(suppl):448S–451S, 1996.
11. Snead, D. B., Birges, S. J., and Kohrt, W. M. Age-related differences in body composition by hydrodensitometry and dual-energy X-ray absorptiometry. J. Appl. Physiol. 74:770–775, 1993.
12. Bouchard, C., Tremblay, A., Després, J.-P., et al. The response to long-term feeding in identical twins. N. Engl. J. Med. 322:1477–1482, 1990.
13. Conway, J. M. Ethnicity and energy stores. Am. J. Clin. Nutr. 62(suppl): 1067S–1071S, 1995.
14. Dietz, W. H. Periods of risk in childhood for the development of adult obesity—what do we need to learn? J. Nutr. 127:1884S–1886S, 1997.
15. National Institutes of Health, National Heart, Lung, and Blood Institute. Clinical guidelines on the identification, evaluation, and treatment of overweight and obesity in adults. Executive summary, June 1998. Available online at: **http://www.nhlbi.nih.gov/guidelines/obesity/ob_home.htm** Accessed 5 Jan 2001.
16. Fields, D. A., Hunter, G. R., and Goran. M. I. Validation of the BOD POD with hydrostatic weighing: influence of body clothing. Int. J. Obes. Relat. Metab. Disord. 24:200–205, 2000.
17. Plourde, G. The role of radiologic methods in assessing body composition and related metabolic parameters. Nutr. Rev. 55:289–296, 1997.
18. Leibel, R. L., Rosenbaum, M., and Hirsch, J. Changes in energy expenditure resulting from altered body weight. N. Engl. J. Med. 332:622–628, 1995.
19. Peters, J. C., Kriketos, A. D., and Hill, J. O. Control of energy balance. In *Biochemical and Physiological Aspects of Human Nutrition*. Stipanuk, M. H., ed. Philadelphia: W.B. Saunders Company, 2000, 425–438.
20. Schwartz, M. W., Baskin, D. G., Kaiyala, K. J., and Woods, S. C. Model for the regulation of energy balance and adiposity by the central nervous system. Am. J. Clin. Nutr. 69:584–596, 1999.
21. Friedman, M. I. Control of energy intake by energy metabolism. Am. J. Clin. Nutr. 62(suppl):1096S–1100S, 1995.
22. Smith, G. P. Control of food intake. In *Modern Nutrition in Health and Disease*, 9th ed. Shils, M. E., Olson, J. A., Shike, M., and Ross, A. C., eds. Baltimore: Williams & Wilkins, 1999. 631–644.
23. Woods, S. C., Seeley, R. J., Porte, D., and Schwartz, M. W. Signals that regulate food intake and energy homeostasis. Science 280:1378–1383, 1998.
24. Anderson, G. H. Regulation of food intake. In *Modern Nutrition in Health and Disease*, 8th ed. Shils, M. E., Olson, J. A., and Shike, M., eds. Philadelphia: Lea & Febiger, 1994. 524–536.
25. Friedman, J. M. The alphabet of weight control. Nature 385:119–120, 1997.
25. Spiegelman, B. M., and Flier, J. S. Adipogenesis and obesity: rounding out the big picture. Cell 87:377–389, 1996.
26. Gura, T. Tracing leptin's partners in regulating body weight. Science 287:1738–1741, 2000.
28. Drewnowski, A., Krahn, D. D., and Demitrack, M. A. Naloxone, an opiate blocker, reduces the consumption of high-fat foods in obese and lean binge eaters. Am. J. Clin. Nutr. 61:1201–1206, 1995.

29. Rolls, B. J., and Hammer, V. A. Fat, carbohydrate and the regulation of food intake. Am. J. Clin. Nutr. 62(suppl):1086S–1095S, 1995.
30. Tremblay, A., Després, J-P., Thriault, G., et al. Overfeeding and energy expenditure in humans. Am. J. Clin. Nutr. 56:857–862, 1992.
31. Diaz, E. O., Prentice, A. M., Goldberg, G. R., et al. Metabolic response to experimental overfeeding in lean and overweight healthy volunteers. Am. J. Clin. Nutr. 56:641–655, 1992.
32. Hirsch, J., Hudgins, L. C., Liebel, R. L., and Rosenbaum, M. Diet composition and energy balance in humans. Am. J. Clin. Nutr. 67(suppl):551S–555S, 1998.
33. Gura, T. Uncoupling proteins provide new clues to obesity's causes. Science 280:1369–1370, 1998.
34. Levine, J. A., Eberhardt, N. L., and Jensen, M. D. Role of nonexercise activity thermogenesis in resistance to fat gain in humans. Science 283:212–214, 1999.
35. Hill, J. O., and Peters, J. C. Environmental contributions to the obesity epidemic. Science 280:1371–1374, 1998.
36. Cutting, T. M., Fisher, J. O., Grimm-Thomas, K., and Birch, L. L. Like mother, like daughter: familial patterns of overweight are mediated by mothers' dietary disinhibition. Am. J. Clin. Nutr. 69: 608–613, 1999.
37. Lisette, C. P., de Groot, G. M., and van Staveren, W. A. Reduced physical activity and its association with obesity. Nutr. Rev. 53:11–18, 1995.
38. Flagel, K. M., Carroll, M. D., Kuczmarski, R. J., and Johnson, C. L. Overweight and obesity in the United States: prevalence and trends, 1960–1994. Int. J. Obesity 22:39–47, 1998.
39. Norman, R. A., Thompson, D. B., Foroud, T., et al. Genomewide search for genes influencing percent body fat in Pima Indians: suggestive linkage at chromosome 11q21-q22. Am. J. Human Genet. 60:166–173, 1997.
40. Esparza, J., Fox, C., Harper, I. T., et al. Daily energy expenditure in Mexican and USA Pima Indians: low physical activity as a possible cause of obesity. Int. J. Obes. Relat. Metab. Disord. 24:55–59, 2000.

8 Weight Management: Body Weight and Health

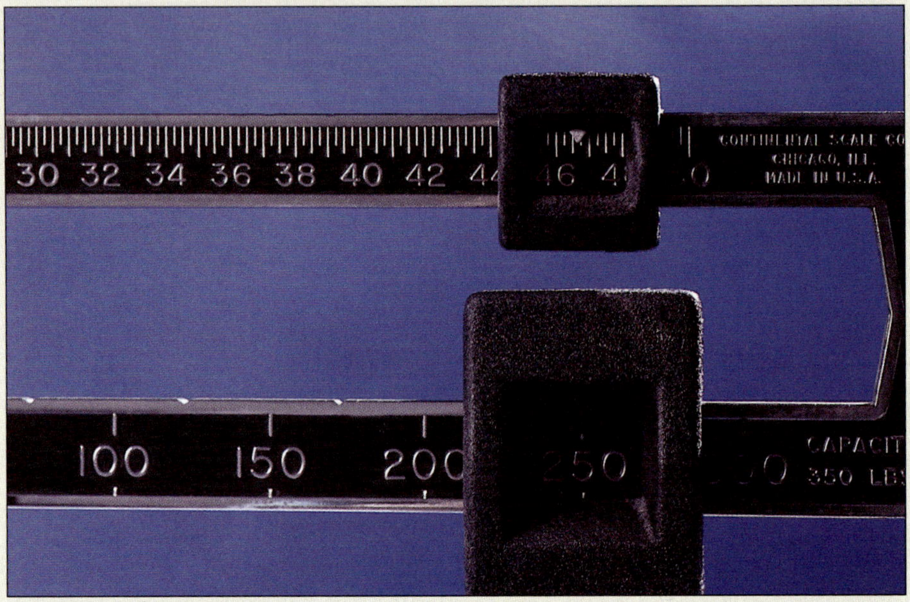

Learning Objectives

After reading this chapter, students should be able to:

1. Discuss the incidence of obesity and its associated health problems.
2. Define "healthy weight."
3. List the factors that should be considered when assessing the risks associated with excess body weight.
4. Explain how the principle of energy balance applies to weight loss.
5. Discuss the concept of weight management and the recommendations for weight loss.
6. Explain why behavior change is important in weight management.
7. Evaluate the appropriateness of a weight-loss program.
8. Describe the roles of drugs and surgery in weight management.
9. Explain the medical consequences of being underweight.
10. Compare and contrast anorexia nervosa, bulimia nervosa, and binge-eating disorder.

Walter had tried everything. He had been on and off diets since he was 19. He had tried the grapefruit diet, the Atkins' diet, the Beverly Hills diet, the fiber diet, the Zone, and a hundred more. Most of them worked for a while. He lost some weight, but then, when he could no longer limit himself to the foods allowed by the current diet, the weight came rushing back. It seemed the more he dieted the more he gained. Every time he lost weight, he gained it all back plus a few more pounds. He once calculated that during his lifetime he had lost (and regained) 600 pounds! Now, at 5 feet 8 inches tall, he weighed over 350 pounds—more than twice his goal weight.

At his last physical his physician told him that his blood cholesterol was 240 mg/100 ml and his blood pressure and blood glucose levels were slightly elevated. The prospects of heart disease and diabetes were scary, but he didn't have to think about these every day. What he did have to deal with every day was the pain in his knees and back from carrying an extra 100+ pounds everywhere he went. He also had to deal with judgmental stares every time he put food in his mouth in a public place, and looks of scorn from fellow bus passengers when he overflowed onto two seats. He was more desperate than ever. With his health risks on the rise, he made an appointment with a physician to discuss prescription weight-loss drugs and the possibility of obesity surgery—so he could lose the weight for good.

Managing weight is a lifelong pursuit. It is best addressed by preventing weight gain in the first place. Just as a family history of heart disease or an increase in blood cholesterol should set in motion dietary and lifestyle changes to maintain health, a family history of obesity or an increase in body weight should trigger dietary and lifestyle changes that maintain weight at a healthy level.

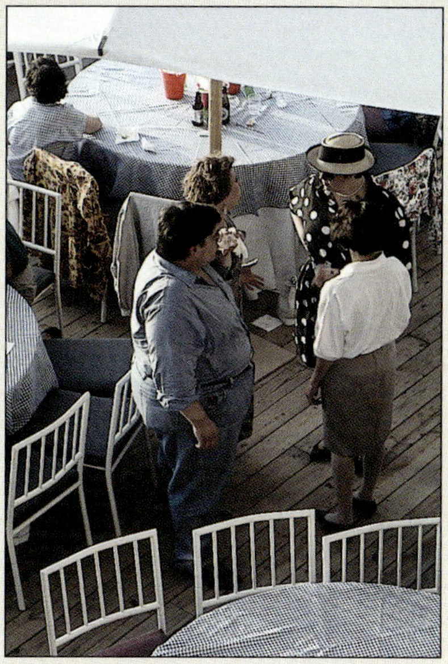

Overweight and Obesity: A Growing Problem

Obesity has been called "one of today's most blatantly visible—yet most neglected—public health problems."[1] Carrying excess body fat contributes to a number of health problems and increases the risk of developing chronic diseases such as diabetes, heart disease, and cancer.[2] Nevertheless, more people around the globe, and particularly in developed countries such as the United States, are **overweight** or obese than ever before. Currently, about 60% of all adult Americans are considered overweight, and almost a quarter (22.5%) are classified as obese.[3,4,5] These percentages have increased continually over the last 40 years (Figure 8.1).[3] Weight problems are also increasing among children and adolescents.[6]

One explanation for this increasing incidence of overweight and obesity is the modern lifestyle, which offers a plentiful and varied diet along with conveniences that reduce energy expenditure. Once weight is gained, it is not easy to lose. Every year about 44% of American women and 29% of American men try to lose weight.[7] Many never lose any weight at all, and most people who lose weight

Obesity A condition characterized by excess body fat. It is defined as a body mass index of 30 kg/m^2 or greater or a body weight that is 20% or more above the healthy body weight standard.

Overweight A body mass index of 25 to 29.9 kg/m^2 or a body weight 10 to 19% above the healthy body weight standard.

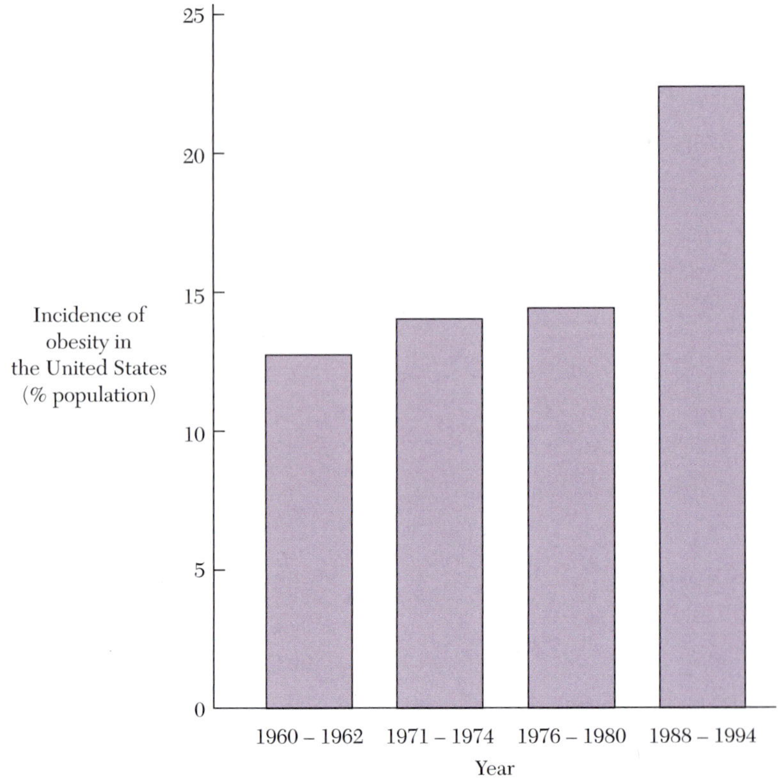

FIGURE 8.1 More Americans than ever are overweight or obese. According to the NHANES surveys conducted approximately every ten years, the prevalence of obesity defined as a BMI of greater than or equal to 30 has increased over the last 40 years, particularly in the last 10 years. (*Source: CDC, National Center for Health Statistics)*

eventually regain it.[8] This generates a ready supply of customers for the thousands of weight-loss plans offered by commercial ventures, physicians, and support groups. It is estimated that Americans spend $30 to $50 billion each year on diet clubs, weight-loss programs, special foods, and over-the-counter weight-loss remedies[9] (Figure 8.2).

The increasing prevalence of obesity and the failure of most attempts at weight loss have created a major public health problem. Estimates suggest that the obesity-related health-care costs in the United States exceed $70 billion per

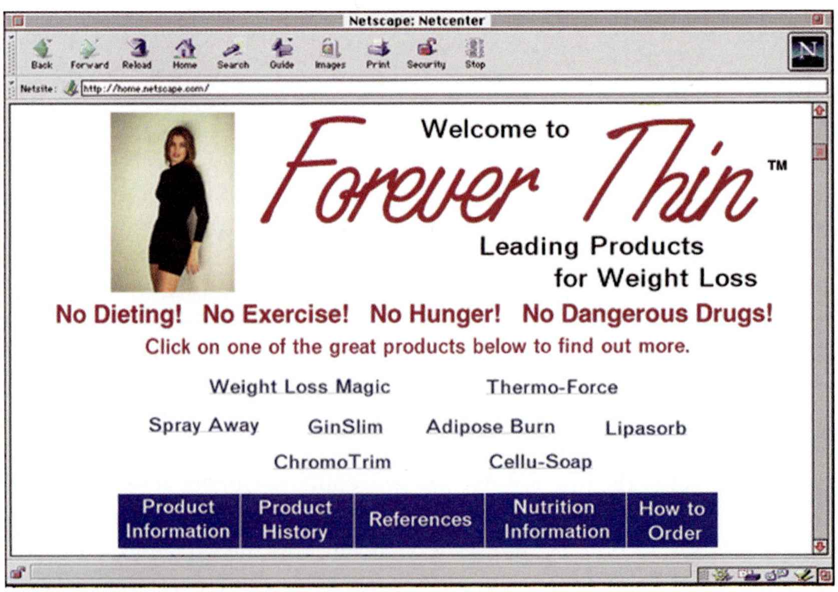

FIGURE 8.2 There are countless weight-loss plans and products available. The Internet makes it possible to purchase these without even getting out of your chair.

year.[10] In response, public health campaigns such as Healthy People 2010 and the Dietary Guidelines for Americans, 2000, stress the importance of achieving and maintaining a healthy weight for all Americans (Figure 8.3).

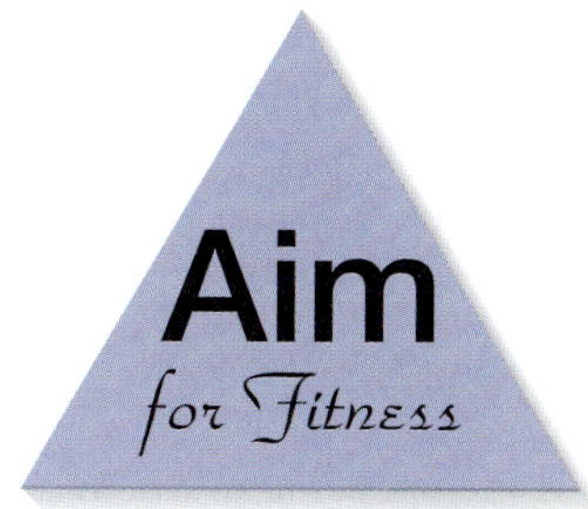

▲ Aim for a healthy weight

FIGURE 8.3 The Dietary Guidelines for Americans, 2000, advise us to "Aim for a healthy weight."

THE HEALTH RISKS OF OBESITY

The risks associated with obesity are related to the degree of excess weight or fat, the distribution of the excess body fat, and the presence of other diseases or risk factors that often accompany the obesity.

A Healthy Weight

Guidelines for a healthy level of body fat or body weight are based on the weight at which the risk of death is lowest (Figure 8.4). The health risks associated with being overweight increase as the degree of overweight increases.

As discussed in Chapter 7, BMI correlates well with body fat and is the currently accepted measure of body weight and fat. It is calculated by dividing weight in kilograms by the square of height in meters. The BMI range associated with the lowest risk of mortality is between 19 and 25 kg/m^2. A BMI below this is classified as **underweight.** A BMI of 25 or over is considered overweight, 30 or over is considered obese, and 40 or over is classified as **extreme** or **morbid obesity.** Figure 8.5 can be used to determine if one's BMI falls in the healthy weight category.

Underweight A body mass index of less than 18.5 kg/m^2 or a body weight 10% or more below the healthy body weight standard.

Extreme or **morbid obesity** A condition in which body weight is 100 pounds (45.5 kg) above healthy body weight or body mass index is greater than 40 kg/m^2.

Even though BMI correlates well with body fat, it is not a perfect tool for evaluating the health risk associated with obesity. An individual with a BMI in the overweight range who consumes a healthy diet and exercises regularly may be more fit than an individual with a BMI in the healthy range who is sedentary and eats a poor diet. Or, an individual may have a high BMI but not have excess body fat. For example, body builders may have a high BMI because they have a high lean body mass. Although BMI is high, their disease risk is low (Figure 8.6).

Distribution of Body Fat

In overweight individuals, the distribution of body fat as well as the amount of excess fat affects the risk of developing chronic diseases. Some people carry their excess fat around and above the waist in the abdominal region; they have more visceral fat. Others carry their extra fat below the waist in the hips and thighs; they have more subcutaneous fat. These body types have been dubbed apples and

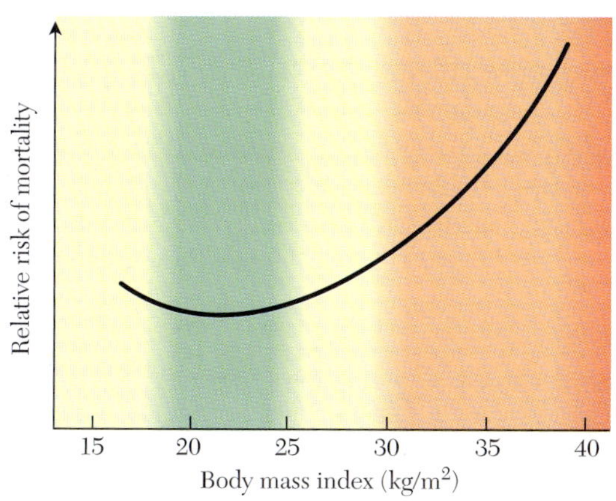

FIGURE 8.4 The overall risk of dying, or risk of mortality, is lowest in individuals with a BMI between about 20 and 25 kg/m^2. The risk of mortality begins to increase more sharply at BMIs near 30 and continues to rise as BMI increases further.

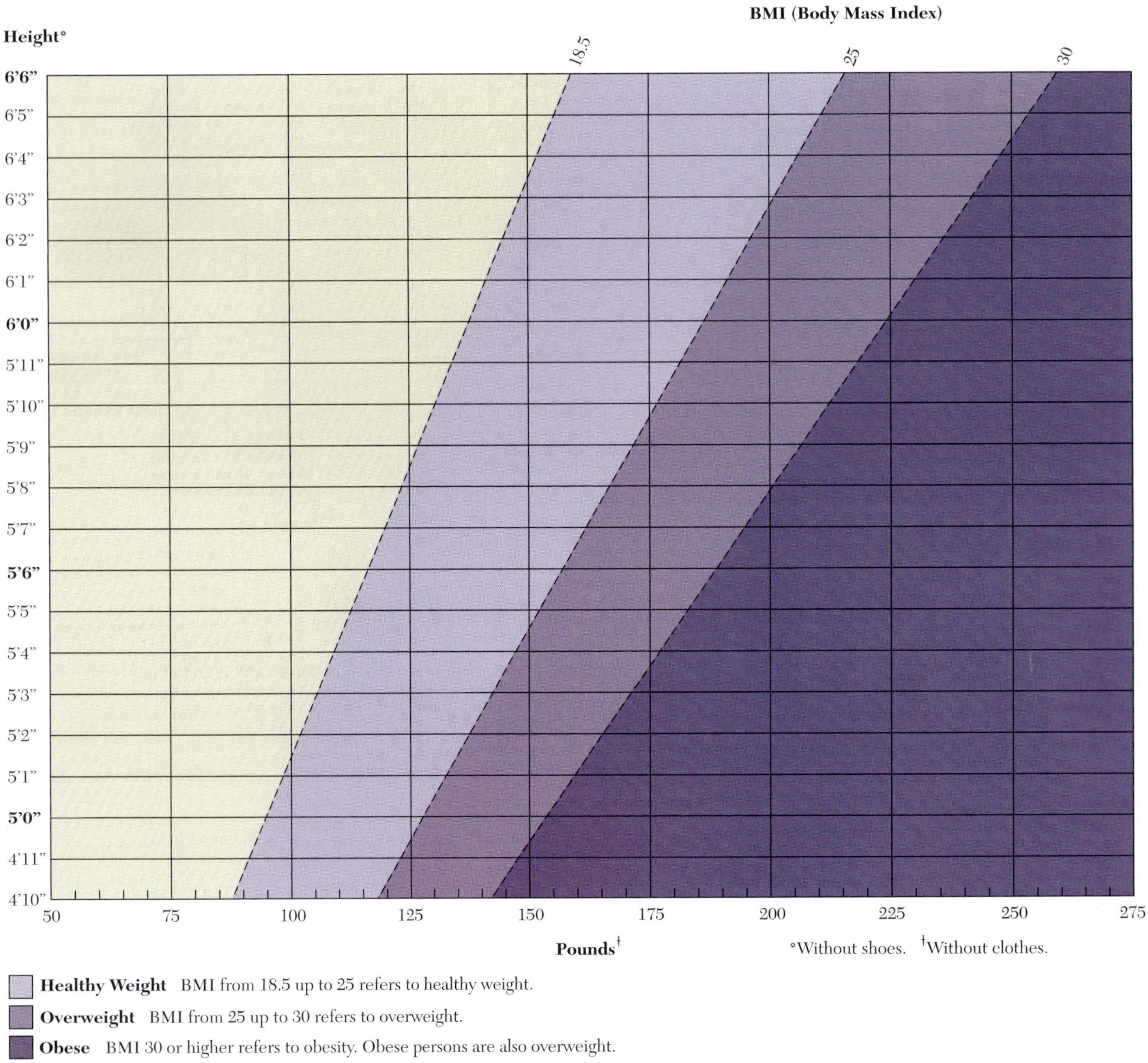

FIGURE 8.5 To determine your BMI range, locate the point that lines up with your weight (in pounds) on the bottom scale and draw a vertical line up from this point. Locate your height (in feet and inches) on the left-hand scale and draw a horizontal line that extends into the graph. The point where these two lines meet indicates your BMI status. *(Report of the Dietary Advisory Committee on the Dietary Guidelines for Americans, 2000)*

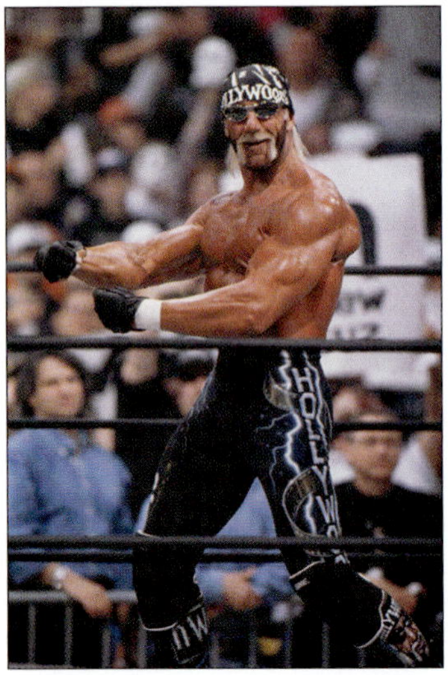

pears, respectively, by the popular literature (Figure 8.7). Health risks increase with increasing visceral fat.

The amount of visceral fat an individual carries can be estimated by measuring waist circumference. For males, a BMI of 25 to 34.9 kg/m^2 and a waist circumference greater than 40 inches is associated with increased risk. For females in this BMI range, waist circumference of greater than 35 inches increases risks.

FIGURE 8.6 Wrestler/actor Hulk Hogan, at 6 feet 8 inches tall and 275 pounds, has a BMI of 30.3, which falls into the category of obese. However, it is unlikely that his high BMI is due to excess body fat or that it indicates an increased risk of disease.

In individuals with a BMI greater than or equal to 35 these cut-off points do not predict risk (see Table 8.1). In order to monitor body weight and risk, the Dietary Guidelines for Americans, 2000, recommend that all Americans keep track of their weight and their waists and avoid increases in both.

Chronic Disease and Body Weight

Heart disease, high blood cholesterol, high blood pressure, stroke, diabetes, gallbladder disease, sleep disorders, respiratory problems, arthritis, and cancers of the breast, uterus, prostate, and colon all occur more frequently in overweight individuals.[5] And, the presence of these diseases increases the risk of illness and premature death that is associated with being overweight. Weight loss can reduce the incidence of these diseases. Benjamin Franklin summed this up when he said, "To lengthen thy life, lessen thy meals."

Web Menu For more information on body weight and health in the United States, go to www.nhlbi.nih.gov/subsites/ and click on Aim for a Healthy Weight. For more information on body weight and health around the world, go to the World Health Organization at www.who.int/nut/.

Heart Disease Obesity is considered a primary risk factor for cardiovascular disease. Carrying excess body fat increases the amount of work required by the heart and the risk of developing high blood pressure and high blood lipid levels. A reduction in body weight and fat has been shown to reduce blood cholesterol levels, blood pressure, and heart disease risk.[11] Regular exercise decreases heart disease risk by promoting the maintenance of a healthy body composition as well as increasing blood HDL (good) cholesterol levels and reducing blood pressure.[12]

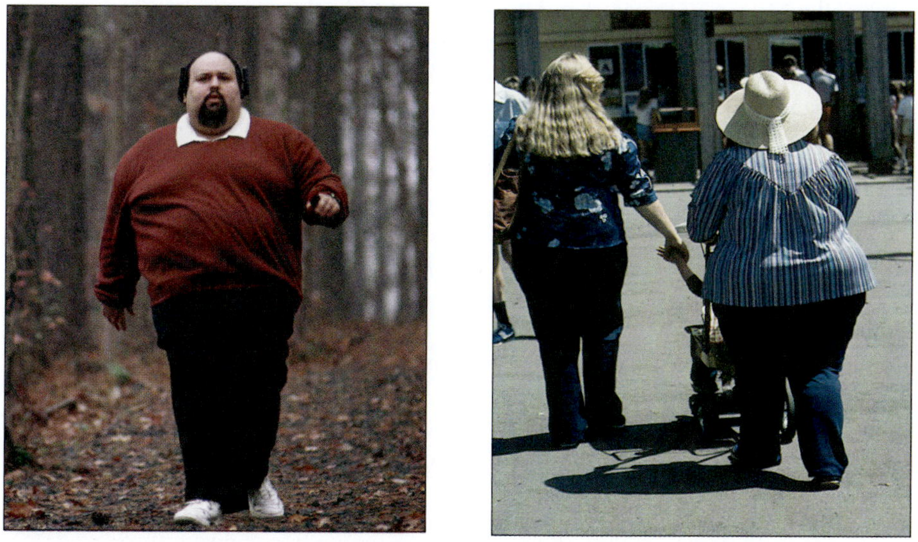

(a) (b)

FIGURE 8.7 (a) Overweight individuals with an "apple" shape deposit fat in the abdominal region and are at greater risk of developing heart disease and diabetes. (b) Overweight individuals with a "pear" shape deposit fat in the hips and thighs where it is primarily subcutaneous. *(a, Corbis; b, ©Tom McHugh/Photo Researchers, Inc.)*

TABLE 8.1 BMI, Waist Circumference, and Disease Risk

		Disease Risk†	
	BMI (kg/m²)*	*Men, waist ≤ 40inches, and women, waist ≤ 35inches*	*Men, waist > 40 inches, and women, waist > 35 inches*
Underweight	< 18.5		
Normal weight	18.5 to 24.9		
Overweight	25.0 to 29.9	Increased	High
Obesity (class I)	30.0 to 34.9	High	Very high
Obesity (class II)	35.0 to 39.9	Very high	Very high
Extreme or morbid obesity (class III)	≥ 40	Extremely high	Extremely high

*BMI = body weight (kg)/ height squared (m²)

†Disease risk for type 2 diabetes, hypertension, and cardiovascular disease relative to individuals with a normal weight and normal waist circumference.

National Institutes of Health, National Heart, Lung, and Blood Institute. Clinical Guidelines on the Identification, Evaluation, and Treatment of Overweight and Obesity in Adults. Executive summary, June 1998. Available online at: **http://www.nhlbi.nih.gov/guidelines/obesity/ob_home.htm**.

Diabetes Excess body fat, particularly when the excess is in the abdominal region, increases the risk of type 2 diabetes. Diabetes, in turn, increases the risks of heart disease and stroke.[13] Atherosclerosis is the most common long-term complication of diabetes and cardiovascular risk factors including hypertension, which predisposes to stroke, are more frequent in diabetics. In overweight individuals who have diabetes, weight loss can help maintain blood glucose levels in the normal range.[14]

Gallbladder Disease Obesity is associated with an increase in gallstone formation. Gallstones are clumps of solid material that form in the gallbladder. They are typically composed mostly of cholesterol and may form as a single large stone or many small ones. Gallstones often cause no symptoms but if they lodge in the bile ducts they can cause pain and cramps. If the passage of bile is blocked lipid absorption in the small intestine is impaired and the gallbladder can become inflamed.

The more obese a person is, the greater his or her risk is of developing gallstones. Women with a BMI of 30 or higher have about twice the risk of developing gallstones as women with a BMI of less than 25. Gallstones are reported in up to 45% of individuals who are more than 100 pounds overweight.[15] The reason that obesity increases the risk of gallstones is unclear, but researchers believe that in obese people, the liver produces too much cholesterol, which deposits in the gallbladder and forms stones. Although the risk of gallstones decreases with a lower body weight, weight loss, in particular rapid weight loss, increases the risk of gallbladder disease because as lipids are released from body stores, cholesterol synthesis increases, increasing the tendency for cholesterol stone formation. Gallstones are one of the most medically important complications of voluntary weight loss.[16]

Other Conditions Obesity can affect many other aspects of health. It increases the incidence and severity of infectious disease and has been linked to poor wound healing and surgical complications.[17] It increases pregnancy risks both for the mother and child.[18] In addition obesity increases the risk of a variety of other diseases including sleep apnea, cancer, and arthritis.[19]

Sleep apnea is a serious, potentially life-threatening condition characterized by brief interruptions of breathing during sleep. In obese individuals, weight loss may decrease both the frequency and severity of sleep apnea symptoms.[20]

Excess body weight and fat affect the risks of certain forms of cancer. In obese men, cancers of the prostate and colon are increased. In women, being overweight seems to protect against the form of breast cancer that occurs in the childbearing years but it increases the risks of postmenopausal breast cancer.[21]

Excess weight and fat can also increase the risk of developing osteoarthritis. This is a type of arthritis that occurs when the cartilage cushioning the joints breaks down and gradually becomes rougher and thinner. As the process continues, a substantial amount of cartilage wears away so the bones in the joint rub against each other causing pain and reducing movement. Being overweight is the most common cause of excess pressure on the joints and it can speed the rate at which the cartilage wears down. Losing weight reduces the pressure and strain on the joints and slows the wear and tear of cartilage. Weight loss can also help reduce pain and stiffness in the affected joints, especially those in the hips, knees, back, and feet.[22]

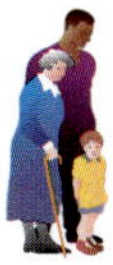

In addition to the physical problems associated with being overweight, there are psychological and social concerns. Obese individuals of every age are more likely to experience depression.[23] Overweight children are often teased and ostracized and frequently find themselves isolated socially from their peers. Overweight individuals face discrimination just about everywhere—in school, in the workplace, even on public transportation.[24]

Assessing the Risks of Excess Body Weight

An assessment of the risks associated with excess body fat must consider not only BMI but also waist circumference, as well as the presence of disease conditions such as cardiovascular disease and diabetes, and the presence of risk factors for these conditions such as high LDL cholesterol and elevated blood glucose. An overweight person is classified as being at high risk if they have two or more of the risk factors listed in Table 8.2.[5] Weight loss is recommended for individuals who are obese and for those with a BMI in the overweight range, if they have a high waist circumference or have two or more other risk factors.[5]

TABLE 8.2 Factors That Increase the Risks of Obesity

Factors
Increasing BMI
Excess visceral fat
Disease conditions
Established coronary heart disease
Other cardiovascular diseases
Type 2 diabetes
Sleep apnea
Other obesity-associated diseases
Gynecological abnormalities
Osteoarthritis
Gallstones
Stress incontinence
Cardiovascular risk factors
Cigarette smoking
Hypertension (systolic blood pressure ≥ 140 or diastolic ≥ 90 mm Hg, or individual taking blood pressure medication)
High LDL cholesterol (>130 mg/dL)
Low HDL cholesterol (< 40 mg/dL)
Impaired fasting glucose (fasting plasma glucose of 110 to 125 mg/dL)
Family history of premature coronary heart disease (before age 55 in father or other male relative or before age 65 in mother or other female relative)
Age (men ≥ 45 and women ≥ 55 years)

National Institutes of Health, National Heart, Lung, and Blood Institute. Clinical Guidelines on the Identification, Evaluation, and Treatment of Overweight and Obesity in Adults. Executive summary, June 1998. Available online at: **http://www.nhlbi.nih.gov/guidelines/obesity/ob_home.htm**.

Weight Management

Weight management programs can help overweight individuals reduce their body weight to a healthy level. For some overweight individuals, who do not have two or more risk factors or a high waist circumference, weight loss may not be necessary to maintain good health.[5]

Managing Weight at a Healthy Level

For more information on healthy weight management, go to the Weight Control Information Network at www.niddk.nih.gov/health/nutrit/win.htm.

The increasing incidence of obesity, along with the alarming failure rate of long-term weight loss, have caused researchers and physicians to reevaluate the way they think about treating overweight individuals. Rather than focusing on reaching a specific weight goal, weight management efforts should focus on achieving a healthier weight and level of fitness that can be maintained for a lifetime. Preventing weight gain and the diseases associated with excess weight may be more important goals than reaching a specific weight.

Weight management is a process that begins during childhood with the development of sound eating and activity habits.[24] Adults who are at a healthy weight should strive to avoid weight gain. For those who are already overweight, the goal of weight management should be to reduce body weight to a level that decreases the health risks associated with being overweight.

Reducing Weight to Reduce Risk For most people, a loss of 5 to 15% of body weight, most of which is fat, significantly reduces disease risk.[25] The initial goal of weight loss should therefore be to reduce body weight by approximately 10% over a period of about 6 months.[5] To accomplish this, a safe rate of weight loss is 1/2 to 2 pounds per week, depending on how much needs to be lost.[25] After this initial weight loss, risks can be re-assessed to determine if additional weight loss would be beneficial.

A slow loss of 10% of body weight is considered achievable for most individuals and is easier to maintain than larger weight losses. Most people who lose large amounts of weight or lose weight rapidly eventually regain all that they have lost. Repeated cycles of weight loss and regain, referred to as **weight cycling,** increase the proportion of body fat with each successive weight regain and cause a decrease in RMR, making subsequent weight loss more difficult (Figure 8.8).[26] Even if an individual has lost and subsequently regained weight in the past, weight loss is recommended if they are still obese or overweight and have two or more risk factors.[25]

Weight cycling The repeated loss and regain of body weight.

The Mathematics of Weight Loss The goal of weight loss is to lose excess body fat without losing lean tissue. Body fat is approximately 15% water and 85% fat, with small amounts of protein and carbohydrate. A pound of body fat therefore contains about 390 g of fat (1 pound = 450 g; 85% of 450 g = 390 g). Because fat provides about 9 kcalories per gram, a pound of fat is equal to about 3500 kcalories (390 g × 9 kcal/g). Therefore, to lose a pound in a week, an average individual must reduce intake and/or increase activity by 500 kcalories per day (3500 kcal/7 days = 500 kcal/day). This is the predicted average weight loss at this energy deficit. However, the actual amount of weight lost per week may vary over time.

Many weight-loss programs and products promise a weight loss of 5 pounds or more per week. Applying the foregoing equations shows that to lose 5 pounds of fat, one's energy expenditure would have to exceed intake by 17,500 kcalories a week (3500 kcal/lb × 5 lb) or 2500 kcalories a day. Because most people expend only about 2500 kcalories each day, creating an energy deficit of 2500 kcalories would require either maintaining normal activity while consuming nothing at all or adding about 10 hours of moderate exercise daily without increasing intake.

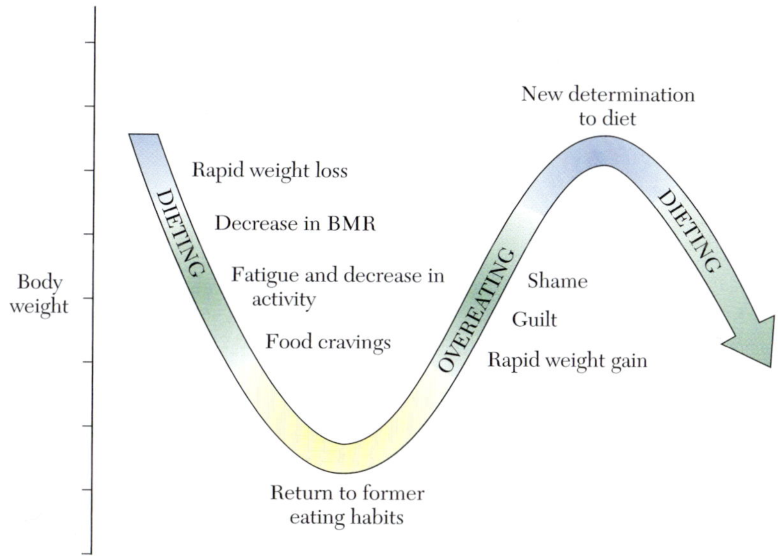

FIGURE 8.8 Weight cycling refers to the repeated loss and regain of body weight.

Despite these daunting figures, many people who start a diet do lose as much as 5 pounds the first week. This is because the weight lost is not all due to fat loss. During rapid initial weight loss, glycogen and muscle tissue are broken down and used for energy, and water is lost. Because muscle is about 80% water, a pound of muscle provides only about 500 kcalories.* Therefore if you are losing muscle rather than fat, an energy imbalance of only 500 kcalories could cause the scale to register a one-pound weight loss—most of which is water.

To promote the loss of fat and not lean tissue, a weight-loss program should encourage the loss of only 1/2 to 2 pounds per week.[25] If weight is lost more rapidly, the loss is less likely to be maintained and the additional loss will be from fluid, glycogen, and muscle protein.

Strategies for Weight Loss and Weight Maintenance

The arithmetic of weight loss is simple, but achieving and maintaining a reduction in body weight is not easy. There are regulatory mechanisms at work to keep body weight stable. As weight decreases, so does RMR, which means that as an individual loses weight they need to eat fewer kcalories to continue their weight loss. In addition, the inclination to exercise may be reduced in overweight individuals and in those consuming reduced-energy diets (see *Research Discoveries:* "Starvation or Intentional Weight Loss?").

Despite hundreds of research studies that address weight loss and management, no one method has been determined to be the most effective. Nonetheless, weight reduction can be accomplished by reducing energy intake and/or increasing energy output by increasing physical activity (Figure 8.9). Applying techniques to change eating behaviors can improve the long-term success rate. In an evaluation of data collected from the National Weight Control Registry, a database of information on individuals who have successfully lost a minimum of 30 pounds and maintained their loss for at least five and a half years, participants reported that they succeeded by limiting their fat intake, eating a variety of foods, and limiting their portion sizes. Seventy-two percent of participants also increased their level of physical activity to a minimum of 30 minutes of moderate physical activity daily. These individuals reported that they were motivated to lose weight by both health and social reasons.[27]

---

*Protein inside the body supplies about 5.6 kcal/g, so a pound of muscle, which is about 20% protein, would supply only about 500 kcal (90 g × 5.6 kcal/g).

RESEARCH DISCOVERIES

Starvation or Intentional Weight Loss?

Starvation is the lack of sufficient energy to maintain life. When the body experiences this lack of energy, a variety of adaptations occurs to promote survival. Unfortunately, these adaptations occur whether you are struggling to survive a famine or trying to lose 10 pounds to look better in a bathing suit. These physiological and psychological changes that occur in response to starvation have implications for the treatment and management of obesity and eating disorders.[a]

Most of what we know about the physiology and psychology of starvation comes from a landmark study conducted by Ancel Keys at the University of Minnesota over 50 years ago.[b] This study investigated the effect of food deprivation on 36 young, healthy, normal-weight men who volunteered to participate in the study as an alternative to military service. The first three months of the study comprised a control period during which the subjects ate normally while their behavior, personality, and eating patterns were observed. During the next six months, energy intake for each subject was restricted to half of his normal intake (an average of about 1570 kcalories per day). This "starvation" period was followed by three months of rehabilitation during which the men were gradually re-fed.

The amount of weight lost during the starvation period varied among the subjects; the average loss was about 25% of original body weight. As the subjects lost weight, their bodies seemed to adapt to prevent further losses by decreasing energy needs. Basal metabolic rates decreased by an average of 39% after six months on the starvation regimen. This was reflected by decreases in body temperature, heart rate, and respiration. When the men were re-fed, their BMR increased; the larger the amount of food consumed, the larger the increase in BMR.

In addition to changes in energy expenditure, subjects experienced dizziness, headaches, reduced strength, poor motor control, edema, hair loss, cold intolerance, tingling in the hands and feet, visual and auditory disturbances, gastrointestinal upsets, and a decreased need for sleep. Most subjects also experienced some emotional changes due to the semistarvation. Depression and mood swings were common, as were irritability, anger, and apathy. There were also changes in social behavior. Most stopped dating and had no interest in sex. This makes sense from an evolutionary standpoint because, during times of famine, energy should be spent looking for food rather than reproducing.

Some of the most striking observations made in this study involved the subjects' relationship with food. The men became preoccupied with food. They had difficulty concentrating on daily tasks because all they could think about was food. Some hoarded food and ate in a ritualized fashion. Three subjects became chefs after the study was over. The consumption of coffee and tea increased so much that it had to be limited to 9 cups per day. Gum chewing also became excessive with some and had to be limited. Binge eating occurred in some men who had no previous history of disordered eating, and periods of overconsumption continued for many into and beyond the re-feeding period.

This work did much to enhance our understanding of the physiological, psychological, and behavioral consequences of energy restriction. The dramatic changes observed in this study occurred in people eating over 1500 kcalories per day, an energy intake that only produces slow weight loss in many people. How can these physical and psychological changes be any different from what people experience on a weight-loss diet? An individual consuming a low-kcalorie weight-loss diet becomes obsessed with food because that is what their biology dictates. When early humans did not have enough to eat, their biology forced them to think about nothing else to ensure survival. People who "cheat" on diets do not lack will power but are simply responding to their biology. The obsessions with food and rituals in food consumption reported in this study are similar to those seen in individuals with anorexia nervosa. How many of the symptoms of eating disorders are the result of the starvation rather than the obsession with body weight and size?

If you consider the findings of the Minnesota starvation study, it is easier to understand why dieters are often unsuccessful in the long term. More research needs to be done into the physical and psychological consequences of intentional starvation. The results might someday help us overcome the body's natural tendency to prevent weight loss and develop weight-loss techniques that are effective and not torturous in the long term.

References

[a] Garner, D. M. The effects of starvation on behavior: implications for dieting and eating disorders. Healthy Weight Journal, September/October 1998, 68–72.

[b] Keys, A., Brozek, J., Henschel, A., et al. *The Biology of Human Starvation*, vols. 1 and 2. Minneapolis: University of Minnesota Press, 1950.

Decreasing Energy Intake Weight loss can be accomplished by reducing energy intake to a level below that needed for energy balance. Reducing energy intake by 250 to 500 kcal/day should produce a weight loss of 1/2 to 1 pound per week in most individuals. The most realistic way to reduce intake is simply to reduce portion sizes and eliminate high-kcalorie foods. To be healthy, the diet must provide for all the body's nutrient needs except for energy. Nutrient density becomes more important as energy intake is reduced. Choosing foods that are low in fat and added sugars will increase the nutrient density of the diet. With intakes of fewer than 1200 kcalories per day, it is difficult to meet the requirements for mi-

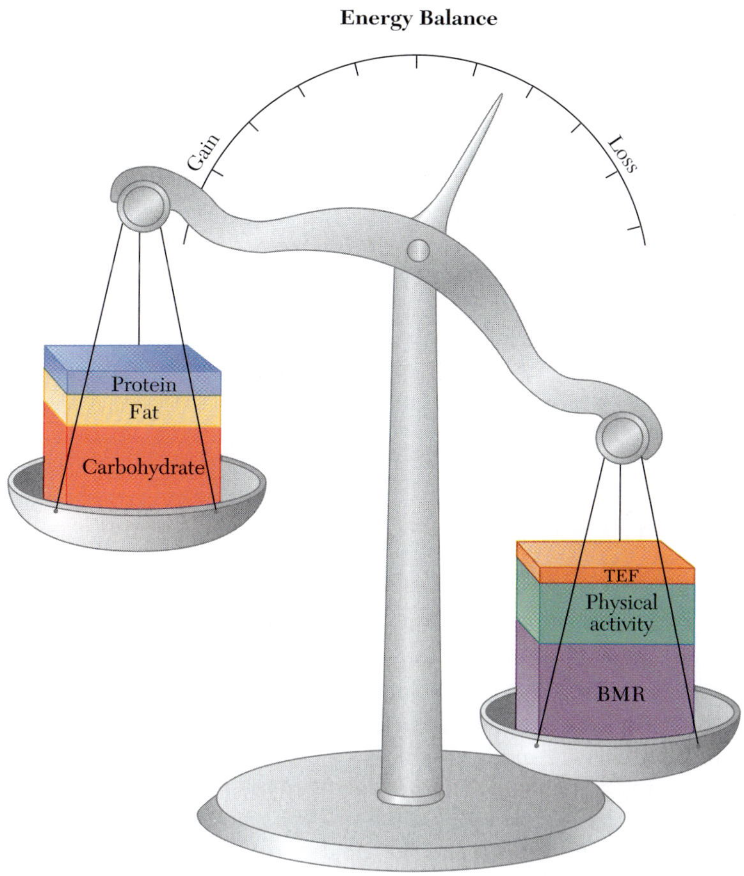

FIGURE 8.9 The mathematics of weight loss is simple. If the total amount of energy entering the body from food is less than the amount expended by BMR, physical activity, and TEF, then energy balance will tip in the direction of weight loss.

cronutrients, so a multivitamin and mineral supplement is also recommended. Medical supervision is also recommended if energy intake is 800 kcalories or less per day.[28,29]

Increasing Energy Expenditure Physical activity is an important component of any well-designed weight-management program. Exercise promotes fat loss and weight maintenance. It increases energy expenditure, so if intake remains the same, energy stored as fat is used for fuel. When beginning an exercise program, individuals should start with small changes and increase activities as fitness level rises. Even small changes in activity can produce weight loss if energy intake is not increased. For example, as shown in Table 8.3, if you replace an hour of watching TV with an hour of slow walking, you will expend about 163 extra kcalories. If you do this every day, it will result in the loss of a pound in about three weeks.

In addition to expending extra energy, exercise promotes muscle development. Because muscle is more metabolically active than adipose tissue, increasing muscle mass helps to increase RMR and prevent the drop in RMR that occurs as body weight decreases. In addition to increasing energy expenditure and muscle mass, physical activity improves overall fitness and relieves boredom and stress. Thus, weight loss is better maintained when physical activity is included in the weight-management program.[30] The benefits of exercise are discussed further in Chapter 14.

Modifying Behavior to Maintain Weight Loss In order to keep weight at a new lower level, food consumption and exercise patterns must be changed for life. Changing these behaviors requires identifying the old patterns that led to weight

TABLE 8.3 Small Increases in Activity Add Up*

Daily activity (replacing one hour of sitting)	Extra energy expended per day (kcal/hour)	Extra energy expended per week (kcal/week)†	Extra energy expended per year (kcal/year)†	Theoretical weight loss (lb/year)†
Walking slowly	163	1141	59,495	17.0
Dancing, slow	237	1659	86,505	24.7
Stair climbing	857	5999	312,805	89.3
Golf, with power cart	192	1344	70,080	20.0
Golf, walking with bag	857	5999	312,805	89.3
Lawn mowing, push	798	5586	291,270	83.2
Lawn mowing, riding	192	1344	70,080	20.0
Light gardening	266	1862	97,090	27.7

*Values are for a 130-pound person.

†This assumes that an hour of sitting is replaced by an hour of this activity every day and that energy intake does not change.

Behavior modification A process used to gradually and permanently change habitual behaviors.

gain and replacing them with new ones to maintain weight loss. This can be accomplished through a process called **behavior modification,** which is based on the theory that behaviors involve (1) antecedents or cues that lead to the behavior, (2) the behavior itself, and (3) consequences of the behavior. These are referred to as the ABCs of behavior modification.

The first step in a behavior modification program is to identify the cues or antecedents. This can be done by keeping a log of eating and exercise patterns and what motivated them. The log can then be analyzed to determine what led to the behavior, whether it was excessive eating or inadequate exercising, and what the consequences of the behavior were. The key to modifying the behavior is to recognize the antecedent, so that the behavior and consequences can be changed (Table 8.4). For example, you are hungry and you smell fresh-baked cookies while shopping at the mall. You buy a dozen cookies and eat half of them; you feel bad because you have blown your diet, so you eat the other half-dozen. The antecedents to this behavior are being hungry while shopping and walking past the bakery smelling the cookies. The behavior is eating half a dozen cookies, and the consequence is the guilt and disappointment you feel, which leads to your consuming more cookies. This behavior pattern can be changed by avoiding shopping when you are hungry, taking a different route through the mall to avoid the food section, or planning ahead to buy only one cookie. That way, you avoid eating more than planned, do not gain weight, and feel a sense of accomplishment. Applying behavior modification techniques to change eating behaviors has been shown to improve long-term weight maintenance.

TABLE 8.4 Behavior Modification in Weight Management

Determine antecedents and behaviors

Buying too much because you are hungry when shopping.

Consuming high-kcalorie snacks because they are in the house.

Grabbing an unplanned snack because it is in sight.

Overeating because you are distracted by watching TV.

Having "seconds" because there is only a little left in the serving bowl.

Alter behaviors

Shop right after eating to avoid snacking while shopping.

Shop from a list to avoid impulse buys.

Keep food out of sight, in the cupboard.

Eat only at a specified location and without other activities.

Leave serving dishes off the table.

Provide positive consequences

Keep track of successes.

Plan nonfood rewards.

Weight Loss at Different Stages of Life

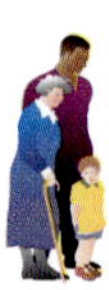

Obesity and overweight is a growing problem among children (Figure 8.10). It is estimated that between 11 and 24% of American children and adolescents are overweight and at higher risk of becoming overweight adults.[6] This growing trend is the result of both excessive intake of foods high in fat and energy, and inadequate physical activity. However, strict weight-loss diets are generally not recommended for children or adolescents because a reduction in intake can interfere with growth. The preferred technique is to encourage physical activity, along with a moderate energy-intake restriction, allowing the child to grow in height with little additional weight gain (see Chapter 16).

Weight-loss diets are also not recommended during pregnancy. Even women who are overweight at the start of pregnancy should gain at a slow, steady rate to

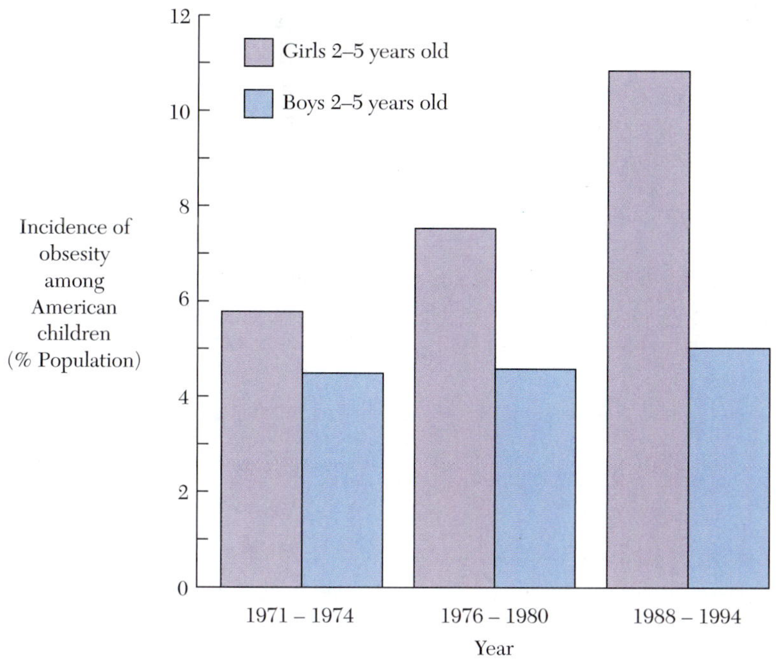

FIGURE 8.10 According to the NHANES surveys conducted approximately every ten years, the prevalence of obesity in American children ages two through five has increased over the last 30 years, particularly in girls. Obesity was defined as a weight for stature at or above the 95th percentile on the NCHS growth charts of weight for stature and age. *(Adapted from WINS Notes, Spring Summer 1997, NIDDK, National Institutes of Health.)*

accumulate about 15 to 25 pounds over the course of pregnancy. A weight-loss program can be initiated after the baby is born and the mother has recovered (see Chapter 15). Slow weight loss is appropriate during lactation, but rapid weight loss can decrease milk production.

For older adults, the risks associated with excess body fat are lower than they are for younger adults.[31] However, the decision to treat obesity should not be based on age alone. Weight loss can enhance day-to-day functioning and improve cardiovascular disease risk factors at all ages.[5] Older people tend to lose muscle and replace it with fat; therefore, weight-training activities are an important part of a weight loss program in the elderly (see Chapter 17).

Options for Reducing Energy Intake

There are thousands of diets and programs to promote weight loss. They vary in their approach, their intensity, and the extent to which health-care practitioners are involved. An ideal weight-management program should provide for a reduction in energy intake along with education about meeting nutrient needs, an increase in energy expenditure, and lifestyle modifications to change the patterns that led to weight gain. When selecting an approach to weight management, an individual should find a plan that is based on sound nutrition and exercise principles, suits their individual food preferences, promotes long-term lifestyle changes, and meets their needs for structure and social support (see Table 8.5). If the program's approach is not one that can be followed for a lifetime, it is unlikely to promote successful weight management. Cost, convenience, and the time commitment required by the program are also important considerations.

Web Menu: For more information on evaluating weight-loss programs, go to the American Dietetic Association at www.eatright.org/ and search for weight loss.

The following sections discuss some of the more common diet plans for reducing energy intake. The advantages and disadvantages of a number of commercial weight-management programs are given in Table 8.6. Pharmaceutical and surgical approaches to reducing intake are also discussed.

TABLE 8.5 What to Look for in a Weight-Management Program

A healthy dietary pattern that can be followed for life

Does the diet plan meet all nutrient needs?

Can the diet plan meet individual health needs? (For example, can it be used by someone who has diabetes or high blood cholesterol?)

Does the program include an education component to teach participants how to make healthy food choices?

Does the program take into consideration a participant's eating habits and preferences?

Is the diet plan flexible enough to be followed in different settings and on different occasions?

Does the diet require the purchase of special foods or supplements?

Reasonable weight loss

Does the program set realistic weight-loss goals in the range of 1/2 to 2 pounds per week?

Physical activity

Does the program stress the need to increase physical activity?

Behavior change

Does the program include some type of social support?

Does the program promote changes in behavior that can be maintained over the long term?

Scientifically sound

Is the program based on sound scientific principles?

Are the personnel monitoring the weight management program health professionals?

Adapted from the American Heart Association's Web site at **http://www.amhrt.org/Health/Risk_Factors/Overweight/Fad_Diets/fadguide.html**.

TABLE 8.6 Advantages and Disadvantages of Some Commercial Weight Management Programs

Program	Approach	Advantages	Disadvantages
Weight Watchers	Low energy, social support	Safe, inexpensive, flexible	Requires group participation
Jenny Craig	Low energy	Safe, convenient	Expensive; relies on purchase of special foods
SlimFast	Low energy	Safe	Does not promote long-term behavior change
The New Beverly Hills Diet	Low energy	Inexpensive	Does not promote long-term behavior change; nutritionally unsound
Optifast	Very low-kcalorie formula	Rapid weight loss	Expensive; dangerous if does not include medical supervision
Fit or Fat	Increased exercise	Safe, inexpensive	No social support
The Zone (and Mastering the Zone) Diet	Low carbohydrate (40% of energy	Inexpensive, flexible	Based on questionable principles; no social support
Eating Thin for Life	Moderation—written as weight-loss success stories, recipes, and menu ideas	Inexpensive	No social support
Dieting with the Duchess	Simple nutrition and exercise tips	Inexpensive, flexible	No social support
Cabbage Soup Diet	Unlimited amounts of cabbage soup, fruit, coffee, and tea	Rapid weight loss	No social support; does not promote long- term behavior change; lack of variety
Sugar Busters	Eliminates sugar; low kcalorie—1200 kcal a day	Inexpensive	No social support; based on unsound principles; insufficient carbohydrate
Volumetrics Weight Control Plan	Emphasizes foods high in water, fiber, and air to promote fullness with few kcalories	Safe, inexpensive	No social support or exercise component
Atkins' Diet	Very low carbohydrate	Inexpensive; rapid initial weight loss	Based on unsound principles; no group support; insufficient carbohydrate

Low-Energy Diets

Weight-loss plans based simply on reducing energy intake are the most common. Many options are available for planning and monitoring a reduced-kcalorie diet. Some simply recommend energy reduction without restricting the types of foods selected, some use exchange systems to plan energy and nutrient intake, and others provide low-kcalorie packaged meals and formulas.

Free Choice Diets Free choice diets monitor only energy intake. They offer flexibility and variety, and can suit the food preferences of any consumer. The disadvantage is that these diets can be difficult to plan and may not meet nutrient needs unless they are based on some type of food selection guidelines. The Food Guide Pyramid can provide the structure necessary to plan a balanced low-kcalorie diet. A diet with as few as 1200 kcalories can be planned by using the low end of the range of suggested servings and making low-kcalorie choices.

Food labels can be used to help select packaged foods that are appropriate for a low-kcalorie diet. The Nutrition Facts portion of a food label lists the kcalories per serving, but it is important to check the serving size (Figure 8.11). Food labels are required to use standard serving sizes, but their "standard" may be different from the consumer's. For instance, the standard serving of cookies is usually one ounce, or about three cookies. If you consume 12 cookies, you are consuming four times more energy than is listed on the label. Nutrient content descriptors such as "low-calorie," "calorie-free," and "light" may also be helpful in selecting foods that are low in energy (Table 8.7). The terms "light" and "lite" can also be used to describe food properties such as texture and color. For example, a label that says "light in texture" means just that; it does not mean that the kcalories are reduced. The term "light" may also appear without explanation on foods like brown sugar, cream, or molasses that have traditionally included the term as part of their name.

Exchange Plans Some diet plans use exchanges to assure nutritional adequacy along with reduced energy. They may use either the Exchange Lists established by the American Diabetes and American Dietetic Associations (see Table 7.2 and Appendix I) or similar plans that recommend a set number of servings from each of several food groups. Diets based on exchanges are more likely to meet nutrient needs than free choice plans and still offer variety from meal to meal and from day to day. In addition, they teach meal-planning skills that are easy to apply away from home and can be used over the long term.

Fixed Meal Diets Fixed meal plans allow only a defined set of foods. Some fixed diet plans sell prepackaged meals with a set number of kcalories. Others provide defined lists of foods allowed at each meal. For instance, a fixed meal plan might specify a cup of corn flakes with a banana for breakfast, ham salad and an apple for lunch, and broiled chicken with broccoli for dinner. These diets are easy to follow but can be boring and are not practical in the long term; they don't teach

Nutrition Facts
Serving Size 2 crackers (14 g)
Servings Per Container About 21

Amount Per Serving
Calories 60 Calories from Fat 15

	% Daily Value*
Total Fat 1.5g	**2%**
Saturated Fat 0g	**0%**
Polyunsaturated Fat 0g	
Monounsaturated Fat 0.5g	
Cholesterol 0mg	**0%**
Sodium 70mg	**3%**
Total Carbohydrate 10g	**3%**
Dietary Fiber Less than 1g	**3%**
Sugars 0g	
Protein 2g	

Vitamin A 0% • Vitamin C 0%
Calcium 0% • Iron 2%

*Percent Daily Values are based on a 2,000 calorie diet. Your daily values may be higher or lower depending on your calorie needs:

	Calories:	2,000	2,500
Total Fat	Less than	65g	80g
Sat Fat	Less than	20g	25g
Cholesterol	Less than	300mg	300mg
Sodium	Less than	2400mg	2400mg
Total Carbohydrate		300g	375g
Dietary Fiber		25g	30g

FIGURE 8.11 Food labels are required to list the energy content per serving of food. Energy is expressed in calories, which really refers to kcalories. Labeling regulations standardize the serving sizes.

TABLE 8.7 Energy Descriptors on Food Labels

Descriptor	Definition
Calorie-free	Contains fewer than 5 kcalories per serving.
Low-calorie	Contains no more than 40 kcalories per serving.
Reduced-calorie or fewer calories	Contains at least 25% fewer calories per serving than an appropriate reference food.
Light or lite	Contains one-third fewer kcalories or half the fat of a comparable product.

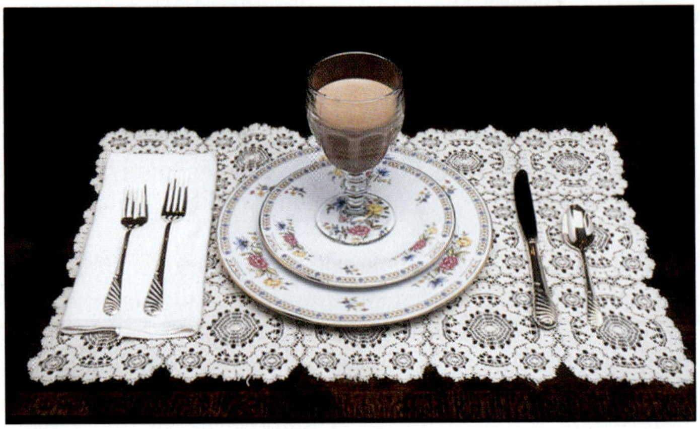

FIGURE 8.12 Liquid diets are easy to follow because there are no food selections to make. Although they may result in weight loss, they do nothing to change eating habits. *(Gregory Smolin)*

food selection skills because the meals are standardized. Similarly, plans that sell prepackaged meals at a set energy level may be easy to follow in the short term, but they can be expensive, they don't teach individual food selection skills, or how to select a nutritionally balanced diet, and they are difficult to follow when traveling or eating out.

Formula Diets Liquid diets can make dieting easier for some people because the problem of choosing a low-energy diet is eliminated (Figure 8.12). Liquid weight-loss diets that are available over-the-counter recommend a combination of food and formula to provide a daily energy intake of about 800 to 1200 kcalories. These formulas can be effective as long as the foods eaten with them are low in kcalories. Although over-the-counter formulas are easy to use and relatively inexpensive, they do little to change eating habits for life. Most diet programs that rely exclusively on liquid formulas have high dropout rates and poor long-term weight-maintenance results. Weight-loss regimens that rely exclusively on liquid formulas should not be used without medical supervision.[28]

Very-Low-Kcalorie Diets

Very-low-kcalorie diet A weight-loss diet that provides fewer than 800 kcalories per day.

Protein-sparing modified fast A very-low-kcalorie diet with a high proportion of protein designed to maximize the loss of fat and minimize the loss of protein from the body.

Very-low-kcalorie diets are defined as those containing fewer than 800 kcalories per day. They became popular in response to a desire for rapid weight loss. These diets are generally a variation of the **protein-sparing modified fast,** a diet providing little energy and a high proportion of protein. The concept behind this is that the protein in the diet will be used to meet the body's protein needs and will, therefore, prevent excessive loss of body protein. Frequently, very-low-kcalorie diets are offered as a liquid formula. These formulas provide from 300 to 800 kcalories and 50 to 100 g of protein per day and meet all other nutrient needs.

Initial weight loss is rapid with very-low-kcalorie diets—3 to 5 pounds per week. This can provide a psychological boost and motivate the dieter to continue losing weight; however, in most cases almost 75% of this initial weight loss is from water loss. Once the initial water loss ends, weight loss slows. The dieter's RMR decreases to conserve energy and physical activity decreases because the dieter often does not have the energy to continue their typical level of physical activity.

Very-low-kcalorie diets are no more effective than other methods in the long term and carry more risks. At these low-energy intakes, body protein is broken down and potassium is excreted. Depletion of potassium can result in an irregular heartbeat and is potentially deadly. Other side effects include gallstones, fatigue, nausea, cold-intolerance, light-headedness, nervousness, constipation or diarrhea, anemia, hair loss, dry skin, and menstrual irregularities. These diets are not recommended for people who are less than 30 to 40% above their healthy body weight, for pregnant or breast-feeding women, or for children, adolescents, or those with severe medical problems.[29] Since 1984, the FDA has required that all very-low-kcalorie diet formulas carry a warning that they can cause serious illness and should be used only under medical supervision.

Diets That Modify Macronutrient Intake

Rather than focusing on counting kcalories as a way of reducing body weight, some diets concentrate on modifying the proportions of energy-containing nutrients.

Low-Fat Diets Because fat is high in kcalories, consuming a low-fat diet typically reduces energy intake. Low-fat diets provide more food for the same amount of energy than high-fat diets and seem to satisfy hunger after less energy is consumed. For example, when people are fed diets of differing fat composition, energy intake decreases as the percent of fat in the diet decreases.[32] Differences in the way dietary fat and dietary carbohydrate are used by the body also explain why low-fat diets are more effective for weight loss. Excess dietary fat kcalories are stored more efficiently than excess carbohydrate kcalories, so consuming excess energy from fat leads to a greater accumulation of body fat than consuming excess energy as carbohydrate (see Chapter 7).[33]

Despite the advantages, low-fat diets are not always low in energy; even a diet low in fat will result in weight gain if energy intake exceeds energy output. This is illustrated by the fact that the percent of kcalories as fat in the typical American diet has decreased while the number of people who are overweight continues to increase. Even individual low-fat foods may not be low in energy. When fat is removed from processed foods, it must be replaced with something—most often with carbohydrates, which contribute kcalories to the food. Thus, one should compare the kcalories in a serving of a low-fat product to the kcalories in a serving of the regular product to be sure that the substitution will decrease the energy content of the diet.

Low-Carbohydrate Diets The popularity of low-carbohydrate diets as a method of weight loss has come and gone and come again. In addition to promising weight loss, these diets claim to improve athletic performance and promote health. Some of these diets severely restrict carbohydrate intake by prohibiting foods such as breads, grains, and fruits, and limiting vegetable intake. They allow high-protein foods such as eggs, red meat, fish, and poultry in unlimited amounts. Other low-carbohydrate diets are less restrictive and limit carbohydrate intake to 40% of energy. Low-carbohydrate diets are based on the premise that excessive carbohydrate intake causes an increase in insulin, which promotes fat accumulation. Restricting carbohydrate is hypothesized to reduce insulin and promote fat loss. It is true that blood insulin levels do rise when carbohydrate is consumed, and insulin can promote fat storage, but the regulation of body fat stores involves more than a single hormone (see Chapter 7 and Chapter 4: *Making Decisions* "Should You Be Eating a Low Carbohydrate Diet?").

Despite the claims that allowable foods are unlimited, weight loss occurs on these diets because intake is reduced. In some cases, weight is lost because the total amount of food allowed by the diet plan is limited; in other cases, it is lost because boredom with the limited food choices causes a reduction in food intake. There is an initial rapid weight loss, most of which is water. This occurs because when carbohydrate intake is low, glycogen stores, along with the water they hold, are lost quickly. Ketones are produced because fat is not completely broken down in the absence of carbohydrate. Excretion of these ketones causes additional water loss. In addition, there is some evidence that ketones in the blood suppress appetite, making it easier to reduce food intake.

While these diets do cause weight loss in the short term, they are not palatable enough to be adhered to for long periods (Figure 8.13). Also, the risks associated

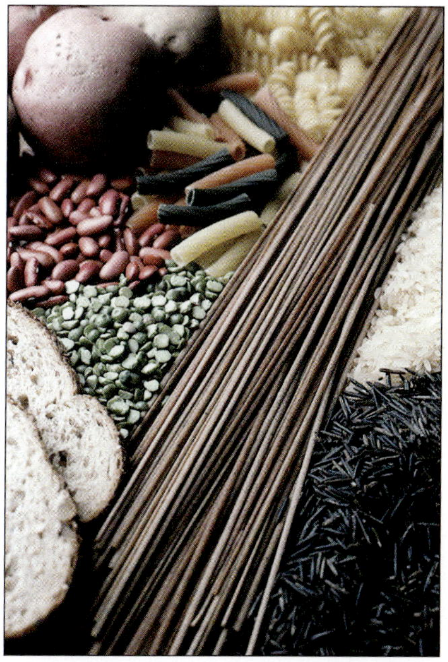

FIGURE 8.13 Diets that are very low in carbohydrate lack variety. When following such a diet, a person must eliminate or restrict the kinds of foods pictured here. *(© Felicia Martinez/Photo Edit)*

with severe carbohydrate restriction are dehydration, potassium depletion, and ketosis. In addition, these diets are high in saturated fat, which promotes heart disease.

Other Approaches to Reducing Intake

Overweight people, desperate to lose weight, are prey to all sorts of products and procedures that promise quick fixes. They have their jaws wired shut, eat a single-food diet for days at a time, select foods based on special fat-burning qualities, and consume odd combinations of foods at specific times of the day.

Jaw-wiring is a temporary procedure that restricts intake to liquids that can be taken through a straw. Weight is generally lost with this procedure and there are few risks, but long-term success is low because without continued weight management, patients may resume their normal diets when the wires are removed.

Diets that emphasize eating primarily a single food such as rice or fruit rely on short-term energy deficits to promote weight loss. They do nothing to change long-term dietary habits. The limited food choices these diets offer can also result in nutrient deficiencies.

Some fads emphasize the supposed magical qualities of food. The grapefruit diet was based on the myth that grapefruit stimulates the breakdown of body fat. In reality, weight loss on such diets is due to the reduction in energy intake and not the magical interaction of specific foods.

Another common diet approach focuses on food combinations and timing of intake. This approach is based on the faulty premise that foods should be eaten only in certain combinations (see Chapter 3) and that, if eaten in the wrong combination, they will not be digested properly, resulting in weight gain and disease.

Fad diets, in general, may promote weight loss over the short term, but since they are not nutritionally sound, they cannot be consumed safely for long periods. They do not encourage the exercise or promote the changes in eating behavior that affect body weight over the long term (see *Critical Thinking*: "Will This Weight-Loss Plan Work?").

Critical Thinking

Will This Weight-Loss Plan Work?

Fat-Away Diet Program

A Fast, Sensible, Three-Step Approach to Weight Loss

Step 1: Replace breakfast and lunch with Fat-Away's scrumptious, nutrient-dense chocolate, vanilla, peach, or strawberry shake. Each shake provides 200 kcalories, 15 grams of protein, and 50% of the Daily Value for vitamins and minerals.

Step 2: For dinner, eat a well-balanced meal, limiting kcalories to 500, including 3 ounces of lean meat, 1 cup of nonfat milk, and 1/2 to 1 cup each of starchy foods, fruits, and vegetables.

Step 3: Before going to bed, take Fat-Away's unique nighttime complex of amino acids. They help convert fat into energy, curb cravings for carbohydrate, and control appetite and satisfy hunger during the day.

Following these easy steps should result in a weight loss of 3 to 5 pounds per week and costs only $39.95 for one week's supply. You should consult your physician before trying this or any other diet.

Does this diet meet all nutritional needs except energy?

Probably. The combination of the nutritionally fortified shake and a variety of solid foods for one meal a day can provide a diet adequate in protein, vitamins, and minerals, although it is probably low in fiber and phytochemicals. Most diets providing fewer than 1200 kcalories do not meet micronutrient needs. This diet can because it includes the nutrient-fortified liquid meal.

Does the program provide a wide variety of obtainable foods with no special products to buy?

No. Although variety is encouraged in the one 500-kcalorie meal, the dieter is required to purchase the powdered liquid-meal formula as well as an amino acid supplement at a cost of about $5.70 per day.

Does the plan offer a reasonable rate of weight loss?

No. It promises a weight loss of 3 to 5 pounds per week. At this rate, muscle as well as fat will probably be lost.

Is the diet flexible enough to account for individual tastes, and is it adaptable to social settings?

Possibly. This plan allows some flexibility because individuals are free to choose what they will eat for one meal a day. However, it is not flexible enough for occasions such as holidays when traditional foods are served at more than one meal.

Is the diet based on scientifically sound principles?

Not entirely. Reducing energy intake below needs will result in weight loss, but an amino acid supplement will do little to curb appetite or convert fat into energy as you sleep. It is supposed to help convert fat into energy, but there is little evidence to support this claim.

Does this program include an exercise component?

Answer:

Does the program promote changes in eating habits and lifestyle that will encourage achieving and maintaining a healthy weight?

Answer:

Making Decisions

Weight-Loss Drugs: Are the Risks Too Great?

Fen-phen was a dream come true—a drug combination that diminished appetite to reduce eating. It made weight loss easy at last. Unfortunately, fen-phen was soon found to be associated with a life-threatening heart valve defect. At that time, more than 18 million people had prescriptions for this drug combination.[a] Some of these individuals were obese, but many were only mildly overweight. The heart valve damage associated with taking fen-phen even for short periods of time could have affected millions. Would it have been better for many of these people to have simply remained slightly overweight? In the same year, a 13-year-old girl weighing 600 pounds died on her living room floor unable to move. Wouldn't drugs have been a better choice for her? As with any treatment, the risks must be weighed against the benefits.

The risks associated with obesity are well documented. Heart disease, hypertension, diabetes, gallbladder disease, and cancer rates all increase. Problems that limit mobility, such as arthritis, increase, as do social problems. It is estimated that obesity-related conditions contribute to 300,000 deaths per year. The risk for overweight individuals depends on how overweight they are, how long they have been overweight, and how old they are. As weight increases, so does mortality but the increase is small until body mass index reaches about 27 kg/m^2 (a 5-ft-5-in. woman who weighs 162 to 168 lb). Risk increases with the length of time that an individual is obese, but as age increases the correlation between body mass index and mortality decreases until it disappears at age 74.[b]

The benefits of weight loss in the obese are clear. Even a reduction of 10 to 15 pounds reduces the risk of disease associated with obesity.[c] Should this loss be accomplished with drugs? Traditional approaches, including reducing energy intake and increasing exercise, chronically fail for many people. For them, drugs may be an option. Unfortunately, there are no perfect weight-loss drugs, nor are any likely to appear in the near future. Over the short term, some weight-loss drugs have been shown to reduce health risks by reducing blood pressure, blood lipid levels, and insulin resistance along with weight. But, no long-term studies have yet been completed to indicate if weight loss accomplished by using drugs can improve health and decrease mortality. Likewise, there is no good information regarding the risks associated with taking these drugs for long periods of time. Obesity is a chronic disease. Taking an obesity drug does not cure the disease but it can reduce body weight. To maintain weight loss, the drug must be continued, and if it is stopped, the weight will return unless changes in intake and expenditure are sustained.

Do the risks of obesity outweigh the risks of obesity drugs? It depends on the individual. For someone who is at significant medical risk due to obesity, or who has a medical condition that increases the risks associated with being overweight, such as cardiovascular disease, the benefits of these drugs may outweigh the risks. On the other hand, for someone with 10 pounds to lose before the holidays, the risks of such drugs probably outweigh the benefits.

References

[a] Frackelmann, K. Diet drug debacle: how two federally approved weight-loss drugs crashed. Science News 152:252–253, 1997.

[b] Stevens, J., Cai, J., Pamuk, E. R., et al. The effect of age on the association between body mass index and mortality. N. Engl. J. Med. 338:1–7, 1998.

[c] Expert Panel on the Identification, Evaluation and Treatment of Overweight in Adults. Clinical guidelines on the identification, evaluation and treatment of overweight and obesity in Adults: Executive summary. Am. J. Clin. Nutr. 68:899–917, 1998.

Drug Therapy

An ideal drug treatment for obesity would permit an individual to lose weight and maintain the loss, be safe when used for long periods of time, have no side effects, and not be addictive. Many attempts have been made to develop such a drug. Extracts of thyroid hormone have been around for 100 years but were taken off the market because they caused hyperthyroidism. Amphetamines, introduced for weight loss in the 1930s, were widely and often indiscriminately used in the 1950s and 1960s. The risk of addiction eventually stemmed their use. During the next 20 years, drug development continued but drug use for obesity declined.[34] In the 1990s, the recognition of obesity as a chronic disease increased interest in prescription and nonprescription weight-loss medications.

Currently, the National Institutes of Health recommends that drug therapy be considered only for individuals with a BMI greater than 30 and for those with a BMI greater than or equal to 27 who have accompanying risk factors or diseases.[5] Nevertheless, many people who do not meet these criteria take medications to lose weight. Some medications may help promote weight loss with little risk; for others, the risks are great (see *Making Decisions*: "Weight-Loss Drugs: Are the Risks Too Great?").

Prescription Medications There are a number of drugs currently on the market that promote weight loss by reducing energy intake. Sibutramine (Meridia) decreases food intake by affecting the activity of brain neurotransmitters that regu-

TABLE 8.8 Prescription Drugs for Weight Loss

Generic name	Trade name	Status	Effect
Dexfenfluramine	Redux	Withdrawn from market	Appetite suppressant
Diethylpropion	Tenuate, Tenuate dospan	Available	Appetite suppressant
Fenfluramine	Pondimin	Withdrawn from market	Appetite suppressant
Phendimetrazine	Bontril Plegine, Prelu-2, X-trozine	Available	Appetite suppressant
Sibutramine	Meridia	Available	Appetite suppressant
Phentermine	Adipex-P, Fastin, Inomin, Obytrim	Available	Appetite suppressant
Orlistat	Xenical	Available	Prevents fat absorption.

late food intake (see Table 8.8). Orlistat (Xenical) reduces fat absorption and therefore energy intake by blocking fat-digesting enzymes in the intestine. Although many drugs have shown promise at promoting weight loss in the short term, weight is regained when the drugs are discontinued. There are also a number of drugs in various stages of development that may someday help reduce body weight by increasing energy expenditure, increasing the release of fat from adipose tissue, or decreasing fat synthesis.[35]

Products Available Without a Prescription There is a variety of products sold over-the-counter to promote weight loss. Some may be moderately effective but, as with prescription medications, the weight is usually regained when the product is no longer taken. Over-the-counter options include nonprescription medications and dietary supplements.

Nonprescription medications are regulated by the U.S. Food and Drug Administration (FDA) and must adhere to strict guidelines regarding the dose per pill and the effectiveness of the ingredients. The FDA does not regulate dietary supplements for weight loss unless they claim to be a substitute for a drug or claim to perform a drug action or therapy (see Chapters 2 and 10 for a discussion of the definition and regulation of dietary supplements). Weight-loss supplements often include herbal sources of compounds contained in prescription medications. Some of these are powerful drugs with dangerous side effects and, because they are not strictly regulated, their safety and effectiveness may not have been carefully tested and doses may vary from tablet to tablet and brand to brand. It cannot be assumed that a product is safe simply because it is labeled "herbal" or "all natural."

Over-the-Counter Medications Only a limited number of substances is approved by the FDA for sale as nonprescription weight-loss medications. Fibers such as methylcellulose and glucomannan are used in weight-loss products because they absorb water to create a feeling of fullness; pills containing them claim to fill the stomach with indigestible bulk so that one feels sated and eats less. The anesthetic benzocaine is included in weight-loss products because it numbs the tongue, making eating a less pleasurable experience. Caffeine, which is a stimulant and a diuretic, is used in many weight-loss products. Stimulants tend to blunt the appetite and diuretics cause the kidneys to increase fluid excretion, resulting in weight loss from water loss. These same effects can be derived from caffeine-containing beverages like coffee, tea, and some soft drinks. Another stimulant that has been sold for many years as an over-the-counter decongestant as well as an appetite suppressant is phenylpropanolamine. In October 2000, after several reports of brain hemorrhages and strokes in individuals taking this drug, the FDA recommended that it no longer be sold over-the-counter or in prescription medications.[36]

Dietary Supplements Common ingredients in weight-loss dietary supplements include the amino acids arginine and ornithine, chromium, and a variety of herbs. Arginine and ornithine are hypothesized to burn fat during sleep because they stimulate the release of growth hormone. Although growth hormone promotes fat loss and muscle growth, research has not found any relationship between body weight and the levels of growth hormone. The mineral chromium is usually included as chromium picolinate. It is claimed to decrease body fat and increase the proportion of lean tissue, but human trials have not consistently demonstrated an effect of supplemental chromium picolinate on body composition or body weight.[37]

Ma huang is an herb that is used in supplements known as herbal fat burners. Ma huang is an herbal source of Ephedra (also called ephedrine, or synphedrine), a central nervous system stimulant that reduces appetite. Ephedra is approved by the FDA for use as a decongestant but not for use in over-the-counter weight-loss medications. Ephedra can be effective at increasing metabolic rate and suppressing appetite, but serious side effects have been reported with its use, particularly in individuals with high blood pressure, diabetes, or thyroid conditions (see Chapter 7, *Making Decisions*: "Fat Burners: The Hot and the Cold").

Other types of herbal products marketed for weight loss are teas and supplements that contain plant-derived laxatives such as senna, aloe, buckthorn, rhubarb root, cascara, and caster oil. Cascara, senna, and caster oil are approved by the FDA and regulated as drugs for use in nonprescription laxatives. These cause weight loss by inducing diarrhea, which causes water loss. They don't lead to fat loss, however, because they do not significantly reduce nutrient absorption. This is because they act in the colon, not in the small intestine, where most absorption occurs. Overuse of herbal laxatives can cause serious side effects, including nausea, diarrhea, vomiting, stomach cramps, chronic constipation, fainting, and severe electrolyte imbalances leading to cardiac arrhythmia and death.[38]

Surgery

Web Menu: For more information on surgery for weight loss, go to the National Institute for Diabetes & Digestive & Kidney Diseases at www.niddk.nih.gov/health/nutrit/pubs/gastsurg.htm.

Surgery is a drastic method of reducing body weight. Obesity surgery involves altering the structure of the gastrointestinal tract to reduce the amount of food that can be consumed and/or the nutrients that can be absorbed. Liposuction is a method for reducing specific fat deposits but it does not significantly affect overall body weight.

Gastrointestinal Surgery Obesity surgery is recommended in cases where the risk of dying from obesity and its complications is great. It is appropriate only for individuals with a body mass index greater than or equal to 40 kg/m^2 (extreme obesity) and in those with a BMI between 35 and 40 kg/m^2 (obesity) who have other life-threatening conditions that could be remedied by weight loss.[5] The success of weight-loss surgery, as with other treatment, depends on the motivation and behavior of the patient. The appropriateness of surgery has to be evaluated on a case-by-case basis by considering the individual's potential risks and benefits[39,40] (see Table 8.9).

Types of Surgery The first surgery that was widely used for severe obesity was the intestinal bypass. This procedure, first used 40 years ago, produced weight loss by bypassing part of the small intestine, thus causing malabsorption. The idea was that patients could eat large amounts of food, which would be poorly digested and pass through the shortened intestine too quickly for the body to absorb much of the energy. The problem with this surgery was that its side effects were unpredictable and sometimes fatal. The original form of the intestinal bypass operation is no longer performed.

TABLE 8.9 Indications for Obesity Surgery

- Severely overweight: BMI of 40 kg/m^2 or greater or 35 to 39.9 kg/m^2 with severe medical conditions such as diabetes, high blood pressure, high blood lipids, sleep apnea, or other cardiopulmonary disorders.
- Tried other methods and failed, and is unlikely to succeed with repeated efforts.
- Physically unable to perform daily activities (work and family-related functions) and quality of life is severely impaired.
- Understands the procedure and its risks; is aware of how life may change after the operation, including the need to chew well and the inability to eat large meals.
- Determined to lose weight and motivated to make a lifelong behavioral commitment that includes well-balanced eating and physical activity.
- Aware of the potential for serious complications, the associated dietary restrictions, and the occasional failures.
- Committed to lifelong medical follow-up.

Adapted from National Institutes of Health, National Heart, Lung, and Blood Institute. Clinical guidelines on the Identification, Evaluation, and Treatment of Overweight and Obesity in Adults. Executive summary, June 1998. Available online at: **http://www.nhlbi.nih.gov/guidelines/obesity/ob_home.htm**.

The most common type of surgery performed today limits stomach capacity by closing off part of the stomach (Figure 8.14). In this procedure, a portion of the stomach is sectioned off, forming a small pouch. Initially this pouch holds about 1 ounce of food and expands to 2–3 ounces with time (a normal stomach holds about a pint). The pouch has a small outlet, which slows the rate at which food leaves the stomach and causes a feeling of fullness. An individual who has this type of surgery must learn to eat small amounts, chew thoroughly, and eat slowly in order to avoid stomach upset, nausea, and vomiting. The procedure leads to weight loss in almost all individuals; about 80% achieve some degree of weight loss, and 50–60% maintain their losses for over five years. An early complication is that the tissue may break down at the staple line, allowing leakage of stomach contents into the abdominal cavity. More long-term side effects include protein and vitamin deficiencies and a breakdown of the bands that section off the stomach, enlarging the pouch.[41]

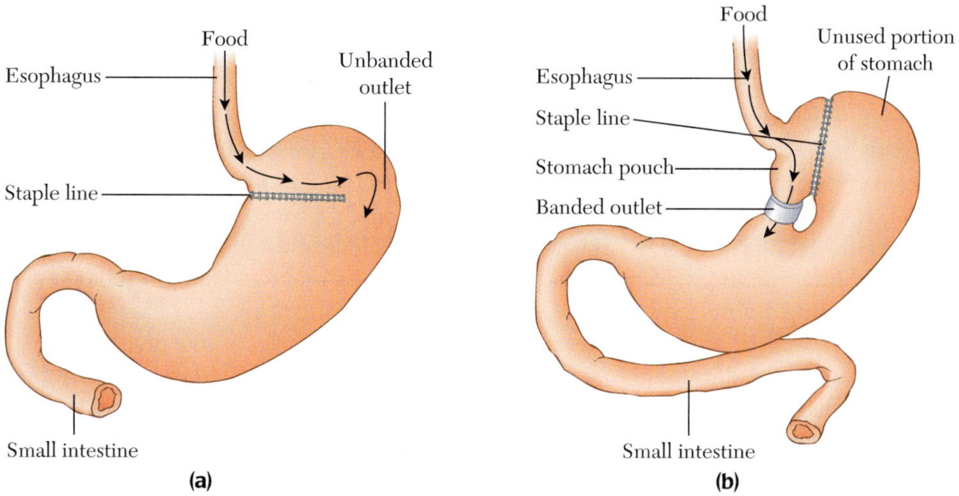

FIGURE 8.14 Gastroplasty (a) and vertical-banded gastroplasty (b) are surgical procedures that reduce the size of the stomach by placing a row of staples across the top of the stomach. The amount the stomach can hold is decreased and stomach emptying is slowed because there is only a small opening at the lower end of the pouch.

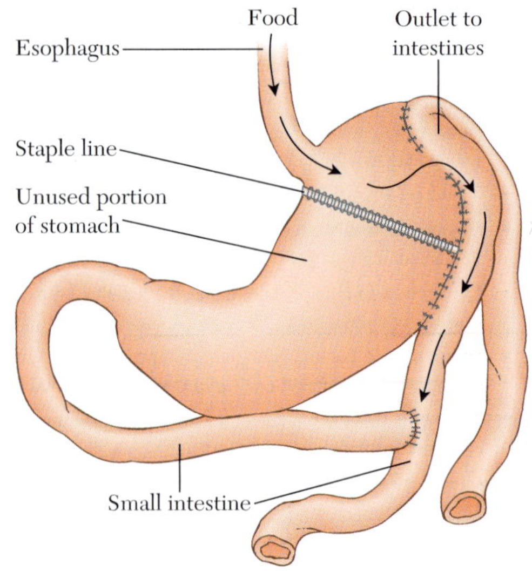

FIGURE 8.15 Gastric bypass surgery reduces the size of the stomach by placing staples across the top of the stomach and attaching the stomach pouch to the small intestine, allowing a portion of the intestine to be bypassed.

Other common surgeries involve bypassing part of the stomach and intestine. These procedures combine the creation of a stomach pouch to restrict food intake with bypassing a segment of the small intestine to reduce absorption (Figure 8.15). Because these operations restrict food intake and cause malabsorption, they produce more weight loss than procedures that only limit stomach size. Individuals generally lose two-thirds of their excess weight within two years of surgery. Because these procedures bypass part of the stomach, they limit the absorption of vitamin B_{12}. Because they bypass the duodenum, there is a risk for iron and calcium deficiencies. Malabsorption of vitamin B_{12} and iron may result in anemia and decreased absorption of calcium may bring on osteoporosis and metabolic bone disease. To prevent these deficiencies, patients who have these surgeries must take nutritional supplements. Another complication that may occur after surgery is "dumping syndrome"—a condition in which food moves too rapidly through the small intestine, causing nausea, weakness, sweating, faintness, and, occasionally, diarrhea after eating. The more of the intestine that is bypassed, the greater the risk for complications and nutritional deficiencies. Patients with extensive bypasses require not only close monitoring but also lifelong use of special foods and medications.

Risk/Benefit Analysis Surgical treatment is a drastic measure that involves permanent changes in the structure and function of the gastrointestinal tract. The potential benefits include weight loss that occurs quickly and continues for about two years after surgery. After weight loss, about 60% of patients who were taking medication for diabetes and high blood pressure are able to manage their disease without medication. Other benefits commonly reported include improved mobility and stamina, better mood, and increased self-esteem and interpersonal effectiveness. These benefits, however, do not come without a price. Individuals who have these procedures must make permanent changes in their eating habits and experience permanent changes in their bowel habits. Also, 10 to 20% of individuals require follow-up surgeries to correct complications such as abdominal hernias, the breakdown of the staple line, and stretched stomach outlets. More than one-third of obese patients who have weight-loss surgery develop gallstones; the risk is increased during rapid or substantial weight loss. Nutritional deficiencies such as anemia, osteoporosis, and metabolic bone disease are also common, occurring in almost 30% of patients. Because rapid weight loss and nutritional deficiencies can harm a developing fetus, women who have weight-loss surgery should not become pregnant until their weight is stable.

Liposuction **Liposuction** is primarily a cosmetic procedure that will not significantly reduce overall body weight but may alter fat distribution. This procedure involves inserting a large hollow needle under the skin into a localized fat deposit and literally vacuuming out the fat. It is often advertised as a way to remove cellulite, which is just fat that has a lumpy appearance because of the presence of connections to the tissue layers below. The risks of this procedure include those associated with general anesthesia and the possibility of infection. The benefit is a reduction in the amount of fat in a specific location.

Liposuction A procedure that suctions out adipose tissue from under the skin; used to decrease the size of local fat deposits such as on the abdomen or hips.

Underweight and Health

Although overweight and obesity are the focus of public health agendas, being underweight with too little body fat is also a problem for many. Low fat stores could affect the ability to survive illness and may be indicative of a disease process that is causing weight loss. Just as overweight individuals have difficulty losing weight, those who are underweight have difficulty gaining it.

Health Risks

Some body fat is essential as an insulator and as a reserve for periods of illness. At the very lower extremes of body weight there is an increased risk of early death,[42] but being just slightly on the low side of the body weight standard may reduce the risk of diabetes and even increase longevity.[43,44] However, this only applies to thin people who are healthy. Substantial reductions in body weight that occur due to illness or eating disorders have been shown to decrease the ability of the immune system to fight disease and are associated with increased mortality. In developed countries, socioeconomic conditions may create isolated pockets of undernutrition, but severe cases of wasting are usually a result either of self-starvation due to eating disorders such as anorexia nervosa or of a disease such as AIDS or cancer.

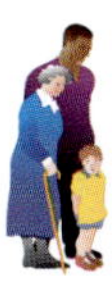

Too little body fat can cause problems at many stages of life. Low weight gains during pregnancy are correlated with an increase in low-birth-weight infants, who are at a higher risk of health complications and death (see Chapter 15). For teenage girls, too little body fat can delay sexual development. In healthy but very lean female athletes, menstrual irregularities are common, increasing the risk of developing osteoporosis (see Chapters 14 and 16).[45] In the elderly, too little body fat increases the risk of malnutrition.

Suggestions for Weight Gain

The first step for someone who wants to gain weight should be a medical evaluation to rule out medical reasons for low body weight. This is particularly important when weight loss occurs unexpectedly.

Low body weight in an otherwise healthy individual is due to a low energy intake and/or a high energy expenditure. Gradually increasing consumption of energy-dense foods is suggested. More frequent meals and high-kcalorie snacks such as milkshakes between meals can help increase energy intake. Replacing low-kcalorie fluids like water and diet beverages with fruit juices and milk may also help. Strength-training exercise should be a component of any weight gain program. This approach requires extra energy to fuel the activity needed to build muscles. These recommendations apply to individuals who are naturally thin and have trouble gaining weight on the recommended energy intake. This dietary approach will not result in weight gain in those who refuse to eat because of an eating disorder.

For more information on eating disorders, go to the American Anorexia Bulemia Association at www.aabainc.org/, the Eating Disorders Prevention Program at www.edap.org/ or to the National Institutes of Mental Health Web site at www.nimh.nih.gov/ and search for eating disorders.

Eating Disorders

In 1988 at a meet in Budapest, a gymnastics judge told Christy Henrich, a world-class athlete from the United States, that she was too fat and needed to lose weight if she wanted to be considered for the Olympic team. In attempts to control her weight, Christy developed the eating disorder anorexia nervosa. Six years later, at the age of 22, weighing less than 50 pounds Christy died of multiple organ failure.[46] How could this happen? How could an individual with the self-discipline to achieve such athletic prowess succumb to such a disease?

Actually, Christy presented what we know to be the typical picture of an anorexic—a hard-working overachiever. Initially she linked her success in gymnastics to her ability to restrict her intake, but at some point she stopped having a realistic perception of her body size and her goal became reducing her weight, not succeeding in her sport (Figure 8.16).

Eating disorders are on the rise among college students whether or not they are athletes. The stresses of school and the responsibilities of growing up may seem overwhelming. To escape, some focus their attention on food intake and body weight, equating control of weight and food intake with accomplishment and success.

Disordered Eating

Anorexia nervosa An eating disorder characterized by self-starvation, a distorted body image, and low body weight.

Bulimia nervosa An eating disorder characterized by the consumption of large amounts of food at one time (bingeing), followed by purging behaviors such as vomiting or the use of laxatives.

Binge-eating disorder An eating disorder characterized by recurrent episodes of binge eating in the absence of purging behavior.

Normal eating patterns are flexible; sometimes people overeat, and sometimes they undereat. What and how much is eaten varies in response to emotions, to time limitations, to hunger, and to the proximity of food. Normal eating must sometimes involve constraint in order to choose foods to maintain weight and meet recommendations for a healthy diet. But generally people eat when they are hungry, choose foods they enjoy, and stop eating when they are satisfied.

The term "eating disorder" is somewhat of a misnomer because it implies that the primary problem is abnormal eating behavior and that learning to eat normally will solve the problem.[47] Unfortunately, this is not true. Eating disorders are a group of conditions that share a pathological concern with body weight and shape. They are primarily psychological disorders that involve nutrition-related behaviors and complications. According to mental health guidelines, there are three categories of eating disorders: **anorexia nervosa, bulimia nervosa,** and eating disorders not otherwise specified, which includes **binge-eating disorder** (see Table 8.10).[48] These illnesses affect over 5 million Americans and thousands of people die annually from their complications.[49]

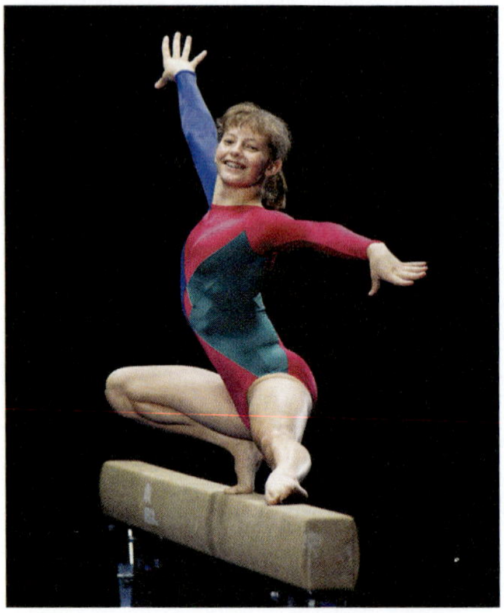

FIGURE 8.16 Eating disorders are common in athletes involved in sports such as gymnastics that require slender bodies and extreme discipline.

Causes and Prevalence

In the search for the cause of eating disorders, psychological, biological, and sociocultural factors have been examined. Certain personality characteristics and psychological problems are common among individuals with eating disorders; the typical picture is an intelligent, adolescent female overachiever who feels ineffective and has low self-esteem and poor self-regulation.[50]

There is some evidence that biology may play a role in the development of eating disorders. Much of the risk of developing anorexia nervosa and bulimia nervosa, including the personality traits that predispose one to these disorders, appears to be inherited.[51] Abnormalities in the levels of neurotransmitters such as serotonin and their metabolites, and in levels of the hormone leptin, have been hypothesized to contribute to the behaviors typical of anorexia and bulimia.[51]

Eating disorders most commonly begin in adolescence, when physical, psychological, and social development is occurring rapidly. While they are

TABLE 8.10 Diagnostic Criteria for Eating Disorders

Anorexia nervosa

Refusal to maintain body weight at or above 85% of normal weight for age and height.

Intense fear of gaining weight or becoming fat, even though underweight.

Disturbance in the way body weight or shape is experienced or denial of the seriousness of the current low body weight.

Absence of at least three consecutive menstrual cycles without other known cause.

Bulimia nervosa

Recurrent episodes of binge eating.

Recurrent inappropriate compensatory behavior to prevent weight gain, such as self-induced vomiting; misuse of laxatives, diuretics, enemas, or other medications; fasting; or excessive exercise.

Occurrence, on average, of binge eating and inappropriate compensatory behaviors at least twice a week for three months.

Undue influence by body shape and weight on self-evaluation.

Disturbance does not occur exclusively during episodes of anorexia nervosa.

Eating disorders not otherwise specified

Criteria for anorexia nervosa are met except the individual menstruates regularly.

Criteria for anorexia nervosa are met except that, despite substantial weight loss, the individual's current weight is in the normal range.

Criteria for bulimia nervosa are met except binges occur at a frequency of less than twice a week and for a duration of less than three months.

Inappropriate compensatory behavior after eating small amounts of food in individuals of normal body weight.

Regularly chewing and spitting out, without swallowing, large amounts of food.

Binge-eating disorder

Recurrent episodes of binge eating in the absence of the regular use of inappropriate compensatory behaviors characteristic of bulimia.

From American Psychiatric Association. Diagnostic and Statistical Manual, 4th ed. Washington, D.C.: American Psychiatric Association, 1994.

more common in young women, males make up 5 to 10% of individuals with eating disorders; male athletes in weight-regulated activities like wrestling are at particular risk. Eating disorders are typically associated with Caucasians of higher socioeconomic class, but they occur in all ethnic groups.[52] They are as common among Hispanic as Caucasian females, and are more frequent among Native Americans and less frequent among African-American and Asian-American females.[53]

Eating disorders are more prevalent in subpopulations that are concerned with weight and body image.[54] For example, the incidence is very low in underdeveloped countries and increases in certain subcultures in developed countries, such as professional dancers and models. Eating disorders are on the rise among athletes, especially those involved in sports that require the athlete to be thin, such as gymnastics and figure skating, or to fit into a particular weight class, such as wrestling. In North America, young women are particularly concerned with body image. Being thin is associated with beauty, success, intelligence, and vitality. What young woman would want to be plump? A young woman facing a future where she must be independent, have a prestigious job, maintain a successful love relationship, bear and nurture children, manage a household, and stay in fashion can become overwhelmed. Unable to master all these roles, she may look for some aspect of her life that she can control. Food intake and body weight are natural choices, because being thin brings the societal associations of success. Young women today too often aspire to the adage that you can never be too rich or too thin.

Anorexia Nervosa

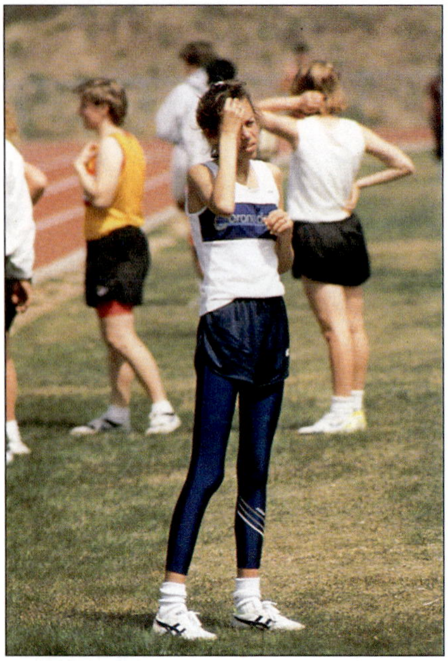

FIGURE 8.17 A person with anorexia nervosa may literally starve herself to death. *(Tony Freeman/PhotoEdit)*

Purging Behaviors such as self-induced vomiting and misuse of laxatives and diuretics to rid the body of energy.

Amenorrhea Delayed onset of menstruation or the absence of three or more consecutive menstrual cycles.

Anorexia nervosa is a life-threatening disorder. It is characterized by extreme weight loss due to behaviors such as self-starvation and excessive exercise, an overwhelming fear of gaining weight, and use of body weight and shape as a means of self-evaluation (see Table 8.10). Anorexia nervosa was originally described over a century ago. The name "anorexia," which means lack of appetite, is a misnomer because it is a desire to be thin rather than a lack of appetite that causes individuals with this disorder to decrease their food intake (Figure 8.17). Anorexia nervosa affects 1% of American girls and approximately 0.5% of women over their lifetime.[51] The average age of onset is 17 years old. There is a 5% death rate in the first two years, and this can reach 20% in untreated individuals.[55]

Although anorexia is a psychological disorder, many of the problems associated with it are nutrition related. Individuals with anorexia may be unable to maintain a minimally healthy body weight; thus show dramatic weight loss, have a fear of gaining weight even when underweight, and display abnormal food consumption patterns. Disturbances in their perception of body size prevent anorexics from seeing themselves as underweight, so they continue to use diets, exercise, or **purging** to remain thin or lose more weight. They often develop a personal diet ritual, limiting certain foods and eating them in specific ways. Anorexics spend an enormous amount of time thinking about food, talking about food, and preparing food for others. Instead of eating, they move the food around the plate and cut it into tiny pieces. Those who use exercise to increase energy expenditure do not stop when they are tired; instead, they train compulsively beyond reasonable endurance. It is estimated that 50% of people with anorexia use purging as a means of weight control.[56]

Consequences of Anorexia The first obvious physical symptom of anorexia is weight loss. As weight loss becomes severe, symptoms of starvation begin to appear. Fat stores are depleted, muscle wasting occurs, and growth decreases. Metabolic rate slows, lowering body temperature and energy expenditure. The reduction in body fat leads to cold intolerance. In females, estrogen levels drop and **amenorrhea** occurs. This affects sexual maturation and can have long-term effects on bone density. Amenorrhea, decreased body weight and fat, and low calcium and vitamin D intake all contribute to decreased bone formation, increased bone loss, and an increased risk of osteoporosis. In males, testosterone levels decrease. Virtually no organ system is unaffected. Heart rate may slow or become irregular and blood pressure may drop. Gastric motility and emptying slow and the incidence of peptic ulcers increases, constipation is common, and pancreatitis (inflammation of the pancreas) may occur. Frequent vomiting brings stomach acid into the mouth, damaging enamel and promoting tooth decay. Kidney damage may occur due to dehydration. The skin may become dry and brittle due to fatty acid deficiency. Hair on the head may become dry, thin, and brittle, and there may be abnormal hair growth on other parts of the body. Immune function may be compromised.

In the final stages of starvation there is abnormal electrolyte balance, dehydration, edema, cardiac abnormalities, absence of ketones due to fat-store depletion, and finally infection, further increasing nutritional needs. Organs shrink due to lack of nutrients and can no longer perform essential functions. Body temperature and blood pressure drop. Heartbeat is irregular and can lead to cardiac arrest.

Treatment of Anorexia Nervosa Early treatment of anorexia is important because starvation may cause irreversible damage. The goal of treatment is to help resolve psychological and behavioral problems while providing for nutritional rehabilitation. Ideally, the treatment of eating disorders involves a team approach, with medical, dental, psychological, and nutritional therapy. If changes in food-intake and other weight-related behavior are the only focus of therapy, interventions are unlikely to be successful and in some cases may be counterproductive.

The goal of nutrition intervention is to promote weight gain by increasing energy intake and expanding dietary choices.[57] The first step is to assess nutritional status and provide a strategy to meet these needs, whether it involves a meal plan, nutritional supplements, or force-feeding techniques such as tube or intravenous feedings. It is generally thought to be counterproductive to use force-feeding methods except in cases where these procedures are required to keep the patient alive.

Medical nutritional therapy for anorexia nervosa involves providing the individual and the family with information on energy needs and normal body weights, as well as on typical food intake patterns. The individual must experiment with eating behaviors to develop healthy patterns that can be maintained over the long term. Self-monitoring techniques, such as food records, tracking laxative use and purging behaviors, and charting weight changes, can be helpful in learning normal eating behaviors. Recovery is a lengthy process involving therapy and experimentation. Occasional relapses to previous behaviors are common.

Medications including antidepressants and tranquilizers are prescribed in some cases to improve mood and reduce anxiety. The effectiveness of these treatments in the acute stages of anorexia is not well documented.[58]

Bulimia Nervosa

Bulimia nervosa is a disorder that involves frequent episodes of **binge eating** or **bingeing** that are almost always followed by purging and other inappropriate compensatory behaviors. A diagnosis of bulimia is based on the frequency with which episodes of binge eating and inappropriate compensatory behaviors occur (see Table 8.10). Bulimia is subdivided into nonpurging and purging types. Nonpurging bulimics use behaviors such as fasting or excessive exercise to prevent weight gain. Purging bulimics regularly engage in behaviors that may include self-induced vomiting and misuse of enemas, laxatives and diuretics, or other medications.

Binge eating or **bingeing** The rapid consumption of a large amount of food in a discrete period of time associated with a feeling that eating is out of control.

During a food binge, a bulimic experiences a sense of lack of control. While a normal teenager may consume 2000 to 3000 kcalories per day, a bulimic may consume over 3400 kcalories in under two hours, and some consume up to 20,000 kcalories in binges lasting as long as eight hours.[59] A binge usually occurs in secrecy and stops only when pain, fatigue, or an interruption intervenes. Bingeing and purging are then followed by intense feelings of guilt and shame.

Bulimia was recognized as a separate eating disorder in the late 1970s and may currently occur in up to 5% of college-age women.[49] Individuals suffering from bulimia are not necessarily underweight and may even be slightly overweight. Bulimia shares with anorexia a preoccupation with body weight and shape. As with anorexics, bulimics have a negative body image accompanied by a distorted perception of their body size. They are preoccupied with the fear that once they start eating they will not be able to stop.

Consequences of Bulimia It is the purging of the binge-purge cycle that is most hazardous to health in bulimia nervosa. Purging by vomiting brings stomach acid into the mouth. Frequent vomiting causes tooth decay and damages the gastrointestinal tract. Gastrointestinal symptoms can include heartburn, sores in the mouth and on the lips, swollen jaws and salivary glands, irritation of the throat, esophageal inflammation, and changes in stomach capacity and stomach emptying.[60] Vomiting can also cause electrolyte imbalance, dehydration, muscle weakness, and menstrual irregularities, and the force of vomiting can result in broken blood vessels in the face and eyes. Laxative and diuretic abuse can cause dehydration and electrolyte imbalance. Rectal bleeding may occur from laxative overuse.

Treatment of Bulimia Nervosa The overall goal of therapy for people with bulimia nervosa is to separate eating from their emotions and from their perceptions of success, and to promote eating in response to hunger and satiety. Psychological issues related to body image and a sense of lack of control over eating must be resolved. Nutritional therapy must address physiological imbalances caused by purging episodes and provide education on nutrient needs and how to meet them. Antidepressant medications have been shown to reduce the frequency of binge episodes. Treatment has been found to speed recovery, but for some women this disorder may remain a chronic problem throughout life.[61]

Other Eating Disorders

A third class of eating disorder, termed "eating disorders not otherwise specified," includes conditions such as weight loss that is less severe than the criteria dictate for anorexia (that is, 15% below healthy body weight) or bingeing and purging that is less frequent than the criteria for bulimia (see Table 8.10).

Binge-Eating Disorder Individuals who suffer from binge-eating disorder engage in recurrent episodes of binge eating but do not regularly engage in purging behaviors such as vomiting, fasting, or excessive exercise. These individuals are likely to have above-normal body weights and may seek help for treatment of obesity rather than for their binge-eating behavior.[47] About one-quarter to one-third of individuals who attend weight-loss clinics meet the criteria for binge-eating disorder.[51]

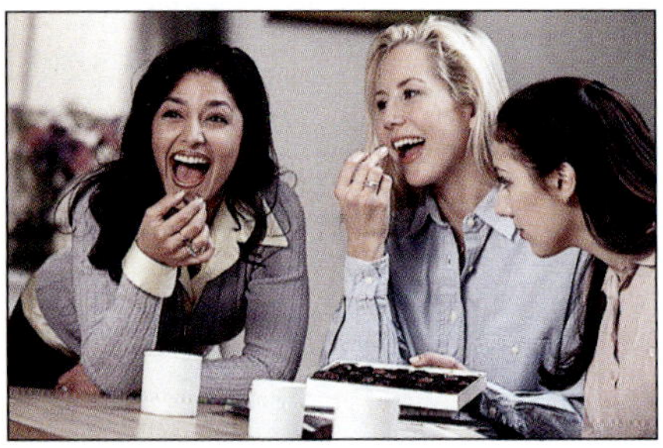

FIGURE 8.18 Fad bulimia is common among sorority members who want to enjoy eating sweets and other snack foods but not gain weight. *(© Tom McCarthy/Photo Edit, Inc.)*

Fad Bulimia Because of the desire of some to have their cake and eat it too, bulimia is "catching on." To those who are concerned about being 10 pounds heavier than they were when they started college, but who don't want to miss out on the food at social gatherings, bulimia may seem like the perfect solution—eat all you want and then purge to eliminate the extra kcalories. This type of bulimia, often termed fad bulimia, is not done in private but takes place among friends. It is particularly common among sorority members (Figure 8.18).[62] It also occurs among male athletes who participate in sports that have competitive weight categories, such as boxing and wrestling.

Despite the attractiveness of being able to eat all you want without gaining weight, purging rituals do not eliminate all the kcalories. Vomiting eliminates 70 to 80% of the ingested energy. The use of laxatives affects the colon, not the small intestine where food is absorbed, so water is lost but most of the energy is not. Diuretics also result in the loss of water, not energy.

The quantities of food consumed by fad bulimics are usually smaller than the amounts eaten by individuals with severe forms of bulimia, and fad bulimics do not exhibit the serious emotional disturbances and shame about the bulimic practices that true bulimics do. Still, fad bulimia is dangerous. If an individual is predisposed to developing an eating disorder, this type of behavior may evolve into

TABLE 8.11 Eating Disorders: How to Help

- Get the person to a doctor; the sooner the illness is treated the more likely there will be a successful outcome.
- Talk to the family (parents, spouse).
- Explain your concerns and the potential hazards of the disease.
- Do not expect the victim to cooperate; denial is common.
- If you work with the person, contact your employee assistance program.

Adapted from Lifescape.com, Toby Goldsmith, M.D. Department of Psychiatry, University of Florida Brain Institute. Available online at **http://www.lifescape.com**.

a more severe eating disorder. Even individuals not predisposed to an eating disorder may learn to use this behavior as a way of dealing with anxiety. The physical damage caused is the same in both fad bulimia and bulimia nervosa. See Table 8.11 for information on how to help someone suspected of having an eating disorder.

Summary

1. More than half of adult Americans are overweight. Most people succeed in short-term weight loss but, in the long term, regain all the weight they have lost.
2. Excess body fat increases the risk of chronic diseases such as diabetes, heart disease, high blood pressure, gallbladder disease, and certain types of cancer.
3. The risks of obesity are related to the degree of overweight, the location of the excess body fat, and the presence of other risk factors and disease conditions. Risk can be assessed by determining BMI, measuring waist circumference, and evaluating other risk factors.
4. Weight management involves adjusting energy intake and expenditure and modifying long-term behaviors. To lose a pound of fat, expenditure must exceed intake by approximately 3500 kcalories. Slow, steady weight loss of 1/2 to 2 pounds per week is more likely to be maintained than rapid weight loss.
5. There are thousands of programs and techniques for weight management. All involve a decrease in energy intake and most also target an increase in energy expenditure. An ideal program involves a decrease in intake, an increase in expenditure, and behavior modification to promote lifestyle change and maintain the loss.
6. Prescription drugs are only recommended for individuals who are significantly overweight or have accompanying health risks. Those currently available act by suppressing appetite or blocking fat absorption. Nonprescription weight-loss medications and dietary supplements are also available. Some herbal weight-loss supplements may cause serious side effects.
7. Surgery is a drastic measure that is considered only for those whose health is seriously at risk because of their obesity. It causes permanent changes in the gastrointestinal tract that affect the amount of food that can be consumed and the absorption of nutrients. Surgery necessitates a lifelong change in eating patterns and behavior.
8. Eating disorders are psychological disorders in which the perception of body size is altered. Anorexia nervosa is characterized by self-starvation and an abnormally low body weight. Bulimia is characterized by repeated cycles of binge eating followed by purging or other behaviors to prevent weight gain. Treatment involves supplying an adequate diet and psychological counseling to change body image and improve eating habits.

Review Questions

1. What health problems are associated with excess body fat?
2. How does the distribution of body fat affect the risks of excess body fat?
3. Define what is meant by a healthy weight.
4. List three risk factors that increase the risks associated with being overweight or obese.
5. By how much energy does expenditure need to exceed intake for a pound of fat to be lost?
6. Describe three approaches to reducing energy intake.
7. What is the best approach to weight management? Why?
8. List some risks and benefits of weight-loss drugs.
9. How does weight-loss surgery cause negative energy balance?
10. What are the characteristics of anorexia nervosa and bulimia nervosa?
11. How is nutrition involved in the treatment of eating disorders?

Applying Critical Thinking Skills

Personal nutrition:

1. Use Figure 8.5 to find your BMI. Are you in the healthy weight range?
   a. If your BMI is in the overweight range, measure your waist circumference. Does it indicate visceral fat storage?
   b. Even if you are not overweight, fill out the table below to see how many factors you have that may increase your risk of obesity-related complications if you become overweight.

Do you have a personal family history of heart disease?	
Are you a male older than age 45?	
Are you a postmenopausal female?	
Do you smoke cigarettes?	

Do you have a sedentary lifestyle?	
Do you have high blood pressure?	
Do you have high LDL cholesterol, low HDL cholesterol, or high triglycerides?	
Do you have diabetes?	

USDA, DHHS, Dietary Guidelines for Americans, 2000.

2. Imagine you have a BMI of 30 kg/m^2.
   a. Use your own height and Figure 8.5 or the equation for BMI (see Chapter 7) to determine about how many pounds you need to lose to get your BMI into the healthy range.
   b. How much weight should you lose per week?
   c. Choose a weight-loss method that best suits your individual needs and explain why you chose this method.
   d. Review the criteria for choosing a weight-management plan listed in Table 8.5. Does your plan meet each of these guidelines?
   e. Should you consider surgery or drugs? Why or why not?

General nutrition issues:

1. Roger just celebrated his 40th birthday. He is about 40 pounds heavier than he was on his 30th birthday. At his current rate of weight gain he will be 80 pounds overweight when he reaches age 50. Roger is 5 feet 8 inches tall and weighs 190 pounds. He has three young children at home and works full time as a salesperson. His day starts at about 6 A.M. when he gets up and has breakfast with his wife and children. He spends most of the morning in his car traveling to visit his accounts. He usually has at least one doughnut-and-coffee break. Lunch is fast food if he is alone or a restaurant meal if he is with clients. Most evenings he is home for dinner. By the time his children are in bed it is about 8 P.M. He sits down with his wife for a glass of wine or a bowl of ice cream.
   a. Design a weight-loss and exercise regimen for Roger. Assume that his wife and children are supportive regarding dietary changes at home.
   b. Does the program you designed fit in with Roger's schedule? Why or why not?
   c. If he follows your suggestions, how long will it take him to lose 40 pounds?
2. Go to the grocery store and select five to ten products labeled "light," "reduced-calorie," "low-calorie," or "calorie-free." Record the number of kcalories and the amount of fat per serving.
   a. Would any of these products be useful for someone on a weight-loss diet?
   b. Can they be consumed in unlimited amounts without significantly increasing energy intake?
   c. Rate these foods in terms of their nutrient density.

REFERENCES

1. Global Database on Obesity and Body Mass Index (BMI) in Adults. Available online at **http://www.who.int/nut/db_bmi.htm**. Accessed 5 Jan 2001.
2. Wickelgren, I. Obesity: how big a problem? Science 280:1364–1367, 1998.
3. Taubes, G. As obesity rates rise, experts struggle to explain why. Science 280:1367–1368, 1998.
4. Flegal, K. M., Carroll, M. D., Kuczmarski, R. J., and Johnson, C. L. Overweight and obesity in the United States: prevalence and trends, 1960–1994. Int. J. Obes. Relat. Metab. Disord. 22:39–47, 1998.
5. National Institutes of Health, National Heart, Lung, and Blood Institute. Clinical Guidelines on the Identification, Evaluation, and Treatment of Overweight and Obesity in Adults. Executive summary, June 1998. Available online at: **http://www.nhlbi.nih.gov/guidelines/obesity/ob_home.htm**. Accessed 5 Jan 2001.
6. Troiano, R. P., and Flegal, K. M. Overweight prevalence among youth in the United States: why so many different numbers? Int. J. Obes. Relat. Metab. Disord. 23(Suppl 2):S22–S27, 1999.
7. Serdula, M. K., Mokdad, A. H., Williamson, D. F., et al. Prevalence of attempting weight loss and strategies for controlling weight. JAMA 282:1353–1358, 1999.
8. Jeffery, R. W. Does weight cycling present a health risk? Am. J. Clin. Nutr. 63(suppl):452S–455S, 1996.
9. Kassirer, J. P., and Angell, M. Losing weight—an ill-fated New Year's resolution. N. Engl. J. Med. 338:52–54, 1998.
10. Committee to Develop Criteria for Evaluating Outcomes of Approaches to Prevent and Treat Obesity, Food and Nutrition Board, Institute of Medicine, National Academy of Sciences. Criteria for evaluating outcomes and approaches to obesity. J. Am. Diet. Assoc. 95:1–10, 1995.
11. Eckel, R. H., and Krauss, R. M. American Heart Association call to action: obesity is a major risk factor for coronary heart disease. AHA Nutrition Committee. Circulation 97:2099–2100, 1998.
12. Sagiv, M., and Goldbourt, U. Influence of physical work on high-density lipoprotein cholesterol: implications for the risk of coronary heart disease. Int. J. Sports Med. 15:261–266, 1994.
13. Leontos, C., Wong, F., and Gallivan, J., for the National Diabetes Education Program Planning Committee. National Diabetes Education Program: opportunities and challenges. J. Am. Diet Assoc. 98:73–75, 1998.
14. Schafer, R. G., Bohannon, B., Franz, M., et al. Translation of the diabetes nutrition recommendations for health care institutions: technical review. J. Am. Diet. Assoc. 97:43–51, 1997.
15. Oria, H. E. Pitfalls in the diagnosis of gallbladder disease in clinically severe obesity. Obes. Surg. 8:444–451, 1998.
16. NIDDK Weight Control Information Network. Dieting and gallstones. Available online at **http://www.niddk.nih.gov/health/nutrit/pubs/dietgall.htm#whatare**. Accessed 11 May 2000.
17. Nieman, D. C., Hensen, D. A., Nehlsen-Cannarella, S. L., et al. Influence of obesity on immune function. J. Am. Diet. Assoc. 99:294–299, 1999.
18. Bongain, A., Insard, V., and Gillet, J. V. Obesity in obstetrics and gynecology. Eur. J. Obstet. Gynenecol. Reprod. Biol. 77:217–228, 1998.
19. Khaidhiar, L., McCowen, K. C., and Blackburn, G. L. Obesity and its co-morbid conditions. Clin. Cornerstone 2:17–31, 1999.

20. Phillps, B. G., Hisel, T. M., Kato, M., et al. Recent weight gain in patients with newly diagnosed obstructive sleep apnea. J. Hypertens. 17:1297–1300, 1999.
21. McTiernam, A. Associations between energy balance and body mass index and the risk of breast carcinoma in women from diverse racial and ethnic backgrounds in the U.S. Cancer 88:1248–1255, 2000.
22. McCabe, S. H. Arthritis: living with your symptoms. American Medical Association. Available online at **http://www.sleepfoundation.org/publications/sleepap.html#1**. Accessed 5 Jan. 2001.
23. Cassell, J. A. Social anthropology and nutrition: a different look at obesity. J. Am. Diet. Assoc. 95:424–427, 1995.
24. Robison, J. I., Hoerr, S. L., Petersmarck, K. A., and Anderson, J. V. Redefining success in obesity intervention: the new paradigm. J. Am. Diet. Assoc. 95:422–423, 1995.
25. U.S. Department of Agriculture and U.S. Department of Health and Human Services. *Nutrition and Your Health: Dietary Guidelines for Americans*, 5th ed. Home and Garden Bulletin No. 232. Hyattsville, Md.: U.S. Government Printing Office, 2000.
26. American Dietetic Association. Position of the American Dietetic Association: weight management. J. Am. Diet. Assoc. 97:71–74, 1997.
27. Klem, M. L., Wing, R. R., McGuire, M. T., et al. A descriptive study of individuals successful at long-term maintenance of substantial weight loss. Am. J. Clin. Nutr. 66:239–246, 1997.
28. Wadden, T. A., Stunkand, A. J., and Brownell, K. D. Very-low-calorie diets: their efficacy, safety and future. Ann. Int. Med. 99:675–684, 1983.
29. American Dietetic Association. Position of the American Dietetic Association: very-low-calorie weight-loss diets. J. Am. Diet. Assoc. 90:722–726, 1990.
30. Wilmore, J. H. Increasing physical activity: alterations in body mass and composition. Am. J. Clin. Nutr. 63(suppl):456S–460S, 1996.
31. Stevens, J., Cai, J., Pamuk, E. R., et al. The effect of age on the association between body mass index and mortality. N. Engl. J. Med. 338:1–7, 1998.
32. Stubbs, R. J., Harbron, C. G., Murgatroyd, P. R., and Prentice, A. M. Covert manipulation of dietary fat and energy density: effect on substrate flux and food intake in men eating ad libitum. Am. J. Clin. Nutr. 62:316–329, 1995.
33. Horten, T. S., Drougas, H., Brachey, A., et al. Fat and carbohydrate overfeeding in humans: different effects on energy storage. Am. J. Clin. Nutr. 62:19–29, 1995.
34. National Task Force on the Prevention and Treatment of Obesity. Long-term pharmacotherapy in the management of obesity. JAMA 276:1907–1915, 1996.
35. Campfield, L. A., Smith, F. J., and Burn, P. Strategies and potential molecular targets for obesity treatment. Science 280:1383–1387, 1998.
36. Food and Drug Administration Science Background: safety of phenylpropanolamine. November 6, 2000. Available online at **http:www.fda.gov/cder/drug/infopage/ppa/science.htm**. Accessed 3 Jan 2001.
37. Anderson, R. A. Effects of chromium on body composition and weight. Nutr. Rev. 56:266–270, 1998.
38. Kurtzweil, P. Dieter's brews make tea time a dangerous affair. FDA Consumer 31: July–August, 1997. Available online at **http://www.fda.gov/fdac/features/1997/597_tea.html/**. Accessed 18 Feb 2001.
39. NHLBI Obesity Education Initiative Expert Panel on the Identification, Evaluation and Treatment of Obesity. *Clinical Guidelines on the Identification, Evaluation and Treatment of Obesity in Adults: The Evidence Report*. Washington, D.C.: U.S. DHHS, 1998.
40. National Institutes of Health Consensus Development Conference Statement: Gastrointestinal surgery for severe obesity. March 25–27, 1991, 1–20. Available online at **http://odp.od.nih.gov/consensus/cons/084/084_statement.htm**. Accessed 18 Feb 2001.
41. NIH Publication No. 96-4006, April 1996, e-text posted 20 February 1998: **http://www.niddk.nih.gov/health/nutrit/pubs/gastsurg.htm**. Accessed 5 Jan 2001.
42. Casper, R. C. Nutrition and its relation to aging. Exp. Gerontol. 30:294–314, 1995.
43. Williamson, D. F. Intentional weight loss: patterns in the general population and its association with morbidity and mortality. Int. J. Obes. Relat. Metab. Disord. 21:(suppl)S14–S19, 1997.
44. Bosello, O., Armellini, S., Zamboni, M., and Fitchet, M. The benefits of modest weight loss in type II diabetes. Int. J. Obes. Relat. Metab. Disord. 21(suppl):S10–S13, 1997.
45. Arena, B., Maffulli, N., Maffulli, F., and Morleo, M. A. Reproductive hormones and menstrual changes with exercise in female athletes. Sports Med. 19:278–287, 1995.
46. Thompson, C. Athletes and eating disorders. Available online at **http:www.mirror-mirror.org/athlete.htm**. Accessed 2 Jan 2001.
47. American Dietetic Association. Position of the American Dietetic Association: nutrition intervention in the treatment of anorexia nervosa, bulimia nervosa and binge eating. J. Am. Diet. Assoc. 94:902–907, 1994.
46. American Psychiatric Association. *Diagnostic and Statistical Manual*, 4th ed. Washington, D.C.: American Psychiatric Association, 1994.
49. American Anorexia Bulimia Association, Inc. Available online at **http://www.aabainc.org/general/index.html**. Accessed 3 Jan 2001.
50. Leon, G. R., Keel, P. K., Klump, K. L., and Fulkerson, J. A. The future of risk factor research in understanding the etiology of eating disorders. Psychopharmacol. Bull, 33:405–411, 1997.
51. Walsh, B. T., and Devlin, M. J. Eating disorders: progress and problems. Science 280:1387–1390, 1998.
52. Gard, M. C., and Freeman C. P. The dismantling of a myth: a review of eating disorders and socioeconomic status. Int. J. Eat. Disord. 20:1–12, 1996.
53. Crago M., Shisslak, C. M., and Estes, L. S. Eating disturbances among American minority groups: a review. Int. J. Eat. Disord. 19:239–248, 1996.
54. Hsu, L. K. Epidemiology of the eating disorders. Psychiatr. Clin. North Am. 19:681–700, 1996.
55. Foreyt, J. P., Poston, W. S. C., II, and Goodrick, G. K. Future directions in obesity and eating disorders. Addict. Behav. 21:767–778, 1996.
56. Medical Sciences Bulletin. Seratonin and eating disorders. Available online at **http://www.pharminfo.com/pubs/msb/serotonin.html**. Accessed 18 Apr 2000.
57. Rock, C. L., and Curan-Celentano, J. Nutritional management of eating disorders. Psychiatr. Clin. North Am. 19:701–713, 1996.
58. Sullivan, P. F., Bulik, C. M., Fear, J. L., and Pickering, A. Outcome of anorexia nervosa: a case-control study. Am. J. Psychiatry 155:939–946, 1998.
59. Farley. D. Eating disorders require medical attention. FDA Consumer 26:27–29, March 1992.
60. Anderson, L., Shaw, J. M., and McCargar, L. Physiological effects of bulimia nervosa on the gastrointestinal tract. Can. J. Gastroenterol. 11:451–459, 1997.
61. Keel, P. K., and Mitchell, J. E. Outcome in bulimia nervosa. Am. J. Psychiatry 154:313–321, 1997.
62. Crandall, C. S. Societal contagion of binge eating. J. Pers. Soc. Psychol. 55:589–599, 1988.

9 The B Vitamins and Choline

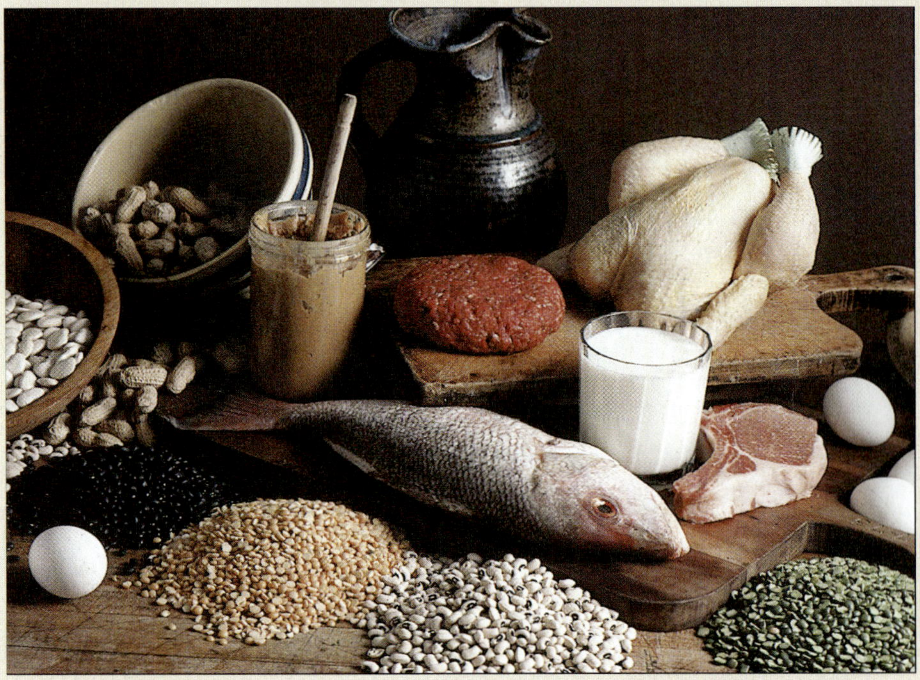

Learning Objectives

After reading this chapter, students should be able to:

1. Define the term "vitamin."
2. Give examples of water-soluble and fat-soluble vitamins and discuss differences in their absorption, storage, and excretion.
3. Describe the factors that affect the amount of a vitamin that is available to the body.
4. Explain the statement "more is not always better" in terms of nutrition.
5. Discuss the similarities in the functions of thiamin, riboflavin, niacin, biotin, and pantothenic acid.
6. Describe the role of vitamin B_6 in amino acid metabolism.
7. Explain why folate is important in cells that are rapidly dividing.
8. Compare the roles of vitamin B_6, folate, and vitamin B_{12} in homocysteine metabolism and discuss how they affect the risk of heart disease.
9. List two food sources for each of the B vitamins.
10. Discuss why choline is not currently classified as a vitamin.

Gordon is 65 years old and generally in good health. He and his wife exercise regularly, watch their weight, and eat a healthy diet. Recently he experienced a few episodes of forgetfulness but laughed it off as old age. Then he began having numbness and tingling in his hands and feet and problems with muscle coordination. Fearing the worst, he made an appointment to see his doctor.

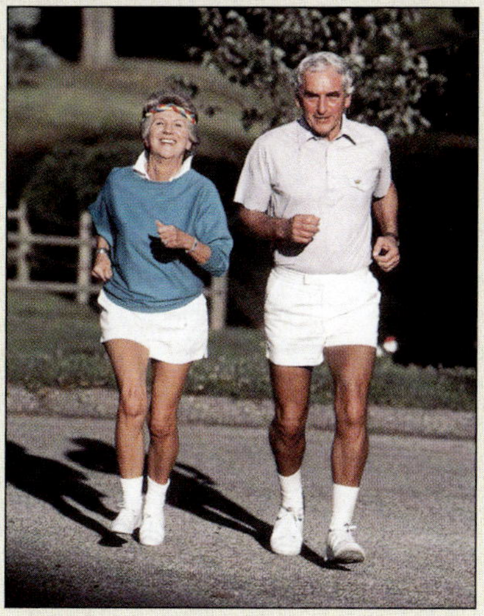

A medical history revealed that, in addition to his other symptoms, Gordon had had episodes of stomach pain that seemed to go away without treatment. Laboratory tests showed that his serum levels of vitamin B_{12} were low but his folate levels were normal. A diet history revealed that he ate very little meat but had a good, balanced diet that included lots of grains, fruits, and vegetables. In addition, he was taking supplements of vitamin B_6 and folate because he read that they could help prevent heart disease. His total intake of B_6 was 80 mg, a dose below the Tolerable Upper Intake Level, or UL, which is set at 100 mg. But totaling the amount of folate provided by fortified grains and supplements revealed that he was consuming almost 2000 μg of folic acid per day, or twice the UL.

When all the testing was done, Gordon's doctor told him he suspected that his problems were caused by a deficiency of vitamin B_{12}. An infection had damaged glands in his stomach, causing a reduction in the amount of stomach acid produced. As a result, the vitamin B_{12} he consumed in his diet was poorly absorbed. His neurological symptoms were likely due to a B_{12} deficiency. The deficiency would also have caused anemia, but his high folate intake masked this symptom. Gordon's doctor gave him an injection of vitamin B_{12} and recommended that he stop taking the folic acid supplement. He recommended a supplement containing vitamin B_{12} to prevent future problems. Gordon was lucky because his symptoms disappeared completely after the injection of B_{12}. If he had waited longer, some of the symptoms may have become permanent.

What Are Vitamins?

The term "vitamin" was coined in 1912 by Polish biochemist Casimir Funk, who originally used the word "vitamine" to refer to substances that are amines (compounds containing an amino group, NH_2) that are also vital to life (vital + amine). Today we know vitamins are vital to life, but they are not all amines, so the "e" has been dropped.

Vitamins are organic compounds that are essential in the diet in small amounts to promote and regulate body functions necessary for growth, reproduction, and the maintenance of health. An organic compound is classified as a vitamin if a lack of the compound in the diet results in deficiency symptoms that are relieved by its addition to the diet. Although vitamins do not provide energy, many aid in the chemical reactions that produce energy from carbohydrate, fat, protein, and alcohol. The general properties of vitamins, as well as specific information about the B vitamins and choline, will be discussed in this chapter; vitamins A, D, K, E, and C will be discussed in Chapter 10.

Vitamins Organic compounds required in the diet in small amounts to promote and regulate the chemical reactions and processes needed for growth, reproduction, and maintenance of health.

Water-soluble vitamins Vitamins that are soluble in water. These include the B vitamins and vitamin C.

Fat-soluble vitamins Vitamins that are soluble in fat. These include vitamins A, D, E, and K.

Coenzymes Small nonprotein organic molecules that act as carriers of electrons or atoms in metabolic reactions and are necessary for the proper functioning of many enzymes.

Fortification A term used generally to describe the addition of nutrients to foods, such as the addition of vitamin D to milk.

Enrichment A term used to describe the addition of specific nutrients to foods in order to restore some of those lost in processing to a level equal to or higher than that originally present.

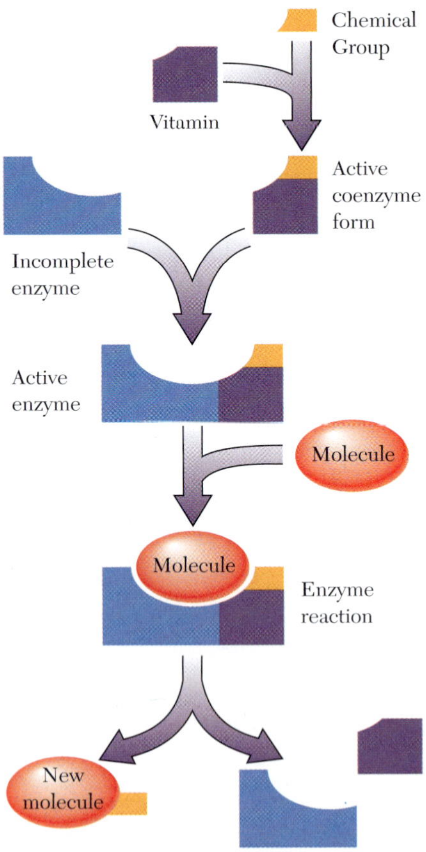

FIGURE 9.1 Many vitamins act as coenzymes. The active coenzyme form of a vitamin serves as a carrier of electrons or chemical groups (shown here in yellow). The coenzyme combines with the incomplete enzyme to form the active enzyme. When the enzyme functions in a reaction, the chemical group (or electrons) is transferred from the coenzyme to a molecule to form a new molecule. The enzyme and coenzyme are then released and can be reused in subsequent reactions.

TABLE 9.1 Vitamins with Common Functions

Vitamins	Function
Thiamin, riboflavin, niacin, pantothenic acid, biotin, vitamin B_6, folate, vitamin B_{12}, vitamin C, vitamin K	Coenzyme
Thiamin, riboflavin, niacin, pantothenic acid, biotin, vitamin B_6	Metabolism of energy-yielding nutrients
Vitamin B_6, folate, vitamin B_{12}	Red blood cell synthesis
Vitamin B_6, folate, vitamin B_{12}	Amino acid/homocysteine metabolism
Biotin, pantothenic acid, niacin	Fatty acid synthesis
Vitamin C, vitamin E	Antioxidant protection
Thiamin, vitamin B_6, vitamin B_{12}	Nerve transmission
Vitamin A, vitamin D	Gene expression

Classification of Vitamins

Initially, the vitamins were named alphabetically in approximately the order in which they were identified: A, B, C, D, and E. The B vitamins were first thought to be one chemical substance but were later found to be many different substances, so the alphabetical name was broken down by number. For example, thiamin, riboflavin, and niacin were originally referred to as vitamins B_1, B_2, and B_3, respectively. Vitamins B_6 and B_{12} are the only ones that are still commonly referred to by their numbers.

Vitamins have traditionally been grouped based on their solubility in water or fat. This chemical characteristic allows generalizations to be made about how they are absorbed, transported, excreted, and stored in the body. The **water-soluble vitamins** include the B vitamins and vitamin C. The **fat-soluble vitamins** include vitamins A, D, E, and K. More recently, with the development of the Dietary Reference Intakes (DRIs), vitamins (along with minerals and other health-promoting food components) are being grouped based on shared functions (Table 9.1). For example, the B vitamins all act as **coenzymes** or components of coenzymes (Figure 9.1). (DRIs for the B vitamins and choline were released together.) Vitamin C is also a water-soluble vitamin that functions as a coenzyme; however, because it is also an antioxidant, the DRI committee chose to evaluate it along with the antioxidant nutrients. The discussion of vitamin C is therefore included in Chapter 10 along with other antioxidant nutrients.

Sources of Vitamins

Almost all foods contain some vitamins (Figure 9.2). Grains are good sources of thiamin, riboflavin, niacin, pantothenic acid, and biotin. Meat and fish are good sources of all of the B vitamins. Milk provides riboflavin, vitamin A, and vitamin D; leafy greens provide folate, vitamin A, vitamin E, and vitamin K; citrus fruit provides vitamin C; and vegetable oils are high in vitamin E.

The vitamin content of foods can be affected by cooking, storage, and processing. Vitamins naturally present in foods can be washed away or destroyed by cooking. Exposure to light and oxygen during food storage and preparation also causes vitamin losses, and processing can either remove or add nutrients. For example, the milling of wheat into white flour causes the loss of the nutrients contained in the bran and germ of the wheat kernel. Further processing may restore these lost nutrients and add others.

The addition of nutrients to foods is called **fortification**. The added nutrients may or may not have been present in the original food. **Enrichment** is a type of fortification in which specific nutrients are added for the purpose of restoring those lost in processing to the same or a higher level than originally present. Enrichment of grain products adds back the vitamins thiamin, niacin, and riboflavin and the mineral iron that are removed in milling, but not all the nutrients lost in processing are restored by enrichment (Figure 9.3). Foods that are staples of the diet are often fortified to prevent vitamin or mineral deficiencies and promote health in the population. For example, milk is fortified with vitamin D to promote bone health, and grains are fortified with folic acid to reduce the incidence of birth defects. Some foods are fortified because they are used in place of other foods that are good sources of an essential nutrient. Margarine, for example, is fortified with vitamin A because it is often used instead of butter, which naturally contains vitamin A.

Supplements are another source of vitamins. Although supplements can provide specific nutrients, they cannot provide all the benefits of foods (Figure 9.4). Even supplements that meet vitamin needs do not provide the energy, protein, minerals, fiber, or phytochemicals that would have been supplied by food sources of these vitamins. In addition, because they provide such a concentrated source of nutrients, they can easily be consumed in toxic doses. The role of supplements will be discussed with each nutrient in this chapter and in greater depth in *Making Decisions*: "Supplementing Safely".

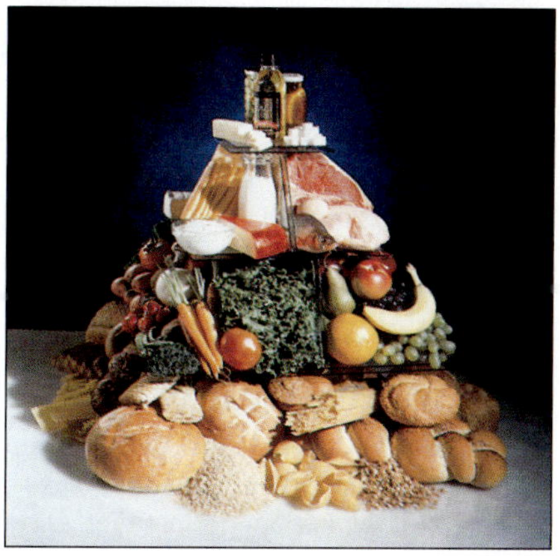

FIGURE 9.2 All the food groups of the Food Guide Pyramid contain choices that are good sources of vitamins. *(© Gary Buss/FPG International)*

Vitamins in the Digestive Tract

About 40 to 90% of the vitamins in food are absorbed, primarily in the small intestine (Figure 9.5). The composition of the diet and conditions in the body, however, may influence **bioavailability**—the amount of a nutrient that can be absorbed and utilized by the body. For example, the amount of fat in the diet affects the bioavailability of fat-soluble vitamins because they are absorbed along with dietary fat. Fat-soluble vitamins are poorly absorbed when the diet is very low in fat. The mechanism by which vitamins are absorbed also determines the amount that enters the body. Fat-soluble vitamins are easily absorbed by simple diffusion. Many of the water-soluble vitamins depend on energy-requiring transport systems or binding molecules in the gastrointestinal tract in order to be absorbed. For example, thiamin and vitamin C are absorbed by energy-requiring transport systems, riboflavin and niacin require carrier proteins for absorption, and vitamin B_{12} must be bound to a protein produced in the stomach in order to be efficiently absorbed in the intestine.

Bioavailability A general term that refers to how well a nutrient can be absorbed and used by the body.

Some vitamins are absorbed in inactive **provitamin** or **vitamin precursor** forms that must be converted into active vitamin forms once inside the body.

Provitamin or **vitamin precursor** A compound that can be converted into the active form of a vitamin in the body.

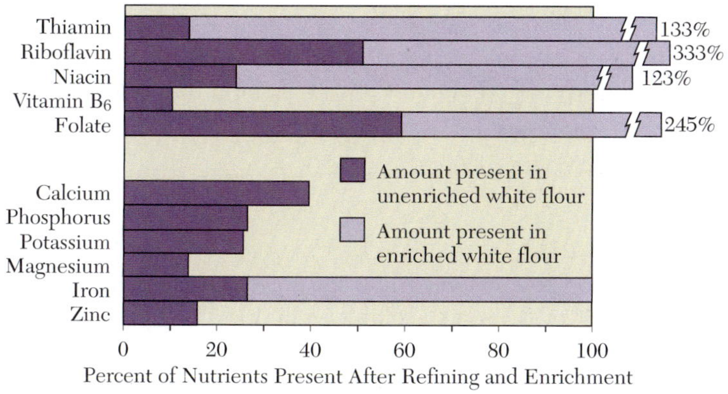

FIGURE 9.3 Many of the nutrients in whole grains are lost in refining, but only a few are added back in enrichment. This figure compares the amounts of some nutrients found in enriched and unenriched white flour with the amount in the whole-wheat grain. The nutrients present in whole durum wheat are represented as 100%. Values for folate are included because enriched grains are also fortified with folic acid.

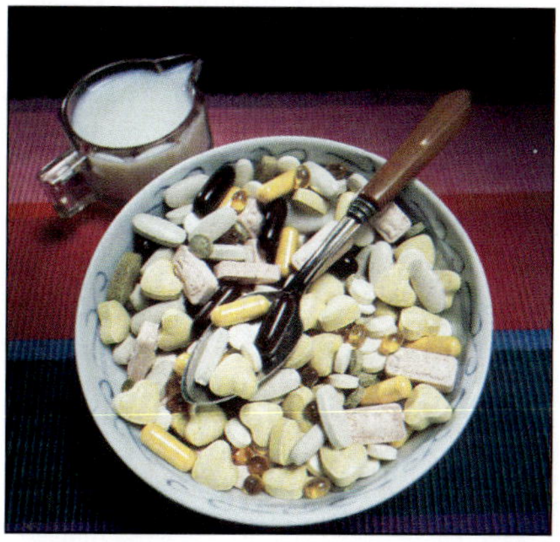

FIGURE 9.4 Vitamin supplements cannot take the place of a balanced diet. *(Charles D. Winters)*

Making Decisions

Supplementing Safely

Half of all American adults take vitamin and mineral supplements regularly.[a] Are you one of them? Should you be? Generally healthy individuals who eat a varied, balanced diet do not need supplements to meet nutrient needs. Why, then, do so many people take them? Many people think of supplements as diet insurance—to make up for a less than perfect diet. Others take supplements in the hope that they will prevent diseases or cure other conditions. Although supplements may provide some of these benefits, nutrient excesses can be toxic. For individuals who choose to take a vitamin and/or mineral supplement, it is important to choose one that is safe. But, choosing a supplement can be confusing.

The FDA estimates that there are 25,000 different products available as dietary supplements.[b] Some claim to have special formulations designed to alleviate stress or maximize antioxidant protection. Others target the needs of women, men, athletes, or seniors. Some claim to be all-natural, others add herbal ingredients that promise everything from a better memory to a reduced risk of cancer. They entice you with terms like "mega," "advanced formula," "high potency," and "ultra." Are these really better than a plain old multivitamin/multimineral supplement?

Selecting a supplement was made somewhat less confusing by the Dietary Supplement Health and Education Act of 1994. This law standardized the information that can be included on supplement labels. Each product must carry a "Supplement Facts" panel similar to the "Nutrition Facts" panel found on processed foods (see Chapter 2). This panel lists the recommended serving size and the name and quantity of each ingredient per serving (see figure). The nutrients for which Daily Values have been established are listed first, followed by other dietary ingredients for which no Daily Value has been established.

Supplement labels make it easier to tell what is supposed to be in supplements, but products do not always provide the amounts that the label declares. This is because dietary supplements are defined as foods and not drugs, so their manufacture is not strictly regulated. The amount contained in each dose and how well it dissolves may vary. Products labeled USP (United States Pharmacopeia) follow a set of voluntary standards for manufacturing.

The Supplement Facts panel on supplement labels can be helpful in determining how much of each nutrient or other

Supplement Facts

Serving Size 1 Tablet

Each Tablet Contains	% DV
Vitamin A 5000 IU (20% as Beta Carotene)	100%
Vitamin C 60 mg	100%
Vitamin D 400 IU	100%
Vitamin E 30 IU	100%
Vitamin K 25 mcg	31%
Thiamin 1.5 mg	100%
Riboflavin 1.7 mg	100%
Niacin 20 mg	100%
Vitamin B_6 2 mg	100%
Folic Acid 400 mcg	100%
Vitamin B_{12} 6 mcg	100%
Biotin 30 mcg	10%
Pantothenic Acid 10 mg	100%
Calcium 162 mg	16%
Iron 18 mg	100%
Phosphorus 109 mg	11%
Iodine 150 mcg	100%
Magnesium 100 mg	25%
Zinc 15 mg	100%
Selenium 20 mcg	29%
Copper 2 mg	100%
Manganese 2 mg	100%

Each Tablet Contains	% DV
Chromium 120 mcg	100%
Molybdenum 75 mcg	100%
Chloride 72 mg	2%
Potassium 80 mg	2%
Boron 150 mcg	*
Nickel 5 mcg	*
Silicon 2 mg	*
Tin 10 mcg	*
Vanadium 10 mcg	*
Lutein 250 mcg	*

* Daily Value (%DV) not established.

SUGGESTED USE:
Adults - One tablet daily.

WARNING: Accidental overdose of iron-containing products is a leading cause of fatal poisoning in children under 6. Keep this product out of reach of children. In case of accidental overdose, call a doctor or poison control center immediately.

Keep bottle tightly closed.
Store at room temperature.

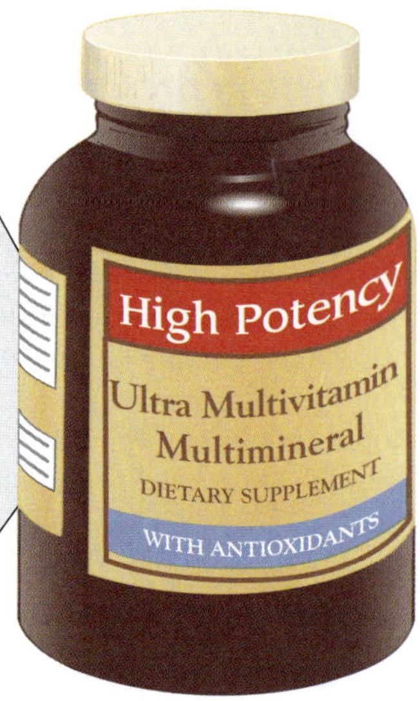

How much of each provitamin can be converted into the active vitamin and the rate at which this occurs determine the amount of the vitamin that is available to function in the body.

Vitamins in the Body

Once absorbed into the blood, vitamins must be transported to the cells. Despite their solubility in water, most of the water-soluble vitamins are bound to blood proteins for transport. Fat-soluble vitamins must be incorporated into lipoproteins or bound to transport proteins in order to be transported in the aqueous environment of the blood. For example, vitamins A, D, E, and K are all incorporated into chylomicrons for transport from the intestine. Vitamin A is stored in the liver, but it must be bound to a specific transport protein to be transported from the liver to other tissues; therefore, the amount delivered to the tis-

substance is in a daily dose (see table). Products that provide no more than 100% of the Daily Value are generally safe and adequate. The nutrients most likely to be present in amounts greater than 100% of the Daily Value are the B vitamins. These are inexpensive and many, but not all, are safe in higher doses. When a product provides nutrients in amounts greater than 100% of the Daily Value, the amounts should be compared to the UL (see inside back cover). Taking any nutrient in amounts that exceed this value significantly increases the risk of potentially serious toxicity symptoms.

Although the amounts of the nutrients in a product may be safe, the product may not provide all the nutrients consumers are seeking to supplement. Some products provide vitamins but not minerals. And some provide only a small proportion of the requirement. For example, most vitamin/mineral supplements contain 100–200 mg of calcium; the requirement is 1000 mg or more. Many products claim to be special formulas for men, seniors, or women, but these may not necessarily provide all the nutrients appropriate for the group they target. Individuals with medical conditions and those taking medications need to consider potential interactions with supplements. For example, individuals taking anticoagulant medications should not take supplements containing vitamin E. People who tend to get kidney stones should avoid vitamin C supplements. Those with iron storage disorders should not take iron supplements.

Another concern with choosing a supplement is the nonvitamin and nonmineral ingredients. Even standard brands are now offering formulations with added herbal ingredients. There are no Daily Values for herbs, carotenoids, flavonoids, isoflavones, and other phytochemicals, so it is difficult to assess whether the amount in a supplement is high or low. A supplement that has a complete assortment of vitamins and minerals does not have much room for large amounts of other ingredients. Often the amounts of these substances added to multivitamin/multimineral supplements are too small to be significant. In addition, the presence of these ingredients, or a label term such as "natural," may increase the cost more than the ingredients contained in the formula.

Finally, dietary supplements should be stored safely and used properly. Products should not be used past their expiration date because some vitamins will degrade over time. Serving recommendations should be followed. For some products the serving size may be six or more tablets per day; for others it may be one tablet. More is not always better when it comes to supplements. Harmful effects or illnesses related to the use of supplements can be reported to FDA MedWatch by calling 1-800-FDA-1088 or going into the MedWatch Web site.

Choosing a Dietary Supplement

- Does it meet your needs? Decide why you want a supplement. If you are taking it for insurance, does it provide both vitamins and minerals? If you want to supplement specific nutrients, are they contained in the product?
- Does it contain potentially toxic levels of any nutrient? Check the % DV for any nutrients that exceed 100%. If they do, do they exceed the UL (see inside back cover)?
- Does it contain any nonvitamin/nonmineral ingredients? If so, have any been shown to be toxic to someone like you (see Chapter 10)?
- Do you have a medical condition that recommends against certain nutrients or other ingredients? Are you a smoker? (You may need more vitamin C, but this increases your risks if you take large amounts of beta-carotene.)
- Are you taking prescription medication with which an ingredient in the supplement may interact? Check with your physician, dietitian, or pharmacist to help identify these interactions.
- Consider the costs—just as more isn't always better, more expensive is not always better, either. Compare costs and ingredients before you buy.

References

[a] Nutrition and You: Trends 2000. American Dietetic Association Available online at **www.eatright.org/pr/2000/010300A.html.** Accessed 4 Jun 2000.

[b] NPR/Kaiser Family Foundation/Kennedy School of Government. Survey of Americans on Dietary Supplements. February 1999. Available online at **www.npr.org/programs/specials/survey/memo.html**. Accessed 5 Jun 2000.

sues depends on the availability of the transport protein. When protein is deficient, sufficient amounts of the vitamin A transport protein are not available, so vitamin A cannot be delivered to the cells where it is needed, even if it is adequate in the diet.

The ability to store and excrete vitamins helps to regulate the amount present in the body. With the exception of vitamin B_{12}, the water-soluble vitamins are easily excreted from the body in the urine. Because they are not stored to any great extent, supplies of water-soluble vitamins are rapidly depleted and they must be consumed regularly in the diet. Nevertheless, it takes more than a few days to develop deficiency symptoms even when these vitamins are completely eliminated from the diet. Fat-soluble vitamins, on the other hand, are stored in the liver and fatty tissues and cannot be excreted in the urine. In general, because they are stored to a larger extent, it takes longer to develop a deficiency of fat-soluble vitamins when they are no longer provided by the diet.

FIGURE 9.5 An overview of vitamins in the digestive tract.

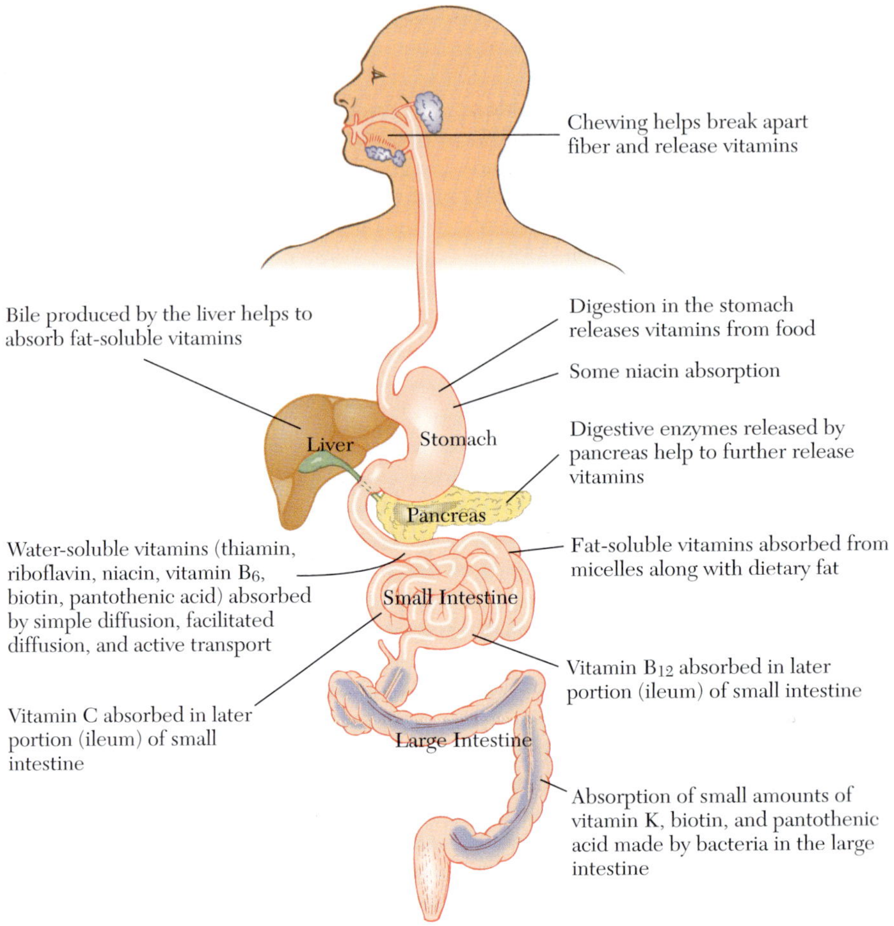

Recommended Intakes

Recommendations for vitamin intake for healthy populations in the United States and Canada are made by the DRIs (see Chapter 2). For each vitamin, scientists review epidemiological data on current dietary intakes in North American populations and data from clinical trials, depletion-repletion studies, nutrient-balance studies, and biochemical and molecular biological studies.

Before an Estimated Average Requirement (EAR) and Recommended Dietary Allowance (RDA) or an Adequate Intake (AI) can be established, specific criteria upon which to base the adequacy of the nutrient are selected. These may include any parameter related to health and nutrient function, such as the amount of a nutrient or metabolite excreted in the urine, the level of a nutrient in the blood, or the activity of an enzyme dependent on that nutrient. The role of the nutrient in reducing disease risk is also taken into account. For example, the amount of a vitamin considered adequate may be defined as the amount that maintains normal blood levels and provides protection from a chronic condition such as cardiovascular disease. The requirements of each life stage and gender are considered separately.

The DRIs consider each vitamin's criteria of adequacy and bioavailability to estimate the average requirement for the population—the EAR. The EAR value is designed to meet the needs of 50% of the healthy population. This value is used to establish an RDA by increasing it to a level that will meet the needs of 97 to 98% of the healthy population. If sufficient information is not available to determine an EAR, an AI is set based on observed or experimentally determined estimates of the average intake in the healthy population. Therefore, for each vitamin and life stage, the DRIs include either an RDA value when sufficient information is available, or an AI when a recommendation is estimated from population data. Either of these values can be used as a goal for dietary intake by individuals.

The DRIs also establish Tolerable Upper Intake Levels (ULs) as a guide to the maximum amount of a vitamin that is unlikely to cause adverse health effects. For some vitamins the UL refers to total intake from foods, fortified foods, and nutrient supplements, for others, it refers to intake from supplements alone.

Vitamins and Health

Vitamins were first discovered when diseases that seemed incurable, and were often fatal, were cured by changes in diet. In 1885 it was discovered that beriberi, a disease that killed thousands of sailors in the Orient, could be prevented by adding meat and whole grains to the usual shipboard diet. In 1913, a fat-soluble factor that allowed animals to grow better was identified in butter, and in 1915, pellagra, a disease that filled psychiatric hospitals in the southern United States, was cured by yeast or liver extract. Discoveries such as these helped scientists connect specific diseases with dietary deficiencies.

Even though the last of the 13 compounds recognized as vitamins today was characterized in 1948, vitamin deficiencies remain a major public health problem in many parts of the world. Thousands of children in developing nations go blind due to vitamin A deficiency and have malformed bones from vitamin D deficiency. In industrialized countries, a more varied food supply, along with the fortification and enrichment of foods, has almost eliminated vitamin-deficiency diseases in the majority of the population. Concern in these countries now focuses on meeting the needs of high-risk groups, evaluating the effects of marginal deficiencies, and assessing the risk of consuming toxic amounts from fortified foods and supplements.

Deficiency Groups at risk of deficiency include those whose requirements are increased, such as pregnant women and children; those whose intake is limited by financial or dietary restrictions; and those whose absorption or utilization is limited by a disease state. But mild deficiencies may also affect the general public. For example, mild deficiencies of vitamin B_6, folate, and vitamin B_{12} have been implicated as factors that increase the risk of cardiovascular disease. Low intakes of fruits and vegetables that provide much of the vitamin C, vitamin E, beta-carotene, and phytochemicals in the diet may be increasing the rates of certain cancers and cardiovascular disease.

Web Menu: For more information on the use and safety of dietary supplements, go to the National Institutes of Health Office of Dietary Supplements at dietary-supplements.info.nih.gov/.

Toxicity The principle of "some is good, so more must be better" does not universally apply in nutrition. Just as there is a minimum amount of a vitamin necessary to prevent deficiency, there is a maximum level above which symptoms of toxicity are likely to occur. For years it was thought that only the fat-soluble vitamins could build up to toxic levels in the body and that excesses of water-soluble vitamins were merely excreted in the urine and could not reach toxic levels. However, as nutrient supplements became more popular, reports of toxicities due to water-soluble vitamins, such as niacin and vitamin B_6, began to appear. If the popularity of vitamin supplements continues, toxicity symptoms are likely to become more common.

THIAMIN

More than 4000 years ago, affluent members of Far Eastern societies began the practice of removing the outer hulls of rice to produce white or "polished" rice (Figure 9.6). As polished rice became the staple of the diet, the prevalence of the

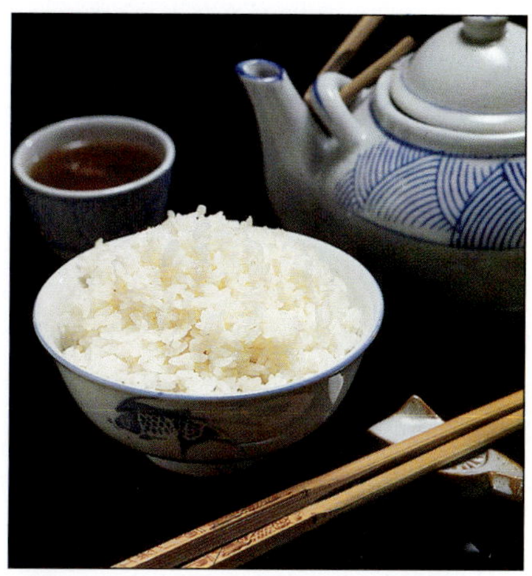

FIGURE 9.6 Unenriched white rice is a poor source of thiamin. *(Charles D. Winters)*

Beriberi The disease resulting from a deficiency of thiamin.

disease **beriberi** increased. The first descriptions of beriberi were made in the mid–17th century by Dutch physicians who treated a young Dutchman who had returned from the East Indies suffering from what the natives called beriberi, or "the lameness." These physicians had no idea that it was due to a dietary deficiency. A connection between diet and beriberi was not made until the late 19th century, when a surgeon in the Japanese navy demonstrated that shipboard beriberi could be prevented by the addition of meat and whole grains to the diet. These foods are now known to be good sources of thiamin.

Sources of Thiamin

Thiamin is widely distributed in foods. A large proportion of the thiamin consumed in the United States comes from enriched grains used in foods such as breakfast cereals and baked goods. Pork, whole grains, legumes, nuts, seeds, and organ meats (liver, kidney, heart) are also good sources (Figure 9.7).

Thiamin in foods may be destroyed during cooking or storage because it is sensitive to heat, oxygen, and low-acid conditions. Thiamin availability is also affected by the presence of antithiamin factors that destroy the vitamin. For instance, there are enzymes in raw shellfish and freshwater fish that degrade thiamin during food storage and preparation and during passage through the gastrointestinal tract. These enzymes are destroyed by cooking, so they are only a concern in foods consumed raw. Tea, coffee, betel nuts, blueberries, and red cabbage contain antithiamin factors that are not inactivated by cooking. Because these make thiamin unavailable to the body, habitual consumption of foods containing antithiamin factors increases the risk of thiamin deficiency.[1]

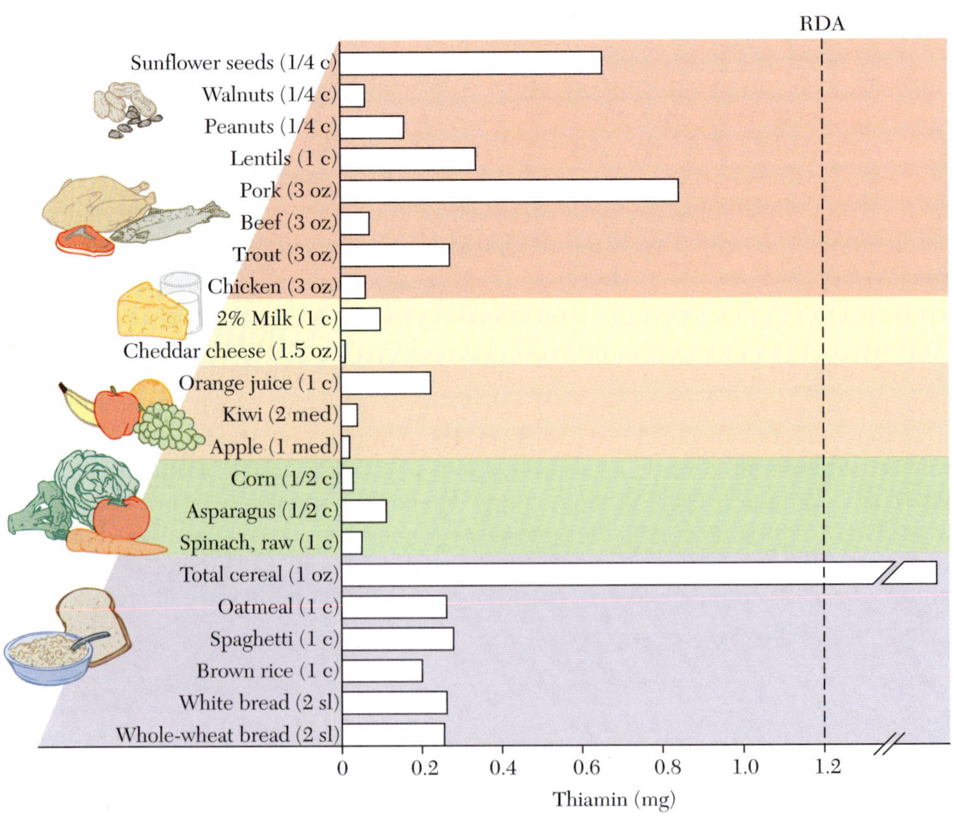

FIGURE 9.7 Thiamin content of selections from each food group of the Food Guide Pyramid. The dashed line represents the RDA for adult men. Pork is an exceptionally good source of thiamin, but other meats are not as good. Whole and fortified grain products are also good sources.

Thiamin in the Body

Thiamin does not provide energy, but it is important in the energy-producing reactions in the body. The active form, **thiamin pyrophosphate**, is a coenzyme in reactions in which carbon dioxide is lost from larger molecules. For instance, the reaction that forms acetyl-CoA from pyruvate and one of the reactions of the citric acid cycle both require thiamin pyrophosphate. Thiamin is therefore essential to the production of energy from glucose. Figure 9.8 illustrates the metabolic reactions that require thiamin as well as those that need the B vitamins riboflavin, niacin, biotin, and pantothenic acid as coenzymes.

Thiamin pyrophosphate The active coenzyme form of thiamin. It is the predominant form found inside cells, where it aids reactions in which a carbon-containing group is lost as CO_2.

Thiamin is also needed for the metabolism of other sugars and certain amino acids, for the synthesis of the neurotransmitter acetylcholine, and for the production of the sugar ribose, which is needed to synthesize RNA (ribonucleic acid).

Recommended Intakes

The RDA for thiamin for adult men age 19 and older is set at 1.2 mg per day and for adult women 19 and older, at 1.1 mg per day. The RDA is based on the amount of thiamin needed to achieve and maintain normal activity of a thiamin-dependent enzyme found in red blood cells and normal urinary thiamin excretion.[2] For an average adult, half of the RDA can be obtained from 3 to 4 ounces (85 to 115 g) of pork or one-quarter cup of shelled sunflower seeds.

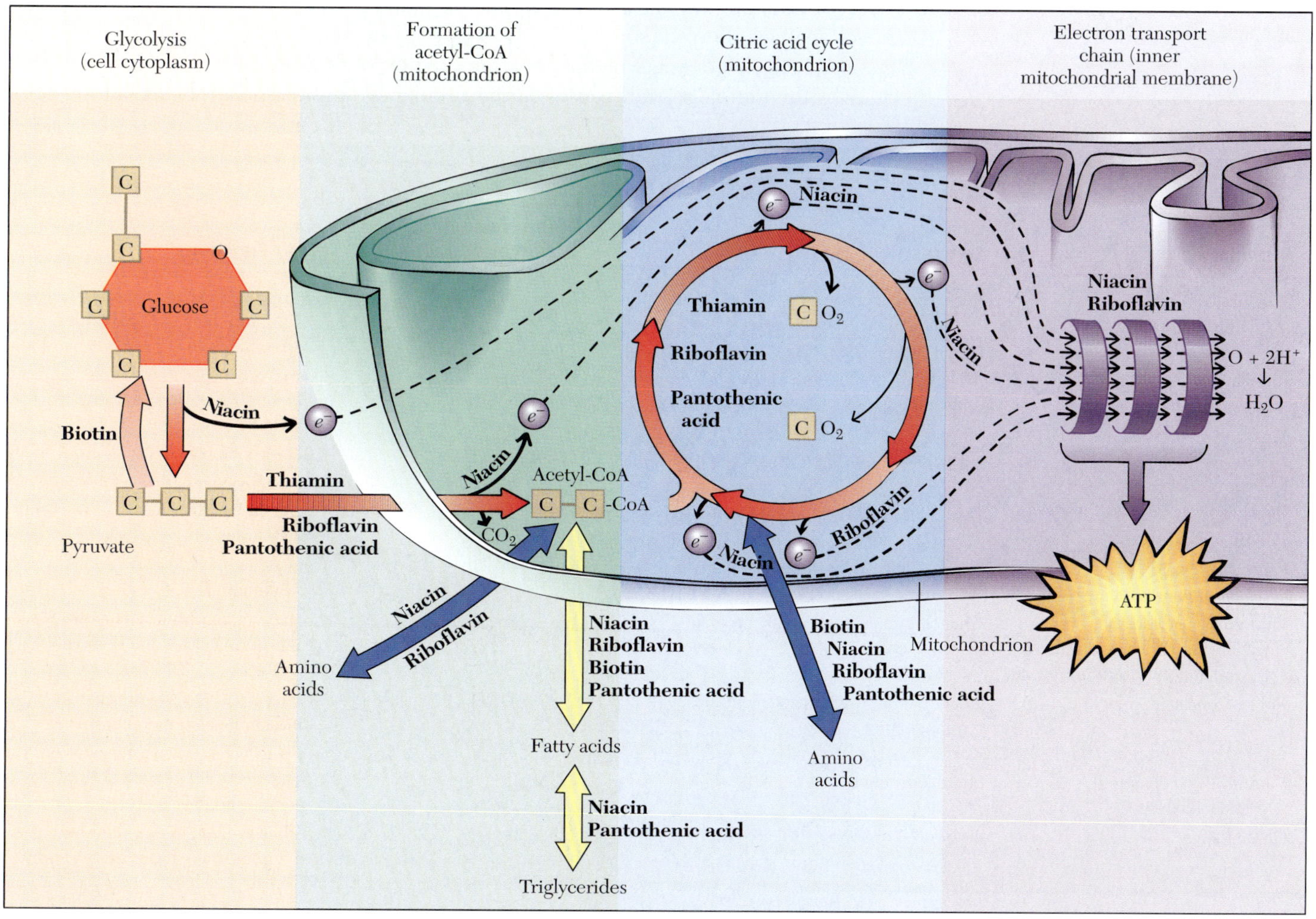

FIGURE 9.8 Many metabolic reactions require the active coenzyme forms of the vitamins thiamin, riboflavin, niacin, biotin, or pantothenic acid. These enzymatic reactions are particularly important for the production of energy from carbohydrate, fat, and protein.

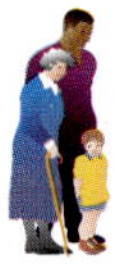

The requirement for thiamin is increased during pregnancy to accommodate the needs of growth and energy utilization, and during lactation to meet the need for increased energy for milk production and to replace the thiamin secreted in milk. There is not enough information to establish an RDA for infants, so an AI has been set based on the thiamin intake of infants fed human milk (see inside front cover).

Thiamin and Health

In the United States today, neither thiamin deficiency nor toxicity is common in the general population. Thiamin deficiency is most often seen in chronic alcoholics.

Thiamin Deficiency Thiamin deficiency results in the disease beriberi. In Sri Lanka, the word "beriberi" literally means "I cannot," describing the extreme weakness and lassitude that occurs with this disease and reflecting the importance of this vitamin in energy metabolism. Beriberi affects the nervous and cardiovascular systems. Some, but not all, of its symptoms can be explained by the roles of thiamin in glucose metabolism and in the synthesis of acetylcholine. The earliest symptoms, depression and weakness, which occur after only about ten days on a thiamin-free diet, are probably related to the inability to completely use glucose. The brain and other nerve tissue rely on glucose for energy. For pyruvate from glucose breakdown to enter the citric acid cycle, it must be converted to acetyl-CoA by a thiamin-dependent enzyme. When thiamin is deficient, the inability to form acetyl-CoA limits energy production and affects nervous system activity. Poor coordination, tingling in the arms and legs, and paralysis may be caused by the lack of acetylcholine. In some cases of beriberi, referred to as wet beriberi, symptoms also include edema, which is an accumulation of fluid in the tissues. It is not clear why thiamin deficiency causes cardiovascular symptoms such as heart failure.

TABLE 9.2 A Summary of the B Vitamins and Choline

Vitamin	Sources	Recommended Intake for Adults*†	Major Functions
Thiamin (vitamin B_1, thiamin mononitrate)	Pork; sunflower seeds; whole, enriched, and fortified grains; legumes	1.1–1.2 mg	Coenzyme in the formation of acetyl-CoA, and the citric acid cycle; nerve function
Riboflavin (vitamin B_2)	Milk, leafy greens, enriched and fortified grains	1.1–1.3 mg	Coenzyme in citric acid cycle, fat metabolism, electron transport chain
Niacin (nicotinamide, nicotinic acid)	Enriched and fortified grains, peanuts, tuna, chicken, beef	14–16 mg NE	Coenzyme in glycolysis, electron transport chain, fat metabolism
Biotin	Liver, egg yolks, synthesized in the gut	30 μg*	Coenzyme in glucose production and fat synthesis
Pantothenic acid (calcium pantothenate)	Meat, whole grains, legumes	5 mg*	Coenzyme in citric acid cycle; fat metabolism
Vitamin B_6 (pyridoxine, pyridoxine HCl, pyridoxal phosphate, pyridoxamine)	Meat, legumes, seeds, leafy greens, whole grains	1.3–1.7 mg	Coenzyme in protein metabolism, neurotransmitter and hemoglobin synthesis
Folate (folic acid, folacin)	Leafy greens, organ meats, legumes, orange juice	400 μg DFE	Coenzyme in DNA synthesis and amino acid metabolism
Vitamin B_{12} (cobalamin, cyanocobalamin)	Animal products	2.4 μg	Coenzyme in folate metabolism; nerve function
Choline	Egg yolks, organ meats leafy greens, nuts	425–550 mg*	Synthesis of cell membranes and the neurotransmitter acetylcholine

*Values with an asterisk (*) represent Adequate Intakes (AI). All other values are Recommended Dietary Allowances (RDA).

†Recommended intakes and UL values for all age groups and stages of life are given on the inside covers.

‡From fortified foods and/or supplements.

ND = insufficient data to determine a UL.

Although overt beriberi is usually thought of as a disease of 19th-century Asia, there are population groups in North America today that are at a high risk for developing thiamin deficiency. Alcoholics are particularly vulnerable because thiamin absorption is decreased due to the effect of alcohol on the gastrointestinal tract. In addition, the liver damage that occurs with chronic alcohol consumption reduces conversion of thiamin to active coenzyme forms. Thiamin intake also may be low due to a diet high in alcohol and low in nutrient-dense foods.[1] Thiamin-deficient alcoholics may develop a neurological condition known as **Wernicke-Korsakoff syndrome**, characterized by mental confusion, psychosis, memory disturbances, and eventually coma.

Wernicke-Korsakoff syndrome A condition involving loss of specific functions in the brain and in nerves throughout the body, due to malnutrition, specifically thiamin deficiency. It develops gradually and is most common in alcoholics.

Thiamin Toxicity Because no toxicity has been reported when excess thiamin is consumed from either food or supplements, not enough information is available to establish a UL for thiamin intake.[2] This does not mean that high intakes are necessarily safe. Intakes of thiamin above the RDA have not been shown to provide health benefits.

Thiamin Supplements Thiamin supplements containing up to 50 mg per day are widely available and are marketed with the promise that they will provide "more energy." Although thiamin is needed to produce energy, it does not provide energy or stimulate energy production. Unless thiamin is deficient, increasing thiamin intake does not increase the ability to produce energy. Because thiamin deficiency causes mental confusion and damages the heart, supplements often promise to improve mental function and prevent heart disease. However, in the absence of a deficiency, supplements do not have these effects.

A summary of the sources, recommended intakes, functions and deficiency and toxicity symptoms of thiamin, other B vitamins, and choline is provided in Table 9.2.

Deficiency Diseases and Symptoms	Groups at Risk	Toxicity	Tolerable Upper Intake Levels (UL)†
Beriberi: nerve tingling, poor coordination, weakness, heart changes	Alcoholics, those in poverty	None reported	ND
Inflammation of mouth and tongue	None	None reported	ND
Pellagra: dermatitis, diarrhea, dementia	Those consuming a limited diet high in corn products; alcoholics	Flushing, nausea, rash, tingling extremities	35 mg/d‡
Dermatitis, nausea, depression, hallucinations	Those consuming large amounts of raw egg whites	Unknown	ND
Fatigue, rash	Alcoholics	Diarrhea, water retention	ND
Headache, neurologic symptoms, nausea, poor growth, anemia	Women, alcoholics	Nerve destruction	100 mg/d
Macrocytic anemia, inflammation of tongue, diarrhea, poor growth, neural tube defects	Women of childbearing age, alcoholics	High doses mask B_{12} deficiency	1000 μg/d‡
Pernicious anemia, macrocytic anemia, poor nerve function	Vegans, elderly, those with stomach or intestinal disease	None reported	ND
Liver dysfunction	None	Sweating, reduced growth, low	3500 mg/d

Riboflavin

While searching for a cure for beriberi, scientists also isolated riboflavin and several other B vitamins as well as thiamin. This occurred because the extracts they made from vegetables and grains could be separated into two components. One contained thiamin, the antiberiberi factor they sought, and the other was a mix of B vitamins that was later determined to contain riboflavin along with vitamin B_6, niacin, and pantothenic acid.

Sources of Riboflavin

Milk is the best source of riboflavin in the North American diet. Other major sources include liver, red meat, poultry, fish, and whole and enriched grain products. Vegetable sources include asparagus, broccoli, mushrooms, and leafy green vegetables such as spinach (Figure 9. 9). Because riboflavin is destroyed by exposure to light, poor handling decreases a food's riboflavin content. This is a problem when milk is stored in clear containers and exposed to light. Cloudy plastic milk bottles block some light, partially protecting the riboflavin, but opaque milk containers are better at preventing losses.

Riboflavin in the Body

Flavin adenine dinucleotide (FAD) and **flavin mononucleotide (FMN)** The active coenzyme forms of riboflavin. The structure of these molecules allows them to pick up and donate hydrogens and electrons in chemical reactions.

Riboflavin forms the active coenzymes **flavin adenine dinucleotide (FAD)** and **flavin mononucleotide (FMN)**. FAD functions in the citric acid cycle and is important for the breakdown of fatty acids. Both FAD and FMN are able to pick up

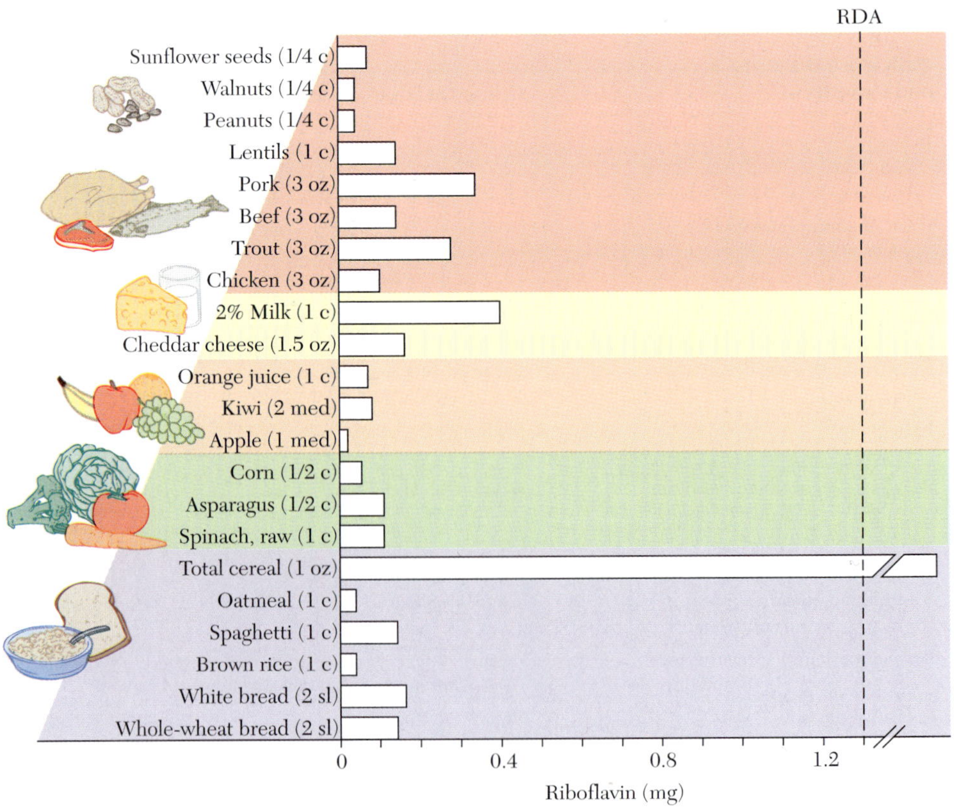

FIGURE 9.9 Riboflavin content of selections from each food group of the Food Guide Pyramid. The dashed line represents the RDA for adult men. Milk is an excellent source of riboflavin, as are fortified cereals.

and release hydrogens and electrons and function as electron carriers in the electron transport chain (see Figure 9.8). Therefore, adequate riboflavin is crucial in producing energy from carbohydrate, fat, and protein. Riboflavin is also involved directly or indirectly in converting a number of other vitamins, including folate, niacin, vitamin B_6, and vitamin K, into their active forms.

Recommended Intakes

The RDA for riboflavin for adult men age 19 and older is 1.3 mg per day and for adult women 19 and older, 1.1 mg per day. This recommendation is based on the amount of riboflavin needed to maintain normal activity of a riboflavin-dependent enzyme in red blood cells and normal riboflavin excretion in the urine.[2] Two cups of milk provide about half the amount of riboflavin recommended for a typical adult. The recommended intake can be met without milk if the daily diet includes two to three servings of meat and four to five servings of enriched grain products and high-riboflavin vegetables, such as spinach.

Additional riboflavin is recommended during pregnancy to support growth and increased energy utilization, and during lactation to allow for the riboflavin secreted in milk. There is not enough information to establish an RDA for infants, so an AI has been set based on the amount of riboflavin consumed by breast-fed infants.

Riboflavin and Health

For the average healthy American, there is little risk of either riboflavin deficiency or toxicity. Worldwide, minor signs of deficiency are seen, usually in combination with other water-soluble vitamin deficiencies.[3]

Riboflavin Deficiency When riboflavin is deficient, injuries heal poorly because new cells cannot grow to replace the damaged ones. Tissues that grow most rapidly, such as the skin and the linings of the eyes, mouth, and tongue, are the first to be affected by a deficiency. Symptoms of riboflavin deficiency, called **ariboflavinosis**, include inflammation of the eyes, lips, mouth, and tongue; scaly, greasy skin eruptions; cracking of the tissue at the corners of the mouth; and confusion. Deficiency symptoms may develop after approximately two months of a riboflavin-poor diet (see Table 9.2).

Ariboflavinosis The condition resulting from a deficiency of riboflavin.

A deficiency of riboflavin is rarely seen alone. It usually occurs in conjunction with deficiencies of other B vitamins. One reason is that the food sources of B vitamins are similar, so a poor diet will likely lead to multiple vitamin deficiencies. Because riboflavin is needed to convert other vitamins into their active forms, some of the symptoms seen with riboflavin deficiency are actually due to deficiencies of these other nutrients.

Riboflavin Toxicity No adverse effects have been reported from overconsumption of riboflavin from foods or supplements, and there are not sufficient data to establish a UL for this vitamin. Large doses of riboflavin are not well absorbed and it is readily excreted in the urine. A harmless side effect of high riboflavin intakes, such as may be obtained from over-the-counter supplements, is bright yellow urine.

Riboflavin Supplements As with thiamin, the role of riboflavin in energy production has led to claims that supplements containing riboflavin will provide an energy boost. Although riboflavin is needed for energy production, it does not provide energy. Because a deficiency causes skin and eye symptoms, riboflavin has also been suggested as a cure for eye diseases and skin disorders. However, in the absence of a deficiency, supplementation does not affect the eyes or skin.

Niacin

Pellagra The disease resulting from a deficiency of niacin.

A deficiency of niacin results in a disease called **pellagra**, which causes progressive physical and mental deterioration. It was first observed in Europe in the 18th century, and in the early 20th century it became endemic in the southeastern United States (see *Research Discoveries*: "Pellagra: Infectious Disease or Dietary Deficiency?"). The appearance of pellagra can be traced to the cultivation of corn as a staple grain in the diet.[4] It primarily affects the poor who eat the cheapest and least varied diet.

Sources of Niacin

Meat and fish are good sources of niacin (Figure 9.10). Other sources include legumes, mushrooms, wheat bran, asparagus, and peanuts. Niacin added to enriched flours and baked goods provides much of the usable niacin in the North American diet. Niacin can also be synthesized in the body from the essential amino acid tryptophan (Figure 9.11). In a diet that contains high-protein foods such as milk and eggs, which are poor sources of niacin but good sources of tryptophan, much of the need for niacin can be met by tryptophan. Tryptophan, however, is only used to make niacin if enough is available to first meet the needs of protein synthesis. When the diet is low in tryptophan, it is not used to synthesize niacin. Food composition tables and databases list only preformed niacin in a food, not the amount of niacin that can be made from tryptophan contained within the food.

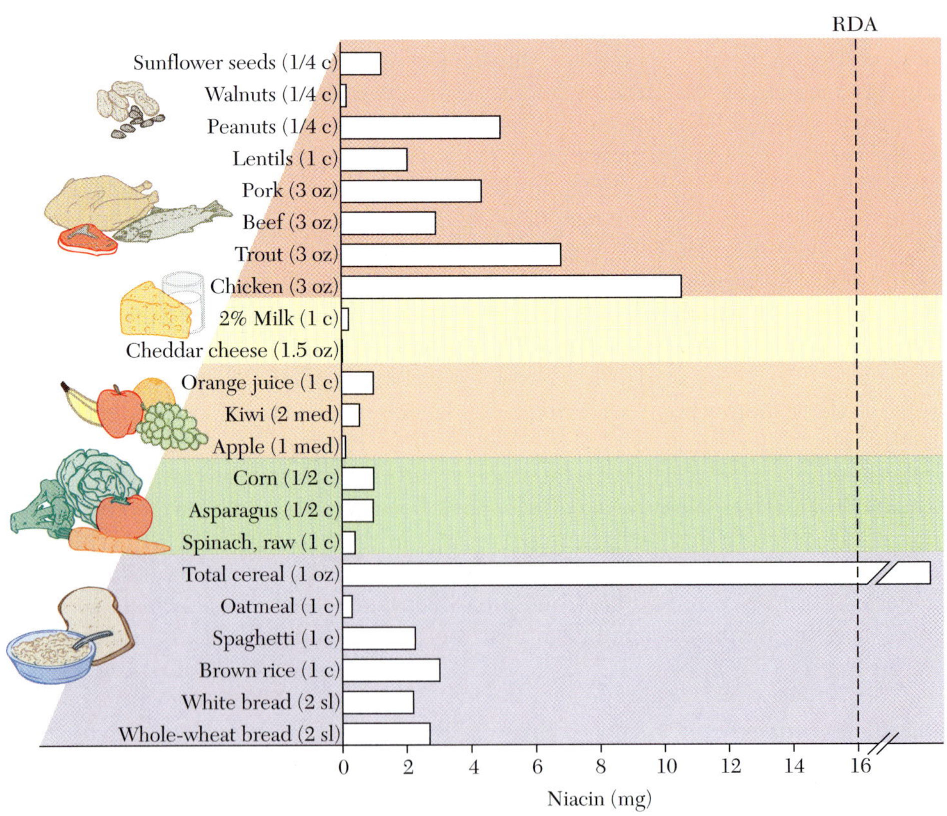

FIGURE 9.10 Niacin content of selections from each food group of the Food Guide Pyramid. The dashed line represents the RDA for adult men. Meats, legumes, and whole and fortified grains are good sources of niacin.

RESEARCH DISCOVERIES

Pellagra: Infectious Disease or Dietary Deficiency?

In the early 1900s, psychiatric hospitals in the southeastern United States were filled with patients with dementia due to a disease called pellagra. Although we now know pellagra is due to niacin deficiency, at the time it was thought to be caused by an infectious agent or toxin. As many as 100,000 people were affected by pellagra and upward of 10,000 deaths resulted per year. In response to this epidemic, the government set up the Thompson-McFadden Pellagra Commission and the U.S. Public Health Service sent Dr. Joseph Goldberger to investigate.

Between 1912 and 1916 investigators with the Pellagra Commission conducted epidemiological and bacteriological studies. Monkeys and baboons were injected with blood, urine, and other extracts from patients with pellagra; they were fed feces and skin scrapings. None of the animals developed the disease. Although these results supported the view that pellagra was not an infection, many questioned whether animal studies could be applied to humans. Perhaps monkeys and baboons were not susceptible to pellagra? The commission still believed that pellagra could be transmitted in some way from a pellagrous to a nonpellagrous person.[a]

Goldberger spent two years studying the communities and institutions where pellagra was common (see figure). He noticed that pellagra was prevalent among people in institutions but that the attendants and nurses never contracted the disease—a fact that did not support an infectious nature. Looking for factors that distinguished the patients from the staff, he noted that the patients were fed the typical diet of the Southern poor; it consisted primarily of corn meal, molasses, and fatback or salt pork. The staff ate a more varied diet. So, Goldberger began experimenting with diet. In an orphanage and a state hospital, he was able to cure pellagra and prevent recurrences by adding milk, eggs, and more meat to the diet. The next step in providing evidence to support his hypothesis was to produce pellagra in healthy people by feeding them a diet similar to the institutional diet. In 1915, at a work farm affiliated with the Mississippi State Penitentiary, twelve convicts volunteered to participate in the experiment in exchange for pardons. They were fed a diet consisting of corn meal, grits, cornstarch, white wheat flour, white rice, cane syrup, sugar, sweet potatoes, small amounts of turnip greens, cabbage, and collards, and a liberal amount of pork fat. After about six months, six men had developed pellagra. Goldberger concluded that the cause was a deficiency of an amino acid, a mineral, a fat-soluble vitamin, or some as yet unknown vitamin factor.

To provide the final proof that pellagra was not due to an infectious agent, Goldberger and 15 of his colleagues voluntarily injected themselves with blood, swabbed their throats with nasal secretions, and swallowed urine, feces, and skin cells from patients that were severely ill with pellagra (later in the experiment they put the feces and other materials in capsules). After six months, none had become ill. Goldberger had proven that pellagra was not an infectious disease but he continued to search for the dietary cause.

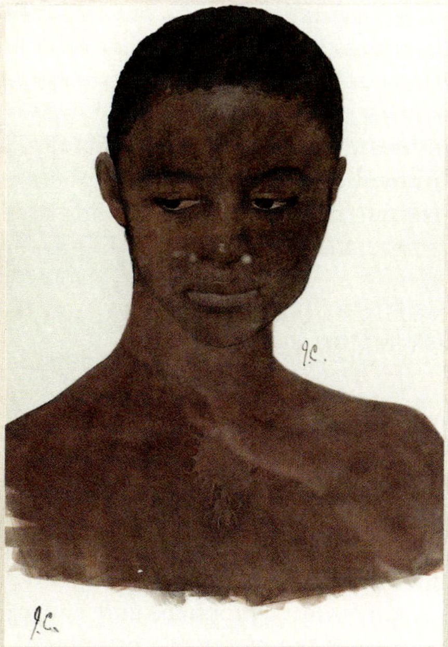

During the summer of 1919, a young artist named John Carroll was assigned to work with Joseph Goldberger's pellagra study. He produced 41 drawings of pellagra patients. The drawing shown here depicts a female pellagra patient in the Georgia State Sanitarium in 1919.

In 1922, a diet comparable to that used to produce pellagra in Goldberger's experiment caused a similar disease in dogs, called black tongue. Subsequent food experiments found that yeast and liver contained a pellagra-preventative factor. These foods could be used to prevent pellagra and cure mild cases. However, despite Goldberger's efforts, the epidemic raged on. Even though it had been demonstrated that yeast and liver could cure pellagra, nothing had been done to change the Southern diet that produced the disease. And, in serious cases of the disease, providing food sources of niacin was often ineffective because inflammation of the gastrointestinal tract, lack of appetite, and vomiting made it difficult for patients to ingest and absorb enough of the pellagra-preventative factor to cure the deficiency. Joseph Goldberger died in January of 1929, the year the epidemic reached its peak.

In 1937, another research team identified the pellagra-preventative factor as nicotinic acid. With this form of the vitamin isolated, it could be given intravenously, bypassing the digestive tract, and saving the lives of pellagra victims. Despite this advance in treatment, pellagra remained a problem among the Southern poor who consumed a diet of primarily corn meal, molasses, and fatback—all poor sources of niacin. Poor dietary habits, poverty, and chronic malnutrition made it a difficult problem to address.[b] Finally, the economic boom created by World War II, combined with a federally sponsored enrichment program, added enough niacin to the diet to end the pellagra epidemic in the United States.

References

[a] Roe, D. A., *A Plague of Corn: The Social History of Pellagra*. Ithaca, N.Y.: Cornell University Press, 1973.

[b] Syndenstricker, V. P. The history of pellagra, its recognition as a disorder of nutrition and its conquest. Am. J. Clin. Nutr. 6:409–441, 1958.

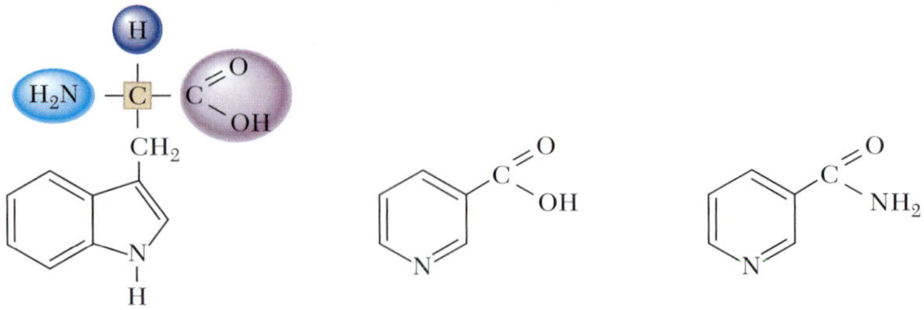

(a) Tryptophan (b) Nicotinic acid (c) Nicotinamide

FIGURE 9.11 (a) The structure of the amino acid tryptophan. Tryptophan can be used to synthesize a metabolite of nicotinic acid that can be converted to nicotinamide and active coenzyme forms of niacin. (b) The nicotinic acid form of niacin. (c) The nicotinamide form of niacin.

The association of niacin deficiency with a limited diet that is based on corn and low in animal products has been attributed to the low-tryptophan content of corn and the fact that the niacin found naturally in corn (and to a lesser extent in other cereal grains) is bound to other molecules and therefore not well absorbed. The treatment of corn with lime water (water and calcium hydroxide), as is done in Mexico and Central America when making tortillas, enhances the availability of niacin (Figure 9.12). As a result, populations that consume corn treated with lime water rarely suffer from pellagra. Today, pellagra remains common in India and parts of China and Africa. Efforts to eradicate this deficiency include the development of new varieties of corn that provide more available niacin and greater amounts of tryptophan than traditional varieties.

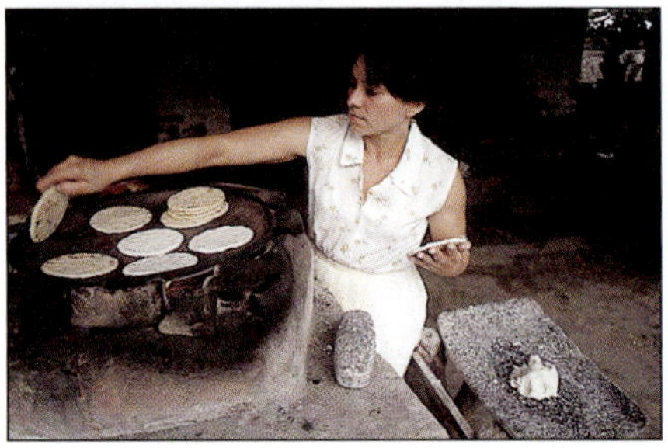

FIGURE 9.12 The treatment of corn with lime water during the preparation of tortillas makes niacin available and is one reason that pellagra has not been prevalent in Mexico and other Latin American countries. *(© Wesley Boyce/Photo Researchers, Inc.)*

Niacin in the Body

Niacin is important in the production of energy from the energy-containing nutrients as well as in reactions that synthesize other molecules. There are two forms of niacin: nicotinic acid and nicotinamide (see Figure 9.11). Either form can be used by the body to make the two active coenzymes **nicotinamide adenine dinucleotide (NAD)** and **nicotinamide adenine dinucleotide phosphate (NADP)**. NAD functions in glycolysis and the citric acid cycle, accepting released electrons and passing them on to the electron transport chain where ATP is formed (see Figure 9.8). NADP acts as an electron carrier in reactions that synthesize fatty acids and cholesterol. The need for niacin is so widespread in metabolism that a deficiency causes major changes throughout the body.

Nicotinamide adenine dinucleotide (NAD) and **nicotinamide adenine dinucleotide phosphate (NADP)** The active coenzyme forms of niacin that are able to pick up and donate hydrogens and electrons. They are important in the transfer of electrons to oxygen in cellular respiration and in many synthetic reactions.

Recommended Intakes

An RDA for niacin has been established based on urinary excretion of niacin metabolites. The RDA for niacin is expressed as **niacin equivalents (NEs)**. One NE is equal to 1 mg of niacin or 60 mg of tryptophan. This allows for the fact that some of the requirement for niacin can be met by the synthesis of niacin from tryptophan, and approximately 60 mg of tryptophan is needed to make 1 mg of niacin. To estimate the niacin contributed by high-protein foods, protein is considered to be about 1% tryptophan. The RDA for adult men and women of all ages is 16 and 14 mg NE per day, respectively.[2] A meal including a medium chicken breast and a cup of steamed asparagus provides this amount (see Table 9.2).

Niacin equivalents (NEs) The measure used to express the amount of niacin present in food, including that which can be made from its precursor, tryptophan. One NE is equal to 1 mg of niacin or 60 mg of tryptophan.

Niacin needs are increased during pregnancy to account for the increase in energy expenditure, and during lactation to account for both the increase in energy expenditure and the niacin secreted in milk. There is not enough information to establish an RDA for infants, so an AI has been set based on the amount of niacin found in human milk.

Niacin and Health

Niacin deficiency is no longer of public health concern in the United States, and excessive intakes of niacin can be toxic. Despite this, niacin is a commonly used vitamin supplement.

Niacin Deficiency The early symptoms of pellagra include fatigue, decreased appetite, and indigestion, followed by the three Ds: dermatitis, diarrhea, and dementia. If untreated, a fourth "D" results—death. The dermatitis resembles sunburn and strikes parts of the body exposed to sunlight, heat, or injury. Gastrointestinal symptoms include a bright-red tongue and may include vomiting, constipation, or diarrhea. Mental symptoms begin with irritability, headaches, loss of memory, insomnia, and emotional instability, and progress to psychosis, acute delirium, and eventually coma and death.

Niacin Toxicity There is no evidence of any adverse effects from consumption of niacin naturally occurring in foods, but supplements can be toxic. The adverse effects of high intakes of niacin include flushing of the skin, a tingling sensation in the hands and feet, a red skin rash, nausea, vomiting, diarrhea, high blood sugar levels, abnormalities in liver function, and blurred vision.[5] Because flushing is the first toxicity symptom to appear as the dose is increased, the UL for adults was set at 35 mg, the highest level that is unlikely to cause flushing in the majority of healthy people. This value applies to the forms of niacin contained in supplements and fortified foods, but does not include niacin naturally occurring in foods.

Niacin Supplements Unlike thiamin and riboflavin, which are touted for enhancing energy and mental capacity, high doses of niacin have been promoted to treat elevated blood cholesterol and to prevent or delay type 1 diabetes.

Niacin and Heart Disease Doses of 50 mg per day or greater of the nicotinic acid form of niacin have been found to decrease blood levels of LDL cholesterol and triglycerides and increase HDL cholesterol.[6] They are also associated with a reduction in recurrent heart attacks and deaths in individuals with cardiovascular disease.[7] Unfortunately, many people cannot take niacin to treat high blood cholesterol because they experience toxicity symptoms such as gastrointestinal distress, skin flushing, and liver abnormalities. Time-release niacin supplements have been developed to reduce these side effects.[8] Supplements containing high doses of niacin should be used only with medical supervision (see Chapter 5, *Making Decisions:* "Dietary Supplements to Reduce Blood Cholesterol").

Web Menu

For more information on niacin and cholesterol, go to the Heart Information Network at www.heartinfo.org or the National Heart, Lung, and Blood Institute's Cholesterol Counts site at www.nhlbi.nih.gov/chd/.

Niacin and Diabetes Large doses (about 1–2 g/day) of the nicotinamide form of niacin are currently under investigation for preventing or delaying the onset of type 1 diabetes.[9] Type 1 diabetes is an autoimmune disease in which the body's immune system destroys the insulin-producing cells in the pancreas. Some but not all studies completed thus far have indicated that nicotinamide is beneficial in preserving pancreatic cell function, thus delaying the onset of type 1 diabetes.[10,11,12] Nicotinamide may also have beneficial effects in the treatment of type 2 diabetes.[13]

BIOTIN

Biotin was discovered in the 1920s and 1930s when rats fed protein derived from raw egg white developed a syndrome of hair loss, dermatitis, and neuromuscular dysfunction. A protein in raw egg white, called avidin, which tightly binds biotin and prevents its absorption, was the cause of the biotin deficiency in these rats.

Sources of Biotin

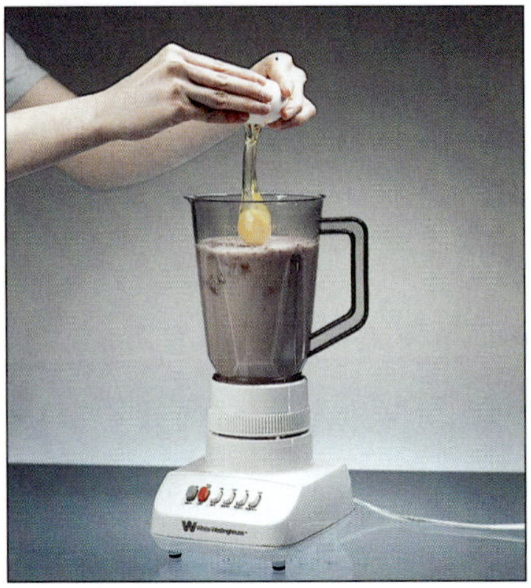

FIGURE 9.13 Raw eggs are a common ingredient in high-protein shakes. Raw egg whites contain a protein that binds biotin, making it unavailable to the body. Raw eggs may also contain bacteria that cause foodborne illness. *(Charles D. Winters)*

Good sources of biotin include liver, egg yolks, yogurt, and nuts. Fruit and meat are poor sources (see Table 9.2). Foods containing raw egg whites should be avoided not only because avidin binds biotin and prevents its absorption, but because raw eggs also may be contaminated with bacteria that can cause foodborne illness (Figure 9.13). Thoroughly cooking eggs destroys bacteria and denatures avidin so that it cannot bind biotin. Biotin is also sensitive to exposure to heat.

Biotin in the Body

Biotin is a coenzyme for a group of enzymes that add the acid group COOH to molecules. It functions in energy production because it is needed to make oxaloacetate, the 4-carbon molecule necessary in the citric acid cycle and in glucose synthesis. Biotin is also important in the metabolism of fatty acids and amino acids (see Figure 9.8).

Recommended Intakes

It is difficult to estimate a biotin requirement because some biotin is produced by bacteria in the gastrointestinal tract and absorbed into the body. No RDA could be determined for biotin, but an AI of 30 μg per day has been established for adult men and women based on the amount of biotin found in a typical North American diet.

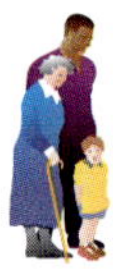

No additional biotin is recommended for pregnancy, but the AI is increased during lactation to account for the amount secreted in milk. The AI for infants is based on the amount of biotin consumed by breast-fed infants.

Biotin and Health

Although biotin deficiency is uncommon, it has been observed in people with malabsorption or protein-energy malnutrition, in those receiving tube feedings or total parenteral nutrition without biotin, in those taking anticonvulsant drugs for long periods, and in those frequently consuming raw egg whites.[14,15] When biotin intake is deficient, symptoms including nausea, thinning hair, loss of hair color, a red skin rash, depression, lethargy, hallucinations, and tingling of the extremities gradually appear.

No toxicity has been reported in patients given 200 mg per day of biotin to treat various disease states, and sufficient data are not available to establish a UL.[2]

Pantothenic Acid

Pantothenic acid, which gets its name from the Greek word *pantos* (meaning "from everywhere"), is widely distributed in foods.

Sources of Pantothenic Acid

Pantothenic acid is particularly abundant in meat, eggs, whole grains, and legumes. It is found in lesser amounts in milk, vegetables, and fruits (Figure 9.14). Pantothenic acid is susceptible to damage by exposure to heat and low- or high-acid conditions.

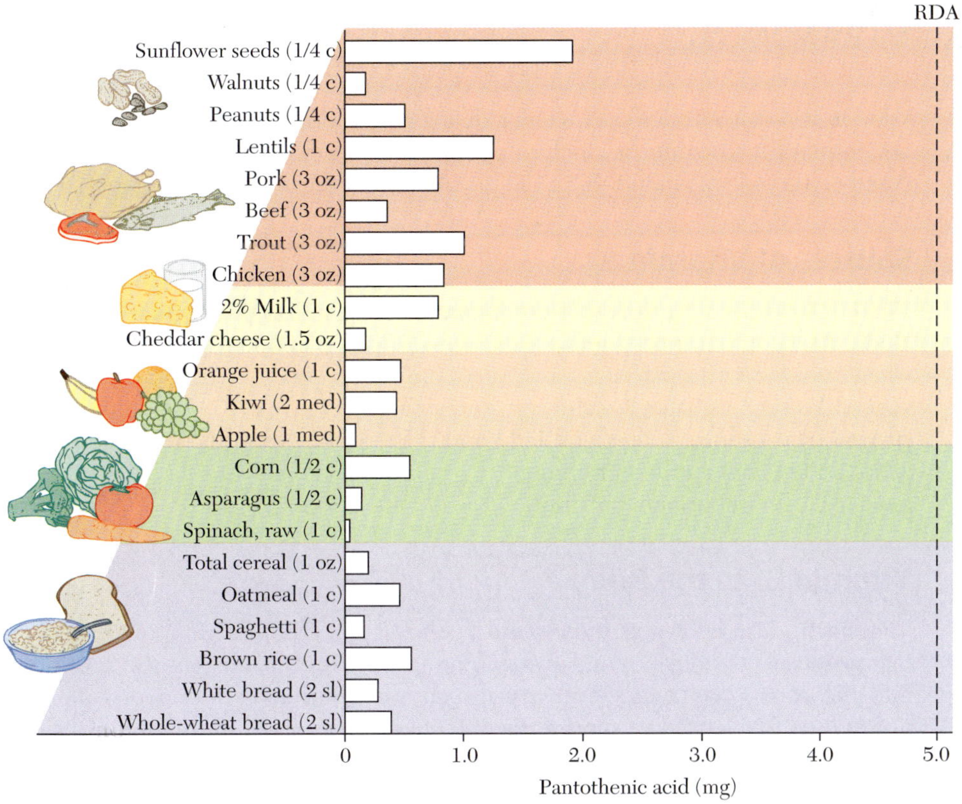

FIGURE 9.14 Pantothenic acid content of selections from each food group of the Food Guide Pyramid. The dashed line represents the RDA for adult men and women. Good sources can be found in all groups of the Pyramid.

Pantothenic Acid in the Body

Pantothenic acid is a component of coenzyme A (CoA), which is part of acetyl-CoA, a molecule formed during the breakdown of carbohydrates, fatty acids, and amino acids. Pantothenic acid is also needed to produce acyl carrier protein needed for the synthesis of cholesterol and fatty acids (see Figure 9.8).

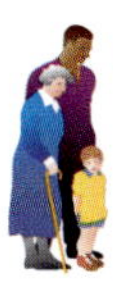

Recommended Intakes

There is no RDA for pantothenic acid, but an AI of 5 mg per day has been recommended for adult men and women.[2] This value is based on the intake of pantothenic acid sufficient to replace urinary losses. The AI is increased to 6 and 7 mg per day to meet the needs of pregnancy and lactation, respectively.

Pantothenic Acid and Health

The wide distribution of pantothenic acid in foods makes deficiency rare in humans. A deficiency of this vitamin alone has not been reported, but it may occur as part of a multiple B-vitamin deficiency resulting from malnutrition or chronic alcoholism.

Pantothenic acid is relatively nontoxic. No toxic symptoms were reported in a study that fed young men 10 g of pantothenic acid per day for 6 weeks. Another study found that doses of 10 to 20 g per day may result in diarrhea and water retention.[16] Data are not sufficient to establish a UL for pantothenic acid (see Table 9.2).

VITAMIN B_6

Vitamin B_6 was identified only when a deficiency syndrome was discovered that did not respond to thiamin or riboflavin supplementation. Recently, interest has focused on the role of vitamin B_6 in the metabolism of the amino acid homocysteine.

Sources of Vitamin B_6

Vitamin B_6 is found in foods of both animal and plant origin. Animal sources include chicken, fish, pork, and organ meats. Good plant sources include whole-wheat products, brown rice, soybeans, sunflower seeds, and some fruits and vegetables such as bananas, broccoli, and spinach (Figure 9.15). Vitamin B_6 is destroyed by exposure to heat and light and is therefore easily lost in processing. It is not added back in the enrichment of grain products, but fortified breakfast cereals make an important contribution to vitamin B_6 intake.[17]

Vitamin B_6 in the Body

Pyridoxine The chemical term for vitamin B_6.

Pyridoxyl phosphate The major coenzyme form of vitamin B_6 that functions in more than 100 enzymatic reactions, most of which involve amino acid metabolism.

Vitamin B_6, also known as **pyridoxine**, comprises a group of compounds including pyridoxal, pyridoxine, and pyridoxamine. All three forms can be converted into the active coenzyme form, **pyridoxal phosphate**. Pyridoxal phosphate is needed for the activity of more than 100 enzymes involved in the metabolism of carbohydrate, fat, and protein. It is particularly important for protein and amino acid metabolism (Figure 9.16). Without pyridoxal phosphate, the nonessential amino acids cannot be synthesized and the semiessential amino acid cysteine can-

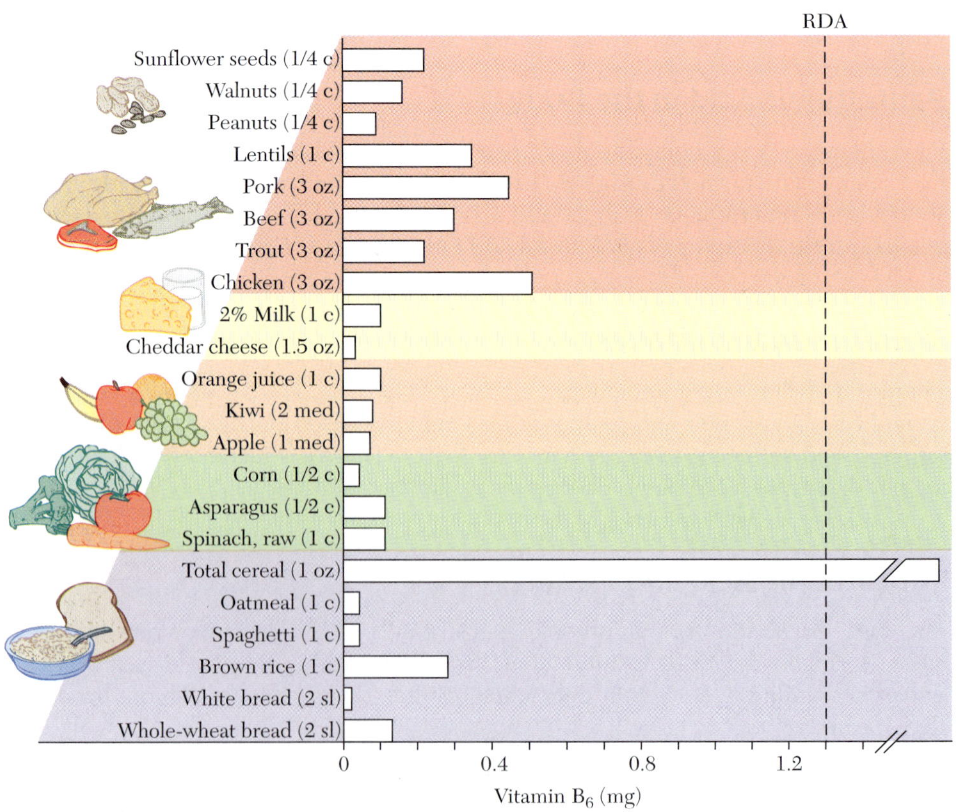

FIGURE 9.15 Vitamin B_6 content of selections from each food group of the Food Guide Pyramid. The dashed line represents the RDA for adult men and women age 50 and younger. The best sources are meats, whole or fortified grains, and legumes.

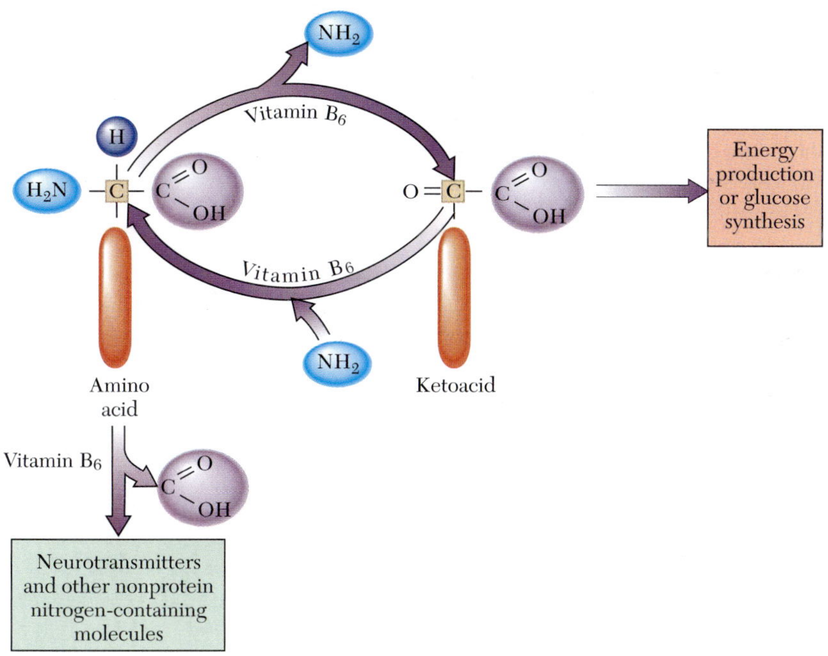

FIGURE 9.16 Vitamin B_6 is needed as a coenzyme for many reactions involved in amino acid metabolism. These include transamination reactions, which transfer amino groups from amino acids to ketoacids to produce new amino acids; deamination reactions, which remove the amino group from amino acids so they can be used to produce energy or to synthesize glucose; and decarboxylation reactions, which remove the acid group (COOH) from amino acids so the remaining molecule can be used to synthesize neurotransmitters and other nonprotein molecules that contain nitrogen.

not be synthesized from methionine. Pyridoxal phosphate is needed to synthesize hemoglobin, the oxygen-carrying protein in red blood cells. Pyridoxal phosphate is important for the immune system because it is needed to form white blood cells. It is also needed for the conversion of tryptophan to niacin, the metabolism of glycogen, the synthesis of certain neurotransmitters, and the synthesis of the lipids that are part of the myelin coating on nerves (see Table 9.2).

Recommended Intakes

The RDA for vitamin B_6 is 1.3 mg per day for both adult men and women 19 to 50 years of age.[2] This is the amount needed to maintain adequate blood concentrations of the active coenzyme form, pyridoxal phosphate. In adults 51 years and older, the RDA is increased to 1.7 mg per day in men and 1.5 mg per day in women to maintain normal blood pyridoxal phosphate. A 3-ounce (85-g) serving of chicken, fish, or pork, or half a baked potato, provides about a quarter of the RDA for an average adult; a banana provides about one third.

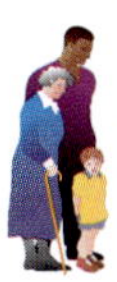

The RDA for vitamin B_6 is increased during pregnancy to allow for metabolic needs and growth of the mother and fetus. Because the vitamin B_6 concentration in breast milk is dependent on the mother's intake, the RDA is increased during lactation to assure adequate levels are supplied to the infant.[18] There is no RDA for infants, but an AI has been established based on the vitamin B_6 content of human milk.

Vitamin B_6 and Health

A vitamin B_6 deficiency syndrome was defined in 1954 when an infant formula was overheated in manufacture, destroying the vitamin B_6. The infants who consumed only this formula developed abdominal distress, convulsions, and other neurological symptoms.[19] No adverse effects have been associated with high intakes of vitamin B_6 from foods, but large doses found in supplements can cause serious toxicity symptoms.

Vitamin B_6 Deficiency Vitamin B_6 deficiency causes neurological symptoms including depression, headaches, confusion, numbness and tingling in the extremities, and seizures. These may be related to the role of vitamin B_6 in neurotransmitter synthesis and myelin formation. Anemia also occurs in vitamin B_6 deficiency due to impaired hemoglobin synthesis; red blood cells are small (microcytic) and pale (hypochromic) due to the lack of hemoglobin. Other deficiency symptoms such as poor growth, skin lesions, and decreased antibody formation may occur because vitamin B_6 is important in protein and energy metabolism. Because vitamin B_6 is needed for amino acid metabolism, the onset of a deficiency can be hastened by a diet that is low in vitamin B_6 but high in protein.

Vitamin B_6 status in the body can be affected by a number of drugs, including alcohol and oral contraceptives. Alcohol decreases the formation of the active coenzyme pyridoxal phosphate and makes it more susceptible to breakdown. Oral contraceptive use has been associated with small decreases in blood levels of pyridoxal phosphate. But, vitamin B_6 supplements are not routinely recommended for women taking oral contraceptives.[2]

Vitamin B_6 and Cardiovascular Disease It has been hypothesized that vitamin B_6 affects the risk of heart disease through its role in the breakdown of homocysteine, an intermediate in methionine metabolism (Figure 9.17). Individuals with a rare genetic disorder that causes chronically high blood levels of homocysteine develop atherosclerosis at an early age. Large doses of vitamin B_6 (100–1000 mg/day) have been shown to reduce elevated homocysteine levels and the risk of atherosclerosis in these patients.[20]

In the normal population, a mild elevation in blood homocysteine has been shown to be a risk factor for cardiovascular disease.[21,22] It has been proposed that a deficiency of vitamin B_6, vitamin B_{12}, or folate, the latter two of which are also involved in homocysteine metabolism, may cause homocysteine accumulation and eventually lead to atherosclerosis. A study that examined the effect of folate and vitamin B_6 intake in women found that those with the highest levels of folate and vitamin B_6 in their diets (from food and supplements) had about half the risk of coronary heart disease as women with the lowest levels.[23] Supplements of all three of these vitamins have been shown to reduce homocysteine levels in individuals with mild homocysteine elevation.[24] At this time, however, DRI scientists have concluded that it is premature to recommend that increased intakes of vitamin B_6, vitamin B_{12}, or folate may reduce the risk of cardiovascular disease.[2]

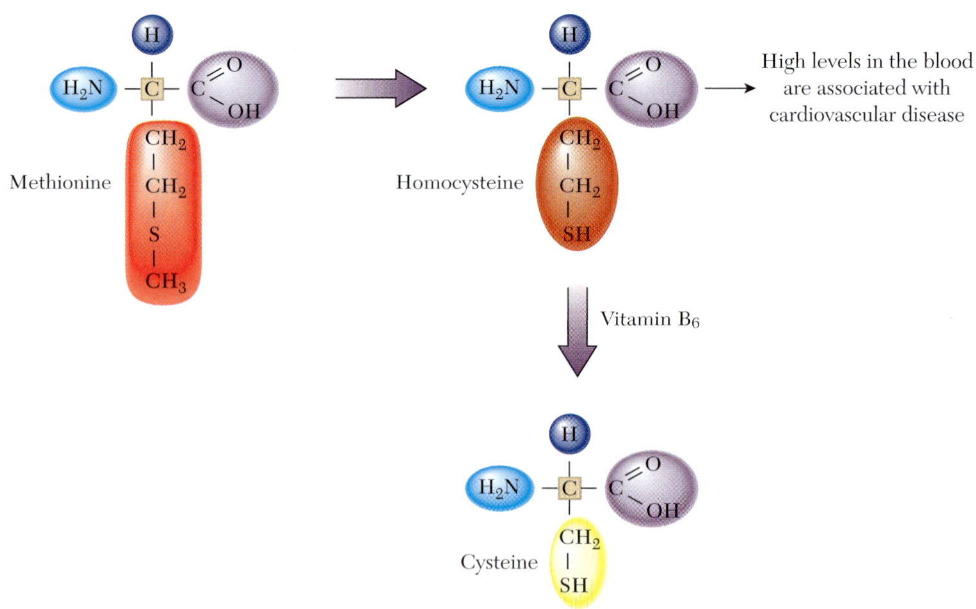

FIGURE 9.17 Vitamin B_6 is needed in methionine metabolism to convert the amino acid homocysteine to cysteine. If vitamin B_6 is deficient, homocysteine can accumulate, increasing the risk of cardiovascular disease.

Vitamin B_6 Toxicity In the 1980s, there were reports of severe nerve impairment in individuals taking 2 to 6 g of vitamin B_6 per day.[25] Some subjects were unable to walk. These symptoms improved when the pyridoxine supplements were stopped. The UL is based on a level of intake that does not cause nerve damage in the majority of healthy people. For adults, the UL is set at 100 mg per day from food and supplements.[2] Because high-dose supplements of vitamin B_6 containing 100 mg per dose (5000% of the Daily Value) are available over the counter, it is easy to obtain a dose that exceeds the UL.

Vitamin B_6 Supplements Supplements of vitamin B_6 are claimed to help a wide variety of ailments ranging from carpal tunnel syndrome to premenstrual syndrome (PMS) and poor immune function. Some of these marketing claims are founded in science, but the role of vitamin B_6 may be exaggerated to sell products. Whatever the reason for considering vitamin B_6 supplements, one should use them with care to reduce the risk of toxicity.

Carpal Tunnel Syndrome Vitamin B_6 has been suggested to be useful in treating a condition called carpal tunnel syndrome, in which pressure on the nerves in the hand causes pain and weakness. Studies have not shown a relationship between carpal tunnel syndrome and vitamin B_6 status.[26] In some patients, supplements have been found to reduce pain, but there is little evidence to support the use of vitamin B_6 supplements as a treatment for carpal tunnel syndrome. Treatment with high doses of B_6 can be toxic.

Premenstrual Syndrome Premenstrual syndrome (PMS) causes mood swings, food cravings, bloating, tension, depression, headaches, acne, breast tenderness, anxiety, temper outbursts, and over 100 other symptoms. Supplements of vitamin B_6 are frequently taken in attempts to alleviate these symptoms.[28] The proposed connection is the fact that vitamin B_6 is needed for the synthesis of the neurotransmitters serotonin and dopamine. Insufficient vitamin B_6 has been suggested to reduce levels of these neurotransmitters, causing the anxiety, irritability, and depression associated with PMS. Numerous studies have evaluated the effect of supplements of 50 to 500 mg of vitamin B_6 per day on PMS symptoms. Although many of these studies involved only small sample sizes and others were poorly controlled, a review of the published results suggests that low doses may be effective at reducing symptoms of PMS.[29]

Web Menu: For more information on vitamin B_6 and premenstrual syndrome, go to the Onhealth with Web MD site at onhealth.webmd.com/ and search for PMS.

Immune Function Immune function can be impaired by a deficiency of any nutrient that hinders cell growth and division. Therefore, one of the most common claims for vitamin supplements in general is that they improve immune function. Vitamin B_6 is no exception. Vitamin B_6 supplements have been found to improve immune function in older adults.[30] However, because the elderly frequently have low intakes of vitamin B_6, it is unclear whether the beneficial effects of supplements are due to an improvement in vitamin B_6 status or to immune system stimulation.

Folate or Folic Acid

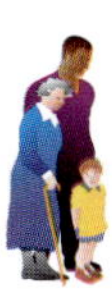

It has been known for over a hundred years that anemia often occurs during pregnancy. In 1937, anemia in a pregnant woman was successfully treated with a yeast preparation named Wills Factor, after Dr. Lucy Wills, who treated this patient. The Wills Factor was later isolated from spinach and named folate, after the Latin word for foliage. Research today focuses on the role of this vitamin in reducing the incidence of birth defects that affect the brain and spinal cord.

Forms of Folate

Folate A general term for the many forms of this B vitamin. The majority of folate found naturally in foods is in the polyglutamate form, which contains a string of glutamate molecules called a polyglutamate tail.

Folic acid The monoglutamate form of folate, which is present in the diet in fortified foods and dietary supplements. Its structure contains only one glutamate molecule.

Folate is a general term for the many chemical forms of this vitamin. Most folate found naturally in foods (food folate) is bound to a string of glutamate molecules. Glutamate is an amino acid, and folate bound to many glutamates is referred to as the polyglutamate form of folate. Before this form can be absorbed, all but one of the glutamate molecules must be removed by enzymes in the brush border of the small intestine, to yield the monoglutamate form. **Folic acid** is a stable monoglutamate form of folate that rarely occurs naturally in food but is used in vitamin supplements and fortified foods. Because folic acid does not have a polyglutamate tail, it is better absorbed. The bioavailability of food folate is only about half that of the synthetic folic acid found in supplements and fortified grains.

Sources of Folate

Web Menu: For more information on folic acid fortification, go to the FDA Center for Food Safety and Applied Nutrition at www.cfsan.fda.gov/ and search for folic acid fortification.

C 62 00 00 00 00 00 27 15

Excellent sources of food folate include liver, spinach, asparagus, oranges, and legumes. Good sources include vegetables such as corn, snap beans, mustard greens, and broccoli, as well as some nuts. Small amounts are found in meats, cheese, milk, fruits, and other vegetables. Cereal grains are also a good source of folate due to fortification (Figure 9.18). The mandatory fortification of enriched grain products with folic acid began in 1998. Labels on foods and supplements that are good sources of folate may include the health claim that consumption of folate has been linked to a decreased risk of neural tube defects. Folate is sensitive to exposure to heat, air, light, and acid conditions.

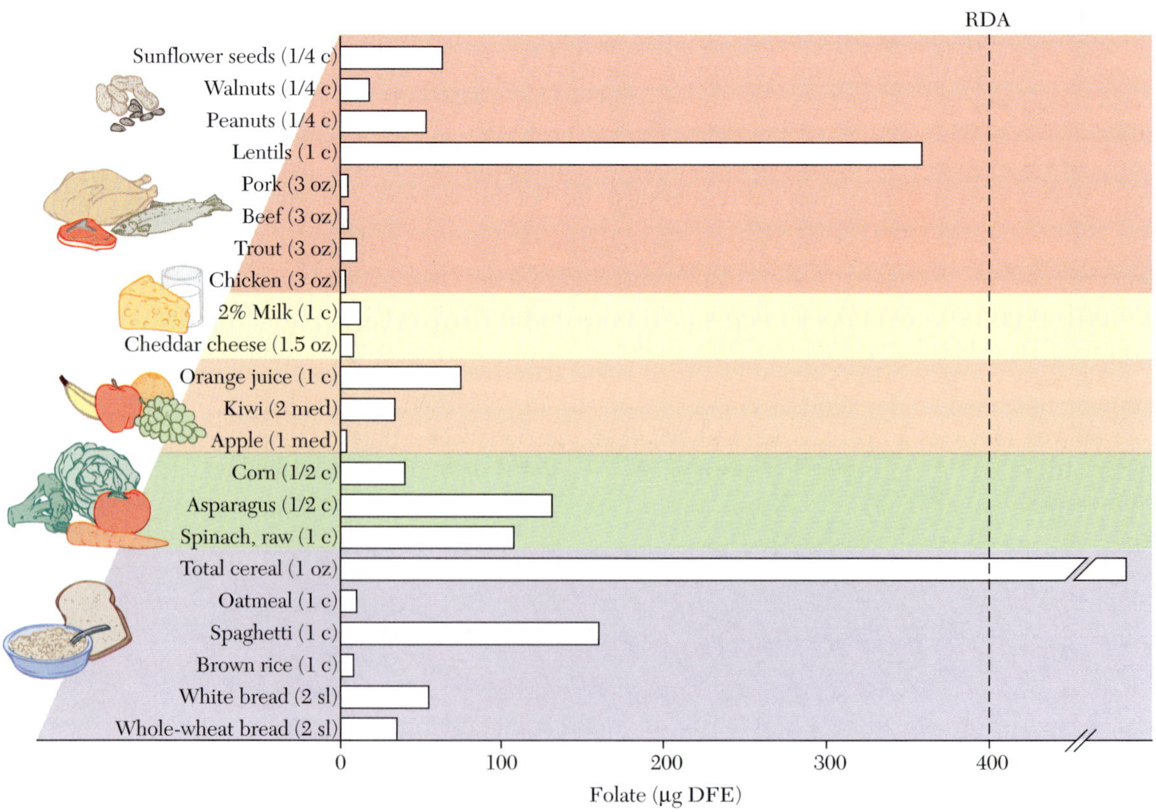

FIGURE 9.18 Folate content of selections from each food group of the Food Guide Pyramid. The dashed line represents the RDA for adult men and women. Legumes, fortified foods, and some fruits and vegetables are good sources.

Folate in the Body

There are a number of different active coenzyme forms of folate that are involved in reactions that transfer chemical groups containing a single carbon atom. Folate coenzymes are needed for the synthesis of DNA and the metabolism of some amino acids. Before a cell divides, its DNA must replicate. Therefore, the role of folate in DNA synthesis makes it particularly important in rapidly growing cells, such as those in the embryo, the bone marrow (where red blood cells are made), the intestinal mucosa, and the skin (see Table 9.2).

Recommended Intakes

The adult RDA for folate is set at 400 μg **dietary folate equivalents (DFEs)** per day for adult men and women. The unit DFE was introduced in order to correct for the bioavailability of the different forms of the vitamin. One DFE is equal to 1 μg of food folate, 0.6 μg of synthetic folic acid from fortified food or supplements consumed with food, or 0.5 μg of synthetic folic acid consumed on an empty stomach. In order to reduce the risk of neural tube defects, a special recommendation is made for women capable of becoming pregnant: a daily intake of 400 μg of synthetic folic acid from fortified foods and supplements is recommended in addition to the food folate consumed in a varied diet. Therefore, the total folate intake of this group should exceed the RDA.

Dietary folate equivalents (DFEs) The unit used to express the amount of folate present in food. One DFE is equivalent to 1 μg of folate naturally occurring in food, 0.6 μg of synthetic folic acid from fortified food or supplements consumed with food, or 0.5 μg of synthetic folic acid consumed on an empty stomach.

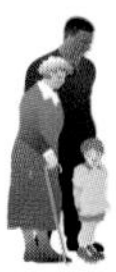

The RDA for folate during pregnancy is increased to 600 μg DFE per day due to the increase in cell division. Although this level can be met by a carefully selected diet, folate is typically supplemented during pregnancy. The RDA is also increased during lactation to account for folate secretion in milk. Needs are high for infants and children because of their rapid growth. Human and cow's milk provide enough folate to meet infant needs, but goat's milk does not. Infants and children given goat's milk may not receive adequate folate unless it is provided from other sources.

Folate and Health

A severe deficiency of folate results in anemia, and low intakes of folate have been associated with an increased risk of neural tube defects, heart disease, and certain types of cancer. An excess of folate can mask the symptoms of vitamin B_{12} deficiency.

Folate Deficiency A deficiency of folate leads to a drop in blood folate levels and a rise in blood homocysteine followed by changes that affect rapidly dividing cells. Deficiency symptoms include poor growth, problems in nerve development and function, diarrhea, inflammation of the tongue, and anemia. Anemia results when folate is deficient because cells in the bone marrow that develop into blood cells cannot duplicate their DNA, and so cannot divide. Instead, they just grow bigger. These large immature cells are known as **megaloblasts** and can be converted into large red blood cells called **macrocytes**. The result is that fewer mature red cells are produced, and the oxygen-carrying capacity of the blood is reduced. This condition is called **megaloblastic** or **macrocytic anemia** (Figure 9.19).

Megaloblasts Large, immature red blood cells that are formed when developing red blood cells are unable to divide normally.

Macrocytes Larger-than-normal mature red blood cells that have a shortened life span.

Megaloblastic or **macrocytic anemia** A condition characterized by abnormally large immature and mature red blood cells and a reduction in the total number of red blood cells.

Groups at risk of folate deficiency include pregnant women and premature infants because of their rapid rate of cell division and growth; the elderly because of their limited intake of foods high in folate; alcoholics because alcohol inhibits folate absorption; and tobacco smokers because smoke inactivates folate in the cells lining the lungs.[31,32]

FIGURE 9.19 Macrocytic anemia occurs when developing blood cells are unable to divide, producing large immature red blood cells (megaloblasts) and large mature red blood cells (macrocytes).

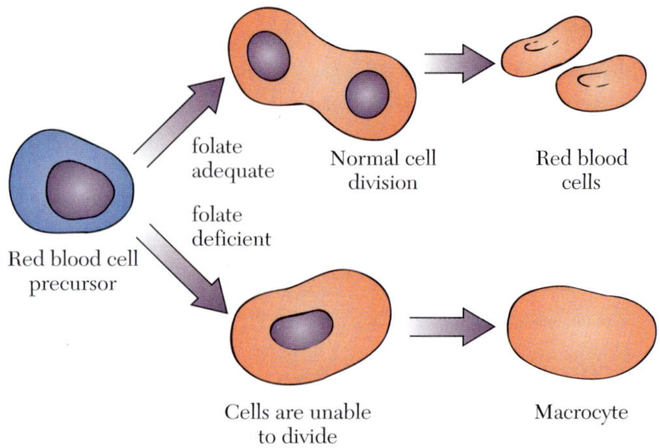

For more information on folic acid and preventing birth defects, go to the March of Dimes at www.modimes.org/ and click on folic acid, or go to the Spina Bifida Association of America at www.sbaa.org/.

Neural tube defects Abnormalities in the brain or spinal cord that result from errors that occur during prenatal development.

Folate and Neural Tube Defects In the United States, about 4000 pregnancies annually result in a baby with a neural tube defect. **Neural tube defects**, such as spina bifida and other birth defects that affect the brain and spinal cord (Figure 9.20), are not true folate deficiency symptoms because not every pregnant woman with inadequate folate levels will give birth to a child with a neural tube defect. Instead, neural tube defects are probably due to a combination of factors that include low folate levels and a genetic predisposition. The exact role of folate in neural tube development is not known, but it is necessary for a critical step called neural tube closure. Neural tube closure occurs only 28 days after conception; therefore, folate status should be adequate even before a pregnancy begins to assure an adequate supply during early development (see Chapter 15). Studies in which supplemental folic acid was given to women before and during early pregnancy showed that 360 to 800 μg per day of synthetic folic acid in addition to food folate was associated with a reduced incidence of neural tube defects.[2,33] Because it is not known whether a diet naturally rich in folate offers the same protection as supplements, and because folate must be adequate before most women are aware that they are pregnant, synthetic folic acid from supplements or fortified foods is recommended for all women of childbearing age.

Folate and Heart Disease The association between low folate stores and an increased risk of heart disease is related to the role of folate in the metabolism of the amino acid methionine. When folate is lacking, homocysteine, produced during methionine metabolism, accumulates because it cannot be converted back to methionine (Figure 9.21). The risk of cardiovascular disease increases with elevated blood homocysteine concentration, and homocysteine concentration in-

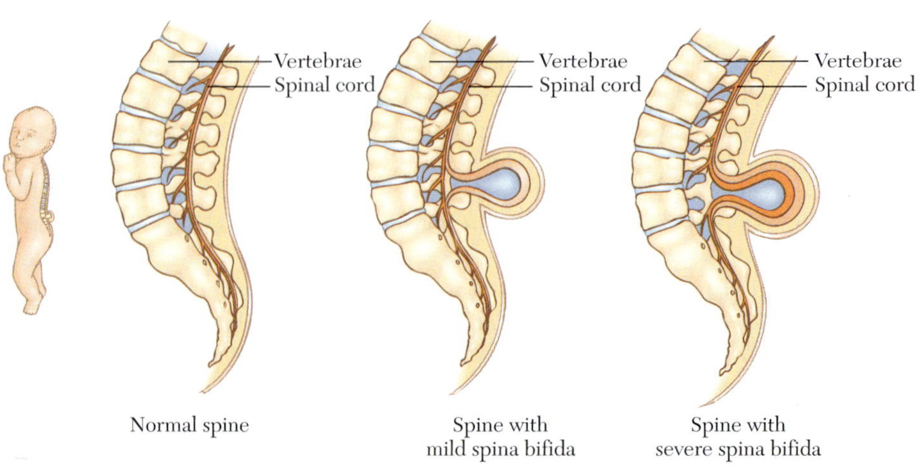

FIGURE 9.20 In an embryo, the neural tube develops into the brain and spinal cord. If folate is inadequate during neural tube closure, neural tube defects such as spina bifida, shown here, are more likely to occur.

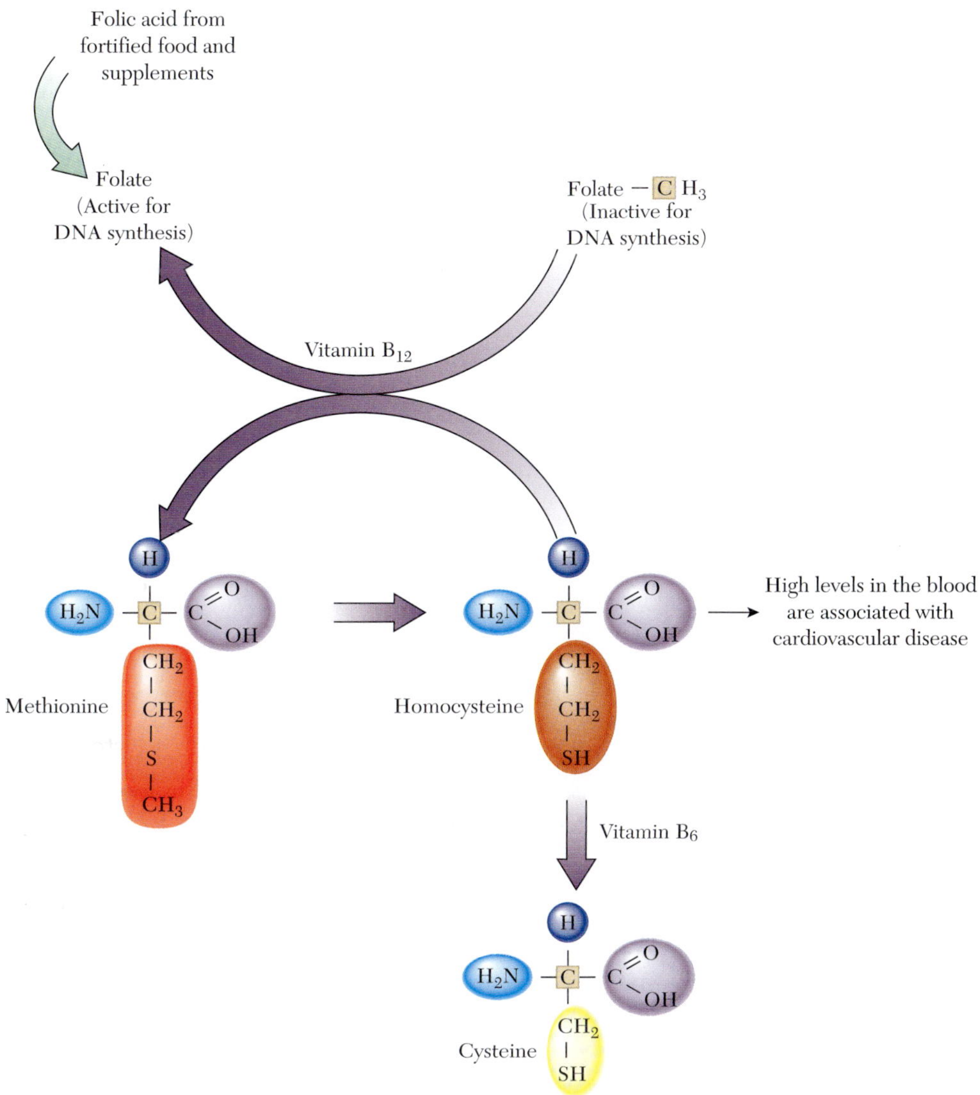

FIGURE 9.21 Coenzyme forms of folate and vitamin B_{12} are needed to convert homocysteine to methionine by adding a methyl group (CH_3). This reaction also converts folate into a coenzyme form that is active for DNA synthesis. This form can also be supplied by supplements. A deficiency of folate, vitamin B_{12}, or vitamin B_6 can lead to the accumulation of homocysteine, which is associated with an increased risk of cardiovascular disease.

creases with folate deficiency (see preceding discussion of vitamin B_6 and cardiovascular disease).[24] Homocysteine concentration and the risk of cardiovascular disease are reduced by increasing intakes of folate.[23,24] The levels added in fortification are likely to have a positive impact on blood homocysteine and the risk of heart disease.[34,35]

Folate and Cancer Low folate status increases the risk of developing cancers that affect epithelial tissues such as those of the uterus, cervix, lung, stomach, esophagus, and colon. Although folate deficiency does not cause cancer, it has been hypothesized that low folate intake enhances an underlying predisposition to cancer. Data supporting the effects of folate intake on cancer risk are strongest for colon cancer. Epidemiological studies show a higher incidence of colon cancer in populations with a low folate intake.[36] It is still not clear how much folate is needed to minimize cancer risk and whether food folate and supplemental folic acid are equally effective. Over a 15-year period, women who consumed greater than 400 μg of folate per day were found to have a reduced colon cancer risk compared to women who consumed 200 μg per day or less. The reduction in risk was greatest among women who took vitamin supplements containing folic acid.[37]

Folate Toxicity Although there is no known folate toxicity, a high intake may mask the early symptoms of vitamin B_{12} deficiency, allowing irreversible nerve damage to occur. Some policy makers question the wisdom of fortifying foods with folate because of the risk of increasing the damage done by vitamin B_{12} deficiency.[38]

The UL for folic acid for adults is set at 1000 μg of folic acid per day from supplements and fortified foods. This value was determined based on the progression of neurological symptoms seen in patients who were deficient in vitamin B_{12} and taking folic acid supplements.

Meeting Folate Needs with Food and Supplements It is estimated that adult women in the United States consume an average of 400 μg DFE from natural and fortified foods daily. This level of intake meets the RDA but falls short of the recommendation for women of childbearing age to consume 400 μg of folic acid from fortified foods and supplements in addition to food folate. Depending on food choices, including 400 μg of synthetic folic acid from fortified foods would mean eating about one to four servings of fortified breakfast cereal or four to six servings of other fortified grain products each day. If it is not possible for a woman of childbearing age to consume 400 μg of folic acid from fortified foods, supplements should be used (see *Critical Thinking*: "Figuring Out Fortified Folate").

Because the fortification of grain products with folic acid is relatively recent, there are some discrepancies in how folate values are expressed in food composition tables and databases. These may provide values that include fortification for some products but not for others, making it difficult to calculate actual folate content of a food or diet. (Appendix A includes fortified values for all nonbrand name items.) Adding to the confusion is the fact the Daily Values on food labels are listed as μg total folate, not as μg DFE. The term μg DFE was developed to correct for differences in the bioavailability of the various forms of folate. For foods that are natural sources of folate, the folate content can be determined by multi-

TABLE 9.3 Calculating Vitamin and Mineral Content from Food Labels

Determine the Daily Value

- Look up the Daily Value for the nutrient of interest (the Daily Value is equal to the Reference Daily Intake values given in Table 2.3).

Determine the % Daily Value

- Find the % Daily Value for that nutrient on your food label.
- Food labels are required to provide the % Daily Values for vitamin A, vitamin C, iron, and calcium. The % Daily Value for folate and other nutrients is voluntarily provided on many product labels.

Calculate the Amount of the Nutrient

- Multiply the % Daily Value by the Daily Value to determine the amount of the nutrient in a serving.
- Example:

The Daily Value for folate is 400 μg.

A serving of canned garbanzo beans provides 20% of the Daily Value for folate. So:

400 μg × 20% of Daily Value = 400 × 0.2 = 80 μg folate

Consider Your Serving Size

- This is the value per serving. Be sure you consider differences between your serving size and the serving size listed on the label.

TABLE 9.4 Calculating Dietary Folate Equivalents in Fortified Foods

The amount of folate in foods fortified with folic acid is equal to the folate naturally present in the food plus the amount of folic acid added. The % Daily Value on food labels is calculated assuming that all of the folate is the naturally occurring form, which is less well absorbed than the folic acid form. Therefore, in order to correctly account for the amount of folate that is available to the body from fortified foods, the % Daily Value must be corrected. This calculation assumes that all of the folate in fortified foods is from added folic acid.

- Determine the amount of folic acid in the fortified food as shown in Table 9.3.
- Multiply the μg folic acid by 1.7, because folic acid added in fortification provides 1.7 times more available folate than folate naturally present in foods.*
- Example:

The Daily Value for folate is 400 μg.

A serving of breakfast cereal provides 50% of the Daily Value for folate. So:

400 μg × 50% = 200 μg folic acid

200 μg folic acid × 1.7 = 340 μg DFE

*To reduce the risk of neural tube defects, it is recommended that women capable of becoming pregnant consume 400 μg of folic acid per day from fortified foods or supplements. Because the recommendation is for 400 μg of folic acid rather than 400 μg DFE, no conversion to DFEs is needed when assessing whether this recommendation has been achieved.

plying the Daily Value (400 μg) by the % Daily Value listed on the label (see Table 9.3). To calculate the folate in a package of frozen spinach that provides 25% of the Daily Value, you would multiply 400 μg folate × 25% = 100 μg DFE. In foods fortified with folic acid, the amount of folate indicated by the % Daily Value must be corrected to account for the greater availability of the folic acid form of the vitamin (see Table 9.4).

Critical Thinking

Figuring Out Fortified Folate

Marcia is considering having a child and wants to be sure she is as healthy as possible before trying to conceive. She consults her physician, who gives her a clean bill of health but suggests she evaluate the amount of folate in her diet. A daily intake of 400 μg of synthetic folic acid from fortified foods and/or supplements is recommended in addition to the food folate consumed in a varied diet.

Why do women capable of becoming pregnant need so much folate?

Research has shown that women who consume extra folate as synthetic folic acid have a reduced risk of having a baby with a neural tube defect, a type of birth defect that affects the brain or spinal cord. The extra folate is therefore only beneficial in women who actually become pregnant. The period of time that this intake is beneficial is short (about one month before to one month after conception). These research studies were done by supplementing the diet with folic acid rather than increasing the intake of folate-rich foods. It is uncertain whether folate found naturally in foods will have the same effect. Because many pregnancies are not planned, it is recommended that 400 μg of folic acid from fortified foods or supplements be included routinely in the diets of women of childbearing age.

Marcia records a typical day's food intake:

Food	Servings	Food	Servings
Breakfast		*Dinner*	
Kix cereal	1 cup	Chicken	3 oz
Milk, reduced-fat	1 cup	Pasta	1 cup
Banana	1 medium	Spaghetti sauce	1/2 cup
Orange juice	8 oz	Roll	1
Coffee	1 cup	Margarine	2 tsp
Lunch		Spinach salad	1 cup
Flour tortilla	1 10-inch	Salad dressing	1 Tbsp
Ground beef	2 oz	Milk, reduced-fat	1 cup
Refried beans	1/2 cup	Ice cream	1/2 cup
Lettuce	2 Tbsp		
Cheese	2 Tbsp		
Tomato	1 Tbsp		
Coke	12 oz		
Apple	1 medium		

Which foods in her diet provide natural sources of folate?

The best sources of naturally occurring folate in Marcia's diet are the orange juice, beans, and spinach. Other fruits, vegetables, and dairy products contribute smaller amounts. Meats contribute little folate. Together, the sources of naturally occurring folate provide about 350 μg DFE.

Which foods are fortified with folic acid?

As of 1998, all enriched grain products must be fortified with folic acid. Fortified foods can be identified because folic acid is included in the ingredient list on food labels. The grain products in Marcia's diet, including the cereal, tortilla, pasta, and roll, are all fortified.

Marcia checks the labels on the fortified foods she eats and finds that they provide the following percent of the Daily Value for folate:

Kix	25%	Flour tortilla	20%
Pasta	30%	Roll	8%

Does Marcia consume 400 μg of synthetic folic acid?

The amount of folate in unfortified grain products is low so it can be assumed that all of the folate in these products is from folic acid. To determine the amount of folic acid per serving, Marcia multiplies the Daily Value (400 μg) by the % DV on the label:

Kix	400 μg × 25% = 100 μg folic acid
Pasta	400 μg × 30% = 120 μg folic acid
Flour tortilla	400 μg × 20% = 80 μg folic acid
Roll	400 μg × 8% = 32 μg folic acid
Total	**= 332 μg folic acid**

Would you recommend Marcia take a folic acid supplement? Why or why not?

Answer:

VITAMIN B_{12}

In 1820, **pernicious anemia**, a fatal form of anemia that did not respond to iron supplementation, was described. Pernicious anemia is caused by an inability to absorb sufficient vitamin B_{12}. In 1926, Drs. Minot and Murphy were awarded the Nobel Prize for curing the disease with a diet containing large quantities of liver, which is a good source of vitamin B_{12}. The vitamin itself was not isolated until 1948. Today, concern focuses on the effects of marginal deficiencies of this vitamin and the potential masking of B_{12} deficiency by high intakes of folic acid.

Pernicious anemia An anemia resulting from an autoimmune disorder in which parietal cells are destroyed, decreasing the production of intrinsic factor. This reduces the absorption of vitamin B_{12}, gradually resulting in deficiency.

Sources of Vitamin B_{12}

Vitamin B_{12} can be synthesized by bacteria but not by plants and animals. Animal tissues accumulate the vitamin from ingestion in the diet or from synthesis by bacterial microflora. The bacteria in the guts of ruminants such as cows synthesize substantial amounts of vitamin B_{12}. The bacteria that reside in the human colon also produce vitamin B_{12}, but it cannot be absorbed. In our diet, vitamin B_{12} is found almost exclusively in animal products. Meats, such as beef and poultry, are excellent sources. Vitamin B_{12} is not supplied by plant-based foods unless they have been contaminated with bacteria, soil, insects, or other sources of the vitamin, or have been fortified with it (Figure 9.22). Vegans seeking nonanimal sources of vitamin B_{12} sometimes consume spirulina algae or miso and tempeh, which are soybean products fermented by microorganisms, but these foods contain almost no usable vitamin B_{12}.[39] Diets that do not include animal products must include supplements or foods fortified with vitamin B_{12} in order to meet needs.[40] Vitamin B_{12} is susceptible to destruction by exposure to air and light.

Vitamin B_{12} in the Digestive Tract

Naturally occurring vitamin B_{12} is bound to protein in food and must be released before it can be absorbed. It is released in the stomach by stomach acid and the protein-digesting enzyme pepsin. The released vitamin B_{12} then binds to proteins called R proteins that are present in saliva, gastric juice, and other body fluids and cells. The R protein–bound vitamin B_{12} travels to the small intestine where pancreatic enzymes free it from the R proteins and it binds to **intrinsic factor**, a protein secreted by the **parietal cells** in the lining of the stomach. The intrinsic factor–vitamin B_{12} complex binds to receptor proteins in the ileum of the small intestine, allowing the vitamin to be absorbed (Figure 9.23). Vitamin B_{12} absorption can be disrupted by reduced stomach acid, insufficient pancreatic secretions, and low levels of intrinsic factor. A small amount of vitamin B_{12} can be absorbed by passive diffusion without these, but this accounts for only about 1 to 2% of the amount of the vitamin that is consumed. Vitamin B_{12} is efficiently recycled. It is secreted into the GI tract in bile and most of it is reabsorbed. Because of this, it can take many years of a deficient diet before the symptoms of vitamin B_{12} deficiency appear.

Intrinsic factor A protein produced by the parietal cells in the stomach lining that functions in the absorption of vitamin B_{12}.

Parietal cells Large cells in the stomach lining that produce and secrete intrinsic factor and hydrochloric acid.

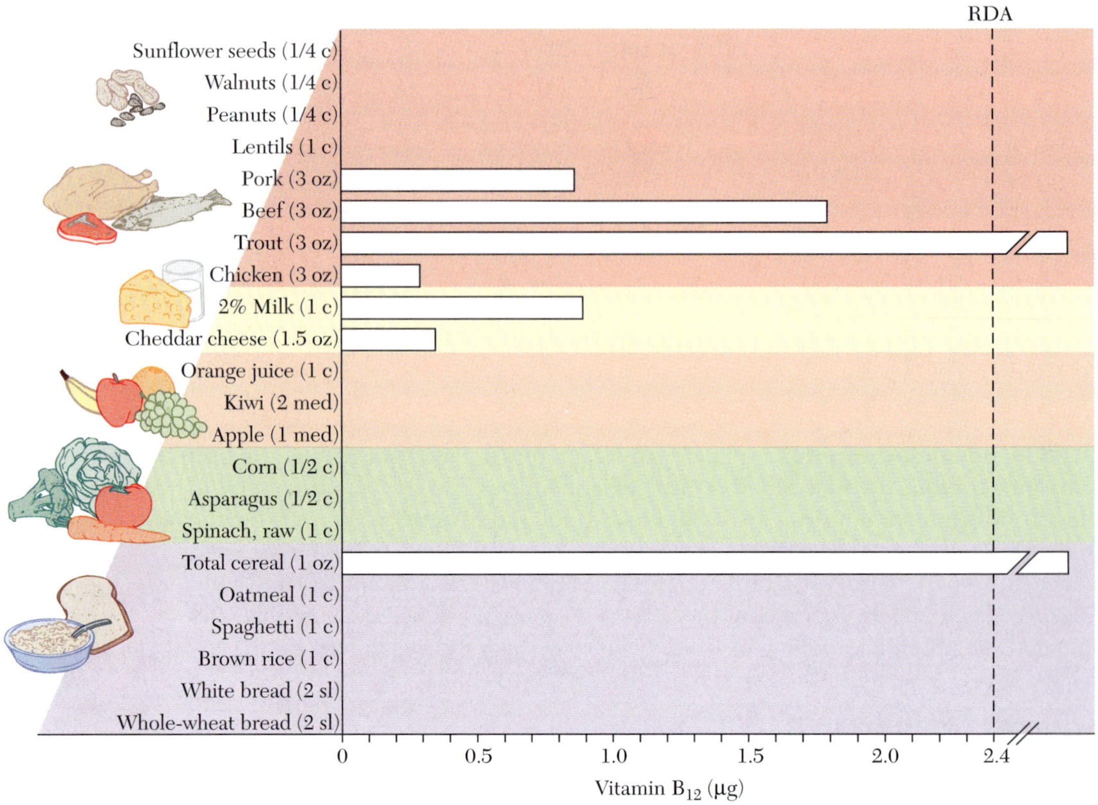

FIGURE 9.22 Vitamin B_{12} content of selections from each food group of the Food Guide Pyramid. The dashed line represents the RDA for adult men and women. Vitamin B_{12} is only found in foods of animal origin or foods that have been fortified with the vitamin.

Cobalamin The chemical term for vitamin B_{12}.

Methylcobalamin and **adenosylcobalamin** The coenzyme forms of vitamin B_{12} that are active in metabolism.

Vitamin B_{12} in the Body

Vitamin B_{12}, or **cobalamin**, is a cobalt-containing compound. Vitamin B_{12} is necessary for the maintenance of myelin, which insulates nerves and is essential for proper nerve transmission. Vitamin B_{12} can be converted into the active coenzyme forms **methylcobalamin** and **adenosylcobalamin**. One B_{12}-dependent reaction rearranges carbon atoms so that the breakdown products of fatty acids can be used to generate energy via the citric acid cycle. A second reaction synthesizes the amino acid methionine from homocysteine. This reaction also regenerates the active coenzyme form of folate that functions in DNA synthesis (see Figure 9.21).

Recommended Intakes

The RDA for vitamin B_{12} for adults of all ages is 2.4 μg per day.[2] This is the amount needed to maintain normal red blood cell parameters and blood vitamin B_{12} concentrations. It is assumed that only 50% of the vitamin B_{12} ingested is absorbed. Average intake in the U.S. population exceeds the RDA for both adult men and women.

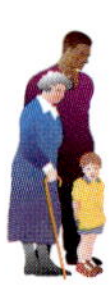

The RDA for vitamin B_{12} is increased during pregnancy, and during lactation, to account for the amount secreted in milk. Pregnant and lactating vegans, like anyone who does not eat animal products, are advised to take a supplement or consume fortified foods to provide the recommended intake for vitamin B_{12}.

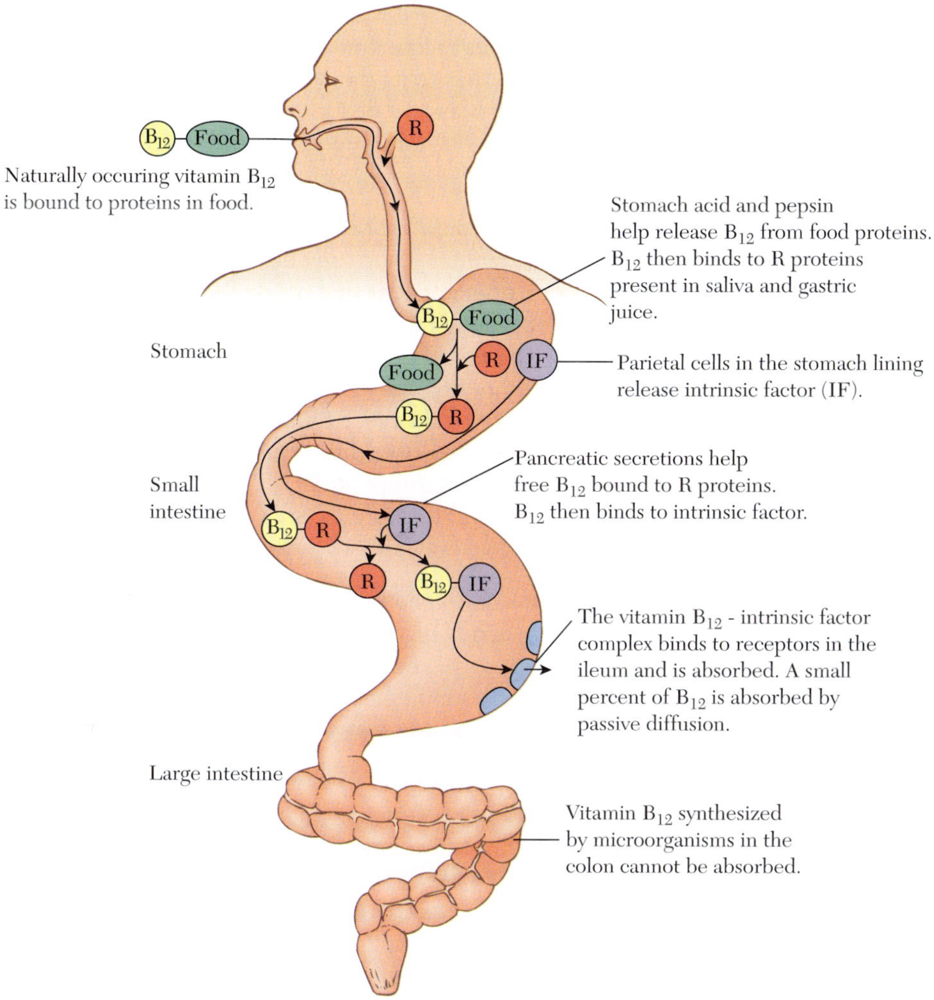

FIGURE 9.23 Normal absorption of vitamin B_{12} requires a healthy stomach, pancreas, and small intestine. In the stomach, intrinsic factor (IF) is produced and acid and pepsin release vitamin B_{12} bound to food proteins. The released B_{12} binds to R proteins. In the small intestine, enzymes from the pancreas release B_{12} from R proteins and it binds intrinsic factor. The vitamin B_{12}–intrinsic factor complex binds to receptors in the ileum of the small intestine, allowing absorption. Although the majority of vitamin B_{12} is absorbed by this mechanism, a small percentage of vitamin B_{12} can be absorbed by passive absorption.

Vitamin B_{12} and Health

Blatant deficiencies of vitamin B_{12} are rare because the body stores and recycles it. However, marginal vitamin B_{12} status is of public health concern particularly for older adults (because they absorb the vitamin poorly) and for vegetarians who consume no animal products.

Vitamin B_{12} Deficiency Because of the efficient recycling of vitamin B_{12}, it can take many years of a deficient diet before the symptoms of deficiency appear. However, when absorption is impaired, the vitamin B_{12} secreted in bile is not reabsorbed so recycling is reduced and deficiency symptoms appear more rapidly. This occurs in both individuals with pernicious anemia, an autoimmune disease in which the parietal cells that produce intrinsic factor are destroyed, and in those with **atrophic gastritis**, an inflammation of the stomach lining that results in a reduction in stomach acid and bacterial overgrowth.

Atrophic gastritis An inflammation of the stomach lining that causes a reduction in stomach acid and allows bacterial overgrowth.

Symptoms of vitamin B_{12} deficiency include an increase in blood homocysteine levels and a macrocytic, megaloblastic anemia that is indistinguishable from that seen in folate deficiency. Neurological symptoms including tingling and numbness, abnormalities in gait, memory loss, and disorientation also occur due to degeneration of the myelin sheath that coats the nerves, spinal cord, and brain. If left untreated, this can lead to paralysis and death (see Table 9.2). Vitamin B_{12} deficiency can be treated by injections of the vitamin or oral megadoses, which can be absorbed by passive diffusion.

Web Menu

For more information on vitamin B_{12} and the elderly, go to the American Dietetic Association at www.eatright.org/positions.html and click on aging.

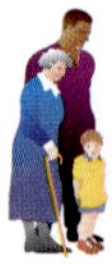

Vitamin B_{12} in Older Adults About 10 to 30% of individuals over 50 years of age are unable to absorb food-bound vitamin B_{12} normally because they have atrophic gastritis.[2,41] With the reduction in stomach acid that accompanies this condition, the enzymes that release protein-bound vitamin B_{12} cannot function properly and the bound vitamin B_{12} cannot be released and absorbed. In addition, microbes in the gut reduce absorption by competing for available vitamin B_{12}. It is recommended that individuals over the age of 50 meet their RDA for vitamin B_{12} by consuming fortified foods such as fortified breakfast cereals and soy-based products or by taking a vitamin B_{12}-containing supplement.[2] The vitamin B_{12} in fortified foods and supplements is not bound to proteins, so it is absorbed even when stomach acid is low.

Vitamin B_{12} in Vegans Deficiency is also a concern among vegan vegetarians because vitamin B_{12} is only found in foods of animal origin. Severe deficiency has been observed in breast-fed infants of vegan women, but marginal deficiency in vegetarians of all ages is a concern if supplements or fortified foods are not included in the diet.

Vitamin B_{12} Deficiency and Folate If individuals with vitamin B_{12} deficiency consume enough folate, they will not develop anemia, which is a reversible symptom of vitamin B_{12} deficiency. Without this symptom, diagnosis can be delayed, allowing more serious and irreversible symptoms, such as nerve damage, to progress. Although the fortification of enriched grain products with folic acid has raised concern that additional folate in the food supply could delay diagnosis of vitamin B_{12} deficiency in some individuals, the total amounts consumed in fortified foods are unlikely to be high enough to be a problem.[42] Large doses consumed in supplements are more likely to exceed the UL for folic acid and mask the anemia due to vitamin B_{12} deficiency.

Vitamin B_{12} Toxicity In healthy individuals no adverse effects have been reported with excess vitamin B_{12} intakes from food and supplements.[2] There are not sufficient data to establish a UL for vitamin B_{12}.

Vitamin B_{12} Supplements Supplements of vitamin B_{12} are available as cyanocobalamin in both oral and injectable forms. Because vitamin B_{12} deficiency causes anemia, supplements of the vitamin, particularly as injections, have been promoted as a pick-me-up for tired, run-down individuals. However, there are no proven benefits of vitamin B_{12} supplementation in individuals who are not deficient. Oral supplements may be of benefit for those at risk for vitamin B_{12} deficiency, such as vegans and individuals over age 50 who may poorly absorb the vitamin from foods.

Choline: Is It a Vitamin?

Choline is needed to synthesize a number of important molecules, including a phospholipid found in cell membranes, the neurotransmitter acetylcholine, and a molecule that can donate methyl groups in chemical reactions. It is also an important source of carbon atoms in biochemical reactions. Choline can be synthesized to a limited extent by humans and is not currently classified as a vitamin. However, there is evidence that it is essential in healthy men.[43] There is not enough information to determine if choline is also essential in the diets of women, infants, children, or older adults.[2]

Choline is widely distributed in foods. Particularly good sources include egg yolks, organ meats, spinach, nuts, and wheat germ (see Table 9.2). Average daily choline intake is estimated to be about 600 to 1000 mg per day. An AI of 550 mg per day for men and 425 mg per day for women has been established based on the amount needed to prevent liver damage. There are few data to assess whether dietary choline is needed at all stages of life. At some stages, requirements may be met by synthesis in the body.

Choline deficiency causes liver abnormalities. Although unlikely in healthy humans, deficiency has been observed in individuals fed a choline-deficient diet and in those receiving total parenteral nutrition without choline.[44] Choline is required by human cells grown in culture, and prolonged deficiency in animals leads to fat accumulation in the liver and may contribute to liver cancer.

Intakes of choline that are much higher than those that can be obtained from foods can cause body odor, sweating, reduced growth rate, low blood pressure, and liver damage. A UL for adults of 3.5 g per day has been set based on the occurrence of low blood pressure.

Summary

1. Vitamins are essential organic nutrients that are required in small quantities in the diet to promote and regulate body processes needed for growth, reproduction, and tissue maintenance. They do not provide energy.
2. Vitamins are naturally present in foods, added to foods by fortification and enrichment, and contained in supplements. The amount of a vitamin that is available to the body is regulated by vitamin absorption, transport, activation, storage, and excretion.
3. Vitamin deficiencies remain a major health problem worldwide. In industrialized countries, marginal dietary deficiencies and toxicities from supplements are a growing concern.
4. Recommended intakes for vitamins are established by evaluating the results from many different kinds of research. The DRIs express recommended intakes as RDAs or AIs.
5. Thiamin in its active coenzyme form is required for the generation of energy from carbohydrate, fat, and protein and for the synthesis of the neurotransmitter acetylcholine. The best food sources are lean pork, legumes, and whole or enriched grain products. The thiamin-deficiency disease beriberi causes nervous system abnormalities. Deficiencies are common in alcoholics. No toxicity has been identified.
6. Riboflavin coenzymes are needed for the generation of energy. Riboflavin deficiency is rarely seen alone because food sources of riboflavin are also sources of other B vitamins and because riboflavin is needed to activate several other vitamins. Milk, meat, and enriched grain products are the best food sources. No toxicity has been identified.
7. Niacin coenzymes are important in the breakdown of carbohydrate, fat, and protein and in the synthesis of fatty acids and sterols. A deficiency results in pellagra, which is characterized by dermatitis, diarrhea, and dementia, and is fatal if untreated. Beef, chicken, turkey, fish, and enriched grain products are the best food sources. The amino acid tryptophan can be converted into niacin, so dietary tryptophan can meet some of the niacin requirement. Supplements of the nicotinic acid form of niacin can lower elevated blood cholesterol but frequently cause toxicity symptoms such as flushing, tingling sensations, nausea, and a red skin rash.
8. Biotin is needed for the synthesis of glucose and fatty acids and the metabolism of certain amino acids. It is difficult to set a dietary requirement for biotin because some of our biotin need is met by bacterial synthesis in the gastrointestinal tract. Therefore, an AI rather than an RDA has been established. Liver and egg yolks are good sources. Toxicity has not been reported.
9. Pantothenic acid is part of coenzyme A (CoA), which is required for the production of energy from carbohydrate, fat, and protein and the synthesis of cholesterol and fat. It is abundant in the food supply, and deficiency is rare. There is no RDA, but an AI has been established.
10. Pyridoxal phosphate, the coenzyme form of vitamin B_6, is needed for the activity of more than 100 enzymes involved in the metabolism of carbohydrate, fat, and protein. Vitamin B_6 is particularly important for amino acid metabolism. Adequate amounts are necessary to keep levels of the methionine metabolite, homocysteine, low and reduce the risk of heart disease. Food sources include chicken, fish, liver, eggs, and whole grains. Large doses of vitamin B_6 can cause nervous system abnormalities.
11. Folate is necessary for the synthesis of DNA, so it is especially important for rapidly dividing cells. Folate

deficiency results in macrocytic anemia. Low levels of folate before and during early pregnancy are associated with an increased incidence of neural tube defects. It is recommended that women of childbearing age consume 400 μg of folic acid from fortified foods and supplements in addition to the folate found in a varied diet. Food sources include liver, legumes, oranges, leafy green vegetables, and fortified grains. Low folate can increase blood homocysteine levels; a high intake of folate can mask the early symptoms of vitamin B_{12} deficiency.

12. Vitamin B_{12} is needed for the metabolism of folate and fatty acids and to maintain the insulating layer of myelin surrounding nerves. Deficiency results in anemia and nerve damage. Vitamin B_{12} is found almost exclusively in animal products. Its absorption from food requires adequate levels of stomach acid, intrinsic factor, and pancreatic secretions. Marginal deficiency is a concern in vegans, who consume no animal products, and in older individuals in whom stomach acid secretion is reduced. Vitamin B_{12} supplements or fortified foods are recommended for these groups.
13. Choline is a substance necessary for metabolism and is not currently classified as a vitamin. It may be required in the diet at certain stages of life, so an AI has been established.

Review Questions

1. What is a vitamin?
2. List four factors that affect how much of a vitamin is available to the body.
3. What do enrichment and fortification mean?
4. Name a function common to all of the B vitamins.
5. In what population groups is thiamin deficiency a concern?
6. Why should milk not be packaged in clear containers?
7. What is pellagra?
8. How is vitamin B_6 involved in protein metabolism?
9. Explain why a deficiency of vitamin B_6, folate, or vitamin B_{12} can cause anemia.
10. Why is low folate intake of particular concern for women of childbearing age?
11. Why are vegans and the elderly at risk for vitamin B_{12} deficiency?
12. Does choline fit the definition of a vitamin? Why or why not?

Applying Critical Thinking Skills

Personal nutrition:

1. Use your food intake record from Chapter 2 to answer the following:
   a. How much folate does your diet contain?
   b. How does your intake compare with the RDA?
   c. If your diet doesn't meet recommendations, suggest modifications to meet the RDA for folate.
   d. List several sources of natural folate in your diet and several foods that are fortified with folic acid.
2. Use your food intake record from Chapter 2 to answer the following:
   a. How much vitamin B_{12} does your diet contain?
   b. How does your intake compare with the RDA?
   c. If your diet doesn't meet recommendations, suggest modifications to meet the RDA for vitamin B_{12}.
   d. List sources of vitamin B_{12} in your diet that are both natural and from fortification.
   e. If you were 60 years old, would your diet meet the recommendation for vitamin B_{12} intake?

General nutrition issues:

1. Evaluate each of the following supplements:

Supplement	Ingredients	Dose
Pyridoxine	100 mg pyridoxine	2 tablets daily
Stress tab	35 mg pyridoxine 1 mg thiamin 1.1 mg riboflavin 30 mg niacin 500 mg choline	3 times daily
Folic acid	800 μg folic acid	Once daily

   a. Do any of them create a risk for toxicity when taken at the recommended dosage? Which ones and why?
   b. Would you recommend them for everyone? For a specific group? Why or why not?
2. Using the Internet, find a link to a manufacturer who sells B vitamin supplements.
   a. What is the highest dose of pyridoxine that you see included in one of its products? Is this a safe dose? What advertising promises are included with supplements containing pyridoxine? Evaluate these claims for accuracy.
   b. What forms of niacin are in supplements marketed by this company? How much niacin is included per dose? Is this a safe level of intake?

References

1. Tanphaichitr, V. Thiamin. In *Modern Nutrition in Health and Disease*, 9th ed. Shils, M. E., Olson, J. A., Shike, M., and Ross, A. C., eds. Baltimore: Williams & Wilkins, 1999, 381–389.
2. Institute of Medicine, Food and Nutrition Board. *Dietary Reference Intakes for Thiamin, Riboflavin, Niacin, Vitamin B_6, Folate, Vitamin B_{12}, Panthothenic Acid, Biotin, and Choline.* Washington, D.C.: National Academy Press, 1998.
3. McCormick, D. B. Riboflavin. In *Modern Nutrition in Health and Disease*, 9th ed. Shils, M. E., Olson, J. A., Shike, M., and Ross, A. C., eds. Baltimore: Williams & Wilkins, 1999, 391–399.
4. Roe, D. A. *A Plague of Corn: The Social History of Pellagra*. Ithaca, N.Y.: Cornell University Press, 1973.
5. McKenney, J. M., Proctor, J. D., Harris, S., and Chinchili, V. M. A comparison of the efficacy and toxic effects of sustained- versus immediate-release niacin in hypercholesterolemic patients. JAMA 271:672–677, 1994.
6. Guyton, J. R., Blazing, M. A., Hagar, J., et al. Extended-release niacin versus gemfibrozil for the treatment of low levels of high-density lipoprotein cholesterol. Niaspan-Gemfibrozil Study Group. Arch. Intern. Med. 160:1177–1184, 2000.
7. Guyton J. R. Effect of niacin on atherosclerotic cardiovascular disease. Am. J. Cardiol. 17:18–23, 1998.
8. Morgan, J. M., Capuzzi, D. M., and Guyton, J. R. A new extended-release niacin (Niaspan): efficacy, tolerability, and safety in hypercholesterolemic patients. Am. J. Cardiol. 82:29U–34U, 1998.
9. Pozzilli, P. Prevention of insulin-dependent diabetes mellitus. Diabetes Metab. Rev. 14:69–84, 1998.
10. Gale, E. A. Molecular mechanisms of beta-cell destruction in IDDM: the role of nicotinamide. Horm. Res. 45(Suppl. 1):39–43, 1996.
11. Lampeter, E. F., Klinghammer, A., Scherbaum, W. A., et al. The Deutsche Nicotinamide Intervention Study: an attempt to prevent type 1 diabetes. DENIS Group. Diabetes 47:980–984, 1998.
12. Pozzilli, P., Brown, P. D., and Kolb, H. Meta-analysis of nicotinamide treatment in patients with recent-onset IDDM. The Nicotinamide Trialists. Diabetes Care 19:1357–1363, 1996.
13. Polo, V., Saibene, A., and Pontiroli, A. E. Nicotinamide improves insulin secretion and metabolic control in lean type 2 diabetic patients with secondary failure to sulphonylureas. Acta. Diabetol. 35:61–64, 1998.
14. Velazquez, A., Teran, M., Baez, A., et al. Biotin supplementation affects lymphocyte carboxylases and plasma biotin in severe protein energy malnutrition. Am. J. Clin. Nutr. 61:385–391, 1995.
15. Mock, N. I., Malik, M. I., Stumbo, P. J., et al. Increased urinary excretion of 3-hydroxyisovaleric acid and decreased urinary excretion of biotin are sensitive to early indicators of decreased biotin status in experimental biotin deficiency. Am. J. Clin. Nutr. 65:951–958, 1997.
16. Food and Nutrition Board, National Research Council. *Recommended Dietary Allowances*, 10th ed. Washington, D.C.: National Academy Press, 1989.
17. USDA Agricultural Research Service. Results from USDA 1994–1996 CSFII. 1997.
18. Borschel, M. W. Vitamin B_6 in infancy: requirements and current feeding practices. In *Vitamin B_6 Metabolism in Pregnancy, Lactation and Infancy*. Raiten, D. J., ed. Boca Raton, Fla.: CRC Press, 1995, 109–124.
19. Bessey, O. A., Adam, D. J., and Hansen, A. E. Intake of vitamin B_6 and infantile convulsions: a first approximation of requirements of pyridoxine in infants. Pediatrics 20:33–44, 1957.
20. Wilcken, D. E., and Wilcken, B. The natural history of vascular disease in homocystinuria and the effects of treatment. J. Inherit. Metab. Dis. 20:295–300, 1997.
21. Mayer, E. L., Jacobsen, D. W., and Robinson, R. Homocysteine and coronary atherosclerosis. J. Am. Coll. Cardiol. 27:517–527, 1996.
22. Graham, I. M., Daly, L. E., Refsum, H. M., et al. Plasma homocysteine as a risk factor for vascular disease. The European Concerted Action Project. JAMA 227:1775–1781, 1997.
23. Rimm, E. B., Willett, W. C., Hu, F. B., et al. Folate and vitamin B_6 from diet and supplements in relation to risk of coronary heart disease among women. JAMA 279:359–364, 1998.
24. Refsum, H., Ueland, P. M., Nygard, O., and Vollset, S. E. Homocysteine and cardiovascular disease. Annu. Rev. Med. 49:31–62, 1998.
25. Schaumburg, H., Kaplan, J., Windebank, A., et al. Sensory neuropathy from pyridoxine abuse. N. Engl. J. Med. 309:445–448, 1983.
26. Keniston, R. C., Nathan, P. A., Leklem, J. E., and Lockwood, R. S. Vitamin B_6, vitamin C, and carpal tunnel syndrome: a cross-sectional study of 441 adults. J. Occup. Environ. Med. 39:949–959, 1997.
27. Jacobson, M. D., Plancher, K. D., and Kleinmen, W. B. Vitamin B_6 (pyridoxine) therapy for carpal tunnel syndrome. Hand. Clin. 12:253–257, 1996.
28. Campbell, E. M., Peterkin, D., O'Grady, K, and Sanson-Fisher, R. Premenstrual symptoms in general practice patients: prevalence and treatment. J. Reprod. Med. 42:637–646, 1997.
29. Wyatt, K. M., Dimmock, P. W., Jones, P. W., and Shaughn O'Brien, P. M. Efficacy of vitamin B_6 in the treatment of premenstrual syndrome: systematic review. BMJ 318:1375–1381, 1999.
30. Lesourd, B. M., Mazari, L., and Ferry, M. The role of nutrition in immunity in the aged. Nutr. Rev. 56(II):S113–S125, 1998.
31. Bailey, L. B. Evaluation of a new Recommended Dietary Allowance for folate. J. Am. Diet. Assoc. 92:463–468, 1992.
32. Keane, E. M., O'Broin, S., Kelleher, B., et al. Use of folic acid-fortified milk in the elderly population. Gerontology 44:336–339, 1998.
33. Czeizel, A. E., and Dudas, I. Prevention of the first occurrence of neural tube defects by periconceptional vitamin supplementation. N. Engl. J. Med. 327:1832–1835, 1992.
34. Schorah, C. J., Devitt, H., Lucock, M., and Dowell, A. C. The responsiveness of plasma homocysteine concentrations. N. Engl. J. Med. 340:1449–1454, 1999.
35. Schorah, C. J., Devitt, H., Lucock, M., and Dowell, A. C. The responsiveness of plasma homocysteine to small increases in dietary folic acid: a primary care study. Eur. J. Clin. Nutr. 52:407–411, 1998.
36. Mason, J. B., and Levesque, T. Folate: effects on carcinogenesis and the potential for cancer chemoprevention. Oncology (Huntingt) 10:1727–1736, 1742–1743, 1996.
37. Giovannucci, E., Stampfer, M. J., Colditz, G. A., et al. Multivitamin use, folate, and colon cancer in women in the Nurses' Health Study. Ann. Intern. Med. 129:517–524, 1998.
38. Cuskelly, G. J., McNulty, H., and Scott, J. M. Fortification with low amounts of folic acid makes a significant difference in folate status of young women: implications for the prevention of neural tube defects. Am. J. Clin. Nutr. 70:234–239, 1999.
39. Miller, D. R., Specker, B. L., Ho, M. L., and Norman, E. J. Vitamin B_{12} status in a macrobiotic community. Am. J. Clin. Nutr. 53:524–529, 1991.
40. Messina, V. K., and Burke, K. I. Position of the American Dietetic Association: vegetarian diets. J. Am. Diet Assoc. 97:1317–1321, 1997.
41. Van Asselt, D. Z., van den Broek, W. J., Lamers, C. B., et al. Free and protein-bound cobalamin absorption in healthy middle-aged and older subjects. J. Am. Geriatr. Soc. 44:949–953, 1996.
42. Keohler, K. M., Pareo-Tubbeh, S. L., Romero, L. J., et al. Folate nutrition and older adults: challenges and opportunities. J. Am. Diet. Assoc. 97:167–173, 1997.
43. Zeisel, S. H., Da Costa, K. A., Franklin, P. D., et al. Choline, an essential nutrient for humans. FASEB J. 5:2093–2098, 1991.
44. Zeisel, S. H. Choline and phosphatidylcholine. In *Modern Nutrition in Health and Disease*, 9th ed. Shils, M. E., Olson, J. A., Shike, M., and Ross, A. C., eds. Baltimore: Williams & Wilkins, 1999, 513–523.

10 Vitamins A, D, K, E, and C and Meeting Needs: Food Versus Supplements

Vitamin A

Forms of Vitamin A
Sources of Vitamin A
Vitamin A in the Digestive Tract
Vitamin A in the Body
Recommended Intakes
Vitamin A and Health

Vitamin D

Forms and Sources of Vitamin D
Vitamin D in the Body
Recommended Intakes
Vitamin D and Health

Vitamin K

Forms and Sources of Vitamin K
Vitamin K in the Body
Recommended Intakes
Vitamin K and Health

Antioxidants

Antioxidants, Pro-Oxidants, and Health
Dietary Antioxidants

Vitamin E: A Fat-Soluble Antioxidant

Forms of Vitamin E
Sources of Vitamin E
Vitamin E in the Body
Recommended Intakes
Vitamin E and Health

Vitamin C: A Water-Soluble Antioxidant

Sources of Vitamin C
Vitamin C in the Body
Recommended Intakes
Vitamin C and Health

Benefits of Food Versus Supplements

A Diet to Meet Vitamin Needs
Other Health Benefits of Food
Dietary Supplements

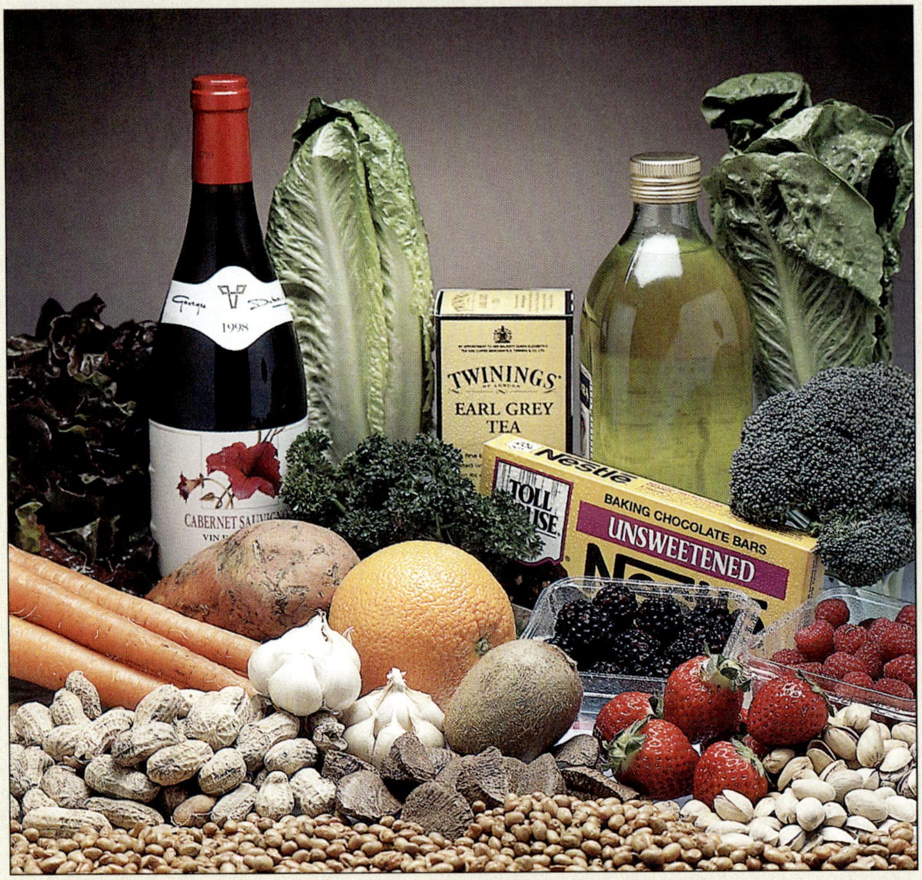

Learning Objectives

After reading this chapter, students should be able to:

1. Compare the sources and potential toxicity of retinoids and carotenoids.
2. Describe the role of vitamin A in vision.
3. Discuss how vitamin A and vitamin D affect gene expression.
4. Explain why vitamin D is known as the sunshine vitamin.
5. Relate the functions of vitamins A, D, and K to their deficiency symptoms.
6. Define "antioxidant" and compare the antioxidant roles of vitamin E and vitamin C.
7. Explain the role of vitamin C in the maintenance of connective tissue.
8. Discuss why variety is important in choosing foods to meet vitamin needs.
9. Compare the health benefits of meeting nutrient needs with food and supplements.
10. Define "dietary supplement" and discuss the potential risks of these products.

Ana will be two years old next week. She is a happy, healthy toddler; you would never know she had been diagnosed with rickets a year ago. Ana was adopted from an orphanage in central China when she was about a year old. After she arrived in the United States, her pediatrician became concerned because she had only one tooth. After examining Ana's ribs and legs, the doctor told her parents that she wanted to draw a blood sample to test for rickets. The pediatrician was concerned because rickets is common in children adopted from China. What is rickets, and what information can such a blood test provide?

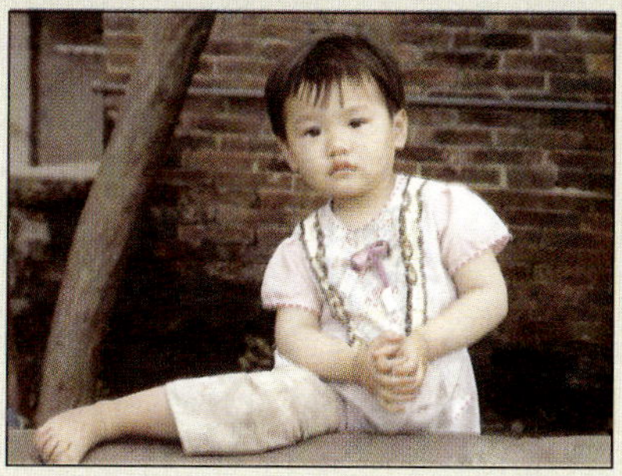

The pediatrician explained that rickets is a condition caused by inadequate vitamin D—due either to a dietary deficiency or to low exposure to sunlight. Vitamin D is needed for proper formation and maintenance of bones and teeth.

Rickets can cause a child's legs to bow and bony bumps to appear on each of the ribs. These poorly formed bones break easily. The teeth erupt late and are very prone to decay. The rickets blood test evaluates levels of calcium and phosphorus in the blood as well as the hormones that regulate calcium and phosphorus concentrations.

Rickets was first recognized in the 1600s. It was common during the Industrial Revolution when people moved into smoggy cities in search of work. Tall buildings and smog-filled air reduced children's exposure to sunlight. With adequate exposure to sunlight, enough vitamin D can be made in the body to meet needs, but with only limited sunlight, vitamin D must be consumed in the diet. Today, children in orphanages in China often do not get enough sun exposure or dietary vitamin D to prevent this deficiency.

VITAMIN A

In ancient times, the Egyptians knew that eating liver could treat night blindness, a difficulty in adjusting from bright light to dim light, such as when a bright light strikes the eyes at night. In 1968, George Wald earned the Nobel Prize in medicine for identifying the mechanism by which vitamin A is involved in vision. Although this is a key function of vitamin A, attention today is focused more on how vitamin A interacts with genes to regulate growth and cell differentiation. Despite our expanding understanding of its functions, vitamin A deficiency remains a world health problem.

Forms of Vitamin A

Vitamin A is found preformed and in precursor, or provitamin, forms in the diet. Preformed vitamin A compounds are known as **retinoids.** The retinoids include retinal, retinol, and retinoic acid. Retinol and retinal can be interconverted from one to the other (Figure 10.1). Yellow-orange pigments called **carotenoids** are precursor forms of vitamin A. About 50 of the 600 carotenoids that have been identified provide vitamin A activity. **Beta-carotene (β-carotene)** is the most potent precursor (see Figure 10.1). Other carotenoids that provide some provitamin A activity and have been analyzed in the food supply include alpha-carotene (α-carotene) and β-cryptoxanthin. These can be converted to vitamin A in the intestinal mucosa and in the liver. Lycopene, lutein, and zeaxanthin are carotenoids that have no vitamin A activity.

Retinoids The chemical forms of preformed vitamin A: retinol, retinal, and retinoic acid.

Carotenoids Natural pigments synthesized by plants and many microorganisms. They give yellow and red-orange fruits and vegetables their color.

Beta-carotene (β-carotene) A carotenoid found in carrots and leafy greens that has more provitamin A activity than other carotenoids. It also acts as an antioxidant.

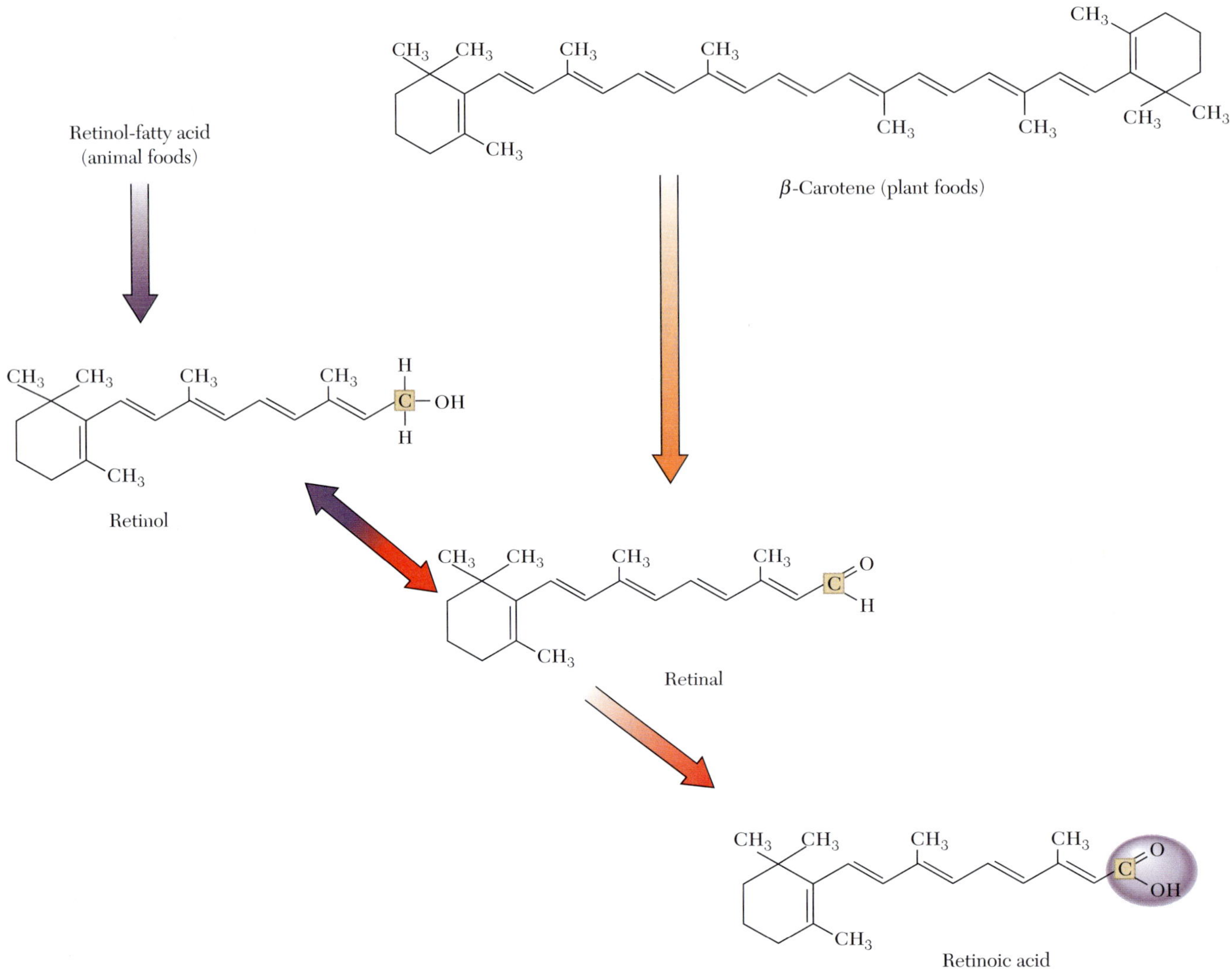

FIGURE 10.1 In the diet, preformed vitamin A is present primarily as retinol bound to fatty acids (retinyl esters). In the body, retinol and retinal can be interconverted, but once retinoic acid has been formed, it cannot be converted back to retinal or retinol. Beta-carotene from plant foods can be converted into retinal in the intestinal mucosa and in the liver. Cleaving a molecule of β-carotene in half theoretically yields two molecules of retinal; however, because β-carotene is not as well absorbed as preformed vitamin A and may not be efficiently converted to retinal, it takes about 12 μg of dietary β-carotene to yield 1 μg of retinol.

Sources of Vitamin A

Preformed vitamin A is found in animal foods such as liver, fish, egg yolks, and dairy products. Margarine and nonfat and reduced-fat milk are fortified with vitamin A because they are often consumed in place of butter and whole milk, which are good sources of this vitamin.

Plant sources of vitamin A contain yellow-orange carotenoid pigments. Beta-carotene is plentiful in carrots, squash, and other red and yellow vegetables and fruits as well as in leafy greens in which the yellow-orange pigment is masked by green chlorophyll (Figure 10.2). Alpha-carotene is found in leafy green vegetables, carrots, and squash; β-cryptoxanthin is in corn, green peppers, and lemons.[1]

To help consumers identify food sources of vitamin A, labels on packaged foods must list the vitamin A content as a percentage of the Daily Value. All forms of vitamin A in the diet are fairly stable when heated but may be destroyed by exposure to light and oxygen.

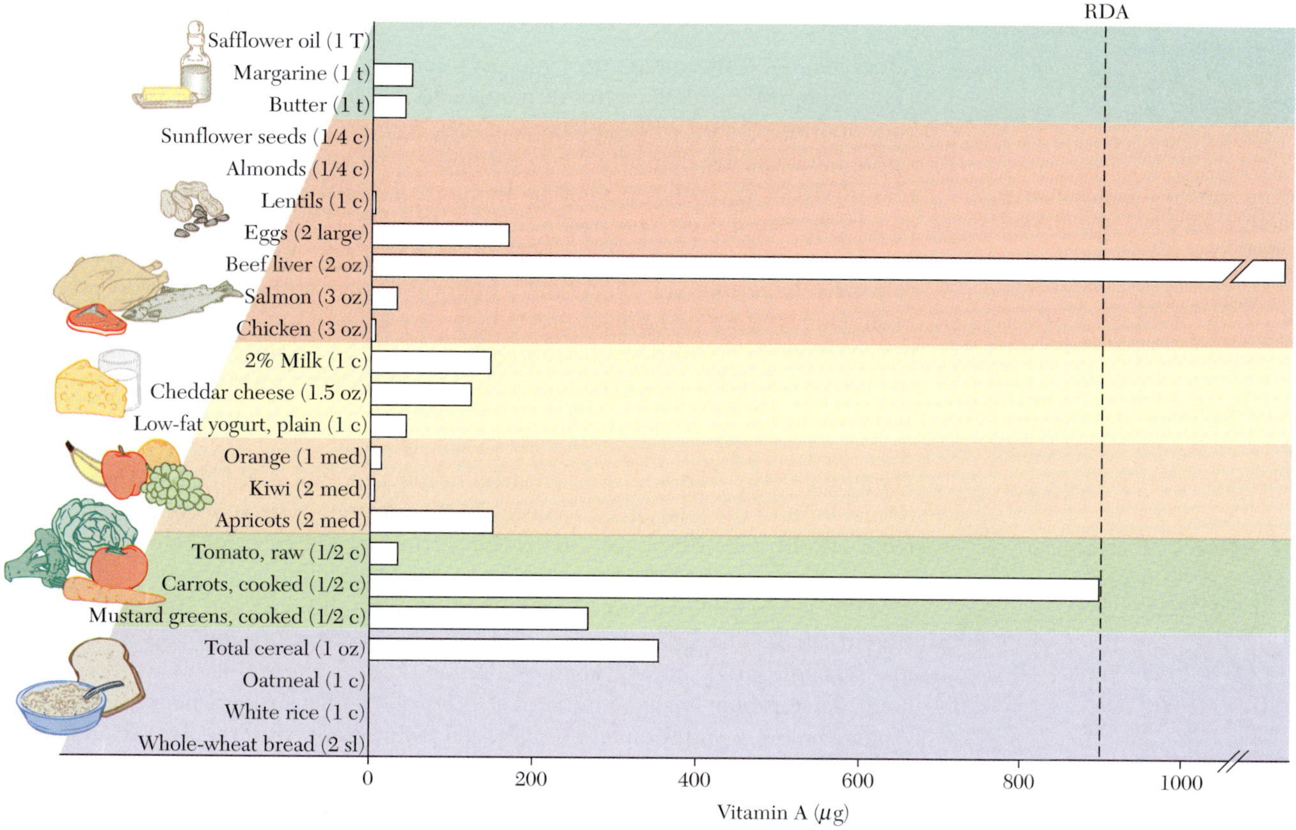

FIGURE 10.2 Vitamin A content of selections from each food group of the Food Guide Pyramid. The dashed line represents the RDA for adult men. Both plant and animal foods are good sources of vitamin A.

Vitamin A in the Digestive Tract

Both retinoids and carotenoids are bound to proteins in foods. To be absorbed, they must be released from the protein by pepsin and other protein-digesting enzymes. In the small intestine, the released retinoids and carotenoids combine with bile acids and other fat-soluble food components to form micelles, which facilitate their diffusion into mucosal cells.[1] Retinoids are present in the diet primarily as retinol bound to fatty acids (retinyl esters). Within the micelle, the fatty acid is removed. Retinol is then absorbed into the mucosal cell, where a fatty acid is reattached. Absorption of preformed vitamin A is efficient, estimated to be 70 to 90% of what is consumed. Carotenoids are less well absorbed than retinoids, so more of this form must be consumed to meet needs.[2] The efficiency of carotenoid absorption decreases as intake increases, so large amounts are not well absorbed. Once in the mucosal cells, much of the β-carotene is converted to retinal and then to retinol.

Vitamin A absorption is reduced in diets low in fat (less than 10 g/day). This is rarely a problem in industrialized countries, where typical fat intake ranges from 50 to 100 g per day. However, in populations with low dietary fat intakes, vitamin A deficiency may occur due to poor absorption. Diseases that cause fat malabsorption also interfere with vitamin A absorption and can cause a deficiency. Consumption of large amounts of the artificial fat Olestra interferes with vitamin A absorption. Olestra cannot be digested and absorbed in the human digestive tract. As it passes through the intestine, it takes fat-soluble substances with it, thereby decreasing the absorption of the fat-soluble vitamins A, D, E, and K as well as carotenoids. Foods containing Olestra are fortified with vitamins A, D, E, and K but not with carotenoids (see Chapter 5).

Vitamin A in the Body

Retinol-binding protein A protein that is needed to transport vitamin A from the liver to tissues in need.

Retinoids and carotenoids are transported from the intestine in chylomicrons. These lipoproteins deliver the retinoids and carotenoids to body tissues such as bone marrow, blood cells, spleen, muscles, kidney, and liver. In the liver, some carotenoids can be converted into retinol. To move from liver stores to the tissues, preformed vitamin A must be bound to **retinol-binding protein.** There is no specific blood transport protein for carotenoids.

The different forms of vitamin A have different functions. Retinol can be converted to retinal, the form that is important for vision. Retinoic acid, which is made from retinol or retinal, affects gene expression and is responsible for vitamin A's role in cell differentiation, growth, and development.[3] Carotenoids that are not converted to retinoids may provide antioxidant functions or other biological activities.

Rhodopsin A light-sensitive compound found in the retina of the eye that is composed of the protein opsin loosely bound to retinal.

The Visual Cycle Vitamin A is involved in the perception of light. In the eye, the retinal form of the vitamin combines with the protein opsin to form the visual pigment **rhodopsin.** Rhodopsin helps transform the energy from light into a nerve impulse that is sent to the brain. This nerve impulse allows us to see.

The visual cycle begins when light passes into the eye and strikes rhodopsin (Figure 10.3). The light changes the retinal in rhodopsin from a curved molecule to a straight one by converting a *cis* double bond in the retinal to a *trans* double bond. This change in shape initiates a series of events causing a nerve signal to be sent to the brain and retinal to be released from opsin. After the light stimulus has passed, the *trans* retinal is converted back to its original *cis* form and is recombined with opsin to regenerate rhodopsin. Each time this cycle occurs, some retinal is lost and must be replaced by retinol from the blood. The retinol is

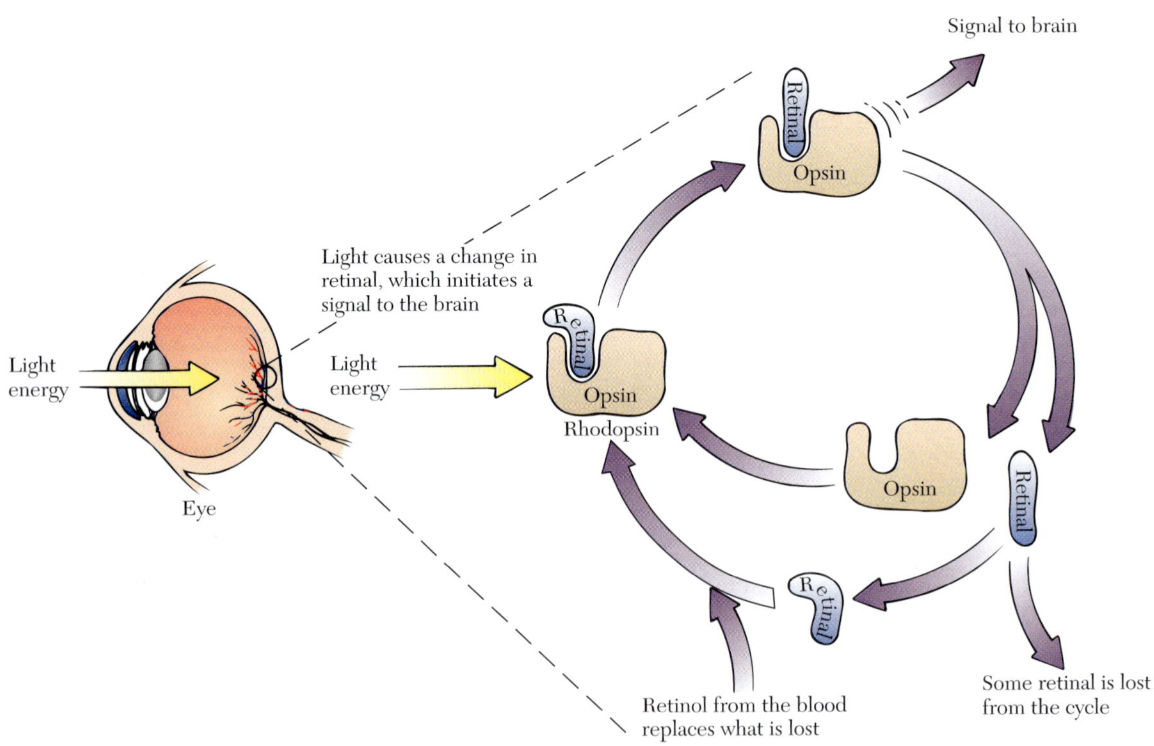

FIGURE 10.3 In the eye, retinal binds to the protein opsin to form rhodopsin. When light strikes rhodopsin, it causes the *cis* form of retinal to be converted to the *trans* form. This change in shape from a curved to a straight molecule sends a nerve signal to the brain and causes retinal to be released from opsin. Some retinal is converted to its original *cis* form and binds opsin to begin the visual cycle again. With each cycle, some retinal is lost and retinol from the blood must be converted to replace it.

converted into retinal in the eye. When vitamin A is deficient, there is a delay in the regeneration of rhodopsin, which causes difficulty in adapting to dim light after experiencing a bright light—the condition called night blindness. Night blindness is one of the first and more easily reversible symptoms of vitamin A deficiency.

Regulating Gene Expression: Cell Differentiation **Cell differentiation** is the process whereby immature cells change in structure and function to become specialized. For instance, in the bone marrow, some cells differentiate into white blood cells, whereas others differentiate to form red blood cells. Vitamin A affects cell differentiation through its impact on gene expression. This means that it can turn on or turn off the production of certain proteins that regulate functions within cells and throughout the body. By affecting gene expression, vitamin A can also determine what type of cell an immature cell will become.

Cell differentiation Structural and functional changes that cause cells to mature into specialized cells.

In order to affect gene expression, the retinoic acid form of vitamin A enters specific target cells. Inside the nucleus of these target cells, retinoic acid binds to protein receptors; this retinoic acid–protein receptor complex then binds to regulatory regions of DNA. This binding changes the amount of messenger RNA (mRNA) that is made by the gene. This in turn changes the amount of the protein that is produced (Figure 10.4). This turning on (or turning off) of the gene increases (or decreases) the production of proteins and thereby affects various cellular functions. For example, vitamin A turns on a gene that makes an enzyme in liver cells that enables the liver to make glucose by gluconeogenesis.

Maintenance of Epithelial Tissue Vitamin A is necessary for the maintenance of epithelial tissue. This type of tissue covers external body surfaces and lines internal cavities and tubes. It includes the skin and the linings of the eyes, intestines, lungs, vagina, and bladder. When vitamin A is deficient, epithelial cells do not differentiate normally because vitamin A is not there to turn on or turn off the production of particular proteins. For example, the epithelial tissue on many body surfaces contains cells that produce mucus for lubrication. When mucus-secreting cells die, new cells differentiate into mucus-secreting cells to replace them. When vitamin A is deficient, the new cells do not differentiate properly and instead become cells that produce a protein called **keratin.** Keratin is the hard protein that makes up hair and fingernails. As the mucus-secreting cells die and are replaced by keratin-producing cells, the epithelial surface becomes hard and dry. This process is known as keratinization. The hard, dry surface does not have the

Keratin A hard protein that makes up hair and fingernails.

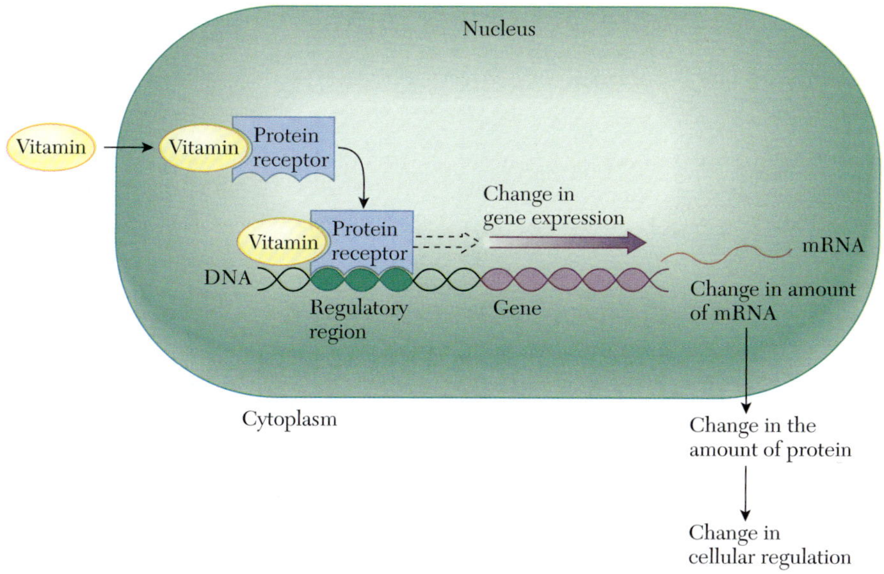

FIGURE 10.4 The retinoic acid form of vitamin A (shown here as the yellow vitamin) functions by entering the nucleus and binding to a protein receptor. The complex then binds to a regulatory region of DNA to change the expression of a gene and hence the amount of a protein synthesized. This in turn alters the cellular functions and body processes that are affected by this protein.

protective capabilities of normal epithelium and increases the likelihood of infection. The risk of infection is compounded by the fact that vitamin A deficiency also decreases immune function.

All epithelial tissues are affected by vitamin A deficiency, but the eye is particularly susceptible to damage. The mucus in the eye normally provides lubrication, washes away dirt and other particles, and also contains a protein that helps destroy bacteria. When vitamin A is deficient, the lack of mucus and the buildup of keratin cause the cornea to dry and leave the eye open to infection. A spectrum of eye disorders, known as **xerophthalmia,** is associated with vitamin A deficiency. In its early stages xerophthalmia can be treated by increasing vitamin A intake, but if left untreated, it can result in a softening of the cornea called **keratomalacia** and permanent blindness.

Xerophthalmia A spectrum of eye conditions resulting from vitamin A deficiency that may lead to blindness. An early symptom is night blindness, and as deficiency continues, a lack of mucus leaves the eye dry and vulnerable to cracking and infection.

Keratomalacia A softening of the cornea that leads to irreversible blindness.

Reproduction, Growth, and Immunity The ability of vitamin A to regulate the growth and differentiation of cells makes it essential throughout life for normal reproduction, growth, and immune function. In reproduction, vitamin A is hy-

TABLE 10.1 Summary of Vitamins A, D, K, E, and C

Vitamin	Sources	Recommended Intake for Young Adults*†	Major Functions
Fat Soluble			
Vitamin A (vitamin A acetate, vitamin A palmitate, retinol, retinal, retinoic acid, retinyl palmitate, provitamin A, carotene, β-carotene, carotenoids)	Liver, fish, carrots, peaches, leafy greens, fortified milk, sweet potatoes, broccoli	700–900 μg	Vision, growth, cell differentiation, reproduction, immune function
Vitamin D (cholecalciferol, ergocalciferol)	Egg yolk, liver, fish oils, tuna, salmon, fortified margarine and milk, sunlight	5 μg (200 IU)*	Absorption of calcium and phosphorus, maintenance of bone
Vitamin K (phylloquinone, menaquinone)	Leafy greens, vegetable oils, intestinal bacterial synthesis	90–120 μg*	Blood clotting
Vitamin E (alpha-tocopherol acetate, alpha-tocopherol)	Vegetable oils, leafy greens, nuts, peanuts	15 mg α-tocopherol	Antioxidant, protects cell membranes
Water Soluble			
Vitamin C (ascorbate, ascorbic acid)	Citrus fruit, strawberries, broccoli, greens	75–90 mg	Collagen synthesis, hormone and neurotransmitter synthesis, antioxidant

*Values with an asterisk (*) represent Adequate Intakes (AI). All other values are Recommended Dietary Allowances (RDA).

†Recommended intakes and UL values for all age groups and stages of life are given on the inside front and back covers.

ND=Insufficient evidence to determine a UL.

pothesized to play a role during early embryonic development by directing cells to form the shapes and patterns needed for a completely formed organism.[4] Poor overall growth is an early sign of vitamin A deficiency in children. Vitamin A affects the activity of cells that form and break down bone, and a deficiency early in life can cause abnormal jawbone growth, resulting in crooked teeth and poor dental health. In the immune system, vitamin A is needed for the differentiation that produces the different types of immune cells. When vitamin A is deficient, the activity of specific immune cells cannot be stimulated. This impaired immune function increases the risk of illness and infection due to defective epithelial tissue barriers.

Recommended Intakes

The recommended intake for vitamin A is based on the amount needed in the diet to maintain normal body stores. The RDA is set at 900 μg of vitamin A per day for adult men and 700 μg per day for adult women (Table 10.1).[2] There is no

Deficiency Diseases and Symptoms	Groups at Risk	Toxicity	Tolerable Upper Intake Levels (UL)†
Night blindness, xerophthalmia, poor growth, dry skin, impaired immunity	Those who live in poverty (particularly children and pregnant women), those consuming very low-fat or low-protein diets	Headache, vomiting, hair loss, liver damage, skin changes, birth defects, bone pain	3000 μg of preformed vitamin A (for adults 19 years and older)
Rickets in children, osteomalacia in adults	Breast-fed infants, children, and elderly (especially with dark skin and little sun exposure), people with kidney disease	Calcium deposits in the soft tissues, growth retardation, kidney damage	50 μg/day (2000 IU)
Hemorrhage	Those taking long-term antibiotics, newborns (especially premature)	Anemia, brain damage	ND
Hemolyzed red blood cells, nerve damage	Those with poor fat absorption, premature infants	Hemorrhage, inhibition of vitamin K activity	1000 mg of any form of supplemental α-tocopherol
Scurvy: poor wound healing, bleeding gums	Alcoholics, elderly men	Diarrhea and other GI distress	2000 mg

TABLE 10.2 Converting Vitamin A Units into μg Vitamin A

Form and source	Amount equal to 1μg vitamin A
Preformed vitamin A in food or supplements	1 μg = 1μg vitamin A
	1 RAE = 1 μg vitamin A
	1 μg RE = 1 μg vitamin A
	3.3 IU = 1 μg vitamin A
β-carotene in food*	12 μg = 1 μg vitamin A
	1 RAE = 1 μg vitamin A
	2 μg RE = 1 μg vitamin A
	20 IU = 1 μg vitamin A
α-carotene or β-cryptoxanthin in food	24 μg = 1 μg vitamin A
	1 RAE = 1 μg vitamin A
	2 μg RE = 1 μg vitamin A
	40 IU = 1 μg vitamin A

*Beta-carotene in supplements may be better absorbed than β-carotene in food and so provides more vitamin A activity. It is estimated that 2 μg of β-carotene dissolved in oil provides 1 μg of vitamin A activity.

recommendation to increase intake above this level for older adults. The RDA is increased in pregnancy to account for the vitamin A that is transferred to the fetus and during lactation to account for the vitamin A secreted in milk. The RDA for children is set lower than that for adults based on their smaller body size. For infants, an AI has been set based on the amount of vitamin A consumed by an average healthy, breast-fed infant.

Recommendations for vitamin A intake are expressed in μg of retinol. This can be supplied by both retinol and carotenoids in the diet. Because carotenoids are less well absorbed and not completely converted to vitamin A, a correction factor must be applied to carotenoids to determine the amount of usable vitamin A, referred to as **retinol activity equivalents (RAE),** provided by the food. Twelve μg of β-carotene provide 1 RAE of vitamin A, and 24 μg of α-carotene or β-cryptoxanthin provide 1 RAE.[2]

Retinol Activity Equivalent (RAE) The amount of retinol, β-carotene, α-carotene, or β-cryptoxanthin that must be consumed to equal the vitamin A activity of 1 μg of retinol. One μg of retinol, 12 μg of β-carotene, or 24 μg α-carotene or β-cryptoxanthin is equal to 1 RAE.

As our understanding of vitamin A has increased, the units in which recommended intakes have been expressed have changed. Older values are still found in food composition databases and tables. The 1989 RDAs used units called retinol equivalents (RE) to account for differences in absorption between retinoids and carotenoids. However, REs are now known to have overestimated carotenoid absorption. For foods containing carotenoids, RE values can be corrected by dividing them in half. Prior to 1980, vitamin A was also expressed in international units (IUs). These units are still often seen on supplement labels. Factors for converting REs and IUs to usable vitamin A are given in Table 10.2.

Web Menu: For more information on the problems of vitamin A deficiency worldwide, go to the World Health Organization at www.who.int/nut/vad.htm.

Vitamin A and Health

Vitamin A deficiency is a world health problem responsible for growth failure, blindness, increased susceptibility to infection, and death. Consumption of too much preformed vitamin A, however, can also be deadly.

Vitamin A Deficiency: A World Health Problem Vitamin A deficiency is a threat to the health, sight, and lives of millions of children in the developing world.[5] Children deficient in vitamin A have poor appetites, are anemic, and grow poorly. They are at increased risk for contracting infections, such as respiratory infections, diarrheal diseases, and measles, and these infections are more severe when they occur.[2,6] Vitamin A–deficient children are more likely to die in childhood than their peers.[6] It is estimated that 3 to 10 million children worldwide have xerophthalmia and 250,000 to 500,000 go blind annually due to vitamin A deficiency

(Figure 10.5).[2] It is most common in India, Africa, Latin America, and the Caribbean.

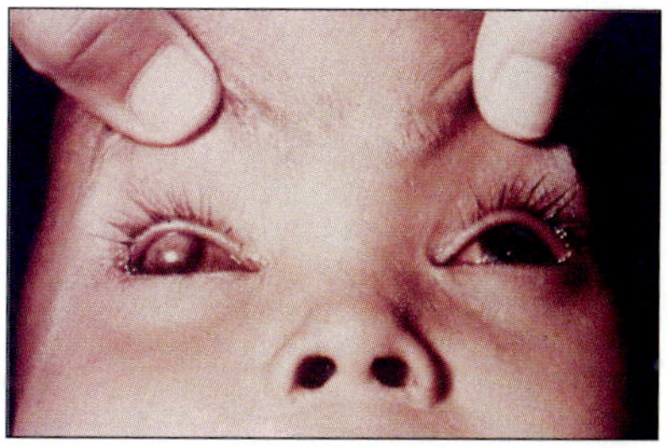

FIGURE 10.5 Vitamin A deficiency, as shown here in a child with xerophthalmia, is a major cause of blindness worldwide. *(L. V. Bergman/The Bergman Collection)*

Vitamin A deficiency can be caused by insufficient intakes of vitamin A, fat, protein, or the mineral zinc. A diet very low in fat can cause a deficiency by reducing vitamin A absorption. Protein deficiency can cause vitamin A deficiency because the retinol-binding protein needed to transport vitamin A from the liver cannot be made in sufficient quantities. The importance of zinc for vitamin A utilization is believed to be due to its role in protein synthesis. When zinc is deficient, proteins needed for vitamin A transport and metabolism are lacking.

Vitamin A deficiency is not common in developed countries, but estimates of typical dietary intakes indicate that between 25 and 50% of adults aged 50 to 70 years have vitamin A intakes that are below a level that assures adequate vitamin A stores. Intakes below the RDA may be caused by poor food choices. In the United States, the intake of fresh fruits and vegetables, many of which are good sources of provitamin A, does not meet recommendations. A typical fast-food meal of a hamburger and french fries provides almost no vitamin A.

Toxicity and Supplements Preformed vitamin A can be toxic. Acute toxicity has been reported in Arctic explorers who consumed polar bear liver, which contains about 60,000 μg of vitamin A in just 3 ounces. Although polar bear liver is not a common dish at most dinner tables, supplements of preformed vitamin A do have the potential to deliver a toxic dose. Signs of acute toxicity include nausea, vomiting, headache, dizziness, blurred vision, and a lack of muscle coordination. Chronic toxicity occurs when preformed vitamin A doses as low as ten times the RDA are consumed for a period of months to years. The symptoms of chronic toxicity include weight loss, muscle and joint pain, liver damage, bone abnormalities, visual defects, dry and scaling lips, and skin rashes. Excess vitamin A has been shown experimentally to stimulate bone resorption and inhibit bone formation. It has therefore been hypothesized that slightly elevated vitamin A intake may contribute to osteoporosis.[7] Birth defects are also associated with high dietary intakes of preformed vitamin A.[8]

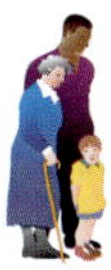

The Tolerable Upper Intake Level (UL) for women of childbearing age is set at a level that is unlikely to have teratogenic effects. For females aged 14 to 18 years, intake of preformed vitamin A from the diet and from supplements should not exceed 2800 μg per day. For women aged 19 to 50 years, intake should not exced 3000 μg per day. The UL for adult men and older women is set at a level that is unlikely to cause liver damage (3000 μg per day). ULs have also been established for infants and children (see inside back cover).

Because preformed vitamin A can be toxic, most supplements contain vitamin A precursors. Carotenoids do not cause the toxicity symptoms seen with preformed vitamin A. Their absorption from the diet decreases at high doses, and once in the body, their conversion to active vitamin A is limited. Large daily intakes of carotenoids—usually in the form of carrot juice or β-carotene supplements—do, however, lead to a condition known as **hypercarotenemia.** In this condition, the carotenoids stored in the adipose tissue make the skin look yellow-orange. This is particularly apparent on the palms of the hands and the soles of the feet. It is not known to be dangerous, and when intake decreases, the skin returns to its normal color.

Hypercarotenemia A condition caused by an accumulation of carotenoids in the adipose tissue, causing the skin to appear yellow-orange.

The DRI committee has evaluated the risks associated with consumption of high doses of carotenoids. Although a UL has not been established for β-carotene or other carotenoids, supplement use is not advised other than for the prevention and control of vitamin A deficiency. High-dose supplements of β-carotene have not been shown to provide any additional benefits and may be harmful to some, including individuals who smoke cigarettes. Two clinical research trials showed an increased incidence of lung cancer in cigarette smokers who took β-carotene supplements.[9] Even though other trials have not shown this effect, until more information is available, smokers are advised to avoid β-carotene supplements and rely on food sources to obtain carotenoids in their diet. The small amounts found in standard-strength multivitamin supplements are not likely to be harmful for any group[10] (see *Critical Thinking:* "Evaluating Vitamin Supplements").

Critical Thinking

Evaluating Vitamin/Mineral Supplements

Miguel is halfway through his freshman year at college. He has been feeling run-down and tired and has had two colds already this semester. When he describes his concerns to the clerk at a local health-food store, she recommends several supplements to keep him healthy and to help him withstand the stresses of school. These include a vitamin C supplement, a stress-formula B-vitamin supplement called B50, Brain Booster, and Prevention Plus. However, after taking a nutrition class, Miguel begins to wonder if he really needs all these and if some could actually be harmful. He evaluates their benefits and risks. Using information from each product's Supplement Facts label, Miguel compiles a list of the amounts of each ingredient in his supplements to compare them with the Daily Values.

Supplement	Ingredient	Dose	% Dv/ dose	Frequency	Total amount (% DV)
Vitamin C	Vitamin C	500 mg	833%	3/day	1500 mg (2500%)
B50	Thiamin	50 mg	3333%	3/day	150 mg (10,000%)
	Niacin	50 mg	250%		150 mg (750%)
	Vitamin B_6	60 mg	2500%		180 mg (7500%)
	Riboflavin	50 mg	2941%		150 mg (8823%)
	Biotin	50 μg	16.66%		150 μg (50%)
	Pantothenic Acid	50 mg	500%		150 mg (1500%)
	Folic Acid	50 μg	12.5%		150 μg (38%)
	Vitamin B_{12}	50 μg	833%		150 μg (2500%)
Brain Booster	Choline	100 mg	—	2/day	200 mg (—)
	Niacin	50 mg	250%		100 mg (500%)
Prevention Plus	Vitamin E	400 IU	1333%	1/day	400 IU (1333%)
	Vitamin C	1000 mg	1667%		1000 mg (1667%)
	Zinc	15 mg	100%		15 mg (100%)

How can Miguel determine if he is consuming potentially dangerous amounts of any of the substances in these supplements?

When he totals the amounts of nutrients in all the supplements, Miguel finds that he is exceeding the recommended intake for vitamin E, vitamin C, and all the B vitamins except biotin and folate. To determine if these amounts might be dangerous, he compares them to the UL values that are given in his nutrition book (see inside back cover). He discovers that there is a UL value for choline even though no Daily Values are available for labeling. He also realizes that the UL for vitamin E is given as mg α-tocopherol and his supplement lists vitamin E in IUs. To evaluate his vitamin E intake, he converts IUs to mg α-tocopherol using the following formula: IU of natural α-tocopherol $\times$ 0.67 = mg α-tocopherol (400 IU $\times$ 0.67 = 268 mg α-tocopherol). This dose is well below the UL of 1000 mg α-tocopherol.

Is he taking any nutrients in amounts that exceed the UL?

- Vitamin C: The three vitamin C supplements containing 500 mg each plus the 1000 mg of vitamin C in Prevention Plus add up to 2500 mg per day, which exceeds the UL of 2000 mg/day
- Niacin: The B50 and Brain Booster both contribute niacin. If he takes the doses recommended by the manufacturers, he will be consuming 250 mg daily. This is well in excess of the UL of 35 mg.
- Vitamin B_6: By taking three tablets of B50 a day, his intake will be 180 mg and will exceed the UL of 100 mg.

Will any of these vitamins cause toxicity symptoms?

- The symptoms that Miguel is most likely to experience from the 2500 mg of vitamin C he is taking are diarrhea, nausea, and abdominal cramps.
- His niacin intake may cause a rash and flushing.
- His intake of vitamin B_6 puts him at risk for nerve damage.

The ULs are set at a level that will not cause an adverse reaction in the majority of healthy people. However, there is no known benefit to consuming an amount of a nutrient above the RDA.

Will any of these prevent Miguel from getting sick or help boost his energy level?

Answer:

Would you suggest that Miguel stop taking any of these supplements? Why or why not?

Answer:

VITAMIN D

Vitamin D is known as the sunshine vitamin because it can be produced in the skin by exposure to ultraviolet light. Because it can be made in the body, there is a long-standing debate as to whether vitamin D is a vitamin or a hormone. By definition, vitamins are dietary essentials. However, vitamin D can be formed in the skin, so it is only essential in the diet when exposure to sunlight is limited or the body's ability to synthesize the vitamin is reduced. Vitamin D acts like a hormone because it is produced in one organ—the skin—and affects other organs, primarily the intestine and bone.

Forms and Sources of Vitamin D

Cholecalciferol The chemical name for vitamin D_3. It can be formed in the skin of animals by the action of sunlight on a form of cholesterol called 7-dehydrocholesterol.

Only a few foods are natural sources of vitamin D. These include liver, fatty fish such as salmon, and egg yolks (Figure 10.6). These foods contain **cholecalciferol,** also known as vitamin D_3. Cholecalciferol is the form of vitamin D that is made in the skin of animals by the action of sunlight on a compound made from cholesterol called 7-dehydrocholesterol (Figure 10.7). Foods fortified with vitamin D include milk and margarine. These may contain vitamin D_3 or vitamin D_2, another active form of the vitamin. Food labels are not required to include the amount of vitamin D, but vitamin D is listed in the ingredient list of fortified foods such as low-fat milk. Vitamin D is destroyed by exposure to air, light, heat, and low-acid conditions.

Vitamin D in the Body

Vitamin D from the diet and from synthesis in the skin is inactive until it is chemically altered in the liver and then in the kidney. In the liver, a hydroxyl group (OH) is added to vitamin D to form 25-hydroxy vitamin D_3, which then travels to the kidney, where another hydroxyl group is added to make the active form of vitamin D: 1,25-dihydroxy vitamin D_3 (Figure 10.8).

Parathyroid hormone (PTH) A hormone released by the parathyroid gland that acts to increase blood calcium levels.

The principal function of vitamin D is to maintain normal blood levels of calcium and phosphorus. When blood calcium levels drop too low, the parathyroid gland releases **parathyroid hormone (PTH),** which stimulates enzymes in the kidney to convert 25-hydroxy vitamin D_3 to the active form of the vitamin.

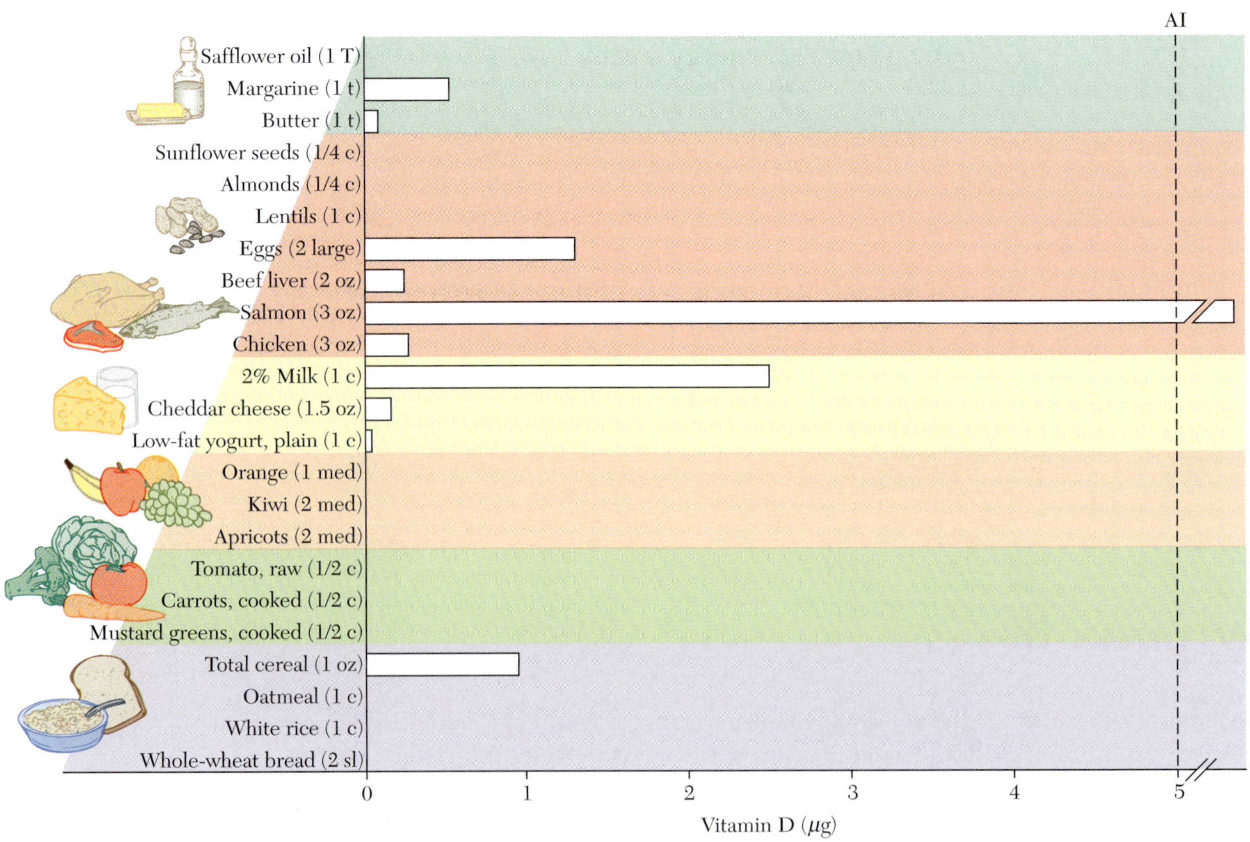

FIGURE 10.6 Vitamin D content of selections from each food group of the Food Guide Pyramid. The dashed line represents the AI for adults 19 through 50 years of age. Only a few foods, such as salmon and eggs, are natural sources of vitamin D; others are fortified with the vitamin.

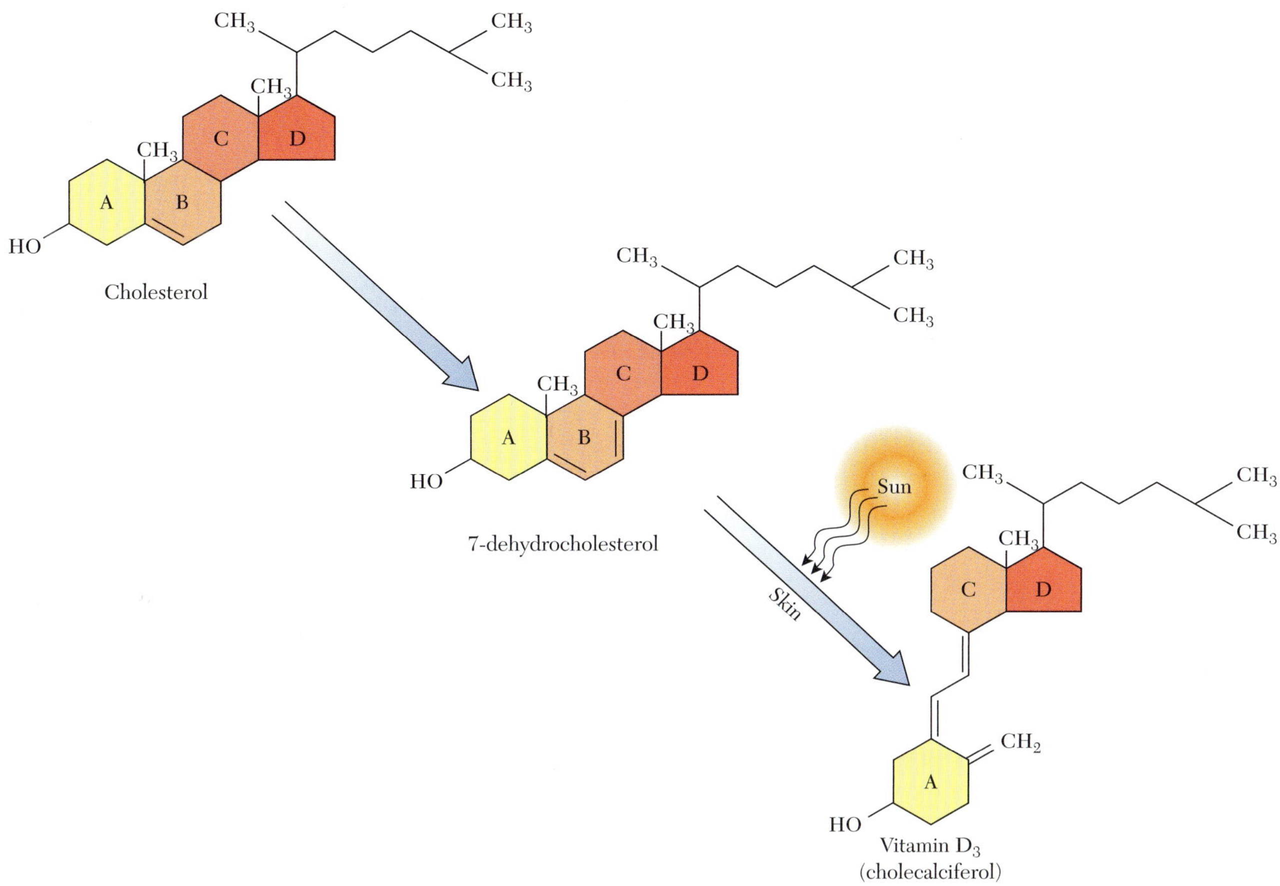

FIGURE 10.7 In the body, 7-dehydrocholesterol can be made from cholesterol and vitamin D_3 (cholecalciferol) can be formed by the action of sunlight on 7-deyhydrocholesterol in the skin.

Active vitamin D regulates calcium and phosphorus balance by altering gene expression in cells at the intestine and bone. At the intestine, vitamin D increases the absorption of calcium and phosphorus because it increases the expression of genes that code for intestinal calcium transport proteins. The mechanism whereby vitamin D affects gene expression is similar to that of vitamin A (see Figure 10.4). At the bone, vitamin D works in conjunction with PTH to increase bone breakdown, releasing calcium and phosphorus into the blood. This occurs because vitamin D causes precursor cells in the bone to differentiate into cells that break down bone.[11] Vitamin D also acts with PTH to increase the amount of calcium retained by the kidneys. Receptors for active vitamin D have been found not only in the bone, intestine, and kidney, but also in the pancreas, parathyroid gland, immune system cells, reproductive organs, and skin.[12] The effect of vitamin D in these tissues is under investigation.

Recommended Intakes

The recommended intake for vitamin D is based on the amount needed in the diet to maintain normal blood levels of 25-hydroxy vitamin D_3. The AI for adults is set at 5 μg per day.[13] The AI is expressed in μg, but the vitamin D content of foods and supplements may also be given as International Units (IUs); one IU is equal to 0.025 μg of vitamin D_3 (40 IU = 1 μg of vitamin D). The AI for vitamin D for adults can be obtained by consuming about 2 cups of vitamin D–fortified milk (see Figure 10.6 and Table 10.1).

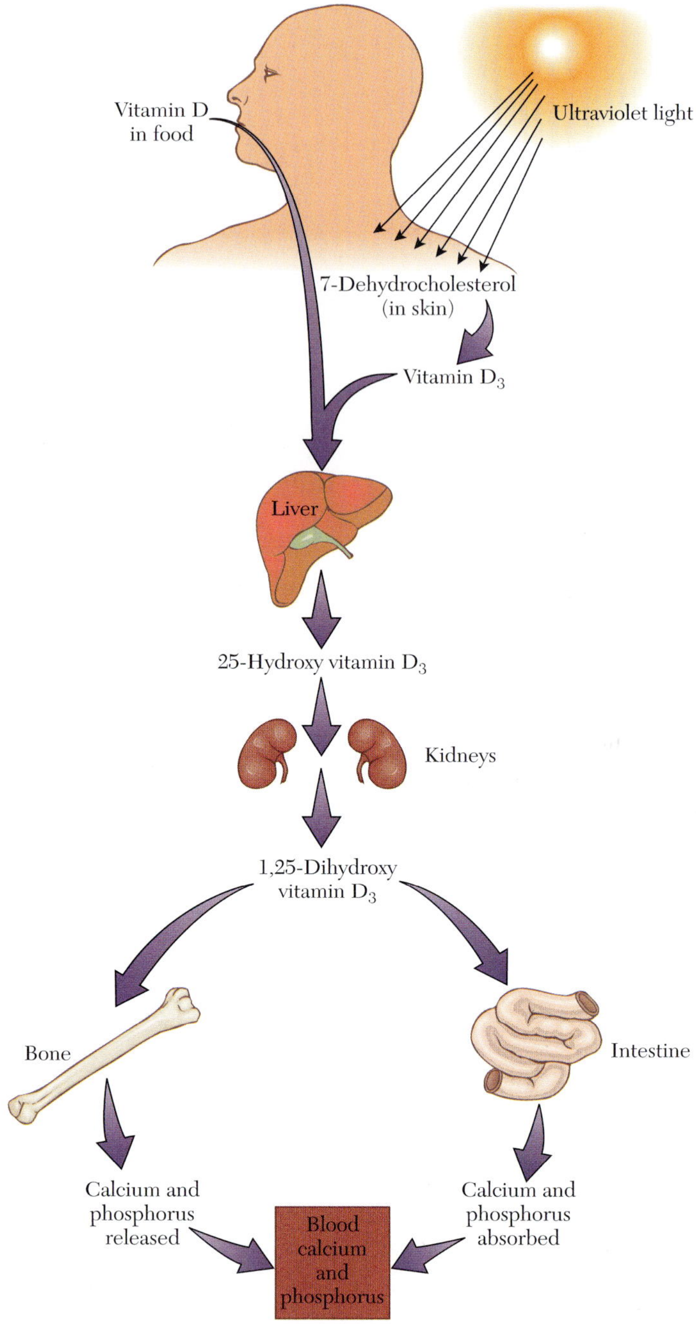

FIGURE 10.8 Vitamin D comes from food and from synthesis in the skin. In order to function, it must have hydroxyl groups (OH) added by chemical reactions that occur in the liver and kidney. Active vitamin D then functions in maintaining calcium and phosphorus balance by stimulating the release of these minerals from bone and their absorption from the intestine.

The AI is based on the assumption that no vitamin D is synthesized in the skin. This assumption is made because of the variation in the extent to which synthesis from sunlight meets the requirement. If there is sufficient sun exposure, dietary vitamin D is not needed. Skin pigmentation, climate, season, clothing, the presence of pollution and tall buildings that block sunlight, and the use of sunscreens all affect the amount synthesized in the skin. Although sunscreens prevent the formation of vitamin D in the skin, children and active adults usually spend enough time outdoors without sunscreens to provide their vitamin D requirement.

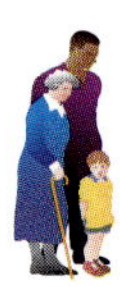

Despite the smaller body size of infants and children, the AI for vitamin D for this age is the same as that for adults. This is to allow for sufficient vitamin D for bone development during periods of rapid growth. Although breast milk is low in vitamin D, infants who are exposed to sunlight for about a half-hour per day do not require supplemental vitamin D. The AI for adults 50 to 70 years of age is increased to 10 μg per day to prevent bone loss during periods of low sun exposure. In adults 70 and older the AI is further increased to 15 μg per day to maintain blood levels of vitamin D and prevent skeletal fractures. The AIs for pregnancy and lactation are not increased above young adult levels.

Vitamin D and Health

Vitamin D is essential for bone health. A deficiency causes improper bone development in children and weakened bones in adults. However, too much vitamin D can be toxic.

Vitamin D Deficiency When vitamin D is deficient, dietary calcium cannot be absorbed efficiently. As a result, calcium is not available for proper bone mineralization, and abnormalities in bone structure occur.

Children who are deficient in vitamin D have weak bones because they do not contain enough calcium and phosphorus. This syndrome, called **rickets,** is characterized by short stature and bone deformities such as narrow rib cages (known as pigeon breasts), enlargement of the joints, and bowed legs. The legs bow because the bones are too weak to support the weight of the body (Figure 10.9). Even though the fortification of milk with vitamin D has helped to greatly reduce rickets in most developed countries, it is still a problem in children who have a poor diet and whose exposure to sunlight is limited, particularly during the winter months.[14] Dark-skinned children are more likely to be vitamin D–deficient than those with lighter skin because dark skin pigment prevents the UV light rays from penetrating into the dermis of the skin, thereby reducing the formation of vitamin D. Rickets is also seen in children with disorders that affect fat absorption and in vegetarian children who do not drink milk.

Rickets A vitamin D deficiency disease in children that is characterized by poor bone development due to inadequate calcium deposition.

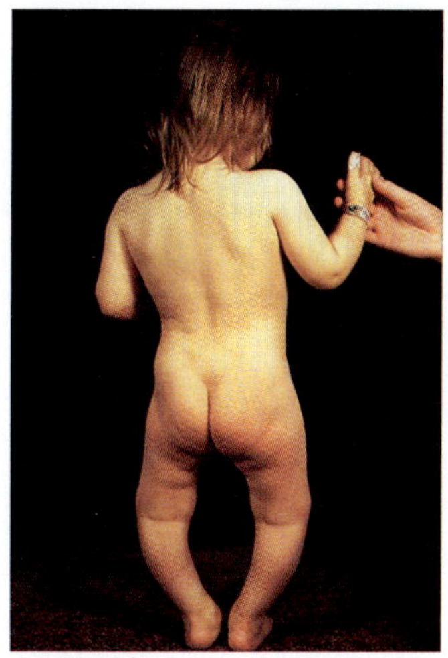

FIGURE 10.9 Bowed legs are characteristic of rickets. *(© Biophoto Associates/Photo Researchers, Inc.)*

In adults, the disease comparable to rickets is called **osteomalacia.** Because bone growth is complete in adults, the bone deformities characteristic of rickets are not seen with osteomalacia, but it does result in the weakening of bones because not enough calcium is available to form the mineral deposits needed to maintain healthy bone. Osteomalacia is characterized by an increase in the amount of nonmineralized bone, which leads to fractures of weight-bearing bones such as those in the hips and spine. This is not to be confused with a condition called osteoporosis, a more common cause of fractures, which is due to a loss of total bone mass (not just minerals) and is discussed in Chapter 12.

Osteomalacia is common in adults with kidney failure because the conversion of vitamin D from the inactive to the active form is reduced. The elderly are also at risk for vitamin D deficiency because the ability to produce vitamin D in the skin decreases with age, and older adults typically cover more of their skin with clothing and spend less time in the sun than their younger counterparts.[15] In addition, the elderly tend to have a lower intake of dairy products. In a study of postmenopausal women, 50% of those with hip fractures were found to have deficient levels of vitamin D, suggesting that low vitamin D status could be contributing to bone loss in postmenopausal women.[16]

Osteomalacia A vitamin D deficiency disease in adults characterized by a loss of minerals from the bone matrix. It causes weak bones and increases the likelihood of bone fractures.

Vitamin D Toxicity and Supplements Consumption of natural food sources of vitamin D does not cause toxicity. And, synthesis of vitamin D from exposure to sunlight does not produce toxic amounts because vitamin D formation is carefully regulated by the body. However, oversupplementation and overfortification do pose a risk. One case of accidental overfortification of milk resulted in the hospitalization of 56 individuals and the deaths of two.[17] Symptoms of vitamin D toxicity include high calcium concentrations in the blood and urine, deposition of calcium in soft tissues such as the blood vessels and kidney, and cardiovascular damage. A UL of 50 μg has been established for adults.

Vitamin K

Coagulation The process of blood clotting.

Vitamin K is one of the few vitamins about which extravagant claims are not made. Like the other fat-soluble vitamins, it was discovered inadvertently by feeding animals a fat-free diet. In this case, researchers in Denmark noted that chicks fed such a diet developed a type of bleeding disorder that was cured by feeding them a fat-soluble extract from green plants. Vitamin K was named for *koagulation,* the Danish word for **coagulation,** or blood clotting.

Forms and Sources of Vitamin K

Phylloquinone Originally called vitamin K_1. The form of vitamin K found in plants.

Menaquinones Originally called vitamin K_2. The forms of vitamin K synthesized by bacteria and found in animals.

As with all the fat-soluble vitamins, vitamin K is found in several forms. **Phylloquinone** is the form found in plants and the primary dietary form of vitamin K. A group of vitamin K compounds, called **menaquinones,** are found in fish oils and meats and are synthesized by bacteria, including those in the human intestine. Menaquinones are the form used in supplements.

Only a relatively small number of foods provide significant amounts of vitamin K. The best dietary sources are liver and leafy green vegetables such as spinach, broccoli, Brussels sprouts, kale, and turnip greens. These leafy green vegetables provide 40 to 50% of the vitamin K in the typical American diet.[18] Certain vegetable oils, such as soybean, cottonseed, canola, and olive oil, are also good sources. Milk, meats, eggs, and cereals contain smaller amounts (Figure 10.10). Some of the vitamin K produced by bacteria in the human gastrointestinal tract is also absorbed. Vitamin K is destroyed by exposure to light and low- or high-acid conditions.

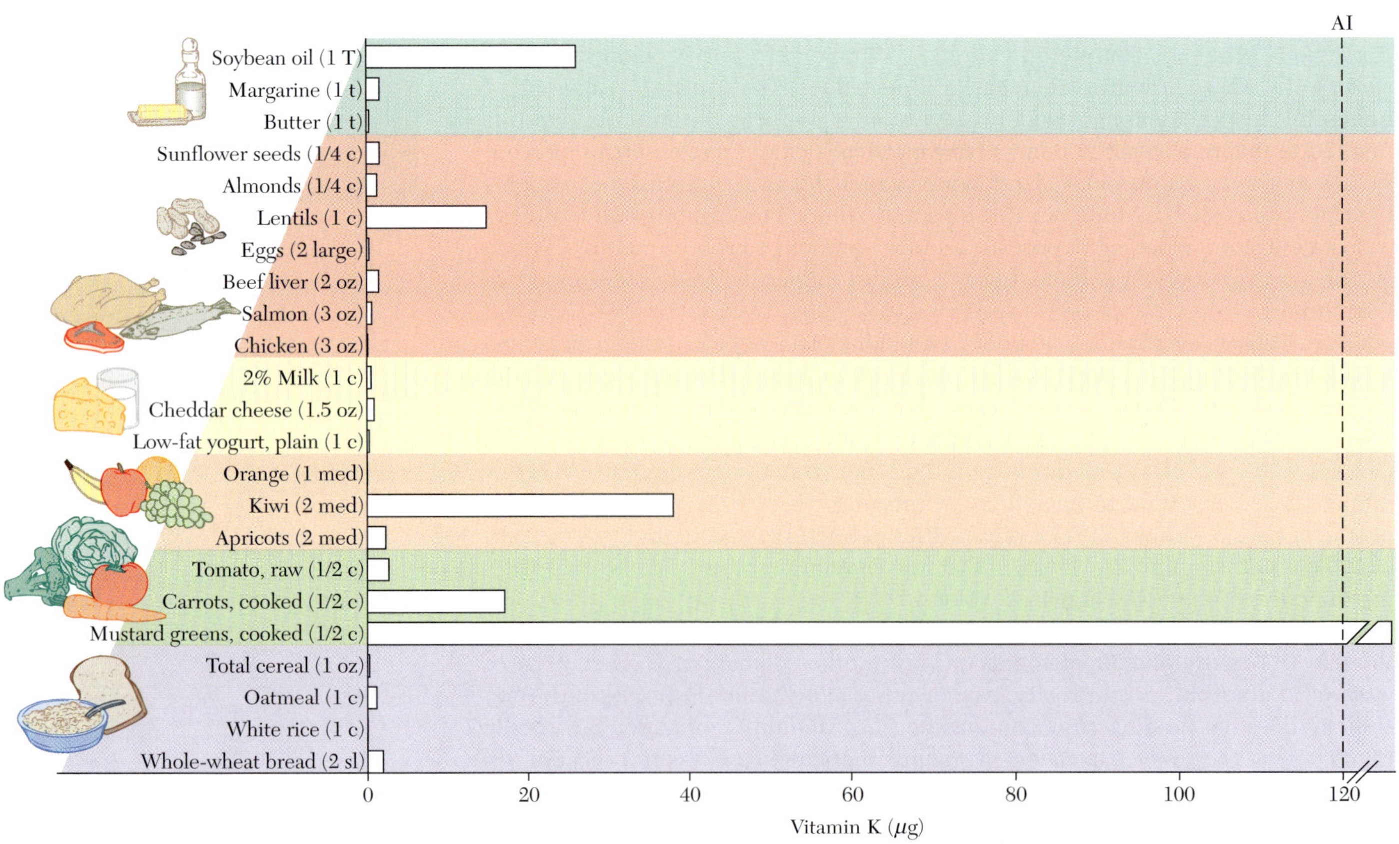

FIGURE 10.10 Vitamin K content of selections from each food group of the Food Guide Pyramid. The dashed line represents the AI for adult men. The best sources of vitamin K are leafy green vegetables and some plant oils.

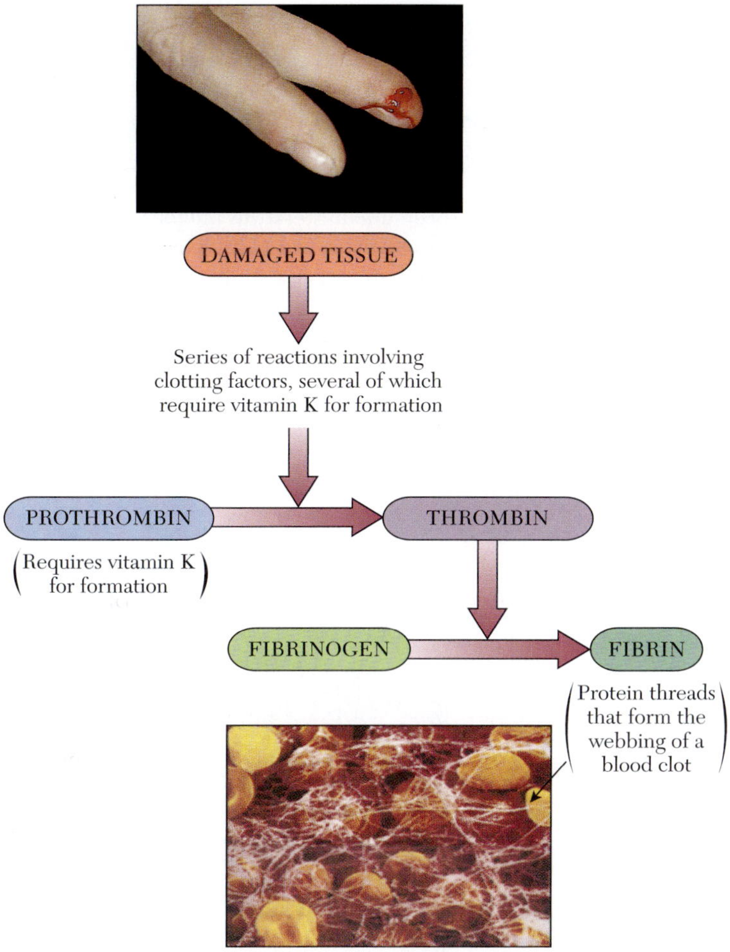

FIGURE 10.11 For a blood clot to form, clotting factors must be activated. Several clotting factors, including prothrombin, require vitamin K for synthesis. Without them, fibrinogen cannot be converted into its active form, fibrin, which is a structural component of blood clots. *(top, © Amethyst/Custom Medical Stock Photo; bottom, CNRI/Science Photo Library/Custom Medical Stock Photo)*

Vitamin K in the Body

Vitamin K is needed for the production of the blood-clotting protein **prothrombin** and other specific blood-clotting factors. These proteins are needed to produce fibrin, the protein that forms the structure of a blood clot (Figure 10.11). Injuries, as well as the normal wear and tear of daily living, produce microscopic tears in blood vessels. To prevent blood loss, these tears must be repaired with blood clots. Other roles for vitamin K are less well understood. For example, there are several vitamin K–dependent proteins in bone that may be involved in bone mineralization and demineralization.[19]

Prothrombin A blood protein required for blood clotting.

Recommended Intakes

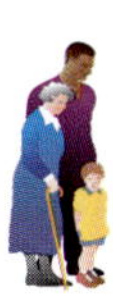

Unlike other fat-soluble vitamins, vitamin K is used rapidly by the body, so a constant supply is necessary. The DRI committee determined that there is not sufficient data to set an RDA for vitamin K. An AI of 120 μg per day for adult men and 90 μg/day for adult women has been established based on the amounts consumed by apparently healthy populations (see Table 10.1).[2] The typical dietary intakes in North America are close to this, but many individuals fail to meet this level on a daily basis.[20] Bacteria in the gastrointestinal tract provide additional vitamin K. Although the form produced by intestinal bacteria is less well absorbed than that from plant sources and is not alone sufficient to meet vitamin K needs, it is an important source of this vitamin. No increase is recommended for pregnant or lactating women or older adults. The AI for infants was determined based on the amount of the vitamin consumed by average healthy breast-fed infants.

RESEARCH DISCOVERIES

Cows, Clover, and Coagulation

One snowy night in 1933, a disgruntled farmer delivered a bale of moldy clover hay, a pail of unclotted blood, and a dead cow to the laboratory of Dr. Carl Link at the University of Wisconsin. Link, the University's first professor of biochemistry, was already making a name for himself in the scientific community when he was presented with the farmer's challenge to speed the typically deliberate pace of research. Why were his cows dying? What could he do to stop the bleeding disease that was killing them? Link had just begun to research hemorrhagic sweet clover disease, the condition that was killing the farmer's cows, but at the time the only advice he could offer was to find alternative feed and try blood transfusions to save the other animals. Link and his colleagues began a line of inquiry that ultimately led to the development of an anti-blood-clotting factor that today saves the lives of hundreds of thousands of people.

In the 1930s, hemorrhagic sweet clover disease was killing cows across the Midwestern prairies of the United States and Canada. It occurred in cattle that were fed moldy, spoiled, sweet clover hay. These animals died because their blood did not clot. Even a minor scratch from a barbed wire fence could be fatal; once bleeding began, it did not stop. Six years after the farmer's challenge, Link and colleagues had isolated the anticoagulant dicumarol from moldy clover. Dicumarol is a derivative of coumarin, which gives clover its sweet scent; mold converts coumarin to dicumarol. Cows fed moldy clover consume dicumarol, which interferes with vitamin K activity and consequently prevents normal blood clotting.

The discovery of dicumarol enhanced our understanding of the blood-clotting mechanism and led to the development of anticoagulant drugs. These drugs help eliminate blood clots and prevent their formation. In carefully regulated doses, they are used to treat heart attacks, which occur when blood clots block one or more of the vessels in and leading to the heart. Dicumarol, first synthesized in 1940, was the first anticoagulant that could be administered orally to humans. Further work with dicumarol led Link to propose the use of a more potent derivative, called warfarin, as rat poison. When rats consume the odorless, colorless warfarin, their blood fails to clot, and they bleed to death. Warfarin was used as a rodenticide for nearly a decade before it was introduced into clinical medicine in 1954. Sodium warfarin soon became the most widely prescribed anticoagulant drug in the nation. In 1955 President Dwight D. Eisenhower was treated with sodium warfarin after suffering a heart attack.

Sodium warfarin and dicumarol have been administered to millions of patients to prevent blood clots, which, by causing heart attacks and strokes, are the number one cause of death in this country. It is ironic that a substance that killed hundreds of cattle across the Great Plains and that efficiently kills rodents in our homes has saved so many human lives.

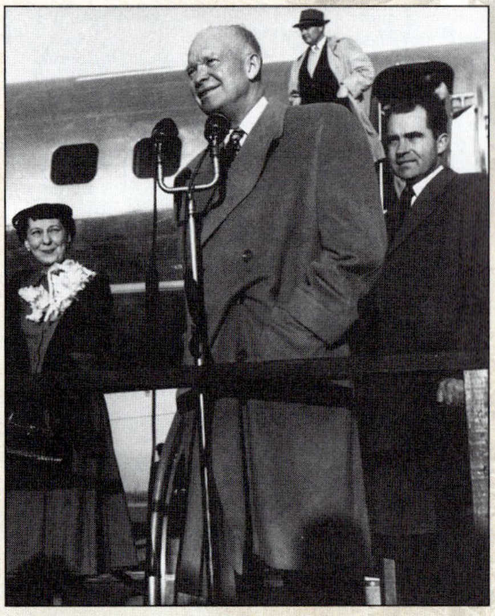

President Eisenhower suffered a heart attack in September 1955. His recovery was aided by treatment with the anticoagulant sodium warfarin. In November of the following year he was elected to his second term.

Vitamin K and Health

The inability to form blood clots due to vitamin K deficiency or drugs that interfere with vitamin K activity can cause death from excess blood loss. Conversely, drugs that inhibit blood from clotting by interfering with vitamin K activity can save lives by preventing the blood clots that cause heart attacks and strokes (see *Research Discoveries:* "Cows, Clover, and Coagulation").

Vitamin K Deficiency Abnormal blood coagulation is the major symptom of vitamin K deficiency. A deficiency is very rare in the healthy adult population, but it may result from fat malabsorption syndromes or the long-term use of antibiotics, which can kill the bacteria in the gastrointestinal tract that are a source of the vitamin. In combination with an illness that reduces the dietary intake of vitamin K, this may precipitate a deficiency. Injections of vitamin K are typically administered before surgery to aid in blood clotting.

Vitamin K deficiency is most common in newborns. There is little transfer of this vitamin from mother to fetus, and because the infant gut is free of bacteria, none is made there. Further, breast milk is low in vitamin K. Therefore, to prevent uncontrolled bleeding, infants are typically given a vitamin K injection within 6 hours of birth.

Vitamin K Toxicity and Supplements A UL has not been set for vitamin K because there are no well-documented reports of adverse effects. This is based on reports that considered intakes of up to 370 μg/day from food or supplements. But because vitamin K functions in blood clotting, high doses can interfere with prescribed **anticoagulant** drugs. Therefore, individuals taking these medications are advised to consult their physicians before using supplements containing vitamin K.

Anticoagulant A substance that delays or prevents blood coagulation.

ANTIOXIDANTS

Oxygen is needed in the body for energy production, but some of this inhaled oxygen can form reactive molecules such as **free radicals,** which contain unpaired electrons. Free radicals of oxygen include the superoxide radical, the hydroxyl radical, and peroxyl radicals. Other reactive oxygen species that are not free radicals include singlet oxygen and hydrogen peroxide. There are also free radicals of nitrogen, carbon, and sulfur that can form and damage cells. Free radicals and other reactive molecules are generated by metabolic reactions inside the body and come from environmental sources such as air pollution and cigarette smoke. If these reactive compounds are not neutralized, they can snatch electrons from DNA, proteins, carbohydrates, or unsaturated fatty acids, causing changes in the structure and function of these molecules. These changes, which can interrupt normal body processes, are referred to as **oxidative damage.** It is hypothesized that the cumulative effect of oxidative damage plays a role in the aging process and in the development of chronic diseases. **Antioxidants** help neutralize highly reactive molecules before they can do damage. There are a number of nutrients that have antioxidant functions in the body.

Free radical A type of highly reactive molecule that contains an atom with an unpaired electron. Many of these cause damage to biological molecules.

Oxidative damage Damage caused by highly reactive oxygen molecules that steal electrons from other compounds, causing changes in structure and function.

Antioxidants Substances that are able to neutralize reactive molecules and hence reduce the amount of oxidative damage that occurs.

Antioxidants, Pro-Oxidants, and Health

The body is equipped with many types of antioxidant defenses to protect against oxidative damage. Some of these are vitamins or vitamin precursors—vitamin C, vitamin E, and β-carotene. Others are enzymes—catalase, glutathione peroxidase, and superoxide dismutase, which rely on minerals such as zinc, iron, and selenium for activity. Each acts under specific conditions at specific locations inside the body to destroy particular types of reactive compounds (Figure 10.12). Some directly destroy damaging free radicals while others neutralize superoxide radicals or hydrogen peroxide before they can form more reactive compounds. Vitamin C can inactivate free radicals, singlet oxygen, and hydrogen peroxide. Vitamin E and β-carotene can inactivate free radicals in lipid membranes. Selenium is a part of the antioxidant enzyme glutathione peroxidase, which neutralizes peroxides before they can form dangerous free radicals. The molecule glutathione, which is made of three amino acids, plays an antioxidant role by participating in this reaction and by helping to regenerate vitamin C. Catalase is an iron-containing enzyme that can also destroy peroxides. Zinc, copper, and manganese are necessary for forms of the enzyme superoxide dismutase, which destroys superoxide radicals.

Several antioxidants typically work together to protect cellular molecules. For example, the enzyme superoxide dismutase converts superoxide radicals into hydrogen peroxide. Other antioxidants are then needed to eliminate the hydrogen peroxide before it causes damage.

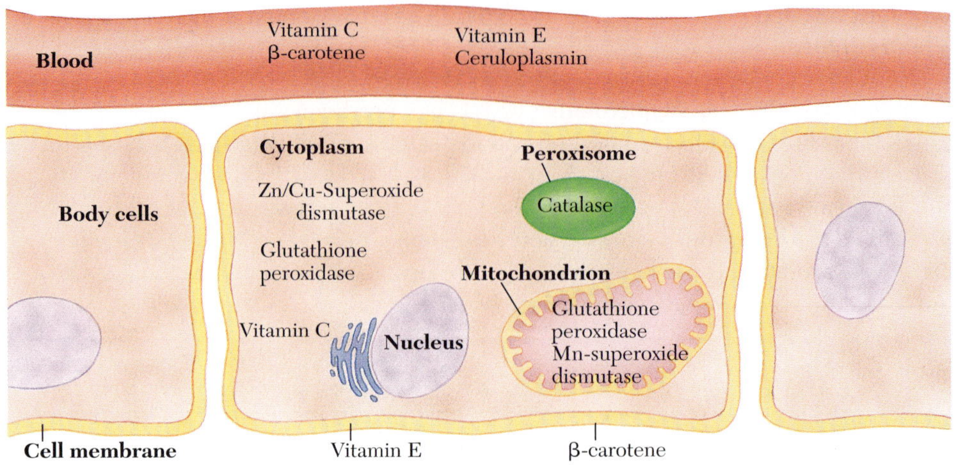

FIGURE 10.12 Antioxidants act at specific locations inside the body or cell. Antioxidant enzymes are located primarily inside cells, where each functions in a specific cellular compartment. For example, zinc/copper-superoxide dismutase and glutathione peroxidase act in the cytoplasm, along with vitamin C. Glutathione peroxidase also functions inside the mitochondria, along with manganese-superoxide dismutase. Catalase acts inside another organelle, the peroxisome. Vitamin E and β-carotene are fat-soluble nutrients that protect cell membranes. Vitamin C, vitamin E, and the copper-containing protein ceruloplasmin function outside the cells by inactivating free radicals circulating in the blood and body fluids

Pro-oxidants Substances that promote oxidative damage.

Oxidative stress A condition that occurs when there are more reactive oxygen molecules than can be neutralized by available antioxidant defenses. It occurs either because excessive amounts of reactive oxygen molecules are generated or because antioxidant defenses are deficient.

If the body's antioxidant defense mechanisms become overwhelmed by **pro-oxidants, oxidative stress** results. Sometimes a cell in oxidative stress adapts and increases the production of antioxidant defenses, making it more resistant. If the stress is too great or lasts too long, oxidative damage to DNA, proteins, carbohydrates, and lipids occurs and cell death or tissue damage can result. DNA damage is hypothesized to be a major reason for the increase in cancer incidence that occurs with age. Damage to proteins can alter the activity of enzymes and interfere with other protein functions. Damage to large carbohydrate molecules, such as those in connective tissue, can decrease the amount of material that cushions joints, contributing to arthritis.[21] And free radical damage to lipoproteins and lipids in membranes is implicated in the development of atherosclerosis.[22]

Dietary Antioxidants

Dietary antioxidant A substance in food that significantly decreases the adverse effects of reactive species, such as reactive oxygen and nitrogen species, on normal physiological function in humans.

The DRIs have defined a **dietary antioxidant** as a substance present in the diet that decreases the adverse effects of reactive species, such as free radicals, in the living human body.[23] It was concluded that vitamin C (a water-soluble vitamin), vitamin E (a fat-soluble vitamin), and the mineral selenium (see Chapter 13) met these criteria as well as providing other functions. Beta-carotene and other carotenoids were considered for inclusion in this group because they act as antioxidants in the laboratory and influence biochemical reactions that involve the oxidative process. However, it was concluded that they do not fit the definition of a dietary antioxidant because the evidence that they decrease the adverse effects of reactive species in the living body is not strong enough. No quantitative recommendations have been made for β-carotene and other carotenoids discussed by the DRI report.

Vitamin E: A Fat-Soluble Antioxidant

Tocopherol The chemical name for vitamin E.

Vitamin E is a fat-soluble vitamin with an antioxidant function. It was first identified as a fat-soluble component of grains that was necessary for fertility in laboratory rats. It took almost 30 years to isolate this vitamin and to determine that it is also necessary for reproduction in humans. The chemical name for vitamin E, **tocopherol,** is from the Greek *tos,* meaning childbirth, and *phero,* to bring forth.

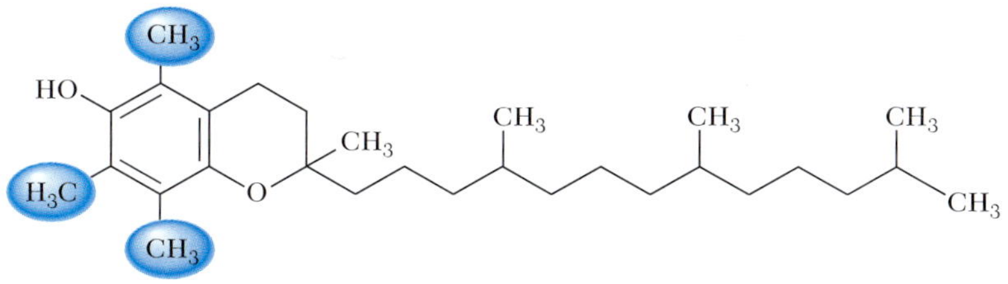

FIGURE 10.13 The structure of α-tocopherol. The structure of other tocopherols (β-tocopherol, γ-tocopherol, and δ-tocopherol) are similar, but one or more of the $-CH_3$ groups highlighted in blue is replaced with a hydrogen atom.

Vitamin E has been promoted as a cure for infertility, an antiscar medication, a defense against air pollution, and a fountain of youth.

Forms of Vitamin E

There are several naturally occurring forms of vitamin E in food, but only the **alpha-tocopherol (α-tocopherol)** form can meet vitamin E requirements in humans (Figure 10.13). The other forms do not meet vitamin E needs because they are not converted to α-tocopherol in humans and cannot be transported by the α-tocopherol transfer protein.

Alpha-tocopherol (α-tocopherol) The only form of tocopherol that provides vitamin E activity in humans.

There are also differences between naturally occurring α-tocopherol and the synthetic form found in dietary supplements and fortified foods. Synthetic α-tocopherol is composed of eight different **isomers.** Only half of these appear in the bloodstream after consumption and so are considered active in the body. Therefore, synthetic α-tocopherol provides half of the biological activity of natural α-tocopherol; 10 mg of synthetic α-tocopherol provides the function of 5 mg of natural α-tocopherol.

Isomers Molecules with the same molecular formula but a different arrangement of molecular groups.

The determination that only the alpha form of tocopherol provides vitamin activity is relatively recent. Prior to this finding, all forms of tocopherol were included in calculations of vitamin E content. Vitamin E content used to be expressed as either International Units (IUs) or α-tocopherol equivalents (α-TEs). An IU is defined as 1 mg of synthetic α-tocopherol. Alpha-TEs are based on an analysis done in rats that found some forms of tocopherol had biological activity that could be expressed as a fraction of that found in α-tocopherol. Most nutrient databases and nutrition labels still use these older units and may therefore overrepresent the amount of functional vitamin E in foods. Equations for converting IUs and α-TEs into mg of α-tocopherol are provided in Table 10.3.

TABLE 10.3 Converting Vitamin E Values into mg α-Tocopherol

To estimate the α-tocopherol intake from foods:

- If values are given as mg α-TEs:

$$\text{mg } \alpha\text{-TE} \times 0.8^{*} = \text{mg } \alpha\text{-tocopherol}$$

- If values are given as IUs:

  First, determine if the source of the α-tocopherol is natural or synthetic.

  - For natural α-tocopherol:

$$\text{IU of natural } \alpha\text{-tocopherol} \times 0.67 = \text{mg } \alpha\text{-tocopherol}$$

  - For synthetic α-tocopherol (dl-α-tocopherol):

$$\text{IU of synthetic } \alpha\text{-tocopherol} \times 0.45 = \text{mg } \alpha\text{-tocopherol}$$

*Based on dietary data from the NHANES III study, approximately 80% of the α-tocopherol equivalents from food are from α-tocopherol and can thus contribute to the body's requirement for vitamin E.

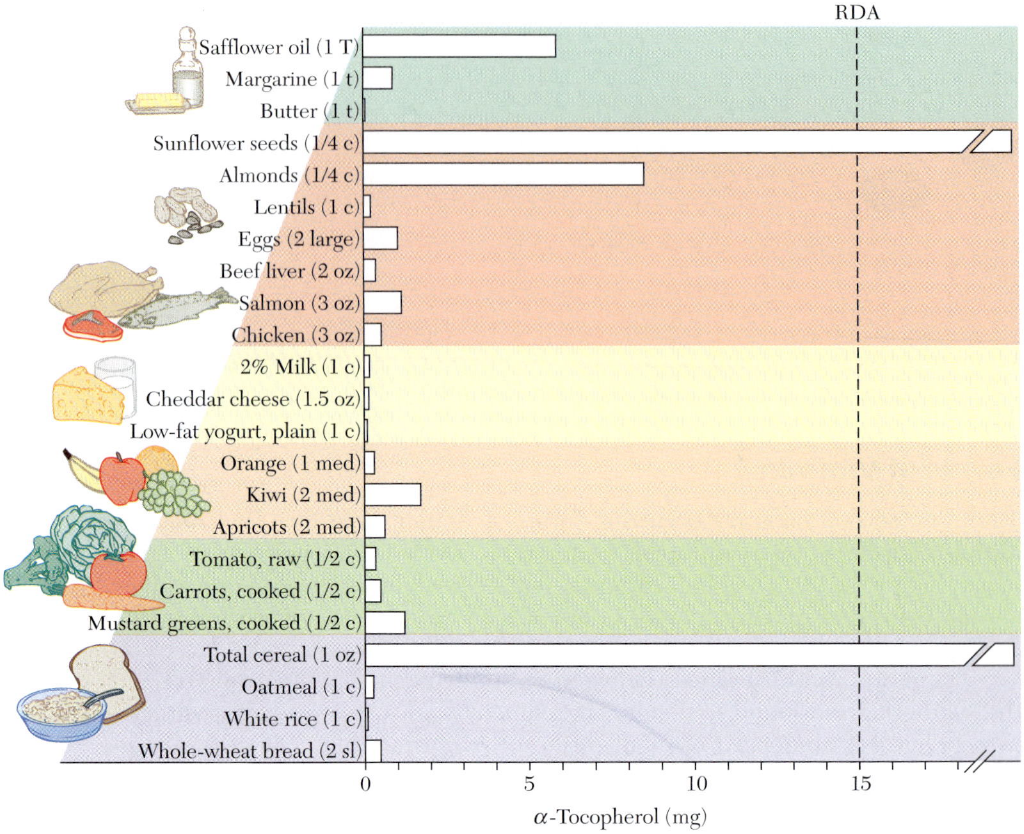

FIGURE 10.14 Vitamin E content of selections from each food group of the Food Guide Pyramid. The dashed line represents the RDA for adults. Vitamin E is found in plant oils, nuts and seeds, leafy green vegetables, and fortified cereals.

Sources of Vitamin E

Dietary sources of vitamin E include nuts and peanuts; plant oils such as soybean, corn, and sunflower oils; leafy green vegetables; wheat germ; and fortified breakfast cereals (Figure 10.14). Vitamin E is listed on some food labels, but its inclusion is not required.

Because vitamin E is sensitive to destruction by oxygen, metals, light, and heat, some is lost during food processing, cooking, and storage. Although it is relatively stable at normal cooking temperatures, the high temperatures used in deep-fat frying and repeated heating of the same oil tend to destroy most of the vitamin E.

Vitamin E in the Body

Vitamin E absorption depends on normal fat absorption. Once absorbed, vitamin E is incorporated into chylomicrons. As chylomicrons are broken down, some vitamin E is distributed to other lipoproteins and delivered to tissues, but most remains in chylomicron remnants. Vitamin E in chylomicron remnants is taken up by the liver, where α-tocopherol is incorporated into very-low-density lipoproteins (VLDLs) for release into the blood. The α-tocopherol in VLDLs is distributed to other plasma lipoproteins. Vitamin E is transferred to tissues from VLDLs with the help of lipoprotein lipase and from LDLs with the help of LDL receptors.

Vitamin E functions primarily as a fat-soluble antioxidant that neutralizes reactive oxygen compounds before they damage unsaturated fatty acids in cell membranes (Figure 10.15). By protecting cell membranes, vitamin E is important

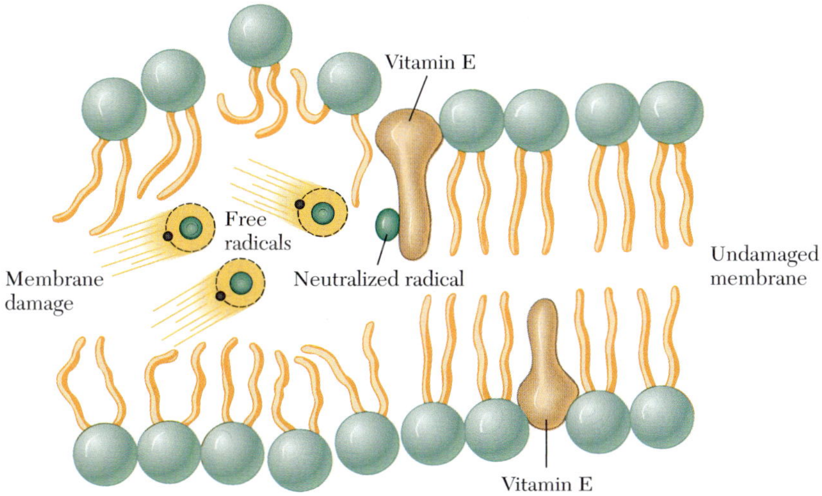

FIGURE 10.15 Vitamin E functions as an antioxidant that neutralizes free radicals, thereby protecting the unsaturated fatty acids in cell membranes.

in maintaining the integrity of red blood cells, cells in nervous tissue, and cells of the immune system. It can defend these cells from damage by heavy metals, such as lead and mercury, and from toxins, such as carbon tetrachloride, benzene, and a variety of drugs. It also protects against some environmental pollutants such as ozone. Because polyunsaturated fats are particularly susceptible to oxidative damage, the requirement for vitamin E increases as the polyunsaturated fat content of the diet increases. After vitamin E donates electrons to neutralize free radicals, its antioxidant function can be restored by vitamin C (Figure 10.16).

Vitamin E may also help reduce the risk of heart disease. As an antioxidant, it inhibits LDL oxidation in cells grown in the laboratory.[24] In addition, vitamin E has other biological actions that may affect the risk of heart disease. For example, it inhibits the activity of an enzyme called protein kinase C, which is needed for the proliferation and differentiation of smooth muscle cells, platelets, and white blood cells—all of which are involved in the formation of atherosclerotic plaque.[23] Vitamin E has also been shown to reduce the synthesis of molecules that cause cells to stick to the lining of blood vessels and to increase the synthesis of enzymes needed for the production of eicosanoids, hormone-like molecules that help lower blood pressure and reduce blood clot formation.[23,25,26]

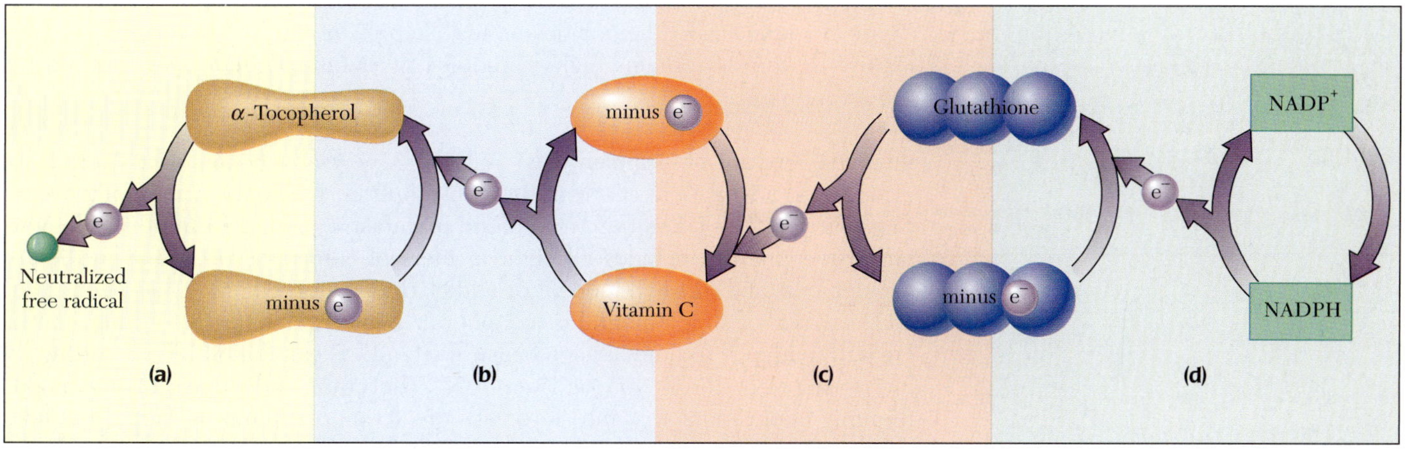

FIGURE 10.16 (a) Vitamin E neutralizes free radicals by donating electrons. Then vitamin E must be regenerated to restore it to the form that can act as an antioxidant. (b) This regeneration requires vitamin C, which acts as an electron donor to restore vitamin E to its original form. (c) Vitamin C is then regenerated by picking up an electron from the antioxidant molecule glutathione. (d) Glutathione then picks up an electron from NADPH, an active coenzyme form of niacin.

Recommended Intakes

Because of the importance of vitamin E in protecting red blood cell membranes, the criteria of adequacy used to establish an RDA for vitamin E is the level of plasma α-tocopherol that protects red blood cells from breaking. This is measured by exposing cells to hydrogen peroxide in the laboratory. The RDA for α-tocopherol for adult men and women is set at 15 mg/day. The RDA does not change with advancing age.

For infants, an AI for vitamin E has been set based on the amount consumed by infants fed principally with human milk. EARs and RDAs for children and adolescents have been estimated from adult values.

There are no reports of vitamin E deficiency during pregnancy, and supplementation with vitamin E does not prevent deficiency in premature offspring. Therefore, the RDA for pregnancy is not increased above nonpregnant levels. To estimate the requirement for lactation, the amount secreted in human milk is added to the requirement for nonlactating women.

Vitamin E and Health

Although vitamin E deficiency is uncommon, supplements claim to grow hair; restore, maintain, or increase sexual potency and fertility; alleviate fatigue; maintain immune function; enhance athletic performance; reduce the symptoms of PMS and menopause; slow aging; prevent heart disease and cancer; and treat a host of other medical problems.

Vitamin E Deficiency Vitamin E deficiency is rare because vitamin E is plentiful in the food supply and is stored in many of the body's tissues. Deficiencies have been identified in premature infants and in individuals with protein energy malnutrition, fat malabsorption, or genetic abnormalities in the α-tocopherol transfer protein. Because vitamin E protects membranes, a deficiency causes membrane changes. Red blood cells and nerves are particularly susceptible. In individuals with cystic fibrosis, a condition that reduces fat absorption, deficiency can develop rapidly, causing serious neurological problems that, if untreated, can become permanent.

All newborn infants have low blood tocopherol levels because there is little transfer of vitamin E from mother to fetus until the last weeks of pregnancy. The levels are lower in premature infants who are born before much vitamin E is transferred from the mother. In these infants, ruptured red blood cells may cause a type of anemia called hemolytic anemia. To prevent this, infant formula for premature newborns contains higher amounts of vitamin E than does formula for full-term infants.

Vitamin E Toxicity and Supplements Vitamin E is relatively nontoxic. There is no evidence of adverse effects from the consumption of vitamin E naturally occurring in foods. The UL is therefore based on intake from any form of supplementary α-tocopherol (includes all eight isomers of α-tocopherol) found in dietary supplements and fortified foods. For adults, the UL for vitamin E has been set at 1000 mg/day of supplemental α-tocopherol. Doses above this level cause an increased tendency to hemorrhage because vitamin E can inhibit blood clotting by interfering with the action of vitamin K. Therefore, individuals taking blood-thinning medications that interfere with the action of vitamin K should not take vitamin E supplements.

Vitamin E Supplements and Cardiovascular Disease In epidemiological studies, intakes of vitamin E greater than 100 IU per day have been associated with a reduced risk of heart disease in both men and women.[27,28] However, the results of human intervention trials that supplemented vitamin E are mixed. One study, which was done in patients with proven coronary artery disease, demonstrated a significant reduction in heart attacks.[29] In contrast, the Heart Outcomes Prevention Evaluation Study, which examined nearly 10,000 adults aged 55 years or older who were at high risk for heart attack or stroke, found that after 4 1/2 years there was no difference in the rate of stroke or heart attack between the control group and the group given vitamin E supplements.[30] Because the results of intervention trials are inconsistent, and because the association between vitamin E intake and heart disease observed in epidemiological studies may be due to substances in the diet other than vitamin E, additional studies are needed before vitamin E supplements can be recommended to the general public to decrease the risk of heart disease.

Vitamin C: A Water-Soluble Antioxidant

Vitamin C deficiency has been the scourge of armies, navies, and explorers throughout history. This deficiency, known as **scurvy,** was described by ancient Greeks, Egyptians, and Romans. In the mid-1500s, the Indians of eastern Canada knew that an extract from white cedar needles would cure the disease. In the 17th century, Sir Richard Hawkins observed on his voyage to the South Seas that this sickness could be cured by including citrus fruit in the diet. Despite his observation, 10,000 British sailors died of scurvy that same year. Over 100 years later, James Lind, a Scottish physician serving in the British navy, tested various agents for their effectiveness at curing scurvy and reported that two patients given citrus fruits recovered within six days. However, it was another 48 years before it was required that lime or lemon juice be included in the rations of the mercantile service, earning British sailors the name "limeys." Unfortunately, the rest of the world did not heed the lesson of the limeys. In the mid-19th century, during the American Civil War, scurvy was rampant.

Web Menu For more information on the history of vitamin C and scurvy, go to pc-78-120.udac.se:8001/WWW/Nautica/Medicine/Medicine.html.

C 62 00 00 00 00 00 27 76

Scurvy A vitamin C deficiency disease.

Sources of Vitamin C

Citrus fruits, such as oranges, lemons, and limes, are an excellent source of vitamin C. Other fruits that are high in vitamin C include strawberries and cantaloupe. Vegetables in the cabbage family, such as broccoli, cauliflower, bok choy, and Brussels sprouts, as well as green leafy vegetables, green and red peppers, okra, tomatoes, and potatoes, are good sources (Figure 10.17). Meat, fish, poultry, eggs, dairy products, and grains are poor sources. The amount of vitamin C in packaged foods must be listed on food labels as a percentage of the Daily Value. Vitamin C is unstable and is destroyed by oxygen, light, and heat, so it is readily lost in cooking. This loss is accelerated by contact with copper or iron cooking utensils and by low-acid conditions.

Vitamin C in the Body

Vitamin C, known as **ascorbate,** or **ascorbic acid,** is a water-soluble vitamin that donates electrons in biochemical reactions (Figure 10.18). Vitamin C also has a more general role as an antioxidant that protects the body from reactive oxygen molecules, helps maintain the immune system, and aids in the absorption of iron.

Ascorbate or **ascorbic acid** Chemical terms for vitamin C.

Reactions Requiring Vitamin C Many of the reactions requiring vitamin C add a hydroxyl group (OH) to other molecules. Two such reactions are essential for the formation of **collagen,** the protein that forms the base of all connective tissue in the body. The hydroxyl groups are necessary for the formation of chemical bonds

Collagen The major protein in connective tissue.

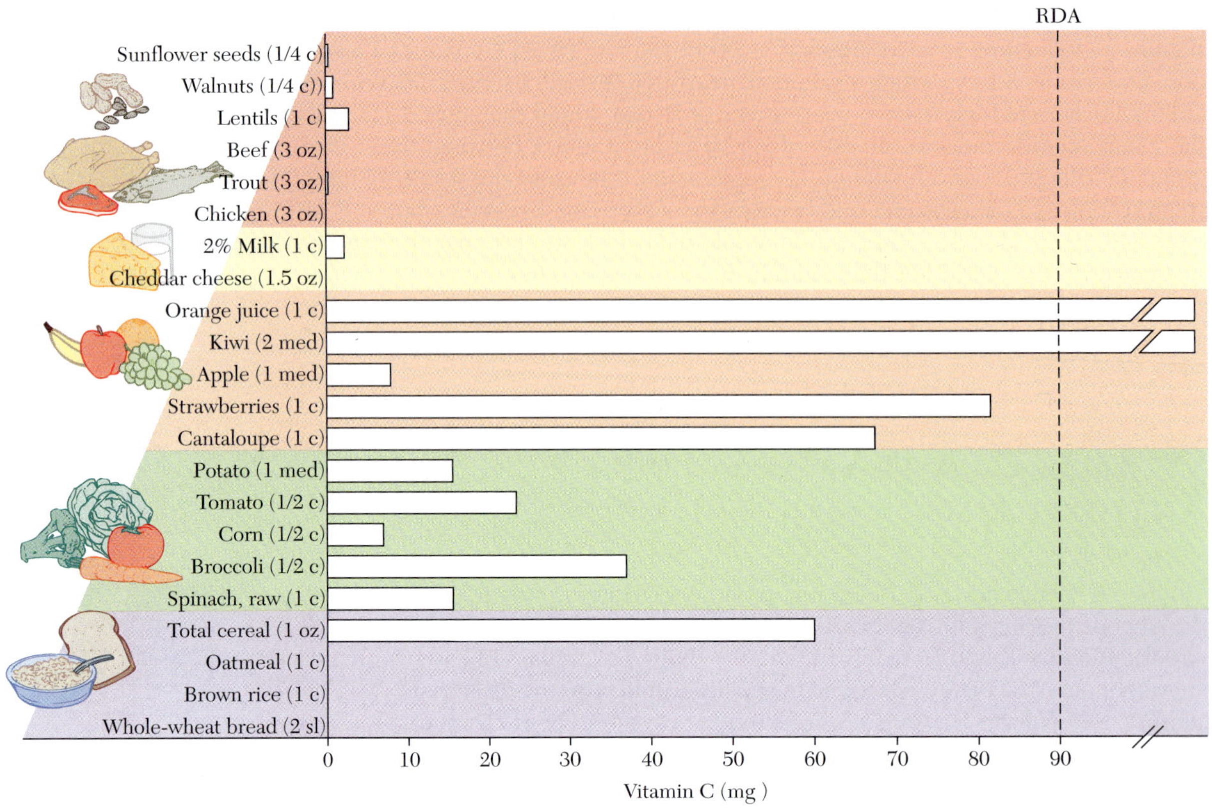

FIGURE 10.17 Vitamin C content of selections from each food group of the Food Guide Pyramid. The dashed line represents the RDA for adult men. Fruits and vegetables are the best sources of vitamin C.

that cross-link strands of collagen to give it strength (Figure 10.19). Vitamin C also serves in reactions needed for the synthesis of other compounds, including neurotransmitters, hormones such as the thyroid and steroid hormones, bile acids, and carnitine needed for fatty acid breakdown.

Vitamin C As an Antioxidant Vitamin C acts as an antioxidant in the blood and other body fluids. It can destroy superoxide radicals and other free radicals before they can damage lipids and DNA (Figure 10.20). Vitamin C has also been shown to scavenge reactive molecules in white blood cells, in the lung, and in the stomach mucosa.[23] The antioxidant properties of vitamin C also affect other nutrients. It regenerates the active antioxidant form of vitamin E (see Figure 10.16) and enhances iron absorption by keeping iron in its more readily absorbed form. When about 50 mg of vitamin C—the amount contained in 3.5 fluid ounces of orange juice—is consumed in a meal containing iron, iron absorption is enhanced (see Chapter 13).

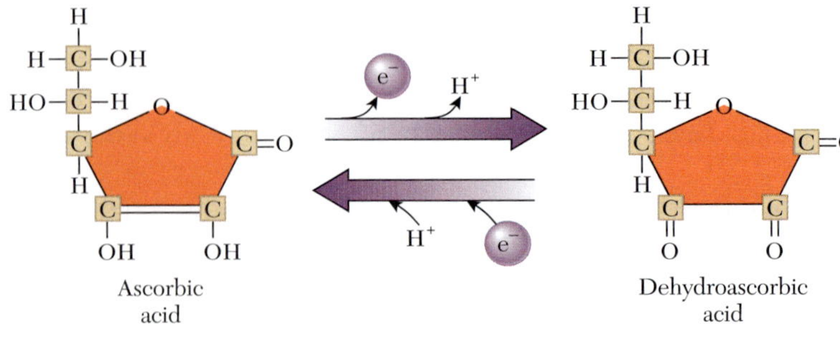

FIGURE 10.18 When ascorbic acid donates electrons and hydrogens in chemical reactions the structure changes to form a molecule of dehydroascorbic acid. This reaction is reversible and vitamin C can be restored by other antioxidants such as glutathione (see Figure 10.16).

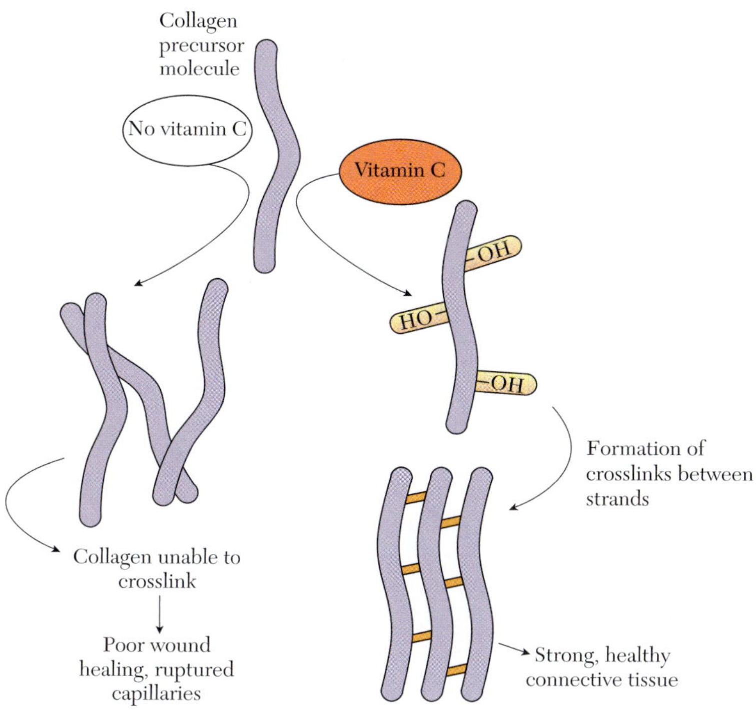

FIGURE 10.19 Vitamin C is needed for the formation of chemical bonds that link collagen molecules together to give connective tissue strength and stability.

Vitamin C may also act as a pro-oxidant by converting iron and copper to reduced forms that can then generate free radicals. There is some evidence that vitamin C supplements could lead to oxidative damage to DNA.[31] However, results of studies on the pro-oxidant effects of vitamin C are inconsistent.[32,33] More research is needed to determine what factors influence whether the antioxidant or pro-oxidant properties of vitamin C predominate.

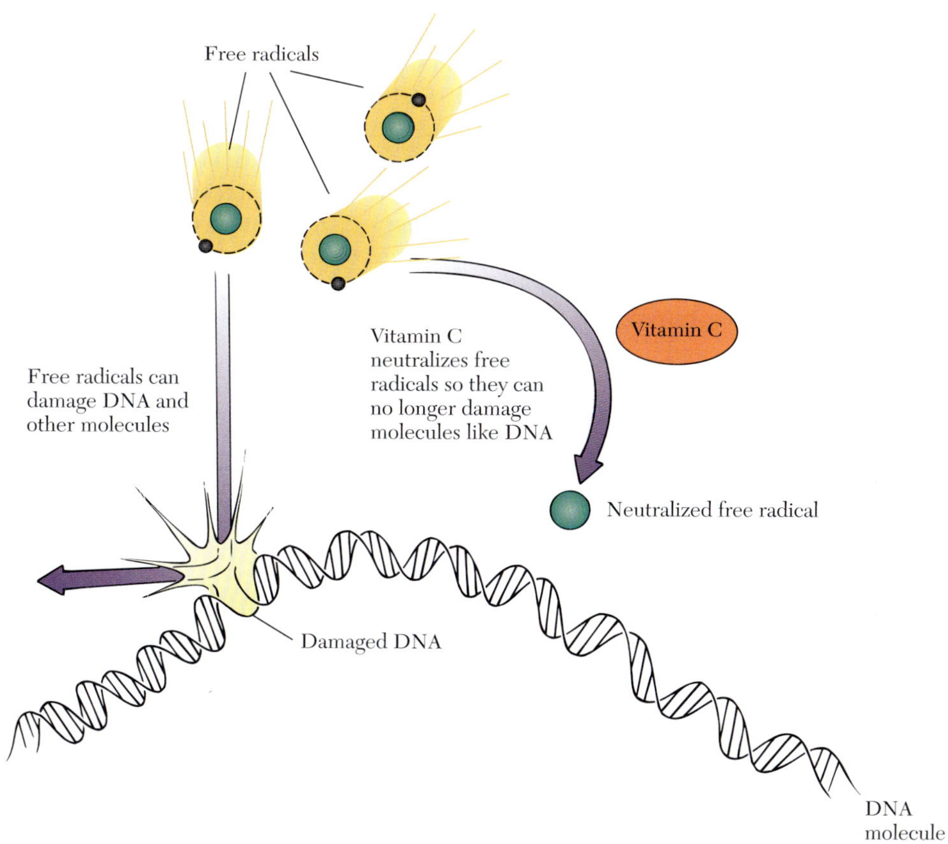

FIGURE 10.20 Vitamin C functions as an antioxidant that donates electrons to neutralize free radicals so that they are no longer damaging.

Recommended Intakes

Humans are one of only a few animal species that require vitamin C in the diet. Most animals can synthesize vitamin C in their bodies. For example, a pig makes 8 g a day. The recommendations for vitamin C intake are based on the amount needed to achieve maximum saturation in the body and to provide antioxidant protection. The antioxidant function of vitamin C in white blood cells is particularly important, and concentrations in these cells reflect body levels. Recommendations have therefore been set at a level that will both minimize urinary excretion and maintain near-maximal concentration of ascorbate in neutrophils, a type of white blood cell.

The RDA for adult men is set at 90 mg/day and for adult women 75 mg/day.[23] These amounts do not change with advancing age (see Table 10.1). This amount is easily obtained by drinking an 8-ounce glass of orange juice.

Infants thrive on the amount of vitamin C they obtain from human milk, so an Adequate Intake (AI) is set based on the mean intake of infants who are fed breast milk. RDAs were established for children and adolescents by extrapolating from adult requirements.

During pregnancy, the RDA is increased by 10 mg/day above the nonpregnant requirement. During lactation, the RDA increases to 120 mg/day for women 19 years of age and older to reflect the amount that is secreted in human milk.

It is estimated that smoking cigarettes uses up about 35 mg of vitamin C daily. It is therefore recommended that smokers consume an extra 35 mg/day. Exercise and mental and emotional stress were not found to affect the requirement for vitamin C.

Vitamin C and Health

In the United States today, vitamin C deficiency is rare, but vitamin C is still the most frequently consumed vitamin supplement.

Vitamin C Deficiency When vitamin C intake is below 10 mg per day, the symptoms of scurvy may appear. These symptoms reflect the role of vitamin C in the maintenance of connective tissue. Without vitamin C, the bonds holding adjacent collagen molecules together cannot be formed and maintained, resulting in poor wound healing, the reopening of previously healed wounds, bone and joint aches, bone fractures, and improperly formed and loose teeth. Connective tissue is also important for blood vessel integrity. A vitamin C deficiency therefore causes weakened blood vessels and ruptured capillaries, which leads to symptoms such as small skin discolorations, bleeding gums, and easy bruising. Anemia may also occur from impaired iron absorption. The psychological manifestations of scurvy include depression and hysteria.

Two centuries ago, fruits containing vitamin C saved the lives of thousands of sailors by preventing scurvy. In the United States, severe vitamin C deficiency leading to scurvy is uncommon, but marginal vitamin C deficiency is a concern for individuals who consume few fruits and vegetables. Scurvy can occur in infants fed diets consisting exclusively of cow's milk and in alcoholics and elderly individuals consuming nutrient-poor diets.

Vitamin C Toxicity Vitamin C is generally considered nontoxic. Large increases in intake do not cause large increases in the amount of vitamin C in body fluids because absorption decreases as the dose increases, and excess vitamin C is excreted by the kidney.[34] However, excessive doses can cause unpleasant side effects. The most common symptoms in healthy individuals consuming high doses of vitamin C are diarrhea, nausea, and abdominal cramps. These are caused when unabsorbed vitamin C draws water into the intestine. Another concern with vitamin C supplements is damage to teeth; the acid in chewed vitamin C tablets is strong enough to dissolve tooth enamel. High intakes of vitamin C should also be avoided by individuals prone to kidney stones, because it can promote stone formation; by those who are unable to regulate iron absorption, because it increases iron absorption (see Chapter 13); and by individuals with sickle-cell anemia, because it can worsen symptoms. Because the structure of vitamin C is similar to that of glucose, it may also interfere with urine tests used to monitor glucose levels in diabetics.

The UL for adults for vitamin C has been set at 2000 mg/day; above this level, the incidence of diarrhea and gastrointestinal disturbance increases in healthy individuals. This value is based on intake from both dietary vitamin C and supplements.

Vitamin C Supplements One third of the population of the United States takes supplements of vitamin C in the hope that it will prevent or reduce symptoms of the common cold. More recently, however, the role of vitamin C as an antioxidant has been used to promote vitamin C supplements as protection against cardiovascular disease and cancer.

Vitamin C and the Common Cold Studies examining the relationship between vitamin C and the common cold date back to the 1930s. A review of placebo-controlled trials that supplemented diets with 1 g (or more) per day found that vitamin C does not reduce the incidence of colds but does moderately reduce the duration and severity of cold symptoms.[23,35] The effect of vitamin C on cold symptoms may be due to its antioxidant effect, its role in stimulating various aspects of immune function, its ability to increase the breakdown of histamine (a molecule that causes inflammation), or a combination of these.[36,37]

Vitamin C and Cardiovascular Disease Vitamin C supplements have been suggested to reduce the risk of cardiovascular disease by reducing blood pressure, blood cholesterol levels, and the formation of oxidized LDL cholesterol. Several studies have suggested that blood pressure is inversely related to vitamin C status; however, the data are not conclusive.[38] It has been hypothesized that vitamin C reduces blood cholesterol because it is involved in the synthesis of bile acids from cholesterol in the liver. Adequate vitamin C would therefore allow cholesterol to be used for bile synthesis, possibly reducing the amount of cholesterol in the blood. Because it is an important plasma antioxidant that can prevent the oxidation of lipids, it has been proposed that vitamin C delays atherosclerosis by preventing the oxidation of LDL cholesterol (see Chapter 5). Of 13 studies examining the effect of vitamin C supplementation on markers of LDL oxidation, 7 showed that supplementation decreased LDL oxidation.[23] Despite these important roles of vitamin C in modulating blood cholesterol levels and protecting LDL cholesterol from oxidation, data thus far from epidemiology and human intervention trials have provided little evidence to support the use of vitamin C supplements in preventing atherosclerosis in humans.[39]

Vitamin C and Cancer It has been suggested that high doses of vitamin C both treat and prevent cancer. Although controlled trials have not found any benefits of vitamin C in the treatment of patients with advanced cancer,[40] there is evidence supporting a role for vitamin C in cancer prevention. Epidemiological studies have found inverse relationships between dietary vitamin C intake and cancers of the bladder, breast, cervix, lungs, gastrointestinal tract, prostate, and pancreas.[41] As an antioxidant, vitamin C may protect against cancer caused by oxidative damage to DNA. In the intestine, vitamin C may prevent cancer by inhibiting the formation of carcinogenic nitrosamines (see Chapter 19). However, despite the association between higher intakes of vitamin C and a lower incidence of various cancers, other factors found in fruits and vegetables might be responsible for the protective effect.[42]

Benefits of Food Versus Supplements

Vitamins are needed in small amounts, but when not enough of one or more is consumed, debilitating deficiency diseases occur, and in some cases the risk for chronic disease increases. By consuming a well-planned and varied diet, most people can meet their vitamin needs. A diet including a variety of foods also provides health benefits beyond those provided by essential nutrients. But for those who cannot meet their needs with food, supplements of vitamins and minerals are available. Also, in addition to nutrient supplements, many other types of dietary supplements are currently popular.

A Diet to Meet Vitamin Needs

To meet requirements, a diet does not need to provide exactly the recommended amount of each vitamin every day. It is the average intake—that consumed over a period of days or weeks—that is important. Almost every food contains some vitamins—in varying amounts and combinations. One simple way to consume a diet that meets needs is to follow the recommendations of the Food Guide Pyramid.

Web Menu For more information on meeting your vitamin needs with the Food Guide Pyramid, go to the USDA Center for Nutrition Policy and Promotion at www.usda.gov/cnpp/pyramid2.htm.

Food Guide Pyramid The Food Guide Pyramid is designed to promote the selection of a diet that meets nutrient needs. A diet that follows the Pyramid serving recommendations and consists of a variety of nutrient-dense choices from within each group will meet vitamin needs.

Serving Recommendations It is important to balance the diet by choosing foods from all groups of the Food Guide Pyramid. No single food group provides all needed vitamins. For example, whole grains are good sources of vitamin E and most of the B vitamins but are poor sources of vitamin C. Therefore, to consume a balanced diet, it is important to consume the recommended number of servings from each group of the Pyramid. Meats provide thiamin, vitamin B_6, and vitamin B_{12}; leafy green vegetables provide vitamin A, folate, vitamin E, and vitamin K; citrus fruits provide vitamin C; whole grains are good sources of many of the B vitamins; milk contains riboflavin, vitamin A, and vitamin D; and vegetable oils contain vitamin E (Figure 10.21).

Choices from Within Food Groups When making selections from each group of the Food Guide Pyramid, variety and nutrient density are both important considerations. Variety is important because different choices from within each food group provide different amounts and types of nutrients. For example, white potatoes and carrots are both in the vegetable group of the Food Guide Pyramid, but they provide very different nutrients. White potatoes are a good source of vitamin C

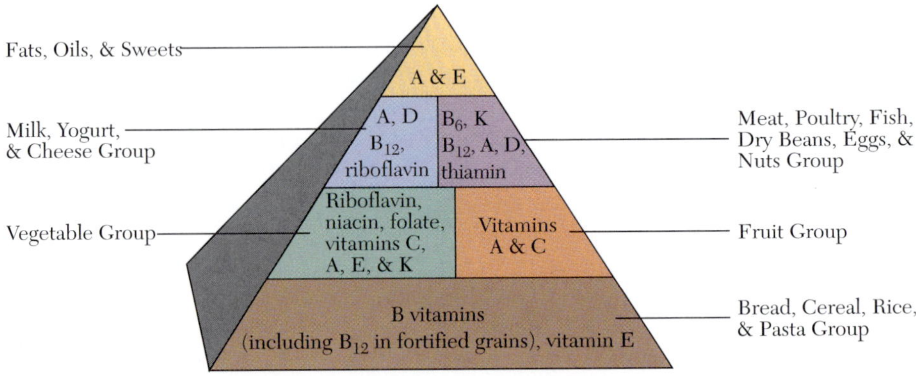

FIGURE 10.21 Each group of the Food Guide Pyramid provides sources of vitamins, but no one group can meet all vitamin needs.

but contain almost no vitamin A; carrots are high in β-carotene (a vitamin A precursor) but have little vitamin C. If your three vegetable choices each day are all potatoes, you will be missing out on vitamin A and other nutrients that you would have consumed in a more varied diet. Choosing a varied diet is also important because nutrients and other food components interact. Interactions may be positive, enhancing nutrient utilization, or negative, inhibiting nutrient use. Variety averages out these interactions. In addition, foods may contain toxic substances such as pesticides, fertilizers, and natural toxins. Different foods contain different amounts of different substances, so a variety of foods ensures you will not get too much of any harmful substance.

Nutrient density—the amounts of essential nutrients in a food relative to the energy provided—is another important factor in choosing foods. For instance, you can get 50% of your RDA for thiamin and niacin from a Big Mac or from a turkey sandwich. Choosing the turkey sandwich, which is more nutrient-dense (the Big Mac contains over 500 kcalories, whereas the turkey sandwich contains about 300 kcalories), allows you to eat more of other foods, which contain other nutrients, without exceeding your energy requirements. The Food Guide Pyramid provides selection tips on food choices from within each group (see Table 2.1).

The Effects of Processing and Storage Heat, light, air, and the passage of time all cause vitamin loss from foods (Table 10.4). Therefore, it is important to consider the nutritional effects of food choices and preparation techniques. Fresh-picked vegetables are less available but provide more nutrients than frozen or canned vegetables. However, if the "fresh vegetable" has actually been a week in transport and another week in the refrigerator, frozen vegetables may actually supply more vitamins. Manufacturers of frozen vegetables often freeze their produce in the fields where they were grown, thereby maintaining most of the nutrients. The processing and heating of canned foods reduces their nutrient content. However, because canned foods keep for a long time, do not require refrigeration, and are often less expensive than fresh or frozen varieties, they provide an available, affordable source of nutrients that may be the best choice in some situations.

TABLE 10.4 Vitamin Losses in Handling

Vitamin	Causes of Loss
Thiamin	Exposure to heat, air, and neutral or low-acid conditions
Riboflavin	Exposure to light, especially in moist and low-acid environments Also destroyed by heat. When it is dry or in a food, it is more stable.
Niacin	Stable
Biotin	Exposure to heat
Pantothenic acid	Exposure to heat and low- or high-acid conditions
Vitamin B_6	Exposure to heat and light
Folate	Exposure to heat, air, light, and acid conditions
Vitamin B_{12}	Exposure to air and light
Vitamin C	Exposure to light and heat and contact with iron or copper cooking utensils. More stable in the presence of acid than in neutral or low-acid conditions, so citrus fruits maintain their vitamin C content longer than other sources. One of the most easily destroyed vitamins
Vitamin A and β-carotene	Exposure to air, light, and acid. Fairly stable in cooking
Vitamin D	Exposure to air, light, heat, and low-acid conditions
Vitamin E	Exposure to high-temperature frying, light, air, and freezing
Vitamin K	Exposure to light and low- or high-acid conditions

Because heat increases vitamin losses, foods, whether canned or fresh, should be stored in a cool location. Even canned foods continue to lose vitamins on the shelf, especially at high temperatures. Fresh produce should be refrigerated and wrapped tightly to retain moisture and decrease exposure to air. For long storage, freezing is best. Fresh vegetables should be blanched before freezing to retain flavor and to stop enzyme activity that destroys vitamins.

Preparation techniques can also have a major impact on nutrient losses. Oxygen, light, and heat inactivate nutrients and water washes them away. To minimize exposure to oxygen and light, vegetables should not be cut up or cooked until the last minute. Also, the smaller the pieces into which they are cut before cooking, the greater the surface area exposed—and the greater the nutrient loss. To prevent water-soluble vitamins from being washed down the drain, vegetables should not be soaked before cooking. Likewise, rice should not be washed before cooking because the water-soluble vitamins added in enrichment will be washed away. Frozen vegetables should not be thawed or washed before cooking.

Cooking technique, time, and temperature can also affect nutrient loss; the higher the temperature and the longer the heat is applied, the greater the loss. Cooking techniques that do not bring food into direct contact with water, such as steaming and pressure cooking, or that use dry heat, such as roasting, grilling, stir-frying, or baking, are best. Vegetables should be cooked minimally so they remain slightly crisp. Pressure cookers can decrease cooking times for foods such as cabbage and beans that require longer cooking times. If foods are cooked in water, some of the vitamins can be retrieved by using the cooking water to make soups and sauces. Microwave cooking is another option. Microwave cooking times are shorter and minimal water is used, both of which help preserve nutrients. For this reason, vitamin retention in microwaved vegetables is often higher than with conventional cooking.

Vitamins on Food Labels Food labels can be helpful in determining vitamin intake from packaged foods. Any vitamin that is added in processing must be listed in the ingredient list, although the amounts are not included. The Nutrition Facts section must list the amount of vitamin A and vitamin C as a percentage of the Daily Value. The listing of other vitamins is voluntary, but many foods, such as fortified breakfast cereals, provide this information. The % Daily Values on labels helps consumers determine whether a food makes a significant contribution to their needs. Table 9.3 illustrates how the actual amount of a vitamin or mineral in a food can be calculated by multiplying the % Daily Value by the Daily Value for that nutrient (see Table 2.3 or Appendix J for the Reference Daily Intakes used to establish Daily Values for vitamins and minerals). Fresh vegetables and fruits rarely come with labels, but nutritional information about these foods is usually provided at the produce counter.

Functional foods Foods that provide a health benefit beyond that provided by the traditional nutrients they contain.

Zoochemicals Substances found in animal foods (*zoo* means animal) that are not essential nutrients but have health-promoting properties.

Phytochemicals Substances found in plant foods (*phyto* means plant) that are not essential nutrients but have health-promoting properties.

Web Menu For more information on functional foods, go to the American Dietetic Association at www.eatright.org/nfs/ and look for the nutrition fact sheet on vitamins, minerals, and functional foods.

Other Health Benefits of Food

Food provides nutrients in infinite combinations and with unlimited variety. In addition, food can provide other health benefits. Foods that provide health benefits beyond basic nutrition have been termed **functional foods.** The substances in foods that provide these benefits include both **zoochemicals,** health-promoting compounds found in animal foods, and **phytochemicals,** health-promoting compounds found in plant foods. Most of the research that has been done in this area has focused on phytochemicals (Figure 10.22). The following sections discuss the general issues related to functional foods and phytochemicals.

Functional Foods In the broadest interpretation of the definition, almost any food can be considered a functional food. The simplest functional foods are unmodified whole foods that naturally contain substances that provide a physi-

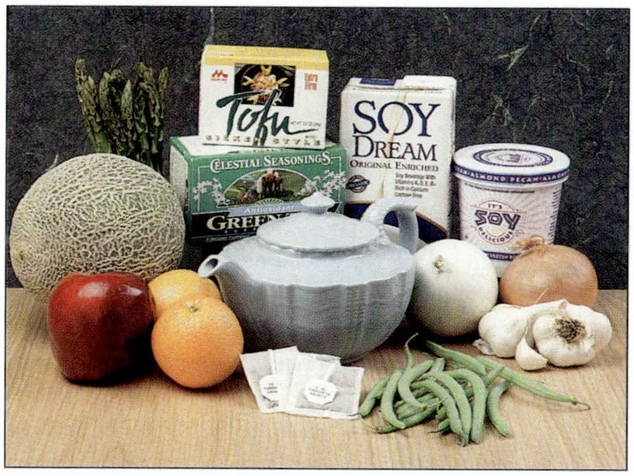

FIGURE 10.22 These plant foods contain a vast assortment of phytochemicals that have health-promoting properties. These properties bring to mind the doctrine of Hippocrates: "Let food be thy medicine and medicine be thy food." *(George Semple)*

ological benefit beyond that provided by the nutrients they contain (see *Making Decisions:* "Chocolate: High-Fat Treat or Functional Food?"). Many fruits and vegetables fit into this category. For instance, broccoli and other cruciferous vegetables have been associated with a decreased cancer risk in epidemiological studies. Further research has shown that these vegetables contain a number of phytochemicals that have anticancer properties. There are also animal products that can be considered functional foods. For example, fish is functional; consumption of a diet high in fish has been related to a reduced risk of heart attacks.[43] The omega-3 fatty acids in fish are believed to play a role. Other functional foods are manufactured or fortified to contain specific health-promoting properties or substances. For example, some orange juice is fortified with calcium to promote healthy bones and some margarines are enriched with plant sterols (Benecol and Take Control) to help lower blood cholesterol (see Chapter 5, *Making Decisions:* "Dietary Supplements to Reduce Blood Cholesterol"). These modified foods have also been called designer foods or nutraceuticals.[44]

Food and supplement labels can be helpful in determining the health-related functions that these products provide (see Chapter 2). Health claims on food labels are one source of this information. Functional foods that contain nutrients or other substances that have been demonstrated by careful research to affect a disease or health-related condition may carry a health claim on their labels. For example, oats contain a soluble fiber that helps lower cholesterol. The evidence supporting this effect was strong enough for the FDA to permit foods containing oats to claim that it helps reduce blood cholesterol. Other foods may contain substances that have been associated with health benefits, but the evidence is not strong enough for a health claim to have been approved. Foods and substances sold as dietary supplements may also include structure/function claims on the label. These claims simply describe how something affects the structure and/or function of the body. For example, the phytochemical lutein has been advocated to prevent the eye disorder macular degeneration. Foods containing lutein may not make such a health claim on the label, but dietary supplements containing lutein may make the structure/function claim that lutein is needed to maintain healthy eyes. Structure/function claims are based on the manufacturer's review of the scientific literature and are easy to identify on the label because they must be accompanied by the disclaimer, "This statement has not been evaluated by the Food and Drug Administration. This product is not intended to diagnose, treat, cure, or prevent any disease." Table 10.5 lists some examples of foods that can be considered functional foods.

Phytochemicals The term "phytochemical" technically means any chemical found in plants. In the plants, phytochemicals serve as protection. For example, the allium compounds in onions and garlic serve as natural pesticides, protecting

Making Decisions

Chocolate: High-Fat Treat or Functional Food?

Chocolate—much praised and often maligned. Few foods conjure up so many mixed messages. It is offered as a reward or treat. It is consumed for comfort. It has been hailed as everything from an antidepressant to an aphrodisiac and been accused of causing acne, weight gain, and tooth decay. Yet, we consume it with vigor—the chocolate industry sells $5 billion worth of chocolate a year in the United States and the Swiss consume 21 pounds per person per year.[a] What makes it so irresistible? Is it simply the seductive flavor of chocolate that lures us into consuming this high-kcalorie, high-fat treat, or are there other benefits that contribute to our attraction to this confection? Should we try to resist, or give in to indulgence?

Chocolate is produced from the seeds of the *Cacao theobroma* tree, which grows only within 10 to 20 degrees of the equator. Christopher Columbus first encountered cocoa beans in 1502 and they were later brought back to Europe by his son Ferdinand as well as by the conquistador Cortez and other Spanish explorers. Mayan Indians consumed a drink, called cacao, made from ground cocoa beans and chilies. This beverage was thought to cure diarrhea and dysentery and to be an aphrodisiac. In Spain, the cacao drink was modified by eliminating the chilies and adding sugar. It became a prized drink among Spanish royalty. Chocolate was not widely available in Europe until the Industrial Revolution. The first chocolate produced in the United States was in the Massachusetts Bay Colony in 1765.

The chocolate we consume today is made from cocoa beans that grow in pods on the cacao tree. The beans are taken from the pod and allowed to ferment. They are then roasted. The hard outer hulls are removed, leaving the "nibs," which are used to produce chocolate liquor. This bitter form of chocolate is used to make what we know as baking chocolate. Eating chocolate is made by mixing the chocolate liquor with sugar and additional cocoa butter, which is the fat that is found in the chocolate liquor. Milk is added to make milk chocolate.

Why do we crave chocolate with such an addiction? There are times when nothing tastes—or makes us feel—as good. Chocolate contains several chemical compounds that may be responsible for the good feelings it induces. One study found that consuming chocolate causes the brain to produce natural opiates, which dull pain and increase feelings of well-being.[a] Other studies found that chocolate could mimic the effects of tetrahydrocannabinol (THC)—the active chemical in marijuana—causing a chocolate "high." This effect was actually found to be due not to THC but to a compound called anandamide, which stimulates a feeling of well-being. Anandamide is produced naturally in the brain, and chocolate contains anandamide as well as compounds that reduce anandamide breakdown, allowing its effects to last longer. Chocolate also contains phenylethylamine, an amphetamine-like compound that causes blood pressure and blood sugar levels to rise, increasing sensations of alertness and contentment. Caffeine and the caffeine-related compounds theobromine and methylxanthine give chocolate a stimulant effect. The amount of caffeine in chocolate (3 to 28 mg/ounce) is small compared to that in coffee (65–150 mg/8 fl oz) and caffeinated carbonated beverages (45 mg/12 fl oz), but, in combination with theobromine and methylxanthine, is enough to make us feel more alert.

So, there are lots of reasons why chocolate makes us feel good, and it makes a nutritional contribution as well by providing small amounts of the essential minerals copper, magnesium, iron, and zinc. But what about all that fat and sugar that come with it? About 50% of the energy in chocolate is from fat and 30% is from saturated fat, but in terms of heart health it may not be as bad as those numbers look. Much of the saturated fat is from stearic acid—a saturated fatty acid that has been shown to have no effect on blood cholesterol levels (although it may increase the risk of cardiovascular disease in other ways). Some of the fat is the monounsaturated fatty acid oleic acid, which has been shown to be beneficial to heart health.[b] And, chocolate contains antioxidants that may offer further protection against heart disease and other health problems. An ounce of milk chocolate contains as many antioxidant polyphenols as a glass of red wine and dark chocolate contains more. The carbo-

plants from insects. When consumed in the diet, most phytochemicals have no effect on health, while some promote health, and others can be toxic. For example, some wild mushrooms contain chemicals that can be deadly to humans. However, we generally use the term "phytochemical" to refer to those substances found in plants that have health-promoting properties.

Food, Phytochemicals, and Health Phytochemicals that have health-promoting properties have been recognized because of epidemiological observations that identified relationships between diets high in certain plant foods and a reduction in chronic disease. Further evaluation of these foods has led researchers to specific phytochemicals that may be responsible for the health benefits. Foods such as garlic, soybeans, cruciferous vegetables, legumes, onions, citrus fruits, tomatoes, whole grains, and a variety of herbs and spices have been found to be excellent sources of these health-promoting compounds.[45] The phytochemicals found in these foods include allium compounds, isoflavones, saponins, indoles, isothiocyanates, dithiolthione, ellagic acid, polyacetylenes, flavonoids, carotenoids, phytates, lignans, glucarates, phthalides, and terpenoids.[46]

hydrate in chocolate is mostly sugar, which can contribute to tooth decay by supporting the growth of acid-producing bacteria in the mouth. But, the fat in chocolate coats the teeth, preventing cavity-causing plaque from forming. Chocolate is energy-dense, providing about 150 kcalories per ounce. Although weight-conscious consumers may avoid it because it adds energy to the diet, data from food surveys indicate that chocolate contributes only 2% of the energy in the American diet. It is therefore unlikely to be a significant reason for the increasing girth of American waistlines. Studies of chocolate's effect on acne showed no connection. It is, however, a cause of headaches in individuals who are sensitive to tyrosine, but the number of people affected is small.

So chocolate provides essential minerals and antioxidants, it doesn't cause acne, and it is no more likely to cause tooth decay than other carbohydrate-containing foods. Should it be a mainstay of the diet? The answer is no—it cannot really be called a nutrient-dense food. But in moderation, it is a treat that may have some positive health effects and therefore can be considered a functional food.

References

[a] Kuwana, E. Discovering the sweet mysteries of chocolate. Available online at **http://faculty.washington.edu/chudler/choco.html.** Accessed 18 Jan 2001.

[b] American Dietetic Association. Chocolate: fact or fiction. Available online at **http//www.eatright.com/nfs/nfs0200a.html.** Accessed 1 Jan 2001.

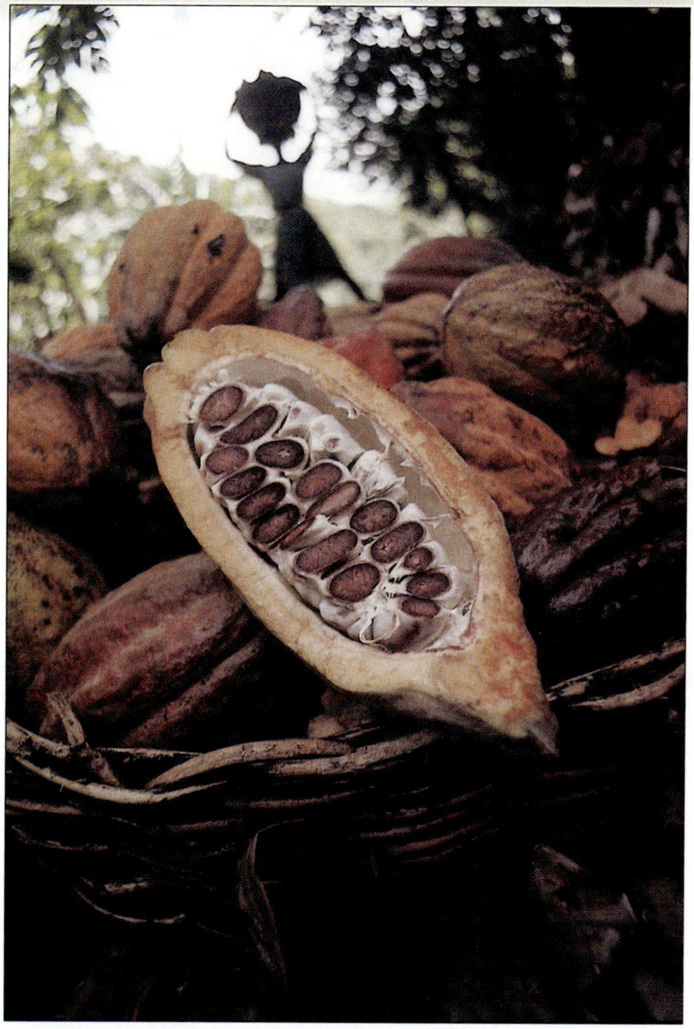

(© James V. Elmore/Peter Arnold, Inc.)

Most phytochemicals are found in more than one type of plant food and many have multiple actions within the body. Carotenoids, polyphenols, and saponins act as antioxidants that scavenge reactive oxygen and nitrogen compounds.[47] Sulfides and isothiocyanates stimulate the activity of enzymes that help deactivate carcinogens. Phytosterols and saponins bind to other molecules, such as cholesterol, and alter their metabolism. Phytoestrogens have structures similar to hormones and act by blocking or mimicking hormone function. Other phytochemicals are health-promoting due to their ability to inhibit the metabolic activation of carcinogens, alter cell-to-cell communication, affect DNA repair mechanisms, or influence other cell processes that may affect cancer development, such as cell proliferation or spontaneous cell death.[47,48] Some classes of phytochemicals, their mechanism of action, and their food sources are given in Table 10.6, and a few of the better studied phytochemcials are discussed here.

Carotenoids Carotenoids are a group of more than 600 compounds found in living organisms including plants, animals, and bacteria. The most prevalent ones in the North American diet include β-carotene, α-carotene, β-cryptoxanthin, lycopene,

TABLE 10.5 Examples of Functional Foods

Functional Food	Key Component	Potential Benefit
Whole-grain products	Fiber	Reduced risk of cancer and heart disease
Oatmeal	Beta glucan soluble fibers	Reduced blood cholesterol
Low-fat products	Reduced fat content	Reduced risk of cancer and heart disease
Grape juice	Phenols	Improved cardiovascular health
Tea	Tannins, catechins	Reduced cancer and heart disease risk
Fish	Omega-3 fatty acids	Reduced heart disease risk
Soy	Phytoestrogens, soy protein	Reduced risk of cancer and heart disease, reduced menopause symptoms
Garlic	Organic sulfur compounds	Reduced risk of cancer and heart disease
Foods containing sugar alcohols	Sugar alcohols	Reduced risk of tooth decay
Cereal fortified with folate	Folic acid	Reduced risk of neural tube defects
Juice fortified with calcium	Calcium	Reduced risk of osteoporosis
Modified margarine	Plant sterols, plant stanol esters	Reduced blood cholesterol
Juices and soups with herbal additives	Echinacea, St. John's wort	Enhanced immune function, improved mood

lutein, and zeaxanthin. The major sources of carotenoids in the diet are fruits and vegetables.

Carotenoids are phytochemicals that have antioxidant properties.[10] The intake of carotenoid-containing fruits and vegetables has been associated with a reduced risk of certain cancers, cardiovascular disease, and age-related eye diseases such as cataracts and macular degeneration.[49] The antioxidant properties of carotenoids are believed to be responsible for some of these effects. Beta-carotene is the best-known carotenoid, but it may be a less effective antioxidant than others.[22] Lycopene, the carotenoid that gives tomatoes their color, is a more potent scavenger of oxygen radicals than other dietary carotenoids.[50] The carotenoids lutein and zeaxanthin are most strongly associated with reduced risk of macular degeneration. Some carotenoids may also promote oxidation depending on the particular carotenoid as well as the amount of oxygen present, the amount of the carotenoid, and interactions with other antioxidants. Some studies show that when β-carotene is added to a vitamin E–deficient diet, it acts as a pro-oxidant.[51] But in the presence of vitamin E, β-carotene acts as an antioxidant. One explanation for the increase in the incidence of lung cancer among smokers supplemented with β-carotene is that pro-oxidant activity prevails over antioxidant activity.

Flavonoids Flavonoids are found in fruits, vegetables, wine, grape juice, and tea. One of the most abundant types of flavonoids is the anthocyanins, which are pigments that give the blue and red colors to blueberries, raspberries, and red cabbage. These compounds are strong antioxidants and have anticancer properties and protect against cardiovascular disease by inhibiting the oxidation of LDL cholesterol and affecting platelet function. The pigments that give the pale yellow color to potatoes, onions, and orange rinds are also flavonoids. Citrus fruits contain about 60 flavonoids that inhibit blood clotting and that have antioxidant, anti-inflammatory, and anticancer properties.[46]

TABLE 10.6 Examples of Phytochemicals

Phytochemical Name or Class	Biological Activities and Possible Effects	Food Sources
Carotenoids (α-carotene, β-carotene, β-cryptoxanthin, lutein, lycopene, zeaxanthin)	Vitamin A precursors (some), antioxidants; increase cell-cell communication; decrease risk of macular degeneration (some)	Yellow-orange-colored fruits and vegetables (apricots, carrots, cantaloupe, broccoli, tomatoes, sweet potatoes), leafy greens such as spinach, dairy products, eggs, and margarine
Flavonoids (Quercetin, kaempferol, myricetin), flavones (apigenin), flavonols (catechins)	Decrease capillary fragility and permeability; block carcinogens and slow growth of cancer cells	Fruits, vegetables, berries, citrus fruits, onions, purple grapes, tea, red wine
Phytoestrogens (isoflavones such as genistein, biochanin A and daidzein, lignins)	Metabolized to estrogen-like compounds in the GI tract; induce cancer cell death; slow the growth of cancer cells; reduce the risk of cancers of the breast, ovaries, colon, and prostate; inhibit cholesterol synthesis; may reduce risk of osteoporosis	Isoflavones are in soybeans, and soy-based foods Lignins are in flax, rye, some berries, and vegetables
Phytosterols (beta-sitosterol, stigmasterol, and campesterol)	Decrease cholesterol absorption from the GI tract; decrease proliferation of colonic cells	Vegetable oils, nuts, seeds, cereals, legumes
Saponins (Soyasaponins, soyasapogenols)	Bind bile acids and cholesterol in the GI tract to reduce absorption; toxic to tumor cells; antioxidant	Soybeans, modified margarines
Glucosinolates (Glucobrassicin), Isothiocyanates (sulphorophane), Indoles (indole-3-carbinol)	Increase the activity of enzymes that deactivate carcinogens; alter estrogen metabolism; affect the regulation of gene expression	Cruciferous vegetables (broccoli, Brussels sprouts, cabbage), horseradish, mustard greens
Sulfides and thiols (dithiolthiones and allium compounds such as diallyl sulfides, allyl methyl trisulfides)	Increase the activity of enzymes that deactivate carcinogens; decrease conversion of nitrates to nitrites in the intestine; may lower cholesterol, blood clotting, and blood pressure	Sulfides are in onions, garlic, leeks, scallions Dithiolthiones are in cruciferous vegetables
Inositol phosphates (Phytate, inositol, pentaphosphate)	Bind metal ions and prevent them from generating free radicals, protect against cancer	Cereals, soybeans, soy-based foods, cereal grains, nuts and seeds (especially abundant in sesame seeds and soybeans)
Phenolic acids (Caffeic and ferulic acids, ellagic acid)	Anticancer properties; prevent the formation of carcinogens in the stomach	Blueberries, cherries, apples, oranges, pears, potatoes Ellagic acid is in berries and nuts
Protease inhibitors	Bind to trypsin and chymotrypsin; decrease growth of cancer cells, inhibit malignant changes in cells; inhibit hormone binding; may aid DNA repair, which can slow cancer cell division and help return a cell to its normal state; prevent tumors from releasing proteases that destroy neighboring cells	Soybeans, other legumes, cereals, vegetables
Tannins	Antioxidants; may inhibit activation of carcinogens and cancer promotion	Grapes, tea, lentils, red and white wine, black-eyed peas
Capsaicin	Modulates blood clotting	Hot peppers
Coumarin (phenolic)	Promotes functions of enzymes that protect against cancer	Citrus fruits
Curcumin (phenolic)	Inhibits enzymes that activate carcinogens; antiinflammatory and antioxidant properties	Turmeric, mustard
Monoterpene (limonene)	Triggers production of enzymes to detoxify carcinogens; inhibits cancer promotion and cell proliferation; affects blood clotting and cholesterol levels	Citrus fruit peels and oils, garlic

Phytoestrogens Besides scavenging for free radicals, some phenolic compounds, often referred to as phytoestrogens, appear to interrupt cancer development and affect health by interfering with the action of the hormone estrogen. Phytoestrogens include isoflavones (also a flavonoid) and lignins. These compounds are structurally modified by the microflora in the intestines to form compounds that are structurally similar to estrogen. They are suspected of blocking estrogen function by tying up estrogen receptors on cells. Isoflavones, the best known of which is genistein, are found in soybeans and are believed to affect hormone-related cancers, including breast and prostate cancer.[46] They are also hypothesized to decrease hot flashes and other symptoms of menopause, although most of the evidence thus far is anecdotal (see Chapter 6, *Making Decisions:* 'Should You Increase Your Intake of Soy Protein?"). Flax seed is rich in lignins. Lignin metabolites are structurally similar to estrogen and have been shown to inhibit the growth of estrogen-stimulated breast cancer.[46]

Phytochemicals That Mimic Cholesterol Phytosterols and saponins are classes of phytochemicals that have structures resembling cholesterol. They decrease cholesterol absorption from the GI tract and therefore lower blood cholesterol—a major risk factor for cardiovascular disease. The phytosterols and saponins in soybeans are believed to contribute to its cholesterol-lowering effect. Phytosterols such as β-sitosterol are the compounds added to margarine to help lower cholesterol.

Sulfur-Containing Phytochemicals Isothiocyanates, dithiolthiones, and sulfides all contain sulfur in their structure. These classes stimulate the activity of enzymes that detoxify carcinogens. Cruciferous vegetables such as broccoli, cauliflower, Brussels sprouts, and cabbage are particularly good sources of isothiocyanates and dithiolthiones. Sulforaphane, an isothiocyanate found in high concentrations in broccoli, is particularly effective at boosting the activity of enzyme systems that detoxify carcinogens, and it has been shown to protect animals from breast cancer.[52] Sulfides include the allium compounds found in garlic, onions, leeks, chives, and shallots. Allium compounds such as diallyl sulfide and allyl methyl trisulfide also act by boosting the activity of cancer-destroying enzyme systems. In addition, these compounds prevent bacteria in the gut from converting nitrates into nitrites that can form carcinogens.

Web Menu: For information on consuming the recommended amounts of fruits and vegetables go to the National Cancer Institute's Five-a-Day program at www.5aday.gov/.

Is There a Recommended Intake for Phytochemicals? The concept that dietary recommendations should be made for substances in foods that are not essential nutrients is relatively new. Choline, which has not yet been determined to be a dietary essential, was included along with the DRIs for B vitamins in 1998 and carotenoids were considered along with the antioxidant nutrients in 2000.[23] No specific recommendations currently exist for the amounts of phytochemicals that should be consumed in the diet, but a set of DRIs that will consider phytochemical intake has been proposed.

Even though there are no quantitative recommendations for phytochemical intake, following recommendations for a healthy diet such as those of the Food Guide Pyramid, which suggests that at least five servings of fruits and vegetables be consumed daily, will provide a diet high in phytochemicals.[54] For example, consuming five fruits and vegetables a day can provide enough carotenoids to keep plasma β-carotene in the range associated with lower chronic disease risk. The concept of choosing a varied diet that will meet nutrient needs and provide a plentiful supply of phytochemicals is emphasized in the recommendations of the "Build a Healthy Base" section of the Dietary Guidelines (Figure 10.23). These emphasize the consumption of plenty of grain products, vegetables, and fruits.

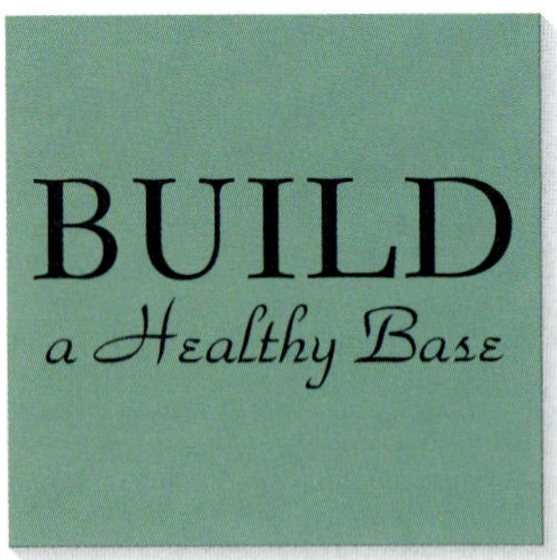

- Let the Pyramid guide your food choices.
- Choose a variety of grains daily, especially whole grains.
- Choose a variety of fruits and vegetables daily.

FIGURE 10.23 Three of the recommendations of the Build a Healthy Base section of the Dietary Guidelines emphasize variety, balance, and the consumption of grains, fruits, and vegetables.

Despite these recommendations, the average American eats only about 1.5 servings of vegetables and 1 serving of fruit each day; only 1 in 11 Americans meets the recommendations of at least three vegetables and two fruits daily.[46] As a result, there are numerous public education campaigns designed to promote "Five a Day"—that is, consumption of at least five fruit and vegetable servings daily. Table 10.7 includes some suggestions for increasing the intake of foods that provide a variety of phytochemicals.

The effects of preparation on the phytochemical content of foods vary. Most phytochemicals are heat stable and so are not destroyed by cooking or lost in cooking water. An exception is allium compounds in onions and garlic, which may be lost in cooking. Cooking may also increase the availability of some phytochemicals, such as the carotenoids and indoles in broccoli.[46]

TABLE 10.7 Suggestions for Increasing Fruit, Vegetable, and Grain Intake

Try a new fruit or vegetable each week.
Eat fruits and vegetables for snacks.
Put fruit on your cereal in the morning or vegetables in your eggs.
Try dried fruit instead of candy.
Drink fruit or vegetable juices instead of soft drinks.
Try baked fruit for dessert.
Double your typical serving of vegetables.
Increase your use of herbs and spices such as garlic, basil, turmeric, parsley, oregano, and hot peppers.
Eat a vegetarian dinner at least once a week.
Add vegetables to your favorite entrees such as spaghetti sauces and casseroles.
Try tofu in cooking.

Dietary Supplements

About half of the adults in the United States use dietary supplements.[54] If foods provide all the nutrients as well as other health benefits, why then are dietary supplements such big sellers? People take supplements to energize themselves, to protect themselves from disease, to cure their illnesses, to enhance what they get in food, and simply to ensure against deficiencies. Although dietary supplements may be beneficial to some individuals under certain circumstances, they can also carry risks. Concentrated doses of vitamins and minerals can result in toxicity and supplements of other substances, such as herbs, may have side effects that outweigh any benefits they may provide.

Regulating Dietary Supplements Dietary supplements are regulated by the Dietary Supplement Health and Education Act of 1994. As defined by this law, a dietary supplement includes any product intended for ingestion as a supplement to the diet and may contain one or more of the following ingredients: vitamins; minerals; herbs, botanicals, or other plant-derived substances; amino acids; enzymes; concentrates; and extracts. In the following discussion, dietary supplements are divided into those that provide essential vitamins and minerals and those that contain primarily nonvitamin, nonmineral substances. Many products contain a combination of these two categories.

According to the Dietary Supplement Health and Education Act, products intended for ingestion as supplements must include the words "dietary supplement" on the label and carry a standardized label similar to food labels (see Chapter 2). Information that may be contained in advertising and in package inserts and literature is also regulated. But, manufacturers are responsible for monitoring the safety of their products. The FDA is only involved if a problem is reported once the product has been marketed. The FDA has the authority to remove a product from the market if it can prove that the product carries significant risk.

Vitamin and Mineral Supplements Eating a variety of foods is the best way to meet nutrient needs, and most healthy adults who consume a reasonably good diet do not need supplements. An argument against the use of supplements is that it gives people a false sense of security, causing them to pay less attention to the nutrient content of the foods they choose. Individuals who are concerned about their nutrient intake should have their diet and nutritional status assessed by a dietitian and a physician.[55] Some individuals cannot meet their requirements with food, either because they have increased needs or excess losses. These people can benefit from vitamin and mineral supplements. Groups who typically

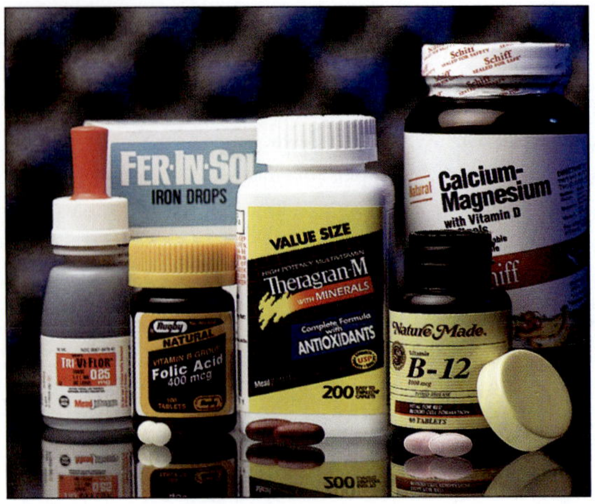

FIGURE 10.24 Many vitamin and mineral supplements are targeted to groups with increased needs for certain nutrients. *(George Semple)*

need vitamin and mineral supplements include dieters, vegans, and groups who are nutritionally vulnerable because of chronic disease; use of medications, cigarettes, or alcohol; or life stage (Figure 10.24).

Dieters Individuals following weight-loss diets restrict the amount of energy in their diet and consequently reduce their intake of micronutrients. It is difficult to consume the recommended amounts of all vitamins and minerals if energy intake is less than 1200 kcalories per day, no matter how well planned the diet is. Therefore, it is important to supplement diets that contain fewer than 1200 kcalories (see Chapter 8).

Vegans Vegan diets must be supplemented with vitamin B_{12} in order to meet needs. Although vegetarian diets are generally high in micronutrients, a vegan diet, which excludes all animal food products, will be deficient in vitamin B_{12}. Vegans need to obtain vitamin B_{12} from fortified foods or from supplements (see Chapters 6 and 9).

Nutritionally Vulnerable Populations Individuals with chronic diseases that affect nutrient utilization, or those taking certain medications, may require vitamin and mineral supplements. For instance, individuals with pernicious anemia require injections of vitamin B_{12} or megadoses of oral supplements to meet their needs. Individuals who are lactose-intolerant may not be able to consume enough dairy products to meet their need for calcium and vitamin D and may therefore benefit from fortified foods and supplements. Individuals who take certain blood pressure medications (thiazide diuretics) may require supplemental potassium (see Chapter 11). Individuals who routinely take medications should discuss nutrient-drug interactions and the need for specific vitamin and mineral supplementation with their doctor or pharmacist (see Chapter 17).

The use of cigarettes and alcohol also affects vitamin requirements. Heavy cigarette smokers, for instance, require more vitamin C to maintain the blood concentrations of vitamin C found in nonsmokers.[57] Individuals who consume more than two alcoholic beverages per day may require supplemental thiamin, niacin, vitamin B_6, and folate because alcohol inhibits the absorption of these vitamins and may affect their metabolism (see Chapters 16 and 17).

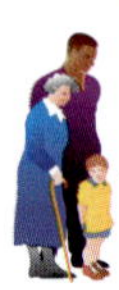

Pregnant women and older adults may need supplements to meet their micronutrient needs. Although a well-planned diet can meet the needs of pregnant women, supplements of iron and folate are recommended, and multivitamin and mineral supplements are usually prescribed (see Chapter 15). In addition, women who are planning a pregnancy should consume supplemental folic acid in fortified foods or supplements (see Chapter 9). A vitamin and mineral supplement may also benefit elderly individuals because the capacity to absorb or utilize vitamins may decrease with aging. For example, many individuals over age 50 do not absorb vitamin B_{12} bound in food. Foods fortified with B_{12} or supplements are recommended for this age group (see Chapters 9 and 17).

How to Choose a Supplement For individuals with limited dietary intakes, a multivitamin and mineral supplement that supplies no more than 100% of the Daily Values may be necessary to meet nutrient needs. Those who decide to take a micronutrient supplement should choose with care to assure that nutrient needs are met and the possibility of toxicity is minimal. The pros and cons of specific vitamin supplements and the risks of toxicity have been reviewed in the Critical Thinking exercise in this chapter and the Making Decisions feature in the previous chapter (see Chapter 9, *Making Decisions:* "Supplementing Safely"). In addition, information on supplements is included in the discussion of each vitamin and mineral in Chapters 9–13.

Nonvitamin/Nonmineral Supplements The use of dietary supplements that contain substances not classified as either vitamins or minerals is increasing dramatically (Figure 10.25). Sales data suggest that there was a 70% increase in sales between 1994 and 1997, and, depending on how the surveys were conducted, that the percent of adults who are using nonvitamin/nonmineral supplements is somewhere between 20 to 68%.[57] Some of these supplements contain nutrients, such as protein and amino acids (see Chapters 6 and 14) and carbohydrates (see Chapters 4 and 14). Some contain compounds that are found in the body but are not considered essential in the diet, and others include compounds found in plants. Because dietary supplements are regulated by the FDA as food and not drugs, their efficacy and safety do not need to be established prior to their sale. A brief discussion of some of these supplements is included here, and individual supplements are discussed throughout the text.

Compounds Found in the Body Some of the ingredients in supplements are substances that are found in the body or that are their precursors or metabolites. These are not dietary essentials because they are synthesized in the body in sufficient quantities to meet needs, and no deficiency symptoms occur when they are absent from the diet. However, some consumers take these supplements because they believe that body levels may not be sufficient for optimal health. Substances that fit into this category include enzymes, hormones, and vitamin-like substances that function in metabolism. The risks of each need to be considered individually.

Supplements of enzymes and hormones frequently do not reach the target organs they are supposed to affect. Because enzymes are proteins, most will be digested into amino acids before they reach cells inside the body (see Chapter 6). Some hormones, such as DHEA and melatonin taken in the hope that they will delay aging, are lipids rather than proteins and may reach the bloodstream intact and affect function.

Supplements also contain other structural or regulatory molecules. Glucosamine and chondroitin sulfate provide substances needed for the formation of healthy joints and are sold to alleviate the pain and progression of arthritis (see

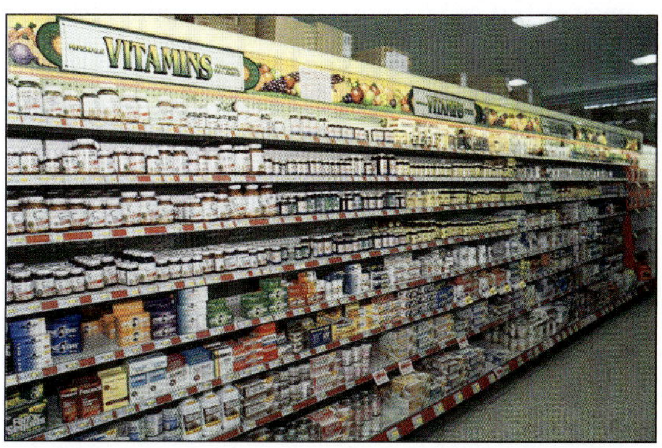

FIGURE 10.25 There are thousands of different types of dietary supplements available on the shelves of health food stores, drug stores, and grocery stores. *(George Semple)*

Making Decisions

Herbal Risk or Herbal Benefit?

Herbal supplements are becoming increasingly popular. They are taken to cure a variety of ailments such as colds, arthritis, depression, and menopausal symptoms as well as to slow aging, improve memory, and enhance well-being. Many herbs have been used medicinally for thousands of years. Because they are "natural"—that is, they are not processed or altered from their original plant sources—herbs are often viewed as harmless. Natural, however, is no guarantee of safety. Why are herbs so popular? How can you tell whether you are choosing an herbal risk or an herbal benefit?

Herbal supplements are readily available and relatively inexpensive. They can be purchased without either a trip to the doctor or a prescription. Although this may be viewed as beneficial by consumers who want to manage their own health, it can also cause problems. When a drug is prescribed to treat a condition, we assume that it will have a beneficial effect on our ailment, that each dose will contain the same amount of drug, that the physician or pharmacist has considered other medications we are taking and other medical conditions that affect us, and that the drug itself will not cause a severe side effect. These assumptions cannot be made with herbs. Some herbs are sold as parts of the raw plant; these may be toxic themselves or may contain bacteria or other contaminants. Those pressed and packaged into pills may also cause problems because their manufacture is not strictly regulated and not all pills provide the same dose. For example, in a study that examined the amount of ephedra in ephedra-containing dietary supplements, it was found that the content often differed by 20% or more from label claims and was inconsistent between two lots of some products.[a] Also, because consumers decide what to treat, herbal remedies can be used inappropriately or can be used instead of needed medical intervention. And there is no guarantee that the herb will not be toxic, either alone or in combination with other drugs and herbs being consumed.

Consumers who choose to use herbal remedies should use them with care. The first step before taking any dietary supplement is to consult your physician or dietitian; often, however, these individuals are not trained in the use of herbal medicines. What about the clerk in the health food store? Sometimes they are knowledgeable, but for many, selling supplements is just an after-school job. The safest advice is to do your own research. Know what you are taking and why. Go beyond the label on the bottle.

Use the suggestions for judging nutrition claims discussed in Chapter 1 of this text to evaluate herbs before you take them. Does the information you have on the herb make sense? Is it too outrageous to believe? For example, a product advertised to cure arthritis overnight is unlikely to fulfill its promise. Where does the information come from? Is it in the ad for the product or a suggestion from the clerk who is selling the herbs? Or did it come from a source not involved in the sale of the product? Is the claim based on scientific research? Who did the research and were the studies done correctly? Were the results interpreted accurately? Can the results be applied to people with your condition or in your life stage? Vague claims that are hard to measure, such as "energize," "detoxify," or "purify," are unlikely to be backed up by scientific research. Check out the product's safety record. Many studies have been done to assess the safety and effectiveness of herbs.

Do a risk-benefit analysis before you buy. For example, echinacea is an herbal immune enhancer often taken to prevent or treat cold symptoms. The proposed benefit is a reduction in cold symptoms. There is research in humans that supports the claim that this herb enhances the immune response. And research has shown it to be relatively nontoxic in healthy adults. A bottle of capsules costs about $5.00. So for most people, the risks are small and the benefits may be real. However, individuals with the disease lupus, in which the immune system attacks body tissues, should not take this supplement because echinacea can worsen symptoms of the disease.

For some herbs, the risks outweigh the benefits. Serious side effects from excessive doses or unusual combinations of herbs and medications are not uncommon. For example, herbs such as comfrey and chamomile, which are consumed in tea, can be toxic in high doses. The use of herbal supplements also may be inappropriate at certain times. For example, St. John's wort can prolong and intensify the effects of narcotic drugs and anesthetic agents, so it should not be taken before surgery.[b] It is recommended that herbal products not be used for two to three weeks prior to surgery.

Some guidelines to follow if you are considering taking herbs or herbal supplements are listed below:

- If you are ill or taking medications, consult your physician before taking herbs.
- Do not take herbs if you are pregnant.
- Do not give herbs to children.
- Do not assume herbal products are safe.
- Do not take herbs with known toxicities.
- Read label ingredients and the list of precautions.
- Start with low doses, and stop taking any product that causes side effects.
- Do not take combinations of herbs.
- Do not use herbs for long periods.

The accompanying table lists some of the suggested benefits and potential risks associated with popular herbal supplements.

Chapter 17, *Research Discoveries*: "Glucosamine and Chondroitin Sulfate: A Meta-Analysis").[58] Inositol is a component of phospholipids in cell membranes, where it plays a role in relaying messages to the inside of the cell. Inositol can be synthesized from glucose. There is no evidence that it is essential in the human diet, but it may have some clinical value in treating diseases such as diabetes and kidney failure.[59] Para-aminobenzoic acid (PABA) is a part of the folate molecule

Potential Benefits and Side Effects of Common Herbal Ingredients

Product	Suggested Benefit	Side Effects
Astralagus (Huang ch'i)	Immune stimulant	Low blood pressure, dizziness, fatigue
Cat's Claw (una de gato)	Relieves arthritis and indigestion, immune stimulant	Should not be taken by individuals with thrombocytopenia (a blood disorder)
Chamomile[c]	Aids indigestion, promotes relaxation	Allergy possible
Chaparral[d,e]	Traditional Native American medicine	Liver damage, possibly irreversible*
Comfrey (borage, coltsfoot)[d,e]	As a poultice for wounds and sore joints; as a tea for digestive disorders	Do not take orally, even as a tea; obstruction of blood flow to liver resulting in liver failure and possibly death*
Dong Quai[e]	Increases energy	May cause birth defects
Echinacea[d,f] (purple cone flower, snake root, Indian head)	Topically for wound healing, internally as an immune stimulant, cold remedy	Allergy possible, adverse effects in pregnant women and people with autoimmune disorders
Ephedra (Ma Huang, Chinese ephedra, epitonin)[d,e]	Relieves cold symptoms, weight loss	High blood pressure, irregular heartbeat, heart attack, stroke, death*
Ginger[c]	Relieves motion sickness and nausea	Irregular heartbeat with large doses
Ginkgo biloba[d,c] (maiden hair, kew tree, Pak ko)	Improved memory and mental function, improved circulation	GI distress, headache, allergic skin reactions
Ginseng[d]	Enhanced immunity, improved sexual function	High blood pressure
Germander[e]	Weight loss, increased energy	Liver disease, possibly death
Kombochu tea[d] (mushroom tea, kvass tea, kwassan, kargasck)	General well-being	GI upset, liver damage, possibly death
Lobelia[d,e] (Indian Tobacco)	Relaxation; respiratory remedy	Breathing problems, rapid heartbeat, low blood pressure, convulsions, coma, death*
Milk thistle[c]	Protects against liver disease	May decrease effectiveness of some medications
Saw palmetto[d]	Improves urinary flow with enlarged prostate	Stomach upset
St. John's wort[d] (hypericum)	Promotes mental well-being	Contains similar ingredients as the antidepressant drug fluoxetine (Prozac) and should not be used by people taking antidepressants
Stephania[d,e] (magnolia)	Weight loss	Kidney damage, including kidney failure resulting in transplant or dialysis*
Valerian[c]	Mild sedative	GI upset, headache, restlessness
Willow bark[d,e]	Pain and fever relief	Reye's syndrome, allergies*
Wormwood[e]	Relieves digestive ailments	Numbness or paralysis of legs, delirium, paralysis*
Yohimbe[d]	Aphrodisiac	Tremors, anxiety, high blood pressure, rapid heart beat, psychosis, paralysis*

*Has been shown to have serious side effects and should be avoided.

References

[a]Gurley, B. J., Gardner, S. F., and Hubbard, M. A. Content versus label claims in ephedra-containing dietary supplements. Am. J. Health Syst. Pharm. 57:963–969, 2000.

[b]Jones, D. M., and Weintraub, P. S. Anesthesiologists warn: if you're taking herbal products, tell your doctor before surgery. Available online at **http://www.asahq.org/PublicEducation/herbal.html.** Accessed 25 May 2000.

[c] Mayo Clinic. Blurbs on Herbs. Available online at **http://www.mayohealth.org/mayo/9703/htm/herb_sb.htm.** Accessed 15 May 2000.

[d] Mayo Clinic. Herbs can have many health effects—some beneficial, some dangerous. Available online at **http://www.mayohealth.org/mayo/9707/htm/me_6sb.htm.** Accessed 1 Apr 2000.

[e]Kurtzweil, P. An FDA guide to dietary supplements. FDA Consumer 32:28–35, Sept./Oct., 1998.

[f] Bartels, C. L., and Miller, S. J. Herbal and related remedies, NCP 13:5–14, 1998.

but has no vitamin activity on its own and cannot be used by humans to synthesize folate. Although topical PABA is used as a sunblock, there is no evidence that oral PABA offers protection from the sun or anything else, and in large doses it may cause liver damage. Carnitine is needed to transport fatty acids into the mitochondria where they are broken down to generate ATP (see Chapters 5 and 14). SAMe, chemically known as S-adenosyl-methionine, is present in the body normally as an intermediate in the metabolism of methionine. SAMe is claimed to be effective for treating such diverse conditions as depression, arthritis, and liver disease. Although there is preliminary evidence that SAMe may be somewhat beneficial in individuals with depression and arthritis, the results of large, well-controlled studies are not yet available and the risks of taking this supplement have not been adequately assessed.[60]

Some supplements contain substances with coenzyme activity. Lipoic acid is a coenzyme needed for the conversion of pyruvate into acetyl-CoA and for a reaction of the citric acid cycle. Although essential to energy production, lipoic acid can be synthesized in adequate amounts by human cells. Ubiquinone, or coenzyme Q, is important for the production of energy from carbohydrate, fat, and protein because it is one of the electron carriers in the electron transport chain. As its name implies, it is present ubiquitously, in animals, plants, and microorganisms, and it is synthesized in the human body. Supplements of ubiquinone have been reported to improve reproductive performance in rats fed a diet deficient in vitamin E, but there is no evidence that it is needed in the diet of healthy humans.

Web Menu: For more information on the risks and benefits of dietary supplements, go to the government nutrition Web site at www.nutrition.gov/, to the FDA Center for Food Safety and Applied Nutrition at www.cfsan.fda.gov/ and click on dietary supplements, or to the NIH office of Dietary Supplements at dietary-supplements.info.nih.gov/.

Herbs, Botanicals, and Other Plant-Derived Substances Technically, an herb is a nonwoody seed-producing plant that dies at the end of the growing season. However, the term is generally used to refer to any botanical or plant-derived substance. Throughout human history, herbs have been used as medicine. This herbal or phytomedicine is an ancient art based in folklore and culture. Herbal products available today, such as Dong Quai, Indian Tobacco, and St. John's wort, borrow from the traditional medicine of many cultures (see *Making Decisions*: "Herbal Risk or Herbal Benefit?") These herbal supplements are offered to improve general well-being as well as for their specific medicinal functions. The physiological effects of some of these are rooted in tradition and anecdote. For others, scientific research has determined that the plant has an effect on human physiology. Supplements that are currently popular include garlic, ginseng, ginkgo biloba, St. John's wort, and echinacea, as well as a variety of phytochemicals.

Garlic has been used medicinally for centuries, and recent research has shown that it may lower blood cholesterol (see Chapter 5, *Making Decisions*: "Dietary Supplements to Reduce Blood Cholesterol"). Garlic supplements allow consumers to increase garlic intake without eating the spice at every meal; some preparations contain a deodorized form. Ginseng has been used in Asia for centuries for its energizing, stress-reducing, and aphrodisiac properties. High doses may cause nervousness and heart palpitations. Ginkgo biloba, also called "maiden hair," is an herb that has been used to enhance memory and to treat a variety of circulatory ailments. Consumption of the leaves may cause side effects such as headaches, gastrointestinal upset, and dizziness. Consumption of other parts of the plant can cause allergic skin reactions. St. John's wort is an herb taken to promote mental well-being. Analysis reveals that it contains low doses of the chemical found in the antidepressant drug fluoxetine (Prozac). Individuals taking antidepressant drugs should not take St. John's wort. Petals of the echinacea plant were used by Native Americans as a treatment for colds, flu, and infections. Today, it is a popular herbal cold remedy. Studies have documented that it is an immune system stimulant. Although side effects have not been reported, allergies are possible.[61] In some countries, such as Germany, echinacea and other herbal remedies are available from pharmacists in prescription doses (Figure 10.26).

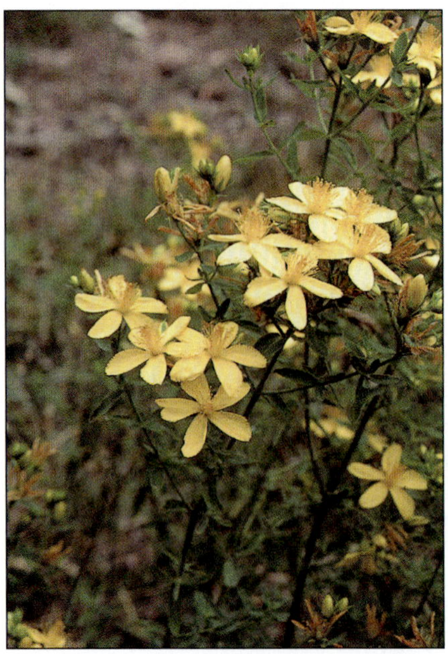

FIGURE 10.26 Just because herbs such as this St. John's wort are natural doesn't mean they are safe for everyone at any dose. *(© Michael P. Gadomski/Photo Researchers, Inc.)*

As already discussed, plants contain hundreds of phytochemicals. Some products try to bottle the health-promoting properties of phytochemicals by extracting them and pressing them into pills or capsules. Popular phytochemical supplements include flavonoids, such as rutin, hesperidin, and pycnogonol. As discussed earlier, flavonoids and bioflavonoids are antioxidants. Supplements containing them are advertised as cures for arthritis, heart disease, high blood pressure, and colds. Although the foods containing these phytochemicals have been shown to have health-promoting properties, supplements of these may not have any health effect.

SUMMARY

1. Vitamin A is needed for vision and for the growth and differentiation of cells. It affects epithelial tissue, reproduction, and immune function by altering gene expression. It is found in the diet both preformed as retinoids and in precursor forms called carotenoids. Preformed vitamin A can be toxic and can increase the risk of birth defects. The major food sources of preformed vitamin A include liver, eggs, fish, and fortified dairy products. Carotenoids are found in fruits and vegetables such as mangoes and carrots. β-carotene is the most potent precursor. Vitamin A deficiency is a world health problem that causes blindness and death.
2. Vitamin D is essential for maintaining proper levels of calcium and phosphorus in the body. It functions by promoting calcium and phosphorus absorption from the intestines and release from bone. Vitamin D can be made in the skin by exposure to sunlight, so dietary needs vary depending on the amount synthesized. In the diet, it is found in fish oils and fortified milk. A deficiency in children results in a condition called rickets; in adults, vitamin D deficiency causes osteomalacia.
3. Vitamin K is essential for blood clotting. Since vitamin K deficiency is a problem in newborns, they are routinely given vitamin K injections at birth. Dicumarol, a substance that inhibits vitamin K activity, is used medically as an anticoagulant. Vitamin K is found in plants and is synthesized by bacteria in the gastrointestinal tract.
4. Antioxidants are substances that help neutralize highly reactive forms of oxygen and nitrogen such as free radicals before they can do damage. Free radicals and other reactive molecules are generated inside the body from normal metabolic reactions and may also come from the environment. They cause oxidative damage by stealing electrons from DNA, proteins, carbohydrates, and unsaturated fatty acids. The body is equipped with a variety of antioxidant defenses, including vitamins and phytochemicals consumed in the diet and enzymes synthesized in the body, many of which rely on minerals for activity.
5. Vitamin E functions primarily as a fat-soluble antioxidant. It is necessary for reproduction and protects cell membranes from oxidative damage. Good dietary sources include nuts, plant oils, green vegetables, and fortified cereals.
6. Vitamin C is a water-soluble antioxidant that donates electrons in biochemical reactions, including those needed for the synthesis and maintenance of connective tissue. A deficiency of vitamin C results in the disease scurvy. Large doses can result in gastrointestinal symptoms.
7. Vitamin needs can be met by a carefully selected diet that follows the recommendations of the Food Guide Pyramid. The diet can be balanced by choosing foods from all groups. From within each group a variety of nutrient-dense foods should be selected. Food processing, storage, and preparation can cause vitamin losses. Food labels can be used to select packaged foods that are good sources of vitamins A and C, and others when voluntarily included on the label.
8. Functional foods are foods that provide physiological benefits beyond that of simply meeting nutrient needs. Some foods are considered functional because they are good sources of phytochemicals. "Phytochemicals" is a term used to refer to the chemicals found in plants. Many of these have health-promoting properties and are associated with reductions in the risk of cancer and other degenerative diseases. Some act as antioxidants, some affect the activity of enzymes or hormones, and others work by other mechanisms. Dietary recommendations advise Americans to increase their consumption of fruits and vegetables because these foods are sources of phytochemicals.
9. Over half the adult population in the United States takes some type of dietary supplement. Dietary supplements may contain vitamins; minerals; herbs, botanicals, or other plant-derived substances; amino acids; enzymes; concentrates or extracts. The FDA regulates dietary supplements, but since they are classified as foods and not drugs, regulations are not as strict.
10. Vitamin supplements are recommended for some groups of individuals such as dieters, vegetarians, and nutritionally vulnerable groups.
11. Many substances that are not nutrients are available as supplements. Some dietary supplements contain compounds that are already present in the body but are not essential in the diet. Others contain plant extracts and herbs. These products may have beneficial physiological actions, but they can also have dangerous side effects.

REVIEW QUESTIONS

1. List two food sources of preformed vitamin A and two sources of provitamin A.
2. List three functions of preformed vitamin A.
3. What are the symptoms of vitamin A deficiency?
4. Can vitamin A be toxic? Can β-carotene be toxic?
5. Why is vitamin D called the sunshine vitamin?
6. Name two sources of vitamin D in the diet.
7. What is the function of vitamin D?
8. What is the main function of vitamin K?
9. What is an antioxidant?
10. What is the function of vitamin E?
11. Name two sources of vitamin E in the diet.
12. What is the function of vitamin C?
13. List three sources of vitamin C in the diet.
14. What is the function of phytochemicals in plants and what effects do they have on people?
15. How can you ensure that your diet is plentiful in phytochemicals?
16. For whom are vitamin and mineral supplements recommended?
17. Are dietary supplements safe? Why or why not?

Applying Critical Thinking Skills

Personal nutrition:

1. Using the three-day food intake record you kept in Chapter 2:
   a. Calculate your average daily intake of vitamin A.
   b. How does your vitamin A intake compare to the RDA for someone of your age and sex?
   c. What are three major food sources of vitamin A in your diet?
   d. Do the major food sources of vitamin A in your diet contain preformed vitamin A or provitamin A carotenoids?
2. Using the food intake record you kept in Chapter 2, evaluate your antioxidant vitamin intake:
   a. Calculate your average intake of vitamin E and correct this value to account for the fact that α-tocopherol makes up about 80% of the total tocopherols in a mixed diet.
   b. Calculate your average intake of vitamin C.
   c. How does your intake of these antioxidant vitamins compare with the RDAs?
   d. If your diet does not meet the RDA for either of these, suggest modifications that will allow your diet to meet the RDA without exceeding your energy needs.

General nutrition issues:

1. Use the Internet to identify several supplements on the market that contain phytochemicals.
   a. What health promises are made about these supplements?
   b. Do they contain a single compound or are they a plant extract containing multiple compounds?
   c. What are the advantages and disadvantages of these supplements? Would you recommend them to a friend? Why or why not?
2. Do a survey of ten people.
   a. Record all of the dietary supplements they take including the number of doses taken per day as well as the reason they chose to take each supplement.
   b. Tabulate the total amount of each vitamin, mineral, or other component each person takes.
   c. Are any of the survey subjects consuming nutrients in excess of the recommendation (RDA or AI)?
   d. Are any nutrients consumed in excess of the UL?
   e. Do you think these supplements will fulfill the expectations of the consumers? Why or why not?

References

1. Furr, H. C., and Clark, R. M. Intestinal absorption and tissue distribution of carotenoids. Nutr. Biochem. 8:364–377, 1997.
2. Food and Nutrition Board, Institute of Medicine. *Dietary Reference Intakes: Vitamin A, Vitamin K, Arsenic, Boron, Chromium, Copper, Iodine, Iron, Manganese, Molybdenum, Nickel, Silicon, Vanadium, and Zinc.* Washington, D.C.: National Academy Press, 2001.
3. Ross, A. C. Vitamin A and retinoids, In *Modern Nutrition in Health and Disease,* 9th ed. Shils, M. E., Olson, J. A., Shike, M., and Ross, A. C., eds. Baltimore: Williams & Wilkins, 1999, pp. 305–327.
4. Maden, M. Vitamin A in embryonic development. Nutr. Rev. 52:S3–S12, 1994.
5. Ross, D. A. Vitamin A and public health. Proc. Nutr. Soc. 57:159–165, 1998.
6. Underwood, B. A. Micronutrient malnutrition: is it being eliminated? Nutr. Today 33:121–129, 1998.
7. Binkley, N., and Krueger, D. Hypervitaminosis A and bone. Nutr. Rev. 58:138–144, 2000.
8. Collins, M. D., and Mao, G. E. Teratology of retinoids. Ann. Rev. Pharmacol. Toxicol, 39:399–430, 1999.
9. Cooper, D. A., Eldridge, A. L., and Peters, J. C. Dietary carotenoids and lung cancer: a review of recent research. Nutr. Rev. 57:133–145, 1999.
10. Pryor, W. A., Stahl, W., and Rock, C. L. Beta carotene: from biochemistry to clinical trials. Nutr. Rev. 58(I):39–53, 2000.
11. Holick, M. F. Vitamin D. In *Modern Nutrition in Health and Disease,* 9th ed. Shils, M. E., Olson, J. A., Shike, M., and Ross, A. C., eds. Baltimore: Williams & Wilkins, 1999, pp. 329–345.
12. DeLuca, H. F., and Zierold, C. Mechanisms and functions of vitamin D. Nutr. Rev. 56(II):S4–S10, 1998.
13. Food and Nutrition Board, Institute of Medicine, *Dietary Reference Intakes: Calcium, Phosphorus, Magnesium, Vitamin D, and Fluoride.* Washington, D.C.: National Academy Press, 1997.
14. Pugliese, M. T., Blumberg, D. L., Hludzinski, J., and Kay, S. Nutritional rickets in suburbia. J. Am. Col. Nutr. 17:637–641, 1998.
15. Jacques, P. F., Felson, D. T., Tucker, K. L., et al. Plasma 25-hydroxyvitamin D and its determinants in an elderly population sample. Am. J. Clin. Nutr. 66:929-936, 1997.
16. DeBoff, M. S., Kohlmeier, L., Hurwitz, S., et al. Occult vitamin D deficiency in postmenopausal U.S. women with acute hip fracture. JAMA 281:1505–1511, 1999.
17. Blank, S., Scanlon, K. S., Sinks, T. H., and Falk, H. An outbreak of hypervitaminosis D associated with the overfortification of milk from a home-delivery dairy. Am. J. Public Health 85:656–659, 1995.
18. Booth, S. L., Pennington, J. A. T., and Sadowski, J. A. Food sources and dietary intakes of vitamin K_1 (phylloquinone) in the American diet: data from the FDA Total Diet Study. J. Am. Diet. Assoc. 96:149–154, 1996.
19. Olson, R. E. Vitamin K. In *Modern Nutrition in Health and Disease,* 9th ed. Shils, M. E., Olson, J. A., Shike, M., and Ross, A. C., eds. Baltimore: Williams & Wilkins, 1999, pp. 363–380.
20. Booth, S. L., and Suttie, J. W. Dietary intake and adequacy of vitamin K. J. Nutr. 128:785–788, 1998.
21. Thomas, J. A. Oxidative stress and oxidative defense. In *Modern Nutrition in Health and Disease,* 9th ed. Shils, M. E., Olson, J. A., Shike, M., and Ross, A. C., eds. Williams & Wilkins, Baltimore, MD, 1999, pp. 751–760.
22. Halliwell, B. Antioxidants and human disease: a general introduction. Nutr. Rev. 55(II):S44–S52, 1997.
23. Food and Nutrition Board, Institute of Medicine. *Dietary Reference Intakes for Vitamin C, Vitamin E, Selenium, and Carotenoids.* Washington, D.C.: National Academy Press, 2000.
24. Abbey, M. The importance of vitamin E in reducing cardiovascular risk. Nutr. Rev. 53:S28–S32, 1995.
25. Steiner, M. Vitamin E, a modifier of platelet function: rationale and use in cardiovascular and cerebrovascular disease. Nutr. Rev. 57:306–309, 1999.
26. Emmert, D. H., and Kirchner, J. T., The role of vitamin E in the prevention of heart disease. Arch. Family Med. 8:537–542, 1999.

27. Rimm, E. B., Stampfer, M. J., Ascherio, A., et al. Vitamin E consumption and the risk of heart disease in men. N. Engl. J. Med. 328:1450–1456, 1993.
28. Stampfer, M. J., Hennekens, C. H., Manson, J. E., et al. Vitamin E consumption and the risk of heart disease in women. N. Engl. J. Med. 328:1487–1489, 1993.
29. Stephens, N. G., Parsons, A., Schofield, P. M., et al. Randomized controlled trial of vitamin E in patients with coronary disease: Cambridge Heart Antioxidant Study (CHAOS). Lancet 347:781–786, 1996.
30. Yusuf, S. Vitamin E supplementation and cardiovascular events in high-risk patients. The Heart Outcomes Prevention Evaluation Study Investigators. N. Engl. J. Med. 342:154–160, 2000.
31. Podmore, I. D., Griffiths, H. R., Herbert, K. E., et al. Vitamin C exhibits pro-oxidant properties. Nature 392:559, 1998.
32. Carr, A., and Frei, B. Does vitamin C act as a pro-oxidant under physiological conditions? FASEB J. 13:1007–1024, 1999.
33. Halliwell, B. Vitamin C: poison, prophylactic or panacea? Trends Biochem. Sci. 24:255–259, 1999.
34. Blanchard, J., Tozer, T. N., and Rowland, M. Pharmacokinetic perspectives on megadoses of ascorbic acid. Am. J. Clin. Nutr. 66:1165–1171, 1997.
35. Hemilä, H. Vitamin C supplementation and common cold symptoms: factors affecting the magnitude of the benefit. Med. Hypotheses 52:171–178, 1999.
36. Jari, R. J., and Harakeh, S. Antiviral and immunomodulatory activities of ascorbic acid. In *Subcellular Biochemistry*, vol. 25: *Ascorbic Acid: Biochemistry and Biomedical Cell Biology*. Harris, J. R., ed. New York: Plenum Press, 1996, pp. 215–231.
37. Johnston, C. S. The antihistamine action of ascorbic acid. In *Subcellular Biochemistry*, vol. 25: *Ascorbic Acid: Biochemistry and Biomedical Cell Biology*. Harris, J. R., ed. New York: Plenum Press, 1996, pp. 189–231.
38. Lynch, S. M., Gaziano, M., and Frei, B. Ascorbic acid and atherosclerotic cardiovascular disease. In *Subcellular Biochemistry*, vol. 25: *Ascorbic Acid: Biochemistry and Biomedical Cell Biology*. Harris, J. R., ed. New York: Plenum Press, 1996, pp. 331–367.
39. Lonn, E. M., and Yusuf, S. Is there a role for antioxidant vitamins in the prevention of cardiovascular diseases? An update on epidemiological and clinical trials data. Can. J. Cardiol. 13:957–965, 1997.
40. Shklar, G., and Schwartz, J. L. Ascorbic acid and cancer. In *Subcellular Biochemistry*, vol. 25: *Ascorbic Acid: Biochemistry and Biomedical Cell Biology*. Harris, J. R., ed. New York: Plenum Press, 1996, pp. 233–247.
41. Head, K. A. Ascorbic acid in the prevention and treatment of cancer. Altern. Med. Rev. 3:174–186, 1998.
42. van Poppel, G., and van den Berg, H. Vitamins and cancer. Cancer Lett. 19:195–202, 1997.
43. Albert, C. M., Hennekens, C. H., O'Donnell, C. J., et al. Fish consumption and risk of sudden cardiac death. JAMA 279:23–28, 1998.
44. American Dietetic Association. Position of the American Dietetic Association: functional foods. J. Am. Diet. Assoc. 99:1278–1285, 1999.
45. Fund, W. C. R. Food, nutrition, and the prevention of cancer: a global perspective. Washington D.C.: American Institute for Cancer Research, 1997.
46. Craig, W. J. Phytochemicals: guardians of our health. J. Am. Diet. Assoc. 97:199–204, 1997.
47. Beecher, G. R. Phytonutrients' role in metabolism: effects on resistance to degenerative processes. Nutr. Rev. 57(II):S3–S6, 1999.
48. Steinmetz, K. A., and Potter, J. D. Vegetables, fruit, and cancer prevention: a review. J. Am. Diet. Assoc. 96:1027–1039, 1996.
49. Cooper, D. A., Eldridge, A. L., and Peters, J. P. Dietary carotenoids and certain cancers, heart disease, and age-related macular degeneration: a review of recent research. Nutr. Rev. 57:201–214, 2000.
50. Miller, N. J., Sampson, J., Candeias, L.P., et al. Antioxidant activities of carotenes and xanthophylls. FEBS Lett. 384:240–246, 1996.
51. Palozza, P. Prooxidant actions of carotenoids in biologic systems. Nutr. Rev. 56:257–265, 1998.
52. Fehey, J. W., Zhang, Y., and Talalay, P. Broccoli sprouts: an exceptionally rich source of inducers of enzymes that protect against carcinogens. Proc. Natl. Acad. Sci. USA 94:10367–10372, 1997.
53. American Dietetic Association. Position of the American Dietetic Association: phytochemicals and functional foods. Am. J. Diet. Assoc. 95:493–496, 1995.
54. American Dietetic Association. Americans' Food and Nutrition Attitudes and Behaviors—Nutrition and You: Trends 2000. Available online at **http://www.eatright.org/pr/2000/010300a.html.** Accessed 11 Nov 2000.
55. American Dietetic Association. Position of the American Dietetic Association: vitamin and mineral supplementation. J. Am. Diet. Assoc. 96:73–77, 1996.
56. Bui, M. H., Sauty, A., Collet, F., and Leuenberger, P. Dietary vitamin C intake and concentrations in the body fluids and cells of male smokers and nonsmokers. J. Nutr. 122:312–316, 1992.
57. Radimer, K. L., Subar, A. F., and Thompson, F. E. Nonvitamin, nonmineral dietary supplements: issues and findings from NHANES III. J. Am. Diet. Assoc. 100:447–454, 2000.
58. Kelly, G. S. The role of glucosamine sulfate and chondroitin sulfates in the treatment of degenerative joint disease. Altern. Med. Rev. 3:27–39, 1998.
59. Aukema, H. M., and Holub, B. J. Inositol and pyrroloquinoline quinone. In *Modern Nutrition in Health and Disease*, 8th ed. Shils, M. E., Olson, J. A., and Shike, M., eds. Philadelphia: Lea & Febiger, 1994, pp. 449–458.
60. Ramos L. Beyond the headlines: SAMe as a supplement. J. Am. Diet. Assoc. 100:414, 2000.
61. Bartels, C. L., and Miller, S. L. Herbal and related remedies. NCP 13:3–18, 1998.

11 Water and the Electrolytes

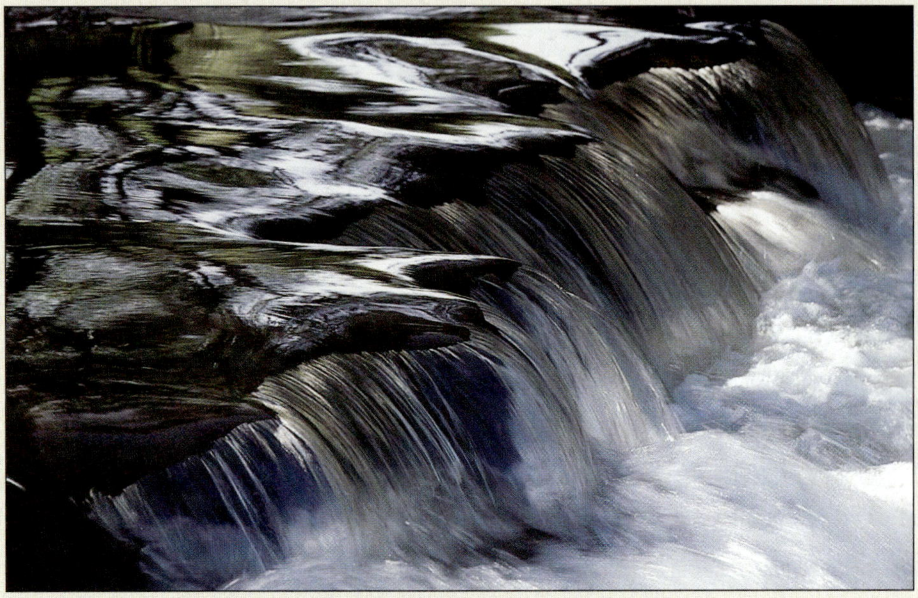

Learning Objectives

After reading this chapter, students should be able to:

1. Explain what is meant by the internal sea.
2. List and describe the sources of body water and the routes by which water is lost.
3. Describe five functions of water in the body.
4. Explain the role of the kidneys in regulating the amount of water in the body.
5. Discuss the effects of dehydration.
6. Define the term "electrolyte" and discuss the functions of electrolytes in the body.
7. Explain how blood pressure is regulated.
8. Define "hypertension" and list its symptoms and consequences.
9. Discuss the effect of dietary salt intake on blood pressure.
10. Describe the DASH diet and how it affects blood pressure.

When Gabriele Andersen-Scheiss emerged from the tunnel into the Olympic stadium in 1984 for the final lap of the women's marathon, she didn't look much like a world-class athlete. The 37-year-old runner staggered around the track as if drunk, her left arm limp, her right leg stiff. What was wrong with this athlete? She had completed about 26 of the 26.2 miles of the marathon and now it wasn't clear she could negotiate a single lap around the track. Should someone stop her?

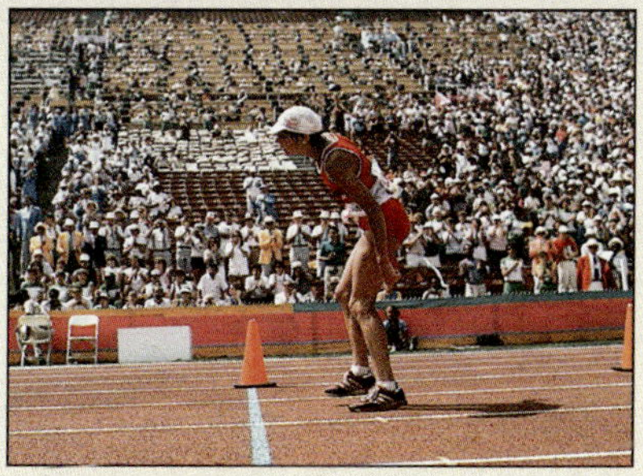

Medical officers rushed over to help but she waved them off. After observing her as she proceeded around the track, doctors made the decision to allow her to continue unaided. Andersen-Scheiss demonstrated the signs of serious dehydration, but because the medics could see that she was sweating profusely, they concluded that she was not yet suffering from heat stroke, the most severe and life-threatening stage of thermal distress. The gold medalist in this race, Joan Benoit, had crossed the finish line 20 minutes earlier, so Andersen-Scheiss struggled simply to finish, not to win. One minute the crowd cheered her on, and the next they pleaded for the medics to stop her. Her final staggering lap around the track to the finish line lasted 5 minutes and 44 seconds. Medics immediately treated her for heat exhaustion. She recovered rapidly, was released from the hospital after only two hours, and returned to the Olympic village to grab a bite to eat. She had finished 37th in the first women's Olympic marathon.

This case illustrates how important water is in maintaining body systems. Dehydration can be devastating and can come on rapidly, but it can be alleviated faster than any other nutrient deficiency. If not treated, however, dehydration can be fatal.

The Internal Sea

The complex molecules necessary for the emergence of life were forged in the earth's first seas. These primordial seas supported life because they were rich in inorganic minerals as well as organic substances (Figure 11.1). As organisms grew

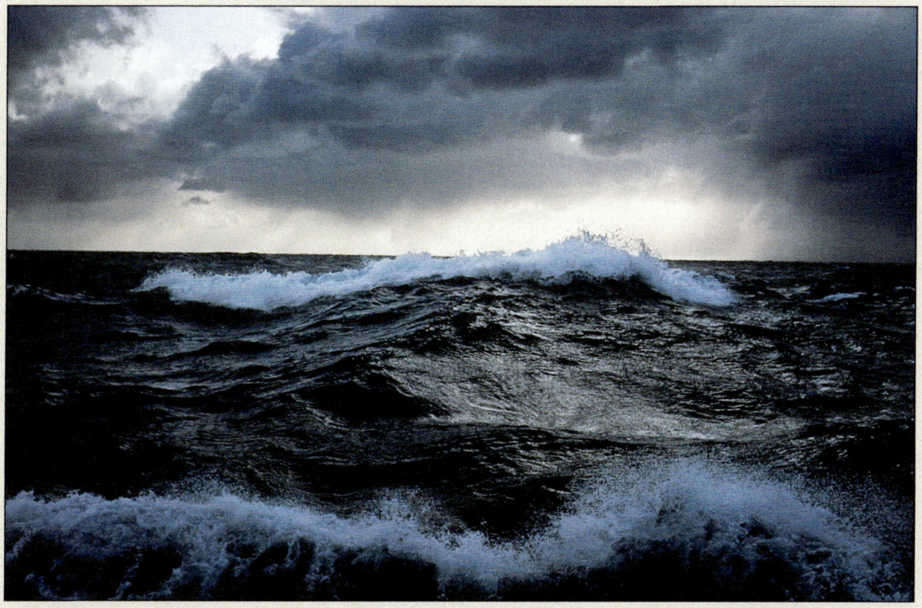

FIGURE 11.1 Seawater, rich in minerals, is similar in composition to blood plasma. (© *Kim Westerskov/Tony Stone Images*)

in complexity, the chemicals critical to their survival were incorporated into an "internal sea" of water and dissolved substances.

Minerals Elements needed by the body in small amounts for structure and to regulate chemical reactions and body processes.

Just as the right combination of water, organic molecules, and **minerals** was necessary for the beginning of life, the right combination is necessary inside the body for the maintenance of life. Scientists are still researching the exact mixture of minerals and other substances necessary for this internal sea to sustain life. The requirements for water and some of the minerals have long been known, but for others our understanding is just emerging. The next three chapters will present the sources, functions, and requirements of the inorganic components of the internal sea—water and minerals.

WATER

Web Menu: For more information on safe sources of drinking water, go to the EPA Office of Water at www.epa.gov/ow. For information on water ecology, go to Environment Canada at www.ec.gc.ca/water/en/nature/e_nature.htm.

Water is essential to survival. An average individual can live for about eight weeks without food, but a lack of water reduces survival to only a few days. Within the body, the amount and distribution of water are highly regulated, and even minor changes in these parameters can be life-threatening. Because water cannot be stored, water intake must be balanced with water losses to meet needs over the short term. When water losses are increased, as they are in hot weather and during exercise, intake must increase to maintain homeostasis.

Sources of Water

Water in the body comes from water in the diet—mostly as water itself and other fluids but also from solid food. For example, low-fat milk is 90% water, apples are about 85% water, and roast beef is about 50% water (Figure 11.2). A small amount of water is generated inside the body by metabolism, but this is not significant in meeting body water needs.

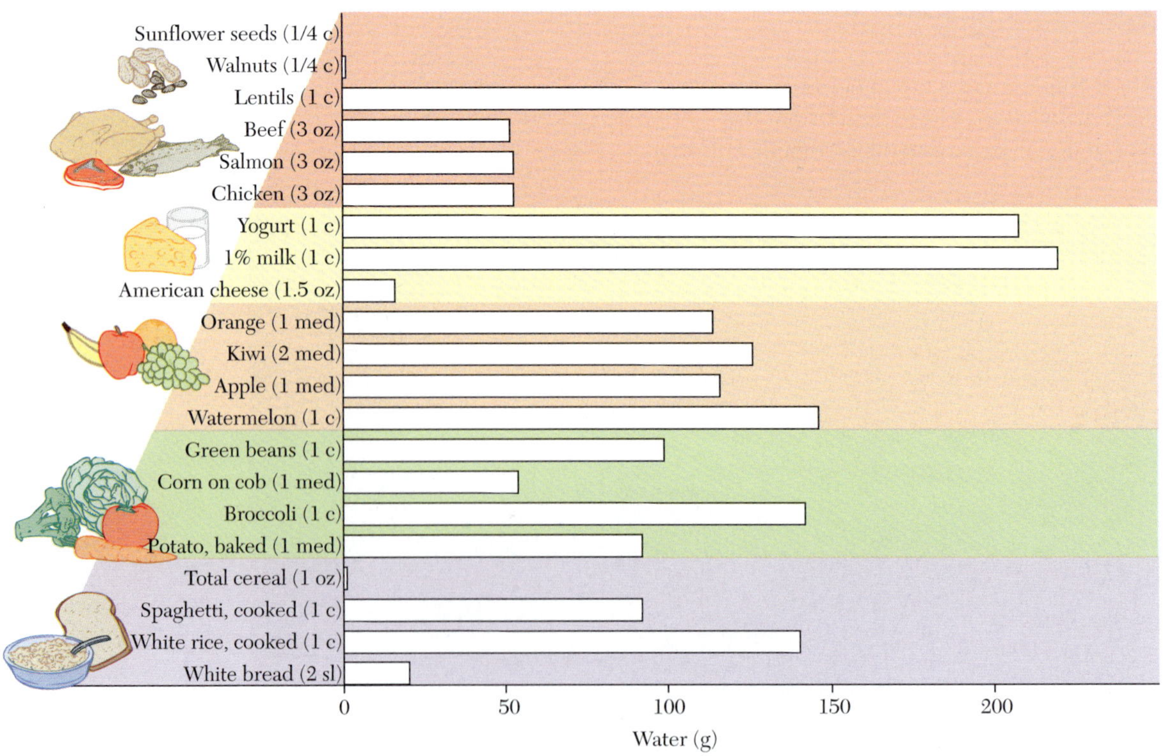

FIGURE 11.2 The body's need for water is met by the water consumed in fluids and food. Fruits and vegetables as well as many choices from other food groups have a high water content.

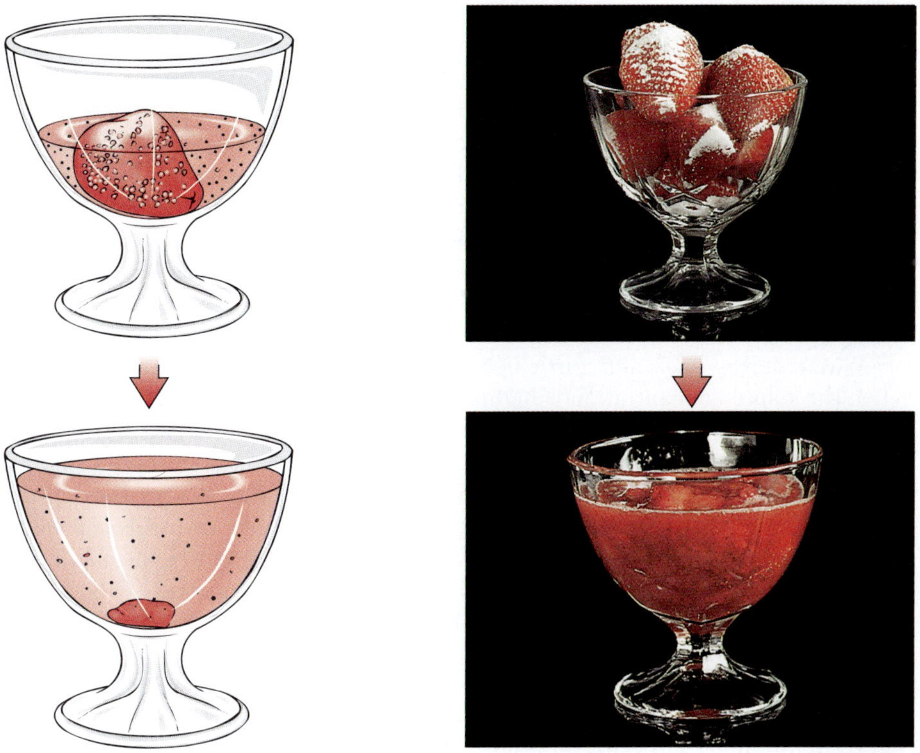

FIGURE 11.3 Osmosis is the process by which water moves across a membrane from an area of lower solute concentration to an area of higher solute concentration. When sugar is sprinkled on strawberries, osmosis draws water out of the strawberries to dilute the concentrated sugar solution on the surface. (*Photos, Dennis Drenner*)

Water in the Digestive Tract

Osmosis The passive movement of water across a semipermeable membrane to equalize the concentration of dissolved solutes on both sides.

Solute A dissolved substance.

Water is absorbed passively by a special type of diffusion called **osmosis**. Osmosis is the diffusion of water across a membrane from an area with a lower **solute** concentration to an area with a higher solute concentration. Osmosis occurs across a selectively permeable membrane, such as a cell membrane, which allows water to pass freely but regulates the passage of dissolved substances. Water moves across this membrane in a direction that will equalize the solute concentration on both sides. For example, when sugar is sprinkled on fresh strawberries, the water inside the strawberries moves across the skin of the fruit to equalize the sugar concentration on each side, causing the fruit to shrink (Figure 11.3).

The absorption of water from the digestive tract occurs because of the osmotic gradient created by the absorption of nutrients from the lumen into the plasma. In other words, as nutrients are absorbed, the solute concentration in the lumen decreases. Water moves with the absorbed nutrients toward the area with the highest solute concentration.

About 1.7 liters of water enter the GI tract each day from the diet. Another 7 liters comes from saliva and other gastrointestinal secretions. Most of this fluid is absorbed in the small intestine; a small amount is absorbed in the colon. The rate of absorption is influenced by the volume of water and the density of nutrients consumed with it. Consuming a large volume of water increases its rate of absorption; increasing the nutrients it contains decreases the rate of absorption.[1]

Water in the Body

The amount and distribution of water in the body is tightly regulated. Water balance is essential to maintaining homeostasis because of the many and varied functions that water serves in the body.

Distribution of Body Water In adults, about 60% of body weight is water. The percentage is higher in infants and in adults decreases with age primarily due to a decline in muscle mass. Water is found in varying proportions in all the tissues of the body; blood is about 90% water, muscle about 75%, and bone about 25%. Adipocytes have a low water content—only about 10%. Because women typically have a higher percentage of body fat than men, they have less body water, and obese individuals have a proportionally lower water content than their lean counterparts.

About two thirds of body water is found inside cells; this is known as **intracellular fluid**. The remaining one third is outside cells, as **extracellular fluid**. Extracellular fluid includes primarily blood plasma and the fluid between cells, called **interstitial fluid**. Interstitial fluid makes up about three fourths of the extracellular fluid and plasma about one fourth. Other extracellular fluids include lymph and fluids in cavities, such as that inside the lumen of the GI tract, the eyes, joints, and spinal cord (Figure 11.4).

Intracellular fluid The fluid located inside cells.

Extracellular fluid The fluid located outside cells. It includes fluid found in the blood, lymph, gastrointestinal tract, spinal column, eyes, and joints, and that found between cells and tissues.

Interstitial fluid The portion of the extracellular fluid located in the spaces between cells.

Blood pressure The amount of force exerted by the blood against the artery walls.

Water moves back and forth between these different fluid compartments. When the solute concentration is higher in one compartment than another, water moves by osmosis. For example, if the concentration of solutes in the blood is high, water from the interstitial fluid is drawn into the blood diluting the solutes. This increases the blood volume and **blood pressure**, that is, the pressure of the blood against the blood vessel walls. This pressure in the blood vessels can cause water to move into the interstitial fluid. Much of this water reenters the capillaries by osmosis. The small amount that remains in the tissues is removed by the lymph vessels. Lymph is therefore composed of interstitial fluid that has been drained away from the tissues for return to the plasma.

Water Losses Water is lost from the body in urine, feces, and through evaporation from the lungs and skin (see Figure 11.4). As shown in Figure 11.5, a typical young man loses about 2.75 liters of water daily through urine, feces, and evaporation. This amount must be replaced through consumption of food and fluids in order to maintain water balance.

Typical urine output is 1 to 2 liters per day, but this varies depending on the amount of fluid consumed and the amount of waste to be excreted. The waste products that must be excreted in urine include urea and other nitrogen-containing products from protein breakdown, ketones from fat breakdown, phosphates, sulfates, and other minerals. The amount of urea that must be excreted is increased when dietary protein intake or body protein breakdown is increased. Ketone excretion is increased when body fat is broken down. In both cases, the need for water increases in order to produce more urine to excrete the extra wastes.

The amount of water lost in the feces is usually small, only about 100 to 200 ml per day (less than a cup). This is remarkable because every day about 9 liters of fluid enter the gastrointestinal tract via food, water, and gastrointestinal secre-

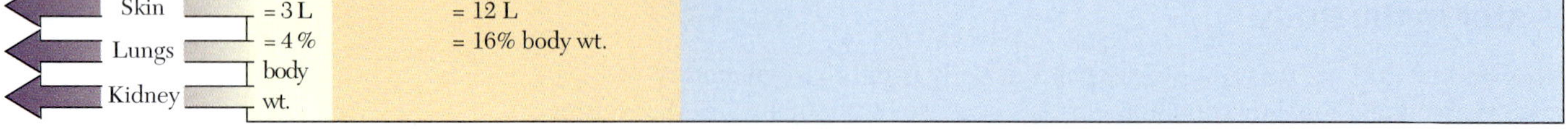

Total body water = 40 L = 60% body wt.
Extracellular fluid = 15 L = 20% body wt.
Intracellular fluid = 25 L = 40% body wt.
GI tract
Plasma = 3 L = 4% body wt.
Interstitial fluid = 12 L = 16% body wt.
Skin
Lungs
Kidney

FIGURE 11.4 This figure indicates the approximate amounts of water in the intracellular and extracellular (plasma and interstitial) fluid compartments of a 70-kg man. Water enters the body primarily through the gastrointestinal tract and is lost in the urine and through evaporation from the skin and lungs. Most body water is located intracellularly but can move back and forth between the intracellular and extracellular compartments.

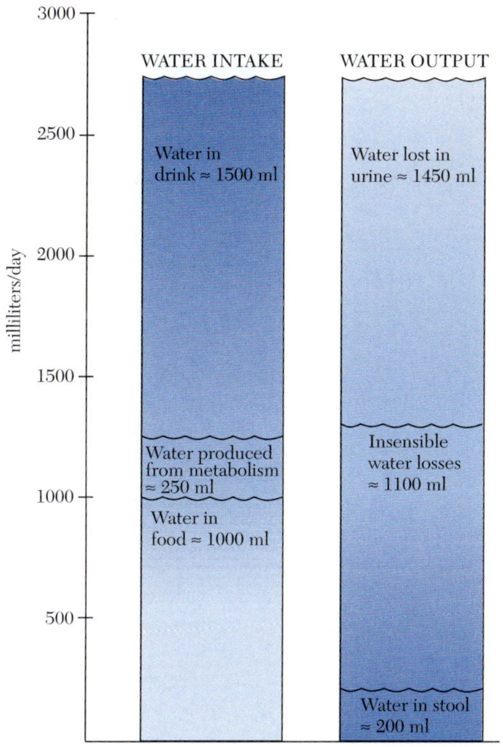

FIGURE 11.5 To maintain water balance, intake must equal output. This figure shows the sources of water intake and output in a 70-kg adult who is not losing water in sweat.

tions. Under normal conditions, more than 95% is reabsorbed before the feces are eliminated. However, in cases of severe diarrhea, large amounts of water can be lost through the gastrointestinal tract.

Water loss due to evaporation from the skin and respiratory tract takes place continuously. Because the individual is unaware that this is occurring, such losses are referred to as **insensible losses**. An inactive person at room temperature loses about 1000 ml per day through insensible losses, but the amount varies depending on body size, environmental temperature and humidity, and physical activity. For example, a very dry environment, such as that in an airplane or in the desert, increases evaporative losses.

Insensible losses Fluid losses that are not perceived by the senses, such as evaporation of water from the skin and lungs.

Water lost in sweat is distinct from insensible losses because it is a detectable loss. The amount of water lost through sweat is extremely variable depending on the individual as well as their environment and degree of physical activity. An individual doing light work at a temperature of about 84°F will lose about 2 to 3 liters of sweat per day. Strenuous exercise in a hot environment can cause water losses in sweat to be as high as 2 to 4 liters in an hour.[2] Even when endurance athletes consume fluids while exercising, they cannot compensate for all water lost in sweat. Water loss can be estimated by comparing body weight before and after exercise. Lost weight can be replaced by consuming the equivalent weight in fluids. For instance, an athlete who loses 2 pounds during a workout should consume an extra 2 pints or a liter of fluid (1 lb = 1 pint = 1/2 liter) (see Chapter 14).

Regulation of Body Water The essential functions of water in the body require that there be a constant supply without excess or deficiency. Because water cannot be stored in the body, intake and excretion must be carefully regulated in order to maintain water balance—that is, the state in which water losses are replaced by water intake over the short term.

Thirst: Regulating Fluid Intake The need to consume water or other fluids is signaled by the sensation of thirst. Thirst is triggered by the thirst center in the hypothalamus when it senses a decrease in plasma volume and an increase in the concentration of dissolved substances in the plasma. A decrease in plasma volume

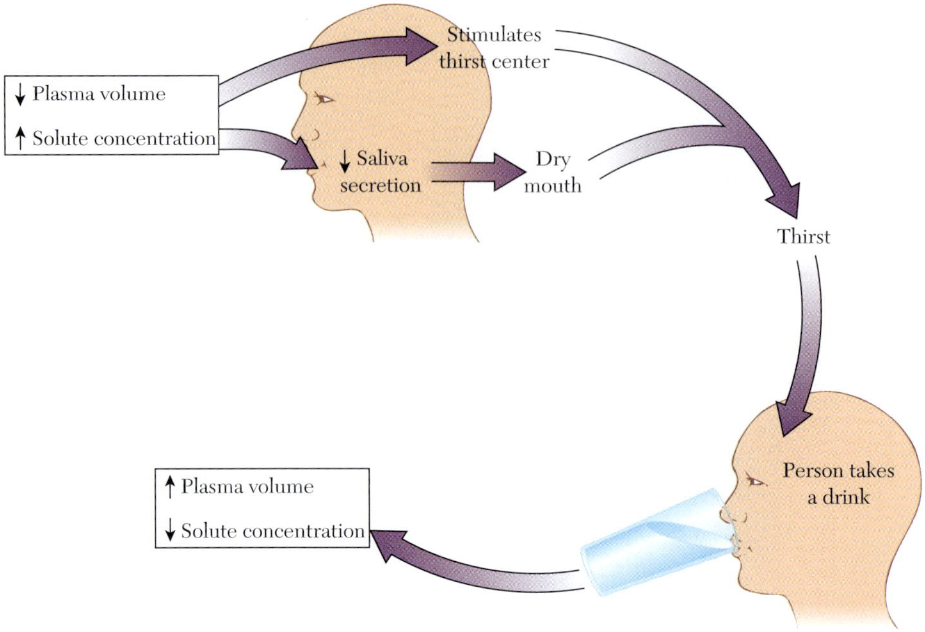

FIGURE 11.6 When an individual hasn't consumed enough fluid, plasma volume decreases and the concentration of solutes in the plasma increases. There is a decrease in saliva, which causes a dry mouth and sends signals to the brain to stimulate thirst. When fluid is consumed, plasma volume increases and solute concentration decreases.

also causes a dry mouth. This is because less water is available to the salivary glands, causing saliva secretion to decrease. Together, signals from the hypothalamus and a dry mouth cause the sensation of thirst and motivate the consumption of fluid (Figure 11.6).

Thirst is not a perfect regulator of water intake, however. It is quenched almost as soon as fluid is consumed and long before water balance has been restored. Also, the sensation of thirst often lags behind the need for water. For example, athletes exercising in hot weather lose water rapidly but do not experience intense thirst until they have lost so much body water that their physical performance is compromised.[3] A person with fever, vomiting, or diarrhea may also be losing water rapidly and thirst mechanisms may not be adequate to replace the fluid. In the elderly, the thirst mechanism often becomes unreliable, so an individual may not be thirsty even though body water is depleted. Also, being thirsty does not mean that the individual will take a drink. Because people cannot and do not always respond to thirst, water loss from the body is regulated by the kidneys to prevent dehydration.

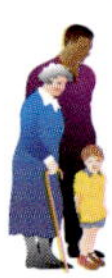

Kidneys: Regulating Water Excretion The kidneys serve as a filtering system that regulates the amount of water and dissolved substances retained in the blood and excreted in urine. As blood flows through the kidneys, water and small molecules are filtered out of the blood vessels. Some of the water and molecules are reabsorbed and the rest are excreted in the urine. The amount of water that is reabsorbed depends on conditions in the body. When the concentration of solutes in the blood is high, the pituitary gland secretes **antidiuretic hormone (ADH)**, which signals the kidneys to reabsorb water, reducing the amount lost in the urine. This reabsorbed water is returned to the blood, decreasing the solute concentration to normal (Figure 11.7). When the solute concentration in the blood is low, ADH levels decrease so less water is reabsorbed and more is excreted in the urine, allowing blood solute concentration to increase to normal. The amount of sodium in the blood, blood volume, and blood pressure also play a role in regulating body water, as discussed later.

Antidiuretic hormone (ADH) A hormone secreted by the pituitary gland that increases the amount of water reabsorbed by the kidney and therefore retained in the body.

Functions of Water Water performs many functions in the body. It serves as a medium in which chemical reactions take place; it transports nutrients; it provides protection; and it helps regulate temperature. It also participates in chemical reactions and is important for regulating acid-base balance within the body (Table 11.1).

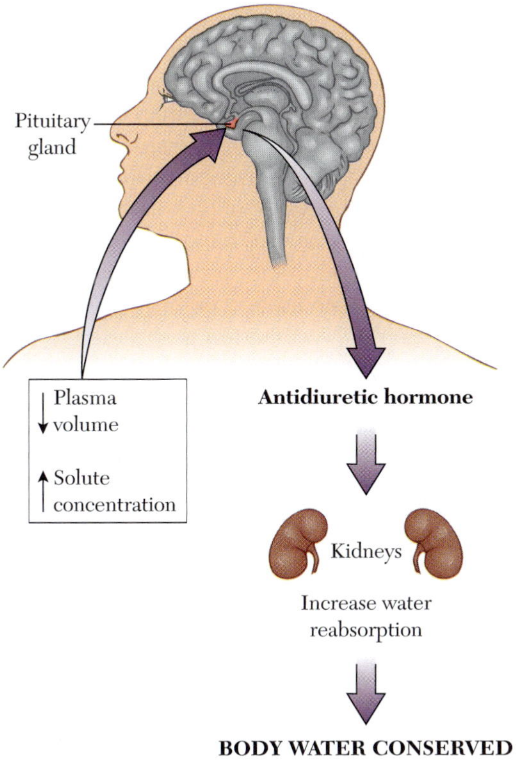

FIGURE 11.7 When an individual hasn't consumed enough fluid, plasma volume decreases and solute concentration increases, signaling the pituitary gland to secrete antidiuretic hormone, which acts on the kidneys to increase water reabsorption thereby decreasing water losses.

Water As a Solvent One of the key functions of water in the body is as a **solvent**, which is a fluid in which solutes can dissolve to form a solution. Water is an ideal solvent for some substances because it is **polar**—that is, the two sides or poles of the water molecule have different electrical charges. The polar nature of water comes from its structure, which consists of two hydrogen atoms and one oxygen

Solvent A fluid in which one or more substances dissolve.

Polar Used to describe a molecule that has a positive charge at one end and a negative charge at the other.

TABLE 11.1 A Summary of Water and the Electrolytes

Nutrient	Sources	Recommended Intake for Adults	Major Functions	Deficiency Symptoms	Groups at Risk	Toxicity	Tolerable Upper Intake Levels (UL)
Water	Food and beverages	1ml/kcal of intake	Solvent, reactant, protector, transporter, temperature regulator	Thirst, weakness, confusion, disorientation	Infants, athletes, elderly, those with fever or diarrhea	Unlikely; confusion, coma, convulsions	N/A
Sodium	Table salt, processed foods	500–2400 mg	Major extracellular ion, nerve transmission, muscle contraction, fluid balance	Muscle cramps	Those consuming a very low sodium intake	High blood pressure in sensitive individuals	N/A
Potassium	Grains, vegetables, fruits	At least 1600–3500 mg	Major intracellular ion, nerve transmission, muscle contraction	Irregular heartbeat, fatigue, muscle cramps	Those consuming a diet high in processed foods, those taking thiazide diuretics	Abnormal heartbeat	N/A
Chloride	Table salt	750–3400 mg	Major extracellular ion	Unlikely	None	None likely	N/A

N/A = No UL established at time of publication.

Dissociate To separate into two charged ions.

Electrolytes Substances that separate in water to form positively and negatively charged ions and are able to conduct an electric current. In nutrition, this term refers to sodium, potassium, and chloride.

Hydrolysis reactions Chemical reactions that break large molecules into smaller ones by the addition of water.

Condensation reactions Chemical reactions that join two molecules together. Hydrogen and oxygen are lost from the two molecules to form water.

pH A measure of the level of acidity or alkalinity of a solution.

Acid A substance that releases hydrogen ions when in solution.

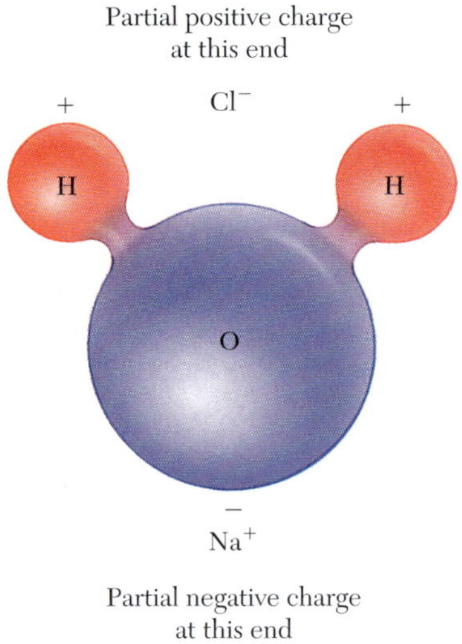

FIGURE 11.8 Two hydrogen atoms share electrons with one oxygen atom to form a molecule of water. The electrons spend more time around the oxygen atom, giving it a slightly negative charge, while the side of the molecule with the two hydrogens has a slightly positive charge. When salt (sodium chloride) is added to water the positive sodium ion is attracted to the negative pole of the water molecule and the negative chloride ion is attracted to the positive pole.

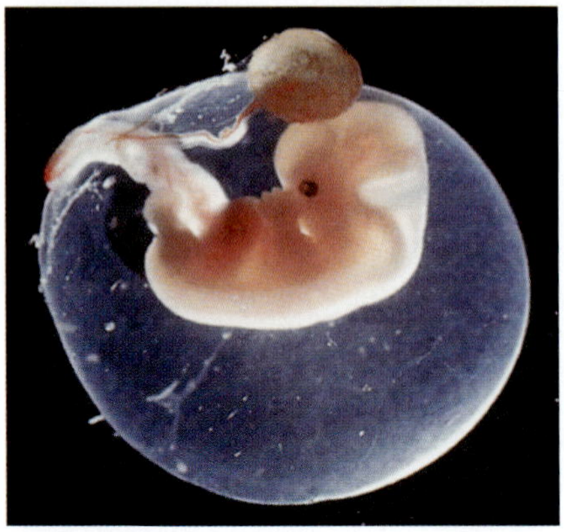

FIGURE 11.9 During development, a watery cushion of amniotic fluid provides protection. (*© Petit Format/Nestle SS/Photo Researchers, Inc.*)

atom. These atoms, like all atoms, are made up of a positively charged central core, or nucleus, with negatively charged electrons orbiting around it. To form a water molecule, the two hydrogen atoms move close enough to share their electrons with an atom of oxygen. But the sharing is not equal. The shared electrons spend more time around the oxygen atom than around the hydrogen atoms, giving the oxygen side of the molecule a slightly negative charge and the hydrogen side a slightly positive charge. The polar nature of water allows it to surround other charged molecules and disperse them. For example, table salt, which dissolves in water, consists of a positively charged sodium ion bound to a negatively charged chloride ion. When placed in water, the sodium and chloride ions move apart, or **dissociate**, because the positively charged sodium ion is attracted to the negative pole of the water molecule and the negatively charged chloride ion is attracted to the positive pole (Figure 11.8). Substances such as sodium chloride that dissociate in water to form positively and negatively charged ions are known as **electrolytes**. Electrolytes got their name because they are capable of conducting an electrical current when dissolved in water. In a solution of electrolytes, the number of positive and negative charges is equal. In nutrition, sodium, chloride, and potassium are referred to as electrolytes.

Water As Transport Blood, which is 90% water, transports oxygen and nutrients to cells. It then carries carbon dioxide and waste products away from the cells. Water in urine transports waste products, such as urea and ketones, out of the body.

Water As Protection Water functions as a lubricant and cleanser. Watery tears lubricate the eyes and wash away dirt, synovial fluid lubricates the joints, and saliva lubricates the mouth, making it easier to chew and swallow food. Water inside the eyeballs and spinal cord acts as a cushion against shock. Similarly, during pregnancy, water in the amniotic fluid provides a protective cushion for the fetus (Figure 11.9).

Water As a Regulator of Temperature Body temperature is closely regulated at about 98.6°F (37°C). If the body temperature rises above 108°F or falls below 80°F, death is likely. The fact that water changes temperature slowly in response to changes in the external environment helps the human body resist temperature change when the outside temperature fluctuates. The water in blood actively regulates body temperature. When body temperature starts to rise, the blood vessels in the skin dilate, causing blood to flow close to the surface of the body and release some of the heat to the environment. This occurs with fevers as well as when environmental temperature rises. In a cold environment, blood vessels in the skin constrict, restricting the flow of blood near the surface and conserving body heat. The most obvious way that water helps regulate body temperature is through the evaporation of sweat. When body temperature increases, the sweat glands in the skin secrete this watery substance. As the sweat evaporates from the skin, heat is lost.

Water in Chemical Reactions Water is involved in chemical reactions in the body. **Hydrolysis reactions** break large molecules into smaller ones by the addition of water. For example, water is added in the reaction that breaks a molecule of maltose into two glucose molecules. Water is also involved in reactions that join two molecules. These reactions are referred to as **condensation reactions**. The formation of a dipeptide from two amino acids requires the removal of a water molecule (Figure 11.10).

Acid-Base Balance The chemical reactions that occur in the body are very sensitive to acidity. Water and the dissolved substances it contains are important for maintaining the proper level of acidity. Acidity is expressed in units of **pH**, which is a measure of the hydrogen ion concentration of a solution. A molecule that dissociates while in solution to release hydrogen ions is called an **acid**. As the hydrogen ion concentration increases, the pH decreases and the solution is said to

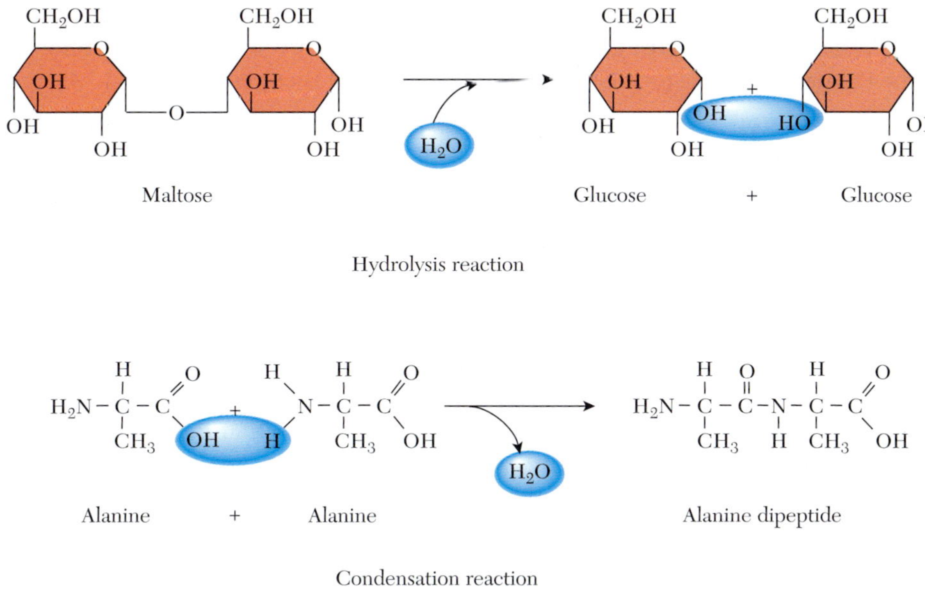

FIGURE 11.10 The cleavage of the disaccharide maltose into two molecules of glucose is an example of a hydrolysis reaction. The formation of a dipeptide is an example of a condensation reaction.

become more acidic. Lemon juice (pH 2.2) and vinegar (pH 3) are examples of acidic solutions. A solution that accepts hydrogen ions is called a **base**. When the hydrogen ion content is low, pH is high and the solution is said to be basic or alkaline. Ammonia (pH 11) and baking soda (pH 9) are both basic. The range of pH units is from 1 to 14, with 1 being very acidic, 14 being very basic, and 7 being neutral. Most reactions in the body occur in slightly basic solutions, around pH 7.4. If body solutions become too acidic or too basic, chemical reactions cannot proceed efficiently (Figure 11.11).

Base A substance that accepts hydrogen ions when in solution.

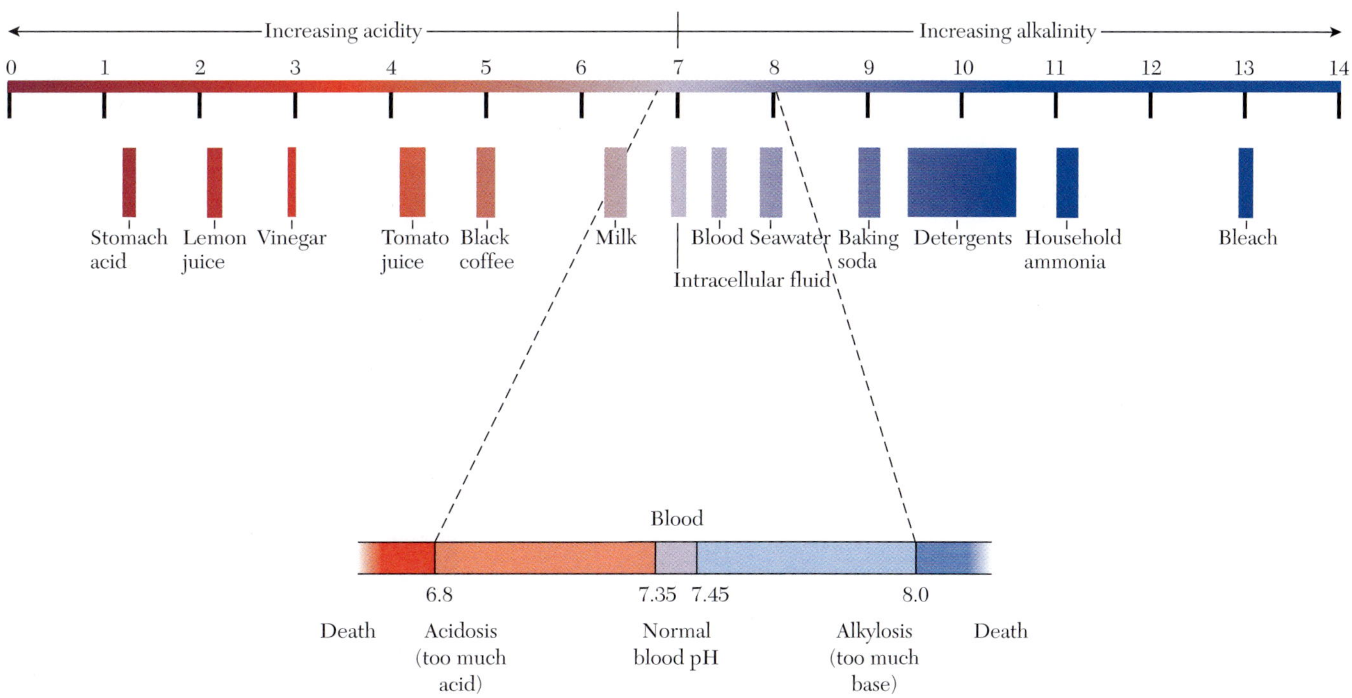

FIGURE 11.11 pH values of common fluids. Fluctuations from the normal blood pH range of between 7.35 and 7.45 lead to acidosis or alkylosis and, if severe, can be fatal.

Acid-base balance in the body is regulated by three types of controls: chemical buffers in body fluids, gas exchange in the respiratory system, and filtration in the kidneys. Water plays an important role in each of these controls.

Chemical Buffers A substance that resist changes in pH by accepting or donating hydrogen ions is called a **buffer**. One of the most important buffer systems involves the reaction of carbon dioxide (CO_2) with water to form a bicarbonate ion (HCO_3^-). Other important buffers in the body include phosphate (see Chapter 12) and blood proteins. Buffer systems work rapidly (in a fraction of a second) and are the body's first line of defense against changes in pH.

Buffer A substance that prevents changes in pH by picking up or releasing hydrogen ions to prevent changes in pH.

Respiratory System The respiratory system affects acid-base balance by eliminating CO_2 from the body. When the amount of acid (H^+) is high, the respiration rate—or number of breaths per minute—increases and more CO_2 is lost in expired air. When CO_2 is lost, the hydrogen ion concentration decreases, causing the pH to increase (Figure 11.12). When the H^+ concentration is low, breathing slows down so less CO_2 is lost and the pH decreases. The respiratory system can cause a change in pH within a few minutes.

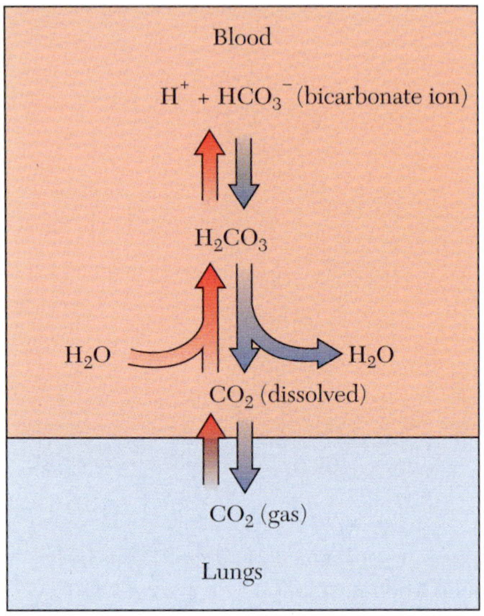

FIGURE 11.12 The respiratory system helps to regulate acid-base balance by increasing or decreasing the loss of CO_2. When the respiratory rate increases so does the amount of CO_2 exhaled. This causes the reactions to move in the direction of the blue arrows so more H^+ combines with HCO_3^- (bicarbonate ion), reducing the amount of H^+ in the blood and thereby reducing acidity (pH increases). When the respiration rate decreases, less CO_2 is lost and the reactions favor the red arrows, so H^+ concentration increases (pH decreases).

Kidneys The kidneys can affect pH by regulating the amount of H^+ and bicarbonate ions that are lost in the urine or retained in the blood. If the blood is too acidic, the kidney can excrete H^+ in the urine and reabsorb bicarbonate (a base) to raise the blood pH. The regulation of pH by the kidney is slower, taking several hours to days.

Water Requirements

Adults need about 1 ml of water per kcalorie of energy requirement, or about 2 to 3 liters per day. This amount is sufficient under average conditions, but needs can be increased by variations in activity, environment, and diet. For instance, a person exercising in a hot climate can require an additional 4 liters or more per day to replace water lost through sweating (Figure 11.13). Water needs are also affected by the composition and adequacy of the diet. For example, a low-energy diet increases water needs because water losses increase

Web Menu

For more information on fluid needs, go to the American Bottled Water Association at www.bottledwater.org/ and click on the hydration calculator.

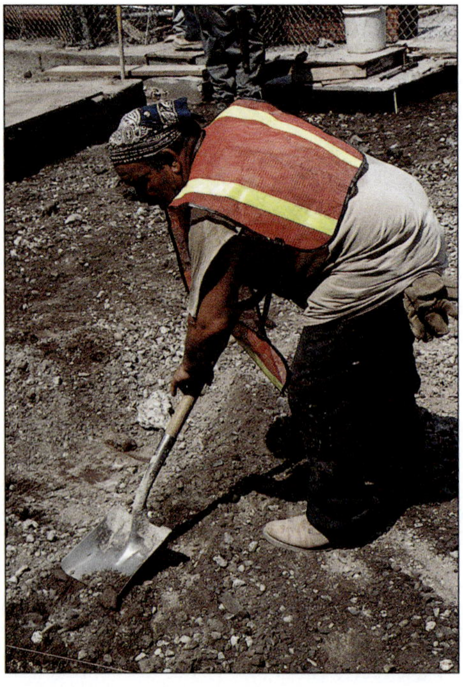

FIGURE 11.13 Physical work in a hot environment can dramatically increase water losses in sweat. (© *Robert Brenner/Photo Edit*)

TABLE 11.2 Factors That Increase Water Needs

Diet

High-protein diet—increases urinary losses to excrete excess nitrogen
Low-energy diet—increases urinary losses to excrete ketones produced
High-sodium diet—increases urinary losses to excrete excess sodium
High-fiber diet—increases fecal losses
Caffeinated beverages—increases urinary losses due to diuretic effect
Alcoholic beverages—increases urinary losses due to diuretic effect

Activity

Exercise—increases sweat and evaporative losses through the respiratory tract

Environment

Low humidity—increases evaporative losses through the skin and respiratory tract
High temperature—increases sweat and evaporative losses
High altitude—increases evaporative losses

Medications

Diuretics—increases urinary losses
Caffeine—increases urinary losses

Medical conditions

Early renal disease—increases urinary losses because kidneys cannot reabsorb water
Diabetes—increases urinary losses to excrete the excess blood glucose
Fever—increases evaporative losses
Diarrhea—increases losses through the gastrointestinal tract
Vomiting—increases losses through the gastrointestinal tract
Burns—increases losses due to fluid lost from burned areas

to excrete the ketones produced by fat breakdown. A high-protein diet increases the amount of nitrogen that must be excreted. A high-sodium diet increases water needs because the excess salt must be excreted in the urine. Caffeine is a **diuretic**, so a diet that is high in caffeine increases water loss from the kidneys and therefore increases water needs. A high-fiber diet also increases water needs because more fluid is retained in the gastrointestinal tract (see Table 11.2).

Diuretic A substance that promotes water loss from the body by increasing the volume of urine.

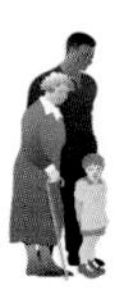

Water needs also increase during pregnancy and lactation. In pregnancy, water is needed to increase blood volume, produce amniotic fluid, and nourish the fetus. During lactation, the fluid secreted in milk, about 750 ml or 3 cups per day, must be restored by the mother's fluid intake.

The fluid requirements for infants are higher than those for adults. One reason is that the infant's kidneys cannot concentrate urine as efficiently as adult kidneys, so water loss is greater. Moreover, insensible losses are more significant in infants and children because body surface area relative to body weight is much greater than in adults. In addition to having greater water needs, infants are susceptible to dehydration because they cannot ask for a drink when they are thirsty. An intake of 1.5 ml per kcalorie of energy expenditure, or about 3 cups (750 ml) a day for a six-month-old infant, is recommended. This is the water-to-energy ratio in human milk.

Water and Health

A deficiency of water can cause clinical symptoms more rapidly than any other nutrient deficiency. Likewise, health can be restored in a matter of minutes or hours when fluid is replaced. An excess of body water, called water toxicity, rarely occurs in healthy individuals.

Dehydration A decrease of 1% or more of body fluids.

Dehydration When water loss exceeds water intake, **dehydration** results. Dehydration occurs when water loss is great enough for blood volume to decrease, thereby reducing the ability to deliver oxygen and nutrients to cells and remove waste products. Even mild dehydration—a body water loss of 1 to 2% of body weight—can impair physical and cognitive performance.[4] Early symptoms of dehydration include headache, fatigue, loss of appetite, dry eyes and mouth, and dark-colored urine. A loss of 5% body water can cause nausea and difficulty concentrating. When water loss approaches 7%, confusion and disorientation may occur. A loss of about 10 to 20% can result in death (Figure 11.14).

Thermal Distress Fluid imbalance in a hot environment or during strenuous exercise can lead to thermal distress, which includes dehydration as well as heat cramps, heat exhaustion, and heat stroke. Heat cramps are involuntary muscle cramps and spasms that are caused by an imbalance of the electrolytes sodium and potassium at the muscle cell membranes. They occur during prolonged strenuous physical activity in a hot environment. They often result when a large amount of water and electrolytes are lost in sweat and replaced with plain water rather than water plus electrolytes. Heat exhaustion occurs when fluid loss causes blood volume to decrease so much that it is not possible to both cool the skin and deliver oxygen to active muscles. Heat exhaustion is characterized by a rapid weak pulse, low blood pressure, fainting, profuse sweating, and disorientation. Heat stroke, the most serious form of thermal distress, occurs when the temperature regulatory center of the brain fails. Heat stroke is characterized by elevated body temperature, hot dry skin, extreme confusion, and unconsciousness. It requires immediate medical attention.

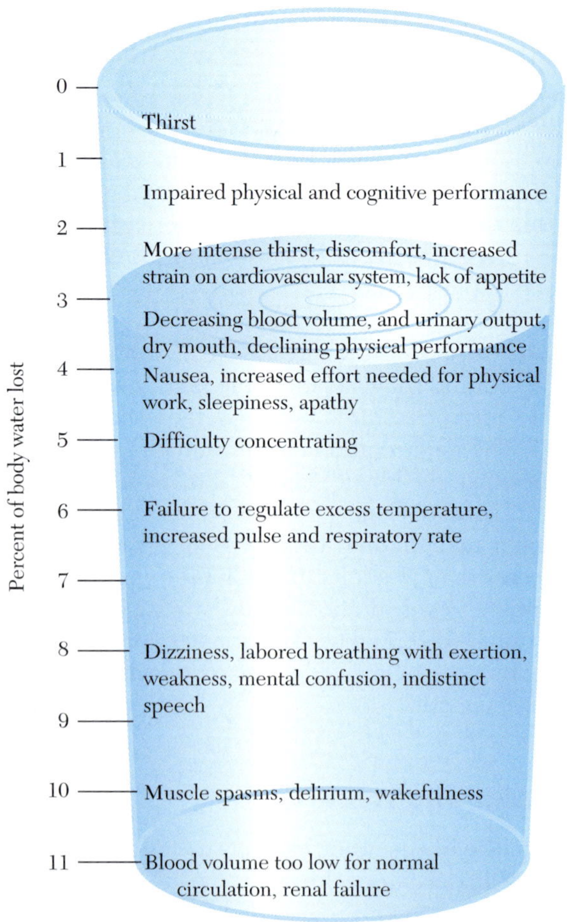

FIGURE 11.14 As the degree of dehydration increases, the adverse effects of dehydration increase in severity. This can occur rapidly if water losses are excessive as may occur with profuse sweating, vomiting, or diarrhea.

Water Intake and Cancer Low fluid intake has been linked to bladder cancer. It is theorized that increased fluid intake reduces exposure of bladder cells to carcinogens by diluting the urine. A study that examined fluid intake and bladder cancer in men found that water intake of 6 or more cups per day was associated with a 51% reduction in bladder cancer risk when compared to those who drank only 1 cup per day.[5]

Water Toxicity An excess of water, or water toxicity, is rare because of the kidneys' ability to regulate how much water is excreted. However, it can occur due to illness or improper administration of intravenous fluids. Symptoms of water toxicity include mental dulling, confusion, coma, convulsions, and even death.

Meeting Fluid Needs

Most adults can meet their water needs by consuming about 8 eight-ounce cups of fluid per day. This does not all need to be consumed as water; other hydrating fluids such as juice, milk, and noncaffeinated beverages can also meet needs. Beverages that contain caffeine or alcohol, such as coffee, tea, caffeinated soda, beer, and wine, are considered dehydrating fluids. Such beverages provide fluid, but they act as diuretics—which actually increase water loss—so they are not effective at maintaining water balance and may increase the need for hydrating fluids. Because a third of the fluids Americans drink every day are dehydrating fluids, the intake of hydrating fluids often may not be sufficient to maintain adequate hydration. Studies suggest that a proportion of the population is chronically slightly dehydrated. One survey found that each day Americans drink about 11.7 cups of hydrating fluids and 5.9 cups of dehydrating fluids.[6] This survey also found that many Americans experience health problems that could be due to dehydration, such as frequent tiredness, dry and itchy skin, headaches, indigestion, lapses in concentration, and constipation (see *Making Decisions:* "Is Bottled Water Better?").

Web Menu: For more information on meeting fluid needs during exercise, go to the Medicine and Science in Sports and Exercise Position stands at www.ms-se.com/ and click on exercise and fluid replacement.

Electrolytes: Salts of the Internal Sea

Electrolytes are elements that conduct electricity when dissolved in water. In nutrition, the term is used to refer to the minerals sodium, potassium, and chloride—the principal electrolytes in body fluids. The modern diet is typically low in potassium and high in sodium and chloride, which are generally consumed together as sodium chloride, or table salt. This is a change from the diets of prehistoric hunter-gatherers, which consisted of plant foods such as nuts, berries, roots, and greens that are high in potassium and low in salt (Figure 11.15). Most of this change is due to the use of salt as a food additive. Salt is used as a preservative in food because it inhibits bacterial growth; it is also used to add flavor and to heighten existing flavors. It was highly prized by ancient cultures in Asia, Africa, and Europe, where it was used in rituals as well as in the preservation of food. Roman soldiers were paid in *sal*, the Latin word for salt, from which we get our word "salary."

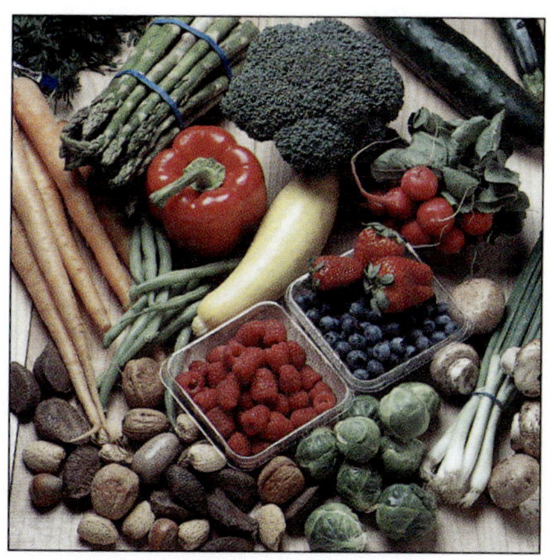

FIGURE 11.15 Foods in their natural state are usually low in sodium. (© *Charles D. Winters)*

Today, rather than a prized commodity, salt is a substance we attempt to limit in the diet. The reason is that diets high in salt have been implicated as a risk factor for high blood pressure.

Making Decisions

Is Bottled Water Better?

We need to consume water to survive. We want it to be safe and taste good. In general the water supply in the United States is safe, but water is not risk-free. Our drinking water is potentially exposed to hundreds of different contaminants, including pesticides, nitrates from fertilizers, microorganisms, metals such as lead and iron, and radioactive compounds. Sometimes a problem arises because contamination has entered a municipal water supply, and sometimes the source of contamination is an individual well or household. For example, *Cryptosporidium*, a parasite that is commonly found in rivers and lakes, has found its way into municipal water supplies and caused several large outbreaks of gastrointestinal illness.[a] Well water can be contaminated with pesticides and fertilizers from agricultural runoff, and lead, leaching from old household plumbing, can contaminate water after it enters the home. Although water contamination is rare, consumers have become concerned about the safety of the water supply and many now use bottled water. But is bottled better?

Bottled water or drinking water is defined as water that is intended for human consumption sealed in bottles or other containers with no added ingredients except safe and suitable antimicrobial agents.[b] Bottled water comes in many forms—spring water, drinking water, purified water, well water. There are over 700 different brands available in the United States. Consumers who assume that buying water in a bottle is a guarantee of purity may be wasting their money. In reality, the jug at the water cooler and the Evian that you guzzle at the gym may not be any safer than tap water. Standards for the purity of municipal water systems are set by the Environmental Protection Agency (EPA). These same standards are used by the FDA to ensure that the minimum quality of bottled water is comparable with that of tap water.[c] Because the standards that regulate bottled water are no more rigid than those regulating tap water, it is not surprising that some bottled water actually is tap water.

About 75% of bottled water comes from protected wells and springs, but the other 25% is from municipal water supplies. To help consumers identify the source of their bottled water and make labeling consistent from state to state, the FDA established standard definitions for all bottled water products.[d] Under these regulations, bottled water that comes directly from tap water must be clearly labeled as such and indicate the municipality from which the water was taken. However, water that has been taken from a municipal water supply and then treated—for example, filtered or disinfected—need not indicate that it is tap water. "Distilled water" and "purified water" are examples of water taken from municipal water supplies and then treated. If you want water that did not come from the tap, select artesian water, spring water, well water, or mineral water. These come from underground water sources (see table).

Water from all of these sources, as well as the water used in certain types of flavored bottled waters, must comply with the bottled water standards set by the FDA. The FDA has also established Current Good Manufacturing Practice (CGMP) regulations for processing and bottling drinking water.[b] According to these regulations, the source of the water to be bottled must be approved and in compliance at all times with the applicable laws and regulations. CGMP regulations require that bottled water be processed, packaged, transported, and stored under safe and sanitary conditions. They also require that bottled water producers monitor the source of their water and their finished products for contaminants to ensure that their products comply with the quality standards for bottled water. Beverages containing flavors in amounts greater than one-percent-by-weight and products labeled as seltzer water, soda water, and tonic water are classified as soft drinks, which are regulated as food, not as water.

Individuals who are concerned about their tap water, but who do not want to carry water home from the grocery store, may choose a home water-treatment system. There are many different kinds. Faucet filters remove chlorine and other substances that make the water taste bad. More elaborate filter units, distillation units, and water softeners remove contaminants but may also

Sources of Electrolytes

The typical American diet contains about 9 g of salt. Salt is 40% sodium and 60% chloride by weight, so 9 g contain 3.6 g of sodium ($9 \times 40\% = 3.6$ g) and 5.4 g of chloride. Most of the salt in the Western diet comes from processed foods. Only 10% comes from salt found naturally in food, while 15% is from that added in cooking and at the table, and 75% is from that added during processing and manufacturing. Most of the sodium in processed foods is from sodium chloride, but other sodium salts, such as sodium bicarbonate, sodium citrate, and sodium glutamate, are also used as food additives and contribute to the sodium content of the diet. These sodium-containing additives are used as preservatives and leavening agents. Drinking water from community water supplies contributes less than 10% of our sodium intake.[7] Softened water or mineral water is often higher in sodium than tap water and, if consumed in large quantities, can contribute significantly to daily sodium intake.

In contrast to sodium and chloride, the richest sources of potassium are unprocessed foods such as fruits, vegetables, whole grains, and fresh meats. Bananas, oranges, potatoes, and tomatoes are some of the best sources. Processed foods are generally low in potassium (Figure 11.16).

change the mineral content of the water. For example, an ion exchange unit, or water softener, removes some minerals, mainly calcium and magnesium, from water and replaces them with sodium. Because minerals in hard water stain tubs, clog water heaters, and cause soap to form a film that is difficult to remove from laundry, softened water makes life easier at home. But, there may be health benefits to hard water. The incidence of heart attacks is lower in areas of the country that have hard water.[e] In addition, softened water has about twice the amount of sodium—about 94 mg per liter. If you are following a sodium-restricted diet, you may need to bypass the water softener when it comes to drinking water.

When choosing your water, you must weigh the benefits against the risks. Bottled water and water-treatment systems cost money, and, whether you are drinking your tap water straight, filtering it with a home water-treatment system, or buying bottled water, contamination is possible. The safest alternative is to buy distilled water. In the distillation process, nonvolatile chemicals are removed and the heat destroys bacteria and other biological contaminants. The resulting water is probably free of contaminants, but it is tasteless and lacking in essential dietary minerals that water usually supplies. Before making a choice, take a look at the results of water-monitoring tests your water company is required to perform and compare them with the legal limits of contaminants set by the EPA. This should help you decide. For information, call the FDA, the International Bottled Water Association, or the EPA Hotline, or look for their sites on the World Wide Web.

References

[a]EPA and CDC Office of Ground Water and Drinking Water. Guidance for people with severely weakened immune systems. June 17, 1998. Available online at **http://www.epa.gov/safewater/crypto.html.** Accessed 14 Jan 2001.

[b] Requirements of laws and regulations enforced by the U.S. Food and Drug Administration. Available online at **http://www.fda.gov/opacom/morechoices/smallbusiness/blubook.htm#btlwater.html.** Accessed 14 Jan 2001.

[c] Notebook. FDA Consumer 29:27, March 1995.

[d] FDA Talk. Paper No. 2 (T95–59), November 7, 1995.

[e] Rubenowitz, E., Axelsson, G., and Rylander, R. Magnesium in drinking water and death from acute myocardial infarction. Am. J. Epidemiol. 143:456–462, 1996.

Types of Bottled Water

Artesian/Artesian well: Water that comes from a well.

Drinking: Water that is sold for human consumption in sanitary containers and contains no added sweeteners or chemical additives (other than flavors, extracts, or essences). It must be kcalorie-free and sugar-free.

Mineral: Water that contains a constant level and relative proportions of minerals at the point of emergence from the source. No minerals can be added to this product.

Purified: Water that has been produced by distillation, deionization, reverse osmosis, or other suitable processes.

Distilled: Water produced by distillation, a process that heats the water to produce steam and then recondenses the steam into liquid water that is free of nonvolatile substances including minerals.

Deionized: Water produced by deionization or reverse osmosis (called reverse osmosis water) to reduce its mineral content.

Sparkling: Water, that after treatment and possible replacement of carbon dioxide, contains the same amount of carbon dioxide that it had at emergence from the source.

Spring: Water that is derived from an underground formation from which water flows naturally to the surface of the Earth. Spring water must be collected only at the spring or through a bore hole tapping the spring.

Well: Water from a hole bored, drilled, or otherwise constructed in the ground that taps the water of an aquifer.

Adapted from the International Bottled Water Association. Available online at **http://www.bottledwater.org/public/faqs.htm#2.**

Electrolytes in the Body

Almost all of the sodium, chloride, and potassium consumed in the diet is absorbed. In the body, electrolytes help regulate fluid balance and are important for nerve conduction, muscle contraction, and transport (see Table 11.1).

Electrolytes and Fluid Balance The distribution of fluid in the body compartments depends on the concentration of electrolytes and other solutes. Water moves by osmosis in response to solute concentration. All body fluids are in osmotic balance so a change in blood volume, for example, also affects interstitial fluid and intracellular fluid volumes. Sodium plays a pivotal role in controlling extracellular fluid volume and water distribution in the body.

The concentration of specific electrolytes in body compartments differs dramatically. Potassium is the principal positively charged ion inside cells, where it is 30 times more concentrated than outside the cell. Sodium is the most abundant positively charged electrolyte in the extracellular fluid and chloride is the principal negatively charged extracellular ion.

The concentration of these electrolytes is regulated, often by active transport. For example, cell membranes are not very permeable to sodium or potassium,

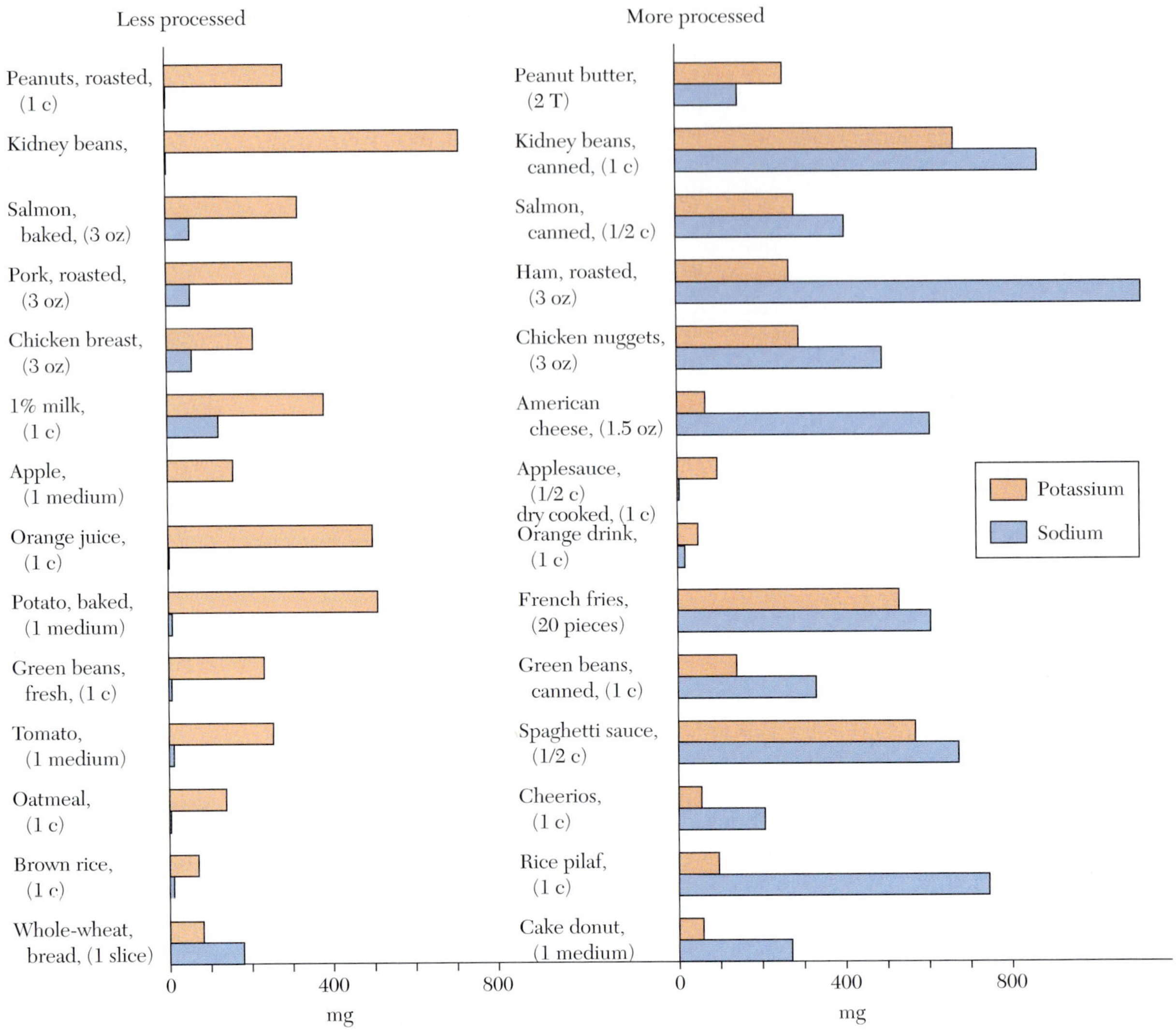

FIGURE 11.16 Less processed foods tend to be low in sodium and good sources of potassium. More processed foods are generally higher in sodium and may also be lower in potassium.

but some does leak across membranes. The sodium-potassium-ATPase is an active transport system that keeps the concentration of potassium higher inside the cells and that of sodium higher outside the cells (Figure 11.17). Maintaining this concentration gradient of electrolytes is important for nerve conduction and muscle contraction. It requires a great deal of energy: It is estimated that the sodium-potassium-ATPase accounts for 20 to 40% of resting energy expenditure in an adult. The pumping of Na^+ across cell membranes is also linked to nutrient transport. For example, glucose and amino acids are transported by systems that depend on the movement of sodium ions across cell membranes.

Nerve Conduction and Muscle Contraction Sodium and potassium are important for the conduction of nerve impulses. An electrical charge, or membrane potential, exists across nerve cell membranes because the number of negative ions just inside the cell membrane is greater than the number outside. This occurs because the cell membrane allows more positively charged ions to leak out of the cell than to leak into the cell. Nerve impulses are created by a change in the electrical charge across cell membranes. Stimuli, such as touch or the presence of neurotransmitters, change the cell membrane's permeability to sodium, allowing sodium to rush into the cells. This reverses, or depolarizes, the charge of the cell

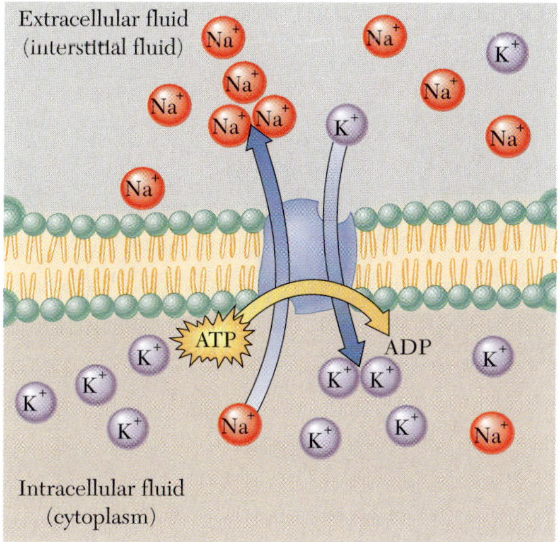

FIGURE 11.17 The sodium-potassium-ATPase pump uses the energy in ATP to pump potassium ions into the cell and sodium ions out. This keeps the concentration of sodium outside the cell higher and the concentration of potassium inside the cell higher. Each cycle of the pump brings two potassium ions into the cell and expels three sodium ions.

membrane at that location, and an electrical current is generated. The nerve impulse travels along the nerve cell as an electrical current. Once the nerve impulse passes, the original membrane potential is rapidly restored by another change in cell membrane permeability; then the original distribution of sodium and potassium ions across the cell membrane is restored by the sodium-potassium-ATPase pump in the cell membrane. A similar mechanism causes the depolarization of the muscle cell membranes, leading to muscle contraction.

Electrolyte Balance Despite large variations in dietary intake, homeostatic mechanisms act to regulate the concentrations of these electrolytes in the body. For example, in northern China, sodium chloride intake is greater than 13.9 g per day; in the Kalahari Desert, it is less than 1.7 g per day; and in an Indian population in Brazil, consumption may be less than 0.06 g of salt per day. However, blood levels of sodium are not significantly different among these groups.[7]

Regulating Electrolyte Intake Sodium and chloride homeostasis is regulated to some extent by the intake of both water and salt. When salt intake is high, thirst is stimulated to increase water intake. When salt intake is very low, a salt appetite causes the individual to seek out the mineral. These mechanisms help ensure that appropriate proportions of salt and water are taken in.

The Kidney: Regulating Electrolyte Excretion Sodium, chloride, and potassium are excreted via the kidney, the skin, and the digestive system. In the absence of profuse sweating or diarrhea, losses through the skin and GI tract are small. The kidneys are the primary regulator of electrolyte balance in the body. Excretion of electrolytes in the urine is decreased when intake is low and increased when intake is high.

Sodium is the primary determinant of extracellular fluid volume. When the concentration of sodium in the blood increases, water follows, causing an increase in blood volume. Changes in blood volume can change blood pressure. This is sensed by pressure sensors throughout the vascular system. These sensors send excitatory or inhibitory signals to the brain to trigger the production and release of proteins and hormones that affect the amount of sodium, chloride—and hence water—retained by the kidneys. For example, when blood pressure decreases, the kidneys release the enzyme **renin**, beginning a series of reactions leading to the formation of **angiotensin II** (Figure 11.18). Angiotensin II increases blood pressure both by causing the blood vessel walls to constrict and by stimulating the release of the hormone **aldosterone**, which acts on the kidneys to increase the amount of sodium (and chloride) reabsorbed from the filtrate. Water follows the reabsorbed sodium, resulting in an increase in blood volume and,

Renin An enzyme produced by the kidney that aids in the conversion of angiotensin to its active form, angiotensin II.

Angiotensin II A compound that causes blood vessel walls to constrict and stimulates the release of the hormone aldosterone.

Aldosterone A hormone that increases sodium reabsorption and therefore enhances water retention by the kidney.

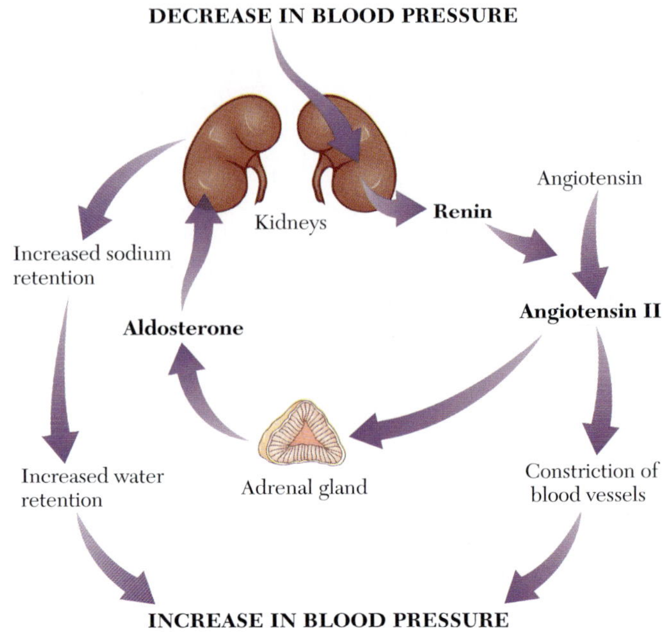

FIGURE 11.18 When blood pressure decreases, a series of events occurs to return it to the normal range. Renin is secreted, which stimulates the conversion of angiotensin to angiotensin II. Angiotensin II constricts blood vessels, thereby increasing blood pressure. It also acts at the adrenal gland to promote aldosterone production, which stimulates the kidney to increase sodium retention, and hence increase water retention, causing an increase in blood volume and blood pressure.

consequently, blood pressure. The increase in blood pressure then inhibits the release of renin and aldosterone so that blood pressure does not continue to rise.

As with sodium and chloride, the kidneys regulate potassium excretion to maintain a relatively constant amount of potassium in the body. If blood levels begin to rise, mechanisms are activated to stimulate the cellular uptake of potassium. This short-term regulation prevents the amount of potassium in the extracellular fluid from getting lethally high. The long-term regulation of potassium balance depends on aldosterone. Aldosterone causes the kidney to secrete potassium into the urine and retain sodium. Aldosterone release is triggered by high plasma potassium, low sodium, or angiotensin II.

Electrolyte Requirements

There is no 1989 RDA for sodium, and DRI values have not yet been established. The National Research Council has, however, estimated a minimum requirement of 500 mg of sodium per day for healthy adults.[7] The Daily Reference Value used to determine a Daily Value for food labels recommends consuming no more than 2400 mg of sodium per day. This is below the typical intake in the United States of about 3600 mg per day of sodium. Because of the effect of sodium on blood pressure in some individuals, the Dietary Guidelines for Americans recommend that salt and sodium be consumed in moderation.

There is also no 1989 RDA for chloride, nor have DRI values yet been established. The estimated minimum requirement is 750 mg per day for adults. The Daily Value used on food labels is 3400 mg.

Likewise, no 1989 RDA or DRI values have been established for potassium, but the National Research Council has recommended a minimum intake of 1600–2000 mg per day to maintain normal body stores and fluid concentrations. The Daily Reference Value recommends at least 3500 mg per day of potassium for adults. Potassium intakes vary greatly depending on food selection. Diets containing few fruits and vegetables provide about 2000 mg of potassium per day, and those high in fruits and vegetables provide 8000 to 11,000 mg.[8]

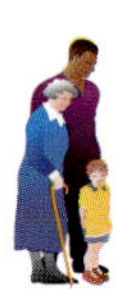

Pregnancy slightly increases sodium needs because the extracellular fluid volume increases. Pregnant women are advised to follow the sodium intake recommendation for the general population (see Chapter 15).[9] At one time, a dietary salt restriction was common during pregnancy to prevent a syndrome known as pregnancy-induced hypertension. The cause of pregnancy-induced hypertension is not known, but salt restriction is no longer recommended. During lactation, sodium needs are increased to replace the amount secreted in milk. This is equal to about 135 mg per day. In infants, sodium needs are estimated from the amount consumed in human milk, which contains more chloride than sodium. This same chloride-to-sodium ratio has been recommended for infant formulas.

Potassium is needed to build new cells, so its requirement increases during times of growth. In pregnancy, extra potassium is needed to build new tissue. During lactation, the increased need is to replace losses in milk. In children, potassium is needed for growth; required amounts can be met by following the recommendations of the Food Guide Pyramid.

Electrolytes and Health

In general, levels of electrolytes in the body are carefully regulated. However, deficient intakes and a number of disease states can affect levels in the body.

Electrolyte Deficiency Deficiencies of sodium and chloride are rare in healthy individuals. Although the taste for salt that triggers your desire to plunge into a bag of salty chips is a learned preference rather than a response to physiological need, humans with very low salt intakes do have a true physiological drive to consume salt. Conditions that cause sodium and chloride depletion include heavy and persistent sweating, chronic diarrhea or vomiting, and kidney disease. A sodium or chloride deficiency can cause disturbances in acid-base and electrolyte balance.

Symptomatic potassium deficiency is also uncommon. It occurs as a result of vomiting, diarrhea, increased urinary losses, and excessive sweating. Individuals at risk include those with eating disorders who may vomit frequently or abuse laxatives, those consuming very-low-energy diets, and those taking thiazide diuretic medications to treat hypertension. Generally, potassium supplements are prescribed along with or incorporated into medications that cause potassium loss. Potassium deficiency results in poor appetite, muscle cramps, confusion, apathy, constipation, and, eventually, an irregular heartbeat.

Electrolyte Toxicity Toxicities are also rare in healthy individuals. Excessive sodium intake has been related to hypertension in salt-sensitive individuals, but, for individuals without salt-sensitive hypertension, no toxic level of sodium intake has been documented as long as water needs are met and the kidneys are functioning properly. However, a high sodium intake increases calcium excretion and has been related to an increased risk of osteoporosis.[10]

Potassium toxicity from the diet is rare because urinary excretion is proportional to intake when kidney function is normal. If supplements are consumed in excess or kidney function is compromised, blood levels of potassium can increase and can eventually cause death due to an irregular heartbeat.

Web Menu: For more information on the incidence, causes, and treatment of high blood pressure, go to the National Heart, Lung, and Blood Institute site index at www.nhlbi.nih.gov/siteindex and look under high blood pressure, or to the American Heart Association Heart and Stroke Guide at www.americanheart.org/Heart_and_Stroke_A_Z_Guide/.

HYPERTENSION

Electrolytes in the body are carefully regulated and, in turn, help regulate fluid volume. As the extracellular fluid volume increases, blood pressure increases. A certain level of blood pressure is necessary to ensure that blood is delivered to all tissues. A healthy blood pressure is 120/80 mm of mercury (mm Hg) or less. The first and larger number is the systolic blood pressure and represents the highest pressure reached during a heart contraction. The lower number is diastolic pressure and represents the blood pressure in the vessels between heart beats. An increase in blood volume or a narrowing of the blood vessels can cause high blood pressure, or

Hypertension Blood pressure that is consistently elevated to 140/90 mm of mercury or greater.

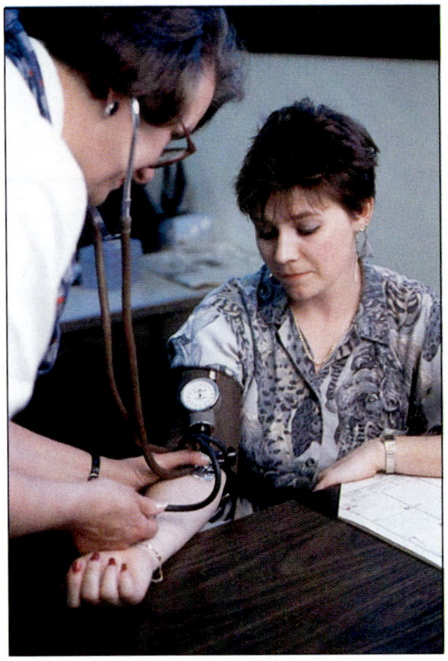

FIGURE 11.19 Blood pressure should be monitored regularly because high blood pressure has no obvious symptoms. Blood pressure measurements consist of two numbers. The top number is the systolic blood pressure, which represents the highest blood pressure reached during heart contraction. Systolic blood pressure should be about 120. The bottom number is the diastolic blood pressure, which indicates the pressure between heartbeats. Diastolic blood pressure should be about 80. *(Charles D. Winters)*

hypertension, generally defined as a blood pressure that is consistently 140/90 mm Hg or greater. This is the level that is associated with increased risk of cardiovascular diseases such as atherosclerosis, heart attack, and stroke.[11] It also increases the risks for kidney disease and early death. It is estimated that 20% of adult Americans have a blood pressure in this range.[11] Approximately 50 million Americans are at increased risk of illness and early death because of hypertension[12,13](Figure 11.19).

Causes of Hypertension

Most people with high blood pressure have essential hypertension, or hypertension with no obvious external cause. It is a complex disorder involving both genetic and environmental factors and is most likely the result of disturbances in one or more of the mechanisms that control body fluid and electrolyte balance. High blood pressure that occurs as a result of other disorders is referred to as secondary hypertension.

There is a genetic predisposition to hypertension, so a family history of high blood pressure increases one's risk of developing this disorder. It is more common in African Americans, Puerto Ricans, and Cuban and Mexican Americans than in non-Hispanic whites.[13] The increased incidence among African Americans is reflected in their 80% higher rate of death from stroke, 50% higher rate of death from heart disease, and 320% greater rate of hypertension-related kidney failure compared to Caucasians.[14] The risk of hypertension increases with age regardless of ethnicity or race. Hypertension occurs more frequently in individuals who have diabetes. Risk increases with obesity, and weight loss can prevent or delay the onset of hypertension in obese individuals.[15] Lifestyle factors also contribute to hypertension. A lack of physical activity, heavy alcohol consumption, and stress can increase blood pressure.[15] Blood pressure is also affected by diet.

Diet and Blood Pressure

Diets high in salt are associated with a higher incidence of hypertension, whereas diets high in fiber, potassium, calcium, and magnesium are associated with a lower incidence of hypertension. Higher intakes of omega-3 fatty acids may also lower blood pressure.[16] A dietary pattern that incorporates a low to moderate sodium intake and larger amounts of these other nutrients has a greater impact than that of any single nutrient.[17,18]

Sodium and Sodium Chloride The Intersalt study, which examined the incidence of hypertension in different populations, found that in populations consuming less than 4.5 g of salt per day, average blood pressure was low and hypertension was rare or absent. In populations consuming 5.8 g of salt or more per day, blood pressure increased with sodium intake.[19] As a result of epidemiological studies such as this one, a restriction of dietary sodium is commonly prescribed to reduce blood pressure in all hypertensive individuals. In addition, to decrease the incidence of hypertension in the population as a whole, moderate sodium intake is recommended by the Dietary Guidelines for Americans (Figure 11.20).

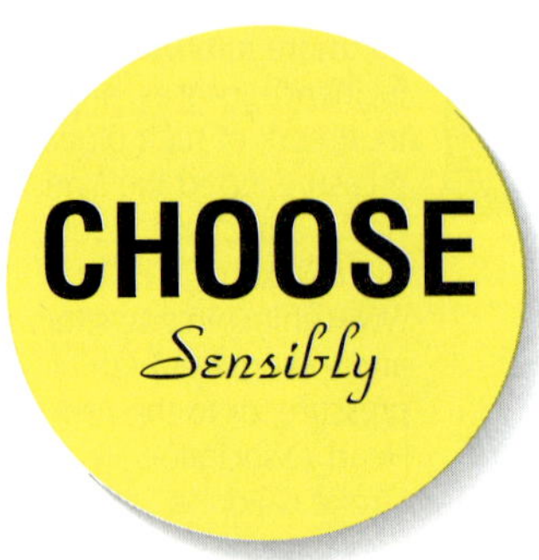

- Choose and prepare foods with less salt

FIGURE 11.20 The Dietary Guidelines for Americans, 2000, recommends that Americans "Choose and prepare foods with less salt."

Whether the intake of sodium or salt affects blood pressure in all individuals is controversial.[20] Some research suggests that the impact of sodium intake on blood pressure depends on whether or not the individual is salt sensitive. In salt-sensitive individuals, a reduction in salt intake will cause a decrease in blood pressure. Of individuals with hypertension, about half are salt sensitive—that is, their hypertension is aggravated by a high-salt diet. In the other half, dietary salt does not affect blood pressure.[21] In individuals who are salt sensitive, sodium has been shown to have little effect on blood pressure unless it is consumed with chloride as salt.[22] However, data from a recent trial has questioned the theory of salt-sensitivity. In this trial, the results showed that the lower the amount of sodium in the diet, the lower the blood pressure. An intake of 2400 mg of sodium (the amount recommended by the Dietary Guidelines) reduced blood pressure in those with and without hypertension, and even more significant reductions were seen when sodium intake was reduced to 1500 mg of sodium per day.[18]

Other Dietary Components That Affect Blood Pressure Nutrients other than sodium and chloride also play a role in maintaining blood pressure in a healthy range. Epidemiology has shown that dietary patterns with high intakes of fiber and the minerals potassium, magnesium, and calcium are associated with lower blood pressure. For example, populations and individuals consuming vegetarian diets, which are high in these nutrients, generally have lower blood pressure than nonvegetarians.[23]

Potassium Intake Primitive cultures worldwide and vegetarians in industrialized countries whose diets are high in potassium have a low incidence of hypertension, whereas groups that have low potassium intakes have a high incidence of hypertension.[24] The risk of stroke, which is associated with hypertension, was found to be lower in men who consumed about 4.3 g of potassium per day compared to those consuming 2.4 g per day.[25] Because populations that have high intakes of sodium generally have low intakes of potassium, it is difficult to tell if the hypertension associated with a high-sodium diet is due to the high sodium or the low potassium. The fact that a high dietary sodium intake increases the excretion of potassium suggests that low levels of potassium in the body affect hypertension. In addition, potassium supplements have been shown to decrease blood pressure.[26] Because excessive potassium intakes can cause an irregular heartbeat, potassium supplements are not recommended unless taken under the supervision of a physician. Increasing consumption of potassium-rich foods such as bananas, oranges, and potatoes is a safer way to increase potassium intake (Figure 11.21).

Calcium and Magnesium Epidemiology also supports a role for calcium and magnesium in regulating blood pressure. Numerous studies have found that individuals with low calcium intakes are more likely to have hypertension.[27] Calcium supplementation has been shown to lower blood pressure slightly in individuals with hypertension, and some analyses have also shown an effect in those with normal blood pressure.[28,29] Low dietary magnesium has also been associated with hypertension; dietary magnesium intakes are inversely correlated with blood pressure.[30,31] High intakes of dietary magnesium have been associated with a reduced risk of stroke in men.[25]

Web Menu

For more information on the DASH diet, go to the DASH diet site at the NHLBI at www.nhlbi.nih.gov/health/public/heart/ and click on DASHing with less salt, or go to the DASH site at dash.bwh.harvard.edu/.

The Total Dietary Pattern: The DASH Diet Studies looking at the effect of individual minerals and other dietary components on blood pressure have produced mixed results. This may be because the impact of each individual nutrient is small and a significant effect is seen only when several components of the diet are modified simultaneously. The Dietary Approaches to Stop Hypertension (DASH) trial published in 1997 examined the effect of dietary patterns on blood pressure and demonstrated that modifying the dietary pattern has a greater impact on blood pressure than modifying the intake of individual nutrients.[17]

In this trial, participants were fed one of three diets, all containing 3000 mg of sodium, an amount somewhat greater than the Daily Value of 2400 mg per day.

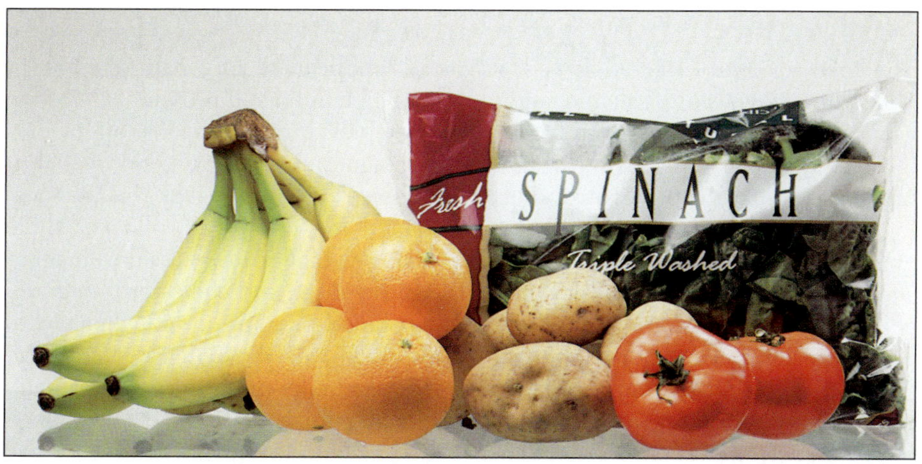

FIGURE 11.21 These foods are rich in potassium. *(George Semple)*

RESEARCH DISCOVERIES

A Total Dietary Approach to Reducing Blood Pressure

For over 25 years, the National Heart, Lung, and Blood Institute (NHLBI) of the National Institutes of Health has been making recommendations for the treatment of high blood pressure. However, their education program had been in operation for 15 years and produced 4 reports before diet was seriously considered in their treatment recommendations. In their 1988 review, the committee determined that there was enticing but conflicting evidence on the effects of dietary modification on blood pressure. Four years later in 1992, the NHLBI requested proposals for a feeding trial that would examine the effects of dietary patterns, rather than single nutrients, on blood pressure in a large sample of individuals. The result of this request, the DASH trial, finally provided conclusive evidence that dietary changes can be effective in lowering blood pressure.[a]

Rationale

Before the DASH trial began there was strong epidemiological evidence correlating a high salt intake, excess body weight, and excess alcohol consumption with increasing blood pressure, and conversely, a vegetarian diet with lower blood pressure. In addition, there was evidence of associations between blood pressure and fat and cholesterol intake, protein intake, fiber intake, and the intake of the minerals potassium, calcium, and magnesium. However, clinical trials that examined the effect of individual nutrients such as calcium, magnesium, fat, saturated fat, cholesterol, and plant versus animal protein on blood pressure were equivocal. Even the effect of sodium intake on blood pressure was considered controversial. These inconsistent and often conflicting results led the NHLBI to consider proposals that would evaluate the effects of dietary patterns rather than individual dietary components on blood pressure.[b]

A Multicenter Feeding Trial

In order to show definitive results, the DASH study needed to define several dietary patterns and then have participants consume these diets for a long enough period of time to determine if they had an effect. Doing an animal study of this sort is relatively easy; the diets are prepared and fed to the caged animals. Because the animals do not have access to other food choices, it is easy to monitor what and how much they consume. The same study is far more difficult in humans, who have access to a wide variety of foods. One approach is to house the study subjects in a research hospital and provide a defined diet while controlling their access to all other food. This approach is frequently used in human nutrition research but was impractical for a study with such large numbers of subjects. An alternative that was considered was to teach the study subjects how to select diets that corresponded to the dietary patterns used in the trial. This would require a large investment of time in counseling participants and in monitoring their intake to be sure that they were compliant with the new dietary pattern. A third approach, which was adopted by the DASH trial, was to allow the study subjects to live at home but provide all their meals and snacks. This approach is not as tightly controlled as housing the subjects in a hospital ward, but is more practical for studying a large group of subjects in which a well-controlled diet is required.

Because of the large number of subjects needed to detect small changes in blood pressure, the study was performed at a number of centers throughout the United States, making it a multicenter feeding study. A central protocol that included specifics about the diets was designed and followed at each of several centers.[b] Participants consumed one meal a day five days a week at the research centers. Other meals were picked up from the centers to be consumed at home. Participants were also required to keep a daily diary of any nonstudy items consumed.

Trial Design

The DASH study population included free-living individuals 22 years of age and older with slightly elevated blood pressure who were not taking blood pressure medications. Study subjects were provided with a control diet for the first three weeks of the study and their blood pressure was monitored. After three weeks, they were randomly assigned to one of three dietary groups for a period of eight weeks. During this intervention period, blood pressure was measured by individuals who did not know to which dietary groups the participants had been assigned (see figure).

The study diets included a control diet, a "fruits and vegetables" diet, and a "combination" diet. Each contained about 3000 mg of sodium, slightly lower than the U.S. average but more than the Daily

---

DASH diet A dietary pattern that is plentiful in fruits and vegetables as well as low-fat dairy products, whole grains, and lean meat, fish, and poultry, making it high in potassium, magnesium, calcium, and fiber, and low in saturated fat and cholesterol.

The first, a control diet, followed a typical American dietary pattern—low in potassium, magnesium, calcium, and fiber, and high in fat and protein. One of the experimental diets was high in fruits and vegetables, providing eight to ten servings per day, making it higher in potassium, magnesium, calcium, and fiber, but otherwise similar to the control diet. The other experimental diet was not only high in fruits and vegetables, it also contained low-fat dairy products, whole grains, and lean meat, fish, and poultry, making it higher in potassium, magnesium, calcium, and fiber, and lower in fat, saturated fat, and cholesterol than the control diet. Both experimental diets lowered blood pressure in individuals with both hypertension and normal blood pressure. However, the effect was most dramatic in the diet that emphasized fruits and vegetables as well as low-fat dairy products, whole grains, and lean meats—a dietary pattern that has become known as the **DASH diet**.[17] The reduction in blood pressure occurred after only two

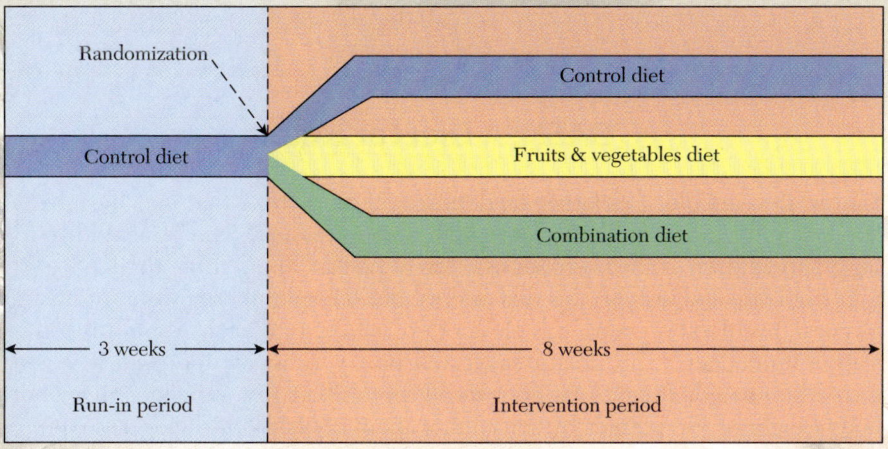

Participants in the DASH trial consumed a control diet for three weeks during what is called the run-in period. They were then randomly assigned to one of three experimental diets for the eight-week intervention period.

Value of 2400 mg. The control diet was designed to match the average intake in the Unites States except for potassium, magnesium, and calcium, which were set at the 25th percentile for intake in the population. The 25th percentile is a level of nutrient intake set such that only 24% of the population consume less than this, whereas about 75% consume more. The fruits and vegetables diet increased servings of fruits and vegetables and decreased sweets; the potassium, calcium, and magnesium were set at the 75th percentile of the typical intake (a level such that 74% of the population consume less than this whereas only about 25% consume more). The combination diet increased fruits and vegetables and low-fat dairy products, included whole grains, poultry, fish, and nuts, and was reduced in sweets, red meats, and fats; it provided potassium, calcium, and magnesium at the 75th percentile of the typical intake.

DASH Results

A total of 459 participants were randomized to the various diet groups. After two weeks, those consuming the combination diet had a reduction in systolic blood pressure of 5.5 mm Hg and diastolic by 3 mm Hg compared to the control group. Those in the fruits and vegetables group had a blood pressure reduction of 2.8 mm Hg systolic and 1.1 mm Hg diastolic. Although these changes seem small, it is estimated that if the American population adopted the DASH combination diet, there would be a 15% reduction in the incidence of coronary heart disease and a 27% reduction in stroke incidence.

Conclusions from a Feeding Trial

Nutrition scientists learn a great deal about the physiological and biochemical roles of nutrients by studying them individually. When too many dietary factors are modified at the same time, it is impossible to determine which ones are the cause of the effects seen. Before the DASH trial was completed, researchers knew that some nutrients sometimes had an effect on blood pressure but the effects were often small and inconsistent. The results of the DASH trial do not tell us which nutrients or dietary components affect blood pressure. Although the combination diet was high in potassium, magnesium, and calcium, the results do not indicate which, if any, of these is responsible for lowering blood pressure. It could be that other dietary factors or combinations of nutrients and dietary components are responsible for the overall effect. However, people eat combinations of foods, not individual nutrients, so although the information provided by the DASH trial tells us less about the physiology of hypertension than studies that look at individual factors, it provides more information about what to eat every day to prevent it.

References

[a] Obarzanek, E., and Moore, T. J. Using feeding studies to test the efficacy of dietary interventions: lessons from the Dietary Approaches to Stop Hypertension trial. J. Am. Diet. Assoc. 99:9s–10s, 1999.

[b] Vogt, T. M., Appel, L. J., Obarzanek, E., et al. Dietary Approaches to Stop Hypertension: rationale, design and methods. J. Am. Diet. Assoc. 99:12s–18s, 1999.

weeks of consuming this diet and persisted throughout the trial. Reductions were similar to that seen with drug therapy or diets that restrict sodium to very low levels of 1100 to 1800 mg per day[32] (see *Research Discoveries:* "A Total Dietary Approach to Reducing Blood Pressure").

The DASH trial did not explore the effect of sodium on blood pressure but a second trial—called DASH-Sodium—compared the effect of the DASH diet to a control diet at three different levels of sodium intake.[18] The high-sodium diet provided 3300 mg sodium per day (slightly less than the average American intake), the intermediate diet provided 2400 mg sodium per day (the current government recommendation), and the low-sodium diet provided 1500 mg sodium per day. Reducing sodium intake reduced blood pressure for both the DASH and control diets. The combination of the DASH diet and the lowest sodium intake reduced blood pressure more than either the DASH diet or low sodium alone.

The results of the DASH and DASH-Sodium trials demonstrate that changing the dietary pattern can lower blood pressure. In addition, the DASH dietary pattern may also reduce cancer risk, prevent osteoporosis, and protect against heart disease (see *Critical Thinking:* "DASH: A Diet for Health").

Critical Thinking

DASH: A Diet for Health

Sam is 48 years old. His father died at age 50 of a stroke that may have been related to undiagnosed and untreated high blood pressure. Sam wants to live to see his grandchildren, so he exercises as often as he can, about three times a week, has quit smoking, and watches his diet and weight. Despite these efforts, at his recent physical, his blood pressure was elevated to 144/92. Rather than start him on medication immediately, his doctor suggested he try a dietary approach first and referred him to a dietitian. A 24-hour recall reveals that Sam is maintaining a normal body weight of 175 pounds by consuming about 2500 kcalories per day. After evaluating his current diet, the dietitian recommends he follow the DASH diet and reduce his sodium intake to lower his blood pressure. Sam is distressed because he already works hard to meet the recommendations of the Food Guide Pyramid.

Current Diet		**Modified Diet**	
Breakfast		*Breakfast*	
Orange juice	3/4 cup	Orange juice	3/4 cup
1% low-fat milk	1 cup	1% low-fat milk	1 cup
Oat flakes with 1 tsp sugar	1 cup	Oat flakes with 1 tsp sugar	1 cup
		Banana	1 medium
Whole-wheat bread with jelly	2 slices	Whole-wheat bread with jelly	2 slices
Margarine	1 tsp	Margarine	1 tsp
Lunch		*Lunch*	
Ham salad	3/4 cup	Tuna salad	3/4 cup
Whole-wheat bread	2 slices	Whole-wheat bread	2 slices
		Carrot sticks	1/2 cup
		Bell pepper strips	1/2 cup
Potato chips	1 oz	Fruit cocktail (in light syrup)	1/2 cup
Cola	1 can	1% low-fat milk	1 cup
Dinner		*Dinner*	
Breaded baked chicken	3 oz	Stir-fry:	
		Chicken	3 oz
		Almonds	10
		Broccoli	1/2 cup
		Mushrooms	1/2 cup
Rice-a-Roni	1 cup	Steamed rice	1 1/2 cups
Salad	1 cup	Salad	1 cup
Light salad dressing	1 Tbsp	Light salad dressing	1 Tbsp
Dinner roll	1	Dinner roll	1
Margarine	2 tsp	Margarine	2 tsp
Green beans	1/2 cup	Cantaloupe	1/2 cup
1% low-fat milk	1 cup	1% low fat-milk	1 cup
Snacks		*Snacks*	
Cookies	2 large	Frozen yogurt	1/2 cup
Dried apricots	5	Dried apricots	5
Milky Way candy bar	1	Graham crackers	2
Cola	1 can		

How does Sam's original diet compare to the recommendations of the Food Guide Pyramid?

His original diet does meet the recommendations of the Food Guide Pyramid. But studies have shown that increasing the number of fruit, vegetable, and low-fat dairy servings to the upper end (and above) of that suggested by the Food Guide Pyramid can help reduce blood pressure.

How does his modified diet compare to the recommendations of the Food Guide Pyramid?

Answer:

How do these changes affect the sodium and potassium content of Sam's diet?

His original diet was fairly high in sodium, containing about 4600 mg, which is above the Daily Value of 2400 mg. Sam learns to check food labels to determine the sodium content of packaged foods. He notes that ham is high in sodium and realizes he can reduce his sodium intake by almost 1000 mg if he has a tuna sandwich instead. He also eliminates highly processed foods like Rice-a-Roni and potato chips that are high in salt and reduces the amount of salt he adds when cooking. These changes reduce his sodium to 2450, close to the Daily Value. Sodium intakes below this offer even greater benefits in terms of blood pressure reduction. The dietary changes have also increased his potassium intake from about 3000 mg to 5000 mg and increased the amount of calcium and magnesium in his diet.

Sam's wife Sara is 42 years old. Although she is not concerned about her blood pressure, her family background and other factors put her at risk for heart disease and osteoporosis.

Will the DASH diet meet her health needs?

Yes, the DASH diet is low in saturated fat and high in fiber and antioxidants from whole grains, fruits, and vegetables to help reduce her risk of cardiovascular disease. The DASH diet also has plenty of calcium to promote bone health.

Sara only weighs 110 pounds and requires about 1800 kcal to maintain her body weight.

How could this diet be changed to reduce the energy content while still including eight servings of fruits and vegetables and three dairy servings per day?

Answer:

TABLE 11.3 Suggestions for Keeping Blood Pressure in a Healthy Range

- Choose and prepare foods with less salt.
- Aim for a healthy weight: Blood pressure increases with increases in body weight and decreases when excess weight is reduced.
- Increase physical activity: It helps lower blood pressure, reduce risk of other chronic diseases, and manage weight.
- Eat fruits and vegetables: They are naturally low in salt and kcalories. They are also rich in potassium, which may help decrease blood pressure.
- If you drink alcoholic beverages, do so in moderation. Excessive alcohol consumption has been associated with high blood pressure.

USDA, DHHS. Dietary Guidelines for Americans, 2000.

Choosing a Diet to Reduce Blood Pressure

Reducing the incidence of hypertension in the United States is a goal of several public health campaigns. Healthy People 2010 addresses high blood pressure by setting a goal to reduce the proportion of adults with high blood pressure and increase the proportion of adults with high blood pressure who are taking action to help control their condition by losing weight, increasing physical activity, and reducing sodium intake. The Dietary Guidelines for Americans, 2000, includes a recommendation to choose sensibly to reduce salt and sodium intake (see Figure 11.20). The Dietary Guidelines 2000 also makes some additional lifestyle suggestions to help keep blood pressure in a healthy range (see Table 11.3). Although the level of sodium consumption recommended by the Dietary Guidelines and the Daily Values used on food labels may not provide the maximum reduction in blood pressure, it encourages the consumption of fresh fruits, vegetables, grains, meats, and dairy products, which are low in sodium—a dietary pattern that may provide more health benefits than just lowering blood pressure.[33]

Selecting a DASH Diet The DASH diet pattern can be achieved by using the Food Guide Pyramid as a guide and aiming toward the high end of the recommended number of servings of vegetables, fruits, dairy products, and grains. Dry beans and nuts should be frequent choices from the Meat, Poultry, Fish, Dry

TABLE 11.4 Daily Serving Recommendations for the DASH Diet

Food Group	Number of Servings per Day*			
Kcalorie level	***1600***	***2000***	***2600***	***3100***
Grains	6–7	7–8	10–11	12–13
Vegetables	3–4	4–5	5–6	6–7
Fruits	3–4	4–5	5–6	6–7
Low-fat dairy	2–3	2–3	3–4	3–4
Meats, fish, poultry	1–2	1–2	2	2–3
Beans, nuts, and seeds	1/3	1/2	2/3	3/4
Limit fats and sweets				

*Serving sizes correspond to the Food Guide Pyramid serving sizes.

TABLE 11.5 Suggestions for Reducing Sodium Intake

Reduce the salt in your diet gradually so that you learn to enjoy the unsalted flavors in foods.

When shopping:

- Use food labels to select foods low in sodium.
- Choose unprocessed foods—they have less sodium than processed foods.
- Choose fresh or frozen vegetables rather than canned.

When cooking:

- Prepare meals from scratch so you control the amount of salt added.
- Do not add salt to the water when cooking rice, pasta, and cereals.
- Flavor foods with ingredients such as lemon juice, onion or garlic powder (not salt), pepper, curry, dill, basil, oregano, or thyme rather than salt.

When eating:

- Limit use of salt at the table.
- Limit salted snack foods like potato chips, salted nuts, salted popcorn, and crackers, and replace them with fresh fruits and vegetables.
- Limit cured, salted, or smoked meats such as bologna, corned beef, hot dogs, and smoked turkey to a few servings a week or less. Substitute sliced roasted turkey, chicken, or beef.
- Limit salty or smoked fish such as sardines, anchovies, or smoked salmon (lox).
- Limit foods prepared in salt brine such as pickles, olives, and sauerkraut.
- Cut down on cheeses, especially processed cheeses.
- Limit the amounts of soy sauce, Worcestershire sauce, barbecue sauce, ketchup, and mustard you add to food.

When eating out:

- Choose foods without sauces, or ask for them to be served on the side.
- Ask that food be prepared without added salt.

Beans, Eggs, and Nuts Group. Nutrient-dense choices from each group will ensure that the energy content of the diet does not exceed needs. Table 11.4 gives the number of servings recommended for the DASH diet at several different energy levels. The risk of hypertension is minimized by combining this dietary pattern with the following suggestions for reducing sodium intake.

Reducing Sodium Intake To reduce sodium intake, consumers need to be aware of the sources of salt in the diet. Dietary sodium comes from food, water, and medications. In general, processed foods are high in sodium. Reducing sodium intake involves limiting the intake of processed foods as well as reducing the amount of salt added to food in cooking and at the table (Table 11.5).

Food labels can be helpful in identifying packaged foods that are high in sodium (Figure 11.22). The total sodium content per serving is included in the Nutrition Facts section, and sodium-containing food additives are itemized in the ingredient list. To help assess how the amount of sodium in a food fits into the recommended diet, food labels also give the sodium content of a serving as a percent of the Daily Value. The 2400-mg Daily Value for sodium is considered the upper limit that is desirable in the diet. Additional information can be obtained from nutrient claims relating to the salt or sodium content of a product. Products with reduced salt content may be labeled as "low salt," "less salt," or "unsalted" (Table 11.6).

Generally, water provides only a small amount of sodium, but some bottled waters and water treated with "softeners" are higher. Over-the-counter medications such as cough medicine and laxatives also can contain large amounts of sodium; many are now available in low-sodium formulas.

FIGURE 11.22 This Nutrition Facts label indicates that a serving of spaghetti sauce light in sodium contains 250 mg of sodium, or about 10% of the Daily Value.

Nutrition Facts
Serving Size 1/2 cup (125g)
Servings Per Container about 3½

Amount Per Serving	
Calories 50	Calories from Fat 10
	%Daily Value**
Total Fat 1g	**2%**
Saturated Fat 0g	**0%**
Cholesterol 0mg	**0%**
Sodium 250mg	**10%**
Potassium 530mg	**15%**
Total Carbohydrate 9g	**3%**
Dietary Fiber 1g	**4%**
Sugars 7g	
Protein 2g	
Vitamin A 10% •	Vitamin C 25%
Calcium 2% •	Iron 10%

*Percent Daily Values are based on a 2,000 calorie diet. Your daily values may be higher or lower depending on your calorie needs.

	Calories:	2,000	2,500
Total Fat	Less than	65g	80g
Sat Fat	Less than	20g	25g
Cholesterol	Less than	300mg	300mg
Sodium	Less than	2,400mg	2,400mg
Potassium		3,500mg	3,500mg
Total Carbohydrate		300g	375g
Dietary Fiber		25g	30g

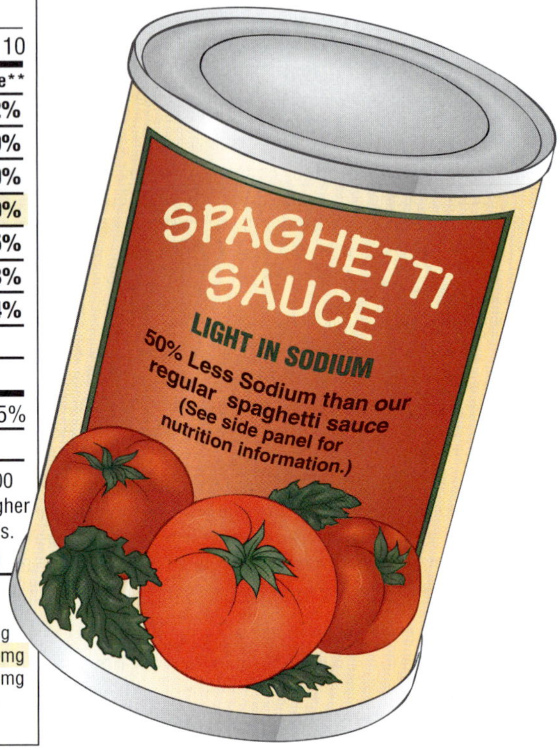

Light Spaghetti Sauce, 250 milligrams (mg) per serving
Regular Spaghetti Sauce, 500mg per serving

TABLE 11.6 Salt and Sodium Content Descriptors on Food Labels

Descriptor	Definition
Sodium-free	Contains less than 5 mg of sodium per serving.
Salt-free	Must meet criterion for "sodium-free."
Very low sodium	Contains 35 mg or less of sodium per serving.
Low sodium	Contains 140 mg or less of sodium per serving.
Reduced or less sodium	Contains at least 25% less sodium per serving than a reference food.
Light in sodium	Contains at least 50% less sodium per serving than the average reference amount for same food with no sodium reduction.
No salt added, without added salt, and unsalted	No salt added during processing, and the food it resembles and for which it substitutes is normally processed with salt. (If the food is not "sodium-free," the statement "not a sodium-free food" or "not for control of sodium in the diet" must appear on the same panel as the Nutrition Facts panel.)
Lightly salted	Contains at least 50% less sodium per serving than a reference amount. (If the food is not "low in sodium," the statement "not a low-sodium food" must appear on the same panel as the "Nutrition Facts" panel.)

Summary

1. Water is an essential nutrient that constitutes about 60% of the adult body weight. It is consumed in beverages and food, and a small amount is produced by metabolism.
2. Body water is distributed between intracellular and extracellular compartments. The amount in each compartment depends largely on the concentration of solutes. Because water will diffuse by osmosis from a compartment with a lower concentration of solutes to one with a higher concentration, the body regulates the distribution of water by adjusting the concentration of electrolytes and other solutes in each compartment.
3. Fluid intake is stimulated by the sensation of thirst, which occurs in response to a decrease in body water. Water is lost from the body in urine and feces and through evaporation from the skin and lungs. The kidney is the primary regulator of water output. If water intake is low, antidiuretic hormone (ADH) will cause the kidney to conserve water. If water intake is high, more water will be excreted in the urine. The amount of water required by the body, about 1 ml per kcalorie of intake, may vary depending on environmental conditions and activity level.
4. The polar structure of the water molecule allows it to function as a solvent for the molecules and chemical reactions involved in metabolism. Water helps to transport other nutrients and waste products within the body and to excrete wastes from the body. It helps to protect the body, regulate body temperature, and lubricate areas such as the eyes and the joints. Water is also involved in the regulation of acid-base balance.
5. Dehydration can occur if water intake is too low or output is excessive. Mild dehydration can cause headache, fatigue, loss of appetite, dry eyes and mouth, and dark-colored urine. Severe dehydration can be fatal. Many Americans do not consume enough fluid.
6. The minerals sodium, chloride, and potassium are electrolytes that are important in the maintenance of fluid balance and the formation of membrane potentials. The North American diet is abundant in sodium and chloride from processed foods and table salt but generally low in potassium, which is high in unprocessed foods such as fruits and vegetables.
7. Electrolyte and fluid homeostasis is regulated primarily by the kidneys. A decrease in blood pressure or blood volume signals the release of the enzyme renin, which helps form angiotensin II. Angiotensin II causes blood vessels to constrict and the hormone aldosterone to be released. Aldosterone causes the kidneys to reabsorb sodium and hence water, thereby increasing blood volume. Failure of these regulatory mechanisms may be a cause of hypertension.
8. Public health guidelines recommend consuming no more than 2400 mg of sodium per day and at least 3500 mg of potassium per day in order to promote a healthy blood pressure.
9. Hypertension, or high blood pressure, is common in the United States. A diet high in sodium increases blood pressure in some if not all individuals. Other nutrients, including potassium, magnesium, and calcium, also affect blood pressure.
10. To reduce the risk of hypertension, public health recommendations suggest a low to moderate intake of salt and sodium. The adoption of the DASH diet—a dietary pattern high in fruits, vegetables, low-fat dairy products, whole grains, and lean meat, fish, and poultry—is also recommended. This diet is rich in potassium, magnesium, calcium, and fiber, and low in fat, saturated fat, and cholesterol.

Review Questions

1. How is the amount of water in the body regulated?
2. Describe the functions of water in the body.
3. What is the recommended water intake for adults?
4. List three fluids that contribute to hydration and three fluids that can contribute to dehydration.
5. List three factors that increase water needs.
6. What physiological factors stimulate thirst?
7. What is an electrolyte? Which minerals are considered nutritional electrolytes?
8. How do electrolytes function in the body?
9. What types of foods contribute the most sodium to the North American diet?
10. What types of foods are good sources of potassium?
11. How is blood pressure regulated?
12. What is the relationship between dietary sodium and blood pressure?
13. What is the DASH diet and how does it affect blood pressure?

Applying Critical Thinking Skills

Personal nutrition:

1. Keep a log of all the fluids you consume in one day.
   a. Calculate your fluid intake. Include water, beverages, and foods that are liquid at room temperature, such as soup and ice cream.
   b. How much of your intake was from dehydrating fluids (those that contain caffeine or alcohol)?
   c. How does your total intake on this day compare with your estimated requirement? How does your intake of hydrating fluids compare with your estimated requirement?

2. Use one day of the food record you kept in Chapter 2 to see how your diet compares to the DASH diet.
   a. Tally the number of servings from each of the food groups in your diet and compare them to the recommended servings for your energy needs as shown in Table 11.4.
   b. Suggest modifications to your diet so that it will meet DASH guidelines.
   c. What difficulties or inconveniences do you see with following this dietary pattern?
   d. What other dietary or lifestyle changes might you make if you are at high risk of hypertension?
3. Processed foods provide about 75% of the sodium in the American diet.
   a. Using food labels, estimate the amount of sodium you consume from processed foods each day.
   b. Make a list of the processed foods in your diet that contain more than 10% of the Daily Value for sodium per serving.
   c. Read the labels of common medications such as antacids and cough medications. Which are high in sodium?

General nutrition issues:

1. Virginia's mother has high blood pressure and has had several strokes. A recent physical exam indicated that Virginia also has high blood pressure. Her physician prescribed medication to lower her blood pressure, but he believes that with some changes in diet and lifestyle Virginia's blood pressure could be brought into the normal range without drugs. Virginia works at a desk. The only exercise she gets is when she takes care of her nieces and nephews one weekend a month. Her typical diet includes a breakfast of cereal, tomato juice, and coffee. She has a snack of donuts and coffee at work, and for lunch she joins coworkers for a fast-food cheeseburger, fries, and milkshake. When she gets home she has a soda and snacks on peanuts or chips. Dinner is usually a TV dinner with milk.
   a. What dietary changes would you recommend for Virginia?
   b. What lifestyle changes would you recommend?

References

1. Maughan, R. J., and Leiper, J. B. Limitations to fluid replacement during exercise. Can. J. Appl. Physiol. 24:173–187, 1999.
2. Shen, H-P. Body fluids and water balance. In *Biochemical and Physiological Aspects of Human Nutrition*. Stipanuk, M., ed. Philadelphia: W. B. Saunders, 2000, pp. 843–865.
3. Askew, E. W. Nutrition and performance in hot, cold, and high-altitude environments. In *Nutrition in Exercise and Sport*, 3rd ed. Wolinsky, I., ed. Boca Raton, Fla.: CRC Press, 1998, pp. 597–619.
4. Armstrong, L. E., and Epstein, Y. Fluid-electrolyte balance during labor and exercise: concepts and misconceptions. Int. J. Sport Nutr. 9:1–12, 1999.
5. Michaud, D. S., Spiegelman, D., Clinton, S. K., et al. Fluid intake and the risk of bladder cancer in men. N. Engl. J. Med. 340:1390–1397, 1999.
6. International Bottled Water Association and Rockefeller University. Americans' poor drinking habits contradict knowledge of health risks. Available online at **http:www.bottledwater.org/public/InfoForRepNatFactSheettest.htm.** Accessed 14 Jan 2001.
7. National Research Council, Food and Nutrition Board. *Recommended Dietary Allowances*, 10th ed. Washington, D.C.: National Academy Press, 1989.
8. National Research Council. *Diet and Health: Implications for Reducing Chronic Disease Risk*. Washington, D.C.: National Academy Press, 1989.
9. Committee on Nutritional Status During Pregnancy and Lactation, National Academy of Sciences. *Nutrition During Pregnancy*. Washington, D.C.: National Academy Press, 1990.
10. Antonios, T. F., and MacGregor, G. A. Salt intake: potential deleterious effects excluding blood pressure. J. Hum. Hypertens. 9:511–515, 1995.
11. Brown, M. J., and Haydock, S. Pathoeatiology, epidemiology and diagnosis of hypertension. Drugs 59:1s–12s, 2000.
12. Burt, V. L., Whelton, P., Roccella, E. J., et al. Prevalence of hypertension in the U.S. adult population: results from the third National Health and Nutrition Examination Survey, 1988–1991. Hypertension 25:305–313, 1995.
13. American Heart Association. High blood pressure statistics. Available online at **http://www.americanheart.org/Heart_and_Stroke_A_ZGuide/hbps.html**. Accessed 14 Jan 2001.
14. Sixth Report of the Joint National Committee on Prevention, Detection, Evaluation, and Treatment of High Blood Pressure. Arch. Intern. Med. 157:2413–2446, 1997.
15. Mikhail, N., Golub, M. S., and Tuck, M. L. Obesity and hypertension. Prog. Cardiovasc. Dis. 42:39–58, 1999.
16. Nurminen, M. L., Korpela, R., and Vapaatalo, H. Dietary factors in the pathogenesis and treatment of hypertension. Ann. Med. 30:143–150, 1998.
17. Appel, L. J., Moore, T. J., Obarzanek, E., et al. A clinical trial of the effects of dietary patterns on blood pressure. N. Engl. J. Med. 336:1117–1124, 1997.
18. Greenland, P. Beating high blood pressure with low-sodium DASH. N. Engl. J. Med. 344:53–55, 2001.
19. Carvalho, J. J., Baruzzi, R. G., Howard, P. F., et al. Blood pressure in four remote populations in the Intersalt study. Hypertension 14:238–246, 1989.
20. Graudal, N. A., Galloe, A. M., and Garrod, P. Effects of sodium restriction on blood pressure, renin, aldosterone, catacholamines, cholesterols, and triglyceride: a meta-analysis. JAMA 279:1383–1391, 1998.
21. Luft, L. C., and Weinberger, M. H. Heterogeneous responses to changes in dietary salt intake: the salt sensitivity paradigm. Am. J. Clin. Nutr. 65(suppl):612S–617S, 1997.
22. Kotchen, T. A., and Kotchen, J. M. Dietary sodium and blood pressure: interactions with other nutrients. Am. J. Clin. Nutr. 65(suppl):708S–711S, 1997.
23. Vogt, T. M., Appel, L. J. Obarzanwk, E., et al. Dietary approaches to stop hypertension: rationale, design and methods. DASH Collaborative Group. J. Am. Diet. Assoc. 99:s12–s18, 1999.
24. Young, D. B., Lin, H., and McCabe, R. D. Potassium's cardiovascular protective mechanisms. Am. J. Physiol. 268:R825–R837, 1995.
25. Ascherio, A., Rimm, E. B., Hernan, M. A. et al. Intake of potassium, magnesium, calcium, and fiber and risk of stroke among U.S. men. Circulation 98:1198–1204, 1998.

26. Whelton, P. K., He, J., Cutler, J. A., et al. Effects of oral potassium on blood pressure: meta-analysis of randomized controlled clinical trials. JAMA 227:1624–1632, 1997.
27. Hamet, P. The evaluation of the scientific evidence for a relationship between calcium and hypertension. J. Nutr. 125(suppl):311S–400S, 1995.
28. Allender, P. S., Cutler, J. A., Follmann, D., et al. Dietary calcium and blood pressure: a meta-analysis of randomized clinical trials. Ann. Intern. Med. 124:825–831, 1996.
29. Dwyer, J. H., Dwyer, K. M., Scribner, R. A., et al. Dietary calcium, calcium supplementation, and blood pressure in African-American adolescents. Am. J. Clin. Nutr. 68:648–655, 1998.
30. Singh, R. B., Niaz, M. A., Moshiri, M., et al. Magnesium status and risk of coronary artery disease in rural and urban populations with variable magnesium consumption. Magnes. Res. 10:205–213, 1997.
31. Ma, J., Folsom, A. R., Melnick, S. L., et al. Associations of serum and dietary magnesium with cardiovascular disease, hypertension, diabetes, insulin, and carotid arterial wall thickness: the ARIC study. Atherosclerosis Risk in Community Study. J. Clin. Epidemiol. 48:927–940, 1995.
32. Zemel, M. B. Dietary pattern and hypertension: the DASH diet. Nutr. Rev. 55:303–305, 1997.
33. Kaplan, N. M. The dietary guideline for sodium. Am. J. Clin. Nutr. 71:1020–1026, 2000.

12 Major Minerals and Bone Health

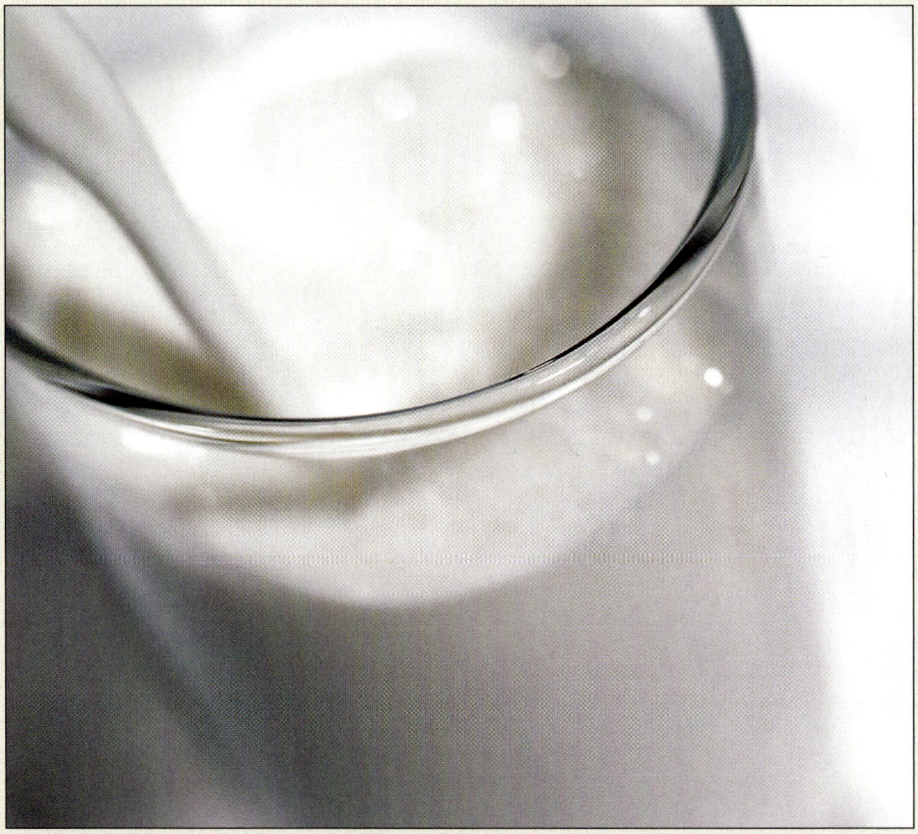

Learning Objectives

After reading this chapter, students should be able to:

1. Define the term "mineral" in the context of nutrition.
2. Describe how interactions among minerals and other dietary components affect mineral bioavailability.
3. Explain the functions of calcium in the body.
4. Describe the roles of parathyroid hormone, calcitonin, and vitamin D in the regulation of blood calcium levels.
5. Discuss the relationships among calcium, peak bone mass, and osteoporosis.
6. List dietary and lifestyle factors that reduce the risk of osteoporosis.
7. Describe the functions of phosphorus in the body.
8. Design a diet that meets the recommended intakes for calcium and phosphorus.
9. Describe the functions of magnesium in the body and name three foods that are good sources of magnesium.
10. Discuss the role of sulfur in the body and where it is found in the diet.

Margie was in a hurry. Her grandchildren would be arriving soon and she was rushing back from the corner store. As the walk light changed, she stepped off the curb to cross the street to her apartment. But when her foot struck the pavement there was a searing pain in her hip, and the next thing she knew she was lying in the street. The visit with her grandchildren would take place in the hospital, rather than her home. She had broken her hip.

At 75 years old, Margie had been relatively healthy and independent. She lived alone in her apartment and did all of her own shopping, laundry, and housework. Now she was facing a nursing-home stay. How could a step off the curb cause her hip to break? How long would it take to heal? Would she ever be independent again?

Margie's hip broke because the bone had been weakened by osteoporosis, which is a disease characterized by low bone density. Osteoporosis leads to fragile bones and an increased susceptibility to fractures. A hip fracture such as Margie's almost always requires hospitalization, major surgery, and a long period of rehabilitation. It can impair a person's ability to walk unassisted and may cause prolonged or permanent disability and even death. Many older adults who experience a hip fracture from osteoporosis require long-term nursing-home care and never regain their independence; 24% die in the year following their injury.

Osteoporosis is a major public health problem in the United States. It is responsible for 1.5 million fractures annually, including 300,000 hip fractures. There are many causes and no cure at this time. The risk of osteoporosis is affected by the intake of calcium and other dietary components as well as by exercise patterns throughout life. The best treatment is prevention.

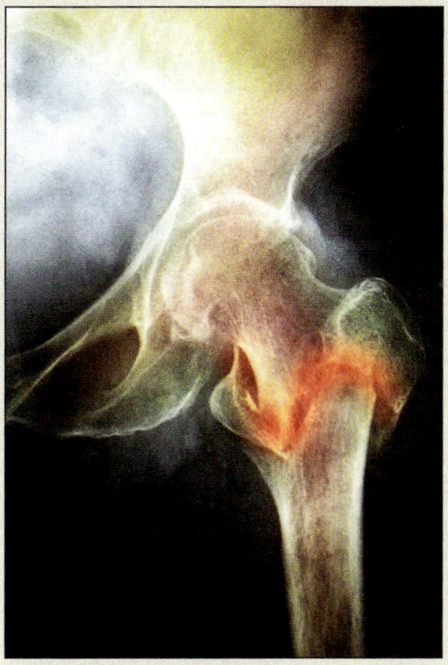

What Are Minerals?

Minerals are inorganic elements that function in the body as structural components and regulators of body processes. Minerals may combine with other elements in the body but they retain their chemical identity. Unlike vitamins, they are not destroyed by heat, oxygen, or acid; the ash that remains after a food is combusted in a bomb calorimeter contains the minerals that were present in that food. Minerals have traditionally been categorized based on the amounts needed in the diet or present in the body. The **major minerals** include those needed in the diet in amounts greater than 100 mg per day or present in the body in amounts greater than 0.01% of body weight. The **trace elements** or **trace minerals** are those minerals required by the body in an amount of 100 mg or less per day or present in the body in an amount of 0.01% or less of body weight (Figure 12.1).

The major minerals include the electrolytes sodium, chloride, and potassium, which were discussed in Chapter 11. Calcium, phosphorus, and magnesium, discussed in this chapter, are major minerals that play a role in bone health, and sulfur is a major mineral that functions in association with other molecules, such as vitamins and amino acids. The trace elements, including iron, zinc, copper, manganese, selenium, iodine, fluoride, chromium, and molybdenum, as well as several others that are needed in minute quantities, are discussed in Chapter 13.

Mineral In nutrition, an element needed by the body in small amounts for structure and to regulate chemical reactions and body processes.

Major minerals Minerals needed in the diet in amounts greater than 100 mg per day or present in the body in amounts greater than 0.01% of body weight.

Trace elements or **trace minerals** Minerals required in the diet in amounts of 100 mg or less per day or present in the body in amounts of 0.01% of body weight or less.

FIGURE 12.1 Minerals are chemical elements found in the periodic table. The major minerals are shown in purple and the trace elements are shown in blue.

H																	He
Li	Be											B	C	N	O	F	Ne
Na	Mg											Al	Si	P	S	Cl	Ar
K	Ca	Sc	Ti	V	Cr	Mn	Fe	Co	Ni	Cu	Zn	Ga	Ge	As	Se	Br	Kr
Rb	Sr	Y	Zr	Nb	Mo	Tc	Ru	Rh	Pd	Ag	Cd	In	Sn	Sb	Te	I	Xe
Cs	Ba	La	Hf	Ta	W	Re	Os	Ir	Pt	Au	Hg	Tl	Pb	Bi	Po	At	Rn
Fr	Ra	Ac	Unq	Unp	Unh	Uns		Une									

Sources of Minerals

Minerals in the diet come from both plant and animal sources. In some foods, the amounts of minerals are predictable because the minerals are regulated components of the plant or animal. For instance, iron is a component of muscle tissue; therefore, it is found in consistent amounts in meat. Magnesium is a component of chlorophyll, so it is found in consistent amounts in leafy greens. In other foods the amounts of minerals vary depending on the mineral concentration in the soil and water at the food's source (Figure 12.2). For example, the soil content of iodine is high near the ocean but usually quite low in inland areas. Therefore, foods grown near the ocean are better sources of iodine than those grown inland. In developed countries, modern agriculture and transportation systems make foods produced in many locations available, so the diet is unlikely to be deficient in trace elements. In countries where the diet consists predominantly of locally grown foods, individual trace element deficiencies and excesses are more likely to occur.

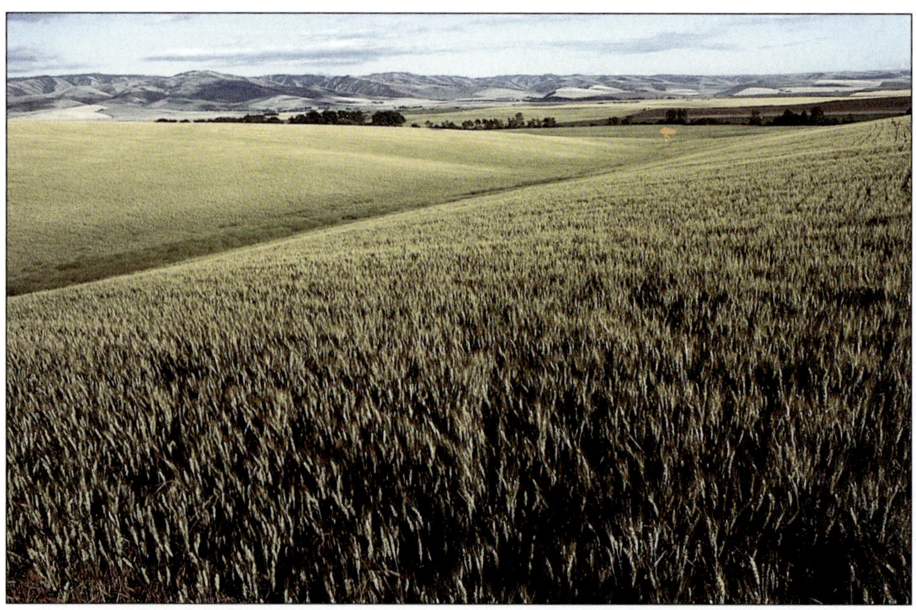

FIGURE 12.2 The amounts of some minerals found in plants varies with the mineral content of the soil in which they are grown. *(© Earl Roberge/Photo Researchers, Inc.)*

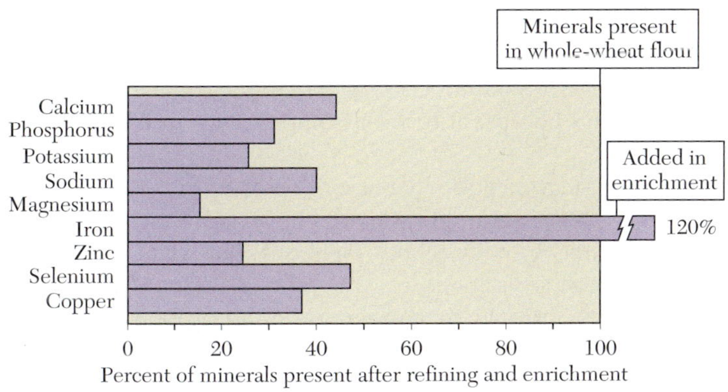

FIGURE 12.3 Some of the minerals in whole grains are lost in refining, but only iron is added back in enrichment. This figure illustrates the minerals present in enriched white flour as a percent of those found in whole-wheat flour.

Food processing and refining also affect the mineral content of foods. Some types of processing such as cooking and the refining of grains can cause minerals to be lost. Boiling, for example, causes a decrease in the potassium content of foods. Peeling off the skins of produce and removing the bran and germ from grains during refining both cause minerals to be lost. For example, iron, selenium, zinc, and copper are lost when flour is refined. But iron is the only mineral replaced by enrichment (Figure 12.3). Other types of processing add minerals to foods. Some are added inadvertently through contamination. For example, the iodine content of dairy products is increased by contamination from the cleaning solutions used in milking machines. Other minerals are added intentionally. For example, preserving foods can increase the sodium or sulfur content of the food and the fortification of breakfast cereals can add calcium and iron (Figure 12.4).

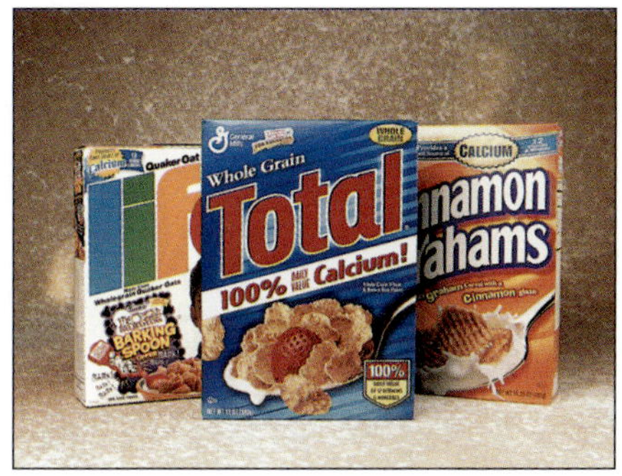

FIGURE 12.4 Many breakfast cereals are fortified with calcium and other minerals. *(George Semple)*

Bioavailability A measure of how well a nutrient can be absorbed and used by the body.

Phytic acid or **phytate** A phosphorus-containing storage compound found in seeds and grains that can bind minerals and decrease their absorption.

Tannins Substances found in tea and some grains that can bind certain minerals and decrease their absorption.

Oxalates Organic acids found in spinach and other leafy green vegetables that can bind certain minerals and decrease their absorption.

Minerals in the Digestive Tract

The degree to which minerals are absorbed from the digestive tract varies dramatically. Almost 100% of the sodium consumed in the diet is absorbed, whereas calcium absorption is typically about 25% and iron absorption may be as low as 5%. For some minerals, the amount absorbed depends primarily on the amount that is consumed. For others, absorption is regulated; these require energy and carrier molecules to be absorbed. The **bioavailability** of minerals is also affected by other nutrients and food components in the diet as well as the nutritional status and life stage of the consumer. Some interactions decrease absorption and others increase it.

Mineral ions that carry the same charge compete for absorption in the gastrointestinal tract. Calcium, magnesium, zinc, copper, and iron all carry a 2^+ charge, and a high intake of one may reduce the absorption of others. For example, a high intake of calcium in a meal containing iron may reduce the absorption of the iron.

Mineral bioavailability is also affected by the binding of minerals to other substances in the GI tract. **Phytic acid**, or **phytate**—an organic compound containing phosphorus that is found in whole grains, bran, and soy products—binds calcium, zinc, iron, and magnesium, limiting their absorption. Phytic acid can be broken down by yeast, so the bioavailability of minerals is increased in yeast-leavened foods such as breads. **Tannins**, found in tea and some grains, can interfere with iron absorption, and **oxalates**, which are organic acids found in spinach, rhubarb, beet greens, and chocolate, have been found to interfere with calcium and iron absorption (Figure 12.5). Dietary fiber also interferes with mineral absorption. Although North Americans generally do not consume enough of any of these components to cause trace element deficiencies, problems occur in developing countries. For example, in some populations the intake of phytate, which decreases zinc absorption, is high enough to increase the requirement for zinc.

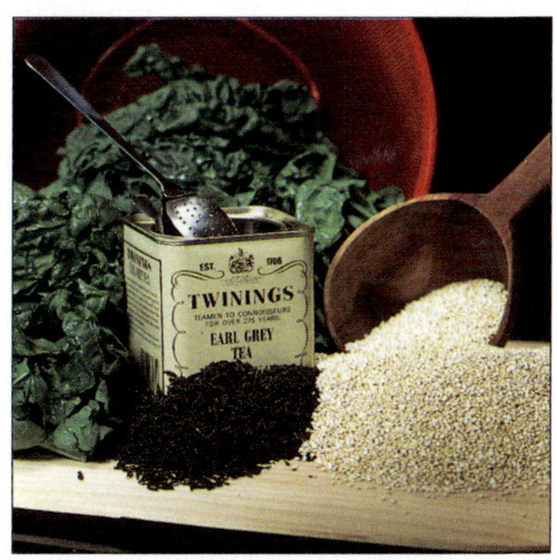

FIGURE 12.5 Compounds such as phytate, oxalates, and tannins found in these foods decrease mineral absorption. *(Charles D. Winters)*

There are also substances in the diet that promote mineral absorption. For example, when iron is consumed with acidic foods, the low pH helps to keep it in its more absorbable chemical form. Vitamin C in the diet enhances the absorption of iron because it is an acid and because it forms a complex with iron that makes the iron more easily absorbed.

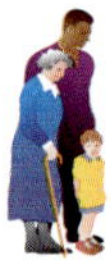

Nutritional status and life stage can also increase or decrease mineral bioavailability. For example, when iron stores are low, the ability of the body to transport iron from intestinal mucosal cells to body tissues increases, but when iron stores are high, iron stays in the mucosal cells and is lost when the cells die. During pregnancy, increased calcium needs are met by an increase in absorption. In the elderly, a decrease in stomach acid may decrease the absorption of some minerals.

Minerals in the Body

Minerals are transported in the blood bound to plasma proteins or specific transport proteins. The binding of minerals to transport proteins helps regulate their absorption and prevents reactive minerals from forming free radicals that could cause oxidative damage. Nutrient intake can affect mineral transport in the body. For instance, when protein intake is deficient, transport proteins (and proteins in general) cannot be synthesized. Therefore, even if a mineral is adequate in the diet, it cannot be transported to the cells where it is needed. In other cases the intake of one mineral can affect how much of another is able to leave the mucosal cell and bind to a transport protein in the plasma. For example, a deficiency of copper can decrease available iron by reducing the amount of iron that can bind to plasma iron transport proteins.

Minerals perform a wide range of vital structural and regulatory roles in the body. Many serve complementary and interdependent roles. For example, phosphorus, magnesium, and fluoride work with calcium to affect the structure and strength of bones; sodium and potassium ions, which both carry a 1^{+} charge, are exchanged across cell membranes to regulate fluid balance and the electrical charge of the membrane. Others have separate and unique roles. For example, chromium plays a role in regulating blood glucose levels, zinc plays an important role in gene expression, and iodine as a component of thyroid hormones helps to regulate metabolic rate. Often minerals function in association with enzymes and other proteins. For example selenium, copper, zinc, iron, and manganese are minerals that each function as enzyme **cofactors** (Figure 12.6).

Cofactor An inorganic ion or coenzyme required for enzyme activity.

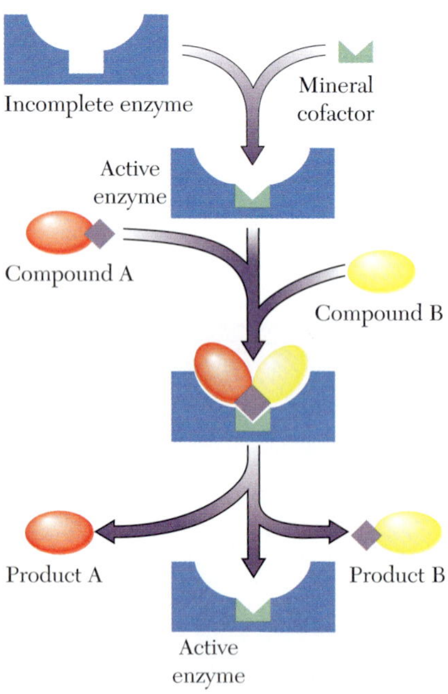

FIGURE 12.6 Many enzymes require mineral ions as cofactors. The cofactor is needed for the active form of the enzyme. In this example, the mineral cofactor is needed for an enzymatic reaction that transfers a chemical group (shown as a purple diamond) from compound A to compound B.

Recommended Intakes

The DRI recommendations for mineral intakes are based on evidence from many types of research studies, ranging from laboratory studies done in animals and clinical trials in humans to epidemiological observations—and, in some cases, from inadvertent findings from rare diseases and medical interventions.

Depletion-repletion studies are often used to assess mineral essentiality and determine mineral requirements. Like other nutrients, minerals are considered essential if a deficiency consistently results in less than optimal biological function and is preventable or reversible by supplementation of that nutrient at levels similar to those found normally in the diet. In a depletion-repletion study, the subject is depleted of a nutrient until symptoms of a deficiency appear; then the nutrient is repleted to a level at which symptoms resolve. However, because of the many potential interactions among minerals and other dietary components, the need for any one mineral must be examined within the context of the total diet, and thus studied along with known amounts of the other dietary components that interact with it. Depletion-repletion studies are particularly difficult to conduct with trace elements because requirements are so small that trace elements present in the environment and those already in the body can meet needs and obscure experimental results.

As with other nutrients, when no other data are available on mineral requirements, needs are estimated by evaluating the intake in a healthy population. It is assumed that if there are no deficiency symptoms, the diet must meet the requirement for that nutrient. One problem with this approach, however, is that deficiency symptoms may become apparent only when the deficiency is severe. Subtle signs of a mineral deficiency in a population may be difficult to detect.

In addition to planned experiments, information about trace element needs has come from the study of diseases related to trace element utilization and from the study of deficiency symptoms in individuals fed solely by **total parenteral nutrition (TPN)** for long periods of time. For example, much of our knowledge about copper comes from studying Menkes' kinky hair syndrome, an inherited condition in which copper absorption and metabolism are abnormal (Figure 12.7). The symptoms of this syndrome are manifestations of a copper deficiency. Observations of a patient receiving a TPN solution deficient in selenium helped establish the essentiality of this mineral. The patient developed symptoms that resolved when selenium was added to the solution.

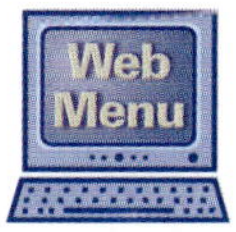

For more information on total parenteral nutrition, go to the American Society for Parenteral and Enteral Nutrition at www.nutritioncare.org/.

Total parenteral nutrition (TPN) A method of providing complete nutrition by infusing nutrients into a large central vein.

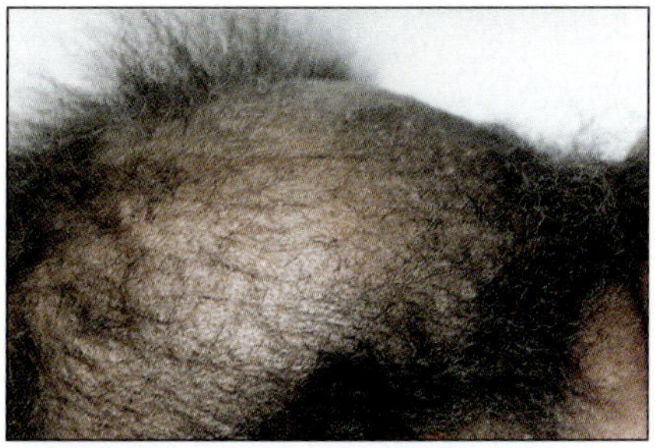

FIGURE 12.7 Much of our understanding of copper deficiency has come from studying individuals with Menkes' kinky hair syndrome, characterized by abnormal hair structure. *(Courtesy of the National Institutes of Health Clinical Center)*

Minerals and Health

The right amount of each mineral is needed in the correct proportions in order to maintain health. Both deficiencies and excesses cause changes in body function. For some minerals, too little or too much causes obvious symptoms that impact short-term health. For others, underconsumption or overconsumption has few immediate symptoms but may affect the risk of chronic disease later in life. Due to the many interactions among minerals, a deficiency or excess of one can affect the status of another.

Deficiency Deficiencies of iron, iodine, and calcium are world health problems. Iron deficiency affects people in both the developed and the developing world. After only a few months of inadequate iron intake there is a decrease in the number and size of red blood cells, reducing the blood's capacity to deliver oxygen. Iodine deficiency disorders are a problem primarily in developing countries, where they impact individuals at every stage of life. Like iron deficiencies, iodine deficiency causes symptoms over a relatively short period of time. Low calcium intake poses a problem in both developed and developing countries. There are no short-term consequences, but a diet deficient in calcium can reduce bone density and impact bone health later in life. Many people in the United States, particularly women, have a low calcium intake and low bone density, and low bone density due to low calcium intake is an emerging problem in developing nations.

Deficiencies of most other minerals are rare, occurring only when the food supply is particularly limited. For example, in certain rural areas of China, selenium deficiency is common because the selenium content of the soil is extremely low and the diet is based on locally grown food.

Toxicity Mineral toxicity occurs most often as a result of environmental pollution or excessive use of supplements. For example, zinc toxicity has occurred with consumption of foods and beverages contaminated with zinc leached from galvanized containers. Trace element supplements pose a risk of toxicity because elements that are essential in small doses may be toxic when consumed in larger amounts. For instance, iron is essential yet can be deadly at high doses. The body's regulatory mechanisms control the absorption and excretion of minerals but have evolved to deal with the amounts of these elements that occur naturally in the diet. Large doses of mineral supplements may override this regulation, causing toxicity.

Supplements can also cause problems because of the complex interactions among minerals. Taking high doses of one can compromise the bioavailability of others, creating a mineral imbalance that can interfere with functions essential to human health.

Calcium (Ca)

Calcium is the most abundant mineral in the body, accounting for 1 to 2% of adult body weight. Adequate calcium intake throughout life is essential for the formation and maintenance of bone. Inadequate intakes over the long term can ultimately result in low bone mass and an increased risk of osteoporosis later in life.

Sources of Calcium

The main source of calcium in the North American diet is dairy products such as milk, cheese, and yogurt. Chocolate milk is a good source of calcium despite the fact that chocolate contains oxalates that bind some of the calcium in the milk and prevent its absorption. Fish that are consumed in their entirety, including the bones, such as sardines and canned salmon, provide a good source of calcium. Legumes and some green vegetables such as broccoli, Chinese cabbage, and kale are also good sources of calcium (Figure 12.8). However, in vegetables that are high in oxalates, the oxalates bind the calcium so it is excreted in the feces. For example, only about 5% of the calcium in spinach is absorbed.[1] Seeds, nuts, and grains provide calcium despite the fact that they contain phytic acid, which reduces calcium absorption.

Some foods are good sources of calcium because it is added during processing. Baked goods such as breads, rolls, and crackers, to which nonfat dry milk powder has been added, provide calcium. Tortillas that are treated with lime water (calcium hydroxide) and tofu that is processed with calcium are good sources of dietary calcium. In addition, there are products on the market, such as orange juice and breakfast cereals, that are fortified with calcium.

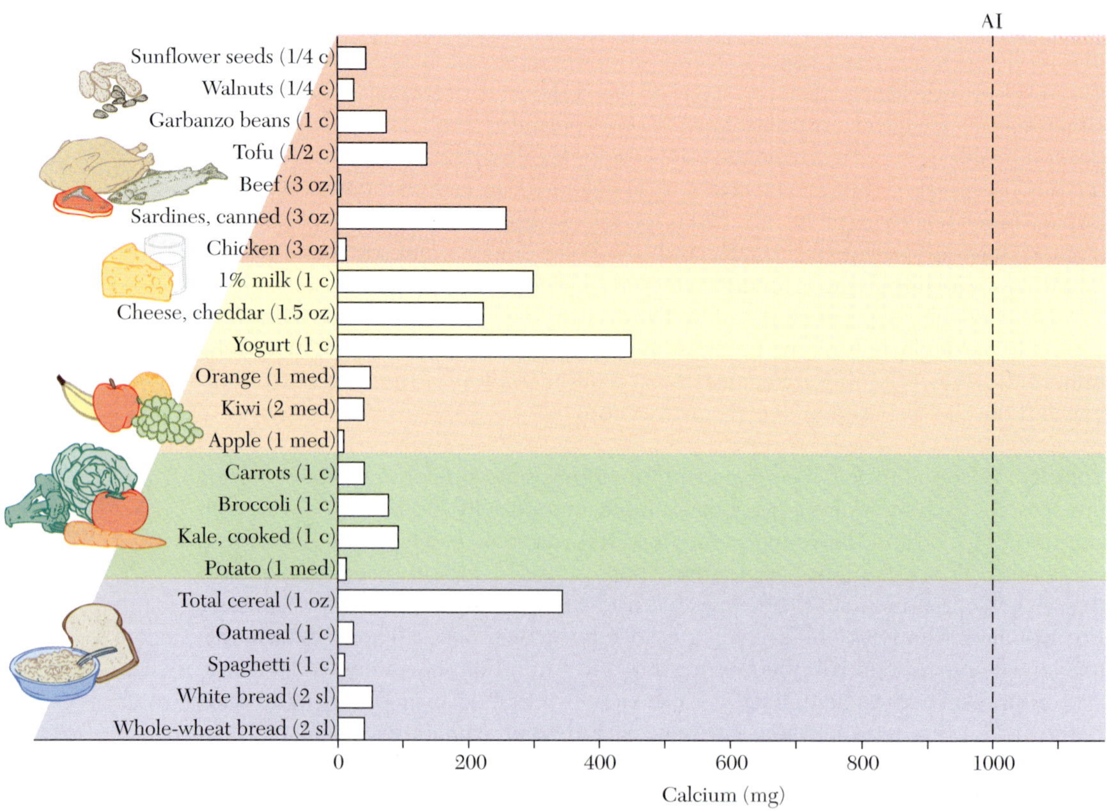

FIGURE 12.8 Calcium content of selections from each food group of the Food Guide Pyramid. The dashed line represents the AI for men and women 19 to 50 years of age.

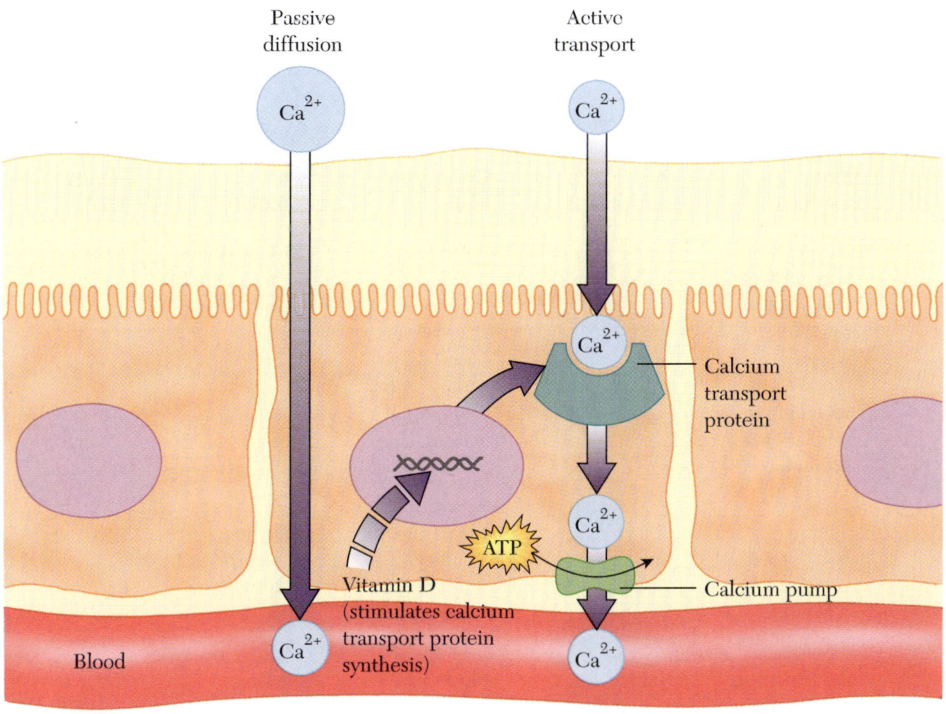

FIGURE 12.9 Some calcium can be absorbed by passive diffusion, particularly when calcium concentrations are high. At lower calcium concentrations, absorption occurs primarily by an active transport mechanism that requires vitamin D. Vitamin D turns on the synthesis of calcium transport proteins that shuttle the calcium across the mucosal cell. A protein pump that requires ATP then moves calcium from the mucosal cells to the bloodstream.

Calcium in the Digestive Tract

To be absorbed, calcium must be in solution. Acid in the stomach helps to get calcium in a soluble form. It is then absorbed by both active transport and passive diffusion (Figure 12.9). When calcium intake is low to moderate, most absorption occurs by active transport, which requires the active form of vitamin D. If vitamin D is deficient, absorption decreases dramatically. At high intakes, passive transport becomes more important. As calcium intake increases, the percentage that is absorbed declines.

The bioavailability of calcium is affected by other dietary components. For instance, lactose consumed with calcium enhances its absorption. On the other hand, tannins, fiber, phytate, and oxalates consumed with calcium decrease absorption. When calcium intake is low, dietary components that alter absorption may affect calcium status, but when calcium intake is adequate, these factors have little effect.[2]

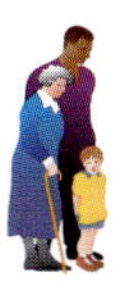

The efficiency of calcium absorption also varies with life stage. During infancy, about 60% of the calcium that is consumed is absorbed, but by young adulthood, absorption is reduced to about 25%. During pregnancy, when calcium need is high, elevated estrogen helps increase calcium absorption. In older adults, absorption declines due to a decrease in blood levels of the active form of vitamin D.[3] An additional decrease in calcium absorption occurs in women after **menopause** due to the decrease in estrogen.

Menopause The physiological changes that mark the end of a woman's capacity to bear children.

Calcium in the Body

Over 99% of the calcium in the body is found in the solid mineral deposit in bones and teeth.[4] The remaining 1% is present in intracellular fluid, blood, and other extracellular fluids, where it plays vital roles in nerve transmission, muscle contraction, blood pressure regulation, and the release of hormones (see Table 12.1).

Calcium in Bones and Teeth Bone is composed of a protein framework, or matrix, that is hardened by deposits of minerals. The most abundant protein in this matrix is collagen. The mineral portion of bone is composed mainly of calcium associated with phosphorus as solid mineral crystals known as **hydroxyapatite**. In

Hydroxyapatite A crystalline compound composed of calcium and phosphorus that is deposited in the protein matrix of bone to give it strength and rigidity.

TABLE 12.1 A Summary of Calcium, Phosphorus, Magnesium, and Sulfur

Mineral	Sources	Recommended Intake for Adults*†	Major Functions	Deficiency Diseases and Symptoms	Groups at Risk	Toxicity	Tolerable Upper Intake Levels (UL)†
Calcium	Dairy products, bony fish, legumes, leafy green vegetables	1000–1200 mg*	Bone and tooth structure, nerve transmission, muscle contraction, blood clotting, blood pressure regulation, hormone secretion	Increased risk of osteoporosis	Postmenopausal women, children, adolescents, elderly, those with kidney disease	Kidney stones in susceptible individuals	2500 mg
Phosphorus	Meat, dairy, cereals, baked goods	700 mg	Structure of bones, teeth, membranes; ATP and DNA; buffer	Bone loss, weakness, lack of appetite	Premature infants, alcoholics, elderly	Calcium resorption from bone	4000 mg
Magnesium	Nuts, greens, whole grains, seeds	310–420 mg	Bone structure, ATP reactions, nerve and muscle function	Nausea, vomiting, weakness, heart changes	Alcoholics, those with kidney and gastrointestinal disease	Nausea, vomiting, low blood pressure	350 mg (nonfood)
Sulfur	Protein foods, preservatives	None specified	Part of amino acids and vitamins, buffer	None when protein needs are met	None	None likely	N/A

*Values with an asterisk (*) represent Adequate Intakes (AI). All other values are Recommended Dietary Allowances (RDA).

†Recommended intakes and UL values for all age groups and stages of life are given on the inside cover.

N/A = No UL established at time of publication.

addition to calcium and phosphorus, bone contains magnesium, sodium, fluoride, and a number of other trace minerals.

There are two types of bone in the skeleton: **cortical** or **compact bone**, which makes up about 80% of the skeleton and forms the sturdy, dense outer surface layer, and **trabecular** or **spongy bone**, which forms an inner spongy lattice that supports the cortical shell (Figure 12.10). Trabecular bone is found in the knobby ends of the long bones, the pelvis, wrists, vertebrae, scapulas, and the areas of the bone that line the bone marrow.

Cortical or **compact bone** Dense, compact bone that makes up the sturdy outer surface layer of bones.

Trabecular or **spongy bone** The type of bone that forms the inner spongy lattice that lines the bone marrow cavity and supports the cortical shell.

Bone Remodeling Bone is a living, metabolically active tissue that is constantly being broken down and reformed in a process called **bone remodeling**. It is formed by cells called **osteoblasts** and is broken down or resorbed by cells called **osteoclasts**. During bone formation, the activity of the bone-building osteoblasts exceeds that of the osteoclasts. When bone is being broken down, the osteoclasts resorb bone more rapidly than the osteoblasts can rebuild it.

Both cortical and trabecular bone tissue undergo remodeling, but it occurs to a greater extent in trabecular bone. Remodeling can be stimulated by dietary intake, mechanical stress on the skeleton, microscopic bone fractures that need repair, and the need to maintain set levels of calcium in extracellular fluids.

Bone remodeling The process whereby bone is continuously broken down and reformed to allow for growth and maintenance.

Osteoblasts Cells responsible for the deposition of bone.

Osteoclasts Large cells responsible for bone breakdown.

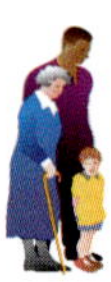

Changes in Bone Throughout Life Most bone is formed early in life. In the growing bones of children, bone formation occurs more rapidly than bone breakdown. Even after growth stops, bone density continues to increase into young adulthood when **peak bone mass** is achieved, somewhere between the ages of 16 and 30.[5]

Peak bone mass The maximum bone density attained at any time in life, usually occurring in young adulthood.

In healthy adults, bone turnover—that is, the ratio of bone breakdown to formation—is in balance, so bone mass remains relatively constant (Figure 12.11). After about age 35 to 45, the amount of bone broken down begins to exceed that which is formed. Although both types of bone are lost with age, the loss of spongy trabecular bone begins earlier than does cortical bone loss.[6] If enough bone is lost, the skeleton is weakened and fractures occur easily. This condition is known as **osteoporosis**. It usually occurs in individuals over 50 years of age.

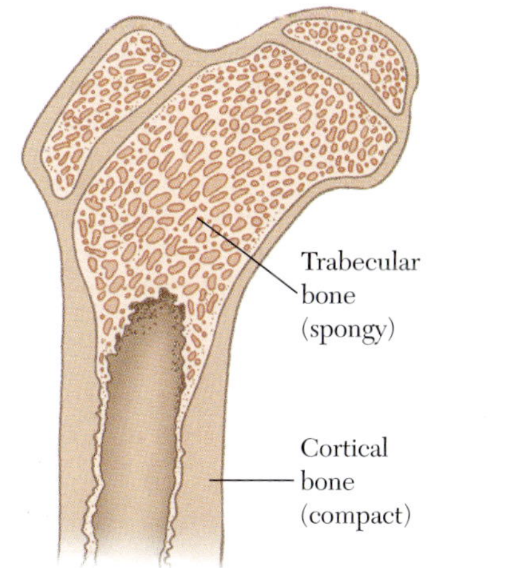

FIGURE 12.10 The compact bone that forms the outer layer of bone is called cortical bone and the spongy interior is referred to as trabecular bone.

Calcium in Body Fluids In addition to maintaining bones and teeth, calcium plays extremely important roles in cell communication and the regulation of body processes. Calcium helps regulate enzyme activity, is needed for the secretion of certain hormones, and is necessary in blood clotting. It is involved in transmitting chemical and electrical signals in nerves and muscles. It is necessary for the release of neurotransmitters, which allow nerve impulses to pass from one nerve to another and from nerves to other tissues. Inside the muscle cells, calcium allows the two muscle proteins, actin and myosin, to interact to cause muscle contraction. Calcium also plays a role in blood pressure regulation, possibly by controlling the contraction of muscles in the blood vessel walls and signaling the secretion of substances that regulate blood pressure.[7]

Osteoporosis A bone disorder characterized by a reduction in bone mass, increased bone fragility, and an increased risk of fractures.

Parathyroid hormone (PTH) A hormone secreted by the parathyroid gland that increases blood calcium levels.

Calcitonin A hormone secreted by the thyroid gland that reduces blood calcium levels.

Calcium Homeostasis The functions of calcium are so vital to survival that there are powerful regulatory mechanisms that maintain constant intracellular and extracellular concentrations. Slight changes in blood calcium levels trigger responses that quickly return levels to normal. This homeostasis is maintained by the hormones **parathyroid hormone (PTH)**, which raises blood calcium, and **calcitonin**, which lowers blood calcium (Figure 12.12).

If the level of blood calcium falls too low, parathyroid hormone is released. PTH acts primarily at the bone and kidney. In bone, it stimulates bone breakdown and the release of calcium and other minerals into the blood. At the kidney PTH interacts with kidney cells to promote the reabsorption of calcium into the blood, reducing urinary calcium excretion. PTH also stimulates the kidney to convert inactive 25-hydroxyvitamin D to active 1,25-dihydroxyvitamin D. This activated vitamin D increases the amount of calcium absorbed from the gastrointestinal tract and, with

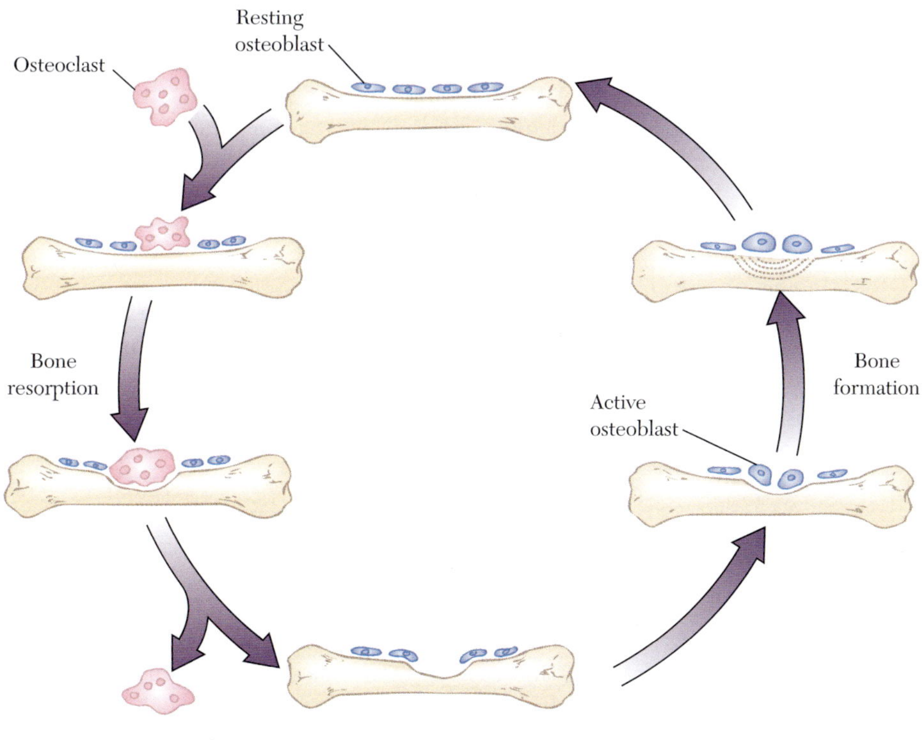

FIGURE 12.11 Bone continuously undergoes remodeling. Osteoclasts resorb bone and osteoblasts build bone. When the amount of bone resorption is equal to the amount of bone formation, the total amount of bone does not change. At any one time about 4% of the total bone surface is involved in bone remodeling.

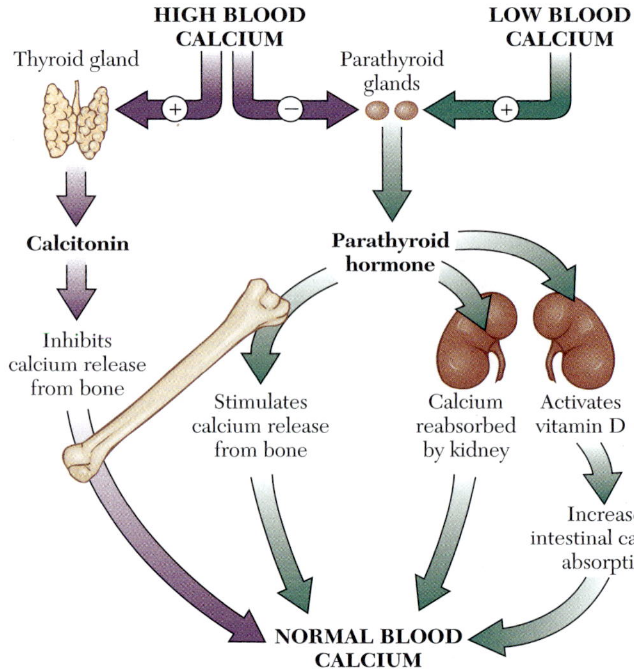

FIGURE 12.12 Levels of calcium in the blood are very tightly regulated by parathyroid hormone and calcitonin. Low blood calcium levels stimulate the release of parathyroid hormone, which increases blood calcium levels by increasing the release of calcium from bone, increasing the reabsorption of calcium at the kidney, and stimulating the formation of active vitamin D, which increases the absorption of dietary calcium from the intestine. High levels of blood calcium inhibit the release of parathyroid hormone and stimulate the release of calcitonin, which inhibits calcium release from bone helping to restore blood calcium to normal.

parathyroid hormone, stimulates calcium release from the bone. The overall effect is to rapidly increase blood calcium levels. If blood calcium levels become too high, the secretion of parathyroid hormone is shut off and calcitonin is secreted. Calcitonin acts primarily on osteoclasts in bone to inhibit bone breakdown and the release of calcium into the blood, resulting in a decrease in blood calcium levels.

The ability to maintain blood calcium levels by removing calcium from bone is beneficial over the short term, but if continued over the long term, it results in progressive loss of bone mass and bone weakening.

Recommended Intakes

A healthy level of calcium intake is the amount necessary to develop and maintain bone and prevent osteoporosis later in life. Unfortunately, it has not been possible to determine how much calcium is needed at each life stage to prevent osteoporosis in later life. Therefore, DRI values for calcium intakes have been set at amounts that allow maximum calcium retention. Increasing dietary calcium above this level will not increase the amount of calcium retained in the body. Adults may continue to lose bone mass at this intake level due to other causes such as loss of estrogen, smoking, and a sedentary lifestyle, but this loss is not due to inadequate calcium intake.

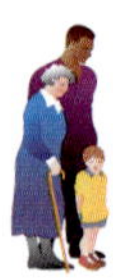

Rather than an RDA, an AI has been determined for calcium because it was not possible to precisely estimate the dietary intake needed for maximum retention. The AI for adults ages 19 through 50 years is 1000 mg per day.[4] Because absorption decreases with age, the AI for men and women age 51 and older is increased to 1200 mg per day. In children and adolescents, the AI is set at a level that will support bone growth. For adolescents, the AI is higher than for adults—1300 mg per day for boys and girls ages 9 through 18.

For infants, an AI is set based on the mean calcium intake of breast-fed infants. Because calcium is not as well absorbed from infant formulas, formula-fed infants require more. There is no special AI for formula-fed infants, but formulas are higher in calcium than breast milk to compensate for the reduced absorption.

The AI for calcium during pregnancy is not increased above nonpregnant levels. This is because there is an increase in maternal calcium absorption during pregnancy that helps to supply the calcium needed for the fetal skeleton. In addi-

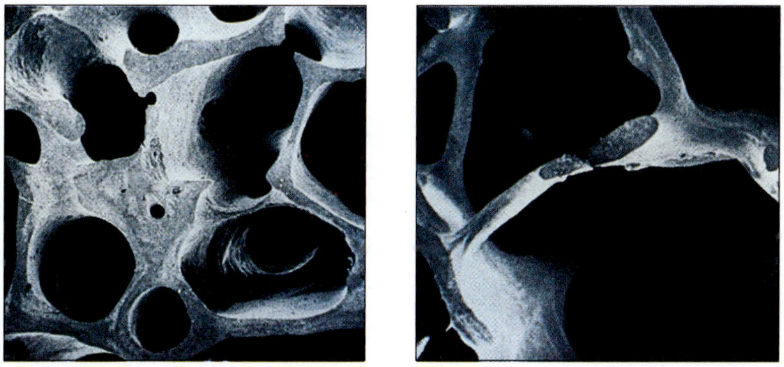

FIGURE 12.13 Osteoporosis causes a decrease in bone density and increases the risk of fractures. Healthy trabecular bone *(left)*. Trabecular bone weakened by osteoporosis *(right)*. *(Courtesy of Wyeth-Ayerst Laboratories)*

tion, because there is no correlation between the number of pregnancies a woman has had and the density of her bones, it has been determined that the maternal skeleton is not used as a supply of calcium for the fetus during pregnancy. However, during lactation, the source of the calcium secreted in milk does appear to be the maternal skeleton.[8] Despite this, the AI is not increased during lactation because increasing dietary calcium does not prevent the loss of maternal skeleton, and because the calcium lost appears to be regained following weaning.

Calcium and Osteoporosis

Osteoporosis occurs when both the protein matrix and the mineral deposits in bone are decreased, resulting in a decrease in the total amount of bone (Figure 12.13). As bone mass decreases, the likelihood of fractures increases. In the United States, about 28 million people have osteoporosis or are at risk due to low bone mass, and 80% of them are women.[9,10] Bone fractures due to osteoporosis account for $10 to $15 billion per year in medical costs.[9,11]

Web Menu: For more information on the incidence and risks of osteoporosis, go to the National Institutes of Health Osteoporosis and Related Bone Disease National Resource Center at www.osteo.org/.

Factors Affecting Osteoporosis Risk The risk of osteoporosis depends on the level of peak bone mass achieved and the rate at which bone is lost. These are affected by age, gender, genetics, and lifestyle. Disease conditions and medications can also cause osteoporosis; this is referred to as secondary osteoporosis (Table 12.2).

TABLE 12.2 Risk Factors for Developing Osteoporosis

Primary Osteoporosis

Sex: Female

Race: White or Asian

Age: Significant increase after age 60

Body Size: Low body weight and BMI

Medical History: Family history of osteoporosis, history of previous fractures, estrogen depletion due to menopause or other causes

Lifestyle: Lack of exercise throughout life, cigarette smoking, excessive alcohol consumption, inadequate calcium and vitamin D intakes

Secondary Osteoporosis

Genetic disorders

Endocrine disorders: low testosterone, hyperthyroidism, hyperparathyroidism

Connective tissue disease

Gastrointestinal disease

Blood disorders

Other diseases that affect bone metabolism: chronic renal failure, diabetes, chronic obstructive lung disease, congestive heart failure, alcoholism

Drugs: especially anticonvulsants and glucocorticoids such as prednisone

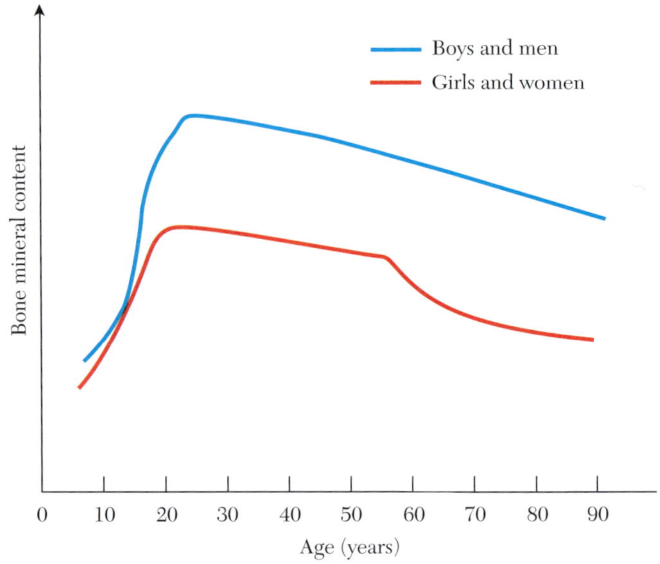

FIGURE 12.14 Men have a higher bone mineral content than women. Although both men and women lose bone after about age 35, women experience an accelerated bone loss for a period following menopause.

Age The risk of osteoporosis increases with age. This is because bones become progressively less dense after about age 35 when bone breakdown begins to exceed bone formation. Other factors that increase bone loss in older adults include a decline in calcium and vitamin D intake, a decrease in physical activity, and a decrease in the efficiency of vitamin D activation by the kidney. In addition, older adults typically spend less time in the sun and wear more clothing to cover the skin when outdoors, which may reduce the amount of vitamin D synthesized in the skin.

Gender and Hormonal Factors Osteoporosis-related fractures occur in one out of every two women over age 50 and in about one in every eight men over 50.[9] The risk of osteoporosis is greater in women than men because men have a higher peak bone mass to begin with and because bone loss is accelerated in women for about five years after menopause (Figure 12.14).[12] This **postmenopausal bone loss** is related to the drop in estrogen levels that occurs around menopause. Declining estrogen affects bone cells and decreases intestinal calcium absorption. During this period, women lose a disproportionate amount of trabecular bone.[13] Because increasing calcium intake has not been shown to prevent postmenopausal bone loss, the AI has been set at the same level for women and for men. After the postmenopausal period, women continue to lose bone but more slowly. This **age-related bone loss**, which also occurs in men, involves the loss of both the compact cortical bone and the spongy trabecular bone (Figure 12.15).

Postmenopausal bone loss The accelerated bone loss that occurs in women for about five years after estrogen production decreases.

Age-related bone loss The bone loss that occurs in both cortical and trabecular bone of men and women as they advance in age.

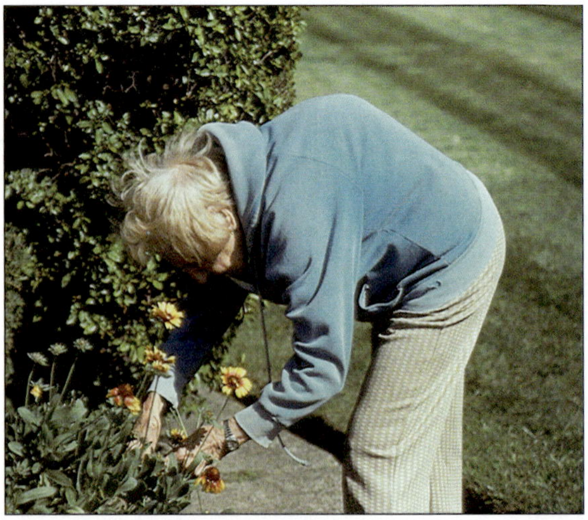

FIGURE 12.15 The bone loss due to osteoporosis can cause a stooped posture and a decrease in stature. *(© Larry Mulvehill/Science Source/Photo Researchers, Inc.)*

Genetics Twin and family studies have shown that genetics is an important determinant of bone density, bone size, and bone turnover. Genetic factors are believed to account for as much as 70% of the variation in bone density and osteoporosis risk.[14] Hormonal and environmental factors such as nutrition, activity level, smoking, and alcohol consumption interact with genetic factors over time to determine actual bone density. Genetic differences among racial groups lead to differences in the risk of osteoporosis. For example, the incidence of osteoporosis in African-American women is half that of Caucasian women despite similar environmental risk factors. The reason for this lower risk of fractures is that African-American women begin menopause with higher bone density and have lower rates of postmenopausal bone loss.[15] Bone density varies in different parts of the skeleton among Asians, Hispanics, and Caucasians, but is generally similar and lower than in African Americans.[16]

Lifestyle Factors Exercise and diet are important determinants of bone density. Other lifestyle factors that affect bone mass include cigarette smoking and alcohol consumption, both of which can decrease bone mass. Studies have shown that smoking is associated with greater bone loss in men.[17] Women who smoke have slightly lower bone mass, some of which may be due to lower body weight in smokers.[18] Excessive alcohol consumption also accelerates bone loss, possibly through a direct effect of alcohol on bone cells or an effect of alcohol on the action of vitamin D, PTH, and calcitonin.[19]

Exercise Weight-bearing exercise, such as walking and jogging, that puts direct weight over the skeleton, increases bone mass.[20] Exercise during childhood and adolescence is thought to be particularly important for achieving a high peak bone mass. In adults who exercise regularly, there is a high correlation between muscle mass and bone mass, and both bone and muscle mass decrease with disuse.[21] A greater body weight also increases bone mass because it increases the amount of weight-bearing exercise that the individual gets in day-to-day activities.[22] In addition, adipose tissue produces estrogen, which helps maintain bone mass and enhances calcium absorption. Therefore, the risk of osteoporosis is decreased in individuals with higher body weight and fat (see *Research Discoveries*: "Bone Loss in Space").

Web Menu For more information on exercise and bone health, go to www.allhealth.com/ and select osteoporosis in the health concerns box.

Diet Diet, particularly calcium intake, can have a significant effect on osteoporosis risk. Calcium is necessary for bone development. Adequate calcium intake during childhood and adolescence is an important factor in maximizing bone density; low calcium intakes during the years of bone formation result in a lower peak bone mass. If calcium intake is low after peak bone mass has been achieved, the rate of bone loss may be increased and, along with it, the risk of osteoporosis.

Although low calcium intake is the most significant dietary factor contributing to osteoporosis, calcium intake alone does not predict the risk of osteoporosis. Other dietary components affect bone mass and bone health by affecting calcium absorption, urinary calcium losses, and bone physiology. Low intakes of vitamin D reduce calcium absorption, thereby increasing the risk of osteoporosis. Diets high in phytate, oxalates, and tannins also reduce calcium absorption. Some studies have demonstrated a connection between dietary sodium intake and calcium loss in the urine, but the impact of sodium on osteoporosis is still controversial.[23,24] Adequate protein is necessary for bone health, but increasing protein intake increases urinary calcium losses. Despite this, high protein intakes are generally not associated with a higher risk of osteoporosis. This is because diets higher in protein are typically higher in calcium, and bone mass depends more on the ratio of calcium to protein than the amount of protein alone. High levels of protein therefore do not have a negative effect on bone mass when calcium intake is adequate.[25] Higher intakes of zinc, magnesium, potassium, fiber, and vitamin C—nutrients that are plentiful in fruits and vegetables—are associated with greater bone mass.[26]

RESEARCH DISCOVERIES

Bone Loss in Space

In 1962 when John Glenn became the first American to orbit the Earth, there was little concern about the effect that his 5-hour flight would have on his bones. By 1997, when Shannon Lucid set the U.S. single-mission space-flight endurance record by spending 188 days aboard the Russian Mir space station, the effect of weightlessness on bone health had become a serious concern. The basis for this concern is that weight-bearing activities such as walking, jogging, and weight training are important for the maintenance of bone health. Under the force of Earth's gravity, these activities cause mechanical stresses on the bones, which stimulate the deposition of calcium into bone. Increasing the amount of exercise increases the stress and consequently bone mass; decreasing exercise causes bone density to revert to the preexercise level.[a] When an astronaut goes into space, the near absence of gravity eliminates the stimulus for bone remodeling and calcium is lost from bone. This elevates calcium levels in the rest of the body and may lead to kidney stones and calcification of the soft tissues. Unless researchers can identify some way of preventing bone loss in space, prolonged space flights may significantly impair skeletal function and cause other health problems. Although the bone loss that occurs in space is a disadvantage for astronauts, it may benefit those on Earth because it has been proposed as a model for studying how osteoporosis occurs with aging.

Studies in the 1960s and early '70s during the Gemini and Apollo space missions showed that astronauts lost calcium from their bones during space travel. Skylab missions then offered an opportunity to study the effects of more extended periods in zero gravity. In one experiment, astronauts maintained a constant dietary calcium intake and made continuous urine and fecal collections for three weeks before their flight, during the 60-day Skylab mission, and for 17 days after returning to Earth. The results showed that urinary calcium losses were increased during the flight. These losses occurred despite vigorous

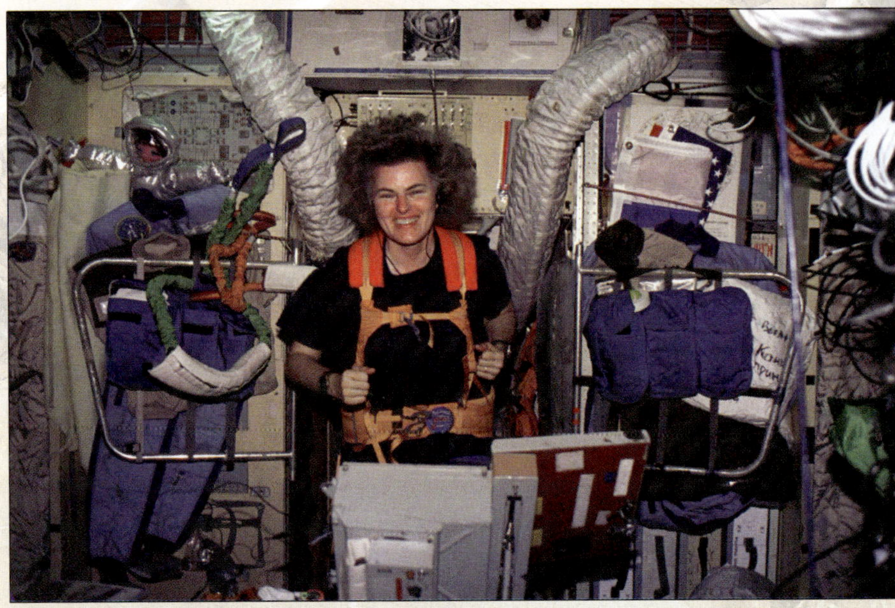

Shannon Lucid exercising on a treadmill aboard the Mir space station. *(© NASA)*

For more information on prevention, diagnosis, and treatment of osteoporosis, go to the Endocrine Society at www.endocrineweb.com/ and click on the osteoporosis center or to the National Osteoporosis Foundation at www.nof.org/.

Preventing and Treating Osteoporosis The best treatment for osteoporosis is to prevent it by achieving a high peak bone mass. Maximizing calcium deposition into bone is especially important during childhood and adolescence. Individuals with the highest peak bone mass after adolescence have a protective advantage over bone loss later in life.[9]

The risk of osteoporosis can be minimized by following appropriate dietary and lifestyle patterns throughout life. A diet rich in fruits and vegetables that is adequate in calcium and vitamin D and not excessive in phosphorus, protein, or sodium will reduce risk. Maintaining an active lifestyle that includes weight-bearing exercise and limiting smoking and alcohol consumption will help to further improve bone density. Once osteoporosis has occurred, it is difficult to restore lost bone.

Calcium Supplements Individuals who do not meet their calcium needs with diet alone can benefit from calcium supplementation. However, because high calcium intake can interfere with the absorption of other minerals, supplements should be

exercise regimens while in flight and were comparable to losses seen in normal adults subjected to prolonged bed rest.[b,c,d]

The study of bone loss in space continued with joint Russian-American studies, many done in astronauts who spent long periods on the Mir space station. Techniques used to study bones in space included measuring hormones and other indicators of bone metabolism in blood and urine samples before and after flights; measuring muscle strength and bone density before, during, and after return to Earth's gravity; and taking X-ray scans to determine total body bone mass as well as bone mass in certain body regions.[e,f] Results indicated that the most significant bone loss occurred in weight-bearing parts of the skeleton. Astronauts lost bone mass from the lower vertebrae, hips, and upper femur at a rate of about 1% per month, and some bones, such as the heel bone, lost calcium even faster. This rate of bone loss is more rapid than that seen under the force of Earth's gravity; as people age they lose bone at a rate of about 1% per year, and even the rapid bone loss that occurs during the postmenopausal period reaches only about 5% a year. In space, bone loss continues at a constant rate throughout a six-month or longer space flight. Once the astronauts have returned to Earth, calcium loss stops within a month, but scientists still don't know if the bone recovers completely. A long space flight may leave astronauts more prone to bone fractures for the rest of their lives.

To try to counteract the effects of weightlessness, astronauts exercise in space on stationary bikes and on treadmills, and pull against bungee cords to simulate gravitational forces. NASA researchers have conducted several studies to evaluate the effects of different types of physical activity (walking, cycling, swimming, etc.) on the body's bones in zero gravity. These studies concluded that walking exercises, and exercises that do not provide high loads to the lower extremities, did not really contribute to the maintenance or buildup of bone density. Exercises that provide higher loads can counteract bone loss to some degree but do not provide sufficient mechanical loads to mimic weight-bearing exercise on Earth.

Astronauts in space and elderly or bedridden persons on Earth all lose bone due to inactivity. Better insight into the relationship between exercise and bone density may lead to the development of exercises and activity patterns that can increase, or at least minimize the decrease in bone mineral density and bone strength seen in these individuals. The research done on mineral loss in zero gravity will help astronauts remain healthy during long-term space flights as well as benefit those at risk for osteoporosis on Earth.

References

[a]Drinkwater, B. L. Weight-bearing exercise and bone mass. In *Physical Medicine and Rehabilitation Clinics of North America: Osteoporosis*. V. Matkovic, ed. Philadelphia: W. B. Saunders Company, 1995, 567–578.

[b]Whedon, G. D., Lutwak, L., Rambaut, P. C., et al. Mineral and nitrogen balance study observations: the second manned Skylab mission. Aviat. Space Environ. Med. 47:391–396, 1976.

[c]Wronski, T. J., and Morey, E. R. Alterations in calcium homeostasis and bone during actual and simulated space flight. Med. Sci. Sports Exerc. 15:410–414, 1983.

[d]LeBlanc, A., Shackelford, L., and Schneider, V. Future human bone research in space. Bone 22(5 suppl): 113S–116S, 1998.

[e]NASA. Bone Mineral Loss and Recovery after Shuttle/Mir Flights. Available online at **http://spaceflight.nasa.gov/history/shuttle-mir/science/shuttmir/shutmir/exphis/musbone.htm**. Accessed 17 Jan 2001.

[f]NASA. Dynamics of Calcium Metabolism and Bone Tissue. Available online at **http://spaceflight.nasa.gov/history/shuttle-mir/science/shuttmir/shutmir/exphis/musdynam.htm.** Accessed 17 Jan 2001.

taken with care. Supplemental calcium can increase peak bone mass in young individuals who do not meet their calcium needs with food. In postmenopausal women, calcium supplements have been found to reduce bone loss, but not to increase bone mass.[27] Calcium supplements are more effective at reducing cortical than trabecular bone loss, and their ability to decrease calcium loss in postmenopausal women is greatest after the first five years of menopause.[4] Treatment of osteoporosis with calcium combined with vitamin D has been shown to prevent bone loss, increase bone density, and decrease the frequency of bone fractures (see *Making Decisions:* Calcium Supplements: Do You Need One? Which One Should You Choose?").[28]

Other Treatments Other treatments for osteoporosis include the hormones estrogen and calcitonin and drugs known as bisphosphonates as well as exercise and diet. Replacing the estrogen lost in menopause has been shown to reduce bone loss and restore some lost bone.[29,30] Calcitonin, administered by injection or nasal spray, can reduce bone resorption.[31] The effects of calcitonin are enhanced by

Making Decisions

Calcium Supplements: Do You Need One? Which Should You Choose?

A carefully planned varied diet that includes three glasses of milk a day will easily provide enough calcium to meet needs. But, many people choose to take a supplement rather than balance their diet. Do calcium supplements provide the same benefits as calcium from foods? Are there any risks? If you choose to take a calcium supplement, which one should you take?

Supplements are not a substitute for foods. Food sources of calcium provide many nutrients other than calcium. For example, milk is an excellent source of high-quality protein and provides riboflavin and vitamins A and D. However, for those concerned just about calcium intake, supplements do provide an easy way to assure that intake meets needs. The supplements are relatively inexpensive, the calcium is well-absorbed, and the risks are minimal.

There are many types of calcium supplements. The most common and least expensive contain calcium carbonate. This form provides the greatest concentration of calcium per gram. Studies have shown that the calcium in calcium carbonate supplements is absorbed as well as the calcium from milk.[a] Other calcium compounds used in supplements include calcium citrate, calcium gluconate, calcium lactate, calcium citrate-malate, and calcium phosphate. A study that compared the absorption of a supplement containing calcium carbonate to one containing calcium citrate found that the calcium citrate was absorbed two and a half times better than the calcium carbonate.[b]

The absorption of calcium from supplements, like the absorption of calcium in foods, can be affected by other food components and nutrients consumed with it. Acidic foods, lactose, and fat, which prolongs transit time, increase calcium absorption from supplements. Oxalate, phytates, and fiber inhibit calcium absorption. Absorption from supplements also depends on how quickly the product dissolves in the stomach. In individuals with low stomach acid, calcium carbonate dissolves very slowly, so absorption is decreased.[c] Other calcium compounds are better absorbed when stomach acid is low but contain less calcium per gram of supplement. In addition, a high-dose supplement may be poorly absorbed because absorption decreases when 400 mg or more is taken in a single dose.[d]

When selecting a supplement, choose one that contains a calcium compound alone, such as calcium citrate or calcium carbonate. Calcium-containing antacids are popular as calcium supplements. For instance, Tums, which contain calcium carbonate, are often used as a calcium supplement because they are inexpensive and taste good. Multivitamin and mineral supplements typically contain only a small portion of the AI for calcium—they would have to be the size of a marble to contain 1000 mg of calcium plus other nutrients. And if supplements containing vitamin D are used, consumers should monitor the amount of vitamin D they are consuming because it is toxic in large doses.

The calcium in preparations such as bone meal, powdered bone, dolomite (limestone), and oyster shell are not different from other supplements in terms of calcium, but they may contain enough lead to be a health hazard if consumed routinely.[e]

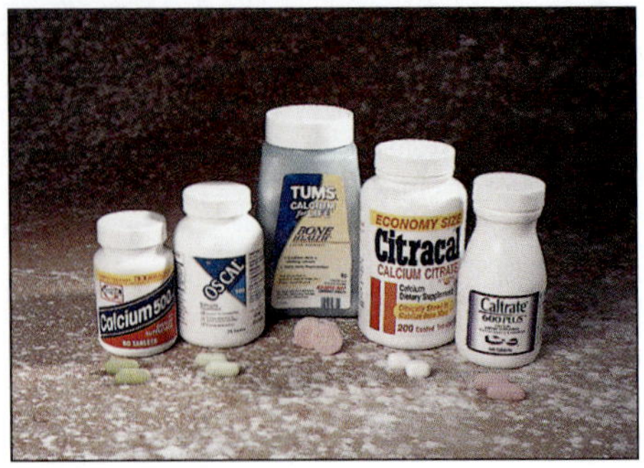

(George Semple)

References

[a]Mortensen, L., and Charles, P. Bioavailability of calcium supplements and the effect of vitamin D: comparisons between milk, calcium carbonate, and calcium carbonate plus vitamin D. Am. J. Clin. Nutr. 63:354–357, 1996.

[b]Heller, H. J., Stewart, A., Haynes, S., and Pak, C. Y. Pharmacokinetics of calcium absorption from two commercial calcium supplements. J. Clin. Pharmacol. 39:1151–1154, 1999.

[c]Whiting, S. J., Wood, R., and Kim, K. Calcium supplementation. J. Am. Acad. Nurse Pract. 9:187–192, 1997.

[d]Heaney, R. P., Weaver, C. M., and Fitzsimmons, M. L. Influence of calcium load on absorption fraction. J. Bone Miner. Res. 5:1135–1138, 1990.

[e]Bourgoin, B. P., Evans, D. R., Cornett, J. R. et al. Lead content in 70 brands of dietary calcium supplements. Am. J. Public Health 83: 1155–1160, 1993.

calcium supplementation. Bisphosphonates act by inhibiting bone resorption and have been shown to prevent postmenopausal bone loss and increase bone mineral density in patients with osteoporosis.[32,33] Exercise can also be helpful in treating osteoporosis.[24] Minerals other than calcium that have been used to prevent and treat bone loss include magnesium, fluoride, and boron, but results with these have been equivocal.

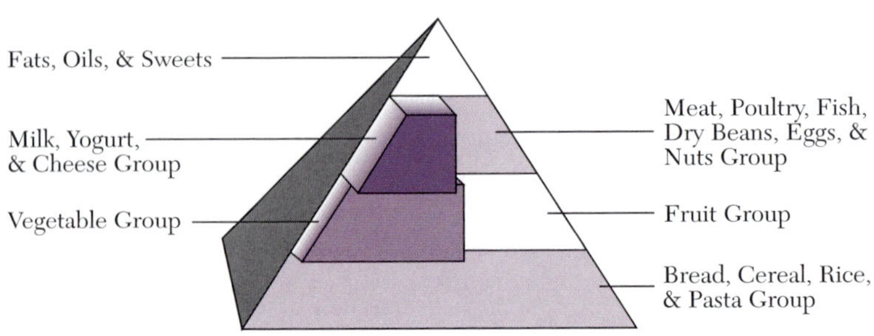

FIGURE 12.16 The food groups that are sources of calcium are raised and colored purple. The darker the shade, the more calcium-rich foods the group contains.

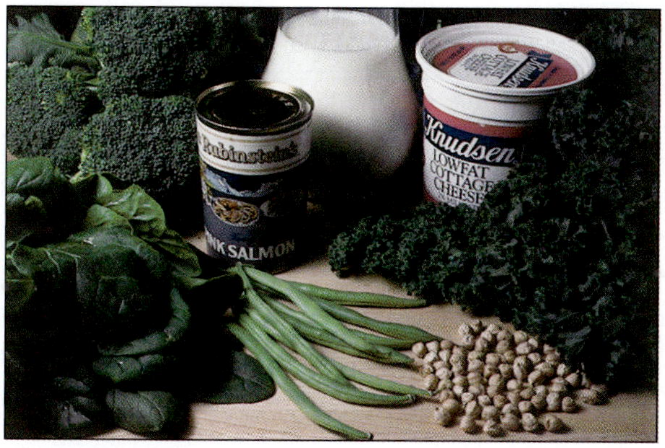

FIGURE 12.17 Dairy products, fish consumed with bones, leafy greens, and legumes are good sources of calcium *(© Felicia Martinez/PhotoEdit)*

Calcium Toxicity

Adverse effects associated with high calcium intake are usually related to intake from supplements. Too much supplemental calcium can cause kidney stone formation and kidney insufficiency, and may interfere with the absorption of other minerals. Calcium interacts with iron, zinc, magnesium, and phosphorus. Although calcium supplements inhibit iron absorption, there is no evidence that the long-term use of calcium supplements with meals affects iron status.[34] High intakes of calcium from supplements have also been found to reduce zinc absorption and thereby increase zinc needs in the diet.[35] There is no evidence of depletion of phosphorus or magnesium associated with calcium intake. A UL of 2500 mg per day from food and supplements has been set for adults ages 19 to 70 years.

Meeting Calcium Needs

Americans typically do not consume enough calcium. It is estimated that only 25% of boys and 10% of girls ages 9 to 17 meet the recommendation of 1300 mg of calcium per day, and only 50 to 60% of adults meet the recommendation of 1000 to 1200 mg per day.[9] Adequate calcium intake can be achieved by following the Food Guide Pyramid recommendation of two to three servings of milk, yogurt, or cheese plus three to five servings of vegetables daily (Figure 12.16). Ice cream, puddings, and soups made with milk are good calcium sources.

Lactose-free sources of calcium include dark-green leafy vegetables such as kale, broccoli, turnip and mustard greens; legumes; soy products processed with calcium; and fish consumed with the bones (Figure 12.17). Fortified foods also provide calcium. Many breakfast cereals and juice products are now fortified with calcium in an effort to increase the typical calcium intake. For packaged foods, nutrient content descriptors help identify good sources of calcium (Table 12.3), and the Nutrition Facts section of the label must provide the percent Daily Value of calcium in a serving (Table 12.4).

Web Menu: To estimate your calcium intake using food frequency, go to www.calciuminfo.com/ and click on the calcium calculator.

TABLE 12.3 Calcium Descriptors on Food Labels

Descriptor	Definition
High-calcium, rich in calcium, excellent source of calcium	Contains 200 mg of calcium or more per serving.
Good source of calcium	Contains at least 100 mg of calcium per serving.
More or added calcium	Contains at least 100 mg more per serving than reference food.

TABLE 12.4 Calculating Calcium Content from Food Labels

Determine:

- The Daily Value for calcium using Table 2.3 or Appendix J
- The % Daily Value for calcium per serving from your food label

Calculate the amount of calcium in grams:

- Multiply the % Daily Value by the Daily Value
- Multiply this amount by the number of servings consumed

For example:

The Daily Value for calcium is 1000 mg. A one cup serving of yogurt provides 25% of the Daily Value for calcium and you ate one cup.

1000 mg × 25% of Daily Value × 1 serving = 1000 × 0.25 × 1 = 250 mg of calcium

Critical Thinking

Meeting Calcium Needs

Laura is nearly 50. Although she has no symptoms, she is worried about her risk for osteoporosis. Her mother is 75 and recently suffered a fractured hip due to reduced bone density caused by osteoporosis. Her previously independent mother is now living in a nursing home and struggling to return to her former life. Laura is frightened that she will face the same future. She finds the following osteoporosis risk factor questionnaire in a health magazine and fills it out.

Gender	☐ Male ☒ Female
How old are you?	☐ 12 to 18 ☐ 19 to 30 ☒ 31 to 50 ☐ 51 to 70 ☐ > 70
Have you ever broken a bone?	☐ Yes ☒ No
What is your bone density?	☒ Never been measured ☐ Normal ☐ Low density
What is your Body Mass Index?	☐ < 18.5 kg/m^2 ☐ 18.5 to 24.9 ☒ 25.0 to 29.9 ☐ 30.0 to 34.9 ☐ ≥ 35
Do you smoke cigarettes?	☒ Yes ☐ No
How much alcohol do you drink?	☐ > 2 drinks/day ☐ 1–2 drinks/day ☒ Several drinks per week ☐ None

How much milk do you drink?	☐ None ☒ 2 or fewer glasses a day ☐ 3 or more glasses a day
How much milk did you drink as a child?	☐ None ☒ 2 or fewer glasses a day ☐ 3 or more glasses a day
How much milk did you drink as an adolescent?	☒ None ☐ 2 or fewer glasses a day ☐ 3 or more glasses a day
How often do you exercise?	☒ Less than 3 times a week ☐ 3 or more times a week
What types of activities do you participate in?	☐ None ☒ Walking, jogging, tennis ☐ Swimming, bicycling
What is your exercise history?	☐ I have been active all my life. ☒ I was active as a child but no longer exercise often. ☐ I recently started exercising.
If you are female, are you currently menstruating?	☒ Yes ☐ No
If you are postmenopausal, how long ago did menopause occur?	☐ Less than 5 years ago ☐ More than 5 years ago
Do you have a family history of osteoporosis	☒ Yes ☐ No

Which of Laura's answers on the questionnaire suggest that she has an increased risk for osteoporosis?

▼

Answer:

Laura is confused about how her milk intake and activity level as a child can affect her osteoporosis risk now. What would you tell her?

▼

Peak bone mass is achieved by about age 35. Because bone development depends on calcium intake and weight-bearing exercise, these are essential early in life to increase peak bone mass. A child who does not get adequate calcium and exercise may have a low peak bone mass, which increases the risk of osteoporosis later in life.

▼

Although Laura does not drink a lot of milk, she knows that other dairy products and many other foods are good sources of calcium. These were not addressed by this questionnaire, so she records what she eats and drinks for a day to estimate her typical calcium intake.

▼

Food	Energy (kcals)	Calcium (mg)
BREAKFAST		
Eggs (2 large)	150	5
Toast with margarine (2 slices)	200	50
Orange juice (3/4 cup)	80	15
Coffee with cream (1 cup)	45	35
LUNCH		
Bologna sandwich on white bread with mayonnaise	260	60
Lettuce and tomato (2 slices)	10	5
Milk (1 cup)	120	300
Apple (1 medium)	80	10
SNACK		
Chips (1 oz)	150	10
Beer (12 fl oz)	140	20
DINNER		
Roast beef (3 oz)	225	5
Mashed potatoes and gravy (1 cup)	350	50
Green beans (1 cup)	35	60
Iced tea (12 oz)	4	0
Ice cream (1/2 cup)	140	70
TOTAL	*1889*	*695*

How does her intake compare to the recommendations for calcium intake?

Answer:

How can she increase her calcium without increasing her energy intake?

At breakfast she could have cereal with milk rather than eggs. She could select cereals that are fortified with calcium and drink calcium-fortified orange juice. At lunch, she could __________

For a snack, she could __________

At dinner, she could __________

Do you think she should take a calcium supplement? Why or why not?

Answer:

Phosphorus (P)

Phosphorus makes up about 1% of the adult body by weight and 85% of this is found as a structural component of bones.[4] The phosphorus in soft tissues has both structural and regulatory roles. In nature, phosphorus is most often found in combination with oxygen as phosphate (Figure 12.18).

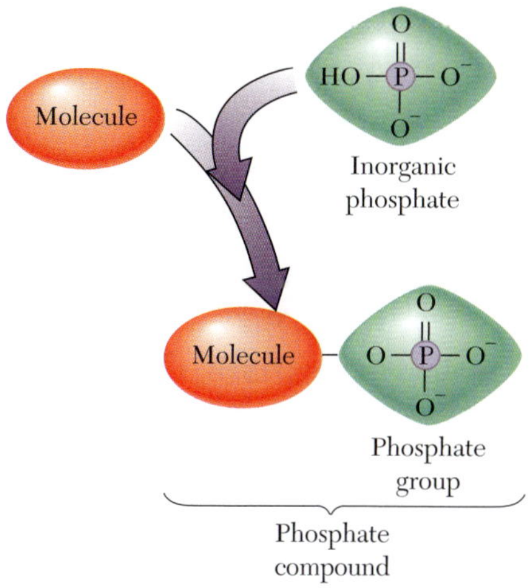

FIGURE 12.18 Inorganic phosphate is phosphorus combined with oxygen. Inorganic phosphate can join with other molecules as a phosphate group. Phosphate compounds are extremely important in the body.

Sources of Phosphorus

Phosphorus is more widely distributed in the diet than calcium. Like calcium, it is found in dairy products such as milk, yogurt, and cheese, but meat, cereals, bran, eggs, nuts, and fish are also good sources (Figure 12.19). Food additives used in baked goods, cheeses, processed meats, and soft drinks also contribute to dietary phosphorus.

Phosphorus in the Digestive Tract

Phosphorus is more readily absorbed than calcium. About 60 to 70% is absorbed from a typical diet. There is no evidence that the efficiency of absorption is affected by the amount in the diet. Vitamin D does aid phosphorus absorption but to a lesser extent than calcium absorption. Phosphorus absorption also occurs by a vitamin D–independent mechanism. Therefore, when vitamin D is deficient, phosphorus can still be absorbed, but its absorption is reduced.

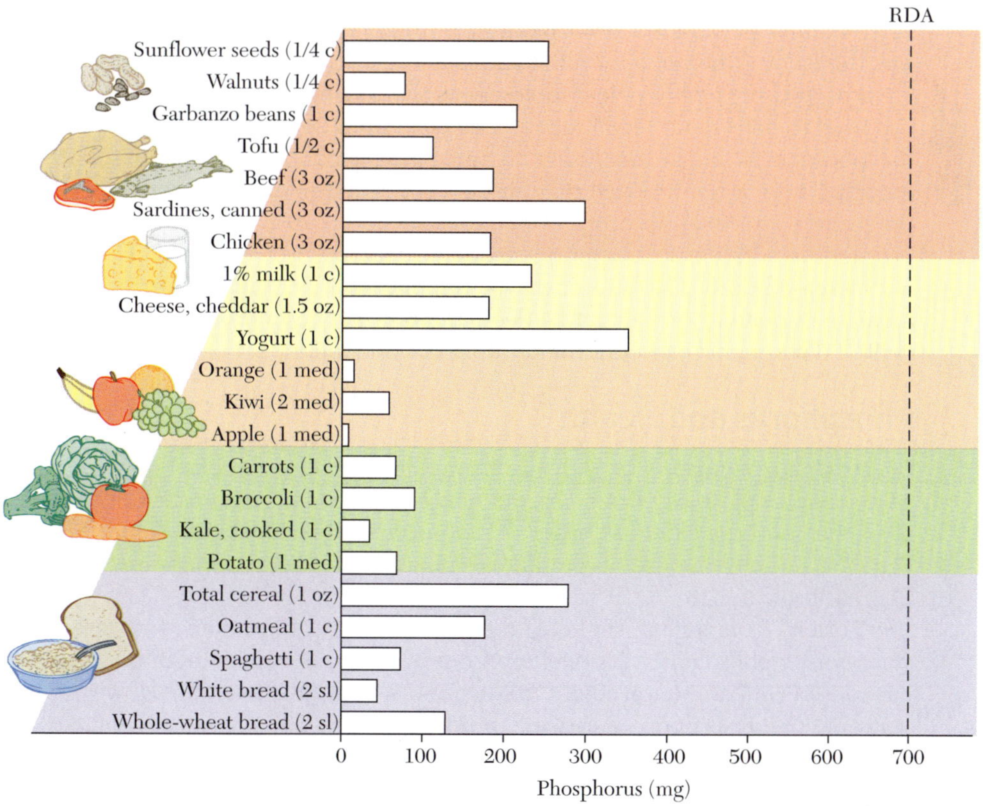

FIGURE 12.19 Phosphorus content of selections from each food group of the Food Guide Pyramid. The dashed line represents the RDA for adults.

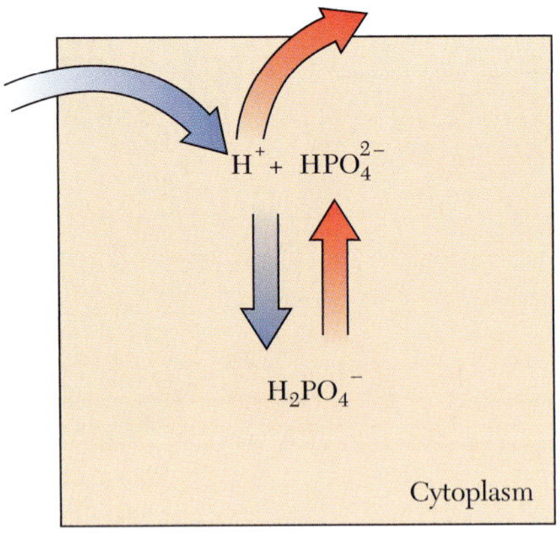

FIGURE 12.20 Phosphate provides a buffer system to help prevent pH changes in the cytoplasm of cells. When H^+ ions are added to the cytoplasm, they combine with HPO_4^{2-} to form $H_2PO_4^-$, and when H^+ ions are lost from the cytoplasm, $H_2PO_4^-$ will release H^+ to keep the hydrogen ion concentration, or pH, in the optimal range.

Phosphorus in the Body

Phosphorus is an important component of a number of molecules with structural or regulatory roles. Phosphorus, along with calcium, forms hydroxyapatite crystals that provide rigidity to the structure of bones. Phosphorus is also a component of the water-soluble head of phospholipids, which form the structure of cell membranes, and is a major constituent of the genetic material DNA and RNA. It is essential for energy production and storage because the high-energy bonds of ATP are formed between phosphate groups. It is also a component of other high-energy compounds, including creatine phosphate, which provides energy to exercising muscles. Phosphorus-containing molecules are important in relaying signals to the interior of cells to mediate hormone action and other metabolic activities. Phosphorus is involved in regulating enzyme activity because the addition of a phosphate group can activate or deactivate certain enzymes. It is also part of the phosphate buffer system that helps regulate the pH in the cytoplasm of all cells so that chemical reactions can proceed normally (Figure 12.20).

Blood levels of phosphorus are not as strictly controlled as those of calcium, but the level is maintained in a ratio with calcium that allows bone mineralization. When blood levels of phosphorus are low, the active form of vitamin D is synthesized. This increases the absorption of both phosphorus and calcium from the intestine and increases their release from bone. With high-phosphorus intakes, more is lost in the urine, so plasma levels rise only slightly. A rise in serum phosphorus indirectly stimulates parathyroid hormone release, causing phosphorus excretion and calcium retention by the kidney as well as calcium and phosphorus release from bone. When parathyroid hormone is not secreted (such as when calcium levels rise), phosphorus is retained by the kidney and calcium is excreted.

Recommended Intakes

For men and women 19 to 50 years of age, the RDA for phosphorus is set at 700 mg.[4] This is the amount needed to maintain normal blood phosphorus levels. Because neither phosphorus absorption nor urinary losses change significantly with age, the RDA is the same for older adults.

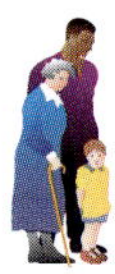

For growing children and adolescents, the accumulation of body phosphorus was used to determine recommended intakes. An RDA was established based on the phosphorus intake necessary to meet the needs for bone and soft tissue growth. There is no evidence that phosphorus requirements are increased during pregnancy; intestinal absorption increases by about 10%, which is sufficient to provide the additional phosphorus needed by the mother and fetus. The RDA is not increased during lactation because the phosphorus in milk is provided by an increase in bone resorption and a decrease in urinary excretion that are independent of dietary intake of either phosphorus or calcium.

Phosphorus and Health

Because phosphorus is so widely distributed in food, dietary deficiencies are rare. Marginal phosphorus deficiencies are most common in premature infants, vegans, alcoholics, and the elderly. Causes of marginal phosphorus status include chronic diarrhea and chronic use of aluminum-containing antacids, which prevent phosphorus absorption.

Toxicity from high phosphorus intake is rare in healthy adults. Increased consumption of phosphorus, particularly from phosphorus-containing food additives, has caused concern that it might have an impact on bone health.[36] However, in a study of bone resorption, increasing phosphorus from 800 mg to 1600 mg per day did not increase resorption.[37] Levels of phosphorus intake typical in the United States are not believed to affect bone health as long as calcium intake is adequate.[4] Based on the upper level of normal serum phosphate, a UL for phosphorus of 4.0 g per day has been set for adults ages 19 to 70.

Magnesium (Mg)

There are approximately 25 g of magnesium in the adult human body. Magnesium is a mineral that affects the metabolism of calcium, sodium, and potassium.

Sources of Magnesium

Magnesium is found in leafy greens such as spinach and kale because it is a component of the green photosynthetic pigment chlorophyll. The germ and bran of whole grains, nuts, seeds, and bananas are also good sources, but fruits, fish, meat, and milk are poor sources (Figure 12.21). Refined foods are generally low in magnesium. In areas with "hard" water, which is high in calcium and magnesium, the water supply may provide a significant amount of magnesium.

Magnesium in the Digestive Tract

About 50% of the magnesium in the diet is absorbed through both active and passive transport mechanisms, and the percentage absorbed decreases as intake increases. The active form of vitamin D can enhance magnesium absorption to a small extent, and the presence of phytate decreases absorption. As calcium in the diet increases, the absorption of magnesium decreases, so the use of calcium supplements can reduce the absorption of magnesium.

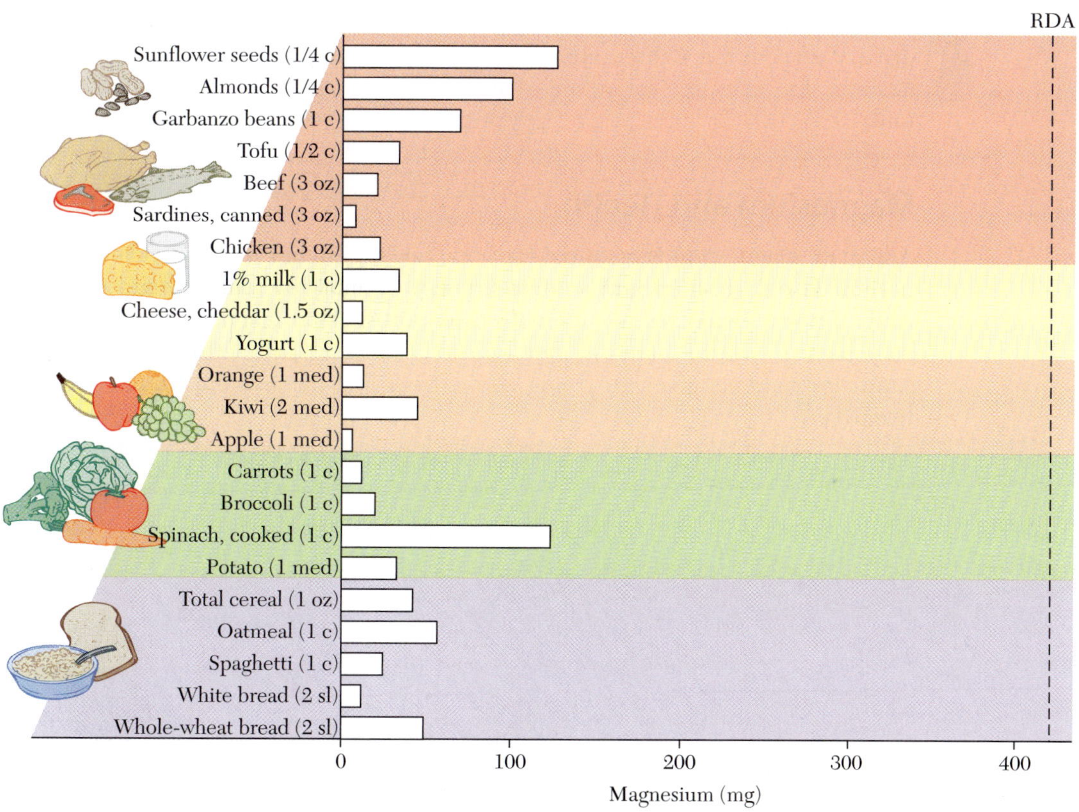

FIGURE 12.21 Magnesium content of selections from each food group of the Food Guide Pyramid. The dashed line represents the RDA for adult men age 31 and older.

Magnesium in the Body

About 50 to 60% of the magnesium in the body is in bone, where it is essential for the maintenance of structure. Most of the remaining body magnesium is present inside cells, where it is the second most abundant positively charged intracellular ion (after potassium). Magnesium is associated with the negative charge on phosphate-containing molecules such as ATP (Figure 12.22). Magnesium is also involved in regulating calcium homeostasis and is needed for the action of vitamin D and many hormones including parathyroid hormone.[38]

Magnesium is a cofactor for over 300 enzymes. It is necessary for the generation of energy from carbohydrate, lipid, and protein (see Table 10.1). In some of these reactions it is involved indirectly as a stabilizer of ATP, and in some directly as an enzyme activator. Magnesium is needed for the activity of sodium-potassium-ATPase, which is responsible for the active transport of sodium and potassium across cell membranes. It is therefore essential for maintenance of electrical potentials across membranes and proper functioning of the nerves and muscles, including those in the heart. Magnesium is important for DNA and RNA synthesis and for almost every step in protein synthesis. Therefore, magnesium is particularly important for growing cells.

Blood levels of magnesium are closely regulated by the kidney. When magnesium intake is low, excretion in the urine is decreased. As intake increases, urinary excretion increases to maintain normal blood levels. This efficient regulation permits homeostasis over a wide range of dietary intakes.

Recommended Intakes

The RDA for magnesium is 400 mg per day for young men and 310 mg per day for young women.[4] This is based on the amount needed to maintain total body magnesium balance. The RDA is slightly higher for adults age 31 and older.

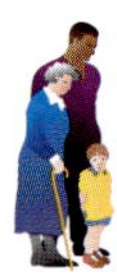

The requirement for pregnancy is increased by 35 mg per day to account for the addition of lean body mass. No increase is provided for lactation because urinary excretion is decreased and bone resorption is increased, releasing magnesium. An AI is set for infants based on the magnesium content of human milk.

Magnesium and Health

Adequate magnesium is essential for bone health. Higher intakes of dietary magnesium in elderly men and women are associated with greater bone density.[39] And, in postmenopausal women with osteoporosis, oral magnesium supplements have been shown to increase bone density and decrease fracture rate.[38] Magnesium supplements given to young adults have had inconsistent effects on bone turnover.[40,41]

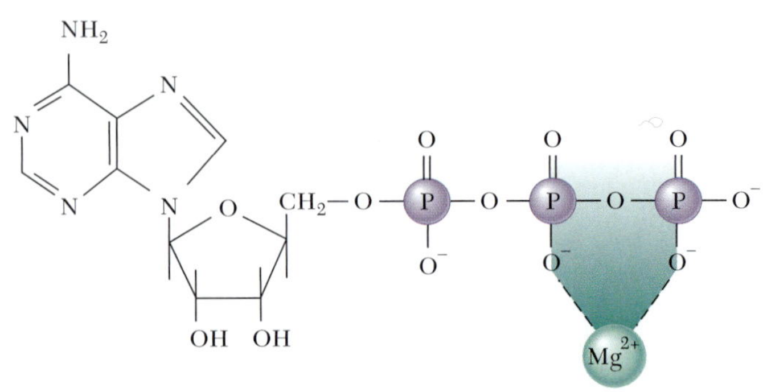

Mg^{2+}– ATP Complex

FIGURE 12.22 The addition of magnesium to ATP stabilizes its structure by forming a magnesium-ATP complex.

Magnesium may also play a role in cardiovascular health. Epidemiological evidence suggests that humans with adequate magnesium status are at a lower risk of atherosclerosis, and supplements improve blood lipid levels.[42] Areas with hard water that is high in magnesium tend to have lower rates of death from cardiovascular disease.[43] Magnesium may also be involved in blood pressure regulation; individuals with higher dietary magnesium intakes have lower blood pressure levels.[44]

Magnesium Deficiency Magnesium deficiency is rare in the general population. However, it does occur in those with alcoholism, malnutrition, kidney disease, and gastrointestinal disease, as well as in those who use diuretics that increase magnesium excretion in the urine. Deficiency symptoms include nausea, muscle weakness and cramping, irritability, mental derangement, and changes in blood pressure and heartbeat. Low blood magnesium levels affect blood calcium and potassium concentrations; therefore, some of these symptoms may be due to alterations in the levels of these other minerals.

Magnesium Toxicity No adverse effects have been observed from ingestion of magnesium in foods, but toxicity can occur from concentrated sources such as magnesium-containing drugs and supplements. Magnesium toxicity is characterized by nausea, vomiting, low blood pressure, and other cardiovascular changes. It has been reported in elderly patients with impaired kidney function who frequently use magnesium-containing laxatives and antacids such as milk of magnesia. There is no evidence that large intakes of magnesium are harmful to people with normal kidney function. The UL for adults and adolescents over nine years of age is 350 mg per day of nonfood magnesium.

Sulfur (S)

Sulfur in the diet comes from organic molecules such as the sulfur-containing amino acids in proteins and the sulfur-containing vitamins. It is also found in some inorganic food preservatives such as sulfur dioxide, sodium sulfite, and sodium and potassium bisulfite, which are used as antioxidants. In the body, the sulfur-containing amino acids methionine and cysteine are needed for protein synthesis. Cysteine is also part of the compound glutathione, which is important in detoxifying drugs and protecting cells from oxidative damage. The vitamins thiamin and biotin, which are essential for energy production, also contain sulfur. Sulfur-containing ions are a part of an important buffer system that regulates acid-base balance.

There is no recommended intake for sulfur, and no deficiencies are known when protein needs are met (see Table 12.1).

Summary

1. Minerals are elements needed by the body to regulate chemical reactions and provide structure. They come from plant and animal sources, and their bioavailability is affected by interactions with other minerals, vitamins, and other dietary components such as fiber, phytates, oxylates, and tannins. For some minerals, bioavailability is affected by body need.
2. Most of the calcium in the body is in bone as a component of hydroxyapatite. Calcium not found in bone is essential for nerve transmission, muscle contraction, blood clotting, and blood pressure regulation. Blood levels of calcium are regulated by parathyroid hormone and calcitonin. Parathyroid hormone stimulates the release of calcium from bone, decreases calcium excretion by the kidney, and activates vitamin D to increase the amount of calcium absorbed from the gastrointestinal tract and released from bone. Calcitonin blocks calcium release from bone.
3. Bone is a living tissue that is constantly being broken down and reformed in a process known as bone remodeling. Early

in life, bone formation occurs more rapidly than bone breakdown to allow bone growth and an increase in bone mass. Peak bone mass usually occurs in young adulthood. With age, bone breakdown begins to outpace formation, causing a decrease in bone mass; this is accelerated in women at menopause.

4. The AI for calcium ranges from 1000 to 1200 mg per day for adults and is 1300 mg per day in adolescents. Sources of calcium in the American diet include dairy products, fish consumed with bones, legumes, and leafy green vegetables.
5. Osteoporosis is a condition in which loss of bone mass increases the risk of bone fractures. The risk of osteoporosis is related to the level of peak bone mass acheived and the rate of bone loss. These are affected by genetics as well as lifestyle factors such as diet and exercise. The best treatment for osteoporosis is prevention. An adequate diet with plenty of calcium and regular exercise help increase bone mass during childhood and adolescence and decrease bone loss in adulthood. Once the disease occurs, treatment may include calcium and vitamin D supplements, exercise, hormone replacement therapy, and other medications.
6. Phosphorus plays a structural role in bones and teeth. Phosphorus is also part of a buffer system that helps prevent changes in pH and is an essential component of phospholipids, ATP, and DNA. Good sources of phosphorus include dairy products, meats, and grains. The RDA for adults is 700 mg per day.
7. Magnesium is important for bone health and it is needed as a cofactor for numerous reactions throughout the body. In reactions involved in energy production it acts as an enzyme activator and stabilizer of ATP. It is also needed to maintain membrane potentials; thus it is essential for nerve and muscle conductivity. Homeostasis is regulated by the kidney. Deficiency is rare, and the best dietary sources are whole grains, nuts, seeds, and green vegetables.
8. Sulfur is needed in the diet as preformed organic molecules such as the amino acids methionine and cysteine, which are needed to synthesize proteins and glutathione, and the vitamins thiamin and biotin, needed for energy metabolism. Sulfur is also part of a buffer system that regulates acid-base balance. A dietary deficiency is unknown in the absence of protein malnutrition.

Review Questions

1. List four factors that can affect mineral bioavailability.
2. What is the major source of calcium in the North American diet?
3. What is the function of calcium in bones and teeth?
4. What is the function of calcium in body fluids?
5. How are blood calcium levels regulated?
6. How is calcium intake related to the risk of osteoporosis?
7. List factors other than calcium that are related to the risk of osteoporosis.
8. What is the function of phosphorus in the body?
9. What foods are good sources of phosphorus?
10. What is the function of magnesium in the body?
11. List foods that are good sources of magnesium.
12. Where is sulfur found in the body?

Applying Critical Thinking Skills

Personal nutrition:

1. Using the food record you kept in Chapter 2, calculate your average calcium intake.
   a. How does your intake compare with the AI for calcium for someone of your age and sex?
   b. If your calcium intake is below the AI, suggest modifications to increase the amount of calcium in your diet without significantly increasing your energy intake.
2. Use food labels and a food composition database to evaluate five foods that are fortified with calcium.
   a. How much calcium is in a serving of each of these foods?
   b. How many servings per day of each would you need to consume to meet your calcium needs?
   c. Are there other dietary components in any of these foods that would interfere with calcium absorption or utilization?

General nutrition issues:

1. Design a diet to meet the energy, protein, and calcium requirements of a 65-year-old woman who is 5 feet 5 inches tall, weighs 130 pounds, and is lactose intolerant.
   a. What are her energy and protein needs?
   b. What are her calcium needs?
   c. List one day's food for this diet.
   d. Is this a reasonable diet to follow every day? Would you recommend fortified foods or calcium supplements? Why or why not?
2. You are a scientist with the U.S. Department of Agriculture and you have been assigned the task of deciding on a food or group of foods that will be fortified with calcium to assure that the population meets their calcium needs. What food or group of foods would you recommend?
   Consider the following factors:
   a. Does the food contain dietary components that interfere with calcium absorption?
   b. Would the amount consumed meet recommendations but not put the population at risk of calcium toxicity?
   c. Is this a food or group of foods that is consumed by the majority of the population?

REFERENCES

1. Heaney, R. P., Weaver, C. M., and Recker, R. R. Calcium absorption from spinach. Am. J. Clin. Nutr. 47:707–709, 1988.
2. Bronner, F., and Pansu, D. Nutritional aspects of calcium absorption. J. Nutr. 129:9–12, 1999.
3. Bouillon, R., Carmeliet, G., and Boonen, S. Ageing and calcium metabolism. Baillieres Clin. Endocrinol. Metab. 11:341–365, 1997.
4. Institute of Medicine, Food and Nutrition Board. *Dietary Reference Intakes for Calcium, Phosphorus, Magnesium, Vitamin D, and Fluoride*. Washington, D.C.: National Academy Press, 1997.
5. Teegarden, D., Lyle, R. M., McCabe, G. P., et al. Dietary calcium, protein, and phosphorus are related to bone mineral density content in young women. Am. J. Clin. Nutr. 68:749–754, 1998.
6. Groff, J. L., Gropper, S. S., and Hunt, S. M. *Advanced Nutrition and Human Metabolism*, 2nd ed. St. Paul, Minn.: West Publishing Company, 1995.
7. Hamet, P. The evaluation of the scientific evidence for a relationship between calcium and hypertension. J. Nutr. 125(suppl):311S–400S, 1995.
8. Affinito, P., Tommaselli, G. A., DiCarlo, C., et al. Changes in bone mineral density and calcium metabolism in breast-feeding women: a one year follow-up study. J. Clin. Endocrinol. Metab. 81:2314–2318, 1996.
9. National Institutes of Health. Consensus Development Conference Statement: Osteoporosis Prevention, Diagnosis, and Therapy, March 27–29, 2000 Available online at **http://odp.od.nihgov/consensus/cons/111/111_intro.htm**. Accessed 17 Jan 2001.
10. Osteoporosis and Related Bone Diseases National Resource Center. Osteoporosis Overview. Available online at **http://www.osteo.org/osteo.html**. Accessed 19 Jan 2001.
11. Riggs, B. L., and Melton, L. J. III. The worldwide problem of osteoporosis: insights afforded by epidemiology. Bone 17:505S–511S, 1995.
12. Reeker, R. R., Davies, K. M., Hiners, S. M., et al. Bone gain in young adult women. JAMA 268:2403–2408, 1992.
13. Riggs, B. L., Khosla, S., and Melton, L. J. A unitary model for involutional osteoporosis: estrogen deficiency causes both type I and type II osteoporosis in postmenopausal women and contributes to bone loss in aging men. J. Bone Miner. Res. 13:763–773, 1998.
14. Eisman, J. A. Genetics of osteoporosis. Endocr. Rev. 20:788–804, 1999.
15. Bohannon, A. D. Osteoporosis and African American women. J. Womens Health Gend. Based Med. 8:609–615, 1999.
16. Bachrach, L. K., Hastie, T., and Wang, M. C. Bone mineral acquisition in healthy Asian, Hispanic, Black, and Caucasian youth: a longitudinal study. J. Clin. Endocrinol. Metab. 84:4702–4712, 1999.
17. Hannan, M. T., Felson, D. T., Dawson-Hughes, B., et al. Risk factors for longitudinal bone loss in elderly men and women: the Framingham Osteoporosis Study. J. Bone Miner. Res. 15:710–720, 2000.
18. Hermann, A. P., Brot, C., Gram, J., et al. Premenopausal smoking and bone density in 2015 perimenopausal women. J. Bone Miner. Res. 15:780–787, 2000.
19. Sampson, H. W. Alcohol, osteoporosis, and bone regulating hormones. Alcohol Clin. Exp. Res. 21:400–403, 1997.
20. Ernst, E. Exercise for female osteoporosis: a systematic review of clinical trials. Sports Med. 25:359–368, 1998.
21. Anderson, J. J. B. The important role of physical activity in skeletal development: how exercise may counter low calcium intake. Am. J. Clin. Nutr. 71:1384–1386, 2000.
22. Melton, L. J. Epidemiology of spinal osteoporosis. Spine 22:2S–11S, 1997.
23. Burger, H., Grobbee, D. E., and Drueke, T. Osteoporosis and salt intake. Nutr. Metab. Cardiovasc. Dis. 10:46–53, 2000.
24. Dawson-Hughes, B., Fowler, S. E., Dalsky, G., and Gallagher, C. Sodium excretion influences calcium homeostasis in elderly men and women. J. Nutr. 126:2107–2112, 1996.
25. Heaney, R. P. Excess dietary protein may not adversely affect bone. J. Nutr. 128:1054–1057, 1998.
26. New, S. A., Robins, S. P., Campbell, M. K., et al. Dietary influences on bone mass and bone metabolism: further evidence of a positive link between fruit and vegetable consumption and bone health. Am. J. Clin. Nutr. 71:142–151, 2000.
27. Riggs, B. L., O'Fallon, W. M., Muhs, J., et al. Long-term effects of calcium supplementation on serum parathyroid hormone level, bone turnover, and bone loss in elderly women. J. Bone Miner. Res. 13:168–174, 1998.
28. Reid, I. R. The roles of calcium and vitamin D in the prevention of osteoporosis. Endocrinol. Metab. Clin. North Am. 27:389–398, 1998.
29. Mizunuma, H., Okano, H., Soda, M., et al. Calcium supplements increase bone mineral density in women with low serum calcium levels during long-term estrogen therapy. Endocr. J. 43:411–415, 1996.
30. Devine, A., Dick, I. M., Heal, S. J., et al. A 4-year follow-up study of the effects of calcium supplementation on bone density in elderly postmenopausal women. Osteoporos. Int. 7:23–28, 1997.
31. Nieves, J. W., Komar, L., Cosman, F., and Lindasya, R. Calcium potentiates the effect of estrogen and calcitonin on bone mass: review and analysis. Am. J. Clin. Nutr. 67:18–24, 1998.
32. McClung, M., Clemmesen, B., Daifotis, A., et al. Alendronate prevents postmenopausal bone loss in women without osteoporosis: a double-blind, randomized, controlled trial. Alendronate Osteoporosis Prevention Study Group. Ann. Intern. Med. 128:253–261, 1998.
33. Wimalawansa, S. J. A four-year randomized controlled trial of hormone replacement and bisphosphonate, alone or in combination, in women with postmenopausal osteoporosis. Am. J. Med. 104:210–226, 1998.
34. Minihane, A. M., and Fairweather-Tait, S. J. Effect of calcium supplementation on daily nonheme-iron absorption and long-term iron status. Am. J. Clin. Nutr. 68:96–102. 1998.
35. Wood, R. J., and Zheng, J. J. High dietary calicum intakes reduce zinc absorption and balance in humans. Am. J. Clin. Nutr. 65:1803–1809, 1997.
36. Calvo, M. S., and Park, U. K. Changing phosphorus content of the U.S. diet: potential for adverse effect on bone. J. Nutr. 126:1168S–1180S, 1996.
37. Bizik, B. K., Ding, W., and Cerklewski, F. L. Evidence that bone resorption of young men is not increased by high dietary phosphorus obtained from milk and cheese. Nutr. Res. 16:1143–1146, 1996.
38. Sojka, J. E., and Weaver, C. M. Magnesium supplementation and osteoporosis. Nutr. Rev. 53:71–74, 1995.
39. Tucker, K. L., Hannan, M. T., Chen, H., et al. Potassium, magnesium, and fruit and vegetable intakes are associated with greater bone mineral density in elderly men and women. Am. J. Clin. Nutr. 69:727–736, 1999.
40. Dimai, H. P., Porta, S., Wirnsberger, G., et al. Daily oral magnesium supplementation suppresses bone turnover in young adult males. J. Clin. Endocrinol. Metab. 83:2742–2748, 1998.
41. Doyle, L., Flynn, A., and Cashman, K. The effect of magnesium supplementation on biochemical markers of bone metabolism or blood pressure in healthy young adult females. Eur. J. Clin. Nutr. 53:255–261, 1999.
42. Dreosti, I. E. Magnesium status and health. Nutr. Rev. 53:S23–S27, 1995.
43. Rubenowitz, E., Axelsson, G., and Rylander, R. Magnesium in drinking water and death from myocardial infarction. Am. J. Epidemiol. 143:456–462, 1996.
44. Ma, J., Folsom, A. R., Melnick, S. L., et al. Associations of serum and dietary magnesium with cardiovascular disease, hypertension, diabetes, insulin, and carotid arterial wall thickness: the ARIC study. Atherosclerosis Risk in Community Study. J. Clin. Epidemiol. 48:927–940, 1995.

13 The Trace Minerals

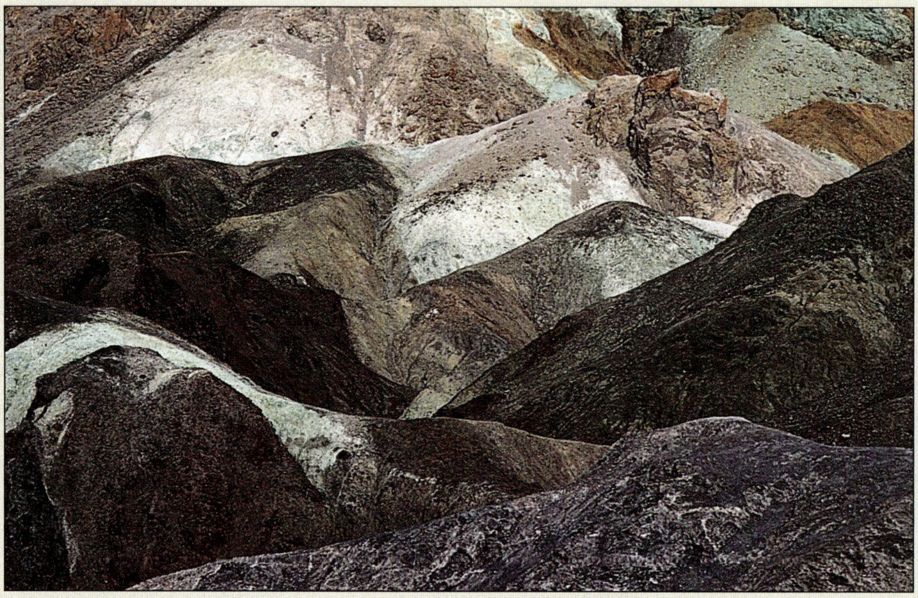

Learning Objectives

After reading this chapter, students should be able to:

1. Describe the primary function of iron and the physiological effects of iron deficiency and iron toxicity.
2. Explain how the amount of iron in the body is regulated.
3. Explain why copper deficiency can lead to anemia.
4. List the functions of zinc.
5. Explain why high intakes of zinc affect copper absorption.
6. Discuss the antioxidant function of manganese.
7. Compare the antioxidant functions of selenium and vitamin E.
8. Discuss the function of iodine and iodinization of foods as a means of preventing deficiency.
9. Discuss the role of fluoride in maintaining dental health.
10. Explain the relationship between blood glucose levels and chromium.

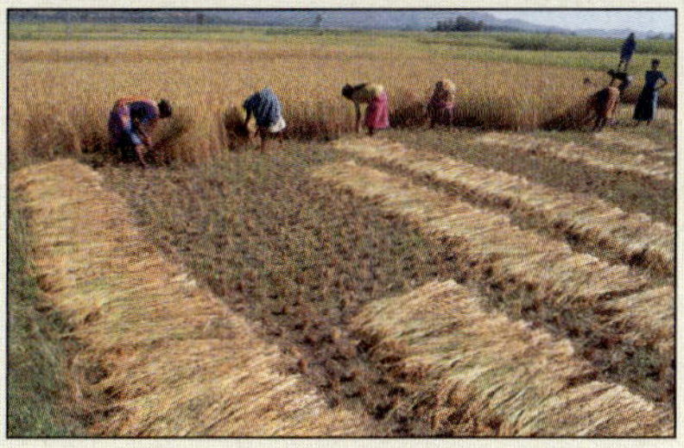

Nissi is a young girl who lives in a village in India. For generations her family has farmed the flood plains of the Ganges River valley. They are subsistence farmers—that is, the crops they grow are used primarily to feed their family. Nissi's diet is made up almost entirely of these homegrown foods that include grains, pulses (seeds, beans, and lentils), and vegetables. A typical meal consists of flat fried bread called chapattis, a porridge made with lentils called dahl, vegetables such as potatoes and cauliflower, and yogurt. Recently Nissi has felt tired all the time and has noticed a lump in her neck that seems to be getting bigger. A visit to the clinic determines that her malaise and the lump in her neck are caused by an iodine deficiency. She is given an injection of iodine in oil and soon not only does she have more energy, but the bulge at the front of her neck begins to disappear.

How could this apparently healthy, well-nourished young woman be suffering from a nutritional deficiency? Despite the small amounts of iodine needed in the diet—only about 150 μg per day—iodine deficiency is a problem for Nissi and her village, as well as for other villages and cities throughout India, because the repeated flooding of the Ganges River valley over the centuries has washed the iodine out of the soil. Food grown in this soil is therefore low in iodine, and a diet based solely on local foods does not provide enough of this essential mineral to meet needs. Left untreated, Nissi's symptoms would have continued to worsen. If she had children, they would be at risk of being born with cretinism—a form of retardation caused by iodine deficiency during pregnancy.

One way to prevent iodine deficiency is to change the diet to include foods that are higher in iodine. However, in Nissi's case, this is not practical because all of the food grown in the region is deficient in iodine. The alternative for Nissi's family is to use iodized salt—salt to which iodine has been added. In the early 1900s, the use of iodized salt virtually eradicated iodine deficiency in the United States and Canada. Today, in developed and developing nations the fortification of commonly consumed foods or condiments is helping to prevent deficiencies of iodine and other nutrients.

IRON (Fe)

Iron was identified as a major constituent of blood in the 18th century. By 1832, iron tablets were used to treat young women in whom "coloring matter" was lacking in the blood. Today we know that the red color in blood is due to the iron-containing protein **hemoglobin**, and that a deficiency of iron decreases hemoglobin production. Despite the fact that iron is one of the best understood of the trace elements, iron deficiency remains the most common nutritional deficiency in North America and worldwide.[1,2]

Hemoglobin An iron-containing protein in red blood cells that binds and transports oxygen through the bloodstream to cells.

Heme iron A readily absorbed form of iron found in animal products. This form of iron is present in proteins as a chemical complex in which the iron is associated with four nitrogen atoms.

Myoglobin An iron-containing protein in the cytoplasm of muscle cells.

Forms and Sources of Iron

Iron in the diet comes from both plant and animal sources (Figure 13.1). Much of the iron in animal products is **heme iron**—iron that is part of a chemical complex found in certain proteins, such as **myoglobin** in muscle and hemoglobin in blood

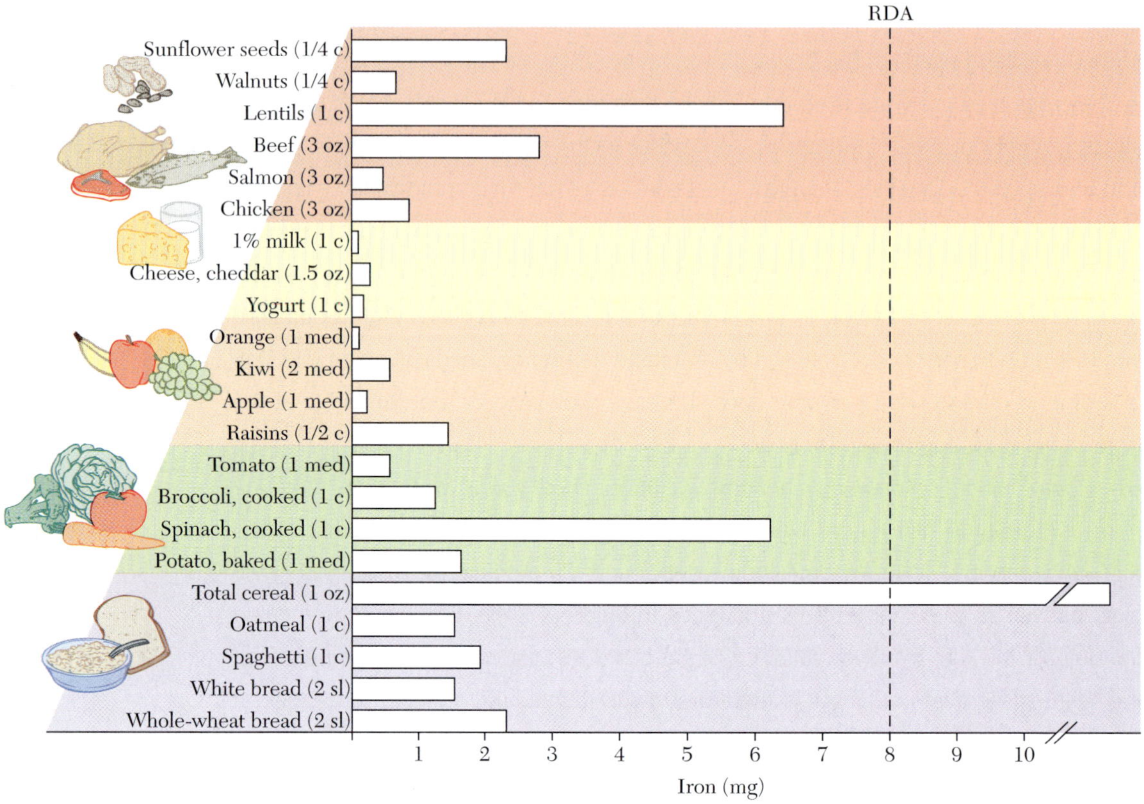

FIGURE 13.1 Iron content of selections from each food group of the Food Guide Pyramid. The dashed line represents the RDA for adult men and postmenopausal women. The RDA for premenopausal women is more than double this at 18 mg/day. Fortified grains and other plant foods are good sources of nonheme iron and meats provide a source of heme iron.

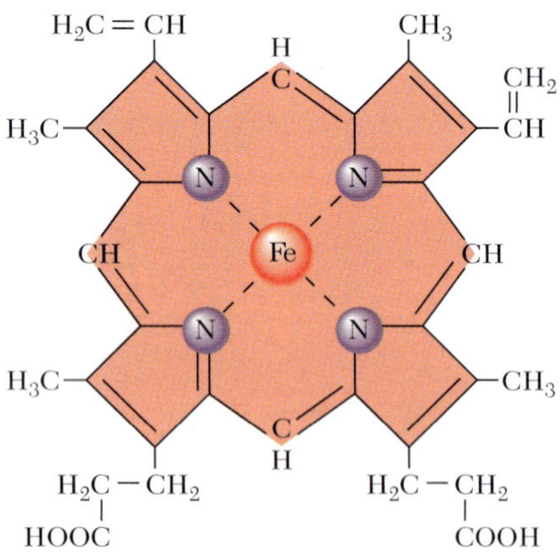

FIGURE 13.2 The iron-containing heme group contains four five-membered nitrogen-containing rings that form a cage around a central iron ion. In hemoglobin and myoglobin the iron ion is in the Fe^{2+} state.

Nonheme iron Iron that is not associated with proteins or that is present in proteins that do not contain heme groups. This form of iron is less well absorbed than heme iron and is found in both animal and plant foods.

(Figure 13.2). Heme iron accounts for about 10 to 15% of the dietary iron in industrialized countries.[3] Meat, poultry, and fish are good sources of heme iron, which is absorbed more than twice as efficiently as **nonheme iron**.

Leafy green vegetables, legumes, meats and whole and enriched grains are good sources of nonheme iron. Iron cooking utensils contribute nonheme iron to the diet because the iron leaches from the cookware into food. Leaching is enhanced by acidic foods. For example, spaghetti sauce cooked in a glass pan contains about 3 mg of iron per serving, but the same sauce cooked in an iron skillet may contain more than 80 mg, depending on how long it is cooked.

Iron in the Digestive Tract

Iron from the diet is absorbed into the intestinal mucosal cells. The bioavailability of nonheme iron is determined by overall meal composition. Some dietary components enhance absorption and some inhibit it.

Absorption of Nonheme Iron When nonheme iron is consumed, stomach acid helps convert the ferric form (Fe^{3+}) to the ferrous form (Fe^{2+}). The ferrous form of iron remains more soluble when it enters the intestine and therefore enters the mucosal cells more readily. The presence of acids, such as ascorbic acid (vitamin C), citric acid, and lactic acid, enhances iron absorption by helping to keep it in the ferrous form. The best studied of these acids is vitamin C, which, when consumed in the same meal as iron, can enhance nonheme iron absorption up to sixfold.[3] In addition to keeping iron in the ferrous form, vitamin C combines with iron and prevents it from forming inabsorbable complexes.[4] Amino acids and sugars also increase nonheme iron absorption by combining with ferrous iron.

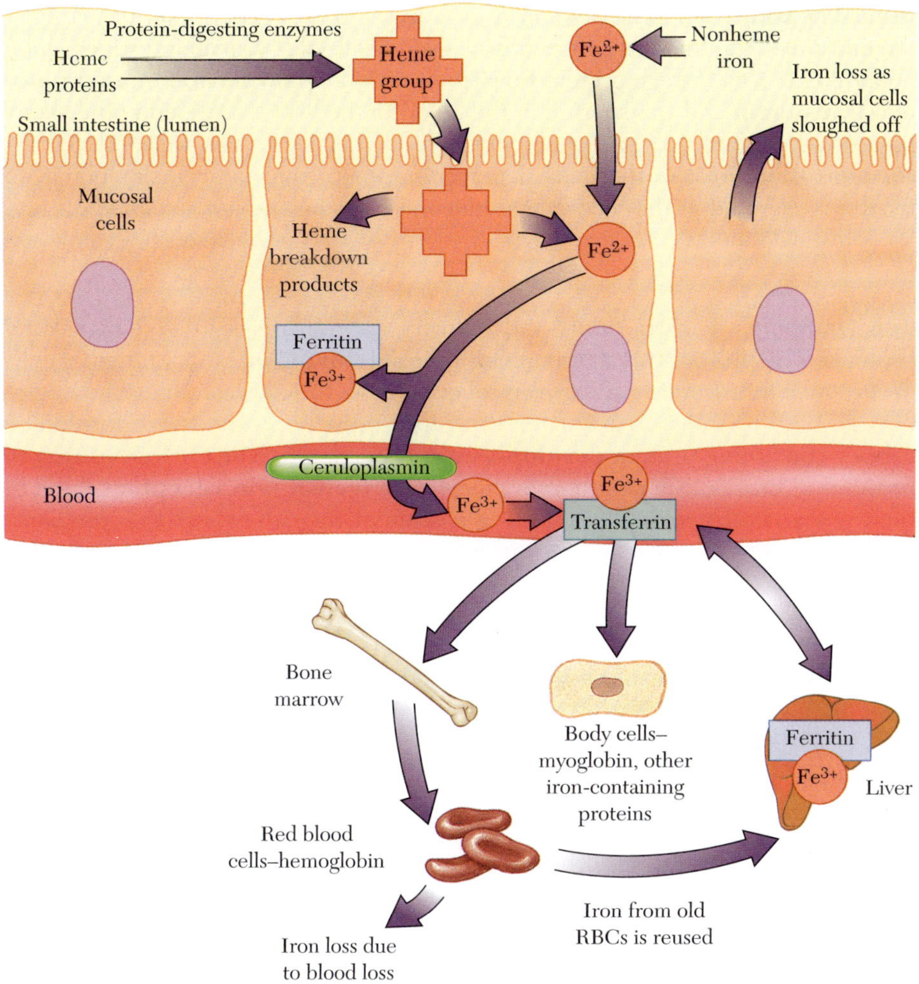

FIGURE 13.3 In the digestive tract, protein-digesting enzymes release the iron-containing heme group from proteins. The heme group enters the mucosal cell where the iron is released. Nonheme iron is absorbed in the ferrous form (Fe^{2+}). Once inside the mucosal cell, some iron may be bound to ferritin for storage. When the mucosal cells die, iron that remains bound to ferritin is excreted in the feces. Iron that enters the blood is converted to ferric iron (Fe^{3+}) by ceruloplasmin and binds to transferrin for transport. Transferrin transports iron to bone, where it is needed to synthesize hemoglobin for red blood cells, and to other body cells, where it is used to synthesize myoglobin and other iron-containing proteins. When red blood cells die they are broken down by cells in the liver, spleen, or bone marrow and the iron is released for reuse. Excess iron is stored primarily in the liver, bound to ferritin.

Consuming animal tissue proteins from sources such as beef, fish, or poultry increases the absorption of nonheme iron as well. For example, a small amount of hamburger in a pot of chili will enhance the body's absorption of iron from the beans.

Dietary factors that interfere with the absorption of nonheme iron include fiber, phytate found in cereals, tannins found in tea, and oxalates found in some leafy greens such as spinach. These prevent absorption by binding iron in the gastrointestinal tract. Some vegetable proteins, including soy protein, also have an inhibitory effect on nonheme iron absorption, and the presence of other minerals may decrease iron absorption. For instance, calcium supplements decrease iron absorption, particularly when both are consumed at the same meal.[5]

Absorption of Heme Iron When heme proteins are consumed, the iron-containing heme group is released from the proteins by protein-digesting enzymes. The heme binds to receptors on the surface of mucosal cells, allowing it to enter the cells, where the iron is released from the heme group (Figure 13.3). Heme iron absorption is not increased by vitamin C, nor is it decreased by substances such as phytates.

Iron in the Body

Iron is essential for life but in excess it is toxic. To protect against the toxic effects of iron, the body regulates the amount that enters from the gastrointestinal tract and has evolved ways to safely transport and store it.

Regulating Body Iron The amount of iron in the body is controlled primarily at the intestine. Iron that has entered the mucosal cells of the small intestine can be bound to the iron storage protein **ferritin** or picked up by the iron transport protein **transferrin** and transported in the blood to the liver, bones, and other body tissues (see Figure 13.3). The amount of iron that leaves the mucosal cell for transport to the rest of the body depends on need. Iron that remains bound to ferritin is excreted in the feces when mucosal cells die and are sloughed off into the intestinal lumen.

Ferritin The major iron storage protein.

Transferrin An iron transport protein in the blood.

Iron Transport The transport and delivery of iron are regulated by several proteins. The protein transferrin picks up iron from the intestinal mucosal cells in the small intestine as well as iron released from the degradation of hemoglobin. To bind to transferrin (or ferritin), iron must be in the ferric form. The copper-containing protein **ceruloplasmin** is needed to convert ferrous iron to ferric iron. Proteins on cell membranes, called **transferrin receptors**, bind to the transferrin-iron complex, allowing it to enter the cell, where the iron is released for use. When iron stores are low, a greater percentage of the iron that has been absorbed into the mucosal cells is transported to other tissues. In this case, less of the iron-storage protein ferritin is made and the number of transferrin receptors increases, allowing more iron to be transported into the cells.[6] When iron is plentiful, more ferritin is made to increase storage capacity and the number of transferrin receptors decreases, so the transport of iron to body cells is reduced. More iron is then left in the mucosal cells and is lost when they die.

Ceruloplasmin A copper-containing protein that converts iron to the ferric form, which can bind to iron storage and iron transport proteins.

Transferrin receptors Proteins found in cell membranes that bind to the iron-transferrin complex and allow it to be taken up by cells.

Iron Stores Iron that is absorbed in excess of immediate needs can be stored in ferritin located primarily in the liver, spleen, and bone marrow. It can be mobilized from body stores as needed. Deficiency signs will appear only after stores are depleted. Levels of ferritin in the blood can be used to estimate iron stores. When ferritin concentrations in the liver become high, some is converted to an insoluble storage protein called **hemosiderin**.

Hemosiderin An insoluble iron-protein compound formed in the liver when the iron storage capacity of ferritin is exceeded.

Iron Losses Iron is not readily excreted. Even when red blood cells die, the iron in their hemoglobin is not lost from the body. The cells are removed from the blood by cells in the liver, spleen, or bone marrow and degraded; the iron is then attached to transferrin for transport back to the bone where it can be incorporated into new red blood cells. Most iron loss even in healthy individuals occurs through blood loss, such as that lost during menstruation and the small amounts lost from the gastrointestinal tract. Some iron is also lost through the shedding of cells from the intestine, skin, and urinary tract.[4]

Functions of Iron Iron in the body is essential for the delivery of oxygen to cells. It is a component of two oxygen-carrying proteins, hemoglobin and myoglobin (Table 13.1). Most of the iron in the body is part of hemoglobin in red blood cells. Hemoglobin transports oxygen to body cells and carries carbon dioxide away from cells for elimination by the lungs. Myoglobin is found in the muscle, where it enhances the rate that oxygen diffuses from the blood into muscle cells, allowing more oxygen to be available for muscle contraction. Iron is also essential for energy production as a part of a key enzyme in the citric acid cycle and of several proteins involved in the electron transport chain. Iron-containing proteins are also involved in drug metabolism and the immune system, and iron is part of the enzyme catalase, which protects the cell from oxidative damage by destroying hydrogen peroxide before it can form free radicals.

TABLE 13.1 A Summary of the Trace Elements

Mineral	Sources	Recommended Intake for Young Adults*†	Major Functions	Deficiency Diseases and Symptoms	Groups at Risk	Toxicity	Tolerable Upper Intake Levels (UL)†
Iron	Red meats, leafy greens, dried fruits, whole and enriched grains	8–18 mg	Part of hemoglobin, which delivers oxygen to cells, myoglobin, which binds oxygen in muscle, and electron carriers in the electron transport chain	Iron deficiency anemia, weakness, lethargy	Infants and preschool children, adolescents, women of childbearing age, pregnant women, athletes	Liver damage	45 mg
Copper	Organ meats, nuts and seeds, whole grains, seafood	900 μg	Functions in proteins in iron and lipid metabolism, superoxide dismutase (SOD), nerve and immune function, collagen synthesis	Anemia, poor growth, bone abnormalities	Those who over-supplement zinc	Vomiting	10 mg
Zinc	Meat, seafood, milk, whole grains, eggs	8–11 mg	Regulates protein synthesis; functions in growth, development, wound healing, immunity, and SOD	Poor growth and development, dermatitis, decreased immune function	Vegetarians, low-income children, elderly	Decreased copper absorption	40 mg
Manganese	Nuts, legumes, whole grains, tea	1.8–2.3 mg*	Functions in carbohydrate and lipid metabolism, SOD	Growth retardation	None	Nerve damage	11 mg
Selenium	Organ meats, eggs, and seafood	55 μg	Antioxidant as part of glutathione peroxidase, spares vitamin E, synthesis of thyroid hormones	Muscle pain and weakness, Keshan disease	Populations in areas with low-selenium soil	Nausea, diarrhea, vomiting, fatigue, hair changes	400 μg
Iodine	Iodized salt, saltwater fish, and seafood	150 μg	Needed for synthesis of thyroid hormones	Goiter, cretinism, mental retardation, growth and developmental abnormalities	Populations living where soil is iodine deficient and iodized salt is not used	Enlarged thyroid	1110 μg
Fluoride	Fluoridated water, tea, fish, toothpaste	3–4 mg*	Strengthens tooth enamel, enhances remineralization of tooth enamel, reduces bacterial acid production	Increased risk of dental caries	Populations in areas with unfluoridated water	Mottled teeth, kidney damage, abnormal bones	10 mg
Chromium	Liver, brewer's yeast, nuts, grains	25–35 μg*	Glucose tolerance	Impaired glucose metabolism	Malnourished children	None reported	ND
Molybdenum	Milk, organ meats, grains, legumes	45 μg	Cofactor for many enzymes	Unknown in humans	None	Arthritis and joint inflammation	2 mg

* Values with an asterisk (*) represent Adequate Intakes (AI). All other values are Recommended Dietary Allowances (RDA).

†Recommended intakes and UL values for all age groups and stages of life are given on the inside cover.

ND = Insufficient evidence to determine a UL.

Recommended Intakes

The RDA for iron is based on the amount needed to maintain a normal functional level of iron but only minimal iron stores. A recommendation for each gender and life-stage group was determined by considering the percentage of dietary iron absorbed, iron losses from the body, and conditions that increase needs, such as growth and pregnancy. The RDA is set at 8 mg per day for adult men age 19 and older and for postmenopausal women.[7] For menstruating women, the RDA is 18 mg per day; the additional 10 mg is recommended to make up for menstrual losses. An RDA of 10.9 mg per day has been set for adult women taking oral contraceptives because these drugs reduce menstrual blood losses and hence iron requirements. An RDA value has also been set for vegetarians because the nonheme iron in plant foods is less well absorbed than heme iron (Table 13.2).

The recommended intake during pregnancy is increased to 27 mg per day to account for the iron deposited in the fetal and maternal tissues. The RDA during lactation is set lower than the RDA for menstruating women because little iron is lost in milk and menstruation is usually absent. The RDA for infants, children, and adolescents considers the additional iron needed for growth. An AI has been set for infants from newborn to six months old based on the mean iron intake of infants principally fed human milk. Because the iron in human milk is more bioavailable than that in infant formula, the American Academy of Pediatrics recommends that infants who are not fed human milk or are only partially nourished with human milk should be fed iron-fortified formula.[8]

TABLE 13.2 Dietary Reference Intake Values for Iron

Gender/Life Stage	AI	RDA	UL
Infants			
0–6 months	0.27 mg	—	40 mg
7–12 months	—	11 mg	40 mg
Children			
1–3 years	—	7 mg	40 mg
4–8 years	—	10 mg	40 mg
Males			
9–13	—	8 mg	40 mg
14–18	—	11 mg	45 mg
≥ 19	—	8 mg	45 mg
Females			
9–13	—	8 mg	40 mg
14–18	—	15 mg	45 mg
19–50	—	18 mg	45 mg
≥ 51	—	8 mg	45 mg
Females taking oral contraceptives			
14–18	—	11.4 mg	45 mg
19–50	—	10.9 mg	45 mg
Pregnancy		27 mg	45 mg
Lactation			
≤ 18	—	10 mg	45 mg
19–50	—	9 mg	45 mg
Vegetarians			
Men ≥ 19	—	14 mg	45 mg
Menstruating women	—	33 mg	45 mg
Adolescent girls	—	26 mg	45 mg

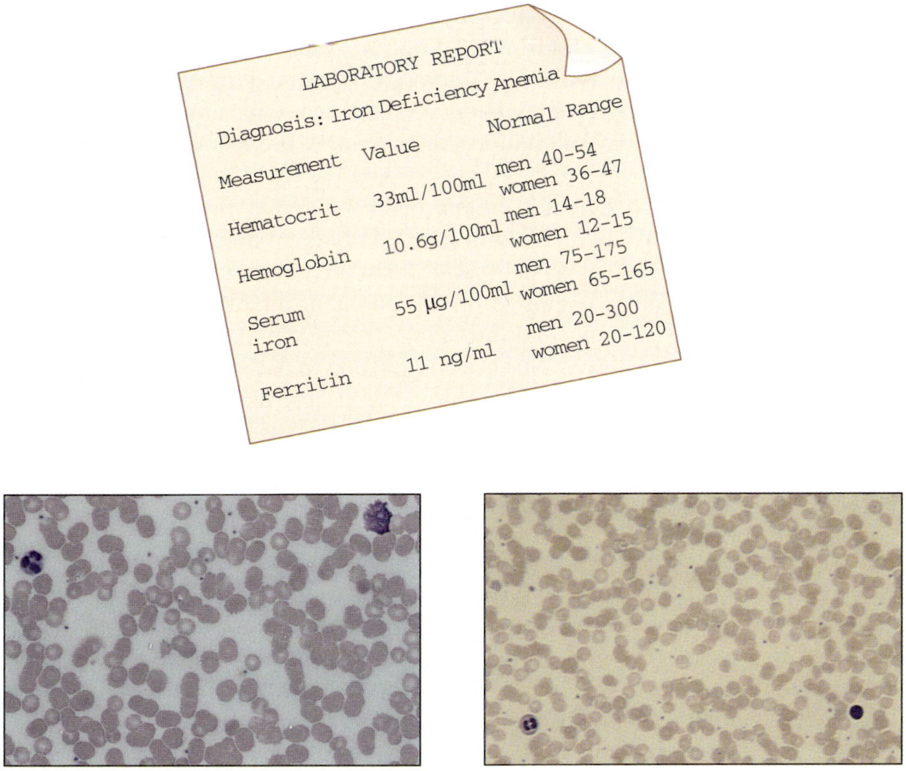

(a) (b)

FIGURE 13.4 Iron deficiency anemia is diagnosed when levels of red blood cells or proteins containing iron are low. It causes the red blood cells to become small and pale. (a) Normal red blood cells. (b) Iron deficiency anemia. *(a, © B & B Photos/Custom Medical Stock Photo; b, © Custom Medical Stock Photo)*

Iron and Health

Iron deficiency and toxicity are both health concerns. Iron deficiency is the most common nutritional deficiency in the United States, affecting 7.8 million adolescent girls and women of childbearing age and 700,000 children aged one to two years.[2] But, when iron accumulates in the body, it can damage tissues, and a single large dose can poison a child.

For more information on iron deficiency anemia worldwide, go to the World Health Organization nutrition page at www.who.int/nut/ and look under micronutrient deficiencies.

Iron Deficiency When iron is deficient, hemoglobin cannot be produced. When not enough hemoglobin is available, the red blood cells that are formed are small and pale and unable to deliver adequate oxygen to the tissues (Figure 13.4). This is known as **iron deficiency anemia**; iron deficiency anemia is the last stage of iron deficiency. Earlier stages may have no symptoms but can be detected with blood tests (Figure 13.5). It is estimated that about 10% of

Iron deficiency anemia A condition that occurs when the oxygen-carrying capacity of the blood is decreased because there is insufficient iron to make hemoglobin. It is diagnosed in adults when hemoglobin concentration is less than 11 g per 100 ml of blood.

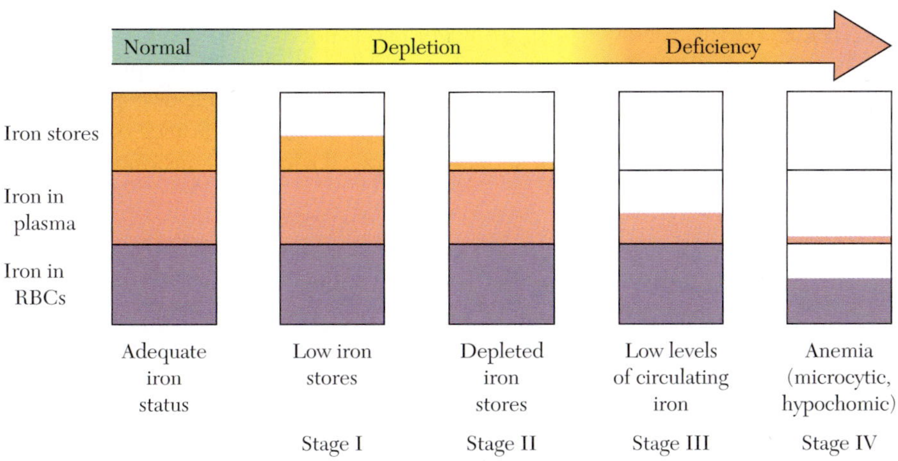

FIGURE 13.5 A negative iron balance first causes a decrease in iron stores. This can be detected by decreases in plasma levels of ferritin (Stage I). Once stores have been depleted (Stage II), plasma iron and the amount of iron bond to transferrin decrease (Stage III). In the final stage, the clinical symptoms of anemia occur and the red blood cells appear small and pale (Stage IV).

women of childbearing age have insufficient iron stores and 3 to 5% have iron deficiency anemia. Among children aged one to three years, 9% are iron deficient and 3% have iron deficiency anemia.[2] The incidence is even greater among low-income and minority women and children. Only about one fourth of adolescent girls and women of childbearing age meet the RDA for iron through their diet.[2]

Symptoms of iron deficiency anemia include fatigue, weakness, headache, decreased work capacity, an inability to maintain body temperature in a cold environment, changes in behavior, decreased resistance to infection, adverse pregnancy outcomes, impaired cognitive development in infants, and an increased risk of lead poisoning in young children. One strange symptom thought to be related to iron deficiency is **pica**. This is a compulsion to eat nonfood items such as clay, ice, paste, laundry starch, paint chips, and ashes. Pica can cause the consumption of substances containing toxic minerals, such as lead-based paints, and it can introduce substances into the diet that inhibit mineral absorption (see Chapter 15).

Pica The compulsive ingestion of nonfood substances such as clay, laundry starch, and paint chips.

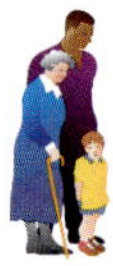

Women of reproductive age are at risk for iron deficiency anemia because of iron loss due to menstruation. Iron deficiency is common among pregnant women, even in industrialized countries, and can lead to premature delivery, low infant birth weight, increased infant mortality, and greater risk to the mother.[7,9] The need for iron is increased during pregnancy to support fetal growth, the increase in maternal blood volume, and the growth of other maternal tissues. Iron deficiency is common in infants and children from four months to six years of age because their rapid growth increases iron needs. Iron stores at birth are sufficient to meet iron needs for the first four to six months of life; after this, infants should consume formula or cereal fortified with iron to ensure an adequate intake. Toddlers with finicky eating habits should be monitored to ensure they are consuming adequate iron from foods such as meats, leafy green vegetables, and fortified cereals (see Chapters 15 and 16).

Adolescents are also at risk for iron deficiency anemia. In adolescent boys, rapid growth and an increase in muscle mass and blood volume increase iron need. In adolescent girls, iron needs are increased because weight gain is almost as great as in boys and iron losses are increased with the onset of menstruation (see Chapter 16).

Athletes are another group susceptible to iron deficiency. This may be due to a low iron intake as well as increases in iron losses due to prolonged training. Based on the amount of iron lost with prolonged training the EAR (Estimated Average Requirement) for those who engage in regular intense physical activity may be 30 to 70% greater than in the general population.[7] If the deficiency progresses to anemia, it can impair athletic performance (see Chapter 14).

Iron Toxicity Iron toxicity can be acute, resulting from ingestion of a single large dose at one time, or chronic, due to the accumulation of iron in the body over time (referred to as iron overload). Iron overload is not likely to result from a high dietary iron intake, but it does occur in individuals with hereditary abnormalities in iron absorption, diseases requiring frequent blood transfusions, or conditions in which red blood cell synthesis is abnormal.[10] Based on the appearance of gastrointestinal symptoms, a UL has been set at 45 mg per day of iron consumed from all sources.

Acute Toxicity Iron is toxic in large amounts causing damage to the intestinal lining, abnormalities in body pH, shock, and liver failure. Even a single large dose can be life threatening. Iron toxicity from supplements is one of the most common forms of poisoning among children under age six, and is the leading cause of liver transplants in children. To alert caretakers to the potential for accidental poisoning from iron-containing drugs and supplements, these products display a

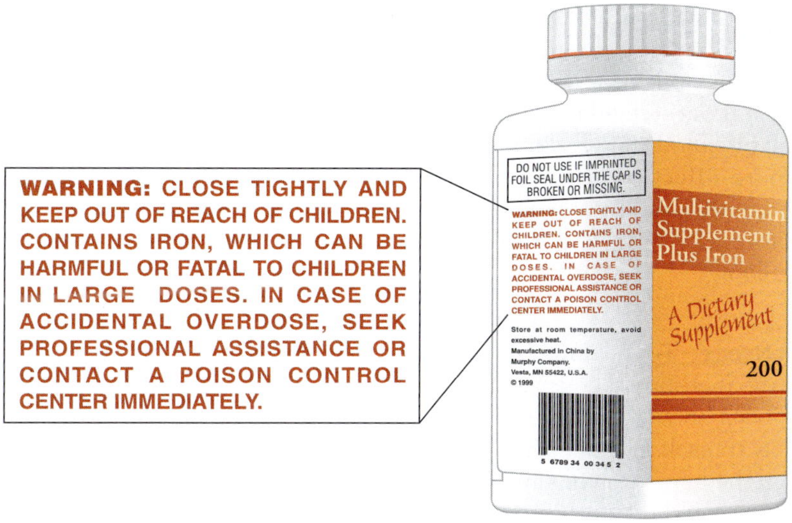

FIGURE 13.6 Labels on iron-containing supplements and medications must carry a toxicity warning.

warning on the label (Figure 13.6). In addition, because most cases of serious iron poisoning have occurred with products containing 30 mg or more per dose, these products are packaged in individual doses to make consumption of many pills difficult for a young child.[11]

Chronically Elevated Iron Stores Iron stores that are above normal but below toxic levels have been hypothesized to be associated with a greater risk of both heart disease and cancer. The relationship between iron and heart disease was originally suggested because heart disease occurs less frequently in premenopausal women, who lose iron in menstrual fluid, than in postmenopausal women and men. A relationship is supported by the fact that blood donation, which depletes iron stores, has also been associated with a reduced risk of heart attacks. One study found that elevated serum ferritin, an indicator of high iron status, is related to an increased risk of heart attacks.[12] Because iron can act as a pro-oxidant, it is hypothesized that it increases the formation of oxidized LDL cholesterol, which then leads to atherosclerosis.[13] However, despite these connections, there is not sufficient evidence to conclusively support or dispute a cause-and-effect relationship between iron and cardiovascular disease.[7]

Excess iron is suggested to increase cancer incidence by boosting the formation of free radicals, suppressing the activity of the immune system, and promoting cancer cell multiplication. However, evidence for a relationship between dietary iron intake and cancer in the general population is inconclusive.[10]

Hereditary Hemochromatosis The most common cause of chronic iron overload is the genetic disorder **hemochromatosis**, which is a condition that is characterized by excessive iron absorption. Hemochromatosis afflicts about 1.5 million Americans. It is the most common inherited disease in Caucasian populations in North America, Australia, and Europe, occurring in about 1 in 300 individuals.[14] Although more frequent in Caucasian populations, it also occurs in African Americans and Hispanics.[15] The accumulation of excess iron that occurs in hemochromatosis causes oxidative changes that result in heart and liver damage, diabetes, and certain types of cancer. Iron deposits also darken the skin. To have these symptoms, an individual must inherit the hemochromatosis gene from both parents. The one in ten people who inherit the gene from only a single parent lack these serious symptoms but do absorb iron more efficiently than people who do not have the gene at all.

Hemochromatosis An inherited condition that results in increased iron absorption and leads to iron deposits and tissue damage.

The public health impact of hemochromatosis is potentially significant. The availability of red meat and the prevalence of iron-fortified foods in the

American diet virtually assure that individuals with two genes for hemochromatosis will eventually accumulate damaging levels of iron. Individuals with only one gene may also be at risk. If individuals with hemochromatosis can be identified, treatment—regular blood withdrawal, the equivalent of the ancient treatment of bloodletting—is simple and prevents the complications of iron overload. To be effective, it must be started before organs are damaged, so screening to identify and treat young healthy individuals is essential in preventing complications.[16] The gene for this disorder has been identified and genetic testing is available.[17]

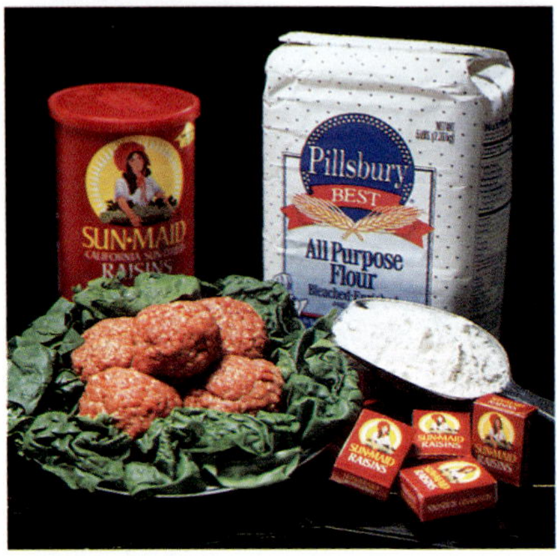

FIGURE 13.7 Iron in our diets comes from both animal and plant sources, but bioavailability from plant sources is often low. *(Charles D. Winters)*

Meeting Iron Needs To meet iron needs, both the amount and the bioavailability of iron from the diet should be considered. The best sources of iron are red meats and organ meats such as liver and kidney. Good vegetable sources are leafy greens such as spinach and kale, although the nonheme iron in plants is less well absorbed than the heme iron in animal sources (Figure 13.7). Iron absorption can be enhanced by including meat, fish, poultry, and foods rich in vitamin C in meals containing iron, and by decreasing the consumption of dairy products, which are high in calcium, at these meals.[5]

Because iron is a nutrient at risk for deficiency in the American diet, the iron content of packaged foods must be listed on food labels. It is given as a percent of the Daily Value for iron, which is 18 mg for adults. Therefore, if your breakfast cereal provides 10% of the Daily Value for iron, it contains about 1.8 mg of iron per serving.

Although diet is the ideal way to meet iron needs, supplements are often recommended for groups at risk for deficiency, such as small children, women of childbearing age, and pregnant women. Iron is commonly available as an individual supplement or as part of multivitamin and mineral supplements. These contain nonheme iron in either the ferrous or ferric form; the ferrous form (Fe^{2+}), such as ferrous sulfate, is more readily absorbed than the ferric form (Fe^{3+}). To enhance absorption, iron supplements should be consumed with foods containing vitamin C, such as orange juice; taken with a meal containing meat, fish, or poultry; and not taken with dairy products or substances that bind iron. Iron supplements should not be taken at the same meal as calcium supplements. Large intakes of iron from supplements can interfere with the absorption of zinc and copper. Iron-containing supplements should be taken only as suggested on the label and stored out of the reach of children or others who could consume them in excess (see *Critical Thinking:* "Increasing Iron Intake").

Critical Thinking

Increasing Iron Intake

Odelia is a twenty-three-year-old college sophomore. She has been feeling tired and run-down all semester. She recently read an article about iron deficiency in young women and became concerned about her iron status. She decides to go to the health center where she is evaluated, completes a diet history, and has her blood drawn.

Her diet history indicates that her iron intake is low and her lab results, shown in Figure 13.4, show that she has iron deficiency anemia. She is given information on increasing iron intake and taking iron supplements.

Odelia decides to try to increase the amount of iron she gets from her diet before considering iron supplements. Since Odelia is originally from Ghana, she enjoys many native foods and consumes a primarily vegetarian diet. A typical day's intake is shown below.

Food	Amount	Iron (mg)
Breakfast		
Grits with butter	1 cup	0.5
Plantain	1	0.9
Whole-wheat toast	1 slice	1.2
Apple juice	3/4 cup	0.7
Tea with sugar	1 cup	0
Lunch		
Apple	1 medium	0.2
Cornbread with butter	1 piece	1.5
Yogurt	1 cup	0.2
Tomato	1 medium	0.5
Tea with sugar	1 cup	0
Dinner		
Rice	1 cup	2.4
Peanuts	1/3 cup	0.9
Kale	1 cup	1.2
Yams	1 cup	1.1
Apple juice	3/4 cup	0.7
Tea with sugar	1 cup	0
Total		*12.0*

At home in Ghana her mother prepared meals in iron cookware. Since moving to the United States, Odelia has used stainless steel cookware and she believes that this may have contributed to her anemia.

Why would switching from iron to stainless steel cookware affect iron status?

Answer:

What other dietary factors could contribute to Odelia's poor iron status?

1. Her total iron intake is low at 12 mg per day compared with the RDA for a young female vegetarian of ______.
2. The iron in her diet comes from plant sources. This might contribute to iron deficiency because ______________________________.
3. The diet is low in vitamin C–rich foods. This might contribute to iron deficiency because ______________________________.
4. Answer: ______________________________.

How could Odelia's breakfast and lunch be modified to increase her iron intake?

Odelia is a vegetarian, so her iron sources are limited to plant foods. There are, however, good plant sources of naturally occurring iron as well as sources fortified with iron. For instance, switching from the half cup of grits, containing about 0.5 mg of iron, to a fortified cereal will greatly increase her intake. Adding 2 tablespoons of raisins to the hot cereal contributes another 0.4 mg. Another good vegetarian source of iron is beans. A bowl of chili with beans at lunch will add 8 mg of iron.

What modifications could Odelia make to increase the iron content of her dinner?

Answer:

Does Odelia's diet meet the recommendations of the Food Guide Pyramid for vegetarians?

Answer:

Are there other nutrient deficiencies for which she may be at risk?

Answer:

Zinc (Zn)

Evidence for the essentiality of zinc in animals was demonstrated in 1934, but the importance of zinc in human nutrition did not attract attention until 1961, when a syndrome of growth depression and delayed sexual development was alleviated by supplemental zinc.[18] This syndrome was seen in Iran and Egypt where the diet is based on vegetable protein. Although not low in zinc, the diet was high in grains containing phytate, which interfered with zinc absorption, causing a deficiency. Zinc is now known to be so ubiquitous in cellular metabolism that even a subtle deficiency may have multiple biological effects and clinical implications.

Sources of Zinc

Zinc is found in both plant and animal foods. Zinc from animal sources is better absorbed than that from plants because the zinc in plant foods is often bound by phytate. Zinc is abundant in red meat, liver, eggs, dairy products, vegetables, and some seafood (Figure 13.8). Whole grains are a good source but refined grains are

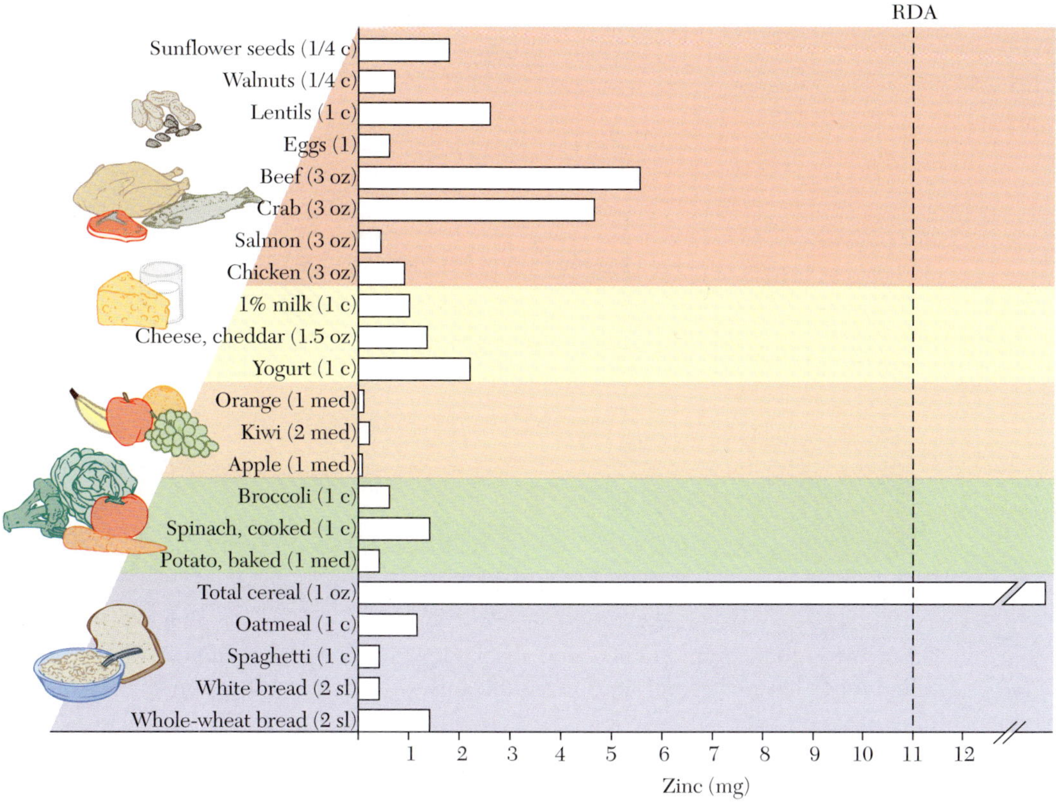

FIGURE 13.8 Zinc content of selections from each food group of the Food Guide Pyramid. The dashed line represents the RDA for adult men. Meat, seafood, and dairy products are good sources of zinc. Zinc is not added during the enrichment of grains but some products are fortified with zinc.

not, because zinc is lost in milling and not added back in enrichment. Grain products leavened with yeast provide more zinc than unleavened products because the yeast leavening of breads reduces the phytate content.[19]

Zinc in the Digestive Tract

The amount of zinc in the body is regulated in part by the amount that is absorbed. Zinc entering the mucosal cells of the intestine may be used by the mucosal cell itself, pass through the mucosal cell into the blood, or be bound by the protein **metallothionein**, which helps regulate the amount of zinc that reaches body tissues. Zinc in the mucosal cells stimulates the synthesis of metallothionein, so when zinc intake is high more metallothionein is made. Zinc bound to metallothionein is not easily transported out of the muscosal cell and is lost when the cells die (Figure 13.9). Conversely, when zinc intake is low, metallothionein synthesis is not stimulated, so concentrations drop and zinc is readily transferred from the mucosal cells to the blood. Metallothionein does not completely prevent zinc transfer to the blood, and high intakes can override this regulatory mechanism.

Metallothionein A protein that binds zinc and copper in intestinal cells and limits their absorption into the blood.

As with iron, the physiological state of the individual affects zinc absorption. When requirements are high, such as during infancy, pregnancy, and lactation, absorption is increased. The efficiency of zinc absorption is also affected by the amount of zinc in a meal as well as a number of other dietary factors. As zinc intake increases, the percentage that is absorbed decreases. Phytate found in corn, cereals, rice, and legumes bind zinc and inhibit absorption. Animal proteins are good sources of zinc and increase absorption by counteracting the inhibitory effect of phytates.[20] Iron also affects zinc absorption. When a high ratio of iron to

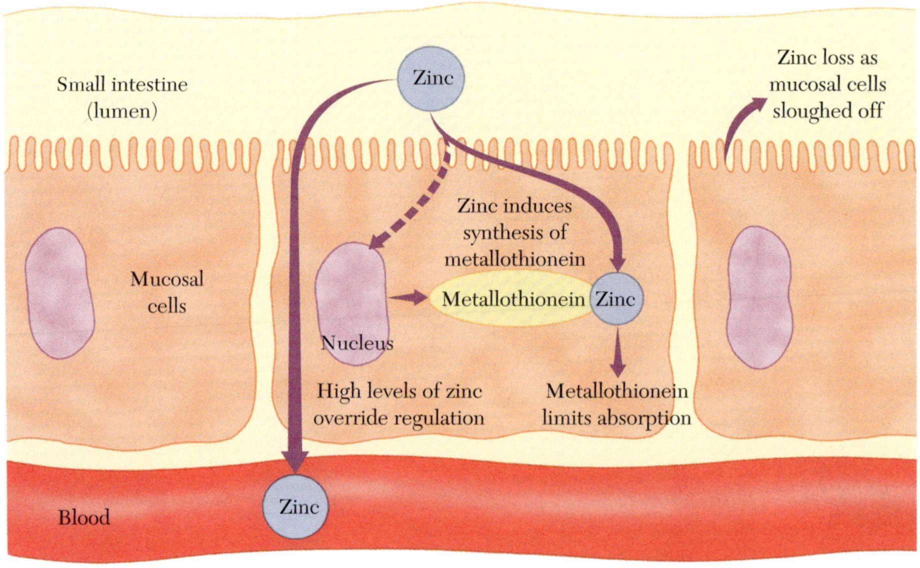

FIGURE 13.9 Zinc absorption is regulated by the protein metallothionein in intestinal mucosal cells. High levels of zinc stimulate the synthesis of metallothionein, which binds zinc, inhibiting its absorption. When zinc levels are low less metallothionein is made so a greater proportion of the zinc is absorbed.

zinc is found in supplements, zinc absorption is reduced, but the use of iron-fortified foods has not been found to significantly affect zinc absorption.[20]

Zinc in the Body

Once zinc has been absorbed, it is bound to albumin in the plasma and transported to the liver. Zinc leaves the liver bound to another protein for transport to other cells. Zinc homeostasis depends not only on regulating absorption but also on regulating excretion. Zinc is excreted in pancreatic juice and intestinal cell secretions, which enter the lumen of the intestine. When zinc levels are low, the zinc excreted into the gastrointestinal tract can be reabsorbed and recycled. When levels are high, it is not reabsorbed and is therefore eliminated in the feces. Additional zinc losses occur from sweat, sloughed skin cells, semen, menstrual fluids, and hair and nail growth.

Zinc Functions Zinc is the most abundant intracellular trace element. It is found in the cytosol, in cellular organelles, and in the nucleus. Zinc is involved in the functioning of nearly 100 different enzymes, including a form of **superoxide dismutase (SOD)**, which is vital for protecting cells from free radical damage. Zinc is also needed by enzymes that function in the synthesis of DNA and RNA, in carbohydrate metabolism, in acid-base balance, and in the removal of the polyglutamate tail from natural forms of folate (a step that is necessary for folate absorption).

Superoxide dismutase (SOD) An enzyme that protects the cell from oxidative damage by neutralizing superoxide free radicals. One form of the enzyme requires zinc and copper for activity and another form requires manganese.

Zinc also plays a role in the storage and release of insulin, the mobilization of vitamin A from the liver, and the stabilization of cell membranes. It influences hormonal regulation of cell division and is therefore needed for the growth and repair of tissues, the activity of the immune system, and the development of sex organs and bone.

Zinc and Gene Expression Some of the functions of zinc can be traced to its role in gene expression. As discussed earlier, zinc stimulates the production of metallothionein by binding to a regulatory factor and activating the transcription of the gene for this protein. Zinc may activate a number of other genes in a similar way.

Zinc also plays a structural role in proteins essential for gene expression. Proteins containing zinc fold around the zinc atom to form a loop, or "finger." This structure allows protein receptors to bind to regulatory regions of DNA, stimulat-

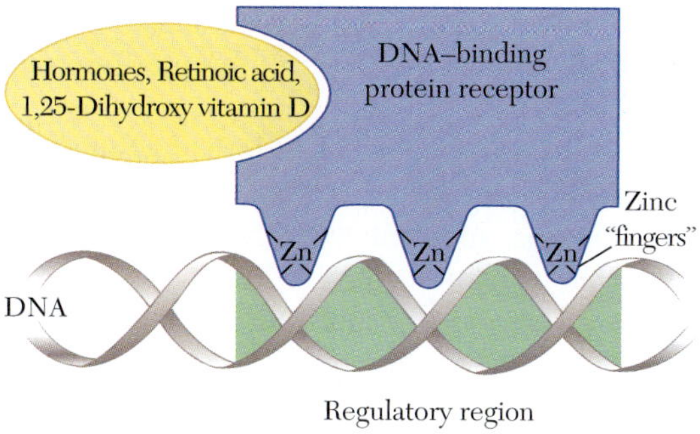

FIGURE 13.10 When zinc is incorporated into proteins it forms a finger-like structure (zinc fingers). This structure allows nuclear protein receptors that bind to hormones, retinoic acid, and 1,25-dihydroxy vitamin D to interact properly with the regulatory region of a gene. This binding affects the expression of the gene.

ing the transcription of a gene (Figure 13.10). Proteins containing zinc fingers are needed for the activity of vitamin A, vitamin D, and a number of hormones including thyroid hormones, estrogen, and testosterone. Without zinc, these nutrients and hormones cannot bind to DNA to increase or decrease gene expression and, hence, the synthesis of certain proteins.

Recommended Intakes

The RDA for zinc is 11 mg per day for adult men and 8 mg per day for adult women.[7] This is based on the amount of zinc needed to replace daily losses from the body.

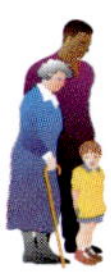

During pregnancy, the recommendation for zinc is increased to account for the zinc that accumulates in maternal and fetal tissues. During lactation, the RDA is increased to compensate for zinc secreted in breast milk. For infants from newborn to six months of age, an AI has been established based on the zinc intake of breast-fed infants. RDAs have been established for older infants, children, and adolescents based on the amount of zinc lost from the body, the need for growth, and absorption of zinc from the diet. Although the RDA for older adults is the same as that for younger adults, the elderly population may be at risk for zinc deficiency because of low intakes.[21]

Zinc and Health

The symptoms of zinc deficiency reflect its importance in protein synthesis and gene expression. Because it is needed for the proper functioning of vitamins A and D and the activity of numerous enzymes, deficiency symptoms can resemble deficiencies of other essential nutrients. Its role in immune function has made it a popular supplement for treating the common cold.

Zinc Deficiency Zinc deficiency has been seen in individuals with a genetic defect in zinc absorption and metabolism called acrodermatitis enteropathica, in those fed TPN solutions lacking zinc, and in individuals consuming low-protein, high-phytate diets. It may also occur in a number of disease states including kidney disease, sickle cell anemia, alcoholism, cancer, and AIDS. The symptoms of zinc deficiency include growth retardation, loss of appetite, taste changes, delayed sexual maturation, dermatitis, hair loss, skeletal abnormalities, malabsorption, night blindness, and depressed immunity.[22] The biochemical mechanism responsible for most of these has not been identified. In addition, because zinc is required for vitamin A transport, a deficiency can affect vitamin A status.[23]

One of the main concerns with even moderate zinc deficiency is altered immune defenses. The impact of zinc deficiency on immune function is rapid and extensive. It results in atrophy of the thymus, a gland involved in maturation of certain types of lymphocytes (immune system cells), and a decrease in the number and function of lymphocytes in the blood. The drop in immune function can lead to an increased incidence of infections.

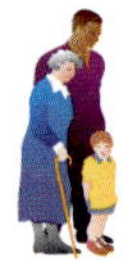

The risk of zinc deficiency is greater in groups such as the elderly, low-income children, and vegetarians—particularly female vegans, and in areas of the world where the diet is high in phytate, fiber, tannins, and oxalates. Groups most likely to be at risk of deficiency in the United States include children from 1 to 3 years of age, adolescent females, and adults 71 years of age and older.[24] Suboptimal zinc intakes have been observed in the United States among low-income children, children with diarrhea, low-birth-weight infants, frail elderly, and pregnant teens. Symptomatic zinc deficiency is relatively uncommon in North America, but in developing countries it has important health and developmental consequences.[25,26] Supplements have been shown to reduce the incidence of diarrhea and infections in children in developing nations.[27]

Zinc Toxicity Zinc can be toxic when consumed in excess of recommendations. A single dose of 1 to 2 g can cause gastrointestinal irritation, vomiting, loss of appetite, diarrhea, abdominal cramps, and headaches. This has occurred with consumption of foods and beverages contaminated with zinc that has leached from galvanized containers. Intakes in the range of 50 to 300 mg per day have been shown to decrease rather than enhance immune function and to reduce HDL cholesterol, the type of cholesterol that has a protective effect against heart disease.[28] Supplements providing 50 mg per day of zinc have been shown to interfere with the absorption of copper.[34] When high zinc intake inhibits copper absorption, it leads to a reduction in the activity of the copper-dependent enzyme copper-zinc superoxide dismutase in red blood cells. A UL has been set at 40 mg per day from all sources based on the adverse effect of excess zinc on copper metabolism.

Zinc Supplements Zinc is often marketed as a supplement to improve immune function, enhance fertility and sexual performance, and cure the common cold. For individuals consuming adequate zinc, there is no evidence that extra is beneficial. In individuals with a mild zinc deficiency, supplementation may result in improved wound healing, immunity, and appetite; in children it can result in improved growth and learning. In healthy older adults, supplements of zinc have been shown to improve the immune response (see Chapter 17).[29]

Zinc added to throat lozenges has been suggested to reduce cold symptoms. The zinc in these lozenges is believed to have its effect by coming in contact with mucosal surfaces where it may block the inflammatory response by complexing with proteins on the cold virus and on human cells.[30] In contrast, the zinc swallowed in a daily vitamin and mineral supplement will not have any effect because this zinc goes to the stomach and doesn't contact the mucosal surfaces affected by cold viruses. A recent review of the effectiveness of zinc lozenges failed to find evidence of a significant reduction in cold duration with zinc lozenges.[31]

Copper (Cu)

The ability of copper to treat certain types of anemia helped establish the essentiality of copper in human nutrition.[32] Further understanding of the impact of copper deficiency in humans came from studying individuals who were inadvertently fed intravenous (TPN) solutions deficient in copper and those with a rare genetic disease in which there is a defect in copper utilization.

Sources of Copper

The richest dietary sources of copper are organ meats such as liver and kidney, shellfish, legumes, nuts and seeds, the bran and germ of grains, and chocolate. Most meats, grain products, fruits, and vegetables are also good sources (Figure 13.11). As with many other trace elements, soil content affects the amount of copper in plant foods.

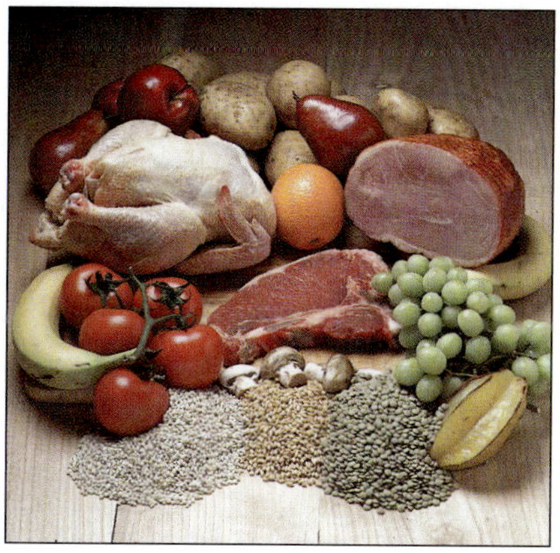

FIGURE 13.11 These foods are good sources of copper. *(Charles D. Winters)*

Copper in the Digestive Tract

About 30 to 40% of the copper in a typical diet is absorbed.[33] The absorption of copper is reduced by high intakes of zinc as well as iron, manganese, and molybdenum. Zinc is particularly important because when intake is high, it stimulates the synthesis of the protein metallothionein in the mucosal cells. Metallothionein helps regulate zinc absorption; however, it preferentially binds copper rather than zinc. Therefore, when metallothionein is synthesized, it binds copper, preventing it from being moved out of mucosal cells into the blood (Figure 13.12).[34] The antagonism between copper and zinc is so great that phytates, which inhibit zinc absorption, actually increase the absorption and utilization of copper.

Other factors that affect copper absorption include vitamin C, which decreases absorption,[33] and large doses of antacids, which inhibit copper absorption and can over the long term cause copper deficiency.

Copper in the Body

Once absorbed, copper binds to albumin, a protein in the blood, and travels to the liver, where it binds to the protein ceruloplasmin, which is involved in the transport of copper to other tissues. Copper must be transported bound to proteins such as albumin and ceruloplasmin because free copper ions can cause cellular damage. Copper can be removed from the body by secretion in the bile and subsequent elimination in the feces.

Copper functions in a number of important proteins and enzymes that are involved in iron and lipid metabolism, connective tissue synthesis, maintenance of heart muscle, and function of the immune and central nervous systems.[35] The copper-containing protein ceruloplasmin converts Fe^{2+} to Fe^{3+}, the form that can bind to transferrin for transport. Copper is also an essential component of the antioxidant enzyme superoxide dismutase (SOD). Copper plays a role in cholesterol and glucose metabolism, and elevated blood cholesterol levels have been

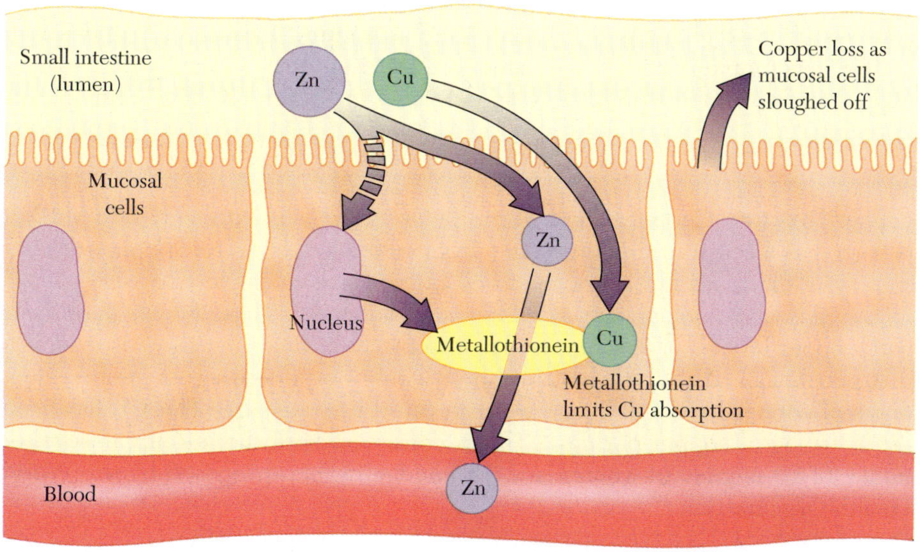

FIGURE 13.12 High levels of zinc can inhibit copper absorption by stimulating the synthesis of metallothionein, which then preferentially binds copper and limits its absorption.

reported in copper deficiency. Copper is also needed for the synthesis of the neurotransmitters norepinephrine and dopamine and several blood clotting factors. It may be involved in the synthesis of myelin, which is necessary for transmission of nerve signals.

Recommended Intakes

An RDA of 900 μg of copper per day has been established for adult men and women. These recommendations are based on the amount of copper needed to maintain plasma copper and ceruloplasmin concentrations, platelet copper concentration, and superoxide dismutase activity in red blood cells.

An AI for infants has been established based on the copper intake of breastfed infants. RDAs for children and adolescents are extrapolated from adult values. During pregnancy, the RDA is increased to 1000 μg per day to account for the copper that accumulates in the fetus and pregnancy-related tissues. During lactation, the RDA is increased to 1300 μg to account for the copper secreted in human milk.[7]

Copper and Health

The amount of copper in North American diets is slightly above the RDA.[7] It has been suggested that the consumption of foods such as breakfast cereals that are fortified with iron and zinc—minerals that interfere with copper absorption—may have an impact on copper status.[36] Despite this, severe copper deficiency is relatively rare, occurring most often in preterm infants and patients fed incomplete TPN. Marginal copper deficiency may be more prevalent but has been difficult to diagnose.[37]

Copper Deficiency The most common manifestation of copper deficiency is anemia. This is due primarily to the fact that the copper-containing protein ceruloplasmin is needed for iron transport. Thus, in copper deficiency, even if iron is sufficient in the diet, it cannot be transported out of the intestinal mucosal cells. Copper deficiency also causes skeletal abnormalities that mimic those observed with vitamin C deficiency (scurvy).[35] This occurs because the enzyme needed for the cross-linking of the connective tissue proteins collagen and elastin requires copper for activity. When copper is deficient, these proteins do not form properly. Copper deficiency has also been associated with impaired growth, degeneration of the heart muscle, degeneration of the nervous system, and changes in hair color and structure. Because of copper's role in the development and maintenance of the immune system, a diet low in copper decreases the immune response and may increase the incidence of infection.[38,39]

Copper Toxicity Copper toxicity from dietary sources is extremely rare but has occurred as a result of drinking water from contaminated water supplies or consuming acidic foods or beverages stored in copper containers. Excessive copper intake causes abdominal pain, vomiting, and diarrhea.[34] These effects may occur with copper intakes of 4.8 mg per day in some individuals but there is evidence that people can adapt to higher exposures without experiencing symptoms. High doses of copper have also been shown to cause liver damage. The UL has been set at 10 mg of copper per day.[7] This is consistent with the safe upper level of intake of 10 mg/day in women and 12 mg/day in men proposed by the World Health Organization.[40]

Manganese (Mn)

Manganese deficiency was described in laboratory animals in 1931. A few cases of manganese deficiency have been reported in humans.

Sources of Manganese

The best dietary sources of manganese are whole grains, legumes, nuts, and tea. Fruits and vegetables are fair sources; refined grains, dairy products, meat, fish, and poultry are poor sources.

Manganese in the Body

Manganese homeostasis is maintained by regulating both absorption and excretion. As with iron, manganese absorption increases when intake is low and decreases when intake is high. The presence of phytate may decrease manganese absorption and animal protein may enhance it. Iron stores may also affect the amount of manganese absorbed. One study found that women with large iron stores as indicated by high serum ferritin levels absorb less manganese.[41] Manganese is eliminated by excretion into the intestinal tract in bile. It is needed as a constituent of some enzymes and an activator of others. Manganese-requiring enzymes are involved in amino acid, carbohydrate, and cholesterol metabolism; cartilage formation; urea synthesis; and antioxidant protection. Like copper and zinc, manganese protects against oxidative damage by functioning in superoxide dismutase. The form of the enzyme that requires manganese is located inside the mitochondria.

Recommended Intakes

There was not sufficient evidence to set an EAR and RDA for manganese; the AI was set at 2.3 mg for adult men and 1.8 mg for adult women based on how much is typically consumed in a healthy population.[7] Recommended intakes are higher both during pregnancy and lactation.

Manganese and Health

Manganese deficiency in animals results in growth retardation, reproductive problems, congenital malformations in the offspring, and abnormalities in brain function, bone formation, glucose regulation, and lipid metabolism.

Because of the varied food supply, manganese deficiency is unlikely in North America. A naturally occurring manganese deficiency has never been reported in humans.[42] A deficiency was observed when a man participating in a study of vitamin K was inadvertently fed a diet deficient in manganese for six months. He lost weight, his black hair turned a red color, and he developed dermatitis and low blood cholesterol. Manganese deficiency was further studied in young male volunteers fed a manganese-deficient diet. After 35 days, 5 of the 7 subjects developed dermatitis and had altered blood levels of cholesterol, calcium, and phosphorus.[43]

Toxic levels of manganese result in damage to the nervous system. This is an occupational hazard for people who inhale manganese dust, and there is evidence that oral manganese can be toxic to the nervous system. The UL for adults has been set at 11 mg per day from all sources.

Selenium (Se)

Although selenium was discovered about 180 years ago, its essential role in human nutrition was not recognized until the 1970s when selenium supplements were found to prevent a heart disorder in children living in regions of China with low soil-selenium levels. Selenium is known to be important in the body's antioxidant defenses, and attention today is focused on the role of selenium in cancer prevention.

Sources of Selenium

Foods of animal origin generally have more consistent amounts of selenium than do plant foods. Seafood, kidney, liver, and eggs are excellent sources of selenium (Figure 13.13); fruits, vegetables, and drinking water are generally poor sources. Grains and seeds can be good sources depending on the selenium content of the soil where they are grown. For example, wheat grown in Kansas has a different selenium content than wheat grown in Michigan. Thus, soil-selenium content can have a significant impact on the selenium intake of populations consuming primarily locally grown food. Selenium intakes vary with geographic location, but intakes in both the United States and Canada appear to meet the RDA.

Selenium in the Body

Selenium absorption is efficient and does not appear to be regulated. Once selenium is absorbed, homeostasis is maintained by regulating the amount excreted in the urine. Selenium is a mineral that functions mostly through

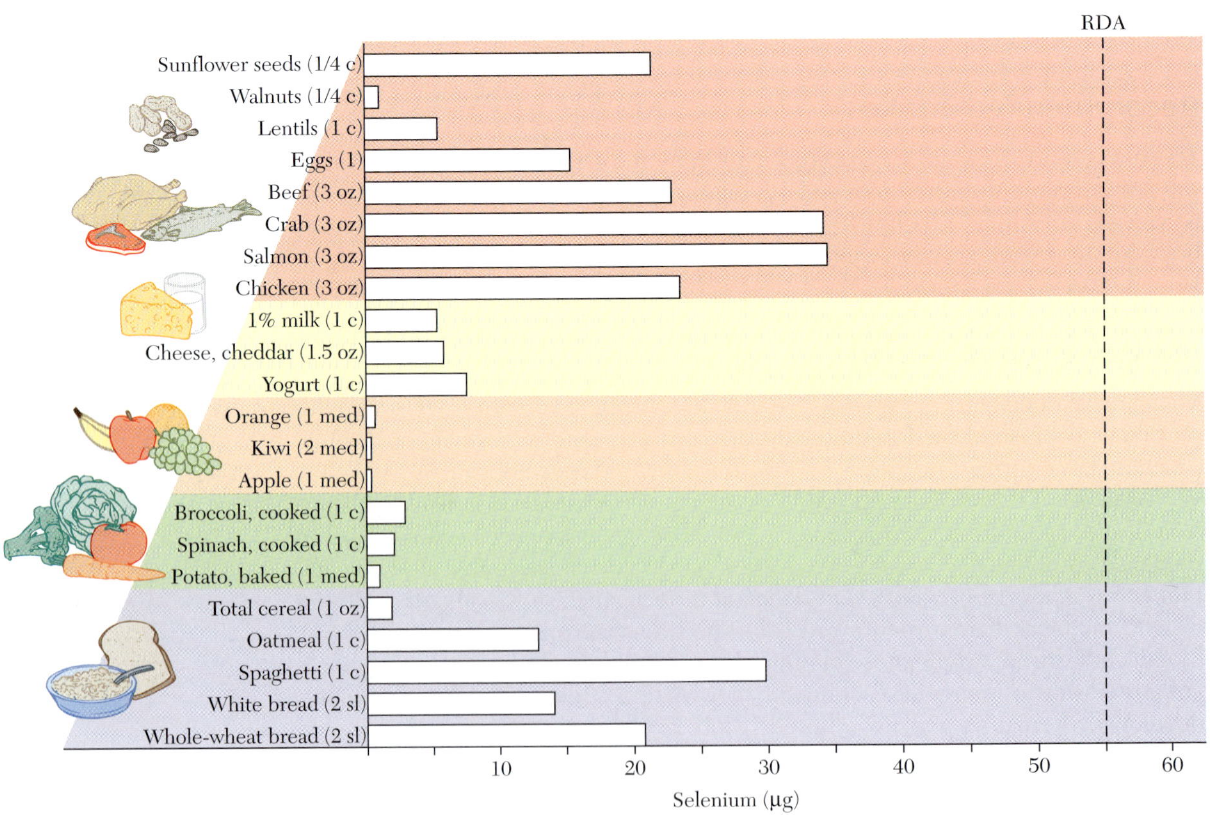

FIGURE 13.13 Selenium content of selections from each food group of the Food Guide Pyramid. The dashed line represents the RDA for adults. Seafood, meats, and eggs are excellent sources of selenium. Fruits and vegetables are generally poor sources and grains and seeds can be good sources depending on the selenium content of the soil where they were grown.

association with proteins called **selenoproteins**. Several of these, including forms of **glutathione peroxidase**, are enzymes that help protect cells from oxidative damage. Glutathione peroxidase neutralizes peroxides so they no longer form free radicals. By reducing free-radical formation, selenium in glutathione peroxidase can spare some of the requirement for vitamin E, because vitamin E is used to stop the action of free radicals once they are produced (Figure 13.14). Selenium is also an essential component of an enzyme needed for the synthesis of the thyroid hormones, which regulate basal metabolic rate.

Selenoproteins Proteins that contain selenium as a structural component of their amino acids. Selenium is most often found as selenocysteine, which contains an atom of selenium in place of the sulfur atom.

Glutathione peroxidase A selenium-containing enzyme that protects cells from oxidative damage by neutralizing peroxides.

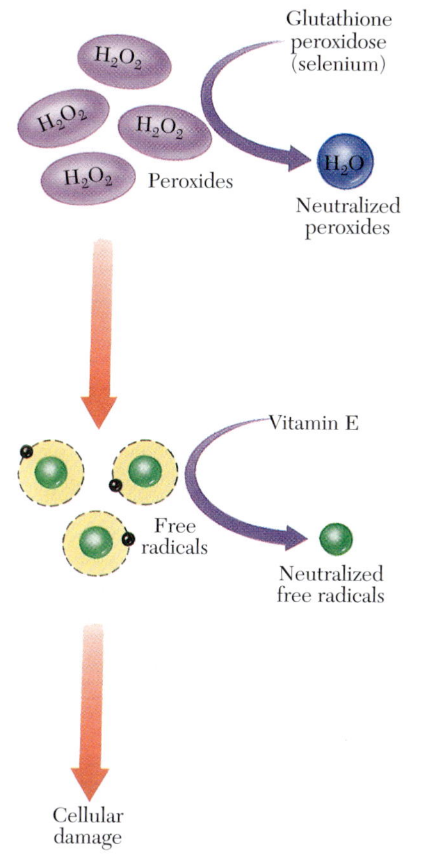

FIGURE 13.14 Selenium is a part of the enzyme glutathione peroxidase, which neutralizes peroxides before they form free radicals. This can spare some of the need for vitamin E.

Recommended Intakes

The RDA for selenium for adults is based on the amount needed to maximize the activity of the enzyme glutathione peroxidase in plasma. For adult men and women of all ages the RDA is set at 55 μg/day.[44]

For infants, an AI for selenium is based on the selenium intake of breast-fed infants. The RDAs for children and adolescents were determined by extrapolation from adult values.

The RDA for pregnancy is increased to 60 μg per day based on the amount of selenium transferred to the fetus. During lactation, the RDA is increased to 70 μg per day to account for the amount of selenium secreted in milk.

Selenium and Health

Low selenium intakes have been related to the incidence of a number of diseases, particularly cancer. But, as with many other nutrients, too much can have toxic effects.

Selenium Deficiency Because of the similar roles of selenium and vitamin E, it has been difficult to separate symptoms of selenium deficiency from those of vitamin E deficiency. A role for selenium was first recognized by studying animals deficient in both vitamin E and selenium. Selenium deficiency was not identified in humans until the late 1970s, when it was observed in patients fed TPN solutions inadvertently deficient in selenium. The deficiency symptoms observed in these individuals included muscular discomfort and weakness. At the same time scientists in China described a disease of the heart muscle called **Keshan disease** that was linked to selenium deficiency. Keshan disease was endemic in regions of China where the diet was restricted to locally grown food and the soil was deficient in selenium (Figure 13.15). It affected primarily women of childbearing age and children. Selenium supplements were found to dramatically reduce the incidence of Keshan disease, but it could not reverse heart damage once it had occurred. Although this disease is now virtually eliminated by selenium supplementation, selenium deficiency is not believed to be the only cause. It is hypothesized that it is due to several interacting factors that include selenium deficiency, other nutritional factors, and an infectious agent.[45] The role of an infectious agent in this disease is supported by studies that have isolated a virus from the hearts of patients who died of Keshan disease. A possible explanation for the role of selenium comes from research done in mice. In these animals, a virus that causes heart damage is more damaging in selenium-deficient mice than in supplemented mice.[46]

Keshan disease A type of heart disease that occurs in areas of China where the soil is very low in selenium.

Selenium and Cancer Animal studies demonstrating that high selenium intake reduces the incidence of cancer as well as observations that the incidence of certain human cancers is increased in regions where selenium intake is low led to the hypothesis that selenium protects against cancer. Interest in the role of selenium in cancer prevention intensified when an intervention trial that provided supplements of 200 μg per day to skin cancer patients found that,

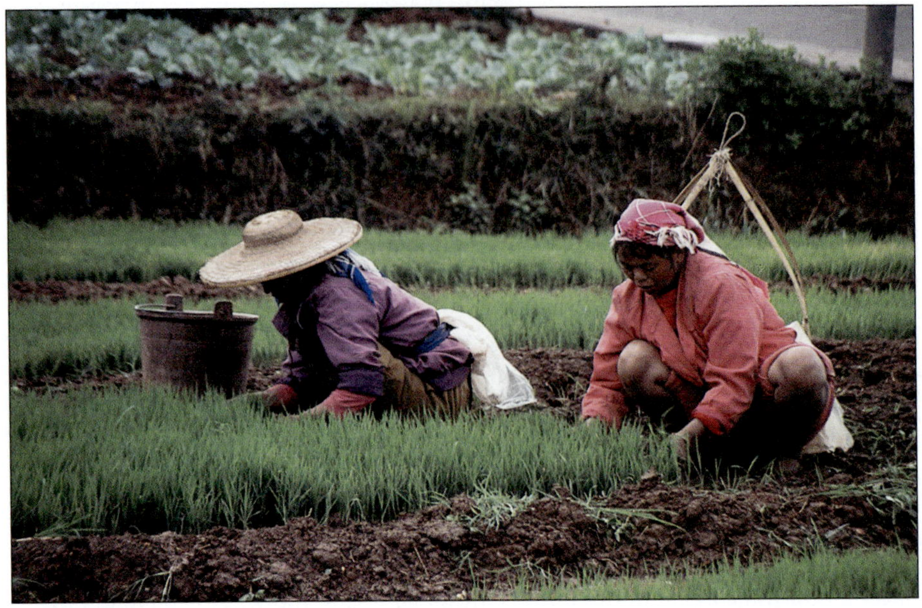

FIGURE 13.15 Because the soil content of many trace elements affects the mineral content of crops grown in the soil, deficiencies of trace elements such as selenium are most common in regions where all food is grown locally. *(© Images International/Visuals Unlimited)*

although skin cancer recurrence was not reduced, total cancer incidence, cancer mortality, and cases of lung, prostate, and colon cancer all decreased in the selenium-supplemented group.[47] The reduction in prostate cancer is supported by a study that found that men with higher selenium intakes, based on the selenium content of toenail clippings, had a reduced risk of prostate cancer.[48] The mechanism of cancer protection is hypothesized to be selenium's ability to turn on the self-destruct mechanism in cancer cells and therefore eliminate cancers before they spread.[49]

Selenium Toxicity In a region of China with very high selenium in the soil, an intake of 5 mg per day resulted in fingernail changes and hair loss. Selenium toxicity has also been reported in the United States because of a manufacturing error that created mineral supplements containing a dose of 27 mg of selenium per tablet (182 times higher than the amount specified on the label). The individuals who used these supplements had symptoms that included nausea, diarrhea, abdominal pain, fingernail and hair changes, nervous system abnormalities, fatigue, and irritability.[50] Adverse effects such as hair loss, fingernail loss, and gastrointestinal upset have been reported at much lower levels. The UL for adults for selenium has been set at 400 μg/day.[44] This includes selenium intake from the diet and from supplements.

Web Menu For more information about selenium supplements, go to the NIH Clinical Center at www.cc.nih.gov/ccc/supplements/ and click on selenium.

Selenium Supplements Selenium supplements are marketed with claims that they will protect against environmental pollutants, prevent cancer and heart disease, slow the aging process, and improve immune function. Although selenium does play a role in these processes, supplements of selenium have not been shown to be of benefit in the general populaiton.

IODINE (I)

Iodine is needed for the synthesis of thyroid hormones. In the early 1900s, iodine deficiency was common in the central United States and Canada, but it has virtually disappeared due to the addition of iodine to table salt in the 1920s. Iodine deficiency, however, remains a world health problem.

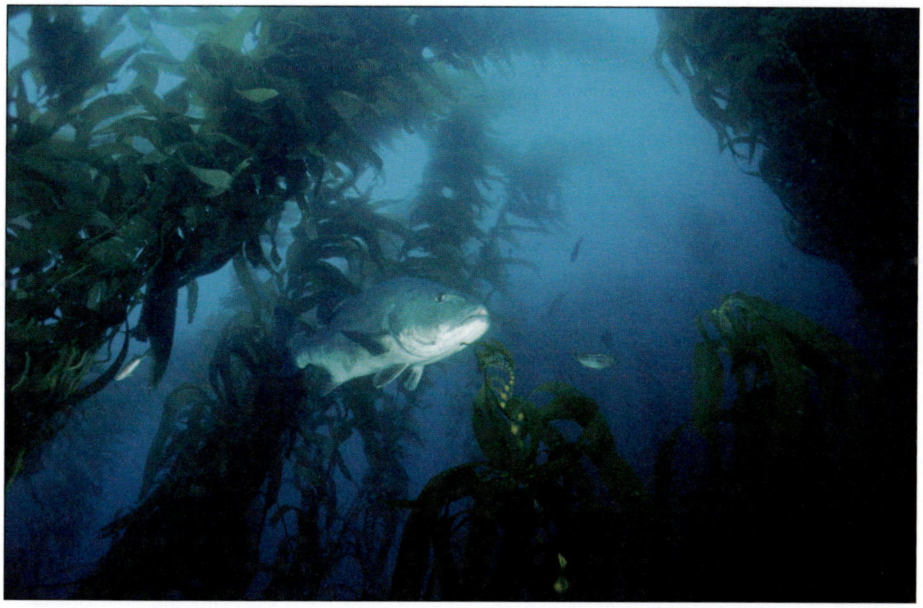

FIGURE 13.16 Most of the iodine in our diet comes from the sea. *(© Rulph A. Clevenger/Corbis)*

Sources of Iodine

Most of the iodine in foods comes from the sea. There are high concentrations of iodine in seawater and seafood (Figure 13.16). Plants grown close to the sea are high in iodine. The amount of iodine in plants grown inland depends on the iodine content of the soil.

Much of the iodine in the North American diet comes from salt fortified with iodine, referred to as iodized salt. Iodized salt contains about 100 μg of iodine per gram. It is commonplace in the United States, and only iodized salt is sold in Canada. Iodized salt should not be confused with sea salt, which is a poor source of iodine because the iodine is lost in the drying process.

Iodine in the diet also comes from contaminants and additives in foods. Dairy products, meat, and eggs may contain iodine because of the iodine-containing additives used in cattle and chicken feed and the use of iodine-containing disinfectants on cows, milking machines, and storage tanks. Iodine-containing sterilizing agents are also used in fast-food restaurants, and iodine is used in dough conditioners and some food colorings.

Iodine in the Body

Iodine is absorbed completely and rapidly from the gastrointestinal tract in the form of iodide ions. Iodine is eliminated from the body by excretion in the urine. Iodine accumulates in the thyroid gland where it is used to synthesize the thyroid hormones thyroxine (T_4) and triiodothyronine (T_3) (Figure 13.17). T_4 is the

T_4

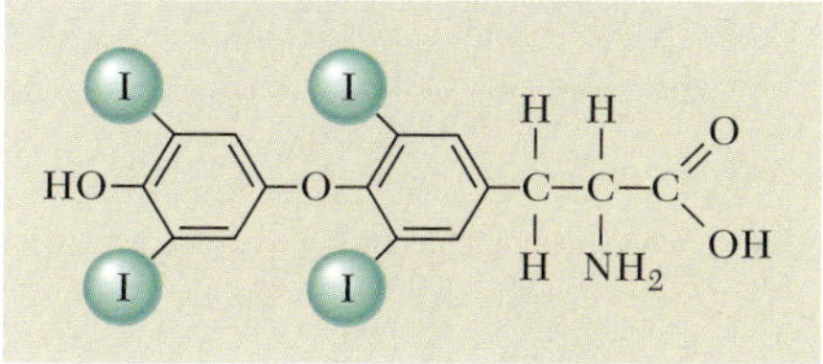

T_3

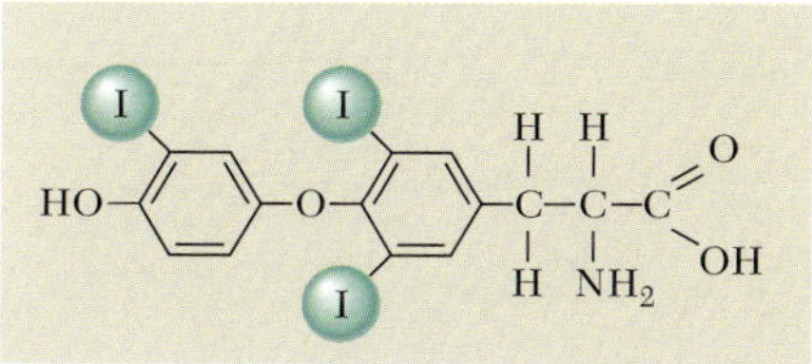

FIGURE 13.17 The thyroid hormones T_3 and T_4 are made from the amino acid tyrosine.

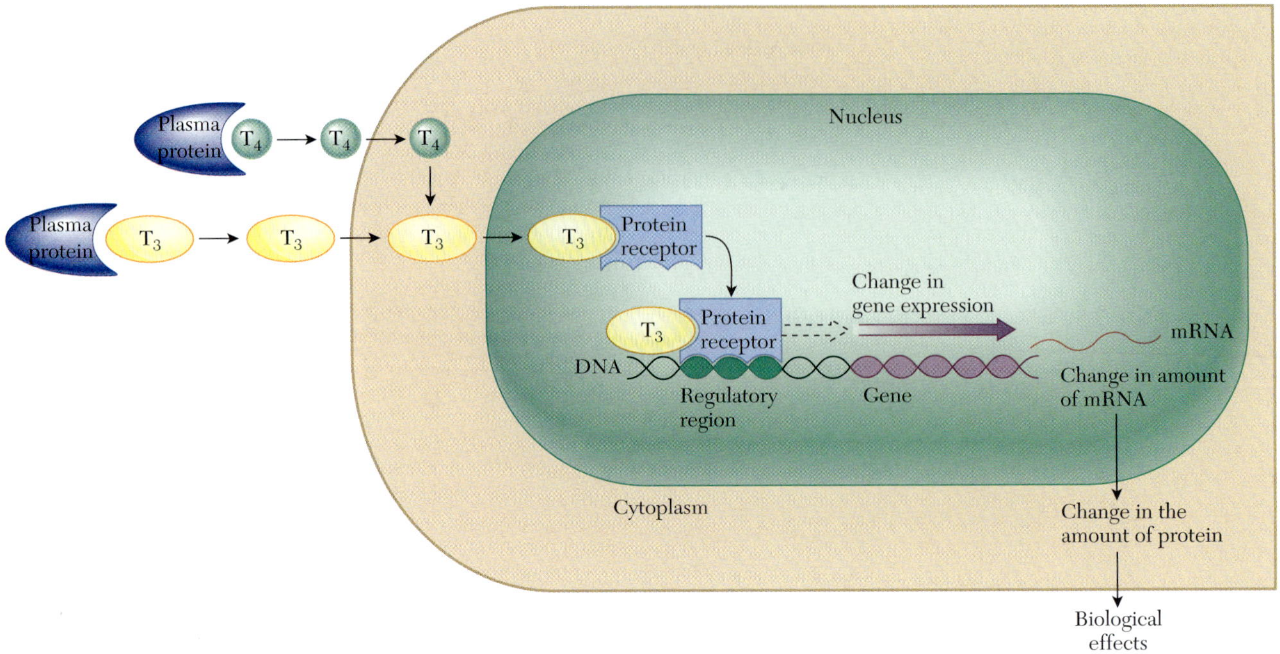

FIGURE 13.18 Thyroid hormones circulate in the blood bound to plasma proteins. Inside the cells an enzyme converts T_4 to T_3. T_3 enters the nucleus and binds to a nuclear protein receptor. The T_3-protein receptor complex binds to a regulatory region of a target gene and effects gene expression.

predominant form in the blood and is converted into the active T_3 form by a selenium-containing enzyme. The thyroid hormones act by affecting gene expression in target cells in a manner similar to vitamins A and D (Figure 13.18). Through gene expression, thyroid hormones regulate basal metabolic rate, growth and development, and promote protein synthesis.

Levels of thyroid hormones are carefully controlled. If blood levels drop, thyroid-stimulating hormone (TSH) is released. This hormone signals the thyroid gland in the neck to take up iodine and synthesize thyroid hormones. When the supply of iodine is adequate, thyroid hormones can be made and their presence turns off the synthesis of thyroid-stimulating hormone (Figure 13.19).

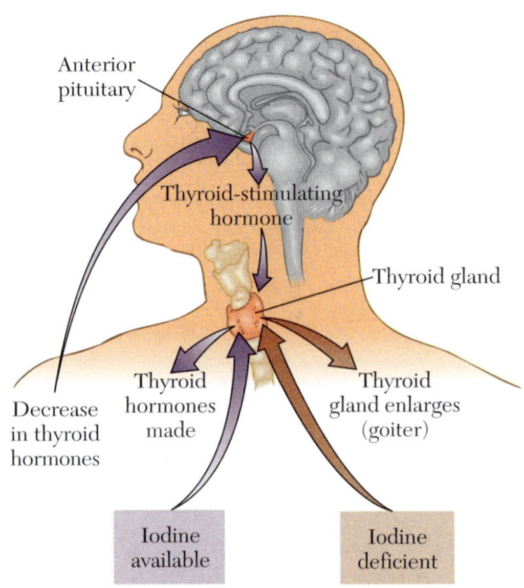

FIGURE 13.19 When thyroid hormone levels drop too low, thyroid-stimulating hormone stimulates the thyroid gland to take up iodine and synthesize more hormones. If iodine is not available, the stimulation continues and the thyroid enlarges, forming a goiter.

Recommended Intakes

The RDA for iodine is based on the amount of dietary iodine needed to achieve normal levels of iodine accumulation and turnover in the thyroid gland. It is set at 150 μg per day for adult men and women.[7] Since the introduction of iodized salt, the intake of iodine in North America has met or exceeded the RDA.

The RDA is higher during pregnancy to account for the iodine that is taken up by the fetus and during lactation to account for the iodine secreted in milk. An AI for infants has been set based on the iodine intake of breast-fed infants. RDAs for children are based on extrapolation from adult data or data from balance studies.

Iodine and Health

Salt fortified with iodine is widely used to increase iodine intake. However, high levels of iodine can be toxic.

Iodine Deficiency Iodine deficiency reduces the production of thyroid hormones. Metabolic rate slows with insufficient thyroid hormones, causing fatigue and weight gain. The most obvious outward sign of deficiency is an enlarged thyroid gland called a **goiter** (Figure 13.20). A goiter forms when reduced thyroid hormone levels cause thyroid-stimulating hormone to be released, stimulating the thyroid gland to make more thyroid hormones. Because iodine is unavailable, the hormones cannot be made and the stimulation continues, causing the gland to enlarge (see Figure 13.19). In milder cases of goiter, treatment with iodine causes the thyroid gland to return to normal size, but this result is not consistent in more severe cases.

A number of other iodine-deficiency disorders occur because of the effect of iodine on growth and development. If iodine is deficient during pregnancy, it increases the risk of stillbirth and spontaneous abortion. Deficiency can also cause a condition called **cretinism** in the offspring. Cretinism is characterized by symptoms such as mental retardation, deaf mutism, and growth failure. Iodine deficiency during childhood and adolescence can result in goiter and impaired mental function.

The risk of iodine deficiency is increased by consuming **goitrogens**, substances in food that interfere with the utilization of iodine or with thyroid function. Goitrogens are found in turnips, rutabaga, cabbage, and cassava. Most are destroyed in cooking or are present in foods that do not play an important role in human diets. However, in African countries where cassava is a dietary staple, high goitrogen intake may play a role in the development of iodine deficiency disorders.[51]

Iodine Fortification Since it was first used in Switzerland in the 1920s, iodized salt has been the major means of combating iodine deficiency. Because of the fortification of table salt with iodine, cretinism and goiter are now rare in North America, but worldwide 600 million people have goiter and 1.5 billion people are at risk for iodine deficiency.[52] At the recommendation of the United Nations Joint Committee on Health Policy, salt iodinization is now being used in most countries where iodine deficiency diseases are a significant public health problem.[53] For groups who do not have access to iodized salt or who will not use it, other forms of iodine supplementation, such as injections or oral doses of iodized oil, can be effective for control of iodine deficiency (see *Making Decisions*: "Should You Choose Iodized Salt?").[54]

Iodine Toxicity Chronically high intakes of iodine can cause impaired thyroid function and an enlargement of the thyroid gland that resembles goiter. A UL for adults has been set at intakes of 1100 μg of iodine per day from all sources.[7] Goiter from excess iodine can also occur if iodine intake changes drastically. For

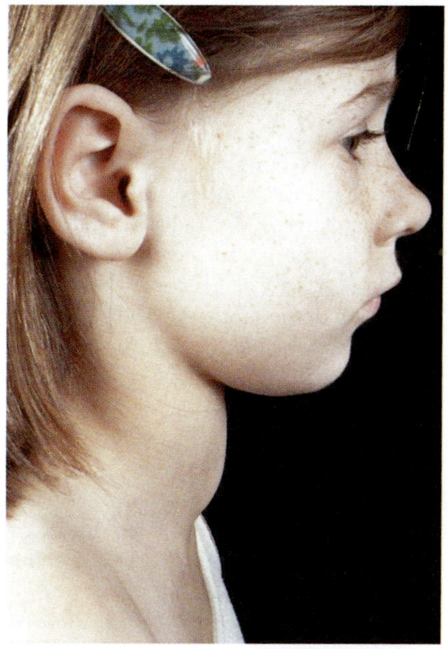

FIGURE 13.20 Iodine deficiency causes enlargement of the thyroid gland, a condition called goiter. *(© Biophoto Associates/Photo Researchers, Inc.)*

Web Menu

For more information on iodine deficiency diseases, go to the International Council for the Control of Iodine Deficiency Disorders at www.people.virginia.edu/~jtd/iccidd/ or to the WHO nutrition site at www.who.int/nut/ and look under micronutrient deficiencies.

Goiter An enlargement of the thyroid gland caused by a deficiency of iodine.

Cretinism A condition resulting from poor maternal iodine intake during pregnancy that causes stunted growth and poor mental development in offspring.

Goitrogens Substances that interfere with thyroid hormone production or utilization.

Making Decisions

Should You Choose Iodized Salt?

When selecting a box of salt for the kitchen cupboard, you can buy plain salt or a product labeled "iodized salt." Iodized salt is salt to which the trace element iodine has been added. In Canada there is no choice; all salt is iodized. In the United States, both are available. Which should you choose?

Iodine is an essential nutrient. The amount consumed in the diet depends as much on where foods are grown as on which foods are chosen. Foods produced in regions where the soil is rich in iodine are better sources of iodine than foods produced in regions where the soil is iodine-poor. The iodine content of plants grown in iodine-deficient soil may be 100 times less than those grown in iodine-rich soil.[a] When the Earth was formed, all soils were high in iodine, but today iodine is most plentiful in areas close to the sea. Mountainous areas and river valleys have little iodine left in the soil because it has been washed out by glaciers, snow, rain, and flood waters. The iodine washed from the soil has accumulated in the oceans, where it is present as iodide ions (I^-). When these ions come in contact with sunlight, they are oxidized to form iodine, which can escape into the air. Every year approximately 400,000 tons of iodine escapes into the atmosphere from the ocean surface. The iodine in the atmosphere is returned to the soil in rain, but the return is slow and the amounts returned to the soil are small. In areas where the forces of nature have resulted in iodine-deficient soil, these same forces will again wash away the iodine deposited from rain. Therefore, iodine-deficient soil will remain deficient.

Iodine-depleted soil is not new to the planet's ecology. Its effect on human health is part of history in many areas. In Europe, the presence of iodine deficiency was recorded by classical art, which portrayed even the wealthy with goiter and cretinism. Leonardo da Vinci is said to have been more knowledgeable about goiter than the medical professors of his time.[b] A century ago goiter was endemic in the central regions of North America. Today, iodine deficiency remains a major public health problem in some parts of the world.

In the United States, Switzerland, and some other European countries, iodine deficiency was virtually eliminated in the early 20th century by the iodinization of salt. Salt was selected as the vehicle for added iodine because iodine could be added to it uniformly, inexpensively, and in a form that was well utilized by the body and because salt was a food item consistently consumed by the majority of the population. Iodine could be added in amounts that would eliminate deficiency when typical quantities of salt were consumed by the population, but would not cause toxicity in those consuming larger amounts of iodized salt or in those who already met their iodine needs from other sources. People did not need to change their eating habits to include the fortified product in their diet. Today, in developing nations where iodine deficiency is still a public health problem, iodized salt as well as iodine-fortified fish sauce, sugar, and drinking water have been used experimentally to increase the iodine content of the diet.[c,d,e,f]

For about 50 years the average intake of iodine in the United States has exceeded the RDA and iodine deficiency has been rare.[g] The typical diet includes iodized salt as well as foods from many sources across the country and around the world. However, recent data from NHANES III has shown a significant reduction in the average American iodine intake. The average intake is still considered sufficient, but the drop has increased the number of people who are at risk of deficiency. The reasons for the decrease in iodine intake are unknown but several possibilities have been suggested.[h] As food patterns change, so has iodine intake. Egg yolks are rich in iodine, but egg consumption has declined due to concerns about dietary cholesterol intake. The amount of salt added in the home may also have declined due to recommendations regarding blood pressure. And, most of the salt in the American diet comes from processed foods, which contain noniodized salt. There have also been changes in the additives and contaminants in foods. The dairy industry has made an effort to reduce the iodine content of milk. The baking industry has replaced some of the iodine-containing dough conditioners with bromine salts, thus reducing the iodine content of commercially manufactured breads.

The decrease in iodine intake in the United States doesn't mean that Americans should sprinkle more iodized salt on their meals. Most people get plenty of iodine, even without iodized salt, especially if they live on the coast or buy food in a supermarket. However, for those who live inland where the soil is deficient in iodine, eat little seafood, and consume primarily foods grown locally, iodized salt is a choice that will ensure their iodine needs are met.

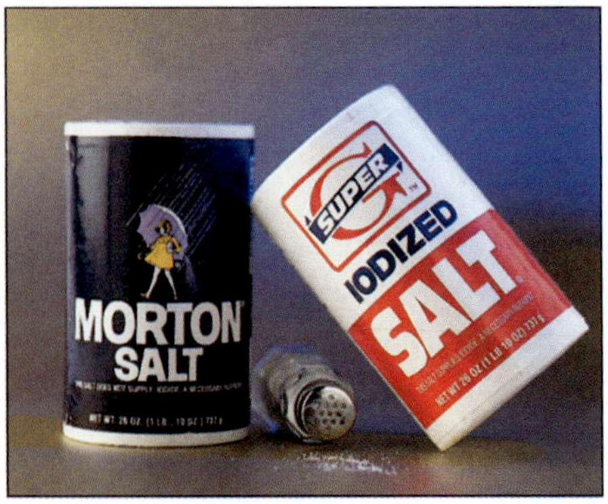

(George Semple)

References

[a] Hertzel, B. S., and Clugston, G. A. Iodine. In *Modern Nutrition in Health and Disease*, 9th ed. Shils, M. E., Olson, J. A., Shike, M., and Ross, A. C., eds. Baltimore: Williams & Wilkins, 1999, 253–264.

[b] Underwood, B. A. Micronutrient malnutrition: is it being eliminated? Nutr. Today 33:121–129, 1998.

[c] Melse-Boonstra, A., Rosendaal, M., Rexwinkel, H., et al. Determination of discretionary salt intake in rural Guatemala and Benin to determine the iodine fortification of salt required to control iodine deficiency disorders: studies using lithium-labeled salt. Am. J. Clin. Nutr. 68:636–641, 1998.

[d] Ranganathan, S., and Reddy, V. Human requirements of iodine and safe use of iodized salt. Indian J. Med. Res. 102:227–232, 1995.

[e] Eltom, M., Elnagar, B., Sulieman, E. A., et al. The use of sugar as a vehicle for iodine fortification in endemic iodine deficiency. Int. J. Food Sci. Nutr. 46:281–289, 1995.

[f] Saowakhontha, S., Sanchaisuriya, P., Pongpaew, P., et al. Compliance of population groups of iodine fortification in endemic areas of goiter in northeast Thailand. J. Med. Assoc. Thai. 77:449–454, 1994.

[g] Hollowell, J. G., Staehling, N. W., Hannon, W. H., et al. Iodine nutrition in the United States. Trends and public health implications: iodine excretion data from National Health and Nutrition Examination Surveys I and III (1971–1974 and 1988–1994). J. Clin. Endocrinol. Metab. 83:3401–3408, 1998.

[h] Lee, K., Bradley, R., Dwyer, J., and Lee, S. L. Too much versus too little: the implications of current iodine intake in the United States. Nutr. Rev. 57:177–181, 1999.

example, in a population with a marginal intake, a large increase in intake due to supplementation can cause thyroid enlargement even at levels that would not be toxic in a healthy population.[55]

Fluoride (F)

The importance of fluoride for dental health has been recognized since the 1930s, when an association between the fluoride content of drinking water and the prevalence of dental caries was noted.

Sources of Fluoride

Fluoride is present in small amounts in almost all soil, water, plants, and animals. The richest dietary sources of fluoride are fluoridated water, fluoridated toothpastes, tea, and marine fish consumed with their bones (Figure 13.21). In the United States, most of the fluoride in the diet comes from toothpaste and from fluoride added to the water supply—usually 0.7 to 1.2 mg per liter. (Water companies often report fluoride levels in parts per million [ppm]; 1 mg/liter = 1 ppm.) Because food readily absorbs the fluoride in cooking water, the fluoride content of food can be significantly increased when it is handled and prepared using fluoridated water. Worldwide, tea contributes significantly to total fluoride intake, particularly in countries that consume large amounts of the beverage. Brewed tea contains 1 to 6 mg of fluoride per liter depending on the amount of dry tea used, the brewing time, and the fluoride content of the water.[56] Cooking utensils also affect food fluoride content. Foods cooked with Teflon utensils can pick up fluoride from the Teflon, whereas aluminum cookware can decrease fluoride content. Fluoride is absorbed into the body in proportion to its content in the diet.

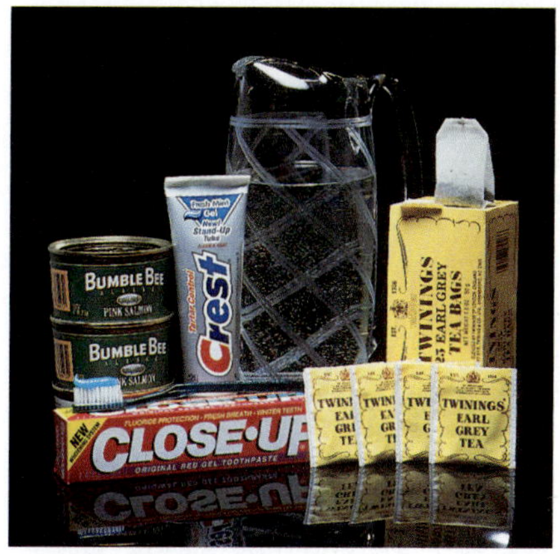

FIGURE 13.21 Dietary sources of fluoride include water, tea, fish eaten with bones, and toothpaste. *(Charles D. Winters)*

Fluoride in the Body

About 80 to 90% of ingested fluoride is absorbed. When taken with milk or other high-calcium foods, absorption is reduced. Fluoride has a high affinity for calcium, so in the body it is usually associated with calcified tissues such as bones and teeth. It is incorporated into bone and tooth enamel crystals, where it forms the compound fluorhydroxyapatite, which replaces hydroxyapatite.

Recommended Intakes

The criterion used to establish an AI for fluoride was the estimated intake shown to reduce the occurrence of dental caries maximally without causing unwanted side effects. The AI for fluoride from all sources is set at 0.05 mg per kg per day for all ages six months and older.[56] Thus, for children aged four through eight years, the AI is set at 1.1 mg per day using a reference weight of 22 kg. For adult men aged 19 and older, the AI is 3.8 mg per day based on a weight of 76 kg; for women, it is 3.1 mg per day based on a weight of 61 kg. The AI is not increased in pregnancy or lactation.

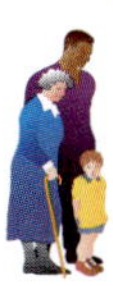

Breast milk is low in fluoride and ready-made infant formulas are prepared with unfluoridated water. Unless infant formula is prepared at home with fluoridated water, it contains little fluoride. The American Academy of Pediatrics suggests a supplement of 0.25 mg per day for children 6 months to 3 years of age, 0.5 mg per day for ages 3 to 6 years, and 1.0 mg per day for ages 6 to 16 who are receiving less than 0.3 mg per liter of fluoride in the water supply.[57] These supplements are available by prescription for children living in areas with low water

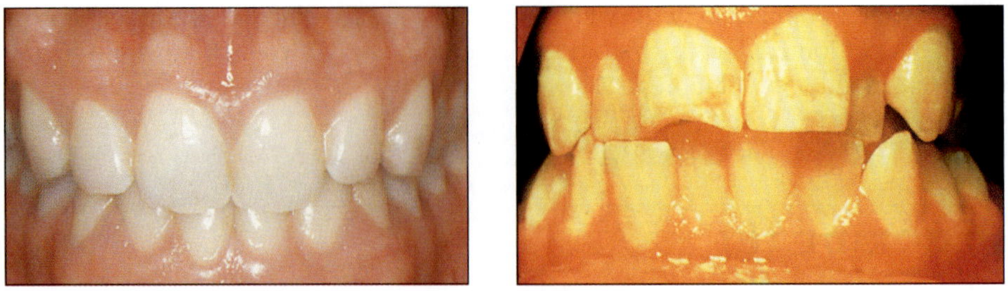

(a) (b)

FIGURE 13.22 Too much dietary fluoride causes the teeth to appear mottled (enamel fluorosis). (a) Normal teeth. (b) Teeth showing enamel fluorosis. *(a, © Edward H. Gill/Custom Medical Stock Photo; b, © NIH/Custom Medical Stock Photo)*

fluoride concentrations. Swallowed toothpaste is estimated to contribute about 0.6 mg per day of fluoride in young children.[56]

Fluoride and Health

Adequate dietary fluoride is important for bone and dental health. There is evidence that fluoride stimulates new bone formation and has therefore been suggested to strengthen bones in adults with osteoporosis. Slow-release fluoride supplements have been shown to increase bone mass and prevent new fractures.[58]

Web Menu For more information on fluoride and dental caries, go to the American Dental Association Oral Health Topics A–Z at www.ada.org/public/topics/ and click on fluoride.

Fluoride and Dental Caries Epidemiology has confirmed the effectiveness of fluoridated water in reducing dental cavities (see *Research Discoveries:* "From Colorado Brown Stain to Water Fluoridation").[59] Fluoride has its greatest effect on dental caries prevention early in life, during maximum tooth development up to the age of thirteen, but it has also been shown to have some beneficial effects in adults.[60] The incorporation of fluoride into tooth enamel during tooth development makes the enamel more resistant to acid. In addition to this effect, research now suggests that much of the benefit of fluoride on caries prevention is due to topical effects that occur in children and adults after the teeth have erupted.[61] Topical fluoride inhibits the dissolution of the tooth minerals by acid. It also enhances the remineralization of tooth enamel by sticking to the tooth surface and attracting calcium ions in the saliva. Finally, when taken up by the bacteria that cause tooth decay, fluoride reduces the amount of acid the bacteria produce.[61]

Fluoride Toxicity Fluoride can cause adverse effects in high doses. Fluoride intakes of 2 to 8 mg per day can cause mottled teeth in children (Figure 13.22). A recent increase in the prevalence of this condition in the United States has occurred due to the chronic ingestion of toothpaste containing fluoride. In adults, doses of 20 to 80 mg per day can result in changes in bone health that can be crippling, as well as changes in kidney function and possibly nerve and muscle function. Death was reported with an intake of 5 to 10 g per day. Due to concern over excess fluoride intake, a new warning is now required on fluoride-containing toothpastes. The label must state, "If you accidentally swallow more than used for brushing, seek professional help or contact a poison control center immediately."

The UL for fluoride is set at 0.1 mg per kg per day for infants and children less than 9 years of age, and at 10 mg per day for people aged 9 through 70.[56]

Chromium (Cr)

It has been known since the 1950s that chromium is needed for normal glucose utilization, but only recently have scientists begun to understand how chromium has this effect.

RESEARCH DISCOVERIES

From Colorado Brown Stain to Water Fluoridation

In 1901, when Dr. Fredrick McKay set up a dental practice in Colorado Springs, Colorado, he noticed that many of his patients had stained or mottled tooth enamel. McKay noted that those with stained teeth, a condition that was termed "Colorado brown stain," seemed to be less susceptible to tooth decay.[a] At the time, dental caries were extremely prevalent, there was no known way to prevent the disease, and the most common way to treat it was to extract the affected tooth.

McKay believed that Colorado brown stain was due to something in the water supply. In 1930 he sent water samples to be analyzed by a chemist working for an aluminum manufacturing company in Bauxite, Arkansas. Using a new methodology called spectrographic analysis, the chemist was able to identify high levels of fluoride in McKay's samples. The identification of high fluoride as a cause of Colorado brown stain led to the establishment of the Dental Hygiene Unit at the National Institutes of Health. It was headed by Dr. H. Trendley Dean, who was presented with the task of investigating the association between fluoride and mottled enamel, which Dean termed "fluorosis."

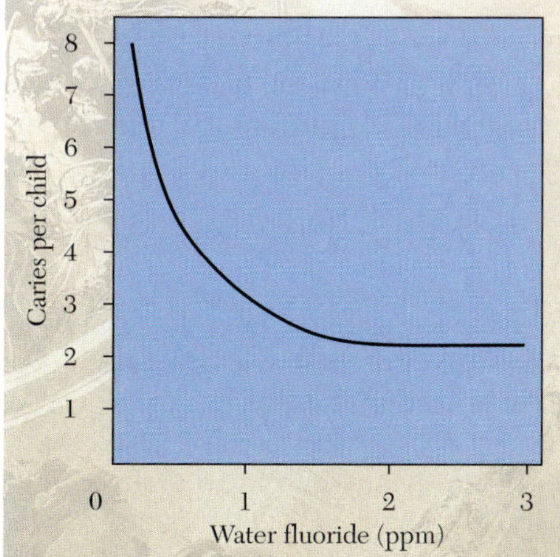

This graph illustrates the effect of water fluoride level on the incidence of dental caries in children 12 to 14 years of age. *(Food and Nutrition Board, Institute of Medicine.* Dietary Reference Intakes for Calcium, Phosphorus, Magnesium, Vitamin D, and Fluoride. *Washington, D.C.: National Academy Press, 1997)*

Dean conducted epidemiological surveys to establish the prevalence of fluorosis across the country. When he compared the prevalence of fluorosis with the prevalence of dental caries among children, he noted a strong inverse relationship.[b] In other words, children with fluorosis had fewer dental caries. Further studies revealed that the protective effect of fluoride on dental caries was seen at water fluoride levels of 1 ppm, a level low enough to cause little fluorosis (see figure). Work designed to identify the harm caused by too much fluoride had discovered the benefits of enough fluoride.

The first intervention trial to test the effectiveness of community water fluoridation began in 1945 and included four pairs of cities: Grand Rapids and Muskegon, Michigan; Newburgh and Kingston, New York; Evanston and Oak Park, Illinois; and Brantford and Sarnia, Ontario, Canada. One city of each pair received the intervention—fluoridated water—and the second city served as a control. Over a 13- to-15 year period, surveys found that caries was reduced 50 to 70% among children in the communities with the fluoridated water.[c] In 1962 epidemiological studies of water consumption patterns and caries incidence in different climates and geographical locations across the country were used to make the first recommendation for an optimal range of fluoride concentration in the water supply. A range of 0.7 to 1.2 ppm was recommended, with the lower range suggested for warmer climates where more water is consumed and the higher range for colder climates.[c]

Despite demonstrated benefits, some people believe that water fluoridation represents a public health hazard and increases the risk of cancer. These beliefs are not supported by scientific facts. The safety and effectiveness of water fluoridation has been assessed frequently. Based on epidemiological data and available evidence related to the adverse effects of fluoride, the small amounts consumed in drinking water do not pose a risk for health problems such as cancer, kidney failure, or bone disease.[d]

As of 1992, about 56% of the population in the United States was receiving fluoridated water either through community water fluoridation or from natural fluoride levels in the water. Fluoride intake has also increased from the widespread use of fluoride toothpaste and the use of fluoridated water in foods and beverages that are distributed in nonfluoridated areas. Although dental caries remain a public health problem affecting about 94% of people 18 or older,[e] increased fluoride intake, combined with advances in dental care, have dramatically improved the dental health of the American public. During both World Wars, the main reason men were rejected for military service was failure to meet the minimum standard of having six opposing teeth.[f] Today, with proper dental care, most people keep their teeth well into old age.

References

[a] McKay, F. S. Relation of mottled enamel to caries. J. Am. Dent. Assoc. 15:1429–1437, 1928.

[b] Dean, H. T. Endemic fluorosis and its relation to dental caries. Public Health Rep. 53:1443–1452, 1938.

[c] Achievements in public health, 1900–1999: Fluoridation of drinking water to prevent dental caries. MMWR, Morb. Mortal. Wkly. Rep. 48:933–940, 1999.

[d] National Research Council. The health effects of ingested fluoride: report of the Subcommittee on the Health Effects of Ingested Fluoride, Committee on Toxicology, Board of Environmental Studies and Toxicology, Commission on Life Sciences. Washington, D.C.: National Academy Press, 1993.

[e] Winn, D. M., Brunelle, J. A., Selwitz, R. H., et al. Coronal and root caries in the dentition of adults in the United States, 1988–1991. J. Dent. Res. 75:642–651, 1996.

[f] Britten, R. H., and Perrott, G .S. J. Summary of physical findings on men drafted in world war. Pub. Health. Rep. 56:41–62, 1941.

Sources of Chromium

Dietary sources of chromium include liver, brewer's yeast, nuts, and whole grains. Milk, vegetables, and fruit are poor sources. Refined carbohydrates such as white breads, pasta, and white rice are also poor sources because chromium is lost in milling and not added back in the enrichment process. Chromium intake can be increased by cooking in stainless steel cookware because chromium leaches from the steel into the food.

Chromium in the Body

In general, chromium is poorly absorbed; however, absorption varies depending on the form of the chromium and other substances present in the intestine. After absorption, chromium is bound to the iron transport protein transferrin or to albumin for transport in the blood.

Chromium is involved in carbohydrate and lipid metabolism. When carbohydrate is consumed, blood glucose levels rise and insulin is released in order to transport the glucose into cells. Insulin binds to protein receptors in cell membranes. This binding triggers the uptake of glucose by the cell, an increase in protein and lipid synthesis, and other effects. Chromium acts as part of a small peptide that binds to the insulin receptors after insulin has bound.[62] This chromium-containing peptide stabilizes insulin and amplifies its effects.[62] When chromium is deficient, this peptide cannot be made and it therefore takes more insulin to produce the same effect.

Recommended Intakes

Based on the chromium content of a well-balanced diet, an AI has been set at 35 μg per day for young men and 25 μg per day for young women.[7] The AI for chromium is increased during pregnancy and lactation. The AI for older adults is slightly lower because energy intakes decrease with age.

Chromium and Health

Overt chromium deficiency is not a significant problem in the United States population, but excessive intake of chromium as **chromium picolinate** has raised toxicity concerns.

Chromium picolinate A well-absorbed form of chromium sold as a dietary supplement that is advertised to promote fat loss and increase lean body tissue.

Chromium Deficiency Deficiencies have been reported in patients receiving long-term TPN that does not contain sufficient chromium and in malnourished children. Symptoms include impaired glucose tolerance with diabetes-like symptoms, such as elevated blood glucose levels and increased insulin levels. Chromium deficiency may also cause elevated blood cholesterol and triglyceride levels. However, the role of chromium in lipid metabolism is not fully understood.[63] There is some evidence that dietary chromium deficiency may play a role in the development of type 2 diabetes, but the significance of this role is not clear.[64] Older adults may be more vulnerable to chromium deficiency than younger adults.[7] A contributing factor may be the use of medications that affect chromium absorption.

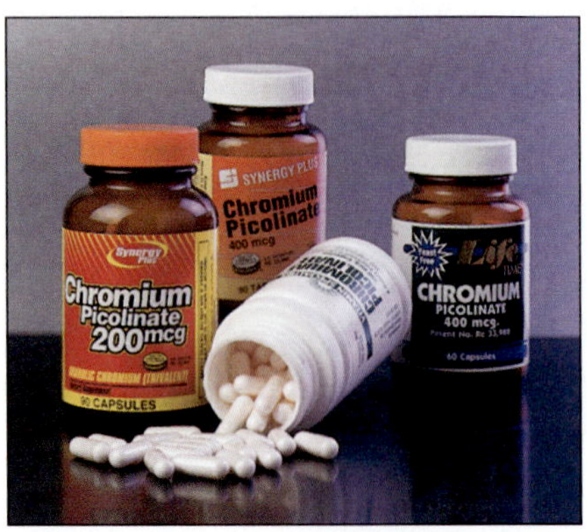

FIGURE 13.23 Chromium supplements are marketed to increase lean body mass and decrease body fat. *(George Semple)*

Chromium Supplements and Toxicity Chromium supplementation of 200 to 1000 μg per day has been shown to have beneficial effects on blood glucose, insulin, and cholesterol levels in individuals with type 2 diabetes.[65] Chromium supplements, particularly as chromium picolinate, are also marketed to reduce body fat and increase lean body tissue (Figure 13.23). This appeals to individuals wanting to lose weight as well as to athletes trying to build muscle. Because chromium is needed for insulin action and insulin promotes protein synthesis, it is likely that adequate chromium is necessary to increase lean body mass. However, most recent studies on the effects of chromium picolinate or other chromium supplements in healthy human subjects have found no beneficial effects on muscle strength, body composition, weight loss, or other aspects of health.[66]

Controlled trials have reported no dietary toxicity in humans, and oral chromium picolinate at doses containing 1.0 mg of chromium per day has produced no adverse effects.[67] Despite the apparent safety of chromium supplements, a few concerns have been raised. Two cases of renal failure have been associated with chromium picolinate supplements, but both of these individuals were taking other drugs known to cause renal toxicity, so it is unclear that the effect was due to the chromium supplement.[67] The safety of chromium picolinate has also been questioned because of studies in cell culture that suggest it may cause DNA damage.[68] This effect is specific to the picolinate form of chromium and may be due to the ability of this form to generate DNA-damaging free radicals.[69] Human studies using the standard supplemental doses of chromium picolinate have not detected an increase in DNA damage, but more work is needed to completely rule out any risk.[70] Despite these concerns, the DRI committee concluded that there was insufficient data to establish a UL for chromium.[7]

Molybdenum (Mo)

Like many other trace elements, molybdenum is needed to activate certain enzymes. The molybdenum content of food varies with the molybdenum content of the soil where the food is produced. The most reliable sources include milk and milk products, organ meats, breads, cereals, and legumes.

Molybdenum is readily absorbed from foods. The amount in the body is regulated by excretion in the urine and bile. Molybdenum is a cofactor for enzymes necessary for the metabolism of the sulfur-containing amino acids methionine and cysteine and of the nitrogen-containing compounds present in DNA and RNA, for the production of uric acid, and for the oxidation and detoxification of various other compounds.

Although molybdenum deficiency in humans has been reported as a result of long-term TPN, a naturally occurring deficiency has never been reported. Deficiency has been induced in laboratory animals by feeding them high doses of the element tungsten, which inhibits molybdenum absorption. The resulting deficiency caused growth retardation, decreased food intake, impaired reproduction, and decreased life expectancy.

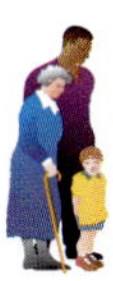

Based on the results of molybdenum balance studies and the bioavailability of molybdenum in the diet, an RDA has been set at 45 μg per day for adult men and women.[7] The RDA is increased during pregnancy and lactation. An AI has been established for infants based on the molybdenum consumed by breast-fed infants. RDA values for children were extrapolated from adult data.

There are few data that show adverse health effects of excess molybdenum in humans. Molybdenum interacts with copper, but a human study using doses up to 1.5 mg of molybdenum per day showed no adverse effects on copper utilization.[71] A UL was set at 2000 μg per day of molybdenum from all sources based on impaired reproduction and growth in animals.

Other Trace Elements

Many other trace elements are found in minute amounts in the human body. Some of these may be essential for human health and others may be present only as a result of environmental exposure.[72] There is sufficient evidence of a role for

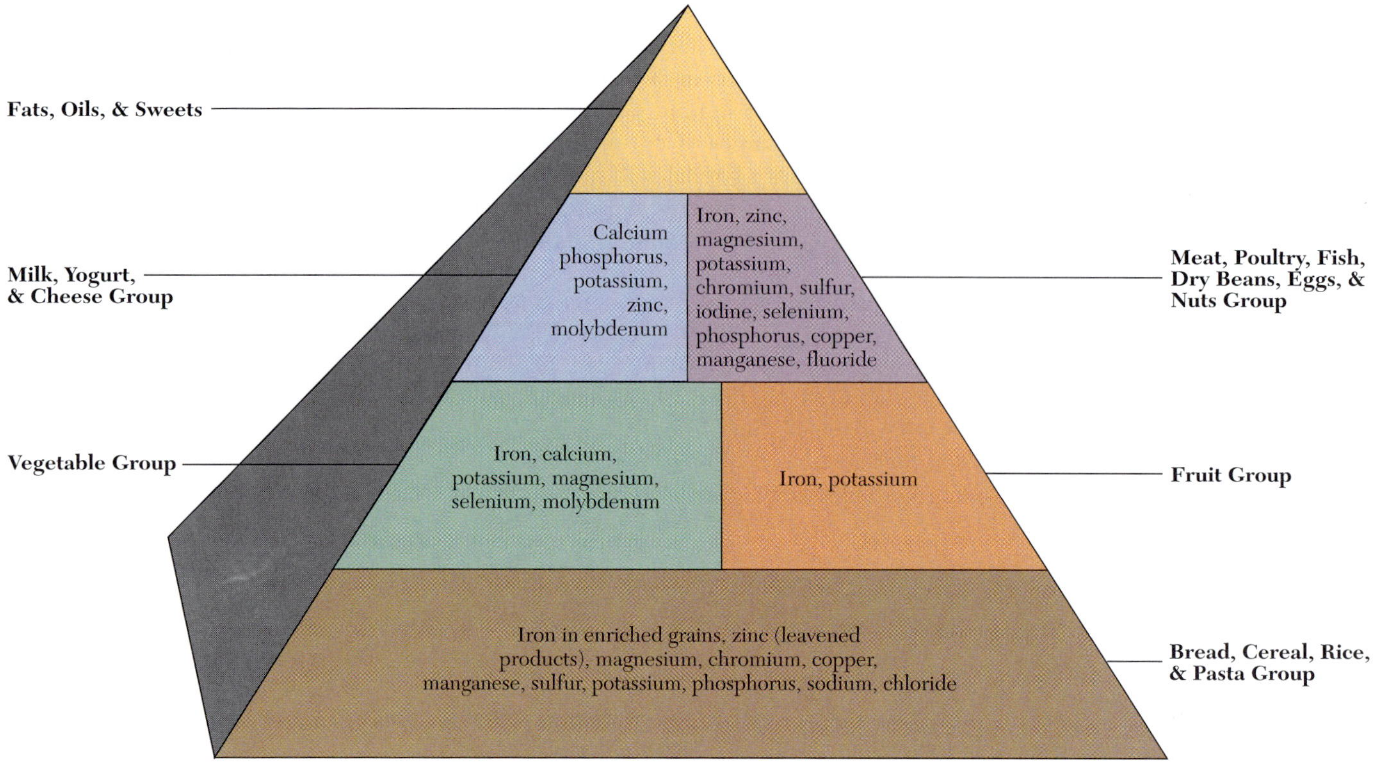

FIGURE 13.24 Each group of the Food Guide Pyramid includes foods that are good sources of minerals; good sources of all minerals are not found within any one group. The Meat, Poultry, Fish, Dry Beans, Eggs, and Nuts Group contributes the greatest variety of minerals because of the diverse types of foods—ranging from beef to legumes and nuts—found in this group.

arsenic, boron, nickel, silicon, and vanadium in human health for these to have been reviewed by the DRI committee.[7] Other trace elements that play a physiological role include aluminum, bromine, cadmium, germanium, lead, lithium, rubidium, and tin. The specific functions of these have not been defined and they have not been evaluated by the DRI committee. All the minerals, both those known to be essential and those that are still being assessed for their role in human health, can be obtained by choosing a variety of foods from each of the groups of the Food Guide Pyramid (Figure 13.24).

Arsenic (As)

Although we usually think of arsenic as a poison, the organic forms of arsenic that occur in foods are nontoxic. Dairy products, fish, meats, grains, cereal products, and fats and oils contribute to the arsenic content of the diet. It is hypothesized that arsenic is involved in the conversion of the amino acid methionine into compounds that affect heart function and cell growth.[73] A deficiency of arsenic depresses growth and impairs reproduction in several species of animals, and in humans it has been correlated with nervous system disorders, blood vessel diseases, and cancer.[74] There is not sufficient evidence to support a recommendation for arsenic intake and no UL has been set.[7]

Boron (B)

Boron in the forms of borax and boric acid was used as a preservative in fish, meats, and ham from the 1870s until the 1950s. It has been known to be essential in plants for almost 70 years, but only since the early 1980s has boron been recognized for its possible essentiality in the human diet. Foods of plant origin such as fruits, leafy vegetables, nuts, tubers, and legumes are rich sources of boron. Cider, wine, and beer are also high in boron, whereas meat, fish, and dairy products are poor sources. Drinking water can also contribute significant amounts of boron, depending on the geographical location.

Although the biochemical function of boron in humans is unknown, studies suggest that it is involved in vitamin D and estrogen metabolism. It has also been hypothesized that boron is involved in the maintenance of cell membranes and in cell communication. Boron deficiency symptoms have been demonstrated in animals and humans.[75] In the young, a deficiency retards growth. In adults, boron deficiency increases urinary excretion of calcium and magnesium and affects the levels of certain steroid hormones. However, there is not enough information available to make a recommendation for dietary intake.

Nutritional supplements containing boron are marketed as protection against osteoporosis. Because our understanding of the role of boron in bone formation and breakdown is in its infancy, a balanced diet, rather than supplements, is a safer way to ensure adequate boron intake. Surveys indicate that the average daily intake of boron is in the range of 1 to 2 mg per day.[75] No RDA or AI has been established. A UL has been set at 20 mg per day for adults based on the appearance of reproductive and developmental effects in animals.[7]

Nickel (Ni)

Good dietary sources of nickel include chocolate, nuts, legumes, and grains. Diets high in fat and foods of animal origin may be low in nickel. Nickel is thought to function in enzymes involved in the metabolism of certain fatty acids and amino acids, and it may play a role in folate metabolism.[76] It also affects the distribution and functioning of a number of other nutrients, including calcium, iron, zinc, and vitamin B_{12}. Nickel deficiency has been demonstrated in a number of animal species and results in depressed growth, impaired reproductive performance, and decreased plasma glucose levels.[77] Human intakes of nickel are generally less than 150 μg per day.[77] No RDA or AI has been established; the UL for adults has been set at 1 mg per day of soluble nickel salts.[7]

Silicon (Si)

Dietary silicon sources include whole-grain products and root vegetables. In animals silicon is involved in the synthesis of collagen and the calcification of bone, possibly by aiding in collagen cross-linking and in the initiation of bone mineralization.[73] Silicon deficiency has been reported in chickens and rats and results in abnormalities in bone and connective tissue, but there is not sufficient evidence to set a requirement for humans. No adverse health effects have been associated with the consumption of silicon that occurs naturally in food and water, so no UL has been set.[7]

Vanadium (V)

Food sources of vanadium include mushrooms, shellfish, black pepper, parsley, processed foods, grains, and grain products. Vanadium has been shown to have an insulin-like action and to stimulate cell proliferation and differentiation. In animals, deficiency has been shown to affect thyroid hormone metabolism and to increase abortion rates and decrease milk production in lactating animals. A requirement has not been established for humans.

Vanadium mimics insulin, and in patients with type 1 diabetes, high dose supplements have been shown to decrease insulin requirements. Supplements are also taken by athletes to increase muscle mass, but there is no good evidence of beneficial effects on body composition. In patients with type 1 diabetes, supplements decreased insulin requirements. The UL has been set at 1.8 mg per day of elemental vanadium.[7]

Summary

1. The amount of iron that is absorbed from the diet depends on the type of iron, other dietary components, and the body's need for iron. Much of the iron in animal-based food products is heme iron, an easily absorbable form. Nonheme iron, which is not well absorbed, comes from both animal and plant sources. If body iron stores are low, more iron is transported from the intestinal mucosa to body cells. When body stores are adequate, less iron is transported from the mucosa.
2. Iron functions as part of hemoglobin, which transports oxygen in the blood, and myoglobin, which enhances the amount of oxygen available for use during muscle contraction. When iron is deficient, adequate hemoglobin cannot be made, resulting in iron deficiency anemia—the most common nutritional deficiency worldwide. Iron is also a component of many other proteins, including some in the electron transport chain and the antioxidant enzyme catalase.
3. Iron can be toxic. Ingestion of a single large dose can be fatal. The accumulation of iron in the body over time causes heart and liver damage. The most common cause of chronic iron overload is hemochromatosis, a genetic disorder in which too much iron is absorbed.
4. Zinc absorption is regulated by metallothionein, a protein that binds zinc in the mucosal cells and limits how much can enter the blood. Since copper binds the same protein, an excess of zinc can stimulate metallothionein synthesis and trap copper in the mucosal cells, causing a copper deficiency.
5. Zinc is needed for the activity of many enzymes, including a form of the antioxidant enzyme superoxide dismutase that also requires copper. Many of the functions of zinc are related to its role in gene expression. Zinc is needed for tissue growth and repair, development of sex organs and bone, proper immune function, storage and release of insulin, mobilization of vitamin A from the liver, and stabilization of cell membranes. Good sources of zinc include red meats, eggs, dairy products, and whole grains. Zinc deficiency results in poor growth, delayed sexual maturation, skin changes, hair loss, skeletal abnormalities, and depressed immunity.
6. Copper functions in a number of important proteins that affect iron and lipid metabolism, synthesis of connective tissue, and antioxidant protection. The copper-containing protein ceruloplasmin is needed to convert iron into the form that can be transported. The richest sources of copper in the diet are organ meats. A copper deficiency can cause anemia and bone abnormalities.
7. Manganese is necessary for the activity of some enzymes, including a form of the antioxidant enzyme superoxide dismutase. Manganese is involved in carbohydrate and lipid metabolism and brain function. Good dietary sources include whole grains and nuts.
8. Selenium is necessary for the activity of the antioxidant enzyme glutathione peroxidase. Glutathione peroxidase destroys peroxides before they can form free radicals. Adequate dietary selenium reduces the need for vitamin E because it reduces free radical formation. Dietary sources include seafood, eggs, organ meats, and plant foods grown in selenium-rich soils. Severe selenium deficiency is rare except in regions with very low soil-selenium content and limited diets. In China, selenium deficiency is associated with a heart condition known as Keshan disease. Low selenium intake has been linked to increased cancer risk.
9. Iodine is an essential component of thyroid hormones, which control basal metabolic rate, growth, and development. The best sources of iodine in the diet are seafood, foods grown near the sea, and iodized salt.
10. When iodine is deficient, continued release of thyroid-stimulating hormone causes the thyroid gland to enlarge, forming a goiter. Iodine deficiency during pregnancy causes a condition in the offspring known as cretinism, which is characterized by growth failure and mental retardation. Iodine deficiency during childhood and adolescence can impair mental function. Although iodine deficiency is a world health problem, it has been virtually eliminated in North America through the use of iodized salt.
11. Fluoride is necessary for the maintenance of bones and teeth. Adequate dietary fluoride helps prevent dental caries. Most of the fluoride in the diet in the United States comes from fluoridated drinking water and toothpaste. Tea is a major source of fluoride around the world.
12. Chromium is needed for normal insulin action and glucose utilization. It is found in liver, brewer's yeast, nuts, and whole grains.
13. Molybdenum is a cofactor for enzymes involved in the metabolism of amino acids and other nitrogen-containing compounds such as DNA and RNA.
14. There is evidence that arsenic, boron, nickel, silicon, and vanadium may be essential in humans as well as animals. These trace elements may be necessary in small amounts but can be toxic if consumed in excess.

Review Questions

1. List several good sources of iron in the diet. Which contain heme iron?
2. Discuss three factors that affect iron absorption.
3. Explain why iron deficiency causes red blood cells to be small and pale.
4. List three life-stage groups at risk for iron deficiency anemia.
5. What is hemochromatosis?
6. Why is zinc important for protein synthesis?
7. Explain why a copper deficiency can contribute to anemia.
8. What is the role of selenium in the body?
9. Why does selenium decrease the need for vitamin E?
10. What is a goiter and why does it form?
11. How does fluoride function in dental health?
12. What is the role of chromium in the body?

Applying Critical Thinking Skills

Personal nutrition:

1. Using the three-day food intake record you kept in Chapter 2:
   a. Calculate your average daily intake of iron.
   b. How does your iron intake compare with the recommendation for someone of your age and sex?
   c. If your intake is low, suggest modifications to your diet that will increase intake to meet the RDA for someone your age and sex.
   d. If your diet already meets the recommendations for iron, make a list of foods you like that are good sources of iron.
   e. Identify the major food sources of iron in your diet and indicate whether they contribute heme iron.
2. Using the three-day food intake record you kept in Chapter 2:
   a. Calculate your average daily intake of zinc.
   b. If you eliminated meat from your diet, would you meet the RDA for zinc?
   c. What foods could you substitute for meat that are good sources of zinc?
3. Using the Internet, search for information on a supplement discussed in this chapter—for instance, zinc lozenges or chromium picolinate.
   a. How does the information compare to the discussion in the text?
   b. Who provided the information? Does it promote the sale of a product?
   c. Is the information supported by scientific studies?

General nutrition issues:

1. A hospitalized patient is receiving a TPN solution containing the recommended amounts of all the vitamins and major minerals as well as the trace elements iron, zinc, iodine, manganese, chromium, and molybdenum.
   a. For which trace element deficiencies is the patient at risk if he needs to remain on TPN for an extended period of time?
   b. For each nutrient for which the patient is at risk of deficiency, indicate what symptoms might appear.
2. A researcher asked his new technician to prepare a diet for his laboratory animals. The technician is interrupted several times while mixing the diet and is unfamiliar with the scale he is using to weigh the diet ingredients. After the diet is fed to the animals for several months they begin to show signs of anemia. An error in diet preparation is suspected. The diet ingredients are:

   Starch, Sucrose, Casein (protein), Corn oil, Mixed plant fibers, Vitamin A, Vitamin D, Vitamin E ,Vitamin K, B vitamin mix, Calcium, Sodium, Potassium, Magnesium, Chloride, Zinc, Iron, Iodine, Selenium, Copper, Manganese, Chromium, Molybdenum

   a. What trace element deficiencies can cause anemia?
   b. What trace element excess could cause anemia?
   c. What vitamin deficiencies can cause anemia?
   d. What dietary components can affect the absorption of trace elements?

References

1. Underwood, B. A. Micronutrient malnutrition: is it being eliminated? Nutr. Today 33:121–129, 1998.
2. Centers for Disease Control and Prevention. Recommendations to prevent and control iron deficiency in the United States. MMWR Morb. Mortal. Wkly. Rep. 47:1–29, 1998. Available online at **http://www.cdc.gov/mmwr/mmwr_wk.html**. Accessed 20 Jan 2001.
3. Lynch, S. R. Interaction of iron with other nutrients. Nutr. Rev. 55:102–110, 1997.
4. Bothwell, T. H. Overview and mechanisms of iron regulation. Nutr. Rev. 53:237–245, 1995.
5. Whiting, S. J. The inhibitory effect of dietary calcium on iron bioavailability: a cause for concern? Nutr. Rev. 53:77–80, 1995.
6. Kuhn, L. C. Iron and gene expression: molecular mechanisms regulating cellular iron homeostasis. Nutr. Rev. 56:S11–S19, 1998.
7. Food and Nutrition Board, Institute of Medicine. *Dietary Reference Intakes: Vitamin A, Vitamin K, Arsenic, Boron, Chromium, Copper, Iodine, Iron, Manganese, Molybdenum, Nickel, Silicon, Vanadium, and Zinc*. Washington, D.C: National Academy Press, 2001.
8. AAP (American Academy of Pediatrics). Iron fortification of infant formulas. Pediatr. 104:119–123, 1999.
9. Allen, L. H. Pregnancy and iron deficiency: unresolved issues. Nutr. Rev. 55:91–101, 1997.
10. Guthrie, J. F., and Achwenk, N. E. Current issues related to iron status: implications for nutrition education and policy. USDA, Family Economics and Nutrition Review 9:2–19, 1996.
11. Iron-containing supplements and drugs: label warning statements and unit-dose packaging requirements. Federal Register, January 1997.
12. Klipstein-Grobusch, K., Koster, J. F., Grobbee, D. E., et al. Serum ferritin and the risk of myocardial infarction in the elderly: The Rotterdam Study. Am. J. Clin. Nutr. 69:1231–1236, 1999.
13. Corti, M. C., Gaxiano, M., and Hennekens, C. H. Iron status and risk of cardiovascular disease. Ann. Epidemiol. 7:62–68, 1997.
14. Halliday, J. W. Hemochromatosis and iron needs. Nutr. Rev. 56(II):S30–S37, 1998.
15. Iron overload disorders among Hispanics—San Diego, California, 1995, MMWR Morb. Mortal. Wkly. Rep. 45:991–993, 1996.
16. Edwards, C. Q., Griffin. L. M., Ajioka, R. S., and Kushner, J. P. Screening for hemochromatosis: phenotype versus genotype. Semin. Hematol. 35:72–76, 1998.
17. Hollan, S. Iron overload in light of the identification of a haemochromatosis gene. Haematologia (Budap) 28:109–116, 1997.
18. Prasad, A. S. Discovery of human zinc deficiency and studies in an experimental human model. Am. J. Clin. Nutr. 53:403–412, 1991.
19. King, J. C., and Keen, C. L. Zinc. In *Moderan Nutrition in Health and Disease*, 9th ed. Shils, M. E., Olson, J. A., Shike, M., and Ross A. C., eds. Baltimore: Williams & Wilkins, 1999, 223–239.
20. Lönnerdal, B. Dietary factors influencing zinc absorption. J. Nutr. 130:1378S–1383S, 2000.
21. Leonard, B. M. Nutrition and immunity in the elderly: modification of immune responses with nutritional treatments. Am. J. Clin. Nutr. 66(suppl):478S–484S, 1997.
22. Shankar, A. H., and Prasad, A. S. Zinc and immune function: the biological basis of altered resistance to infection. Am. J. Clin. Nutr. 68(suppl):447S–463S, 1998.

23. Christina, P., and West, K. P. Interactions between zinc and vitamin A: an update. Am. J. Clin. Nutr. 68(suppl.):435S–441S, 1998.
24. Briefel, R. R., Bialostosky, K., Kennedy-Stephenson, J., et al. Zinc intake of the U.S. population: findings from the Third National Health and Nutrition Examination Survey, 1988–1994. J. Nutr. 130:1367S–1373S, 2000.
25. Aggett, P. J., and Comerford, J. G. Zinc and human health. Nutr. Rev. 53:S16–S22, 1995.
26. Black, R. E. Preface: zinc for child health. Am. J. Clin. Nutr. 68(suppl):409S, 1998.
27. Fraker, P. J., King, L. E., Laakko, T., and Vollmer, T. L. The dynamic link between the integrity of the immune system and zinc status. J. Nutr. 130: 1399S–1406S, 2000.
28. Sandstead, H. H. Requirements and toxicity of essential trace elements, illustrated by zinc and copper. Am. J. Clin. Nutr. 61(suppl):621S–624S, 1995.
29. Bogden, J. D. Studies on micronutrient supplements and immunity in older people. Nutr. Rev. 53:S59–S65, 1995.
30. Novick, S. G., Godfrey, J. C., Pollack, R. L., and Wilder, H. R. Zinc-induced suppression of inflammation in the respiratory tract caused by infection with human rhinovirus and other irritants. Med. Hypotheses 49:347–357, 1997.
31. Jackson, J. L., Lesho, E., and Peterson, C. Zinc and the common cold: a meta-analysis revisited. J. Nutr. 130:1512S–1515S, 2000.
32. Mills, E. S. The treatment of idiopathic (hypochromic) anemia with iron and copper. Can. Med. Assoc. J. 22:175–178, 1930.
33. Wapnir, R. A. Copper absorption and bioavailability. Am. J. Clin. Nutr. 67(suppl):1054S–1060S, 1998.
34. Turnlund, J. R. Copper. In *Modern Nutrition in Health and Disease*, 9th ed. Shils, M. E., Olson, J. A., Shike, M., and Ross, A. C., eds. Baltimore: Williams & Wilkins, 1999, 241–252.
35. Uauy, R., Olivares, M., and Gonzales, M. Essentiality of copper in humans. Am. J. Clin. Nutr. 67(suppl):952S–959S, 1998.
36. Johnson, M. A., Smith, M. M., and Edmonds, J. T. Copper, iron, zinc, and manganese in dietary supplements, infant formulas, and ready-to-eat breakfast cereals. Am. J. Clin. Nutr. 67(suppl):1035S–1040S, 1998.
37. Milne, D. B. Copper intake and assessment of copper status. Am. J. Clin. Nutr. 67(suppl):1041S–1045S, 1998.
38. Kelley, D. S., Daudu, P. A., Taylor, P. C., et al. Effects of low-copper diets on human immune response. Am. J. Clin. Nutr. 62:412–416, 1995.
39. Percival, S. S. Copper and immunity. Am. J. Clin. Nutr. 67(suppl): 1064S–1068S, 1998.
40. World Health Organization. Copper. In *Trace Elements in Human Nutrition and Health*. Geneva: World Health Organization, 1996, 123–143.
41. Finley, J. Manganese absorption and retention by young women is associated with serum ferritin concentration. Am. J. Clin. Nutr. 70:37–43, 1999.
42. Finley, J. W., and Davis, C. D. Manganese deficiency and toxicity: are high or low dietary amounts of manganese cause for concern? Biofactors 10:15–24, 1999.
43. Friedman, B. J., Freeland-Graves, J. H., Bales, C. W., et al. Manganese balance and clinical observations in young men fed a manganese-deficient diet. J. Nutr. 117:133–143, 1987.
44. Food and Nutrition Board, Institute of Medicine. *Dietary Reference Intakes for Vitamin C, Vitamin E, Selenium, and Carotenoids*. Washington, D.C.: National Academy Press, 2000.
45. Levander, O. A., and Beck, M. A. Interacting nutritional and infectious etiologies of Keshan disease: insights from coxsackie virus B-induced myocarditis in mice deficient in selenium or vitamin E. Biol. Trace Elem. Res. 56:5–21, 1997.
46. Levander, O. A., and Beck, M. A. Selenium and viral virulence. Br. Med. Bull. 55:528–533, 1999.
47. Clark, L. C., Combs, G. F. Jr., Turnbull, B. W., et al. Effect of selenium supplementation for cancer prevention in patients with carcinoma of the skin. JAMA 276:1957–1968, 1996.
48. Yoshizawa, K., Willett, W. C. Morris, S. J., et al. Study of prediagnostic selenium level in toenails and the risk of advanced prostate cancer. J. Natl. Cancer Inst. 90:1219–1224, 1999.
49. Harrison, P. R., Lanfear, J., Wu, L., et al. Chemopreventive and growth inhibitory effects of selenium. Biomed. Environ. Sci. 10:235–245. 1997.
50. Helzlsouer, K., Jacobs, R., and Morris, S. Acute selenium intoxication in the United States. Fed. Proc. 44:1670, 1985.
51. Rao, P. S., and Lakshmy, R. Role of goitrogens in iodine deficiency disorders and brain development. Indian J. Med. Res. 102:223–226, 1995.
52. Underwood, B. A. From research to global reality: the micronutrient story. J. Nutr. 128:145–151, 1998.
53. van der Haar, F. The challenge of the global elimination of iodine deficiency disorders. Eur. J. Clin. Nutr. 51(suppl):S3–S8, 1997.
54. Furnee, C. A. Prevention and control of iodine deficiency: a review of a study on the effectiveness of oral iodized oil in Malawi. Eur. J. Clin. Nutr. 51(suppl):S9–S10, 1998.
55. Stanbury, J. B., Ermans, A. E., Bourdoux, P., et al. Iodine-induced hyperthyroidism: occurrence and epidemiology. Thyroid 8:83–100, 1998.
56. Food and Nutrition Board, Institute of Medicine. *Dietary Reference Intakes for Calcium, Phosphorus, Magnesium, Vitamin D, and Fluoride*. Washington, D.C.: National Academy Press, 1997.
57. ADA (American Dental Association) Council on Dental Therapeutics. New Fluoride guidelines proposed. J. Am. Dent. Assoc. 125:366, 1994.
58. Pak, C. Y., Sakhaec, K., and Zerwekh, J. E. Sustained-release sodium fluoride in the management of established menopausal osteoporosis. Am. J. Med. Sci. 313:23–32, 1997.
59. Horowitz, H. S. The effectiveness of community water fluoridation in the United States. J. Pub. Hlth. Dent. 56:253–258, 1996.
60. American Dental Association. Fluoridation facts. Available online at **http://www.ada.org/public/topics/fluoride/facts-intro.html**. Accessed 1 Jan 2001.
61. Featherstone, J. D. Prevention and reversal of dental caries: role of low level fluoride. Community Dent. Oral. Epidemiol. 27:31–40, 1999.
62. Vincent, J. B. The biochemistry of chromium. J. Nutr. 130:715–718, 2000.
63. Anderson, R. A. Recent advances in the clinical and biochemical manifestations of chromium deficiency in human and animal nutrition. J. Trace Elem. Exp. Med. 11:241–250, 1998.
64. Anderson, R. A. Chromium as an essential nutrient for humans. Regul. Toxicol. Pharmacol. 26:S35–S41, 1997.
65. Anderson, R. A., Cheng, N., Bryden, N. A., et al. Elevated intakes of supplemental chromium improve glucose and insulin variables in individuals with type 2 diabetes. Diabetes 46:1786–1791, 1997.
66. Lukaski, H. C. Chromium as a supplement. Ann. Rev. Nutr. 19:279–301, 1999.
67. Jeejeebhoy, K. N. The role of chromium in nutrition and therapeutics and as a potential toxin. Nutr. Rev. 57:329–335, 1999.
68. Stearns, D. M., Wise, J. P. Sr., Patierno, S. R., and Wetterhahn, K. E. Chromium (III) picolinate produces chromosome damage in Chinese hamster ovary cells. FASEB J. 9:1643–1648, 1995.
69. Speetjens, J. K., Collins, R. A., Vincent, J. B., and Woski, S. A. The nutritional supplement chromium (III) tris(picolinate) cleaves DNA. Chem. Res. Toxicol. 12:483–487, 1999.
70. Kato, I., Vogelman, J. H., Dilman, V., et al. Effect of supplementation with chromium picolinate on antibody titers to 5-hydroxymethyl uracil. Eur. J. Epidemiol. 14:621–626, 1998.
71. Turnland, J. R., and Keys, W. R. Dietary molybdenum: effect on copper absorption, excretion, and status in young men. In *Trace Elements in Man and Animals 10*. Roussel, A. M., Anderson, R. A., and Favier, A., eds. New York: Kluwer Academic, 2000.
72. Mertz, W. Risk assessment of essential trace elements: new approaches to setting recommended dietary allowances and safe limits. Nutr. Rev. 53:179–185, 1995.

73. Uthus, E. O., and Seaborn, C. D. Deliberations and evaluations of the approaches, endpoints and paradigms for dietary recommendations of other trace elements. J. Nutr. 126:2452S–2459S, 1996.
74. Mayer, D. R., Kosmus, W., Beyer, W., et al. Serum arsenic and selenium concentrations in hemodialysis patients: correlations to associated diseases. In *Trace Elements in Nutrition and Health*. Abdulla, M., Vohora, S. B., and Athar, M., eds. New Delhi: Wiley Eastern Limited, 1995, 41–48.
75. Hunt, C. D., and Stoecker, B. J. Deliberations and evaluations of the approaches, endpoints and paradigms for boron, chromium, and fluoride dietary recommendations. J. Nutr. 126:2441S–2451S, 1996.
76. Uthus, E. O., and Poellot, R. A. Dietary folate affects the response of rats to nickel deprivation. Biol. Trace Elem. Res. 52:23–35, 1996.
77. Nielsen, F. H. Other trace elements. In *Present Knowledge in Nutrition*, 7th ed. Ziegler, E. E., and Filer, L. J. Jr., eds. Washington, D.C.: ILSI Press, 1996, 353–377.

14 Nutrition and Exercise

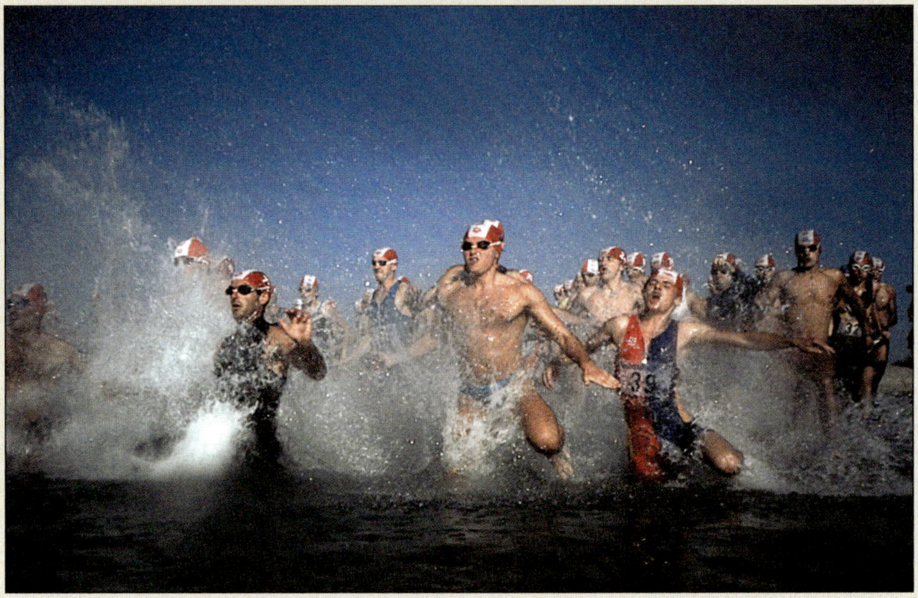

Learning Objectives

After reading this chapter, students should be able to:

1. Discuss the interactions among nutrition, exercise, and fitness.
2. Define fitness and describe the characteristics of a fit individual.
3. Describe the components of a well-planned exercise regimen.
4. Explain why the availability of oxygen determines which nutrients are used to produce ATP.
5. Discuss how the intensity and duration of exercise affect nutrient utilization.
6. Compare nutrient utilization during exercise in well-trained athletes with that of sedentary individuals.
7. Contrast the macronutrient intake recommended for athletes with that for sedentary individuals.
8. List the nutrients at risk for deficiency in athletes and discuss why they are likely to be deficient.
9. Explain the recommendations for fluid intake during exercise.
10. Discuss how nutrient intake before, during, and after competition can affect athletic performance.
11. Do a risk/benefit analysis of an ergogenic aid.

As Tour de France champion Lance Armstrong pedaled his bicycle up the last 6 kilometers of a mountain in the French Alps, his normally smooth pedal stroke became choppy. Other riders caught him and passed him and he did not respond. He later called this "the hardest day of my life on the bike."

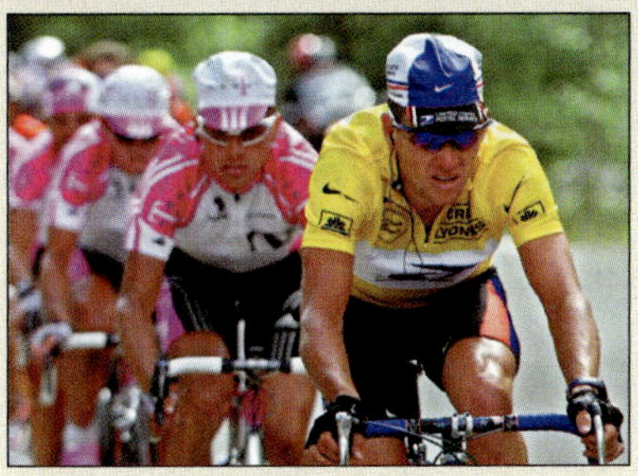

Just seven days earlier he had taken the lead while climbing the last mountain of a ride that included four such climbs. In the final 12 miles of that ascent, which rose up a 7.9% grade, he had amazed sports enthusiasts by accelerating past the best cyclists in the world as if they were standing still. Through the next five days in the mountains he continued at a strong pace, gaining time over his closest rivals. But on this day and this climb he was exhausted and falling farther behind as he pedaled along in low gear. What was wrong with the defending champion and leader of the 2000 Tour de France? The key to understanding his difficulty came in an interview after the day's ride, when he said, "I didn't eat enough, and I had no energy."

The Tour de France requires cyclists to ride over 2000 miles in 23 days with only 2 days' rest. The route climbs through the Pyrenees and the Alps. Tour de France athletes spend 5 or 6 hours on the bike, often riding 100 to 150 miles a day. It is arguably the most grueling sports event on the planet.

What does an athlete need to eat and drink to fuel such intense, prolonged activity? When the cook for the U.S. Postal Service team that Armstrong rides with was asked what they eat, his answer was "pasta and more pasta." The cook had 88 pounds of pasta with him and would need to buy more along the way. To meet the energy demands of the Tour, cyclists consume 6000–7000 kcalories per day. All that pasta may indeed be an important part of their success, but peak performance also depends on when the food and drink is consumed. What an athlete eats before the event, during the event, and afterward affects performance, particularly in a competition like the Tour de France, in which athletes need to perform strenuous endurance exercise day after day. Adequate nutrition is needed both to fuel the day's activity and to ensure success the following day. On this particular day in the Alps, Armstrong was low on energy. But he recovered by refueling and rehydrating, and the next day he again looked like the leader of the Tour. He ultimately rode victorious into Paris as the winner of his second consecutive Tour de France. Most of us will never participate in an event as demanding as this, but proper nutrition is important for ensuring the fuel and fitness levels needed for the events of our daily lives.

Nutrition, Exercise, and Fitness

Fitness is defined as the ability to perform routine physical activity without undue fatigue. For some, fitness means being able to easily walk around the block, mow the lawn, or play with their children. For others, fitness means optimal performance of strenuous exercise. For everyone, nutrient intake and exercise affect fitness and, in turn, fitness affects nutrient needs, exercise ability, and overall health. The right mixture of nutrients is essential to performance whether you are a marathon runner or a mall walker. For every exerciser, the diet must

Fitness The ability to perform routine physical activity without undue fatigue.

provide sufficient energy from the appropriate sources to fuel activity, protein to maintain muscle mass, micronutrients to allow the utilization of energy-containing nutrients, and water to transport nutrients and cool the body. By increasing energy output exercise increases energy needs. The additional food consumed to meet these needs also increases micronutrient intake. Exercise improves overall health by strengthening the cardiovascular system and helping to maintain muscle tone at a level that optimizes function and prevents injury.

Parameters of Fitness

Being fit means maintaining cardiorespiratory endurance, muscle strength and endurance, flexibility, and a healthy body composition. These parameters are important to every aspect and task of daily life and help to define an individual's level of overall fitness.

Cardiorespiratory system The circulatory and respiratory systems, which together deliver oxygen and nutrients to cells.

Aerobic exercise Exercise such as jogging, swimming, or cycling that increases heart rate and requires oxygen in metabolism. This type of exercise improves cardiovascular fitness.

Stroke volume The volume of blood pumped by each beat of the heart.

Resting heart rate The number of times that the heart beats per minute while a person is at rest.

Maximum heart rate The maximum number of beats per minute that the heart can attain. It declines with age and can be estimated by subtracting age in years from 220.

Maximal oxygen consumption or **VO_2 max** The maximum amount of oxygen that can be consumed by the tissues during exercise.

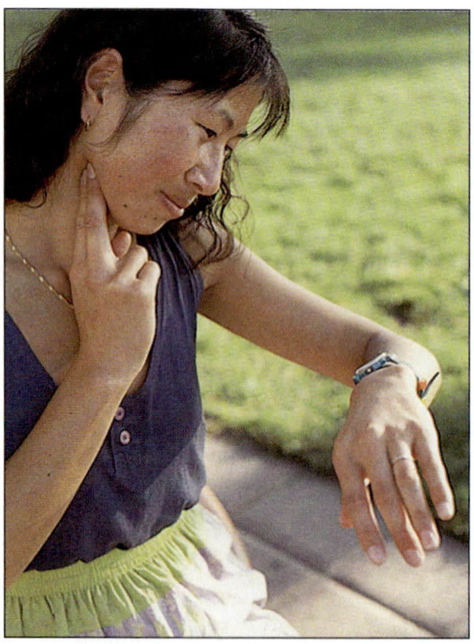

FIGURE 14.1 Heart rate can be estimated by feeling the pulse at the side of the neck just below the jaw bone. A pulse is caused by the heart beating and forcing blood through the arteries. The number of pulses per minute equals heart rate. (*© Michael Newman/PhotoEdit*)

Cardiorespiratory Endurance Cardiorespiratory endurance determines how long one can continue a task, whether it is climbing stairs, raking leaves, or running a race. It requires muscle strength but also involves the cardiovascular and respiratory systems, referred to jointly as the **cardiorespiratory system.** Endurance is increased by **aerobic exercise,** the type of exercise that increases the heart rate and uses oxygen.

Regular aerobic exercise strengthens heart muscle and increases **stroke volume,** which is the amount of blood pumped with each beat of the heart. As the amount pumped with each beat increases, the number of times per minute the heart needs to beat to deliver the same amount of blood decreases. This in turn decreases the **resting heart rate,** which is the rate at which the heart must beat to supply blood to the tissues at rest. Resting heart rate can be measured by counting the number of pulses, or heartbeats, per minute while at rest (Figure 14.1). An average adult has a resting heart rate of about 70; conditioned athletes have a resting heart rate of about 50. The more fit a person is, the lower their resting heart rate and pulse are and the more activity they can perform before reaching **maximum heart rate.** Maximum heart rate is the maximum number of beats per minute that the heart can attain. It is dependent on age and can be estimated by subtracting one's age from 220.

By strengthening the heart, aerobic exercise also increases **maximal oxygen consumption,** or **VO_2 max,** which is the maximum amount of oxygen that can be consumed by the body's cells during exercise. VO_2 max is dependent on the ability of the cardiorespiratory system to deliver oxygen to the cells and the ability of the cells to use oxygen to produce energy. The greater the VO_2 max, the more intense the activity a person can engage in before a lack of oxygen affects performance. VO_2 max can be determined in an exercise laboratory by measuring oxygen uptake during exercise. To perform this measurement, an individual may be asked to run on a treadmill while the air breathed is measured (Figure 14.2). Oxygen consumption or uptake is calculated by subtracting the amount of oxygen exhaled from the amount of oxygen inhaled. The workload is then increased by increasing the speed and/or grade of the treadmill until the individual is too fatigued to continue. The amount of oxygen consumed at the highest workload achieved is the VO_2 max. A trained athlete will have a greater VO_2 max than an untrained individual.

In order to increase cardiorespiratory endurance, exercise should be performed at a heart rate of 60 to 90% of maximum (maximum heart rate = 220 − age). For example, a 40-year-old person would need to exercise at an intensity that keeps the heart rate between 108 and 162 beats per minute (Figure 14.3). A good rule of thumb for determining if an activity is at an aerobic intensity is that the exerciser should be able to carry on a conversation but not sing while exercising. Potentially aerobic activities include walking, dancing, jogging, cross-country skiing, cycling, and swimming. The intensity at which these activities need to be

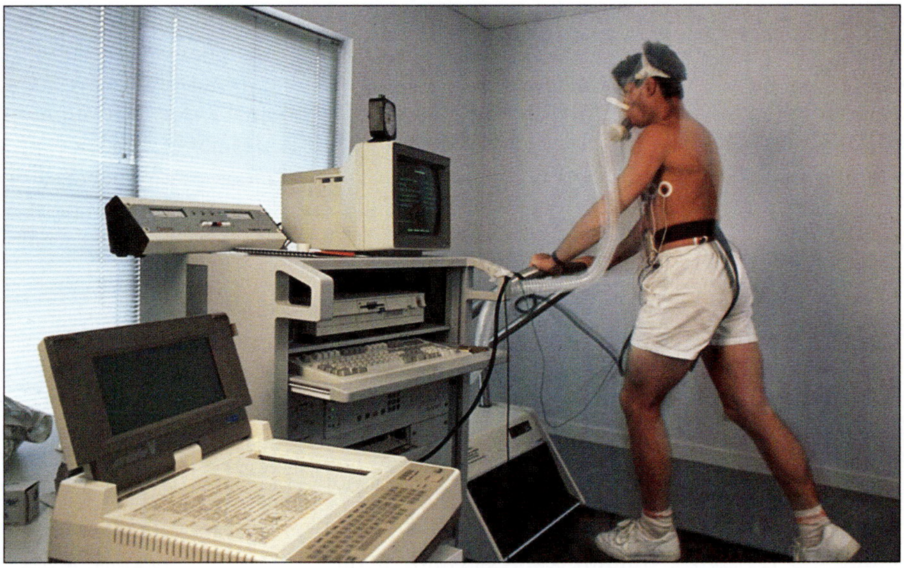

FIGURE 14.2 Maximal oxygen consumption can be estimated by measuring oxygen uptake while running to exhaustion on a treadmill. *(© Jon Love/The Image Bank)*

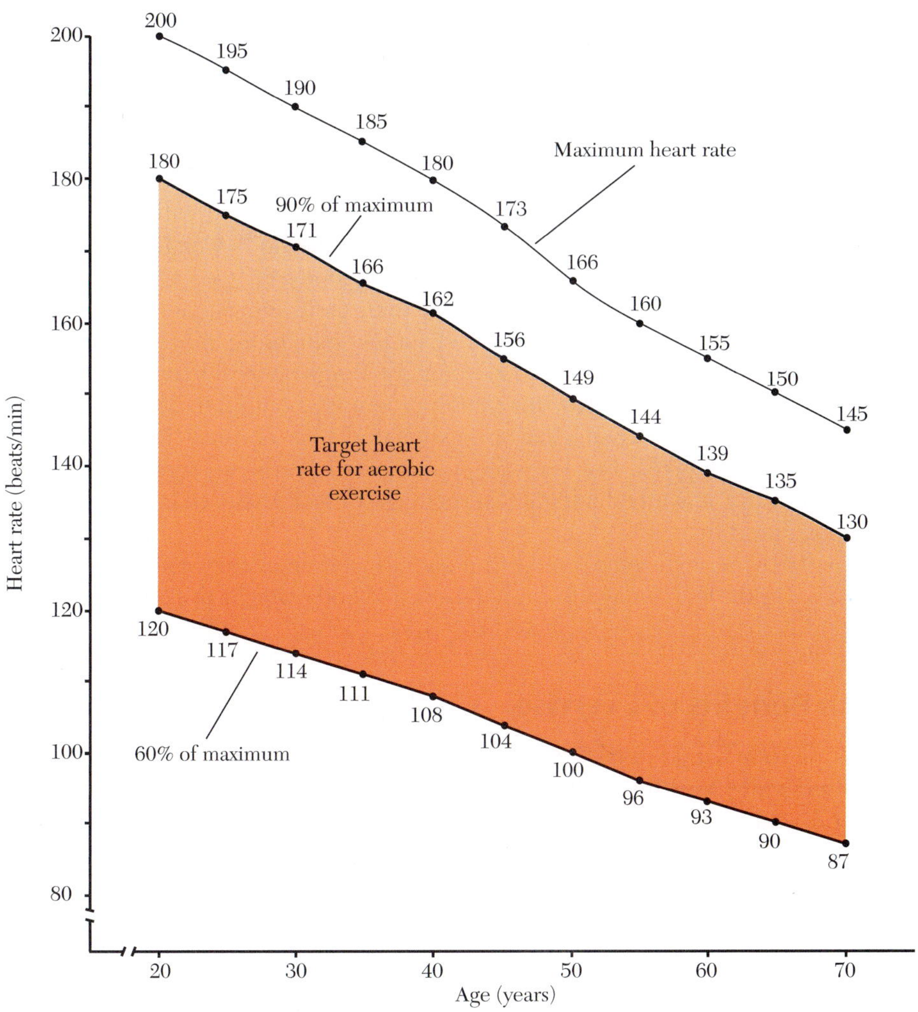

FIGURE 14.3 The orange area represents the target heart rate for aerobic exercise—between 60 and 90% of maximum heart rate. Exercise performed at this level will benefit cardiovascular health. (Adapted from McArdle, W. D., Katch, F. I., and Katch, V. L. *Exercise Physiology: Energy, Nutrition, and Human Performance,* 3rd ed. Philadelphia: Lea & Febiger, 1991.)

performed to be aerobic depends on the individual and how well trained they are. An individual beginning an exercise program might easily get an aerobic workout from a walk around the neighborhood, but this would barely raise the heart rate of a seasoned athlete. If the intensity of the activity is too low, it does not improve cardiorespiratory fitness. If the activity is too intense, it is also not aerobic because oxygen cannot be delivered and used quickly enough to meet energy needs. For example, running at a pace of 6 minutes per mile may keep the heart rate of a marathon runner in the aerobic range but would exceed the VO_2 max of a weekend jogger.

Muscle Strength and Endurance Muscle strength and endurance enhance the ability to perform tasks such as pushing or lifting. In daily life, this could mean lifting a bag of groceries, unscrewing the lid of a jar, or shoveling snow. For an athlete, this can mean being able to lift a greater amount of weight, apply more force to a bicycle pedal, or pull harder in a swimming stroke. Muscle strength and endurance are increased by repeatedly using muscles in activities that require moving against a resisting force. This type of exercise is called strength-training or resistance-training exercise and includes activities such as weight lifting.

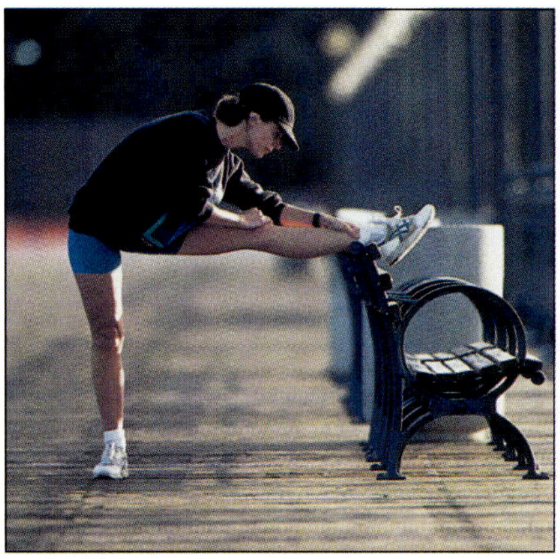

FIGURE 14.4 Stretching muscles to increase and maintain flexibility is an important component of any exercise regimen. *(© David Madison/Tony Stone Images)*

Flexibility Flexibility determines range of motion—how far one can bend and stretch muscles and ligaments. If flexibility is poor, one cannot bend easily to tie shoelaces or stretch to remove packages from the car. Increased flexibility makes day-to-day tasks easier and reduces the risk of injury. Regularly moving the limbs, neck, and torso through their full ranges of motion helps increase and maintain flexibility (Figure 14.4).

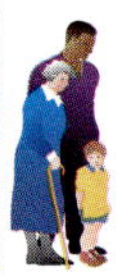

Body Composition Individuals who are physically fit have a greater proportion of lean body tissue than unfit individuals of the same body weight. Lean body mass can be assessed by measuring the percent body fat (see Chapter 7). In general, women have more stored body fat than men. During adolescence, females gain proportionately more fat and males gain more muscle mass. For young adult women, the desirable percent of body fat is 20 to 30% of total weight; in young adult men, the desirable percent is about 12 to 20%.[1] The proportions of lean and fat tissue that are associated with optimal fitness also depend on individual goals. For example, a competitive athlete, such as a runner or a weight lifter, may need a higher percentage of lean tissue than a nonathlete to be considered fit.

Lean body mass decreases in both men and women as they age, and there is an increase in the percentage of body fat even if body weight remains the same. Some of this change can be prevented by physical activity.

Health Benefits of Exercise

In addition to making the tasks of everyday life easier, fitness through regular activity offers many health benefits (Table 14.1). A regular exercise program makes it easier to maintain a healthy body weight; helps to maintain muscles, bones, and joints; and reduces the risk of osteoporosis. It can also help to prevent or delay the onset of cardiovascular disease, hypertension, diabetes, and cancer. And, it can improve mood and prevent depression.[2]

Healthy Body Weight A regular program of balanced physical activity increases the amount of energy expended in activity and helps to limit or reduce body fat and maintain or increase the proportion of lean tissue. Because lean body tissue is more metabolically active than adipose tissue, having more lean body mass increases the energy needed for resting metabolic rate (Figure 14.5). The combination of increased energy needs for physical activity and a rise in

TABLE 14.1 The Benefits of Fitness

- Increases endurance by increasing the amount of blood and consequently oxygen delivered to the tissues.
- Strengthens the heart muscle and increases stroke volume.
- Decreases resting heart rate and consequently the amount of work required by the heart at rest.
- Increases the amount of activity that can be performed before reaching maximum heart rate.
- Increases VO_2 max, which enables more intense activity to be performed before a lack of oxygen affects performance.
- Improves circulation.
- Increases the amount of weight that can be lifted or pushed, the number of times a movement can be repeated without fatigue, and how far muscles and ligaments can comfortably be stretched.
- Increases energy expenditure, making it easier to maintain a healthy body weight and composition.
- Lowers blood pressure and increases HDL cholesterol levels in the blood, both of which reduce the risk of cardiovascular disease.
- Increases peak bone mass and prevents bone loss.
- Improves glucose tolerance and insulin sensitivity, which can reduce the risk of diabetes and help reduce medication dose in those who have the disease.
- Helps arthritic joints move more easily.
- Reduces the risk of certain types of cancer.
- Improves sleep patterns and reduces depression.

RMR increases the amount of energy one can consume while maintaining a healthy body weight. Resting metabolic rate also rises for a number of hours after an exercise session; however, the increase in RMR after light to moderate exercise is too small to have a significant effect on energy balance or weight loss.[3]

Exercise is an essential component of any weight-reduction program. It increases energy needs, promotes the loss of body fat, and slows the loss of lean tissue that can occur with energy restriction. Individuals who participate in regular moderate-intensity physical activities lose weight more rapidly than those who diet without exercising.[4]

Cardiovascular Disease Exercise reduces the risk of cardiovascular disease.[5] Aerobic exercise strengthens the heart muscle, thereby reducing resting heart rate and decreasing the heart's workload. Exercise may also lower blood pressure and increase HDL cholesterol levels in the blood, both of which reduce the risk of cardiovascular disease.[6]

Diabetes People with excess body fat are more likely to develop type 2 diabetes. By keeping body fat within the normal range, aerobic exercise can decrease the risk of developing diabetes. Physical activity that includes both aerobic exercise and strength training is also important in the treatment of type 2 diabetes. It is recommended that people with type 2 diabetes expend 1000 kcalories per week in physical activity.[7] This amount of exercise can improve glucose tolerance and insulin sensitivity, enhance muscle strength and endurance, flexibility, and body composition, and decrease risk factors for cardiovascular disease.[7] Exercise can also reduce or eliminate the need for medication to maintain normal blood glucose levels. Regular, rather than sporadic, physical activity is necessary because the effects of exercise on blood glucose levels and insulin sensitivity disappear within 72 hours of the last exercise session. Because exercise can affect energy requirements and medication needs, individuals with diabetes should develop exercise programs with the help of physicians and dietitians.

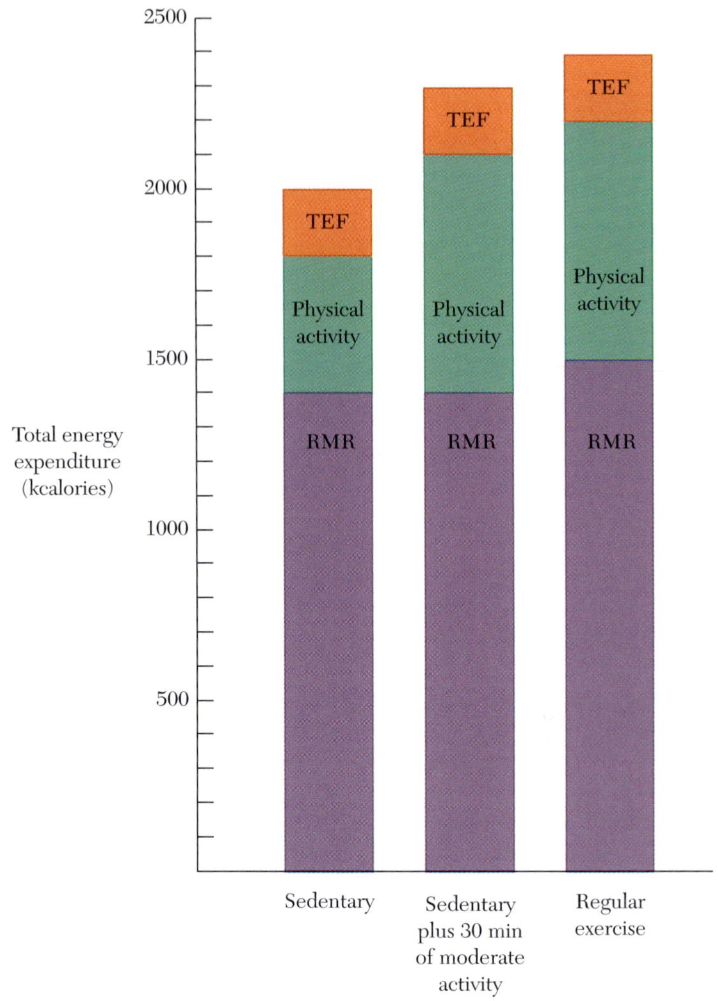

FIGURE 14.5 Total energy expenditure is the sum of resting metabolic rate (RMR), physical activity, and the thermic effect of food (TEF). Exercise increases energy expenditure. When a sedentary individual adds 30 minutes of moderate-intensity exercise, their total energy expenditure may increase by as much as 300 kcalories per day. When this individual continues the added exercise as part of their daily routine, their muscle mass increases causing a rise in resting metabolic rate, which further increases total energy expenditure. If energy intake does not increase, weight loss will occur.

Osteoporosis and Joint Disorders Exercise reduces the risk of osteoporosis. One of the causes of bone loss is lack of use; therefore, weight-bearing exercise such as walking, running, and aerobic dance can increase peak bone mass and also prevent bone loss (see Chapter 12). Exercise can also benefit individuals with arthritis because the strength and flexibility promoted by exercise help arthritic joints move more easily.

Cancer Individuals who exercise regularly may be reducing their cancer risk. There is some evidence that exercise reduces breast cancer risk, but it is not clear whether risk reduction is related to exercise intensity or duration, or to the age at which the exercise is performed.[8] The evidence that exercise reduces colon cancer risk is stronger; active individuals are less likely to develop colon cancer than their sedentary counterparts.[9] When evaluating the impact of exercise on cancer risk, diet and other lifestyle factors must also be considered. It is possible that some of the effect is due to the fact that people who exercise regularly are more likely to have healthier overall diets and lifestyles.

Psychological Benefits In addition to its other benefits, exercise can improve sleep patterns and overall outlook on life. One way that exercise benefits psychological health is that it stimulates the release of chemicals called **endorphins,** which are thought to trigger what athletes describe as an "exercise high." Endorphins are also thought to aid in relaxation, reduce anxiety, and improve mood, pain tolerance, and appetite control.

Endorphins Peptides that act as natural euphorics and reduce the perception of pain under certain stressful conditions.

Exercise Recommendations

Based on the evidence that increasing exercise reduces the incidence of chronic disease, many public health organizations are recommending that Americans increase their activity level. Recommendations on how much exercise is enough vary depending on who is making the recommendation. Some recommendations are based on the energy expended. For instance, the Surgeon General's Report on Physical Activity and Health recommends that Americans expend at least 150 kcalories a day or 1000 kcalories a week through exercise.[2] Other recommendations are based on the amount of time spent in activity. For example, the Dietary Guidelines recommend that Americans engage in at least 30 minutes of moderate activity daily (Figure 14.6).[10] Healthy People 2010 recommends 30 minutes of vigorous activity daily and suggests that for most people this will increase energy expenditure by about 1050 kcalories per week.[11] No matter how the recommendation is worded, each acknowledges that there is a significant health benefit to including a moderate amount of physical activity on most if not all days of the week. Despite this, most Americans include very little activity in their daily lives—only one third of Americans spend 30 minutes or expend 150 kcalories per day engaged in activity.[12]

In applying exercise recommendations, the fitness level of the individual and that individual's exercise goals must be considered. What is best for a middle-aged man trying to reduce his risk of chronic disease is different from what is best for an 18-year-old college basketball player, and different still from that for an octogenarian trying to continue living independently. Almost everyone can participate in some form of exercise, no matter where they live, how old they are, or what physical limitations they have. Exercise classes are held in nursing homes. Heart patients, amputees, the blind, and those in wheelchairs compete in athletic events. Even a small amount of exercise is better than none, and, within reason, more exercise is better than less. Whether you are 16 or 60, a couch potato or a Lance Armstrong, regular exercise can improve fitness and consequently overall health.

For more information on exercise recommendations and the health benefits of exercise, go to the Dietary Guidelines for Americans at www.health.gov/dietaryguidelines/.

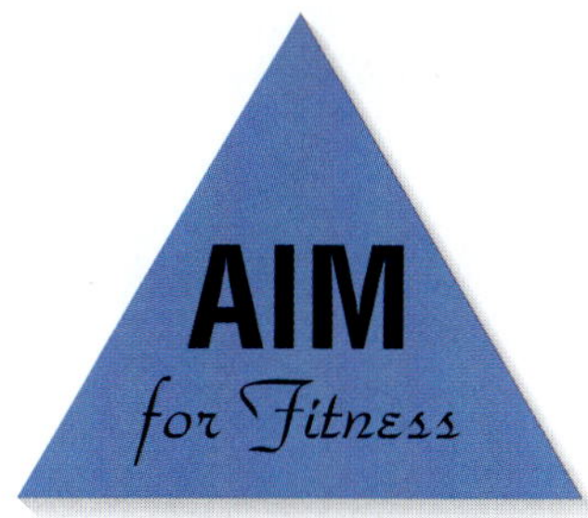

▲ Be physically active each day

FIGURE 14.6 The Dietary Guidelines, 2000, recommend that Americans "Be physically active each day."

Improving Fitness

Cardiorespiratory fitness, flexibility, and body composition as well as muscle strength can be improved by exercise training. The body adapts to perform the task demanded, whether it is to lift a heavier weight, stretch a millimeter farther, or continue for a few minutes longer. When a muscle is exercised, the stress or overload causes the muscle to adapt by increasing in size and strength—a process referred to as **hypertrophy.** By progressively increasing the amount or intensity of exercise at each exercise session, the muscle slowly hypertrophies. The greater the increase in exercise, the larger the training effect. Conversely, if a muscle is not used, it becomes smaller and weaker, a process called **atrophy.** For example, when an individual is bedridden and unable to move about, the muscles atrophy. Once the individual is up and active again, muscles regain strength and size. Everyone can increase their strength by challenging the muscles with exercise. Even elderly sedentary individuals have been found to increase muscle strength dramatically with weight training.[13]

Hypertrophy The increase in the size or bulk of an organ that may occur due to an increase in usage.

Atrophy A reduction in the size of a structure that may occur from disuse.

Structuring a Fitness Program A well-planned exercise regimen includes aerobic exercise, strength training, and stretching. Regardless of how long, how intense, and how often an individual exercises, an appropriate warm-up and cool-down period, including flexibility exercises, is recommended.

Aerobic Activities Aerobic exercise, such as walking, bicycling, skating, swimming, or jogging, should be performed for about 20 to 60 minutes three to five days per week. For optimal benefit, aerobic activity should be performed at a level that raises the heart rate to 60 to 90% of its maximum (see Figure 14.3). For a sedentary individual beginning an exercise program, mild exercise such as walking can raise the heart rate into this range. As fitness improves, exercisers must perform more intense activity to raise their heart rates to this level.

For more information on planning a healthy exercise program, go to Canada's physical activity guide at www.paguide.com/, the Washington Coalition for Promoting Physical Activity at www.beactive.org/, or go to healthfinder.gov/ and search for exercise.

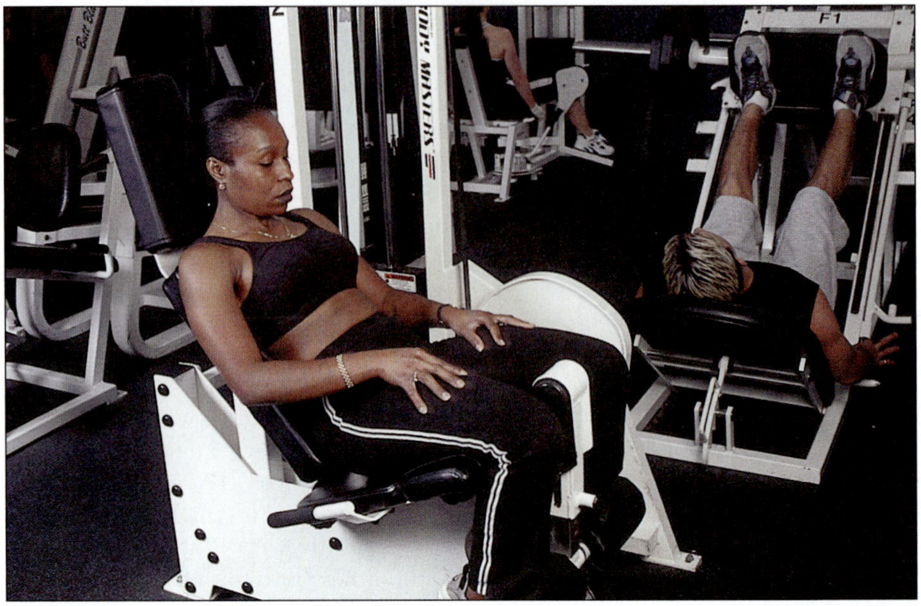

FIGURE 14.7 Strength-training machines provide a safe way to improve muscular strength. *(© Rachel Epstein/Photo Edit)*

Strength Training Strength training, such as weight lifting, should be done two to three days a week at the start of an exercise program, and two days a week after the desired strength has been achieved. This can be done with weights or using resistance-exercise machines (Figure 14.7). Each session should include a minimum of eight to ten exercises that train the major muscle groups. The weights lifted should be heavy enough to cause the muscle to be near exhaustion after repeating each exercise 8 to 12 times. Increasing the amount of weight lifted will increase muscle strength, whereas increasing the number of repetitions will improve endurance (Table 14.2).

Stretching To improve and maintain flexibility, stretching exercises should be done at least three days a week. Muscles should be stretched to a position of mild discomfort and held for 10 to 30 seconds. Each stretch should be repeated three to five times.

Balancing Exercise Intensity, Duration, and Frequency The combination of exercise frequency, duration, and intensity that is needed to achieve a desired fitness level depends on the exerciser. Young healthy athletes may require very intense activity to obtain a training effect. Older adults and those who have not previously

TABLE 14.2 Exercise Recommendations to Improve and Maintain Fitness

Type of Exercise	Examples	Frequency	Duration
Aerobic	Walking, jogging, bicycling, swimming, cross-country skiing	3 to 5 days per week	20 to 60 minutes
Strength training	Weight lifting with free weights or weight machines	2 to 3 days per week	30 minutes
Stretching	Yoga, stretching exercises	3 or more days per week	5 to 10 minutes

been active can increase their fitness by exercising at a lower intensity if the duration and frequency of exercise are increased. However, there is a minimum amount of exercise below which few benefits will be obtained. To provide a stimulus for improving and maintaining fitness in healthy adults, aerobic endurance training must be done two or more days per week at an intensity that is greater than 55 to 65% of maximum heart rate and for a duration of more than 10 minutes.[14] These minimum recommendations can be met in a variety of ways. What works best depends on the participant's needs, goals, and abilities. For example, a short intense workout may suit the needs of some individuals, while others prefer a longer workout at a lower intensity. Some may choose to exercise for a longer period once during the day, while others may spread their exercise throughout the day in shorter bouts of 10-minute duration.

Using the Activity Pyramid When planning an exercise program, emphasis should be placed on making permanent lifestyle changes that will lead to a lifetime of physical activity. One way to organize daily activities to meet these goals is to use the Activity Pyramid shown in Figure 14.8. The base of the pyramid includes simple, everyday activities such as walking the dog, parking the car farther away to increase the walking distance to the office or grocery store, or taking the

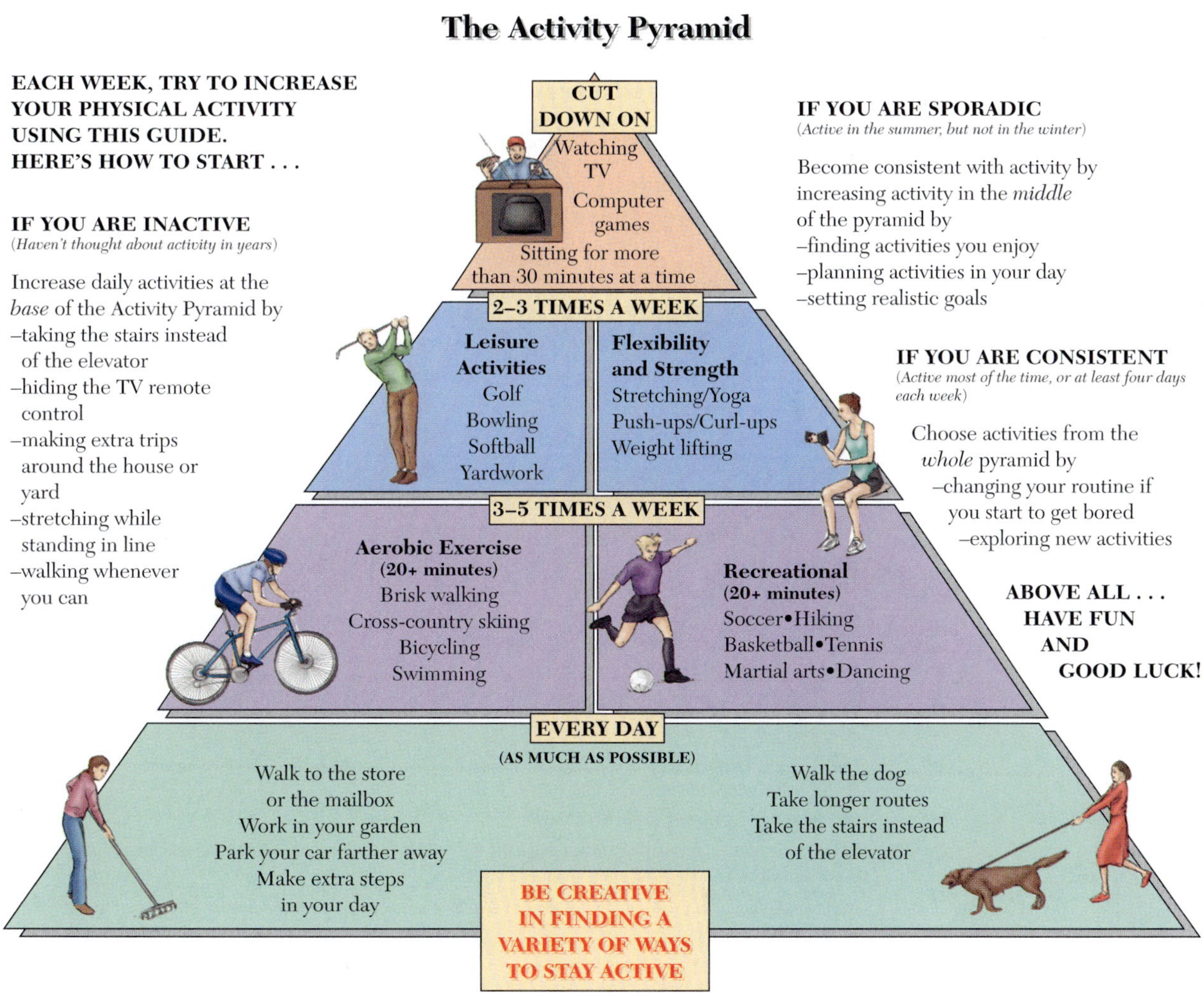

(Copyright © 1996 Park Nicollet HealthSource® Institute for Research and Education. Reprinted with modifications by permission.)

FIGURE 14.8 A pyramid shape can be used to build an active lifestyle. At the base are activities that you do every day. Layered over this base are aerobic exercise, recreational activities, and strength and flexibility exercises. At the very top are sitting activities that should be reduced.

stairs rather than the elevator. At the next level of the pyramid are aerobic activities that should be layered on top of an active base. These focus on improving heart and lung function and include walking, running, swimming, biking, or aerobic recreational activities such as basketball, soccer, or hiking. These should be done three to five times a week for 20 minutes or longer. The third level of the pyramid includes activities to increase flexibility and build muscle strength. The exercise at this level should take place two to three times a week and include leisure activities such as golf or bowling and flexibility and strength activities such as yoga and weight lifting. The narrow tip of the Activity Pyramid focuses on activities that should be decreased, such as sitting, watching TV, and playing computer games. Long periods of sitting (more than 30 minutes) should be interrupted by getting up and moving for a few minutes. This could mean standing while talking on the phone, stretching while sitting in traffic, or getting up from your desk occasionally to use the water fountain two floors up. Even small amounts of exercise contribute to overall fitness.

Getting Started Incorporating exercise into day-to-day life requires a behavior change, and changing behavior is not easy. The first step in beginning an exercise program is to recognize the reasons for not exercising and identify ways to overcome them. There are many reasons people avoid exercise: They do not enjoy it, they feel they have to join an expensive health club, they have little motivation to do it alone, or they find it inconvenient and uncomfortable. Finding a type of exercise that is enjoyable, a time that is realistic and convenient, and a place that is appropriate and safe are important first steps in adopting a pattern of increased exercise. Special clothes and large amounts of time and money are not needed. Riding a bike to class or work rather than driving or taking the bus, taking a walk at lunch time, and enjoying a game of catch are all effective ways to increase everyday activity level. Behavioral strategies such as those listed in Table 14.3 may help promote regular exercise.

Exercising Safely Safety should be a concern in planning any exercise regimen. Personal medical history as well as the exercise environment must be considered. Those embarking on an exercise program should check with their physician to be

TABLE 14.3 Suggestions for Beginning and Maintaining an Exercise Program

- Start slowly—Instead of planning to run three miles a day, five days a week, plan to start with a 20-minute walk three days a week.
- Make it fun—Choose activities you enjoy and find a partner with whom to exercise.
- Set specific attainable goals—"I will walk for 20 minutes after dinner three days a week."
- Make it convenient—Plan to walk early in the morning, during your lunch hour at work, or after dinner.
- Include a warm-up and a cool-down period—Warming up helps prepare muscles, ligaments, and tendons for the upcoming activity and mobilizes fuel supplies needed for activity. A cool-down helps to prevent muscle cramps.
- Challenge your strength or endurance once or twice a week and do more moderate workouts on other days.
- Include at least one day of rest each week—If it's easier to exercise on weekends, plan to take Monday off.
- Record your progress—Keep a record of your activity so you can track your progress and keep yourself motivated.
- Listen to your body—Symptoms such as lightheadedness or chest pain or pressure require immediate attention. Paying attention to more minor aches and pains allows you to stop before an injury occurs.
- Reward yourself—Plan to reward yourself when you succeed at your goal: a new book, a movie.

sure that their exercise plans are safe in relation to their medical history. To decrease the risk of injury, each exercise session should begin with a warm-up to increase blood flow to the muscles. This might include a few minutes of mild stretching and some walking, easy jogging, or cycling. A cool-down after the workout helps prevent muscle cramps and slowly brings heart rate down. An appropriate cool-down might include 5 to 10 minutes of light activity such as walking or stretching.

Weather conditions can be a health concern. Physical activity produces heat, which normally is dissipated to the environment, partly by the evaporation of sweat. When the environmental temperature is high, heat is not efficiently transferred to the environment, and when humidity is high, sweat evaporates slowly, making it difficult to cool the body. Thus, exercise should be reduced or curtailed in unusually hot and humid conditions. Cold environments can also pose problems for the outdoor exerciser. In general, cold does not impair exercise capacity, but the numbing of exposed flesh and the bulk of extra clothing can cause problems for joggers and bicyclists. Because exercise produces heat, clothing must allow for evaporation of sweat while providing protection from the cold. For swimmers, cold water can cause performance to deteriorate.

Avoiding Overtraining To improve muscle strength and cardiorespiratory fitness, the body must be stressed and respond to the stress by increasing muscle size and strength. Initially, training can cause fatigue and weakness, but during rest the body rebuilds to become stronger. If not enough rest occurs between exercise sessions, there is no time to regenerate so fitness and performance do not improve. In athletes, excessive training can lead to **overtraining syndrome,** which involves emotional, behavioral, and physical symptoms that persist for weeks to months. It is caused by repeatedly training without sufficient rest to allow for recovery. The most common symptom of overtraining syndrome is fatigue that limits workouts and is felt even at rest. Some athletes experience a decrease in appetite and weight loss as well as muscle soreness, increased frequency of viral illnesses, and increased incidence of injuries. They may become moody, easily irritated, depressed, have altered sleep patterns, or lose their competitive desire and enthusiasm. Overtraining syndrome occurs only in serious athletes who are training extensively, but rest is essential for anyone working to increase their fitness (see *Research Discoveries:* "Training: Sometimes Less Is Better").

Overtraining syndrome A collection of emotional, behavioral, and physical symptoms that occur when training without sufficient rest persists for weeks to months.

Web Menu: For more information on sports and exercise recommendations for children, go to Kidshealth at www.kidshealth.org/parent/nutrition_fit/.

Exercise Benefits at Different Life Stages

Exercise and fitness are important at all stages of life. However, the type of activity that is appropriate for children, pregnant women, and older adults differs.

Exercise Benefits Children Healthy children should be encouraged to engage in regular physical activity with the goal of adopting appropriate lifelong exercise behaviors. Children who learn to enjoy physical activity are more likely to become active adults who maintain a healthy body weight and have a lower risk of cardiovascular disease, diabetes, osteoporosis, and certain types of cancer. However, modern lifestyles do not promote activity in children; television, computers, and video games are often chosen over physical activity. Studies have found that children who watch 4 or more hours of television per day have more body fat and a greater body mass index than those who spend fewer than 2 hours watching TV.[15]

The Dietary Guidelines recommend that children and adolescents spend at least 60 minutes per day in developmentally appropriate exercise.[10] Activity for young children should be intermittent, with periods of moderate to vigorous activity lasting 10 to 15 minutes or more along with periods of rest and recovery. To promote this amount of exercise, a variety of enjoyable activities should be stressed and competition deemphasized (Figure 14.9). Learning by example is always best; children who have physically active parents are the leanest and the fittest.

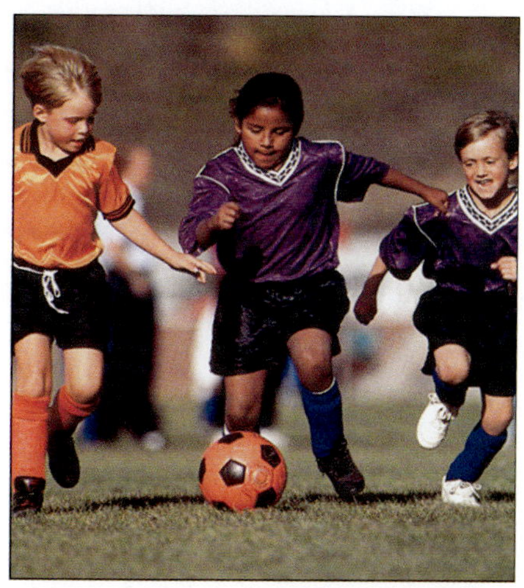

FIGURE 14.9 Children who participate in and enjoy exercise are more likely to have active lifestyles as adults. *(© Lori Adamski Peek/Tony Stone Images)*

RESEARCH DISCOVERIES

Training: Sometimes Less Is Better

The Ball State University swim team was talented. They trained long and hard. Why then couldn't they perform consistently well? In search of an answer, the coach enlisted the help of Dr. David Costill, director of the Human Performance Laboratory at the school. Costill began by assessing the condition of the swimmers. He attached monitors to measure heart rates and took blood samples to measure lactic acid levels. These measurements would help assess how well the athletes' bodies were responding to their training schedule. With continued training, heart rates and lactic acid accumulation were expected to decrease. However, Costill found that many of the swimmers had high lactic acid levels after practice despite the fact that they were well-trained.[a] Perhaps they were training too long and too hard.

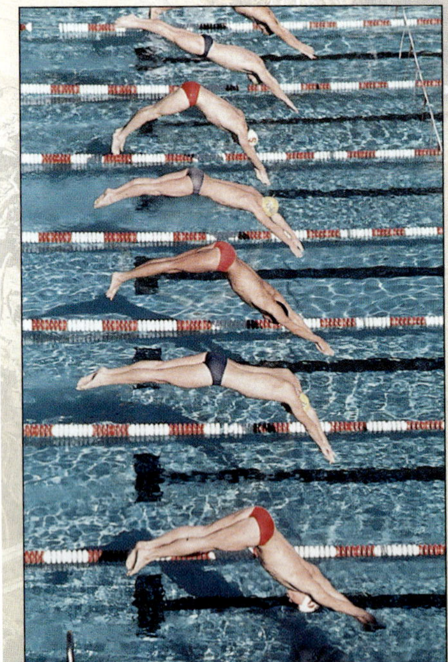

(© Tim Davis/Photo Researchers, Inc.)

Further studies helped to clarify the problems and suggest some solutions. Costill studied the swimmers on an increased training schedule; they swam at their normal pace but doubled the distance.[b] Some of the swimmers were unable to tolerate the heavier training schedule. Costill took muscle biopsies and found that muscle glycogen was depleted in these swimmers, indicating that they were running out of fuel. Their carbohydrate intake was not sufficient to meet the needs of the increased training, and their performance was suffering.[b] Other swimmers were able to tolerate the heavier training but it was not enhancing their performance. In addition, the extra training had other negative consequences. The swimmers' ratings of their muscle soreness, depression, anger, fatigue, and overall mood disturbances increased and they reported a reduction in their general sense of well-being.[c] Could cutting down on training actually improve performance?

Traditionally, it was believed that increased training increases strength and endurance. However, Costill hypothesized that the swimmers were overtrained. To test his hypothesis, he divided the team into two groups. One group of swimmers trained for 1.5 hours in the morning and 1.5 hours at night. A second group participated only in the afternoon session. Costill found that the group that trained the most experienced a decline in speed, whereas the second group showed an improvement.

So doubling the training time did not enhance performance.[d] Costill suggested that the Ball State swimming coach cut training time in half: Instead of working out twice a day, they cut out the morning workout. The team now consisted of more rested swimmers who swam faster than before; they ended with their best season in 10 years.

Costill's work suggested that when athletes train too much they are not able to maintain muscle glycogen, and increases in the amount of energy and carbohydrate in the diet may not be able to keep up. This work helped solidify the recognition that fitness is a combination of proper diet and the right amount of exercise. Just as dietary excesses and deficiencies can hurt performance, too little or too much training can result in less-than-peak performance. When excessive training continues over a period of three weeks or more, athletes are at risk for overtraining syndrome.[e] Overtraining syndrome is characterized by underperformance, persistent fatigue, altered mood, and increased rates of infection. To avoid overtraining, athletes should have one day of rest each week, alternate hard and easy training days, and optimize their nutrition, especially carbohydrate and energy intake.

References

[a] *The Champion Within.* Infinite Voyage Video Series, Intellimation, Inc. Santa Barbara, Calif.: QED Communications, Inc., and the National Academy of Sciences, 1991.

[b] Costill, D. L., Flynn, M. G., and Kirwan, J. P. Effects of repeated days of intensified training on muscle glycogen and swimming performance. Med. Sci. Sports Exerc. 20:249–254, 1988.

[c] Morgan, W. P., Costill, D. L., Flynn, M. G., et al. Mood disturbances following increased training in swimmers. Med. Sci. Sports Exerc. 20:408–414, 1988.

[d] Costill, D. L., Thomas, R., Robergs, R. A., et al. Adaptations to swimming training: influence of training volume. Med. Sci. Sports Exerc. 23:371–377, 1991.

[e] Lehmann, M. J., Lormes, W., Opitz-Gress, A., et al. Training and overtraining: an overview and experimental results in endurance sports. J. Sports Med. Phys. Fitness 37:7–17, 1997.

Exercise During Pregnancy Exercise can be beneficial during pregnancy as long as it is performed in a way that limits the risks to the mother and fetus. Exercise that is too intense has the potential to harm the fetus by reducing the amount of oxygen and nutrients it receives or by increasing body temperature. Pregnant women should not participate in activities that have a risk of abdominal trauma, falls, or joint stress, such as contact and racquet sports.[16] Outdoor exercise in hot, humid weather should also be avoided. To prevent overheating, plenty of fluids should be consumed and exercise should be carried out in a well-ventilated environment.

Women who were physically active before their pregnancy can often continue their exercise programs; women who begin an exercise program after becoming pregnant should start slowly, with low-intensity, low-impact activities such as walking.[17] When performed safely, exercise during pregnancy can improve overall fitness, reduce stress and lower back pain, prevent excess weight gain, improve digestion, reduce constipation, reduce the risk of developing gestational diabetes, improve mood and body image, and speed recovery from childbirth.

Exercise and Aging Many physiological changes occur with increasing age, including a decrease in lean body mass, muscle strength and endurance, and cardiorespiratory endurance (see Chapter 17). Regular physical activity can prevent or slow some of these changes.[6] For example, a program of regular exercise that includes strength training can prevent some of the reduction in lean body mass and maintain muscle strength and endurance, and regular aerobic exercise can increase or maintain cardiorespiratory endurance (Figure 14.10). Stretching can help maintain flexibility into old age. Exercise can also help to promote better balance and reduce the likelihood of falls (see *Critical Thinking:* "A Sensible Exercise Strategy").

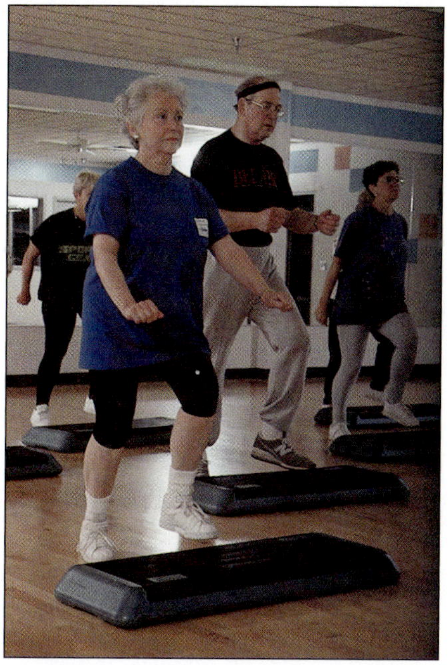

FIGURE 14.10 Exercise offers benefits at any age. Older adults who exercise regularly can prevent some of the decline in muscle mass that occurs with age, maintain cardiorespiratory endurance, and stay independent longer. *(© Jerry Wachter/Photo Researchers, Inc.)*

Critical Thinking

A Sensible Exercise Strategy

At this year's Memorial Day picnic, Fred found that he was exhausted from just running the bases during the company softball game. He realized that he needed to get back in shape. He is 40 years old, 5 feet 10 inches tall, and weighs 185 pounds. He played sports in college, but now he rarely exercises, and when he does he is sore for a few days afterward. He would like to lose a few pounds, but most of all he would like to increase his fitness level by increasing his strength and endurance.

Fred's fitness plan

Fred decides he will follow the exercise schedule he used in college. He joins a gym. Every night after work he lifts weights for 30 minutes and then does an hour of aerobic exercise outdoors, either jogging or riding a bicycle. After a week on his new schedule, Fred realizes that he is tired, sore, and discouraged. He still can't run more than a block without being winded. And, his family is upset that he has missed dinner every night.

Where did he go wrong?

It is unrealistic to go from almost no exercise to more than an hour of exercise five days a week. Fred needs an exercise program that will fit easily into his daily routine without drastically changing his schedule.

He consults with a trainer at the gym to help him design a plan that is more likely to work for him. The trainer shows Fred the Activity Pyramid (Figure 14.8) and talks about the components of a good exercise regimen and the principles of training. He suggests a program that will modify Fred's overall lifestyle while improving his cardiorespiratory endurance, strength, and flexibility. Fred needs to start slow but can increase the frequency and duration of his exercise as his strength and endurance improve.

Aerobic Activity

Just because Fred was a runner in high school doesn't mean he can just start a running program at age 40 after years of inactivity. The trainer explains target heart rate and suggests that Fred start with walking and progress to a combination of walking and jogging 3 days a week for 20 minutes at a level of 60% of his maximum heart rate. The trainer also suggests that Fred make alternative plans for when the weather is bad and he can't exercise outdoors.

What is Fred's target heart rate?

Maximum heart rate = 220 − age = 220 − 40 = 180 beats per minute:

60% of maximum = 180 × 0.6 = 108 beats per minute
90% of maximum = 180 × 0.9 = 162 beats per minute

He should exercise at a level that brings his heart rate up to 108 but not more than 162 beats per minute. As he becomes more fit, Fred will have to jog more and walk less to keep his heart rate at this level.

Flexibility and Strength

To improve his flexibility and strength, the trainer designs a program of stretching and weight-lifting exercises. He recommends that Fred stretch for a few minutes before and after he works out and that he do the weight lifting twice a week, adding slowly to the weight as his strength improves.

Lifestyle

The trainer also suggests that Fred try to make his overall lifestyle more active. Fred decides to make family time more active by replacing TV shows and movies with hikes and bike rides.

How has this change in activity affected Fred's energy needs for the week?

On the three days a week when he walks, he replaces 1/2 hour of sitting with 1/2 hour of walking, increasing his energy expenditure by 117 kcalories (see Table 14.4).

1 hour of walking = 328 kcal/ hour = 164 kcal/30 min
1 hour of sitting = 93 kcal/ hour = 47 kcal/30 min
Increase in energy expenditure = 164 kcal − 47 kcal = 117 kcal

On days that Fred goes to the gym he spends 15 minutes and 109 kcalories weight lifting (434 kcal per hour × 0.25 hour = 109 kcal). This replaces 15 minutes of sitting at only about 24 kcalories, so he expends an extra 85 kcalories. During the week he therefore expends an extra 521 kcalories (117 kcal × 3 days of walking + 85 kcal × 2 days of weight lifting).

If Fred's food intake does not change, how long will it take for him to lose 5 pounds?

Answer:

Metabolism During Exercise

The body runs on energy from the carbohydrate, fat, and protein consumed in food and contained in body stores. Exercise duration and intensity and the physical conditioning of the exerciser affect which of these nutrients are used for energy and how efficiently they are metabolized.

Fuels for Activity

To be used by the body, the energy contained in carbohydrate, fat, and protein must be converted into the high-energy compound ATP, the immediate source of energy for all body functions. In a resting muscle, there is enough stored ATP to sustain intense activity for a few seconds. As the ATP in muscle is used, enzymes break down another high-energy compound, **creatine phosphate,** to replenish the ATP supply. As with ATP, the amount of creatine phosphate stored in the muscle at any time is small. The energy in stored ATP and creatine phosphate is enough to fuel muscle activity for the first 10 to 15 seconds of exercise. Activity of longer duration requires that the body replenish ATP from the metabolism of the energy-yielding nutrients (Figure 14.11).

Creatine phosphate A compound found in muscle that can be broken down to generate ATP.

The availability of oxygen in muscle cells is key to determining which macronutrients will be used to produce ATP. Oxygen availability is determined both by how quickly the heart can deliver blood from the lungs—where it picks up oxygen—to the muscle cells, and by the amount of hemoglobin in the blood, which determines how much oxygen the blood can carry. When oxygen is available, carbohydrate, fat, and protein can all be used to produce ATP via **aerobic metabolism.** When oxygen is unavailable, ATP must be generated by **anaerobic metabolism** or **anaerobic glycolysis,** which can use only carbohydrate as a fuel.

Aerobic metabolism Metabolism in the presence of oxygen. In aerobic metabolism, glycolysis, the citric acid cycle, and the electron transport chain break down carbohydrates, fatty acids, and amino acids into carbon dioxide and water to produce ATP.

Anaerobic metabolism or **anaerobic glycolysis** Metabolism in the absence of oxygen. Two molecules of ATP are produced from each molecule of glucose.

Carbohydrate As an Energy Source The carbohydrate fuel used for activity is glucose. It can be used as a fuel source regardless of whether oxygen is available at the cells. The glucose used to power muscle activity may come from glycogen inside the muscle or from glucose delivered via the bloodstream. The glucose delivered in the blood comes from that released by the liver or absorbed from the diet.

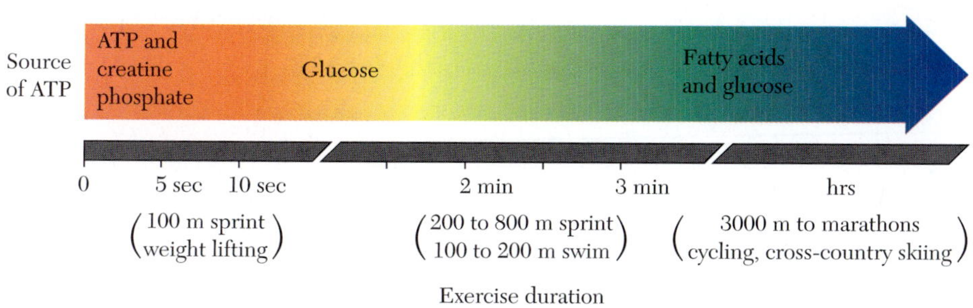

FIGURE 14.11 When exercise begins, ATP and creatine phosphate stored in the muscle provide ATP for muscle contraction. As creatine phosphate stores become depleted, anaerobic glycolysis, which breaks down glucose from the blood or from muscle glycogen, becomes the predominant source of ATP. After about 3 minutes, aerobic metabolism, which uses fatty acids and glucose to produce ATP, takes over as the predominant means of energy production.

Lactic acid A compound produced from pyruvate when glucose is metabolized in the absence of oxygen.

The first stage of glucose metabolism, anaerobic glycolysis, does not require oxygen. It breaks down glucose to form pyruvate, releases electrons, and produces two molecules of ATP. At this point if oxygen is not available, the metabolism of carbohydrate stops and the pyruvate and released electrons combine to form **lactic acid.** If oxygen is available, the pyruvate and electrons proceed through aerobic metabolism, producing more ATP along with carbon dioxide and water. Aerobic metabolism includes the conversion of pyruvate to acetyl-CoA; the citric acid cycle, which breaks down acetyl-CoA, producing some ATP and releasing electrons; and the electron transport chain, which passes electrons down a chain of molecules to oxygen, releasing energy to make ATP. Aerobic metabolism produces ATP more efficiently than anaerobic metabolism. The same molecule of glucose that produces two molecules of ATP in anaerobic glycolysis can produce about 36 to 38 molecules of ATP when metabolized aerobically (Figure 14.12).

Fat As an Energy Source Stored fat accounts for 90% of stored energy in a typical adult. It provides a lightweight, energy-dense fuel supply. Fatty acids from the diet and from stored triglycerides provide an important fuel for muscular activity.[18] Oxygen must be present for fatty acids to be metabolized, and some carbohydrate is needed to completely metabolize fatty acids for energy.

During exercise, triglycerides in adipose tissue and in muscle fibers are broken down into fatty acids and glycerol. Fatty acids from adipose tissue are released into the blood and are then taken up by the muscle cells. Inside the muscle

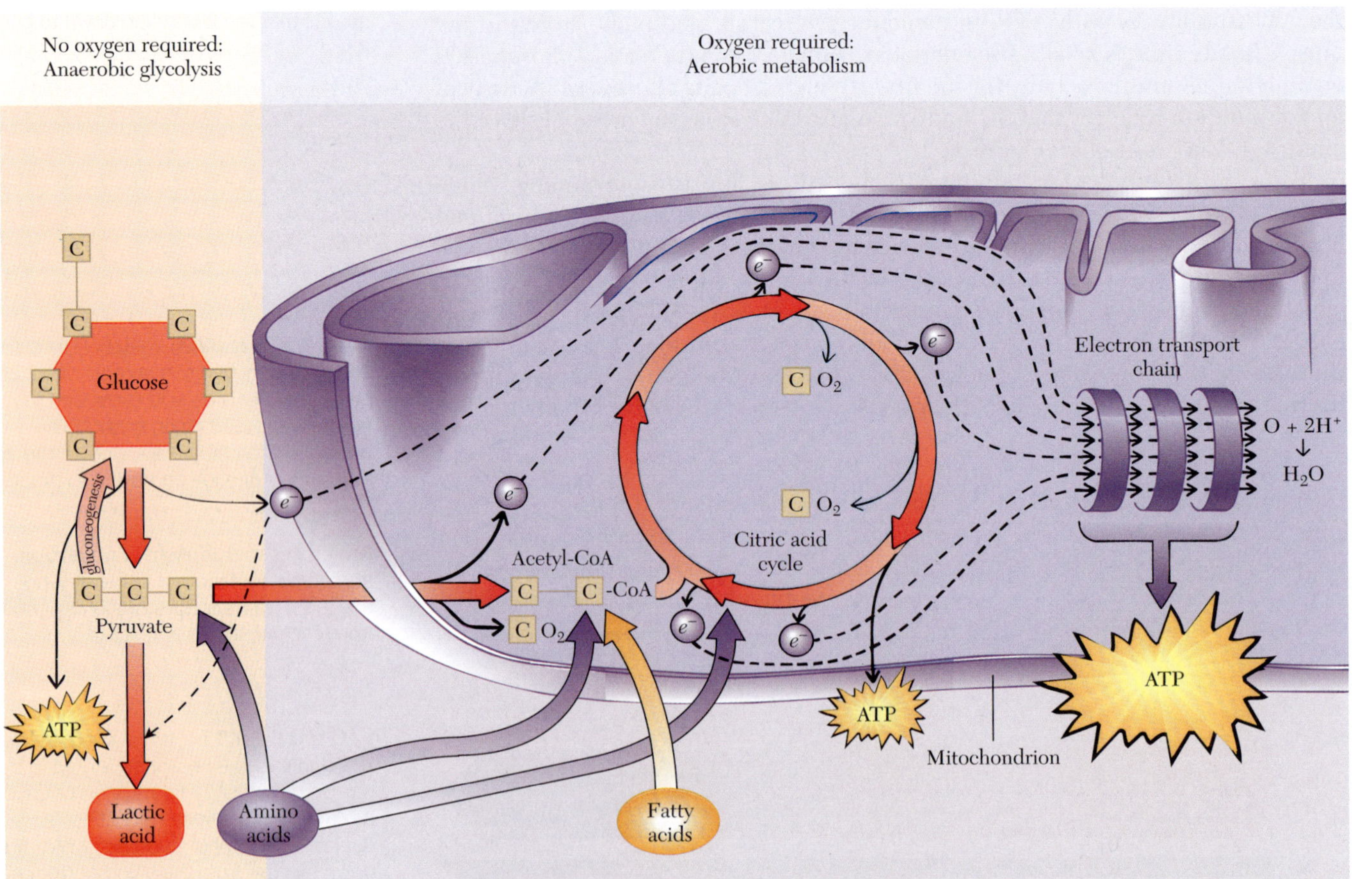

FIGURE 14.12 In the absence of oxygen, ATP is produced from glucose by anaerobic glycolysis. When oxygen is present, ATP is produced by aerobic metabolism of glucose, fatty acids, and amino acids. Aerobic metabolism is more efficient, producing more ATP from the same amount of glucose as anaerobic metabolism.

cell, fatty acids from triglycerides within the muscle and those delivered by the blood must be transported into the mitochondria to produce ATP. Inside the mitochondria, fatty acids are broken into two-carbon units to form acetyl-CoA. Acetyl-CoA is metabolized via the citric acid cycle and electron transport chain to produce ATP, carbon dioxide, and water (see Figure 14.12).

The rate at which fatty acids can be used by the muscle depends on how quickly they can be delivered to mitochondria in the muscle cell. To enter the mitochondria, fatty acids must be activated with the help of **carnitine,** a molecule that is produced in liver and kidney cells from the amino acids lysine and methionine. Because it is made in the body, carnitine is not an essential nutrient. Nevertheless, carnitine supplements are marketed to athletes with the promise that they will enhance the utilization of fat during exercise. This appeals to endurance athletes because the ability to use more fatty acids spares carbohydrate and therefore allows athletes to exercise for a longer time before exhaustion. It also appeals to those who want to reduce body fat by burning more fat. Studies that examined the effect of carnitine supplements in healthy individuals found that they did not affect the utilization of fat as fuel during exercise or improve exercise endurance.[19]

Carnitine A molecule synthesized in the body that is needed to transport fatty acids and some amino acids into the mitochondria for metabolism. Supplements of carnitine are marketed to athletes to enhance performance.

Protein As an Energy Source Protein can be broken down into amino acids, which can be used to produce ATP when oxygen is available. At rest and during most types of exercise, protein breakdown only contributes about 2 to 5% of the body's total energy requirement. Protein becomes an important source of energy during endurance exercise—exercise that continues for many hours. Endurance exercise increases the use of amino acids both as an energy source and as a raw material for glucose production via gluconeogenesis. To be used for energy or to make glucose, amino acids must first be deaminated. In the muscle, the carbon skeleton can enter the citric acid cycle to produce ATP. In the liver, the carbon skeleton can produce glucose via gluconeogenesis.

Effect of Exercise Intensity and Duration

Both the intensity and duration of exercise can affect the contributions that carbohydrate and fat make as fuels for energy production. Fuel utilization in turn affects how long exercise can continue before **fatigue** sets in.

Fatigue The inability to continue an activity at an optimal level.

While at rest, the cardiorespiratory system is able to deliver adequate blood, and, consequently, oxygen, to the muscles to allow aerobic metabolism of fatty acids.[20] During exercise, however, the delivery of oxygen to tissues can become limiting, causing the muscle cells to rely at least partially on the anaerobic metabolism of glucose. Generally, the more intense the exercise, the more the muscles rely on glucose to provide energy (Figure 14.13). Thus, with low-intensity exercise, the cardiorespiratory system can deliver enough oxygen to muscles to allow aerobic metabolism to predominate, so fatty acids and some glucose are used as fuel. When intensity reaches the VO_2 max, most energy is derived from anaerobic metabolism of glucose.

ATP production via anaerobic metabolism is rapid, but it is not efficient. When glucose is metabolized anaerobically, muscle glycogen is used 18 times faster than when the glucose is fully oxidized by aerobic metabolism. Because the amount of stored glycogen available to produce glucose during exercise is limited, intense exercise cannot be continued for long periods of time before glycogen is depleted and the athlete becomes fatigued. Lower-intensity exercise can continue for longer periods because aerobic metabolism predominates after the first few minutes of exercise (Figure 14.14). Aerobic metabolism is more efficient and uses both glucose and fatty acids for energy. However, even aerobic metabolism uses some glucose, so if exercise continues long enough, glycogen stores will eventually be depleted.

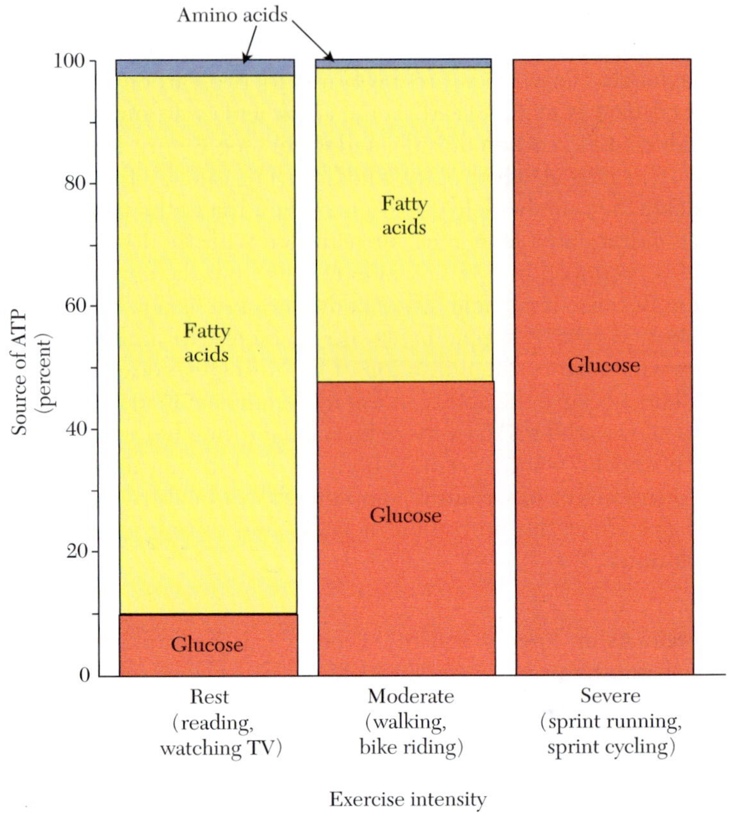

FIGURE 14.13 As exercise intensity increases, the proportion of energy supplied by glucose increases. During exercise, the total amount of energy expended is greater than that at rest. *(Adapted from Horton, E. S. Effects of low-energy diets on work performance. Am. J. Clin. Nutr. 35:1228–1233, 1982.)*

Exercise fatigue occurs because of the depletion of liver and muscle glycogen and the accumulation of lactic acid. When athletes run out of glycogen, they experience a feeling of overwhelming fatigue that is sometimes referred to as "hitting the wall" or "bonking." During intense exercise that relies on anaerobic metabolism, fatigue occurs quickly because of rapid glycogen depletion and also because pyruvate is converted to lactic acid (see Figure 14.12). The accumulation of lactic acid changes the acidity of the muscle, reducing its ability to contract. Lactic acid also inhibits the mobilization of fat from adipose tissue, forcing the muscle to rely more on glycogen, thus depleting it even faster. When exercise stops and oxygen is available again, lactic acid can be either carried away by the blood to other tissues to be broken down, or metabolized aerobically in the muscle. After intense exercise, a mild cool-down, such as walking, may allow enough blood flow to the muscle to remove built-up lactic acid and prevent cramping.

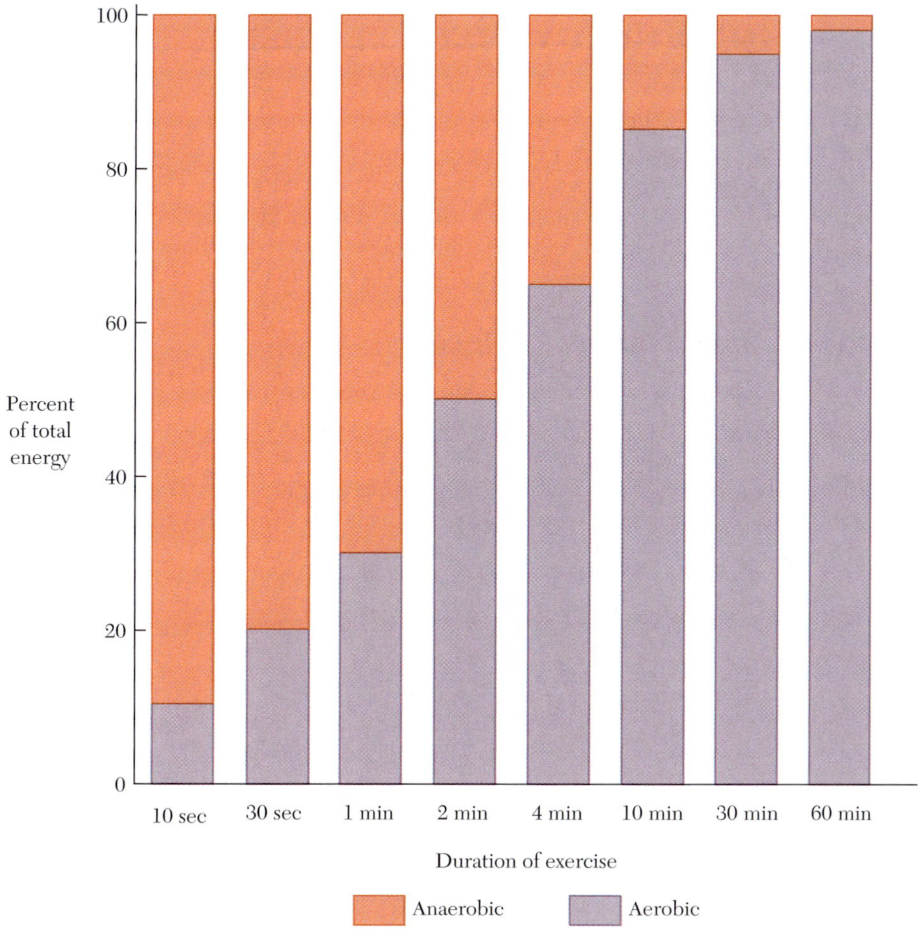

FIGURE 14.14 Exercise of long duration relies primarily on aerobic metabolism. During the first few minutes of exercise, most energy is derived from the anaerobic metabolism of glucose, but as exercise continues, aerobic metabolism makes a greater contribution to energy production. By 30 minutes, over 90% of the energy needed to fuel activity is obtained aerobically. *(Adapted from Astrand, P. O., and Rodahl, K.* Textbook of Work Physiology. *New York: McGraw-Hill, 1977.)*

Effect of Training

Training with repeated aerobic exercise causes physiological changes that increase VO_2 max—the amount of oxygen that can be delivered to and used by the muscle cells. This in turn affects which fuels can be used by the exercising muscle cells.

As already discussed, aerobic training affects the cardiorespiratory system. The heart becomes larger and stronger so that the stroke volume is increased, allowing more blood to be delivered to the body with each beat. The number of capillary blood vessels in the muscles increases, allowing more efficient delivery of blood—and consequently oxygen and fuels—to muscle cells. The total blood volume and number of red blood cells—hence the amount of hemoglobin—increase, allowing more oxygen to be delivered to the cells. Living and working at high altitudes, where the atmosphere contains less oxygen, also causes adaptations that improve the capacity of the cardiorespiratory system to deliver oxygen. Therefore, endurance athletes often train at high altitudes to enhance their aerobic capacity.

At the cellular level, training produces an increase in the ability to store glycogen and an increase in the number and size of muscle-cell mitochondria (Figure 14.15). Because aerobic metabolism occurs in the mitochondria, this increases the cell's capacity to burn fatty acids to produce ATP. The use of fatty acids spares glycogen, which delays the onset of fatigue. Because trained athletes store more glycogen and use it more slowly, they can sustain aerobic exercise for longer periods at higher intensities without experiencing fatigue than can untrained individuals. A trained athlete can also exercise at a higher percentage of their VO_2 max before lactic acid begins to accumulate.

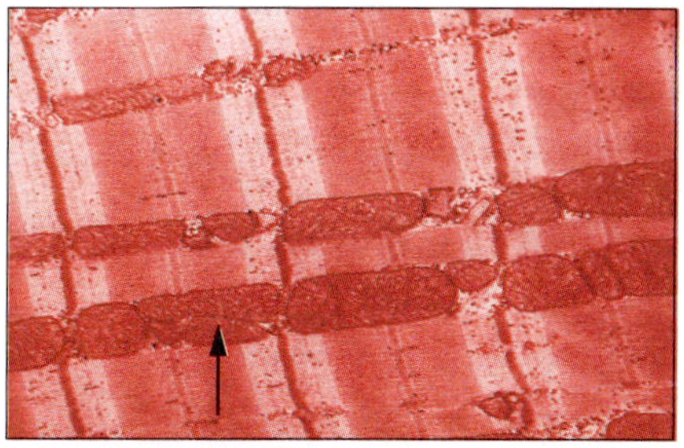

FIGURE 14.15 Mitochondria are the site of aerobic metabolism. In trained athletes, the number of mitochondria in muscle cells increases. The arrow indicates one of the many muscle cell mitochondria seen in this magnification of a stained section of skeletal muscle fibers. *(Don W. Fawcett/Visuals Unlimited)*

PROVIDING ENERGY FOR EXERCISE

Energy needs include those required for basal metabolic rate, physical activity, and the thermic effect of food. For a casual exerciser, the energy needed for activity may increase energy expenditure by a few hundred kcalories a day. For an endurance athlete, such as a marathon runner, the energy needed for training may increase expenditure by 2000 to 3000 kcalories per day. Some athletes require 6000 kcalories a day or more to maintain their body weight.

Factors That Affect Energy Needs

The more intense an activity, the more energy it requires. Likewise the more time spent exercising, the more energy it requires. For example, riding a bicycle for 10 minutes requires ten times the energy needed to ride for 1 minute. Also, moving a heavier body requires more energy than moving a lighter one. Therefore, more energy is required for a 250-pound woman to walk for 5 minutes than for a 120-pound woman to do the same (see Table 14.4 and Appendix K).

TABLE 14.4 Energy Expended for Activity

	Kcalories per Hour by Body Weight						
Activity	**50 kg 110 lb**	**57 kg 125 lb**	**64 kg 140 lb**	**70 kg 155 lb**	**77 kg 170 lb**	**84 kg 185 lb**	**91 kg 200 lb**
Aerobics (moderate)							
Male	455	480	506	531	556	582	607
Female	394	413	433	453	472	492	511
Biking (12 mph)							
Male	380	401	422	443	464	486	507
Female	329	345	361	378	394	410	427
Bowling (recreational)							
Male	121	128	135	142	148	155	162
Female	105	110	115	121	126	131	136
Dancing (recreational)							
Male	364	384	405	425	445	465	486
Female	315	331	346	362	378	393	409
Gardening (moderate)							
Male	303	320	337	354	371	388	405
Female	263	276	289	302	315	328	341
Golf (walking with bag)							
Male	425	448	472	496	519	543	567
Female	368	386	404	422	441	459	477
Jumping rope (moderate speed)							
Male	595	628	661	694	727	760	793
Female	515	540	566	591	617	642	668
Running (10 min/mi)							
Male	619	653	688	722	757	791	826
Female	536	562	589	615	642	669	695
Sitting at ease							
Male	73	77	81	85	89	93	97
Female	63	66	69	72	76	79	82
Swimming (moderate speed)							
Male	364	384	405	425	445	465	486
Female	315	331	346	362	378	393	409
Walking (15 min/mi)							
Male	257	271	285	300	314	328	342
Female	222	233	244	255	266	277	288
Weight lifting							
Male	340	359	378	397	415	434	453
Female	294	309	323	338	352	367	382

ESHA Research, Salem, OR.

There are also some special considerations that affect the energy needs for activity. For example, although an obese woman would expend more energy walking a mile than a lighter counterpart, she may expend less energy when swimming because the buoyancy of her adipose tissue reduces the amount of work required to swim. If a lean individual and an obese individual were in the weightlessness of space, it would require no more energy for one to leap across the room than for the other. A paraplegic in a wheelchair may have lower energy needs because many of the major muscles in the body are always inactive; on the other hand, a person with the form of cerebral palsy that causes uncontrolled muscle movements may have higher energy needs because the muscles never stop moving.

Weight Loss in Athletes

Athletes involved in activities where small, light bodies offer an advantage—such as ballet, gymnastics, and certain running events—may restrict energy intake to maintain a low body weight. However, while a slightly leaner physique may be beneficial in the activity, dieting to maintain an unrealistically low weight may threaten health and performance.

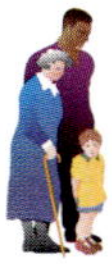

In adolescents, athletic activities combined with weight loss may affect the maturation process and increase the risk of developing anorexia or bulimia.[21] Female ballerinas and gymnasts who maintain extremely low levels of body fat often have delayed menses and delayed sexual maturation.[22] To fit into a specific weight class, athletes in sports such as wrestling sometimes use sporadic diets that severely restrict fluid and energy intake (see discussion of fluid needs). Such dietary practices may be detrimental to health and performance.[23]

An athlete who needs to lose weight should do so in advance of the competitive season to prevent the restricted diet from affecting performance. The general guidelines for healthy weight loss should be followed: Reduce energy intake, increase activity, and change the behaviors that led to weight gain (see Chapter 8). To preserve lean body mass and enhance fat loss, weight should be lost at a rate of about 1/2 to 1 pound per week. This can be accomplished by reducing total energy intake by 200 to 500 kcalories per day and increasing exercise.

If weight gain is desired, 200 to 500 extra kcalories should be consumed per day. Exercise training should accompany weight gain to promote an increase in lean tissue.

Energy Sources

The source of dietary energy is often as important as the amount of energy. In general, the diet of physically active individuals should contain the same proportion of carbohydrate, fat, and protein as is recommended to the general public.

Carbohydrate A healthy diet provides 55 to 60% of energy as carbohydrate. Most of this should come from foods high in complex carbohydrates and unrefined sugars such as whole grains, legumes, vegetables, fruits, and milk. These foods provide vitamins, minerals, phytochemicals, and fiber as well as energy. For athletes in training, adequate carbohydrate is necessary to rapidly replace muscle and liver glycogen stores depleted by daily exercise.

Fat A diet that provides 30% or less of its energy from fat is recommended for athletes as well as the general population. Fat is an important source of energy for exercise, but excess dietary fat is unnecessary. Body stores of fat provide enough energy to support the requirements of even the longest endurance events. Excess energy consumed as fat, carbohydrate, or protein can cause an increase in body fat.

Protein Dietary protein is essential to maintain muscle mass and strength. However, muscles grow in response to exercise, not in response to additional dietary protein (Figure 14.16). A diet that contains the 1989 RDA for protein (0.8 g/kg)

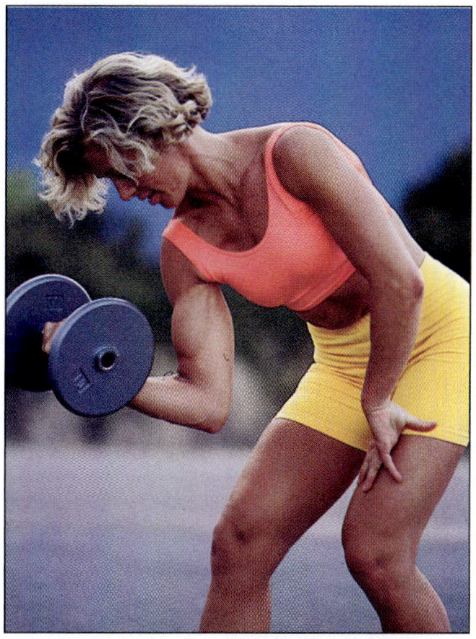

FIGURE 14.16 Increasing muscle size involves time and hard work. It is accomplished by increasing resistance exercise, not by increasing protein intake. *(© Marc Romanelli/The Image Bank)*

Making Decisions

Ergogenic Hormones: What Athletes Will Do for an Edge

"Citius, altius, fortius"—faster, higher, stronger—the Olympic motto. For as long as there have been competitions, athletes have yearned for something—anything—that would give them the competitive edge. Everything from desiccated liver to bee pollen and shark cartilage has been used as an ergogenic aid. The majority of these potential performance boosters have turned out to offer more of a psychological edge than a physiological one. However, when athletes from Eastern European nations began to dominate international strength events, the athletic community became aware of the muscle-building effects of large doses of anabolic steroids. Finally, an effective ergogenic aid had been found. Since then, anabolic steroids have been determined to be dangerous and their use is now illegal. They are regulated as controlled substances under the 1988 Anti–Drug Abuse Act and the Anabolic Steroids Act of 1990. However, the effectiveness of these hormones in building muscle and improving performance has led athletes to experiment with these and many other hormones in the endless search for a competitive edge.

Anabolic Steroids The term "anabolic steroid" refers to steroid hormones that accelerate protein synthesis and growth. The anabolic steroids used by athletes are synthetic versions of the human steroid hormone testosterone. Natural testosterone stimulates and maintains the male sexual organs and promotes the development of bones and muscles and the growth of skin and hair. The synthetic testosterone used by athletes has a greater effect on muscle development and bone, skin, and hair than it does on sexual organs. When synthetic testosterone is taken in conjunction with exercise and an adequate diet, muscle mass increases. However, these drugs also make the body think testosterone is being produced, and therefore the body reduces its production of natural testosterone. Without natural testosterone, the sexual organs are not maintained; this leads to testicular shrinkage and a decrease in sperm production. In adolescents, the use of synthetic testosterone causes bone growth to stop and height to be stunted. Anabolic steroid use may also cause oily skin and acne, water retention in the tissues, yellowing of the eyes and skin, coronary artery disease, liver disease, and sometimes death. Users may have psychological and behavioral side effects such as violent outbursts and depression, possibly leading to suicide. The dangers of steroid use are increased by the fact that they are illegal, so their manufacturing and distribution procedures are not regulated. Users can never be sure of the potency and purity of what they are taking.

Steroid Precursors Steroid precursors are compounds that can be converted into steroid hormones in the body. These include androstenedione, androstenediol, DHEA, norandrostenediol, and norandrostenedione. Steroid precursors can be sold legally as dietary supplements.

The best known of the steroid precursors is androstenedione, often refered to as "andro." It is a precursor to testosterone that is marketed as an alternative to anabolic steroids to increase levels of testosterone. Andro has been used for years by bodybuilders, but it was launched to public prominence when professional baseball player Mark McGwire announced his use of it during the 1998 major league baseball season when he hit 70 home runs to break the league's single-season home-run record. McGwire has subsequently stopped using andro and it has been banned by the International Olympic Committee, the National Collegiate Athletic Association, and all major international sports federations except major league baseball.

Despite andro's popularity, few studies had until recently examined whether it actually increases blood testosterone or produces anabolic effects. Recent studies have not conclusively answered those questions. One study found no difference between the increase in muscle strength, muscle mass, and lean body mass and the decrease in fat mass that occurred in subjects taking andro and subjects in a control group not taking the supplement after eight weeks of resistance training.[a] In addition to failing to demonstrate anabolic effects, this study found that andro caused a decrease in

provides adequate protein for most active individuals. Competitive athletes participating in endurance and strength sports may require more. In endurance events such as marathons, protein is used for energy and to maintain blood glucose, so these athletes may benefit from 1.2 to 1.4 g of protein per kilogram per day. Strength athletes who require amino acids to synthesize new muscle proteins may benefit from 1.4 to 1.8 g per kilogram per day.[24] This amount, however, is about the same as that contained in the typical American diet—10 to 20% of energy needs. For example, an 85-kg man consuming 3000 kcalories, 18% of which is from protein, would be consuming 135 g, or 1.6 g of protein per kg body weight.

Although protein supplements are often marketed with the promise of enhancing muscle growth or improving performance, the protein provided by expensive supplements will not meet an athlete's needs any better than the protein found in a balanced diet. Supplements of synthetic anabolic steroids are used by some athletes to increase muscle mass; however, these are illegal and have

HDL cholesterol, suggesting that it may increase the risk of heart disease. In a second study, a similar dose of andro was found to raise testosterone levels, but the researchers did not measure muscle strength or mass.[b] Another study found that andro had no anabolic effect on muscle protein metabolism.[c]

As with any dietary supplement, the fact that andro is available over the counter does not guarantee its safety. Scientists still do not know how much androstenedione is absorbed, where it acts, or how much is converted to testosterone. It is not known whether androstenedione will cause testicular shrinkage, liver disease, and heart disease like anabolic steroids. In addition, the purity of what is sold commercially is unknown, unregulated, and probably quite variable.

Peptide Hormones Peptide hormones now compete with anabolic steroids on the black market of alleged tissue-building performance-enhancing drugs. The ability of manufacturers to produce peptide hormones through genetic engineering has increased their availability not only to individuals with conditions that require these hormones, but also to athletes.

Human growth hormone is a peptide hormone that is produced naturally by the pituitary gland. It is important for tissue building during growth in children. Recombinant growth hormone is used to treat children who are small due to growth hormone deficiency. Growth hormone levels decline with age and may account for some of the decrease in fat-free mass that occurs with age. In adults, growth hormone maintains lean tissue, stimulates fat breakdown, increases the number of red blood cells, and boosts heart function. This hormone is appealing to athletes because it increases muscle protein synthesis. But despite these physiological effects, the ergogenic benefits of growth hormone among athletes remain unproven.[d] Increases in muscle strength obtained from resistance training were not improved by growth hormone. Growth hormone did cause a greater increase in fat-free mass, but there was no increase in incorporation of amino acids into muscle suggesting that the increase was likely due to fluid retention or accumulation of connective tissue. More important, prolonged use of growth hormone can cause heart dysfunction and high blood pressure as well as excessive growth of some body parts, such as hands, feet, and facial features. It has been difficult to detect growth hormone use among athletes because it is only detectable in the blood for a short time and does not appear to any great extent in the urine.

Another peptide hormone that is popular among endurance athletes is erythropoeitin, known as EPO. Natural erythropoeitin is produced by the kidneys and stimulates stem cells in the bone marrow to differentiate into red blood cells. Recombinant EPO is used to treat anemia due to kidney disease, chemotherapy, HIV infection, and blood loss. It can enhance the performance of endurance athletes by increasing the ability to transport oxygen to the muscles. It therefore increases VO_2 max and aerobic performance and spares glycogen. However, too much EPO can cause production of too many red blood cells, which can lead to excessive blood clotting, heart attacks and strokes. The International Olympic Committee banned EPO in 1990 after it was linked to the death of more than a dozen cyclists.[f] As with growth hormone, it is difficult to detect whether EPO is being used, and tests currently measure only hematocrit or hemoglobin concentration. Researchers are currently developing tests to detect the use of growth hormone and EPO so the prohibition on the use of these hormones can be enforced.

References

[a] King D. S., Sharp, R. L., Vukovich, M. D., et al. Effect of oral androstenedione on serum testosterone and adaptations to resistance training in young men: a randomized controlled trial. JAMA 28:2020–2028, 1999.

[b] Leder, B. Z., Longcope, C., Catlin, D. H., et al. Oral androstenedione administration and serum testosterone concentrations in young men. JAMA 283:779–782, 2000.

[c] Rasmussen B. B., Volpi, E., Gore, D. C., and Wolfe, R. R. Androstenedione does not stimulate muscle protein anabolism in young healthy men. J. Clin. Endocrinol. Metab. 85:55–59, 2000.

[d] Jenkins, P. J. Growth hormone and exercise. Clin Endocrinol. 50:683–689, 2000.

[e] Frisch, H. Growth hormone and body composition in athletes. J. Endocrinol. Invest. 22(Suppl): 106–109, 1999.

[f] Ritter, S. K. Faster, higher, stronger. Chem. Engineering News 77:42–52, 1999.

dangerous side effects (see *Making Decisions:* "Ergogenic Hormones: What Athletes Will Do for an Edge").

Micronutrient Needs

Exercise increases the need for vitamins and minerals involved in energy production. A balanced diet that meets energy needs generally provides these additional vitamins and minerals. However, this may not be true for exercisers consuming low-energy diets, such as individuals trying to lose weight or athletes such as ballerinas or gymnasts who want to maintain very low body weights. To avoid deficiencies, these individuals must consume carefully planned diets or include a supplement in order to meet their vitamin and mineral needs. For some competitive athletes, particularly females, maintaining adequate iron and calcium status are a concern.

Iron

For most individuals, exercise does not increase iron needs. However, in athletes, particularly female athletes, a reduction in iron stores is common. If this reduction progresses to anemia, it can impair exercise performance as well as reduce immune function and affect other physiologic processes.[25]

Poor iron status may be caused by an inadequate dietary iron intake, an increased demand for iron, increased iron losses, or a redistribution of iron due to exercise training. Dietary iron intake may be limited in athletes who are attempting to keep body weight low, or in those who consume a vegetarian diet and therefore do not eat meat—an excellent source of readily absorbable heme iron. Iron needs may be increased in athletes because exercise stimulates the production of red blood cells, so more iron is needed for hemoglobin synthesis. Iron is also needed for the synthesis of muscle myoglobin and the iron-containing proteins needed for ATP production in the mitochondria. An increase in iron losses with prolonged training, possibly because of increased fecal losses, also contributes to increased iron needs in athletes. Iron balance may also be affected by the breaking of red blood cells from impact in events such as running (foot-strike hemolysis), or by the contraction of large muscles. However, this rarely causes anemia because the breaking of red blood cells stimulates the production of new ones. Although a separate RDA for iron for athletes has not been established it is estimated that the EAR may be 30 to 70% greater for those who engage in regular intense exercise.[26]

Some athletes experience a condition known as **sports anemia,** which is a temporary decrease in hemoglobin concentration that occurs during exercise training. This is an adaptation to training that does not seem to impair delivery of oxygen to tissues. It occurs when blood volume expands to increase oxygen delivery, but the synthesis of red blood cells lags behind the increase in plasma volume.

Sports anemia Reduced hemoglobin levels that occur as part of a beneficial adaptation to aerobic exercise, in which expanded plasma volume dilutes red blood cells.

Female athlete triad The combination of disordered eating, amenorrhea, and osteoporosis that occurs in some female athletes, particularly those involved in sports in which low body weight and appearance are important.

Amenorrhea Delayed onset of menstruation or the absence of three or more consecutive menstrual cycles.

Calcium

Calcium is needed to promote and maintain high bone density, which in turn reduces the risk of osteoporosis. In general, exercise—particularly weight-bearing exercise—increases bone density, thereby reducing the risk of osteoporosis. Studies of bone density in exercising women have shown that athletes generally have a bone density that is 5 to 15% higher than in nonathletes. And, participation in exercise programs that include running or weight training can cause a 1 to 2% increase in bone mineral density.[27,28] However, in female athletes trying to maintain extremely low body weight and fat, calcium status can be at risk.

Female athletes who strive to reduce body weight and fat to improve performance, to achieve an ideal body image, or to meet goals set by coaches, trainers, or parents are at risk for a syndrome of interrelated disorders referred to as the **female athlete triad.** This syndrome includes disordered eating, **amenorrhea,** and osteoporosis (Figure 14.17). Eating disorders can create a physiological condition similar to starvation and contribute to menstrual abnormalities. It is also hypothesized that high levels of exercise affect the menstrual cycle by increasing energy demands or causing stress-related hormonal changes.[29] When combined with disordered eating, high levels of exercise can contribute to amenorrhea—the delayed onset or absence of menses in women. Amenorrhea results in low estrogen levels and interferes with calcium status and consequently causes reductions in bone mass and bone-mineral density. Low estrogen levels reduce calcium absorption and, when combined with poor calcium intake (common in female athletes and females in general), leads to premature bone loss, failure to reach

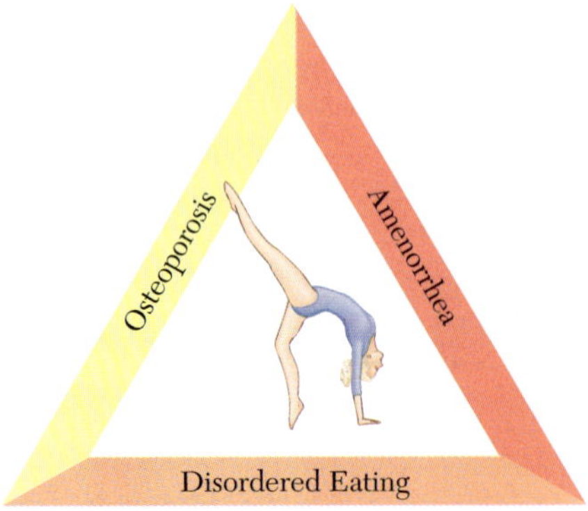

FIGURE 14.17 The female athlete triad includes disordered eating, amenorrhea, and osteoporosis. Women with these conditions typically have low body fat and may experience multiple or recurrent stress fractures. This syndrome is more common in women who are perfectionists, highly competitive, and have a low self-esteem.

maximal peak bone mass, and an increased risk of stress fractures. Neither adequate dietary calcium nor the increase in bone mass caused by weight-bearing exercise can compensate for bone loss due to low estrogen levels. If menses resume, bone loss can be at least partially reversed, but whether these athletes are at greater risk of osteoporosis later in life is not known.[30]

Fluid Needs During Exercise

For more information on hydration for athletic performance, go to www.uoregon.edu/~anelson1/hydrationstart.htm.

Water is needed to regulate body temperature and to transport oxygen and nutrients to the muscles and waste products away from muscles. Failure to consume enough fluid to replace water lost through the lungs and in sweat can be critical to the health and performance of even the most casual exerciser. Anyone exercising should consume extra fluids before, during, and after exercise.

Regulation of Body Temperature

During exercise, the increase in metabolic processes increases the amount of heat produced. It is necessary to dissipate this heat in order to maintain normal body temperature and homeostasis. One cooling mechanism is the diversion of blood flow to the surface of the body. This increase in blood flow to the skin greatly enhances the amount of heat lost to the environment. Another mechanism for heat loss is evaporation of water from the respiratory passages and the skin. When body temperature begins to rise, sweat glands secrete large volumes of a dilute salt solution called sweat. When sweat reaches the skin, it evaporates, cooling the body. For every liter of water that evaporates, 580 kcalories of heat are transferred to the environment.

Thermal Distress If the water lost in sweat and through evaporation from the lungs is not replaced, total body water may be reduced enough to cause some type of **thermal distress** or **heat disorders.** Thermal distress includes dehydration, heat cramps, heat exhaustion, and heat stroke. Dehydration occurs when water loss is great enough for blood volume to decrease, thereby reducing the ability to deliver oxygen and nutrients to exercising muscles. Even mild dehydration—a body-water loss of 1% of body weight—can impair exercise performance (Figure 14.18). Heat cramps are involuntary cramps and spasms in the muscles involved in exercise. They are caused by an imbalance of the electrolytes sodium and potassium at the muscle cell membranes and can occur when water and salt are lost during extended exercise. Heat exhaustion occurs when fluid loss causes blood volume to decrease so much that it is not possible to both cool the skin and deliver oxygen to active muscles. It is characterized by a rapid weak pulse, low blood pressure, fainting, profuse sweating, and disorientation. Heat stroke, the most serious form of thermal distress, occurs when the temperature regulatory

Thermal distress or **heat disorders** Conditions including dehydration, heat cramps, heat exhaustion, and heat stroke that can occur due to a combination of exercise, hydration status, and climatic conditions.

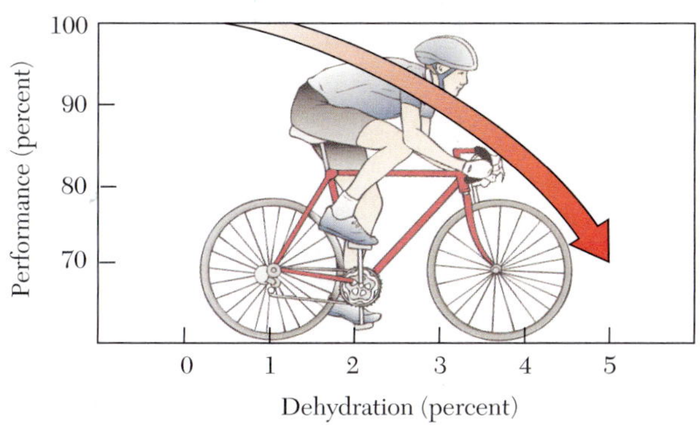

FIGURE 14.18 As the level of dehydration increases, exercise performance declines. *(Adapted from Saltin, B., and Castill, D. I. Fluid and electrolyte balance during prolonged exercise. In* Exercise, Nutrition, and Energy Metabolism. *Horton, E. S., and Tergung, R. I., eds. New York: Macmillan, 1988.)*

center of the brain fails. Heat stroke is characterized by elevated body temperature, hot dry skin, extreme confusion, and unconsciousness. It requires immediate medical attention.

Factors Affecting the Risk of Thermal Distress The risk of thermal distress is affected by ambient temperature and humidity as well as the condition of the exerciser (Figure 14.19). When environmental temperature increases, the amount of heat that can be transferred from the body to the environment decreases and the evaporation of sweat becomes more important for cooling. At rest in a temperate environment, an individual loses about 1.1 liters (about 4.5 cups) of water per day, or 50 ml per hour, from the skin and lungs. Exercise in a hot environment can increase this tenfold. The ability to cool the body by evaporation decreases as the humidity in the surrounding environment increases. Acclimatizing to the heat by repeated bouts of exercise can cause physiological adaptations that improve the capacity to exercise in the heat.

The risk of dehydration is also increased in some cold environments. Cold air, particularly at high altitudes, is less humid, so more water is lost through evaporation from the respiratory tract. Cold stress also stimulates an increase in urine production and therefore in water losses. Dissipating the heat produced while exercising in a cold environment can be difficult. People often overdress, so as exercise proceeds, the excess heat produced cannot be lost to the environment.

Because water helps cool the body, the risk of heat disorders is greatly increased when someone begins exercise in a dehydrated condition. Excess body fat can also increase the risk of thermal distress for several reasons. Carrying a large amount of body fat increases the amount of work and therefore the metabolic cost of weight-bearing activity, so more heat is produced. Fat acts as an insulator and so retards heat conduction to the surface. And, because obese people have a

Heat index (apparent temperature)

Air temperature °F	Relative humidity (%) 40	45	50	55	60	65	70	75	80	85	90	95	100
110	136												
108	130	137											
106	124	130	137										
104	119	124	131	137									
102	114	119	124	130	137								
100	109	114	118	124	129	136							
98	105	109	113	117	123	128	134						
96	101	104	108	112	116	121	126	132					
94	97	100	102	106	110	114	119	124	129	135			
92	94	96	99	101	105	108	112	116	121	126	131		
90	91	93	95	97	100	103	106	109	113	117	122	127	132
88	88	89	91	93	95	98	100	103	106	110	113	117	121
86	85	87	88	89	91	93	95	97	100	102	105	108	112
84	83	84	85	86	88	89	90	92	94	96	98	100	103
82	81	82	83	84	84	85	86	88	89	90	91	93	95
80	80	80	81	81	82	82	83	84	84	85	86	86	87

With prolonged exposure and/or physical activity

Extreme danger	Heat stroke highly likely
Danger	Heat stroke, heat cramps, and/or heat exhaustion likely
Extreme caution	Heat stroke, heat cramps, and/or heat exhaustion possible
Caution	Fatigue possible

FIGURE 14.19 Exercise in extreme conditions increases the risk of thermal distress. This figure demonstrates the risks associated with exercise in weather with a high "heat index." The "heat index" or "apparent temperature" is a measure of how hot it feels when the relative humidity is added to the actual air temperature. To find the heat index, find the intersection of the temperature on the left side of the table and the relative humidity across the top of the table. The shaded zones correspond to heat index levels that may cause increasingly severe heat disorders with continued exposure and/or physical activity. *(Source: National Weather Service, online at http://weather.noaa.gov/weather/hwave.html)*

smaller surface-area-to-body-mass ratio than lean people, they are less efficient at dissipating heat through blood flow to the surface and the evaporation of sweat.[31]

Temperature Regulation in Children Children are at a greater risk for thermal distress because they produce more heat, are less able to transfer heat from muscles to the skin, and sweat less than adults. To reduce risks, children should rest periodically in the shade, consume fluids frequently, and limit the intensity and duration of activities on hot days. Children may also take longer to acclimatize to heat, so they should exercise at a reduced intensity and be given more time to acclimatize than mature competitors. Also, children lose more heat in cold environments than adults because they have a greater surface area per unit of body weight. Therefore, they are more prone to **hypothermia.**

Hypothermia A condition in which body temperature drops below normal. Hypothermia depresses the central nervous system, resulting in the inability to shiver, sleepiness, and eventually coma.

Weight Loss Through Dehydration Athletes involved in sports organized by weight classes, such as wrestling and boxing, sometimes go to unhealthy extremes to keep body weight down so they can compete in lower weight classes (competing at the high end of a weight class is thought to give an advantage over smaller opponents).[23] Frequently, this rapid weight loss is accomplished by dehydration, through such practices as vigorous exercise, fluid restriction, wearing vapor-impermeable suits, and using saunas and steam rooms. More extreme measures include vomiting and the use of diuretics and laxatives. These practices can be dangerous and even fatal. They may impair performance and can adversely affect heart and kidney function, temperature regulation, and electrolyte balance.[32]

Meeting Fluid Needs

Exercising individuals typically consume only about one third to two thirds of the amount of the fluid they lose in sweat.[33] Because thirst is not a reliable indicator of fluid needs, it is important for anyone exercising to consume fluid at regular intervals (Table 14.5). About 2 cups of fluid should be consumed 2 hours before exercise, and, on warm days, an additional 1 to 2 cups about 30 to 60 minutes before exercising is recommended.[34] During exercise, whether casual or competitive, 3 to 6 ounces of fluid should be consumed every 10 to 15 minutes. A good way to prevent dehydration is to consume enough fluid during exercise to minimize weight loss (Figure 14.20). And, immediately after exercise, each pound of weight lost should be replaced with 16 ounces of fluid (16 ounces = 1 pound).

TABLE 14.5 Recommendations for Fluid Intake

Before Exercise
Begin exercise well hydrated by consuming fluids during the 2 hours before exercise.
Consume 14 to 20 ounces of fluid during the 30 minutes before exercise.
During Exercise
Consume 3 to 6 ounces of fluid every 15 minutes.
For exercise lasting less than 60 to 90 minutes, water is the best fluid.
For exercise lasting longer than 60 to 90 minutes, consuming a fluid containing about 6% carbohydrate may improve endurance.*
For exercise lasting longer than 8 hours, a fluid containing carbohydrate and electrolytes may be beneficial.
After Exercise
Begin fluid replacement immediately after exercise.
Consume 16 ounces of fluid for each pound of weight lost.

* This is the amount of carbohydrate contained in a typical sports hydration beverage. On a food label it would be the equivalent of about 14 g/cup.

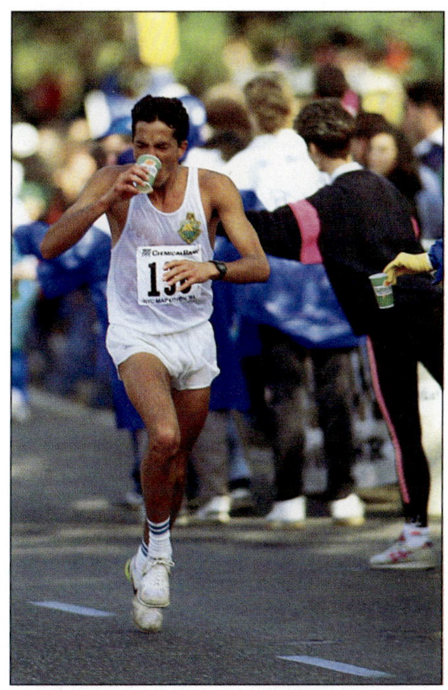

FIGURE 14.20 Fluids should be consumed before, during, and after exercise to maintain adequate hydration. *(© John Kelly/The Image Bank)*

Food and Drink for Competition

For most of us, a trip to the gym requires no special nutritional planning beyond that needed to consume a balanced diet and plenty of water. For more serious athletes, nutrients consumed before, during, and after activity can affect performance, and for competitive athletes, this may give or take away the extra seconds that can mean victory or defeat. Thus far, no magic pill that maximizes performance has been discovered, but there are a number of sound sports nutrition recommendations.

Glycogen Supercompensation

Glycogen supercompensation or **carbohydrate loading** A regimen of diet and exercise training designed to maximize muscle glycogen stores before an athletic event.

Glycogen provides a source of stored glucose. Larger glycogen stores allow exercise to continue for longer periods. Glycogen stores and hence endurance are increased with increasing carbohydrate intake (Figure 14.21). Serious athletes who want to substantially increase their glycogen stores before a competition may choose to follow a regimen of diet and exercise referred to as **glycogen supercompensation** or **carbohydrate loading.** This is more involved than simply eating a large spaghetti dinner before running in a 10-kilometer fun run. It involves depleting glycogen stores by exercising strenuously and then replenishing glycogen by consuming a high-carbohydrate diet for a few days before competition, during which time only light exercise is performed. The current practice is to taper down exercise during the six days before competition while progressively increasing the carbohydrate content of the diet to about 550 g per day, or 70% of energy, during the three days before competition.[35] Because consuming this much carbohydrate can be difficult, there are a number of high-carbohydrate liquid supplements available. These contain about 20 to 25 g of carbohydrate per 100 ml, or 50 to 60 g of carbohydrate in a 1-cup serving. These should not be confused with sports drinks designed to be consumed during competition, which contain only about 4 to 8 g of carbohydrate per 100 ml. A glycogen supercompensation regimen will increase glycogen stores 20 to 40% above the level that would be achieved on a typical diet.[36]

Although glycogen supercompensation is beneficial to endurance athletes, it will provide no benefit and even has some disadvantages for those exercising for periods of less than 90 minutes. For every gram of glycogen in the muscle, 3 g of water are also deposited. Therefore, glycogen supercompensation can cause a 2- to 7-pound weight gain as well as some muscle stiffness. As glycogen is used, the water is released. This can be an advantage when exercising in hot weather, but the extra weight is a disadvantage for those competing in events of short duration.

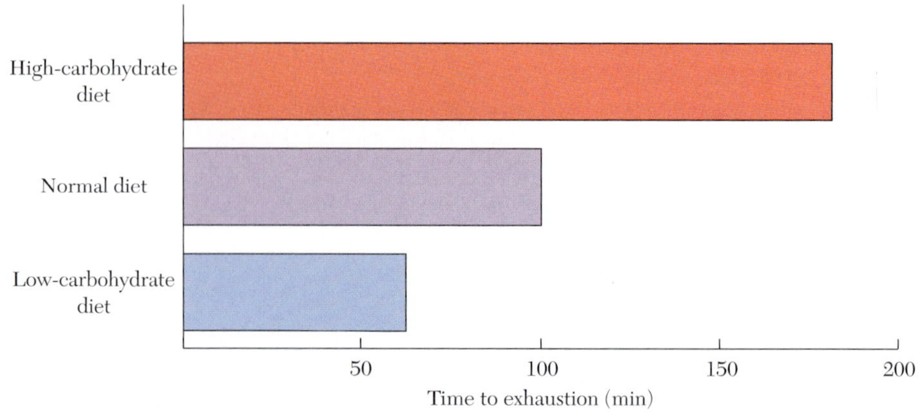

FIGURE 14.21 The amount of carbohydrate consumed in the diet affects the level of muscle glycogen and hence the endurance of the athlete. This graph shows endurance capacity during cycling exercise after three days of a very-low-carbohydrate diet (less than 5% of energy from carbohydrate), a normal diet (about 55% carbohydrate), and a high-carbohydrate diet (82% carbohydrate). *(From Bergstrom, J., Hermansen, L., Hultman, E., and Saltin, B. Diet, muscle glycogen and physical performance. Acta. Physiol. Scand. 71:140–150, 1967.)*

Meals for Competition

The goal of meals eaten before competition is to maximize glycogen stores and provide adequate hydration while minimizing any digestion, hunger, and gastric distress during the competition. The wrong precompetition meal can hinder performance more than the right one can enhance it. The goal for meals after competition is to replenish losses that occurred during the competition, including fluids and electrolytes in sweat.

Precompetition Meals Meals before competition should ensure that liver glycogen stores are full. Muscle glycogen is only depleted by exercise, but liver glycogen is used to supply blood glucose and is therefore depleted even during rest if no food is ingested. A high-carbohydrate meal (60–70%) eaten 2 to 4 hours before the event will fill liver glycogen stores. The meal should be low in fat (10–25%), moderate in protein (10–20%), and provide about 300 kcalories—for example, a cup of pasta with tomato sauce and a slice of bread, or a turkey sandwich and a cup of juice. High-fiber foods should be avoided to prevent feeling bloated during competition. Spicy foods that could cause heartburn, and large amounts of simple sugars that could cause diarrhea, should also be avoided unless the athlete is accustomed to eating these foods.

In addition to providing nutritional clout, a precompetition meal that includes "lucky" foods may impart an added psychological advantage. Some athletes find that in addition to a precompetition meal, a small high-carbohydrate snack or beverage consumed shortly before an event may enhance endurance.[36] Because foods affect people differently, athletes should test the effect of precompetition meals and snacks during training, not during competition.

During Exercise Food consumption during exercise is not necessary except during activities of long duration. However, fluid consumption during exercise is essential even for short-duration activities. For most exercisers, water is the best fluid to drink.[34] Alcohol and beverages containing caffeine, such as colas, iced tea, and coffee, act as diuretics and therefore reduce body fluids rather than increase them.

Exercise lasting longer than 60 to 90 minutes may cause body carbohydrate stores to be depleted. Athletes can benefit from consuming some carbohydrate during exercise of this duration. This carbohydrate is most easily consumed in a beverage. Consuming a fluid containing about 6% carbohydrate—that is, 4 to 8 g of carbohydrate per 100 ml of fluid—is recommended. This is the amount of carbohydrate found in popular sports beverages such as Gatorade and Powerade. The carbohydrate in these beverages helps to maintain blood glucose levels, therefore providing a source of glucose for the muscle and delaying fatigue. As the amount of carbohydrate in the beverage increases, the rate at which the solution leaves the stomach decreases. Water and carbohydrate trapped in the stomach do not benefit the athlete. Therefore, beverages containing larger amounts of carbohydrate, such as fruit juices and soft drinks, are not recommended unless they are diluted with an equal volume of water.

Small amounts of minerals, including sodium and chloride, are lost in sweat, but for most activities, replacing electrolytes is not a primary concern because sweat consists mostly of water. The amounts of sodium and other minerals lost in sweat during exercise lasting even as long as 5 hours are not enough to affect health or performance and can easily be replaced by food eaten after the exercise has stopped. Only in extremely long events lasting longer than 8 hours, such as ultramarathons or Ironman triathalons, are there significant losses of sodium and other minerals in the sweat. If, during one of these endurance events, an athlete were to drink water without electrolytes, the water would dilute the sodium remaining in the blood. When the blood is diluted, it signals the brain to stop the thirst sensation and stimulates the production of urine by the kidneys, increasing water loss and resulting in dehydration. The consumption of fluids containing electrolytes will prevent blood from becoming too diluted.[37] It is recommended that ultraendurance athletes include 0.5 to 0.7 g of sodium per liter (1.2 to 1.8 g of sodium chloride per liter) in their rehydration drinks. Consuming salt alone in pill form is unnecessary and dangerous because the salt will draw water away from the tissues and may cause dehydration, nausea, and vomiting. Therefore, the common belief that salt pills are necessary to replace the sodium lost in sweat and prevent dehydration is a misconception.

Postcompetition Meals When exercise ends, the body must shift from the catabolic state of breaking down glycogen, triglycerides, and muscle proteins for fuel to the anabolic state of restoring muscle and liver glycogen, depositing lipids, and synthesizing muscle proteins. The first priority is to replace fluid losses, but restoration of glycogen stores is also critical to the ability to perform subsequent endurance activities. Appropriate postcompetition intake can replenish muscle and liver glycogen within 24 hours of the athletic event. To maximize glycogen replacement, a high-carbohydrate meal or drink should be consumed as soon as possible after the event and again every 2 hours for 6 hours after the event. Ideally the meals should provide about 0.7 to 1.5 g of carbohydrate per kg of body weight, which is about 50 to 100 g of carbohydrate for a 70-kg person—the equivalent of two pancakes with syrup and a glass of fruit punch.[35] Approximately 600 g of carbohydrate, or about 8 to 10 g per kg, should be consumed during the 24 hours after exercise. The consumption of fructose compared to glucose induces less muscle glycogen synthesis and more liver glycogen synthesis.

Web Menu: For more information on dietary supplements and their potential risks and benefits, go to the Office of Dietary Supplements at dietary-supplements.info.nih.gov/, or to the government nutrition site at www.nutrition.gov/ and click on dietary supplements.

Ergogenic Aids

Athletes use a variety of performance-enhancing, or **ergogenic, aids** (Figure 14.22). Anything designed to enhance performance can be considered an ergogenic aid; running shoes are mechanical aids; psychotherapy is a psychological aid; drugs are pharmacological aids. The following sections discuss dietary supplements that are used as ergogenic aids (Table 14.6). Although many of these

Ergogenic aids Anything designed to increase the ability to work or improve performance.

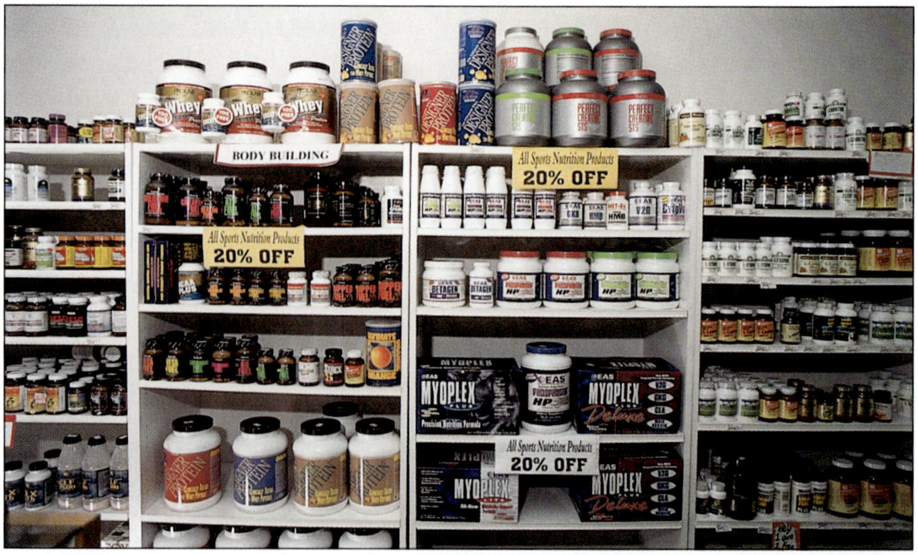

FIGURE 14.22 Many types of supplements are marketed to athletes as ergogenic aids. *(George Semple)*

TABLE 14.6 Claims, Effectiveness, and Risks of Popular Ergogenic Aids

Ergogenic Aid	Claim	Effectiveness	Risk
Androstenedione	Converted to testosterone, which increases muscle growth and strength.	No long-term human studies on safety or ergogenic effects.	May have risks similar to illegal steroids, such as stunted growth, acne, unwanted hair growth, premature baldness, increased blood cholesterol levels, and decreased sperm production.
Arginine, ornithine, and lysine	Cause the release of growth hormone, which stimulates muscle development and decreases body fat.	Most studies show no increase in lean body mass with supplementation.	High levels of one amino acid may interfere with the absorption of others. Cause diarrhea at high doses.
Bee pollen	Causes faster recovery from training workouts, which enables a higher level of training.	No evidence that it improves training level or other parameters of performance.	Some individuals have allergic reactions.
Bicarbonate (sodium bicarbonate, baking soda)	Helps buffer lactic acid produced during exercise, thereby delaying fatigue.	Research demonstrates that supplements increase blood pH and may enhance performance and strength in intense anaerobic activities but not in aerobic exercise.	Causes bloating, diarrhea, and high blood pH.
Branched chain amino acids (leucine, isoleucine, and valine)	Improve endurance and prevent fatigue.	Some studies show improvements in endurance (but no greater than achieved with carbohydrate supplementation) and protection against muscle damage. Others show no effect.	No toxicity reported.
Caffeine	Increases the release of fatty acids from adipose tissue, spares glycogen, and enhances endurance.	Research supports claims of increased endurance, but the effect depends on the individual.	Causes dehydration, nervousness, anxiety, insomnia, digestive discomfort, abnormal heartbeat with doses > 10 mg/kg
Carnitine	Enhances the utilization of fatty acids and spares glycogen.	Most studies show no increase in fatty acid utilization or improvement in exercise performance.	L-Carnitine form has little risk, but D,L-Carnitine and D-carnitine forms can be toxic.
Chromium (chromium picolinate)	Increases lean body mass, decreases body fat, delays fatigue.	Affects glucose utilization, protein synthesis, and lipid metabolism via its effect on insulin action, but there is no evidence that supplements affect these processes unless a deficiency exists.	No toxicity reported in humans, but the chromium picolinate form has been shown to damage DNA in cells grown in the laboratory.
Creatine (creatine monohydrate)	Increases energy production and speeds recovery after high-intensity exercise.	Research suggests that creatine supplements increase muscle creatine and creatine phosphate synthesis after exercise, and enhance strength, performance, and recovery from high-intensity exercise.	Causes stomach pain.
DHEA (dehydro-epiandrosterone)	Converted into testosterone and estrogen inside the body and promises to build muscles, burn fat, and delay chronic diseases associated with aging.	No proven benefits.	May cause acne, oily skin, facial hair, voice deepening, hair loss, mood changes, liver damage, and stimulate existing cancers.
Ephedra (Chinese ephedra, Ma Huang)	Increase time to exhaustion, inhibit hunger, and stimulate energy expenditure and fat breakdown.	Research shows that it causes selective fat breakdown with weight loss and increases in time to exhaustion especially when taken with caffeine.	High doses can lead to heart attack, stroke, seizure, psychosis, and death. Low doses are associated with dizziness, headache, gastrointestinal distress, irregular heartbeat, or heart palpitations.

continued

TABLE 14.6 *continued*

Ergogenic Aid	Claim	Effectiveness	Risk
Ginseng (*P. Ginseng* or Chinese ginseng)	Enhances performance	Evidence that about 2 g of dried root per day taken for 8 to 12 weeks may improve muscle strength and aerobic capacity.	May increase the effects and side effects of other stimulants such as caffeine.
Glutamine	Increases muscle glycogen deposition following intense exercise, enhances immune function, and prevents the adverse effects of overtraining such as fatigue and increased incidence of certain infections.	Little evidence that glutamine supplementation increases immune function or prevents the symptoms of overtraining, no evidence that glutamine increases glycogen synthesis.	No evidence of toxicity shown.
HMB (β-hydroxy β-methyl butyrate)	Increases ability to build muscle and burn fat in response to exercise.	Some studies support an increase in lean body mass and strength.	No toxicity in animals, but little information in humans.
Medium-chain triglycerides (MCT)	Provide energy to bodybuilders without promoting fat deposition; reduce muscle protein breakdown during prolonged exercise.	Studies show that they increase endurance and fatty acid oxidation in mice, but there is no evidence of a benefit in humans.	None known.
Vanadium (vanadyl sulfate)	Aids insulin action; allows more rapid and intense muscle pumping for bodybuilders.	No evidence to support a benefit for bodybuilders.	Reduces insulin production.

supplements are expensive and most have not been shown to improve performance, athletes are vulnerable to their enticements.[38] When considering the use of an ergogenic supplement, an athlete should remember that, as dietary supplements, these products do not have to be proven safe or effective before they can be sold (see Chapter 10). Consumers should weigh health risks against potential benefits prior to using these products (see Table 14.7).

Vitamin Supplements

Many of the B vitamins are promoted as ergogenic supplements. The promises made about these supplements are extrapolated from their biochemical functions. Thiamin, riboflavin, niacin, and pantothenic acid are all involved in muscle energy

TABLE 14.7 Assessing the Risks of Ergogenic Supplements

Why do you want a supplement?

- Has the supplement you are considering been shown to provide these benefits?

What ingredients does the product contain?

- Does it contain any ingredients that have been shown to be toxic to someone like you?
- Do you have a medical condition that recommends against certain nutrients or other ingredients?
- Are you taking prescription medication with which an ingredient in the supplement may interact?

How much of each ingredient does it contain?

- Does it contain potentially toxic levels of any nutrient? Check the % Daily Value. Does the level exceed the UL?
- Don't take more than is recommended on the package. More isn't always better and may cause side effects.

Consider the costs

- More expensive is not always better.
- Compare costs and ingredients before you buy.

metabolism. Thiamin and pantothenic acid are needed for carbohydrate to enter the citric acid cycle for aerobic metabolism. Riboflavin and niacin are needed to shuttle electrons to the electron transport chain so ATP can be formed. Vitamin B_6 is involved in protein and amino acid metabolism. During exercise it is needed to use amino acids for energy, to break down muscle glycogen, and to convert lactic acid to glucose in the liver. Vitamins B_6, B_{12}, and folic acid are promoted for aerobic exercise because they are involved in the transport of oxygen to exercising muscle. Vitamin B_6 is needed for the synthesis of hemoglobin, and folic acid and vitamin B_{12} are both involved in the synthesis of red blood cells. All of these vitamins are indeed needed for energy metabolism, and a deficiency of one or more of these would interfere with energy production and impair athletic performance. Because athletes must consume more food to meet energy needs, more vitamins are consumed as well. A reasonably well-planned diet based on grains, vegetables, and fruits and including some meat and milk provides enough of all the B vitamins to meet an athlete's needs without supplements.

Antioxidant supplements are promoted to athletes because exercise increases oxidative processes, and hence the production of free radicals. Free radicals can damage tissues and have been associated with fatigue during exercise.[19,39] It has been suggested that antioxidant supplements, including vitamin C, vitamin E, and beta-carotene, will prevent free-radical damage and delay fatigue. Vitamin E and vitamin C have been the most extensively studied. Vitamin E is particularly important in maintaining muscle function by protecting muscle cell membranes from free radical damage. Vitamin C acts as a free radical scavenger in aqueous solutions, such as the intracellular fluid and blood. Supplementation with mixtures of antioxidants has been shown to prevent free radical damage but has not been demonstrated conclusively to enhance performance.[40,41] As long as athletes do not consume vitamin E, vitamin C, and beta-carotene supplements in amounts that exceed the Tolerable Upper Intake Levels (ULs) recommended by the DRIs, there is little risk associated with their use; however, a diet that includes plenty of fruits and vegetables will ensure adequate intakes of these nutrients as well as provide other dietary antioxidants.

Mineral Supplements

Some of the minerals advertised as endurance enhancers include chromium, vanadium, selenium, zinc, and iron. Chromium supplements, as chromium picolinate, claim to increase lean body mass and decrease body fat. Chromium is needed for insulin action, and insulin promotes protein synthesis; therefore, adequate chromium status is likely to be important for lean-tissue synthesis. The picolinate form is used because it is believed to be absorbed better than other forms of chromium. Research in pigs has demonstrated that supplemental chromium causes an increase in muscle mass and a decrease in body fat, but most studies on the effects of chromium picolinate or other chromium supplements in healthy human subjects have found no beneficial effects on muscle strength, body composition, weight loss, or other aspects of health.[42] Controlled trials have reported no dietary toxicity in humans, and oral chromium picolinate at doses containing 1.0 mg of chromium per day has produced no adverse effects.[43] Because no adverse effects have been associated with chromium intake from food or supplements, no UL has been established.[26] Despite the apparent safety of chromium supplements, a few concerns have been raised. Two cases of renal failure have been associated with chromium picolinate supplements, but both of these individuals were taking other drugs known to cause renal toxicity so it is unclear if the effect was due to the chromium supplement.[43] The safety of chromium picolinate has also been questioned because of studies in cell culture that suggest it may cause DNA damage.[44] This effect is specific to the picolinate form of chromium and may be due to the ability of this form to generate DNA-damaging free radicals.[45] Human studies using the standard supplemental doses of chromium picolinate have not detected an increase in DNA damage, but more work is needed to completely rule out any risk.[46]

Vanadium, usually as vanadyl sulfate, is another mineral marketed for its ability to assist the action of insulin. Vanadium supplements promise to increase lean body mass, but there is no evidence that they have an anabolic effect, and toxicity is a concern.[40] A UL of 1.8 mg per day of elemental vanadium has been set for adults age 19 and older.[26]

Selenium is marketed for its antioxidant properties and zinc for its role in protein synthesis and tissue repair, but neither of these supplements has been found to improve athletic performance in individuals with adequate mineral status. Iron is also marketed as an ergogenic mineral because it is needed for hemoglobin synthesis. If an iron deficiency exists, as it frequently does in female athletes, supplements can be of benefit.

Amino Acid Supplements

Amino acid supplements are also promoted to athletes. Supplements of some single amino acids affect hormone levels and muscle physiology, but their effect on exercise performance is unclear. Glycine supplements are promoted because glycine is a precursor to creatine, but it does not provide the ergogenic effects that creatine supplements do (see next section). The amino acids ornithine, arginine, and lysine are marketed with the promise that they will stimulate the release of growth hormone and, in turn, enhance the growth of muscles. Large doses of these amino acids have been shown to stimulate growth hormone release, but in the amounts typically supplemented, serum growth hormone levels are not increased and there is no effect on muscle growth or strength in weight lifters.[40]

Glutamine supplements promise to increase muscle glycogen deposition following intense exercise, to enhance immune function, and to prevent the adverse effects of overtraining such as fatigue and increased incidence of certain infections. Glutamine supplementation has not been found to increase glycogen synthesis.[47] Glutamine is important for immune system cells, and decreases in the plasma glutamine have been reported following prolonged exercise; however, the effects of glutamine supplementation on immune function or the symptoms of overtraining are inconsistent.[40]

The branched-chain amino acids (leucine, isoleucine, and valine) are the predominant amino acids used for fuel during exercise. Supplements of these are promoted to improve performance in endurance athletes. The results of studies examining the effect of branched-chain amino acids on endurance performance have found that they do not enhance performance, particularly when compared to the endurance-enhancing effect of carbohydrate supplementation.[48]

There is little evidence to support the use of amino acid supplements by athletes, and in general these supplements are not recommended. High doses of individual amino acids may interfere with the absorption of other amino acids from the diet (see Chapter 6). And, there have been several reports of illness caused by contaminants in the supplements. Like any dietary supplement, amino acid supplements should be taken with caution and the risks weighed against potential benefits.

Other Ergogenic Aids

Substances that are not nutrients are also marketed as ergogenic aids. Creatine, bicarbonate, and caffeine are nonnutrients that can have an ergogenic effect for some types of activity. Many herbal preparations are also marketed to athletes; some, such as ginseng and ephedra, may have ergogenic effects, but in the case of ephedra, the risk of serious side effects is great. Many other supplements that are sold to enhance performance, such as bee pollen, wheat germ oil, brewer's yeast, royal jelly, DNA, and RNA, have not been found to be ergogenic.

Creatine Creatine supplements promise to replenish creatine phosphate for quick energy and to increase muscle mass (Figure 14.23). Creatine is a nitrogen-containing compound found in the body, primarily in muscle, where it is used to make creatine phosphate. It is synthesized by the kidney, liver, pancreas, and other tissues and is consumed in the diet in muscle meats and milk. The more creatine in the diet, the greater the muscle stores. Individuals who consume diets low in creatine, such as vegetarians, have lower body stores. Supplements of creatine monohydrate have been shown to increase levels of both creatine and creatine phosphate in muscle.[49,50] Once muscle creatine levels have increased, they remain elevated for several weeks after the supplement is stopped.

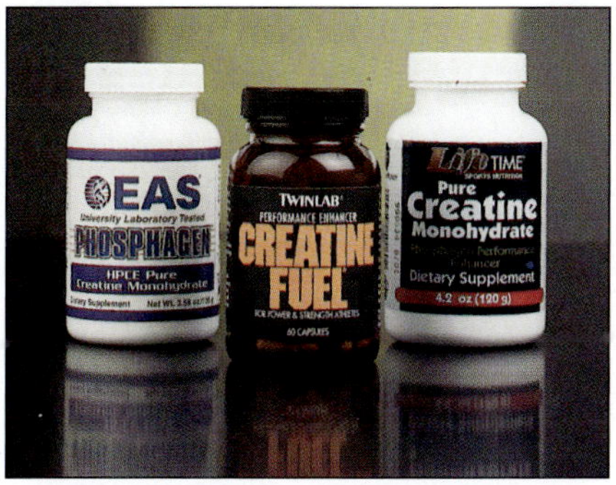

FIGURE 14.23 Creatine supplements are marketed to athletes to delay fatigue and increase muscle mass. *(George Semple)*

Increasing muscle creatine and creatine phosphate provides muscles with more quick energy for activity, delays fatigue, and allows creatine phosphate to be regenerated more quickly after exercise. And, it prevents the accumulation of lactic acid, which impairs performance.[49] These effects make creatine supplementation beneficial for exercise that requires explosive bursts of energy, such as sprinting and weight lifting, but do not enhance performance in long-term endurance activities such as marathons. Creatine supplements have also been found to increase body mass mostly through lean tissue. This increase is believed to be due to water retention related to creatine uptake in the muscle. An increase in muscle mass and strength may also occur in response to the greater amount and intensity of training that may be achieved.[50] Although creatine supplements have been demonstrated to be effective in the short term, there are little data on whether chronic use further increases performance.

A number of studies have suggested that creatine supplements are safe, but controlled toxicology studies have not been done and the safety and efficacy of the long-term use of high-dose supplements is unknown.[51] There are anecdotal reports of muscle cramps, tears, pulls, dehydration, and gastrointestinal distress among users. Research studies have not confirmed that creatine supplementation causes muscle cramps or gastrointestinal complications, and the acute effects of high-dose creatine supplementation on body fluid balance have not been fully investigated.[49] Product purity is also a concern. Because large doses of 5 to 30 g (1 to 6 teaspoons) are needed to be effective, even a minor contaminant might be consumed in significant amounts. Ingestion of creatine before or during exercise is not recommended, and the FDA has advised consumers to consult a physician before using creatine.

Bicarbonate Bicarbonate ions act as buffers in the body. It is hypothesized that bicarbonate supplements neutralize the lactic acid produced by anaerobic exercise and thus delay fatigue and allow improved performance. Taking bicarbonate before exercise has been found to improve performance and delay exhaustion in sports such as sprint cycling, which involve intense exercise lasting for only 1 to 7 minutes, but it is of no benefit for lower-intensity aerobic exercise.[40]

Caffeine Some athletes may try to enhance endurance by consuming caffeine before an event. Caffeine has been shown to enhance performance during prolonged moderate-intensity endurance exercise and short-term intense exercise.[52] It is hypothesized that this occurs because caffeine enhances the release of fatty acids, and when fatty acids are used as a fuel source, glycogen is spared, delaying the onset of fatigue. The effect may vary, depending on the type of activity and the athlete. Athletes who are unaccustomed to caffeine respond better than those who routinely consume it. In some athletes caffeine may impair performance by increasing water loss in the urine or by causing gastrointestinal upset. Regardless of its effectiveness, athletes should know that excess caffeine is illegal. The International Olympic Committee prohibits athletes from competing when urine caffeine levels are 12 μg per ml or greater. For urine caffeine to reach this level, an individual would need to drink 6 to 8 cups of coffee within about a 2-hour period. Caffeine is also found in pill form in products such as NoDoz, which contains about 100 mg of caffeine per tablet—about the same amount as that in a cup of coffee (Table 14.8).

TABLE 14.8 The Caffeine Content of Foods and Medications

Food or Medication	Amount	Caffeine (mg)
Coffee, regular	1 cup (240 ml)	139
Coffee, espresso	4 fluid ounces	200
Coffee, decaffeinated	1 cup	3
Tea, brewed	1 cup	45
Pepsi Cola	12 oz (1 can)	37
Diet Pepsi	12 oz (1 can)	50
Mountain Dew	12 oz (1 can)	54
Hot chocolate	1 cup	7
Brownie	1	14
Chocolate bar	1 oz	15
NoDoz	1 tablet	100
Excedrin	1 tablet	65
Empirin, Anacin	1 tablet	32

Herbal Supplements Most herbs that are used as ergogenic aids are poorly researched so the evidence for their benefits is only anecdotal. Ginseng and ephedra are the best studied of herbal ergogens.[53]

Ginseng is promoted to increase endurance. There are many different varieties of ginseng (American, Chinese, Japanese, Siberian) and it comes in many forms (tinctures, whole root, powdered root, teas, and extracts). Human clinical trials of Chinese ginseng (*P. ginseng*) have shown that when taken in appropriate doses for long enough by individuals engaged in physical activity of sufficient intensity, it may increase muscle strength and aerobic capacity.[53] The benefits may be greater for untrained or older subjects. Ginseng supplements are generally considered safe based on over 2000 years of use with few reported side effects. Side effects may, however, occur in some individuals, and it has been shown to increase the effects and side effects of other stimulants such as caffeine.[53,40]

Ephedrine, also called ephedra, Chinese ephedra, or Ma Huang, is also taken to improve performance. Unlike other herbal supplements the active ingredient, ephedrine, is well characterized; ephedrine is used in many over-the-counter and prescription antihistamine, decongestant, and appetite suppressant products. Ephedrine is a stimulant that mimics the effects of epinephrine. Large doses of ephedrine, about 25 mg, have not been shown to improve athletic performance and when combined with large amounts of caffeine ($>$ 100 mg), have been associated with serious side effects including nervousness, headaches, nausea, hypertension, cardiac arrhythmias, and even death. Lower doses of ephedrine combined with moderate amounts of caffeine have been shown to increase the time to exhaustion in exercise and to promote a reduction in body fat during weight loss. The use of ephedrine, whether herbal or synthetic, has been banned from amateur sporting events.[53]

Other Supplements Bee pollen is a mixture of the pollen of flowering plants, plant nectar, and bee saliva. It contains no extraordinary factors and has not been shown to have any performance-enhancing effects. In addition, ingesting or inhaling bee pollen can be hazardous to individuals allergic to various plant pollens.[54] Brewer's yeast is a source of B vitamins and some minerals, but has not been demonstrated to have any ergogenic properties. Likewise, there is no evidence to support claims that wheat germ oil will aid endurance. As an oil, it is high in fat, but it is no better as an energy source than any other fat. Royal jelly is a substance produced by worker bees to feed to the queen bee. While it helps the queen bee grow to twice the size of worker bees and to live 40 times longer, royal jelly does not appear to enhance athletic capacity in humans. Finally, DNA and RNA are marketed to aid in tissue regeneration. In the body they carry genetic information and are needed to synthesize proteins, but DNA and RNA are not required in the diet, and supplements do not help replace damaged cells (see *Critical Thinking:* "Can Supplements Safely Increase Speed?").

Critical Thinking

Can Supplements Safely Increase Speed?

Diana is on the college track team. She would like to improve her sprint times and is thinking about trying some dietary supplements. Based on articles and advertisements in sports magazines, she selects bicarbonate to improve her sprint times and chromium to reduce her body fat and increase her lean body mass. But before she begins taking them, she wants to explore their risks and benefits. The ads and articles about these supplements make the following claims:

- Bicarbonate will help neutralize lactic acid produced by muscles during anaerobic exercise and therefore improve performance in short-term exhaustive exercise.
- Chromium will increase lean body tissue and enhance fat loss.

Do the claims made for these products make sense?

Bicarbonate is a buffer found naturally in the body that helps keep acidity in the normal range. So the claim that more might help buffer lactic acid is logical, assuming the bicarbonate from the supplement reaches the muscle cells where the lactic acid is produced.

Chromium is a mineral that is needed for insulin to perform its functions. Insulin is needed for many essential roles, including getting glucose into cells, turning on protein synthesis, and stimulating the synthesis of fat. The claim that it will increase lean tissue makes some sense metabolically, but Diana is not sure why taking chromium would enhance only the protein-building aspect of insulin's function.

Is there evidence that these supplements work?

The advertisements show photographs of sprinters and body builders and quote their testimonials on the effectiveness of these products. This type of anecdotal evidence does not convince Diana, so she makes a trip to the library to explore the scientific literature.

Where should Diana look for more information?

In order to find sound scientific studies, Diana should look for articles in well-respected peer-reviewed journals in the field of nutrition and sports, such as the *International Journal of Sport Nutrition* and *Medicine and Science in Sports and Exercise.* She should then look for studies that focus on athletes involved in the types of activities she performs. She can also check the government nutrition site at **www.nutrition.gov** for links to information on dietary supplements.

Do these supplements have scientifically proven benefits?

Diana finds several articles on bicarbonate and chromium. The studies of bicarbonate involve exhaustive exercise lasting 1 to 7 minutes and demonstrate that the performance of sprinters taking bicarbonate is enhanced compared to that of sprinters taking a placebo. For chromium, the studies are contradictory. One shows an increase in the amount of weight gained and a decrease in body fat in college weight trainers, while another study finds no significant effects.

What are the risks of taking bicarbonate and chromium?

Bicarbonate is sold as sodium bicarbonate, so it is high in sodium. Since it is not an essential nutrient, it is difficult to find information on toxicity. One article that Diana read used a dose of 0.3 g per kilogram of body weight 2 to 3 hours before an event. At this dose some subjects experienced nausea, bloating, intestinal cramping, and diarrhea. Large intakes of water were recommended to prevent diarrhea.

Chromium is an essential mineral, but the muscle-building effects of chromium are still questionable. The doses in supplements are about 200 μg per day, well above the AI for chromium of 25 μg/day. Although the evidence for chromium toxicity was not substantial enough to establish a UL, one study found that the picolinate form of chromium caused DNA damage in cells grown in the laboratory.

Diana decides that she will wait for more research to be done before she takes chromium picolinate as an ergogenic aid. Because she eats a balanced diet and takes a multivitamin and mineral supplement that contains chromium, she concludes that she is getting adequate chromium. She is still unsure whether bicarbonate will offer more benefits than risks.

What would you recommend Diana do?

Answer:

SUMMARY

1. Fitness, which is the ability to perform routine physical activity without undue fatigue, is defined by an individual's cardiorespiratory endurance, muscle strength and endurance, flexibility, and body composition.
2. Regular exercise improves fitness in individuals of all ages and can reduce the risk of chronic diseases such as obesity, heart disease, diabetes, and osteoporosis. Exercise can also delay some of the changes in body composition and metabolism that occur with age.
3. A well-designed fitness program involves aerobic exercise, stretching, and strength training. There are numerous recommendations for how much exercise is enough; most agree that a minimum of 30 minutes of moderate activity should be performed on most days of the week. One way to create a more active lifestyle is to choose enjoyable activities and follow the recommendations of the Activity Pyramid.
4. Activity is fueled by ATP. Small amounts of ATP are stored in the muscle and can be replenished by the breakdown of creatine phosphate. ATP and creatine phosphate can power activity that lasts for 10 to 15 seconds. For exercise to continue, additional ATP must be produced from the metabolism of carbohydrate, fat, and protein. When oxygen is limited, anaerobic glycolysis produces ATP from carbohydrate. When oxygen is plentiful, aerobic metabolism generates ATP. Aerobic metabolism is more efficient than

anaerobic glycolysis and can utilize glucose, fatty acids, and amino acids as energy sources.

5. The availability of oxygen and the proportion of carbohydrate and fat used as fuel for a given activity depend on the intensity and duration of the activity and the training of the exerciser. For short-term, high-intensity activity, ATP is generated primarily from the anaerobic metabolism of glucose. For lower-intensity exercise of longer duration, aerobic metabolism predominates, and both glucose and fatty acids become important fuel sources. The proportion of energy generated from fatty acids increases with the duration of low-intensity exercise. Protein becomes an important source of energy only when exercise continues for many hours. Training improves oxygen delivery and utilization, allowing aerobic exercise to be sustained for longer periods at higher intensities.
6. The daily diet of an active individual should provide sufficient energy to fuel activity. In general, it should contain about 55 to 60% of total energy as carbohydrate from whole grains, fruits, vegetables, and milk to ensure that glycogen stores are replenished after daily exercise; less than 30% of energy as fat; and about 10 to 20% of energy as protein.
7. Sufficient micronutrients are needed to generate ATP from macronutrients and to transport oxygen and wastes to and from the cells. Some athletes are at risk for deficiencies of iron and calcium. Female athletes who are concerned about maintaining a low body weight are at risk of developing the female athlete triad: disordered eating, amenorrhea, and osteoporosis.
8. Fluid intake before, during, and after exercise must replace water lost in sweat and from evaporation through the lungs. Water intake during activity must be sufficient to ensure that the body can be cooled and that nutrients and oxygen can be delivered to body tissues. If water intake is inadequate, exercise performance will decrease and thermal distress may occur. Hot and humid environments increase the risk of thermal distress. Plain water is the best fluid to consume for most exercise.
9. Competitive endurance athletes may utilize glycogen supercompensation regimens to maximize glycogen stores before an event.
10. Meals eaten before competition should provide about 300 kcalories; should be high in carbohydrate, low in fat, moderate in protein, and low in fiber; and should satisfy the psychological needs of the athlete. The only thing that needs to be consumed during short duration exercise is water. During exercise lasting longer than 60 to 90 minutes, athletes might benefit from fluids containing glucose. Electrolyte replacement is only necessary during ultraendurance activities lasting more than 8 hours. Postcompetition meals should replace lost fluids and electrolytes and begin restoring muscle and liver glycogen.
11. Many types of ergogenic aids are marketed to improve athletic performance. Some are beneficial for certain types of activity, but many offer little or no benefit. An individual risk-benefit analysis should be used to determine if a supplement is appropriate for you.

Review Questions

1. List the health benefits of fitness.
2. What is aerobic exercise?
3. What is strength training?
4. How does aerobic exercise affect resting heart rate?
5. How much exercise is enough?
6. What is maximal oxygen consumption and how is it affected by aerobic exercise?
7. What fuels are used to produce ATP in anaerobic metabolism? Aerobic metabolism?
8. Which is more efficient, aerobic or anaerobic metabolism? Why?
9. What factors affect the availability of oxygen and the type of fuel used during exercise?
10. What fuels are used in exercise of long duration such as marathon running?
11. What fuels are used for very intense exercise such as sprinting?
12. List some physiological adaptations that occur with training. How do they affect endurance?
13. Why is fluid intake important before, during, and after exercise? What are the recommendations?
14. How does exercise affect protein needs?
15. What is glycogen supercompensation (carbohydrate loading)?
16. Can ergogenic aids enhance exercise performance? How? Are they safe?

Applying Critical Thinking Skills

Personal nutrition:

1. Keep a log of your activity for one day.
   a. Note the number of hours you spend in (1) sleep, (2) very light activity, (3) light activity, (4) moderate activity, and (5) heavy activity (see Chapter 7).
   b. What is your RMR per hour? (Use Table 7.5 or Appendix N.)
   c. What are your energy needs for activity? (Use Table 7.6, Table 14.4, or Appendix K.)
   d. If you replaced one hour of very light activity with a one-hour jog, what would your new energy expenditure be?
   e. What snack could you add to your diet to balance the added expenditure of the jog?
2. Taking into consideration your typical weekly schedule of activities and events, design a reasonable exercise program for yourself using the Activity Pyramid. Include the types of activities, the times during the week you will be involved

in each activity, and the length of time you will engage in each activity. Choose activities you enjoy and schedule them for reasonable lengths of time and at reasonable frequencies.

a. What everyday changes have you made that will increase the energy expended in day-to-day activities?
b. Which activities are aerobic, which improve flexibility, and which are for strength training?
c. Can each of these activities be performed year-round? Suggest alternative activities and locations for inclement weather.

General nutrition issues:

1. Peter is beginning an exercise program. He plans to run before lunch and then play racquetball every night after dinner. Once he begins his exercise program he finds that he feels lethargic and hungry before his late-morning run. After running, he doesn't have much of an appetite, so he saves his fast-food lunch until midafternoon. He is still hungry enough to eat dinner at home with his family, but finds that he is getting stomach cramps and is too full when he goes to play racquetball. His typical diet is listed below:

Typical Diet

Breakfast
Orange juice
Coffee

Lunch
Big Mac
French fries
Milk shake

Dinner
Steak
Baked potato with sour cream and butter
Green beans in butter sauce
Salad with Italian dressing
Whole milk

a. How might Peter change his diet so it is better suited to his exercise program?
b. Does his exercise program include both an aerobic and a strength-training component?
c. Do you think Peter will be able to stick with this exercise program? Why or why not?
d. Suggest some changes that would make Peter's exercise program more balanced.

2. Do a risk-benefit analysis of an ergogenic aid (a quick way to do this is to use the Internet to collect information). List the risks and benefits and then write a conclusion stating why you would or would not take this substance.

References

1. Abernathy, R. P., and Black, D. R. Healthy body weights: an alternative perspective. Am. J. Clin. Nutr. 63(suppl):448S–451S, 1996.
2. U.S. Department of Health and Human Services, Centers for Disease Control and Prevention, and the President's Council on Physical Fitness and Sports. Physical Activity and Health: A Report of the Surgeon General (Executive Summary), 1996.
3. Zelasko, C. J. Exercise for weight loss: what are the facts? J. Am. Diet. Assoc. 95:1414–1417, 1995.
4. Weyer, C., Linkeschowa, R., Heise, T., et al. Implications of the traditional and the new ACSM physical activity recommendations on weight reduction in dietary treated obese subjects. Int. J. Obes. Relat. Metab. Disord. 22:1071–1078, 1998.
5. Physical activity and cardiovascular health. NIH Consensus Development Panel on Physical Activity and Cardiovascular Health. JAMA 276:241–246, 1996.
6. American College of Sports Medicine. American College of Sports Medicine position stand: exercise and physical activity for older adults. Med. Sci. Sports Exerc. 30:992–1008, 1998.
7. Albright, A., Franz, M., Hornsby, G., et al. American College of Sports Medicine position stand. Exercise and type 2 diabetes. Med. Sci. Sports Exerc. 32:1345–1360, 2000.
8. Gammon, M. D., John, E. M., and Britton, J. A. Recreational and occupational physical activities and risk of breast cancer. J. Natl. Cancer Inst. 90:100–117, 1998.
9. Colditz, G. A., Cannuscio, C. C., and Frazier, A. L. Physical activity and reduced risk of colon cancer: implications for prevention. Cancer Causes Control 8:649–667, 1997.
10. U.S. Department of Agriculture, U.S. Department of Health and Human Services. *Nutrition and Your Health: Dietary Guidelines for Americans,* 5th ed. Home and Garden Bulletin No. 232. Hyattsville, Md.: U.S. Government Printing Office, 2000.
11. Healthy People 2010. Available online at **http://www.health.gov/healthypeople/.** Accessed 6 Sept 2000.
12. Jones, D. A., Ainsworth, B. E., Croft, J. B., et al. Moderate leisure-time physical activity: who is meeting the public health recommendations? A national cross-sectional study. Arch. Fam. Med. 7:285–289, 1998.
13. Taaffe, D. R., and Marcus, R. Musculoskeletal health and the older adult. J. Rehabil. Res. Dev. 37:245–254, 2000.
14. ACSM Position Stand on the recommended quantity and quality of exercise for developing and maintaining cardiorespiratory and muscular fitness and flexibility in adults. Med. Sci. Sports Exerc. 30:975–991, 1998.
15. Andersen, R. E., Crespo, C. J., Barlett, S. J., et al. Relationship of physical activity and television watching with body weight and level of fatness among children: results from the Third National Health and Nutrition Examination Survey. JAMA 279:938–942, 1998.
16. Wang, T. W., and Apgar, B. S. Exercise during pregnancy. Am. Fam. Physician 57:1846–1852, 1998.
17. American College of Sports Medicine. *ACSM's Guidelines for Exercise Testing and Prescription,* 5th ed. Baltimore: Williams & Wilkins, 1995.
18. Horowitz, J. F., and Klein, S. Lipid metabolism during endurance exercise. Am. J. Clin. Nutr. 72(suppl):558S–563S, 2000.
19. Brass, E. P. Supplemental carnitine and exercise. Am. J. Clin. Nutr. 72(suppl):618S–623S, 2000.
20. Ratzin Jackson, C. G. Overview of human energy transfer and nutrition. In *Nutrition in Exercise and Sport,* 3rd ed. Wolinski, I., ed. Boca Raton, Fla.: CRC Press, 1998, 159–177.
21. Beals, K. A., and Manore, M. M. Nutritional status of female athletes with subclinical eating disorders. J. Am. Diet. Assoc. 98:419–425, 1998.
22. Arena, B., Maffulli, N., Maffulli, F., and Morleo, M. A. Reproductive hormones and menstrual changes with exercise in female athletes. Sports Med. 19:278–287, 1995.
23. Oppliger, R. A., Case, H. S., Horswill, C. A., et al. American College of Sports Medicine position statement: weight-loss in wrestlers. Med. Sci. Sports Exerc. 28:ix–xii, 1996.
24. Paul, G. L., Gautsch, T. A., and Layman, D. K. Amino acid and protein metabolism during exercise and recovery. In *Nutrition in Exercise and Sport,* 3rd ed. Wolinski, I., ed. Boca Raton, Fla.: CRC Press, 1998, 125–158.

25. Beard, J., and Tobin, B. Iron status and exercise. Am. J. Clin. Nutr. 72(suppl):594S–597S, 2000.

26. Food and Nutrition Board, Institute of Medicine. Dietary Reference Intakes: *Vitamin A, Vitamin K, Arsenic, Boron, Chromium, Copper, Iodine, Iron, Manganese, Molybdenum, Nickel, Silicon, Vanadium, and Zinc.* Washington, D.C.: National Academy Press, 2001.

27. Lohman, T. G., Going, S., Pamenter, R. W., et al. Effects of resistance training on regional and total bone mineral density in premenopausal women: A randomized prospective study. J. Bone Miner. Res. 10:1015–1024, 1995.

28. Friedlander, A. L., Genant, H. K., Sadowsky, A., et al. A two-year program of aerobics and weight training enhances bone mineral density of young women. J. Bone Miner. Res. 10:574–585, 1995.

29. Otis, C. L., Drinkwater, B. L., Johnson, M., et al. American College of Sports Medicine position stand on the female athlete triad. Med. Sci. Sports Exerc. 29:i–ix, 1997.

30. Bennell, K. L., Malcom, S. A., Wark, J. D., and Brukner, P. D. Skeletal effects of menstrual disturbances in athletes. Scand. J. Med. Sci. Sports 7:261–273, 1997.

31. Chung, N. K., and Pin, C. H. Obesity and the occurrence of heat disorders. Mil. Med. 161:739–742, 1996.

32. Remick, D., Chancellor, K., Pederson, J., et al. Hyperthermia and dehydration-related deaths associated with intentional rapid weight loss in three collegiate wrestlers—North Carolina, Wisconsin, and Michigan, November–December, 1997. MMWR 47(06):105–108, 1998. Available online at **http://www.cdc.gov/mmwr/preview/index98.html.** Accessed 5 Feb 2001.

33. Senay, L. C. Water and electrolytes during physical activity. In *Nutrition in Exercise and Sport,* 3rd ed. Wolinski, I., ed. Boca Raton, Fla.: CRC Press, 1998, 257–276.

34. American College of Sports Medicine. Position stand on exercise and fluid replacement. Med. Sci. Sports. Exerc. 28:i–vii, 1996.

35. Wilkinson, J. G., and Liebman, M. Carbohydrate metabolism in sport and exercise. In *Nutrition in Exercise and Sport,* 3rd ed. Wolinski, I., ed. Boca Raton, Fla.: CRC Press, 1998, 63–99.

36. Coyle, E. F. Substrate utilization during exercise in active people. Am. J. Clin Nutr. 61(suppl):968S–979S, 1995.

37. Luetkemeir, M. J., Coles, M. R., and Askew, E. W. Dietary sodium and plasma volume levels with exercise. Sports Med. 23:279–286, 1997.

38. Butterfield, G. Ergogenic aids: evaluating sport nutrition products. Int. J. Sport Nutr. 6:191–197, 1996.

39. Dekkers, J. C., van Doornen, L. J. P., and Kemper, H. C. G. The role of antioxidant vitamins and enzymes in the prevention of exercise-induced muscle damage. Sports Med. 21:213–238, 1996.

40. Williams, M. H. Facts and fallacies of purported ergogenic amino acid supplements. Clin. Sports Med. 18:633–649, 1999.

41. Clarkson, P. M., and Thompson, H. S. Antioxidants: what role do they play in physical activity and health? Am. J. Clin. Nutr. 72(suppl):637S–646S, 2000.

42. Lukaski, H. C. Chromium as a supplement. Ann. Rev. Nutr. 19:279–301, 1999.

43. Jeejeebhoy, K. N. The role of chromium in nutrition and therapeutics and as a potential toxin. Nutr. Rev. 57:329–335, 1999.

44. Stearns, D. M., Wise, J. P. Sr., Patierno, S. R., and Wetterhahn, K. E. Chromium (III) picolinate produces chromosome damage in Chinese hamster ovary cells. FASEB J. 9:1643–1648, 1995.

45. Speetjens, J. K., Collins, R. A., Vincent, J. B., and Woski, S. A. The nutritional supplement chromium (III) tris(picolinate) cleaves DNA. Chem. Res. Toxicol. 12:483–487, 1999.

46. Kato, I., Vogelman, J. H., Dilman, V., et al. Effect of supplementation with chromium picolinate on antibody titers to 5-hydroxymethyl uracil. Eur. J. Epidemiol. 14:621–626, 1998.

47. van Hall, G., Saris, W. H., van de Schoor, P. A., and Wagenmakers, A. J. The effect of free glutamine and peptide ingestion on the rate of muscle glycogen resynthesis in man. Int. J. Sports Med. 21:25–30, 2000.

48. Davis, J. M., Welsh, R. S., De Volve, K. L., and Alderson, N. A. Effects of branched-chain amino acids and carbohydrate on fatigue during intermittent, high-intensity running. Int. J. Sports Med. 20: 309–314, 1999.

49. Feldman, E. B. Creatine: a dietary supplement and ergogenic aid. Nutr. Rev. 57:45–50, 1999.

50. Terjung, R. L., Clarkson, P., Eichner, E. R., et al. American College of Sports Medicine roundtable: the physiological and health effects of oral creatine supplementation. Med. Sci. Sports Exerc. 32:706–717, 2000.

51. Oler, S. M. Creatine is an ergogen for anaerobic exercise. Nutr. Rev. 55:21–25, 1997.

52. Spriet, L. L. Caffeine and performance. Int. J. Sport Nutr. 5(suppl): 84S–99S, 1995.

53. Bucci, L. R., Selected herbals and human exercise performance. Am. J. Clin. Nutr. 72: 624S–636S, 2000.

54. Bauer, L., Kohlich, A., Hirschwehr, R., et al. Food allergy: pollen or bee products? J. Allergy Clin. Immunol. 97:65–73, 1996.

15 Nutrition During Pregnancy and Lactation

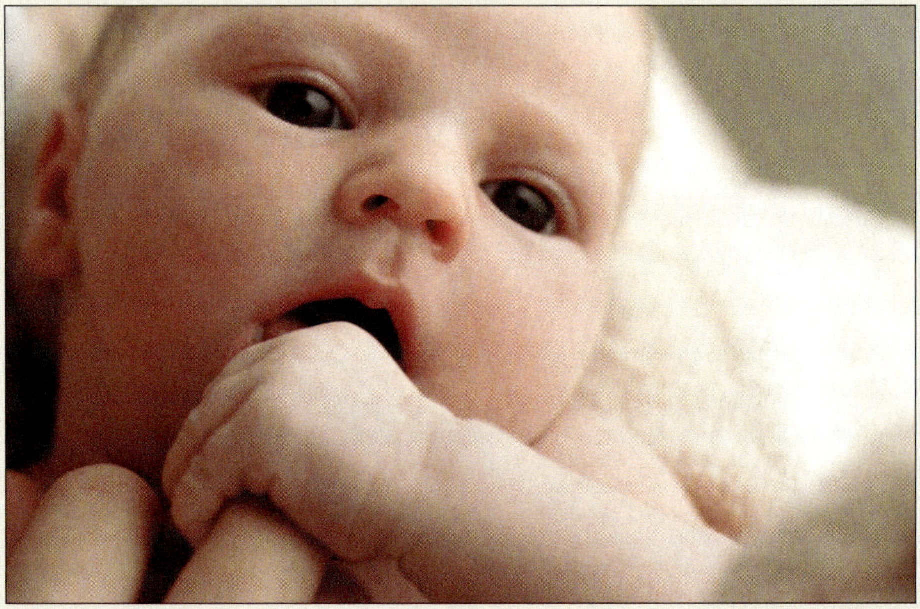

Learning Objectives

After reading this chapter, students should be able to:

1. Explain why a woman's nutrient intake during pregnancy is so important.
2. Describe how the changes that occur in a woman's body during pregnancy affect her nutritional status.
3. Compare the nutrient needs of pregnant women with those of nonpregnant women.
4. Explain the risks associated with gaining too little or too much weight during pregnancy.
5. Explain how maternal age affects nutrient needs and the risks of pregnancy.
6. Describe the effects that drug and alcohol use have on pregnancy outcome.
7. Compare the nutrient needs of lactating women with the needs of nonpregnant nonlactating women of childbearing age.
8. Compare the energy and protein needs of a newborn infant, an older child, and an adult.
9. Indicate the best way to monitor the adequacy of an infant's dietary intake.
10. Compare the benefits of breast-feeding to those of bottle-feeding.

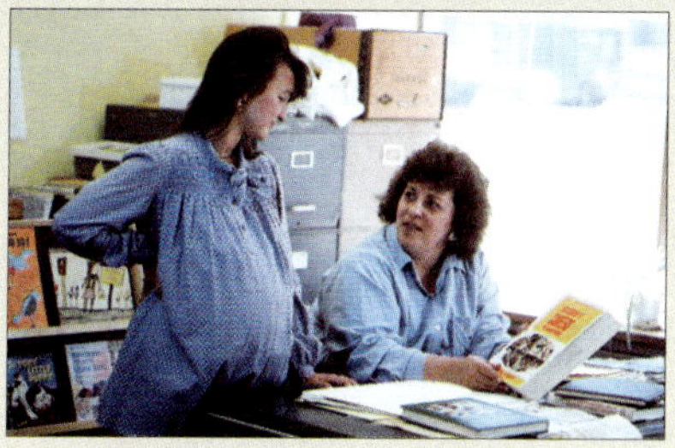

Jasmine is a healthy 26-year-old pregnant woman. At her first visit to the obstetrician, she is told that she and the baby seem healthy except that her iron stores are low. The obstetrician prescribes a prenatal vitamin and gives her a pamphlet on nutrition during pregnancy. Jasmine is concerned because the pamphlet recommends that she gain 20 to 25 pounds over the course of her pregnancy and suggests a dietary intake that includes much more than she usually eats. Because she has always worried about her weight, Jasmine typically skips breakfast and has only pretzels and diet soda for lunch, then eats a big dinner with her husband in the evening. Jasmine's sister, who has three young children, is now 25 pounds heavier than she was before the birth of her first child eight years ago and Jasmine doesn't want to follow in her footsteps. She also remembers her grandmother telling her that gaining too much weight makes the delivery more difficult. So Jasmine decides to continue to follow her usual eating pattern; she believes that because she is taking the supplement, she will get all the nutrients her baby needs.

By the fourth month of her pregnancy, Jasmine has gained only one pound and is feeling tired and run down; she tells the doctor that she stopped taking the supplement because it was making her nauseous and constipated. Her doctor explains that during pregnancy the mother must supply all of the raw materials necessary for the development of the infant. Therefore, the mother's health and nutritional status are crucial to a successful pregnancy outcome. A deficiency or excess of nutrients, as well as the use of alcohol, drugs, and cigarettes, may cause birth defects, premature birth, and low birth weight. If Jasmine continues to restrict her food intake and does nothing to improve her iron status, she may be putting herself and her baby at risk.

Jasmine reevaluates the importance of gaining a few pounds versus the health of her baby. She makes an appointment with a dietitian to help her plan a diet that will supply the nutrients needed to maintain her health, support the physiological changes in her body, and provide for the rapid growth and development of her unborn baby. Jasmine knows that good nutrition cannot guarantee a healthy baby, but adequate nutrition along with consistent prenatal care can reduce the risk of having a baby that is born too soon or too small.

THE PHYSIOLOGY OF PREGNANCY

Pregnancy in humans, from **conception** to birth, usually lasts 40 weeks, or about nine months. During this time, a single cell grows and develops into a complete human infant that is ready for life outside the womb. This development requires a safe environment to which oxygen and nutrients are provided in the right amounts and at the right times and from which waste products are removed. In order to accommodate the growing **fetus,** many physiological changes take place in the mother.

Conception The union of sperm and egg (ovum) that results in pregnancy.

Fetus The developing human from the ninth week to birth. Growth and refinement of structures occur during this time.

For more information on human development, go to the Child Development Institute at www.childdevelopmentinfo.com/development/ and click on prenatal development.

Prenatal Growth and Development

Reproduction requires the fertilization of an egg, or ovum, from the mother by a sperm from the father. **Fertilization,** which occurs in the **fallopian tube** or **oviduct,** produces a single-celled **zygote.** The zygote travels down the mother's fallopian tube into the uterus. Along the way, the zygote divides many times to form a ball of smaller cells sometimes called a preembryo. In the uterus, the preembryo attaches to the uterine lining in a process known as **implantation** (Figure 15.1). Once implantation is complete, about two weeks after fertilization, the preembryo is known as an **embryo.** Beginning at the ninth week of development and continuing until birth, the developing offspring is known as a fetus.

After implantation of the preembryo, two new organs, the **amniotic sac** and the **placenta,** form to provide protection and nourishment. The amniotic sac is a fluid-filled membrane that surrounds the developing embryo and protects it from the bumps and bruises of the outside world. The placenta provides a network of blood vessels that allow nutrients and oxygen to be transferred from mother to fetus and waste products to be transferred from the fetus to the mother's blood for elimination. The placenta is made up of tissue from both the mother and the fetus. The maternal portion of the placenta develops from the uterine lining. The fetal portion of the placenta develops from the outer layer of preembryonic cells. These cells divide to form branchlike projections that grow into the lining of the uterus where they are surrounded by pools of maternal blood. The projections contain blood vessels that supply the developing fetus. Although maternal and fetal blood do not mix, the close proximity of blood vessels that supply the fetus with maternal blood allows nutrients and oxygen to easily pass from mother to baby, and allows carbon dioxide and other wastes to pass from baby to mother for elimination (Figure 15.2). The placenta also secretes hormones that are necessary to maintain pregnancy.

As these structures form, the embryo continues to grow and develop. The cells differentiate to form the multitude of specialized cell types that make up the human body, and arrange themselves in the proper shapes and locations to form body organs and structures. The embryonic stage of development begins about two weeks after fertilization and lasts until the eighth week after fertilization. By the end of the embryonic period, the embryo is approximately 3 cm long (a little more than an inch) and has a beating heart and the rudiments of all major external and internal structures. The fetal period of development then begins at the

Fertilization The union of sperm and egg (ovum).

Fallopian tubes or **oviducts** Narrow ducts leading from the ovaries to the uterus.

Zygote The cell produced by the union of sperm and ovum during fertilization.

Implantation The process by which the developing ball of cells embeds in the uterine lining.

Embryo The developing human from the beginning of the third week to the eighth week after fertilization. All organ systems are formed during this time.

Amniotic sac A membranous sac containing the amniotic fluid, which surrounds the embryo or fetus.

Placenta An organ produced from both maternal and embryonic tissues. It produces hormones and allows for the transfer of nutrients and oxygen from the mother's blood to the fetus and wastes from the fetus to the mother's blood.

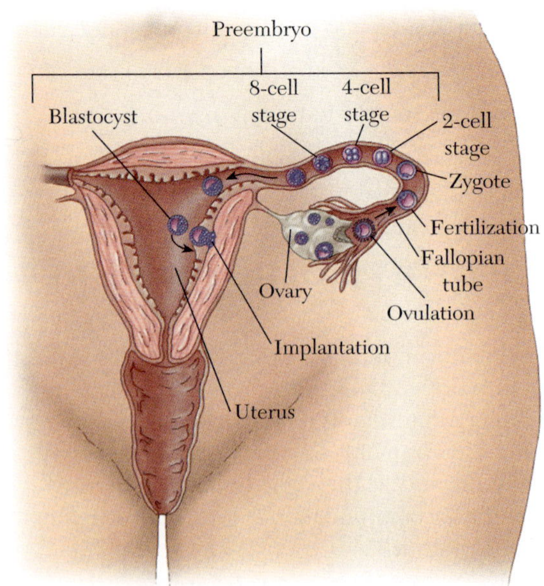

FIGURE 15.1 The mother's egg or ovum is released from the ovary by the process of ovulation. The egg then passes into the fallopian tube where fertilization occurs. After fertilization the zygote continues down the fallopian tube toward the uterus and begins to divide forming the preembryo. By the time the preembryo reaches the uterus, it consists of about 100 cells. Development continues in the uterine cavity, where the preembryo develops a fluid-filled cavity. At this stage it is called a blastocyst. Implantation occurs when the outer layer of blastocyst cells secretes substances that erode the uterine lining, allowing it to become completely embedded.

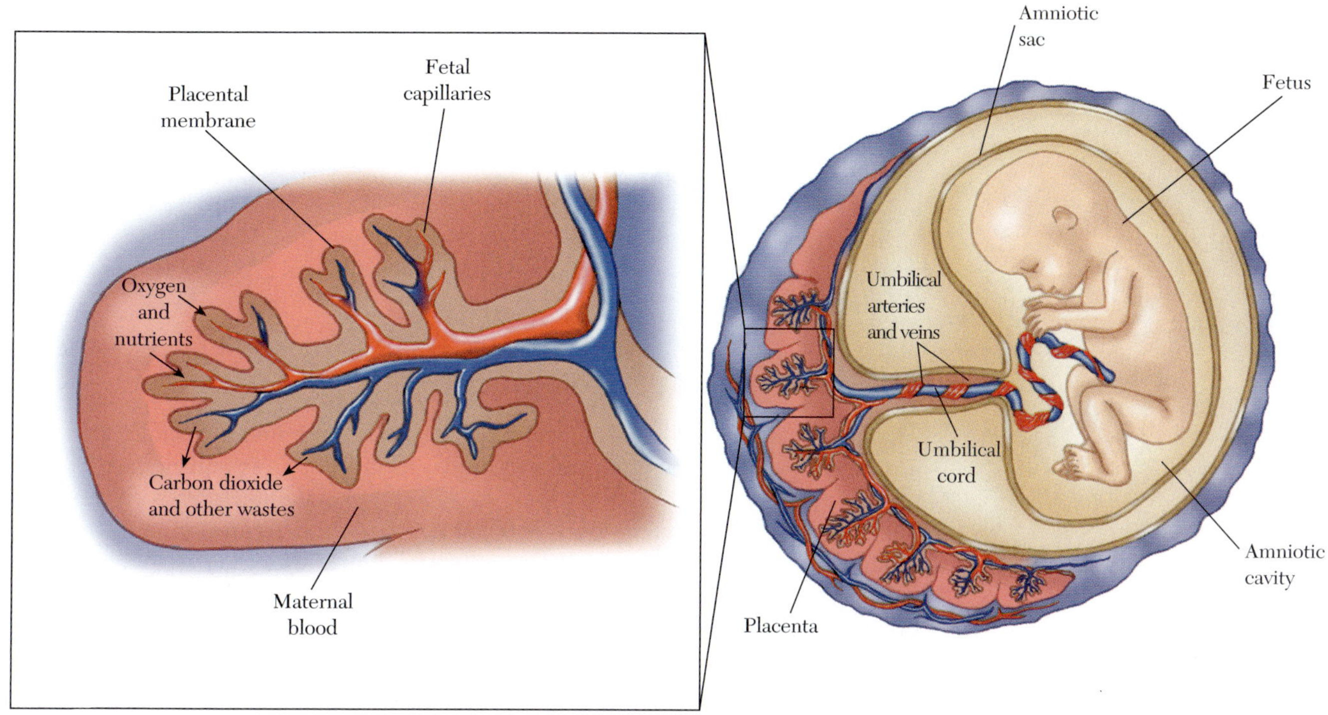

FIGURE 15.2 During pregnancy, the amniotic sac protects the fetus and the placenta allows nutrients and wastes to be transferred between mother and baby. The fetal part of the placenta consists of treelike projections that contain fetal blood vessels. Maternal blood flows into cavities surrounding these fetal structures. This close proximity between maternal and fetal blood allows the transfer of gases, nutrients, and waste products.

ninth week of development and continues until birth (Figure 15.3). During this time, structures that appeared during the embryonic period continue to grow and mature.

The fetal period usually ends after 40 weeks of gestation with the birth of an infant weighing about 3 to 4 kilograms (6.6 to 8.8 lb).[1] Infants who are born on time but have failed to grow well in the uterus are said to be **small-for-gestational-age.**

Small-for-gestational-age An infant born at term weighing less than 2.5 kg (5.5 lb).

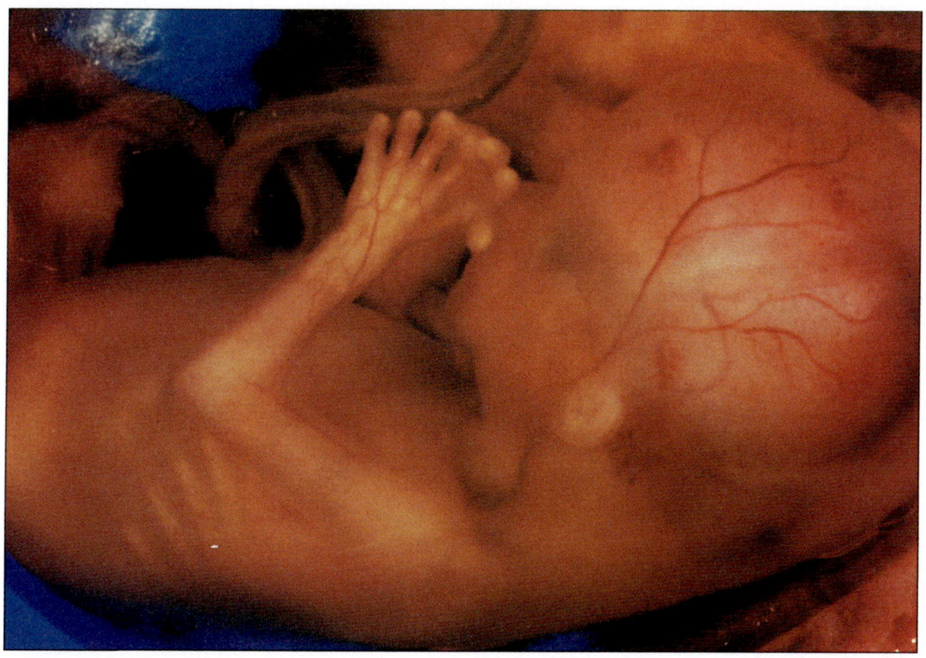

FIGURE 15.3 At 16 weeks the fetus is about 16 cm (6.4 inches) long and structures that formed during the embryonic period are continuing to mature. *(Custom Medical Stock Photo)*

Those born before 37 weeks of gestation are said to be **preterm** or **premature.** Whether born too soon or just too small, **low-birth-weight infants** (those weighing less than 2.5 kg [5.5 lb] at birth) and **very-low-birth-weight infants** (those weighing less than 1.5 kg [3.3 lb]), are at increased risk for illness and early death.[2] To successfully continue to grow and develop, these infants often require special care, including modified feeding methods that employ special formulas, tube feeding, or intravenous feeding. Survival improves with increasing gestational age and birth weight. Today, with advances in medical and nutritional care, infants born at a gestational age of 25 weeks and those weighing as little as 1 kg (2.2 lb) can survive (Figure 15.4).

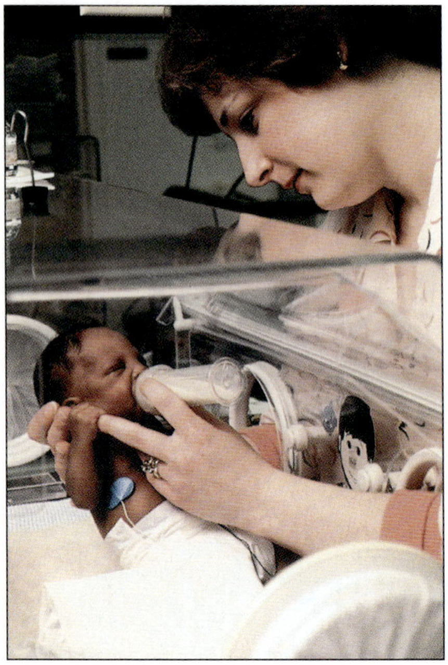

FIGURE 15.4 Even though medical science can help premature infants survive, they are at far greater risk of illness and death than infants born at term. *(© Blair Seitz/Photo Researchers, Inc.)*

Preterm or **premature** An infant born before 37 weeks of gestation.

Low-birth-weight A birth weight less than 2.5 kg (5.5 lb).

Very-low-birth-weight A birth weight less than 1.5 kg (3.3 lb).

Teratogen A substance that can cause birth defects.

Spontaneous abortion or **miscarriage** Interruption of pregnancy prior to the seventh month.

Critical Periods in Development

The developing embryo and fetus are particularly vulnerable to assault when cells are dividing, differentiating, and moving to form structures and organs. During these "critical periods of development," anything that interferes with development can cause irreversible birth defects. Because each organ system develops at a different rate, the timing of the assault determines which organ system is primarily affected. Because the majority of cell differentiation occurs during the embryonic period, this is the time when exposure to **teratogens**—chemical, biological, or physical agents that cause birth defects—can be most damaging (Figure 15.5). Severe damage to an embryo or fetus usually results in a **spontaneous abortion** or **miscarriage.**

Maternal Physiology

To develop and maintain the systems necessary to support the growing fetus, a woman's body undergoes many changes during pregnancy. Her blood volume increases by 50% and her heart, lungs, and kidneys work harder to deliver nutrients and oxygen and remove wastes. The placenta develops, and the hormones produced by it orchestrate other changes, such as uterine growth; relaxation of muscles and ligaments to accommodate the growing fetus and allow for childbirth; breast development; and increased fat deposition to provide the energy stores for late pregnancy and lactation. These changes all result in weight gain and can affect the type and level of physical activity that is safe. In some cases they can also cause side effects that range from mild discomfort to life-threatening complications such as gestational diabetes and hypertension.

Maternal Weight Gain Adequate weight gain during pregnancy is essential to the health of mother and fetus.

Components of Weight Gain Typically the weight of the infant at birth is only about 25% of the total pregnancy weight gain; that of the placenta is about 5%, and that of the amniotic fluid is about 6%. Changes in maternal tissues account for most of the weight gained during pregnancy. This includes increases in the size of the uterus and breasts, in the volume of blood and extracellular fluid, and in fat stores (Figure 15.6).

Recommended Weight Gain The recommended weight gain during pregnancy is 25 to 35 pounds (11.5 to 16 kg) for healthy, normal-weight women. However, the rate of weight gain is as important as the total weight gain. Little gain is expected in the first three months, or trimester, of pregnancy—usually about 2 to 4 pounds (0.9 to 1.8 kg). In the second and third trimesters, when the fetus grows from less than a pound to 6 to 8 pounds, the recommended maternal weight gain is about 1 pound (0.45 kg) per week. Women who are underweight or overweight at conception should also gain weight at a slow, steady rate (Figure 15.7). Weight gains

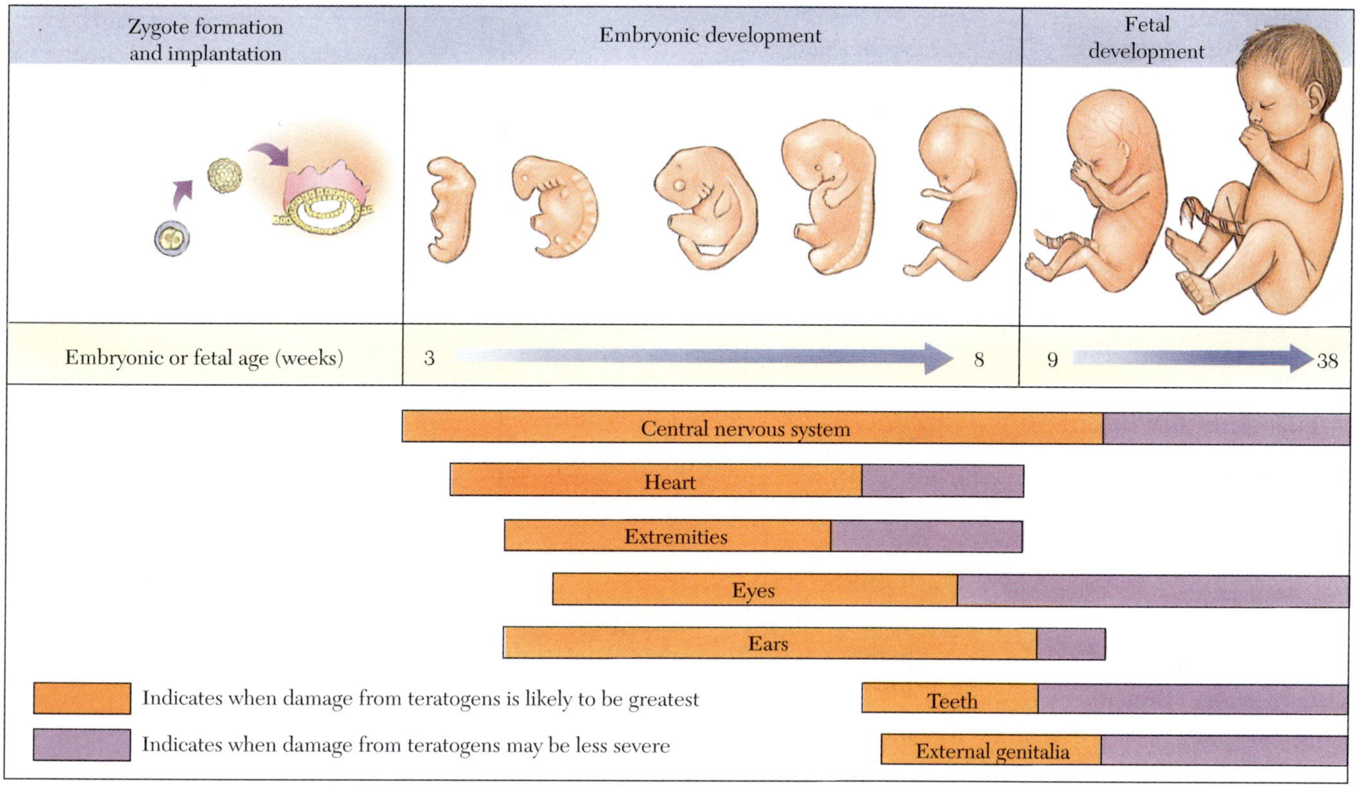

FIGURE 15.5 The periods that are critical for development are different for different body systems. *(Adapted from Moore, K., and Persaud, T.* The Developing Human, *5th ed. Philadelphia: W. B. Saunders Company, 1993.)*

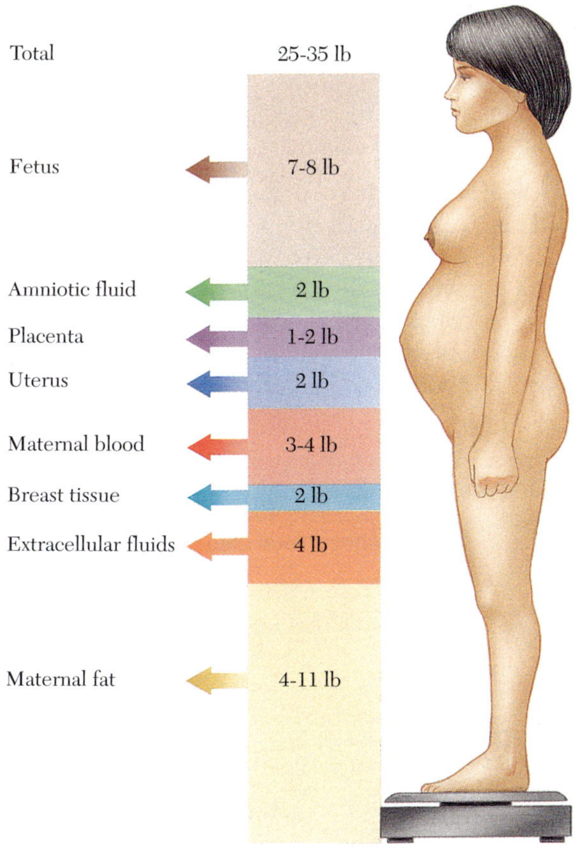

FIGURE 15.6 The weight gained by a woman during pregnancy includes increases in the weight of her tissues as well as in the weight of the fetus, placenta, and the amniotic fluid.

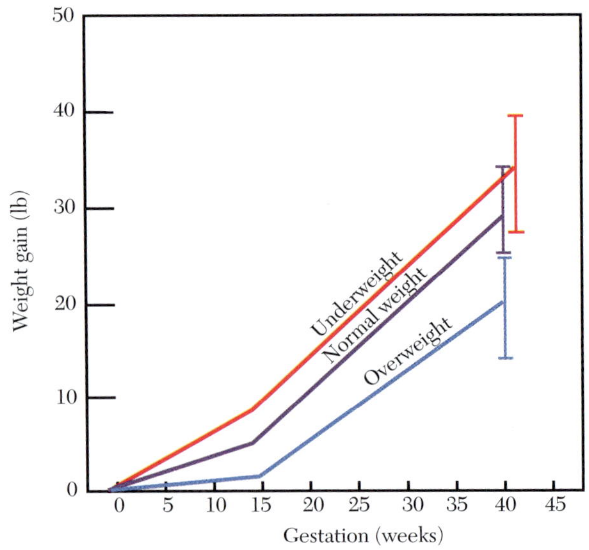

FIGURE 15.7 The same pattern of weight gain is recommended for women who are normal weight, underweight, or overweight at the start of pregnancy, but the recommendations for total weight gain are different. *(Adapted from Committee on Nutritional Status During Pregnancy and Lactation.* Nutrition During Pregnancy. *Washington, D.C.: National Academy Press, 1990.)*

of up to 40 pounds (18 kg) are recommended for women who begin pregnancy underweight. Overweight women should gain less, only about 15 to 25 pounds (7 to 11.5 kg) over the course of pregnancy (Table 15.1).

Risks of Inappropriate Weight Gain Gaining too little or too much weight as well as being underweight or overweight during pregnancy can affect the health of both mother and fetus.[1,3] Being underweight by 10% or more at the onset of pregnancy or gaining too little weight during pregnancy increases the risk of producing a low-birth-weight or preterm baby (Figure 15.8). Excess weight, whether present before conception or gained during pregnancy, can also compromise the outcome of the pregnancy. The mother's risks for hypertension, gestational diabetes, difficult delivery, and cesarean section are increased by excess weight, as is the risk of having a baby with a neural tube defect or a low APGAR score (a five-point evaluation used to assess the health of a newborn baby), or who is **large-for-gestational-age.**[4] However, dieting during pregnancy is not advised even for obese women. If possible, excess weight should be lost before the pregnancy begins or, alternatively, after the child is born and weaned.

Large-for-gestational-age An infant weighing greater than 4 kg (8.8 lb) at birth.

Postpartum Weight Women lose approximately 10 pounds at birth from the weight of the baby, amniotic fluid, and placenta. In the week after delivery, another 5 pounds of fluid are typically lost. Once this initial fluid and tissue weight is lost, further weight loss requires that energy intake be less than energy output. After the mother has recovered from delivery, a balanced diet combined with moderate exercise will promote weight loss and the return of muscle tone. Within a year of delivery most women lose all but about 2 pounds of the weight gained

TABLE 15.1 Recommendations for Pregnancy Weight Gain

Prepregnancy Weight Status*	Recommended Total Gain
Underweight (BMI < 19.8)	28 to 40 lb (12.5 to 18.0 kg)
Normal weight (BMI 19.8 to 26)	25 to 35 lb (11.5 to 16.0 kg)
Overweight (BMI > 26 to 29)	15 to 25 lb (6.8 to 11.5 kg)
Obese (BMI > 29)	15 lb minimum (6.8 kg minimum)

*Note that the BMI ranges used here to define underweight, normal weight, overweight, and obesity differ slightly from the ranges established by the NIH National Heart, Lung, and Blood Institute's Clinical Guidelines on the Identification, Evaluation, and Treatment of Overweight and Obesity in Adults (see Chapters 7 and 8).

From Committee on Nutritional Status During Pregnancy and Lactation. *Nutrition During Pregnancy.* Washington, D.C.: National Academy Press, 1990.

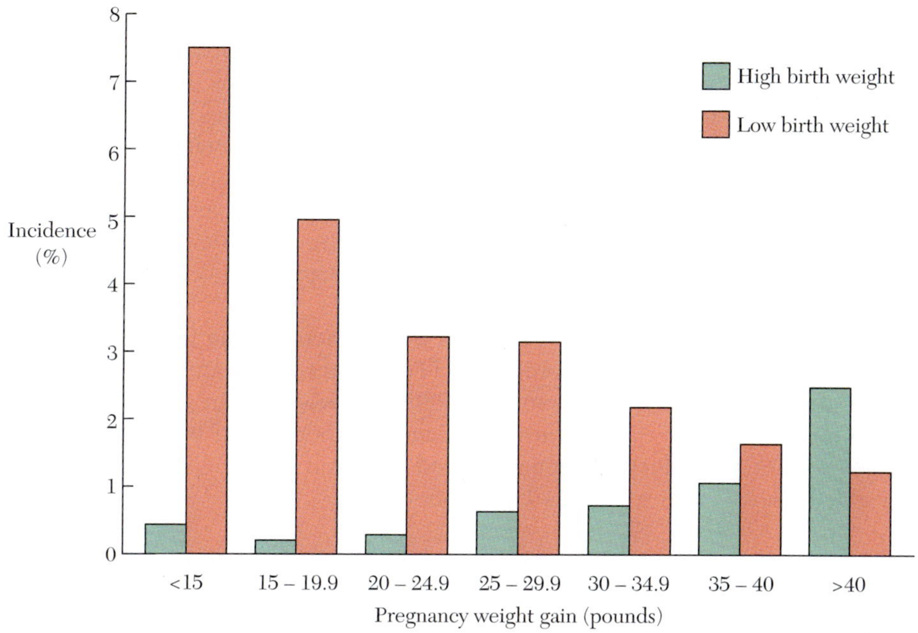

FIGURE 15.8 This graph illustrates that the incidence of low-birth-weight babies increases in women who are of normal weight at the start of pregnancy but gain less than the recommended amount of weight during pregnancy. The incidence of high birth weight increases in women who gain more than the recommended amount during pregnancy. *(Adapted from Cogswell, M., Serdula, M., Hungerford, D., and Yip, R. Gastrointestinal weight gain among average-weight and overweight women—what is excessive? Am. J. Obstet. Gynecol. 172:705–712, 1995.)*

during pregnancy.[5] As discussed later in this chapter, breast-feeding may help to promote weight loss in some women.

Women who gain more than the recommended amount of weight during pregnancy are more likely to retain weight postpartum. African-American women are more likely to retain more weight postpartum than are white women in all weight-gain categories.[3]

Physical Activity During Pregnancy For healthy, well-nourished women, carefully chosen moderate exercise is recommended during pregnancy. Physical activity during pregnancy improves overall fitness, reduces stress, prevents excess weight gain, prevents low back pain, improves digestion, reduces constipation, reduces the risk of gestational diabetes, improves mood and body image, and speeds recovery from childbirth. Too much exercise that is too intense has the potential to harm the fetus by reducing the amount of oxygen and nutrients it receives or by increasing body temperature. Therefore, guidelines have been developed to minimize the risks and maximize the benefits of exercise during pregnancy (Table 15.2). All pregnant women should check with their physicians before engaging in any exercise program.

TABLE 15.2 Guidelines for Physical Activity During Pregnancy

1. Obtain medical permission before beginning an exercise program.
2. Increase activity very gradually if inactive before pregnancy.
3. Regular exercise (at least three times per week) is preferable to intermittent activity.
4. Stop exercising when fatigued and do not exercise to exhaustion.
5. Choose non-weight-bearing activities such as swimming that have minimal risk of falls or abdominal injury.
6. Avoid strenuous exertion during the first trimester; at other times, strenuous exercise should not be continued for more than 15 minutes.
7. Avoid exercise that is performed lying on one's back after the first trimester.
8. Avoid exercising in hot or humid environments.
9. Drink plenty of liquids before, during, and after exercise.
10. Resume prepregnancy exercise routines gradually after the birth of the child.

Modified from Dewey, K. G., and McCrory, M. A. Effects of dieting and physical activity on pregnancy and lactation. Am. J. Clin. Nutr. 59 (suppl):446S–453S, 1994; and American College of Obstetricians and Gynecologists. *Exercise During Pregnancy and the Postpartum Period* (Technical Bulletin #189). Washington, D.C.: ACOG, 1994.

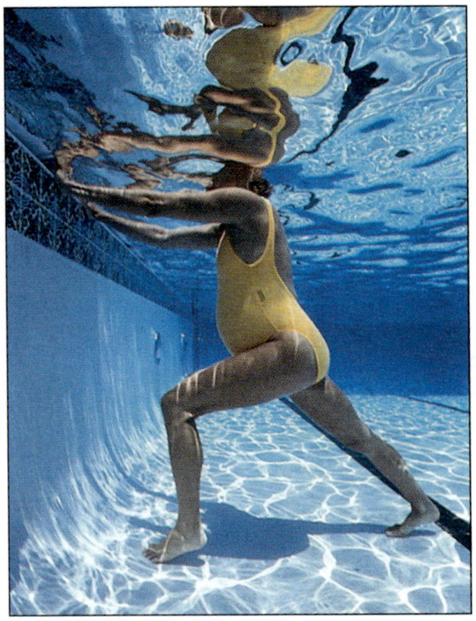

FIGURE 15.9 During pregnancy, exercising in the water can reduce stress on joints and help keep the body cool. *(© Tracy Frankel/The Image Bank)*

Women who were physically active before their pregnancy can usually continue their exercise programs, but women who begin an exercise program after becoming pregnant should start slowly with low-intensity, low-impact activities such as walking.[6] The risk of injury is greater during pregnancy because women weigh more and carry that weight in the front of their bodies where it can interfere with balance and place stress on the bones, joints, and muscles. Activities that have a risk of abdominal trauma, falls, or joint stress, such as contact and racquet sports, should be avoided.[7] Exercise in the water is recommended because the body's buoyancy in water compensates for the changes in weight distribution (Figure 15.9).[8]

To ensure adequate delivery of oxygen and nutrients to the fetus, intense exercise should be limited during pregnancy. To prevent overheating, plenty of fluids should be consumed and exercise should be carried out in a well-ventilated environment. Outdoor exercise in hot, humid weather should be avoided. Also, women who exercise during pregnancy need to consume enough energy to meet the added demands of exercise and pregnancy.

Discomforts of Pregnancy The physiological changes that occur during pregnancy can cause uncomfortable side effects for the mother. Some are caused by changes in fluid distribution, others by hormonal changes that affect the gastrointestinal tract. In most cases, these changes cause discomfort for the mother, but only rarely do they affect the development and well-being of the fetus.

Edema Swelling due to the buildup of extracellular fluid in the tissues.

Edema During pregnancy, blood volume expands to nourish the fetus, but this expansion may also cause the accumulation of extracellular fluid in the mother's tissues known as **edema.** Edema is characterized by swelling, particularly in the feet and ankles. Edema can be uncomfortable but does not increase medical risks unless it is accompanied by a rise in blood pressure. Restriction of dietary sodium below the amount recommended for the general population is not recommended, nor is fluid restriction.

Morning Sickness Morning sickness is a syndrome of nausea and vomiting that occurs during pregnancy. The term is somewhat of a misnomer because symptoms can occur anytime during the day or night. The condition is thought to be related to the hormonal changes of pregnancy and may be alleviated to some extent by eating small, frequent snacks of dry, starchy foods, such as plain crackers or bread. In most women, symptoms decrease significantly after the first trimester, but in some cases the symptoms last for the entire pregnancy and, in severe cases, may require intravenous nutrition to assure that needs are met.

Heartburn Heartburn, a burning sensation caused by stomach acid leaking up into the esophagus, is another common digestive complaint during pregnancy because the hormones produced to relax the muscles of the uterus also relax the muscles of the gastrointestinal tract. This involuntary relaxation of the gastroesophageal sphincter allows the acidic stomach contents to back up into the esophagus, causing irritation. The severity increases as pregnancy progresses because the growing baby crowds the stomach. The fuller the stomach, the more likely that its contents will back up into the esophagus. Consuming small meals throughout the day rather than a few large meals can reduce heartburn. Because high-fat foods, such as fried foods, rich sauces, and desserts, leave the stomach slowly, a low-fat diet of grains, fruits, vegetables, plain meats, and low-fat dairy products is less likely to cause heartburn. Remaining upright rather than reclining after eating also reduces heartburn because acidic juices are less likely to flow into the esophagus. Avoiding substances that are known to cause heartburn, such as caffeine and peppermint, can also be helpful.

Constipation Constipation is a frequent complaint during pregnancy. The pregnancy-related hormones that cause muscles to relax also decrease intestinal motility and slow transit through the gut. Constipation becomes more of a problem late in pregnancy when the weight of the uterus puts pressure on the gastrointestinal tract. Maintaining a moderate level of physical activity and consuming at least one half-gallon of water and other fluids per day as well as high-fiber foods such as whole grains, vegetables, and fruits are recommended to prevent constipation. Hemorrhoids are also more common during pregnancy, as a result of both constipation and physiological changes in blood flow.

Gestational Diabetes A consistently elevated blood glucose level during pregnancy is known as **gestational diabetes.** It occurs in 2 to 6% of all pregnancies and is most common in obese women.[9] This form of diabetes usually resolves when the pregnancy is completed, although the mother remains at higher risk for developing type 2 diabetes (see Chapter 4).

Gestational diabetes A consistently elevated blood glucose level that develops during pregnancy and returns to normal after delivery.

High levels of glucose in the mother's blood can adversely affect the fetus. Glucose passes freely across the placenta, so high maternal blood glucose provides extra energy to the fetus. This extra energy can result in a baby who is large for gestational age and consequently at increased risk for complications. Like other types of diabetes, gestational diabetes requires medical management as well as monitoring of blood glucose levels, consumption of a carefully planned diet eaten at consistent intervals throughout the day, and regular exercise. In some cases insulin or oral medication may be required to maintain normal blood glucose levels.

Pregnancy-Induced Hypertension **Pregnancy-induced hypertension** is a spectrum of conditions involving elevated blood pressure during pregnancy. It can result in preterm labor and low-birth-weight infants, and is a major risk factor for maternal and fetal illness and death. Pregnancy-induced hypertension occurs in about 6 to 8% of pregnancies but accounts for nearly 15% of pregnancy-related maternal deaths in the United States.[10] It is more common in mothers under 20 or over 35 years of age, those in low-income groups, and in women with chronic hypertension or kidney disease.

Pregnancy-induced hypertension A spectrum of conditions involving elevated blood pressure that usually occurs after 20 weeks of gestation. It may be accompanied by protein in the urine, edema, and, rarely, convulsions and coma.

The mildest form of pregnancy-induced hypertension is **gestational hypertension,** which is an abnormal rise in blood pressure that occurs after the 20th week of pregnancy. **Preeclampsia** is a form of pregnancy-induced hypertension that causes an increase in blood pressure, excretion of protein in the urine, and edema. Its onset is often signaled by a weight gain of several pounds within a few days. It can progress to a more severe form, **eclampsia,** in which life-threatening seizures occur.

Gestational hypertension A mild form of pregnancy-induced hypertension involving an elevation in blood pressure that occurs after the 20th week of pregnancy.

Preeclampsia A form of pregnancy-induced hypertension that is characterized by an increase in body weight, elevated blood pressure, protein in the urine, and edema.

Eclampsia The most severe form of pregnancy-induced hypertension involving elevated blood pressure, protein in the urine, convulsions, and coma during pregnancy or shortly after delivery.

The cause of pregnancy-induced hypertension is not known, but research suggests that low calcium intake may be involved. Although some research demonstrates a possible beneficial effect of supplemental calcium in preventing and treating pregnancy-induced hypertension, evidence is not strong enough to support routine supplementation of all pregnant women.[11,12] But pregnant teens, individuals with inadequate calcium intake, and women known to be at risk of developing pregnancy-induced hypertension may benefit from additional dietary calcium.[11] Treatment includes bed rest and careful medical monitoring. A moderate intake of dietary sodium is recommended, but sodium restriction is not a cure. The condition usually resolves after delivery.

Web Menu

For information about prenatal care, risks and problems during pregnancy, and postnatal care, go to the New York Online Access to Health (NOAH) at www.noah-health.org/ and click on pregnancy under health topics.

NUTRITION AND THE RISKS OF PREGNANCY

Most of the 4 million women who give birth every year in the United States are healthy during pregnancy and produce healthy babies. However, childbearing is not without risks. In the United States every year, 300 to 500 women die as a result of childbirth. Eleven percent of babies are born too soon, 7.4 % are low-birth-weight, and 7.2 out of each 1000 born alive die within the first year of life.[13] The reasons for poor pregnancy outcome vary. Some women are at increased risk because of poor nutritional status, some because of health problems that exist before the pregnancy occurs, and others are at risk because of their age or because they have limited access to health care before and during pregnancy, lack a supportive home environment, or lack the money and facilities to purchase, prepare, and consume nutritious foods. Some women are at increased risk because they smoke, drink alcohol, or use illicit drugs (Table 15.3).

TABLE 15.3 Factors That Increase Pregnancy Risks

Maternal Factor	Maternal Risk	Infant/Fetal Risk
Prepregnant BMI < 19.8 or gaining too little weight during pregnancy	Anemia, premature rupture of the membranes, hemorrhage after delivery	Low birth weight, preterm birth
Prepregnancy BMI > 26 or gaining too much weight during pregnancy	Pregnancy-induced hypertension, gestational diabetes, difficult delivery, cesarean section	Large-for-gestational-age, low Apgar scores (a score used to assess the health of a baby in the first minutes after birth), and neural tube defects
Malnutrition	Decreased ability to conceive, anemia	Fetal growth retardation, low birth weight, birth defects, preterm birth, spontaneous abortion, stillbirth; increased risk of chronic disease later in life
PKU	High blood levels of phenylketones	Mental retardation if low phenylalanine diet is not carefully followed by mother
Hypertension	Stroke, heart attack, premature separation of the placenta from the uterine wall	Low birth weight, fetal death
Diabetes	Difficulty adjusting insulin dose, preeclampsia, cesarean section	Large-for-gestational-age, congenital abnormalities, fetal death
Frequent pregnancies: 3 or more during a 2-year period	Malnutrition	Low birth weight, preterm birth
Poor obstetric history or history of poor fetal outcome	Recurrence of problem in subsequent pregnancy	Birth defects, death
Age:		
Teenage	Malnutrition, pregnancy-induced hypertension	Low birth weight
Older than 35	Pregnancy-induced hypertension, gestational diabetes	Down syndrome and other chromosomal abnormalities
Alcohol	Poor nutritional status	Alcohol-related birth defects, fetal alcohol syndrome
Cigarette smoking	Lung cancer and other lung diseases, miscarriage	Low birth weight, miscarriage, stillbirth, preterm birth, sudden infant death syndrome, respiratory problems
Cocaine use	Hypertension, miscarriage premature labor and delivery	Intrauterine growth retardation, low birth weight, preterm birth, birth defects, sudden infant death syndrome

Maternal Nutritional Status

Proper nutrition is important before pregnancy to support conception and maximize the likelihood of a healthy pregnancy. At any time during pregnancy, maternal malnutrition due to an excess or deficiency of energy or individual nutrients can affect pregnancy outcome.

Nutritional Status Before Pregnancy A woman's nutritional status before she becomes pregnant may affect her ability to conceive and successfully complete a pregnancy. For example, starvation diets, anorexia nervosa, and excessive athletic activity, such as marathon running, can interfere with ovulation and therefore make conception less likely. Obesity can alter hormone levels and decrease fertility.

Nutritional status can also be affected by some birth control methods and these can therefore have an impact on a subsequent pregnancy. For example, oral contraceptives are associated with reduced blood levels of vitamin B_6 and vitamin B_{12}.[14,15] If conception occurs soon after oral contraceptive use stops, these levels will not have had time to return to normal.

Malnutrition During Pregnancy Maternal malnutrition can cause fetal growth retardation, low infant birth weight, birth defects, premature birth, spontaneous abortion, and stillbirth. The effect of malnutrition depends on how severe the malnutrition is and when during the pregnancy it occurs. Low energy intake during early pregnancy is not likely to interfere with fetal growth because the energy demands of the embryo are small. However, if the embryo does not receive adequate amounts of the nutrients needed for cell division and differentiation, such as folate and vitamin A, malformations or death can result. Malnutrition after the first trimester is less likely to have teratogenic effects because most organs and structures have already formed, but it will interfere with fetal growth. Malnutrition also interferes with the growth and function of the placenta. A poorly developed placenta cannot deliver sufficient nutrients to the fetus and the result is a small infant that may also have other developmental abnormalities. Even a mild energy restriction during the last trimester, when the fetus is growing rapidly, could affect birth weight. In general, poor nutrition early in pregnancy affects embryonic development and the potential of the embryo to survive and poor nutrition in the latter part of pregnancy affects fetal growth.

Long-Term Effects of Maternal Nutrition It has been proposed that problems in maternal nutrition can cause adaptations that change fetal structure, physiology, and metabolism and can affect the child's risk of developing chronic diseases later in life. Evidence for this comes from epidemiological studies that suggest that individuals who were small at birth or disproportionately thin or short have higher rates of heart disease, high blood pressure, high blood cholesterol, and abnormal glucose/insulin metabolism in middle age.[16] The intake of individual nutrients may also affect chronic disease. For example, in one study the children of women who took a calcium supplement during pregnancy had lower systolic blood pressure than the children of women who did not take a calcium supplement.[12]

Nutrients As Teratogens Deficiencies or excesses of some nutrients can have teratogenic effects. For example, inadequate folate intake may affect neural tube development (see folate below). Excess vitamin D can cause mental retardation. Too much vitamin A is of particular concern because the risk of kidney problems and central nervous system abnormalities in the offspring increases even when maternal intake is not extremely high. Although data strongly support the teratogenic effects of vitamin A, the threshold of intake at which risk increases is unclear. One study found that the consumption of supplements containing 3000 μg/day or more of preformed vitamin A or 4500 μg/day from food and supplements increased the risk of birth defects, whereas others found that supplements in this range of intake did not increase risk.[17,18] A UL for pregnant women 19 to 50 years of age has been set at 3000 μg/day of preformed vitamin A from food and supplements.[19] Supplements consumed during pregnancy can provide vitamin A as beta-carotene, which is not teratogenic.

Maternal Health History

The outcome of a pregnancy can be affected by the health of the mother at the time she becomes pregnant as well as by the frequency and outcomes of her previous pregnancies.

Preexisting Conditions Women with chronic diseases such as hypertension or diabetes, or with genetic abnormalities such as PKU, must be carefully monitored during pregnancy to ensure the health of both mother and fetus.

The effect of hypertension depends on when it develops and how severe it is. As in nonpregnant individuals, high blood pressure in pregnant women increases the risk of stroke and heart attack, but in pregnancy it also increases the risk of low birth weight and premature separation of the placenta from the wall of the uterus, resulting in fetal death.

Women with diabetes must carefully manage diet and medication to ensure that glucose levels stay in the normal range throughout pregnancy. The need for insulin increases during the second and third trimesters, so women with preexisting diabetes may need to adjust their medication dosage. When normal blood glucose is maintained throughout pregnancy, the risk of complications is greatly reduced.[20] When maternal blood glucose is elevated, it provides extra nutrients to the growing fetus, resulting in large-for-gestational-age newborns who are at increased risk. Likewise, low blood glucose during pregnancy can deprive the baby of nourishment.

To prevent brain damage in the fetus, women with PKU must consume a low-phenylalanine diet during pregnancy. This ensures that maternal phenylalanine levels remain low enough that the amounts of phenylalanine and phenylalanine by-products crossing the placenta are not teratogenic. If the mother's levels rise too high, the baby is at risk because the immature enzyme systems in the embryo and fetus cannot break down the metabolic by-products of phenylalanine that cross the placenta from the mother's blood.

Reproductive History Reproductive history is an important predictor of pregnancy risk. Frequent pregnancies, particularly those with little time between them, increase the risk for maternal malnutrition because the mother may not have replenished nutrient stores depleted in the previous pregnancy. A short interval between pregnancies also increases the risk of preterm and low-birth-weight infants. Women with a history of poor pregnancy outcomes are also at increased risk. For example, a women who has had a number of miscarriages is more likely to have another, and a woman who has had one child with a birth defect has an increased risk for defects in subsequent children.

Maternal Age

Women in their teens who are still developing and older women who are more likely to have existing medical conditions are at greater risk of developing complications during pregnancy.

The Pregnant Teenager Teenage pregnancy is a major public health problem. One in every five babies is born to a teenager, and more than 10% of these mothers are age 15 or younger.[22] Economic, social, and medical issues as well as nutritional problems contribute to poor pregnancy outcomes in these girls.

Pregnancy places a nutritional strain on a woman's body at any age, but this stress is compounded when the mother herself is still growing. Adolescent girls continue to grow and mature physically for about four to seven years after menstruation begins. Therefore, the risk associated with a pregnancy is greater during this time than it is in women who have stopped growing. To better assess the nutritional status and nutritional goals of the pregnant teenager, the Dietary Reference Intakes include an age category within pregnancy that focuses on the needs of pregnant teens. For example, the RDA for zinc in pregnant girls age 18 or younger is greater than it is in either pregnant women age 19 or older or nonpregnant girls age 18 or younger.

Consuming a diet that meets a teenage mother's need for growth as well as for pregnancy can be difficult. For example, pregnant teens typically consume a diet that contains less calcium, iron, zinc, magnesium, vitamin D, folate, and vitamin B_6 than is recommended. Teenagers are also at greater risk of pregnancy-induced hypertension and are more likely to deliver preterm and low-birth-weight babies than are more mature women.[21] The pregnant teenager needs early medical intervention and nutritional counseling to produce a healthy baby.[22]

The Older Mother Many women in their thirties and forties are having babies. The nutritional requirements for older mothers during pregnancy are no different than for women in their twenties, but pregnancy after the age of 35 does carry additional risks because older women are more likely to start pregnancy with medical conditions such as cardiovascular disease, kidney disorders, obesity, and diabetes.[23] During pregnancy, older women are also more likely to develop gestational diabetes, pregnancy-induced hypertension, and other complications.[24] There is a higher incidence of low-birth-weight deliveries and of chromosomal abnormalities, especially Down syndrome. Today, careful medical monitoring throughout pregnancy is reducing the risks to older mothers and their babies (Figure 15.10).

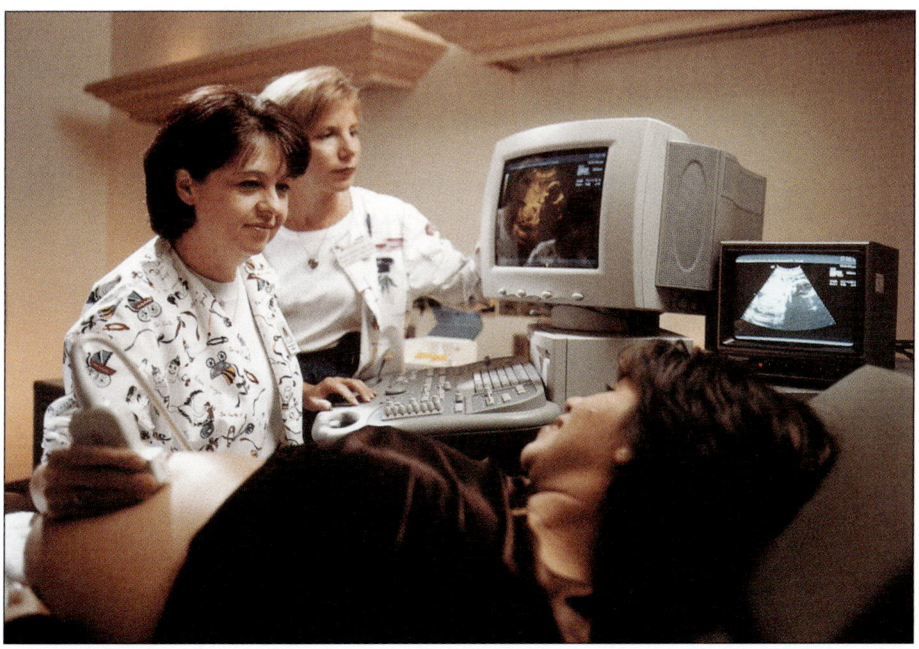

FIGURE 15.10 Prenatal care, including ultrasound monitoring to assess the baby's progress, can help older women have healthy pregnancies and produce healthy babies. *(© Stewart Cohen/Stone)*

Go to the USDA Food and Nutrition Service at www.fns.usda.gov/fns/ for information about programs such as WIC that are designed to improve the nutrition of women and children.

The March of Dimes at www.modimes.org/ provides information on normal development and the prevention of birth defects.

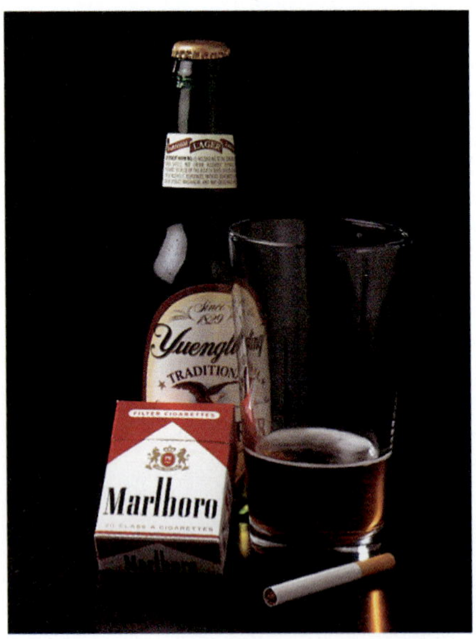

FIGURE 15.11 Women who smoke, drink alcohol, or use illicit drugs during pregnancy put their babies at risk. *(George Semple)*

Alcohol-related birth defects or **fetal alcohol effects** A spectrum of abnormalities including learning and developmental disabilities and behavioral abnormalities in children due to maternal alcohol consumption during pregnancy.

Fetal alcohol syndrome The most severe alcohol-related birth defects, characterized by physical and mental abnormalities.

Socioeconomic Factors

One of the greatest risk factors for poor pregnancy outcome is low income level. Poverty limits access to food, health care, and education.[25] Low-income women have a higher incidence of low-birth-weight and preterm infants.

Ideally, prenatal care should start before conception. Low-income women, however, are unlikely to receive any care until late in pregnancy. One federally funded program that addresses the nutritional needs of pregnant women is the Special Supplemental Nutrition Program for Women, Infants, and Children (WIC). WIC has been shown to reduce health-care costs by providing preventative care to low-income pregnant women through nutrition education and food vouchers.[26] This program provides services to pregnant women, to nonlactating women for 6 months after birth, to lactating women for 12 months after birth, and to infants and children up to 5 years of age, but it does not address the need for good nutrition for women planning a pregnancy.

Substances That Affect Pregnancy Outcome

The placenta prevents some but not all hazardous substances from passing from the mother's blood to the embryonic or fetal blood. The rapidly dividing cells of the embryo and fetus are sensitive to many substances that might normally be a part of a woman's daily routine, including cigarette smoke, alcohol, and drugs (Figure 15.11). Even over-the-counter and prescription medications can affect pregnancy outcome. A woman who is pregnant or considering pregnancy should quit smoking and consult with her physician before taking any medication.

Alcohol Alcohol is a teratogen that impairs fetal growth and development and is the leading cause of preventable birth defects and mental retardation.[27] It is a toxin that reduces blood flow to the placenta, thereby decreasing the delivery of oxygen and nutrients to the fetus. The use of alcohol can also impair maternal nutritional status, further increasing the risk to the embryo or fetus. Alcohol can cause learning and developmental disabilities and behavioral abnormalities referred to as **alcohol-related birth defects** or **fetal alcohol effects.** These occur in 1 out of every 1000 live births in the United States and in 43 of every 1000 babies born to heavy drinkers. They are more common in babies born to minority women and women of lower socioeconomic status.[28]

More severe alcohol-related damage during pregnancy is called **fetal alcohol syndrome.**[27] Fetal alcohol syndrome is a pattern of facial deformities, growth retardation, and permanent brain damage that causes problems throughout the child's lifetime. Mental retardation is the most common and most serious effect. The most notable physical effects of fetal alcohol syndrome are visible in the head and face: The head circumference is small, the cheekbones are poorly developed, the nose is short with a low nasal bridge between the eyes, the area under the nose is flat, and the upper lip is thin (Figure 15.12a). Growth retardation either during gestation or after birth is common. Newborns with the syndrome may be shaky and irritable, and have poor muscle tone and alcohol withdrawal symptoms. Other problems include heart and urinary tract defects, impaired vision and hearing, and delayed language development.

Debilitating behavioral problems, such as poor concentration and poor social and communication skills, plague adolescents and adults diagnosed with fetal alcohol syndrome. These problems interfere with their ability to hold jobs and live independently. Because alcohol consumption in each trimester has been associated with abnormalities, and because there is no level of alcohol consumption that is known to be safe during pregnancy, complete abstinence from alcohol during pregnancy is recommended. Warning labels to this effect appear on containers of beer, wine, and hard liquor (see Figure 15.12b).

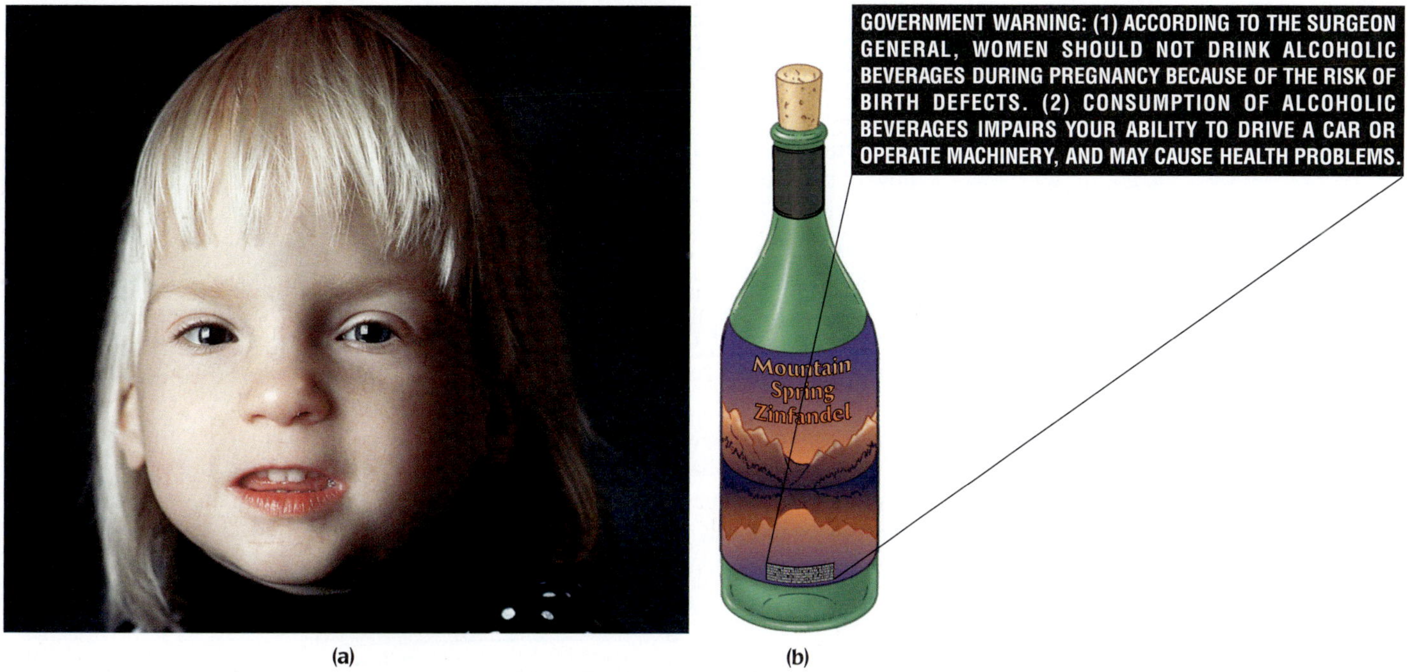
GOVERNMENT WARNING: (1) ACCORDING TO THE SURGEON GENERAL, WOMEN SHOULD NOT DRINK ALCOHOLIC BEVERAGES DURING PREGNANCY BECAUSE OF THE RISK OF BIRTH DEFECTS. (2) CONSUMPTION OF ALCOHOLIC BEVERAGES IMPAIRS YOUR ABILITY TO DRIVE A CAR OR OPERATE MACHINERY, AND MAY CAUSE HEALTH PROBLEMS.
Mountain Spring Zinfandel
(a)
(b)

FIGURE 15.12 (a) Children with fetal alcohol syndrome have common facial characteristics, including a low nasal bridge, a short nose, distinct eyelids, and a thin upper lip. (b) Alcoholic beverage packages include a warning against alcohol consumption during pregnancy. *(a, © George Steinmetz)*

Cigarettes It is estimated that 14.6% of pregnant women smoke cigarettes. Exposure to cigarette smoke affects the baby before birth and throughout life.[29] Compounds in tobacco smoke bind to hemoglobin and reduce oxygen delivery to fetal tissues. In addition, the nicotine absorbed from cigarette smoke constricts arteries and limits blood flow, reducing both oxygen and nutrient delivery to the fetus. Low-birth-weight babies are common among smokers; it is estimated that 20% of all such births could be prevented if women stopped smoking while pregnant. The risks of miscarriage, stillbirth, and premature birth are also increased in mothers who smoke.[30]

The risk of **sudden infant death syndrome (SIDS),** or **crib death,** and respiratory problems are increased in children exposed to cigarette smoke both in the uterus and after birth.[31] Thus, the effects of maternal smoking follow children throughout life. Children whose mothers smoked while pregnant may have impaired intellectual development and a greater risk of developing lung disease in their youth.[32]

Sudden infant death syndrome (SIDS) or **crib death** The unexplained death of an infant, usually during sleep.

Caffeine Caffeine is a natural component of coffee, tea, and chocolate and is added to some soft drinks and medications (see Table 14.8). Caffeine has not been found to be a teratogen in humans, but consumption of more than 300 mg per day by the mother during pregnancy has been associated with small reductions in birth weight and an increase in the risk for spontaneous abortion.[33] A typical "cup" of American coffee contains about 140 mg of caffeine, so this amount would be equivalent to about 2 1/2 cups of coffee per day.

Illicit Drug Abuse Substance abuse during pregnancy is a national health issue. Exposure to cocaine, opiates, or amphetamines has been shown to affect infant behavior and impact learning and attention span during childhood.[34]

Cocaine abuse during pregnancy has increased dramatically in the last decade. The health-care cost of treating cocaine-addicted infants is estimated at more than $500 million annually.[35] Cocaine increases the risk of complications to the mother and creates problems for the infant before, during, and after delivery. Cocaine use during pregnancy is associated with a high rate of miscarriages, intrauterine growth retardation, premature labor and delivery, low birth weight, birth defects, and sudden infant death syndrome.[36] This drug easily crosses the placenta and causes damage by constricting blood vessels, thereby reducing the flow of oxygen and nutrients to the rapidly dividing fetal cells.[37]

At birth, cocaine-exposed babies are small and overly excitable. They have a small head circumference, which is associated with lower IQ scores. Cocaine also affects brain chemistry by altering the action of neurotransmitters. This may cause the impulsiveness and moodiness characteristic of some cocaine-exposed children. Some of these babies also have physical deformities, and most suffer from behavioral problems severe enough to sabotage their education and social development.

Marijuana also crosses the placenta and enters fetal blood. Thus far, studies on the effect of marijuana use on pregnancy outcome have been conflicting—some found no negative effects while others found that marijuana-exposed infants are shaky and easily startled.[38]

Nutritional Needs of Pregnancy

Pregnancy involves a series of small, continuous physiological adjustments that affect the metabolism of nutrients. For some nutrients, absorption is increased; for others excretion is reduced. Some nutrients accumulate in new tissues where they serve structural or regulatory roles. Some are deposited in maternal stores to help meet the energy and nutrient demands of the pregnancy and subsequent lactation. Nutrients may also be redistributed among tissues, and for some the rate of metabolism or turnover is increased.[39] During pregnancy, maternal intake must supply all the nutrients needed to provide for the growth and development of the fetus while continuing to meet the mother's needs. Because the increased need for energy is proportionately smaller than the increased need for protein, vitamins, and minerals, a well-balanced, nutrient-dense diet is required.

Energy and Macronutrients

A typical pregnancy requires a total of about 55,000 additional kcalories.[1] Although this number may seem staggering, it amounts to only about an extra sandwich and glass of milk, or about 300 kcalories, per day during the second and third trimesters of the pregnancy (Figure 15.13). During the first trimester the additional energy required is small, and the 1989 recommended energy allowance is not increased.

Carbohydrate The carbohydrate composition of the diet during pregnancy should be about the same as that recommended for the general population—55 to 60% of energy. If carbohydrate intake is less than 100 g per day, ketosis may occur. Although the fetus can metabolize low levels of ketones, prolonged ketosis may be harmful.[40]

Fat There is evidence that the need for essential fatty acids and for fatty acids synthesized from the essential fatty acids, such as eicosapentaenoic acid and docosahexaenoic acid, is increased during pregnancy. The essential fatty acid status of the fetus depends on the status of the mother. During pregnancy, there is a decrease in maternal levels of some fatty acids, particularly for docosahexaenoic acid. It is hypothesized that this may decrease the amounts of these fatty acids

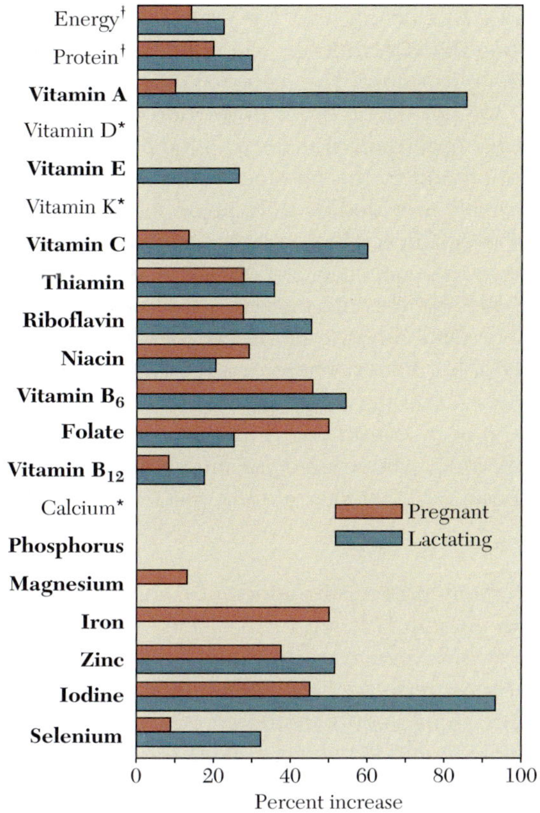

FIGURE 15.13 This graph illustrates the percentage increase in recommended nutrient intakes for a 25-year-old woman during pregnancy and lactation. Nutrients in bold have Dietary Reference Intake RDA values; nutrients followed by an asterisk have AIs, and those followed by a single dagger have 1989 RDAs. (The RDA for iron during lactation is equal to half the RDA for nonlactating nonpregnant women.)

available to the fetus.[41] However, the recommended 30% of energy as fat can easily supply more than enough of these fatty acids to meet needs.

Protein Protein needs are increased during pregnancy (see Figure 15.13). Protein is needed for the structure of all new cells in both the mother and the fetus. An increase of 10 g of protein per day above the 1989 RDA for nonpregnant women is recommended throughout pregnancy to provide for the increase in maternal blood volume; for the development of the placenta, breasts, uterus, and uterine muscles; and for the development and growth of all fetal structures. For a woman weighing 136 pounds (62 kg), this increases protein needs to about 60 g per day. Most women already consume this amount or more.

Water The need for water is increased during pregnancy because of the increase in blood volume, the production of amniotic fluid, and the needs of the fetus. This requires the consumption of only an extra 30 ml (1 fluid ounce) per day. Adequate total fluid consumption, about 2 liters per day, should be maintained throughout pregnancy to prevent constipation.

Micronutrients

The need for many vitamins and minerals is increased during pregnancy. Due to growth in maternal and fetal tissues as well as increased energy utilization, the requirements for the B vitamins, such as thiamin, niacin, and riboflavin, increase. To meet the needs for increased protein synthesis in fetal and maternal tissues, the requirements for vitamin B_6 and zinc increase. The needs for calcium, vitamin D, and vitamin C increase to provide for the growth and development of bone and connective tissue. To form new fetal and maternal cells, the needs for folate, vitamin B_{12}, zinc, and iron are increased.

Calcium The fetus retains about 30 g of calcium over the course of gestation. Most of the calcium is deposited during the last trimester when the fetal skeleton is growing most rapidly and the teeth are forming. The maternal demand for calcium is increased by as much as 300 mg per day in order to provide for mineralization of the fetal skeleton. The normal expansion of maternal blood volume and an increase in urinary calcium excretion add to the physiologic demand for calcium.[42] The additional calcium is normally provided by an increase in the absorption of calcium from the diet during pregnancy, which may be due in part to an increase in estrogen and an increase in the concentration of active vitamin D in the blood.[42] The increased need for calcium does not increase maternal bone resorption and studies have found no correlation between the number of pregnancies a woman has had and the density of her bones. Therefore, the AI for calcium for pregnant women age 19 and older—1000 mg a day—is not increased above nonpregnant needs.[43] This AI can be met by consuming three to four servings of milk or other dairy products daily. Women who are lactose intolerant can meet their calcium needs with yogurt, cheese, reduced-lactose milk, calcium-rich vegetables, and calcium-fortified foods.

Vitamin D Adequate vitamin D is essential to ensure efficient calcium absorption, but the recommended intake for vitamin D is not increased above nonpregnant levels. When pregnant women receive regular exposure to sunlight, vitamin D supplements are unnecessary. If exposure to sunlight is limited and sufficient vitamin D is not consumed in the diet, supplements should be considered. Most prenatal supplements provide 10 μg of vitamin D, which is twice the AI but well below the UL for pregnancy of 50 μg.[43] Inadequate vitamin D may be a particular problem in African-American women because their calcium and vitamin D intake is often low due to lactose intolerance, which limits dairy product consumption, and their darker pigmentation reduces the synthesis of vitamin D in the skin.

Neural tube A portion of the embryo that develops into the brain and spinal cord.

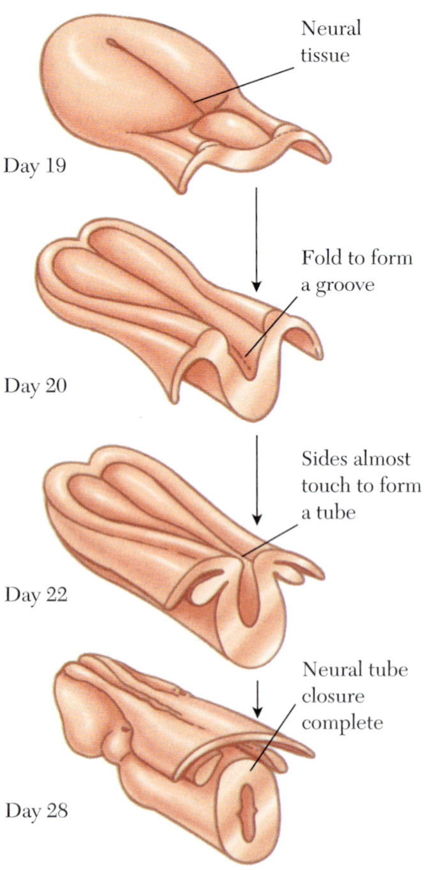

FIGURE 15.14 The neural tube forms early during the embryonic period of development. It develops from a flat plate of neural tissue. First a groove appears and then the edges fold up and join to form the neural tube, which will become the brain and spinal cord.

Vitamin C Vitamin C is important for bone and connective tissue formation because it is needed for the synthesis of collagen, the major protein in connective tissue, which gives structure to skin, tendons, and the protein matrix of bones. Vitamin C deficiency during pregnancy increases the risk of infections, premature rupture of the membranes, premature birth, and eclampsia. Plasma vitamin C levels decline as pregnancy progresses due to expansion of plasma volume and the transfer of vitamin C to the fetus. To allow adequate vitamin C transfer, the RDA is increased by 10 mg above the RDA for nonpregnant women.[44] The requirement for vitamin C can easily be met with foods such as citrus fruit or juice, and supplements are generally not necessary.

Folate Folate is needed for the synthesis of DNA and thus for cell division. During pregnancy, cells multiply to form the placenta, expand maternal blood, and allow for fetal growth. Adequate folate intake is crucial even before conception because rapid cell division occurs in the first days and weeks of pregnancy.

Folate is believed to be essential for proper formation of the **neural tube,** which is the portion of the embryo that develops into the brain and spinal cord. During development, neural tissue forms a groove; the groove closes when the sides fold together to form a tube (Figure 15.14). This neural tube closure occurs between 21 and 28 days of development. If it does not occur normally, the infant will be born with a neural tube defect, such as spina bifida (see Chapter 9). The mechanism whereby folate reduces neural tube defects is unknown. It has been hypothesized that folate might overcome a deficit in the production of DNA or protein at a critical time in neural tube closure, or that it selectively increases the spontaneous abortion rate of affected fetuses.[45]

Because the neural tube closes so early in development, often before a woman even knows she is pregnant, the DRIs recommend that women capable of becoming pregnant consume 400 μg daily of synthetic folic acid from fortified

TABLE 15.4 Calculating Dietary Folate Equivalents in Fortified Foods

The folate listed on labels of fortified foods is primarily folic acid, which is more available than natural forms of folate. In order to compare the folate content of these foods to recommendations, the amount of folic acid must be converted to dietary folate equivalents, expressed as μg DFE. This calculation assumes that all of the folate in these foods is from added folic acid.

Determine the amount of folic acid in the fortified food:

- Multiply the Daily Value for folate by the % Daily Values listed on the label.
- The Daily Value is 400 μg.

Convert the μg folic acid into μg DFE:

- Multiply the μg folic acid by 1.7.
- Folic acid added to a food in fortification provides 1.7 times more available folate per μg than folate naturally present in foods.

For example:

- A serving of English muffins provides 6% of the Daily Value for folate:
  To find the μg folic acid: 400 μg × 6% = 24 μg folic acid
  To convert to μg DFE: 24 μg folic acid × 1.7 = 40 μg DFE

foods, supplements, or a combination of the two, in addition to consuming a varied diet rich in natural sources of folate (see Chapter 9, *Critical Thinking*: "Figuring Out Fortified Folate"). To help women obtain adequate folic acid, enriched grain products in the United States are fortified with folic acid (see Table 15.4 and *Research Discoveries*: "The Folate Link: From Epidemiology to Public Health Policy").

Adequate folate continues to be important even after the neural tube closes. Cell division continues in both embryonic and fetal development and folate is central because of its role in DNA synthesis. Marginal folate status can impair cell growth and replication in both the fetus and the placenta. If folate is inadequate during pregnancy, megaloblastic anemia—the type of anemia in which blood cells do not mature properly—may result (see Chapter 9). Low dietary folate intakes and circulating folate levels are associated with increased risk of preterm delivery, low birth weight, and fetal growth retardation.[46] Thus, to maintain red blood cell folate levels in pregnant women, the RDA for folate is set at 600 μg dietary folate equivalents per day.[14] Natural sources of folate include orange juice, legumes, leafy green vegetables, and organ meats. Fortified sources include enriched breads, cereals, and other grain products. Folic acid supplements can also be used to meet this goal. Most prenatal supplements contain 400 μg of folic acid.

Vitamin B_{12} Vitamin B_{12} is essential for the regeneration of active forms of folate, so a deficiency of vitamin B_{12} can also result in megaloblastic anemia. Based on the amount of vitamin B_{12} transferred from the mother to the fetus and the increased efficiency of B_{12} absorption that occurs during pregnancy, the RDA for pregnancy is set at 2.6 μg per day.[14] This amount is easily met by a diet containing animal products. Deficiency has been observed in infants of vegan mothers. Vegans must consume foods fortified with vitamin B_{12} or take vitamin B_{12} supplements to meet their needs.

Zinc Zinc is involved in the synthesis and function of DNA and RNA and the synthesis of proteins. It is therefore extremely important for growth and development. Low zinc status during pregnancy is associated with an increased risk of fetal malformations, low birth weight, and preterm delivery. Complications in the mother include an increased risk of pregnancy-induced hypertension, hemorrhage,

RESEARCH DISCOVERIES

The Folate Link: From Epidemiology to Public Health Policy

Neural tube defects (NTDs), such as spina bifida and anencephaly, affect approximately 3900 pregnancies in the United States each year. Since the 1950s, researchers suspected that this type of birth defect might be related to the dietary intake of the mother. Epidemiological studies showed that NTDs were more common in women in lower socioeconomic groups who were more likely to consume a poor diet. Studies also showed that babies conceived in the winter and early spring were more likely to have these defects, possibly because at this time the diet would be lower in fruits and vegetables that are good sources of folate. Today, half a century later, public health policies mandate the fortification of food with the synthetic form of folate, folic acid.

The Folate/NTD Link A specific link between NTDs and folate was identified in the 1970s when lower concentrations of red-blood-cell folate during the first trimester were found in women who later gave birth to neural tube defect–affected babies.[a] Several observational studies also supported the hypothesis that consumption of adequate folate before conception prevented NTDs, but conclusive data were lacking.[b,c,d,e] In order to prove that folate was involved in the development of NTDs, controlled studies of folate supplementation were needed. The first intervention study of folate supplementation showed that supplementation in early pregnancy reduced the incidence of NTDs in women who had previously given birth to a baby with an NTD.[f] However, this finding was criticized because the subjects were not randomly assigned to the control and experimental groups. A second large-scale multicenter double-blind study was begun that did randomly assign nonpregnant women to receive either folic acid or a placebo.[g] This trial also studied women who had already had an infant with an NTD. Participants were randomly assigned to four study groups that received various combinations of folic acid and multivitamin supplements. The original study was to include 2000 women; however, after only 1195 pregnancies, the study was stopped because researchers were able to conclude at that point that folic acid supplementation alone reduced NTD recurrence by 71%. The link between the occurrence of NTDs and folate was clear but there were still many unanswered questions and concerns.

Safety and Efficacy The amount of folic acid supplemented in these studies was very high. Was this dose safe? Could a smaller amount be as effective? These trials of folate supplementation were performed in women who had already had a neural tube defect–affected pregnancy. But 95% of babies with NTDs are born to women who have no previous NTD offspring. Would folic acid supplements prevent the first occurrence of NTDs? Another intervention trial helped to answer these questions. Women planning a pregnancy who had no history of NTDs were randomly assigned to receive a multivitamin including either 800 μg of folic acid or a placebo for at least one month before conception and until at least the date of the second missed menstrual cycle.[h] The study evaluated 5453 pregnancies. In the 2391 women receiving the placebo, there were six babies born with NTDs, but in the 2471 women in the multivitamin group, there were no NTDs.[i] This and other studies helped determine the amount of supplemental folic acid and the maternal blood level of folate needed to reduce the incidence of NTDs. One study showed that a daily intake of only 400 μg of folic acid, an amount typically found in over-the-counter multivitamin preparations, reduced the occurrence of NTDs by 60%.[j] A subsequent study that treated a group of women of childbearing age with 0, 100, 200, or 400 μg of folic acid for six months found that women receiving 200 μg reached a blood folate level that would prevent 41% of NTDs and women who received 400 μg reached a blood folate level that decreased NTD risk by 47%.[k]

Research Leads to Recommendations The results of these trials led the Centers for Disease Control and Prevention and the U.S. Public Health Service to recommend that all women of childbearing age who are capable of becoming pregnant consume 400 μg per day of folic acid.[l] The recommendation was based on strong scientific evidence but presented some practical problems. How could the population's folate be increased? Education was considered, but it was felt that educating women to consume foods high in folate would be costly and ineffective. Folic acid supplements were

infection, and prolonged labor.[47] Because zinc absorption is inhibited by high iron intakes, iron supplements may compromise zinc status if the diet is low in zinc. The RDA during pregnancy is increased above the nonpregnant level to account for the amount of zinc that accumulates in maternal and fetal tissues during pregnancy. For pregnant women age 19 and older, the RDA is 11 mg per day.[19]

Iron Iron deficiency anemia is common during pregnancy. It has been associated with an increased risk of low-birth-weight and preterm delivery, and possibly impaired health of the infant.[48] Because low iron stores are so common among women of childbearing age, many women start pregnancy with diminished iron stores and quickly become deficient. This occurs despite the fact that iron absorption is increased during pregnancy and iron losses are decreased due to the cessation of menstruation.

recommended, but after five years it was determined that only one third of women of childbearing age were consuming a supplement containing the recommended amount of folic acid.[m] Therefore, it was concluded that the most reliable way to ensure that women of childbearing age obtained this amount of folate was through food fortification.

Fortifying the Food Supply Fortification of the food supply with folate would have a number of benefits. Preventing NTDs would have great medical, ethical, and economic advantages. And, increased folate intake would also reduce the risk of heart disease in the general population. However, there were also risks. A high folic acid intake can mask the symptoms of vitamin B_{12} deficiency, allowing it to go untreated while irreversible neurological changes progress. This was a concern because one in five people over 65 years of age are at risk of vitamin B_{12} deficiency. What was needed was a level of food fortification that would increase folate intake to a level that would prevent NTDs but would not be high enough to mask vitamin B_{12} deficiency.

In addition to deciding how much folic acid to add, public health officials needed to determine to which foods it should be added. Typically, foods selected for fortification are foods that are commonly consumed in regular amounts by the population at risk of deficiency. If an unpopular food was fortified, it would not provide the needed benefit. On the other hand, if too much of the fortified food is consumed by a segment of the population, it could result in dangerously high levels of the nutrient. In this case, the target population was women of childbearing age of all races and cultures. The goal was to find a food that was uniformly consumed by this population and not overconsumed by others. The foods chosen were enriched grain products such as bread, flour, corn meal, pasta, grits, rice, and other grains. The folic acid could be added to these grains during the enrichment process. The amount to be added was 140 μg per 100 g of grain product. This amount is probably too small for a women to obtain all 400 μg from this source, but it was also felt to be low enough that it did not pose a risk to those who were deficient in vitamin B_{12}.

In 1998, a U.S. Food and Drug Administration regulation mandated the fortification of enriched grain products with folic acid. The level of fortification chosen balanced the need to provide enough folic acid to reduce the risk of neural tube defects with the possibility of masking vitamin B_{12} deficiency. Studies are underway to determine the effects that this public health mandate will have on the incidence of neural tube defects.

References

[a] Smithells, R. W., Sheppard, S., and Schorah, C. J. Vitamin deficiencies and neural tube defects. Arch. Dis. Child. 51:944–949, 1976.

[b] Mulinare, J., Cordero, J. F., Erickson, J. D., and Berry, R. J. Periconceptional use of multivitamins and the occurrence of neural tube defects. JAMA 260:3141–3145, 1988.

[c] Milunsky, A., Jick, H., Jick. S. S., et al. Multivitamin/folic acid supplementation in early pregnancy reduces the prevalence of neural tube defects. JAMA 262:2847–2852, 1989.

[d] Bower, C., and Stanley, F. J. Dietary folate as a risk factor for neural tube defects: evidence from a case-controlled study in Western Australia. Med. J. Aust. 150:613–618, 1989.

[e] Mills, J. L., Rhoads, G. G., Simpson, J. L., et al. The absence of a relation between the periconceptional use of vitamins and neural-tube defects. N. Engl. J. Med. 321:430–435, 1989.

[f] Smithells, R. W., Sheppard, S., Schorah, C. J., et al. Possible prevention of neural tube defects by periconceptional vitamin supplementation. Lancet 1:339–340, 1980.

[g] MRC Vitamin Study Research Group. Prevention of neural tube defects: results of the MRC vitamin study. Lancet 338:131–137, 1991.

[h] Czeizel, A. E., and Dudás, I. Prevention of the first occurrence of neural-tube defects by periconceptional vitamin supplementation. N. Engl. J. Med. 327:1832–1835, 1992.

[i] Czeizel, A. E. Folic acid and the prevention of neural tube defects. J. Pediatr. Gastroenterol. Nutr. 20:4–16, 1995.

[j] Werler, M. M., Shapiro, S., and Mitchell, A. A. Periconceptional folic acid exposure and the risk of occurrent neural tube defects. JAMA 269:1257–1261, 1993.

[k] Daly, S., Mills, J. L., Molloy, A. M., et al. Minimum effective dose of folic acid for food fortification to prevent neural-tube defects. Lancet 350:1666–1669, 1997.

[l] Centers for Disease Control and Prevention. Recommendations for the use of folic acid to reduce the number of cases of spina bifida and other neural tube defects. MMWR 41:2133–2138, 1992.

[m] Use of folic acid–containing supplements among women of childbearing age—United States, 1997. MMWR 47:131–134, 1998. Available online at **http://cdc.gov/mmwr/preview/mmwrhtml/00051435.htm**. Accessed 10 Feb 2001.

Iron needs are high during pregnancy to provide for the synthesis of hemoglobin and other iron-containing proteins in both maternal and fetal tissues. The fetus draws iron from the mother to ensure adequate fetal hemoglobin production, mostly during the last trimester. Babies born prematurely may not have had time to accumulate sufficient iron, but babies born at term usually have adequate iron stores even if the mother is deficient.

The RDA for iron during pregnancy is 27 mg per day, compared to 18 mg per day for nonpregnant women.[19] It takes an exceptionally well-planned diet to meet iron needs during pregnancy. Red meats, leafy green vegetables, and fortified cereals are good sources of iron. Foods that enhance iron absorption, such as citrus fruit or meat, should also be included in the diet. Iron supplements are often recommended during the second and third trimesters (see *Critical Thinking:* "Nutrient Needs for a Successful Pregnancy").

Web Menu For more information on nutrition during pregnancy and lactation, go to the Food and Nutrition Information Center of the USDA at www.nal.usda.gov/fnic/pubs/bibs/topics/ and click on Nutrition During Pregnancy and Breast-Feeding.

Meeting Nutrient Needs During Pregnancy

The energy and protein needs of pregnancy can be easily met by following the Food Guide Pyramid recommendations for pregnant women (Figure 15.15). The additional servings recommended from the Bread, Cereal, Rice, and Pasta Group and the Vegetable Group provide energy, protein, micronutrients, and fiber, particularly if whole grains are chosen. The extra serving of milk that is recommended provides energy, protein, calcium, vitamin D, and riboflavin. The additional ounce of meat provides energy, protein, vitamin B_6, vitamin B_{12}, iron, and zinc. These recommendations can be met by adding a snack such as a roast beef sandwich with lettuce and tomato and a glass of milk.

Food Cravings and Aversions Most women change their diets during pregnancy. Some changes are made in an effort to improve nutrition to ensure a healthy infant, but other changes are based on cravings, aversions, or cultural or family traditions. Foods that are commonly craved include sweets and dairy products. Common aversions include coffee and other caffeinated drinks, highly seasoned foods, or fried foods.[49] It has been suggested that hormonal or physiological changes during pregnancy—in particular, changes in taste and smell—may be the cause of such cravings and aversions.

Pica An abnormal craving for and ingestion of unusual food and nonfood substances.

An unusual type of food craving that is more common in pregnancy is **pica.** This is an abnormal craving for and ingestion of unusual food or nonfood substances having little or no nutritional value. Commonly consumed substances include clay, laundry starch, ice and freezer frost, baking soda, cornstarch, and ashes.[50] Pica is more common in African-American than Caucasian women, in rural than urban women, and in women with a family history of the practice.

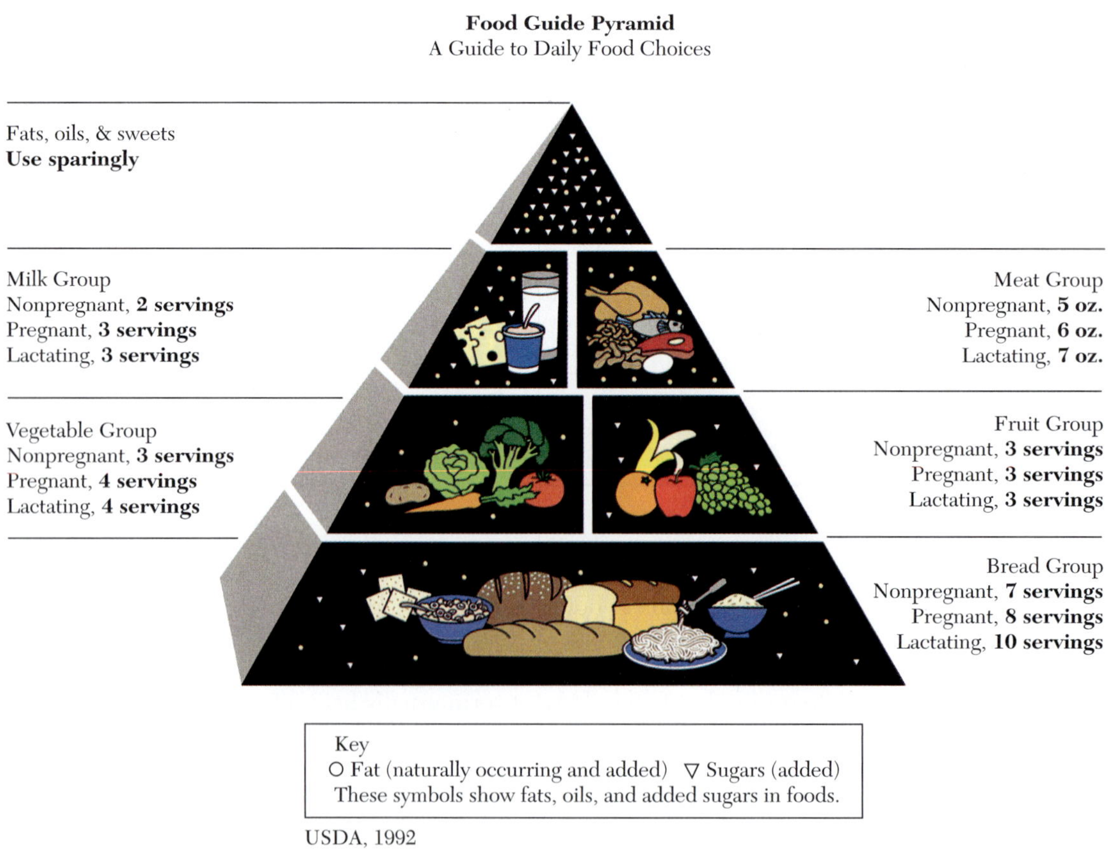

FIGURE 15.15 The recommendations of the Food Guide Pyramid can be applied during pregnancy and lactation. Shown here are the recommended servings for a 25-year-old woman before pregnancy and during pregnancy and lactation. *(U.S. Department of Agriculture, Home and Garden Bulletin No. 252, 1992.)*

Pica during pregnancy is potentially dangerous. The consumption of large amounts of some substances may cause micronutrient deficiencies by reducing the intake of nutrient-dense foods and by reducing nutrient absorption from food. The substances consumed could also cause intestinal obstruction or perforation and may contain toxins or parasites. Consumption of large amounts of starch provides kcalories and may cause excess weight gain.[49]

Anemia and pregnancy-induced hypertension are more common in mothers who practice pica, but it is not clear if pica is a result of these conditions or a cause. In newborns, anemia and low birth weight are often related to pica in the mother. Because of the association of these conditions with micronutrient intake, it was once thought that pica was an attempt to meet micronutrient needs. It is now believed that pica may be more related to cultural factors than the need for micronutrients.

Vitamin and Mineral Supplements Meeting the increased micronutrient needs of pregnancy requires a very carefully planned nutrient-dense diet. Supplements that are generally recommended include folic acid before and during pregnancy and iron during the second and third trimesters.[1] A multivitamin and mineral supplement may also be necessary in women whose food choices are limited, such as vegetarians, or in those whose needs are very high, such as pregnant teenagers.

The supplements prescribed by physicians contain iron and folate, but they also contain about 15 other vitamins and minerals. There is nothing wrong with taking a multivitamin and mineral supplement during pregnancy as long as the recommended dosage is not exceeded. The concern of public health agencies is that individuals taking supplements may ignore other components of their diet, thinking that the supplement will meet all their needs. Prenatal vitamin and mineral supplements do supply many nutrients at levels that meet or slightly exceed the recommended intake for pregnancy, but some nutrients are present in amounts that do not meet the needs of pregnancy, and others are missing altogether. For example, the ingredients listed in Table 15.5 illustrate that this prenatal supplement contains only 200 mg of calcium, which is only 20% of the AI for a pregnant woman age 19 or older.[43] The reason it does not contain more is that the

TABLE 15.5 Nutrients in a Typical Prenatal Supplement

Nutrient	Amount per Tablet	Recommendations for Pregnancy
Vitamin A (μg)	800	770
Vitamin D (μg)	10	5*
Vitamin E (mg α-tocopherol)	11–15	15
Vitamin C (mg)	80–120	85
Folate (μg DFE)	680–1700	600
Thiamin (mg)	1.5	1.4
Riboflavin (mg)	1.6–3.0	1.4
Niacin (mg)	17–20	18
Vitamin B_6 (mg)	2.6–10	1.9
Vitamin B_{12} (μg)	2.5–12	2.6
Biotin (μg)	30	30*
Pantothenic acid (mg)	7	6*
Calcium (mg)	200	1000*
Iron (mg)	60–65	27
Magnesium (mg)	100	350
Copper (mg)	2–3	1.0
Zinc (mg)	25	11

Values given are for a pregnant woman 19 to 30 years of age during her third trimester.
Unless indicated, values represent Dietary Reference Intake RDA values.
*Adequate Intake (AI).

tablet would have to be very large to provide the recommendation of 1000 mg. To meet her needs, a pregnant woman would need to consume this tablet plus the amount of calcium in about three glasses of milk. For similar reasons, the tablet doesn't meet the recommendation for magnesium. Even if all the calcium and magnesium needed for pregnancy could be packed into a little pill, it still would not provide an adequate diet. Prenatal supplements do not contain the protein needed for tissue synthesis or the complex carbohydrates needed for energy. They lack fiber, which helps prevent constipation, and they do not contain fluid for expanding tissues and blood volume and maintaining normal bowel function. They are also lacking in food components such as the phytochemicals that are supplied by a diet rich in whole grains, fruits, and vegetables.

Prenatal supplements are not absolutely necessary to meet the nutrient needs of pregnancy, but a very carefully planned diet is necessary to provide all the nutrients needed to produce a healthy baby. If a prenatal supplement is taken, it should be included as part of a healthy diet.

Critical Thinking

Nutrient Needs for a Successful Pregnancy

Alice is a 25-year-old woman who is four months pregnant. From the start—before she tried to conceive—she has been careful about her nutritional health. To obtain enough folate, she took care to consume plenty of fortified grain products and foods that are naturally high in folate. Now that she is in her second trimester, her doctor is concerned about her intake of iron and other nutrients and has prescribed a prenatal supplement. Alice follows his advice and takes the supplement, but she is curious about whether her diet could meet the nutrient needs of pregnancy without supplements. She records her intake for a typical day:

Food	Food Guide Pyramid Group	Iron (mg)
Breakfast		
1 cup corn flakes	1 grain	8.7
with 1/2 cup reduced-fat milk	1/2 milk	0
3/4 cup orange juice	1 fruit	0.8
1 cup decaffeinated coffee		0.1
with sugar and cream	fats, oils, and sweets	0
Lunch		
Tuna sandwich		
3 oz tuna	1 meat	1.3
2 tsp mayonnaise	fats, oils, and sweets	0
2 slices white bread	2 grain	1.5
20 french fries	2 vegetable	0.5
1 can orange soda	fats, oils, and sweets	0.2
3 chocolate chip cookies	1 grain	0.8
1 apple	1 fruit	0.3
Dinner		
3-oz chicken leg	1 meat	2.5
1/2 cup peas	1 vegetable	1.3
1 piece corn bread	2 grain	1.4
1 tsp margarine	fats, oils, and sweets	0
1 cup lettuce and tomato salad	1 vegetable	0.4
1 Tbsp dressing	fats, oils and sweets	0
1 cup reduced-fat milk	1 milk	0.1

Does her diet meet the Food Guide Pyramid recommendations for a pregnant woman? If not, what food groups does she need to increase or decrease?

Answer:

Alice was about 10 pounds overweight when she started her pregnancy. How does this affect her energy and nutrient needs during pregnancy?

Answer:

What substitutions would you suggest to increase her iron intake? With these substitutions, will Alice's diet meet the iron needs of pregnancy without supplements?

Answer:

Lactation

The nutrient requirements of pregnancy include those needed to prepare for **lactation.** During pregnancy, body fat is deposited to provide energy for lactation. After childbirth, the breast-feeding mother's nutrient intake must support milk production and can influence the nutrient composition of her milk.

The Physiology of Lactation

During pregnancy, hormones prepare the breasts for lactation by stimulating the enlargement and development of milk ducts and the milk-producing glands, called alveoli (Figure 15.16). Lactation involves both the synthesis of the milk components, such as milk proteins, lactose, and milk lipids, and the movement of these milk components through the milk ducts to the nipple. During the first few days after childbirth, the breasts produce and secrete a small amount of a clear yellow fluid called **colostrum.** Colostrum is an immature milk that is rich in protein, including immune factors that help protect the newborn from disease. Within about a week of childbirth, there is a rapid increase in milk secretion, and its composition changes from colostrum to mature milk.

Milk production is stimulated by the pituitary hormone **prolactin,** which is released in response to the suckling of the infant. The more the infant suckles, the more milk is produced. The ejection of milk from the milk-producing glands and its movement through the ducts and storage sinuses to the nipple are referred to as **let-down.** Let-down occurs in response to release of a second pituitary hormone, **oxytocin.** Oxytocin, like prolactin, is released in response to the suckling

Lactation Milk production and secretion.

Colostrum The first breast milk, which is secreted in late pregnancy and up to a week after birth. It is rich in protein and immune factors.

Prolactin A hormone released by the anterior pituitary that acts on the milk-producing glands in the breast to stimulate and sustain milk production.

Let-down A hormonal reflex triggered by the infant's suckling that causes milk to be released from the milk glands and flow through the duct system to the nipple.

Oxytocin A hormone produced by the posterior pituitary gland that acts on the uterus to cause uterine contractions and on the breast to cause the movement of milk into the secretory ducts that lead to the nipple.

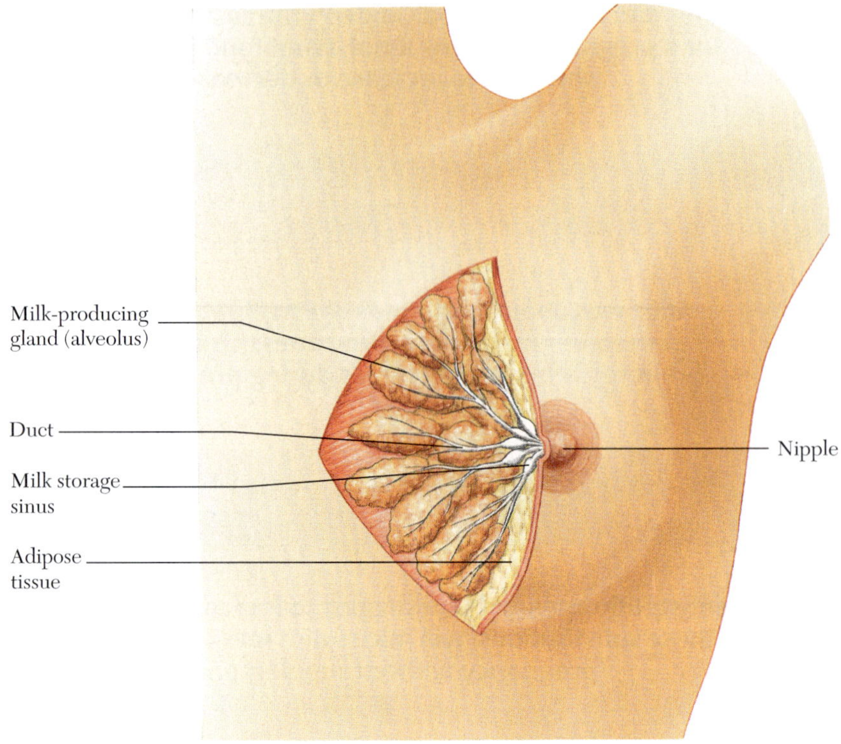

FIGURE 15.16 During lactation, milk travels from the milk-producing glands through the ducts to milk storage sinuses and then to the nipple.

of the infant (Figure 15.17). As nursing becomes more automatic, oxytocin release and the let-down of milk may occur in response to the sight or sound of an infant. It can be inhibited by nervous tension, fatigue, or embarrassment. The let-down response is essential for successful breast-feeding and makes suckling easier for the child. If let-down is slow, the child can become frustrated and difficult to feed.

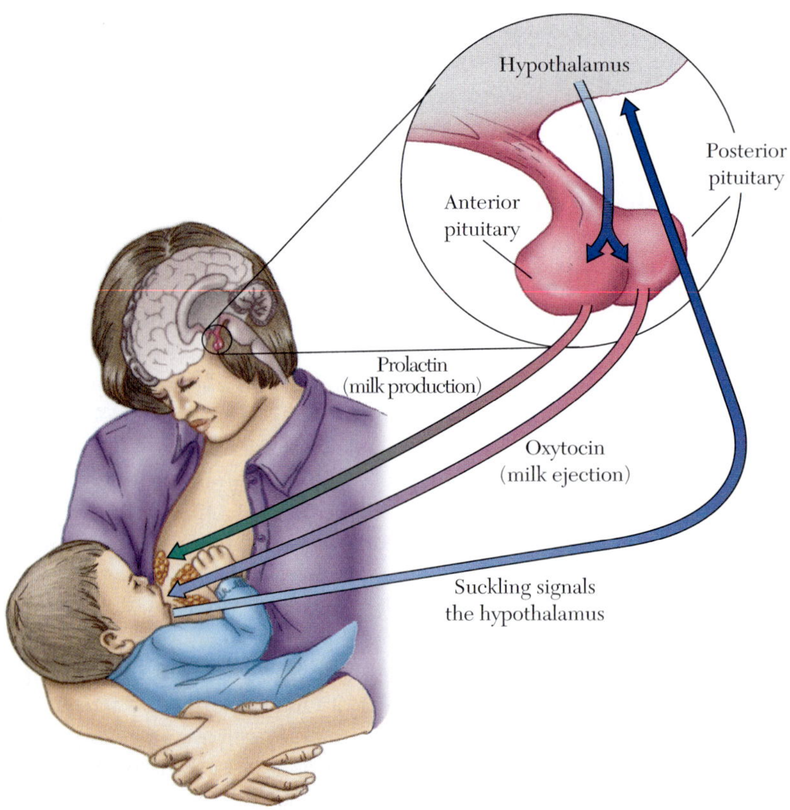

FIGURE 15.17 When the infant suckles, nerve receptors in the nipple send signals to the hypothalamus in the brain. The hypothalamus signals the release of prolactin from the anterior pituitary and oxytocin from the posterior pituitary. Prolactin stimulates milk production and oxytocin triggers the flow of milk from the glands through the duct system to the nipple.

Maternal Nutrient Needs During Lactation

The need for energy and many nutrients is even greater during lactation than during pregnancy. This is because the mother is providing for all of the nutrient needs of the infant, who is growing faster and is more active than he or she was in the womb. The newborn also has greater energy and nutrient needs for processes such as body temperature regulation and digestion that were partially or completely managed by the mother when the fetus was still in the womb.

Energy and Macronutrient Needs During Lactation During the first six months of lactation, approximately 600 to 900 ml, or 2.5 to 3.75 cups, of milk are produced daily. This amount may be higher or lower depending on the amount that the infant consumes.

Energy Needs During Lactation Producing a cup (240 ml) of breast milk requires about 225 kcalories. The milk itself contains approximately 175 kcalories, and the additional 50 kcalories are needed to synthesize the components of the milk. Providing an infant with 750 ml of milk would require approximately 700 kcalories from the mother. It is estimated that fat stored during pregnancy will provide 200 to 300 kcalories per day during the first three months of lactation. The remainder must be supplied by the diet. Therefore, an increase of about 500 kcalories per day over nonpregnant needs is recommended during early lactation.

It is normal to lose weight during the first six months after delivery. Beginning one month after birth, most lactating women lose 1 to 2 pounds (0.5 to 1 kg) per month for six months. Some women will lose more and others may maintain or even gain weight regardless of whether or not they breast-feed. Some studies report that breast-feeding does not affect the amount of weight lost,[51] whereas others suggest it does so initially[52] or if breast-feeding continues for at least six months.[53] Rapid weight loss is not recommended during lactation because it can decrease milk production. Regular exercise may speed weight loss and does not impair milk production.[54]

Protein Needs During Lactation The protein needed to produce milk increases maternal protein needs; therefore, the 1989 RDA recommends an increase in protein intake of about 15 to 20 g per day above nonpregnant needs.

Water Needs During Lactation To avoid dehydration and ensure adequate milk production, fluid intake should be increased by about 1 liter per day during lactation. This can be done by consuming an extra glass of milk, juice, or water at every meal and whenever the infant nurses. When fluid intake is low, the mother's urine will become more concentrated to conserve water for milk production.

Micronutrient Needs During Lactation The recommended intakes for several vitamins and minerals are increased during lactation to meet the metabolic needs of synthesizing milk and to replace the nutrients secreted in the milk itself (see Figure 15.13). Maternal intake of some vitamins can affect milk composition. This is particularly true of vitamins C, B_6, B_{12}, and D. When maternal intake is low, the amounts in milk are decreased.

For other nutrients, including calcium and folate, levels in the milk are maintained at the expense of maternal stores. To provide the calcium secreted in human milk, there is an increase in maternal bone resorption and a decrease in urinary calcium excretion.[42] However, the AI for calcium is not increased above nonlactating levels because the loss of calcium from maternal bones is not prevented by increases in dietary calcium. Calcium supplements during lactation also do not affect the concentration of calcium in the milk or maternal bone mineral changes.[55] Although lactation is associated with maternal bone loss, the calcium lost is replaced after weaning.[56] Folate needs are increased during lactation to account for the amount needed to replace folate secreted in milk and the amount needed by nonlactating women to maintain folate status.[14]

Iron needs during lactation are low because little iron is lost in milk, and, in most women, iron losses are decreased because menstruation is absent. The RDA for lactating women age 19 and older is 9 mg/day, half that of nonpregnant non-lactating women of childbearing age.[19]

Meeting Maternal Nutrient Needs During Lactation Meeting the needs of lactation requires a varied nutrient-dense diet that follows the Food Guide Pyramid recommendations for lactating women (see Figure 15.15). The need for calcium can be met by consuming three servings of dairy products, and additional nutrients and energy are obtained from extra servings of vegetables and grains and a larger serving of meat or meat substitutes. Most lactating women can meet all their needs without supplements.

Nutrition for the Infant

When a child is born and the umbilical cord is cut, he or she suddenly becomes actively involved in obtaining nutrients rather than being passively fed through the placenta (Figure 15.18). Nutrient needs are high to support growth, development, and activity. Suckling from either the breast or bottle must satisfy all nutrient needs.

Nutrient Needs of the Newborn

During the first few months after birth, growth is more rapid than at any other time of life. Many of the infant's organ systems and metabolic processes are still developing. Since infants' digestive abilities are limited and they have no teeth, a special type of diet is required.

Energy and Macronutrient Needs Energy requirements per unit of body weight are about three times greater in newborns than in adults (Table 15.6). The 1989 recommended energy allowances for infants from newborn to 6 months of age and from 6 to 12 months of age are 108 and 98 kcalories per kilogram of body weight, respectively, whereas adults require only 30 to 40 kcalories per kilogram.

Fat About 40 to 50% of the energy in an infant's diet should come from fat, with 3% from essential fatty acids. Breast milk and formulas contain approximately 50% of energy as fat. This high energy density allows the infant's small stomach to hold enough food to meet energy needs. A sufficient supply of docosahexaenoic acid (an omega-3 fatty acid) and arachidonic acid (an omega-6 fatty acid) are important for nervous system development. These fatty acids are constituents of cell membranes

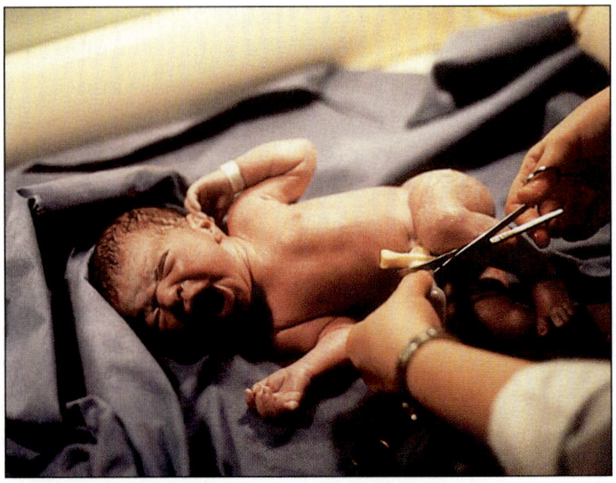

FIGURE 15.18 At birth the umbilical cord is cut and the child must obtain nutrients orally. *(© Jerry Cooke/Photo Researchers, Inc.)*

TABLE 15.6 Energy and Nutrient Needs of Infants Compared to Adults

Nutrient/Energy	Newborn Recommendation	Adult Recommendation
Energy	108 kcal/kg body weight	35 kcal/kg body weight
Protein	2.2 g/kg body weight	0.8 g/kg body weight
Carbohydrate	40% of energy intake	55–60% of energy intake
Fat	50% of energy with sufficient amounts of the essential fatty acids linoleic and alpha-linolenic acids and an increased need for docosahexaenoic and arachidonic acids	30% or less of energy with sufficient amounts of the essential fatty acids linoleic and alpha-linolenic acids
Fluid	150 ml/kg	35 to 40 ml/kg

and are incorporated into the retina of the eye and brain tissue. Infants can synthesize docosahexaenoic acid and arachidonic acid from their precursors, alpha-linolenic acid and linoleic acid respectively, but the rate of conversion is not great enough to meet the need for optimal retinal and brain formation.[57] The need for these fatty acids is even greater in preterm infants. Rapid development of the retina and brain continue to increase the need for these two fatty acids for about two years after birth. They are found in both breast milk and infant formulas.

Carbohydrate Carbohydrate is a major contributor to energy intake in the infant. The source of carbohydrate in breast-fed infants and most bottle-fed infants is lactose. About 39% of the energy in breast milk is from lactose. As the infant grows and solid foods are introduced, carbohydrates other than lactose are consumed, the percentage of energy from carbohydrate in the diet increases, and the percentage from fat decreases.

Protein As with energy, the infant's protein requirement per unit of body weight is very high compared with the adult requirement: The 1989 RDA is 2.2 g per kilogram from birth to six months of age, compared with 0.8 g per kilogram for an adult. The ideal protein source for newborns is human milk. Infant formulas are designed to mimic its amino acid pattern. The more closely the protein resembles that in human milk, the better it meets needs. A diet too high in protein may lead to dehydration because the excretion of metabolic wastes produced when excess protein is consumed increases water loss.

Water The fluid requirements of infants are also very high compared with those of adults. Infant kidneys are poorly developed and unable to reabsorb much of the water that is filtered out of the blood. Therefore, infants lose proportionately more water in their urine than adults. Infants also lose proportionately more water through evaporation than do adults because they have a large surface area compared with their total body weight. These factors, in addition to the fact that infants cannot express that they are thirsty, puts them at risk for dehydration. They rely on their caregivers to provide them with enough fluid. It is recommended that infants consume 150 ml of water per kilogram of body weight. Usually the amount of water in breast milk or formula is enough to meet needs. Hot weather, fever, diarrhea, and vomiting increase water loss and therefore require that additional water be provided.

In the developing world, diarrhea is the most common cause of infant death, and in the United States it kills one child each day. The cause of the diarrhea is usually a bacterial or viral infection; the cause of death is dehydration. The fluid intake of infants with diarrhea should be monitored carefully and a pediatrician should be contacted. Mixtures of sugar, water, and electrolytes are available to replace lost fluids.

Micronutrients There are several vitamins and minerals that may be limited in the unsupplemented infant diet. These include iron, vitamin D, vitamin K, fluoride, and vitamin B_{12}. Nutrient supplements should be given to infants only when recommended by a pediatrician and only in the amounts prescribed. Vitamin B_{12} is not known to be toxic, but iron, vitamin D, vitamin K, and fluoride are toxic at high doses.

Iron Iron deficiency is a concern in infants after the first four to six months of life. It is not a problem before this because infants are born with large iron stores and a high hemoglobin concentration. The iron in human milk, though not particularly abundant, is very well absorbed and is, along with the iron mobilized from the infant's stores, sufficient to meet needs. The AI for infants from birth to 6 months old is therefore only 0.27 mg per day, based on the amount of iron provided by human milk.[19] After four to six months, the infant's iron stores decrease but iron needs remain high to provide for hemoglobin synthesis, tissue growth, and iron storage. The RDA for infants 7 to 12 months old is set at 11 mg per day.[19] The diets of breast-fed infants should contain solid foods that are good sources of iron, such as iron-fortified rice cereal. Bottle-fed babies can obtain iron from iron-fortified infant formulas.

Vitamin D Newborns are also potentially at risk for vitamin D deficiency. Breast milk is relatively low in this vitamin, so breast-fed infants who do not receive adequate exposure to sunlight, such as those living in cold climates, may not obtain adequate vitamin D. To synthesize adequate vitamin D, about 15 minutes per day of sun exposure, with only the face exposed, is needed for light-skinned babies; a longer time is required for darker-skinned babies. An AI of 5 μg of vitamin D has been set for infants from birth to 12 months of age. This may be provided as a supplement for breast-fed infants. Infant formulas contain 10 μg of vitamin D per liter of formula; therefore, formula-fed infants can meet their needs without supplements.

Vitamin K Vitamin K, important in blood clotting, is another nutrient for which newborns are at risk of deficiency. Little of this vitamin crosses the placenta from mother to fetus, and because the gut is sterile at birth, no microbial vitamin K synthesis occurs. Breast milk is also low in vitamin K, so breast-fed infants are at risk of hemorrhage due to vitamin K deficiency. Today, most newborns receive a vitamin K injection at birth to prevent the possibility of hemorrhage. This provides them with enough vitamin K to last until their intestines are colonized with the bacteria that synthesize it. The AI for infants from birth to 6 months old is set at 2.0 μg per day based on the amount of vitamin K consumed by breast-fed infants and assuming the infant has received a prophylactic vitamin K injection at birth.[19]

Fluoride Fluoride is important in the development of teeth even before they erupt. Breast milk is low in fluoride and formula manufacturers use unfluoridated water in preparing liquid formula. Therefore, breast-fed infants, infants fed premixed formula, and those fed formula mixed with low-fluoride water are often supplemented beginning at six months of age. In areas where the drinking water is fluoridated, infants fed formula reconstituted with tap water should not be given fluoride supplements.

Vitamin B_{12} Vitamin B_{12} may be deficient in the breast milk of vegan mothers. Therefore, infants of vegan mothers should be supplemented with vitamin B_{12}.

Monitoring Infant Growth

Although nutrient needs for infants are fairly well defined, it is difficult to calculate an infant's actual nutrient intake. The best indicator of adequate nourishment is normal growth. Most healthy infants follow standard patterns of growth, so an infant's growth can be monitored by comparing length, weight, and head circumference to standards for infants of the same age.

Growth Charts Growth charts plot typical growth patterns of infants, children, and adolescents in the United States based on data from five national surveys collected between 1963 and 1994. Charts for infants from birth to 36 months of age and children and adolescents from 2 to 20 years of age are included in Appendix B.[58] For infants from birth to 36 months of age, charts are available to monitor weight-for-age, length-for-age (measured in a supine, or lying down, position), head-circumference-for-age, and weight-for-length (Figure 15.19). (See Chapter 16 for discussion of growth patterns in older children.)

Using growth charts, an infant's pattern of growth can be monitored and compared with other infants of the same age. The resulting ranking, or percentile,

Web Menu For information about infant growth patterns and the development of growth charts, go to the National Center for Health Statistics at www.cdc.gov/growthcharts/.

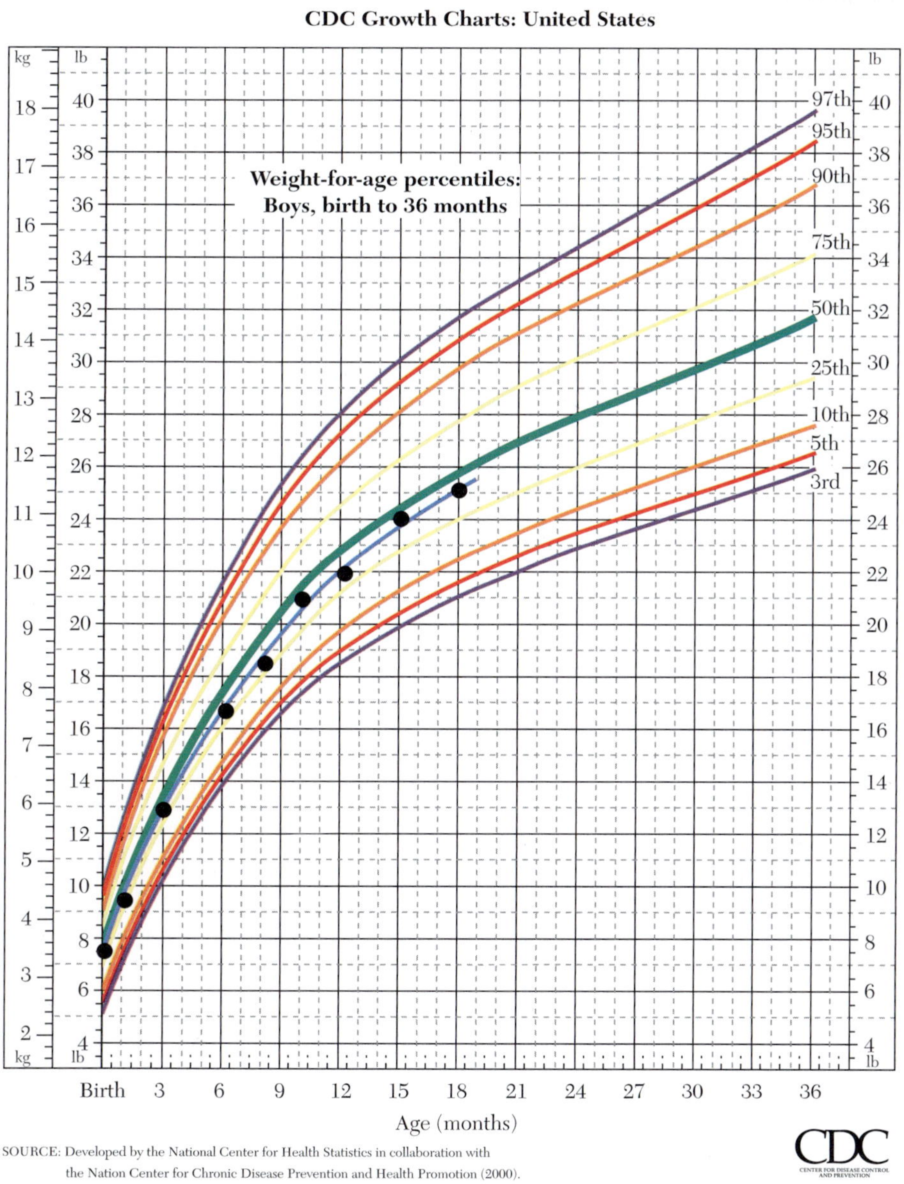

FIGURE 15.19 Growth charts, such as this one, which shows weight-for-age percentiles for boys from birth to 36 months of age, demonstrate typical patterns of growth. For example, shown in blue is the growth curve of a baby whose birth weight was at the 40th percentile and continued to grow along this percentile curve. *(Developed by the National Center for Health Statistics in collaboration with the National Center for Chronic Disease Prevention and Health Promotion, 2000.)*

indicates where the infant's growth falls in relation to population standards. For example, if a newborn boy is at the 20th percentile for weight, it means that 19% of newborn boys weigh less and 80% weigh more. Children usually continue at the same percentiles as they grow. For instance, a child who is at the 50th percentile for length and 25th percentile for weight should continue to follow approximately these length and weight curves. A dramatic deviation from the pattern could indicate overnutrition or undernutrition.

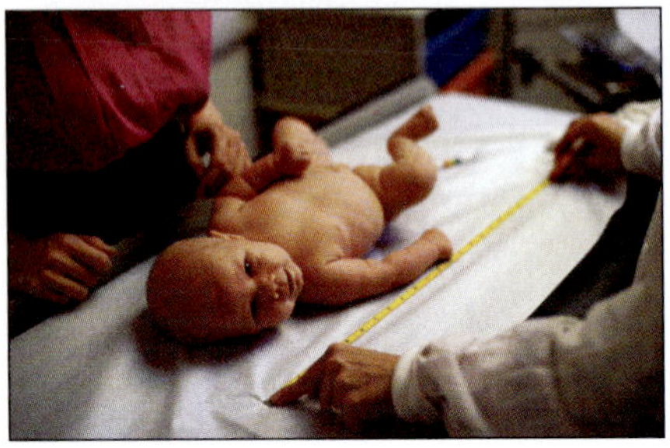

FIGURE 15.20 Infant length is measured in the supine position. *(© Doug Wilson/Corbis)*

Growth Rates Whether an infant is 6 pounds or 8 pounds at birth, the rate and pattern of growth should be approximately the same—rapid initially and slowing slightly as the infant approaches one year of age. A rule of thumb is that an infant's birth weight should double by four months and triple by one year of age. In the first year of life, most infants increase their length by 50% (Figure 15.20). Breast-fed and bottle-fed infants have similar growth for the first three to four months, but after this, bottle-fed infants grow at a faster rate. Small infants and premature infants often follow a pattern parallel to but below the growth curve for a period of time and then experience catch-up growth that brings them onto the growth curve in a place compatible with their genetic growth potential. Slight fluctuations in growth rate are normal, but a consistent pattern of not following the growth curve or a sudden change in growth pattern is cause for concern.

A rapid increase in weight without an increase in height may be an indication that the infant is being overfed. Growth that is slower than the predicted pattern indicates **failure to thrive.** This is a catch-all term for any type of growth failure in a young child. The cause may be a congenital condition or the presence of disease, poor nutrition, neglect, abuse, or psychosocial problems. Whatever the cause, the treatment is usually an individualized plan that includes adequate nutrition and careful monitoring by physicians, dietitians, and other health-care professionals. Just as there are critical periods in embryonic and fetal life, there are critical periods for growth and development during infancy. For example, the brain is growing rapidly at birth, and undernutrition at this time can permanently affect brain development.

Failure to thrive The inability of a child's growth to keep up with normal growth curves.

Feeding the Newborn

Newborns have small stomachs, can consume only liquids, and have high nutrient requirements. They should be fed on demand throughout the day and night, about eight times during a 24-hour period. The ideal food for the newborn is breast milk, but infant formula can also meet a newborn's needs. Solid food should not be introduced into the diet until the child is at least four to six months of age. Introducing solid food before four months is not recommended because the infant's feeding abilities and gastrointestinal tract are not mature enough to handle foods other than breast milk or formula.

Meeting Nutrient Needs with Breast-Feeding Breast milk is designed specifically for the human newborn, it requires no special preparation, and the amount available varies with demand. Thus, breast-feeding is the preferred form of infant nutrition and is usually the recommended choice for feeding the newborn of a healthy, well-nourished mother.[59] Public health programs promote breast-feeding, and, as a result, the percentage of infants who are breast-fed has increased from 20% in 1970 to 59.4% in 1995. Breast-feeding is most common among college-educated women over the age of 30, but the greatest increases in breast-feeding incidence have occurred among groups that historically have not had high rates, such as African Americans, women with low incomes, those less educated, those employed full-time, those less than 25 years of age, and women participating in the WIC program.[60]

Advantages of Breast-Feeding Breast-feeding has nutritional, immunological, physiological, and psychological benefits for both mother and child.[59] Breast milk provides protection against infection early in life by passing immune factors from the mother to the infant. Breast-fed babies have fewer allergies, ear infections, respiratory illnesses, and urinary tract infections than formula-fed babies, and they have fewer problems with constipation and diarrhea. There is also evidence that breast-feeding protects against sudden infant death syndrome, diabetes, and chronic digestive diseases.[61] The strong suckling required by breast-feeding aids in the development of facial muscles, which help in speech development and the correct formation of teeth. Breast-fed babies are also less likely to be overfed, because the amount of milk consumed cannot be monitored visually. With bottle-feeding, it is often tempting to encourage the baby to finish the entire bottle whether or not he is hungry.

For the mother, breast-feeding has the advantage of providing a readily available and inexpensive source of nourishment for her infant. Breast-feeding has been estimated to save more than $400 per child in food purchases during the first year. It requires no preparation or bottles and nipples that must be washed. It is more ecological because it doesn't require energy for manufacturing or generate waste from discarded packaging. Physiologically, breast-feeding causes contractions that help the mother's uterus return to size more quickly and may promote weight loss in some women, especially when continued for more than six months.[62] Women who breast-feed have a lower risk of developing osteoporosis and breast and ovarian cancers.[61] Lactation also inhibits ovulation, lengthening the time between pregnancies; however, it does not reliably prevent ovulation and so cannot be effectively used for birth control. Oral contraceptives can be used immediately postpartum, but formulations containing only progestin are preferable because they do not affect milk volume or composition. Oral contraceptives containing estrogen may decrease milk volume.[63] Psychologically, breast-feeding can be a relaxing, emotionally enjoyable interaction for both mother and infant (Table 15.7).

Web Menu

For information on lactation and breast-feeding, go to the La Leche League at www.lalecheleague.org/.

How Long Should Breast-Feeding Continue? Physiologically, lactation can continue as long as suckling is maintained. Nutritionally, breast-feeding alone is sufficient to support optimal growth for about six months, and the American Academy of Pediatrics recommends breast milk along with supplemental feeding of solids for the first year of life—and longer—as mutually desired by mother and child.[61] After 12 months the baby no longer needs breast milk to meet nutrient needs. As the infant obtains more and more of its energy from solid foods, milk production decreases due to reduced demand. However, breast-feeding beyond 12 months continues to provide nutrition, comfort, and an emotional bond between mother and child. The length of time a woman breast-feeds is up to her and her baby. In most cultures it is acceptable to breast-feed for two to three years. As part of its Integrated Management of Childhood Illness Program, the World Health Organization recommends that infants in developing nations be breast-fed for two years.[64] In the United States, because of social pressures and convenience issues, few women continue for more than six months.

How Much Is Enough? A strong, healthy baby will be able to suckle shortly after birth. Within a week, milk production and breast-feeding are usually fully established (Figure 15.21). Infants should be fed on demand every 1.5 to 3 hours. A feeding should last approximately 8 to 12 minutes at each breast. Although it is difficult to measure the amount of milk an infant takes from the breast, a well-fed newborn should urinate enough to soak six to eight diapers a day and gain about 1/3 to 1/2 pound per week.

Practical Aspects of Breast-Feeding Breast-feeding does not always come naturally to mother or infant and can require practice and patience. Effective suckling by the infant and relaxation of the mother are essential to successful

TABLE 15.7 Risks and Benefits of Breast- and Bottle-Feeding

Risk/Benefit	Breast-Feeding	Bottle-Feeding
Nutrients	Ideal food for human babies. Composition changes over time.	Modeled after human milk, but certain components cannot be duplicated. Composition does not change with time. Must be prepared carefully to supply the correct nutrient mix and ratio of nutrients to fluid.
Amount	Underfeeding can be a problem in newborns if the mother is not well-versed in breast-feeding and monitoring the infant for signs of dehydration.	Overfeeding is a risk because of the desire of caregivers to have the baby empty the bottle.
Immunity	Immune factors are transferred from mother to infant.	There are no immune factors in formula.
Allergies	Allergies to breast milk are rare and the risk of food allergies is reduced.	There are a variety of choices if the infant is allergic to one type of formula.
Risk from mother	Certain contaminants such as environmental pollutants, medications, illicit drugs, and disease-causing organisms such as HIV can pass from mother to baby.	None.
Environmental contamination	Breast milk is sterile, but pumped milk can become contaminated if handled improperly.	Bacterial contamination is a risk if formula is prepared under unsanitary conditions or stored improperly.
Ease for caregivers	No equipment to wash, always available, but may require more time from the mother.	Requires more preparation and washing, but other family members can share responsibility for feeding.
Ease for baby	Suckling is harder for the baby but aids in development of teeth and facial muscles needed for speech. Pumped breast milk can be easily consumed by weak or sick infants.	Easier for baby, which is especially important for weak or sick infants.
Benefit to mother	Promotes uterine contractions which help the uterus return to prepregnancy size. May promote loss of weight and body fat if continued for more than six months. May reduce risk of breast cancer.	May allow more sleep.
Cost	Cheaper, but the mother must be well-nourished.	More expensive when including the cost of formula and equipment as well as energy used in preparation and clean up.

breast-feeding. Some foods and other substances in the mother's diet, such as garlic or spicy foods, contain chemicals or flavors that pass into breast milk and cause adverse reactions in some babies. These reactions seem to be individual to the mother and child. As long as a food does not affect the infant's response to feeding, it can be included in the mother's diet. Caffeine in the mother's diet can make the infant jittery and excitable, so large amounts should be avoided while breast-feeding. Alcohol, which is harmful for infants, passes into breast milk. It is most concentrated an hour to an hour and a half after consumption and is cleared from the milk at about the same rate it disappears from the bloodstream. Therefore, occasional limited alcohol consumption while breast-feeding is probably not harmful if intake is timed to minimize the amount present in milk when the infant is fed.

Breast-feeding does not mean that a mother must be available for every feeding. Milk may be pumped from the breast and stored for later feedings. A working mother can nurse her baby in the morning and evening and provide formula or pumped breast milk to be fed from a bottle while she is away from home. A mother taking prescription drugs for only a short time can use a breast pump to maintain milk production (discarding the milk) until the medication is no longer needed (Figure 15.22). Because pumped milk is exposed to pumps and bottles, care must be taken to avoid bacterial contamination. If not immediately fed to the baby, pumped milk should be refrigerated. It can be kept refrigerated for 24 to 48 hours, but if it will not be used within that period, it should be frozen in a clean container. Warming breast milk in a microwave is not recommended, because this destroys some of its immune properties and may cause some portions of the milk to be dangerously hot. The best way to warm milk is by running warm water over the bottle.

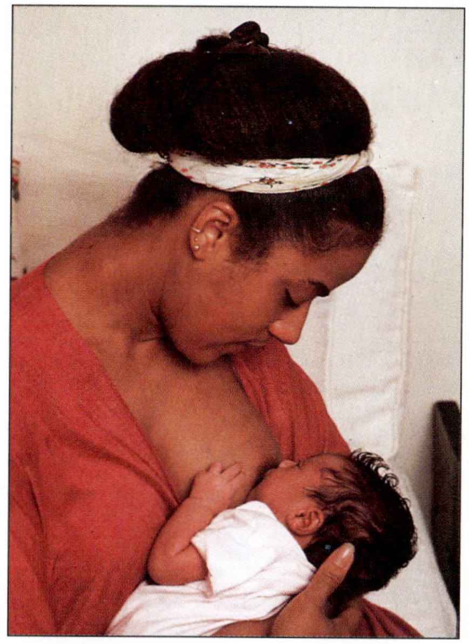

FIGURE 15.21 By the time the infant is a week old, mother and child have usually adjusted to breast-feeding. *(© Erika Stone/Photo Researchers, Inc.)*

Composition of Human Milk The nutrient composition of breast milk is specifically designed for the human infant and changes as the infant develops. As discussed above, colostrum is higher in water, protein, immune factors, minerals, and some vitamins than mature milk. It is produced for up to a week after delivery. While colostrum is produced, it may seem that the newborn is not receiving enough to eat; however, supplemental bottle feedings are not necessary. The nutrients in colostrum meet infant needs until mature milk production begins. During the first few months of life, the immune factors provided first by colostrum, and later by mature milk, compensate for the infant's immature immune system. Colostrum also has beneficial effects on the gastrointestinal tract, acting as a laxative that helps the baby excrete the thick, mucousy stool produced during life in the womb.

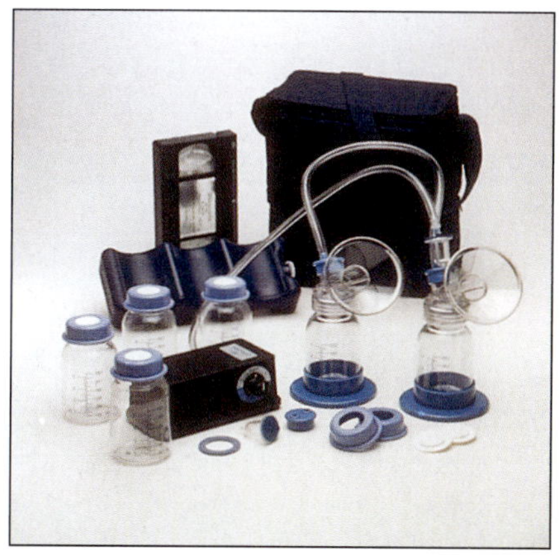

FIGURE 15.22 Breast pumps can be used to pump milk, which can be fed to infants in a bottle. This can relieve the mother from having to be responsible for all feedings. *(Bailey Medical Engineering)*

The composition of mature human milk changes over time, meeting the nutrient needs for up to the first year of life. Mature human milk contains about 175 kcalories per cup (240 ml) and is a good source of protein, fat, magnesium, and calcium. When compared with cow's milk, it is very different in both appearance and composition. Human milk looks thin and watery and has less protein and minerals than cow's milk. Lactalbumin, the predominant protein in human milk, forms a soft, easily digested curd in the infant's stomach. The amino acids methionine and phenylalanine, which are difficult for the infant to metabolize, are present in lower amounts in human milk proteins than in cow's milk proteins. Human milk is also a good source of taurine, an amino acid needed for bile salt formation and eye and brain function.

The fat in human milk is more easily digested than that in cow's milk. Human milk is higher in cholesterol and the essential fatty acid linoleic acid. It is also higher in the long-chain polyunsaturated fatty acids arachidonic acid and docohexaenoic acid, which are essential for normal brain development, eyesight, and growth.[65] The fat content of breast milk changes throughout a feeding, gradually increasing during the nursing session. Thus, for the baby to attain satiety and obtain adequate energy, it is important for nursing to continue long enough for the infant to obtain the higher-fat milk.

Lactose is the primary carbohydrate in human milk. It is digested slowly, and it stimulates the growth of acid-producing bacteria. It also promotes the absorption of calcium and other minerals and provides a source of galactose for nervous system development.

Human milk is low in iron, but the iron present is easily absorbed. About 50% of the iron in human milk is absorbed, compared with only 2 to 30% from many other foods.

Human milk also contains a number of other substances that protect the infant from disease. Antibody proteins and immune system cells pass from the mother into her milk to provide the infant immune protection. A number of enzymes and other proteins prevent the growth of harmful microorganisms. Several carbohydrates have been identified that protect against disease-causing organisms, including viruses that cause diarrhea.[66] One substance in breast milk favors the growth of the beneficial bacterium *Lactobacillus bifidus* in the infant's colon, which inhibits the growth of disease-causing organisms (see *Critical Thinking:* "Nourishing a New Baby").

Meeting Nutrient Needs with Bottle-Feeding A hundred years ago a baby who could not be breast-fed had little chance of survival. Today infants who cannot breast-feed can still thrive. When breast-feeding is not the choice, there are many commercially available infant formulas modeled after the nutrient content of breast milk. Unmodified cow's milk should never be fed to infants; its higher protein and mineral content taxes the kidneys and predisposes the infant to dehydration. Young infants may also become anemic if fed cow's milk because it contains little absorbable iron and can lead to iron loss by causing small amounts of gastrointestinal bleeding.

When Is Bottle-Feeding Best? Despite efforts to increase the number of women who breast-feed, the infant formula business is booming. Many women prefer not to breast-feed at all, and many breast-feed for only a short time. Sometimes this is a lifestyle choice, and in some cases breast-feeding is not the best choice for health reasons. Bottle-feeding is easier for the infant; less strength is needed to consume the same nutrients. An infant who is small or weak may not have the strength to receive adequate nutrition from breast-feeding. In this case, formula, which provides almost the same nutrients as breast milk, can be used, or pumped breast milk can be offered to the infant in a bottle.

In some cases bottle-feeding is the best choice because it reduces the transmission of disease and drugs via breast milk. Hepatitis and HIV infection, which causes AIDS, can be transmitted to the infant in breast milk, but common illnesses such as colds, flu, and skin infections should not interfere with breast-feeding.[67] In the United States, women who are infected with HIV are advised not to breast-feed, but in developing nations, the risks of malnutrition associated with not breast-feeding outweigh the risk of passing this infection on to the infant. Women who are taking medications should check with their physician about whether it is safe to breast-feed. Because alcohol and drugs such as cocaine and marijuana can be passed to the baby in breast milk, alcoholic and drug-addicted mothers are counseled not to breast-feed. Nicotine from cigarette smoke is also rapidly transferred from maternal blood to milk, and heavy smoking may decrease the supply of milk.[68] Also, secondhand exposure to smoke may be damaging to the infant's lungs and may increase the risk of sudden infant death syndrome.[31]

How Much Is Enough? As with breast-fed infants, formula-fed infants should be fed on demand every few hours. Newborns have small stomachs, so at each feeding they may consume only a few ounces of formula. As the infant grows, the amount consumed at each feeding will increase to 4 to 8 ounces. Caregivers should respond to cues from the infant that hunger is satisfied, even if a bottle of formula is not finished. Encouraging infants to finish every bottle can result in overfeeding and excess weight gain. As with breast-fed infants, adequate intake can be judged from the amount of urine produced and the amount of weight gained.

Practical Aspects of Bottle-Feeding Infant formula must be prepared carefully in order to avoid mixing errors and contamination. If the proper measurements are not used in preparing formula, the child can receive an excess or deficiency of energy and nutrients and an improper ratio of nutrients to fluids. If the water and all the equipment used in preparing formula are not clean or if the prepared formula is left unrefrigerated, foodborne illness may result. Because sanitation is often a problem in developing nations, infections that lead to diarrhea and dehydration occur more commonly in formula-fed than in breast-fed infants. Commercially prepared formulas are sterile and powdered formulas contain no harmful microorganisms. To avoid introducing harmful microorganisms, the water used to mix powdered formula should be boiled for one to two minutes and allowed to cool before mixing.[69] Hands should be washed before preparing formula, and bottles and nipples should be washed in a dishwasher or placed in a pan of boiling water for 5 minutes. Formula should be prepared immediately before a feeding, and any excess should be discarded. Opened cans of ready-to-feed and liquid concentrate formula should be covered and refrigerated and used within the time indicated on the can. Formula may be fed either warm or cold, but the temperature should be consistent.

Nursing bottle syndrome Extreme tooth decay in the upper teeth resulting from putting a child to bed with a bottle containing milk or other sweetened liquids.

The position of the child is important during feeding. The infant's head should be higher than the stomach, and the bottle should be tilted so that there is no air in the nipple (Figure 15.23). If the hole in the nipple is too large, the infant may swallow air with the formula and feel full before receiving adequate nutrition. If the hole is too small, the infant may tire before nutrient needs are met. Just as breast-fed infants alternate breasts, bottle-fed infants should be held alternately between the left and right arms to promote equal development of the head and neck muscles.

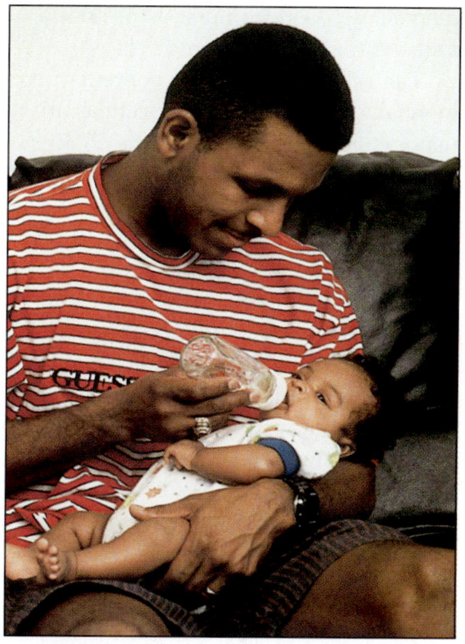

FIGURE 15.23 The position of the baby and the bottle are both important during feeding. *(© Erika Stone/Photo Researchers, Inc.)*

Infants should never be put to bed with a bottle of formula. At night, while the child sleeps, the flow of saliva is decreased and the sugar in the liquid is allowed to remain in contact with the teeth for many hours. This causes the rapid and serious decay of the upper teeth referred to as **nursing bottle syndrome.** Usually, the lower teeth are protected by the tongue and are unaffected (Figure 15.24).

Formula Choices The modern era of infant formulas began with the development of artificial milk made from skimmed cow's milk to which homogenized animal and vegetable fats were added to approximate the fatty acid composition of human milk. Over the past 30 to 40 years, very few problems have resulted from inadequate or imbalanced formulas. In the 1950s, a few cases of vitamin A deficiency were seen in infants receiving formula made from defatted soy flour, and skin lesions have been seen in infants fed formulas low in linoleic acid. In 1978, a company accidentally left chloride out of two of its formulas, and infants fed these developed symptoms that included poor muscle control, delayed speech development, and slowed growth. Infant formulas can never duplicate the living cells, active hormones, enzymes, and immune system molecules in human milk, but formulas today try to replicate human milk as closely as possible in order to match the growth, nutrient absorption, and other parameters obtained with breast-feeding. Formula is available in ready-to-feed, liquid concentrate, or powdered forms (see *Making Decisions:* "Choosing an Infant Formula").

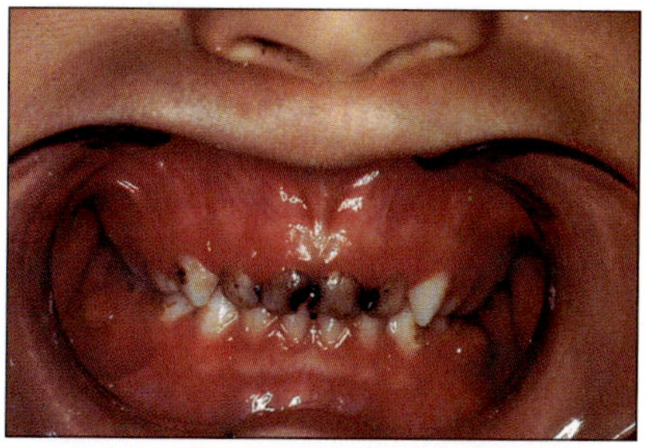

FIGURE 15.24 Nursing bottle syndrome causes rapid decay of the upper front teeth. *(K. L. Boyd, D.D.S./Custom Medical Stock Photo)*

Special Formulas for Special Needs There are a number of conditions, including allergies, prematurity, and genetic abnormalities, that alter the nutrient needs of newborns. To meet these unusual needs, special formulas are available. Milk allergy is an example of a relatively rare nutrition-related problem that can be life-threatening but is easily treated with a modified diet. There are over 25 proteins in milk that can be the cause of a milk allergy. Many, but not all, are inactivated by scalding the milk. For infants who cannot tolerate human or cow's milk, soy protein formulas are available. And for those who cannot tolerate soy protein, formulas made from predigested proteins, called protein hydrolysates, are an option.

Making Decisions

Choosing an Infant Formula

Which infant formula is best? Infants are often formula-fed from birth, and many are formula-fed after a few months of breast-feeding. Selecting an infant formula can be confusing. Is one safer or more nutritious than the other? Is a less expensive formula likely to be missing certain nutrients? Is cow's milk–based formula better than a soy-based formula? Is premixed formula better than powdered?

The safety and nutrient content of commercially prepared infant formulas are not major considerations in formula choices because they are regulated by the FDA. The FDA guidelines for the amounts of nutrients in infant formulas are based on the composition of human milk from a healthy mother and follow the recommendations of the American Academy of Pediatrics Committee on Nutrition.[a] Quality control is strictly regulated, requiring that each batch of formula be tested for stability and analyzed to ensure it contains the appropriate amounts of required nutrients.

Cow's milk is the standard base for infant formula. When modified to more closely match breast milk, it provides a nutritious and easily absorbed product. Hydrolysed cow's-milk formula and soy-based formula are available if cow's-milk formula is not well tolerated by an infant. Cow's-milk hydrolysates are usually recommended over soy formula because they provide higher quality protein and the calcium they contain is better absorbed. Soy-based formulas are necessary for infants who are lactose intolerant because soy formula contains sucrose or corn syrup instead of lactose.

Formulas are marketed in three basic forms: ready-to-feed, liquid concentrates, and powdered. Ready-to-feed formulas require no preparation and are available in sizes ranging from 4-ounce bottles to 32-ounce containers. Liquid concentrates are prepared for use by mixing equal amounts of the concentrate and water. Powdered formulas are prepared by mixing 1 tablespoon of powder for every 2 ounces of water. When properly prepared, all of these provide the needed nutrients in an appropriate concentration. Problems arise when formulas are mixed incorrectly or when the water used to prepare them is contaminated. Incorrect mixing can result from a lack of understanding, poor measuring techniques, the addition of extra water to make the formula last longer, or the belief that a more concentrated formula will make the baby grow better. Even correctly mixed formula is a health hazard if the water used to mix it contains contaminants such as lead or disease-causing microorganisms. Water for formula should come from a safe source and be boiled before use.

Because the composition and safety of infant formulas is regulated, the major considerations when choosing one are cost, ease of transport, and convenience of preparation. Ready-to-feed formulas are easiest to use but may cost more and are heavier and bulkier to carry home from the store. Liquid concentrates are a good compromise because they provide more formula for less weight and are easy to mix. Powders are the least expensive and the easiest to transport home in a grocery bag but require more measuring and mixing. Since all of these products are nutritionally comparable, the choice depends on the needs of the caregivers.

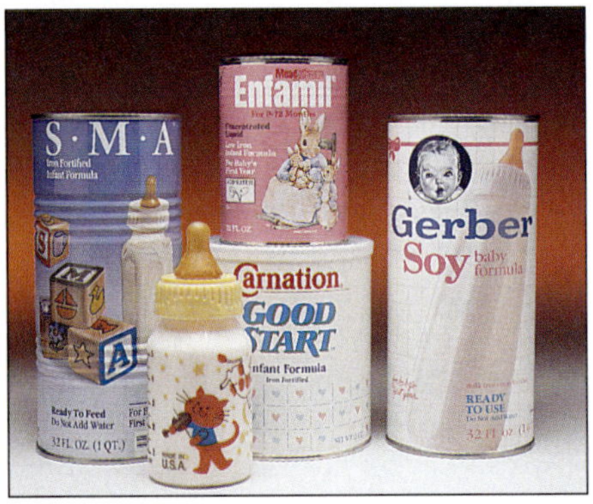

(Charles D. Winters)

Reference

[a] Stehlin, I. B. Infant formula: second best but good enough. FDA Consumer 29:17–20, June 1996.

Premature infants have special needs because they do not have fully developed organ systems or metabolic pathways. If they are too small or weak to nurse or take a bottle, pumped breast milk or formula can be fed through a tube. In some cases, very small infants must be fed intravenously.

Some nutrients that are produced in the bodies of full-term infants are essential in the diets of premature infants. For example, preterm infants are less able to synthesize the amino acids tyrosine and cysteine and the fatty acid docosahexaenoic acid. These and other substances, such as taurine and carnitine, are needed in higher amounts by premature babies. The energy, protein, and micronutrient requirements of preterm infants are also higher due to their rapid growth and development. Preterm infant formulas are available to meet the needs of premature babies.

Genetic abnormalities that prevent the normal metabolism of specific nutrients may alter dietary needs. For instance, infants with the genetic disease phenylketonuria (PKU) lack an enzyme needed to metabolize the amino acid phenylalanine (see Chapter 6). If a child with PKU is fed breast milk or a formula that contains phenylalanine, the by-products of phenylalanine metabolism accumulate and can cause brain damage. This can be prevented by feeding infants with PKU a special formula that provides only enough phenylalanine to meet the need for protein synthesis. Because this special diet must be started as soon as possible, infants born in the United States and Canada are tested for PKU at birth.

A relatively common but not life-threatening problem in infants is **colic.** Colic involves daily periods of inconsolable crying that cannot be stopped by holding, feeding, or changing the infant. Colic usually begins at a few weeks of age and continues through the first two to three months. It occurs in both breast- and bottle-fed infants. Although its cause is unknown, it is hypothesized that colic is related to intestinal gas caused by milk intolerance, improper feeding practices, or immaturity of the central nervous system.

Colic Inconsolable crying that is believed to be due either to pain from gas buildup in the gastrointestinal tract or immaturity of the central nervous system.

Critical Thinking

Nourishing a New Baby

Tamika had a baby last week. He is a healthy 6-pound, 19-inch-long boy named Henry. Her grandmother has come to stay for a while to help with the baby. Tamika is breast-feeding. After three weeks, the baby still wakes up at night to eat. Grandma says to give him a bottle of formula mixed with cereal before bed to help him sleep through the night.

Will this help the baby sleep?

There is no evidence that babies who consume cereal in their bottles sleep better. Henry is still too young to need any food other than breast milk or formula and may have difficulty digesting the cereal.

When Henry is six weeks old, Tamika must return to work. She would like to continue breast-feeding even though Henry will be home with Grandma while she is at work across town.

What options does she have?

Answer:

Grandma says that Henry is so big that he can't possibly meet his needs from breast milk alone. He is hungry every 3 hours and Grandma says babies should not be fed any more than every 4 to 5 hours. So, she decides to make him some concentrated formula to increase his energy intake.

How often should infants be fed? What problems could be caused by feeding a formula that is too concentrated?

Answer:

SUMMARY

1. Pregnancy begins with the fertilization of an egg by a sperm, producing a zygote. About two weeks after fertilization, the embryonic period of development begins. The embryo grows and the cells differentiate and move to form the organs and structures of a human body. At nine weeks, the fetal period of development begins. The fetus grows and the organs formed during the embryonic period mature. The fetal period continues until birth, which occurs after about 40 weeks of gestation. Because the embryo and fetus are developing and growing rapidly, they are susceptible to damage from poor nutrition and physical, chemical, or other environmental teratogens.
2. During pregnancy, maternal physiology changes to support the pregnancy and prepare for lactation. The amniotic sac and the placenta develop; maternal blood volume increases; the uterus and supporting muscles expand; body fat is deposited; the heart, lungs, and kidneys work harder; the breasts enlarge; and total body weight increases.
3. Recommended weight gain during pregnancy is 25 to 35 pounds for normal-weight women. All pregnant women, whether normal-weight, underweight, or overweight, should gain weight at a similar rate during pregnancy. If too little weight is gained, the infant may be small at birth and at increased risk for illness and death. Too much weight gain can place both mother and baby at risk, but weight loss should never be attempted during pregnancy.
4. During healthy pregnancies, a carefully planned program of moderate-intensity exercise can be beneficial and safe.
5. The changes in maternal physiology and the growth and development of the fetus sometimes cause unwanted side effects. Digestive system discomforts that are common in pregnancy include morning sickness, heartburn, constipation, and hemorrhoids. Changes in glucose utilization can cause gestational diabetes. An elevation in blood pressure, called pregnancy-induced hypertension, can cause edema, weight gain, and proteinuria (preeclampsia), and in severe cases can be life-threatening (eclampsia).
6. Factors that can increase the risks of pregnancy include the nutritional status of the mother; preexisting maternal health conditions; a maternal age that is under 20 or over 35 years; a short interval between pregnancies; a history of poor reproductive outcomes; poverty; and behaviors such as smoking, alcohol use, and illicit drug use.
7. Nutritional status is important before, during, and after pregnancy. Poor nutrition before pregnancy can decrease fertility or lead to a poor pregnancy outcome. During pregnancy the requirements for energy, protein, water, vitamins, and minerals increase. The B vitamins are needed to support increased energy and protein metabolism; calcium, vitamin D, and vitamin C are needed for bone and connective tissue growth; protein, folate, vitamin B_{12}, and zinc are needed for cell replication; and iron is needed for red blood cell synthesis.
8. During lactation, the need for energy, protein, fluid, and many vitamins and minerals is even greater than during pregnancy.
9. Newborns grow more rapidly and require more energy and protein per kilogram of body weight than at any other time in life. Fat and fluid needs are also proportionately higher than in adults. A diet that is adequate in energy, protein, and fat may not necessarily meet the needs for iron, fluoride, and vitamins D and K.
10. Breast milk is the ideal food for new babies. It is designed specifically for the human newborn, is always available, requires no special equipment, mixing, or sterilization, and provides immune protection. When breast-feeding is not chosen, there are many infant formulas on the market that are patterned after human milk and provide adequate nutrition to the baby.
11. Infant formulas are the best option when the mother is ill or is taking prescription or illicit drugs, or when the infant has special nutritional needs. The major disadvantages of bottle-feeding are the potential for bacterial contamination, overfeeding, and errors in mixing formula.

REVIEW QUESTIONS

1. List three physiological changes that occur in the mother's body during pregnancy.
2. How much weight should a woman gain during pregnancy?
3. How do the recommendations for weight gain differ for overweight and underweight women?
4. What kind of exercise is safe during pregnancy?
5. How does maternal age affect nutrient requirements during pregnancy?
6. How does alcohol consumed by a woman during pregnancy affect the child?
7. How do the requirements for energy and protein change during pregnancy?
8. Why does the mother's recommended intake for iron increase during pregnancy?
9. Are vegetarian diets safe for pregnant women? Why or why not?
10. How do maternal energy and protein requirements change during lactation?
11. What are the advantages of breast-feeding?
12. When is bottle-feeding a better choice?

Applying Critical Thinking Skills

Personal nutrition:

1. Assume that one day of the food record you kept in Chapter 2 is the record of a 25-year-old pregnant woman.
   a. Does this diet meet her energy and protein needs? If not, what foods would you add to the diet to meet the needs of pregnancy?
   b. Does this diet meet the iron and calcium needs of a 25-year-old pregnant woman? List three foods that are good sources of each.
   c. Does this diet meet the folate needs of a 25-year-old pregnant woman? What foods could you add to a diet that is low in folate to meet needs without supplements? What foods in this diet are fortified with folic acid?

General nutrition issues:

1. For each of the following nutrients, describe any differences between the needs of nonpregnant, pregnant, and lactating women. Explain why the requirements for pregnancy and lactation do or do not differ from those for the nonpregnant state.
   a. Energy
   b. Protein
   c. Calcium
   d. Iron
   e. Folate
2. Use the Internet to find out about the WIC program in your area.
   a. Would it be easy for you to use this program if you were a pregnant or lactating woman or had a young child?
   b. What income levels does it serve?
3. Marina is 16 years old and is pregnant with her first child. She is 5 feet 4 inches tall and weighs 110 pounds. She eats breakfast at home with her mother and two brothers and has lunch in the school cafeteria. After school she often has a snack with friends and then has dinner at home. A day's sample diet is listed here:

Sample Diet

Food	Serving Size
Breakfast	
Pastry	1
Fruit punch	6 oz
Lunch	
Hamburger	1
on bun	1
Canned peaches	1/2 cup
Diet cola	12 oz
Snack	
Ice cream cone	1
Dinner	
Chicken	1 drumstick
Rice	1 cup
Refried beans	1/2 cup
Tortillas	3
Fruit punch	12 oz

   a. What is the RDA or AI for folate, vitamin D, calcium, iron, and zinc for a 16-year-old pregnant woman?
   b. Does Marina's diet meet the recommendations for these nutrients?
   c. What is the energy content of this diet?
   d. Will Marina gain the recommended amount of weight if she consumes this diet throughout her pregnancy?
   e. What dietary changes would you make to meet the needs of the second trimester of pregnancy and to ensure a healthy pregnancy for both mother and baby?

References

1. Committee on Nutritional Status During Pregnancy and Lactation, National Academy of Sciences. *Nutrition During Pregnancy.* Washington, D.C.: National Academy Press, 1990.
2. Bryson, S. R., Theriot, L., Ryan, N. J., et al. Primary follow-up care in a multidisciplinary setting enhances catch-up growth of very-low-birth-weight infants. J. Am. Diet. Assoc. 97:386–390, 1997.
3. Abrams, B., Altman, S. L., and Pickett, K. E., Pregnancy weight gain: still controversial. Am. J. Clin. Nutr. 71(suppl):1233S–1241S, 2000.
4. Galtier-Dureure, F., Boegner, C., and Bringer, J. Obesity and pregnancy: complications and cost. Am. J. Clin. Nutr. 71(suppl): 1242S–1248S, 2000.
5. Smith, D. E., Lewis, J. L., Caveny, L. L., et al. Longitudinal changes in adiposity associated with pregnancy: the CARDIA study. JAMA 271:147–151, 1994.
6. American College of Sports Medicine. *ACSM's Guidelines for Exercise Testing and Prescription*, 5th ed. Baltimore: Williams & Wilkins, 1995.
7. Wang, T. W., and Apgar, B. S. Exercise during pregnancy. Am. Fam. Physician 57:1846–1852, 1998.
8. Katz, V. L. Water exercises in pregnancy. Semin. Perinatol. 20:285–291, 1996.
9. Sullivan, B. A., Henderson, S. T., and Davis, J. M. Gestational diabetes. J. Am. Pharm. Assoc. (Wash.) 38:364–371, 1998.
10. Report of the National High Blood Pressure Education Program Working Group on High Blood Pressure in Pregnancy. Am. J. Obstet. Gynecol. 183:S1–S22, 2000.
11. Ritche, L. D., and King, J. C. Dietary calcium and pregnancy-induced hypertension: is there a relation? Am. J. Clin. Nutr. 71(suppl): 1371S–1374S, 2000.
12. Villar, J., and Belizán, J. M. Same nutrient, different hypothesis: disparities in trials of calcium supplementation during pregnancy. Am. J. Clin. Nutr. 71(suppl):1375S–1379S, 2000.
13. Centers for Disease Control and Prevention. Available online at **http://www.cdc.gov/.** Accessed 8 Feb 2001.

14. Food and Nutrition Board, Institute of Medicine. *Dietary Reference Intakes for Thiamin, Riboflavin, Niacin, Vitamin B-6, Folate, Vitamin B-12, Pantothenic Acid, Biotin, and Choline.* Washington, D.C.: National Academy Press, 1998.
15. Green, T. J., Houghton, L. A., Donovan, U., et al. Oral contraceptives did not affect biochemical folate indexes and homocysteine concentrations in adolescent females. J. Am. Diet. Assoc. 98:49–54, 1998.
16. Godfrey, K. M., and Barker, D. J. P. Fetal nutrition and adult disease. Am. J. Clin. Nutr. 71(suppl):1344S–1352S, 2000.
17. Rothman, K. J., Moore, L. L., Singer, M. R., et al. Teratogenicity of high vitamin A intake. N. Engl. J. Med. 333:1369–1373, 1995.
18. Shaw, G. M., Wasserman, C. R., Block, G., and Lammer, E. J. High maternal vitamin A intake and risk of anomalies of structures with a cranial neural crest cell distribution. Lancet 347:899–900, 1996.
19. Food and Nutrition Board, Institute of Medicine. *Dietary Reference Intakes for Vitamin A, Vitamin K, Arsenic, Boron, Chromium, Copper, Iodine, Iron, Manganese, Molybdenum, Nickel, Silicon, Vanadium, and Zinc.* Washington, D.C.: National Academy Press, 2001.
20. Kitzmiller, J. L., Buchanan, T. A., Kjos, S., et al. Pre-conception care of diabetes, congenital malformations, and spontaneous abortions. Diabetes Care 19:514–541, 1996.
21. Fraser, A. M., Brockert, J. E., and Ward, R. H. Association of young maternal age with adverse reproductive outcomes. N. Engl. J. Med. 332:1113–1117, 1995.
22. American Dietetic Association. Position of the American Dietetic Association: nutrition care for pregnant adolescents. J. Am. Diet. Assoc. 94:449–450, 1994.
23. Prysak, M., and Kisly, A. Age greater than thirty-four years is an independent pregnancy risk factor in nulliparous women. J. Perinatol. 17:296–300, 1997.
24. Bianco, A., Stone, J., Lynch, L., et al. Pregnancy outcome at age 40 and older. Obstet. Gynecol. 87:917–922, 1996.
25. Kramer, M. S., Seguin, L., Lydon, J., and Goulet, L. Socio-economic disparities in pregnancy outcome: why do the poor fare so poorly? Paediatr. Perinat. Epidemiol. 14:194–210, 2000.
26. Owen, A. L., and Owen, G. M. Twenty years of WIC: a review of some effects of the program. J. Am. Diet. Assoc. 97:777–782, 1997.
27. Appelbaum, M. G. Fetal alcohol syndrome: the nurse practitioner's perspective. Nurse Pract. 2:27–33, 1996.
28. Abel, E. L. An update on incidence of FAS: FAS is not an equal opportunity birth defect. Neurotoxicol. Teratol. 17:437–443, 1995.
29. Kendrick, J. S., and Merritt, R. K. Women and smoking: an update for the 1990s. Am. J. Obstet. Gynecol. 175:528–535, 1996.
30. DiFranza, J. R., and Lew, R. A. Effect of maternal smoking on pregnancy complications and sudden infant death syndrome. J. Fam. Pract. 40:385–394, 1995.
31. Klonoff-Cohen, H. S., Edelstein, S. L., Lefkowitz, E. S., et al. The effect of passive smoking and tobacco exposure through breast milk on sudden infant death syndrome. JAMA 273:795–798, 1995.
32. Chomitz, V. R., Cheung, L. W., and Leiberman, E. The role of lifestyle in preventing low birth weight. Future Child 5:121–135, 1995.
33. Hinds, T. S., West, W., Knight, E. M., and Hartland, B. F. The effect of caffeine on pregnancy outcome variables. Nutr. Rev. 54:203–207, 1996.
34. Wagner, C. L., Katikaneni, L. D., Cox, T. H., and Ryan, R. M. The impact of prenatal drug exposure on the neonate. Obstet. Gynecol. Clin. North Am. 25:169–194, 1998.
35. Rizk, B., Atterbury, J. L., and Groome, L. J. Reproductive risks of cocaine. Hum. Reprod. Update 2:43–55, 1996.
36. Fox, C. H. Cocaine use in pregnancy. J. Am. Board Fam. Pract. 7:225–228, 1994.
37. Plessinger, M. A., and Woods, J. R., Jr. Maternal, placental, and fetal pathophysiology of cocaine exposure during pregnancy. Clin. Obstet. Gynecol. 36:267–278, 1994.
38. Lee, M. J. Marijuana and tobacco use in pregnancy. Obstet. Gynecol. Clin. North Am. 25:65–83, 1998.
39. King, J. C. Physiology of pregnancy and nutrient metabolism. Am. J. Clin. Nutr. 71(suppl):1218S–1225S, 2000.
40. Mitchell, G. A., Kassovska-Bratinova, S., Boukaftane, Y., et al. Medical aspects of ketone body metabolism. Clin. Invest. Med. 18:193–216, 1995.
41. Hornstra, G. Essential fatty acids in mothers and their neonates. Am. J. Clin. Nutr. 71(suppl):1262S–1269S, 2000.
42. Ritchie, L. D., Frung, E. B., Halloran, B. P., et al. A longitudinal study of calcium homeostasis during human pregnancy and lactation and after resumption of menses. Am. J. Clin. Nutr. 67:693–701, 1998.
43. Food and Nutrition Board, Institute of Medicine. *Dietary Reference Intakes for Calcium, Phosphorus, Magnesium, Vitamin D. and Fluoride.* Washington, D.C.: National Academy Press, 1997.
44. Food and Nutrition Board, Institute of Medicine. *Dietary Reference Intakes for Vitamin C, Vitamin E, Selenium, and Carotenoids.* Washington D.C.: National Academy Press, 2000.
45. Hook, E. B., and Czeizel, A. E. Can terathanasia explain the protective effect of folic-acid supplementation on birth defects? Lancet 350:513–515, 1997.
46. Scholl, T. O., and Johnson, W. G. Folic acid: influence on the outcome of pregnancy. Am. J. Clin. Nutr. 71(suppl):1295S–1303S, 2000.
47. King, J. C. Determinants of maternal zinc status during pregnancy. Am. J. Clin. Nutr. 71(suppl):1334S–1343S, 2000.
48. Allen, L. H. Anemia and iron deficiency: effects on pregnancy outcome. Am. J. Clin. Nutr. 71(suppl):1280S–1284S, 2000.
49. Mitchell, M. K. *Nutrition Across the Life Span.* Philadelphia: W. B. Saunders, 1997.
50. Rainville, A. J. Pica practices of pregnant women are associated with lower maternal hemoglobin level at delivery. J. Am. Diet. Assoc. 98:293–296, 1998.
51. Potter, S., Hannum, S., McFarlin, B., et al. Does infant feeding method influence maternal postpartum weight loss? J. Am. Diet. Assoc. 91:441–446, 1991.
52. Kramer, E. M., Stunkard, A. J., Marshall, K. A., et al. Breast-feeding reduces maternal lower body fat. J. Am. Diet. Assoc. 93:429–433, 1993.
53. Dewey, K. G., Heinig, M. J., and Nommsen, L. A. Maternal weight-loss patterns during prolonged lactation. Am. J. Clin. Nutr. 58:162–166, 1993.
54. Dewey, K. G. Effects of maternal caloric restriction and exercises during lactation. J. Nutr. 128:386S–389S, 1998.
55. Prentice, A. Calcium requirements of breast-feeding mothers. Nutr. Rev. 56:124–130, 1998.
56. Krebs, N. F., Reidinger, C. J., Robertson, A. D., and Brenner, M. Bone mineral density changes during lactation: maternal dietary and biochemical correlates. Am. J. Clin. Nutr. 65:1738–1746, 1997.
57. Bendich, A., and Brock, P. E. Rationale for the inclusion of long chain polyunsaturated fatty acids and for concomitant increase in vitamin E in infant formulas. Int. J. Vitam. Nutr. Res. 67:213–231, 1997.
58. U.S. Department of Health and Human Services, Centers for Disease Control and Prevention, National Center for Health Statistics CDC growth charts: United States, Advance Data, No. 314, June 8, 2000 (revised). Available online at **www.cdc.gov/growthcharts.** Accessed 8 Feb 2001.
59. American Dietetic Association. Position of the American Dietetic Association: promotion of breast-feeding. J. Am. Diet. Assoc. 97:662–666, 1997.
60. Ryan, A. S. The resurgence of breast-feeding in the United States. Pediatrics 99:596, 1997.
61. American Academy of Pediatrics, Working Group on Breast-Feeding. Breast-feeding and the use of human milk. Pediatrics 100:1035–1039, 1997.

62. Janney, C. A., Zhang, D., and Sowers, M. F. Lactation and weight retention. Am. J. Clin. Nutr. 66:1116–1124, 1997.
63. Kelsey, J. J. Hormonal contraception and lactation. J. Hum. Lact. 12:315–318, 1996.
64. WHO Fact Sheet No. 178: reducing mortality from major childhood killer diseases. September 1997. Available online at **http://www.who.ch/inf/fs/fact178.html.** Accessed 3 Sept 2000.
65. Jensen, C. L., Prager, T. C., Fraley, J. K., et al. Effect of dietary linoleic/alpha-linolenic acid ratio on growth and visual function of term infants. J. Pediatr. 131:200–209, 1997.
66. Newburg, D. S., Peterson, J. A., Ruis-Palacios, G. M., et al. Role of human-milk lactadherin in protection against symptomatic rotavirus infection. Lancet 351:1160–1164, 1998.
67. Williams, R. D. Breast-feeding best bet for babies. FDS Consumer 28:19–23, October 1995.
68. Golding, J. Unnatural constituents of breast milk—medication, lifestyle, pollutants, viruses. Early Hum. Dev. 29(suppl):S29–S43, 1997.
69. Stehlin, I. B. Infant formula: second best but good enough. FDA Consumer 29:17–20, June 1996.

16 Nutrition from Infancy to Adolescence

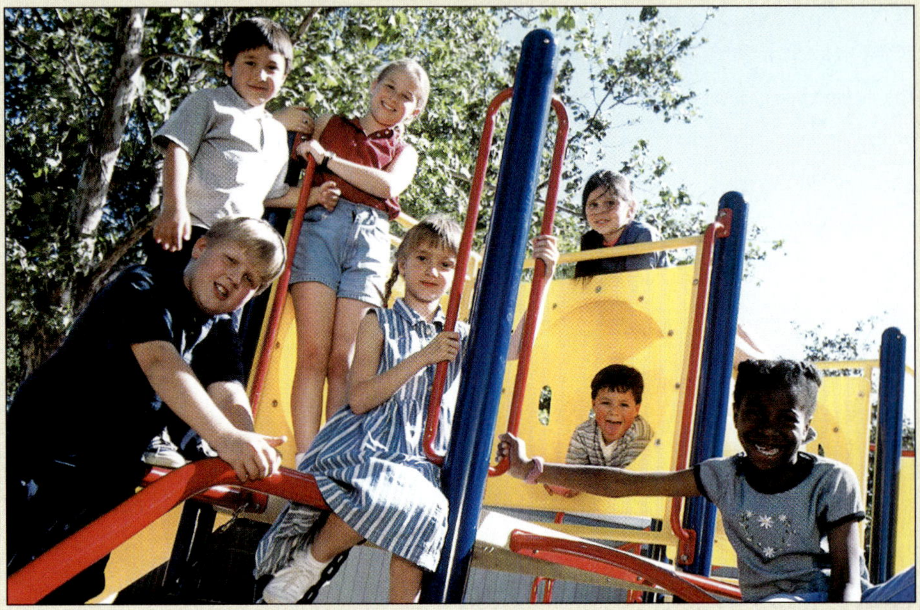

Learning Objectives

After reading this chapter, students should be able to:

1. Explain why growth is the best indicator of nutrient intake in children and teens.
2. Discuss how eating patterns learned in childhood can affect long-term health.
3. Compare the energy and protein requirements of infants, children, adolescents, and adults.
4. Give examples of how children's environments influence their nutrient intake.
5. Explain the recommendations for weight management in children, teens, and teen athletes.
6. Discuss how sexual maturation affects nutrient requirements in males and females.
7. Summarize the recommendations for preventing and managing food allergies.
8. Describe the National School Lunch Program.
9. List three ways in which watching television contributes to childhood obesity.
10. Explain how alcohol consumption affects nutritional status and overall health.

Felicia is 13 years old and just entering the eighth grade. She has been overweight since she was very young, always above the 95th percentile for weight. Currently she is 5 feet 4 inches tall and weighs 180 pounds. At her recent checkup, her physician noted that her blood pressure was elevated and her cholesterol levels were at the high end of the normal range. He recommended that Felicia and her mother meet with a dietitian to discuss ways to manage her weight and improve her diet.

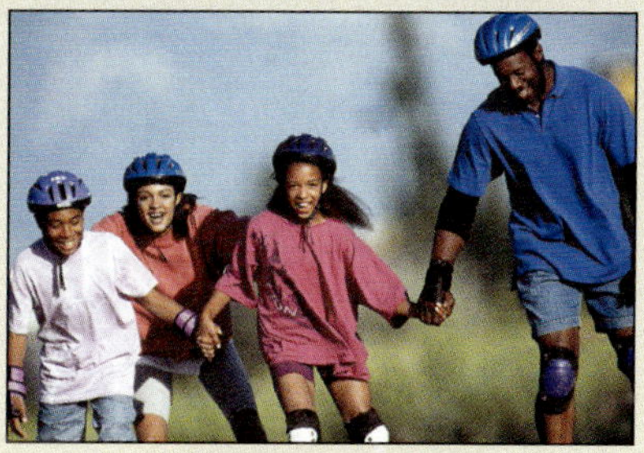

During the meeting, Felicia explains that she knows she should eat less and exercise more but can't find a way to make these changes in her life. She spends most of her day sitting at a desk in school. She has gym class only twice a week and hates to go because she is always chosen last when they pick teams. When she does get a chance to participate she is not very good and feels self-conscious. She eats what is on the school menu because she can purchase it at reduced cost as part of the National School Lunch program. It is difficult for her to exercise after school because she goes to the library study program until her mother gets out of work at 5 P.M.. She gets a little more exercise on weekends by going out with friends, but they frequently go out for ice cream or fast food. She feels like an outcast if she doesn't join them.

The dietitian asks about Felicia's favorite foods and discusses ways to reduce her energy intake without taking away all the foods she loves. They discuss serving sizes and Felicia recognizes that the serving of cereal she has for breakfast each morning is equivalent to about two to three servings according to the food label. The dietitian also works with Felicia's mother to plan economical dinners that the family will enjoy but that are moderate in energy and fat. Felicia and her mother, who also needs to lose a few pounds, decide to get some regular exercise by walking after dinner. Those evening walks soon progress to activities that include the whole family, such as roller blading and bike riding.

Good nutrition and exercise patterns developed early in life are key to health in later years. High-energy diets and low-activity lifestyles have become typical in the United States and contribute to the current obesity crises. Diet and lifestyle changes in childhood can help to stem the tide of obesity and the health problems it promotes. When the entire family becomes involved in modifying diet and exercise patterns, the chances of success are greater and both the children and the adults benefit.

Nutrition Goals and Guidelines for Children and Adolescents

Nutrient intake during childhood helps shape the adult that the child will become. Eating habits developed during childhood and adolescence may last a lifetime. What children eat depends on what they have learned to eat as well as on their personal preferences. Consuming a well-balanced diet allows children to meet their nutrient needs for growth and development and to prevent or delay the onset of the chronic diseases that plague American adults.

Monitoring Growth and Development

Many physical changes occur between infancy and adulthood. During the period from birth to around 18 to 20 years of age, the diet must supply the nutrients needed for rapid growth and development as well as for maintenance and activity. The ultimate size (height and weight) that an individual will attain is affected by genetic, environmental, and lifestyle factors. A child whose parents are 5 feet tall may not have the genetic potential to grow to 6 feet, but when adequately nourished, most children follow standard patterns of growth. A normal growth pattern is the best indicator of adequate nourishment.

Growth Patterns Growth is most rapid in the first year of life, when an infant's length increases by 50%, or about 10 inches. In the second year of life, children generally grow about 5 inches, in the third year 4 inches, and thereafter about 2 to 3 inches per year. During adolescence, there is a period of growth that is almost as rapid as that of infancy.

Children's growth can be monitored by comparing their pattern of growth to standard growth patterns using growth charts (see Appendix B).[1] To account for the variability among ethnic groups and breast-fed and bottle-fed babies, the growth charts were developed using data from all segments of the U.S. population. For infants, charts are available to monitor weight-for-age, length-for-age, and head-circumference-for-age. Weight-for-length tables are available for babies and toddlers 45 to 103 centimeters (18 to 40 inches) in length and weight-for-stature charts are available for children between 77 and 121 cm (30 to 48 inches) in stature. For children and adolescents age 2 to 20 years, charts are available to assess weight-for-age, stature-for-age, weight-for-stature, and BMI-for-age. The BMI-for-age growth chart can help identify children and adolescents who are over- and underweight (Figure 16.1).

Abnormal Growth Growth occurs in spurts and plateaus, but overall growth patterns are predictable. If a child's overall pattern of growth changes, his dietary intake should be evaluated to determine the reason for the sudden change.

Underweight Just as there are critical periods in prenatal development, there are critical periods in childhood when malnutrition can cause lasting damage. Growth and development can occur only when the proper hormonal signals are available; thus, nutrient deficiencies at critical times can prevent cells from dividing and adequate nutrition later on may not be able to compensate. Malnutrition can also have a profound effect on children's physical, emotional, behavioral, and cognitive development.[2]

If sufficient energy is not consumed weight will decrease and if the deficiency continues, growth in height will slow or stop. A child who falls below the fifth percentile of the BMI-for-age distribution is considered underweight and should be evaluated to determine the cause of his or her low body weight. If there is no medical reason for the low body weight and the child is otherwise healthy, nutritional intervention can help increase body weight. Consuming small frequent meals can increase energy intake, but increasing the number of snacks should not decrease the nutrient density of the diet. Caregivers should monitor children to assure they eat nutritious foods first. Adolescents who are underweight can increase their weight by combining muscle-building exercises with increases in energy intake.

Overweight A drastic increase in body weight may be due to an energy intake that exceeds output. Research has found that overweight children and adolescents are more likely than their normal-weight counterparts to be overweight as adults.[3] As with adults, excess body weight in childhood and adolescence increases the risk of chronic disease. A child is considered overweight when BMI falls at or above the 95th percentile and is at risk of being overweight when BMI

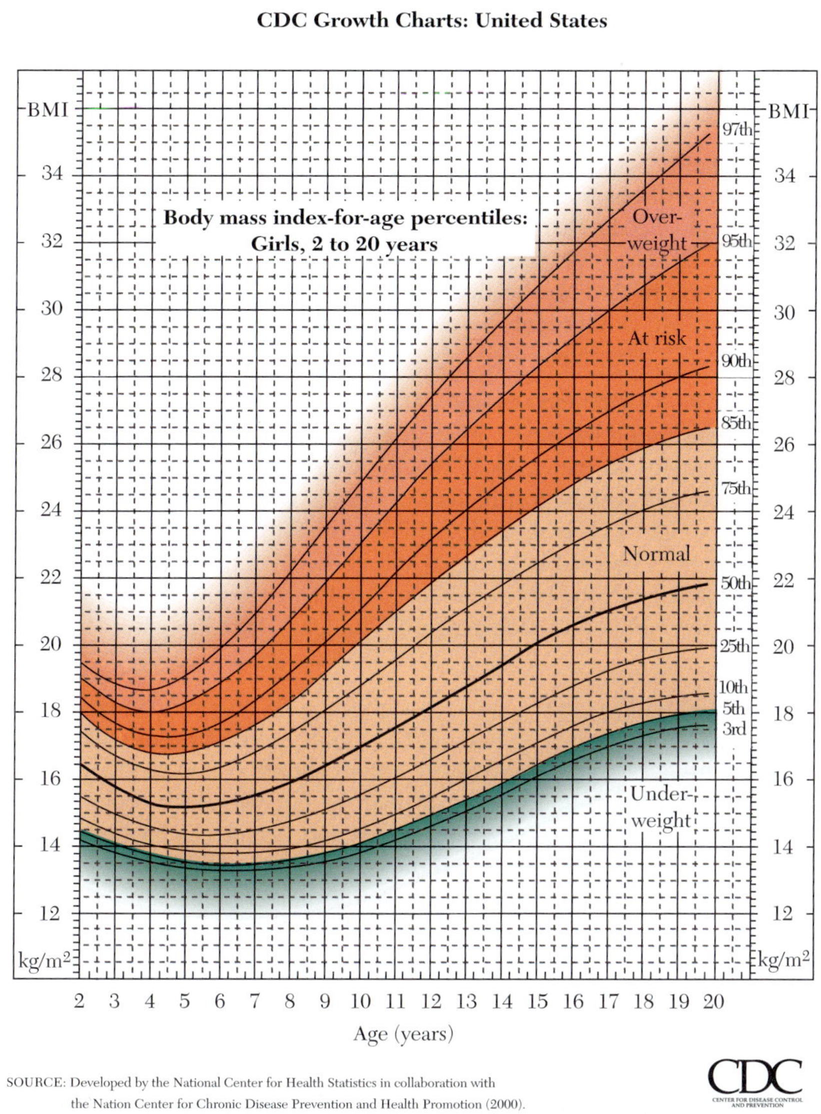

FIGURE 16.1 Growth charts are helpful for monitoring a child's pattern of growth. This example illustrates body mass index-for-age percentiles for girls ages 2 to 20. Body mass index (BMI) can be used beginning at two years of age, when an accurate stature can be obtained. BMI is predictive of body fat and has been recommended to screen for underweight and overweight children, ages two years and older. The colored areas represent BMI values that are associated with underweight, normal weight, at risk of overweight, and overweight. *(Developed by the National Center for Health Statistics in collaboration with the National Center For Chronic Disease Prevention and Health Promotion, 2000.)*

is greater than or equal to the 85th percentile and less than the 95th percentile (see Figure 16.1).

Reducing Chronic Disease Risk

Most children and adolescents in the United States consume more fat, saturated fat, and sodium than is recommended and fail to meet the recommendation for daily physical activity. This lifestyle can affect their health now and in the future.

Obesity Overweight and obesity are major health problems in children in the United States. More than 13% of American children ages 6 to 11 years and 14% of adolescents ages 12 to 19 years are overweight. Heredity, environment, and lifestyle all play a role in childhood obesity. Thus, obese parents are more likely to

Web Menu For more information on obesity and weight management in children, go to the National Institute of Diabetes, & Digestive, & Kidney Diseases at www.niddk.nih.gov/ and click on weight loss and control under health information.

have obese offspring not only because they pass on a genetic tendency to be overweight but also because their children may learn poor eating and exercise habits. Sound nutrition and exercise habits can prevent obesity despite a genetic predisposition.

Consequences of Obesity Being overweight or obese in childhood increases the risk of other chronic diseases. A high BMI in childhood is correlated with elevated levels of blood lipids, insulin, and blood pressure in young adulthood.[4] These risk factors increase the chances of developing heart disease, diabetes, and hypertension. As in adults, the distribution of body fat in the abdominal region in children and adolescents is associated with greater cardiovascular risk.[5]

Preventing and Treating Childhood Obesity Achieving and maintaining a healthy weight requires consuming balanced meals that are moderate in energy and increasing physical activity. In many cases, slowing weight gain to allow children to "grow into" their current weight is sufficient to reduce BMI to a healthy level. As long as the rate of weight gain is slowed, a child at the 95th percentile for BMI at age 7 can be at the 90th percentile by age 9 and at the 85th percentile by age 11. To achieve this, gradual and stepwise changes in diet and exercise that involve the entire family are recommended (see Critical Thinking: "Meeting But Not Exceeding Needs").

Reducing Intake Modifying a child's intake patterns can be difficult. Denying food may promote further overeating by making the child feel that there will not be enough to satisfy hunger. Energy intake restrictions should be relatively mild, allowing adequate nutrition to continue growth in height with little weight gain. Healthy, low-fat foods such as whole-grain breads and cereals, fruits and vegetables, lean meats, and reduced-fat dairy products should be offered at meals and for snacks. Meals should not be skipped because this may actually increase energy intake by increasing the amount of food consumed at other times during the day. Because children, like adults, may overeat for comfort, self-reward, or out of boredom, parental involvement is important in helping the child find other sources of gratification.

When meals and the overall weight-management strategy are planned, social as well as physiological needs should be considered. For example, a teenage girl attempting to manage a weight problem might plan for a pizza party by deciding what she will eat earlier in the day and set a limit on how many slices of pizza she will eat at the party. This plan may also allow for some extra kcalories on that day. Even if she eats more than she planned at the party, she should continue her low-energy eating plan the next day.

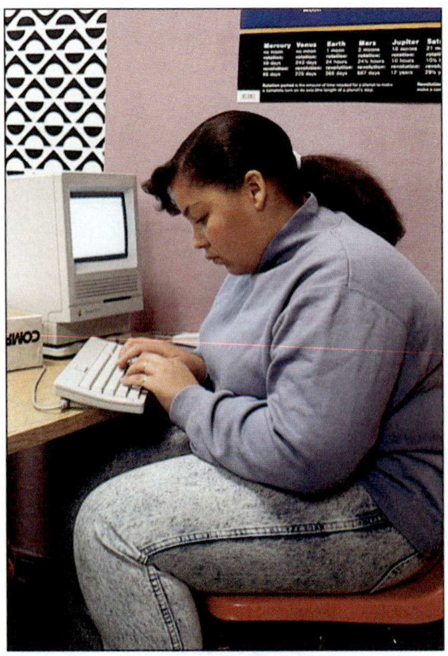

FIGURE 16.2 The prevalence of obesity is increasing among teens in the United States, in part due to an increase in the amount of time spent in sedentary activities such as watching television and working at computers. *(© Lawrence Migdale/Photo Researchers, Inc.)*

Increasing Activity Although energy intake among American children overall is not increasing, they are getting heavier, suggesting that lack of physical activity is a major contributor to the increase in body weight.[6] Watching television, playing video games, and surfing the Web have replaced neighborhood games of tag and soccer for many children and adolescents (Figure 16.2). Increasing activity may therefore be even more important than dietary changes when treating obesity.

Overweight children are less likely to be physically active than lean children. They may be embarrassed by their bodies and shy away from participating in group activities. Increases in physical activity need to be gradual in order to make exercise a positive experience. Activities should be enjoyable and not doled out as punishment. Children should start by engaging in activities such as games, walks after dinner, bike rides, hikes, swimming, and volleyball that can be enjoyed by the whole family. Also, parents who are active, play with their children, watch their children compete or play, or take children to activities or sports events have more active children.[7] Encouraging such activity sends a positive message to "be more active" rather than a negative message to "not eat so much."

Diabetes Type 2 diabetes is a serious disease affecting 15 million adult Americans. Until recently, type 2 diabetes was considered a disease that affected primarily adults over 40, but it is now on the rise among America's youth.[8] The typical picture of type 2 diabetes in this population is a child from age 10 to midpuberty, overweight, with a family history of the disease. Little is known about this disease in children, but based on experience with adults, it is thought to be a progressive disease that increases in severity with time from diagnosis. The longer an individual has the disease the greater their risk of complications that involve the circulatory system or nervous system and that can lead to blindness, kidney failure, heart disease, or amputations (see Chapter 4).[9]

The goal of treatment is to normalize blood glucose levels and treat related conditions such as hypertension and high blood lipid levels. The recommended treatment for children who have elevated blood glucose but are not ill is education about the disease to promote a lifestyle change that includes a balanced diet moderate in energy and increased physical activity. However, due to the progressive nature of diabetes, most will eventually require drug treatment. Preventative measures that may delay or prevent the onset of type 2 diabetes include weight management and increased physical activity for those at risk.

Blood Cholesterol and Heart Disease Children in the United States and Canada currently consume about 33% of their energy from fat, with 11% from saturated fat.[2] This exceeds the amounts recommended for a healthy diet. As in adults, diets high in saturated fat promote elevated blood cholesterol levels in children. The recommended level for blood cholesterol in children ages 2 to 18 is less than 170 mg per 100 ml. In the United States, many children have blood cholesterol levels higher than this.[10] Elevated blood cholesterol levels during childhood and adolescence are associated with higher blood cholesterol and higher mortality rates from cardiovascular disease in adulthood.[11]

Web Menu

For more information on the relationship between diet and heart disease and hypertension, go to the American Heart Association's Web site at www.americanheart.org/.

The American Academy of Pediatrics recommends blood cholesterol monitoring for high-risk children and teenagers. This includes those with parents or grandparents who developed heart disease before age 55, and those whose parents have cholesterol levels over 240 mg per 100 ml. To reduce the risk of developing high blood cholesterol levels and, subsequently, heart disease, the fat content of children's diets should gradually be reduced beginning at the age of two years. After the age of two the recommendations for dietary fat are the same as for adults—no more than 30% of energy from fat.[12] An evaluation of the impact of low-fat diets found that this dietary pattern promoted a reduction in blood cholesterol without interfering with growth and development.[13]

Hypertension High blood pressure or hypertension may also be a concern early in life. Those who have blood pressure at the high end of normal as youngsters are more likely to develop hypertension as adults.[14] Increases in blood pressure are associated with excess body fat, reduced activity level, and a high sodium intake, so attention should be paid to these nutritional and lifestyle factors in children. This is particularly important if there is a family history of hypertension. As in adults, an active lifestyle, maintenance of a healthy body weight, and a diet moderate in sodium and high in grains, fruits, and vegetables is recommended to maintain normal blood pressure.

Providing a Nutritious Diet

The Healthy Eating Index, which scores diet quality based on the recommendations of the Food Guide Pyramid and the Dietary Guidelines with regard to fat, saturated fat, cholesterol, sodium, and variety, reveals that most children and adolescents in the United States consume a diet that needs improvement (Figure 16.3). The typical diet of children and adolescents is low in fruits and vegetables and high in sweet and salty processed foods and provides more than the

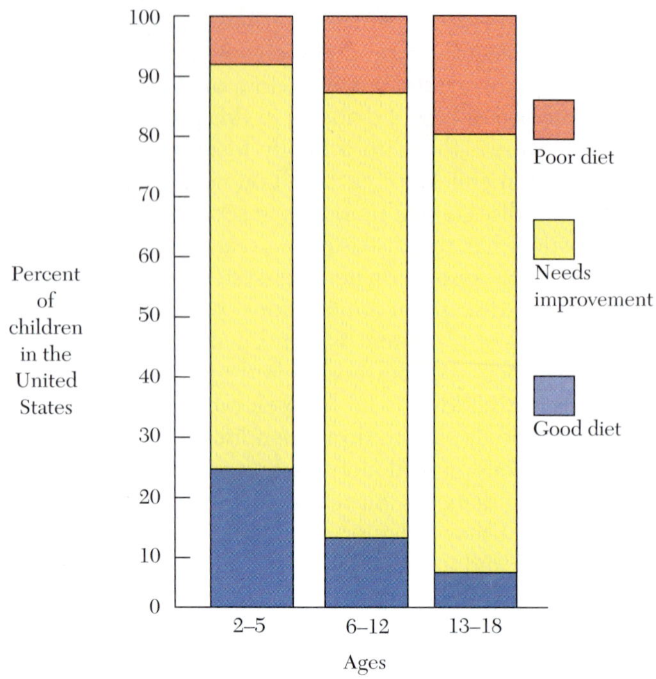

FIGURE 16.3 This graph illustrates the percentage of American children ages 2 to 18 that have a good diet, a diet that needs improvement, and a poor diet. The classification is based on the Healthy Eating Index. A Healthy Eating Index score of 80 implies a good diet. A score between 51 and 80 implies a diet that needs improvement and a score less than 51 indicates a poor diet. As children get older, the percentage that eats a good diet decreases. *(U.S. Department of Agriculture, Center for Nutrition Policy and Promotion. Continuing Survey of Food Intakes by Individuals. 1996.)*

recommended amounts of fat and not enough calcium. As children get older, their diet quality declines; in particular, there are decreases in the amount of fruit and milk consumed.[15]

The development of nutritious eating habits starts with caregivers offering a balanced and varied diet adequate in energy and essential nutrients and appropriate to the child's developmental needs. While caregivers are responsible for deciding what foods should be offered to the child, when they should be offered, and where they should be eaten, the child must decide whether to eat, what foods to eat, and how much to consume.

What and When to Offer? Meals for children should be planned according to the food groups and serving recommendations of the Food Guide Pyramid. Food choices should be developmentally appropriate. Young children have small stomachs and high energy needs, so frequent meals and snacks are necessary. A meal or snack should be offered every 2 to 3 hours, and, because children thrive on routines and feel secure in knowing what to expect, a consistent pattern should be maintained from day to day. The texture of foods should also be appropriate to the child's developmental stage to reduce the risk of choking. Vegetables served to young children should be cooked until soft for easy chewing. Food should not be too hot or too spicy. As children grow, choices should change to meet their developmental abilities.

No matter how erratic children's food intake may be, caregivers should offer a variety of appropriate healthy food choices at each meal and let the children select what and how much they will eat (Figure 16.4). To increase the likelihood that a new food will be accepted, it should be introduced at the beginning of a meal when the child is hungry. If a new food becomes associated with a bad experience, such as burning the mouth, the child will be unlikely to try it again.

A Positive Eating Environment Developing sound eating habits also involves providing companionship, conversation, and a pleasant location at mealtime. Children eat better with company, so caregivers should sit with children and eat what they eat (Figure 16.5).[16] Children also need time to finish eating. Slow eaters are unlikely to finish eating if they are abandoned by siblings who run off to play and adults who leave to wash dishes.

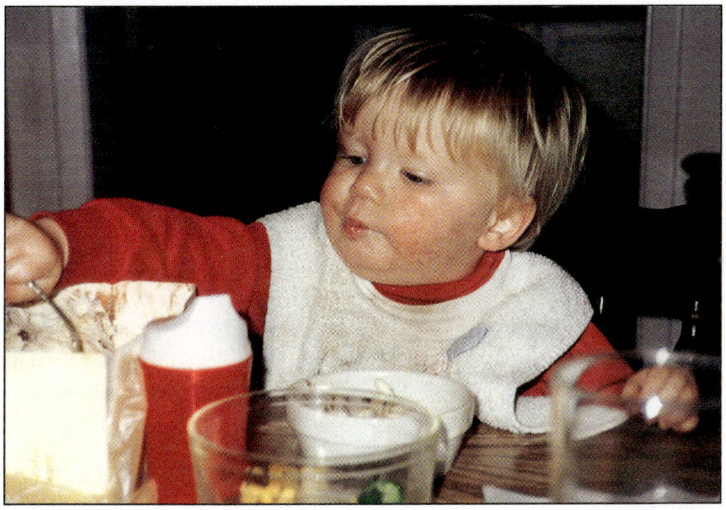

FIGURE 16.4 Caregivers should offer a variety of healthy food choices and allow children to select what they will eat and how much. *(Mary Grosvenor)*

To make mealtime a nutritious, educational, and enjoyable experience, it should not become a battle zone.[16] Threats and bribes are counterproductive and can create problems where none had previously existed. Food is not a reward or a punishment: It is simply nutrition.

Influences on Food Intake Many factors other than nutrient needs determine which foods are consumed. In young children, which foods are offered is a major determinant of what is consumed, but individual taste always plays a role in food choices. As the child grows, influences from the outside world increase. When a child is enrolled in day-care or preschool programs, parents may no longer be in control of—or even aware of—what the child is eating. When the child is in school, carefully packed lunches may be discarded or traded for more appealing foods. During adolescence, physiological changes dictate nutritional needs but peer pressure may dictate food choices.

Family eating habits and dietary patterns have a strong influence on children's food choices; in particular, preferences for high-fat foods have been shown to be associated with parents' intake and body weight.[2] There is also evidence that repeated exposure to foods increases the acceptance of those foods.[17] So, if a child's role models eat a diet high in fat and low in fruits and vegetables, the child will follow suit. Studies have shown that eating habits developed in early childhood persist at least through adolescence.[17]

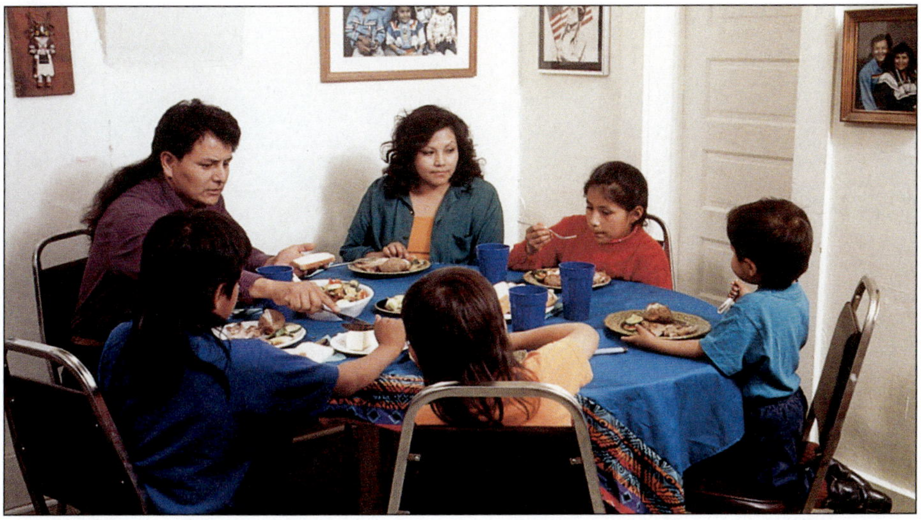

FIGURE 16.5 Companionship and conversation at meals helps create a positive eating environment. *(© Lawrence Migdale/Photo Researchers, Inc.)*

Critical Thinking

Meeting But Not Exceeding Needs

Sage is a busy 15-year-old high school student. Until recently she hadn't paid much attention to her diet because she ate all her meals at home or at school. Now she has a part-time job and frequently eats lunch, dinner, and snacks on her own. Her parents are concerned because Sage seems to be gaining weight and all she wants to do when she isn't working is lie around and watch TV. Previously she would ride her bike to friends' houses or walk over to the field to watch football practice after school. Her parents are both overweight and are concerned that Sage is also developing a weight problem, so they take her to see their doctor.

At the doctor's office, she is weighed and measured and has a blood sample taken. The doctor reports that Sage is healthy except for a low hematocrit, suggesting she is anemic. Her body mass index (BMI) is in the normal range but has increased over the last year. It had been at the 50th percentile and she is now almost at the 75th. The doctor prescribes an iron supplement and suggests that Sage and her parents consult with a dietitian for counseling on iron intake as well as weight management.

The dietitian talks to Sage and her mother to obtain information about her current diet and what she ate before she started working. Sage tells the dietitian that since she has more independence in selecting her meals she is trying to cut her kcalorie intake by eating a smaller breakfast and skipping lunch at school. Her typical diet before she started working and her current diet are shown here.

Sage's Original Diet			Sage's Current Diet		
Food	***Energy (kcals)***	***Iron (mg)***	***Food***	***Energy (kcals)***	***Iron (mg)***
Breakfast			*Breakfast*		
Cornflakes (1 cup) with 2% milk (1/2 cup)	163	8.68			
Orange juice (1 cup)	105	1.10	Orange juice (1 cup)	105	1.10
Toast (2 slices) with margarine	197	1.57	Bagel with cream cheese (1 Tbsp)	245	3.17
Lunch			*Lunch*		
Ham and cheese sandwich with lettuce and mayonnaise	376	2.45			
Corn chips (1 oz)	155	0.76			
Apple	81	0.50			
2% milk (1 cup)	121	0.12			
Snack			*Snack*		
Cheese Pizza (1 slice)	162	1.47	Frozen yogurt (1 cup)	153	0.65
Cola (1 can)	153	0.11			

Sage's Original Diet			Sage's Current Diet		
Food	***Energy (kcals)***	***Iron (mg)***	***Food***	***Energy (kcals)***	***Iron (mg)***
Dinner			*Dinner*		
Baked chicken leg	240	9.24	Fast-food breaded chicken sandwich	507	3.48
Asparagus (6)	18	0.42	Fries (large order)	430	0.87
Rice Pilaf (1 cup)	215	1.83			
Reduced-fat milk (1 cup)	121	0.12	Vanilla shake	370	0.18
Snacks			*Snacks*		
			Chocolate bar with almonds	216	0.67
			Potato chips (1 oz)	156	0.2
Total	*2107*	*28.37*		*2182*	*10.32*

What changes has Sage made in her diet that might contribute to her anemia and weight gain?

- She has reduced the volume of food she eats but has increased the number of high-fat, high-energy foods, making her new diet higher in fat and energy. Her original diet provided 2107 kcalories, 30% of which was from fat, and her current diet has more energy (2182 kcals) and contains 37% fat.
- She now eats less meat (which contains heme iron), and fewer leafy green vegetables (which contain nonheme iron). Her original diet easily met the RDA of 15 mg of iron. Her current diet falls short of the RDA with only 10.3 mg.
- Her fiber intake has decreased because she consumes fewer vegetables and whole grains.
- She has added low-nutrient-density snacks such as candy and chips.

Why might iron deficiency anemia contribute to Sage's weight gain?

Iron deficiency causes fatigue so activity level decreases, reducing the energy output side of the energy balance equation.

Suggest some different meal and snack choices that Sage could eat away from home to increase her iron without increasing her energy intake.

Answer:

Infants, Toddlers, and Young Children

Nourishing a growing child is not always an easy task. Nutrient intake must meet the needs for maintenance and activity as well as growth, but suiting children's tastes as well as meeting their needs can be a challenge to caregivers whether they are feeding infants who are sampling solid foods for the first time (ages four months to one year), toddlers (ages one to three years), or young children (ages four through eight years).

Introducing Solid Food

Although breast milk or formula meets most nutritional needs until one year of age semisolid and solid foods can be gradually introduced into the infant's diet starting between the fourth and sixth months of life. Introducing solid foods earlier provides no nutritional or developmental advantages. Despite this some parents offer semisolid foods before this age because they think the infant is hungry or the added food will help them sleep through the night. Studies have shown that there is no difference in sleeping patterns based on such feeding practices.

Before four to six months of age the infant's feeding abilities and gastrointestinal tract are not mature enough to handle foods other than breast milk or formula. The young infant takes milk by a licking motion of the tongue called suckling, which strokes or milks the liquid from the nipple; solid food placed in the mouth at an early age is usually pushed out as the tongue thrusts forward. By four to six months of age, the early reflex to bring the tongue to the front of the mouth to suckle has diminished, and the tongue is held farther back in the mouth, allowing solid food to be accepted without being expelled. By this age, feeding is easier because infants can hold their heads up steadily and are able to sit, either with or without support. Internally, the digestive tract has developed and enzymes are present for starch digestion. The kidneys are more mature and better able to concentrate urine. With all of these changes, the child is ready to begin a new approach to eating.

What Foods to Introduce First? The most commonly recommended first food is iron-fortified infant rice cereal mixed with formula or breast milk. Rice cereal is recommended because it is easily digested and rarely causes allergic reactions. After rice has been successfully included in the diet, other grains can be introduced, with wheat cereal offered last because it is the grain most likely to cause an allergic reaction. To monitor for food allergies, it is important to introduce new foods one at a time. Each new food should be offered for a few days without the addition of any other new foods. If an allergic reaction occurs, it is most likely due to the newly introduced food. Foods that cause symptoms such as rashes, digestive upsets, or respiratory problems should be discontinued before any other new foods are added.

After cereals are introduced, puréed vegetables or fruits can be offered. Some suggest that vegetables be offered before fruits so that the child will learn to enjoy food that is not sweet before being introduced to sweet foods. At one year of age infants can be given whole cow's milk, which should be continued until two years of age, when lower-fat milks can be used.

Increasing Variety As the child becomes familiar with more variety, food choices should be made from each of the food groups in the Food Guide Pyramid. Once teeth have erupted, foods with more texture can be added. For the 6- to 12-month-old child, small pieces of soft or ground fruits, vegetables, and meats are appropriate (Table 16.1). To avoid the possibility of choking, foods that can easily lodge in the throat, such as carrots, grapes, and hot dogs, should not be offered to infants or toddlers.

TABLE 16.1 Typical Meal Patterns for Infants

		Servings per Day		
Food	***Serving Size***	***4–6 Months (tongue able to stay in back of mouth and not push food out)***	***6–8 Months (can easily move hand to mouth)***	***9–12 Months (can use a cup and easily consume finger foods)***
Formula or breast milk*	8 oz	4	4	4
Dry infant cereal	2 Tbsp	2	2	2
Vegetables	2–3 Tbsp	—	2	3
Fruits	2 Tbsp	—	2	4
Fruit juice	4 oz	—	—	1 (by cup)
Meats (or egg yolk)	1 Tbsp	—	2–4 (strained)	4–6 (chopped)
Finger foods		—	1†	4‡

*Includes that added to cereal.

†Dry toast, teething biscuits.

‡Table foods, except foods in shapes and sizes that are likely to cause choking, such as large pieces of meat, whole grapes, or hot dogs or carrots cut in circular slices.

As children become more independent, they will want to feed themselves. Although this is not always a neat and clean process, it is important for development (Figure 16.6). By the age of eight or nine months, infants can hold a bottle and self-feed finger food such as crackers. By ten months, most infants can drink from a cup.

Children often have periods known as food jags, when they will eat only certain foods and nothing else. The general guideline here is to continue to offer other foods along with those the child is focused on. It is the nutrient content of the total diet averaged over days or weeks that is important, so a few days of a food jag is unlikely to affect the child's overall nutritional health.

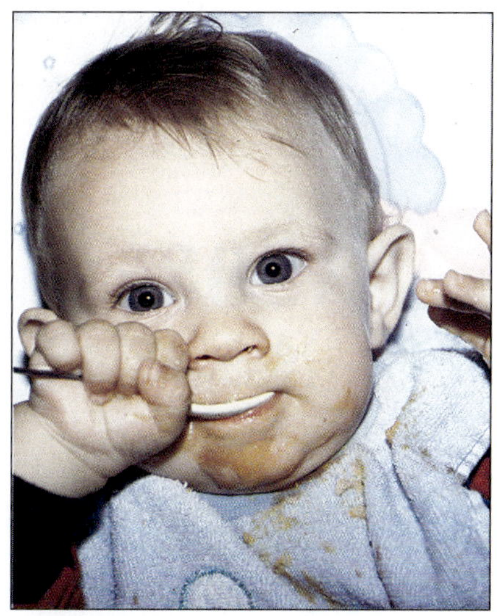

FIGURE 16.6 Self-feeding is important in infant development but is not a tidy process. *(Gregory Smolin)*

Children's Nutrient Needs

Infants grow quickly during the first year. Their energy and nutrient needs are large relative to their small body size (see Chapter 15). As children grow, their nutrient requirements per unit of body weight decrease, but total needs increase because they gain weight and become more active. While a one-year-old will be standing and toddling, a two-year-old will be running, jumping, and climbing. Activity level in preschoolers is highly variable: Some children are relatively inactive, while others never slow down. During a growth spurt, appetites may seem insatiable, while between spurts, children may seem to eat nothing at all.

Recommended intakes are not different for boys and girls until nine years of age, at which time sexual maturation begins to cause differences in nutrient needs. The DRIs group recommended intakes for children into those for toddlers, ages one through three, and for early childhood, ages four through eight. The 1989 RDAs include three age groups: years one through three, four through six, and seven through ten.

Energy, Protein, and Fluid Children need energy and protein for growth as well as to maintain body tissues. Although growth and metabolic rate slow as children mature, the total need for energy and protein increases because body size increases. The average two-year-old needs about 1300 kcalories and 16 g of protein per day. By age eight, that child will need about 2000 kcalories and 28 g of protein per day (Figure 16.7).

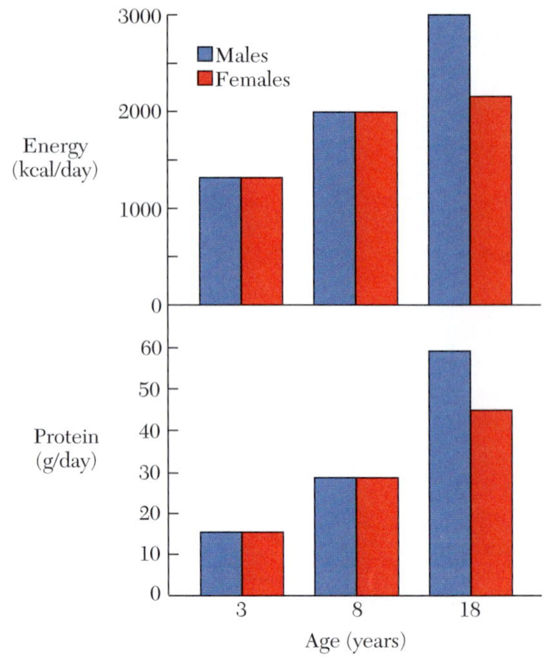

FIGURE 16.7 The total need for both energy and protein increases with age. The needs of males and females do not differ until adolescence.

Fluid requirements increase in proportion to energy requirements. By one year of age, a child's kidneys have matured and the fluid lost through evaporation has decreased, so fluid requirements are similar to those of adults: 1 ml of fluid per kcalorie of energy consumed.

Fat From birth until the age of two, the requirement for dietary fat is greater than that of adults—about 40 to 50% of energy. This relatively high-fat diet is necessary for the development of the nervous system and to provide enough energy in a small volume of food to meet the needs for growth. After the age of two, the fat in children's diets should be gradually reduced to no more than 30% of energy from fat, the same as for adults (Figure 16.8).[12]

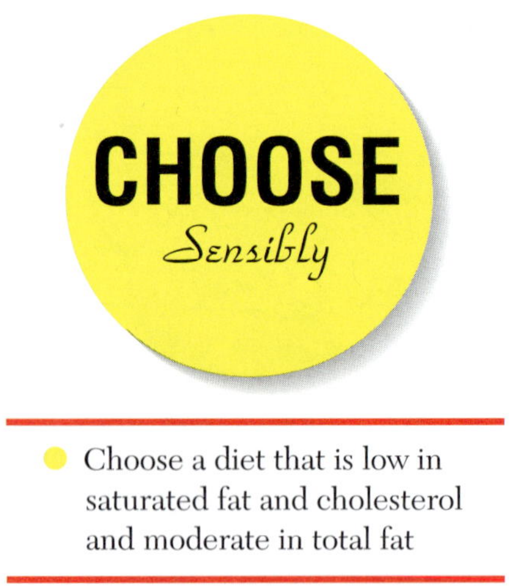

FIGURE 16.8 The Dietary Guidelines recommend that everyone over the age of two years consume a diet that is low in saturated fat and cholesterol and moderate in total fat. *(USDA, DHHS, 2000)*

Carbohydrate and Fiber Carbohydrate recommendations for children over about age two are the same as those for adults: 55 to 60% of energy. As in the adult diet, most of the carbohydrate in a child's diet should be from complex carbohydrate. Foods high in added sugars, such as cookies, candy, and soda, should be limited because they are low in nutrient density. Fruit juice is a good source of naturally occurring simple carbohydrate for young children, but excess quantities of apple and pear juice should be avoided. These contain sorbitol, a poorly absorbed sugar alcohol that can cause diarrhea. Honey and corn syrup should not be served to children less than a year old because these foods may contain spores of *Clostridium botulinum,* the bacterium that causes botulism poisoning (see Chapter 19). Older children and adults are not at risk from botulism spores because the environment in a mature gastrointestinal tract prevents the bacterium from growing.

Specific fiber recommendations have not been made for children, but as a rule of thumb, the number of grams of fiber a child consumes should equal age in years plus 5 g. For example, a five-year-old should consume 10 g of fiber per day ($5 + 5 = 10$ g).[18] Fiber supplements are not recommended for children, since high intakes are filling and can limit the amount of food and, consequently, the nutrients that a small child can consume.

Micronutrient Needs As children grow, so do their vitamin and mineral requirements. Surveys indicate that the diets of children in the United States are likely to be deficient in folate, vitamin A, vitamin B_6, vitamin C, vitamin E, calcium, iron, and zinc.[19] The low intakes of vitamins A, C, and E are most likely due to low intakes of fruits and vegetables.

Calcium Adequate calcium intake is essential for children to achieve maximum peak bone mass, which is important in preventing osteoporosis later in life (see Chapter 12). For toddlers, the AI for calcium is 500 mg per day and for young children the AI is 800 mg per day. Despite the importance of calcium for establishing peak bone mass, calcium intake in American children and adolescents is declining, primarily due to a decrease in the consumption of milk, which is an excellent source of calcium.[2] This decrease in milk consumption has been accompanied by an increase in the consumption of soft drinks, which contain no calcium (Figure 16.9). Children who cannot or do not consume dairy products should meet their calcium needs with fortified foods and calcium-rich vegetables.

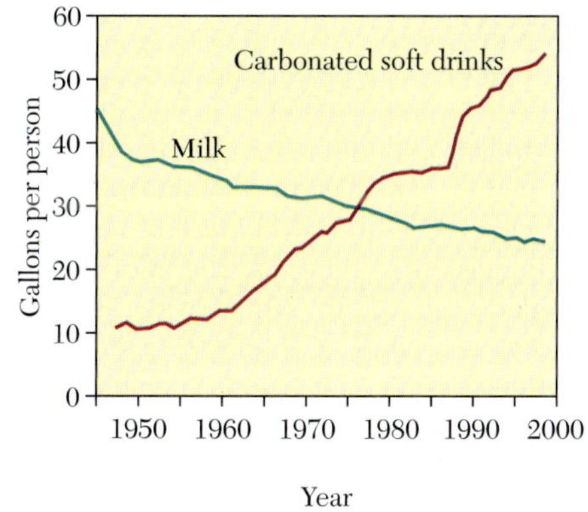

FIGURE 16.9 Consumption of milk, which is a major contributor of dietary calcium, has been declining since the 1940s, whereas the consumption of carbonated beverages, which contain no calcium, has increased over the same period. In 1945, Americans consumed more than four times as much milk as carbonated soft drinks, but by 1998, soft-drink consumption was more than two times greater than milk consumption. *(USDA Economic Research Service. Major trends in the U.S. food supply, 1909–1999. Food Review 23:12, 2000. Available online at* http://www.ers.usda.gov/epubs/pdf/foodrevw/jan2000/.)

Iron Iron deficiency anemia is one of the most prevalent forms of malnutrition in children. Although iron intake by American children has increased over the last 20 years, iron deficiency is still a public health problem.[20] Iron deficiency can affect learning ability, intellectual performance, stamina, and mood.[21] It can also lower the child's resistance to illness and slow recovery time. Good sources of iron that are acceptable to small children include fortified grains and breakfast cereals, raisins, eggs, and lean meats.

If anemia is diagnosed, iron supplements are usually prescribed until iron stores are repleted. These should be kept out of the reach of children. Overdoses of iron-containing supplements are the leading cause of poisoning deaths among children under six years of age.[22] To help protect children, products containing iron include a warning about the hazards to children of ingesting large amounts of iron. Products containing 30 mg or more per dose are packed in individual doses.[23] The time and effort required for a child to open these wrappers may reduce the chances of consuming enough to cause toxicity.

Meeting Children's Nutrient Needs

Children have small stomachs and high nutrient needs; therefore, they should consume nutritious meals and snacks throughout the day. A missed meal or snack can leave a child without sufficient energy to perform optimally at school or play. A good breakfast is particularly important for ensuring optimal performance at school (see *Research Discoveries:* "Is Breakfast Food Really Brain Food?").

A Balanced, Varied Diet Children need a varied diet based on whole grains, vegetables, and fruits, and adequate in milk and other high-protein foods. A version of the Food Guide Pyramid designed to be appealing for children two to six years of age has been developed by the U.S. Department of Agriculture (Figure 16.10). It is suggested that children consume the low end of the range of servings recommended for adults. Recommendations for children four to six years of age are the same as those for adults, but the servings may need to be split between several meals or snacks. For children ages two to three, the serving size should be reduced. For all children two to six years of age, a total of 2 cups of milk (or other choices from the dairy group) are recommended each day. Examples of meal patterns for a three-year-old and an eight-year-old are shown in Table 16.2.

Creativity may be needed to ensure that selections from each of the food groups of the Pyramid are included in children's diets. For instance, if vegetables are refused, they can be added to soups and casseroles. Fruit can be served on cereals or as juice. Milk can be added to hot cereal, cream soups, puddings, and custards. Powdered milk can be used in baking, and cheese can be offered in recipes such as macaroni and cheese, cheese sauce, and pizza. Meats can be used in spaghetti sauce, stews, casseroles, burritos, or pizza.

Food selections from within each Pyramid group are also important for children. High-sugar, high-fat choices need to be balanced with whole grains, fresh

RESEARCH DISCOVERIES

Is Breakfast Food Really Brain Food?

Breakfast is often lost in the shuffle of getting a family up and off to work or school. Children who are not particularly hungry first thing in the morning will gladly go off to school with an empty stomach. Once at school, schedules often don't permit students to eat anything until lunch, several hours later. The result may be a span of 15 or more hours without food. It seems like common sense that a fast of this length would affect both nutrition and performance, but well-designed research studies did not test this hypothesis until recently.

Breakfast, Nutrition, and Performance Breakfast can have a long-term effect on nutritional health and academic performance. A study that evaluated the contribution of breakfast to daily nutrient intake found that children who eat breakfast consume more energy and are more likely to meet the recommended intakes for vitamins and minerals than children who skip breakfast.[a] This is particularly important for children whose typical diets barely meet nutrient requirements, but even well-nourished children benefit from the short-term effects of eating breakfast. Breakfast provides energy and nutrients to the brain. Glucose is the primary energy source for the brain, and blood glucose levels have been found to affect the performance of tasks involving recall and memory.[b] Without breakfast, the brain must rely on energy from body stores for morning activities.

Studies have found that children who eat breakfast perform better on achievement tests and have fewer behavior problems in school. In a study of children in the Philadelphia and Baltimore schools, breakfast eaters had better math grades, less hyperactivity, better psychosocial behaviors, and less absence and tardiness than nonbreakfast eaters.[c] Another study compared children in grades three through six who participated in the National School Breakfast Program with those who were eligible but did not participate in the program. Over the course of the school year, students who participated in the School Breakfast Program showed improvements in cognitive performance and had a reduction in tardiness and absenteeism.[d] Because breakfast consumption improves school attendance, it gives children greater learning opportunities.[e] These studies, which evaluated school performance over the long term, have been criticized because subjects were not randomly assigned to breakfast and no-breakfast groups; this flaw in their design may have interfered with the results.

It is not feasible to keep children in a controlled laboratory setting for weeks or months to study the long-term effects of breakfast, but well-controlled laboratory studies have been used to examine the short-term effects of breakfast on academic performance. In one such study, well-nourished 9- to 11-year-old children were fed a standard dinner and then slept at the research facility overnight. In the morning, half of the subjects had a breakfast of waffles with syrup and margarine, orange juice, and milk (535 kcal); the other half drank a placebo that had no kcalories. Then problem-solving skills were evaluated in both groups. One week later the subjects were crossed-over to the other experimental group: the breakfast eaters on the first admission drank the placebo on the second visit. Comparison of the children's problem-solving performance after the two treatments showed that they performed better on the day they ate breakfast.[f]

The results of these and other studies have shown that breakfast consumption is important. It makes a significant contribution to total daily nutrient intake and provides the brain with a ready supply of glucose for morning activities. The overall effect of a good breakfast is an improvement in school performance. But what constitutes a good breakfast?

A Good Breakfast A good breakfast should provide a quarter to a third of the day's nutrients. For example, a breakfast of orange juice, toast with jelly, and oatmeal with milk and raisins provides about 450 kcalories as well as protein, B vitamins, vitamins C, A, and D, and the minerals calcium and iron. Though not every child will eat this good breakfast, even children who do not like breakfast may be willing to consume a slice of toast with peanut butter or a bowl of cereal. Parents are often concerned that sugared breakfast cereals are not a nutritious choice. Despite the high-sugar, low-fiber content of many breakfast cereals marketed to children, they have few other nutritional strikes against them. For example, although 40% of the energy in Cap'n Crunch comes from simple sugars, it is still low in fat and provides 20% or more of the Daily Value for thiamin, riboflavin, niacin, vitamin B_6, folate, vitamin B_{12}, pantothenic acid, and iron. When 1/2 cup of reduced-fat milk is added to the cereal, it also provides 15% of the Daily Value for calcium. Wheaties and Bran Flakes may be healthier choices, but a breakfast of sugared children's cereal is much better than no breakfast at all.

Children who cannot or will not eat breakfast before they leave the house can take a snack to be eaten on the way to school or during recess if they get hungry before lunch. Fruit, yogurt, a bag of dry cereal, or half a sandwich is certainly a better alternative than a candy bar from a vending machine. Having breakfast at school is also an option. The National School Breakfast Program provides meals free or at a reduced cost for families who meet income guidelines.

Breakfast is brain food, providing the first dietary energy source of the day. Whether the child is in preschool or high school, breakfast is a must.

References

[a] Nicklas, T. A., O'Neil, C. E., and Berenson, G. S. Nutrient contribution of breakfast, secular trends, and the role of ready-to-eat cereals: a review of the data from the Bogalusa Heart Study. Am. J. Clin. Nutr. 67:757S–763S, 1998.

[b] Benton, D., and Parker, P. Y. Breakfast, blood glucose, and cognition. Am. J. Clin. Nutr. 67(suppl)772S–778S, 1998.

[c] Kennedy, E., and Davis, C. USDA School Breakfast program. Am. J. Clin. Nutr. 67:798S–803S, 1998.

[d] Meyers, A. F., Sampson, A. E., Weitzman, M., et al. School breakfast program and school performance. Am. J. Dis. Child. 143:1234–1239, 1989.

[e] Pollitt, E., and Mathews, R. Breakfast and cognition: an integrative summary. Am. J. Clin. Nutr. 67(suppl):804S–813S, 1998.

[f] Pollitt, E., Leibel, R. L., and Greenfield, D. Brief fasting, stress, and cognition in children. Am. J. Clin. Nutr. 34:1526–1533, 1981.

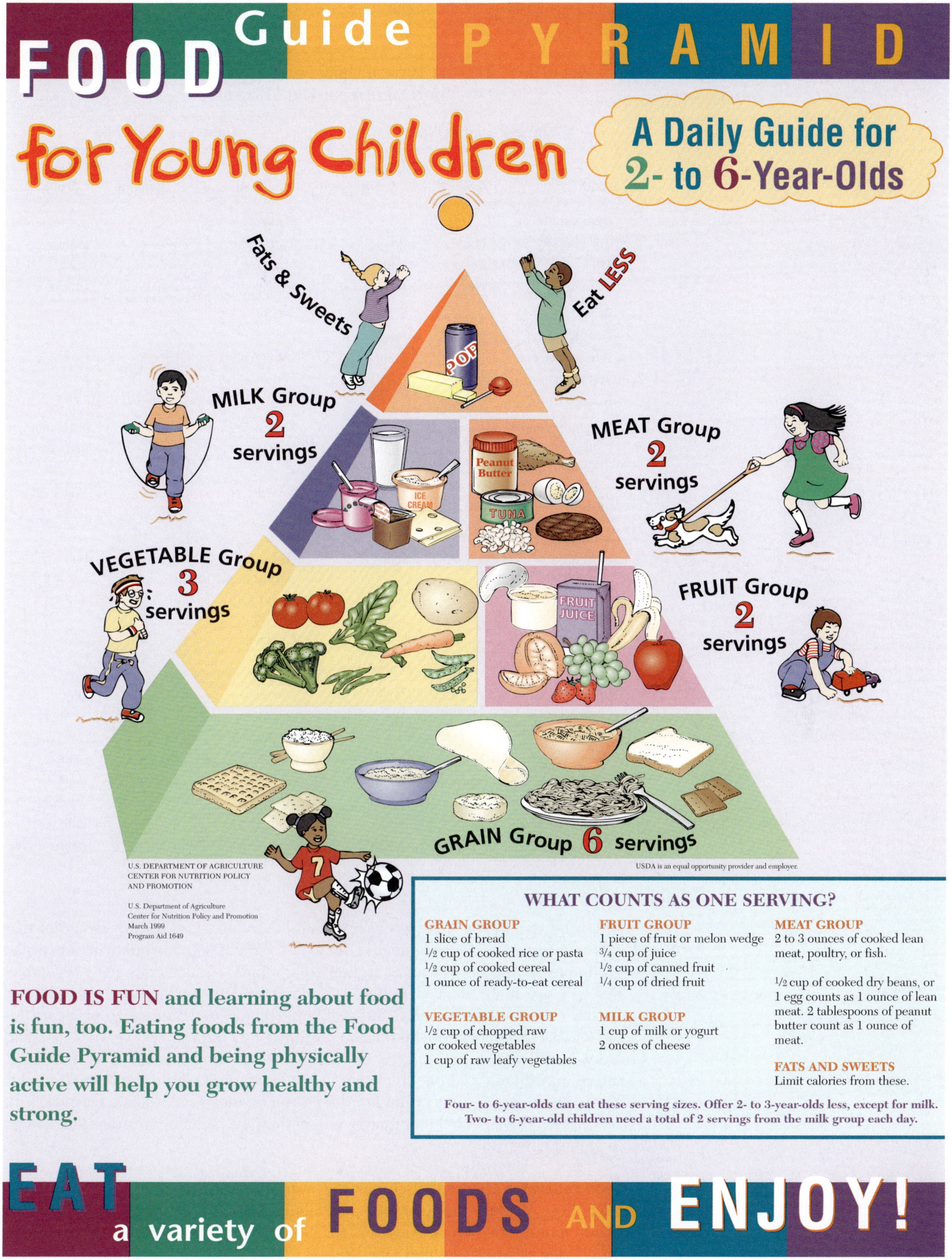

FIGURE 16.10 A version of the Food Guide Pyramid designed to be appealing for children two to six years of age has been developed by the U.S. Department of Agriculture. The serving recommendations of the Food Guide Pyramid can be used to plan children's diets, but the serving sizes may need to be smaller. *(USDA, 1999)*

TABLE 16.2 A Typical Daily Food Intake for Three- and Eight-Year-Old Children

Three-Year-Old Child			Eight-Year-Old Child		
Food	***Amount***	***Food Group***	***Food***	***Amount***	***Food Group***
Breakfast			*Breakfast*		
Corn flakes	3 Tbsp	grain	Corn flakes	3/4 cup	grain
Milk, 2%	1/2 cup	milk	Milk, 2%	3/4 cup	milk
Banana	3 Tbsp	fruit	Banana	1 medium	fruit
Snack			*Snack*		
Peanut butter	1 Tbsp	meat	Pretzels	4	grain
Wheat crackers	3	grain	Orange juice	1/2 cup	fruit
Apple juice	1/2 cup	fruit			
Lunch			*Lunch*		
Vegetable soup	1/4 cup	vegetable	Vegetable soup	1 cup	vegetable
Grilled tuna sandwich	1/2	grain, meat	Grilled tuna sandwich	1	grain, meat
Tomato	1/4	vegetable	Tomato	1/2	vegetable
Milk, 2%	1/2 cup	milk	Milk, 2%	3/4 cup	milk
Snack			*Snack*		
Hot cocoa	1/2 cup	milk	Hot cocoa	3/4 cup	milk
			Peanut butter and jelly sandwich	1	grain, meat
Cookie	1	grain	Cookies	2	grain
Snack					
Pretzels	2	grain			
Orange juice	1/2 cup	fruit			
Dinner			*Dinner*		
Rice	3 Tbsp	grain	Rice	3/4 cup	grain
Chicken	1 drumstick	meat	Chicken	2 drumsticks	meat
Broccoli	1 floret	vegetable	Broccoli	3 florets	vegetable
Milk, 2%	1/2 cup	milk	Milk, 2%	3/4 cup	milk
Ice cream	1/2 cup	milk	Ice cream	3/4 cup	milk

fruits and vegetables, and low-fat meats and dairy products to provide a diet that meets recommendations. Sugared breakfast cereals are included in the bread group but should be consumed in limited amounts. French fries are a vegetable, but they are high in fat and should be consumed in moderation. High-fat and fried meats should be limited and visible fat should be trimmed from meat. Reduced-fat dairy products should be consumed by children two years of age and older in order to maintain their fat intake at the recommended level. However, the composition of the total diet should not be ignored when reducing fat intake. For instance, using reduced-fat hot dogs or lunch meats will reduce fat intake but may not improve overall diet quality unless they are included in a diet that is high in grains, fruits, and vegetables.

Food Labels for Children Because the nutrient needs of children are different from those of adults, there are separate labeling regulations for foods designed for children under two years of age and for those between two and four years (Figure 16.11). The serving sizes and Daily Values on labels of food for young children are based on amounts appropriate for this age group. The FDA has set Daily Values

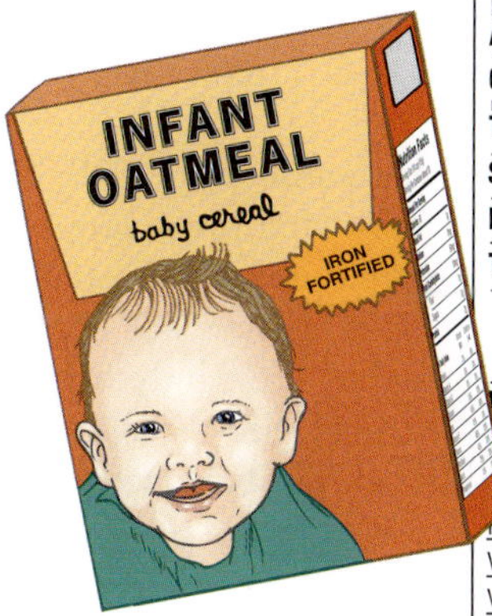

Nutrition Facts
Serving Size 1/4 cup (15g)
Serving Per Container About 30

Amount Per Serving	
Calories 60	
Total Fat	1g
Sodium	0mg
Potassium	50mg
Total Carbohydrate	10g
Fiber	1g
Sugars	0g
Protein	2g

Daily Value	Infants 0-1	Children 1-4
Protein	7%	6%
Vitamin A	0%	0%
Vitamin C	0%	0%
Calcium	15%	10%
Iron	45%	60%
Vitamin E	15%	8%
Thiamin	45%	30%
Riboflavin	45%	30%
Niacin	25%	20%
Phosphorus	15%	10%

(a)

Nutrition Facts
Serving Size 1 jar (140g)

Amount Per Serving	
Calories 110	Calories from Fat 0
Total Fat	0g
Saturated Fat	0g
Cholesterol	0mg
Sodium	10mg
Total Carbohydrate	27
Dietary Fiber	4
Sugars	1
Protein	0

% Daily Value	
Protein 0%	Vitamin A 6%
Vitamin C 45%	Calcium 2%
Iron 2%	

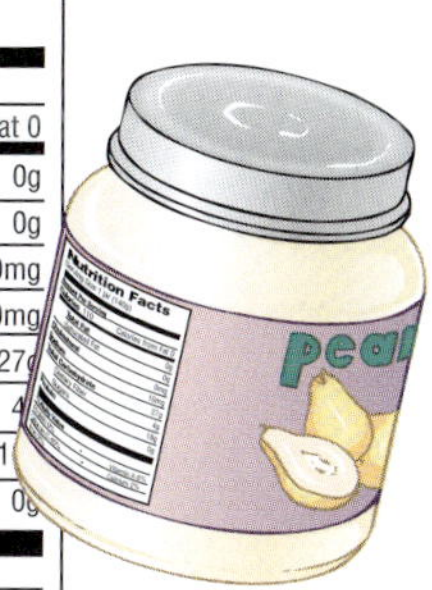

(b)

FIGURE 16.11 Special labeling regulations apply to food designed for children under two years of age (a) and for those between two and four years old (b).

for children for vitamins, minerals, and protein. Labels include the percent Daily Value for these nutrients when they are present in significant amounts. The labels of foods intended for young children provide information needed by caregivers to make wise food selections, but many of the foods consumed by young children do not have special labels because they are also adult foods. When selecting these foods, caregivers need to keep in mind that the needs of young children, especially for fat, are different from the needs of adults.

Daily Values for total fat, saturated fat, cholesterol, total carbohydrate, fiber, and sodium have not been established for children under age four.[24] Because young children have higher fat needs than adults, labels on foods intended for children under age two are not permitted to list the amount of saturated fat, polyunsaturated fat, monounsaturated fat, cholesterol, kcalories from fat, and kcalories from saturated fat on the label. Labels on foods designed for two- to four-year-olds are required to include only the amount of cholesterol and saturated fat per serving but can voluntarily provide information on kcalories from fat and saturated fat and grams of polyunsaturated and monounsaturated fat per serving.

Labels for foods for children under age two are not allowed to carry health claims or most nutrient content claims, such as "low fat."[24] However, claims such as "provides 50% of the Daily Value for vitamin C" that describe the percentage of vitamins or minerals in a food compared to the Daily Value for children under age two are permitted. The descriptors "unsweetened" and "unsalted" are also allowed, but "no sugar added" and "sugar free" are approved only for use on dietary supplements for children.

Do Children Need Vitamin and Mineral Supplements? Children who consume a well-selected, varied diet can meet all their vitamin and mineral requirements without supplements. However, occasional skipped meals and unfinished dinners are a normal part of most children's eating behavior. And, multiple dietary surveys have found that young children have low intakes of both vitamins and minerals.[25] Children who have particularly erratic eating habits, those on regimens to manage obesity, those with limited food availability, and those who consume a vegan diet may benefit from a multivitamin and mineral supplement. However, an analysis of supplement use among children demonstrated that, in general, those who took supplements already consumed a healthier diet than those who did not take supplements.[19]

If a children's supplement is offered, it should provide no more than 100% of the Daily Value for vitamins and minerals. There are many children's supplements available, but they are rarely marketed for their nutrient content. Instead, the sales pitch focuses on their color, flavor, and shape. The choices are enticing—all look and taste like candy, and most children think they are candy. However, supplements can be dangerous and, in the case of iron, life-threatening when taken in excessive doses. The supplements should be administered by caregivers and stored out of the reach of children.

ADOLESCENTS

Once a child has reached about 9 to 12 years of age, the physical changes associated with sexual maturation begin to occur. The maturation process creates differences in the nutrient requirements of males and females. As with children, the nutrient intake of adolescents is also affected by psychosocial development and the environment in which they live. The DRIs begin recommendations for adolescent intake at age nine because the hormonal changes that mark the beginning of adolescence occur by this age in some girls, particularly in African Americans. The DRIs group recommended intakes for adolescents into those for ages 9 through 13 and for ages 14 through 18.[26] Nutrient recommendations for adolescents based on the 1989 RDAs include two groups, ages 11 through 14 and ages 15 through 18.

The Changing Body: Sexual Maturation

Puberty A period in life characterized by rapid growth and physical changes that ends in the attainment of sexual maturity.

Adolescent growth spurt An 18- to 24-month period of peak growth velocity that begins at about ages 10 to 13 in girls and 12 to 15 in boys.

Menarche The onset of menstruation, which normally occurs between the ages of 10 and 15.

During adolescence, organ systems develop and grow, body composition changes, and the growth rates and nutritional requirements of boys and girls diverge. This period of rapid change, which ends in sexual maturation, is called **puberty.** Human growth and development is more rapid in the early teens than at any time except for the first two years after birth. During adolescence, girls and boys grow about 11 inches and gain about 40% of their eventual skeletal mass.[27] From ages 10 to 17, girls gain about 53 pounds and boys about 70 pounds. During adolescence, there is an 18- to 24-month period of peak growth velocity, called the **adolescent growth spurt.** In girls, the growth spurt occurs between the ages of 10 and 13. In boys, it occurs between ages 12 and 15.

The hormonal changes that occur with sexual development orchestrate the type of growth that occurs and the change in body composition that results. During the growth spurt, boys tend to grow taller and heavier than girls and do so at a faster rate. Boys gain fat but also add so much lean mass as muscle and bone that their percentage of body fat actually decreases. In girls, **menarche,** the onset of menstruation, is typically followed by a deceleration in growth rate and an increase in fat deposition. By age 20, females have about twice as much adipose tissue as males and only about two thirds as much lean tissue (Figure 16.12). These physiologic changes affect nutrient needs. Because there is a large individual variation in the age at which these growth changes occur, the stage of maturation is often a better indicator of nutritional requirements than actual chronological age.

Nutrition during childhood and adolescence can affect growth and sexual development. Nutritional deficiencies can cause poor growth and delayed sexual

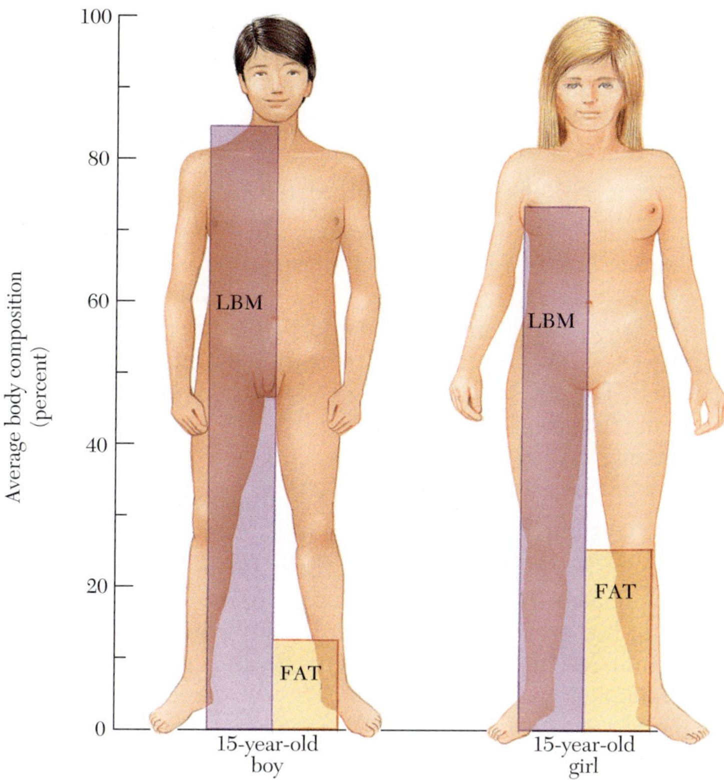

FIGURE 16.12 After puberty, males have a higher percentage of lean body mass and less body fat than females. *(Adapted from Forbes, G. B. Body composition. In* Present Knowledge in Nutrition, *6th ed. Brown, M. L., ed. Washington, D.C.: International Life Sciences Institute, Nutrition Foundation, 1990.)*

maturation. Taller, heavier children usually enter puberty sooner than shorter, lighter ones.[28]

Adolescent Nutrient Needs

Recommendations for nutrient intake in adolescents are based on the needs for growth and development; total nutrient needs are greater at this time than during any other time of life. The best indicators of adequate intake are satiety and growth that follows the curve of the growth charts.

Energy and Macronutrients Energy requirements for boys begin to exceed those for girls as they develop more muscle and a greater body size. Adolescent girls need 38 to 46 kcalories per kilogram of body weight, and boys' requirements range from 40 to 55 kcalories per kilogram (see Figure 16.7). Protein requirements for both groups reach the adult recommendation of 0.8 g per kilogram by about age 19, but because boys are generally heavier, they require more total protein than girls. These higher requirements for males continue throughout life. Adolescents, like adults, should consume a diet containing about 55 to 60% carbohydrate and no more than 30% of energy from fat.

Micronutrients The requirements for many vitamins and minerals increase to adult levels during adolescence. Because data are often not available for this age group, the recommended intakes are often extrapolated from adult values.

Vitamins During adolescence, the need for B vitamins involved in energy metabolism increases because energy expenditure increases. Intake may not meet needs. For example, riboflavin is frequently low in teen diets, especially in those of girls, possibly due to low milk intake. Vitamin B_6 is needed for protein synthesis; therefore, need is increased because of the rapid growth that occurs during adolescence. Folate and vitamin B_{12} needs are increased because of the high rate of cell division. Vitamin B_{12} intake is typically adequate, but folate is a vitamin at risk for deficiency in the adolescent population.[29] Adequate vitamin D is important for skeletal growth; the AI for vitamin D is set at 5 μg per day. In active teens who engage in outdoor activities, much of the requirement is met by synthesis from sunlight. Adequate quantities of vitamins A, C, and E are needed to preserve the structure and function of the newly synthesized cells. These vitamins are generally consumed in sufficient amounts in the teen diet.

Iron Iron deficiency anemia is common in adolescents. Iron is essential for the synthesis of iron-containing proteins needed for the expansion of blood volume and the increase in muscle mass and overall body size. Because blood volume expands at a faster rate in boys than in girls, boys require more iron for tissue synthesis than girls. However, the iron loss due to menstruation makes total need greater in adolescent girls. The RDA for adolescents 14 to 18 years of age is set at 11 mg for boys and 15 mg for girls.[30] Adolescent girls typically consume less than the recommended amount.[29] Good sources of iron acceptable to teens include fortified grains and breakfast cereals and lean red meats.

Calcium Bone contains 99% of the calcium in the body. Although bone mass may continue to increase until age 30, about 45% of the bone present in the adult is laid down during adolescence. The adolescent growth spurt increases both the length and the density of bones; therefore, to form healthy bone, adequate calcium is essential. Calcium retention varies with growth rate, with the fastest-growing adolescents retaining the most calcium. The AI for calcium during adolescence is 1300 mg per day for both sexes. Calcium intake is typically low for adolescent boys and girls.[20] This may compromise the level of peak bone mass achieved, increasing the risk of developing osteoporosis later in life.

The calcium needs for teens can be met by including milk, yogurt and frozen yogurt, and ice cream in the diet, and adding cheese to hamburgers, nachos, and pizza (Figure 16.13). Because many of the major sources of calcium can be high in saturated fat, adolescents should be encouraged to consume reduced-fat dairy products and vegetable sources of calcium. Adolescent girls are likely to skimp on drinking milk, favoring low-kcalorie soft drinks. This may put them in double jeopardy, since diet soda does not supply calcium and some varieties are high both in caffeine, which increases calcium excretion, and in a form of phosphorus that increases calcium losses (Figure 16.14).[31]

Zinc Zinc is important in protein synthesis. During adolescence, the increase in protein synthesis required for the growth of skeletal muscle and the development of organs increases the need for zinc. The RDA for zinc in adolescent boys and girls 14 to 18 years of age is 11 and 9 mg, respectively.[29] Zinc is often deficient in the teen diet.[30] Good sources include meats and whole grains. A long-term deficiency results in growth retardation and altered sexual development. Although severe zinc deficiency is rare in developed countries, even mild deficiency can cause poor growth, affect appetite and taste, impair immune response, and interfere

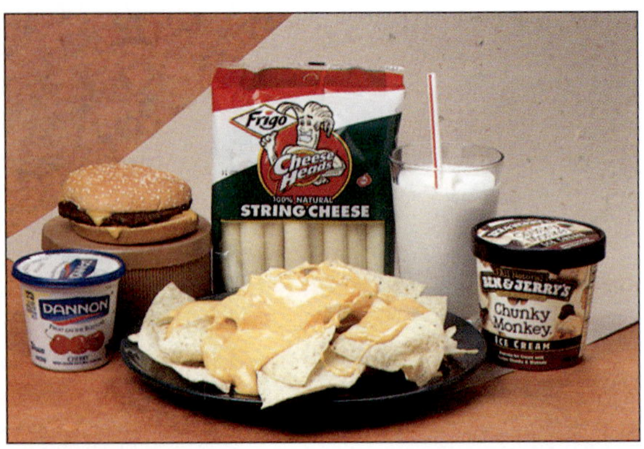

FIGURE 16.13 These foods provide good sources of calcium and are common choices for teens. *(George Semple)*

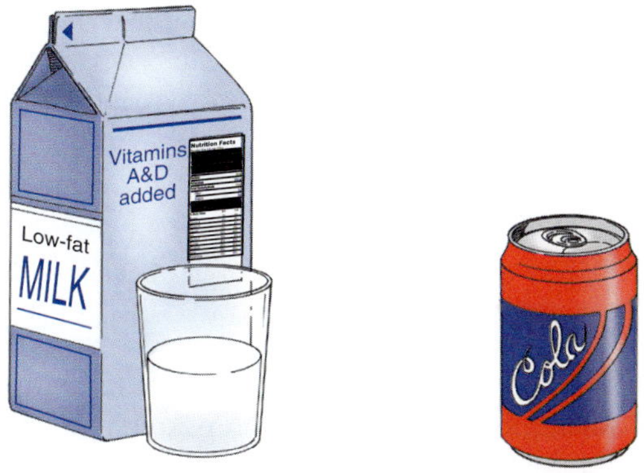

	Low-fat milk	Cola soft drink
Serving size	8 oz	12 oz
Energy (kcal)	102	150
Protein (g)	8	0
Calcium (mg)	300	0
Phosphorus (mg)	235	45
Riboflavin (mg)	0.4	0
Vitamin A (μg)	144	0
Vitamin D (μg)	2.5	0
Caffeine (mg)	0	40

FIGURE 16.14 An 8-ounce glass of milk is a good source of protein, calcium, riboflavin, vitamin A, and vitamin D. A serving of a carbonated beverage (12 fluid ounces) contains more energy, contributes few nutrients, and often contains caffeine.

with vitamin A metabolism. Adequate zinc is essential to meet the needs for rapid growth and sexual maturation in this age group.

Meeting Adolescent Nutrient Needs

No matter when or where foods are consumed, an adolescent's diet should follow the recommendations of the Food Guide Pyramid—with choices made from the high end of the range of serving recommendations. For example, a diet containing 3000 or more kcalories should contain 11 servings of grains. This level may seem difficult to reach, but it is not when it is spread over the course of a day: A large bowl of cereal and two slices of toast for breakfast is four servings; two tacos for lunch and crackers after school is four more servings; and a dinner of spaghetti and garlic bread can add another three or four servings. The diet should also provide five to nine servings of fruits and vegetables. Unfortunately, fruits and vegetables are the food groups most likely to be lacking in the American diet: In a nationwide survey, only 29% of students had eaten five or more servings of fruits and vegetables on the preceding day.[32] French fries, which are high in fat and salt, are the most frequently consumed vegetable. And many people never consume fruit. Sources of fruits and vegetables acceptable to teens include fruit juice, salads, and tomato sauce and vegetables on pizza and spaghetti. Because the teen diet, especially that of boys, is typically high in fat, saturated fat, cholesterol, and sodium,[29] meals offered at home should be low in fat and sodium. This can help to balance the high-fat choices that are made away from home.

Nutrition-Related Concerns in Children and Adolescents

From a child's point of view, nutrition is not a major concern. Social activities and peer pressure, as well as taste and convenience, are important determinants of food intake. Lifestyle choices such as vegetarianism, meals away from home, and time spent in front of television sets and computer screens have more impact on eating habits than do nutrient needs. There is no sense of urgency about consuming a diet to reduce the risk of developing chronic disease. Adolescent concerns focus on appearance, weight, athletic performance, or simply a full stomach. The desire to fit in socially may also contribute to high-risk behaviors that can affect nutritional status.

Dental Caries

Because the primary teeth guide the growth of the permanent teeth, maintaining healthy primary teeth is just as important as preserving permanent ones. Dental caries (cavities) has been called the most common nutrition-related disease in the United States. Decay occurs when there is prolonged contact between sugar and bacteria on the surface of the teeth. Diets high in sugar and carbohydrate and frequent eating promote tooth decay. Preventing tooth decay involves limiting carbohydrate snacks, especially those that stick to teeth; brushing teeth frequently to remove sticky sweets; and consuming adequate fluoride (Figure 16.15; see also Chapters 3, 4, and 13). Children three years of age and over should be seen by a dentist regularly.

Hyperactivity

Hyperactivity is a problem in 5 to 10% of school-aged children, occurring more frequently in boys than in girls. This syndrome involves extreme physical activity, excitability, impulsiveness, distractibility, a short attention span, and a low tolerance for frustration. Hyperactive children have more difficulty learning but usually are of normal or above-average intelligence. Hyperactivity is now considered part of a larger syndrome known as **attention deficit hyperactive disorder (ADHD).**

Attention deficit hyperactive disorder (ADHD) A condition that is characterized by a short attention span and a high level of activity, excitability, and distractibility.

One popular misconception is that hyperactivity is caused by a high sugar intake, but research on sugar intake and behavior has failed to support this hypothesis.[33] Hyperactive behavior that is observed after sugar consumption is likely the result of other circumstances in that child's life. For example, the excitement of a

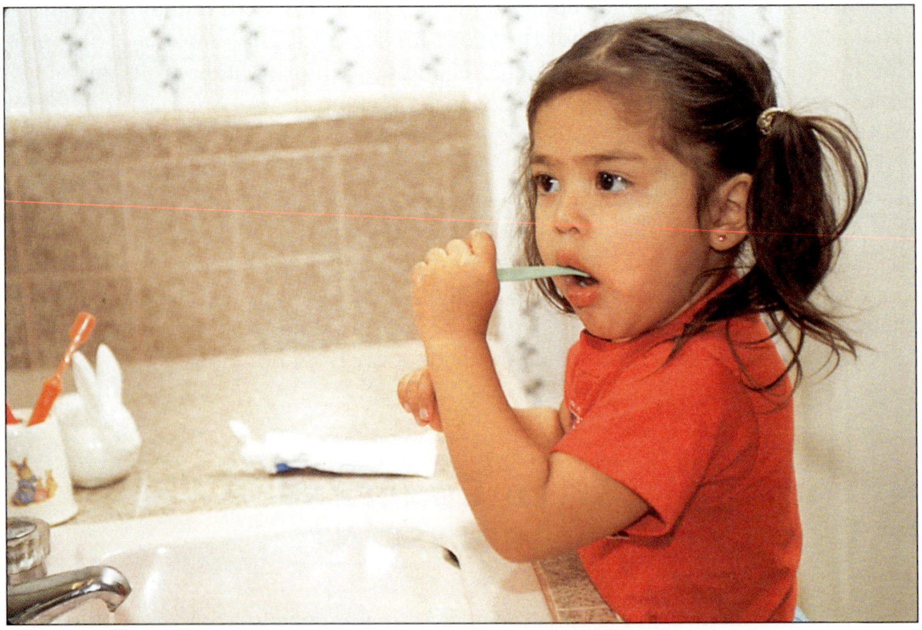

FIGURE 16.15 Frequent supervised toothbrushing by children can help prevent dental caries. *(David Young-Wolff/PhotoEdit)*

birthday party rather than the cake is most likely the cause of hyperactive behavior. Other situations that might cause hyperactivity include lack of sleep, overstimulation, the desire for more attention, or lack of physical activity.

In addition to sugar, other foods and food additives have also been implicated as a cause of hyperactivity. Numerous studies have been done to test the hypothesis that food sensitivities cause hyperactivity, but the results have been inconsistent.[34] Some children with this disorder seem to improve when particular foods or additives are eliminated, while others do not. Hyperactivity should be diagnosed and treated by a physician using behavioral and dietary modification, special educational techniques, counseling, and, in some cases, medication.

Another possible cause of hyperactive behavior in children is caffeine. Caffeine is a stimulant that can cause sleeplessness, restlessness, and irregular heartbeats. Beverages, food, and medicines containing caffeine are often a part of children's diets (see Table 14.8 for the caffeine content of food, beverages, and medications). For example, caffeinated beverages such as Coke and Mountain Dew are often included in children's fast-food meals. A 12-ounce cola contains about 40 to 55 mg of caffeine. Because of children's small size, the same amount of caffeine has a greater effect on a child than it does on an adult.

Food Allergies and Intolerances

Web Menu For information on food allergies, go to the Food Allergy Network at www.foodallergy.org/.

Adverse reactions to foods can be due to food allergies or food intolerances. True allergic reactions to food, or food allergies, are relatively rare, occurring in less than 2% of young children.[35]

Food Allergies An allergic reaction occurs when incompletely digested proteins are absorbed from the intestine, enter the lymph and/or bloodstream, and cause an immune system response. Exposure to an **allergen** for the first time causes the immune system to produce **antibodies** to that allergen. When the allergen is encountered again through consumption of the same food, symptoms result as the immune system battles the allergen. These symptoms, including vomiting, diarrhea, asthma, hives, eczema, runny nose, hay fever, general cramps and aches, and swelling of tissues, may occur almost immediately or take up to 24 hours to appear and can vary from mild to severe and life-threatening.

Allergen A foreign substance, usually a protein, that stimulates an immune response.

Antibodies Protein molecules produced by the immune system that specifically bind antigen.

Foods that commonly cause allergies include wheat, peanuts, eggs, milk, nuts, seafood, soy products, and some meats. Allergies to food are more common in infants because their digestive tracts are not fully mature. After about three months of age, the risk of developing food allergies is reduced because incompletely digested proteins are less likely to be absorbed. Many children who develop food allergies before the age of three will outgrow them. For example, of children allergic to eggs at one year of age, only 4% were still allergic by age five.[35] Allergies that appear after three years are more likely to be a problem for life.

Diagnosing Food Allergies Food allergies can be diagnosed by several laboratory methods. Such tests can identify foods that are likely to cause problems, but they are not 100% reliable. An **elimination diet** and **food challenge** can be used to confirm the cause of a food allergy. An elimination diet involves removing all foods suspected of causing an allergic reaction from the diet. When a diet that causes no symptoms has been established, it is consumed for two to four weeks. Then, in the food challenge, a small portion of the suspected allergen is offered and the individual is monitored for an allergic reaction. If no reaction occurs, then increasing amounts are introduced until a normal portion is offered. If there is still no reaction, then the food can be ruled out as an allergen. Foods such as peanuts, which can cause serious and even deadly reactions, should not be reintroduced into the diet as a food challenge (see *Making Decisions:* "Should Peanut Butter Sandwiches Be on the School Lunch Menu?").

Elimination diet An eating plan that eliminates foods that are suspected to cause an adverse food reaction.

Food challenge The reintroduction of foods into the diet one at a time while the person is carefully observed in a medical setting for the recurrence of allergy symptoms.

Making Decisions

Should Peanut Butter Sandwiches Be on the School Lunch Menu?

The question of whether peanut butter sandwiches should be included in the school lunch menu may seem odd, but some advocates for children who are allergic to peanuts believe that schools should be peanut-free. An allergy to peanuts is one of the most common food allergies. It usually begins in infancy or early childhood, is rarely outgrown, and can cause severe reactions. However, other food allergies, such as those to wheat and seafood, can also cause serious reactions, but these items are not being banned from the school cafeteria. Why all the attention to peanuts?

The main reason that peanut allergies have commanded such particular attention is that reactions can occur with exposure to minute amounts of the allergen and can be fatal. Amounts of peanut protein as low as 100 μg can cause a reaction, whereas for other food allergies, up to a thousandfold more—50 to 100 mg of an allergen—must be eaten before a reaction occurs.[a] And individuals who are allergic to peanuts may be at risk even if the peanuts do not find their way into their mouths. A survey found that 66% of allergic individuals develop symptoms simply from contact with peanuts.[b] Some even experience reactions when peanut allergen is merely inhaled. Allergic symptoms vary but often include skin reactions such as flushing and hives, difficulty breathing, and a drop in blood pressure. When respiratory symptoms occur, the allergic individual must be injected with epinephrine immediately and then treated by a physician.

Individuals with an allergy to peanuts should avoid all contact with peanuts. Peanuts, peanut butter, and peanut butter candy are obvious foods to avoid. Others are not so obvious. Children with peanut allergy and their caregivers must rely on food labels to make safe choices. Labels identify foods, such as cookies and crackers, that contain peanut fragments, peanut flour, and peanut oil. Labels may also state that the product "may contain peanuts" or that it was "manufactured in a facility that processes peanuts." These statements are included because minute amounts of peanut protein may contaminate foods manufactured in the same location as peanut-containing foods. For instance, cheese sandwich crackers seem like a safe snack, but a thorough reading of the ingredient list reveals that the last ingredient is peanuts. This is because the cheese crackers were manufactured in the same processing facility as peanut butter sandwich crackers, so the label reflects the possibility of cross-contamination. This information protects both the company from legal action and the allergic individual from inadvertently consuming a peanut-containing food.

Because peanut allergies can be so severe and occur from such low exposures, some have suggested that peanuts be eliminated from the school lunchroom. As long as peanut butter is around, there is a possibility of cross-contamination. For example, if the same knife that spread peanut butter is dipped into the jelly jar, the allergic child who is served only a jelly sandwich may suffer a peanut reaction. Eliminating peanut butter from the cafeteria would reduce the amount of peanut allergen in the school, but it would not make the school peanut free or guarantee the safety of allergy suffers. Even in a school that doesn't serve peanut butter sandwiches, lunches brought from home will surely contain peanut products. A peanut butter–smeared finger or shirt or a taste of someone else's lunch could cause an allergic reaction.

So, should your school be peanut free? Will prohibition of peanuts prevent allergic reactions? Peanut butter sandwiches are a nutritious staple of many children's diets. Does it violate the rights of those who like peanut butter and jelly sandwiches to force a school to eliminate them from the menu to protect the few children who have this allergy? While this may be decided in the courts, awareness of the problem can protect an allergic child.

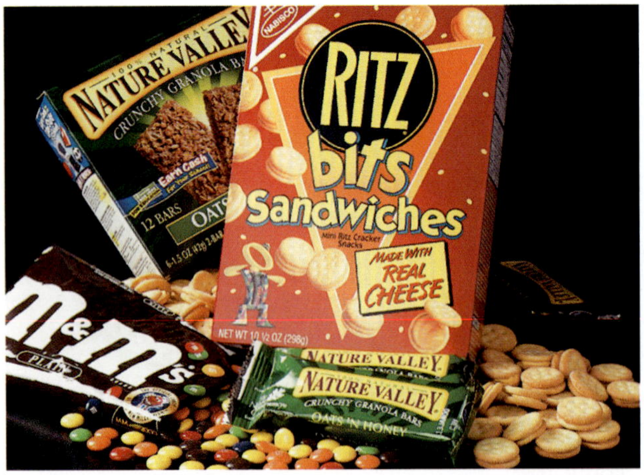

Parents of children with allergies must read labels carefully. These products are all manufactured at facilities that also process peanuts and therefore are labeled to indicate that they may have inadvertently been contaminated with peanuts. *(George Semple)*

References

[a] Hourihane, J. O., Kilburn, S. A., Nordlee, J. A., et al. An evaluation of the sensitivity of subjects with peanut allergy to very low doses of peanut protein: a randomized, double-blind, placebo-controlled food challenge study. J. Allergy Clin. Immunol. 100:596–600, 1997.

[b] Hourihane, J. O., Kilburn, S. A., Dean, P., and Warner, J. O. Clinical characteristics of peanut allergy. Clin. Exp. Allergy 27:634–639, 1997.

Preventing and Managing Food Allergies Breast-feeding is recommended for infants from families with a history of allergies because it reduces the risk of developing food allergies. Infants who are breast-fed are less likely to be exposed to foreign proteins that cause food allergies. In addition, their gut matures earlier and they are protected by antibodies and other components present in human milk. The benefits of breast-feeding are increased if the mother avoids eating common allergy-causing foods such as peanuts, eggs, fish, and dairy products during lactation. To decrease the chances of allergies when solid foods are introduced, wheat, eggs, and fish should not be introduced until the child is 12 months of age, and peanuts should not be given until 36 months.[35]

The best way to manage a food allergy is to avoid consuming the offending allergen. If certain foods must be avoided in the diet, care must be taken to ensure that nutrient needs are met without these foods. The information on food labels can help to identify food sources of an allergy-causing ingredient.

Food Intolerances **Food intolerances** do not involve antibody production by the immune system. Rather, they are caused by foods that are difficult or impossible to digest. Food intolerances can be caused by chemical components in foods, by toxins that occur naturally in foods, by substances added to foods during processing or preparation, or simply by large amounts of foods, such as onions or prunes, that cause local GI irritation.[35] Lactose intolerance is an example of a food intolerance caused by a reduced ability to digest milk sugar. It is not an allergy to milk proteins.

Food intolerance An adverse reaction to a food that does not involve the immune system.

Lead Toxicity

Lead is an environmental contaminant that can be toxic, especially in children under six years of age. Children are particularly susceptible because they absorb lead much more efficiently than do adults. It is estimated that children may absorb as much as 30 to 75% of ingested lead, whereas adults absorb only about 11%.[36] Once absorbed from the gastrointestinal tract, lead circulates in the bloodstream and then accumulates in the bones and, to a lesser extent, the brain, teeth, and kidneys.

Symptoms Lead disrupts neurotransmitters and thus interferes with the functioning of the nervous system. High levels of lead can contribute to iron deficiency anemia, changes in kidney function, nervous system abnormalities, and even seizures, coma, and death.[37] In young children, lead poisoning can cause learning disabilities and behavior problems. High lead levels in the bones of young boys have been linked to attention problems, aggressive behavior, and delinquency.[38] In childhood and adolescence, lead causes an increase in the incidence of dental caries.[39] In adults, lead poisoning can damage the reproductive organs and cause high blood pressure.[40] During pregnancy, lead toxicity can damage the fetal nervous system.

Environmental Exposure Lead is found naturally in the Earth's crust, but over the years industrial activities have redistributed it in the environment. Lead is now found in soil contaminated with lead paint dust; it also enters drinking water from old corroded lead plumbing, lead solder on copper pipes or brass faucets. It is present in polluted air, and its presence in leaded glass and in glazes used on imported and antique pottery can contaminate food and beverages. Because of the risks of lead toxicity from environmental contamination, lead is no longer used in house paint, gasoline, or solder. As a result, the number of children with elevated blood lead levels has decreased by 85% over the last 20 years.[36] Despite these gains, nearly a million children under six years of age have blood lead levels that are high enough to cause damage.[41] The problem is greatest among children living in poverty. These children often live in older houses, which are more likely to

TABLE 16.3 Reducing Lead Exposure

Reducing exposure from lead paint: If you live in a house built before 1978, it may contain lead paint or lead paint may have been sanded or scrapped off at some time.

- Wash floors and other surfaces weekly with warm water and detergent.
- Wipe soil off shoes before entering the house.
- Cover exposed soil in the yard with grass or mulch.

Reducing exposure from tap water: If your home has old plumbing, lead may be leaching into your tap water. More leaches into hot water than cold, and water that has been standing in the pipes has more lead.

- Use cold water for drinking and cooking.
- Allow water to run for 30 seconds before use.

Reducing exposure from food containers: Pottery glazes and lead crystal contain lead. The FDA limits the amount of lead allowed in ceramic foodware, but the lead content of pottery designed for ornamental use is not regulated.

- Look for engraved warnings such as "Not for Food Use—May Poison Food" and "For Decorative Purposes Only" to identify pottery that should not be used to serve food.
- Do not store acidic foods such as fruit juices or tomato juice in ceramic containers.
- Limit the use of antique or collectable tableware for food or beverages to special occasions.
- Use your lead crystal stemware to drink from, but do not store anything in lead crystal.
- Pregnant women should not routinely use lead crystal glasses.
- Infants should not be fed from lead crystal baby bottles.

For additional information: Contact the Centers for Disease Control and Prevention at 1-888-232-6789; the Environmental Protection Agency's Safe Drinking Water Hotline at 1-800-426-4791; the Consumer Product Safety Commission at 1-800-638-CPSC; the National Lead Information Center at 1-800-LEAD-FYI; or access Web sites for these agencies and organizations.

contain lead paint, and children often consume chipped paint as they explore their environments. The old plumbing in these houses may contaminate the water with lead. In addition, children living in poverty are more likely to be malnourished, and malnutrition increases lead absorption because lead is better absorbed from an empty stomach and when other minerals such as calcium, zinc, and iron are deficient. An inverse relationship has been found between blood lead levels and dietary iron intake, suggesting that adequate iron intake prevents lead absorption and can help protect against lead toxicity.[37]

Preventing Toxicity Children should have their blood lead levels monitored.[36] The effects of lead poisoning are permanent, but if high levels are detected early, the lead can be removed with medical treatment. The best way to prevent lead poisoning is to learn how to avoid lead exposure (Table 16.3) and consume a nutritionally adequate diet.

Vegetarian Diets

Many children and adolescents consume vegetarian diets because their families are vegetarians. As children grow into teenagers, they may decide to consume a vegetarian diet even if the rest of the family does not. According to one survey, 37% of teens said they try to avoid red meat,[42] and on any given day, 15% of college students choose vegetarian meals.[43] Some give up meat because they are concerned about animals and the environment, and some do it for health reasons or to lose weight. Although vegetarian diets can be a healthful alternative, foods must be carefully chosen to meet needs and avoid excesses.

Vegan vegetarian diets pose a particular risk of nutrient deficiencies for children. Because children's protein needs per kilogram are greater than in adults, vegan diets pose a potential risk for protein deficiency in small children. Iron and zinc are a particular concern because the best sources of these minerals are red meats and these minerals are poorly absorbed from plant sources. Dairy products are poor sources of iron and zinc, so lacto vegetarians as well as vegans are at risk for deficiencies. Because of the lower bioavailability of iron from plant sources, a special RDA for iron of 14 mg/day for vegetarian men and 26 mg/day for vegetarian adolescent girls has been established.[30] Vitamin B_{12} is found almost exclusively in animal products; therefore, those consuming vegan diets must use supplements or fortified foods to meet needs. The major source of calcium in the North American diet is dairy products, so again, vegan diets must be carefully planned to meet calcium needs. For small children, calcium-fortified foods such as soy milk may be needed because they cannot eat enough calcium-rich vegetables to meet needs. Likewise, most dietary vitamin D comes from fortified dairy products, so vegans must get their vitamin D from sunshine or consume other sources of this vitamin such as fortified soy milk.

Although we think of vegetarian diets as healthy, they are not necessarily high in fruits and vegetables or low in fat, particularly if high-fat dairy products are chosen. For example, a slice of cheese pizza and a can of cola is a vegetarian meal but not a particularly healthy one. However, when chosen carefully, a vegetarian diet can be low in fat, saturated fat, and cholesterol and high in complex carbohydrate, fiber, and micronutrients. For example, a vegetarian lunch of a pita sandwich with hummus (chickpeas), tomatoes, and spinach, along with some dried fruit and a glass of reduced-fat milk, is low in fat and contains good sources of calcium and plant sources of iron.

Meals Away from Home

Forty years ago, mothers had a greater impact on children's food choices because they were home to offer three meals a day. Today, many children live in single-parent households and 60% of women with young children work outside the home.[6] The increase in working mothers and single-parent households means children consume many of their meals away from home—in restaurants and fast-food establishments as well as day-care facilities and schools.

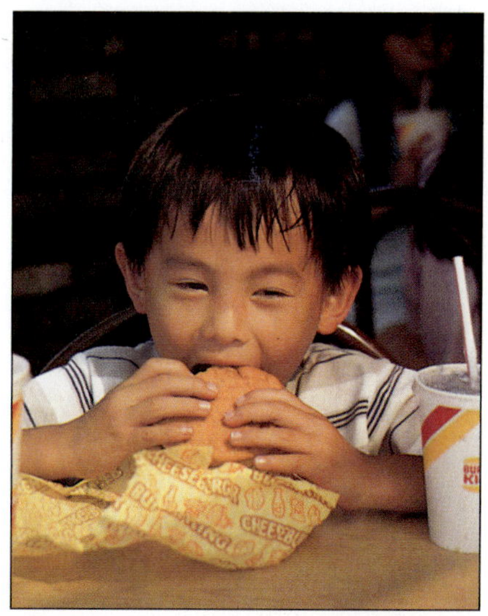

FIGURE 16.16 Children love fast food but it is generally high in fat and low in milk, fruits, and vegetables. *(© Arthur R. Hill/Visuals Unlimited)*

Fast Food Children generally love fast food, and there is nothing wrong with an occasional fast-food meal. But, these meals are typically lacking in milk, fruits, and vegetables. They are high in kcalories and fat and low in calcium, fiber, and vitamins A and C (Figure 16.16). To fit fast food into a healthy diet, more nutrient-dense fast-food choices need to be made and other meals and snacks throughout the day need to supply the missing nutrients. Many fast-food franchises now offer vegetables, salads, and milk. And some of the old standbys are not bad choices. A plain, single-patty hamburger provides a lot less fat and energy than one with two patties and a high-fat sauce. A chicken sandwich can be a low-fat choice if it is grilled or barbecued, not breaded and fried (see Appendix A). French fries are high in fat, but if they are combined with low-fat foods throughout the day, they can still be part of a healthy diet. A fast-food meal is only one part of the overall dietary pattern. If the missing milk, fruits, and vegetables are consumed at other times during the day, the total diet can still be a healthy one.

Web Menu: The USDA's Healthy School Meals Resource System at schoolmeals.nal.usda.gov:8001/ provides resources for healthy school meals and links to other nutrition information.

Meals at School The National School Breakfast and Lunch Programs were designed to improve the dietary intake and nutritional health of America's children. The National School Breakfast Program is available in about half the nation's schools and serves more than 7 million children. The breakfasts served must provide at least 25% of the 1989 RDA for certain nutrients and furnish at least one serving of milk; one serving of fruit, juice, or vegetables; and either two servings of bread, two servings of meat, or one serving of each. Meals are provided free or at a reduced cost for families who meet income guidelines. The National School Lunch Program is mandated to provide nutritious meals and to promote nutrition

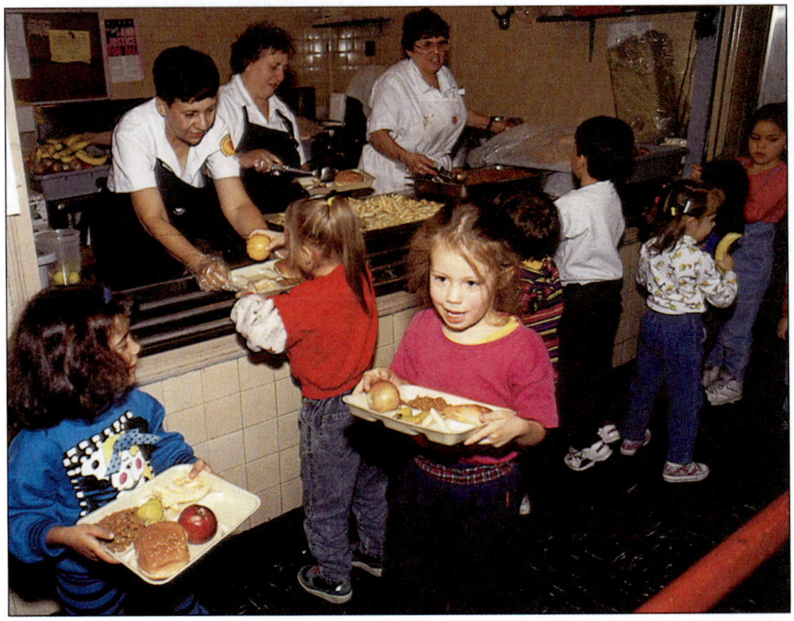

FIGURE 16.17 Participating in the School Lunch Program can improve nutrient intake. *(David M. Grossman/Photo Researchers, Inc.)*

education by teaching children to make appropriate food choices.[44] The program provides meals to school-aged children on a sliding cost scale depending on household income (Figure 16.17). Each lunch meal must provide one third of the 1989 RDA for protein, vitamin A, vitamin C, iron, calcium, and energy and meet the Dietary Guidelines recommendations of no more than 30% of energy from fat and no more than 10% from saturated fat. Within these guidelines, each school or school district can decide which foods to serve and how they are prepared. In addition to lunches, federal guidelines regulate foods sold in snack bars and vending machines that compete with school lunch programs. These must provide at least 5% of the RDA for one or more of the following: protein, vitamin A, vitamin C, niacin, riboflavin, calcium, and iron.

An analysis of the foods students chose to eat from the meal offered found that students who participated in school lunch programs consumed one third of the RDA for energy, protein, vitamin A, vitamin C, vitamin B_6, calcium, iron, and zinc and drank twice as much milk as students not participating in school lunch programs. However, they consumed more fat than is recommended: 37% of the energy they consumed at lunch came from fat. Those who purchased meals from vending machines consumed fewer vitamins and minerals and an even greater percentage of energy from fat.[18]

Activity Level

Most children are naturally active, and extended periods of inactivity are not normal for healthy children. However, modern lifestyles with video games, computers, and television have changed the way children spend their leisure time. Hours spent running and playing outside have been replaced by hours sitting in front of television and computer screens.

The Nutritional Impact of Television Many children today spend more time watching television than they do in any activity other than sleep.[2] One study showed that children who watch four or more hours of TV per day have greater body fat and higher BMI than those who watch fewer than two hours a day.[45] Television affects nutritional status in a number of ways: It introduces children to foods they might otherwise not be exposed to, it promotes snacking, and it reduces physical activity. Through advertising, television has a strong influence on

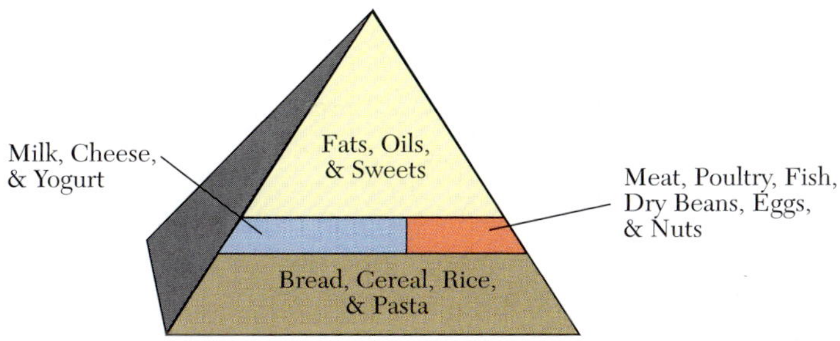

Saturday Morning Pyramid

FIGURE 16.18 The Saturday Morning Pyramid illustrates the percentage of foods in different Food Guide Pyramid groups that is advertised during children's Saturday morning television. Public service announcements and advertisements for fast-food restaurants and frozen meals were not included because they did not logically fit into one Food Guide Pyramid category. This top-heavy pyramid illustrates that a high percentage of the foods advertised are high in fat or sugar and low in nutrient density. No foods fitting into either the vegetable or the fruit groups were advertised. *(Kotz, K., and Story, M. Food advertisements during children's Saturday morning television programming: are they consistent with dietary recommendations? J. Am. Diet. Assoc. 94:1296–1300, 1994.)*

the foods selected by young children (Figure 16.18). A review of commercials broadcast during children's programming found that over 60% were for food products—primarily sweetened breakfast cereals; sweets such as candy, cookies, doughnuts, and other desserts; snacks; and beverages—that are high in sugar, fat, or salt.[46] Also, television promotes snacking behavior. Although snacks are an important part of a growing child's diet, many children snack on sweet and salty foods that are low in nutrient density while watching TV.

Activity Recommendations Physical activity helps promote a healthy body weight, strong bones, and psychological well-being. Nevertheless, a survey of U.S. children showed that 48% of girls and 26% of boys do not exercise vigorously on a regular basis and that participation in daily school-based physical education programs is decreasing.[2] An appropriate level of physical activity is an important factor in maintaining fitness and healthy body weights among American children.

Web Menu: For more information on exercise recommendations for children, go to Kidshealth at www.kidshealth.org/parent/ and click on nutrition and fitness.

Numerous public health agencies have made recommendations to promote physical activity among America's youth. The Centers for Disease Control and Prevention have published guidelines recommending daily physical education in schools. The Dietary Guidelines recommend that children participate in vigorous physical activity for at least an hour per day.[12] Because children have short attention spans, periods of moderate to vigorous activity lasting 10 to 20 minutes each should be interspersed with periods of rest and recovery. Children should be exposed to a variety of different types of activities that are designed to meet their developmental abilities and involve various levels of intensity (Figure 16.19). Learning to enjoy sports and exercise in childhood can set the stage for an active lifestyle in adulthood.

Appearance and Body Image

Adolescence is a time in life when appearance is of particular concern. The hormonal changes of puberty often cause acne, and teens are frequently unhappy with their bodies. Many girls want to lose weight even if they are not overweight. Many boys, on the other hand, want to gain weight to achieve a muscular, strong appearance.

Acne Acne, which is common in adolescence, is triggered by the hormonal changes that occur with the onset of puberty. At one time, acne was believed to be related to diet, and long lists of foods to avoid were doled out to teens with acne. Since then, restrictions on the intake of foods such as chocolate, french fries, and soft drinks have been found to have no effect on the severity of acne. Anxiety, lack of sleep, and hormonal fluctuations of the menstrual cycle are more likely to cause acne flare-ups than specific foods, but a well-balanced diet will ensure that the skin has all the nutrients needed to maintain its integrity. Medications are also available to treat acne. One prescription medication that is a derivative of vitamin A, called 13-*cis*-retinoic acid (Accutane), can be taken orally to treat a severe form of acne called cystic acne. Another prescription vitamin A

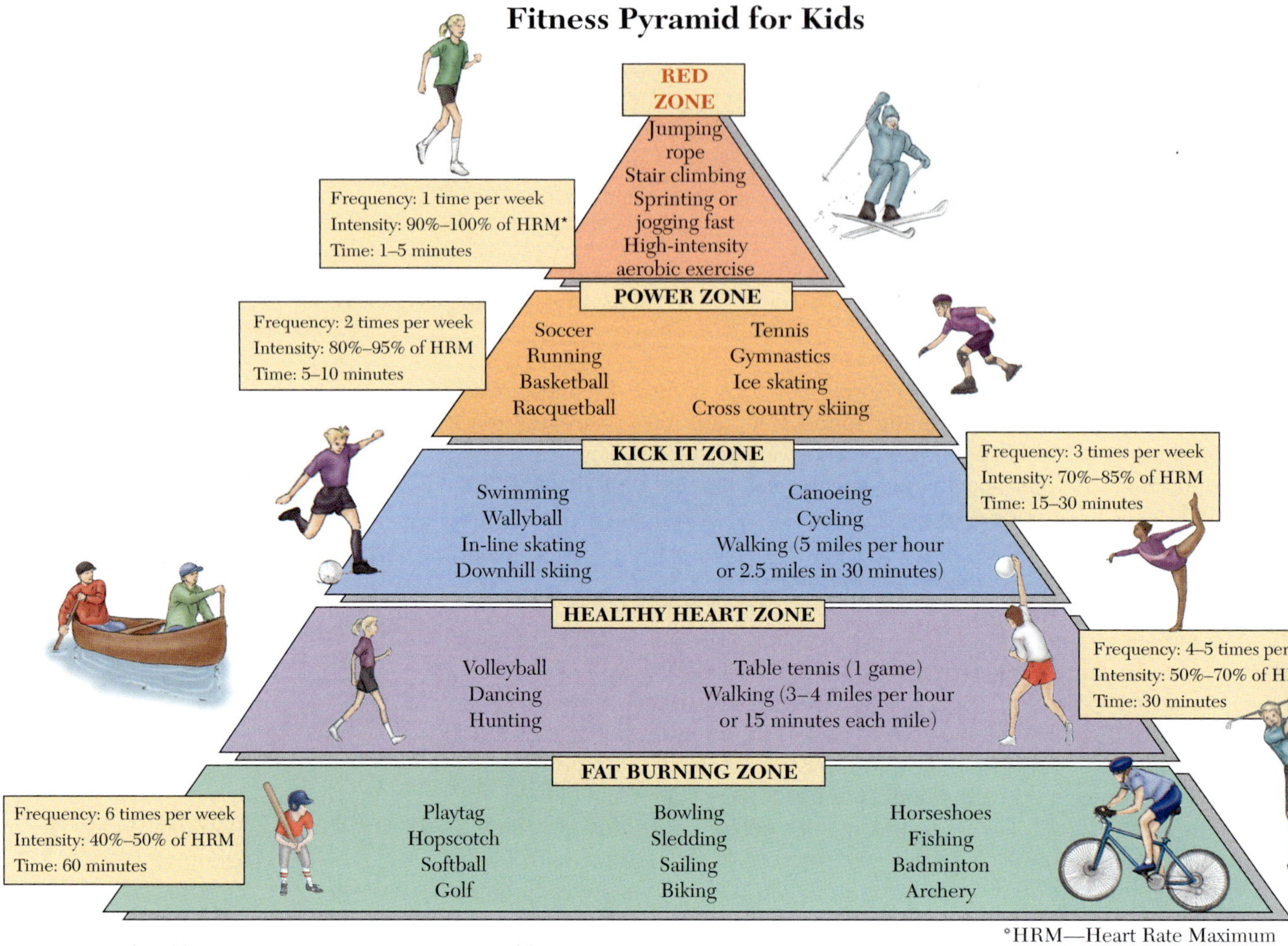

(Adapted from: American Dietetic Association. Position of the American Dietetic Association: Dietary guidance for healthy children ages 2 to 11 years. J. Am. Diet. Assoc. 99:93–101, 1999)

FIGURE 16.19 Children should participate in a variety of activities of varying intensity. The Fitness Pyramid for Kids provides recommendations for the frequency, intensity, and duration of activities that are appropriate for children.

derivative, called Retin-A, is used topically to treat acne. In addition to reducing acne, Retin-A tightens the skin and decreases wrinkles, making it a popular drug with older adults. Neither Accutane nor Retin-A should be used by anyone who is pregnant or planning a pregnancy. Although these drugs are derivatives of vitamin A, vitamin A supplements cannot be substituted as a treatment for acne. In addition, large doses of vitamin A are toxic.

Body Weight and Eating Disorders Because of the importance of physical appearance during adolescence, being overweight or underweight can lead to social and emotional problems. Obese children in the United States are less well accepted by their peers than normal-weight children and are frequently ridiculed and teased; obese adolescents may be discriminated against by adults as well as by their peers. This can lead to feelings of rejection, social isolation, and low self-esteem. The isolation of obese adolescents from teen society results in boredom, depression, inactivity, and withdrawal—all of which can cause an increase in eating and a decrease in energy output, worsening the problem.

Concern about physical appearance can be a precipitating factor in the development of eating disorders. Eating disorders, such as anorexia and bulimia, are more common in adolescence than at any other time in life. The pressure of taking on the responsibilities of adulthood, combined with pressure from peers and society to be thin, may contribute to this high incidence (see Chapter 8). Many individuals with eating disorders feel ineffectual in their lives and may be using food to achieve some measure of self-control. Female teens are particularly at risk, but eating disorders also occur in males and in younger children. The excessive concern about weight and body image that characterizes these conditions may begin as early as the preschool years. These abnormal concerns can lead to battles over food and eating and to excessively finicky eating habits, resulting in poor growth and abnormal development. Disordered eating is often hidden by other eating patterns. For example, vegetarian adolescent females were twice as likely as nonvegetarians to report frequent dieting, four times as likely to report intentional vomiting, and eight times more likely to purge using laxatives.[47]

The Impact of Athletics Exercise has many benefits, but some teen athletes may go to extremes to increase muscle mass or decrease body weight to achieve a desired appearance or performance level. The nutrition misinformation that is common in school athletics, combined with the willingness of young athletes to follow any advice that promises to improve performance, can lead to serious health problems. Excessive use of dietary supplements, inappropriate training diets, and fad diets are of particular concern in this age group (see Chapter 14).

Dietary Supplements Teen athletes require more water, energy, protein, carbohydrate, and micronutrients than their less active peers, but supplements are rarely needed to meet these needs. If the extra energy needs of teen athletes are met with whole grains, fresh fruits and vegetables, and dairy products, their protein, carbohydrate, and micronutrient needs will easily be met. An exception is iron, which may need to be supplemented, particularly in female athletes to prevent anemia (see Chapter 14).[48]

In addition to micronutrient supplements, high school athletes often try to increase muscle mass by using anabolic steroids, androstenedione, and creatine. Anabolic steroids are illegal, and although they do increase muscle mass, the risks far outweigh the benefits (see Chapter 14, *Making Decisions:* "Ergogenic Hormones: What Athletes Will Do for an Edge"). Androstenedione is a testosterone precursor that is legally sold as a dietary supplement, but the long-term health effects of this supplement have not yet been determined. Creatine is an amino acid that is used to synthesize creatine phosphate, which can generate ATP for muscle contraction. Research has supported the benefits of creatine supplementation for short-term anaerobic exercise that requires explosive bursts of energy such as sprinting and weight lifting.[49] Creatine supplements have not been associated with serious side effects, but controlled toxicology studies have not been done, and the safety and efficacy of the long-term use of high dose supplements is unknown.[50] Despite the rising popularity of supplements, the best and safest way for young athletes to increase muscle mass is the hard way: Lift weights and eat more.

Body Weight in Athletes Success in some sports depends on being light and lean. Athletes involved in such sports may restrict their food intake in order to keep their weight low. Weight restriction, however, may affect nutritional status and maturation and increase the risk of developing an eating disorder.[51] In female athletes, the combination of hard training and weight restriction can lead to a syndrome referred to as the female athlete triad, which includes disordered eating, amenorrhea, and osteoporosis (see Chapter 14). In male athletes who participate in sports, such as wrestling, that require athletes to fit into a specific weight class on the day of the event, dangerous methods of quick weight loss are a concern. Severe energy intake restriction, water deprivation, vomiting, and diuretic and laxative abuse are common practice among wrestlers. Low-energy diets can interfere with normal growth and may be too limited in variety to meet these athletes' needs for vitamins and minerals. Even more of a danger is the practice of restricting water intake and encouraging sweat loss to decrease body weight. This may achieve the temporary weight loss necessary to put the athlete in a lower weight class, but dehydration is dangerous and can impair athletic performance.[52]

High-Risk Behaviors

As adolescents search for their place in the world, they are likely to be exposed to and perhaps to participate in high-risk behaviors. Some of these, including teen pregnancy, cigarette smoking, and alcohol consumption, have the potential to affect their nutritional status as well as general health.

Teen Pregnancy As discussed earlier, sexual maturity in girls affects nutrition because it increases body fat and iron needs. The use of oral contraceptives or a pregnancy during adolescence can also affect nutritional status.

Oral Contraceptive Use Oral contraceptives may contain either estrogen or progesterone or a combination of the two. These hormones may be prescribed to adolescent girls for a number of reasons and can affect nutrition because they affect nutrient metabolism. Oral contraceptives may cause a rise in fasting blood sugar and a tendency toward abnormal glucose tolerance in those with a family history of diabetes. They may also cause changes in body composition, including weight gain due to water retention and an increase in lean body mass. Oral contraceptives reduce the need for iron by reducing menstrual flow. Therefore a special RDA has been established for individuals taking oral contraceptives; the RDA for adolescent girls is 11.4 mg of iron per day. Blood levels of vitamins B_6 and B_{12} have been found to be low in oral contraceptive users, although it is not known whether these changes in blood levels reflect an increased need for these nutrients.[53,54]

Pregnancy Because adolescent girls continue to grow and mature for several years after menstruation starts, the pregnant teenager must meet her own nutrient needs for growth and development as well as the needs of pregnancy. This puts the pregnant adolescent at nutritional risk. In order for the mother and fetus to remain healthy, special attention must be paid to all aspects of prenatal care, including nutrient intake (see Chapter 15). Due to the special nutrient needs of this group, the DRIs have included a life-stage group for pregnant girls age 18 or younger. For many nutrients, the recommended intake follows either the needs of adolescence or the needs of pregnancy, but for some, like magnesium and zinc, the needs of pregnant teens exceed the needs of either nonpregnant teens or pregnant women age 19 or older (Figure 16.20).

Cigarette Smoking Approximately 35% of high school students in the United States smoke cigarettes.[55] Many teens start smoking in order to promote weight loss or maintenance. Because smoking is associated with lower body weights in adult women, they believe smoking will curb appetite and help them stay thin or lose weight.[56] However, a comparison of the diets of smokers and nonsmokers revealed that smokers consumed more energy. The diets of smokers were also higher in total fat, saturated fat, cholesterol, and alcohol and lower in polyunsaturated fat, fiber, vitamin C, vitamin E, and beta-carotene.[57] Smoking increases the risk of cardiovascular disease and lung cancer, and this dietary pattern can affect nutritional status and further increase the risk of developing heart disease and cancer. Because smoking increases the requirement for vitamin C, it is recommended that smokers consume an extra 35 mg/day.[58]

Web Menu For information about alcoholism and other drug addictions, go to the National Council on Alcoholism and Drug Dependence (NCADD) at www.ncadd.org/ or the National Institute on Drug Abuse at www.nida.nih.gov/.

C 62 00 00 00 00 00 31 60

C 62 00 00 00 00 00 31 61

Alcohol Use Although it is illegal to sell alcohol to adolescents, this is often the time of life when individuals first experiment with alcohol consumption. Alcoholic beverages are commonly available at teen social gatherings, and the peer pressure

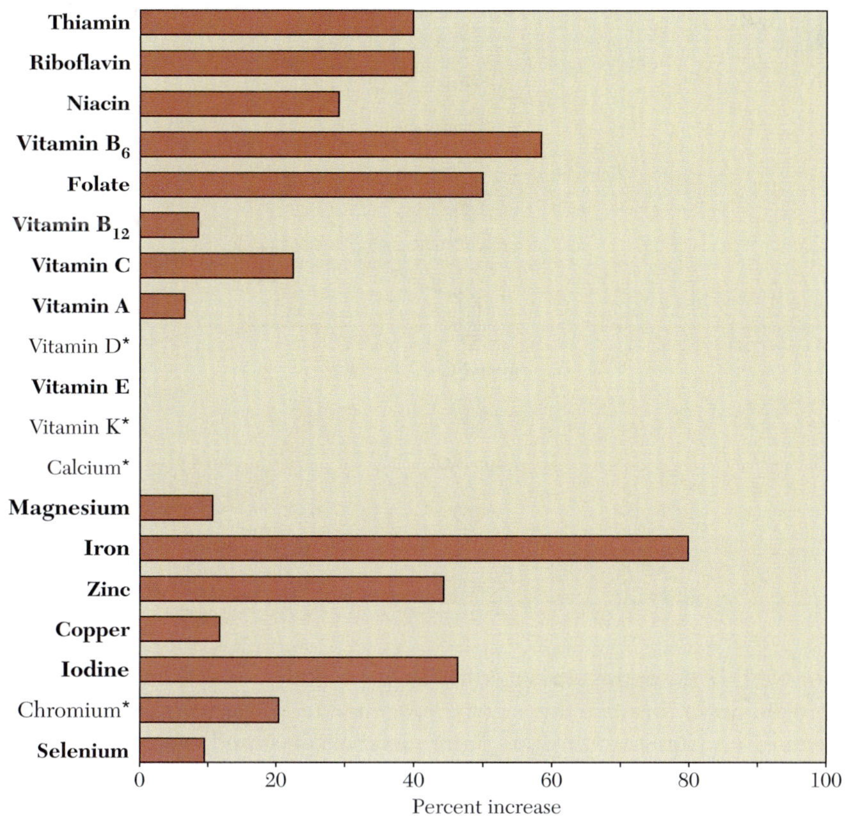

FIGURE 16.20 The needs for most micronutrients increase during pregnancy. The percentage increases in micronutrient needs above nonpregnant levels are shown here for a 14- to 18-year-old teen during pregnancy. Nutrients in bold are RDA values and those in plain text with an asterisk are AI values.

to consume them is strong. Surveys of American youth suggest that about 10.4 million Americans between the ages of 12 and 20 have had at least one drink during the previous month; of these, 6.8 million are **binge drinkers,** and 2.1 million are classified as **heavy drinkers.**[59]

Binge drinker Someone who consumes five or more drinks in a row on a single occasion.

Heavy drinker Someone who consumes five or more drinks per occasion on at least five different days.

Alcohol consumption can affect nutritional status as well as other aspects of health. It adds energy to the diet—7 kcalories per gram, and it is a drug that has effects that occur soon after ingestion and long-term health consequences that are associated with overuse.

Alcohol Absorption and Metabolism Alcohol is a small molecule that is rapidly and almost completely absorbed in the upper gastrointestinal tract. Small amounts are absorbed in the mouth and esophagus. Absorption continues in the stomach and the majority occurs in the small intestine. Because of this rapid absorption, the effects of alcohol consumption are almost immediate, especially if it is consumed on an empty stomach. If there is food in the stomach when alcohol is consumed, less will be absorbed there because less is in contact with the stomach wall. Food also slows stomach emptying and therefore decreases the rate at which alcohol enters the small intestine, where absorption is the most rapid. Some alcohol is metabolized by alcohol dehydrogenase in the stomach. Women tend to have less of this stomach enzyme, which may be one reason women become intoxicated after consuming less alcohol than men.

Absorbed alcohol travels to the liver via the portal circulation. Because alcohol is a toxin and cannot be stored in the body, it is metabolized before other molecules. In the first step of alcohol metabolism, it is converted to acetaldehyde by the liver enzyme alcohol dehydrogenase. Acetaldehyde is a toxic compound that is further degraded to a 2-carbon molecule that forms acetyl-CoA. These reactions release electrons and hydrogen ions that are picked up by NAD, producing NADH. Although these processes produce ATP, they also quickly reduce the amount of available NAD and increase the amount of NADH in the cell. The

FIGURE 16.21 The breakdown of alcohol by alcohol dehydrogenase releases hydrogen ions and electrons, which convert NAD to NADH. The accumulation of NADH slows the citric acid cycle so that little acetyl-CoA can enter and most is instead used for fat synthesis.

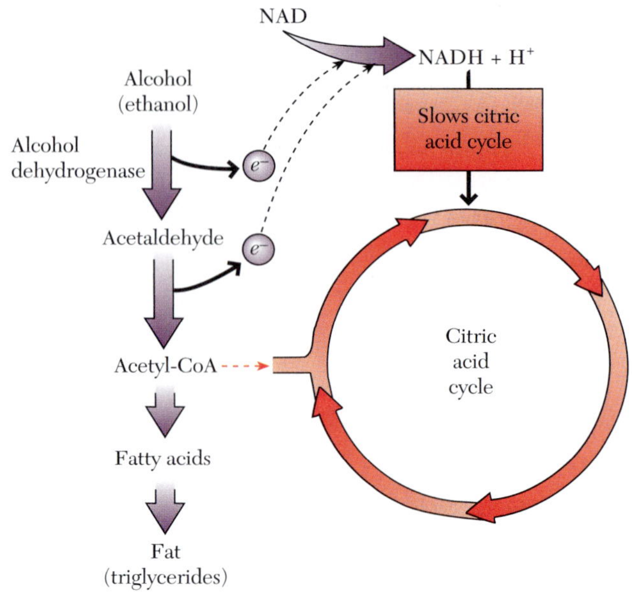

buildup of NADH slows the citric acid cycle, preventing acetyl-CoA from being further broken down. Instead, the acetyl-CoA generated by alcohol breakdown as well as acetyl-CoA from carbohydrate or fat metabolism is used to synthesize fatty acids that accumulate in the liver (Figure 16.21). Fat accumulation can be seen in the liver after only a single bout of heavy drinking.

Immediate Effects of Alcohol Consumption Depending on body size, amount of previous drinking, food intake, and general health, the liver can break down about 0.5 oz of alcohol per hour. This is the amount of alcohol that is considered one drink; it is the amount contained in 5 fluid ounces of wine, 12 fluid ounces of beer, or 1.5 fluid ounces of distilled liquor. When alcohol intake exceeds the ability of the liver to break it down, the excess circulates in the bloodstream until the liver enzymes can metabolize it. At the brain, alcohol acts as a depressant. First, it affects reasoning; if drinking continues, the vision and speech centers of the brain are affected. Next, large-muscle control becomes impaired, causing lack of coordination. Finally, the individual loses consciousness. If drinking were to continue, the anesthetic effects would suppress breathing and heart rate (Table 16.4). It is

TABLE 16.4 Effects of Alcohol on the Central Nervous System

Number of Drinks*	Blood Alcohol† (percent)	Effect on Central Nervous System
2	0.05	Impaired judgment, altered mood, relaxed inhibitions and tensions, increased heart rate
4	0.10	Impaired coordination, delayed reaction time, impaired peripheral vision
6	0.15	Unrestrained behavior, slurred speech, blurred vision, staggered gait
8	0.20	Double vision, inability to walk, lethargy
12	0.30	Stupor, confusion, coma
≥ 14	0.35 to 0.60	Unconsciousness, shock, coma, death

*Each drink contains 0.5 ounces of ethanol and is equivalent to 5 fluid ounces of wine, 12 fluid ounces of beer, or 1.5 fluid ounces of distilled liquor.

†Values represent blood alcohol within approximately one hour after consumption for a 150-pound individual. Actual blood alcohol values depend on the amount of alcohol in the beverage, the rate of consumption, foods consumed with the alcohol, gender, and body weight.

possible for an individual to drink fast enough for alcohol levels to continue to rise after he or she has lost consciousness, resulting in death. This can occur with binge drinking. Binge drinking is a problem on college campuses that causes about 50 deaths and hundreds of cases of alcohol poisoning annually. It is estimated that about 40% of college students "binge" on alcohol at least once during a two-week period.[59]

Alcohol is excreted by the kidney, where it acts as a diuretic, increasing fluid excretion. Therefore, excessive alcohol intake can cause dehydration. Some alcohol is also eliminated by the lungs. The amount lost through the lungs is predictable and reliable enough to be used to estimate blood alcohol level from a measure of breath alcohol. This is the basis of the Breathalyzer tests administered to determine if an individual is driving under the influence of alcohol.

Effects of Chronic Alcohol Use One risk associated with regular alcohol consumption is the possibility of addiction. The risk of addiction is increased in individuals who begin drinking at a younger age.[59] Alcohol addiction, like any other drug addiction, is a physiological problem that needs treatment. Alcoholism is believed to have a genetic component that makes some people more likely to become addicted, but environment also plays a significant role. Thus, someone with a genetic predisposition toward alcoholism whose peers do not consume alcohol is much less likely to become addicted.

Long-term excessive alcohol consumption has serious health implications. Alcohol either directly or indirectly affects every organ in the body and increases the risk of malnutrition and many chronic diseases. Alcohol contributes energy but few other nutrients and replaces more nutrient-dense energy sources in the diet. Alcohol damages the lining of the small intestine, decreasing the absorption of several B vitamins and vitamin C. Thiamin deficiency is a particular concern with chronic alcohol consumption. Alcohol can also alter the storage, metabolism, and excretion of other vitamins and some minerals.

The most significant physiological effects of chronic alcohol consumption occur in the liver. Alcoholic liver disease progresses in a number of phases. The first phase is **fatty liver,** a condition that occurs when alcohol consumption increases the synthesis and deposition of fat in the liver. The second phase, **alcoholic hepatitis,** is an inflammation of the liver. Both of these conditions are reversible if alcohol consumption is stopped and good nutritional and health practices are followed. If alcohol consumption continues, **cirrhosis** may develop. This is an irreversible condition in which fibrous deposits scar the liver and interfere with its function (Figure 16.22). Because the liver is the primary site of many metabolic reactions, cirrhosis is often fatal. In addition to causing liver disease, heavy drinking is associated with hypertension, heart disease, stroke, and other health problems (Table 16.5).

Fatty liver The accumulation of fat in the liver.

Alcoholic hepatitis Inflammation of the liver caused by alcohol consumption.

Cirrhosis Chronic liver disease characterized by the loss of functioning liver cells and the accumulation of fibrous connective tissue.

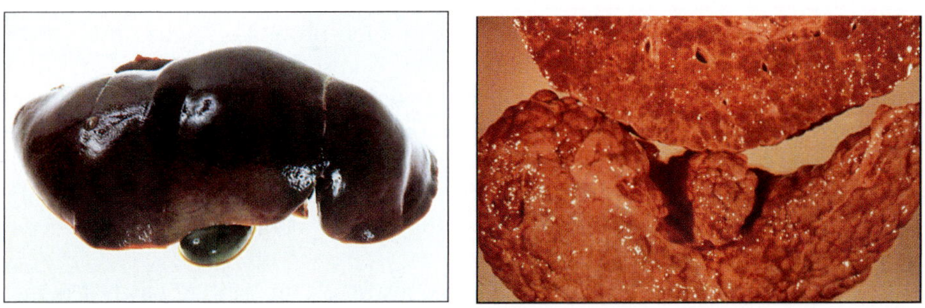

FIGURE 16.22 Chronic alcohol consumption can cause permanent liver damage. A normal liver is shown on the left, and a cirrhotic liver is shown on the right. *(left, Custom Medical Stock Photo; right, Phil Birn/Custom Medical Stock Photo)*

TABLE 16.5 Health Effects of Chronic Alcohol Use

Health Effect	Role of Alcohol
Birth defects	Increases the risk of fetal alcohol effects and fetal alcohol syndrome when consumed during pregnancy.
Gastrointestinal problems	Damages the lining of the stomach and small intestine, and contributes to the development of pancreatitis.
Liver disease	Causes fatty liver, alcoholic hepatitis, cirrhosis.
Malnutrition	Decreases nutrient absorption and alters the storage, metabolism, and excretion of some vitamins and minerals. Associated with a poor diet because alcohol replaces more nutrient-dense energy sources in the diet.
Neurological disorders	Contributes to impaired memory, dementia, and peripheral neuropathy.
Cardiovascular disorders	Associated with cardiovascular diseases such as cardiomyopathy, hypertension, arrhythmias, and stroke.
Blood disorders	Increases the risk of anemia and infection.
Immune function	Depresses the immune system and results in a predisposition to infectious diseases, including respiratory infections, pneumonia, and tuberculosis.
Cancer	Increases the risk for cancer, particularly of the upper digestive tract—including the esophagus, mouth, pharynx, and larynx—and of the liver, pancreas, breast, and colon.
Sexual dysfunction	Can lead to inadequate functioning of the testes and ovaries, resulting in hormonal deficiencies, sexual dysfunction, and infertility. It is also related to a higher rate of early menopause and a higher frequency of menstrual irregularities (duration, flow, or both).
Psychological disturbances	Causes depression, anxiety, and insomnia, and is associated with a higher incidence of suicide.
Mortality	Up to 40,000 deaths per year in the United States are alcohol-related.

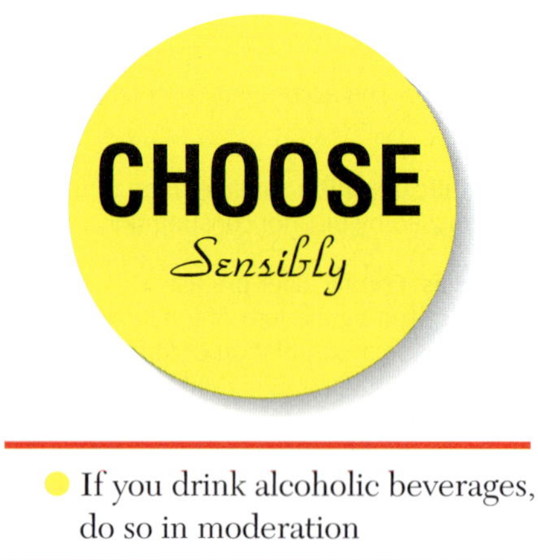
CHOOSE
Sensibly
If you drink alcoholic beverages, do so in moderation

FIGURE 16.23 The Dietary Guidelines for Americans recommend that alcohol be consumed in moderation. *(USDA, DHHS, 2000)*

Safe Drinking In general, the risk of developing chronic alcohol-related diseases is reduced if fewer than two drinks a day are consumed. Although moderate alcohol consumption is associated with a reduction in the risk of heart disease in some individuals, there are certain groups who should not drink, such as children, women who are pregnant or trying to conceive, alcoholics, individuals who plan to drive or engage in another activity that requires attention or skill, and individuals using prescription or over-the-counter medication (see Chapter 17, *Making Decisions:* "The Risks and Benefits of Alcohol Use in Adults").[12] Excess alcohol consumption, whether occasional or chronic, is hazardous to health. Individuals who do drink should not drink in excess (Figure 16.23). Because of the effects of alcohol on reaction time, eye-hand coordination, accuracy, and balance, alcohol should not be consumed before driving an automobile. Not only does alcohol impair one's ability to operate a motor vehicle, but it also impairs one's judgment in the decision to drive.

When alcohol is consumed, it should be consumed slowly with meals. Alcohol absorption is slowed when it is consumed with high-protein or high-carbohydrate foods. Also, the alcohol in an alcoholic punch is absorbed faster if mixed with a carbonated beverage than with a noncarbonated fruit-juice base. It usually takes an hour to metabolize the alcohol in one drink (0.5 oz), so no more than one drink should be consumed every 1.5 hours. Sipping, not gulping, allows the liver time to break down what has already been consumed. Alternating nonalcoholic and alcoholic drinks will also slow down the rate of alcohol intake and prevent dehydration.

Unfortunately, once alcohol has been consumed, the rate at which it is metabolized and eliminated from the body cannot be accelerated. Cold showers, brisk walks, and black coffee may help an individual to wake up, but will not sober them up.

Summary

1. Good nutrition in childhood sets the stage for nutrition and health in the adult years. The diet must meet the needs for growth and development as well as reduce the risk of chronic disease later in life.
2. Growth that follows standard patterns indicates adequate nutrition. Too little weight gain can signal malnutrition or other health problems. Too much weight gain can lead to obesity. Overweight and obesity among children are important health concerns. Obese children are likely to become obese adults and children who are overweight are more likely to have elevated blood pressure, blood glucose, and blood cholesterol.
3. Introducing solid foods between four and six months of age adds iron and other nutrients to the diet and aids in muscle development. Children like to have control over what they eat. In order to meet nutrient needs and develop nutritious habits, a variety of healthy foods should be offered at meals and snacks throughout the day.
4. Energy and protein needs per kilogram of body weight decrease as children grow, but total needs increase because of the increase in total body weight and activity level. Beginning at two years of age, fat intake should be decreased gradually to 30% or less of energy. Dietary carbohydrates should come primarily from whole grains, vegetables, fruits, and milk.
5. Low dietary intakes of vitamin A, vitamin C, calcium, iron, and zinc put some American children at risk of deficiencies.
6. During adolescence, accelerated growth and sexual maturation have an impact on nutrient requirements. Body composition and the nutritional requirements of boys and girls diverge. Males gain more lean body tissue, while females have a greater increase in body fat.
7. During the adolescent growth spurt, total energy and protein requirements are higher than at any other time of life. Young men require more protein and energy than young women.
8. In adolescence, vitamin and mineral requirements increase to meet the needs of rapid growth. The minerals calcium, iron, and zinc are likely to be low in the adolescent diet. Iron deficiency anemia is common, especially in girls as they begin losing iron through menstruation.
9. Dental caries is the most common nutritional disease in the United States.
10. Food allergies are caused by the absorption of allergens, most of which are proteins. Food allergies involve the immune system and are more common in infancy when the gastrointestinal tract is not fully mature and is therefore more likely to absorb whole proteins. An elimination diet and a food challenge can identify specific foods that cause allergies. Unlike food allergies, food intolerances do not involve the immune system. Newly introduced foods should be appropriate to the child's stage of development and offered one at a time to monitor for food allergies.
11. Lead is absorbed more efficiently in small children, so toxicity is of particular concern. Once inside the body, it interferes with nervous system function. Children who consume vegetarian diets are at risk for low intakes of iron, zinc, calcium, vitamin D, and vitamin B_{12}. Meals away from home at school or at fast-food restaurants are common and impact overall nutrient intake. The School Breakfast and Lunch Programs can improve the nutritional intake of students who participate.
12. Psychosocial changes occurring during the adolescent years make physical appearance of great concern. Obesity can be psychologically and socially devastating. Eating disorders are more common in adolescence than at any other time. Adolescent athletes can be influenced by nutrition misinformation, and they may try dangerous practices such as using anabolic steroids to increase muscle mass or following fad diets and using fluid restriction to lose weight.
13. Inactivity is an important factor contributing to the increased incidence of overweight among children and teens. It is recommended that children engage in some type of physical activity for at least an hour and up to several hours per day. Television introduces children to foods they might otherwise not be exposed to, promotes snacking, and reduces physical activity.
14. A pregnant teenager must meet nutrient needs for her own growth and development as well as for her pregnancy.
15. Alcohol has short-term effects on the central nervous system, including the impairment of reasoning, judgment, and coordination, and eventually the loss of consciousness. Chronic alcohol use damages the liver and can cause malnutrition by decreasing nutrient intake and absorption and interfering with nutrient utilization.

Review Questions

1. How does nutrient intake during childhood affect health later in life?
2. What is the best way to determine if a child is eating enough?
3. What impact does a child's BMI have on their future health?
4. What factors influence the maximum height that a child will reach?
5. When should solid and semisolid foods be introduced into an infant's diet?
6. How do the recommendations for fat intake change when a child reaches the age of two years?
7. Why is anemia a problem in young children? In teenage girls?
8. Why are snacks an important part of children's diets?
9. Why is breakfast important?
10. What is the adolescent growth spurt? How does it affect nutrient requirements?
11. Describe two physiological differences between males and females after puberty that affect their nutrient needs.
12. How can fast foods be incorporated into a healthy diet?
13. How should new foods be introduced to monitor for the development of food allergies?
14. Why are teenagers particularly susceptible to eating disorders?
15. How can alcohol consumption affect nutritional status?

Applying Critical Thinking Skills

Personal nutrition:

1. Assume you had a Big Mac, a small order of fries, and a 16-ounce cola for lunch.
   a. How many servings from each food group of the Food Guide Pyramid does this represent?
   b. List the numbers of additional servings from each food group that you would need to satisfy the daily recommendations of the Food Guide Pyramid.
   c. Select foods from each group to complete your intake for the day.
   d. Do the foods you selected meet the selection recommendations of the Food Guide Pyramid and your energy needs?
2. Use the Internet or a diet analysis computer program to look up the nutrient composition of your favorite fast-food meal.
   a. What is the percent of kcalories from carbohydrate in the meal? From fat?
   b. Compare the amount of energy, fat, protein, iron, calcium, vitamin C, and vitamin A in this meal to the recommended amounts of each for a person of your age and gender.

General nutrition issues:

1. The table here gives the height and weight measurements recorded for a girl from age six to age nine.

Age	Height (in.)	Weight (lb)
6	45	44
7	48	53
8	50	77
9	52	97

   a. Calculate her BMI at each age and plot these values on the BMI-for-age growth chart in Figure 16.1.
   b. What recommendations would you have about her weight?
2. What recommendations would you make for each of the following young athletes?
   a. Frank is a wrestler. His usual weight is just at the low end of a weight class and he wants to lose enough weight to be in the next lower class.
   b. Sam is a football player. He has been getting hit hard in the last few games and wants to bulk up. He is looking into taking supplements to speed up the process.
   c. Talia is a dancer who has recently gained a few pounds. Her coach notices that she no longer drinks or snacks during practice.

References

1. U.S. Department of Health and Human Services, Centers for Disease Control and Prevention, National Center for Health Statistics. CDC growth charts: United States. Advance Data, No. 314, June 8, 2000 (revised). Available online at **www.cdc.gov/growthcharts.** Accessed 28 Aug 2000.
2. American Dietetic Association. Position of the American Dietetic Association: dietary guidance for healthy children aged 2 to 11 years. J. Am. Diet. Assoc. 99:93–101, 1999.
3. Shumei, S., and Chumlea, W. Tracking of body mass index in children in relation to overweight in adulthood. Am. J. Clin. Nutr. 70:145S–148S, 1999.
4. Sinaiko, A. R., Donahue, R. P., Jacobs, D. R., et al. Relation of weight and rate of increase in weight during childhood and adolescence to body size, blood pressure, fasting insulin, and lipids in young adults. Circulation 99:1471–1476, 1999.
5. Daniels, S. R., Morrison, J. A., Sprecher, D. L., et al. Association of body fat distribution and cardiovascular risk factors in children and adolescents. Circulation 99:541–545, 1999.
6. Kennedy, E., and Goldberg, J. What are American children eating? Implications for public policy. Nutr. Rev. 53:111–126, 1995.
7. Nutrition and Health Promotion Program, International Life Sciences Institute. A survey of parents and children about physical activity patterns: key findings. September–October 1996. Available online at **http://www.ilsi.org/nhppress.html#2.** Accessed 11 Feb 2001.
8. American Diabetes Association. Type 2 diabetes in children and adolescents. Diabetes Care 23:381–386, 2000.
9. National Institute of Diabetes & Digestive & Kidney Diseases, National Institutes of Health, National Diabetes Information Clearinghouse. Fact Sheet on Diabetes Statistics. NIH Publication No. 98-3926, Nov. 1997; updated Feb. 1998. Available online at **http://www.niddk.nih.gov/health/diabetes/pubs/dmstats/dmstats.htm.** Accessed 27 Nov 2000.
10. Ernst, N., and Obarzanek, E. Child health and nutrition: obesity and high blood cholesterol. Prev. Med. 23:427–436, 1994.
11. Berenson, G. S., Wattigney, W. A., Srinivasan, S. R., and Radhakrishnamurthy, B. Rationale to study the early natural history of heart disease: the Bogalusa Heart Study. Am. J. Med. Sci. 310(suppl): 22S–28S, 1995.
12. U.S. Department of Agriculture and U.S. Department of Health and Human Services. *Nutrition and Your Health: Dietary Guidelines for Americans*, 5th ed. Home and Garden Bulletin No. 232. Hyattsville, Md.: U.S. Government Printing Office, 2000.
13. Obarzanek E., Kimm, S. Y., Barton, B. A., et al. Long-term safety and efficacy of a cholesterol-lowering diet in children with elevated low-density lipoprotein cholesterol: seven-year results of the Dietary Intervention Study in Children (DISC). Pediatrics 107:256–264, 2001.
14. Bao, W., Threefoot, S. A., Srinivasan, S. R., and Berenson, G. S. Essential hypertension predicted by tracking of elevated blood pressure from childhood to adulthood: the Bogalusa Heart Study. Am. J. Hypertens. 8:657–661, 1995.
15. Federal Interagency Forum on Child and Family Statistics. America's Children: Key National Indicators of Well-Being. Third annual report. Available online at **http://childstats.gov.** Accessed 13 Sept 2000.
16. Nahikian-Nelms, M. Influential factors of caregivers' behaviors at mealtime: a study of 24 child-care providers. J. Am. Diet Assoc. 97:505–509, 1997.

17. Lytle, L. In defense of a low-fat diet for healthy children. J. Am. Diet. Assoc. 100:39–41, 2000.
18. American Dietetic Association. Position of the American Dietetic Association: child and adolescent food and nutrition programs. J. Am. Diet. Assoc. 96:913–917, 1996.
19. Stang, J., Story, M. T., Harnack, L., et al. Relationships between vitamin and mineral supplement use, dietary intake and dietary adequacy among adolescents. J. Am. Diet. Assoc. 100:905–910, 2000.
20. Centers for Disease Control and Prevention. Recommendations to prevent and control iron deficiency in the United States. MMWR Morb. Mortal. Wkly. Rep. 47:1–29, 1998. Available online at **http://www.cdc.gov/mmwr/.** Accessed 10 Feb 2001.
21. Pollitt, E. Iron deficiency and educational deficiency. Nutr. Rev. 55:133–141, 1997.
22. Hingley, A. T. Preventing childhood poisoning. FDA Consumer 30:7–11, March 1996.
23. U.S. Food and Drug Administration. Iron-containing supplements and drugs: label warning statements and unit-dose packaging requirements. Federal Register, January 1997.
24. Kurtzweil, P. Labeling rules for young children's foods. FDA Consumer 29:14–18, March 1995.
25. Roberts, S. B., and Heyman, M. B. Micronutrient shortfalls in young children's diets: common, and owing to inadequate intakes both at home and at child care centers. Nutr. Rev. 58:27–29, 2000.
26. Food and Nutrition Board, Institute of Medicine. *Dietary Reference Intakes for Calcium, Phosphorus, Magnesium, Vitamin D, and Fluoride.* Washington, D.C.: National Academy Press, 1997.
27. Mitchell, M. K. *Nutrition Across the Life Span.* Philadelphia: W. B. Saunders, 1997.
28. Slyper, A. H. Childhood obesity, adipose tissue distribution and the pediatric practitioner. Pediatrics 102:1–4, 1998.
29. Food and Nutrition Board, Institute of Medicine. *Dietary Reference Intakes for Vitamin A, Vitamin K, Arsenic, Boron, Chromium, Copper, Iodine, Iron, Manganese, Molybdenum, Nickel, Silicon, Vanadium, and Zinc.* Washington, D.C.: National Academy Press, 2001.
30. U.S. Department of Agriculture, Agriculture Research Service, ARS Food Surveys Research Group. 1997 Results from USDA 1994–1996 CSFII and 1994–1996 Diet and Health Knowledge Survey. Available online at **http://www.bare.usda.gov/bhnrc/foodsurvey/home.htm.** Accessed 10 Feb 2001.
31. Calvo, M. S., and Park, Y. K. Changing phosphorus content of the U.S. diet: potential for adverse effect on bone. J. Nutr. 126:1168S–1180S, 1996.
32. Centers for Disease Control and Prevention. Youth risk behavior surveillance, United States, 1997. CDC Surveillance Summaries, August 14, 1998. MMWR Morb. Mortal. Wkly. Rep. 47:1–89, 1998. Available online at **http://www.cdc.gov//mmwr.** Accessed 10 Feb 2001.
33. Wolraich, M. L., Wilson, D. B., and White, J. W. The effect of sugar on behavior or cognition in children: a meta-analysis. JAMA 274:1617–1618, 1995.
34. Breakey, J. The role of diet and behavior in childhood. J. Paediatr. Child Health 33:190–194, 1997.
35. Chandra, R. K. Food hypersensitivities and allergic disease: a selective review. Am. J. Clin. Nutr. 66(suppl):526S–529S, 1997.
36. Farley, D. Dangers of lead still linger. FDA Consumer 32:16–21, January/February 1998.
37. Hammad, T. A., Sexton, M., and Langenberg, P. Relationship between blood lead and dietary iron intake in preschool children. Annals Epidemiol. 6:30–33, 1996.
38. Needleman, H. L., Reiss, J. A., Tobin, M. J., et al. Bone lead levels and delinquent behavior. JAMA 275:363–369, 1996.
39. Moss, M. E., Lanphear, B. P., and Auinger, P. Association of dental caries and blood lead levels. JAMA 281:2294–2298, 1999.
40. Fackelmann, K. Hypertension's lead connection: does low-level exposure to lead cause high blood pressure? Sci. News 149:382–383, 1996.
41. Update: blood lead levels—United States, 1991–1994. MMWR Morb. Mortal. Wkly. Rep. 46:141–146, 1997.
42. Kaufman, L., Springen, K., Rogers, A., and Gordon, J. Children of the corn. Newsweek:60–62, August 28, 1995.
43. Curcio, B. A. For college students, bulgur beats burgers. Eating Well: 21, September/October 1995.
44. U.S. Department of Agriculture Nutrition Program Facts: National School Lunch Program: Q's and A's on the National School Lunch Program. Available online at **http://www.usda.gov/fcs/cnp/school%7e2htm.** Accessed 11 Feb 2001.
45. Andersen, R. E., Crespo, C. J., Bartlett, S. J., et al. Relationship of physical activity and television watching with body weight and level of fatness among children: results from the third National Health and Nutrition Examination Survey. JAMA 279:938–942, 1998.
46. Sylvester, G. P., Achterberg, C., and Williams, J. Children's television and nutrition: friends or foes? Nutrition Today 30:6–15, February 1995.
47. Neumark-Sztainer, D., Story, M., Resnick, M. D., and Blum, R. W. Adolescent vegetarianism: a behavioral profile of a school-based population in Minnesota. Arch. Pediatr. Adolesc. Med. 151:833–838, 1997.
48. American Dietetic Association. Timely statement of the American Dietetic Association: nutrition guidance for adolescent athletes in organized sports. J. Am. Diet. Assoc. 96:611–612, 1996.
49. Terjung, R. L., Clarkson, P., Eichner, E. R., et al. American College of Sports Medicine roundtable: the physiological and health effects of oral creatine supplementation. Med. Sci. Sports Exerc. 32:706–717, 2000.
50. Oler, S. M. Creatine is an ergogen for anaerobic exercise. Nutr. Rev. 55:21–25, 1997.
51. Beals, K. A., and Manore, M. M. Nutritional status of female athletes with subclinical eating disorders. J. Am. Diet. Assoc. 98:419–425, 1998.
52. Bazzarre, T. L. Nutrition and strength. In *Nutrition in Exercise and Sport,* 3rd ed. Wolinski, I., ed. Boca Raton, Fla.: CRC Press, 1998, 369–419.
53. Green, T. J., Houghton, L. A., Donovan, U., et al. Oral contraceptives did not affect biochemical folate indexes and homocysteine concentrations in adolescent females. J. Am. Diet. Assoc. 98:49–54, 1998.
54. Food and Nutrition Board, Institute of Medicine, *Dietary Reference Intakes for Thiamin, Riboflavin, Niacin, Vitamin B-6, Folate, Vitamin B-12, Pantothenic Acid, Biotin, and Choline.* Washington, D.C.: National Academy Press, 1998.
55. Trends in cigarette smoking among high school students—United States, 1991–1999. MMWR Morbidity and Mortality Weekly Report 49:755–758, 2000.
56. Crisp, A. H., Halek, C., Sedgewick, P., et al. Smoking and pursuit of thinness in schoolgirls in London and Ottawa. Postgrad. Med. J. 74:473–479, 1998.
57. Dallongville, J., Marecaus, N., Fruchart, J. C., and Amouyel, P. Cigarette smoking is associated with unhealthy patterns of nutrient intake: a meta-analysis. J. Nutr. 128:1450–1457, 1998.
58. Food and Nutrition Board, Institute of Medicine. *Dietary Reference Intakes for Vitamin C, Vitamin E, Selenium, and Carotenoids.* Washington, D.C.: National Academy Press, 2000.
59. National Council on Alcoholism and Drug Dependence (NCADD) Youth, alcohol and other drugs. Available online at **http://www.ncadd.org/facts/youthalc.html.** Accessed 24 Apr 2001.

17 Nutrition and Aging

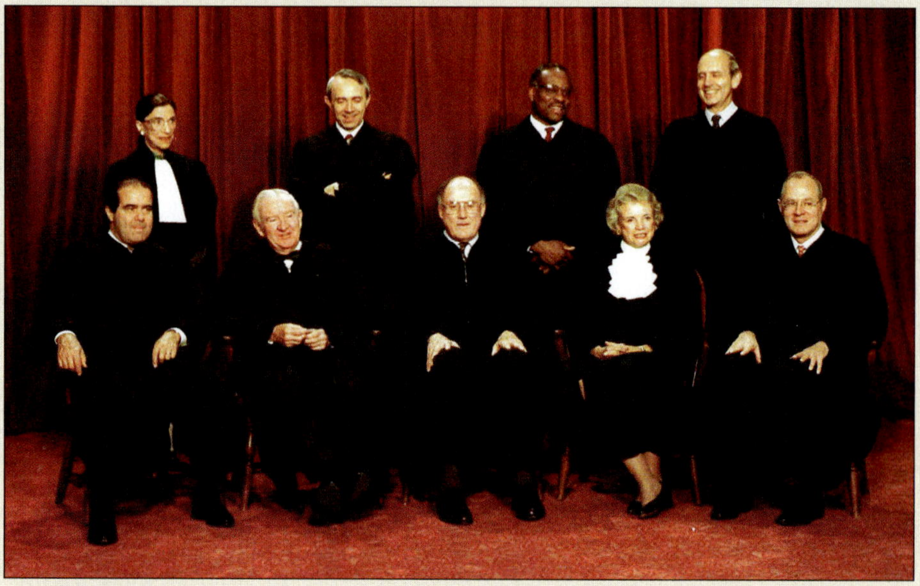

Learning Objectives

After reading this chapter, students should be able to:

1. Define aging and discuss its causes.
2. Explain what is meant by compression of morbidity.
3. List the normal physiological changes that can affect nutritional status.
4. Explain how the nutrient needs of older adults can be affected by their increased frequency of disease and use of medications.
5. Give an example of how diseases that affect mobility or mental status could affect nutrient intake.
6. Explain how the social and economic changes that often occur with increasing age affect the risk of malnutrition.
7. Explain how exercise and a nutritious diet affect the degenerative changes of aging.
8. Compare the nutrient needs of older adults to those of young adults.
9. List nutrients that may need to be supplemented in the diets of older adults.
10. Describe a federal program designed to help older adults meet nutrient needs.

Min has always taken good care of herself. She wants to stay healthy to enjoy and take care of her family. Now at 79 years of age, she is no longer doing such a good job. Min has been living alone for the past year since her husband died. Right after he died, her family spent a lot of time with her. Her daughter or grandchildren visited almost daily, bringing her groceries, helping her cook, or sharing a meal or snack with her. Her son, who lives farther away, visited several times a month to take her out to eat or to the theater. But a few months ago, her daughter moved out of state with her husband and now can no longer visit regularly. Her grandchildren still visit, but not as often. Now Min eats alone. She hates to cook for one person so she often has cereal or a cheese sandwich for dinner. She likes fresh vegetables but won't buy them anymore because they go to waste so quickly.

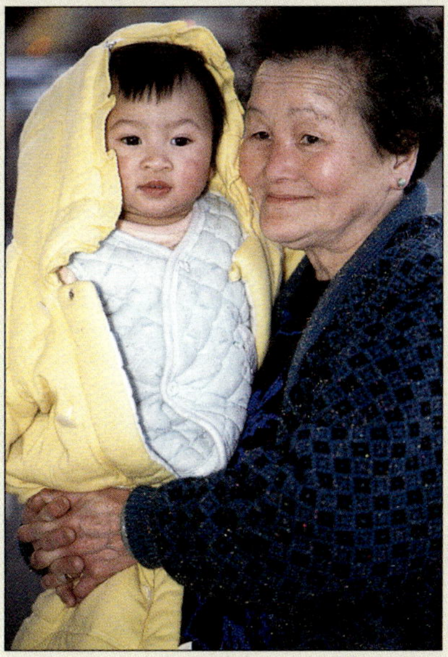

Other aspects of her lifestyle have also changed. She used to walk every morning with her friends, but during the year that her husband was ill, she wasn't comfortable leaving him alone, so she stopped this social exercise. She walked once with her friends a few weeks ago but was embarrassed that she could no longer keep up with them. She has gained a few pounds and is tired all the time. At her last doctor's visit, both her blood pressure and her blood sugar were slightly elevated.

Min knows she should take better care of herself, but depression and loneliness have made it difficult. The birth of her first great-grandchild has finally helped Min reconnect with her family and with the need to take care of herself. She calls an old friend to tell her that she is a great-grandmother and her friend invites her to join her at the local senior center. She soon finds that she is attending the seniors' exercise class regularly and has also signed up for several other activities. She now has more energy and has lost a few pounds. She joins friends for meals at the senior center three times a week, and on Sundays she and one or two friends go out to a restaurant.

What Is Aging?

Aging A process that occurs over a lifetime that is associated with and responsible for an ever-increasing susceptibility to disease and death.

Biologically, **aging** is not something that begins at age 55, 65, or 75; it is a process that begins with conception and continues throughout life. It can be defined as the inevitable accumulation of changes over time associated with and responsible for an ever-increasing susceptibility to disease and death. Although universal to all living things, aging is a process we don't fully understand. We do know that our genetic makeup and the environment and lifestyle in which we spend our years affect both how long we live and how long we remain healthy.

Web Menu: For public health data and statistical information on older adults, go to the Federal Interagency Forum on Aging-Related Statistics at www.agingstats.gov/ or the National Center for Health Statistics at www.cdc.gov/nchs/.

A Growing Population

Currently 13% of the population of the United States is age 65 and older; within the next 50 years, one out of every five people will be over 65 (Figure 17.1). The fastest-growing segment of the population in the industrialized nations is the oldest old—individuals age 85 and older (Table 17.1).[1]

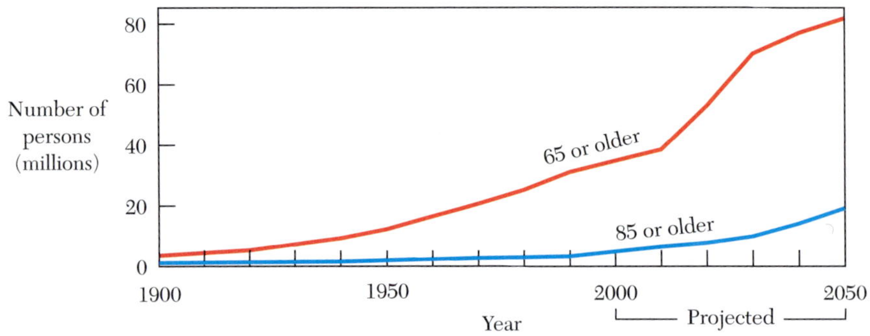

FIGURE 17.1 This graph illustrates the increase over the last century in the total number of persons age 65 or older and 85 or older. Data for the years 2000 to 2050 are based on projections of the population and indicate that in the next few decades there will be almost 80 million people in the United States who are 65 or older. *(U.S. Census Bureau, Decennial Census Data and Population Projections. Available online at* http://www.agingstats.gov.*)*

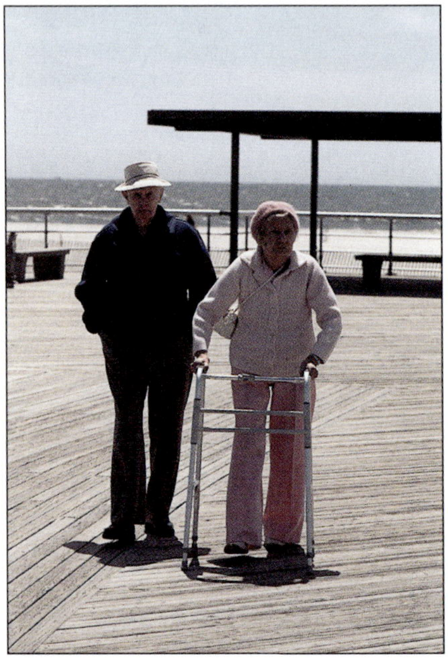

FIGURE 17.2 The diversity of health and abilities is greater in the elderly than among other age groups. *(© Larry Mulvehill/Photo Researchers, Inc.)*

Life span The maximum age to which members of a species can live.

Life expectancy The average length of life for a population of individuals.

Compression of morbidity The postponement of the onset of chronic disease such that disability occupies a smaller and smaller proportion of the life span.

Successful Aging

There is great diversity among older adults. There are 70-year-olds riding bicycles and others in wheelchairs. Some are healthy, independent, and engaged in their communities, while others are chronically ill, dependent, and at high risk for malnutrition (Figure 17.2). Keeping older adults healthy, referred to as successful aging, is a major public health goal in the United States; it has been called one of the greatest social challenges of the next century.[2,3] It will benefit not only aging individuals but also their family members, who must find the time and resources to care for them, and the public health programs designed to meet their needs.

Life Expectancy The maximum age to which humans can live, or **life span,** is about 100 to 120 years. But, most individuals do not live this long. The average length of time that an individual can be expected to live, or **life expectancy,** varies between and within populations. In the United States in 1900, when many children died of childhood illnesses, life expectancy was only 50 years, but today, with advances in technology and improved nutrition and health care, the average is over 76 years.[4] However, even though average life expectancy in the United States is over 76 years, the average *healthy* life expectancy is only about 64 years. Disease and disability, which become more and more common with advancing age, often restrict the last 12 years of life.[3]

The goal of successful aging is to increase not only life expectancy but also the number of years of healthy life that an individual can expect. This is referred to as **compression of morbidity.** It can be achieved by slowing the biological changes that accumulate over time and postponing the diseases of aging long enough to approach or reach the limits of life span before any symptoms appear (Figure 17.3). Nutrition is an important lifestyle factor for successful aging because of its impact on health, self-sufficiency, and the quality of life in older adults.[5]

Nutrition and the Compression of Morbidity Nutrition plays a major role in the compression of morbidity because many of the diseases that are major causes of disability in older adults—cardiovascular disease, hypertension, diabetes, cancer,

TABLE 17.1 Common Age-Group Definitions

Term	Definition
Approaching old age	Individuals 55 to 64 years of age
Older adult	Individuals 65 years of age and older
Young old	Individuals ages 65 to 74
Old	Individuals ages 75 to 84
Oldest old	Individuals 85 years of age and older

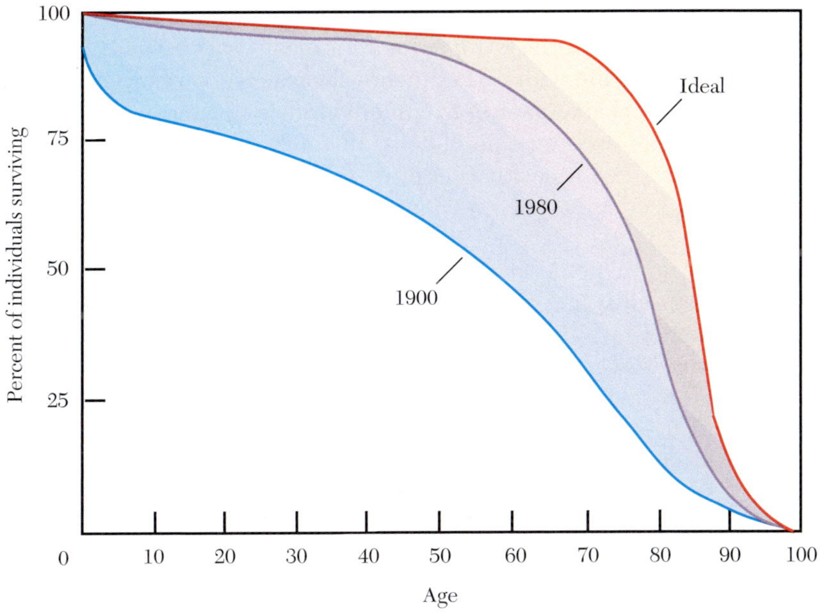

FIGURE 17.3 This graph illustrates the effect of compression of morbidity on survival in a population; the steeper the curve, the greater the compression of morbidity. The decline in deaths from infectious diseases between 1900 and 1980 allowed more people to survive into adulthood. Delaying the onset of chronic diseases will allow more people to remain healthy and survive into their seventies and eighties. *(Adapted from Fries, J. F. Aging, natural death, and the compression of morbidity. N. Engl. J. Med. 303:130–135, 1980.)*

and osteoporosis—are nutrition-related. A healthy diet will not necessarily prevent these diseases, but it may slow the changes that accumulate over time, postponing the onset of disease symptoms. As discussed in Chapters 5 and 14, the risk of developing cardiovascular disease can be decreased by exercise and a diet low in saturated fat and cholesterol and high in whole grains, fruits, and vegetables. As discussed in Chapters 4, 7, and 14, the risks and complications of diabetes are reduced by maintaining a healthy weight and exercising regularly. And as discussed in Chapter 11, hypertension may be reduced by consuming a diet moderate in sodium and high in fruits, vegetables, and low-fat dairy products. As discussed in Chapter 12, osteoporosis may be prevented by adequate calcium intake and exercise throughout life. And, as discussed throughout this text, the likelihood of developing certain types of cancer can be reduced by consuming a diet low in fat and high in whole grains, vegetables, and fruits.

Diet, Lifestyle, and Longevity The discovery of areas of the world where inhabitants supposedly lived to a very old age generated hope that specific foods could extend life. Although the elderly in these regions are now believed to be no older than individuals throughout the rest of the world, they do remain healthier.[6] They are not overweight, hypertension is rare, and the incidence of both heart disease and osteoporosis is low. No one food has been determined to be common among these people, but there are a number of lifestyle similarities: All are societies in which people are physically active, consume largely vegetarian diets, and provide strong psychosocial support for the elderly. This suggests that although life span is not extended by changes in lifestyle, the physiological changes, nutritional problems, and chronic illness common in old age can be postponed by a healthy diet and lifestyle.

What Causes Aging?

As organisms become older, the number of cells they have decreases and the ability of the remaining cells to function declines. As tissues and organs lose cells and cell function, the ability of the organism to perform the physiological functions necessary to maintain homeostasis decreases; disease becomes increasingly common and the risk of malnutrition increases. This loss of cells and cell function occurs throughout life, but the effects are not felt for many years because humans and other organisms begin life with extra functional capacity, or **reserve capacity.** Reserve capacity allows an organism to continue functioning normally despite a decrease in the number and function of cells. In young adults, the reserve capacity of organs is four to ten times that required to sustain life. As a person ages and reserve capacity decreases, the effects of aging become evident in all body systems.[7]

Reserve capacity The amount of functional capacity that an organ has above and beyond what is needed to sustain life.

There are two major hypotheses to explain why aging occurs. One favors the idea of a genetic clock and argues that the cell death associated with aging is a genetically-programmed event. The other views the events of aging as the result of cellular wear and tear. The actual cause of the cell death associated with aging is probably some combination of both of these, and the rate at which cell death occurs and at which aging proceeds is determined by the interplay among genetics, environment, and lifestyle.

Programmed Cell Death

The hypothesis that cell death is triggered when genes that disrupt cell function are activated, causing the selective, orderly death of individual cells or groups of cells, is referred to as **programmed cell death.**[8] This hypothesis is supported by the fact that cells grown in the laboratory divide only a certain number of times before they die. Cells from older individuals will divide fewer times than those from younger individuals, and those from longer-lived species will divide more times than those from shorter-lived species. If cells in an organism stop reproducing and continue to die, the total number of cells will decline, resulting in a loss of organ function.

Programmed cell death The death of cells at specific, predictable times.

Wear and Tear

The second hypothesis suggests that aging is the result of an accumulation of cellular damage. This wear and tear may result from errors in DNA synthesis, increases in glucose levels, or damage caused by free radicals. Free radicals cause oxidative damage to proteins, lipids, carbohydrates, and DNA, and may also indirectly harm cells by producing toxic products. For example, age spots—brown spots that appear on the skin with age—are caused by the oxidation of lipids, which produces a pigment called lipofuscin, or age pigment. The damage done to cells by free radicals is associated with aging and has been implicated in the development of a number of chronic diseases common among the aging, including cardiovascular disease and cancer.

Genetics, Environment, and Lifestyle

The rate at which the changes associated with aging accumulate depends on genetics, environment, and lifestyle. Genes determine the efficiency with which cells are maintained and repaired. Individuals with less cellular repair capacity will lose cells faster, and consequently will age, more quickly. Likewise, genes determine susceptibility to age-related diseases such as cardiovascular disease and cancer. However, individuals who inherit a low capacity to repair cellular damage may live long lives if they are not exposed to factors that damage cells and if they eat well and exercise regularly. In contrast, individuals with exceptional cellular repair ability may still experience rapid cell damage if they smoke cigarettes, consume a diet high in fat and low in antioxidant nutrients, and live sedentary lives. Thus, no matter what individuals' genes predict about how long they will live, their actual longevity is also affected by lifestyle factors and the extent to which they are able avoid accidents and disease (Figure 17.4).

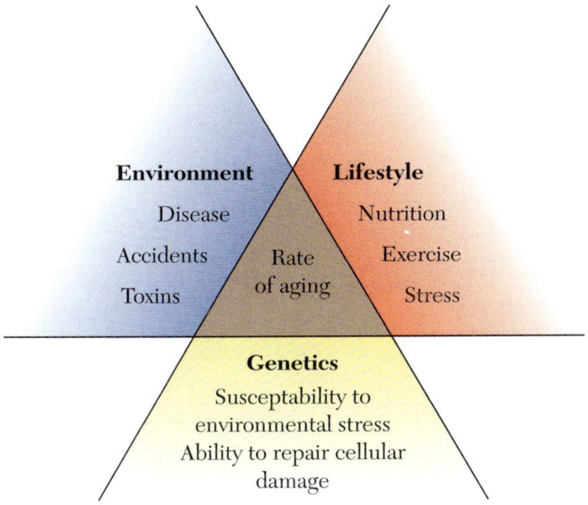

FIGURE 17.4 The rate at which an individual ages is affected by their genetic makeup, the environment in which they live, and the lifestyle choices they make.

Nutrition and the Aging Process

The physiological changes that occur with age can affect nutritional status. Although aging itself does not cause malnutrition in healthy, active adults, nutritional health can be compromised by conditions that become increasingly common with advancing age (see Table 17.2).[9] For example, both the increased frequency of disease with age and the resulting increase in the use of medications can affect nutritional status. Likewise, there are social and economic changes common in older adults that increase the risk of **food insecurity** and, consequently, malnutrition (Figure 17.5).

Food insecurity An inability to acquire appropriate foods in a socially acceptable way.

Table 17.2 Factors That Increase the Risk of Malnutrition Among the Elderly

Reduced intake due to:
Decreased appetite, which may be caused by lack of exercise, depression, or social isolation
Changes in taste, smell, and vision
Dental problems
Limitations in mobility
Medications that restrict mealtimes or affect appetite
Lack of money to buy food
Lack of nutrition knowledge

Reduced absorption and utilization due to:
Gastrointestinal changes
Medications that affect absorption
Diseases such as diabetes, kidney disease, alcoholism, and gastrointestinal disease

Increased requirements due to:
Illness with fever or infection
Injury or surgery

Increased losses due to:
Medications that increase nutrient excretion
Diseases such as gastrointestinal and kidney disease

FIGURE 17.5 The causes and consequences of malnutrition in the elderly are linked.

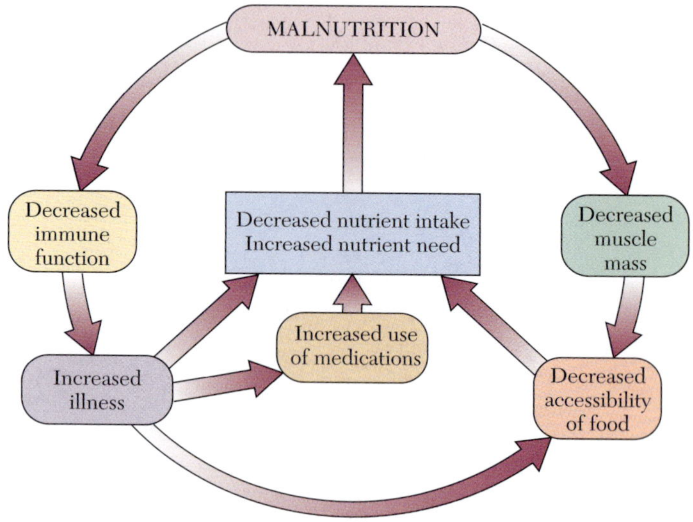

Physiological Changes

It is difficult to determine which of the changes that occur with aging are inevitable consequences of the aging process and which are the effect of disease states. Whether caused by disease or the inescapable loss of cells and cell function, the changes that occur in the functional capacity of organs and organ systems can affect nutritional status by affecting the appeal of food, digestion and absorption, nutritional requirements, and the ability to obtain food.

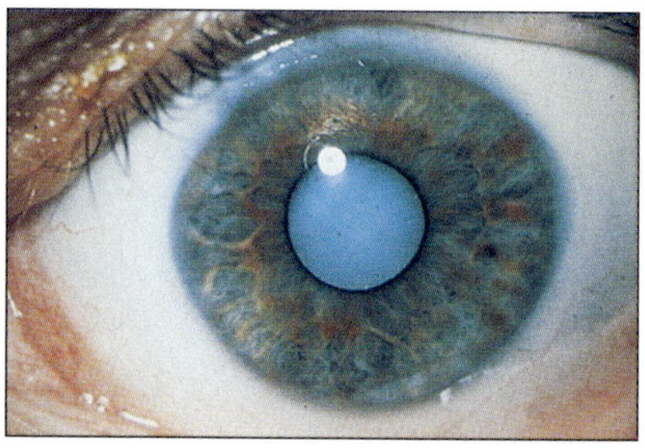

FIGURE 17.6 Cataracts cause the lens of the eye to become cloudy and impair vision. *(© Science VU/Visuals Unlimited)*

For information and resources related to macular degeneration, go to the Macular Degeneration Foundation at www.eyesight.org/ and the National Eye Institute at www.nei.nih.gov/.

Macular degeneration A progressive degeneration of the central portion of the retina, causing gradual loss of central vision.

Cataracts A disease of the eye that results in cloudy spots on the lens (and sometimes the cornea) that obscure vision.

Sensory Changes Beginning at around age 60, there is a progressive decline in the ability to taste and smell that becomes more severe in persons over 70. The decline of these senses can contribute to impaired nutritional status by decreasing both the appeal and the enjoyment of food.[10] Some studies suggest that the decline in taste acuity is due to a reduction in the number of taste buds on the tongue; others suggest that it is the result of changes in sensitivity to specific flavors such as salty and sweet.[11] The sense of smell is important because odors provide important clues to food acceptability before food enters the mouth. Once in the mouth, some molecules reach the nasal cavity, where their odor is detected. It is the blending of the odor message from the nasal cavity and the taste message from the tongue that provides the overall food flavor. When the sense of smell is diminished, food is not as flavorful. Changes in taste and smell have also been related to a greater intake of sweet foods among older adults.[11]

Vision also typically declines with age, making shopping for and preparation of food difficult. **Macular degeneration** is the most common cause of blindness in older Americans. The macula is a small area of the retina of the eye that distinguishes fine detail. With age, oxidative damage reduces the number of viable cells in the macula. As the macula degenerates, visual acuity declines, ultimately resulting in blindness. **Cataracts** are another common reason for declining sight. Of people who live to age 85, half will have cataracts that impair vision (Figure 17.6).

Gastrointestinal Changes Aging causes changes in the gastrointestinal tract and its accessory organs that may alter the palatability as well as the digestion of food and the absorption of nutrients. One change is a decrease in the secretion of saliva into the mouth. Saliva mixes with food to allow it to be tasted and to provide lubrication for easy swallowing. A reduction in the amount of saliva causes dryness, which decreases the taste of food and makes swallowing difficult. Saliva is also an important defense against tooth decay because it contains substances that kill bacteria and it helps wash material away from the teeth. Thus, a dry mouth increases the likelihood of tooth decay and **periodontal disease.** Loss of teeth and improperly fitting dentures also limit food choices and can contribute to poor nutrition in the elderly.

Periodontal disease A degeneration of the area surrounding the teeth, specifically the gum and supporting bone.

Aging may delay stomach emptying and cause changes in gastric secretions. Delayed stomach emptying can reduce hunger and, therefore, nutrient intake.[11] Reduced gastric secretions can affect the absorption of some nutrients. It is estimated that 10 to 30% of American adults over age 50 and 40% of those into their 80s have **atrophic gastritis,** an inflammation of the stomach lining that is characterized by a decrease in the secretion of stomach acid.[12,13] Reduced stomach acid secretion allows microbial overgrowth in the stomach and small intestine.[12,14] Increased populations of microbes in the gut compete with absorption for the available vitamin B_{12}. In addition, when stomach acid is reduced, the enzymes that release vitamin B_{12} from food do not function properly and food-bound vitamin B_{12} cannot be absorbed. Atrophic gastritis may also affect the absorption of iron, folate, calcium, and vitamin K in older adults.[13]

Atrophic gastritis An inflammation of the stomach lining that causes a reduction in stomach acid and allows bacterial overgrowth.

With age there is also a reduction in digestive enzymes from the pancreas and small intestine, but there is enough reserve capacity that this decrease rarely impairs digestion and absorption. There are functional changes in the colon—including decreased motility and elasticity, weakened abdominal and pelvic muscles, and decreased sensory perception—that can lead to constipation. Low fiber and fluid intakes and lack of activity also contribute to constipation. Although constipation occurs in about the same frequency in all age groups,[15] it is estimated that 20 to 30% of individuals over age 65 are dependent on laxatives.[16] Exercising regularly and consuming adequate fluid and fiber are safer ways to prevent constipation.

Changes in Other Organs Age-related changes in other organs may affect nutrient metabolism. Most absorbed nutrients travel from the intestine to the liver for metabolism or storage. The liver has a greater regenerative capacity than most organs, but with age, there is a decrease in liver size and blood flow and an increase in fat accumulation, all of which eventually decrease the liver's ability to metabolize nutrients and break down drugs and alcohol. With age, the pancreas may become less responsive to blood glucose levels, and the body cells may become more resistant to insulin, resulting in diabetes. Changes in the heart and blood vessels reduce blood flow to the kidneys, making waste removal less efficient. The kidneys themselves become smaller, and their ability to filter blood and to excrete the products of protein breakdown declines.[17] In some individuals blood urea levels may increase if protein intake is too high. The kidney's ability to concentrate urine also decreases with age, as does the sensation of thirst, increasing the risk of dehydration.[17]

Changes in Body Weight and Composition Many individuals gain weight as they get older—most gaining more than 10 pounds after adult height is attained.[18] Increases in body weight tend to occur during a person's twenties, thirties, and forties. Then, after age 65, it is more common for individuals to lose weight. In adults under 50 years of age, the increase in body fat that accompanies weight gain increases the risk of chronic disease, but the risks associated with excess body fat are lower for older adults.[19,20]

In addition to changes in total body weight, aging is accompanied by an increase in body fat, especially in the visceral/abdominal area, and a decrease in lean tissue, including a loss in muscle mass and strength and a decrease in bone

FIGURE 17.7 (a) In most individuals, the proportion of muscle mass decreases and body fat increases with age. *(Adapted from Cohen, S. H., et al. Compartmental body composition based on the body nitrogen, potassium, and calcium. Am. J. Physiol. 239:192–200, 1980.)* (b) Magnetic resonance image of a thigh cross section from a 25-year-old man (*left*) and a 65-year-old man (*right*). The thighs are of similar size, but the thigh from the older man has a greater amount of fat (shown in white) around and through the muscle, indicating significant muscle loss. *(S. A. Jubrias and K. E. Conley, University of Washington Medical Center)*

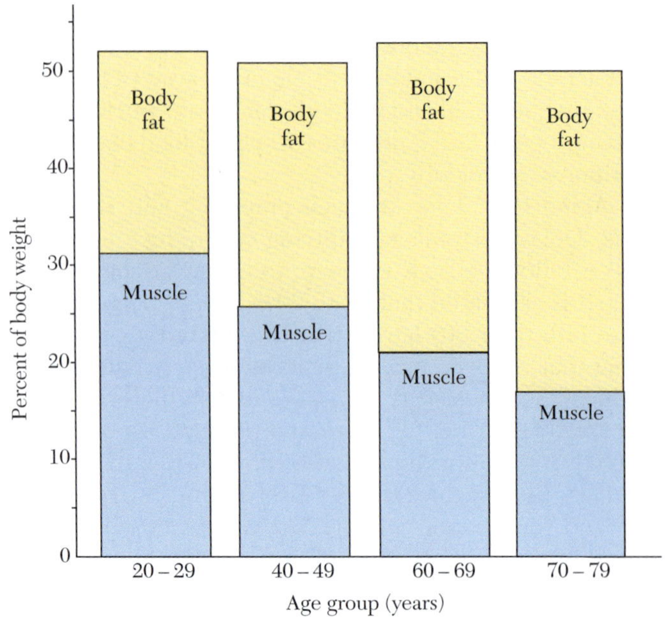

(a)

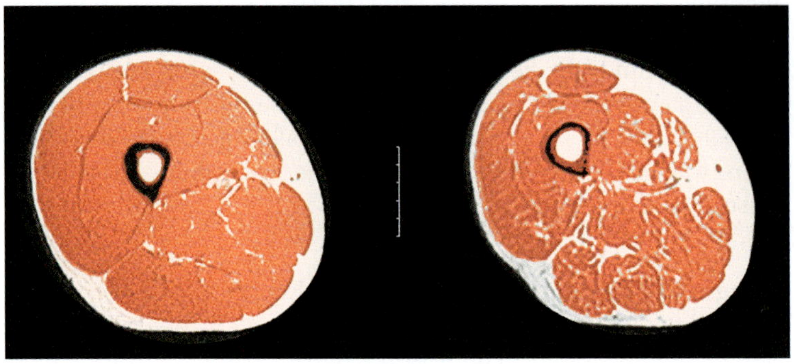
(b)

density (Figure 17.7).[21] This change in body composition occurs even if total body weight remains constant. The decline in muscle size and strength affects both the skeletal muscles needed to move the body and the heart and respiratory muscles needed to deliver oxygen to the tissues. Therefore, both strength and endurance are decreased, making the tasks of day-to-day life more difficult. The changes in muscle strength contribute to physical frailty, which is characterized by general weakness, impaired mobility and balance, and poor endurance. Both muscle weakness and loss of bone mass increase the risk of falls and fractures. In the oldest old, loss of muscle strength becomes the limiting factor in the ability to continue to live independently.

Exercise Some of the reduction in muscle strength and mass that occurs with age is due to changes in hormone levels and in muscle protein synthesis, but a lack of exercise is also an important contributor.[22] A recent survey showed that 40% of adults over the age of 65 are sedentary—that is, they participated in no leisure-time physical activity during a two-week period.[23]

Regular exercise can help maintain muscle mass, bone strength, and cardiorespiratory function and can increase energy needs.[24] For example, when John Glenn returned to space at age 77, exercise training helped his body handle the rigors of space as well as men half his age (Figure 17.8).

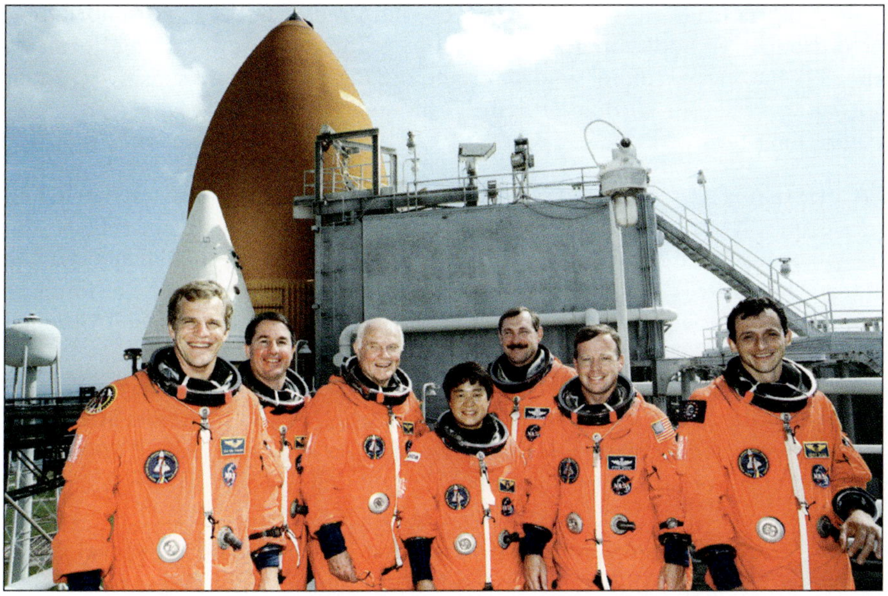

FIGURE 17.8 Exercise helped 77-year-old John Glenn endure the rigors of space flight just as well as his younger crewmates. *(NASA)*

Energy Restriction Laboratory studies in animals have found that a diet deficient in energy can slow aging and extend life span.[25] By restricting the food intake of rats and mice to 50 to 70% of that typically consumed, age-associated longevity is increased, physiological deterioration is retarded, and in some cases age-associated diseases are prevented. This effect has not been demonstrated in humans. In humans, a stable body weight is a sign of good health. Extreme thinness or unintentional weight loss is a health risk, especially among older adults.[26]

Hormonal Changes It has been hypothesized that declining levels of some hormones play a role in the aging process. There are decreases in insulin, growth hormone, dehydroepiandosterone (DHEA), melatonin, estrogen, testosterone, and other hormones. Some of these hormonal changes are partially responsible for the changes in body composition discussed earlier.

Insulin One of the most common hormone-related changes that occurs with aging is elevated blood glucose. This is due to both a decrease in the amount of insulin released by the pancreas and a decrease in insulin sensitivity at the tissues. This decreased insulin sensitivity is related to poor diet, inactivity, increased abdominal fat mass, and decreased lean mass. About 40% of individuals between the ages of 65 and 74 and 50% of those over 80 have type 2 diabetes, and about half of these cases are undiagnosed.[21]

Growth Hormone Growth hormone stimulates growth and protein synthesis; its levels gradually decline with age in both men and women. Many of the age-related changes in body composition (decrease in lean body mass and increase in body fat), blood lipid levels, and aerobic capacity resemble the symptoms of an abnormal condition known as adult growth hormone deficiency. This similarity has led to speculation that normal decreases in growth hormone levels are partially responsible for these age-related changes and that restoring growth hormone to levels seen in younger adults may be beneficial in normal aging. Controlled clinical trials, however, have not supported the benefits of replacing growth hormone.[27] Growth hormone administration does have effects on body composition, but when growth hormone administration was compared to a program of resistance exercises, the resulting increases in muscle mass, muscle protein synthesis, and muscle strength were not greater in the growth hormone-treated group.[28] In addition, growth hormone administration has side effects, including edema, carpal tunnel syndrome, and decreases in insulin sensitivity, and it is not known whether chronic growth hormone treatment affects cancer risk or has other long-term risks.[29]

DHEA DHEA is a precursor to sex hormones such as testosterone, estrogen, and progesterone. Even though low levels of this hormone are not known to be the cause of age-associated disorders, DHEA supplements are available over the counter. Their use is promoted to strengthen bones, muscles, and the immune system, and to prevent diabetes, obesity, heart disease, and cancer. Although some of these effects have been demonstrated when DHEA is administered to animals, beneficial effects of DHEA supplementation in humans have not been clearly established.[30] In addition, it is not clear whether the increases in sex hormones that may occur with DHEA administration create a risk of developing ovarian, prostate, or other types of cancer.[21]

Melatonin Levels of melatonin, a hormone that is secreted by the pineal gland, also decline with age. Melatonin is secreted during the night and is involved in regulating the body's cycles of sleep and wakefulness. It has been hypothesized that the decline in melatonin influences aging by affecting body rhythms and triggering genetically programmed aging at a cellular level.[31] Melatonin is also an antioxidant and may enhance immune function.[32] It is available as a dietary supplement, but its effect on aging in humans has not been determined and little information is available concerning any adverse effects.[33]

Menopause Physiological changes that mark the end of a woman's menstrual cycles and capacity to bear children.

Sex Hormones The most striking and rapidly occurring age-related hormonal change is **menopause,** which normally occurs in women around the age of 50. During menopause, the cyclical release of the female hormones estrogen and progesterone slows and eventually stops, causing ovulation and menstruation to cease. The period of decline in estrogen is accompanied by changes in mood, skin, and body composition (an increase in body fat and a decrease in muscle mass). These hormonal changes also have a powerful impact on the disease risks and nutritional status of older women. The reduction in estrogen decreases the risk of breast cancer but increases the risk of heart disease to a level more similar to that in men. Reduced estrogen also increases the risk of osteoporosis by increasing the rate of bone breakdown and decreasing calcium absorption from the intestine. Menopause is also associated with a higher incidence of mental impairment. These effects can be treated with hormone replacement therapy; restoring estrogen to the levels found in younger women prevents changes in body composition, loss of bone mass, and loss of mental function. Hormone replacement therapy also reduces risk factors for heart disease but does not affect the progression of heart disease in women who have heart disease at the time therapy is initiated.[34] A concern with this therapy is that it may increase the risk of breast cancer.

Menopause does not occur in men, but with age men do experience a gradual decrease in testosterone levels that may contribute to the decrease in muscle mass and strength.

Changes in Immune Function The ability of the immune system to fight disease declines with age.[35] As it does, the incidence of infections, cancers, and autoimmune diseases increases, and the effectiveness of immunizations declines. Some of the decrease in immune function may be due to nutritional deficiencies.[35,36] In turn, the increases in infections and chronic disease that occur can affect nutritional status.

The immune response depends on the ability of cells to differentiate, divide rapidly, and secrete immune factors, so nutrients that are involved in cell differentiation, division, and protein synthesis can influence the immune response. In addition, antioxidants may influence immunity by preventing the free-radical damage that can accelerate aging and decrease the immune response. Supplements of beta-carotene and several micronutrients, including zinc, vitamin E, and vitamin B_6, have been shown to improve immune response in both the healthy and the diseased elderly.[35,37–39] However, these individuals may have been deficient in these nutrients prior to supplementation. And because high doses of some nutrients, including zinc, copper, and iron, depress immune function, supplements should be taken with care.

Medical Conditions

With age there is an increase in the incidence of both acute and chronic illness. The reduction in reserve capacity and decline in immune function make infectious diseases more frequent and more serious in the elderly. In addition, most older adults have at least one chronic medical condition.[1] The incidence of cardiovascular disease, diabetes, kidney disease, osteoporosis, hypertension, cancer, arthritis, periodontal disease, atrophic gastritis, macular degeneration, cataracts, and **Alzheimer's disease** all increase with age. All of these conditions can cause food insecurity. Some change nutrient requirements, some decrease the appeal of food, and some impair the ability to maintain nutritional status by affecting mobility or mental function (Table 17.3). And, the increased incidence of disease increases the need for medications, some of which may further increase the risk of malnutrition.

Alzheimer's disease A disease that results in the relentless and irreversible loss of mental function.

Conditions That Decrease Mobility More than half of the older population suffers from some form of physical disability, and the incidence increases with age. Over 4.4 million older adults have difficulty carrying out the activities of daily life, including shopping, food preparation, and getting around the house.[40] These limitations affect the ability to maintain good nutritional health.

A number of disease conditions can decrease mobility in the elderly. Arthritis, a condition that causes joint pain upon movement, is the most common cause

Web Menu: For more information about arthritis, go to the Arthritis Foundation at www.arthritis.org/.

TABLE 17.3 Medical Conditions Affecting Nutrient Intake

Medical Condition	Nutritional Impact
Periodontal disease, dental caries, ill-fitting dentures	Limits intake of fresh fruits, vegetables, and meats, thus reducing energy, fiber, protein, and micronutrient intake.
Macular degeneration, cataracts	Limits ability to shop for food, read food labels, and prepare food.
Atrophic gastritis	Reduces absorption of vitamin B_{12}, iron, folate, calcium, and vitamin K.
Diverticulitis	Treatment restricts intake of nuts and seeds and certain fibers.
Diverticulosis	Treatment increases fiber intake, thus increasing fluid needs.
Diabetes	Treatment restricts carbohydrates and limits food choices.
Kidney disease	Treatment may restrict protein, phosphorus, sodium, magnesium, and fluid intake, thus limiting food choices.
Hypertension	Treatment may restrict sodium intake, and some drug treatments increase potassium losses.
Arthritis	Limits ability to shop for and prepare foods.
Cardiovascular disease	Treatment may restrict saturated fat and cholesterol, thus reducing protein intake from animal products such as meat and eggs.
Alzheimer's disease, dementia	Limits ability to prepare and consume healthy meals.

RESEARCH DISCOVERIES

Glucosamine and Chondroitin Sulfate: A Meta-Analysis

Osteoarthritis is a painful and disabling degenerative disease of the joints that affects approximately 12% of the U.S. population.[a] It is more common in women, and the incidence increases with advancing age. The joints most frequently involved include those of the hands and the large weight-bearing joints such as the knees and hips. Osteoarthritis occurs when the connective tissue that cushions the ends of bones in the joints degenerates over time; the bones then rub together, causing pain and further damage and limiting motion. Current treatment for this disease involves drugs that relieve pain and reduce inflammation, such as acetaminophen, aspirin, and ibuprofen. Two dietary supplements, glucosamine and chondroitin sulfate, have become popular with arthritis sufferers. Research suggests that these may not only relieve pain but also help repair the damaged tissue.

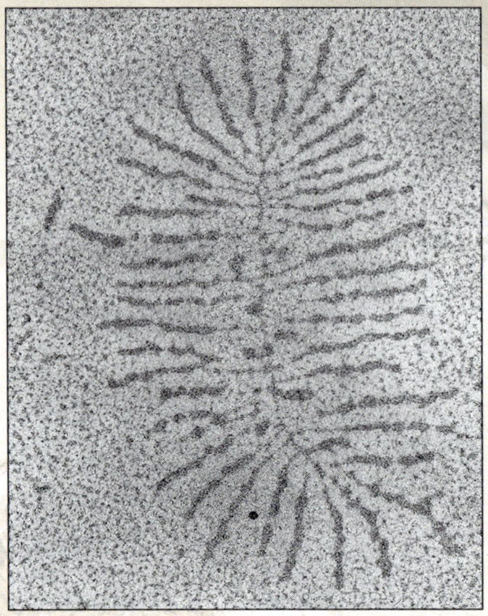

The proteoglycan complex has a large fluffy structure that helps give cartilage its gel-like properties, its resistance to changes in shape, and its ability to distribute force evenly throughout the joint. *(Courtesy of Dr. Joseph A. Buckwalter, The University of Iowa)*

What Are Glucosamine and Chondroitin Sulfate? Glucosamine and chondroitin sulfate are not essential nutrients. They are molecules that are made by our bodies and found in the food supply. In the body, they are found in and around the cells of cartilage, the type of connective tissue that cushions joints. Glucosamine and chondroitin sulfate are needed for the synthesis of molecules called proteoglycans, which are an extracellular component of cartilage. Proteoglycans are very large and bind large numbers of water molecules to form a porous, gel-like material that fills the extracellular space in cartilage (see figure). This gel-like substance acts like a packing material that can resist crushing forces.

One hypothesis as to why glucosamine and chondroitin sulfate supplements may benefit arthritis sufferers is that they provide the raw materials needed to synthesize proteoglycans. Chrondroitin is a large molecule that provides proteoglycans with strength and resilience. Glucosamine sulfate is a small molecule needed as a building block. It is also hypothesized that glucosamine inhibits inflammation and increases the production of hyaluronic acid, another molecule that is a component of the proteoglycan complex and contributes to the lubricating and shock-absorbing properties of cartilage. Supplements of both glucosamine and chondroitin sulfate are said to reduce arthritis pain, stop cartilage degeneration, and possibly stimulate the repair of damaged joint cartilage.

Are They Effective? A Meta-Analysis Much of the research that has been done to test the effectiveness of these supplements indicates that they are safe and beneficial, but how beneficial is unclear. Some studies found large improvements while others found that the supplements had only small effects. The results obtained by

of disability in older individuals, affecting almost 60% of those age 70 and older. Osteoarthritis, the form of arthritis most common in the elderly, is characterized by abnormalities in the joint surfaces and is most likely the result of a lifetime of wear and tear (see *Research Discoveries*: "Glucosamine and Chondroitin Sulfate: A Meta-Analysis"). Osteoporosis and its associated fractures can also affect mobility. Some of the decrease in mobility that is due to disease and normal aging can be prevented by a healthy diet and lifestyle.

Dementia A deterioration of mental state resulting in impaired memory, thinking, and/or judgment.

Conditions That Affect Mental Status Altered mental status can affect nutrition. Although many individuals maintain adequate nervous system function into old age, the incidence of depression and **dementia** increase with age. Depression can decrease social interactions and food consumption. Dementia is an impairment in memory, thinking, and/or judgment that is severe enough to cause personality changes and affect daily activities and relationships with others; about a third of men and women age 85 and older have moderate or severe memory impairment.[41] Causes of dementia include multiple strokes, alcoholism, and Alzheimer's disease. Vitamin B_{12} status may also affect mental function in the elderly. With aging, there is a decrease in blood vitamin B_{12} levels and a rise in

individual subjects are even more contradictory. Some subjects experienced more relief when taking glucosamine or chondroitin sulfate than they did with anti-inflammatory drugs, while others found that these supplements provided no benefits at all. How can these conflicting results be sorted out? One way to evaluate the contradictory results of a large number of trials is to perform a meta-analysis of the data. This type of analysis integrates data from different trials to get an overall assessment of the combined results.

In order to combine data from different studies, certain similar conditions must exist. A recent meta-analysis of the effectiveness of glucosamine and chondroitin sulfate for the treatment of osteoarthritis examined the data from studies that assessed osteoarthritis of the knee or hip, ran for a duration of four weeks or more, and reported data on the effect that the treatment had on symptoms.[b] To be included in this meta-analysis, studies also had to be double-blind, randomized, and placebo-controlled. Fifteen such studies were included in the analysis, six that studied glucosamine and nine that studied chondroitin sulfate. The meta-analysis indicated that these supplements had moderate to large effects on the symptoms of osteoarthritis. These studies were also evaluated for possible bias, trial size, and quality. With all these factors considered, it was concluded that the reports of beneficial effects may have been exaggerated, but were still significant.

What's to Come? Based on the promising results from many small trials, the National Institutes of Health (NIH) has launched a large study to evaluate the effects of glucosamine and chondroitin sulfate. The trial will be conducted in nine centers across the country and is the first multicenter clinical trial in the United States to test the effects of these dietary supplements for treatment of osteoarthritis. It will test the short-term (16 weeks) effectiveness of glucosamine and chondroitin sulfate, given separately and in combination, for reducing pain and improving function in patients with osteoarthritis of the knee.

Is It Too Soon to Try Them? Currently glucosamine and chondroitin sulfate are sold as dietary supplements, not as drugs. Consequently, their manufacture is not carefully regulated and dosages are not standardized. One analysis found that glucosamine supplements generally contain the amount listed on the label but more than half of the samples of chondroitin sulfate supplements contained less than 40% of what was listed on the label.[c] Despite the problem of dosage, no adverse effects have been reported in trials of these compounds or in over-the-counter use. Therefore, the risk seems to be low and the potential benefits real. But until these compounds are fully tested, the Arthritis Foundation and the American College of Rheumatology are urging patients with osteoarthritis to continue proven treatments and disease-management techniques and to inform their physicians if they are considering using these supplements.

References

[a] Barclay, T. S., Tsourounis, C., and McCart, C. M. Glucosamine. Ann. Pharmacother. 32:574–579, 1998.

[b] McAlindon, T. E., LaValley, M. P., Gulin, J. P., and Felson, D. T. Glucosamine and chondroitin for treatment of osteoarthritis: a systematic quality assessment and meta-analysis JAMA 283:1469–1475, 2000.

[c] Eddington, N. Analysis of glucosamine and chondroitin sulfate content in marketed products and the caco-2 permeability of chondroitin sulfate raw materials. J. Am. Nutraceut. Assoc. 3:37–44, 2000.

metabolites indicative of poor B_{12} status. It has been hypothesized that high homocysteine levels from B_{12} deficiency may contribute to small vascular lesions in the brain that lead to dementia.[42] In most cases, vitamin B_{12} supplements do not improve neurological function; however, in some elderly patients with mild dementia and low blood levels of vitamin B_{12}, supplementation was found to improve mental function.[43]

Over half of the cases of dementia in the elderly are due to Alzheimer's disease, which affects 6–8% of all persons over 65. Alzheimer's is a progressive, incurable loss of mental function. The brains of Alzheimer's patients are characterized by the accumulation of an abnormal protein and a loss of certain types of nerve cells.[44] Its cause is currently unknown, but there does appear to be a genetic component in some cases. Many ineffective nutritional cures have been marketed for Alzheimer's disease. For example, supplements of choline and lecithin have been promoted to increase levels of the neurotransmitter acetylcholine, which is deficient in Alzheimer's patients. Oxidative stress and the accumulation of free radicals have been suggested to be involved in the disease and therefore antioxidant nutrients such as vitamins E and C, β-carotene, and zinc have been suggested to play a protective role. Although in individuals consuming

Web Menu

For information about Alzheimer's disease and related disorders, visit the Alzheimer's Disease Education and Referral (ADEAR) Center's Web site at www.alzheimers.org/.

low levels of these nutrients cognitive skills may be impaired, there is little evidence that intakes above the recommendations protect against Alzheimer's disease.[42] Alzheimer's patients typically have low serum concentrations of vitamin B_{12} and elevated levels of homocysteine, but it is unclear whether this is a cause or a consequence of the disease. When high aluminum levels were discovered in the brains of Alzheimer's patients, many people tried to reduce exposure by restricting the use of aluminum cookware and aluminum-containing deodorants. To date, neither nutritional supplements nor aluminum restriction has proved helpful in treating or preventing Alzheimer's disease.

Web Menu: For information about medications and their side effects, go to the U.S. Food and Drug Administration Center for Drug Evaluation and Research at www.fda.gov/cder/drug/ or the National Library of Medicine at medlineplus.gov/ and click on drug information.

Increased Use of Medications Because health problems increase with increasing age, older adults are likely to take medications. Almost half of older Americans take multiple medications daily (Figure 17.9).[45] The use of prescription and over-the-counter medications can affect nutritional status and contribute to malnutrition. The more medications taken, the greater the chance of side effects such as increased or decreased appetite, changes in taste, constipation, weakness, drowsiness, diarrhea, and nausea. Although these medications are necessary and provide beneficial effects, illness related to incorrect doses or inappropriate combinations of drugs is a significant health problem in the elderly, accounting for 5 to 23% of all hospitalizations. Medications commonly used by older individuals include aspirin, antacids, laxatives, diuretics, anticoagulants (blood thinners), anticonvulsants, heart medications, and pain medications. Both the effects of drugs on nutritional status and the effects of nutritional status on the effectiveness of the drugs must be considered.

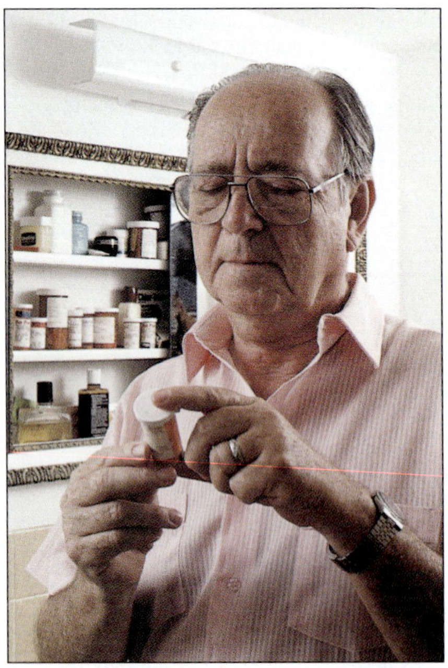

FIGURE 17.9 Many older adults take one or more medications every day. *(© Joseph Nettis/Photo Researchers, Inc.)*

The Effect of Medications on Nutritional Status Medications can affect nutrition by altering appetite or nutrient absorption, metabolism, or excretion (Table 17.4). These effects occur with both prescription and over-the-counter products. In many situations, drugs do not significantly alter overall nutritional status, but they can have a significant impact on the nutritional status of individuals who must take them for extended periods, who take multiple formulations, or who already have marginal nutritional status.

Some medications directly affect the gastrointestinal tract. For example, some alter or diminish taste perception, and more than 250 drugs, including blood-pressure medications, antidepressants, decongestants, and the pain reliever ibuprofen (found in Advil, Motrin, and Nuprin), can cause mouth dryness, which can decrease interest in eating by interfering with taste, chewing, and swallowing. Aspirin is a stomach irritant and can cause small amounts of painless bleeding in the gastrointestinal tract, resulting in iron loss. The heart stimulant digoxin can cause gastrointestinal upset, loss of appetite, and nausea. Narcotic pain medications such as codeine can lead to constipation, nausea, and vomiting.

Other medications can decrease nutrient absorption. Cholestyramine (Questran), which is used to reduce blood cholesterol, can decrease the absorption of fat-soluble vitamins, vitamin B_{12}, iron, and folate. Antacids that contain aluminum or magnesium hydroxide (Rolaids or Maalox) combine with phosphorus in the gut to form compounds that cannot be absorbed; chronic use can result in loss of phosphorus from bone and possibly accelerate osteoporosis. Repeated use of stimulant laxatives can deplete calcium and potassium. Mineral oil laxatives prevent the absorption of fat-soluble vitamins. If it is not possible to prevent constipation by consuming a diet high in fiber and fluid, bulk-forming laxatives are a safer choice.

The metabolism of medications can also affect nutritional status. For example, anticonvulsive drugs taken by people prone to epileptic seizures increase the liver's capacity to metabolize and eliminate vitamin D, therefore increasing the need for vitamin D.

TABLE 17.4 Medications That May Cause Nutrient Deficiencies

Drug Group	Drug	Potential Deficiency
Antacids	Sodium bicarbonate	Folate, phosphorus, calcium, copper
	Aluminum	Phosphorus
Anticonvulsants	Phenytoin, phenobarbital, primidone	Vitamins D and K
	Valproic acid	Carnitine
Antibiotics	Tetracycline	Calcium
Antibacterial agents	Gentamicin	Potassium, magnesium
	Neomycin	Fat, nitrogen
	Boric acid	Riboflavin
	Trimethoprim	Folate
	Isoniazid	Vitamins B_6, D, and niacin
Anti-inflammatory agents	Sulfasalazine	Folate
	Prednisone	Calcium
	Aspirin	Vitamin C, folate, iron
Anticancer drugs	Colchine	Fat, vitamin B_{12}
	Methotrexate	Folate, calcium
Antiocoagulant drugs	Warfarin	Vitamin K
Antihypertensive drugs	Hydralazine	Vitamin B_6
Diuretics	Thiazide	Potassium
	Furosemide	Potassium, calcium, magnesium
Hypocholesterolemic agents	Cholestyramine	Fat, fat-soluble vitamins, iron, folate, vitamin B_{12}
Laxatives	Mineral oil	Fat-soluble vitamins
	Phenolphthalein	Potassium, calcium
	Senna	Fat, calcium, vitamin B_6, folate, vitamin C
Tranquilizers	Chlorpromazine	Riboflavin

Adapted from Roe, D. A. *Diet and Drug Interactions.* New York: Van Nostrand Reinhold, 1989.

Some medications affect nutrient excretion. Diuretics, which are used to treat hypertension and edema, cause water loss, but some types (thiazides) also increase the excretion of potassium. People taking thiazide diuretics are advised to include several good sources of potassium in their diet each day or to take prescribed supplements.

The Effect of Food and Nutritional Status on Medications Food components can either enhance or retard the absorption and metabolism of drugs. Some drugs, such as the pain medication Darvon, are absorbed better or faster if taken with food. Others, such as aspirin and ibuprofen, should be taken with food because they are irritating to the gastrointestinal tract. On the other hand, since food can delay how quickly drugs leave the stomach, some are best taken with just water. Other drugs interact with specific foods. For instance, the antibiotic tetracycline should not be taken with milk because it binds with calcium, making both unavailable.

Nutritional status can also affect drug metabolism. If nutritional status is poor, the body's ability to detoxify drugs may be altered. For example, in a malnourished individual, theophylline, used to treat asthma, is metabolized slowly, resulting in high blood levels of the drug, which can cause loss of appetite, nausea, and vomiting.

Specific nutrients can also affect the metabolism of drugs. High-protein diets enhance drug metabolism in general, and low-protein diets slow it. Vitamin K hinders the action of anticoagulants, taken to reduce the risk of

Making Decisions

The Risks and Benefits of Alcohol Use in Adults

Almost every human culture since the dawn of civilization has produced and consumed some type of alcoholic beverage. It is part of religious ceremonies, social traditions, and even medical prescriptions. Dating back to 2100 B.C., Sumerian clay tablets record physicians' prescriptions for beer, and in ancient Egypt, both beer and wine were prescribed as part of medical treatment. Yet many people refrain from alcohol for religious, cultural, personal, or medical reasons. When consumed in excess, alcohol causes medical and social consequences that affect drinkers and their families. Whether alcohol represents a risk or provides some benefits depends on who is drinking it and how much is consumed.

For some people, the risks of alcohol consumption far outweigh any benefits. Children should not consume alcohol. They are more sensitive than adults to alcohol's toxic effects—drunkenness and poisoning leading to seizures, coma, and death.[a] Women who are pregnant or trying to conceive should not consume alcohol because it may damage the fetus. Individuals who plan to drive or operate machinery should not drink alcohol because it impairs coordination and reflexes. Finally, because alcohol is a drug that interacts with numerous medications, individuals using prescription or over-the-counter drugs should avoid alcohol.[b]

For everyone, the risks of *excess* alcohol consumption outweigh the benefits. The abuse of alcohol contributes to domestic violence and leads to more than 100,000 deaths per year, including 20,000 from traffic accidents. The incidence of alcohol poisoning, especially among college students who binge drink, is on the rise. Many college campuses are now prohibiting the consumption of alcohol and designing safe-drinking campaigns for their students. Alcoholics are ten times more likely to develop cancer of the liver, pancreas, and stomach, and they have an increased risk of cirrhosis, peptic ulcers, and certain types of stroke.

Deciding whether *moderate* alcohol consumption is more of a risk than a benefit is more challenging. Moderate alcohol consumption may increase the risk of obesity.[c] Alcohol suppresses lipid oxidation, and in drinkers, fat is preferentially deposited in the abdominal region. This excess abdominal fat increases the risk of high blood pressure, heart disease, and diabetes. There is also some evidence suggesting that alcohol consumption may increase the risk of breast cancer, but this finding is not consistent, particularly at low levels of alcohol consumption.[d,e] In addition to these health risks, there is concern that recommending moderate drinking may lead to excessive drinking and addiction in susceptible individuals.

Another possible risk associated with drinking alcoholic beverages, even in moderation, is that they may contain chemical contaminants. Lead contamination can be caused by lead foil used to seal older wine bottles and by leaded crystal decanters used to store liqueurs. Urethane is another possible contaminant. It is a carcinogen that contaminates distilled liquors such as bourbon because it is a by-product of the distillation process.[f]

Despite these concerns, moderate alcohol consumption also has benefits. Consumption of alcoholic beverages before or with meals can stimulate appetite and improve mood. It can be relaxing, producing a euphoria that can enhance social interactions. Studies have shown that light drinking is associated with a reduction in mortality.[g] Most of this effect is likely due to the inverse relationship that exists between heart disease and consumption of small amounts

blood clots. On the other hand, omega-3 fatty acids, such as those in fish oils, inhibit blood clotting and may intensify the effect of an anticoagulant drug and cause bleeding. It is safe to eat fish (a source of omega-3 fatty acids) while taking anticoagulant drugs; however, the use of fish-oil supplements is not recommended.

Drugs can also interact with each other. For example, alcohol affects the metabolism of over a hundred medications. Drug interactions can exaggerate or, in some cases, diminish the effect of a medication. Mixing certain drugs can be fatal. Individuals taking any medication should consult their doctor, pharmacist, or dietitian regarding how the drug could affect the action of other drugs they may be taking, how the drug could affect their nutrition, and how their nutrition could affect the action of the drug.

Alcohol Use Alcohol consumption increases the risk of malnutrition in the elderly. Alcohol is high in kcalories and provides few nutrients. Too much damages the brain, heart, liver, and other organs (see Chapter 16). It impairs judgment and balance and it therefore increases the frequency of falls and makes it harder to remember to eat and take medications correctly. Alcohol consumption should be limited to no more than one drink per day for women and two per day for men[45] (see *Making Decisions:* "The Risks and Benefits of Alcohol Use in Adults").

of alcohol.[h] Alcohol consumption increases HDL cholesterol level and may have an effect on the aggregation of platelets. These benefits are stronger when red wine is consumed, likely due to the phenolic phytochemicals in red wine.[i] Wine consumption has been suggested as a reason for the lower incidence of heart disease in certain cultures. For example, the Mediterranean diet, which has been associated with a reduced risk of heart disease, includes daily consumption of wine in moderation, and one explanation for the French paradox—the fact that the French eat a diet that is as high or higher in fat than the American diet but suffer from far less heart disease—is the glass of wine they drink with meals.

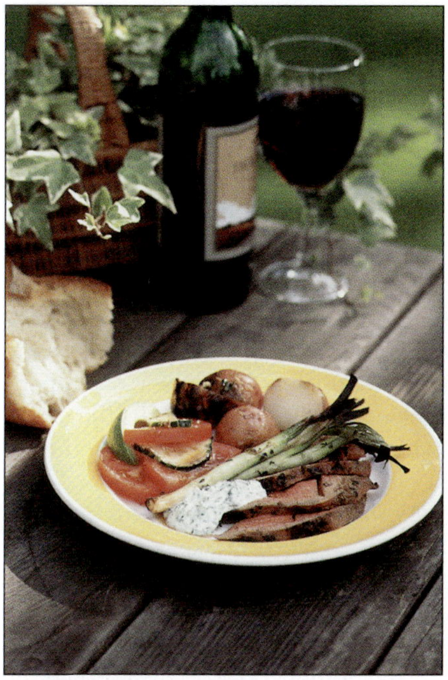

(© Philip Salaverry/Stone)

Whether the benefits of alcohol consumption outweigh the risks, drinking is a personal decision that must take into account medical and social considerations. But those who choose to drink should do so in moderation—about 1 to 2 drinks per day (one drink equals approximately 5 fluid ounces of wine, 12 fluid ounces of beer, or 1.5 fluid ounces of distilled liquor). Alcohol should be consumed slowly. It usually takes an hour to metabolize the alcohol in one drink. Consuming alcohol with meals slows its absorption and may also enhance its protective effects on the cardiovascular system. Like aspirin, alcohol prevents blood clotting, so when it is consumed with a meal, it may counteract the tendency of a large meal to promote blood clotting and therefore reduce the risk of an immediate heart attack. Also, the effect of alcohol on HDL is believed to be greater when the liver is processing nutrients from a meal.

References

[a] Hingley, A. T. Preventing childhood poisoning. FDA Consumer 30:7–11, March 1996.

[b] U.S. Department of Agriculture, U.S. Department of Health and Human Services. *Nutrition and Your Health: Dietary Guidelines for Americans,* 5th ed., 2000. Item Number 147-G. Hyattsville, Md.: U.S. Government Printing Office, 2000.

[c] Suter, P. M., Häsler, E., and Vetter, W. Effects of alcohol on energy metabolism and body weight regulation: is alcohol a risk factor for obesity? Nutr. Rev. 55:157–171, 1997.

[d] Rohan, T. E., Jain, M., Howe, G. R., and Miller, A. B. Alcohol consumption and risk of breast cancer: a cohort study. Cancer Causes Control 11:239–247, 2000.

[e] Garland, M., Hunter, D. J., Colditz, G. A., et al. Alcohol consumption in relation to breast cancer risk in a cohort of United States women ages 25–42. Cancer Epidemiol. Biomakers Res. 8:1017–1021, 1999.

[f] Segal, M. Too many drinks spiked with urethanes. FDA Consumer 32:5–8, April 1998.

[g] Chick, J. Alcohol, health and the heart. Alcohol 33:576–591, 1999.

[h] Cleophas, T. J. Wine, beer and spirits and the risk of myocardial infarction: a systematic review Biomed. Pharmacother. 53:417–423, 1999.

[i] Ruh, J. C. Wine and polyphenols related to platelet aggregation and atherosclerosis. Drugs Exp. Clin. Res. 25:125–131, 1999.

Social and Economic Conditions

There are a variety of social and economic changes that often accompany aging. These factors are all interrelated and affect nutritional status by decreasing the motivation to eat and the ability to acquire and enjoy food.

Income Level About 3.4 million elderly persons live below the poverty level (Figure 17.10).[40] The highest rates of poverty occur among the oldest of the old, minorities, women, persons living alone, and those with disabilities. Many older individuals, regardless of income level, must live on a fixed income as they retire from their jobs. This makes it difficult to afford health care, especially medications, and a healthy diet. Food is often the most flexible expense in the budget, so limiting the types and amounts of foods consumed may be the only option available for older adults trying to meet expenses. Substandard housing and inadequate food preparation facilities can make the situation worse because food cannot easily be prepared and eaten at home.

Dependent Living Most older individuals continue to live in a family setting: 66% of adults over 65 years of age live at home. But this number decreases with age; only 46% of individuals over 85 still live at home.[40] The physical and psychological decline associated with aging causes many older adults to eventually

FIGURE 17.10 Of persons 65 and older, 37% have an income level that is less than $10,000 per year. *(U.S. Bureau of the Census. "Consumer Income." Current Population Reports, P60–200, September, 1998.)*

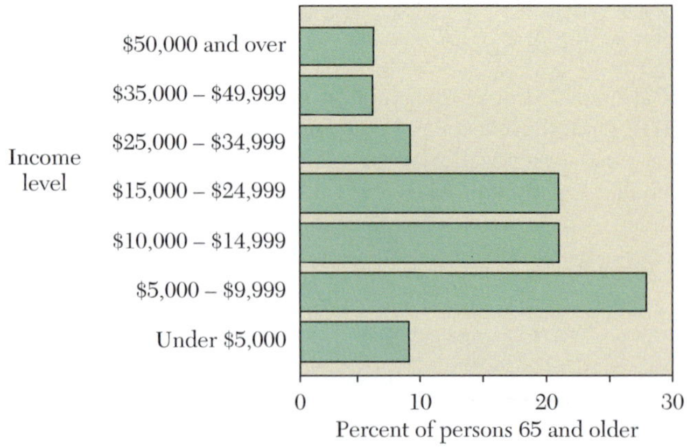

require some assistance in living. Poor eyesight and other physical restrictions can limit the ability to drive a car. Without help, these disabilities would prohibit many older adults from getting to markets and food programs and therefore restrict the types of food available to them. While a social support system consisting of family members, friends, and other caregivers can help many people stay at home, others require assisted-living facilities where they have their own apartments but can obtain assistance around the clock. For some, however, the extent of their disability is great enough that a nursing home is needed to provide the appropriate level of care.

Malnutrition can be a problem among older adults no matter where they live. Even older individuals living independently have reduced intakes of energy and protein. Those in nursing homes are at increased risk for malnutrition because they are more likely to have medical conditions that increase nutrient needs or that interfere with food intake or nutrient absorption, and because they are dependent on others to provide for their care.[46] In addition, 50% of institutionalized elderly suffer from some form of disorientation or confusion that further

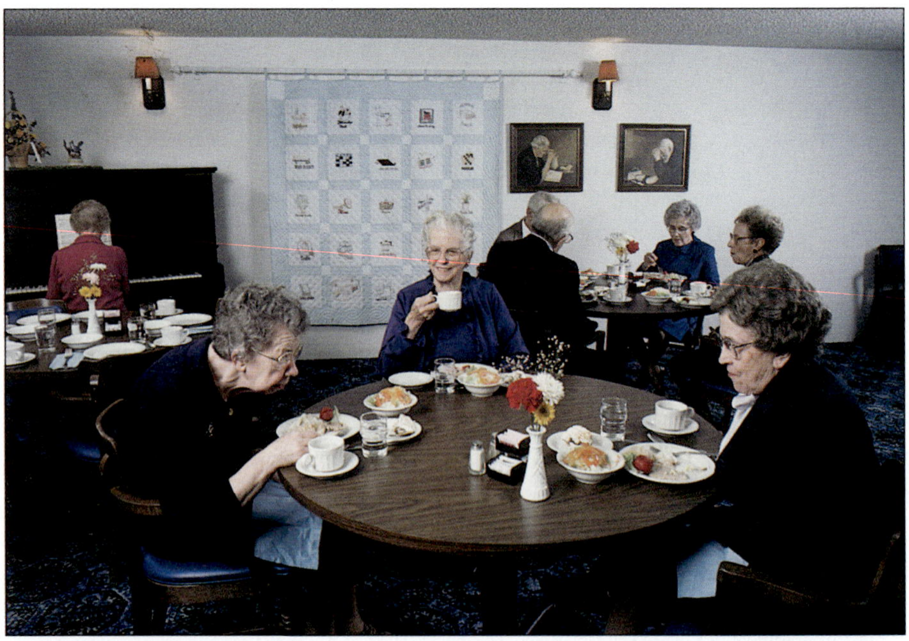

FIGURE 17.11 Social interaction may reduce depression and make eating more appealing, thereby improving nutritional status. *(© Blair Seitz/Photo Researchers, Inc.)*

increases the likelihood of decreased nutrient intake. Even when adequate meals are provided, nursing-home residents frequently do not consume all of the food served, increasing the likelihood of fluid and energy deficits.[47] Whether older adults reside at home, in an assisted-living setting, or in a nursing home, care must be taken to assess their individual needs and to ensure access to appetizing meals that meet these needs.

Depression Social, psychological, and physical factors all contribute to depression in the elderly.[48] Retirement and the death or relocation of friends and family can cause social isolation. Physical disability causes loss of independence. These contribute to depression by decreasing the ability to engage in normal daily activities, easily visit with friends and family, and provide for personal needs. Depression can make meals less appetizing and decrease the quantity and quality of foods consumed, thereby increasing the risk of malnutrition (Figure 17.11). (See *Critical Thinking:* "Meeting the Needs of the Elderly.")

Critical Thinking

Meeting the Needs of the Elderly

Recently, Sasha was introduced to the DETERMINE checklist in her nutrition class (see Table 17.5). As she scanned it, she began to think about her Aunt Pauline, since many of the conditions that predispose elderly people to malnutrition sounded familiar.

Sasha is Pauline's closest relative. She has been helping her every other week by doing some cleaning and grocery shopping. After learning about the problem of malnutrition in the elderly, Sasha decides to take on the responsibility of helping to make sure her great-aunt is adequately nourished. During her next visit, Sasha asks Pauline to be her subject for a class project on nutritional assessment. As they talk, Aunt Pauline explains that she used to eat with a neighbor but that recently her neighbor moved into a nursing home. Pauline knows she doesn't eat well but she hates cooking for herself. Sasha also learns that her aunt's cataracts make it difficult for her to read medicine bottles and food labels. Sasha records the following information about her aunt on the DETERMINE checklist.

Checklist	Aunt Pauline
Disease	She has high blood pressure, arthritis, and cataracts.
Eating poorly	She doesn't keep much food in her refrigerator, and doesn't like to cook for herself.
Tooth loss or mouth pain	None.
Economic hardship	None.
Reduced social support	Her friend moved to a nursing home within the past year; few relatives are nearby.
Multiple medicines	She takes hormones, as well as blood pressure and arthritis medications.
Involuntary weight loss/gain	She thinks she has lost weight—between 5 and 10 pounds.
Needs assistance in self-care	She needs help shopping and cleaning.
Elder above age 80	She is 75.

Six of the nine items on the DETERMINE checklist apply to Aunt Pauline, confirming Sasha's concern that her aunt is at risk of malnutrition. A 24-hour recall of her intake of food and beverages is shown here:

Food	Amount	Food	Amount
Breakfast		*Dinner*	
Bran flakes	3/4 cup	Cottage cheese	1/2 cup
Low-fat milk	1/2 cup	Toast with butter	2 slices
Coffee	1 cup	Apple juice	1 cup
Artificial sweetener	1 tsp		
Lunch			
Chicken noodle soup	1 cup		
Crackers	6		
Applesauce	1/2 cup		
Tea	1 cup		

How does her diet compare to the serving recommendations of the Food Guide Pyramid for people over 70?

- She consumes only 5 cups of fluid and one cup is coffee, which contains caffeine and therefore contributes to fluid loss.
- She consumes 1 dairy serving compared to the recommended 2 servings.
- Other answers____________________________________

Suggest some food choices that would increase Pauline's fiber intake.

Answer:

Would you suggest any food or nutrient supplements for Pauline? If so, which ones?

Answer:

Nutrition for Older Adults

Older adults are a diverse group, which makes defining and meeting nutrient needs challenging. The incidence of diseases that affect nutritional status is increased, and economic and social factors, such as a fixed income and social isolation, affect appetite and food availability. To meet the nutritional needs of the elderly, their individual medical, psychological, social, and economic circumstances must be considered.

Nutrient Needs

General dietary recommendations are difficult to establish for older adults. For instance, the requirements of a wheelchair-bound 70-year-old are different from those of a more active 70-year-old individual. Dietary recommendations are developed to meet the needs of the majority of healthy individuals in a population, but "healthy" is difficult to define in such a diverse group. The 1989 RDAs divide adulthood into three age categories, but the DRIs have expanded this to four: young adulthood, ages 19 through 30; middle age, 31 through 50 years; adulthood, ages 51 through 70; and older adults, those over 70 years of age. This recognizes the possible higher nutrient intake needs of younger adults, the decline with age in the need for nutrients involved in energy metabolism, and the variability in the functional capacity of older adults.

Energy Energy needs are typically reduced in the elderly. This occurs for several reasons. Energy requirements are the sum of the needs for basal metabolic rate (BMR), physical activity, and the thermic effect of food. A change in any one of these alters total energy needs. BMR is influenced by lean body mass, and because lean body mass usually decreases with age, there is a reduction in this component of energy expenditure in the elderly.[49] Physical activity also tends to decline with age. This causes a decrease in the activity component of energy expenditure and contributes to the reduction in lean body mass and BMR. The energy needed for the thermic effect of food does not change as adults age.[50]

The 1989 energy allowances recommend a reduction of 600 kcalories in men age 51 and older and 300 kcalories in women age 51 and older compared to younger age groups. Some of the decrease in energy needs can be prevented by exercise, which increases energy expenditure and helps prevent the loss of lean body mass.[49] Increasing energy needs through exercise also allows an increase in food intake without weight gain so that micronutrient needs are more easily met (Figure 17.12).

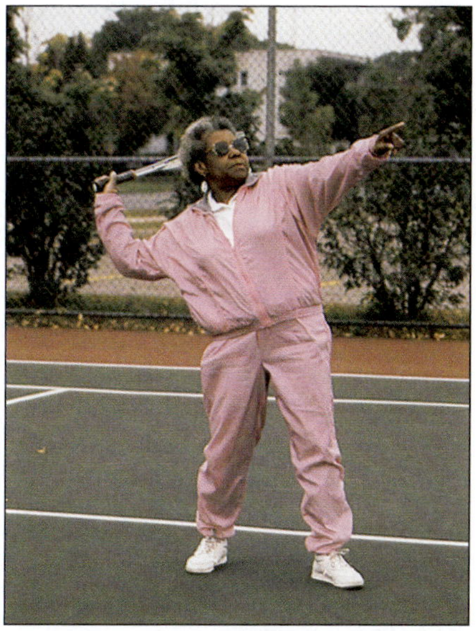

FIGURE 17.12 Exercise increases energy needs and helps to maintain lean body mass. *(© CLEO/PhotoEdit)*

Protein Unlike energy requirements, the need for protein does not decline with age. Therefore, an adequate diet for older adults must be somewhat higher in protein relative to energy intake. Although the 1989 RDA for older adults is no different from that for younger adults, actual need depends on the individual. In some, the protein requirement may be less than the 1989 RDA because there is less lean body mass to maintain, whereas in others it may be greater than the 1989 RDA because protein absorption or utilization is reduced.

Fat The digestion and absorption of fat is no different in older adults and the recommendations regarding dietary fat apply to older as well as younger adults. A diet with no more than 30% of energy from fat that contains less than 10% of energy from saturated fat, 10 to 15% from monounsaturated fat, and no more than 10% from polyunsaturated fat, that limits cholesterol to 300 mg per day, and that is based on grains, fruits, and vegetables may be as important for preventing and managing chronic diseases in the elderly as it is in young adults. Such a diet will also meet the need for essential fatty acids and be nutrient-dense, making it easier to meet nutrient needs despite diminished energy requirements. There are certain situations, such as being underweight, where greater fat intake may be warranted.

Fiber The recommendations for fiber intake for older adults are not different from the rest of the adult population—10 to 13 g per 1000 kcalories of intake. According to NHANES III survey data, the mean dietary fiber intake in men and women 70 years of age and older was below this, at about 14 to 16 g per day. Fiber helps prevent constipation, hemorrhoids, and diverticulosis—conditions that are common in older adults. High-fiber diets are also important in the prevention and management of diabetes, cardiovascular disease, and obesity.

Water Dehydration is a major problem in older adults, especially the oldest old and those who are institutionalized.[5] This occurs because homeostatic mechanisms that regulate fluid balance may be compromised with age. There is a reduction in the sense of thirst, which can decrease fluid intake, and the kidneys are no longer as efficient at conserving water, so water loss increases. Activity level, ambient temperature, kidney function, disease states, and medications affect water intake and losses. For example, depression decreases water intake, diabetes increases urinary water losses, and diseases that cause vomiting or diarrhea increase water loss through the GI tract. Medications such as laxatives and diuretics also increase the risk of dehydration in the elderly by increasing water loss. Changes in mobility may limit access to water even in the presence of thirst. Inadequate fluid along with low fiber intake contributes to constipation.

Micronutrients The recommended intake for most of the micronutrients is not changed for older adults; however, the risk of micronutrient deficiencies increases in this age group due to deficient intakes as well as changes in digestion, absorption, and metabolism (Figure 17.13).

B Vitamins The only B vitamins for which recommendations differ between older and younger adults are vitamins B_6 and B_{12}. The RDA for vitamin B_6 is greater in individuals age 51 and older than for younger adults, and in the older age groups, the RDA for men is higher than for women. This is because higher dietary intakes are needed to maintain the same biochemical indicators of

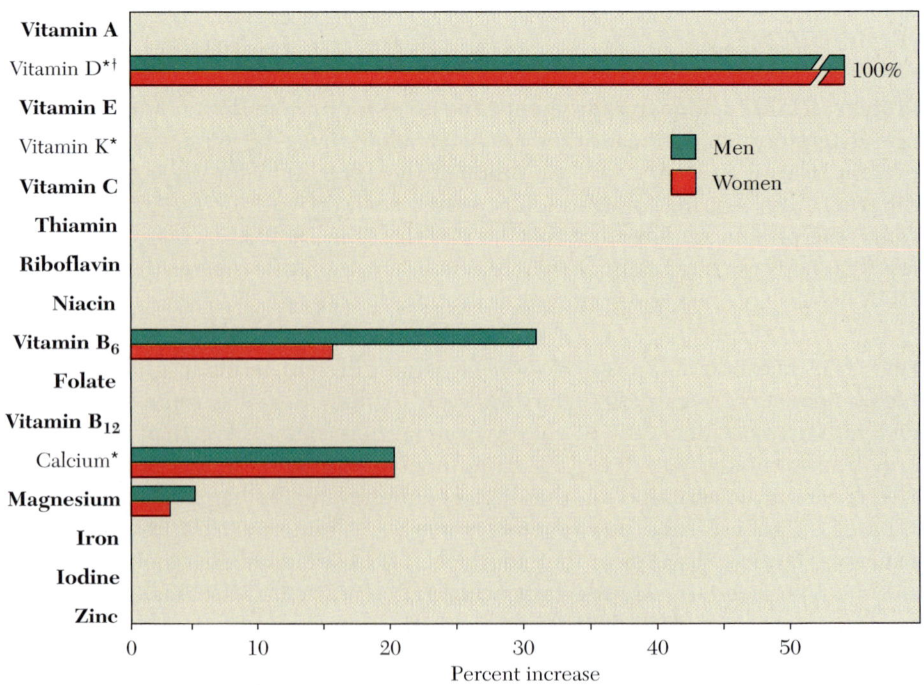

†This represents the AI for individuals 51 to 70 years old. For those over age 70 the AI is increased by 200%

FIGURE 17.13 The nutrient needs of older adults are not drastically different from those of young adults. This graph illustrates the percentage increase in micronutrient recommendations for adults ages 51 and older compared to those of young adults ages 19 through 30. The RDA for vitamin B_{12} is not increased but it is recommended that vitamin B_{12} be obtained from fortified foods or supplements. Nutrients in bold are RDA values and those in plain text with an asterix are AI values. (The RDA for iron for women over 50 years of age is reduced by 56%.)

adequacy. Vitamin B_{12} is a nutrient of concern for older adults because of both reduced absorption of food-bound B_{12} and low dietary intakes, especially among the poor. The RDA for vitamin B_{12} is not increased, but it is recommended that individuals over the age of 50 meet their RDA for vitamin B_{12} by consuming fortified foods such as fortified breakfast cereals or soy-based products, or by taking a supplement containing vitamin B_{12}. This recommendation is made because food-bound vitamin B_{12} is not absorbed efficiently in many elderly due to atrophic gastritis, which affects 10 to 30% of individuals over age 50.[12] The vitamin B_{12} in fortified foods and supplements is not bound to proteins, so it is absorbed even when stomach acid is low.

Vitamin D and Calcium Because vitamin D is necessary for calcium absorption, a deficiency may contribute to osteoporosis. Intakes of this vitamin are often low in the elderly population, usually due to limited consumption of dairy products. In addition, exposure to sunlight, which is necessary for the formation of provitamin D in the skin, is often limited in the elderly because they spend less time outdoors or tend to wear clothing that covers or shades their skin when they go out. Vitamin D deficiency is also a concern because the capacity to synthesize provitamin D in the skin and to form active vitamin D in the kidney decreases with age. Using bone loss as an indicator of adequacy, the AI for men and women ages 51 to 70 has been doubled from that of younger age groups to a value of 10 μg per day. For individuals over age 70, this is further increased to 15 μg per day.

Calcium status is a problem in the elderly because intakes are low and intestinal absorption decreases with age. The current AI for adults ages 51 and older is 1200 mg, an increase from the AI of 1000 mg set for younger adults.[51] Although the decrease in estrogen that occurs at menopause causes bone loss, it cannot be prevented by increasing calcium intake, so the AIs for men and women are not different.

Dietary Antioxidants The hypothesis that aging is caused by oxidative damage has led to the popular conclusion that high dietary intakes of antioxidants will retard the aging process. Although it is an exaggeration to say these nutrients will retard aging, adequate intakes may delay or prevent some of the changes that occur with age. For example, vitamin C, vitamin E, and beta-carotene have been found to improve immune function and may therefore help protect the body from infectious disease.[35] There is also evidence that they may help prevent age-related macular degeneration and cataracts.[52] In addition, high intakes of beta-carotene and vitamin E have been associated with a reduced risk of heart disease.[53,54,55] Diets high in antioxidant nutrients are also associated with a reduced incidence of certain types of cancer. The evidence that antioxidants in supplement form will have these effects is not as strong as the evidence supporting a diet plentiful in foods high in these nutrients. When obtained from foods, these nutrients bring with them phytochemicals, some of which offer additional antioxidant protection and some of which protect us from chronic disease in other ways (Figure 17.14).

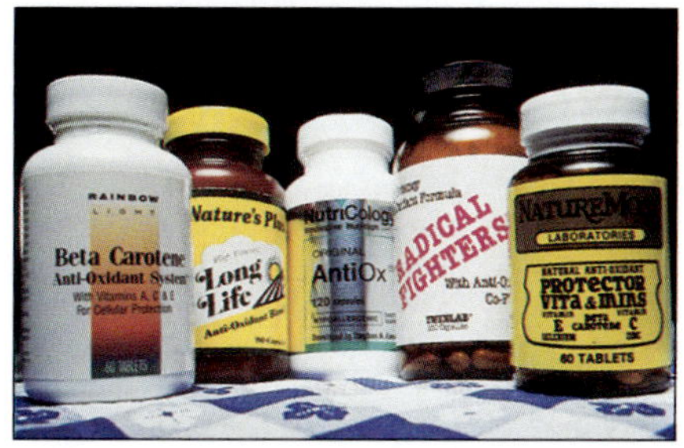

(a)

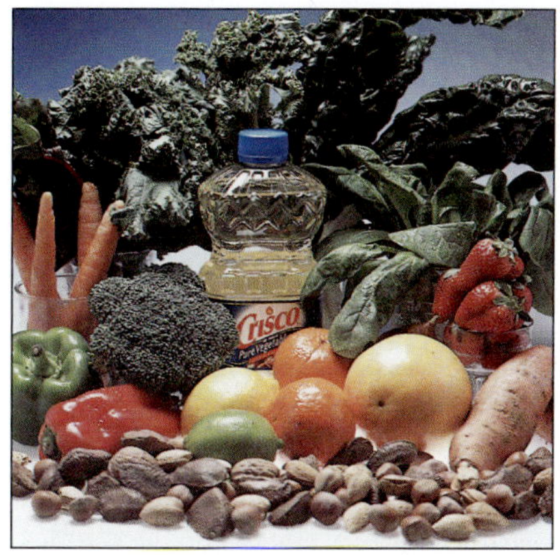

(b)

FIGURE 17.14 (a) Supplements are often consumed to increase antioxidant intake. *(Charles D. Winters)* (b) Foods that are good sources of dietary antioxidants such as beta-carotene, vitamin C, vitamin E, and selenium also provide fiber, energy, other micronutrients, and phytochemicals. *(Charles D. Winters)*

Web Menu: For information about healthy aging and resources for elderly persons and their families, go to the Administration on Aging at www.aoa.dhhs.gov/ and the National Institute on Aging at www.nih.gov/nia/.

Meeting Nutrient Needs

Despite the fact that the nutrient needs of older adults are not drastically different from those of young adults, it is more challenging to meet these needs. One reason for this is that energy needs are reduced while most micronutrient needs remain the same or increase. Changes in health and social and economic conditions also make meeting nutrient needs difficult. A number of programs have been developed to help older adults plan and consume diets that meet their needs.

Planning Diets A modified Food Guide Pyramid has been developed to emphasize the nutrients and food selections that are of particular concern for older adults. In some cases nutrient supplements may be necessary to meet needs.

A Modified Food Guide Pyramid The modified Food Guide Pyramid shown in Figure 17.15 has been designed to plan diets that will meet the special needs of older adults. This modified pyramid is built on a base of water—eight 8-ounce glasses per day. This helps emphasize that dehydration resulting from a decreased sensation of thirst and many medications is a chronic problem and that older adults need to be more conscious of water consumption. This pyramid also has a narrower base than the traditional USDA Food Guide Pyramid to illustrate that energy need is typically reduced among the elderly.[56] The numbers of servings are set at equal to or greater than the minimum recommended by the Food Guide Pyramid, and nutrient-dense choices from each food group are recommended. To highlight the importance of fiber in the diets of older adults, the pyramid for seniors includes a fiber icon in the food groups containing grains, fruits, vegetables, and beans, nuts, and seeds. Another key difference in this pyramid is a flag at the top that indicates the possible need for dietary supplements.

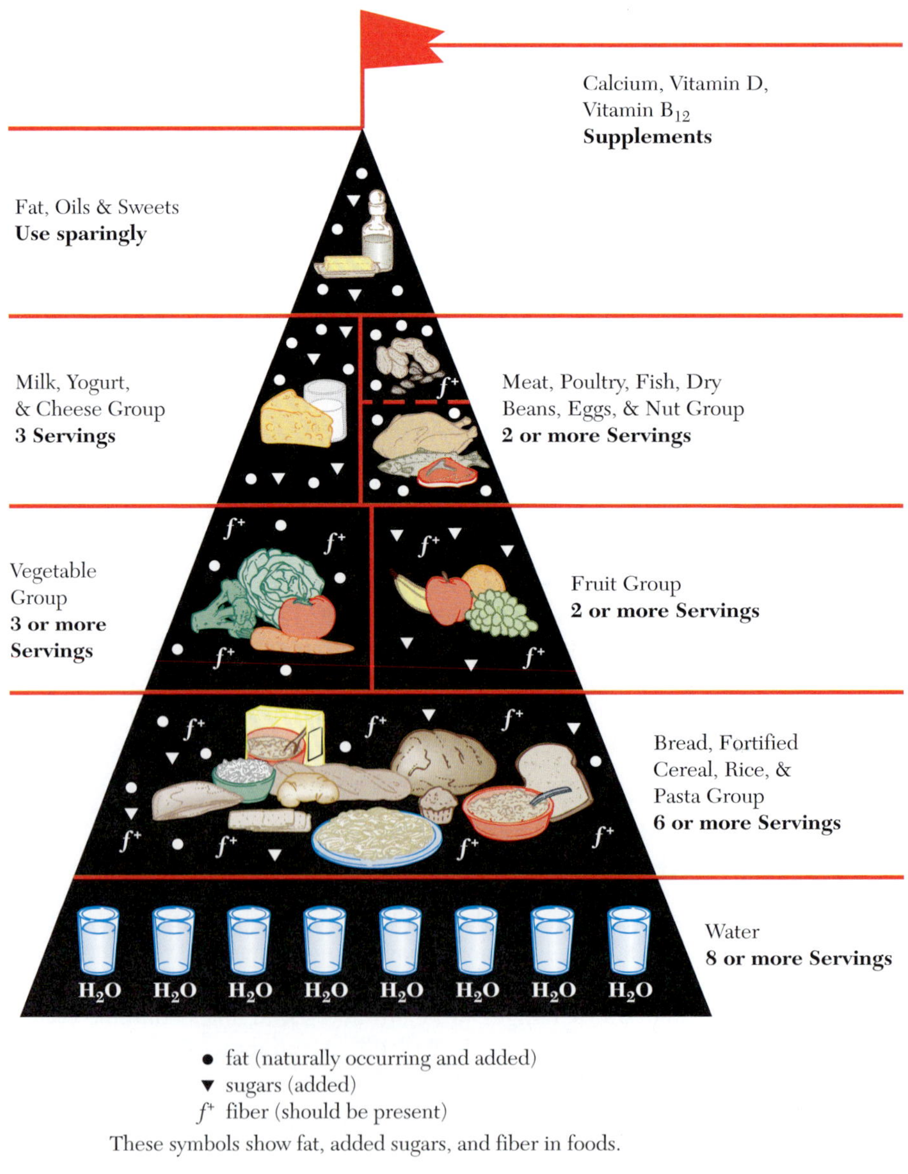

FIGURE 17.15 This modification of the Food Guide Pyramid targets the needs of healthy mobile seniors (over age 70) and is not designed to meet the needs of those with special dietary needs or significant health problems.

Dietary Supplements Although supplements are not usually necessary to meet micronutrient needs, many older adults may benefit from supplementing some nutrients. Vitamin D is a concern because its production in the skin is decreased and exposure to sunlight may be limited. A calcium supplement may be necessary to meet needs particularly in elderly women because it can be difficult to consume 1200 mg of calcium from food without exceeding energy needs. Because the absorption of vitamin B_{12} decreases with age, supplemental vitamin B_{12} from pills or fortified foods is recommended for older adults. However, as with other age groups, older adults should be cautious to avoid overdoses, and the resulting toxicities, when selecting supplements. And, supplements should not take the place of a balanced, nutrient-dense diet high in grains, fruits, and vegetables. These foods also contain phytochemicals and other substances that may protect against disease (see Chapter 10).

A multivitamin and mineral supplement containing no more than 100% of the Daily Value for any nutrient is the safest way to supplement the diet. Supplements containing megadoses or nonnutrient substances should be avoided. Many of these are a waste of money and others can be toxic. For example, lecithin is claimed to lower cholesterol and to treat Alzheimer's, but there is no proof that it does either. RNA is claimed to rejuvenate old cells, improve memory, and prevent wrinkling, but there are no controlled studies to support any of these claims. Superoxide dismutase (SOD), an enzyme that protects against oxidative damage, is said to slow aging and treat Alzheimer's. However, even if higher tissue levels of SOD provided extra antioxidant protection, SOD is a protein that is broken down to amino acids in the GI tract, so oral supplements will not increase blood or tissue levels of this enzyme. Coenzyme Q, a synthetic version of a compound in the electron transport chain, is marketed to older adults as a way to slow aging by enhancing the immune system. However, it does not boost immune function and may be dangerous for people with poor circulation.

Preventing Food Insecurity It is estimated that from 2.5 to 4.9 million older Americans experience food insecurity in any given six-month period.[57] Any factor, whether physical, psychological, emotional, social, or economic, that interferes with the availability of or the ability to acquire desirable foods in socially acceptable ways can lead to food insecurity, and, subsequently, malnutrition. To assure that older adults can meet their needs each case must be handled individually. In some cases, this involves providing meals; in others, it requires providing education about nutrient requirements, economics, and food preparation. For some individuals, assistance with shopping or meal preparation helps eliminate food insecurity.

Economic Factors Being able to afford a healthy diet is a problem for many older individuals. Reduced-cost food and meals at senior centers, food stamps, food banks, soup kitchens, and **commodity foods** are available to people with limited incomes. Programs that provide education about low-cost nutritious food choices can help reduce food costs.

Commodity foods Foods that are purchased and stored by the government to eliminate excess in the marketplace.

Social Factors Loneliness can be a reason for poor nutrient intake. Living, cooking, and eating alone can decrease interest in food (Figure 17.16). This can be a problem not only for the elderly but also for anyone who typically eats alone. Buying single servings of food is an option, although it can be expensive. To avoid spoilage of perishable items, grocers can be asked to break up packages of meat, eggs, fruits, and vegetables so small amounts can be purchased. Large packages can be purchased and shared among friends. Cooking larger portions and freezing meals in single-serving portions can be helpful not only with cost but also in relieving the boredom of eating the same leftovers several days in a row. Creativity and flexibility in what defines a meal can also help. An easy single meal can be prepared by topping a potato with cooked vegetables and cheese, or with leftover

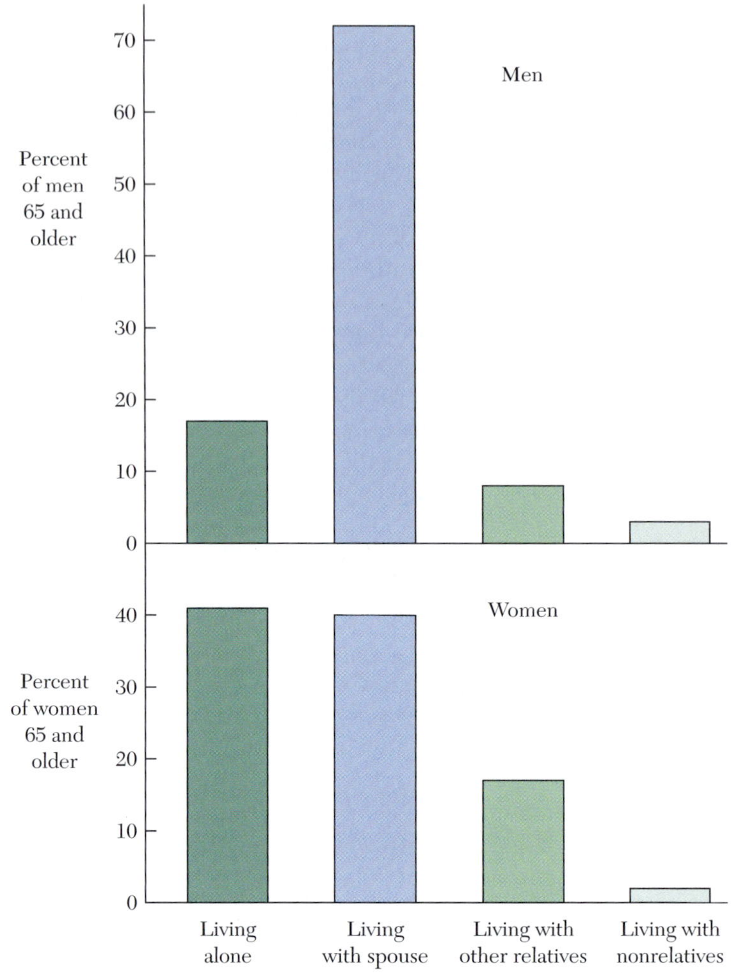

FIGURE 17.16 Many older adults live alone. Loneliness contributes to depression and can decrease the appeal of food and contribute to malnutrition. *(U.S. Bureau of the Census. "Household and Family Characteristics: March, 1997." Current Population Reports, P20–509.)*

chili or spaghetti sauce (Figure 17.17). Yogurt or a bowl of cereal with fruit and milk is also a nutritious dinner option.

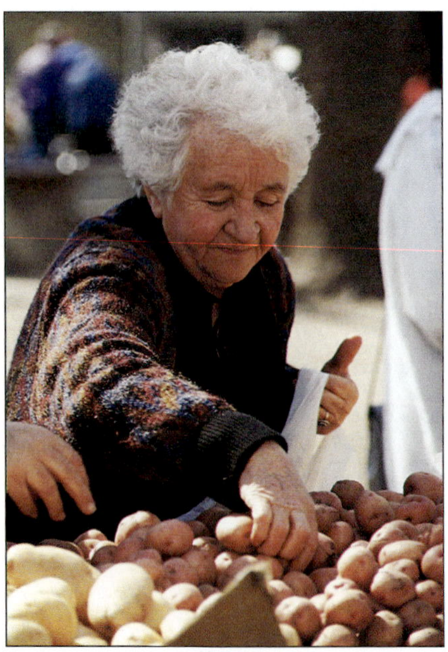

FIGURE 17.17 Selecting acceptable foods that are nutritious and easy to prepare is important in meeting the needs of the elderly. *(©Tony Freeman/PhotoEdit)*

Mobility Food intake may also be reduced if limitations in mobility make it difficult to cook. About 53% of adults 65 and older have some kind of disability and 33.4% have disabilities that are considered severe.[5] Precooked foods, frozen dinners, salad-bar items, and instant foods such as cereals and rice and noodle dishes can provide a meal with almost no preparation. Medical nutritional products, such as Ensure or Boost, can also be used to supplement intake. These are canned and fortified, so a small volume can meet most nutrient needs and they will keep for long periods. Eating at senior centers or sharing shopping and cooking chores with a friend can reduce the amount of cooking required and increase social interaction. Home health services are also available to help with cooking and eating, and most senior centers, health departments, and social service agencies offer meals, rides, and in-home care.

Medical Factors It is estimated that 85% of elderly individuals have nutrition-related diseases.[58] The management of many of these ailments requires restricting or increasing specific foods and nutrients. These diets may contribute to malnutrition if they restrict favorite foods and if the individuals to whom the diet is prescribed do not understand how to substitute foods that will give them adequate energy, nutrients, and eating pleasure. A thorough knowledge of one's dietary prescription and a working knowledge of food labels can enhance one's ability to comply with dietary restrictions and meet nutrient needs while consuming a varied diet. For example, an individual with diabetes who is counting carbohydrates can find the carbohydrate content on the label of almost any packaged food. Individuals with diverticulosis or constipation who are monitoring their fiber intake can use food labels to determine a food's fiber content.

The use of prescription or over-the-counter medications to treat medical conditions can also affect eating habits. Physicians, pharmacists, and dietitians can provide information about possible interactions between foods and mediations. Purchasing all prescription medications from the same pharmacy will help ensure that the pharmacist is aware of all medications taken and their possible interactions.

Nutrition Programs for the Elderly Increasing the number of healthy years that individuals enjoy is a major public health goal for the 21st century. To address this goal, there are many federal, local, and private programs designed to promote nutritional health among older adults. Some of these promote health care and screening for malnutrition; others provide access to food and social interaction.

Nutrition Screening Initiative To address concerns over the nutritional health of the elderly, the federal Nutrition Screening Initiative was developed to promote screening for and intervention in nutrition-related problems in older adults.[59] This program tries to increase awareness of nutritional problems in the elderly by involving practitioners and community organizations as well as relatives, friends, and others caring for the elderly in evaluating the nutritional status of the aging population. This program developed the DETERMINE checklist based on an acronym for the physiological, medical, and socioeconomic situations that increase the risk of malnutrition among the elderly (see Table 17.5). The elderly themselves, family members, and caregivers can use this tool to identify when malnutrition is a potential problem.

Web Menu

For information about having meals delivered to a friend or relative, or to volunteer, visit the Meals on Wheels Association of America at www.projectmeal.org/.

Congregate and Home-Delivered Nutrition Programs The federal Older Americans Act provides nutrition services to older individuals who are in economic need, particularly low-income minorities. Programs that provide nutritious meals in communal settings promote social interaction and can improve nutrient intake. The Congregate and Home-Delivered Nutrition Programs established by the

TABLE 17.5 DETERMINE: A Checklist of the Warning Signs of Malnutrition

Disease	Any disease, illness, or condition that causes changes in eating can predispose one to malnutrition. Memory loss and depression can also interfere with nutrition if they affect food intake.
Eating poorly	Eating either too little or too much can lead to poor health.
Tooth loss or mouth pain	An unhealthy mouth, teeth, or gums interferes with eating.
Economic hardship	Having to or choosing to spend less than $25–$30 per person per week on food interferes with nutrition.
Reduced social support	Being alone has a negative effect on morale, well-being, and eating.
Multiple medicines	The more medicines one takes, the greater the chances of side effects such as weakness, drowsiness, diarrhea, changes in taste and appetite, nausea, and constipation.
Involuntary weight loss/gain	Unintentionally losing or gaining weight is a warning sign that should not be ignored. Being overweight or underweight also increases the risk of malnutrition.
Needs assistance in self-care	Difficulty walking, shopping, and cooking increases the risk of malnutrition.
Elder above age 80	The risks of frailty and health problems increase with increasing age.

TABLE 17.6 National Programs Promoting Better Nutrition Among Older Americans

Older Americans Act–Title III Congregate and Home-Delivered Nutrition Programs

Serves at least one meal five days a week to persons age 60 and older. Meals are served at home or in churches, schools, senior centers, or other facilities.

Older Americans Act–Title VI Congregate and Home-Delivered Nutrition Programs

Provides home-delivered and congregate meals to Native American organizations.

Older Americans Act–Title III Health Promotion and Disease Prevention Program

Provides health-promotion and disease-prevention services in areas where there are large numbers of economically needy older adults.

Nutrition Screening Initiative

Promotes nutritional screening and more attention to nutrition in all health-care and social-service settings that provide for older adults.

Food Stamp Program

Provides food stamps to low-income individuals, including the elderly. These can be used instead of cash to purchase food.

Nutrition Program for the Elderly

Provides grants, cash, and commodity foods to states and tribes to supplement congregate and home-delivered meal programs.

Commodity Supplemental Food Program–Elderly

Provides food, nutrition education, and health-service referrals to individuals with low incomes, including the elderly.

Child and Adult Care Food Program (Adult Day Care)

Provides cash reimbursements and food commodities to community day-care centers that serve meals and snacks to children and elderly with special needs.

Food Distribution Program on Indian Reservations

Distributes commodity foods to low-income persons, including the elderly, living on or near Indian reservations.

Older Americans Act provide congregate meals at locations such as senior centers, community centers, schools, and churches. For those who are unable to attend congregate meals, home-delivered meals are available.

Although such programs are a first step in meeting nutritional needs, currently most provide only one meal a day for five days a week. Each meal served must provide at least a third of the 1989 RDA.[60] In practice, participants in these elder nutrition programs are receiving 40 to 50% of their daily intake from the meal consumed.[61] Studies have shown that individuals who receive these meals have a better-quality diet and fewer hospitalizations than those who do not.[62] These and other programs addressing the nutritional needs of older adults are described in Table 17.6.

SUMMARY

1. Aging is the accumulation of changes over time that results in an ever-increasing susceptibility to disease and death. A combination of genetic, environmental, and lifestyle factors determines how long we live and how long we remain healthy.
2. The elderly are the fastest-growing segment of the American population. As a population, we are living longer but not necessarily healthier lives. Compression of morbidity—that is, increasing the number of healthy years—is an important public health goal.
3. Life span is a characteristic of a species. The average age to which people in a population live, or life expectancy, is a characteristic of a population. An individual's longevity is affected by genetic background, diet, and lifestyle.

4. As the body ages, reserve capacity decreases, causing organ function to decline. There are changes in vision and the sense of smell that affect the ability to eat as well as the appeal of food. Changes in digestion and absorption decrease the intake and absorption of nutrients, changes in metabolism affect nutrient utilization, changes in hormonal patterns affect body function, and changes in mobility and mental capacity limit the ability to acquire, prepare, and consume food.
5. The incidence of disease increases with advancing age. Both infectious and chronic diseases affect nutrient requirements and the ability to consume a nutritious diet. The medications used to treat disease also affect nutrition, especially when they are taken over long periods of time and when multiple medications are taken simultaneously.
6. Energy needs are reduced with age but the requirement for most nutrients remains the same. In addition, the absorption and metabolism of some nutrients change with age, making it more difficult to meet nutrient needs.
7. When planning diets for older adults, their medical, psychological, social, and economic circumstances must be considered. Meals should be economical, convenient to prepare and consume, and nutrient-dense. A modified Food Guide Pyramid is available to help plan diets for this age group.
8. The DETERMINE checklist helps identify older adults who are at risk of malnutrition. The federal Older Americans Act includes programs that provide older adults with low-cost or free meals in their homes or in a social setting. Although these programs are helpful, they do not ensure adequate nutrition for all elderly.

Review Questions

1. How long can each of us expect to live?
2. What is meant by compression of morbidity?
3. Why are older adults at risk for malnutrition?
4. List three physiological changes that occur with aging.
5. List three ways in which the use of medications interacts with nutrition.
6. What social and economic factors increase nutritional risk among the elderly?
7. Why are energy needs decreased in older adults?
8. Why is it so important for elderly individuals to consume a nutrient-dense diet?
9. What nutrients may need to be supplemented in the diets of the elderly? Why?
10. How do recommendations such as the RDAs and the Dietary Guidelines for Americans apply to individuals over the age of 65?

Applying Critical Thinking Skills

Personal nutrition:

1. Use one day of the food record you kept in Chapter 2 and compare it with the recommended energy allowance for a person who is 75 years old. Modify your food choices to meet the recommendations of the senior pyramid shown in Figure 17.15.
2. How might you modify your food choices to accommodate the following medical conditions or dietary modifications:
   a. A low-sodium diet?
   b. A protein restriction of 0.6 g per kilogram of body weight?
   c. A loss of smell and taste?
   d. A dry mouth and poorly fitting dentures?

General nutrition issues:

1. Use the Internet to determine what kind of nutrition information is available to individuals planning for the care of their elderly parents or relatives. What are the costs?
2. Assume that you have an elderly friend who lives and eats alone. Find resources in your area that would be able to provide meals and other services for your friend.
3. Prepare an outline for a 20-minute lecture on nutrition and aging that will be given at a senior center in your area.
   a. Define two goals for the lecture.
   b. Outline five main points that you will discuss.

References

1. U.S. Department of Health and Human Services, Administration on Aging. 1997 Census Estimates of the Older Population. Available online at **http://www.aoa.dhhs.gov/aoa/stats/99pop/default.htm.** Accessed 17 Feb 2001.
2. Hodes, R. J., Cahan, V., and Pruzan, N. The National Institute of Aging at its twentieth anniversary: achievements and promise of research on aging. J. Am. Geriatr. Soc. 44:204–206, 1996.
3. Healthy People 2010: National Health Promotion and Disease Prevention Objectives. Washington, D.C.: U.S. Department of Health and Human Services, 1998. Available online at **http://web.health.gov/healthypeople.** Accessed 17 Feb 2001.
4. National Center for Health Statistics. Table 12: Estimated Life Expectancy in Years by Race and Sex, 1997. National Vital Statistics Report, Vol. 47, No. 28, December 13, 1999. Available online at

http://www.cdc.gov/nchs/fastats/lifexpec.htm. Accessed 17 Feb 2001.

5. American Dietetic Association: Position of the American Dietetic Association: Nutrition, aging and the continuum of care. J. Am. Diet Assoc. 100:580–595, 2000.
6. Mazess, R. B., and Forman, S. H. Longevity and age exaggeration in Vilcabamba, Ecuador. J. Gerontol. 34:94–98, 1979.
7. Young, A. Ageing and physiological functions. Philos. Trans. R. Soc. Lond. B. Biol. Sci. 352:1837–1843, 1997.
8. Kirkwood, T. B. L. Comparative life spans of species: why do species have the life spans they do? Am. J. Clin. Nutr. 55(suppl):1191S–1195S, 1992.
9. Blumberg, J. Nutritional needs of seniors. J. Am. Coll. Nutr. 16:517–523, 1997.
10. Duffy, V. B., Backstrand, J. R., and Ferris, A. M. Olfactory dysfunction and related nutritional risk in free-living elderly women. J. Am. Diet. Assoc. 95:879–884, 1995.
11. Morley, J. E. Anorexia of aging: physiologic and pathologic. Am. J. Clin. Nutr. 66:760–773, 1997.
12. Food and Nutrition Board, Institute of Medicine. *Dietary Reference Intakes for Thiamin, Riboflavin, Niacin, Vitamin B_6, Folate, Vitamin B_{12}, Pantothenic Acid, Biotin, and Choline.* Washington, D.C.: National Academy Press, 1998.
13. Saltzman, J. R., and Russell, R. M. The aging gut. Nutritional issues. Gastroenterol. Clin. North Am. 27:309–324, 1998.
14. van Asselt, D. Z., van den Broek, W. J., Lamers, C. B., et al. Free and protein-bound cobalamin absorption in healthy middle-aged and older subjects. J. Am. Geriatr. Soc. 44:949–953, 1996.
15. Harari, D., Gurwitz, J. H., Avorn, J., et al. Bowel habits in relation to age and gender: findings from the National Health Interview Survey and clinical implications. Arch. Intern. Med. 156:315–320, 1996.
16. Brucker, M. C., and Faucher, M. A. Pharmacologic management of common gastrointestinal health problems in women. J. Nurse-Midwifery 42:145–162, May/June 1997.
17. Lubran, M. M. Renal function in the elderly. Ann. Clin. Lab. Sci. 25:122–133, 1995.
18. Stevens, J., Tyroler, H., Cai, J., et al Body weight change and carotid artery wall thickness. The Atherosclerosis Risk in Communities (ARIC) Study. Am. J. Epidemiol. 147:563–573, 1998.
19. Stevens, J., Cai, J., Pamuk, E. R., et al. The effect of age on the association between body mass index and mortality. N. Engl. J. Med. 338:1–7, 1998.
20. Willett, W. C. Weight loss in the elderly: cause or effect of poor health? Am. J. Clin. Nutr. 66:737–738, 1997.
21. Lamberts, S. W. J., van den Beld, A. W., and van der Lely, A-J. The endocrinology of aging. Science 278:419–424, 1998.
22. Proctor, D. N., Balagopal, P., and Nair, K. S. Age-related saropenia in humans is associated with reduced synthetic rates of specific muscle proteins. J. Nutr. 128:351S–355S, 1998.
23. National Center for Health Statistics. *Health, United States, 1999, with Health and Aging Chartbook.* Hyattsville, MD: National Center for Health Statistics, 1999.
24. Evans, W. J., and Cyr-Campbell, D. Nutrition, exercise and healthy aging. J. Am. Diet. Assoc. 97:632–638, 1997.
25. Masoro, E. J. Caloric restriction and aging: an update. Exp. Gerontol. 35:299–305, 2000.
26. Wallace, J. I., and Schwartz, R. S. Involuntary weight loss in elderly outpatients: recognition, etiologies and treatment. Clin. Geriatr. Med. 13:717–735, 1997.
27. Butler R. N., Fossel M., Pan C. X., et al. Efficacy and safety of hormones and antioxidants. Geriatrics 55:48–52, 2000.
28. Zachwieja, J. J., and Yarasheski, K. E. Does growth hormone therapy in conjunction with resistance exercise increase muscle force production and muscle mass in men and women aged 60 years or older? Phys. Ther. 79:76–82, 1999.
29. Cummings, D. E., and Merriam, G. R. Age-related changes in growth hormone secretion: should the somatopause be treated? Semin. Reprod. Endocrinol. 17:311–325, 1999.
30. Williams. J. R. The effects of dehydroepiandrosterone on carcinogenesis, obesity, the immune system, and aging. Lipids 35:325–331, 2000.
31. Rieter, R. J. The pineal gland and melatonin in relation to aging: a summary of the theories and the data. Exp. Gerontol. 30:199–212, 1995.
32. Maestroni, G. J. P-helper-2 lymphocytes as a peripheral target of melatonin. J. Pineal Res. 18:84–89, 1995.
33. Guardiola-Lemaitre, B. Toxicology of melatonin. J. Biol. Rhythms 12: 697–706, 1997.
34. Herrington, D. M., Reboussin, D. M., Brosnihan, K. B., et al. Effects of estrogen replacement on the progression of coronary-artery atherosclerosis. N. Engl. J. Med. 343:522–529, 2000.
35. Lesourd, B. M., Mazari, L., and Ferry, M. The role of nutrition in immunity in the aged. Nutr. Rev. 56 (II):S113–S125, 1998.
36. Lesourd, B. Protein undernutrition as the major cause of decreased immune function in the elderly: clinical and functional implications. Nutr. Rev. 53:S86–S94, 1995.
37. Meydani, S. N., Meydani, M., Blumberg, J. B., et al. Vitamin E supplemention and *in vivo* immune responses in healthy elderly subjects. JAMA 277:1380–1386, 1997.
38. Meydani, S. N., Wu, D., Santos, M. S., et al. Antioxidants and immune response in aged persons: overview of the present evidence. Am. J. Clin. Nutr. 62(suppl):1426S–1476S, 1995.
39. Bogden, J. D. Studies on micronutrient supplements and immunity in older people. Nutr. Rev. 53:S59–S65, 1995.
40. U. S. Department of Health and Human Services, Administration on Aging. Profile of Older Americans, 1998. Available online at **http://www.aoa.dhhs.gov/aoa/stats/profile/default.htm.** Accessed 17 Feb 2001.
41. National Center for Health Statistics. Older Americans 2000: Key Indicators of Well-Being. Available online at **http://www.agingstats.gov.** Accessed 12 Oct 2000.
42. Nourhashemi, F., Gillette-Guyonnet, S., Andrieu, S., et al. Alzheimer's disease: protective factors. Am. J. Clin. Nutr. 71:643S–649S, 2000.
43. Stabler, S. P., Lindenbaum, J., and Allen, R. H. Vitamin B_{12} deficiency in the elderly: current dilemmas. Am. J. Clin. Nutr. 66:741–749, 1997.
44. Vogel, G. Tau protein mutations confirmed as neuron killers. Science 280:1524–1525, 1998.
45. American Academy of Family Physicians. The Nutrition Checklist. Available online at **http://www.aafp.org/nsi.** Accessed 23 Oct 2000.
46. American Dietetic Association: Position of the American Dietetic Association: liberalized diets for older adults in long-term care. J. Am. Diet. Assoc. 98:201–204, 1998.
47. Chidester, J. C., and Spangler. A. A. Fluid intake in the institutionalized elderly. J. Am. Diet. Assoc. 97:23–28, 1997.
48. Cui, X. J., and Vaillant, G. E. Antecedents and consequences of negative life events in adulthood: a longitudinal study. Am. J. Psychiatry 153:21–26, 1996.
49. Evans, W. J., and Cyr-Campbell, D. Nutrition, exercise and healthy aging. J. Am. Diet. Assoc. 97:632–638, 1997.
50. Young, V. R. Energy requirements in the elderly. Nutr. Rev. 50:95–101, 1992.
51. Food and Nutrition Board, Institute of Medicine. *Dietary Reference Intakes: Calcium, Phosphorus, Magnesium, Vitamin D, and Fluoride.* Washington, D.C.: National Academy Press, 1997.
52. Christen, W. G. Antioxidant vitamins and age-related eye disease. Proc. Assoc. Am. Physicians 111:16–21, 1999.
53. Kohlmeier, L., and Hastings, S. B. Epidemiologic evidence of a role of carotenoids in cardiovascular disease prevention. Am. J. Clin. Nutr. 62(suppl):1370S–1376S, 1995.
54. Rimm, E. B., Stampfer, M. J., Asherio, A., et al. Vitamin E consumption and the risk of heart disease in men. N. Engl. J. Med. 328:1450–1456, 1993.
55. Stampfer, M. J., Hennekens, C. H., Manson, J. E., et al. Vitamin E consumption and the risk of heart disease in women. N. Engl. J. Med. 328:1487–1489, 1993.

56. Russell, R. M., Rasmussen, H., and Lichtenstein, A. H. Modified food guide pyramid for people over seventy years of age. J. Nutr. 129:751–753, 1999.
57. Wellman, N. S., Weddle, D. O., Brain, C. T., and Kranz, S. Elder insecurities: poverty, hunger, and malnutrition. J. Am. Diet. Assoc. 97:S120–S122, 1997.
58. White, J. V., Ham, R. J., Lipschitz, D. A., et al. Consensus of the Nutrition Screening Initiative: risk factors and indicators of poor nutritional status in older Americans. J. Am. Diet. Assoc. 91:783–787, 1991.
59. American Academy of Family Physicians. Nutrition Screening Initiative. Available online at **http://www.aafp.org/nsi/index.html.** Accessed 17 Feb 2001.
60. Fogler-Levitt, E., Lau, D., Csima, A., et al. Utilization of home-delivered meals by recipients 75 years of age or older. J. Am. Diet. Assoc. 95:552–557, 1995.
61. U. S. Department of Health and Human Services, Administration on Aging. Elderly Nutrition Program. Available online at **http://www.aoa.gov/nutrition/default.htm.** Accessed 17 Feb 2001.
62. Roe, D. A. Development and current status of home-delivered meals programs in the United States: are the right elderly served? Nutr. Rev. 52:29–33, 1994.

18 Feeding the World

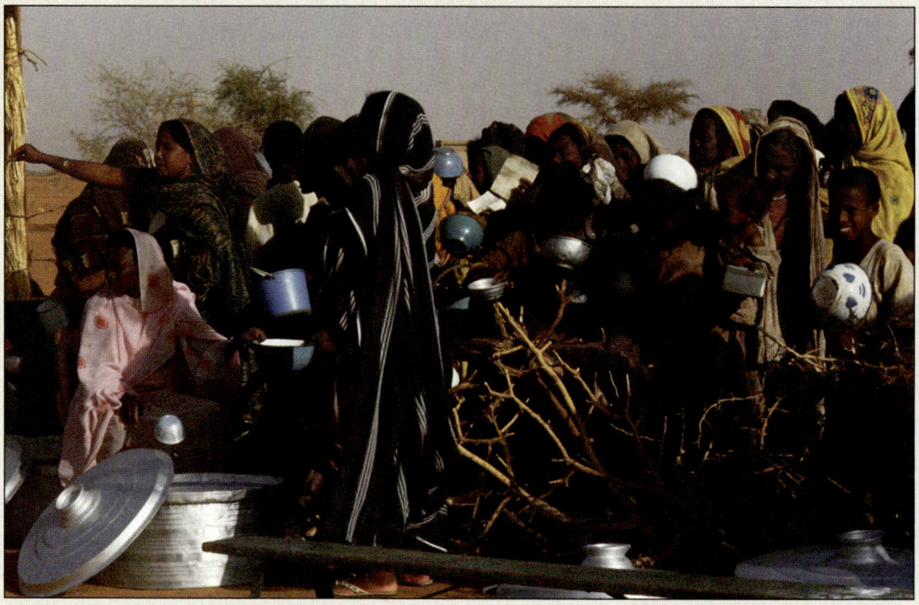

Learning Objectives

After reading this chapter, students should be able to:

1. Compare the prevalence of under- and overnutrition in developed and developing nations.
2. Discuss the impact of undernutrition in the developing world.
3. Describe the cycle of malnutrition.
4. Discuss the causes of food shortages.
5. List the most common nutrient deficiencies worldwide.
6. Propose some solutions to the problems of world hunger.
7. Describe the problem of undernutrition in the United States.
8. Discuss programs designed to address undernutrition in the United States.

For World Food Day, José wanted to prepare a poster to put in the university student union. He decided that a collage of newspaper and magazine headlines would be a good way to illustrate the inadequate food supply and resulting hunger and malnutrition that plagues most of the world. Some research on the Internet turned up a number of stories from around the world.

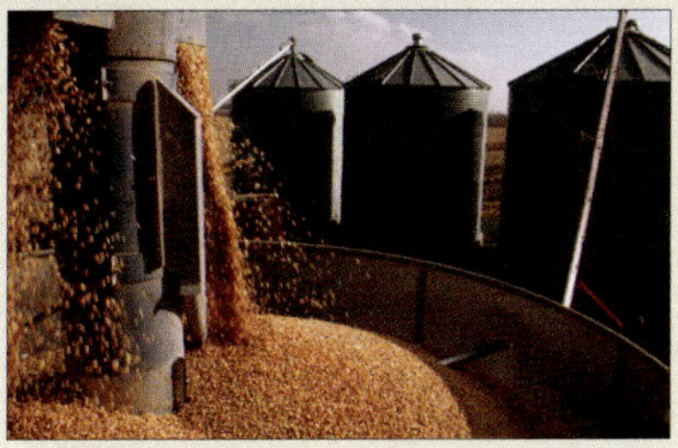

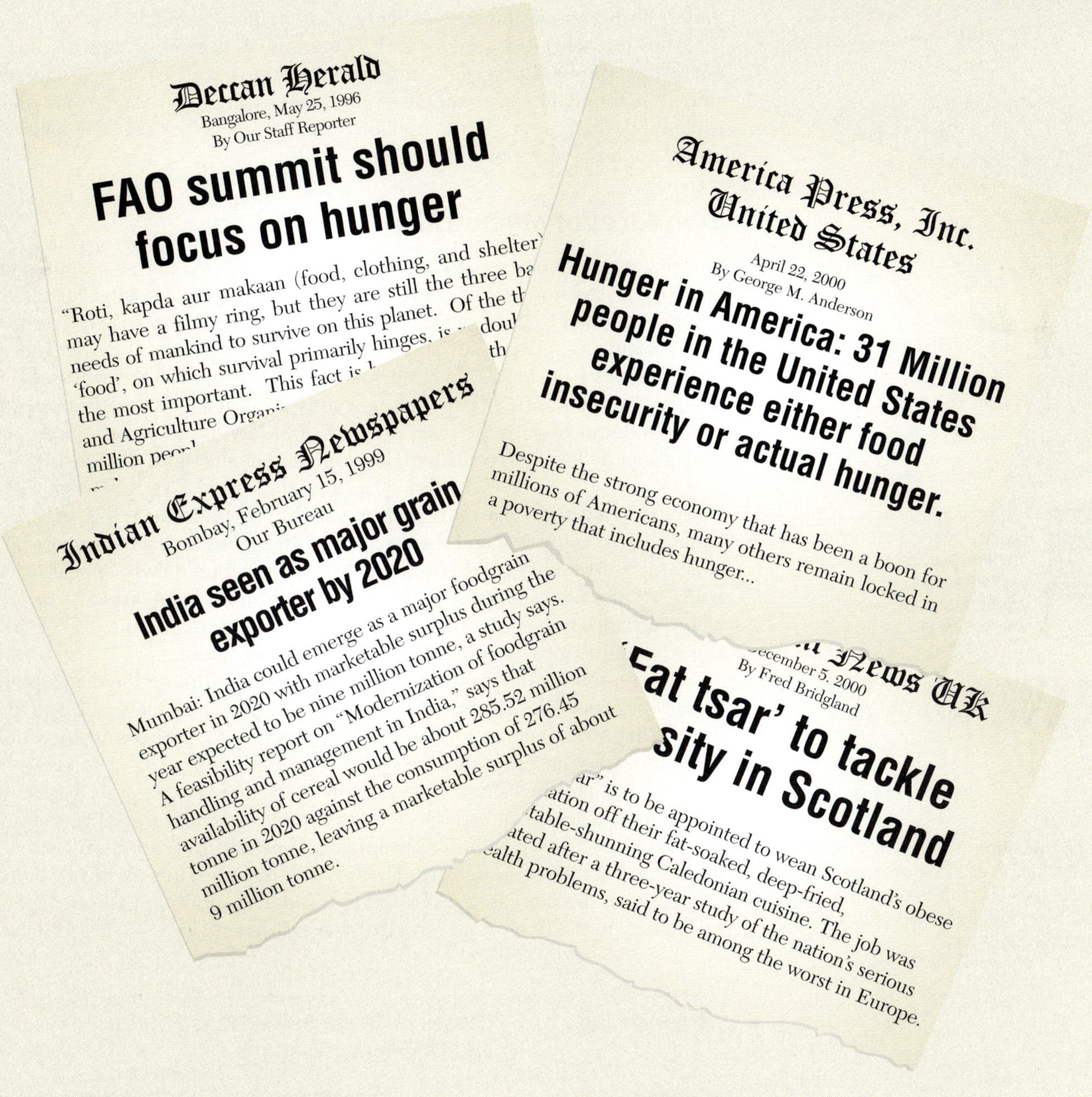

Deccan Herald
Bangalore, May 25, 1996
By Our Staff Reporter

FAO summit should focus on hunger

"Roti, kapda aur makaan (food, clothing, and shelter) may have a filmy ring, but they are still the three ba[sic] needs of mankind to survive on this planet. Of the th[ree] 'food', on which survival primarily hinges, is ... the most important. This fact is ... and Agriculture Orga... million peo...

America Press, Inc.
United States
April 22, 2000
By George M. Anderson

Hunger in America: 31 Million people in the United States experience either food insecurity or actual hunger.

Despite the strong economy that has been a boon for millions of Americans, many others remain locked in a poverty that includes hunger...

Indian Express Newspapers
Bombay, February 15, 1999
Our Bureau

India seen as major grain exporter by 2020

Mumbai: India could emerge as a major foodgrain exporter in 2020 with marketable surplus during the year expected to be nine million tonne, a study says. A feasibility report on "Modernization of foodgrain handling and management in India," says that availability of cereal would be about 285.52 million tonne in 2020 against the consumption of 276.45 million tonne, leaving a marketable surplus of about 9 million tonne.

...News UK
...ecember 5, 2000
By Fred Bridgland

...Fat tsar' to tackle ...sity in Scotland

...ar" is to be appointed to wean Scotland's obese ...ation off their fat-soaked, deep-fried, ...table-shunning Caledonian cuisine. The job was ...ated after a three-year study of the nation's serious ...ealth problems, said to be among the worst in Europe.

When José looked at all of this information together, he realized that his understanding of world hunger was not as complete as he had thought. In India, where José believed malnutrition was common, there was a grain surplus. In the United States, where the grocery-store shelves were always packed, people were going hungry. José began to realize that hunger and malnutrition are complicated problems, and that viewing them as simply a result of a lack of food is inaccurate.

Nutrition and World Health

A well-nourished population consumes a diet that prevents deficiencies and at the same time does not promote conditions related to excess intakes of energy or nutrients. The headlines José gathered suggest that many populations throughout the world are not well nourished and that malnutrition has two faces. In developed nations today there are pockets of undernutrition, but the majority of nutritional problems are related to overconsumption. In developing nations, undernutrition predominates—affecting 840 million people.[1,2]

Why does this dichotomy exist? There are many reasons, but the underlying one is that the food produced around the world is not distributed equitably, resulting in abundance in some places and scarcity in others. And, even when food is plentiful, the types of foods available or the food choices that are made may not provide optimal nutrition.

Two Faces of Malnutrition

Overnutrition—due to a pattern of intake that is high in energy, saturated fat, cholesterol, and sodium, and low in fiber—contributes to the nutrition-related diseases that are common in the United States. Although this dietary pattern is related to a higher incidence of diseases such as cardiovascular disease, obesity, cancer, diabetes, osteoporosis, and other nutrition-related chronic diseases the diet is also plentiful in micronutrients, so deficiency diseases are rare. In developing nations, where undernutrition is the main problem, low energy and protein intakes and micronutrient deficiencies contribute to a high rate of infectious disease (Table 18.1).

Web Menu: For more information on the health impact of economic and nutrition transition, go to the World Health Report at the World Health Organization Web site at www.who.int/.

Nutrition Transition Despite the prevalance of undernutrition in developing countries, overnutrition and the disease risks it carries are an emerging and future concern. Nutrition-related chronic diseases are either newly appearing, rapidly rising, or already established in every country around the world.[3,4] In countries where urbanization is occurring rapidly the incidence of chronic diseases is on the rise while infectious diseases remain a common problem.[5]

The reason for the growing problem of overnutrition in the developing world is that as economic conditions improve access to food increases and diet and lifestyle patterns change to resemble those of developed countries. Traditional diets in developing countries are based on a limited number of foods—primarily starchy roots and high-fiber grains. As incomes increase, the diet becomes more varied and the intake of meat, fish, milk, cheese, eggs, and fresh fruits and vegetables increases.[6] Along with this economic and **nutrition transition** come changes in lifestyle that decrease activity. There is a shift toward less physically demanding occupations, an increased use of motorized transportation, more labor-saving technology in the home, and more passive leisure activities (Figure 18.1).

Nutrition transition The shift in dietary pattern that occurs as incomes increase—from a diet high in complex carbohydrates and fiber to a more varied diet higher in fats, saturated fat, and sugar.

Table 18.1 Causes of Death in the United States and Developing Nations

	United States (% deaths)	Developing Nations (% deaths)
Infectious disease	6	45
Noncommunicable disease	72	36
Injuries	5	11
Other	17	8

World Health Organization, 1999, at **http://www.who.int.infectious-disease-report/pages/graph2.html**, and Centers for Disease Control and Prevention at **http://www.cdc.gov/nchs/data/nvs48_11.pdf.**

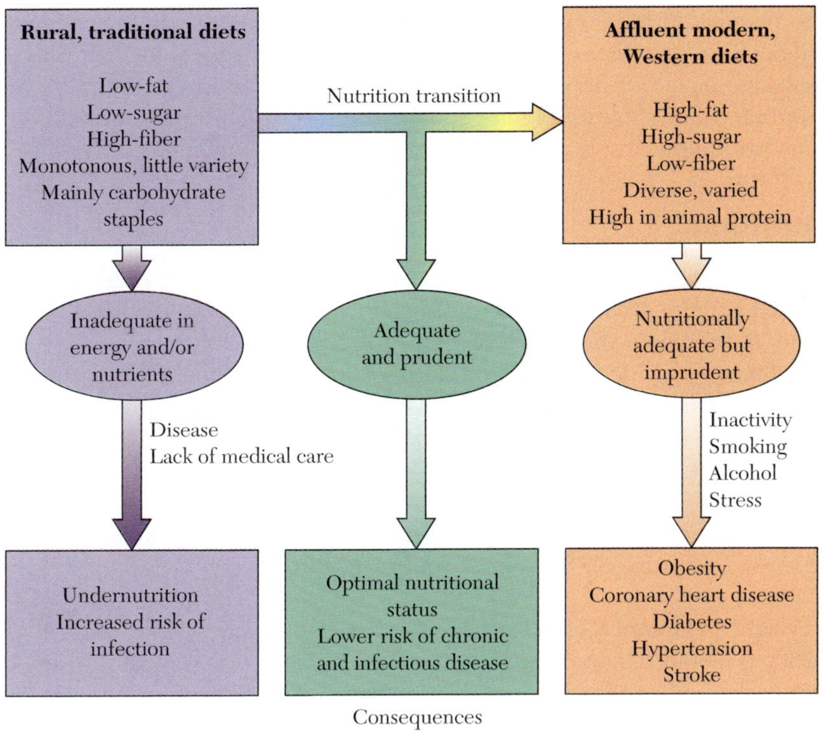

FIGURE 18.1 This schematic represents the dietary changes that occur with nutrition transition and the health consequences associated with these changes. A diet that falls somewhere between the traditional rural diet that may be inadequate in energy, protein, or micronutrients and the affluent Western diet that meets nutrient needs but is high in fat and sugar and low in fiber is optimal for health. *(Adapted from Vorster, H. H., Bourne, L. T., Venter, C. S., and Oosthuizen, W. Contribution of nutrition to the health transition in developing countries: a framework for research and intervention. Nutr. Rev. 57:341–349, 1999.)*

Some of the effects of this transition are positive. Shifts in diet are accompanied by increases in life expectancy and by decreases in birthrate and the incidence of infectious disease and nutrient deficiencies. But many of the effects are negative. The transition in diet and lifestyle is associated with an increase in the rates of heart disease, cancer, diabetes, and adult and childhood obesity.[6] Obesity levels in some developing countries are as high as those in the developed world.[7] Heart disease, stroke, and other chronic diseases now cause 39% of all deaths in developing countries.[8] The goal in developing nations is to promote economic growth and reduce undernutrition and infectious disease, while at the same time preventing overnutrition and delaying the onset of chronic disease.

Preventing Overnutrition A major focus of health and nutrition policies and programs in developing nations is to prevent undernutrition by improving food security, the availability of health services, and economic status. A problem facing international development agencies is how to promote economic growth and at the same time prevent the undesirable effects of nutrition transition. To address these growing health concerns, individual countries have developed public health campaigns and policies that also include strategies to prevent overnutrition and promote healthy lifestyles (see Appendix F). International campaigns also target the prevention and control of chronic diseases.[4] One such program is Interhealth, developed by the World Health Organization (WHO). Each country involved in Interhealth must assess its nutritional behaviors and intakes, physical activity levels, blood pressure and blood cholesterol levels, and other chronic disease risk factors such as smoking, alcohol consumption, and obesity. Then they must implement strategies to reduce these risk factors, monitor trends in mortality, and evaluate the success of their programs. A component of the Interhealth program, called the Interhealth Nutrition Initiative, was developed to collect information about global population and nutrition trends and to evaluate programs related to food and nutrition. Nutrition goals for countries involved must emphasize the availability of a safe and adequate food supply as well as the promotion of dietary practices to reduce chronic disease risk. For countries where chronic disease rates are low and infectious disease rates and undernutrition are high, programs directed toward feeding the population are emphasized. For countries with high chronic disease risks, nutrition recommendations similar to the Dietary Guidelines for Americans encourage maintenance of appropriate body weight; decreased consumption of total fat, saturated fat, cholesterol, and sodium; increased consumption of fiber-rich foods and complex carbohydrates; and moderate alcohol intake.[4]

Undernutrition

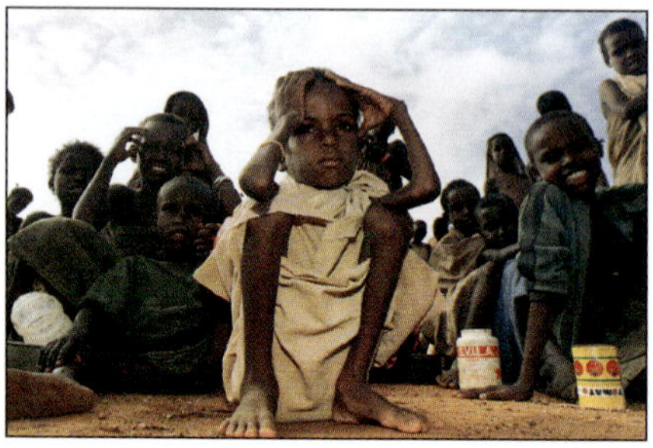

FIGURE 18.2 Undernutrition is more common in developing nations, especially among children because of their high nutrient needs. *(Reuters/Bettmann)*

Hunger is one of the first images that comes to mind when the topic of global nutrition is raised (Figure 18.2). Hunger and malnutrition are devastating problems that continue to dominate the health of the world's poorest nations. Nearly 30% of people in the developing world suffer from one or more of the multiple forms of malnutrition.[9] The undernutrition prevalent in the developing world results from a diet inadequate either in energy or in nutrients or from diseases, such as infections, that increase nutrient needs or interfere with the ability to consume and utilize nutrients. Undernutrition increases the rate of low-birth-weight births and infant mortality, stunts the growth of children, increases the incidence of infectious disease, and promotes a **cycle of malnutrition.**

Cycle of malnutrition A cycle in which malnutrition is perpetuated by an inability to meet nutrient needs at all life stages.

Infant mortality rate The number of deaths during the first year of life per 1000 live births.

Stunting A decrease in linear growth rate, which is an indicator of nutritional well-being in populations of children.

Low Birth Weight and Infant Mortality Low-birth-weight infants—those weighing less than 2500 g (about 5.5 pounds) at birth—are at greater risk of complications, illness, and early death. A higher number of low-birth-weight infants means a higher **infant mortality rate,** which is the number of deaths per 1000 live births in a population. The infant mortality rate and the number of low-birth-weight births are indicators of the health and nutritional status of a population. The average infant mortality rate worldwide is about 64 per 1000, but in developing nations the average rate is 120 per 1000, compared to only 7 per 1000 in more developed countries.[10] Low-birth-weight infants who do survive require extra nutrients, which are usually not available. Malnutrition in infancy and childhood has a profound effect on growth and development as well as on susceptibility to infectious disease (Table 18.2).

Stunting Malnourished children grow poorly. The prevalence of decreased linear growth, referred to as **stunting,** is used as an indicator of the well-being of populations of children.[11] It is estimated that 32.5% of children under age five in developing countries suffer from stunting,[12] which represents a steady improvement since 1980. Deficiencies of energy, protein, iron, and zinc, as well as prolonged infections, have been implicated as causes of stunting. Stunting in childhood produces smaller adults who have a reduced work capacity. Stunted women are more likely to give birth to low-birth-weight babies.

TABLE 18.2 Infant Mortality in Various Countries

Country	Infant Mortality (deaths per 1000 live births)
Finland	4
Italy	5
United States	7
El Salvador	31
China	31
Philippines	32
India	70
Haiti	71
Nigeria	76
Ivory Coast	81

World Bank. World Development Indicators. Available online at **www.worldbank.org/data/wdi2000/pdfs/tab2_18.pdf.**

Infectious Disease Undernourished children have depressed immune systems, which reduces their ability to resist infection. Of the 50 million deaths that occur worldwide each year, 80% are in developing countries, and half of the mortality is due to infectious diseases and parasites.[10] Infections decrease appetite and increase energy requirements and nutrient losses—which further contribute to undernutrition. Undernourished children may die of infectious diseases that would not be life-threatening in well-nourished children (Figure 18.3). Even immunization programs, designed to reduce the incidence of infectious disease, may be ineffective because the immune systems of undernourished individuals cannot respond normally. Mortality from infectious diseases is increased even among children with mild to moderate malnutrition.[13]

The Cycle of Malnutrition In populations where undernutrition is a chronic problem, the cycle of malnutrition prevents the development of a healthy productive population (Figure 18.4). The cycle begins when women consume a deficient diet during pregnancy. These women are more likely to give birth to low-birth-weight

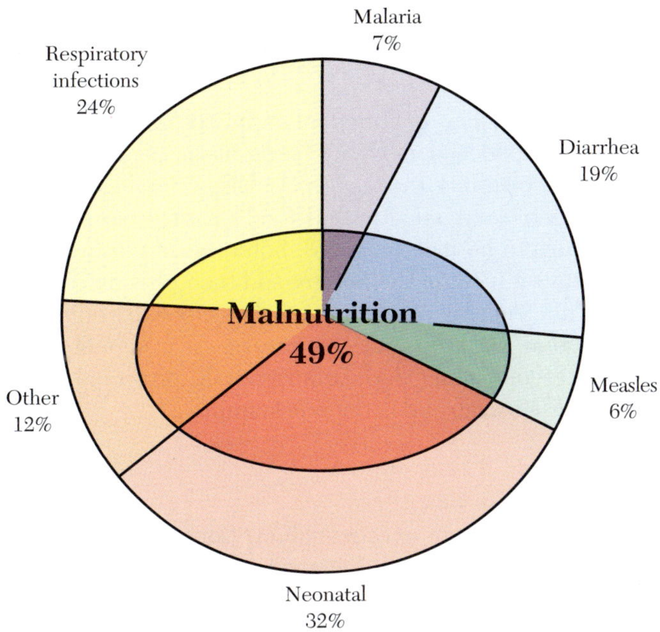

FIGURE 18.3 This diagram illustrates the contribution of malnutrition to childhood death in developing countries. The arcs of the circle show the disease states involved and the inner circle shows the contribution of malnutrition to death from each disease state. *(World Health Organization. Nutrition for Health and Development, 1999. Available online at* http://www.who.int/nut.*)*

infants who are susceptible to illness and early death. The children who do survive may be small and weakened physically and mentally. They grow into undernourished adults unable to contribute optimally to economic and social development. Thus, the women in this next generation also begin their pregnancies poorly nourished and are therefore likely to give birth to low-birth-weight infants. Interruption of this cycle of malnutrition at any point can benefit the individuals and the society. Healthy children can then grow into healthy adults who produce healthy offspring and can contribute fully to society.

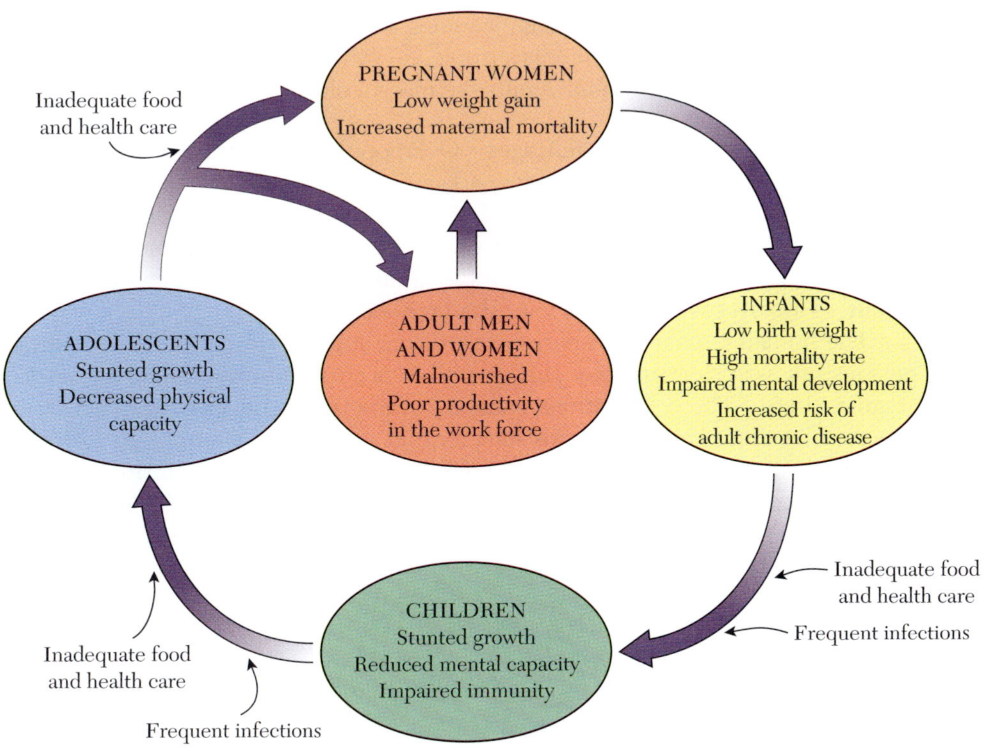

FIGURE 18.4 Malnutrition affects individuals at every stage of life. It often begins *in utero,* continues through infancy and childhood, and extends into adolescent and adult life. This cycle of malnutrition affects both the health and the productivity of a population.

World Hunger: Causes and Solutions

Although much of the world currently has an abundant supply of food, there are areas where the total amount of food and nutrients available is insufficient to nourish the population. Poverty—resulting from overpopulation, inefficient land use, and inequitable distribution of land, wealth, and food—causes populations and individuals within populations to be malnourished. Solutions to the problem of undernutrition must first focus on feeding the hungry and then providing them with the opportunity for self-sufficiency by promoting a balance between the size of the population, the production of food, and the use of environmental resources. Such strategies include controlling population growth, providing food, and changing agricultural, political, social, and economic systems.

Food Shortage

Food shortages cause widespread protein-energy malnutrition in local populations. They occur when the food supply is insufficient to feed the population; when cultural practices limit food choices; when economic inequities result in lack of money, health care, and education for individuals or populations; and when environmental resources are misused, limiting the ability to continue to produce food. Any combination of these factors can result in **food insecurity** within a population or segment of a population.

Food shortage due to **famine** is very visible because it causes many deaths in one area during a short period of time. This widespread failure in the food supply due to a collapse in the food production and marketing systems can be brought on by nature or by humans. Drought, floods, earthquakes, and crop destruction by diseases or pests cause nature-induced famines (Figure 18.5). Man-made famines are caused by wars and civil conflicts. Regions that produce barely enough food for survival under normal conditions are vulnerable to the disaster of famine. Populations living at this level do not have reserves of food, money, or livestock. This situation is analogous to a man standing in water up to his nostrils: If all is calm, he can breathe, but if there is a ripple; he will drown. When a ripple such as a natural or civil disaster occurs, it cuts the margin of survival and creates famine.

Overpopulation Creates Food Shortages Overpopulation exists when a region has more people than its natural resources can support. Some regions can support more people than others before food shortages occur. For example, a fertile river valley can produce more food per acre than can a desert environment. Even in fertile regions of the world, however, if the number of people increases too much, resources are overwhelmed and food shortages occur.

The human population is currently growing at a rate of more than 80 million persons per year, and most of this growth is occurring in developing countries (Figure 18.6). These countries cannot escape from poverty because their economies cannot keep pace with such a rapid population growth.[14] In addition, the growing populations reduce the amount of available agricultural land by using it for housing and industry. Efforts to produce enough food on the available land can damage the soil and deplete environmental resources, further reducing the capacity to produce food in the future. While the problem of hunger today is due primarily to the unequal distribution of resources, it is estimated that, worldwide, food production has begun to lag behind population growth.[15] If this trend continues, there will soon be too little food in the world to feed the population regardless of equality of resource distribution.

Culture Affects Food Availability In some cultures, access to food may be limited for certain individuals within households. For example, women and girls may receive less food than men and boys because culturally they are viewed as less

Web Menu: For more information on the problem of world hunger, go to International organizations that provide information on food and nutrition, such as the World Health Organization at www.who.int/, the Food and Agriculture Organization of the United Nations at www.fao.org/, and UNICEF at www.unicef.org/.

Food shortage Insufficient food to feed a population.

Food insecurity The inability to obtain sufficient food for any reason.

Famine A widespread lack of access to food due to a disaster that causes a collapse in the food production and marketing systems.

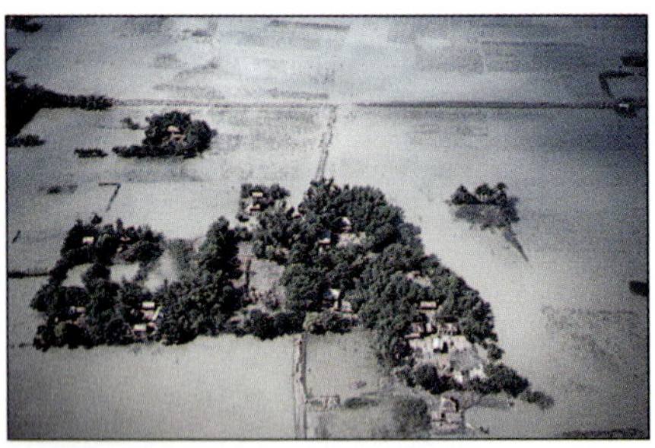

FIGURE 18.5 Natural disasters, such as floods and typhoons, destroy homes, farms, and infrastructure and can lead to famine. *(© Bruce Brander/Photo Researchers, Inc.)*

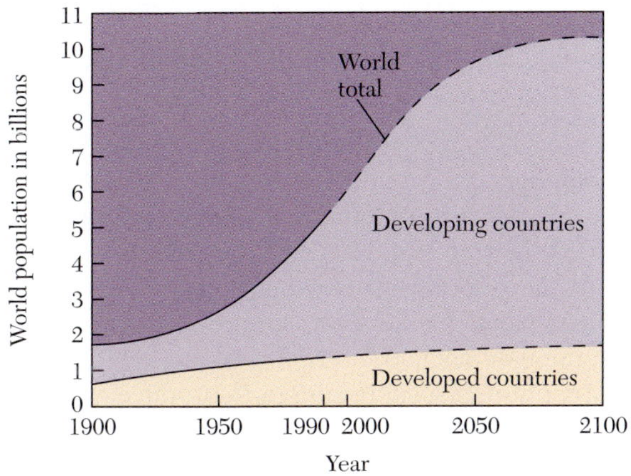

FIGURE 18.6 Most of the increase in world population is occurring in developing countries, and this trend is expected to continue.

important. How much food is available to an individual within such households may depend on gender, control of income, education, age, birth order, or genetic endowments.[16]

The cultural acceptability or unacceptability of foods also contributes to food shortages and malnutrition. If available foods are culturally unacceptable, a food shortage exists unless the population can be educated to use and accept the new food. For example, insects are eaten in some cultures and provide an excellent source of protein, but they are unacceptable to others. Another example is greens, which are often available locally but are underutilized because people have traditionally not eaten them and do not know how to prepare them.

Poverty Reduces Food Availability About a quarter of the world's population lives in poverty, surviving on less than a dollar a day.[1] Poverty is at the root of the problem of undernutrition. The link between hunger and poverty is so strong that in most parts of the world their incidence is almost identical (Figure 18.7). Poverty can be viewed as the cause as well as the result of inadequate food production, distribution, and storage; inappropriate utilization of resources; unsanitary living conditions; and lack of health care and education. Poverty and food insecurity

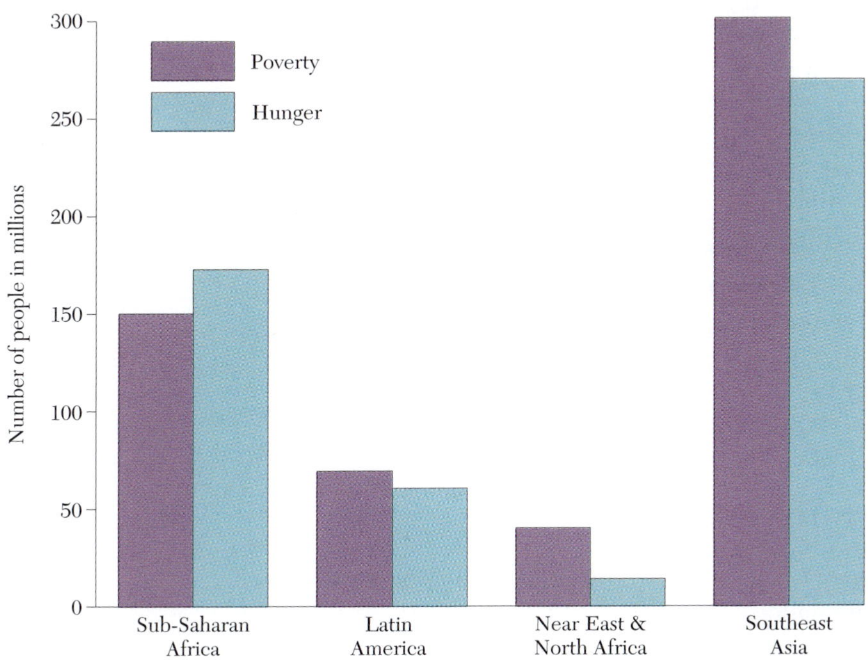

FIGURE 18.7 The incidences of hunger and poverty are almost identical in most parts of the world. *(Adapted from Univ, P. The state of world hunger. Nutr. Rev. 52:151–161, 1994.)*

occur in countries, in households, and among individuals when food and resources are not distributed equitably. And food insecurity increases the risk of malnutrition.

Economic Policies On the national level, lack of money limits the ability to produce, transport, and distribute food. National economic priorities also contribute to food shortages in populations. Most nations traditionally grew **subsistence crops,** the crops they needed to feed their people. However, colonialism, such as that on the African continent, and the development of modern trade practices shifted the emphasis from producing food for local consumption to producing **cash crops,** which can be sold on the national and international market. This improves the cash flow into the country but uses local resources to produce crops for export and leaves the least fertile land to grow food for local consumption.

Subsistence crops Crops grown as food for the local population.

Cash crops Crops grown to be sold (often exported) for monetary return rather than to be used for food locally.

Household and Individual Poverty At the household and individual level, if money is scarce, food cannot be obtained and the incidence of malnutrition increases. The poorest poor do not own land to grow food and do not have money to buy enough food or enough of the right kinds of food to meet nutritional needs. They do not have access to transportation to get to markets and must walk long distances to buy food and collect firewood for cooking.

Malnutrition increases the incidence of disease and disability, and, in turn, disease further increases malnutrition. The poor have less access to health care, so disease goes untreated—which can increase nutrient needs and limit the ability to acquire food. Lack of health care also increases infant mortality and the incidence of low-birth-weight births. Lack of immunizations and treatment for infections and other illnesses result in an increased incidence of and morbidity from infectious disease and a decrease in survival rates from chronic diseases such as cancer.

Lack of education and subsequent illiteracy go hand in hand with poverty, reducing opportunities to escape poverty and increasing the risk of undernutrition and disease (Table 18.3). Insufficient education leads to inadequate care for infants, children, and pregnant women. A lack of education about food preparation and storage can affect food safety and the health of households; unsanitary food preparation increases the incidence of gastrointestinal diseases, which contribute to malnutrition.

TABLE 18.3 Indicators of Poverty and Malnutrition

	Infant Mortality (deaths per 1000 live births)	Life Expectancy (years)	Illiteracy (percent of population)	Access to Medical Care (people per physician)
More Developed Countries	20	76	3	680
Less Developed Countries				
Sierra Leone	182	37.2	66.7	—
Central Africa	113	44.9	57.6	25,920
Ghana	67	60	33.6	22,970
Ivory Coast	81	46.7	57.4	11,739
El Salvador	31	69.6	23	848
Cuba	7	76	4.1	176
Haiti	71	54.1	54.2	4,000
India	70	62.6	46.5	2,459
Bangladesh	79	58.1	61	12,884

Global cardiovascular disease information base: **http://cvdinfobase.ic.gc.ca/gcvi/default/htm,** and World Bank: **http://www.worldbank.org/data/wdi2000/pdfs/tab2_18.pdf.**

Environmental Resources Affect Food Production As discussed, the land and resources available for food production are limited. Some resources, such as minerals and fossil fuels, are present in the earth in limited amounts and are nonrenewable—that is, once used they cannot be replaced in a reasonable amount of time. Technology will need to find substitutes for these resources. Other resources, if they are not damaged, are renewable. **Renewable resources** can be used at a rate at which the Earth can restore them. For example, if agricultural land is used wisely—crops rotated, erosion prevented, contamination limited—it can be reused almost indefinitely. However, if this land is not used carefully, soil erosion, nutrient depletion, and accumulation of pollutants in soil and water may occur at a rate that exceeds the Earth's ability to restore and repair these resources. As agricultural lands are depleted, forests may be cut down to create more agricultural land. This deforestation contributes to soil erosion and, along with air pollution, contributes to global climate changes. Lack of water and pollution of existing water also limit agricultural productivity, and overgrazing destroys rangelands. Whether animal products, agricultural crops, or fish or seafood are being produced and distributed, the environmental cost could be high. To maintain adequate agricultural land and water resources, those available must be used in ways that will sustain them for continued use.

Renewable resources Resources that can be restored and replaced by natural processes and that can therefore be used forever.

Environmental Cost of Meat Production Modern meat production is an example of the inefficient use of natural resources. Modern methods of raising cattle use grain, water, and fossil fuels, and create both air and water pollution. Cattle raised in the United States spend most of their lives eating grass from grazing lands; then, for about their last 100 days, the animals are kept in stockyards and fed grain to increase their body fat. A large proportion of the grain produced in the United States is used for this purpose. To produce this feed grain, fertilizers and pesticides are used, soil is eroded, and groundwater is contaminated. Much of the grain is grown on land that must be irrigated, so water supplies are depleted as well. About 87% of the fresh water in the world today is consumed by agriculture.[17] In addition, the animals themselves produce methane gas in their gastrointestinal tracts; this gas enters the air, contributing to the greenhouse effect and thus to global warming. And when animal sewage is stored in ponds and heaps, it can contaminate waterways and as it decomposes, it produces more methane gas, which pollutes the air (see *Making Decisions:* "Are Vegetarian Diets Better for the Environment?")

Environmental Cost of Agricultural Crops The environmental cost of producing plant-based foods is lower than that of producing animal products, but it may still be substantial. For example, growing a head of lettuce in California using pesticides and fertilizer and then trucking it in a refrigerated car to New York requires a great deal of energy. The price of our food may reflect some of these costs, but the cost of the damage to soil, groundwater, and farm workers caused by pesticides and fertilizers is not included. These and other social, medical, and ecological costs associated with modern agricultural practices are difficult to measure.

Overfishing and Water Pollution Throughout human history fish have been an important source of food. However, increases in population have increased demand for fish to the point that the Earth's oceans are being depleted. Because the ocean is open to fishermen from around the world, its use has been difficult to control. According to the United Nations Food and Agriculture Organization, 70% of the world's fish stocks are currently being fished at or beyond their ability to replenish themselves. Pollution also threatens the world's fishing grounds. Oil spills and deliberate dumping can occur offshore, and sewage, pesticides, organic pollutants, and sediments from erosion wash into coastal waters where most fish spend at least part of their lives. Heavy metals such as lead, cadmium, and mercury can enter the food chain and are toxic to both fish and humans.

Making Decisions

Are Vegetarian Diets Better for the Environment?

One of the reasons people choose to adopt vegetarian diets is concern about the environment. They argue that producing animal products consumes large amounts of energy, destroys forests and grazing lands, and pollutes the air and water. Although these arguments are valid in some instances, the impact of food animals on the ecosystem depends on how they are integrated into the environment.

For thousands of years, animals were raised on small farms or grazed on open land. The drive to produce animals more efficiently and more profitably has moved them off the family farm and into large agribusinesses. This has had an impact on energy use, land and water use, and air quality.

On a small farm, animals can consume crop wastes, kitchen scraps, and cellulose grasses that people cannot eat, and turn them into meat, milk, and eggs that make important contributions to the human diet. But animals raised in agribusinesses are fed grain rather than grasses and kitchen scraps. This is inefficient because humans who eat the animals get back only a fraction of the energy they could have gotten from eating the grain. For every 100 kcalories of plant material a cow eats, only 10 kcalories are stored in the cow and can be consumed by humans.[a] In the United States, 1 pound of pork provides 1000 to 2000 kcalories in the diet and costs 14,000 kcalories to produce. Worldwide, 38% of the total grain produced is fed to chickens, pigs, and cows. In the United States, as much as 70% of grain grown is fed to animals. Livestock production also uses water—430 gallons to produce 1 pound of pork in the United States. For the world to adopt an American-type diet would require "more grain than the world can grow and more energy, water, and land than the world can supply."[b]

Management of animal waste materials also affects the environment. On small farms, manure is used for fertilizer in local fields, but when thousands of animals are confined to a small area, manure builds up rapidly and the runoff may pollute nearby rivers and lakes. This can cause algae overgrowth that kills other aquatic life and causes nitrate pollution of drinking water. Animal wastes also produce gases that are released into the atmosphere, contributing to acid rain and global warming.

The sheer number of domestic animals is also destructive to the environment. When pastures are overstocked and grazing lands are overgrazed, it reduces the potential to continue to use these lands. Forests such as those in the Amazon are being cut down to create new grazing land for cattle. Forests serve to absorb carbon dioxide; therefore, deforestation allows carbon dioxide to accumulate in the atmosphere and contributes to global warming. Whether domestic animals are confined or free, the natural resources of the Earth are no longer able to sustain their increasing numbers without serious ecological consequences. Is the elimination of animal foods the answer to feeding the world and saving the planet?

Animal foods make important contributions to the human diet. In parts of the developing world, small amounts of meat and milk obtained from animals may mean the difference between survival and starvation. Animal products also make important economic contributions. Manure is a valuable fertilizer and a source of cooking fuel. When integrated into farming, animal products provide extra income during good times and insurance during bad times. In the United States, we rely on animal foods to provide vitamin B_{12}, much of our calcium, and highly absorbable sources of iron and zinc. Eliminating animal products entirely would reduce both the variety of food and the nutrient content of the human diet.

The environmental problems caused by animal production occur both because of the way animals are raised and because there are too many of them, not because of their existence. If we are to both feed the world and preserve the environment, sustainable agricultural systems must be adopted. The aim of sustainable agriculture is to produce vegetable and animal foods while preserving the long-term fertility and productiveness of the planet. The natural ecosystems of the Earth include both plants and animals, so it is not surprising that agricultural systems modeled after natural ecosystems would require both. For example, in a sustainable system, cattle and sheep would eat only from grazing lands unsuitable for growing crops, rather than be fed grains that can be consumed by humans. This agricultural method utilizes both unproductive and productive cropland in an ecologically sound manner. Although this type of system uses fewer resources, it also produces many fewer animals than the present system. To absorb the decrease in production, demand for animal products would have to decrease in developed nations. Consuming a diet that is higher in grains, vegetables, and fruits and lower in animal products is therefore a goal that is compatible not only with the recommendations of the Dietary Guidelines but also with the ecology of the planet. Completely eliminating animal products is neither necessary nor beneficial. Both plants and animals are essential for a diversified ecosystem, and both plant and animal foods make valuable contributions to the diet.

References

[a]Raven, P. H., Berg, L. R., and Johnson, G. B. *Environment,* 3rd ed. Philadelphia: Harcourt College Publishers, 2001.

[b]Durning, A. T. Fat of the land. World Watch 4:7–11; 1991.

Nutrient-Poor Diets

An adequate energy intake does not ensure adequate nutrition. The right combination of nutrients is also important for nutritional health. Undernutrition can be caused by a poor-quality diet as well as by a shortage of food.

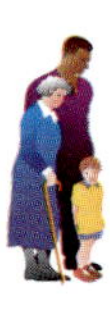

The typical diet in developing countries is based on high-fiber grain products and has little variety. Adults who are able to consume a relatively large amount of this diet may be able to meet their nutrient needs. But those with increased needs or a limited capacity to consume these foods are at risk for nutrient deficiencies. Children, pregnant women, the elderly, and the ill may not be able to eat enough

TABLE 18.4 Malnutrition at Different Life Stages

Life Stage	Common Deficiencies	Consequence
In utero	Energy	Low birth weight
	Iodine	Brain damage
	Folate	Neural tube defects
Infancy/young child	Protein, energy	Growth retardation, increased risk of infection
	Iron	Anemia
	Iodine	Developmental retardation, goiter
	Vitamin A	Infection, blindness
Adolescence	Protein, energy	Stunting, delayed growth
	Iron	Anemia
	Iodine	Delayed/retarded intellectual development, goiter
	Vitamin A	Infection, blindness
	Calcium	Inadequate bone mineralization
Pregnant women	Protein, energy	Intrauterine growth retardation, increased mortality of mother and fetus
	Folate	Maternal anemia, neural tube defect in infant
	Iron	Maternal anemia
	Iodine	Cretinism in infant, goiter in mother
	Vitamin A	Infection, blindness
Adult	Energy, protein	Thinness, lethargy
	Iron	Anemia
Elderly	Energy	Thinness, lethargy
	Calcium and protein	Osteoporosis fractures, falls

World Health Organization. Nutrition for Health and Development, 1999. Available online at **http://www.who.int/nut/.**

of this bulky grain diet to meet their needs. Thus, deficiencies of protein, iron, iodine, and vitamin A are common because of poor-quality diets (Table 18.4).

Protein-Energy Malnutrition Over 200 million children under the age of five suffer from deficiencies of protein and energy.[2] Protein and energy deficiencies usually occur together. However, in individuals with high protein needs—those who are growing, developing, or healing—protein deficiency can predominate (see Chapter 6). Kwashiorkor, a deficiency of protein but not of energy, occurs as a result of the wrong combination of foods rather than a general lack of food. It is common in children over 18 months of age for whom the main energy source is a bulky cereal grain low in high-quality protein. Children have small stomachs and are not able to consume enough of this diet to meet their protein needs (Figure 18.8). Other factors, such as metabolic changes caused by infection, may also play a role in the development of kwashiorkor.[18]

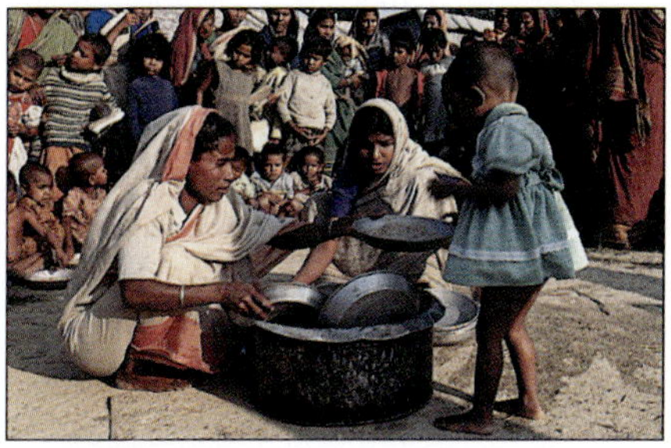

FIGURE 18.8 Small children are often unable to eat enough of a bulky grain diet to meet their high nutrient needs. *(© John Paul Kay/Peter Arnold, Inc.)*

Micronutrient Deficiencies Micronutrient malnutrition affects billions of people worldwide and impacts the mortality, morbidity, reproductive health, growth, and development of individuals and the economic productivity of societies.[19]

Iron Deficiency Anemia Iron deficiency anemia is the most common nutritional problem in both developed and developing nations, but the prevalence is almost fourfold higher in the developing world, where it affects 43% of all women and 34% of all men.[11] When the amount of iron available in the diet does not meet individual needs, it causes iron deficiency, which can lead to anemia (see Chapter 13). It is estimated that a third of the world's population, over 2 billion people, suffer from iron deficiency anemia, and another 5 billion have deficient iron stores.[9] The overall prevalence of iron deficiency anemia among preschool children is 39% and among pregnant women is 52%, but more than 90% of these cases are in developing countries (Figure 18.9).

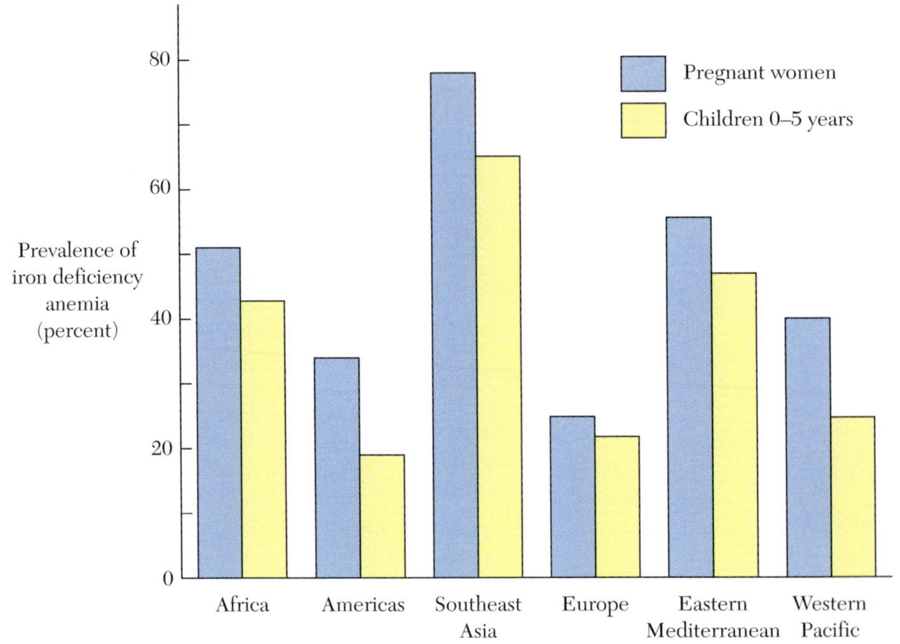

FIGURE 18.9 This graph illustrates the prevalence of iron deficiency anemia among pregnant women and young children (0 to 5 years of age) in different regions of the world. *(WHO.* Global Database on Anaemia. *Geneva: WHO, 1998.)*

Iron deficiency can result from an increased need for iron, a chronic loss of iron due to blood loss, or a diet with inadequate amounts of iron-containing foods or poor iron bioavailability. Nonheme iron from plant sources is the major dietary source of iron in many parts of the developing world where meat consumption is economically unfeasible. This dietary pattern increases the risk of iron deficiency because nonheme iron is poorly absorbed. Also, intestinal parasites, especially hookworm, cause gastrointestinal blood loss, which depletes iron through blood loss and leads to iron deficiency anemia.[11] The greater rates of both acute and chronic infections, such as malaria, in the developing world aggravate dietary iron deficiency.

Iron deficiency can have a major impact on the health and productivity of a population. Anemia during pregnancy increases the risk of maternal and fetal mortality, premature delivery, and low birth weight. Iron deficiency in infants and children can stunt growth and retard mental development, decrease physical activity levels, decrease resistance to infection, and increase morbidity due to disease.[20] In older children and adults it causes fatigue and decreased productivity.

Iodine Deficiency Diseases Iodine is an essential trace element that is a constituent of the thyroid hormones (see Chapter 13). It is estimated that 1.6 billion people live in areas considered to be at risk for iodine deficiency and that about 655 million, or 12% of the global population, have goiter, a symptom of iodine deficiency.[11,21]

During pregnancy, iodine deficiency increases the incidence of stillbirths, spontaneous abortions, and developmental abnormalities in the offspring, such as metal retardation, deaf-mutism, and cretinism.[9] Cretinism is the most severe manifestation of iodine deficiency. It is characterized by irreversible mental and physical retardation. Cretinism is devastating to individuals and families, but the more subtle effects of iodine deficiency on mental performance and work capacity may have a greater impact on the population as a whole. Iodine-deficient children have lower IQs and impaired school performance.[22] Iodine deficiency in children and adults is associated with apathy and decreased initiative and decision-making capabilities. Worldwide iodine deficiency diseases are believed to be the greatest single cause of preventable brain damage in the fetus and infant, and of retarded psychomotor development in young children.[9]

Iodine deficiency occurs in regions with iodine-deficient soil that rely extensively on locally produced food. The Eastern Mediterranean region and Africa have the highest incidence of iodine deficiency disorders (Figure 18.10). Because

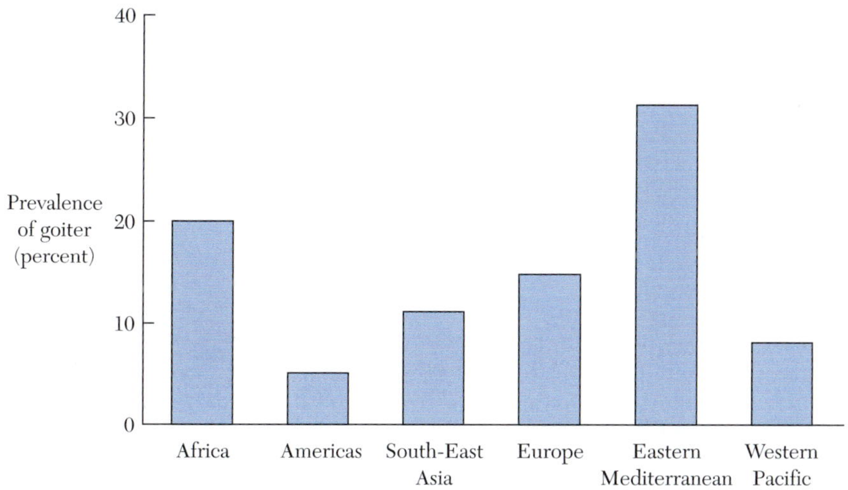

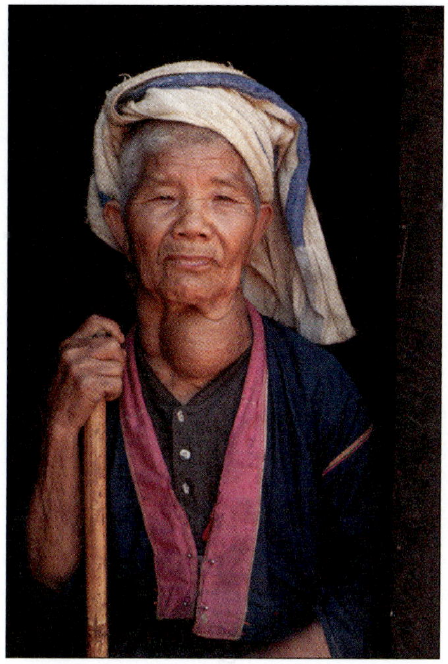

FIGURE 18.10 This graph illustrates the percent of the population affected by goiter (see photo) in different regions of the world. *(WHO/UNICEF/ICCID.* Progress Toward the Elimination of Iodine Deficiency Disorders (IDD). *WHO/NHD/99.4. Geneva: WHO, 1999.) (photo © Alison Wright/Corbis)*

soil iodine is low in regions where deficiency is common, the problem can be solved only by importing foods high in iodine or by adding iodine to the local diet by supplements or fortification.

Vitamin A Deficiency Obtaining sufficient vitamin A is a particular problem during periods of rapid growth and development, such as during infancy, early childhood, pregnancy, and lactation. Frequent infections, such as those causing diarrheal disease and measles, contribute to vitamin A deficiency by increasing need.[11] Deficiencies of other nutrients, including fat, protein, and zinc, can also contribute to vitamin A deficiency by affecting absorption and utilization. Vitamin A cannot be absorbed without fat, so a diet very low in fat can cause a deficiency by preventing absorption. Protein and zinc are needed for the transport and metabolism of vitamin A, so deficiencies of either can make vitamin A unavailable to body tissues.

Control of vitamin A deficiency is a major public health goal of the World Health Organization. It is estimated that 3 to 10 million children worldwide suffer from vitamin A deficiency; the incidence is highest in East and South Africa (Figure 18.11).[9,23,24] Vitamin A deficiency causes blindness; retards growth;

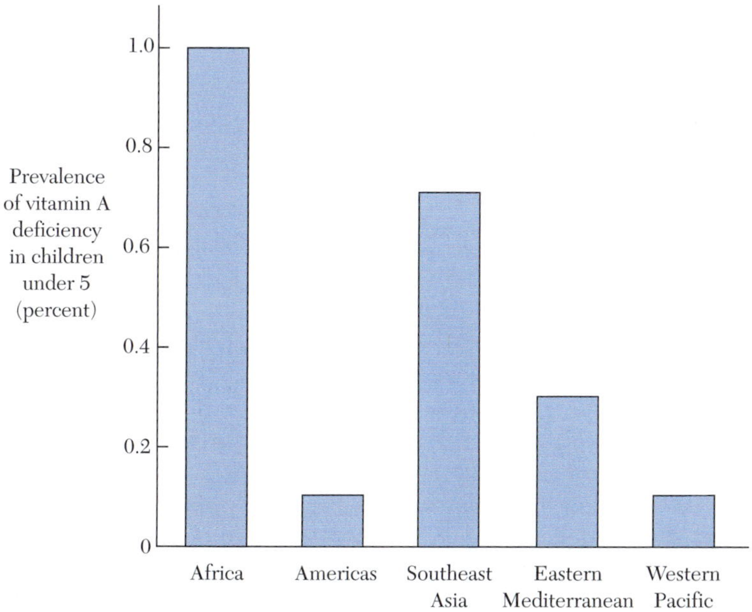

FIGURE 18.11 This graph illustrates the percentage of children under age five who have clinical signs of vitamin A deficiency. Although the highest prevalence of vitamin A deficiency is found in Africa, the highest number of clinically affected children occurs in Southeast Asia. *(World Health Organization. Nutrition for Health and Development, 1999. Available online at* http://www.who.int/nut/.*)*

RESEARCH DISCOVERIES

Vitamin A: The Anti-Infective Vitamin

In the United States in 1910, one out of every four infants died before one year of age. The major causes of death were infectious diseases: epidemics of diarrhea during the summer and respiratory infections during the winter.[a] Similar problems affected children in Europe. Efforts to reduce infant mortality focused on improving hygiene, encouraging breastfeeding, and improving the quality of the milk supply. At about the same time, scientists began to discover vitamins in foods. This led to observations in the early part of the 20th century that nutritional deficiency, particularly vitamin A deficiency, was associated with an increased incidence and severity of infectious disease.[b]

One of the most convincing pieces of evidence that vitamin A helped prevent infections arose from the observations of British scientist Sir Edward Mellanby. In 1925, an epidemic of pneumonia swept through a colony of dogs in a research laboratory. Mellanby observed that the pneumonia occurred almost exclusively in the vitamin A–deficient animals. He hypothesized that the vitamin A deficiency increased susceptibility to respiratory infections and that this may be relevant to infections in children.[c] Subsequent animal experiments confirmed that vitamin A deficiency caused an increase in infections. It was hypothesized that vitamin A increased the body's resistance to infection, and it was dubbed the "anti-infective vitamin."[d]

The theory that vitamin A could be used as anti-infective therapy triggered 20 years of clinical investigations into the effect of vitamin A on the incidence and severity of infectious diseases. Clinical trials were conducted to determine if vitamin A, given as cod liver oil, could reduce morbidity and mortality from respiratory disease, measles, and other infections. The results of these trials were mixed; however, the pharmaceutical industry focused on the positive results and began promoting cod liver oil as a dietary supplement that would decrease the severity of and reduce recovery time from ailments such as whooping cough, measles, mumps, chicken pox, and scarlet fever.[a] The theory that vitamin A was an anti-infective vitamin was widely accepted by the public, and the administration of cod liver oil became a routine for millions of children in the United States and Europe in the 1940s.

Research into the anti-infective properties of vitamin A slowed after the 1940s, in part due to the development of antibiotics to treat infections. Despite the fact that fewer vitamin A trials took place, evidence that nutritional status played a role in susceptibility to infection continued to accumulate. In 1959, the World Health Organization published a paper that reviewed the mounting evidence of a relationship between nutritional status and infection.[e]

Today, antibiotics, vaccinations, and a nutritious and varied diet have reduced infant morbidity and mortality in the United States and other developed na-

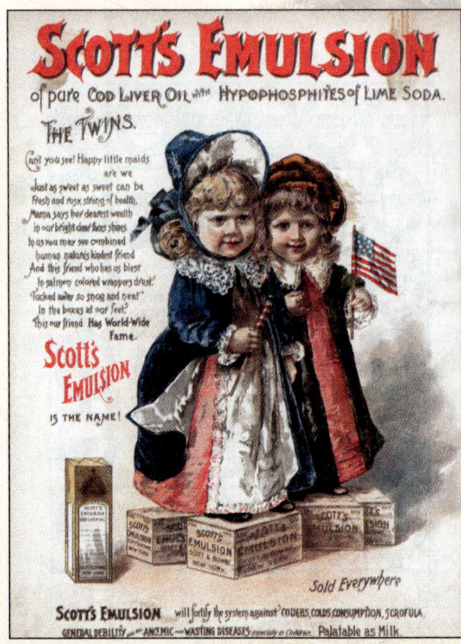

As this 1940s ad shows, cod liver oil was promoted to reduce the incidence and severity of infections in children. *(© Bettmann/Corbis)*

depresses immune function, which increases the risk of infections; and is often accompanied by anemia (see Chapter 10). In communities where vitamin A deficiency exists, supplementation has been shown to significantly reduce childhood deaths due to infection.[25] (See *Research Discoveries:* "Vitamin A: The Anti-Infective Vitamin.")

Other Nutrients of Concern In addition to deficiencies of protein, iron, iodine, and vitamin A, there are several vitamin and mineral deficiencies that have recently emerged or reemerged as problems throughout the world. Beriberi, pellagra, and scurvy, caused by deficiencies of thiamin, niacin, and vitamin C, respectively, are rare in the developed world but still occur among the extremely poor and underprivileged and in large refugee populations. Folate deficiency is also a problem in many parts of the world. It causes megaloblastic anemia during pregnancy and often compounds existing iron deficiency anemia (see Chapter 10). In women of childbearing age, low folate intake increases the risk of having a baby with a neural tube defect. Folate deficiency may also contribute to coronary heart disease and stroke by causing elevated homocysteine levels, and low folate status is

tions. In many developing nations, however, infant mortality from infectious diseases remains high. Interest in the relationship between vitamin A status and infection regained momentum in the 1980s with the observation that Indonesian children with mild vitamin A deficiency had increased mortality.[f] Since then, a large number of controlled clinical trials have demonstrated that vitamin A supplementation reduces morbidity and mortality among children in developing nations. These recent studies have clearly demonstrated that poor nutritional status leads to more frequent and more severe infectious illnesses and that infection triggers a set of metabolic responses that cause nutrient losses. Our understanding of how vitamin A status affects the immune system and of how infection affects vitamin A status is far greater now than it was in the early part of the 20th century.

Both malnutrition and infection negatively affect health. When the two occur together, one condition aggravates the other and the result can be deadly. Infection leads to malnutrition and malnutrition increases the duration and severity of infections. To a well-nourished child, common infectious diseases such as measles are usually a passing illness. To a malnourished child, the same disease can result in life-long disabilities or death. Worldwide, infections kill about 10 million children under age five every year, and about 50% of these deaths are associated with malnutrition.[b] Vitamin A supplementation trials in populations where vitamin A deficiency is common have shown that supplements given between 6 and 72 months of age can reduce overall mortality by 23%. A combined approach of vitamin A supplementation and vaccination, as has been used to combat measles, achieves more than the sum of the benefits of each.

Before the measles vaccine was developed in the 1960s, measles claimed 7 to 8 million lives a year. Vaccination has nearly eliminated measles in many Western countries but it remains a major problem in developing nations due to incomplete immunizations and high fatality rates. The relationship between vitamin A and measles is complicated. A deficiency of vitamin A reduces the ability of the immune system to defend itself against infection and once a measles infection has occurred, it causes loss of vitamin A that could precipitate acute vitamin A deficiency and blindness.[g] When vitamin A is given as part of measles management, the fatality rate is reduced by more than 50%. The WHO and UNICEF currently advise that massive doses of vitamin A be provided to children with measles and that vitamin A be supplemented at the time of measles vaccination. Providing vitamin A supplements is a short-term answer that should accompany long-term solutions to vitamin A deficiency and malnutrition, such as changes in dietary intake patterns and fortification of appropriate foods with vitamin A. A teaspoon of cod liver oil a day will prevent vitamin A deficiency but is not, unfortunately, a manageable long-term solution to the problem of vitamin A deficiency worldwide.

References

[a] Semba, R. D. Vitamin A as "anti-infective" therapy, 1920–1940. J. Nutr. 129:783–791, 1999.

[b] Brundtland, G. H. Nutrition and infection: malnutrition and mortality in public health. Nutr. Rev. 58(II):S1–S4, 2000.

[c] Mellanby, E. Diet and disease, with special reference to the teeth, lungs, and prenatal feeding. Lancet 1:151–519, 1926.

[d] Green, H. N., and Mellanby, E. Vitamin A as an anti-infective agent. Brit. Med. J. 2:691–696, 1928.

[e] Scrimshaw, N. S., Taylor, C. E., and Gordon, J. E. Interaction of nutrition and infection. Am. J. Med. Sci. 237:367–403, 1959.

[f] Sommer, A., Hussaini, F., Tarwotjo, I., and Susanto, D. Increased mortality in children with mild vitamin A deficiency. Lancet 2:585–588, 1983.

[g] West, C. E. Vitamin A and measles. Nutr. Rev. 58(II):S46–S54, 2000.

associated with cancer, especially of the colon.[9] In the United States, enriched grain products are fortified with folic acid to assure adequate intake and to reduce the incidence of neural tube defects.

Deficiencies of the minerals selenium, zinc, and calcium are also of concern.[8] Selenium deficiency has been identified in population groups in China, New Zealand, and the Russian Federation. Selenium deficiency is associated with an increased incidence of Keshan disease, a type of heart disease that affects mainly children and young women. Mild zinc deficiency is now believed to be more widespread than previously thought. Zinc deficiency can cause growth retardation or failure, diarrhea, immune deficiencies, skin and eye lesions, delayed sexual maturation, night blindness, and behavioral changes. It may also contribute to intrauterine growth retardation and neural tube defects in the fetus, and in the elderly it may affect taste acuity and cause dermatitis and impaired immune function. Inadequate calcium intake is also a concern worldwide due to its association with the occurrence of osteoporosis. Although factors other than low calcium intake, such as hormone levels and exercise, play a role in the development of osteoporosis, calcium supplementation has been proposed as a means of combating the high prevalence of spine and hip fractures due to osteoporosis, particularly in postmenopausal women.

Solutions to World Hunger

Solving the problem of world hunger is a daunting task. It involves controlling population growth, meeting the nutritional needs of a large and diverse population with culturally acceptable foods, increasing food production and economic opportunity, and maintaining the global ecosystem. It requires international cooperation, commitment from national and local governments, and the involvement of local populations. The solutions involve economic policies, technological advancement, education, and legislative measures. They require input from politicians, nutrition scientists, economists, and the food industry.

An International View Solving the problem of hunger and malnutrition around the world will require action and commitment at both the national and international level.[26] Plans and policies need to be designed to eradicate poverty, to increase food production in a sustainable manner, to improve access to adequate food, and to develop trade policies that foster food security for all.[27] In 1996 the World Food Summit pledged to cut in half the number of hungry people in the world by the year 2015. Much work is needed if this goal is to be achieved.

Food security has been defined as a condition in which "all people, at all times, have physical and economic access to sufficient, safe, and nutritious food to meet their dietary needs and food preferences for an active and healthy life".[27] Some view food security as a supply problem that could be solved by controlling population growth and increasing agricultural production. Others see food security as a demand problem that could be solved by more equitable food distribution, reducing overconsumption in certain areas, and improving **food self-sufficiency** by reducing the industrialization of farming. However the problem is viewed, programs and policies must first provide food and then establish sustainable programs to allow continued production and distribution.

Food self-sufficiency The ability of an area to produce enough food to feed its population.

Web Menu: For more information on private agencies that work to solve problems related to world hunger, go to the Worldwatch Institute at www.worldwatch.org/, or Food First at www.foodfirst.org/.

Relief Organizations There are many international, national, and private organizations working toward the goal of relieving world hunger. The World Health Organization (WHO), the United Nations' (UN) Food and Agriculture Organization (FAO), and the World Bank provide food and economic relief. The emphasis of the FAO is on the production, intake, and distribution of food. WHO targets community health centers and emphasizes the prevention of nutrition problems, such as micronutrient deficiencies. The World Bank finances projects such as supplementation and fortification to foster economic development. The United Nations Children's Fund (UNICEF), which relies on volunteer support, distributes food to all countries in need with a goal of assisting developing countries that occasionally suffer periods of starvation. The Red Cross, the UN Disaster Relief Organization, and the UN High Commissioner for Refugees concentrate on famine relief. The Peace Corps focuses more on fostering long-range development. More and more agencies and independent organizations are engaging in both development and relief efforts. A few examples include the U.S. Agency for International Development, Oxfam, the Hunger Project, and Catholic Relief Services.

Responding to Emergency Situations The first step toward solving the problem of undernutrition is to stop starvation. Although short-term food and medical aid do little to prevent future hunger, this type of relief is necessary for a population to survive an immediate crisis such as famine. The standard approach has been to bring food into the stricken area (Figure 18.12). These foods generally consist of agricultural surpluses from other countries and often are not well planned in terms of their nutrient content.[28] Famine relief efforts are frequently hindered by

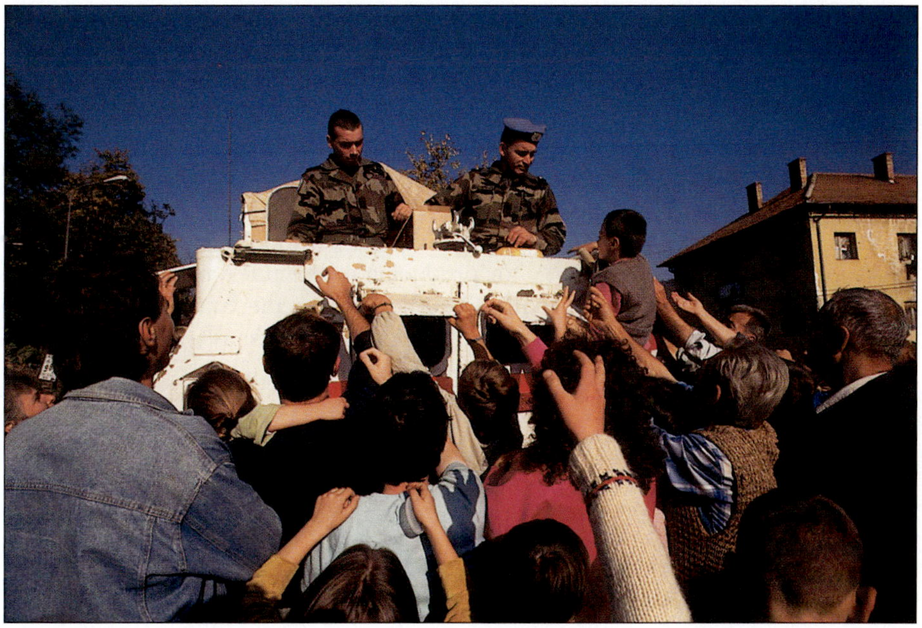

FIGURE 18.12 There are many international relief organizations that provide food to hungry people throughout the world. *(© Wesley Bocxe/Photo Researchers, Inc.)*

war, looting, and the lack of supporting infrastructure, such as roads, bridges, and airports, that is necessary to deliver food.

Increasing the Ratio of Food to People Short-term crises can be solved by international intervention, but long-term solutions need to be based on the cultural and economic needs of the local population. Local governments need to work to increase the ratio of food to people by controlling population growth and increasing food production.

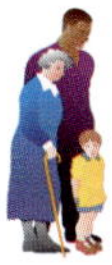

The size of the population needs to be comparable to its ability to produce food. One solution is to decrease the rate of population growth by controlling birthrates. Although the rate of population growth worldwide has slowed from more than 6 children per woman in 1950 to 3.3 in 1998, the world's population is still growing faster than the food supply.[14]

Changes in economic policies can help reduce population growth. In many areas, children provide economic security.[29] They are needed to work the farms, support the elders, and otherwise contribute to the economic survival of the family. With high infant mortality rates, people choose to have many children to ensure that some will survive. They feel safe having fewer children only when they are financially secure and able to acquire the necessities of life. Programs that foster economic development and ensure access to food, shelter, and medical care have been shown to cause a decline in birthrates. For example, a reduction in birthrates occurred along with economic success in South Korea.

Increasing the general level of education has also been shown to reduce population growth.[16] When the social and economic status of women is improved, birthrates decline. Women with more education tend to marry later and have fewer children. Education also increases the likelihood that women will have control over their fertility, provides knowledge to improve family health, decreases infant and child mortality rates, and offers options other than having numerous children. For example in Botswana, women with a secondary-level education have an average of 3.1 children. Those with only a primary-level education have 5.1 children, and women with no education have an average of 5.9 children.[29]

A more direct method of reducing population growth is to encourage family planning. To be successful, family-planning efforts must be acceptable to the population and compatible with their cultural and religious needs. A number of approaches, such as provision of contraceptives, education, and economic incentives, have been used to decrease population growth. In Singapore, Thailand, Colombia, and Costa Rica, programs that provide contraceptive information, services, and supplies have been somewhat successful in slowing population growth. In some countries, population-control education is being integrated into the school curriculum, and in Mexico and Egypt, popular television shows carry family-planning messages.

Better Access to Food In order to provide long-term food security, populations must develop manageable systems for producing acceptable, sustainable sources of food. Increasing the level of food self-sufficiency, or the country's capacity to feed its population, can help to prevent food shortages. To assure that the food produced can be acquired by all, economic solutions must also strive to eliminate poverty.

Trade Policies to Foster Food Self-Sufficiency Trade policies often determine what crops will be grown on a nation's arable land. A decision to grow a cash crop instead of food for local consumption may mean that less food is available for the local diet. For example, if a large portion of the arable land in west Africa is used to grow cash crops such as coffee and cotton, little agricultural land remains to grow grains and vegetables that nourish the local population. If, however, the cash from the crop is used to purchase nutritious foods from other countries, producing cash crops may help alleviate undernutrition.

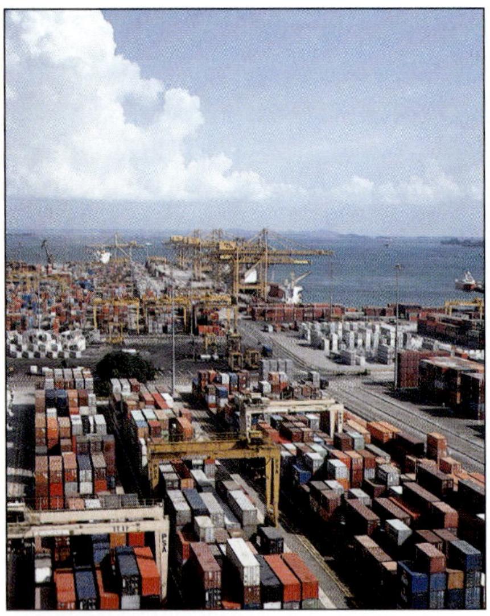

FIGURE 18.13 Many countries rely on imports to meet their local food needs. *(© Rex A. Butcher/Stone)*

Countries that have few natural resources must rely on international trade to distribute world resources more equitably. Trade can provide an economic advantage if food is imported and other products, on which a good monetary return is obtained, are exported. Newly industrialized countries in Asia, such as Korea, have increased food imports to decrease the number of hungry people (Figure 18.13). In general, the countries of the world are becoming more interdependent on food imports and on exports to pay for this food.[30] If this interdependence increases the availability of food for the world population, it is beneficial; but policies and practices in each nation must be developed to ensure that the population can be fed. If only the wealthy portion of the population has access to food imports, hunger and malnutrition will remain a problem.

Alleviating Poverty Although controlling population growth and ensuring adequate food production or importation are essential steps in eliminating world hunger, hunger will still exist as long as there is poverty. Even when food is plentiful in a region, the poor do not have access to enough of the right foods to maintain their nutritional health. Economic development that guarantees safe and sanitary housing, access to health care and education, and the resources to acquire enough food are essential to eliminate hunger. Poor, hungry people have little influence on government policies, but these policies can result in higher incomes, lower food prices, or feeding programs for the poor, all of which can improve food security.

Increasing Food Availability and Safety Educational programs as well as technology may be necessary to make food available and safe. Providing food or technology does little if individuals do not know how to use it. For example, a new crop variety is not beneficial unless local farmers know how to grow it and the population accepts it as a food source and knows how to prepare it for consumption. For instance, white yams are a common food in some regions but are a poor source of beta-carotene. If the yellow yam, which is rich in beta-carotene, became an acceptable choice, the diet would more easily meet vitamin A needs.

Food safety is also a concern when changing traditional dietary practices. For example, introducing papaya to the diet to improve vitamin A status will not improve nutritional status if it is washed in unsanitary water and causes dysentery among the people it is meant to nourish.

Education to encourage breast-feeding can also improve nutritional status and health. Breast-feeding reduces the risk of infectious diseases in infants. When infants are not breast-fed, education about nutritious breast-milk substitutes and safe preparation of formulas is essential. However, this information is often lacking among the poor.

Preserving the Environment The resources needed to support food production depend on the methods used. In developing countries, the resources used by a single person are small, but the numbers of people are so great that in many cases sufficient food cannot be produced without depleting and damaging soil, forests, and water supplies. In developed nations, the population is less dense but the resource demands made by each individual are far greater because of lifestyle and the production methods used. A single child born in the United States uses 10 to 1000 times more resources daily than the average Chilean, Ghanaian, or Yemenite.[17,29]

Solutions to the problem of providing enough food must assure that natural resources are conserved to allow continued food production for future generations. This requires maintaining the earth's renewable resources while developing technologies to increase production. It may require changes in consumption and production patterns. Promoting sustainable use of land and resources requires the support of both consumers and government policy makers (see *Critical Thinking:* "How Can One Person Make a Difference?").

Sustainable Food Production Maintaining the world food supply for the long term requires development of policies that promote sustainable agriculture. Sustainable methods produce food while allowing the environment to restore itself so food can be produced indefinitely. Renewable resources such as fertile agricultural land; grazing land; fish in lakes, rivers, and oceans; fresh water; and clean air can be used forever if they are not exploited. For instance, rotating the crops grown in a field prevents the depletion of specific nutrients in the soil, whereas growing the same crop year after year depletes the soil and increases the need for added fertilizers. Producing these fertilizers uses resources, and applying fertilizers increases water pollution. Pollution of the water reduces the amount available to irrigate the crops and nourish the population. Restoring water once it has become polluted takes long periods of time or expensive treatments.

Techniques of sustainable food production rely on ecological principles and normal biological processes such as natural predator-prey relationships and disease-resistant crops. Chemical fertilizers can be eliminated or minimized by using **integrated pest management** and fertilizing with animal manure. Crop rotation, plowing techniques, and terracing maintain soil fertility and prevent soil erosion (Figure 18.14). Other methods include agroforestry, in which techniques from forestry and agriculture are used together to restore degraded areas; natural systems agriculture, which develops agricultural systems that include many types of plants and which therefore function like natural ecosystems; and the technique of reducing fertilizer use by matching nutrient resources with the demands of the plant.[29,31]

Integrated pest management Agricultural production that combines chemical and nonchemical methods of pest control and emphasizes the use of natural toxins and more effective pesticide application.

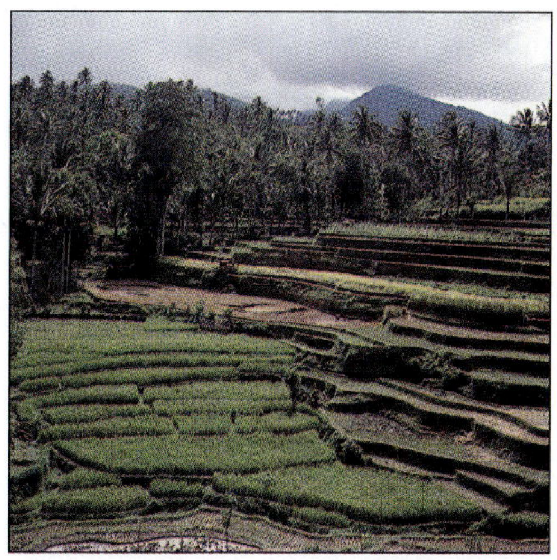

FIGURE 18.14 Agricultural techniques, such as the terracing shown here, help sustain the environment by preventing soil erosion. *(© Christian Grzimek/OKAPIA/Photo Researchers, Inc.)*

Water and energy are conserved by relying more on labor-intensive agricultural methods, which produce less food in the short term but will protect water and land resources in the long term. These methods are often more appropriate in developing nations than are high-technology methods because these areas typically have large populations but little access to modern machinery such as tractors and pumps.

Policies are beginning to reflect environmental issues. For example, concern about pesticides in the environment has led government intervention in the pesticide market to focus on the development of natural means of pest control.[32]

New Technologies to Increase Food Production New technologies are needed to increase food production without damaging the environment. Technological advances such as high-yielding crop varieties, irrigation, and mechanization have dramatically increased our ability to produce food. Corn yields in eastern Colorado, for example, have increased by 400 to 500% since 1940.[31]

Genetic engineering is one technology that is being implemented to increase food production while minimizing environmental damage. It is being used to produce plants and animals with new or more desirable traits. This technology can help meet the world's nutritional needs by creating safer pesticides, disease-resistant crops, foods with greater nutrient density, and products to increase the intake of deficient nutrients. However, in some cases, fear of this new technology has limited its use (see Chapter 20).

In order to increase food production, technological developments need to interface with cultural needs and economic structures. For instance, tractors increase food production in the United States, but providing tractors to developing nations does no good if there is no gas to power them or mechanics or parts to repair them. In addition, technology needs to be evaluated for its impact on the environment in order to maintain high levels of production without further compromising natural resources.

Providing the Right Combination of Nutrients In addition to sufficient energy in the diet, the right mix of nutrients is necessary to ensure the nutritional health of the population. If the foods and crops that are grown or imported do not meet all nutrient needs, the quality of the diet will be poor and malnutrition will occur. If the diet does not provide the right mix of foods, either dietary patterns must be changed or nutrients must be added to the diet by fortifying foods or including dietary supplements. Strategies to reduce micronutrient deficiencies also include control of infectious and parasitic diseases. Consumers must also learn how to choose foods that provide the needed nutrients and how to handle them safely.

Nutrification The process of adding one or more nutrients to commonly consumed foods with the goal of adding to the nutrient intake of a group of people.

Nutrification **Nutrification** is the process of adding one or more nutrients to commonly consumed foods with the goal of increasing the nutrient intake of a population. Nutrification will not provide energy to a hungry population, but it can increase the protein quality of the diet and eliminate micronutrient deficiencies. Nutrification programs have been created by a combination of partnerships among industry, academia, and government.[19] Industry and academia can provide the technology for adding the nutrient and government public health policies can promote the consumption of the nutrified foods.

In order for nutrification to solve a nutritional problem in a population, it must be implemented wisely. Nutrification works if vulnerable groups consume centrally processed foods. The foods selected for nutrification should be among those consistently consumed by the majority of the population so that extensive promotion and reeducation are not needed to encourage their consumption. The nutrient should be added uniformly and in a form that optimizes its utilization. Nutrification has been used successfully in preventing health problems in the United States: The fortification of cow's milk to increase vitamin D intake was a major factor in the elimination of infantile rickets (see Chapter 10), and the enrichment of grains with niacin helped eliminate pellagra. The most recent addition is the fortification of grains with folic acid to reduce neural tube defects in newborns (see Chapters 9 and 15).

Nutrification has also been used successfully in developing countries. The addition of iodine to salt reduced iodine deficiency from 84% to almost zero in school children in Thailand (Figure 18.15). And fortification of sugar with iron has been found to improve iron status in Guatemalan communities.[33] In the Philippines, the fortification of margarine with vitamin A has improved the population's vitamin A status,[34] and the effectiveness of vitamin A–fortified sugar is being evaluated in Bolivia.[35] In Guatemala, where marginal vitamin A status is prevalent, fortification of sugar has moved the country toward adequate vitamin A status.[11] Iron fortification of flour is being pursued in Latin America, the Caribbean, Central and South America, the Middle East, North Africa, and Central Asia. Iron fortification in Venezuela was shown to be effective at reducing the prevalence of anemia in school-aged children.[36]

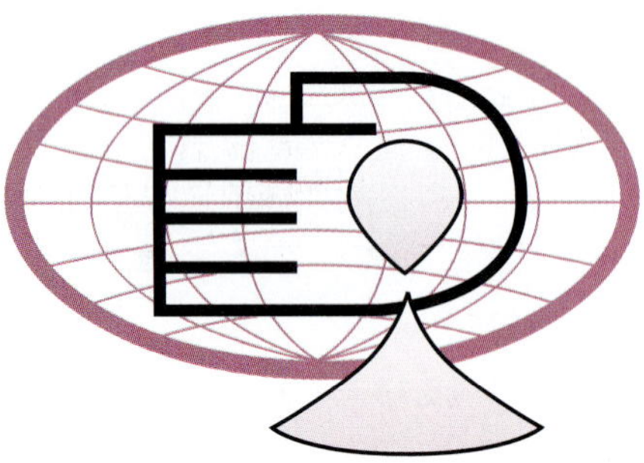

FIGURE 18.15 This logo is used around the world to identify iodized salt.

Supplementation Supplementation can also be used to reduce the prevalence of micronutrient malnutrition. Of countries where vitamin A deficiency is a public health problem, 78% have policies supporting regular vitamin A supplementation in children. Many have also adopted the WHO recommendation to provide all breast-feeding women with a high-dose supplement of vitamin A within eight weeks of delivery. This improves maternal vitamin A status and raises the amount of vitamin A that is in breast milk and therefore passed to the infant.[37] Supplementation, along with regular deworming programs, is also used to reduce iron deficiency anemia. Many countries have adopted programs to supplement children older than six months with iron and pregnant women with iron and folate.

Education To improve the nutritional quality of the diet, consumers have to consume the foods that have been fortified, take the supplements recommended, or change their diets to include natural sources of nutrients that are deficient. Education to modify dietary patterns may promote the use of produce from home gardens. This education must include information about which foods are good nutrient sources so that choices made when purchasing foods or growing vegetables at home can meet micronutrient needs.

Critical Thinking

How Can One Person Make a Difference?

Sandra is concerned about the problems of hunger, malnutrition, and global ecology. Although she is a college student who cannot afford to make monetary contributions to relief organizations, she would like to contribute in other ways. She enjoys working with children, so she arranges to spend one afternoon a week helping with local programs that target child nutrition education. She also volunteers one evening a week in a church soup kitchen near campus, helping to prepare and serve food.

To help maintain global ecology, Sandra makes some lifestyle changes that reduce the impact she has on the environment. When grocery shopping, she brings a canvas bag. This reduces the amount of waste she generates by eliminating the need for a new paper or plastic bag each time she shops. She asks her grocer to wrap the meat and chicken she buys in recyclable paper, and she begins recycling cans, bottles, and paper goods. To reduce the amount of nonrecyclable, nonbiodegradable waste she generates, she tries to avoid purchasing products in nonrecyclable containers. She also takes a number of other steps to protect the environment.

What impact will the following changes have on the environment?

Action	Impact
Instead of driving her car the 2 miles from home to campus, she rides her bike.	This reduces the use of fossil fuels and reduces air pollution.
She contacts her local utility company to come and do an energy audit of her home and make energy-saving suggestions.	This will reduce energy usage in her home.
Instead of buying nonrecyclable juice boxes for her lunch, she brings juice in a Thermos.	Answer:
She decides to begin composting the leftover vegetable scraps and other plant matter from her kitchen.	Answer:
When she can afford it, she chooses organically grown produce.	Answer:
She selects locally grown foods when possible.	Answer:

What other changes could Sandra make to decrease her impact on the environment?

Answer:

Hunger and Food Insecurity at Home

The New York Times

February 7, 2001

Homeless Shelters in New York Fill to Highest Levels Since 80's

By NINA BERNSTEIN

The number of homeless people lodging nightly in the New York City shelter system this winter has risen above 25,000, the most since the late 1980's, city figures show, with the largest increases coming among women and children over the last few years. ...

The increase, Mr. Oesterreich stressed, is part of a national trend. He cited a 25-city survey by the United States Conference of Mayors that calculated a 17 percent rise in the number of families applying for help because of homelessness.

In the United States, most of the nutritional problems are related to overnutrition. It is estimated that more than half of adults in the United States are overweight.[38,39] Heart disease, hypertension, and cancer—all related to obesity—are the leading causes of death. While much of the population is concerned with consuming a diet to lower the risks for these chronic diseases, hungry families are standing in line at food pantries and soup kitchens and living in homeless shelters. It is estimated that 10 million Americans, including 4 million children, do not get enough to eat.[40] Government food and nutrition policy must be concerned with improving economic security as well as providing food to the hungry and maintaining the food supply at an affordable level; at the same time, policy must promote healthy diets to reduce diseases related to overconsumption.

Causes of Food Insecurity

There is adequate food in the United States to feed the entire population, yet food insecurity, hunger, and undernutrition are still problems for vulnerable individuals and groups within the population. In 1999 about 10% of all U.S. households were food-insecure (Figure 18.16).[41] In 3% of households, one or more household members went hungry at least sometime during the course of the year.

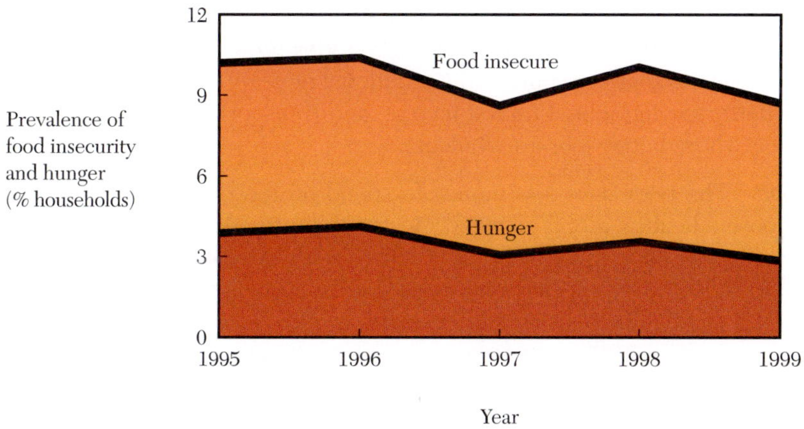

FIGURE 18.16 This graph illustrates the prevalence of food insecurity and hunger in U.S. households between 1995 and 1999. *(Andrews, M., Nord, M., Bickel, G., and Carlson, S. Household Food Security in the* United States, *1999. Food Assistance and Nutrition Research Report No. 8. Food and Rural Economics Division, Economic Research Service, U.S. Department of Agriculture. Available online at* http://www.ers.usda.gov:80/epubs/pdf/fanrr8/.*)*

Households with children experienced double the rate of food insecurity as households without children. Food insecurity is higher in the inner cities than in the suburbs and occurs more often among Hispanic and African-American households. Poverty, the main cause of food insecurity, reduces access to food, education, and health care. Despite the relationship between poverty and food insecurity, it cannot be assumed that everyone living in poverty is food-insecure, or that those above the poverty line have plenty to eat. Illness, disability, a sudden decrease in income, or high living expenses can put anyone at risk for food insecurity.

Poverty About 13.8% of Americans, including 20.8% of children, live at or below the poverty level.[42] Poverty not only limits access to a healthy diet but also to ways of increasing income, creating a cycle of poverty from which it is difficult to escape (Figure 18.17).

As the U.S. economy has shifted from manufacturing- to service-based, many factories have closed and manufacturing facilities have moved abroad where labor costs are lower. Former employees often lack the experience or education to move on to other types of work. Unable to find well-paying jobs, they must work

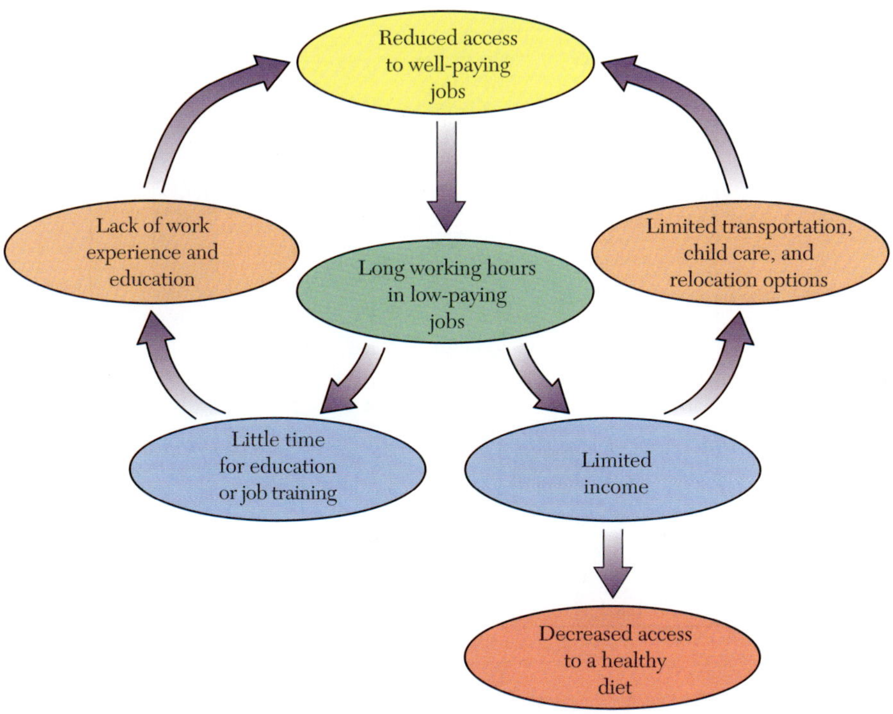

FIGURE 18.17 Many Americans are trapped in a cycle of poverty because they are unable to acquire the education, training, or resources necessary to obtain better-paying jobs.

longer hours at lower-paying jobs. Low incomes reduce access to transportation and childcare, which can also limit access to better jobs. Long work hours reduce the amount of time available to pursue the additional education or training necessary to find better-paying jobs. Limited income and transportation prohibit relocation to areas where better jobs are available.

Access to Food The poor have less money to spend on food and therefore their ability to choose a healthy diet is reduced. Access to more affordable food is limited by a number of factors. Lower profits have driven supermarkets out of the cities and into the suburbs. Because many low-income families do not own cars, they must shop at small, expensive corner stores or pay cab fares to take advantage of the lower prices and greater variety in suburban supermarkets. The poor may also pay more for food because limited cash reserves and lack of food storage facilities prohibit the purchase of bulk quantities of food that save per-item costs. Inadequate food preparation facilities and lack of education about how to select economical nutritious foods also limit access to a nutritious diet.

Access to Education Lack of education, which is a cause and a consequence of poverty, also contributes to hunger and food insecurity. For those at or below the poverty level, educational opportunities are fewer and the quality of education lower than in higher socioeconomic groups (Figure 18.18). Academic traditions can also limit the chances of obtaining higher education. For example, if no one in the family has ever gone to college, an adolescent may not even consider it as an option. In the short term, lack of education about food safety can increase the incidence of foodborne illness and lack of knowledge about how to stretch limited food budgets and select healthy diets can contribute to malnutrition. Too little food may cause the diet to be deficient in energy or particular nutrients, but poor food choices also allow undernutrition to coexist with obesity. In the long term, lack of education prevents people from getting well-paying jobs to allow them to escape from poverty.

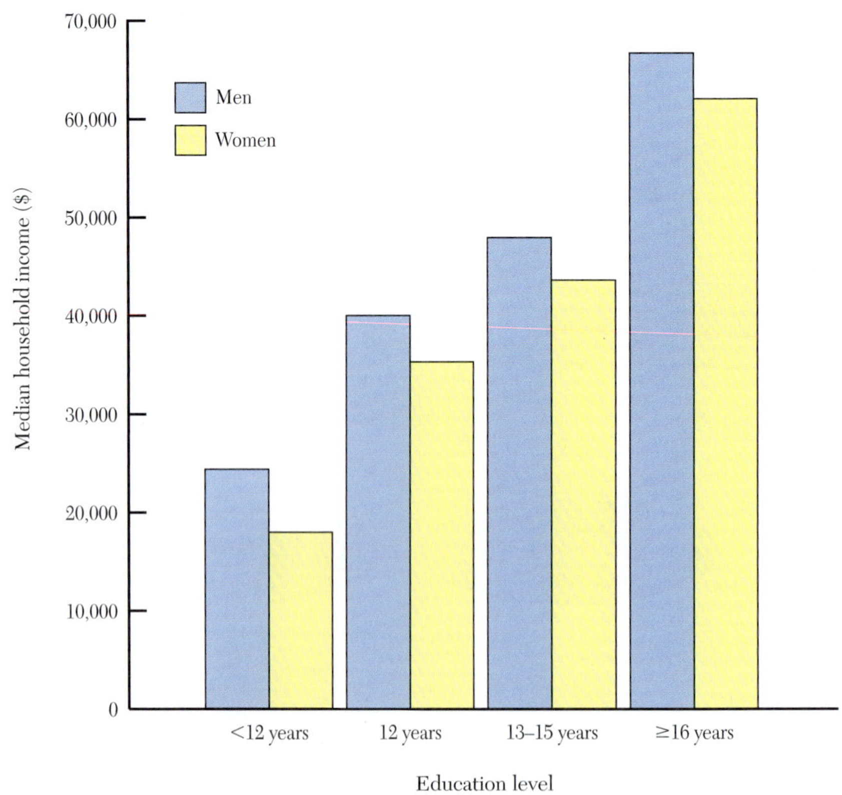

FIGURE 18.18 Income level in the United States is directly correlated with level of education in both men and women. *(U.S. Department of Commerce, Bureau of the Census. Current Population Survey, March 1997.)*

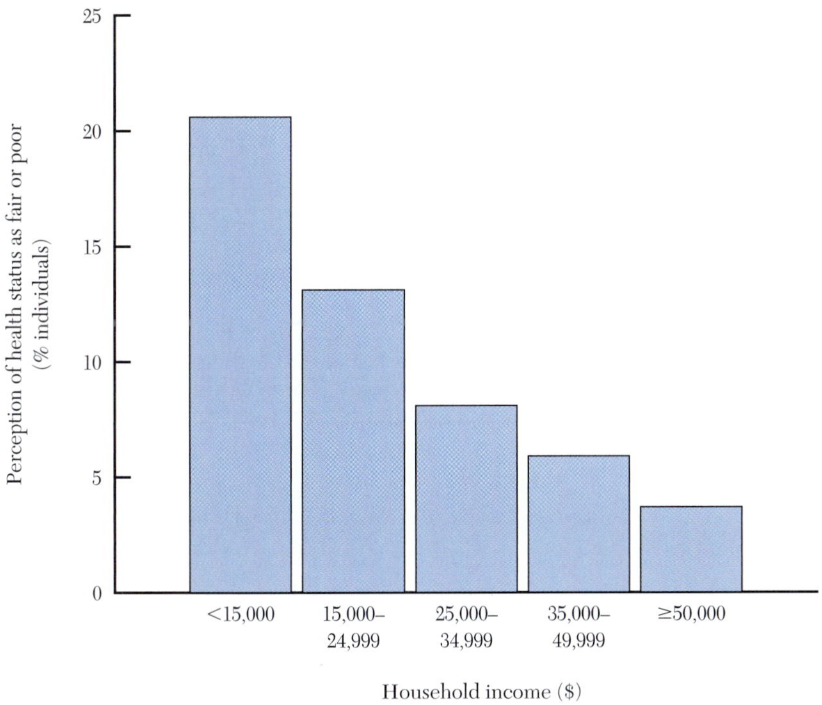

FIGURE 18.19 The percentage of people who report their health status as fair or poor is related to household income. *(Centers for Disease Control and Prevention, National Center for Health Statistics. National Health Interview Survey, 1995.)*

Health Status and Access to Health Care Poverty limits access to health care, leading to poorer health status; people in the lowest income households are more likely than those in higher income households to report their health status as fair or poor (Figure 18.19). Poor health and physical and mental disabilities can lead to food insecurity by affecting nutrient needs and by limiting the ability to acquire and prepare foods. Poverty is linked to undernutrition as well as to diet-related chronic disease. For example, iron deficiency is more than twice as frequent in low-income children, and the incidence of heart disease, cancer, hypertension, and obesity increases with decreasing income.[42]

As in developing nations, poverty is reflected in infant mortality rates. Average infant mortality in the U.S. population is about 7.3 per 1000 live births. However, there are groups within the population that have infant mortality rates as high as those in impoverished nations. Among African Americans, the infant mortality rate is 14.7 per 1000 live births—twice that of the general population.[43] This difference mirrors the higher poverty rate in this group. One of the major goals of Healthy People 2010 is to eliminate health disparities among Americans.[44]

Vulnerable Populations There are subgroups within the U.S. population that are at increased risk of hunger and undernutrition. These include the homeless; women, infants, and children; the elderly; Native Americans and Alaska Natives; and migrant and seasonal workers. According to a 1997 survey by the hunger-relief organization Second Harvest, 62% of people who rely on emergency food assistance are women, 38% are children under age 18, and 16% are over 65.[45] Considering that children make up only 27% of the U.S. population and the elderly 13%, a disproportionate number of children and elderly are seeking food assistance.

The Homeless The poor must use most of their income to pay for shelter. It is estimated that people who live in poverty spend about 80% of their income on housing, which seriously reduces the chances that their families will be adequately fed.[46] The high cost of housing not only limits food budgets but also has created a growing problem of homelessness in the United States. It is estimated that over half a million Americans are homeless, and one of the major health

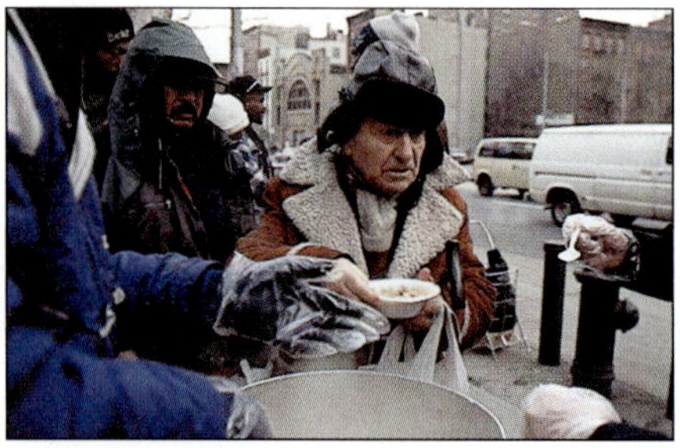

FIGURE 18.20 Soup kitchens and shelters provide meals to the homeless and others in need. *(© Argus Fotoarchiv/Peter Arnold, Inc.)*

problems of the homeless population is malnutrition.[47] Homeless people are at high risk of food insecurity because they lack not only money but also cooking and food storage facilities. Without cooking facilities, they must rely on ready-to-eat foods. Without storage facilities, they cannot use less expensive staples such as rice and dried beans, which can be purchased in bulk.[48] Homeless individuals often rely on soup kitchens and shelters to obtain adequate food (Figure 18.20). A study of homeless preschool children found that several times each month the children did not have enough food to eat and that they rarely consumed the recommended amounts of grains, fruits, vegetables, or dairy products.[49]

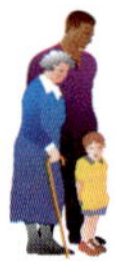

Women and Children Poverty has become a women's issue. Almost 30% of households with children headed by a single woman live below the poverty level.[41] Poverty and food insecurity put these women and children at risk of malnutrition, and their special nutritional needs magnify this risk. Because of their increased need for some nutrients, malnutrition may occur in pregnant women, infants, and children even when the rest of the household is adequately fed. For example, the amount of iron in the family diet may be enough to prevent anemia in all but a pregnant teenager.

The Elderly Due to diseases and disabilities, older adults may be limited in their ability to purchase, prepare, and physically ingest food. This puts the elderly, especially the elderly poor, at risk for malnutrition. A recent survey found that 8 to 14% of older adults experience food insecurity at some point in a six-month period.[47] Greater nutritional risk among older adults is associated with more hospital admissions and hence greater health care costs. The number of individuals over age 85 is expected to quadruple by the year 2050, and although older Americans are more affluent than ever before, the number at risk of food insecurity will increase as their overall number does. Providing food security for older adults improves their quality of life and reduces health-care costs (see Chapter 17).

Native Americans and Alaska Natives Many Native Americans and Alaska Natives live in remote locations, which reduces access to food (Figure 18.21). The unemployment and poverty rates are high among these groups. Unemployment for the United States as a whole was 5.6% in 1995 but was 35% among Native Americans living on or adjacent to reservations; only 29% of those employed earned more than $9048 a year.[42]

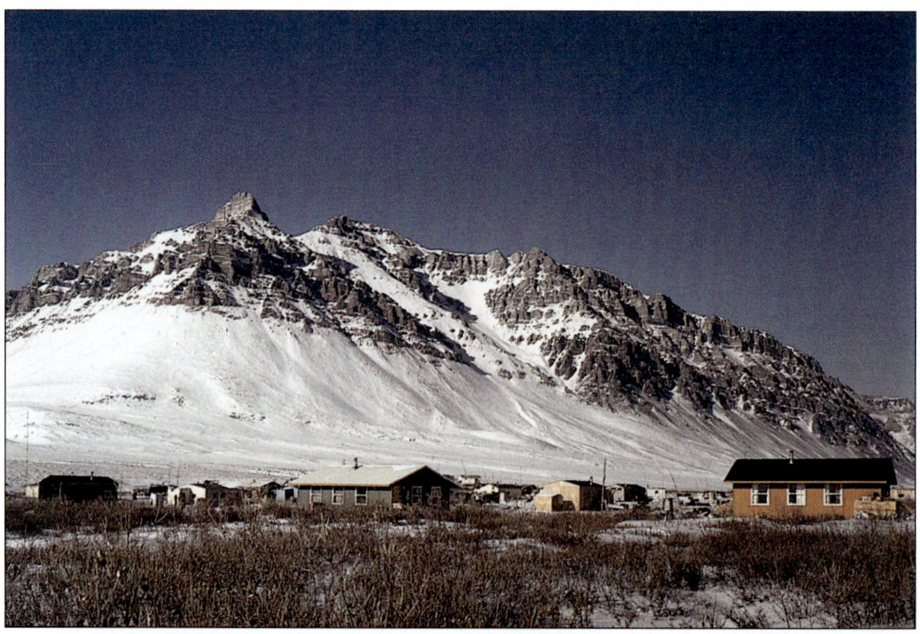

FIGURE 18.21 Living in remote locations limits access to food. *(© McCutcheon/Visuals Unlimited)*

Migrant and Seasonal Farm Workers Migrant workers have limited access to food because labor camps are in remote locations and transportation is limited. Low incomes and difficult working and living conditions limit their ability to purchase food and prepare adequate meals.

Solutions to Food Insecurity

Solving the problem of undernutrition in the United States requires alleviating poverty and providing access to an adequate nutritious food supply at a reasonable cost. Historically, many approaches have been attempted to meet this goal. Some have met with success and others have done little to increase access to a nutritious diet for all. Programs that provide access to affordable food and promote healthy eating have been referred to as a nutrition safety net for the American population.

A Historical Perspective Government response to hunger first occurred in the United States during the Great Depression of the 1930s with the distribution of farm surpluses by the Federal Supplies Relief Corporation.[50] Awareness of undernutrition in the United States was again aroused during World War II, when it was determined that 70% of the men rejected from the military draft had poor nutritional histories. At this time, the School Lunch Program (see Chapter 16) was initiated to improve the nutritional status of American youth and create the potential for a strong military.[47]

Between 1952 and 1960, the government showed little interest in the problems of hunger and malnutrition—an attitude that may have stemmed from the assumption that every citizen was well-fed in a land overflowing with food. In the 1960s, federal programs including the Food Stamp Program and the Commodity Program were developed in response to the hunger witnessed by John F. Kennedy on his travels through the United States during his presidential campaign. At the same time, Martin Luther King Jr.'s Southern Christian Leadership Conference cited areas of hunger in cotton-growing states, where replacement of cotton by corn and soybeans had put many field hands out of work. Reports of hunger also began to appear from other parts of the country, such as Appalachia, northern Maine, Indian reservations in the Southwest, ghettos in large cities, and Native sections of Alaska. In 1967, teams of nutritionists and physicians were sent around the country to assess the problem of hunger. The resulting report indicated widespread malnutrition in every ethnic group in every part of the country, urban and rural. The report was brought to Congress and broadcast on prime-time television in 1968 in the CBS documentary "Hunger in America." It was a rude awakening for the American public, and the awareness prompted interested organizations to coalesce into the National Council on Hunger and Malnutrition in the United States. The U.S. Senate formed the Senate Select Committee on Nutrition and Human Needs, and a White House Conference on Food, Nutrition, and Health was convened in 1969 to develop workable, implementable recommendations. There were 1800 such recommendations relating to poverty programs, diet, health, and consumer concerns. The Commodity Program was expanded, the Food Stamp Program was made permanent, the Special Supplemental Food Program for Women, Infants, and Children (WIC) was developed, child nutrition programs were expanded, and nutrition programs for the elderly were created.[47]

In 1977, a follow-up survey to assess hunger in America found that although poverty had not changed, the number of hungry people had decreased. There had been a major improvement in the diets of poor people from 1965–66 to 1977. This change was attributed solely to federal food assistance programs. This reduction in hunger was a major social advance, but as times change, so do political agendas. Many of the attempted solutions of the 1960s and 1970s fell by the wayside in the 1980s and early 1990s, although a key group of programs still provides the poor and other at-risk groups with access to food and nutrition education. In response to the challenge of the 1996 World Food Summit, several initiatives during the late 1990s helped to strengthen the nutrition safety net in the United States.[51] Among these were the expansion of health care coverage to uninsured children, increased funding for early childhood development programs such as Head Start, and the inclusion in Healthy People 2010 of an objective to cut food insecurity in half by 2010. In addition, nutrition guidelines, such as the Dietary Guidelines and the Food Guide Pyramid, were developed to promote the consumption of not only an adequate diet but one that will reduce the risks of chronic disease.

As we move further into the 21st century, the structure of the nutrition safety net is being influenced by measures designed to reduce the number of welfare recipients in the United States. The federal Personal Responsibility and Work Opportunity Reconciliation Act of 1996 will not affect WIC or the School Breakfast and Lunch Program, but other components of the nutrition safety net will be changed drastically. For instance, the maximum food-stamp benefits that a family can receive will be reduced, and the length of time able-bodied adults can receive food stamps will be limited to 3 months out of every 36 unless the adult is working or engaged in a work-related program.[52] The goal is to encourage welfare recipients to find work, stay employed, and earn enough money to attain self-reliance. However, the success of this program may be limited by the fact that many former welfare recipients can find jobs that pay only minimum wage, making it difficult to move out of poverty. Only time will reveal the effects of these types of changes in federal assistance programs. If net household income is decreased by these changes, the number of individuals who are at risk for food insecurity at any given time may increase. If, on the other hand, these changes move people out of poverty, the result may be to promote long-term food and financial security.

Web Menu: For more information on nutrition programs, go to the U.S. Department of Health and Human Services at www.dhhs.gov/, the USDA Food and Nutrition Service at www.fns.usda.gov/fns/, or Bread for the World at www.bread.org/.

Programs to Provide Access to Food In the United States the two major programs designed to make sure that all people have access to an adequate diet are the Food Stamp Program and the Emergency Food Assistance Program (see Table 18.5). The Food Stamp Program provides monthly benefits in the form of coupons or electronic transfers using a plastic card that can be used to purchase food, thereby supplementing the food budgets of low-income individuals and families. The Food Stamp Program served about 22.9 million people per month in 1997—that is, about one in nine people in the United States.[53] The Emergency Food Assistance Program distributes USDA food commodities to individuals for home use as well as to organized programs. Available commodities vary depending on market conditions. Products that are typically available include canned and dried fruits, canned vegetables, canned meats, peanut butter, butter, cheese and pasta products. This program provided states with about $80 million worth of USDA commodities in 1997.[53]

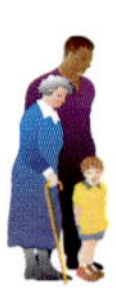

Because women, infants, children, the elderly, and the homeless are at highest risk of malnutrition, a number of programs target these particular groups (see Chapters 15–17). The WIC program provides coupons to purchase nutrient-dense foods to pregnant women, lactating and non–breast-feeding postpartum women, and infants and children who are at nutritional risk (Figure 18.22).[54] Preschool and school meal programs provide meals to children once they reach preschool age. And the Nutrition Program for the Elderly helps prevent malnutrition in the elderly by providing nutritious meals in congregate settings and by home delivery.

There are few specific programs that serve the homeless. In 1991, the Healthy Meals for Healthy Americans Act created the Homeless Children Nutrition Program to provide meals for homeless preschool-aged children living in shelters. Most of the homeless rely on food banks, feeding centers, and other community resource agencies to provide food; however, this does not

TABLE 18.5 Programs to Prevent Undernutrition in the United States

Program	Target Population	Goals and Methods
Food Stamp Program	Low-income individuals	Increases access to food by providing coupons that can be used to purchase food at the grocery store.
Commodity Supplemental Food Program	Low-income pregnant women, breast-feeding and non–breast-feeding postpartum women, infants and children under six years of age, and the elderly	Provides food by distributing USDA commodity foods.
Special Supplemental Nutrition Program for Women, Infants, and Children (WIC)	Low-income pregnant women, breast-feeding and non–breast-feeding postpartum women, infants, and children up to the age of 5	Increases access to the right mix of foods by providing coupons for purchasing foods that are good sources of those nutrients at risk of deficiency in these groups.
WIC Farmers Market Nutrition Program	WIC participants	Increases access to fresh produce by providing coupons to purchase produce at authorized local farmers' markets.
National School Breakfast Program	Low-income children	Provides free or low-cost breakfasts to improve the nutritional status of children.
National School Lunch Program	Low-income children	Provides free or low-cost lunches at school to improve the nutritional status of children.
Special Milk Program	Low-income children	Provides milk for children in schools, camps, and child-care institutions with no federally supported meal program.
Summer Food Service Program	Low-income children	Provides meals for children during the summer months.
Child and Adult Care Food Program	Children up to age 12 and handicapped adults	Provides cash reimbursements and food commodities to child-care programs and community adult day-care centers.
Head Start	Low-income preschool children and their families	Provides education, including nutrition education, to low-income children and their families.
Nutrition Program for the Elderly	Individuals age 60 or over and their spouses	Provides free congregate meals in churches, schools, senior centers, or other facilities, and home-delivers to the homebound.
Homeless Children Nutrition Program	Preschoolers living in shelters	Reimburses providers for meals served to homeless preschool children in shelters.
Emergency Food Assistance Program	Low-income people	Provides commodities to soup kitchens, food banks, and individuals for home use.
Healthy People 2010	U.S. population	Sets national health promotion objectives to improve the health of the U.S. population through health-care system and industry involvement, and individual actions.
Expanded Food and Nutrition Education Program (EFNEP)	Low-income families	Provides education in all aspects of food preparation and nutrition.
Nutrition Education and Training Program (NET)	Children, parents, teachers, and food service personnel	Provides a comprehensive, school-based nutrition education program.
Temporary Assistance for Needy Families (TANF)	Low-income households	Provides money to ensure housing, food, and clothing to low-income families. Exact requirements and provisions are determined by the states.

guarantee an adequate nutrient intake. Often meals at feeding centers are based more on the types of foods donated than the definition of an adequate diet. Innovative approaches are being developed to feed homeless people. One approach is to provide kitchens and cooking facilities in shelters for the homeless. Inhabitants of such shelters have been found to have better nutritional status.[48]

Even with federal assistance programs, many individuals still rely on church, community, and charitable emergency food shelters to provide for their basic nutritional needs. Second Harvest, the nation's largest charitable hunger relief organization, provided food to 21 million people in 1997.[45]

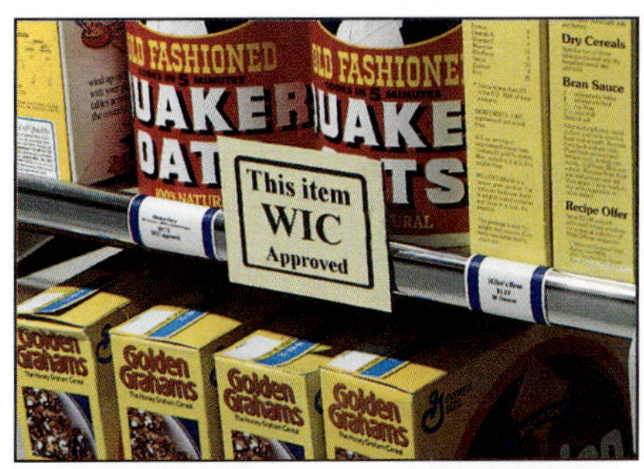

FIGURE 18.22 WIC supplies vouchers for foods that provide nutrients needed for healthy pregnancy and childhood. *(© Tony Freeman/PhotoEdit)*

Nutrition Education The link between nutrition education and diet quality is strong. People with more nutrition information and more awareness of the relationship between diet and health consume healthier diets.[55] Increasing nutrition knowledge can also reduce medical care costs and improve the quality of life.

TABLE 18.6 One Week's Meals for a Family of Four Using the Thrifty Food Plan

Monday	Tuesday	Wednesday	Thursday
Breakfast			
Orange juice (3 c) Ready-to-eat cereal (3 c flakes) Toasted English muffin (4) 1% low-fat milk (2 c)	Orange juice (3 c) Banana (4) Bagel (4) Margarine (4 tsp) 1% low-fat milk (2 c)	Orange Juice (3 c) †Cooked rice cereal Bagel (4) Margarine (4 tsp)	Orange juice (3 c) Scrambled eggs (4) Hash brown potatoes (2 c) 1% low-fat milk (2 c)
Lunch			
*Turkey patties Hamburger bun (4) Orange juice (3 c) Coleslaw (2 c) 1% low-fat milk (2 c)	*Crispy chicken †Potato salad †Orange gelatin salad Peaches, canned (1 c) †Rice pudding	†Turkey chili Macaroni (2 c) *Peach-apple crisp 1% low-fat milk (2 c) Orange juice (3 c)	Turkey ham (11 oz, 2 tbsp) salad dressing) sandwiches (4) †Baked beans Banana, slices (2 c) †Oatmeal cookies Orange juice (3 c) 1% low-fat milk (2 c)
Dinner			
†Beef-noodle casserole Lima beans (2 c) Banana orange salad (2 bananas, 2 oranges) (2 c) 1% low-fat milk (2 c)	*Turkey stir-fry Steamed rice (3 c) White bread (4 slices) *Peach-apple crisp 1% low-fat milk (2 c)	†Baked cod w/cheese *Scalloped potatoes Spinach (1 1/3 c) Margarine (4 tsp) Chocolate pudding (2 c)	*Beef pot roast Egg noodles (4 c) Peas and carrots (1 c) Orange slices (2 c) Biscuits (8) Margarine (4 tsp) †Rice pudding 1% low-fat milk (2 c)
Snack			
White bread (4 slices) †Chickpea dip Lemonade (4 c)	Orange juice (3 c)	*Crispy potatoes	Lemonade (4 c)

*Recipes were tested and sensory-evaluated in the food laboratory and by households.

†Recipes were tested and sensory-evaluated in the food laboratory.

Note: Daily menus are designed in no specific sequence. Amounts of foods that a family is expected to use are shown in parentheses for most foods. Amounts of allowed margarine and milk can be combined or divided differently at meals. Recipes are provided for foods shown with asterisks. Serving sizes are shown on the recipes.

USDA Center for Nutrition Policy and Promotion. The Thrifty Food Plan, 1999. Executive Summary, Aug. 1999. Available online at **www.usda.gov/cnpp/FoodPlans/TFP99/index.htm.**

Education can help individuals with lower incomes stretch limited food dollars by making wise choices at the store and reducing food waste at home. The USDA develops food plans that serve as a standard for a nutritious diet at a minimal cost. By following the menu suggestions of the lowest-cost plan, the Thrifty Food Plan, a family of four (male and female ages 20 to 50 and two children ages 6 to 8 and 9 to 11) can purchase foods for a nutritious diet at a cost of about $101.50 per week (Table 18.6). The Thrifty Food Plan is used as the basis for food stamp allotments.

Education can promote community gardens to increase the availability of seasonal vegetables. It can teach people how to prepare foods that become available through commodity distribution and food banks. It can teach safe food handling and food preparation methods. Knowing which foods to choose and how to handle them safely is as important in preventing malnutrition as having the money to buy enough food.

Friday	Saturday	Sunday
Breakfast		
Orange juice (3 c) Ready-to-eat cereal (3 c flakes) English muffin (4) Margarine (4 tsp) 1% low-fat milk (2 c)	Orange juice (3 c) *Baked French toast Cinnamon-sugar topping (4 tsp) 1% low-fat milk (2 c)	Orange juice (3 c) *Baked potato cakes White toast (4 slices) 1% low-fat milk (2 c)
Lunch		
†Potato soup Snack crackers, low salt (5 each) *Tuna pasta salad Orange slices (2 c) †Oatmeal cookies 1% low-fat milk (2 c)	†Potato soup Snack crackers, low salt (5 each) Apple and orange slices (2 apples, 2 oranges) (2 c) †Rice pudding 1% low-fat milk (2 c)	Baked fish (12 oz, 4 tbsp) salad dressing) sandwiches (4) *Crispy potatoes †Macaroni salad Melon (1 1/3 c) Orange juice (3 c) 1% low-fat milk (2 c)
Dinner		
Beef pot roast (12 oz) Noodles (4 c) Green beans (1 1/3 c) Leaf lettuce (1 1/3 c) Salad dressing (4 tbsp) †Rice pudding 1% low-fat milk (2 c)	*Saucy beef pasta White bread (4) Canned pears (2 c) Orange juice (3 c) 1% low-fat milk (2 c)	*Turkey-cabbage casserole (8 c) Orange slices (2 c) White bread (2 slices) †Chickpea dip 1% low-fat milk (2 c)
Snack		
Biscuits (8) Margarine (4 tsp) Lemonade (4 c)	Lemonade (4 c)	

There are a number of government programs designed to provide nutrition education. One of the goals of Healthy People 2010 is to increase the nutrition education provided by schools as well as by work sites. The Expanded Food and Nutrition Education Program (EFNEP) provides education in all aspects of food preparation and nutrition to low-income families. The Family Nutrition Program provides funding to develop and provide nutrition education programs for people on food stamps. In addition, the Dietary Guidelines for Americans, the Food Guide Pyramid, and food labels educate the general public about making wise food choices.

Policies to Control Food Costs The price of food depends on the amount produced and the consumer demand, so controlling the supply of food is important in determining cost. If the supply is large, prices will be low, but if supply forces prices to drop too much, the profit to the farmer and food industry may be too low to justify harvesting the crop. Government policy has tried to prevent this by controlling agricultural production with programs like the Grain Reserve Program and the Price Support Program. The Grain Reserve Program draws surplus grain off the market when excess is produced or prices decline. This practice keeps grain prices more stable and saves food for times when the harvest is not as plentiful. The Price Support Program also protects farmers from the drop in prices that results from overproduction. While these programs protect farmers, moderate food prices, and limit what reaches the marketplace, they may not provide incentive for farmers to limit production when demand is low. Federal programs also have the potential to support sustainable agriculture by regulating the use of natural resources and agricultural chemicals.

Policies to Affect the Foods Produced Food policy can have an effect on what foods are produced and consumed by the population. For example, the grading of meat is based on the fat content, which is associated with flavor and tenderness. The greater the fat content, the higher the grade and the greater the cost. Beef labeled "prime" is higher in fat and cost than that labeled "choice" or "select." A change in grading policy could encourage the production of lower-fat meats.

An example of how policy can affect production is pricing in the dairy industry. For years the USDA milk pricing system favored the production of milk high in fat. To respond to the health needs of the consumer, the USDA is now changing its policy—lowering the price it pays farmers for butterfat and increasing the price it pays for skim milk. The goal is to provide less of an incentive for farmers to produce milk with a high butterfat content. Thus, changes in technology and policy affect what foods are produced and in turn consumed, which can then affect the nutritional health of the population

Summary

1. Overnutrition coexists with undernutrition in both developed and developing nations. Nutrition and education policies and programs must work to feed the population when hunger and malnutrition are prevalent. At the same time, they must reduce the incidence of chronic diseases where they are a problem and, as the economy grows, prevent the population from adopting dietary and lifestyle patterns that result in an increase in chronic disease.
2. In poorly nourished populations, a cycle of malnutrition exists in which poorly nourished women give birth to low-birth-weight infants at risk of disease and early death. If these children survive, they grow into adults who are physically unable to fully contribute to society. Indicators of the nutritional status of a population are the infant mortality rate and the incidence of low birth weight and stunting.
3. Hunger and undernutrition occur when there is a shortage of food. Short-term food shortage, such as famine, may result from a natural or man-made disaster. Chronic food shortage occurs when overpopulation and limited natural resources create a situation in which there are more people than food. The inequitable distribution of food and resources caused by poverty creates food insecurity within a population even if there is enough total food.
4. Malnutrition occurs when there is not enough food and when the quality of the diet is poor. Protein, iron, iodine, and vitamin A deficiencies are common worldwide. Groups at risk of these nutrient deficiencies include pregnant women, children, the elderly, and the ill.
5. Short-term solutions to undernutrition provide food through relief at the local, national, and international levels. Long-term solutions include control of population growth, economic and agricultural policies that promote self-sufficiency and alleviate poverty, improvements in the quality of the food supply, and the development of sustainable systems and technologies that will provide food and meet nutrient needs without damaging the environment.
6. Undernutrition is associated with poverty. Lack of education and job experience make it difficult to escape poverty. The homeless, women, children, the elderly, and minority groups are most often food-insecure. However, food insecurity can occur even when income is adequate.
7. Nutrition programs in the United States focus on maintaining a nutrition safety net, which will provide access to affordable food and promote healthy eating in the United States. Some programs designed to help feed the hungry address the general population, whereas others focus on specific high-risk groups. Most programs provide access to food and some provide nutrition education.

Review Questions

1. Why is overnutrition a concern in all countries around the world?
2. What segments of the world population are at greatest risk for undernutrition?
3. What is the cycle of malnutrition?
4. How does overpopulation contribute to food shortage?
5. How does poverty contribute to world hunger?
6. How are economic growth and population growth related?
7. List three micronutrient deficiencies that are world health problems.
8. Why are environmental issues important in maintaining the world's food supply?
9. How does sustainable agriculture reduce environmental damage?
10. How can nutrification help eliminate malnutrition?
11. List four groups in the U.S. population that are at risk for undernutrition.
12. List three federal programs that address malnutrition in the United States.

Applying Critical Thinking Skills

Personal nutrition:

1. Keep a record of how much money you spend on food in a day or a week and use this to estimate your monthly food costs.
   a. Suggest specific changes in the foods you choose that will reduce your food costs.
   b. How do these changes affect the nutrient content of your diet?
2. Do a survey to determine least expensive way to buy the following products:

Product	Corner Store ($)	Super-market ($)	Discount/ Warehouse Store ($)
Orange juice (8 fl oz)			
Orange juice (1/2 gal)			
Brand-name cereal (e.g., Kix or Corn Flakes) (15-oz box)			
Box of same cereal (28-oz)			
Bag of chips (1-oz)			
Bag of same brand of chips (15–16-oz)			

   a. Calculate the cost per ounce for each item at each type of store.
   b. Is it consistently cheaper to buy the larger size package?

General nutrition issues:

1. World Food Day is October 16. List some ideas for campus-wide programs to increase awareness of global nutrition issues.
2. Use the Internet to locate Web sites for organizations such as Worldwatch or Bread for the World Institute. Research one area of the world where hunger and undernutrition are a major problem:
   a. What is the cause of undernutrition in this area?
   b. What solutions are in place or proposed to solve these problems?
3. The diet in an underdeveloped country is deficient in iodine. To solve the problem, the government imports iodized salt. When iodine deficiency continues to be a problem, a study of the local diet finds it to be very low in added salt. Not enough of the imported iodized salt was used to have an effect on the iodine status of the population. Use the following information to suggest a way that iodine intake might be increased in this population:

   The following foods are typically consumed:

   Corn and corn tortillas
   Dried beans
   White rice
   Fresh tomatoes
   Fresh vegetables—greens and squash
   Pork
   Fresh fruits

   A typical breakfast is cornmeal and fruit; lunch is a hot meal, usually with some kind of vegetable soup served with tortillas; and dinner is meat, beans, rice, tortillas, and fruit. Most of the food is grown and prepared locally.

References

1. Bread for the World Institute. Executive Summary: Hunger in a Global Economy: Hunger 1998. Available online at **http://www.bread.org/bfwi/summ98.html.** Accessed 12 Dec 2000.
2. Table set thinly as Food Summit pledges to halve world hunger in 20 years. UN Chronicle 33:24–28, 1996.
3. Posner, B. M., Franz, M., Quatromoni, P., and the INTERHEALTH steering committee. Nutrition and the global risk for chronic diseases: the INTERHEALTH Nutrition Initiative. Nutr. Rev. 52:201–207, 1994.
4. Posner, B. M., Quatromoni, P. A., and Franz, M. Nutrition policies and interventions for chronic disease risk reduction in international

settings: the INTERHEALTH Nutrition Initiative. Nutr. Rev. 52:179–187, 1994.

5. Vorster, H. H., Bourne, L. T., Venter, C. S., and Oosthuizen, W. Contribution of nutrition to the health transition in developing countries: a framework for research and intervention. Nutr. Rev. 57:341–349, 1999.
6. Drewnowski, A., and Popkin, B. M. The nutrition transition: new trends in the global diet. Nutr. Rev. 55:31–43, 1997.
7. Popkin, B. M., and Doark, C. M. The obesity epidemic is a worldwide phenomenon. Nutr. Rev. 56:106–114, 1998.
8. World Health Organization. *The World Health Report, 1998: Life in the 21st Century—A Vision for All.* Geneva: World Health Organization, 1–241, 1998.
9. World Health Organization. Nutrition for Health and Development, 1999. Available online at **http://www.who.int.nut/.** Accessed 12 Dec 2000.
10. Bengoa, J. M. A half-century perspective on world nutrition and the international nutrition agencies. Nutr. Rev. 55:309–314, 1997.
11. United Nations Administrative Committee on Coordination, Sub-Committee on Nutrition. *Third Report on the World Nutrition Situation.* Geneva: ACC/SCN, December 1997.
12. United Nations Administrative Committee on Coordination, Sub-Committee on Nutrition. *Fourth Symposium of the World Nutrition Situation: Nutrition Throughout the Life Cycle.* Geneva: ACC/SCN, in collaboration with IFPRI, 2000.
13. Pelletier, D. L. The potentiating effects of malnutrition on child mortality: epidemiologic evidence and policy implications. Nutr. Rev. 52:409–415, 1994.
14. National Geographic Society. Millennium in maps: population. Supplement to National Geographic Magazine, October 1998.
15. International Food Policy and Research Institute (IFPRI). *A 20/20 Vision for Food, Agriculture, and the Environment: The Vision, Challenge, and Recommended Action.* Washington, D.C.: IFPRI, 1995.
16. Beckman, D., Cohen, M. J., and Kennedy, E. Position of the American Dietetic Association: world hunger. J. Am. Diet. Assoc. 95:1160–1162, 1995.
17. Raloff, J. The human numbers crunch. Sci. News 149:396–397, 1996.
18. Torún, B., and Chew, F. Protein-energy malnutrition. *In Modern Nutrition in Health and Disease,* 9th ed. Shils, M. E., Olson, J. A., Shike, M., and Ross, A. C., eds. Baltimore: Williams & Wilkins, 1999, 963–988.
19. Darnton-Hill, I. Developing industrial-government-academic partnerships to address micronutrient malnutrition. Nutr. Rev. 55:76–81, 1997.
20. Pollitt, E. Functional significance of the covariance between protein energy malnutrition and iron deficiency anemia. J. Nutr. 125:2272S–2277S, 1995.
21. Ramalingaswami, V. New global perspectives on overcoming malnutrition. Am. J. Clin. Nutr. 61:259–263, 1995.
22. Hetzel, B. S., and Clugstrum, G. A. Iodine. In *Modern Nutrition in Health and Disease,* 9th ed. Shils, M. E., Olson, J. A., Shike, M., and Ross, A. C., eds. Baltimore: Williams & Wilkins, 1999, 253–264.
23. World Health Organizaiton. Vitamin A—The Good News: Donald McLaren Highlights Recent Developments. Available online at **http://www.who.int/chd/pub/newslet/dialog/9/vitamin_a.htm.** Accessed 12 Dec 2000.
24. Ross, D. A. Vitamin A and public health. Proc. Nutr. Soc. 57:159–165, 1998.
25. West, C. E. Vitamin A and measles. Nutr. Rev. 58(II):S46–S54, 2000.
26. United Nations Food and Agriculture Organization. United Nations World Food Summit Briefing, November 1996. Available online at **http://www.fao.org.** Accessed 12 Dec 2000.
27. United Nations Food and Agriculture Organization. Rome Declaration on World Food Security and World Food Summit Plan of Action, November 13, 1996. Available online at **http://www.fao.org.** Accessed 12 Dec 2000.
28. Sloham, J. Emergency feeding programmes: still not delivering the goods. Br. J. Med. 305:596–597, 1992.
29. Raven, P. H., Berg, L. R., and Johnson, G. B. *Environment,* 3rd ed. Philadelphia: Harcourt College Publishers, 2001.
30. Uvin, P. The state of world hunger. Nutr. Rev. 52:151–161, 1994.
31. Matson, P. A., Parton, W. J., Power, A. G., and Swift, M. J. Agricultural intensification and ecosystem properties. Science 277:504–509, 1997.
32. Waibel, H. Government intervention in crop protection in developing countries. Ciba Found. Symp. 177:76–90, 1993.
33. Viteri, F. E., Alvarez, E., Batres, R., et al. Fortification of sugar with iron sodium ethylenediaminotetraacetate (FeNaEDTA) improves iron status in semirural Guatemalan populations. Am. J. Clin. Nutr. 61:1153–1163, 1995.
34. Solon, F. S., Solon, M. S., Meshansho. H., et al. Evaluation of the effect of vitamin A–fortified margarine on the vitamin A status of preschool Filipino children. Eur. J. Clin. Nutr. 50:720–723, 1996.
35. Arraya, J. C., and Canelas, W. *Assessment of Vitamin A in Fortified Sugar—Simplified.* Abstract, 17th International Vitamin A Consultative Group Meeting, Guatemala City, 1996. Washington, D.C.: International Vitamin A Consultative Group, 1996.
36. Layrisse, M., Chaves, J. F., Mendez-Castellano, H., et al. Early response to the effect of iron fortification in the Venezuelan population. Am. J. Clin. Nutr. 64:903–907, 1996.
37. World Health Organization, United Nation's Children's Fund, International Vitamin A Consultative Group. *Vitamin A Supplements: A Guide to Their Use in the Treatment and Prevention of Vitamin A Deficiency and Xerophthalmia,* 2nd ed. Geneva: WHO, 1997.
38. National Institutes of Health; National Heart, Lung, and Blood Institute. Clinical Guidelines on the Identification, Evaluation, and Treatment of Overweight and Obesity in Adults. Executive Summary, June 1998. Available online at **http://www.nhlbi.nih.gov/nhlbi/cardio/obes/prof/guidelines/ob_xsum.htm.** Accessed 12 Dec 2000.
39. Update: prevalence of overweight among children, adolescents, and adults—United States, 1988–1994. MMWR Morb. Mortal. Wkly. Rep. 46:198–202, 1998.
40. National Center for Health Statistics. Fact Sheets: Ten Million Americans Do Not Get Enough to Eat. Available online at **http://www.cdc.gov/nchswww/releases/98factsheets.** Accessed 12 Dec 2000.
41. Andrews, M., Nord, M., Bickel, G., and Carlson, S. Household Food Security in the United States, 1999. Food Assistance and Nutrition Research Report No. 8. Food and Rural Economics Division, Economic Research Service, U.S. Department of Agriculture. Available online at **http://www.ers.usda.gov:80/epubs/pdf/fanrr8/.** Accessed 11 Dec 2000.
42. U.S. Department of Agriculture, Foreign Agricultural Service. Discussion Paper on Domestic Food Security, February 13, 1998. Available online at **http://www.fas.usda.gov/icd/summit/discussi.html.** Accessed 11 Dec 2000.
43. National Center for Health Statistics, Centers for Disease Control and Prevention. Infant Mortality Rates, Fetal Mortality Rates, and Perinatal Mortality Rates, According to Race: United States, Selected Years, 1950–96. Available online at **http://www.cdc.gov.nchs/datawh/statab/pubd/hus98t23.htm.** Accessed 11 Dec 2000.
44. Healthy People 2010. A Systematic Approach to Health Improvement. Available online at **http://www.health.gov/healthy people/Document/htm1/uih/uih_2.htm.** Accessed 14 Feb 2001.
45. Second Harvest. Hunger: The Faces and Facts—A Profile of Who Is Hungry. Available online at **http://www.secondharvest.org/websecha/d_ffla.htm.** Accessed 12 Dec 2000.
46. Mayer, J. Hunger and undernutrition in the United States. J. Nutr. 120:919–923, 1990.

47. American Dietetic Association. Position on domestic food and nutrition security. J. Am. Diet. Assoc. 98:337–342, 1998.
48. Wiecha, J. L., Dwyer, J. T., Jacques, P. F., and Rand, W. M. Nutritional and economic advantages for homeless families in shelters providing kitchen facilities and food. J. Am. Diet. Assoc. 93:777–783, 1993.
49. Taylor, M. L., and Oblinsky, S. A. Food consumption and eating behavior of homeless preschool children. J. Nutr. Ed. 26:20–25, 1994.
50. Poppendieck, J. Hunger and public policy lessons from the Great Depression. J. Nutr. Ed. 24(Suppl):6S–10S, 1992.
51. U.S. National Progress Report on Implementation of the U.S. Action Plan on Food Security and World Food Summit Commitments, 2000. Available online at **http://www.fas.usda.gov/.** Accessed 11 Dec 2000.
52. Oliveira, V. Cost of food-assistance programs declined slightly in first half of 1996. Food Review 26–33, USDA Food and Consumer Service, September/December 1996.
53. U.S. Department of Agriculture. Food, Nutrition, and Consumer Service Mission. Available online at **http://www.usda.gov/mission/fncs.htm.** Accessed 14 Dec 2000.
54. Owen, A. L., and Owen, G. M. Twenty years of WIC: a review of some effects of the program. J. Am. Diet. Assoc. 97:777–782, 1997.
55. U.S. Department of Agriculture Economic Research Service, Center for Nutrition Policy and Promotion. USDA's Healthy Eating Index and Nutrition Information. Available online at **http://www.ers.usda.gov/epubs/pdf/tbl1866.** Accessed 12 Dec 2000.
56. U.S. Department of Agriculture, Center for Nutrition Policy and Promotions. Official USDA Food Plans: Cost of Food at Home at Four Levels, U.S. Average, October, 2000. Available online at **http://www.usda.gov/cnpp.** Accessed 11 Dec 2000.

19 Food Safety

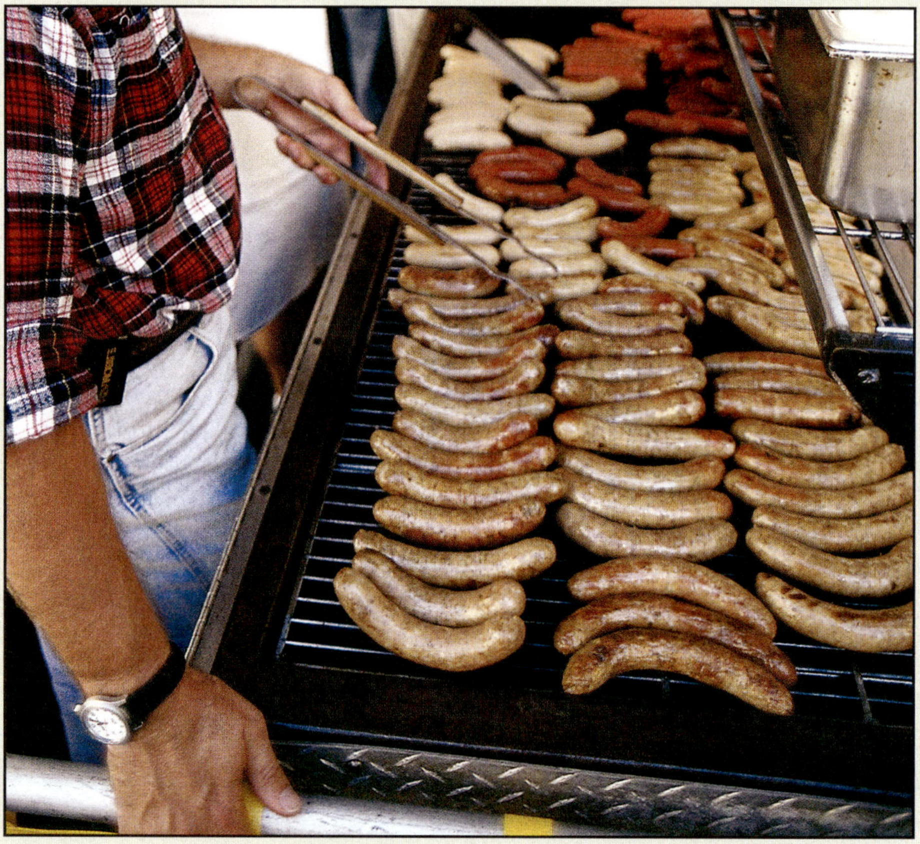

Learning Objectives

After reading this chapter, students should be able to:

1. Name the primary cause of foodborne illness in the United States.
2. Discuss how the dose of a contaminant in food affects the reaction that occurs with exposure.
3. Explain why food safety is a focus of public health programs.
4. Give an example of a bacterium, a virus, a mold toxin, and a parasite that has the potential to cause foodborne illness.
5. Describe how a HACCP program works.
6. Explain how care in choosing, preparing, cooking, handling, and storing food can reduce the risk of foodborne illness.
7. Use a diagram of the food chain to show how chemicals used in agriculture and industry make their way into our food supply.
8. Compare the risks and benefits of food additives.

One hundred children at the elementary school were absent or went home sick that day. Forty of them vomited at school. Was this due to a fast-moving virus? Was it even caused by a virus? Only a few of the teachers and parents became ill, even though they were in contact with the children and presumably were just as likely as the children to catch an intestinal virus.

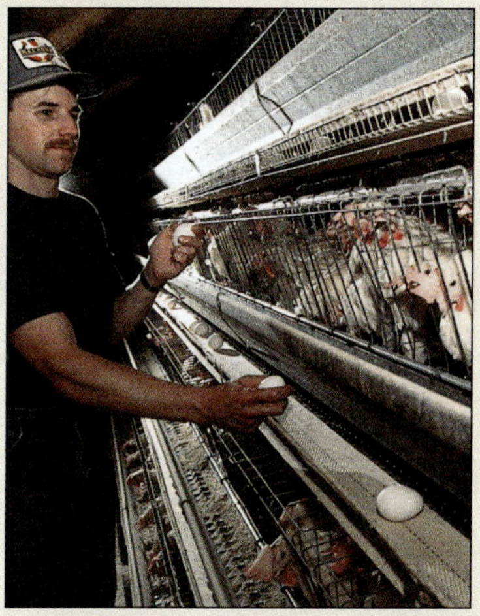

When this number of individuals becomes ill at the same time, a common immediate cause is always a possibility. In such a situation, the local health department must be notified. In the case of the school, the illnesses occurred on a Friday. By Monday, almost everyone had recovered fully. Nonetheless, the health department came to inspect the school and investigate the cause of the illnesses. Within a few weeks they were able to trace the source of the infection. The school had held a "Welcome Back, Spring" celebration the day before everyone became ill. The first graders made cupcakes, the second graders made cookies, the third graders made popcorn balls, and the fourth graders made ice cream. After interviewing the children and adults who got sick, it was determined that only those who ate ice cream became ill. Symptoms included nausea and vomiting, diarrhea, abdominal pain, and fever. All became ill within 72 hours of consuming the ice cream. Many of the ill children were seen by physicians, and the organism *Salmonella enteritidis* was isolated from their stool samples. Further investigation revealed that the recipe used by the fourth graders to make the ice cream included six grade-A raw eggs. The students cranked the ice cream by hand and it took about 2 hours for it to harden. The ice cream was then stored frozen until the picnic. The kids who prepared the ice cream were not ill at the time it was made but became ill 13 to 15 hours after consuming it. Tracking the ingredients used to make the ice cream revealed that the school had purchased the eggs from a distributor in Florida who had bought them from a farm in Maryland. The flock of chickens was tested and found to be the source of the *Salmonella.* The eggs from that farm must now undergo a pasteurization process before they are sold.

Even though everyone who got sick had eaten ice cream, not everyone who ate ice cream got sick. Whether a contaminated food causes illness depends on the consumer, the consumer's body size and health status, and the amount consumed. Fewer adults than children became ill because the adults were larger and tended to eat smaller portions. Also, those who ate the ice cream later in the day after some of it had melted and come to room temperature were more likely to become ill.

A Safe Food Supply

The American food supply is one of the safest in the world; nonetheless, *Salmonella* contaminate chicken sold in the United States, pesticide residues are found on our fruit, and industrial waste has polluted some of our waterways. Headlines announce *E. coli* in meat, bean sprouts, and apple juice; *Salmonella* in eggs, on vegetables, and in cereal; *Cyclospora* on fruit; *Cryptosporidium* in drinking water; hepatitis A in frozen strawberries; and dioxins in fish. Although the American food supply may in fact be the safest in the world, it is not risk free or beyond improvement.

For information on food safety concerns throughout the world, go to the World Health Organization at www.who.int/ and click on health topics; then click on food safety.

Everyone wants to consume food that is safe, but it is nearly impossible to choose a diet that is free of all potential hazards. Food has always carried risks. And today, despite the fact that the causes of **foodborne illness** are understood, more than 70% of the 1.5 billion episodes of diarrhea that occur globally every year, killing 3 million children under the age of five, are estimated to be due to food contaminated by microbes.[1] As science develops tools to combat some of these, new strains of harmful microorganisms are emerging. Changes in agricultural technology, trade patterns, food processing, and dietary habits have increased the risks associated with microbial contamination and introduced new risks. Pesticides used to increase crop yields in South America contaminate fruits and vegetables shipped to New York; materials in food packaging may be leaching into the foods they are designed to protect; and additives used to preserve food may cause allergies and intolerances. Regulatory agencies, food manufacturers, and retailers, as well as consumers, need to work together to maximize the safety of the food supply (Figure 19.1).

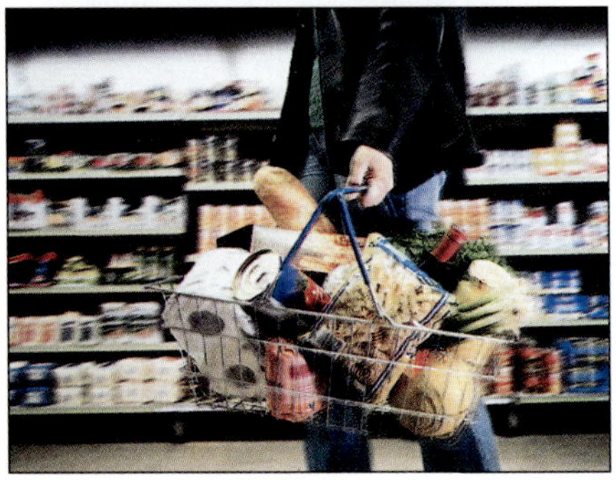

FIGURE 19.1 Choosing safe, nutritious foods is one way that consumers help control the safety of the foods they eat. *(© Ray Botterell/Stone)*

Causes of Foodborne Illness

It is estimated that 76 million people in the United States become ill from foodborne illness each year; 325,000 are hospitalized and 5000 die.[2,3] Foodborne illness can be caused by biological, chemical, or physical contaminants in food. Most of the foodborne illness in the United States is caused by biological contamination of food by **pathogens** such as bacteria, viruses, fungi, and parasites. More than 200 known diseases are transmitted this way. While chemical contaminants such as environmental **toxins** can also increase risk to consumers, the incidence of illness is much lower than that associated with pathogens. Physical contaminants such as glass or animal hair also have the potential to cause foodborne illness. In order for a food to cause foodborne illness, it must be contaminated with a foreign substance, and the contamination must be significant enough to cause symptoms in the individual consuming it.

Foodborne illness An illness caused by consumption of food containing a contaminant such as a toxin or disease-causing microorganism.

Pathogens Organisms capable of causing disease.

Toxins Substances that can cause harm at some level of exposure.

Contamination Some foods naturally contain substances that are toxic to humans, but most cause illness because they are contaminated with foreign pathogens or other substances. This contamination may occur where the food is grown or produced. Eggs, for example, may be contaminated with the bacteria *Salmonella enteritidis* directly from the hen on the farm (Figure 19.2); fish may be contaminated by agricultural runoff into the stream where they live; molds may grow on grains during unusually wet or dry growing seasons; and milk can be contaminated with medications administered to the cows.

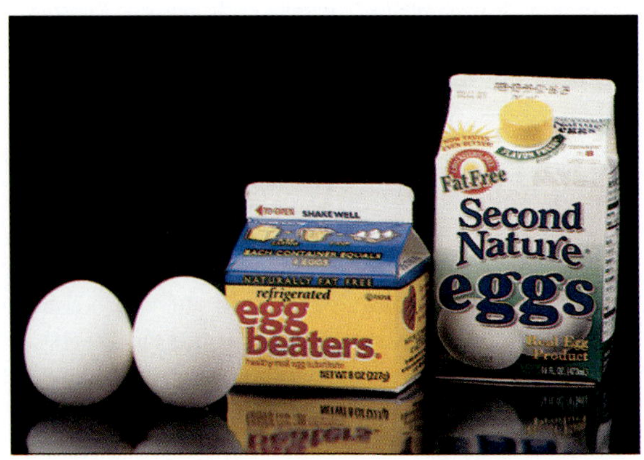

FIGURE 19.2 *Salmonella* contamination is a concern in the production of frozen eggs. *(George Semple)*

Food may also be contaminated during processing, handling, or storage. This often occurs by **cross-contamination,** in which a contaminated food or utensil comes in contact with an uninfected food, resulting in the transfer of the contaminant. This can occur in manufacturing plants, stores, restaurants, or at home. It is a more common occurrence at home, but it affects a larger number of people per incident when it occurs in a retail establishment. For example, *E.coli* O157:H7 from a single cow can be spread during processing to contaminate thousands of pounds of hamburger. However, careful sanitation and food handling by producers, retailers, and consumers can control most of these sources of contamination. In fact, regardless of the original source of contamination, most of the cases of foodborne illness are caused by foods prepared at home and can be prevented by safe food handling procedures.[4]

Cross-contamination The transfer of contaminants from one food to another.

Dose Even though a food is contaminated, it will not cause every individual who consumes it to become ill. Many foods are contaminated with hazardous substances, but most do not cause illness. The potential of a substance to cause harm depends on how potent it is, the amount or dose that is consumed, how frequently it is consumed, and who consumes it. Some contaminants in food can cause harm even when minute amounts are consumed, and almost any substance can be toxic if a large enough amount is consumed. Many substances have a **threshold effect;** that is, they are harmless up to a certain dose or threshold, after which negative effects increase with increasing intake. Body size, nutritional status, and how the body metabolizes a substance also affect the toxicity threshold. Small doses are more dangerous in children because the amount of toxin per unit of body weight is greater. Poor nutritional or health status may decrease the body's ability to detoxify harmful substances.

Threshold effect A reaction that occurs at a certain level of ingestion and increases as the dose increases. Below that level there is no reaction.

The way that a substance is stored in or excreted from the body also determines its potential for harm. Substances that are stored in the body are more likely to be toxic because they accumulate over time. They are deposited in bone, adipose tissue, the liver, or other organs, eventually causing toxicity symptoms. For instance, vitamin A is stored in the liver and can be toxic if excess amounts are consumed over a long period. Substances that are easily excreted when consumed in excess, such as vitamin C, are less likely to cause toxicity.

The interaction of toxins with one another and with other dietary factors also affects toxicity. For example, mercury, which is extremely toxic, is not absorbed well if the diet is high in selenium, and the absorption of lead is decreased by the presence of iron and calcium in the diet.

Safeguarding the Food Supply

Early in the last century, the government became involved in safeguarding the food supply. The first food regulations were outlined in the Pure Food and Drug Act of 1906 and the Meat Inspection Act of 1906. Since then, great strides have been made in protecting the American food supply. In fact, the Centers for Disease Control and Prevention (CDC) has determined that progress in protecting the food supply is one of the ten greatest health-care improvements of the 20th century.[5] Nonetheless, recent media coverage of large outbreaks of foodborne illnesses has heightened concern about food safety and encouraged regulatory agencies and food manufacturers to establish a better system for safeguarding the food supply. The federal government has responded with the National Food Safety Initiative—conceived to reduce the incidence of foodborne illness by improving food safety practices and policies throughout the United States. Because microorganisms are the most common cause of foodborne illness, the focus of this initiative is on reducing the risk of microbial foodborne illness. However, the initiative also recognizes that chemical and physical contaminants can cause foodborne illness.[6]

Web Menu

For more information on the National Food Safety Initiative, organizations that safeguard our food supply, and all aspects of food safety, go to the government's food safety information site at www.foodsafety.gov/.

Table 19.1 Agencies Responsible for Food Safety

Agency	Responsibility
World Health Organization (WHO)	Develops international food safety policies, food inspection programs, and standards for hygienic food preparation; promotes technologies that improve food safety and consumer education about safe food practices.
Food and Drug Administration (FDA) at the Department of Health and Human Services (DHHS)	Ensures the safety and wholesomeness of all foods sold across state lines with the exception of red meat (beef, veal, pork, and lamb), poultry, and egg products; inspects food-processing plants; inspects imported foods with the exception of red meat, poultry, and egg products; sets standards for food composition; oversees use of drugs and feed in food-producing animals; and enforces regulations for food labeling, food and color additives, and food sanitation.
Food Safety and Inspection Service (FSIS) at the U.S. Department of Agriculture (USDA)	Enforces standards for the wholesomeness and quality of red meat, poultry, and egg products, including that imported from other countries. If a food is suspect, it can be tested for contamination, and entry into the country can be denied.
Environmental Protection Agency (EPA)	Regulates pesticide levels and must approve all pesticides before they can be sold in the United States; establishes water quality standards.
National Marine Fisheries Service at the Department of Commerce	Oversees the management of fisheries and fish harvesting. Operates a voluntary program of inspection and grading of fish products.
Animal and Plant Health Inspection Service (APHIS) at the USDA	Monitors disease in food-producing animals.
Centers for Disease Control and Prevention (CDC) at DHHS	Monitors and investigates the incidence and causes of foodborne diseases.
Bureau of Alcohol, Tobacco, and Firearms (ATF) at the Department of the Treasury	Enforces laws regulating the production, distribution, and labeling of alcoholic beverages.
State and local governments	Inspect food-processing plants, grocery stores, restaurants, and institutions such as schools and hospitals.

Monitoring the Safety of the Food Supply The safety of the food supply is monitored by agencies at the international, federal, state, and local levels (Table 19.1). International cooperation on food inspection and regulatory standards helps to ensure the safety of imported food. Approximately 40 different nations are now partners with the United States in ensuring food safety through agreements that regulate a variety of food products.

In the United States, federal agencies monitor various segments of the food supply. These agencies set standards and establish regulations for the safe and sanitary handling of food and water (see Chapter 11, *Making Decisions:* "Is Bottled Water Better?"). They also set standards for both the nutrition and safe-handling information included on food labels. They regulate the use of agricultural chemicals, additives, and packaging materials; inspect food processing and storage facilities; and investigate outbreaks of foodborne illness. They also provide guidelines to state and local governments for regulating dairy products and the food sold in restaurants. The U.S. Food and Drug Administration (FDA) publishes the **Food Code,** which provides recommendations for safeguarding public health when food is offered to the consumer. State agencies have the primary responsibility for milk safety and the inspection of restaurants, retail food

Food Code A set of recommendations published by the FDA for the handling and service of food sold in restaurants and other establishments that serve food.

stores, dairies, grain mills, and other food-related establishments within their borders (Figure 19.3). As a result, regulations vary from state to state.

Consumers must also be actively involved in preventing foodborne illness by following safe food handling, cooking, and storage practices. Individuals must decide what foods they will consume and evaluate the risks involved. A food that has been manufactured, packaged, and transported with the greatest care can still cause illness if it is not carefully handled at home. For example, contaminated foods such as eggs, chicken, or hamburger can cause illness if they are undercooked. Consumers can also protect themselves and others by reporting incidents involving unsanitary or unsafe handling or deceptive or mislabeled food to the appropriate agencies (Table 19.2).

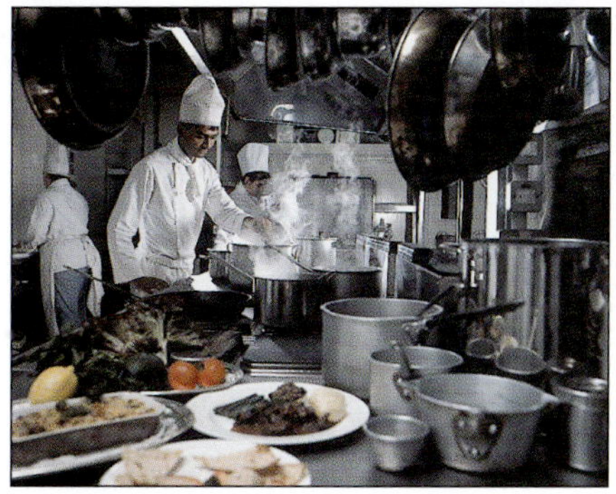

FIGURE 19.3 State and local governments are responsible for regulating the safety of food sold at restaurants. *(© John Miller/Stone)*

Preventing, Controlling, or Eliminating Food Hazards: HACCP Traditionally, methods for monitoring the food supply have involved spot-checks of manufacturing conditions and products (Figure 19.4). These spot-checks often relied only on visual inspection, so contamination was easily missed. More recently, the National Food Safety Initiative has promoted the implementation of a system called **Hazard Analysis Critical Control Point (HACCP)** to improve food safety. HACCP is a systematic approach based on the identification of points in the handling of food, called **critical control points,** at which chemical, physical, or biological hazards can occur. Using HACCP requires establishing a standardized plan to prevent, control, or eliminate the contamination before the food reaches the consumer (Table 19.3).

Web Menu: For more information on safe food preparation and storage at home, go to www.homefoodsafety.org/.

Hazard Analysis Critical Control Point (HACCP) A management system in which food safety is addressed through the analysis and control of biological, chemical, and physical hazards, from raw material production, procurement, and handling to the manufacturing, distribution, and consumption of the finished product.

Critical control points Possible points in food production, manufacturing, and transportation at which contamination can occur or be prevented.

TABLE 19.2 How to Report a Food Hazard

First, get all the facts. Has the product been used as intended and according to the manufacturer's instructions? Has the expiration date passed?

Then, report the item or incident to the appropriate agency as soon as possible. Do not wait.

- Problems relating to any food except meat and poultry, including adverse reactions, should be reported to the FDA Food and Seafood Information line (1–800–332–4010). An emergency requiring immediate action, such as a case of foodborne illness, should be reported to the FDA's emergency number (1–301–443–1240). For a problem not requiring immediate attention, the FDA district office consumer complaint coordinator for your geographic area can be contacted.[a]
- Issues relating to meat and poultry should be reported first to the state's department of health or agriculture and then to the USDA hotline (1–800–535–4555).
- Restaurant food and sanitation problems can be reported directly to local or state health departments.
- Issues related to alcoholic beverages should be reported to the Department of the Treasury's Bureau of Alcohol, Tobacco, and Firearms.
- Accidental poisonings should be reported to state or local poison control centers or hospitals before calling the Centers for Disease Control and Prevention.
- Pesticide, air, and water pollution should be reported first to the state's environmental protection department and then to the EPA.
- Products purchased at the grocery store should be returned to the store. Grocery stores are concerned with the safety of the foods they sell, and they will take the responsibility of tracking down and correcting the problem.
- Hazardous household products are the responsibility of the state department of consumer protection and, federally, the Consumer Product Safety Commission (**http://www.cpsc.gov/**).
- False advertising should be reported first to your state's department of consumer protection and then to the Federal Trade Commission (**http://www.ftc.gov/**). Issues related to food additives are dealt with by the Adverse Reaction Monitoring System (ARMS).
- Unsolicited products received in the mail should be reported to the U.S. Postal Service (**http://www.usps.gov/websites/depart/inspect/**).

[a] U.S. Food and Drug Administration. How to report adverse reactions and other problems with products regulated by FDA. FDA Backgrounder, April 29, 1998. Available online at **http://www.fda.gov/opacom/backgrounders/problem.html.**

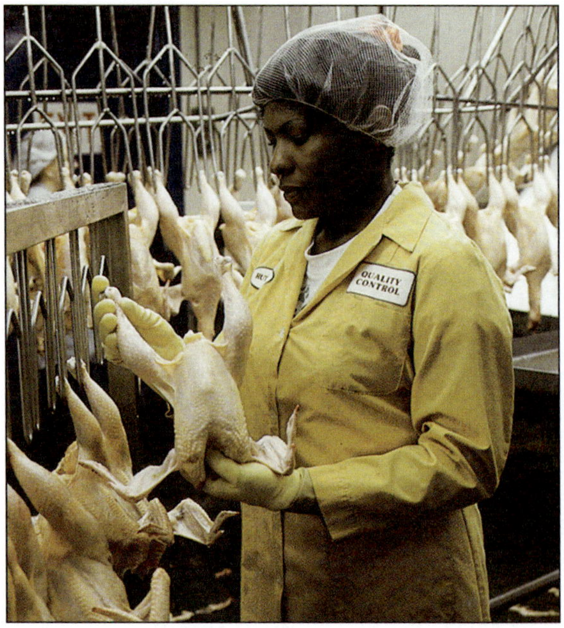

FIGURE 19.4 Traditional methods of protecting the food supply rely on spot-checks by food safety inspectors. *(© Don Smetzer/Tony Stone Worldwide-Click/Chicago Ltd.)*

Pasteurization The process of treating food products to kill disease-causing organisms. Traditional pasteurization relies on heating to kill the microorganisms, but irradiation, referred to as cold pasteurization, can also be used (see Chapter 20).

The HACCP system allows the food manufacturing and food service industries to anticipate where contamination might occur. And, it establishes record-keeping procedures to verify that the system is working consistently. For example, contamination with *Salmonella* has been identified as a risk in the production of shelled frozen eggs. To produce this product, eggs are removed from their shells, mixed together in large vats, heated in a process called **pasteurization** to kill *Salmonella* and other microbial contaminants, packaged, and then frozen. The critical control point for preventing contaminated eggs from getting to consumers is the pasteurization process. To monitor the effectiveness of this process in the frozen egg industry, bacterial tests are performed on samples of eggs following pasteurization. All the eggs are held refrigerated or frozen until the results of the bacterial tests have been obtained. If the samples are *Salmonella*-free, the eggs are released to the market. If they contain *Salmonella,* the entire batch of eggs cannot be sold and pasteurization conditions are adjusted to ensure that the bacteria are killed in the next batch. Keeping records enables manufacturers to trace which eggs were pasteurized when, for how long, and at what temperature, and when and where they were shipped, in the event of an outbreak of foodborne illness (see *Research Discoveries:* "Pasteurization: From Spoiled Wine to Safe Milk").

The advantage of HACCP over standard inspections by the FDA is that it is preventative rather than punitive. It places responsibility for ensuring food safety on the food manufacturer or distributor and permits more efficient and effective government oversight. Currently, HACCP is required in the processing of seafood, meat, poultry, and fruit and vegetable juices.

Monitoring and Responding to Outbreaks of Foodborne Illness Monitoring outbreaks of foodborne illness is key to both reducing the impact of an incident and preventing future incidents. However, tracking foodborne illness is complicated by a number of factors. Underreporting is a major barrier to obtaining accurate information on the actual frequency of foodborne illness. Often individuals believe they have the flu rather than a foodborne illness. Also, many pathogens that are transmitted through food are also spread through water or from person to person; therefore, the incidence that is due to food transmission is difficult to determine. And finally, some foodborne illness is caused by pathogens or agents that have not yet been identified and thus cannot be officially diagnosed as a

TABLE 19.3 Seven Principles of HACCP

1. ***Conduct a hazard analysis.***	Analyze the processes associated with the production of a food, identify the potential hazards (biological, chemical, and physical), and list preventive measures (temperature, pH, moisture level) to control these hazards.
2. ***Identify critical control points.***	Identify steps in a food's production (from the raw state, through processing and shipping, to consumption by the consumer), called critical control points, at which the potential hazard can be prevented, controlled, or eliminated—for example, cooking, cooling, packaging, and metal detection.
3. ***Establish critical limits.***	Establish preventative measures with measurable limits for all critical control points. For example, for a cooked food this might be a minimum cooking time and temperature required to ensure elimination of harmful microbes. If these critical limits are not met, the food safety hazards are not being prevented, eliminated, or reduced to acceptable levels.
4. ***Establish monitoring procedures.***	Establish procedures to monitor the critical limits. For example, how and by whom will the cooking temperature be monitored? Adjustments can be made while continuing the process.
5. ***Establish corrective actions.***	Establish plans to discard the potentially hazardous product and to correct the out-of-control process when monitoring shows that a critical limit has not been met—for example, reprocessing or discarding food if the minimum cooking temperature is not met.
6. ***Establish verification procedures.***	Establish procedures to verify the scientific or technical validity of the hazard analysis, the adequacy of the critical control points, and the effectiveness of the HACCP plan. An example of verification is the testing of time and temperature recording devices to verify that a cooking unit is working properly.
7. ***Establish record-keeping and documentation procedures.***	Prepare and maintain a written HACCP plan. This would include records of hazards and their control methods, the monitoring of each critical control point, and notations of corrective actions taken. Each principle must be backed by sound scientific knowledge—for example, published studies on the time and temperatures needed to control specific foodborne pathogens.

U.S. Food and Drug Administration. HACCP: a state-of-the-art approach to food safety. FDA Backgrounder, August 1999. Available online at **http://www.fda.gov/opacom/backgrounders/haccp.html.**

foodborne illness.[2] Nonetheless, several programs are in place to allow the monitoring of outbreaks of foodborne illness.

In response to the Food Safety Initiative, a national computer network linking public health laboratories is in place.[7] This enables epidemiologists to quickly respond to serious and widespread food contamination problems. With this system, the distinctive DNA fingerprint of a pathogenic strain of a microorganism can be tracked. For example, if outbreaks of foodborne illness in Ohio and Minnesota are both caused by the same strain of an organism, epidemiologists know that the outbreaks were caused by the same food source. They can focus their search for the source of contamination on foods distributed to both locations. To confirm the source, the DNA fingerprint of organisms found in victims can be matched to the DNA fingerprint from a contaminated food source.

RESEARCH DISCOVERIES

Pasteurization: From Spoiled Wine to Safe Milk

In 1857, mutiny was occurring among sailors in Napoleon's navy because wine supplies were spoiling after only a few weeks at sea. Napoleon recognized this spoilage problem as a threat to his hopes for world conquest. He turned to Louis Pasteur for help. To study the problem, Pasteur traveled to a vineyard in Arbois, France, where spoilage was causing considerable economic losses for the wine industry. By examining the spoiled wine under a microscope, Pasteur was able to demonstrate the presence of certain strains of microorganisms. He suggested that spoilage could be prevented by heating the wine to a point that killed harmful microbes but that did not affect the flavor. This experimentation with heating wine revealed that the process worked as Pasteur had predicted and became the foundation for the modern treatment of bottled liquids to prevent their spoilage, a process known as pasteurization.

Pasteurization had a major public health impact, particularly when applied to the milk industry. Between 1880 and 1907, five hundred outbreaks of milk-borne diseases occurred in the United States. Milk from cows suffering from Bang's disease caused undulant fever in humans, a chronic debilitating disease characterized by intermittent fever. Also, milk contaminated after leaving the cow caused typhoid, scarlet fever, diphtheria, and tuberculosis. Pasteurization eliminated these pathogenic organisms. By 1900, pasteurized milk was commonly available, but raw milk was still more popular because the high-temperature pasteurization process used at the time left the milk with a cooked taste.

In 1906, Milton J. Rosenau, director of the U.S. Marine Hospital Service Hygienic Laboratory, established a low-temperature, slow pasteurization process (140°F for 20 minutes) that killed pathogens without changing the taste of the milk. This discovery eliminated the primary obstacle to public acceptance of pasteurized milk. By 1936, pasteurized, certified milk was the standard in most large cities, but over half of all milk consumed in the United States was still raw. More progress toward improving milk safety came in 1924 when the Public Health Service created a document to assist Alabama in developing a statewide milk sanitation program. This document ultimately evolved into the Grade A Milk Pasteurization Ordinance. This voluntary agreement established uniform sanitation standards for the interstate shipment of Grade A milk. It now serves as the basis of milk safety laws in all 50 states and Puerto Rico.[a]

The milk pasteurization process kills pathogenic bacteria and reduces the total number of microorganisms present, but it allows many microbes to survive. Milk is graded on the basis of bacterial count. A maximum of 20,000 bacteria per milliliter is allowed in Grade A milk. The multiplication of the bacteria that remain eventually causes the milk to spoil. To prevent rapid multiplication after pasteurization, the milk must be cooled immediately and remain refrigerated. In addition to killing microorganisms, the heat also destroys enzymes in the milk; the inactivation of lipase extends the shelf life of homogenized milk by preventing it from going rancid. The inactivation of another enzyme called phosphatase is used to gauge the adequacy of pasteurization. Lack of phosphatase activity indicates that the heat treatment has been adequate, but if phosphatase activity remains, it indicates that the milk was not treated adequately and may not be safe.

Today almost all milk sold in the United States is pasteurized, and the same techniques are used to prevent spoilage in many other foods. Thanks to the work of Louis Pasteur, we now enjoy the nutritional benefits of milk with minimal risk of contamination with disease-causing organisms.

Reference

[a] U.S. Public Health Service. 1924. United States Proposed Standard Milk Ordinance, Public Health Reports. Washington, D.C.: Public Health Service, November 7, 1924.

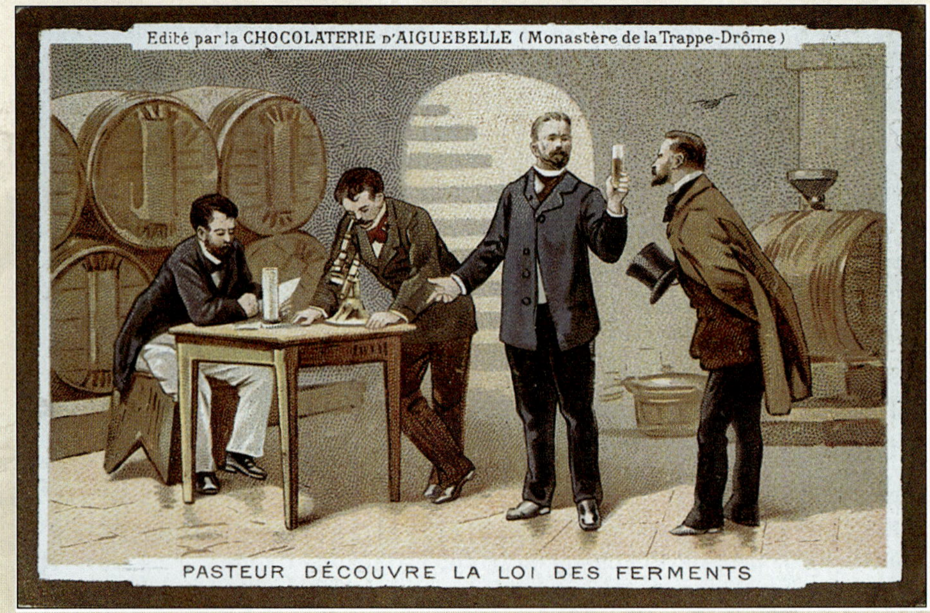

This painting depicts Louis Pasteur studying the souring of wine. *(© Jean-Loup Charmet/Science Photo Library/Photo Researchers, Inc.)*

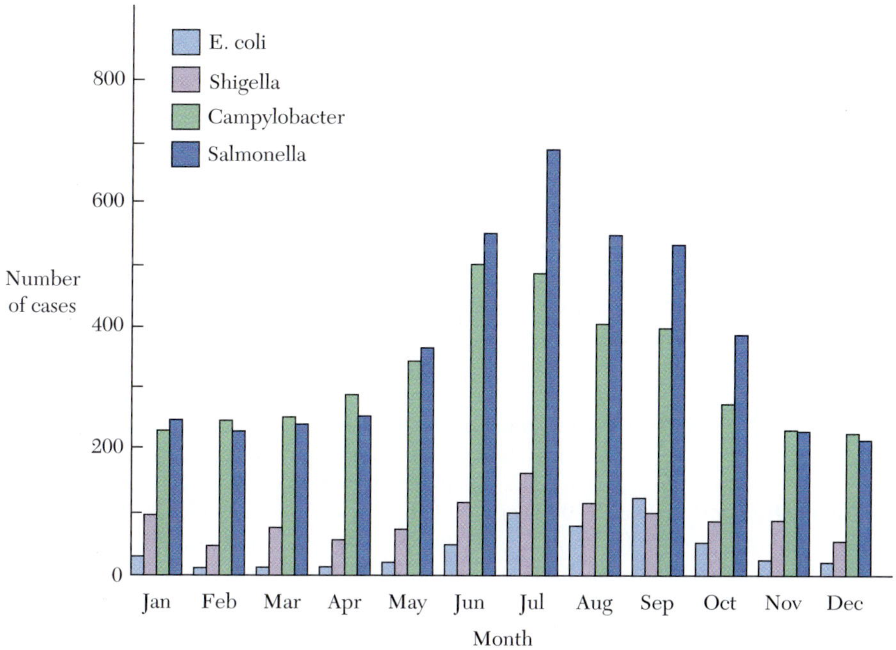

FIGURE 19.5 FoodNet information is used to monitor the incidence of foodborne diseases in the United States. This graph illustrates the number of cases of foodborne illness caused by *Campylobacter, Salmonella, Shigella,* and *E. coli* O157:H7 each month as reported to FoodNet in 1999. *(Foodborne Diseases Active Surveillance Network, CDC Emerging Infections Program.* FoodNet Surveillance Report for 1999. *November 2000. Available online at* www.cdc.gov/foodnet/annuals.htm.*)*

Another program, Foodborne Diseases Active Surveillance Network, or FoodNet, established in 1996, is a collaborative effort by the Centers for Disease Control and Prevention, the U.S. Department of Agriculture, the U.S. Food and Drug Administration, and selected state health departments. FoodNet is designed to actively monitor the incidence of the most common microbial foodborne diseases (Figure 19.5).[8] With a better understanding of the incidence of foodborne illness, systems to prevent outbreaks can be more effectively designed.

Foodborne Pathogens

Foodborne illness can be caused by the consumption of food contaminated with bacteria, viruses, molds, or parasites or with toxins produced by these organisms. Among all illnesses attributable to foodborne pathogens, 67% are caused by viruses, 30% by bacteria, and 3% by parasites (see *Research Discoveries:* "A New Worry: Prions and Mad Cow Disease").[2]

Most cases of microbial foodborne illness are relatively mild, involving short-term abdominal upset. However, symptoms can include life-threatening disorders. For example, foodborne illness can result in spontaneous abortion, hemolytic uremia syndrome (which can cause kidney failure and death), and long-lasting conditions like arthritis and Guillain-Barré syndrome, which is the most common cause of acute paralysis in adults and children. Young children, pregnant women, elderly persons, and individuals with compromised immune systems, such as those with AIDS and cancer patients receiving chemotherapy, are most susceptible to severe reactions. As many as 5000 people in the United States, mostly children and the elderly, die each year as a result of food-related illness.[2] Avoiding microbial foodborne illness requires knowledge of how contamination occurs and how to handle, store, and prepare food safely.

Web Menu: For information regarding foodborne pathogens and natural toxins, click on the FDA's Bad Bug Book at www.cfsan.fda.gov/.

Bacteria

Bacteria are microscopic single-celled organisms. Bacterial cells differ from animal and human cells in a number of ways. They are smaller—about one thousandth the volume of a typical animal cell—and they do not contain a separate

Bacteria Small single-celled organisms that have no nucleus or other membrane-bound organelles.

RESEARCH DISCOVERIES

A New Worry: Prions and Mad Cow Disease

Mad cow disease, or bovine spongiform encephalopathy (BSE), is a neurological disease that affects cattle. It was first diagnosed in England in 1986 and has now spread to other parts of Europe. Within 10 years of its appearance in cattle, a human form of the disease was identified. What causes this untreatable, incurable, and always fatal disease? How concerned should U.S. residents be?

Bovine Spongiform Encephalopathy BSE is a degenerative disease of the nervous system. Symptoms begin with weight loss and changes in temperament. Within weeks or months, the animal is dead. BSE belongs to a group of diseases called transmissible spongiform encephalopathies (TSEs). These include scrapie in sheep, chronic wasting syndrome in elk and deer, and kuru and Creutzfeldt-Jakob Disease (CJD) in humans. These diseases are characterized by a long incubation period, up to 20 years, during which there is no sign of infection. They cause changes that give the brain a spongelike appearance. Epidemiological research has determined that BSE originated from sheep that carried scrapie, which has been present in British sheep for about 200 years. It is believed to have moved into cattle when the remains of slaughtered diseased sheep began to be included in protein supplements that were fed to cattle. These supplements were banned in the UK in 1988 to prevent further spread of BSE. However, due to the long incubation period, the frequency of new cases did not start to decline until late 1993.

From Cows to Humans In March 1996, ten cases of the human disease CJD were reported in Britain. CJD is a degenerative disease of the nervous system that may begin with mood swings and numbness and always progresses to dementia and death.[a] There is a genetic form of CJD, but most cases occur sporadically around the world at a rate of about one case per million per year. The ten British cases resembled classical forms of CJD, but there were differences. This now-termed variant form of CJD (vCJD) affected younger patients (average age of 29 years, as opposed to 65 years), and the course of the disease was slower (a median of 14 months from first symptoms until death as opposed to 4.5 months). In addition, vCJD was linked to exposure to BSE, probably through food. Thus, within ten years, BSE had crossed the species barrier to humans. As of early December 2000, the CJD surveillance unit for the United Kingdom had reported 81 cases of vCJD.[b]

A New Infectious Agent? For many years the cause of TSEs was unknown. In 1972, Dr. Stanley Prusiner at the University of California began searching for the infectious agent that causes CJD. He was expecting to find a virus, but ten years later he had isolated a protein. He called this protein a prion, short for proteinaceous infectious particle. The scientific community did not readily accept his discovery because prions challenge a basic principle of biology—that every entity capable of reproducing itself must contain either DNA or RNA. A prion would have to carry, in a protein alone, information that could be transferred from one protein to another. Prusiner was awarded the 1997 Nobel Prize in Medicine for his work.

Evidence for the theory that TSEs are caused by prions continues to grow. It has been shown that the infectious agent in TSEs is not destroyed by conditions that would damage DNA and RNA. It is stable to freezing, drying, irradiation, and heat-

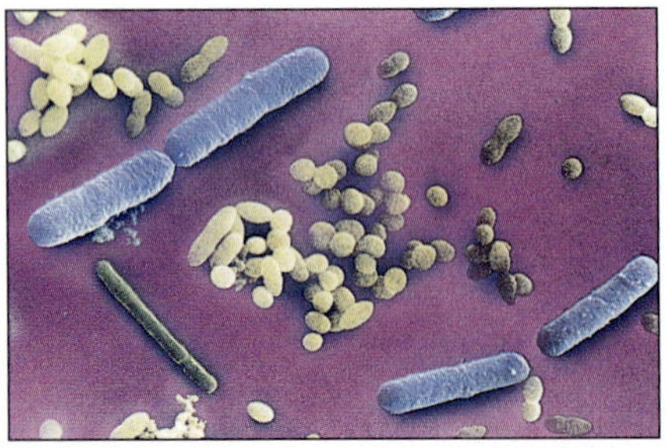

FIGURE 19.6 This color-enhanced micrograph of bacteria found in the human intestine illustrates the diversity of bacterial shapes. *(© David M. Phillips/Photo Researchers, Inc.)*

membrane-bound nucleus or organelles. They come in many different shapes, from spheres and rods to spirals (Figure 19.6). In order to grow and reproduce, bacteria require water and nutrients and specific environmental conditions. Most grow best in the temperature range between 40 and 140° Fahrenheit, but some can survive at temperatures below and above this range (Figure 19.7). Most require a neutral pH (around 7), but some can grow in more acidic or basic conditions. Some require oxygen (aerobic bacteria) while others grow in the absence of oxygen (anaerobic bacteria).

When the environmental conditions are optimal and water and nutrients are available, bacterial cells divide rapidly. Most can divide, forming two cells, in only about 20 to 30 minutes. In another 20 to 30 minutes, each daughter cell divides again. This exponential growth means that a food contaminated with only a few hundred bacteria could have over a hundred thousand bacteria in just 2 hours if left in conditions that favor growth.

Bacteria are ubiquitous in our environment. They are present in the soil, on our skin, on most surfaces in our homes, and in the food we eat. Most of the bacteria in our environment are harmless, and some are beneficial, but some are pathogenic, causing disease. They cause foodborne illness either by growing in the gastrointestinal tract or by producing toxins that are ingested in food.

ing at normal cooking temperatures and those used for pasteurization and sterilization. Also, animals with the disease do not produce antibodies against it as they would to a virus or bacterium.

The aberrant prions identified in TSEs can be thought of as the "evil twin" of a normal protein, called PrP (for prion protein), that is present in healthy nerve cells. The DNA sequence that codes for PrP was identified, and it was discovered that all mammals have the DNA that makes this protein. The difference between the normal protein and its deadly twin lies not in the amino acid sequence, but in the way the protein is folded. It is hypothesized that the abnormal protein reproduces by attaching itself to the normal PrP and converting it into the abnormal prion. The abnormal prion proteins are not degraded normally, so they accumulate, forming clumps called plaques. These plaques damage nerve tissue.

Because the changes in an aberrant prion are passed on to normal PrP proteins, tissue from a diseased animal can pass the disease on to other animals.[c] The most probable cause of vCJD is exposure to the BSE prion, most likely from consumption of a food product containing bovine central nervous system tissue. Thus far, meat and milk have not been demonstrated to transmit the disease and direct transmission from one human to another is thought to be unlikely.

Should We Be Concerned? As of this writing, not a single case of BSE or vCJD has been diagnosed in the United States. The reason for this is a combination of luck and vigilance by government agencies. In the 1950s the United States banned the import of sheep and goats from Britain. This ruling, which was imposed to prevent the spread of scrapie, most likely also prevented BSE from entering the country. In 1989, three years after BSE was identified in Britain, the USDA placed restrictions on the import of all ruminants from countries where BSE was known to exist. And in 1997, the USDA took further steps by restricting the import of ruminants and most ruminant products from all of Europe.[d] In addition to blocking the entry of products potentially carrying this disease, the United States has taken steps to block transmission. To prevent animal-to-animal transmission, mammalian proteins cannot be used in protein supplements for animal feeds. To prevent human-to-human exposure, blood donations are not accepted from individuals who spent substantial time in Europe in the 1980s. In addition, it has been recommended that vaccine manufacturers not use bovine products from countries where BSE has been reported. Because of these precautions, the risk of animals being exposed to BSE and humans contracting vCJD in the United States remains extremely low.

References

[a] U.S. Department of Agriculture Animal and Plant Health Inspection Service. Bovine Spongiform Encephalopathy. Available online at **http://www.aphis.usda.gov/oa/bse.** Accessed 2 Mar 2001.

[b] World Health Organization. Variant Creutzfeldt-Jakob Disease (vCJD) Fact Sheet. Revised December 2000. Available online at **http://www.who.int/inf-fs/en/fact180.html.** Accessed 4 Mar 2001.

[c] Mad cow and human prion disease. Neuro News, May 18, 1998. Available online at **http://neuroscience.about.com/science/neuroscience/library/weekly/aa051898.htm.** Accessed 5 Mar 2001.

[d] Bren, L. Trying to keep mad cow disease out of U.S. herds. FDA Consumer, March/April 2001. Available online at **http://www.fda.gov/fdac/features/2001/201_cow.html.** Accessed 6 Mar 2001.

Foodborne infection Illness produced by the ingestion of food containing microorganisms that can multiply inside the body and produce injurious effects.

Bacterial Foodborne Infection **Foodborne infection** is caused when a food containing pathogenic bacteria is ingested and the bacteria take up residence and reproduce in the gastrointestinal tract. These bacteria may also grow in other tissues or produce toxins within the body. Usually a large number of bacteria must be consumed to cause illness. Some common causes of bacterial infections include *Salmonella, Escherichia coli, Campylobacter jejuni, Listeria monocytogenes,* and *Vibrio vulnificus.* The most frequent sources of foodborne illness and the symptoms associated with them are included in Table 19.4.

Salmonella It is estimated that about 1.4 million people are infected with *Salmonella* each year in the United States.[2] Most of these people experience just diarrhea, but sometimes more serious infections can be fatal. *Salmonella* is found in animal and human feces and infects food through contaminated water or improper handling. *Salmonella* outbreaks can be caused by contaminated meat, meat products, dairy products, seafood, fresh vegetables, and cereal, but poultry and eggs are the most common food sources. Poultry products are often contaminated because poultry farms house large numbers of chickens in close proximity, allowing one infected chicken to infect thousands of others.

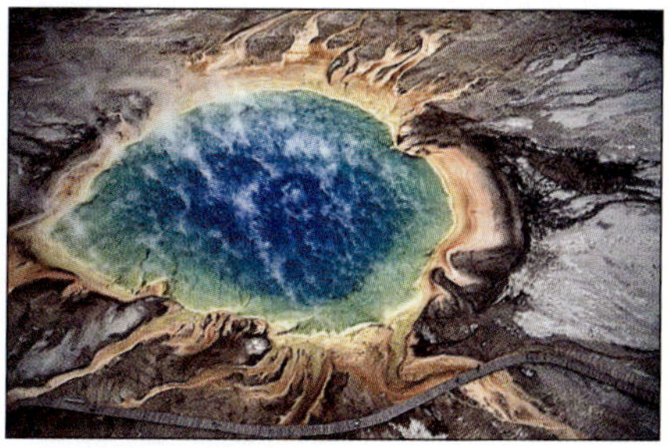

FIGURE 19.7 The colors seen in the hot springs in Yellowstone National Park are due to thermophilic bacteria that thrive at temperatures near the boiling point. The bacteria that grow in the hottest temperatures give the water a bright blue color. The yellow and brown colors are due to bacteria that grow in the cooler waters around the edge. *(© Douglas Faulkner/Photo Researchers, Inc.)*

TABLE 19.4 Examples of Organisms That Cause Foodborne Illness

Microbe	Sources	Symptoms	Onset	Duration
Bacteria				
Salmonella	Fecal contamination, raw or undercooked eggs and meat, especially poultry	Nausea, abdominal pain, diarrhea, headache, fever	6–48 hrs	1–2 days
Campylobacter jejuni	Unpasteurized milk, undercooked meat and poultry	Fever, headache, diarrhea, abdominal pain	2–5 days	1–2 wks
Listeria monocytogenes	Raw milk products, raw and undercooked poultry and meats, raw and smoked fish, produce	Fever, headache, stiff neck, chills, nausea, vomiting	Days to weeks	6 wks
Vibrio vulnificus	Raw seafood from contaminated water	Cramps, abdominal pain, weakness, watery diarrhea, fever, chills	15–24 hrs	2–4 days
Staphylococcus aureus	Human contamination from coughs and sneezes, eggs, meat, potato and macaroni salads	Severe nausea, vomiting, diarrhea	2–8 hrs	24–48 hrs
Escherichia coli O157:H7	Fecal contamination, undercooked ground beef	Abdominal pain, bloody diarrhea, kidney failure	5–48 hrs	3 days to 2 wks or longer
Clostridium perfringens	Fecal contamination, deep-dish casseroles	Fever, nausea, diarrhea, abdominal pain	8–22 hrs	6–24 hrs
Clostridium botulinum	Canned foods, deep-dish casseroles, honey	Lassitude, weakness, vertigo, dizziness, respiratory failure, paralysis	18–36 hrs	10 days or longer (must administer antitoxin)
Shigella	Fecal contamination of water or foods, especially salads such as chicken, tuna, shrimp, and potato	Diarrhea, abdominal pain, fever, vomiting	12–50 hrs	5–6 days
Yersinia enterocolitica	Pork, dairy products, and produce	Diarrhea, vomiting, fever, abdominal pain; often mistaken for appendicitis	24–48 hrs	Weeks
Viruses				
Norwalk virus	Fecal contamination of seafood	Diarrhea, nausea, vomiting	1–2 days	2–6 days
Hepatitis A virus	Human fecal contamination of food or water, raw shellfish	Jaundice, liver inflammation, fatigue, fever, nausea, anorexia, abdominal discomfort	10–50 days	1–2 wks to several months
Parasites				
Giardia lamblia	Fecal contamination of water and uncooked foods	Diarrhea, abdominal pain, gas, anorexia, nausea, vomiting	5–25 days	1–2 wks but may become chronic
Cryptosporidium parvum	Fecal contamination of food and water	Severe watery diarrhea	Hours	2–4 days but sometimes weeks
Trichinella spiralis	Undercooked pork, game meat	Muscle weakness, flu symptoms	Weeks	Months
Anisakis simplex	Raw fish	Severe abdominal pain	1 hr to 2 wks	3 wks
Toxoplasma gondii	Meat, primarily pork	Toxoplasmosis (can cause central nervous system disorders, flulike symptoms, and birth defects in children born of women exposed during pregnancy)	10–23 days	May become chronic carrier

U.S. Food and Drug Administration. Center for Food Safety and Nutrition. Foodborne Pathogenic Microorganisms and Natural Toxins Handbook: The "Bad Bug Book." Available online at **http./www.cfsan.fda.gov/~mow/intro.html.**

A new way to reduce infection is to spray chicks with beneficial bacteria (Figure 19.8). The FDA has approved the use of a spray that includes 29 types of living, nonpathogenic bacteria that are present in the normal gut of adult chickens.[9] The chicks ingest the bacteria when they preen their feathers and the bacteria colonize their digestive tracts, competing with the pathogens and reducing their growth. The spray prevents chicks from being infected with *Salmonella, Listeria,* and *E. coli* O157:H7.

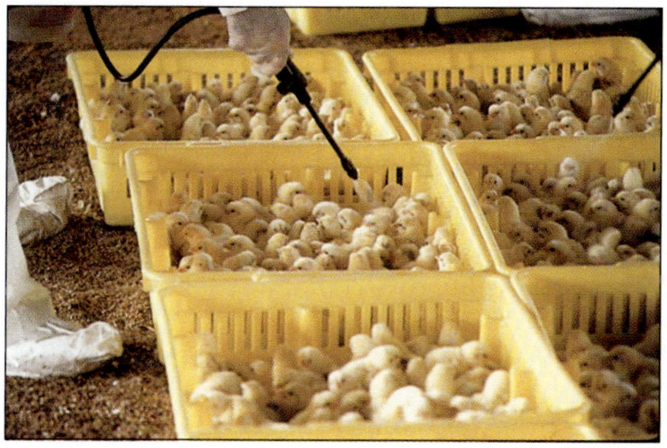

FIGURE 19.8 A shower of beneficial bacteria prevents chicks from being infected with bacteria that are pathogenic to humans. *(Agricultural Research Service/USDA)*

Even when food contaminated with *Salmonella* is brought into the kitchen, careful handling and cooking of the food can prevent the organisms from causing illness. Washing food can remove some of the bacteria, and washing hands, cutting boards, and utensils can prevent cross-contamination. If a contaminated food is stored in the refrigerator, the multiplication of the *Salmonella* will be slowed. If a contaminated food is left at room temperature, the *Salmonella* will multiply rapidly, and when the food is ingested, large numbers of bacteria will be ingested with it. *Salmonella* is killed by heat—so foods likely to be contaminated, such as poultry and eggs, should be cooked thoroughly.

E. coli *Escherichia coli* (*E. coli*) is a bacterium that inhabits the gastrointestinal tracts of humans and other animals. Some strains of *E. coli* are harmless, but others cause infection and produce harmful toxins. One strain of *E. coli,* found in water contaminated by human or animal feces, is the cause of "travelers' diarrhea" and infant diarrhea in developing nations. Another strain, *E. coli* O157:H7, discovered in 1982, causes abdominal pain, bloody diarrhea, and, in severe cases, kidney failure and even death, especially among children.

E. coli comes in contact with food through fecal contamination of water or unsanitary handling of food. *E. coli* can multiply slowly even at refrigerator temperatures, but if a contaminated food is thoroughly cooked to 160°F, both the bacteria and the toxin are destroyed.

Hamburger contaminated with *E. coli* O157:H7 is a risk because the bacteria are mixed throughout the meat during grinding. While the *E. coli* on the outside of the hamburger is quickly killed during cooking, those in the interior survive if the hamburger is not cooked thoroughly. This strain was responsible for the deaths of several children who consumed undercooked, contaminated hamburgers from a fast-food chain in 1993. Fruits and vegetables can also be a source of *E. coli* if they are contaminated by tainted water or manure fertilizers. In 1996, unpasteurized apple juice contaminated with *E. coli* O157:H7 caused illness in 66 people and the death of one child. Transmission of *E. coli* from cross-contamination is a particular risk at day-care centers if caregivers do not carefully wash their hands after diaper changes.

Campylobacter Two species of *Campylobacter, Campylobacter jejuni* and *Campylobacter coli,* also cause foodborne infection. *Campylobacter* is the most frequent cause of acute infectious diarrhea in developed countries.[6] Common sources are undercooked chicken, unpasteurized milk, and untreated water. This organism grows slowly in the cold and is killed by heat, so, as with *Salmonella,* thorough cooking and careful storage help prevent infection.

Listeria Another cause of bacterial infection is *Listeria monocytogenes.* Most cases of listerosis (*Listeria* infection) result in flulike symptoms, but in high-risk groups such as pregnant women, newborns, the elderly, and the ill, it can cause meningitis and serious blood infections and has one of the highest fatality rates of all foodborne illnesses. *Listeria* is a very resistant organism that survives at higher and lower temperatures than most bacteria; it can survive and grow at refrigerator temperatures. It is found in processed ready-to-eat foods such as hot dogs, lunch meats, and some dairy products. Because consumers consider ready-to-eat foods to be safe, they often do not handle them as carefully as raw foods. To prevent listerosis, ready-to-eat foods such as hot dogs and dry sausage should be reheated to steaming, unpasteurized milk and soft cheeses should be avoided, and utensils and cutting boards should be washed to prevent cross-contamination.

Vibrio *Vibrio vulnificus* infection usually causes gastrointestinal upset but can be deadly in vulnerable populations. The bacteria are common in mollusks such as oysters, clams, and mussels harvested from the Gulf of Mexico in the summer when the water is most likely to be contaminated with human fecal matter. Foods that pose a risk include raw and undercooked seafood.

Foodborne intoxication Illness caused by consuming a food containing a toxin.

Bacterial Foodborne Intoxication **Foodborne intoxication** is caused by the consumption of food that contains the toxins produced by microbes. Thus the symptoms of illness are caused by the toxin, not the organism itself. Unlike food infections, which are usually caused by ingesting large numbers of bacteria, intoxication can be caused by only a few microorganisms that have produced a toxin. Although the bacteria are fairly easy to kill, some food toxins are difficult to destroy.

Staphylococcus *Staphylococcus aureus* is a common cause of microbial foodborne intoxication. These bacteria live in the human nose and throat and can be transferred to food through the coughing or sneezing of food handlers. Foods that are common sources include cooked ham, salads, bakery products, and dairy products.

Spore A dormant stage of some bacteria that is resistant to heat but that can germinate and produce a new organism when environmental conditions are favorable.

Clostridium The bacterium *Clostridium perfringens* may cause illness by both infection and intoxication. It is found in soil and in the intestines of animals and humans. It thrives in anaerobic conditions and is difficult to kill because it forms heat-resistant **spores**—a stage of bacterial life that remains dormant until environmental conditions favor growth. *Clostridium perfringens* is often called the "cafeteria germ" because foods stored in large containers have anaerobic centers that provide an excellent growth environment. Sources include improperly prepared roast beef, turkey, pork, chicken, and ground beef.

Another strain of *Clostridium, Clostridium botulinum,* produces the deadliest bacterial food toxin. Although the bacteria themselves are not harmful, a toxin is produced as the spores begin to grow and develop. The toxin blocks nerve function, resulting in vomiting, abdominal pain, double vision, dizziness, and paralysis causing respiratory failure. If untreated, botulism poisoning is often fatal, but today modern detection methods and rapid administration of antitoxin have reduced mortality. Low-acid foods, such as potatoes or stew, that are held in anaerobic conditions provide optimal conditions for botulism spores to germinate. Canned foods, particularly improperly home-canned foods, can also be a source of botulism. Canned foods should be discarded if the can is bulging because this indicates the presence of gas produced by bacteria as they grow. Once formed, botulism toxin can be destroyed by boiling, but if the safety of a food is in question, it should be discarded; even a taste of botulism toxin can be deadly.

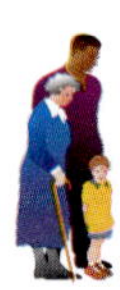

The most common form of botulism is infant botulism.[10] It was first described in 1976 and occurs when botulism spores are ingested and germinate in the intestinal tract. The bacteria produce toxin, some of which is absorbed into the bloodstream, causing symptoms such as generalized weakness, weakened neck muscles, flaccid paralysis, respiratory problems, and impaired sucking ability. Only infants are affected because in adults, well-established competing intestinal microflora prevent the spores from germinating. Because *botulism* spores can contaminate honey, it should never be fed to infants under one year of age.

Viruses

We usually think of **viruses** as the cause of respiratory infections, but they can also cause foodborne illnesses. Viruses are not cells. Rather, they are packets of DNA or RNA in a protein case. Viruses are extremely small, even compared to bacteria, and cannot be seen with a regular light microscope; an electron microscope must be used.

Viruses Minute particles not visible under an ordinary microscope that depend on cells for their metabolic and reproductive needs.

To reproduce, viruses must enter living cells. They can infect animal, plant, or bacterial cells. The type of cell that a virus can infect is specific to the type of virus, so a virus that infects human cells cannot enter and reproduce in plant cells. Although the viruses that cause human disease do not grow and reproduce in foods, they can contaminate foods and then infect the cells of the consumer. Viruses come in contact with food when it is contaminated with human or animal feces. Shellfish are notorious carriers of viral infections (Figure 19.9). Cooking can inactivate viruses in food, and cross-contamination can be prevented by washing and sterilizing food preparation surfaces and utensils.

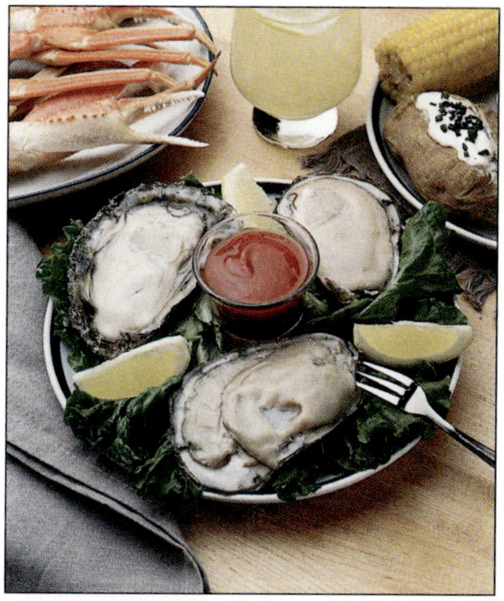

FIGURE 19.9 Consumption of raw shellfish such as oysters is a common cause of viral infections. *(© Larry Lefever/From Grant Heilman)*

Norwalk virus causes almost 60% of all foodborne illness due to pathogens.[2] It was named for an epidemic of gastrointestinal illness that occurred in an elementary school in Norwalk, Ohio, in 1969. The virus is transmitted by consumption of food or water contaminated with human or animal feces. Eating mollusks and other shellfish caught in contaminated water is a common cause.[11] Because cooking destroys Norwalk virus, uncooked foods such as raw shellfish and salads are the most common cause of foodborne illness from this virus.

Hepatitis A is a virus that causes an inflammation of the liver. It can be contracted from food contaminated by unsanitary handling or from eating raw or undercooked shellfish caught in sewage-contaminated waters. Hepatitis A infection can require a long recovery period and, in some cases, results in permanent liver damage. Individuals who have contracted the hepatitis A virus may remain carriers for years; it is also possible to carry the virus without having disease symptoms. In drinking water, hepatitis A is destroyed by chlorination. Cooking destroys the virus in food, and good sanitation can prevent its spread.

Fungi

Fungi A group of organisms that obtains nutrients by secreting enzymes that digest food outside their bodies. The breakdown products are then absorbed into their cells. They are important for the decomposition of organic material.

Molds Multicellular fungi that form a filamentous branching growth.

Mutagen A substance that causes changes in the molecular structure of DNA.

Carcinogen An agent that can cause cancer.

Fungi include **molds,** yeasts, and mushrooms. They are a food safety concern not because they infect people, but because of the toxins they produce. Many types of mushrooms contain dangerous toxins, and molds that grow on foods such as bread, cheese, and fruit produce toxins called mycotoxins. Aflatoxin is a mycotoxin that is one of the most potent **mutagens** and **carcinogens** known. The mold that produces aflatoxin grows on corn, nuts, flour, whole grains, rice, legumes, and peanut butter. These should be discarded if moldy. Another mold toxin that contaminates the grain rye is ergot. Ergot causes convulsions, delusions, and a burning sensation in the hands, and is a natural source of the hallucinogenic drug LSD. Today, modern milling removes the part of the grain that harbors this mold, so the disease ergotism is rare.

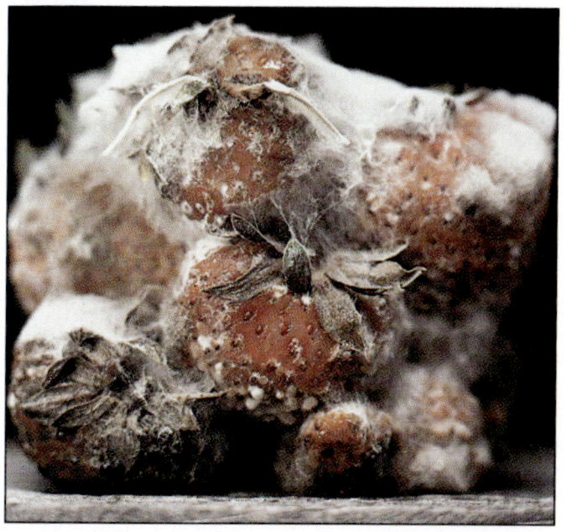

FIGURE 19.10 Mold can grow at refrigerator temperatures and it will grow on almost any food if it sits in the refrigerator long enough. *(© Charles D. Winters)*

Molds require nutrients, including water, to grow. They obtain the nutrients by digesting the food on which they grow and absorbing the resulting nutrients. The water is obtained from the food on which they are growing or from the atmosphere. They can live in a wide range of acidity (from pH 2 to 9) and can grow in concentrated salt and sugar solutions. They also thrive over a wide range of temperatures, including refrigerator temperature. Molds reproduce by forming spores that are dispersed by air, water, and living things. The spores of molds are all around us in the soil, in the air, and on surfaces. When a spore lands on an appropriate food supply, such as some leftovers in the refrigerator, it germinates and begins to grow (Figure 19.10). Cooking and freezing stop fungal growth but do not eliminate the mycotoxins that have already been produced. If a food is moldy, it should be discarded, the area where it was stored should be cleaned, and neighboring foods should be checked to see if they have also become contaminated with mold.

Parasites

Parasites Organisms that live at the expense of others without contributing to the survival of the host.

Many different types of **parasites** can enter the body through the diet. Some are microscopic single-celled animals while others are worms that can be seen with the naked eye. There are only a few that cause problems in the food supply in North America, but foodborne parasitic diseases are a major public health problem worldwide. For example, foodborne trematodes (flukes or flatworms) affect 40 million people, and more than 10% of the world's population is at risk of infection.[1] Most parasitic infections can be avoided by consuming fresh food that has been washed in clean water. Thorough cooking will kill parasites in food.

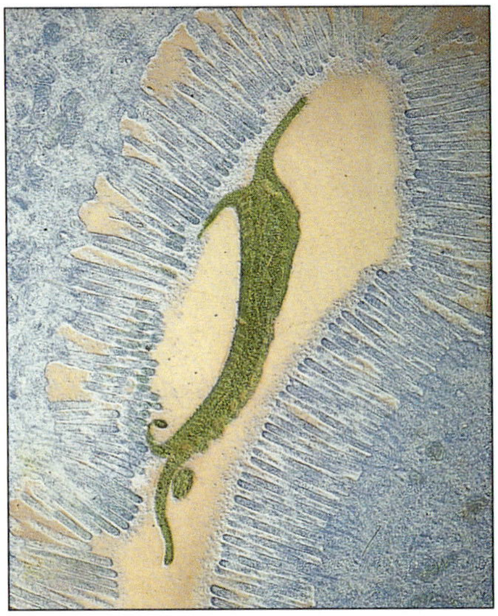

FIGURE 19.11 *Giardia lamblia* is a single-celled organism that infects the intestinal tract. In this electron micrograph, *Giardia* (shown in green) is seen attached to the microvilli of the human small intestine. *(© CNRI/Science Photo Library/Photo Researchers, Inc.)*

Giardia lamblia is a single-celled animal that can infect the gastrointestinal tract through water or food contaminated with human or animal feces (Figure 19.11). It is the most frequent nonbacterial cause of diarrhea.[12] Hikers who drink untreated water from streams contaminated with animal feces sometimes contract *Giardia,* and it is becoming a problem in day-care centers because cross-contamination can easily occur. It exists in two forms—one that grows in the gastrointestinal tract and one that is a resting form called a cyst that is passed from person to person. The cysts are resistant to chlorination and so can contaminate water supplies if they are not filtered. Boiling does destroy the cysts.

Another single-celled animal is *Cryptosporidium parvum.* It causes watery diarrhea and is commonly spread by contaminated water, but cases have also been reported from unpasteurized apple juice and homemade chicken salad.[13,14]

Trichinella spiralis is a parasite found in raw and undercooked pork, pork products, and game meats, particularly bear. Once ingested, these small, wormlike organisms find their way to the muscles, where they grow, causing flulike symptoms, muscle weakness, fever, and fluid retention. Trichinosis, the disease caused by *Trichinella* infection, can be prevented by thoroughly cooking meat to kill the parasite before it is ingested. Curing, smoking, canning, or freezing also destroys the parasites.

Fish are a common source of parasitic infections. Fish can carry the larvae (a wormlike stage of an organism's life cycle) of parasites such as roundworms, flatworms, flukes, and tapeworms. The larval form of the small roundworm *Anisakis simplex,* or herring worm, found in raw fish causes one such infection, called Anisakis disease.[12] Once consumed, these parasites invade the stomach and intestinal tract, causing severe abdominal pain. As the popularity of eating raw fish has increased, so has the incidence of parasitic infections from fish (Figure 19.12). However, the fresher the fish is when it is eviscerated, the less likely it is to cause this disease, because the larvae move from the fish's stomach to its flesh only after the fish dies.

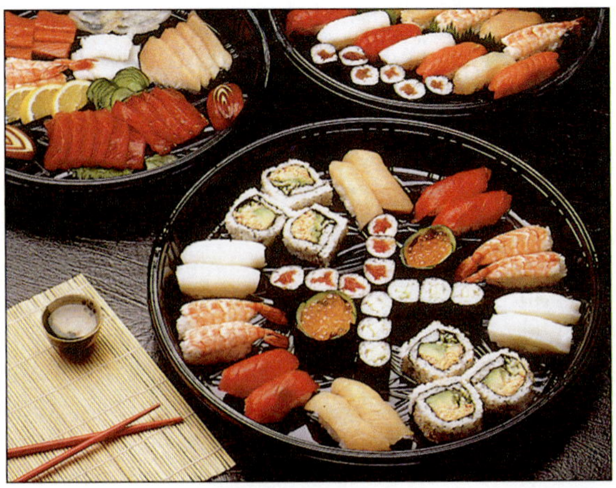

FIGURE 19.12 The incidence of parasitic infections has increased with the popularity of raw fish, such as this sushi. *(R. Pleasant/FPG International)*

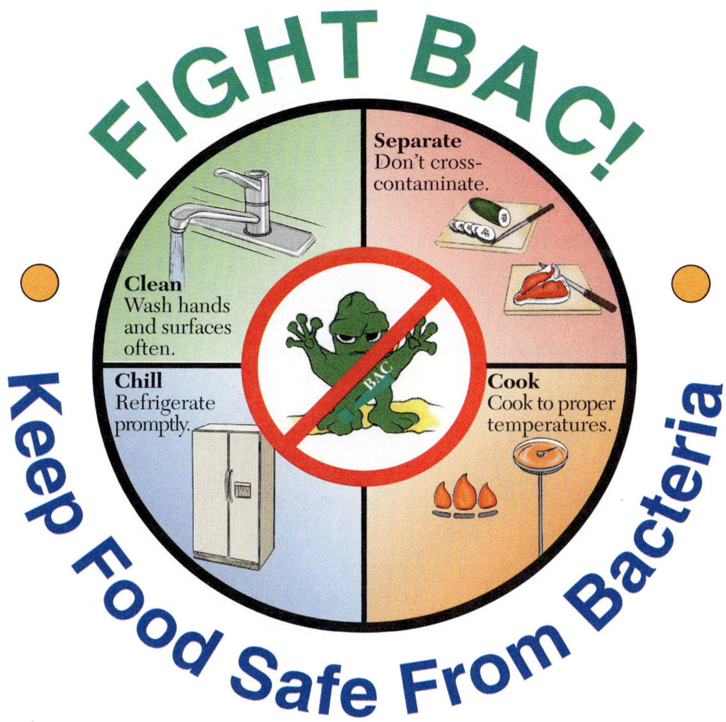
FIGHT BAC!
Separate
Don't cross-contaminate.
Clean
Wash hands and surfaces often.
Chill
Refrigerate promptly.
Cook
Cook to proper temperatures.
BAC
Keep Food Safe From Bacteria

FIGURE 19.13 The Fight Bac! educational campaign recommends that consumers follow four steps—clean, separate, cook, and chill—to prevent foodborne illness.

Reducing Risks

Despite the variety of organisms that can cause foodborne illness, most cases can be avoided if food is handled properly. To help consumers prevent microbial foodborne illness, the Partnership for Food Safety Education has launched an educational campaign called Fight Bac! (Figure 19.13). Just as manufacturers are asked to identify critical control points in food handling at which contamination can be prevented and monitored, consumers can take a similar approach in selecting, storing, preparing, and serving food and leftovers (Table 19.5).

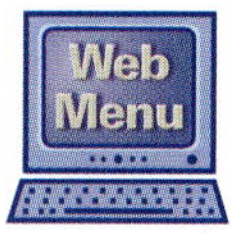

For steps to prevent foodborne illness, go to the Fight Bac! Web site at www.fightbac.org/.

Selecting Safe Foods The first critical control point in preventing foodborne illness is the selection of safe foods at the store to reduce the contaminants that are brought into the home. Food should come from reputable vendors who are known to purchase their stocks with safety in mind. Foods should appear fresh; meat and fish should not be gray or brown. Frozen fish should be in sealed packages. Frozen foods should not contain frost or ice crystals, which may indicate that the product has been stored for a long time or that the food has been thawed and refrozen. Thawing allows food to reach temperatures at which bacteria may grow. Items stored low in the freezer are more likely to remain at a constant temperature.

Food packaging should be secure. Jars should be firmly closed, seals should not be broken, and cans should not be rusty, dented, or bulging. Most packaged products are dated as either "sell by" or "use by." A "sell by" date indicates when the grocery store should take the product off the shelf. A "use by" date indicates the date by which the product should be consumed. Outdated products should not be purchased and store managers should be notified if they are on the shelves. Although dates are helpful, they do not ensure food safety; one food may be safe and wholesome after the expiration date while another, if it has not been handled properly, may be spoiled before it reaches its expiration date. Foods that are discolored or smell contaminated and those in damaged packages should not be purchased or consumed. Generally, grocery stores encourage customers to return damaged or tainted products.

TABLE 19.5 Critical Consumer Control Points

Food choice

- Avoid jars that are open or have broken seals.
- Avoid rusted, dented, or bulging cans.
- Check product expiration dates.
- Select frozen foods from below the frost line in the freezer.

Food storage

- Refrigerate or freeze cold foods immediately.
- Discard food that has been in the refrigerator for longer than is safe.

Sanitation

- Wash hands, cooking utensils, and surfaces with warm soapy water before each food preparation step.
- Wash food preparation items before using for food service.

Cooking

- Use a meat thermometer.
- Thorough cooking destroys most bacteria, toxins, viruses, and parasites (see temperature recommendations).

Refrigeration

- Thaw food in the refrigerator.
- Refrigerate cooked food immediately after service.

Reheating

- Thorough reheating to 165°F will destroy microorganisms that have recontaminated cooked foods and toxins that have been produced.

When in doubt, throw it out.

Safe Food Storage Storage is another critical control point in the home. Proper storage both before and after cooking can reduce the risk of foodborne illness. Consumers need to pay attention to storage as soon as the food leaves the grocery store. Cold foods, which should be selected last when shopping, should be refrigerated or frozen as quickly as possible. Cold foods should be kept cold, at 40°F or less, and hot foods should be kept hot, at greater than 140°F. The goal is to prevent foods from sitting for long periods at temperatures that favor bacterial growth (Figure 19.14). Refrigerator temperature should be set between 38 and 40°F and freezers at 0°F. Produce should be stored in the refrigerator. Fresh meat, poultry, and fish should be frozen immediately if it will not be used within a day or two. Processed meats such as hot dogs and bologna must also be kept refrigerated but can be kept longer than fresh meat (Table 19.6).

Preparing and Serving Food Safely The next critical control point is preparation. Even when microorganisms come into the home, most foodborne illness can be prevented by proper kitchen precautions. A clean kitchen is essential for safe food preparation. Hands, countertops, cutting boards, and utensils should be washed with warm soapy water before each food preparation step. Food should be thawed in the refrigerator, in the microwave oven, or under running water—not at room temperature. Foods that are going to be cooked should not be prepared on the same surfaces as foods that are eaten raw; uncooked meats and poultry may contain microbes that can contaminate any food that touches it or its juices. For example, if a raw chicken contaminated with *Salmonella* is cut up on a cutting board that is then used unwashed to chop vegetables for a salad, the vegetables will become contaminated with the bacteria. When the chicken is cooked, the *Salmonella* will be killed, but the contaminated vegetables are not cooked, so the

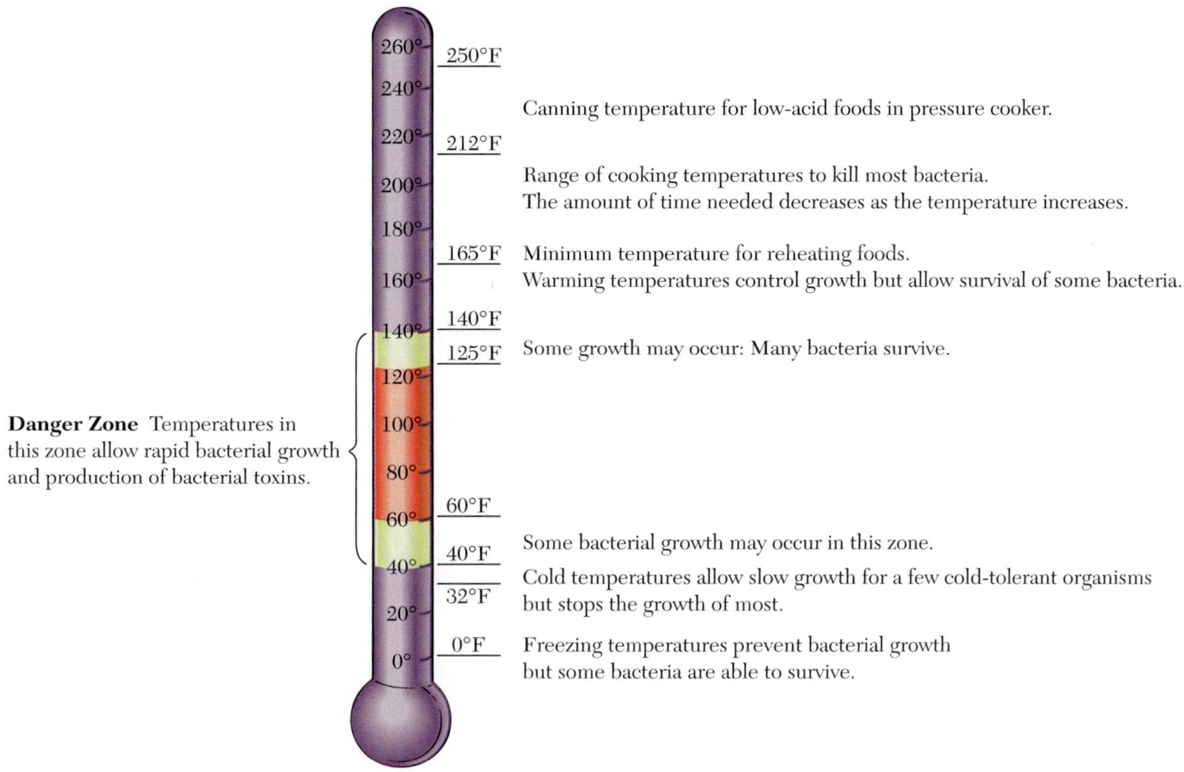

FIGURE 19.14 The effect of temperature on bacterial growth.

bacteria can grow and cause foodborne illness. Cutting boards used to cut raw meat, poultry, or fish should be washed with soap and hot water and then sanitized with a mild bleach solution after each use.[15] Cross-contamination can also occur when uncooked foods containing live microbes come in contact with foods that have already been cooked. Therefore, cooked meat should never be returned to the same dish that held the raw meat, and sauces used to marinate uncooked foods should never be used as a sauce on cooked food. As a precaution, meat packaging in food stores is labeled with safe handling guidelines (Figure 19.15).

Making sure that food is thoroughly cooked is one of the most important control points in the home, because heat will destroy most harmful microorganisms.

TABLE 19.6 General Recommendations for Refrigerating Leftovers

Food Item	Keep Up To
Cooked vegetables	3–4 days
Cooked pasta	3–5 days
Cooked rice	1 week
Deli meats	5 days
Greens	1–2 days
Soup and stews	3–4 days
Stuffing	1–2 days
Meat	
Ham	3–4 days
Cooked beef, poultry, pork, and fish	3–4 days
Cooked seafood	2 days
Meat in gravy	1–2 days

American Dietetic Association. Available online at **http://www.eatright.org.**

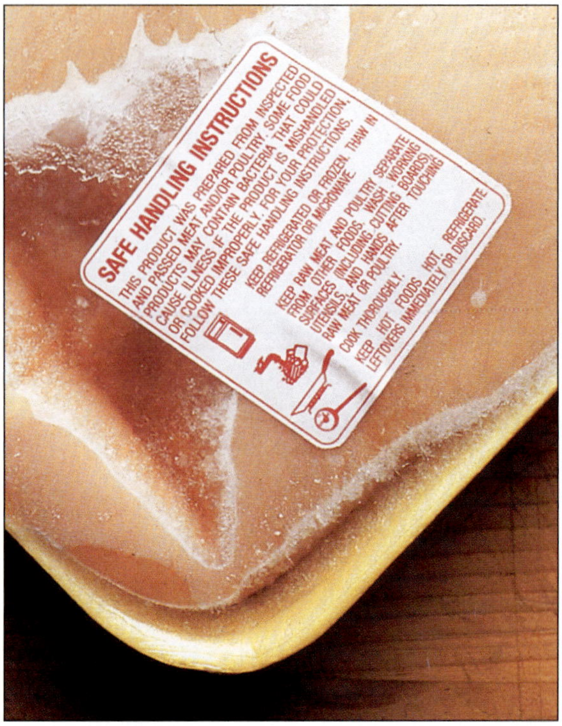
SAFE HANDLING INSTRUCTIONS
THIS PRODUCT WAS PREPARED FROM INSPECTED AND PASSED MEAT AND/OR POULTRY. SOME FOOD PRODUCTS MAY CONTAIN BACTERIA THAT COULD CAUSE ILLNESS IF THE PRODUCT IS MISHANDLED OR COOKED IMPROPERLY. FOR YOUR PROTECTION, FOLLOW THESE SAFE HANDLING INSTRUCTIONS.
KEEP REFRIGERATED OR FROZEN. THAW IN REFRIGERATOR OR MICROWAVE.
KEEP RAW MEAT AND POULTRY SEPARATE FROM OTHER FOODS. WASH WORKING SURFACES (INCLUDING CUTTING BOARDS), UTENSILS, AND HANDS AFTER TOUCHING RAW MEAT OR POULTRY.
COOK THOROUGHLY.
KEEP HOT FOODS HOT. REFRIGERATE LEFTOVERS IMMEDIATELY OR DISCARD.

FIGURE 19.15 Meat carries labels offering safe handling guidelines. *(Dennis Drenner)*

A meat thermometer should be used because color is not a good indicator of safety. Red meat and fish should be cooked to an internal temperature of 160°F and poultry to 180°F. Shellfish should be cooked to an internal temperature of 145°C for 15 seconds. Eggs should not be eaten raw, since *Salmonella* can contaminate the inside of the shell; they should be boiled for 7 minutes, poached for 5 minutes, or fried for 3 minutes on a side. Thorough cooking may be a problem when using a microwave oven, because these appliances do not cook evenly and therefore bacteria may survive in cold pockets in the food (Table 19.7).

TABLE 19.7 Safe Cooking Temperatures

Food Item	Internal Temperature (°F)
Beef, veal, lamb	
Ground products	160
Nonground products	
Medium-rare	145
Medium	160
Well done	170
Poultry	
Ground products	165
Whole bird	180
Breasts and boneless roasts	170
Thighs, wings, drumsticks	180
Duck	180
Stuffing	165
Pork	
Noncured products	
Medium	160
Well done	170
Ham	160
Eggs	160
Leftovers	165

American Dietetic Association. Available online at **http://www.eatright org/.**

Safe Handling of Leftovers Cooked food can be recontaminated, so it must be refrigerated as soon as possible after serving and should not be left out to cool at room temperature. The best temperatures for bacterial growth are the temperatures at which food usually sets between service and storage. Large portions of food should be divided before refrigeration so they will cool quickly and not remain at bacterial growth temperatures for long periods in the refrigerator. When refrigerated leftovers are reheated, they should be heated thoroughly enough to destroy any bacteria that may have grown in them. The National Restaurant Association recommends reheating foods to an internal temperature of 165°F.

Food Safety Away from Home Safe food practices at home will not prevent foodborne illness when eating away from home. Although most of the foodborne illness in the United States is caused by food prepared in homes, an outbreak in a commercial or institutional establishment usually involves more people at a time and is more likely to be reported. Food in retail establishments has many opportunities to be contaminated because of the large volume of food that is handled and the large number of people involved in its preparation. Consumers should choose restaurants with food safety in mind. Restaurants should be clean, and cooked foods should be served hot. Cafeteria steam tables should be kept hot enough that the water is steaming. Cold foods such as salad bar items should be held refrigerated or on ice. The safest salad bar items, as well as the most nutritious, are fresh fruits and vegetables and dried fruits. However, recent incidents of foodborne illness from salad bar fruit have made even these suspect. For example, an outbreak of foodborne illness was caused by cantaloupe that was contaminated with *Salmonella* in the field and cut up before the outer skin was washed. The bacteria were carried onto the fruit, and when it was left at room temperature, enough bacteria grew to cause illness.

Even when a restaurant uses extreme care in food preparation, customers can be a source of contamination. Because customers serve themselves at salad bars, cross-contamination from one customer to another is a risk. Salad and dessert bars in restaurants are usually equipped with "sneeze guards"—clear plastic shields placed above the food to prevent contamination from coughs and sneezes (Figure 19.16). Customers are also asked to use a clean plate if they go back for second helpings.

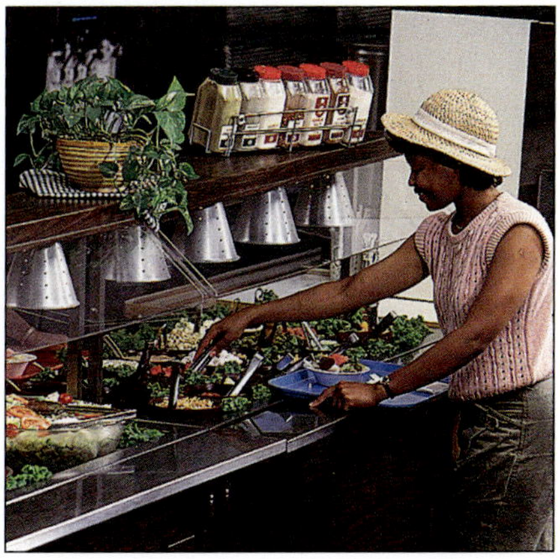

FIGURE 19.16 Clear plastic shields, or "sneeze guards," above salad bars prevent customers from contaminating food with microorganisms transmitted by coughs and sneezes. *(© Charles Gupton/Tony Stone Images)*

Picnics and other large events where food is served provide a prime opportunity for microbes to flourish because food is often left at room temperature or in the sun for hours before it is consumed. Foods that last well without refrigeration, such as fresh fruits and vegetables, breads, and crackers, should be selected for these occasions.

Any food that is transported should be kept cold. Lunches should be transported to and from work or school in a cooler or an insulated bag. They should be refrigerated upon arrival or kept cold with ice packs. Most foods that are brought home from work or school uneaten should be thrown out and not saved for another day.

CHEMICAL CONTAMINANTS IN FOOD

The safety of the food supply can be affected by compounds used in agricultural production and by industrial wastes that contaminate the environment. These chemical contaminants are taken up by plants and consumed by small animals. These plants and animals are then eaten by larger animals, which are in turn eaten by still larger animals, thus passing the contaminants up through the food chain to all levels of the food supply. Contaminants are found in the greatest

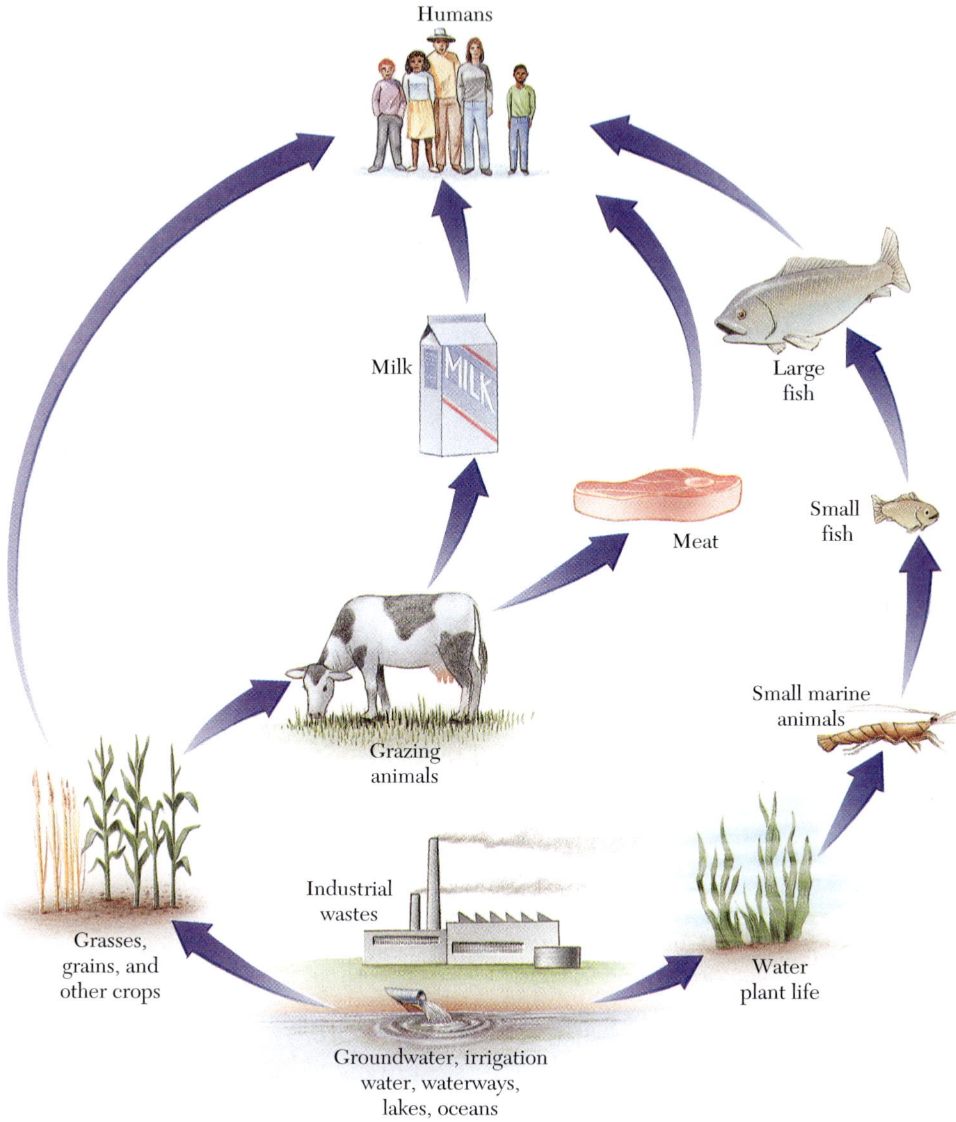

FIGURE 19.17 Industrial pollutants that contaminate the water supply become more and more concentrated as they are passed up the food chain from plants to small animals to larger animals. The largest organisms, such as cattle and large fish, may have high levels of these contaminants in their adipose tissue.

concentration in foods of animal origin because animals are at the top of the food chain (Figure 19.17).

Pesticides

Pesticides are used to prevent plant diseases and insect infestations. They are applied to crops growing in the fields as well as after harvesting to prevent spoilage and extend the shelf life of produce. Crops grown using pesticides generally produce higher yields and look more appealing because insect damage is limited. Some residues of these chemicals remain on the food when it arrives at our tables, and pesticides may travel from the fields into water supplies, soil, and other parts of the environment. For instance, pesticides are found not only on treated produce but also in meat, poultry, fish, dairy products, and lard, and in groundwater.[16]

The potential risks of pesticides to consumers depend on the type and amount consumed as well as who consumes it. Small amounts of pesticides are unlikely to cause an immediate reaction but could cause health problems if routinely consumed over a long period.

Regulation of Pesticides The types of pesticides that can be used on food crops and the residual amounts that can remain when foods reach consumers are regulated. New pesticides are now so carefully tested for safety that years may pass between the time they are developed and when they can be used. The Environmental Protection Agency (EPA) must approve and register pesticides that are used in food production and establish allowable limits, or **tolerances.** The FDA and USDA then monitor pesticide levels in foods. To establish tolerances for pesticides, the risk of toxicity is weighed against the benefit that the pesticide provides. The risks are based on the known incidence of toxicity and the predicted exposure that consumers will have to the toxin. Tolerance levels are then set at the minimum amount of the pesticide needed to be effective; these levels are often several hundred times lower than the level found to cause reactions in test animals.[17]

Tolerances The maximum amount of pesticide residues that may legally remain in food; set by the EPA.

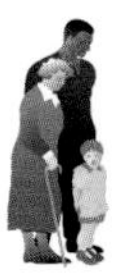

In the past, tolerance levels were set based on body weights and food consumption patterns of adults. However, pesticides may be more of a danger to children than adults. Children are smaller, so the same amount of pesticide provides a larger dose per unit of body weight. And, children often have less varied diets than adults. For example, a two-year-old who drinks nothing but apple juice for weeks at a time would be consuming more than the predicted amount of pesticide residue. The 1996 Food Quality Protection Act requires the EPA to determine that a tolerance level of a pesticide is safe for children as well as adults.[18]

In general, the amounts of pesticides to which people are exposed through foods are small. According to the FDA's pesticide residue monitoring program, the levels of pesticides found in the American food supply are below tolerances. Less than 2% of the food samples studied had residues of pesticides that either exceeded tolerance levels or contained pesticides for which there is no legal tolerance, and the overall incidence was comparable for domestic and imported foods.[19] However, because of country-to-country differences in crops, pests, growing conditions, and pesticide regulations, imported foods may contain pesticides that are not used in the United States and for which the EPA has not set tolerance levels. Nevertheless, a report by the National Research Council in 1996 concluded that the majority of synthetic chemicals, including pesticides, in the diet are present at levels below which any significant adverse biological effect is likely and that they are unlikely to pose a cancer risk.[20] Although special-interest groups concerned with overuse of pesticides disagree with this conclusion,[21] the fact remains that repeated consumption of large doses of any one pesticide is unlikely because most people consume a variety of foods produced in many different locations.

Reducing Exposure In addition to developing safer, more effective chemical pesticides, agricultural production methods are being implemented to make low-pesticide and pesticide-free produce available to the consumer.

Exploiting Natural Toxins Integrated pest management (IPM) is a method of agricultural pest control that reduces pesticide usage by combining chemical and nonchemical techniques. IPM emphasizes the use of natural toxins and more effective pesticide application.

Many toxins occur naturally in plants. These function as natural pesticides that offer protection from bacteria, molds, and insect pests. These naturally pest-resistant crops are advantageous because they thrive without the use of expensive added pesticides. Plants high in natural pesticides can be produced through breeding programs or genetic modification (see Chapter 20). The natural toxins in plants can also be isolated and applied to crops like synthetic pesticides.

Making Decisions
Herbal Tea: Healthy or Hazardous?

For thousands of years, herbs have been used medicinally, and today herbal teas are consumed for their aroma and flavor as well. Although herbal teas are thought to be a healthy alternative to caffeinated beverages, little is really known about the safety of some of the herbs.

Many herbal teas on the market have ingredient lists that look like a garden tour: lemon grass, rosehips, spearmint, raspberry leaves, chamomile flowers. Most of these and other ingredients used in commercially prepared teas have been used for centuries with relative safety. However, problems arise when people consume herbal teas in excessive amounts or concoct their own brews. For example, comfrey tea can cause liver disease. Comfrey roots and leaves contain chemicals that have been found to cause cancer in rats. Lobelia, also known as Indian tobacco, was used in the 19th century to treat asthma, but, when used in large amounts, it can cause vomiting, breathing problems, convulsions, coma, and death. Sassafras tea, which was once used as a stimulant, blood thinner, and reputed cure for rheumatism and syphilis, causes cancer in rats. Oil of sassafras and safrole from sassafras root bark were taken out of root beer over 30 years ago, and today sassafras bark is banned from all food products. There have been reports of illness caused by tea made from the leaves of foxglove plant, from which the heart drug digitalis is derived. Abnormal menstrual bleeding was reported in a woman consuming a homemade brew that included, among other ingredients, tonka beans, melilot, and woodruff. These contain coumarin, which may act as an anticoagulant. Herbal teas containing plant-derived laxatives such as senna, aloe, cascara, buckthorn, rhubarb root, and castor oil are marketed as "dieter's teas." Senna, cascara, and castor oil are found in over-the-counter laxatives and are regulated as drugs. When consumed in excessive amounts, plant-derived laxatives can cause stomach cramps, fainting, vomiting, diarrhea, and even death.[a]

Currently, the regulation of herbal teas depends on the types of claims made about their use. If a tea claims to prevent or cure a disease, the FDA regulates it as a drug, and it must be approved as safe and effective for its intended use. For example, teas claiming to help with smoking cessation, weight loss, constipation, or sore throats are considered drugs. Herbal teas claiming less dramatic effects, such as calming, relaxing, and soothing, are classified as dietary supplements by the FDA and therefore regulated as foods rather than drugs or additives.

Concern about the effects of herbs has prompted the FDA to collect samples of herbal products to determine health hazards and assess unsubstantiated claims. In Canada, an advisory committee was established to review information about herbs and make recommendations. The result was a ban on more than 50 herbs and warning labels on five others that may cause problems during pregnancy. The herb industry itself has also initiated a program to evaluate 200 or so commercially available herbs that currently are not approved for use as food flavorings. Their evaluations include factors such as the use of the herb in other countries, chemical composition, pharmacological properties, reports of adverse reactions, and toxicity studies. Advice for herbal tea drinkers is to stick to commercial varieties, avoid steeping teas too long, and avoid consuming any one variety in excess.

Reference

[a] Kurtzweil, P. Dieter's brews make tea time a dangerous affair. FDA Consumer, July/August 1997; updated December 1997. Available online at **http://www.fda.gov/fdac/features/1997/597_tea.html.** Accessed 7 December 2000.

Web Menu: For information on standards that govern the production and marketing of organic foods, go to the USDA's National Organic Program at www.ams.usda.gov/nop/.

Organic food Food that is produced according to the production and handling standards established by the National Organic Program of the USDA. Food produced using synthetic pesticides and fertilizers, sewage sludge, genetically modified ingredients, and irradiation do not meet the definition of organic.

As with all chemical toxins, natural toxins move through the food supply. For example, a cow that has foraged on toxic plants can pass the toxin into her milk and poison the consumer of the milk. Abraham Lincoln's mother died from drinking milk from a cow that had eaten poisonous snakeroot plants. The potential for toxicity, however, depends on the dose of toxin consumed and the health of the consumer. Most natural toxins in the food supply are consumed in doses that pose little risk to the consumer. For instance, solanine, a neurotoxin found in the green layer under potato skins, is not toxic in amounts typically consumed. But consuming ten times the typical amount of potatoes could cause symptoms (see *Making Decisions:* "Herbal Tea: Healthy or Hazardous?").

Using Organic Techniques **Organic food** production is based on biological methods that avoid the use of synthetic pesticides, herbicides, or fertilizers. Consumer demand for these products has been increasing; sales for organic produce rose from \$78 million in 1980 to \$3.5 billion in 1996.[22] Some of this increase is due to the belief that organic foods are safer or superior in quality, taste, or nutrient content to conventionally grown foods; however, this is not necessarily the case.

The production methods used in organic farming may be more ecologically sound than the standard methods used today. They foster the cycling of resources

TABLE 19.8 Labeling of Organic Foods

Labeling Term	Meaning
100% organic	Contains (by weight or fluid volume, excluding water and salt) 100% organically produced raw or processed ingredients. May display USDA seal.
Organic	Contains (by weight or fluid volume excluding water and salt) not less than 95% organically produced raw or processed agricultural products. May display USDA seal.
Made with organic ingredients (specified ingredients or food groups)	Contains (by weight or fluid volume excluding water and salt) at least 70% organically produced ingredients.

and conserve biodiversity. Organic farming techniques reduce the exposure of farm workers to pesticides and decrease the quantity of pesticides introduced into the food supply and the environment. However, organic foods are not risk-free. Manure is often used for fertilizer. If the manure is not treated properly, it can increase the risks of microbial foodborne illness associated with the food, and runoff can pollute lakes and streams. And irrigation water, rain, or a variety of other sources can introduce traces of synthetic pesticides and other agricultural chemicals not approved for organic use into organically-grown foods. The threshold for pesticide residues in organic foods is set at 5% of the EPA's pesticide-residue tolerance.[23] In addition, they are usually more expensive and available in less variety than conventionally grown foods.

Recently the USDA's National Organic Program developed standards for organic foods.[23] These national standards define both substances approved for use and those prohibited from use in organic food production and handling. For example, an organic food may not include ingredients that are treated with irradiation, produced by genetic modification, or grown using sewage sludge or industrially synthesized fertilizers and pesticides. Certain natural pesticides and other manufactured agents are permitted. Farming and processing operations that produce and process organic foods must be certified by the USDA as meeting regulations for organic production. The National Organic Program has also established standards for the labeling of products that are organically produced or contain organically produced ingredients (Table 19.8). Products meeting the definition of "100% organic" or "organic" may display the USDA "Organic" seal shown in Figure 19.18.

FIGURE 19.18 The USDA organic seal can appear on the label of raw or processed agricultural products that meet the definition of "100% organic" or "organic."

Web Menu: For more information on environmental contaminants, go to the EPA at www.epa.gov/ or the World Health Organization health topics at www.who.int and click on environment.

Environmental Contaminants

Many chemicals that contaminate the environment find their way into our food supply. Fish are a major source of environmental contaminants because they accumulate contaminants when the waters where they live and feed are polluted. Pollutants in water can also contaminate crops and move up the food chain to contaminate other animal products, such as milk and meat.

Dioxins The term **"dioxins"** refers to a group of environmental contaminants that share similar chemical structures. There are three general categories of dioxins—chlorinated dibenzodioxins (CDDs), chlorinated dibenzofurans (CDFs), and polychlorinated biphenyls (PCBs). Sometimes the term "dioxin" is used specifically to refer to the most well-known and best-studied of these compounds, 2,3,7,8,tetrachlorinated dibenzo-p-dioxin. CDDs and CDFs are produced in nature as a result of volcanic eruptions and forest fires, and as a

Dioxins A group of environmental contaminants that are produced naturally and as industrial by-products. Repeated ingestion causes them to accumulate in biological tissues over time, damages body systems, and contributes to the development of cancer. The term "dioxin" is often used to refer to the most well-known and well-studied of these compounds.

by-product of some manufacturing processes, including smelting, bleaching of paper pulp, manufacturing of some chemicals and pesticides, and waste incineration. PCBs are man-made but are no longer produced in the United States. They were used extensively in the manufacture of electrical capacitors and transformers.

Dioxins are found in air, water, soil, and food and are an environmental concern because they break down so slowly that some of the dioxins from past pollution still contaminate the environment and will for many years. For example, the manufacture of PCBs stopped in the United States in 1977. But because PCBs in runoff from manufacturing plants contaminated water, they are still found in the environment and in fish. PCBs accumulate in adipose tissue and become more concentrated as they move up the food chain; humans who consume large quantities of contaminated fish accumulate PCBs in their adipose tissue.

Long-term exposure to dioxins may damage the human immune, endocrine, and reproductive systems as well as contribute to the development of cancer. Dioxins are a particular problem for mothers and infants. Prenatal exposure can damage the nervous system and cause learning deficits in children.[24,25] Because PCBs are secreted in breast milk, the American Academy of Pediatrics recommends that although the benefits of breast-feeding outweigh the risks of low levels of PCBs, in areas where high exposures of PCBs have occurred breast-feeding women should check with their local health department for recommendations on fish consumption.[26]

Overall, the best strategy for lowering the risk presented by dioxins is to choose a diet of lean fish, meat, poultry, and reduced-fat dairy products and to increase consumption of fruits, vegetables, and grain products. These strategies help lower the intake of saturated fats as well as reduce the risk of exposure to dioxins.[27]

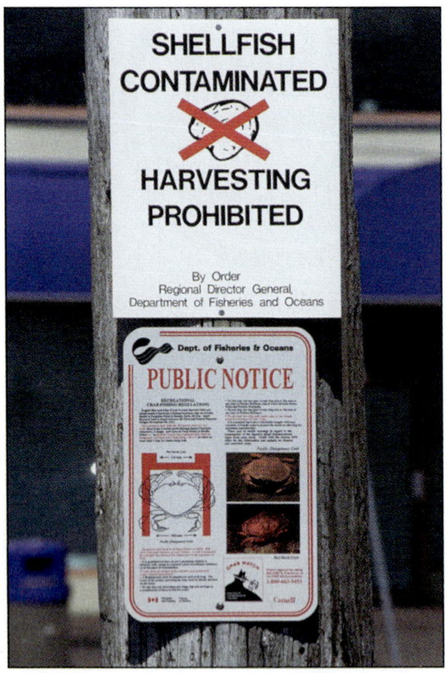
SHELLFISH
CONTAMINATED
HARVESTING
PROHIBITED
By Order
Regional Director General,
Department of Fisheries and Oceans
Dept. of Fisheries & Oceans
PUBLIC NOTICE

FIGURE 19.19 It is unsafe to consume shellfish from contaminated waters. *(Corbis/Paul A. Souders)*

Toxic Metals and Other Contaminants Toxic metals such as cadmium, lead, arsenic, and mercury as well as other contaminants such as the radioactive substance strontium-90 have also found their way into our waterways and consequently into fish and shellfish. Cadmium and lead can interfere with the absorption of other minerals and can have a direct toxic effect: Cadmium can cause kidney damage and lead is a particular problem for children because it can impair brain development (see Chapter 16). Arsenic is believed to contribute to cancer development, and mercury, which has been found in large fish, particularly swordfish and shark, damages nerve cells.[28] Large fish at the top of the food chain are more likely to contain high levels of industrial contaminants, but shellfish also accumulate contaminants because they feed by passing large volumes of water through their bodies (Figure 19.19). Choosing farm-raised fish is one way to reduce exposure to toxins that contaminate our water.

PAHs and Heterocylic Amines **Polycyclic aromatic hydrocarbons (PAHs)** are a class of organic compound that contaminates foods and the environment. PAHs pollute air, water, and soil due to wood-burning stoves, diesel exhaust, and oil-burning heaters and boilers. Because they are produced during roasting, grilling, smoking, and frying, they contaminate foods such as meat, meat products, fish, tea, coffee, and some kinds of cheese and cereal. As early as 1775, PAH-containing soot was linked to cancer in chimney sweeps. Several of the PAHs found in food have been shown to cause cancer in laboratory animals. Grilled meats are high in PAHs because they are formed when fat drips onto the flame below. Therefore, eating grilled fatty meat every day is not recommended, but occasional grilling, particularly with low-fat meat,

Polycyclic aromatic hydrocarbons (PAHs) A class of mutagenic substances produced during cooking when there is incomplete combustion of organic materials—such as when fat drips on a grill.

presents little risk. Foods that are cooked with the heat source at the top are low in PAHs.

Broiled and pan-fried meats contain another potential hazard—**heterocyclic amines (HAs),** such as benzopyrene. HAs are formed from the burning of amino acids and other substances in meats. Well-done meat and meat cooked using hotter temperatures contain greater amounts. The cooking temperatures recommended by the FDA are designed to prevent microbial foodborne illness and minimize the production of HAs. Levels of HAs can be reduced by precooking meat in the microwave and discarding the juice.

Heterocyclic amines (HAs) A class of mutagenic substances produced when there is incomplete combustion of amino acids during the cooking of meats—such as when meat is charred.

Choosing Wisely to Reduce Risks

Even though individual consumers cannot detect chemicals in food, care in selection and preparation of plant and animal food products can reduce the amounts that are consumed. Tips for food choices and preparation steps that help reduce exposure to pesticides and other contaminants are given in Table 19.9. One of the easiest ways to reduce exposure is to choose a variety of different foods avoiding excessive consumption of any one food. Although many consumers consider consumption of pesticides and other contaminants a significant risk, the health risk of eliminating foods from the diet that may contain residues is probably greater than that of the exposure. Fruits and vegetables may contain some pesticide residues but are a major component of a healthy diet. Fish may contain contaminants that enter waterways but provide a source of dietary protein and omega-3 fatty acids

TABLE 19.9 Reducing Exposure to Chemical Contaminants from Food

Choose carefully

- Choose home-grown or locally grown produce. It is likely to contain fewer pesticides because those used to extend shelf life during shipping are not needed.
- Choose foods produced organically or using IPM. Fewer pesticides are used during production, so these foods are likely to contain fewer pesticide residues.
- Pregnant and lactating women and small children should avoid swordfish, shark, king mackerel, and tilefish—these long-lived fish have higher levels of mercury.
- Choose farm-raised fish to reduce exposure to environmental contaminants.
- Choose lean meats. Contaminants accumulate in adipose tissue.
- Choose a variety of foods. This reduces the likelihood of ingesting dangerous amounts of any individual contaminant.

Prepare carefully

- Peel or wash. Contaminants can be removed or reduced by peeling fruits and vegetables or washing them with tap water and scrubbing with a brush if appropriate.
- Remove outer leaves. For leafy vegetables such as lettuce and cabbage, removing and discarding the outer leaves eliminates the leaves with the highest pesticide levels.
- Remove waxes. Waxes added to maintain freshness also seal in pesticides and are often combined with fungicides to inhibit the growth of molds. Wax can be removed by rinsing produce in warm water and scrubbing it with a brush, but to eliminate all wax, the produce must be peeled.
- Remove excess fat and internal organs. Most toxins concentrate in adipose tissue. Removing skin and trimming all fat from fish and meat before cooking or eating can reduce toxin amounts. Internal organs such as the green-colored "tomale" in lobster and the "mustard" in blue crabs should not be consumed because toxins such as PCBs and cadmium accumulate in these organs.
- Use a variety of cooking methods. Avoid frequent grilling, which allows fats to drip into the fire, to reduce exposure to PAHs.

that help reduce the risk of heart disease (see *Critical Thinking:* "Comparing the Risks with the Benefits").

Critical Thinking

Comparing the Risks with the Benefits

After completing a food safety unit in his nutrition class, Eric was afraid to eat just about everything! The next day he ate nothing but cereal and crackers, but then decided take a more rational approach to food safety. He knew that his diet was generally healthy and that he was rarely sick, but he also recognized that a few of the foods he enjoys carry risks. He prefers his meat rare, likes to lick cookie dough containing raw eggs from the bowl while baking, and he and his girlfriend enjoy eating sushi and raw oysters. He makes the following list of foods he typically eats that may pose a risk of foodborne illness and then records the risks and benefits of each:

Food	Risk	Benefit
Hamburger	Can be contaminated with pathogenic *E. coli* O157:H7.	A good source of protein and iron in his diet.
Chicken	Is often contaminated with *Salmonella.*	An economical source of protein that is low in fat.
Fish	Can be contaminated with environmental pollutants such as PCBs and toxic metals.	A low-fat source of high-quality protein and omega-3 fatty acids that have been associated with a reduced risk of cardiovascular disease.
Raw fish and shellfish	Can be a source of bacterial, viral, and parasitic infections.	A low-fat source of high-quality protein and omega-3 fatty acids.
Cookie dough	Contains raw eggs, which may be contaminated with *Salmonella.*	Tastes good.
Fruits and vegetables	May contain pesticide residues and be contaminated with pathogens.	An excellent source of fiber and vitamins in the diet. They also contain health-promoting phytochemicals.

After reviewing the risks and benefits of his diet, Eric decides to wait until cookies are baked before eating them. He also realizes he can minimize the risk associated with eating hamburger and chicken by thoroughly cooking them, because *E. coli* and its toxins and *Salmonella* are destroyed by heat.

What other things can he do to minimize the risks associated with his typical diet while including foods that are beneficial?

Answer:

Eric typically brings a bag lunch from home. What safe food choices could he include?

Answer:

Food Additives

During the processing of foods for transport and distribution, some substances are intentionally added to preserve or enhance their appeal (Figure 19.20). Although these are intended to enhance the quality of the food, in some cases they may also add to the risks.

For more information on food and color additives, go to the government's food safety site at www.foodsafety.gov/~fsg/additive.html.

Defining Food Additives

By legal definition, a **food additive** is a substance that can reasonably be expected to become a component of a food during processing. This includes **direct food additives,** which are intentionally added during the preparation, packaging, transport, and holding of food, and **indirect food additives,** which are substances known to enter food unintentionally during processing, such as a chemical in the packaging that migrates into the food. Direct and indirect food additives are regulated by the FDA. When foods or packaging materials are handled improperly, unexpected substances may accidentally enter food. These **accidental contaminants** are not regulated by the FDA.

Food additives Substances that can reasonably be expected to become a component of a food during processing. The foods that may contain them and the amounts that may be present are regulated by the FDA.

Direct food additives Substances intentionally added to foods. They are regulated by the FDA.

Indirect food additives Substances that are expected to unintentionally enter foods during manufacturing or from packaging. They are regulated by the FDA.

Accidental contaminants Substances that unexpectedly enter foods during manufacturing or from packaging. They are not regulated by the FDA.

Standards of identity Regulations that define the allowable ingredients, composition, and other characteristics of foods.

Regulating Food Additives

The Pure Food and Drug Act of 1906 stated that only additives that were proven to be safe and effective could be used in foods. In 1938, the federal Food, Drug, and Cosmetic Act provided exemptions and safe tolerance levels for additives that were necessary or unavoidable in production. This law established **standards of identity** for foods. These prescribed recipes define exactly the ingredients that can be contained in certain foods such as mayonnaise, jelly, and orange

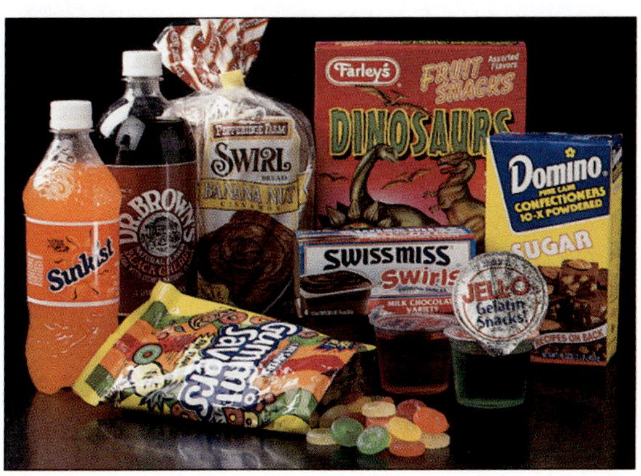

FIGURE 19.20 The additives in these foods prevent the bread from molding, the fruit snacks from hardening, and the powdered sugar from clumping; they also smooth the texture of the pudding and give color to soft drinks and candy. *(George Semple)*

juice. These foods were originally exempt from listing the product's ingredients on the food label; however, today even foods with standards of identity must list ingredients.[29] The Food, Drug, and Cosmetic Act also gave the FDA the responsibility of testing food additives for safety. Because the FDA could not possibly test all additives, the 1958 Food Additives Amendment transferred the responsibility for testing from the FDA to the manufacturer.

Since 1958, all new additives have had to be demonstrated to be safe before they could be added to food. Safety tests must be done using at least two animal species, usually rats and mice. These tests are used to determine the highest level of a substance at which no deleterious effects are observed. The highest amount of the substance that can be added to food is then set at 1/100 of this level.

When a manufacturer wants to use a new food additive, a petition must be submitted to the FDA. The petition describes the chemical composition of the additive, how it is manufactured, and how it is detected and measured in food. The manufacturer must then prove that the additive will be effective for its intended purpose at the proposed levels, that it is safe for its intended use, and that its use is necessary. The burden of proof is placed on the manufacturer, who has the financial incentive to have the compound approved. This often takes years of testing. For example, before the FDA approved the fat replacer Olestra for use in salty snack foods in January 1996, it evaluated more than 150,000 pages of data from over 150 studies that were included in Procter & Gamble's original 1987 food additives petition and several amendments to that petition.

Generally recognized as safe (GRAS) A group of chemical additives that is generally recognized as safe based on their long-standing presence in the food supply without obvious harmful effects.

The GRAS List When the 1958 Food Additives Amendment was passed, over 600 chemicals defined as food additives were already in common use. The amendment added a category of materials that were considered **generally recognized as safe (GRAS).** GRAS substances are exempt from the regulations applied to substances defined as food additives, color additives, or pesticides. If the safety of a substance on the GRAS list is questioned, the FDA must provide evidence that the substance is unsafe before it can be removed from the list. For example, the artificial sweetener cyclamate was removed from the GRAS list because it was found to cause cancer in laboratory animals. Substances on the GRAS list are subject to ongoing review.

Delaney Clause A clause added to the 1958 Food Additives Amendment of the Pure Food and Drug Act that prohibits the intentional addition to foods of any compound that has been shown to induce cancer in animals or humans at any dose.

The Delaney Clause The 1958 Food Additives Amendment also included the **Delaney Clause,** which was designed to protect the public from additives found to be carcinogenic. The Delaney Clause states that a substance that induces cancer in either an animal species or humans at any dosage, no matter how large, may not be intentionally added to food. Currently, support is growing to amend the Delaney Clause to allow the use of substances that are added at a level so low that they would not represent a significant health risk. Like pesticides, food additives found to be carcinogenic at high doses would then be evaluated using a risk-benefit analysis.

Direct Food Additives

Direct food additives enhance the quality, appearance, and flavor of our food supply. Although some have been questioned as potential hazards, additives are used only if it is concluded that the benefits they offer outweigh any risk they might pose. Food additives are used to improve the nutritional quality of food, to preserve foods, to enhance flavor or improve taste, and to aid in processing or preparation. They may not be used to disguise inferior products or to deceive the

TABLE 19.10 Additives Commonly Used in Foods

Additive	Function	Example of Use
Acetic acid	Provides acidity	Gives tartness to dressings and sauces.
Ascorbic acid	Preservative, nutrient	Keeps fruit from darkening, inhibits rancidity in fatty foods, enhances nutritional value of beverages.
Baking soda (sodium bicarbonate)	Leavening agent	Generates gas so ensures baked goods rise.
Beet extract	Natural color	Gives deep red color to foods.
BHA (butylated hydroxyanisole)	Preservative	Acts as an antioxidant to prevent rancidity of fats, oils, and dried meats; keeps baked goods fresh.
BHT (butylated hydroxytoluene)	Preservative	Acts as an antioxidant to prevent rancidity in potato flakes, enriched rice, and shortenings.
Calcium silicate	Anticaking agent	Absorbs moisture to keep powdered foods like baking powder free-flowing
Carrageenan	Stabilizer, texturizer	Improves consistency and texture of chocolate milk, frozen desserts, puddings, and syrup.
Citric acid	Preservative, provides acidity	Provides acidity in beverages and dessert products.
FD&C colors	Color	Adds color to foods, drugs, and cosmetics.
Gelatin	Thickener, gelling agent	Provides texture to desserts, confectionery products, and canned meat products
Glycerides (monoglycerides and diglycerides)	Emulsifier	Prevents ice cream from separating while melting, keeps oil in peanut butter from separating.
Glycerine (glycerol)	Humectant	Binds water to prevent moisture losses in flaked coconut, marshmallows, and toaster foods.
Guar gum	Thickener	Thickens liquids such as gravies and sauces.
Gum arabic	Stabilizer, emulsifier	Keeps butter mixed in buttered syrups and stablilizes flavors in dry-mix food products.
Lactic acid	Preservative	Controls molds in pickles, sauerkraut, cheese, buttermilk, and yogurt.
Lecithin	Emulsifier	Prevents separation of oil and vinegar in mayonnaise.
Magnesium stearate	Anticaking agent	Prevents clumping in flour.
Pectin	Thickener	Gels jams, jellies, and preserves.
Potassium sorbate	Preservative	Controls surface molds on cheese, syrups, margarine, and mayonnaise.
Propylene glycol	Humectant	Improves texture of foods by holding moisture.
Sodium benzoate	Preservative	Controls molds in syrup, margarine, soft drinks, and fruit products.
Sodium chloride	Preservative, flavor agent	Prevents microbial growth in cured meats, adds flavor to soups.
Sodium nitrite	Preservative	Prevents botulism growth in cured meats, fish, and poultry.
Sorbitol	Sweetener, humectant	Keeps fruit snacks and gummy candies soft.
Sulfites (sulfur dioxide, sodium sulfide, sodium and potassium bisulfite, and sodium and potassium metabisulfite)	Preservative	Acts as an antioxidant to prevent discoloration in fruits and vegetables like dried apples and dehydrated potatoes.
Tartaric acid	Increases acidity	Adds tartness to carbonated fruit-flavored drinks.

consumer. They are also not permitted in foods where they significantly destroy nutrients or where the same effect can be achieved by sound manufacturing processes. For example, sulfites cannot be used on meats because they restore the red color, giving a false appearance of freshness, and they cannot be used in foods that are important sources of thiamin, such as enriched flour, because they destroy thiamin. Examples of some food additives and how they are used are given in Table 19.10.

Additives to Maintain or Improve Nutritional Quality Many nutrients are added to foods. As discussed in Chapter 9, refined grains are enriched with iron and some of the B vitamins that are lost in processing. In other cases, food is fortified with nutrients typically lacking in the diet. For instance, enriched grain products are fortified with folic acid and milk is fortified with vitamins A and D.

Preservatives Compounds that extend the shelf life of a product by retarding chemical, physical, or microbiological changes.

Additives to Maintain Product Quality Many different substances are added to foods to maintain their quality. **Preservatives** are added to food to prevent bacteria and molds from causing food spoilage, to extend shelf life, or to preserve natural color and flavor. Sugar and salt are two of the oldest preservatives. They prevent microbial growth by decreasing the water availability in the product; without adequate water, microbes cannot grow. For example, the high concentration of sugar in jams and jellies draws water away from the microbial cells and prevents them from growing.

Nitrosamines Carcinogenic compounds produced by reactions between nitrites and amino acids.

Most preservatives have little documented risk. However, for some, the risks have been carefully weighed against the benefits. For example, nitrites and nitrates are used in cured meats such as ham and hot dogs to retard the growth of bacteria, particularly *Clostridium botulinum,* which causes deadly botulism poisoning. However, they also react with amino acids in the body to form **nitrosamines.** Nitrosamines are known to be carcinogenic in animals, but there is little evidence that nitrites and nitrates pose a serious risk in the amounts consumed in the human diet.[30] To minimize any risk of nitrosamines without increasing the risk of bacterial illness, the FDA has limited the amount of nitrites that can be added to food and has required the addition of antioxidants, which reduce nitrosamine formation, to foods containing nitrites. Consumers can reduce the risk of nitrites by limiting cured meat consumption to 3 to 4 ounces per week and maintaining adequate intakes of vitamins C and E.

Sulfites are another preservative that can be a health risk to consumers. In sensitive individuals exposure can cause symptoms that range from gastrointestinal upset and hives to severe asthmatic reactions.[31] Sulfite use is prohibited on foods intended to be eaten raw, but they may be used to prevent discoloration in dried fruits and fresh-cut potatoes, to control black spots in freshly caught shrimp, and to prevent discoloration, bacterial growth, and fermentation in wine (Figure 19.21). Sulfites are also used to preserve baked goods, canned vegetables, condiments, and maraschino cherries. A packaged food containing sulfites can be identified by the presence of sulfur dioxide, sodium sulfite, sodium or potassium bisulfite, or sodium or potassium metabisulfite in the ingredient list.[31] Individuals sensitive to sulfites should also be aware that foods served in restaurants could contain sulfites. For example, a potato dish served in a restaurant may be prepared using potatoes that were peeled and soaked in a sulfite solution before cooking.

Additives That Aid in Processing or Preparation Many different types of additives are used in product processing and preparation. Emulsifiers improve the homogeneity, stability, and consistency of products such as ice cream. Stabilizers, thick-

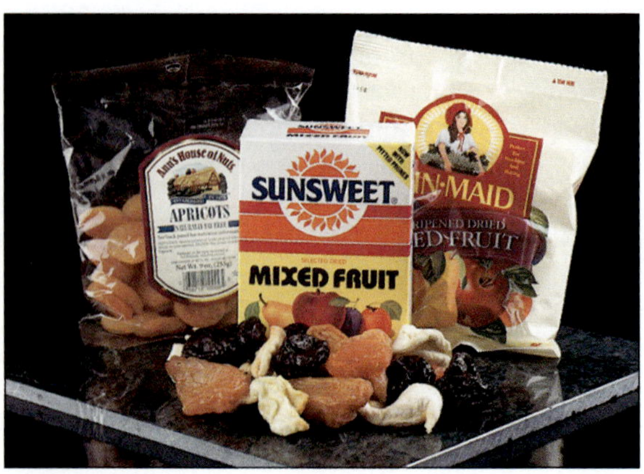

FIGURE 19.21 Sulfites are used in products such as dried fruit, but they can cause deadly reactions in sulfite-sensitive individuals. *(George Semple)*

eners, and texturizers, such as pectins and gums, are used to improve consistency or texture in pudding and to stabilize emulsions in foods such as salad dressing. Leavening agents are added to incorporate gas into breads and cakes, causing them to rise. Acids are added as flavor enhancers, preservatives, and antioxidants. Humectants, such as propylene glycol, cause moisture to be retained so products stay fresh. Anticaking agents prevent crystalline products such as powdered sugar from absorbing moisture and caking or lumping.

Additives That Affect Color and Flavor Additives are also used to enhance the flavor and color of foods. Flavor additives may supplement, magnify, or modify the original taste or aroma of a food. For example, both natural and artificial sweeteners are added to enhance the flavor of foods (see Chapter 4), and fat replacers such as Simplesse and Olestra increase the appeal of fat-free and low-fat foods by adding body, texture, and taste that simulates fat (see Chapter 5).

Colors can be used to make foods appear more appetizing; however, they cannot be used as deception to conceal inferiority. The FDA's list of permitted colors includes two categories: certified food colors and those exempt from certification. Certified food colors are synthetic dyes derived primarily from petroleum and coal sources. Certification means that each batch of the food color is tested to ensure safety, quality, consistency, and strength of color. About 10% of the food consumed in the United States contains certified food colors. Colors derived from plant, animal, and certain mineral sources are exempt from certification. Examples include beet juice, caramel, and paprika extract. The soft drink industry is the single largest user of color additives.

Colors found to be potential hazards have been removed from the list of permissible additives.[32] However, the certified food color FD&C Yellow No. 5 (listed as tartrazine on medicine labels), which may cause itching and hives in hypersensitive individuals, was not considered a great enough risk to be removed from the food supply. It is found in beverages, desserts, and processed vegetables.

The ingredient list of the food label can be used to identify the presence of color additives. All foods that contain FDA-certified color additives must list them by name in the ingredient list. Colors that are exempt from certification, such as dehydrated beets and carotenoids, do not have to be specifically identified and may be listed on the label collectively as "artificial color."[33]

Indirect Food Additives

Indirect additives include any substance that may find its way into a food during production, processing, storage, or packaging. An example of an indirect additive is methylene chloride, which is used in the process of decaffeinating coffee. Methylene chloride is a carcinogen, but the levels found in decaffeinated coffee are too low to be a risk. Urethane is a compound that forms during the fermentation of alcoholic beverages. The concentration increases if the product is heated. It is a cancer-causing substance in animals, but it is unclear if it is a risk in humans. Other indirect additives include bits of plastic, glass, and paper that can enter the food from packaging and medications and hormones that enter food because they are used to treat food-producing animals.

Contamination from Packaging Packaging can protect food from spoilage, but even the best packaging can introduce risk if it becomes a part of the food. A variety of substances leach into foods from plastics, paper, and even dishes. The amounts and types of these indirect additives are regulated by EPA tolerance levels and FDA inspections. For example, dioxin levels in foods are monitored because dioxins can contaminate foods that come in contact with bleached paper products.

Regulations regarding indirect additives from packaging apply only when the product is used as intended. When used improperly, packaging can migrate into food and become an accidental contaminant. For instance, some plastics migrate into food when heated in a microwave oven. Thus, only packages designated for microwave cooking should be used.

Drugs Used in Animal Production Antibiotics and hormones given to animals raised for food can make their way into the food supply. Therefore, the FDA regulates which drugs can be used as well as the residues allowed in the food.

Antibiotics Antibiotics are used in livestock production to treat and prevent disease and to promote growth. Animals treated with antibiotics can produce greater yields at a lower cost, but if improperly used residues of these drugs remain in the meat and can be hazardous to consumers. The FDA is responsible for regulating which antibiotics or other drugs can be used to treat animals designated for food production. Before a drug is used it is evaluated to ensure that it is safe and effective for the animals that receive it and that it has no harmful effect on consumers of the food products.[34] The FDA also specifies the amount of time that must pass between administration of a drug and when meat or milk from the treated animal can be sold to allow the drug to be metabolized and excreted. The USDA monitors tissue samples from slaughtered animals for drug residues.

Perhaps a more important concern raised in relation to antibiotic use in animals is the creation of antibiotic-resistant bacteria. When bacteria are exposed to an antibiotic, those that are resistant to that antibiotic survive and produce new bacteria that are also resistant to the antibiotic. If these resistant bacteria infect humans, the resulting illness cannot be treated with that antibiotic. Since nearly half the antibiotics produced in the United States are used to prevent disease in animals, this use is suspected of being a major contributor to the development of antibiotic-resistant strains of bacteria.[35]

Hormones Certain hormones have been approved for use in small amounts to improve the rate of weight gain in cattle and sheep and milk production in dairy cows. Some, such as testosterone and estrogen, are naturally occurring hormones. Generally, these are administered in a slow-release form and levels in meat are no higher than those found in untreated animals. Before synthetic hormones can be used, it must be demonstrated that the amount that remains in the meat is below the level determined to be safe.

A synthetic hormone that has created public concern is genetically engineered bovine somatotropin (bST). Cows naturally produce somatotropin, a hormone that stimulates milk production. Genetically engineered bST has the same effects as the natural hormone, but it is produced by bacteria and injected into cows to increase their milk production. Consumer groups contend that genetically engineered bST causes health problems for the cows and for humans who consume milk or meat from the cows. An FDA review of the effect of bST concluded that it causes no serious long-term health effects in cows. The only concern is a possible increase in udder infections. Because these infections are often treated with antibiotics, it has been suggested that this could increase the antibiotic residues in the milk from cows treated with bST. Monitoring is currently in place to ensure that this does not occur. The FDA has concluded that milk and meat from bST-treated cows are not health risks to consumers.[36]

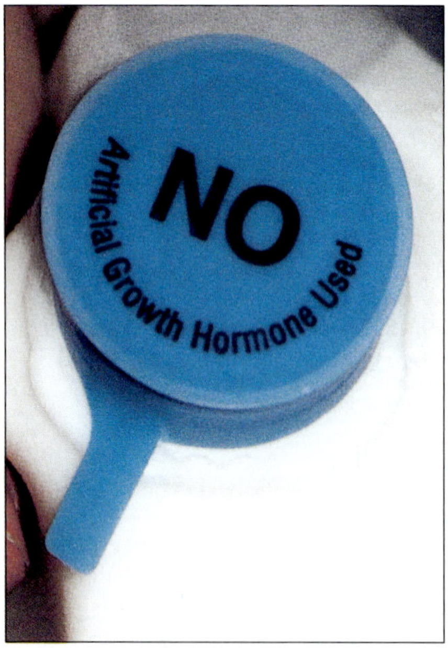

FIGURE 19.22 Milk from cows treated with genetically engineered bovine somatotropin is indistinguishable from other milk, but dairies that do not use bovine somatotropin may choose to indicate this on the label. *(Lori Smolin)*

Cow's milk naturally contains bST, and it is not possible to detect a difference between milk from bST-treated and untreated cows. Pasteurization destroys 90% of bST, and digestion breaks down the rest, so it is unlikely that genetically engineered bST is secreted in milk. There is no difference in the milk from treated and untreated cows, so the FDA does not require milk from bST-treated cows to be specially labeled. Companies may voluntarily label their products as long as the labeling is truthful and not misleading (Figure 19.22).

Summary

1. The safety of the food supply can be affected by biological, chemical, and physical contaminants. Microbial contamination of food is the most common cause of foodborne illness. The harm caused by contaminants in the food supply depends on the type of contaminant, the dose consumed, the length of time over which it is consumed, and the size and health status of the consumer.
2. The food supply is monitored for safety by food manufacturers and regulatory agencies at the international, federal, state, and local levels. Consumers also play an important role in limiting the risks of developing foodborne illness.
3. The use of HACCP (Hazard Analysis Critical Control Point) offers a method for preventing food contamination, monitoring food processing methods, and tracking contaminated foods to prevent foodborne illness.
4. Microbial foodborne illness can be caused by bacteria, viruses, molds, and parasites. Some bacteria cause foodborne infection because they are able to grow in the gastrointestinal tract when ingested. Others produce toxins in food and cause foodborne intoxication when the toxin is ingested. Viruses ingested in contaminated food cause foodborne illness because they can multiply inside human cells. Molds that grow on foods cause illness because they produce toxins that are harmful when consumed. Parasites that contaminate water or food cause illness when they grow and reproduce inside the body.
5. The risk of foodborne illness can be reduced by proper food selection, preparation, and storage. Consumers should choose the freshest meats and produce, select frozen foods that have been kept at constant temperatures, and avoid packages with broken seals or contents that appear spoiled. Once in the home, foods should be cooked thoroughly and leftovers stored properly. Kitchen surfaces, hands, and cooking utensils should be cleaned between preparation steps.
6. Contaminants, such as pesticides applied to crops and industrial wastes that leach into water, may find their way into the food supply. Industrial pollutants such as dioxins, toxic metals, and radioactive substances contaminate the environment and can make their way into the food supply. As these contaminants move up the food chain, their concentrations increase. Some contaminants are formed in food during cooking.
7. To decrease the potential risk of chemical contaminants, safer pesticides are being developed and farmers are reducing the amounts applied by using integrated pest management and organic methods. Other chemicals can enter the food supply because they contaminate the environment. Consumers can reduce the amounts of chemical contaminants in food by careful selection and handling of foods.
8. Food additives include all substances that can reasonably be expected to find their way into a food during processing. These include direct food additives, which are intentionally added to preserve or enhance the appeal of food, and indirect food additives, which are substances known to find their way into food during production, processing, cooking, and packaging. Direct and indirect food additives are regulated by the FDA. Accidental contaminants that enter food when it is used or prepared incorrectly are not regulated by the FDA.

Review Questions

1. What is the major cause of foodborne illness in the United States?
2. List three factors that affect the toxicity of a substance.
3. Explain what HACCP is and how it can prevent food contamination.
4. List three ways in which the federal government is involved in ensuring a safe food supply.
5. List three common bacterial food contaminants. What can be done to avoid the foodborne illnesses they cause?
6. What temperature range allows the most rapid bacterial growth?
7. What is the difference between foodborne infection and foodborne intoxication?
8. How do viruses get into the food supply?
9. How do pesticides applied to crops find their way into animal products?
10. Do food additives reduce or increase the risks associated with foods? Why?
11. What is the GRAS list?

Applying Critical Thinking Skills

Personal nutrition:

1. Evaluate your food safety knowledge by taking the food safety true/false test at **http://vm.cfsan.fda.gov/~dms/fse-t-f.html.**
2. Use the Internet to go to **http://www.fda.gov** and using their search feature find the exercise called "Can Your Kitchen Pass the Food Safety Test?" Complete the exercise and answer the following:
   a. What was your score?
   b. Based on how you answered these questions, what changes should you make in the way you store and handle foods in your kitchen?

c. Based on how you answered these questions, are there foods that you will eliminate from your diet? Why?

General nutrition issues:

1. When 67 people became ill after consuming food at a company picnic, investigators determined that the tossed salad, the egg salad, and the turkey slices were all contaminated with *Salmonella.* Invent a scenario that would explain how all three became contaminated.
2. For each of the foods given below:
   a. Indicate whether it is likely to be a cause of microbial foodborne illness.
   b. Describe a scenario in which the food could become contaminated.
   c. Explain what you could do to avoid contamination and/or foodborne illness in each case.
   Fruit salad
   Home-canned green beans
   Deviled eggs
   Stir-fried chicken with vegetables
   Potato salad served at a summer picnic
   Raw seafood
   Unpasteurized cheese
3. A train crash spills a load of PCBs in a river that feeds into a local reservoir. How would this water contamination affect:
   a. the safety of the drinking water?
   b. the milk from dairy cattle grazing nearby?
   c. the fish that swim in the river?
   d. the crops irrigated by this water?

References

1. World Health Organization. Food Safety: A Worldwide Public Health Issue. Available online at **http://www.who.int/fsf/fctshtfs.htm.** Accessed 19 Oct 2000.
2. Mead, P. S., Slutsker, L., Dietz, V., et al. Food-related illness and death in the United States. Emerg. Infect. Dis. 5:607–625, 1999.
3. National Academy of Sciences. *Ensuring Safe Food from Production to Consumption.* Washington, D.C.: National Academy Press, 1998.
4. Knabel, S. J. Institute of Food Technologists Scientific Status Summary: Foodborne illness: role of home food handling practices. Food Technol. 49:119–131, 1995.
5. Centers for Disease Control and Prevention. Ten Great Public Health Achievements—United States, 1900–1999. Available online at **http://www.cdc.gov/phtn/tenachievements/.** Accessed 15 Dec 2000.
6. U.S. Food and Drug Administration, U.S. Department of Agriculture, and Environmental Protection Agency. Food Safety from Farm to Table: A New Strategy for the 21st Century. February 21, 1997. Available online at **http://www.cfsan.fda.gov/~dms/fs-draft.html.** Accessed 15 Dec 2000.
7. U.S. Department of Health and Human Services. National Computer Network in Place to Combat Foodborne Illness (press release). May 22, 1998. Available online at **http://www.cdc.gov/od/oc/media/pressrel/r980522.htm.** Accessed 15 Dec 2000.
8. Centers for Disease Control and Prevention. FoodNet. Available online at **http://www.cdc.gov/foodnet/.** Accessed 14 Dec 2000.
9. Stephenson, J. Fighting flora with flora: FDA approves an anti-*Salmonella* spray for chickens. JAMA 279:1152, 1998.
10. Cerington, M. Clinical spectrum of botulism. Muscle Nerve 21:701–710, 1998.
11. Kohn, M. A., Farley, T. A., Ando, T., et al. An outbreak of Norwalk virus gastroenteritis associated with eating raw oysters: implications for maintaining safe oyster beds. JAMA 273:466–471, 1995.
12. U.S. Food and Drug Administration, Center for Food Safety and Nutrition. Foodborne Pathogenic Microorganisms and Natural Toxins Handbook: The "Bad Bug Book." Available online at **http://www.cfsan.fda.gov/~mow/intro.html.** Accessed 1 Apr 2001.
13. Outbreaks of *Escherichia coli* O157:H7 infection and cryptosporidosis associated with drinking unpasteurized apple cider—Connecticut and New York, October 1996. MMWR Morb. Mortal. Wkly. Rep. 46:4–8, 1997.
14. Foodborne outbreak of diarrheal illness associated with *Cryptosporidium parvum*—Minnesota, 1995. MMWR Morb. Mortal. Wkly. Rep. 45:783–784, 1996.
15. Kurtzweil, P. Can your kitchen pass the food safety test? FDA Consumer 28:14–18, October 1994.
16. Kolpin, D. W., Barbash, J. E., and Gilliom, R. J. Occurrence of pesticides in shallow groundwater of the United States—initial results from the National Water-Quality Assessment Program. Environ. Sci. Technol. 32:558–566, 1998.
17. Foulke, J. E. FDA reports on pesticides in foods. FDA Consumer 27:29–32, June 1993.
18. Cooney, C. M. New pesticide law drops "zero-tolerence" standard, focuses on exposure to children. Environ. Sci. Technol. 30:380A, September 1996.
19. U.S. Food and Drug Administration. FDA Report: Pesticides in Our Food, 1998. Available online at **http://www.cfsan.fda.gov/~dms/pes97.html.** Accessed 15 Dec 2000.
20. National Research Council, Committee on Comparative Toxicology of Naturally Occurring Carcinogens. Individual chemicals in the diet generally pose no risk to Americans, NRC concludes. Food Chem. News 37:32–33, February 19, 1996.
21. Acquavella, J., Burns, C., Flaherty, D., et al. A critique of the World Resource Institute's report "Pesticides and the Immune System: The Public Health Risks." Environ. Health Perspect. 106:51–54, 1998.
22. U.S. Department of Agriculture. Remarks of Secretary Glickman: Proposed Organic Standards. December 15, 1997. Available online at **http://www.usda.gov/news/releases/1997/12/0443.** Accessed 15 Dec 2000.
23. U.S. Department of Agriculture, Agricultural Marketing Service. National Organic Program: Final Rule. Available online at **http://www.ams.usda.gov/nop/nop2000/nop/finalrulepages/finalrulemap.htm.** Accessed 1 Mar 2001.
24. Clarkson, T. W. Environmental contaminants in the food chain. Am. J. Clin. Nutr. 61(suppl):682S–686S, 1995.
25. Jacobson, J. L., and Jacobson, S. W. Intellectual impairment in children exposed to polychlorinated biphenyls *in utero.* N. Engl. J. Med. 335:783–789, 1996.
26. American Academy of Pediatrics, Committee on Environmental Health. PCBs in breast milk. Pediatrics 84:122–123, 1994.

27. U.S. Food and Drug Administration, Center for Food Safety and Applied Nutrition. Questions and Answers About Dioxins. Available online at **http://www.fda.gov/cvm/index/dioxin/dioxinqa.htm.** Accessed 15 Dec 2000.
28. Foulke, J. E. Mercury in fish: cause for concern? FDA Consumer 28:5–8, September 1994.
29. Segal, M. Ingredient labeling: what's in a food? FDA Consumer 27:14–18, April 1993.
30. Eichholzer, M., and Gutzwiller, F. Dietary nitrates, nitrites, and N-nitroso compounds and cancer risk: a review of the epidemiologic evidence. Nutr. Rev. 56:95–105, 1998.
31. Papazian, R. Sulfites: safe for most, dangerous for some. FDA Consumer 30:11–14, December 1996.
32. U.S. Food and Drug Administration. Food Color Facts. January 1993. Available online at **http://www.cfsan.fda.gov/~lrd/colorfac.html.** Accessed 15 Dec 2000.
33. U.S. Food and Drug Administration, Center for Food Safety and Applied Nutrition. Office of Cosmetics Fact Sheet: Color Additives, February 7, 1995. Available online at **http://www.cfsan.fda.gov/~dms/cos-221.html.** Accessed 15 Dec 2000.
34. U.S. Food and Drug Administration, Center for Veterinary Medicine Communications and Education Branch. Monitoring for Residues in Food Animals. Revised March 1994. Available online at **http://www.fda.gov/cvm/index/memos/cvmm19.html.** Accessed 2 March 2001.
35. Kaneene, J. B., and Miller, R. Problems associated with drug residues in beef from feeds and therapy. Rev. Sci. Tech. 16:694–708, 1997.
36. Ropp, K. L. New animal drug increases milk production. FDA Consumer 28:24–27, May 1994.

20 Food Technology: More and Safer Food

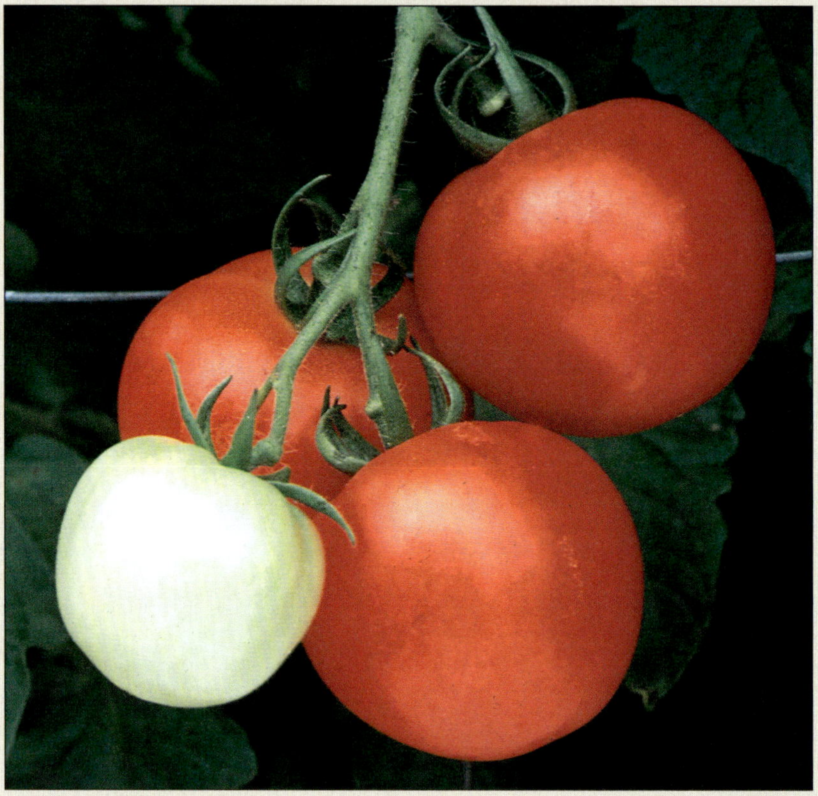

Learning Objectives

After reading this chapter, students should be able to:

1. Discuss the impact of technology on the food supply.
2. List several methods of food preservation.
3. Describe how temperature is used to improve food safety.
4. Define "water activity" and explain how it applies to food preservation.
5. Identify some methods of food packaging that preserve food by reducing exposure to oxygen.
6. Explain how irradiation is used to preserve food.
7. Describe how food irradiation is regulated in the United States.
8. Define "biotechnology" and explain how it is used to improve the food supply.
9. Compare the use of traditional selective breeding and biotechnology for developing new types of plants and animals.
10. Prepare arguments for and against the use of biotechnology in the food and agricultural industry.

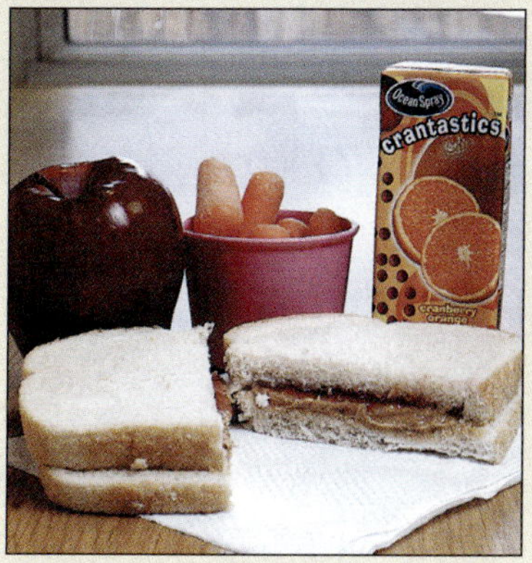

It's called golden rice. And it may be worth its weight in gold. This genetically engineered rice variety will produce a food that has the potential to eradicate vitamin A deficiency, a nutrient deficiency that causes blindness in 500,000 children around the world each year. Simply replacing the staple grain with the new "golden" variety could save the sight and lives of thousands of children.

But this doesn't mean much to Miles. He is a seven-year-old who is severely allergic to peanuts and nuts. He and his family have to be very careful to keep products containing peanuts and nuts out of his diet. They are therefore concerned about the use of genetic engineering to create new food products. This technology combines genes from different organisms, and therefore the new products could contain genetic material from allergy-causing foods. They just read an article about a variety of soybean developed in the mid-1990s. To increase the protein content of the soybeans, a gene from the Brazil nut was introduced. Testing soon revealed that the gene coded for a protein that was an allergen, and the soybeans never reached the marketplace.[1]

Miles's family took particular note of this article because he takes soybutter and jelly sandwiches to school for lunch everyday. This sandwich spread is made from roasted soybeans and contains no peanuts or nuts. If, however, the soybeans in the spread had been replaced with the variety that was genetically altered using genes from Brazil nuts, Miles could suddenly be allergic to his favorite food.

Golden rice is currently being grown at agricultural research stations in the developing world, and many think it will fulfill its promise of significantly reducing vitamin A deficiency. And, to date, no cases have been reported of allergic reactions occurring as a result of genetically modified food. Nonetheless, careful monitoring of this new science will be important to ensure that it enhances the food supply without increasing its potential hazards.

Food and Technology

In the broadest sense, technology refers to any method used to alter our interaction with the environment. Technology has been part of providing a safe and adequate food supply since the earliest times. Some of the oldest food-related technologies include the domestication of animals and the simplest farming techniques. Over the centuries they have also included the development of pesticides and fertilizers, mechanized farm equipment, and breeding methods to enhance certain traits in plants and animals. The technologies used to preserve foods range from ancient methods such as cooking and drying to modern packaging and irradiation. The most recent technologies involve genetically modifying plants to produce high-yielding, nutrient-enhanced crops (Figure 20.1).

Without technology, people are restricted to local foods that must be eaten soon after harvest or slaughter. While this has some appeal, it severely limits the variety of foods in the diet, particularly during the winter months, and increases the risk of malnutrition. Any irregularity, such as a change in climate, could affect the supply of food and result in starvation. Despite the benefits of technology in terms of food safety, quality, and storage, it can also introduce hazards to consumers and to the environment.

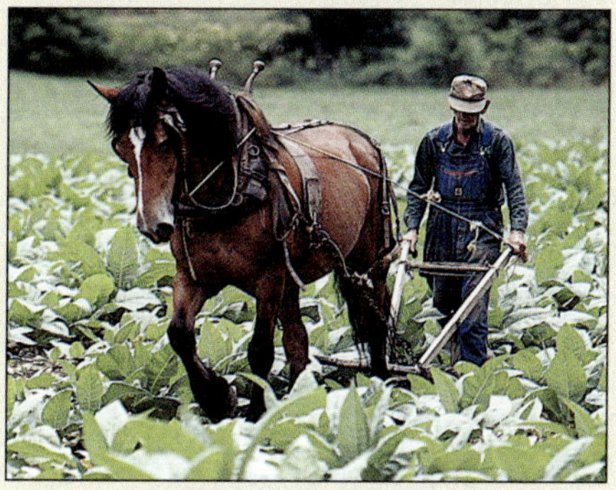

(a)

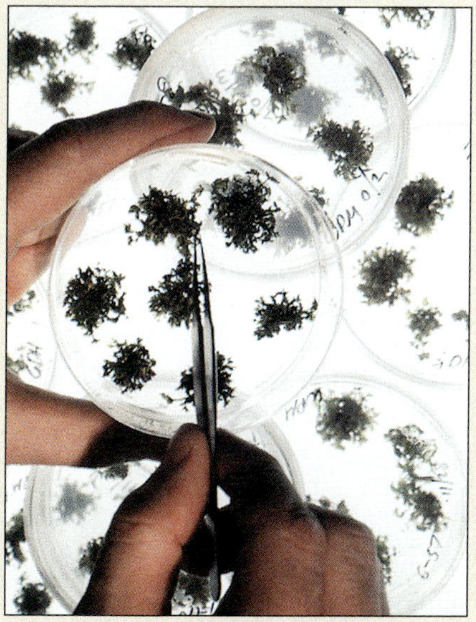

(b)

FIGURE 20.1 Agricultural technology includes traditional farming methods (a) as well as modern laboratory techniques (b). *((a) © William J. Webber/Visuals Unlimited; (b) Roger Tully/Stone)*

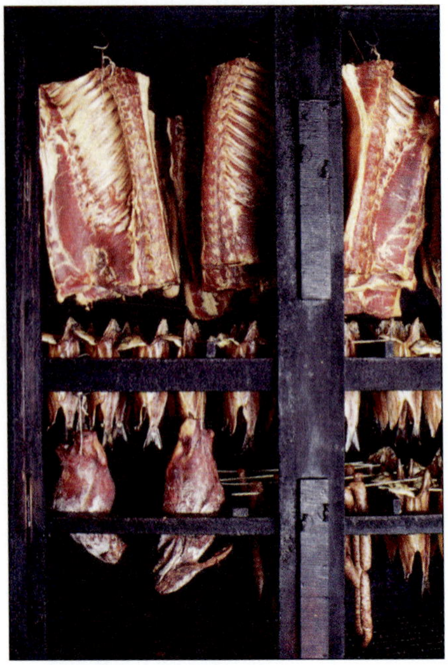

FIGURE 20.2 Smoking meats is a very old method of food preservation. *(© Jacqui Hurst/Corbis)*

Technology to Preserve Food

For thousands of years, humans have been treating food in order to protect it from spoilage. Many of the oldest methods of food preservation—drying, smoking, fermentation, salting, heating, and cooling—are still used today (Figure 20.2). Newer techniques of packaging and the use of chemical preservatives and food irradiation continue to increase the safety and variety of available foods. Most food preservation techniques rely on manipulating the environment by altering its temperature, pH, water content or availability, or the amount of oxygen to make it unfavorable for microbial growth.

Temperature

Microorganisms grow best within specific temperature ranges. Increasing the temperature above this range can kill microbes, and decreasing it below this range can slow or completely stop their growth. But heating and cooling are not guarantees of safety, particularly if used incorrectly. If foods are not heated long enough or to a high enough temperature, or if they are not cooled quickly enough after cooking, there is a risk of foodborne illness.

High Temperatures Cooking food is one of the oldest methods of ensuring food safety. It kills disease-causing organisms and destroys toxins (see Chapter 19). To be effective, cooking must heat food to temperatures high enough and for a long enough period of time that microbes are killed and any toxins they produce are destroyed. For example, it is recommended that eggs be cooked to an internal temperature of 160°F to assure that the *Salmonella* they may carry is killed. Heat treatment is also used in canning, pasteurization, and aseptic processing.

Canning Canning dates back to 19th-century France, where it was developed as a result of Napoleon's effort to keep his army well fed. In 1810, Nicholas Appert was awarded 12,000 francs for preserving food by placing it in a stoppered, airtight bottle and then heating it. The canning process used today involves sealing food in a glass or aluminum container and then heating it to temperatures that destroy bacteria and the spores of *Clostridium botulinum*. The growth of microorganisms in canned goods is also prevented by a lack of oxygen as discussed later in the chapter. When food is canned properly, it is safe for periods up to several years. One disadvantage of canning is that the high temperatures used to kill the microbes also reduce the vitamin content of the food. Vitamin C and the B vitamins are particularly susceptible to damage by heat.

Heat Pasteurization Heat pasteurization is a process that uses relatively mild temperatures to destroy disease-causing microorganisms and extend the shelf life of foods, particularly bottled beverages like milk, beer, and wine. The development of this process by Louis Pasteur was also the result of Napoleon's desire to keep his troops well fed *and* supplied with wine (see Chapter 19, *Research Discoveries*: "Pasteurization: From Spoiled Wine to Safe Milk"). Unlike canning, pasteurization does not kill all the microorganisms in the product. Instead, the food is heated for a set time and temperature that will destroy most disease-causing organisms and reduce the number of microorganisms that cause spoilage while preserving the taste of the product. Because the heating times and temperatures are lower, fewer nutrients are destroyed.

Aseptic processing A method that places already sterilized food in a sterilized package.

Sterilization A process that kills all the living organisms in the treated material.

Aseptic Processing A more recent addition to the technologies that rely on heat to preserve food is **aseptic processing.** This process heats foods to temperatures that result in **sterilization.** The sterilized foods are placed in sterilized packages using sterilized equipment.[2] Because aseptic processing sterilizes the product before it is packaged, the time and temperature of heating can be tailored to the food being packaged. This is an advantage over traditional canning because damage due to heat is reduced and nutrient content is maintained. Aseptic processing is currently used to produce boxed milk and juices that can be stored without refrigeration. These can remain free of microbial growth at room temperature for years (Figure 20.3).

Low Temperatures Cooling food by refrigeration or freezing prevents it from spoiling by slowing or stopping microbial growth. Prehistoric man could preserve his food in the winter by keeping it frozen, but commercial frozen foods are relatively recent (Figure 20.4). The modern frozen food industry owes its beginnings to Clarence Birdseye. His work as a field naturalist in the Arctic showed him that when fish is frozen very quickly, it keeps its fresh characteristics and can be stored frozen for long periods. In the 1920s and '30s, Birdseye developed quick-freezing processes and equipment that launched the frozen foods industry.[3]

To prevent microbial growth, refrigerator temperatures should be set at 40°F or less; this is low enough to stop the growth of most pathogens. However, some bacteria are able to grow at these low temperatures and can eventually result in food spoilage. Almost no microorganisms can grow at freezer temperatures (0°F), and those that do grow extremely slowly. Cooling foods to refrigerator temperatures and freezing them have little effect on nutritive value.

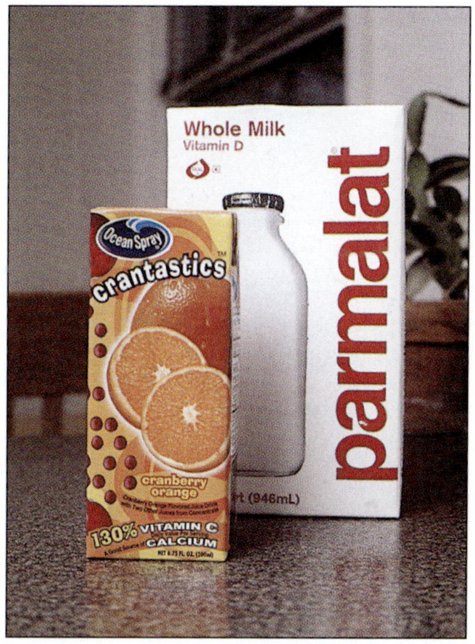

FIGURE 20.3 Milk and juice in aseptic packaging can be stored without refrigeration. *(© George Semple)*

Acidity

Most bacteria grow best in a relatively neutral pH—between 6 and 7.5—and most will not grow below pH 4.5. Therefore, techniques that reduce the pH of foods are used to prevent microbial growth. For example, adding vinegar to cucumbers to make pickles prevents bacterial growth and dramatically extends the shelf life of the cucumber. Low pH also increases the effectiveness of heat treatments, so acidic foods like tomatoes and fruits do not need to be heated to as high a temperature during canning.

Some bacteria produce acid as an end product of metabolism. As they grow, the acid accumulates, lowering the pH of their environment. Their growth is eventually inhibited when the environmental pH gets too low. Food preservation by **fermentation** takes advantage of these microorganisms. For example, lactic acid–producing bacteria are added to milk to produce fermented dairy products such as yogurt and buttermilk. Sausage, such as summer sausage, salami, and Lebanon bologna, are made by using acid-producing microorganisms. The acids preserve the meat and give it a tangy flavor.

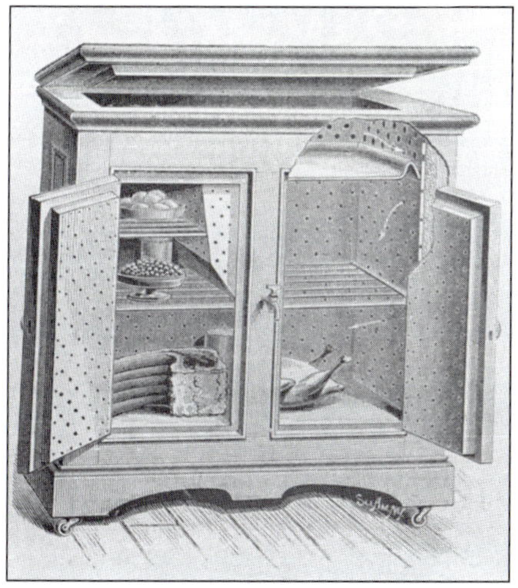

FIGURE 20.4 Before electric refrigerators were common in homes, perishable foods were stored in an insulated ice box. *(© Bettmann/Corbis)*

Water

Water is an essential nutrient for microorganisms. Water makes up a major portion of most foods. Fruits, vegetables, and meats are 70 to over 90% water. Some of the oldest methods of food preservation, such as drying and salting, prevent microbial growth by removing water or making it unavailable to the microbes. The amount of water available for chemical reactions is referred to as **water activity.** It is measured on a scale of 0 to 1.0. Most pathogens require a water activity of between 0.85 and 1.0—the water activity of most fruits, vegetables, meats, and cheeses. Lowering the water activity sufficiently makes it impossible for microorganisms to grow.

Fermentation A process in which microorganisms metabolize components of a food and therefore change the composition, taste, and storage properties of the food.

Water activity A measure of the amount of available water in a food.

Drying Drying removes water. It is used most commonly to preserve fruits and meats. Fruits such as apricots, plums (prunes), and grapes (raisins) are commercially dried in the sun (Figure 20.5). Other foods such as meats are dried by heating and by smoking. Smoking also adds chemicals that provide flavor and inhibit microbial growth. A newer method of drying is **freeze-drying.** In this procedure, the foods are frozen first and a vacuum is then used to remove the water while the

Freeze-drying A process in which substances are frozen and then exposed to a vacuum so the water is removed by sublimation (a change from solid ice to gaseous water vapor).

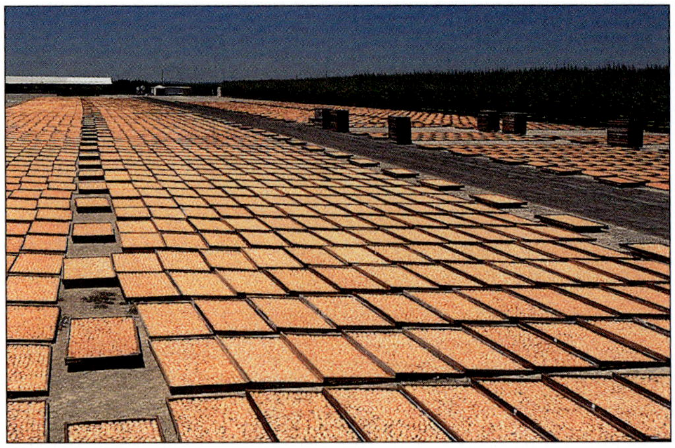

FIGURE 20.5 Drying fruits such as these apricots removes water and therefore prevents bacterial growth. *(© Inga Spence/Visuals Unlimited)*

food remains frozen. Freeze-drying is an expensive procedure; it is used to produce instant coffee and lightweight nonperishable meals such as those for backpackers and the military.

Addition of Solutes Solutes such as salt and sugar are food preservatives that prevent microbial growth by lowering water activity. Solutes reduce the availability of water because the high number of dissolved particles pulls water away from bacteria by osmosis. Salting is often used to preserve meat and fish. Meats preserved with salt are referred to as cured. Cured meats such as ham and salami are common in the modern diet and salt pork was a staple on the American frontier and could be kept through an entire winter. Sugar is also added to preserve foods and is responsible for the low water activity and long shelf life of jams and jellies.

Using food additives such as salt and sugar obviously has an impact on nutritional value, increasing the sodium and refined sugar content of the food. While these additives have increased the shelf life of many foods, they are a public health concern because the refined sugar and sodium content of the American diet exceeds recommendations (Figure 20.6).

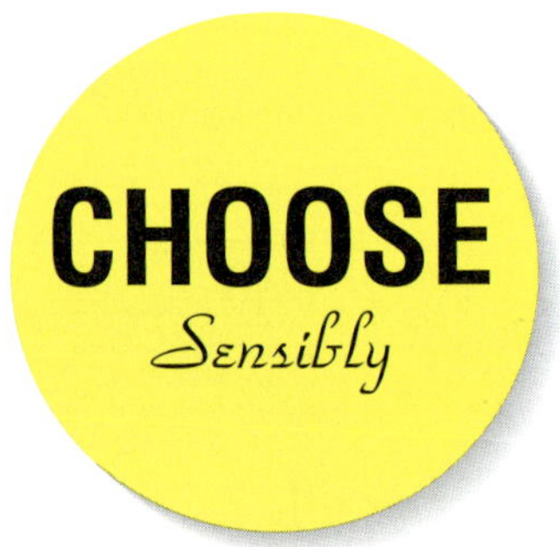

- Choose beverages and foods to moderate your intake of sugars
- Choose and prepare foods with less salt

FIGURE 20.6 The Dietary Guidelines for Americans recommends a diet moderate in sugars and salt.

Oxygen

Another factor that affects microbial growth is the presence of oxygen. Most microbes are aerobic, meaning they require oxygen for growth. Preservation techniques that limit oxygen availability, such as canning, prevent the growth of these microbes.

Canning The canning process places food in an airtight container and then, as discussed earlier, heats the container to a temperature that kills the bacteria in the food. If the container is not heated sufficiently, some bacteria may survive, but most cannot grow or reproduce because they require oxygen to do so. Unfortunately, there are also anaerobic bacteria, such as *Clostridium botulinum*, that grow better in low-oxygen environments. If these are present in a food and are not killed in the canning process, they can grow in the low-oxygen environment, and cause foodborne illness.

Modified Atmosphere Packaging Reducing the availability of oxygen is used to extend the shelf life of fresh refrigerated foods such as pasta, vegetables, fish, chicken, and beef. To make such foods—for example, beef teriyaki—the raw ingredients are sealed in plastic pouches, the air is vacuumed out, and the pouch and its contents are partially precooked and immediately refrigerated. In some products, the oxygen in the package is replaced with a gas such as carbon dioxide or nitrogen, in which microbes are unlikely to grow.[4] This is called **modified atmosphere packaging (MAP).** This type of processing eliminates the need for the extreme cold of freezing or the extreme heat of canning, so flavor and

Modified atmosphere packaging (MAP) A type of food packaging in which the gases inside the package control or retard chemical, physical, and microbiological changes.

nutrients are better preserved. Unlike canned foods, fresh refrigerated products are not heated to sufficient temperatures to kill all bacteria, and unlike frozen foods, they are not kept at temperatures low enough to prevent all bacteria from growing. However, the partial cooking and the removal of oxygen, as well as the fact that they are stored at refrigerator temperatures, prevent the growth of most bacteria. These foods should be used by the expiration date printed on the package, refrigerated constantly until used, and heated according to the time and temperature given on the package directions.

Chemical Preservatives

Chemical preservatives are used in food to maintain freshness and inhibit the growth of microorganisms. These food additives act in a number of different ways and target different types of microorganisms. For example, calcium propionate is an antifungal agent added to bread to prevent the growth of mold. Sodium benzoate is also an antifungal agent but is used in soft drinks, salad dressings, and cheeses. Sodium nitrite is an antibacterial agent that is used in bacon, ham, and hot dogs to prevent *Clostridium botulinum* spores from germinating. A list of chemical preservatives and their functions is included in Chapter 19.

Irradiation

Web Menu: For more information on food irradiation, go to the government food safety site at www.foodsafety.gov/ and search for food irradiation.

Irradiation A process in which foods are exposed to radiation to kill contaminating organisms and retard ripening and spoilage.

Irradiation, also called cold pasteurization, is a process that exposes food to high doses of X rays, gamma radiation, or high-energy electrons to kill microbes and inactivate enzymes thereby increasing safety and shelf life. The food is passed through an enclosed chamber called an irradiator, where it is exposed to a source of ionizing energy. The energy penetrates the food and the packaging, and most of it passes through, leaving no residue. The very small amount of energy that does not pass through the food is retained as heat. The dose of radiant energy used to treat a specific food is set at the lowest level necessary to achieve a specified result.

Irradiation is currently used in more than 40 countries in processing everything from frog legs to rice. It has been endorsed by the United Nations Food and Agriculture Organization, the World Health Organization, and the U.S. Food and Drug Administration (FDA), and it is one of the technologies singled out in the National Food Safety Initiative for its potential to improve the safety of food and reduce the incidence of foodborne illness.

Food irradiation has been used since the 1960s; wheat and wheat powder were approved for irradiation in 1963, and astronauts have eaten irradiated food since Apollo 17 went to the moon in 1972. Despite this, only a limited number of foods treated with irradiation have been sold in the United States; the bulk of what has been available is spices, herbs, and dried vegetable seasonings. Part of the reason for the limited use of irradiation is lack of irradiation facilities, but public fear and suspicion of the technology is also a major factor limiting the availability of irradiated foods. The word "irradiation" fosters the belief that the food itself becomes radioactive. Opponents to food irradiation claim that it introduces carcinogens, reduces the nutritional value of food, and is used to allow the sale of previously contaminated foods. In fact, irradiated food is not radioactive and there is no evidence to support the claim that it causes cancer. Scientific studies conducted over the past 50 years have found that the benefits of food irradiation outweigh any potential risks.[5]

Benefits Irradiation benefits consumers, retailers, and manufacturers by increasing the safety and shelf life of foods. The FDA has approved the use of irradiation to destroy pathogens in red meat and poultry and contaminants in spices; prevent insect infestation in flour and spices; increase the shelf life of potatoes; eliminate *Trichinella* in pork, *E. coli* in meat, and *Salmonella* in eggs; control insects in

TABLE 20.1 Foods Approved for Irradiation in the United States

Approval Year	Food	Purpose
1963	Wheat flour	Control mold
1964	White potatoes	Inhibit sprouting
1986	Pork	Kill *Trichinella* parasites
1986	Fruits and vegetables	Insect control, increase shelf life
1986	Herbs and spices	Sterilization
1990 (FDA)	Poultry	Reduce bacterial pathogens
1992 (USDA)	Poultry	Reduce bacterial pathogens
1997 (FDA)	Meat	Reduce bacterial pathogens
2000 (USDA)	Meat	Reduce bacterial pathogens
2000 (FDA)	Shell eggs	Reduce *Salmonella*

Adapted from Centers for Disease Control and Prevention. Frequently Asked Questions About Food Irradiation. Available online at **http://www.cdc.gov/ncidod/dbmd/diseaseinfo/foodirradiation.htm#whatis.**

fruits, vegetables, and grains; and slow the ripening and spoilage of some produce (Table 20.1). It may, therefore, be used in place of chemicals to reduce insect and microbial contamination and to slow ripening during food storage.[6] Irradiation increases the shelf life of fruits and vegetables by slowing the decay process (Figure 20.7). Irradiation of meat and poultry eliminates 99.9% or more of pathogens, thereby reducing the risk of foodborne illness from cross contamination or undercooking. Pathogens such as *Listeria, E. coli, Salmonella*, and *Staphylococcus aureus* are eliminated by irradiation. However, to destroy viruses such as hepatitis and Norwalk-like viruses that are associated with raw shellfish would require higher doses of irradiation than are currently approved.

Irradiation also benefits the environment. Spices that are not irradiated need to be fumigated with chemicals such as ethylene oxide to eliminate microbes. This chemical is being phased out for environmental and worker safety reasons. Irradiation prevents the spread of harmful insects when fruits and vegetables are transported, and it replaces chemical fumigants used to prevent insect infestation in rice and grains.

Irradiation kills almost all pathogens that are present in foods at the time of irradiation, but that is not a guarantee of safety. Irradiated food, just like any other food, can be unsafe if it is contaminated after it is irradiated or if it is not stored properly. Even when 99.9% of bacteria are killed, 0.1% can survive and

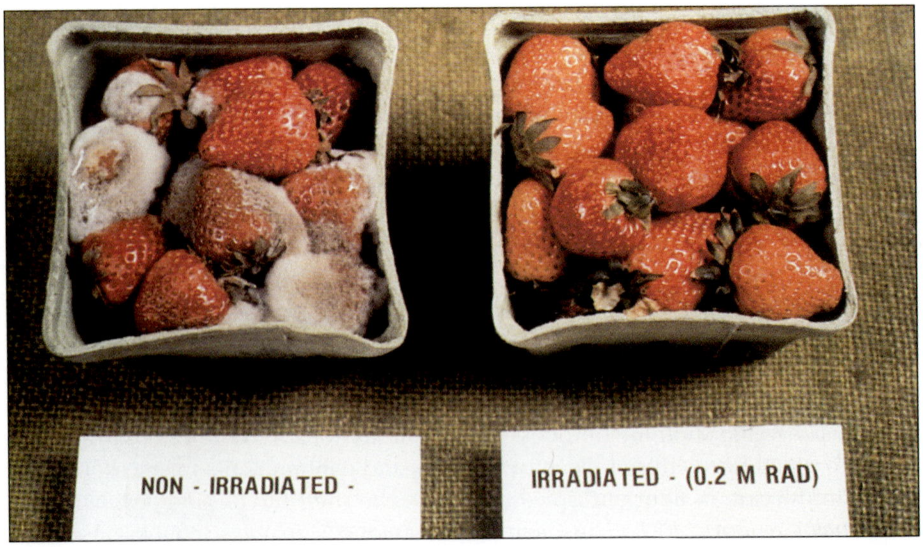

FIGURE 20.7 After two weeks in cold storage, the strawberries treated by irradiation remain free of mold (right), whereas the untreated strawberries picked at the same time are covered with mold (left). *(© Council for Agricultural Science and Technology)*

multiply if the food is stored improperly. For ensuring safe food, irradiation is not a replacement for proper food handling by producers, processors, and consumers.

Effect on Nutritive Value and Quality Irradiation does not compromise nutritional quality or noticeably change food texture, taste, or appearance as long as it is properly applied to a suitable product.[6,7] Because irradiation does not significantly raise the temperature of a food, nutrient losses are small and significantly less than losses that occur with canning, drying, heat pasteurization, and sterilization. Proteins, fats, and carbohydrates are not significantly altered by irradiation. The B vitamins and vitamin C are the nutrients most sensitive to losses. But, studies comparing irradiated with nonirradiated fruits have shown that the increase in losses due to irradiation are too small to affect the overall nutrient content of the diet.

Although the appearance and flavor of foods are generally not affected, irradiation does cause chemical changes to food. Studies done in multiple species and across multiple generations have found these changes to be benign. The free radicals and other compounds formed during irradiation have been determined to be the same as those formed when food is exposed to heat during other processing and cooking methods such as steaming, roasting, heat pasteurization, freezing, and canning.[6] No ill effects have been seen in humans consuming a diet made up almost entirely of irradiated foods.[8]

TREATED BY IRRADIATION

FIGURE 20.8 Foods treated with irradiation must display this symbol on their labels.

Labeling and Regulation Irradiated foods must be labeled with the radura symbol and the statement "treated with radiation" or "treated by irradiation" (Figure 20.8). Products that contain irradiated spices or other irradiated ingredients do not need to display this symbol, and irradiation labeling requirements do not apply to food served in restaurants.[7] Because irradiation produces changes in the chemistry of foods, it is treated as a food additive, and the level of radiation that may be used in the United States is regulated by the FDA and the Department of Agriculture (USDA).

Technology to Enhance the Food Supply

Technology is used to increase the amount of food produced and to improve the quality of food available. Like food preservation techniques, technology to improve the food supply is not new. Selecting and planting only the seeds from the hardiest plants and breeding only the strongest animals were early forms of technology used to enhance the food supply. As knowledge increased, specific plants could be selectively pollinated and animals artificially inseminated to assure the desired mixing of genetic material. More recently, **biotechnology** has been added to the tools available to enhance the food supply.

Biotechnology Processes that involve genetic engineering to alter—and, ideally, to improve—the characteristics of plants, animals, or other life-forms.

Genetics: From Genes to Traits

The characteristics of a plant or animal are carried in its genes. These genes, which are segments of DNA, can be passed from generation to generation. Genes contain the information that directs the synthesis of proteins. The specific proteins that are made then determine the traits that an individual organism displays.

DNA Structure DNA is a long, threadlike molecule consisting of two strands that twist around each other forming a double helix. Each strand has a backbone made up of alternating units of the sugar deoxyribose and phosphate groups. Each deoxyribose sugar is attached to a molecule called a base. There are four different bases that occur in DNA—adenine, thymine, cytosine, and guanine—that are

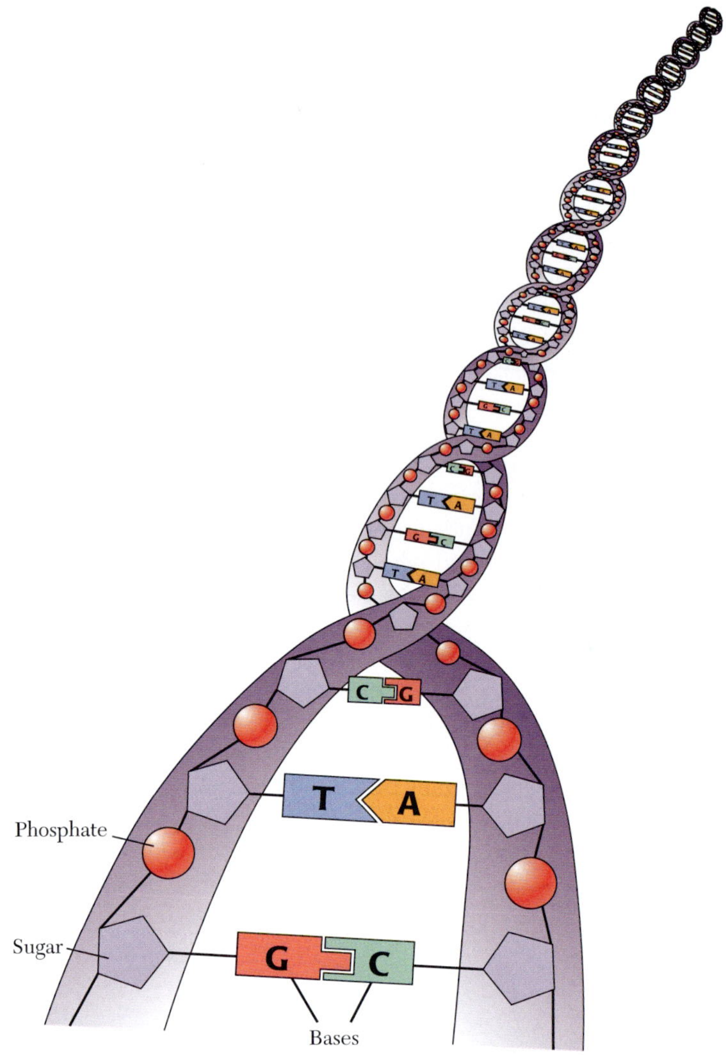

FIGURE 20.9 DNA is a double-stranded molecule. Each strand has a backbone that is made up of phosphate groups and the 5-carbon sugar deoxyribose arranged in an alternating pattern. Each sugar has one of four bases attached to it. The bases are adenine, thymine, cytosine, or guanine. The two strands of the DNA molecule are bonded together by the bases; adenine bonds to thymine and cytosine bonds to guanine. The two strands twist around one another to form a double helix.

usually abbreviated as A,T, C, and G, respectively (Figure 20.9). The bases bind to one another, connecting the two strands. Each base binds only to its complementary base: adenine to thymine and cytosine to guanine.

The DNA of all organisms—plants, bacteria, and animals, including humans—is made up of the same DNA bases. The differences in the sequence of bases are responsible for all of the genetic differences between living things, whether they are differences between species or differences between individuals of the same species. Different individuals of the same species have small differences in the base sequence in their DNA; only identical twins share the same base sequence. Organisms of different species, such as a human and a corn plant, have larger differences in the sequences of DNA bases.

Genes, Proteins, and Traits The sequence of bases present in a gene specifies the sequence of amino acids that will be present in a protein. If the gene is expressed, the protein is made, providing certain characteristics to the organism. For example, if a protein that stimulates growth is made, the organism will be bigger, and if a protein pigment is made, it will affect the color of the plant or animal. The presence or absence of specific proteins determines the traits that an individual organism displays (Figure 20.10).

Even though organisms of different species are very different, they may have genes with similar base sequences if they both need to make the same protein.

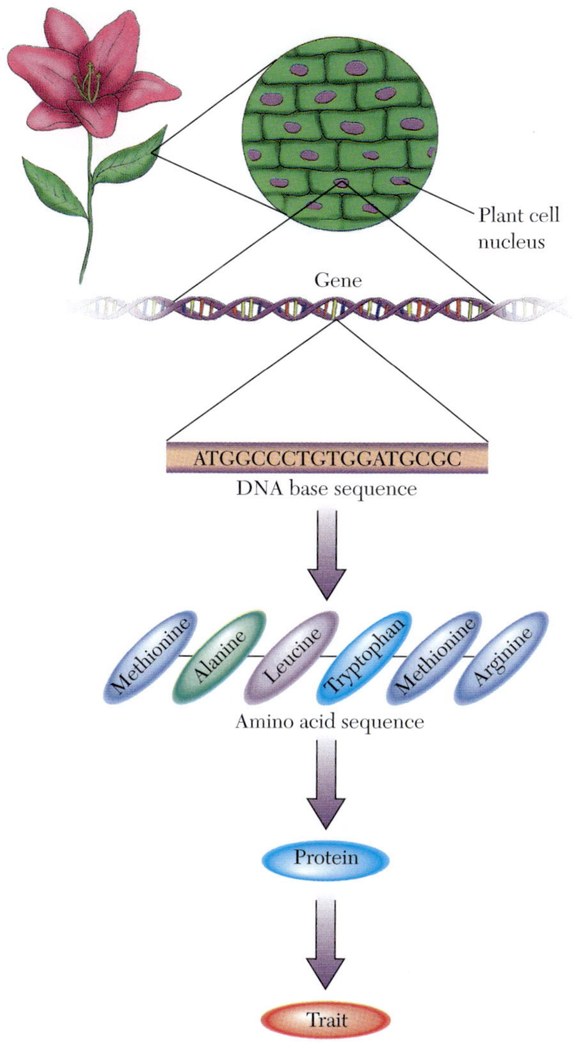

FIGURE 20.10 DNA, containing segments called genes, is located in the nuclei of plant and animal cells. The pattern of bases in genes codes for the sequence of amino acids that are joined to form proteins. These proteins are responsible for the traits an organism possesses.

For example, humans and pigs both rely on the protein hemoglobin to carry oxygen in the blood, so both humans and pigs have a gene with a very similar sequence of bases that codes for the protein hemoglobin. It is estimated that 25% of the genes found in plants are also present in humans, presumably because they code for proteins needed by both organisms.[9]

Traits Are Passed from Parent to Offspring When an organism reproduces, it passes its genes—and thus the instructions to make the protein coded for by each gene—to the next generation. When two organisms breed, some genes from each are passed to the offspring. The result is new combinations of genes and the traits for which they code. Over time, mutations can occur in the sequence of bases that make up the genes. Some of these mutations result in traits harmful to the organism, reducing its ability to survive and reproduce. Because the organism dies or cannot reproduce, the mutations are not passed on to the next generation. Other mutations result in beneficial traits, which allow the organism to survive more easily and thus to reproduce and pass on the altered genes. Over millions of years many genes have been changed by mutations, and those that code for beneficial traits have been passed on because the organisms carrying them have been able to reproduce. Both traditional plant and animal breeding and modern biotechnology take advantage of these natural genetic phenomena (see *Research Discoveries*: "The Birth of Biotechnology").

RESEARCH DISCOVERIES

The Birth of Biotechnology

In a delicatessen in Hawaii in 1972, over hot pastrami and corned beef sandwiches, a collaboration between Stanley Cohen of Stanford University and Herbert Boyer of the University of California at San Francisco was born. From this meeting of the minds and the pooling of research tools, the age of recombinant DNA was begun, and what we know of as the biotechnology industry was launched.[a]

At the time, Cohen's research focused on understanding the biology of plasmids. These small loops of DNA are found in bacteria and are separate from the main piece, or chromosome, of bacterial DNA (see figure). Plasmids can bestow the bacteria with extra traits that are not present in the chromosome, such as the ability to grow in the presence of an antibiotic. Plasmids float in the cytoplasm of bacterial cells and can replicate independently of the chromosome. At a conference in Hawaii, Cohen presented work that demonstrated that bacteria would take up plasmid DNA when treated with calcium chloride. Once inside the cell, the plasmid DNA was capable of reproducing, and when the cell divided, the offspring also contained the plasmid. Because all the descendants of a bacterial cell that takes up a plasmid contain a plasmid identical to the one that originally entered the cell, it was now possible to make copies or clones of the individual plasmid. Cohen could tell which cells contained the plasmid because the plasmids he used carried the trait for antibiotic resistance. When treated with the antibiotic, only the cells that contained the antibiotic resistance plasmid could survive. The trait of antibiotic resistance is still used in biotechnology today as a marker to identify cells that contain a plasmid with other genes of interest.

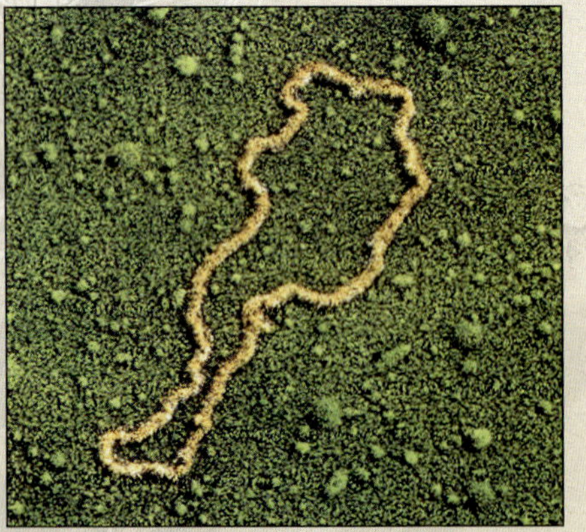

This electron micrograph shows a plasmid, which is a small loop of DNA found in bacterial cells. *(© Professor Stanley N. Cohen/SPL/Photo Researchers, Inc.)*

The work that Boyer presented at the same Hawaiian conference involved restriction enzymes isolated from *E. coli,* a common bacterium found in the gastrointestinal tract. These enzymes had the ability to cut DNA in specific locations in a way that made the ends easy to precisely paste together with the enzyme DNA ligase.

By combining their two techniques, Cohen and Boyer realized that fragments of DNA, produced by cutting DNA with Boyer's restriction enzyme, could be joined to plasmids, which could then be introduced into bacteria using the procedure developed in Cohen's lab. In this way, a new piece of DNA could be introduced into bacterial cells. The concept was straightforward, but no one knew whether DNA molecules constructed artificially would be able to code for proteins or reproduce in living cells.

After the Hawaii meeting, Cohen selected a small plasmid that carried resistance to the antibiotic tetracycline. Using Boyer's restriction enzyme, he cut the plasmid and mixed it with some other DNA fragments. The pieces were joined with DNA ligase to form new plasmids containing DNA from both the original tetracycline-resistant plasmid and from the DNA fragments. They called these recombinant plasmids "chimeras," after the mythical fire-breathing beast that possessed the head of a lion, the body of a goat, and the tail of a serpent. These chimera were then introduced into bacterial cells. By treating the cell culture with tetracycline, Cohen and Boyer were able to kill all bacteria except those that had acquired resistance from the plasmid. As the bacteria multiplied so did the plasmids, making copies of the inserted DNA. This technique of recombining DNA from different sources and cloning, or copying, the DNA is the basis for all genetic engineering.[b]

Cohen and Boyer continued their work and went on to demonstrate that DNA from animal cells could be transferred into bacteria and propagate there.[c] Subsequent work took this a step further, demonstrating that bacteria containing DNA transplanted from a mouse could produce a biologically active mouse cell protein.[d] This established that bacterial cells could be used as molecular manufacturing plants. Within a few years, the technique had been used to clone human insulin, which became the first recombinant DNA drug on the market.

By combining techniques developed in two different research laboratories, this collaboration built the foundation for an entire industry. What followed were multimillion-dollar companies and the development of genetically engineered medications to treat human disease and genetically modified crops and other products that impact the food supply.

References

[a] Access Excellence. Winding Your Way Through DNA, from Corned Beef to Cloning. Available online at **http://accessexcellence.org/AB/WYW/cohen/index.html.** Accessed 31 Oct 2000.

[b] Cohen, S. N., Chang, A. C., Boyer, H. W., and Helling, R. B. Construction of biologically functional bacterial plasmids *in vitro.* Proc. Natl. Acad. Sci. U.S.A. 70:3240–3244, 1973.

[c] Morrow, J. F., Cohen, S. N., Chang, A. C., et al. Replication and transcription of eukaryotic DNA in *Escherichia coli.* Proc. Natl. Acad. Sci. U.S.A. 71:1743–1747, 1974.

[d] Chang, A. C., Nunberg, J. H., Kaufman, R. J., et al. Phenotypic expression in *E. coli* of a DNA sequence coding for mouse dihydrofolate reductase. Nature 275:617–624, 1978.

Traditional Breeding versus Modern Biotechnology

Humans began to direct the genetic modification of plants and animals about 10,000 years ago when they were first domesticated. Almost every fruit, vegetable, or crop grown today has been in some way genetically modified using traditional **selective breeding** techniques. Some of these crops, such as pumpkins, potatoes, sugar beets, and varieties of corn, oats, and rice, would not have developed without human intervention. And this intervention has allowed us to produce more food that is more nutritious and can better withstand harsh environments and resist disease. Biotechnology is a more sophisticated, more powerful approach to genetic modification. While this tool, which rapidly alters the genetic makeup of organisms, has enormous potential for increasing the quantity and quality of the food supply, it has also created safety concerns.

For more information on traditional methods of plant breeding, and to try breeding your own variety of peas, go to www.sonic.net/~nbs/projects/anthro201/exper/.

Selective breeding Techniques to selectively control mating in plants and animals to produce organisms that better serve human needs.

Traditional Breeding Technology Farmers and ranchers have traditionally used the technique of selection to improve crops or livestock. Planting seeds from the best crops and breeding only the strongest animals allows the most desirable traits to be passed on to the next generation.

Plant breeders have also used **hybridization** to improve the characteristics of their crops. Hybridization is a process in which two related plants are cross-fertilized. The resulting offspring has characteristics from both parent plants. These methods introduce the genes for traits that add to the quality and productivity of various plants. For example, a breeder who wanted to produce a variety of wheat that was high-yielding and was resistant to cool temperatures would cross plants with these two traits.

Hybridization The process of cross-fertilizing two related plants with the goal of producing an offspring that has the desirable characteristics of both parent plants.

Crossbreeding of animals has a similar goal. Animal breeders use both inbreeding and outbreeding. Inbreeding involves crosses between closely related animals. It can intensify desirable traits but may also intensify undesirable traits. Outbreeding crosses unrelated animals to reduce undesirable traits, increase variability, and introduce new traits. Today, inbreeding and outbreeding are carried out by artificial insemination.

These techniques work well but they have limitations in terms of both time and outcome. Breeding generations of plants or animals to consistently produce a desired trait is time-consuming; a new trait can only be produced once in the reproductive cycle of the plant or animal. Another limitation is that only plants or animals of the same or closely related species can be interbred. In addition, not every offspring will inherit the desirable traits. Because crossbreeding transfers a set of genes from the parents to the offspring, both desirable and undesirable traits are transferred. Eliminating the undesirable genes while keeping the desirable ones can require many crosses (Figure 20.11).

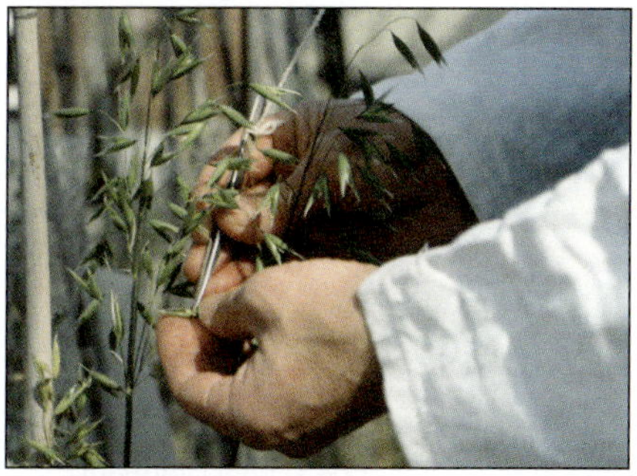

FIGURE 20.11 Cross-pollination, as shown in these oat seedlings, is a traditional method of plant breeding. *(© David Woodfall/Stone)*

Modern Biotechnology Modern biotechnology relies on the techniques of **recombinant DNA,** also referred to as genetic modification or genetic engineering, to alter the DNA of plants and animals to produce new traits or enhance desirable ones (Table 20.2). The techniques of modern biotechnology allow specific traits to be introduced to or eliminated from plants, animals, yeast, or bacteria. It often involves taking the gene for a desirable trait from one organism and transferring it to another.

Recombinant DNA DNA that is produced by joining DNA from different sources to create a unique combination of genes.

Methods of Biotechnology The bulk of biotechnology used in food production involves the genetic modification of plants. The first step in the production of a genetically modified plant is to identify a stretch of DNA, or gene, for a given desirable trait, such as resistance to a particular disease. This gene of interest could be from a plant, an animal, or a bacterial cell. The gene can be clipped out with specific DNA-cutting enzymes called restriction enzymes (see Chapter 6, *Research Discoveries*: "Manipulating Genes"). One of two different

TABLE 20.2 Terms Used in Genetic Engineering

Term	Definition
Biotechnology	Manipulating life-forms via genetic engineering to provide desirable products for human use.
Bioengineered foods	Foods that have been produced using biotechnology.
Chimera	A DNA molecule composed of DNA from two different species, or an organism consisting of tissues of diverse genetic constitution.
Cloning	Producing an exact duplicate of a gene or an organism.
DNA	A long threadlike molecule that carries the genetic information of an organism.
Gene	A unit of DNA that provides genetic information coding for a trait. It is the physical basis for the transmission of the characteristics of living organisms from one generation to another.
Gene splicing	The precise joining of DNA from different sources to create a new gene structure.
Genetic engineering	The selective, deliberate alteration of genes. It can be used to manipulate the genetic material of an organism in such a way as to allow it to produce new and different types of proteins. Other terms applicable to the same process are gene splicing, gene manipulation, genetic modification, or recombinant DNA technology.
Genome	The total complement of genetic information in an organism.
GM crops	Genetically modified crops.
GMO	Genetically modified organism.
Hybridization	The mating of different plants to increase vigor.
Plasmid	An independent, stable, self-replicating piece of circular DNA in bacterial cells. It is not a part of the normal cell genome.
Recombinant DNA	DNA that has been formed by joining the DNA from different sources.
Transgenic	An organism whose sperm or eggs contain genetic material originally derived from an organism other than the parents or in addition to the parental genetic material.

Plasmid A loop of bacterial DNA that is independent of the bacterial chromosome.

techniques can then be used to transfer the clipped gene into cells of the plant that is to be modified.[10] In one method the gene is pasted into, or recombined with, a loop of bacterial DNA called a **plasmid** (Figure 20.12). Plasmids have the ability to carry genes from one place to another. The plasmid, containing the gene of interest, is taken up by a bacterial cell. The bacterial cell can then transfer the gene to a plant cell. Once inside the plant cell, the new DNA migrates to the nucleus, where the gene for the new trait is integrated into the plant's DNA. The DNA is then referred to as recombinant DNA because the DNA from the plasmid has been combined with the plant's DNA. The second method used to get genes into cells involves painting the desired segment of DNA onto microscopic metal particles (see Figure 20.12). These are then loaded into a "gene gun" and shot into the plant cells. Once inside the cells, the DNA is washed off the metal particles by cellular fluids and migrates to the nucleus, where it is incorporated into the plant's DNA, forming recombinant DNA. The modified plant cells produced by either technique are then allowed to multiply. As they do, the new gene is reproduced with them. The cells are then placed in a special culture medium that allows them to differentiate into the different types of cells that make up a whole plant. Each new plant that grows contains the new gene and therefore the trait, such as disease resistance, coded for by that gene.

Advantages Modern biotechnology has two important advantages over traditional breeding techniques. First, it enables breeders to select, modify, and transfer single genes. This speeds up the process by reducing the time and cost of

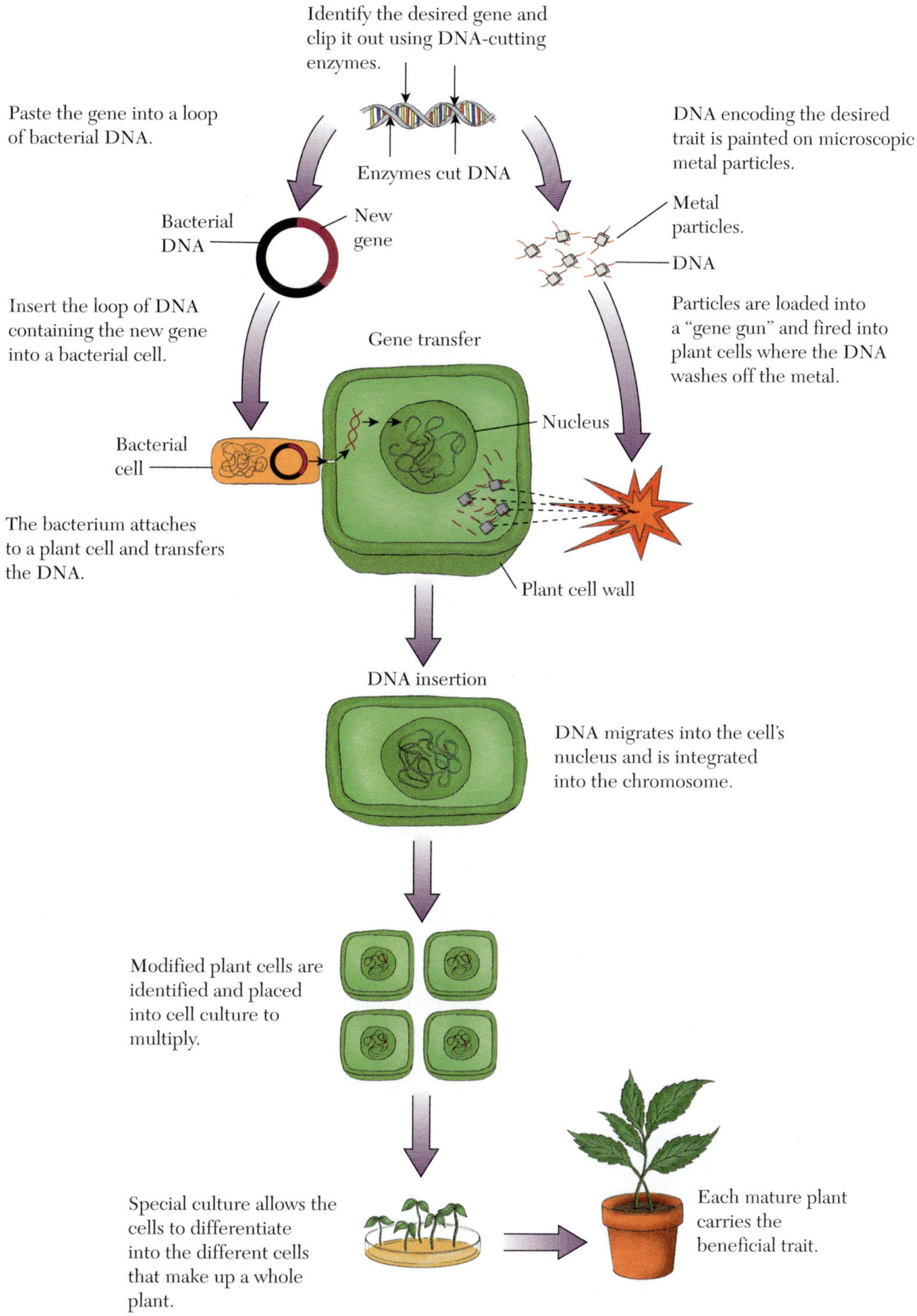

FIGURE 20.12 Two different techniques are used to transfer new genetic information into plant cells. For both, the first step is to isolate the stretch of DNA, or gene, that carries the desirable trait. In the method diagrammed on the left, bacterial plasmids and cells are used to transfer the gene into the plant cell. In the method diagrammed on the right, a "gene gun" is used to physically accelerate the DNA into the plant cells. Both methods can be used to produce plants that have new, beneficial, traits.

breeding the crosses that are needed to select out the undesirable traits. A second important advantage is that biotechnology can select desirable genes from any species because the DNA of plants, animals, yeast, and bacteria is the same. Biotechnology is not limited by whether two animals are capable of crossbreeding. Recombinant DNA allows traits from different species and completely different organisms to be used.

TABLE 20.3 Examples of Crops Produced by Bioengineering

Food	Alteration
Cherry tomato	Taste, color, texture
Flavr Savr tomato	Delayed ripening
Tomato	Thicker skin, altered pectin content
Corn	Insect protection, herbicide resistance
Cotton	Insect protection, herbicide resistance
Squash	Virus resistance
Papaya	Virus resistance
Potatoes	Potato beetle resistance, virus resistance
Soybeans	Herbicide resistance, high oleic content to reduce need for hydrogenation
Sugar beets	Herbicide resistance
Sunflower	High oleic acid content to reduce need for hydrogenation

Applications of Modern Biotechnology

The techniques of biotechnology can be used in a variety of ways in both production and processing to alter the quantity, quality, cost, safety, and shelf life of the food supply. This technology has great potential for addressing the problem of world hunger and malnutrition (Table 20.3). However, while genetic engineering has the potential to significantly improve the quality of the world's food supply, it is worth noting that many have concerns about the rapid advancement of these techniques and their impact on human health.

For more information on the applications, impact, and implications of genetic engineering, go to the Ag Biotech InfoNet at www.biotech-info.net/ or to the Council for Biotechnology Information at www.whybiotech.com/.

Improving Crop Yields Genetic modification of crops can increase yields either directly, by inserting genes that improve the efficiency with which plants convert sunlight into food, or indirectly, by creating plants that are resistant to herbicides, pesticides, and plant diseases, thus reducing crop losses. Scientists are also working to develop plants that can withstand drought, freezing, and salt toxicity. Many attempts in the last century to increase crop yields in developing countries have failed because they require expensive machinery and chemicals. With genetically engineered crops, simply providing a new type of seed can increase food production.

Herbicide Resistance Genes that impart herbicide resistance allow farmers to achieve weed-free fields with fewer pesticides. Crop yields are increased because there is less competition for soil resources. This benefits the farmers because they can produce more per acre, purchase fewer herbicides, and spray less often. It benefits consumers because the lower production costs and higher yields can translate into lower prices at the store. And, it benefits the environment because less tractor fuel is needed to spray herbicides and fewer farm chemicals are used.

Insect Resistance Genetic engineering techniques can increase insect resistance in plants. For example, a gene from the bacterium *Bacillus thuringiensis* produces a protein that is toxic to certain insects but safe for humans and other animals (Figure 20.13). By inserting the gene for this protein into plant cells, scientists have created plants that manufacture their own insecticide. The protein produced by this gene, known as Bt, has been used as an insecticide for over 30 years to control pests. But when plants manufacture their own insecticide, Bt does not need to be sprayed on the plants. This saves the farmer money, fuel, and time. It also benefits the environment because the Bt affects only insects feeding on the crop of interest and is not spread to surrounding foliage. Corn, potatoes, and cotton have been genetically modified to produce the Bt protein. During the first three years of commercial availability, cotton with the Bt gene reduced chemical insecticide use by 2 million pounds. Crops that are genetically modified to produce their own Bt cannot be labeled as organic (see *Critical Thinking*: "Organic versus Biotechnology").

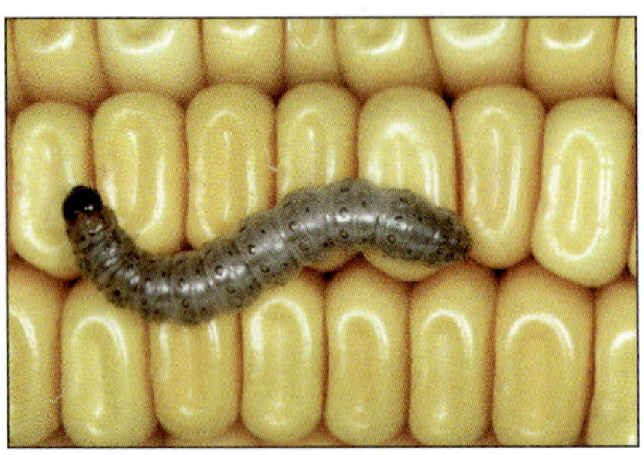

FIGURE 20.13 Biotechnology developments, such as plants containing the Bt protein, can reduce crop losses due to insect pests like this European corn borer. *(© Marlin E. Rice/Iowa State University)*

In addition to creating insect-resistant plants, genetic engineering has been used to create environmentally friendly pesticides. These pesticides are produced by bacteria, which are killed and then sprayed on plants. Thus these bacteria are used as a pesticide.

Disease Resistance Potato, squash, cucumber, watermelon, and papaya have been modified to resist viral infections.[11] This technology has helped to preserve the papaya crop in Hawaii, which was threatened by the ring spot virus. By inserting into the papaya a gene that acted like a vaccine, scientists were able to produce papaya plants that were immune to the virus (Figure 20.14).[12]

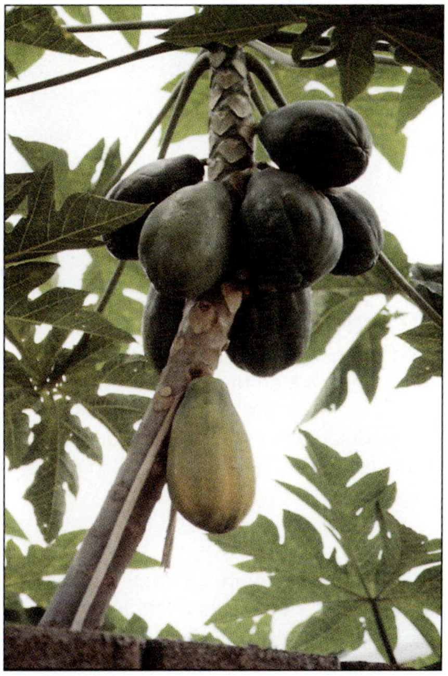

FIGURE 20.14 By inserting a gene that acts like a vaccine into the papaya plant scientists were able to produce plants that were immune to a deadly virus—saving Hawaii's papaya industry. *(© Denny Kaltreider/Visuals Unlimited)*

Improving Nutritional Quality Some of the major nutritional deficiencies worldwide are being addressed using genetically modified crops. To address protein deficiency, varieties of corn, soybeans, and sweet potatoes are being developed with higher levels of essential amino acids. To address iron deficiency, rice has been engineered to contain more iron.[13] To address vitamin A deficiency, genes that code for the production of enzymes needed for the synthesis of the vitamin A precursor beta-carotene have been inserted into rice.[14] Half of the world's population depends on rice as a dietary staple, but it is a poor source of vitamin A. The genetically modified rice, called Golden rice for the bronze color imparted by the beta-carotene pigment (Figure 20.15), provides enough beta-carotene to prevent vitamin A deficiency if just 300 g (about 2 cups) a day are consumed. This new rice is being distributed to public rice breeding institutions where local breeders can incorporate it into rice varieties that are grown for local consumption.[12]

Biotechnology is also being used to provide foods that may help prevent chronic disease. For example, genetic modification has produced a variety of soybeans that have a higher percentage of monounsaturated fat—a type of fat that may help reduce the risk of cardiovascular disease. Vegetable oils that have lower amounts of saturated fat are also being developed, as are oils that contain more of the antioxidant vitamin E than the traditional varieties.[15]

Other qualities that affect a food's role in the diet can also be changed by genetic engineering. For example, potatoes that are denser and have less water have been developed because they absorb less oil when fried—lowering the fat content of an order of french fries.

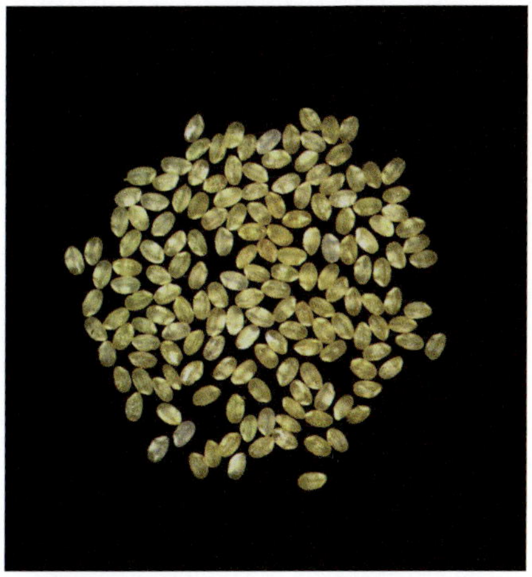

FIGURE 20.15 This genetically modified rice, called Golden rice, contains beta-carotene and could be used to help prevent vitamin A deficiency in regions where rice is a staple in the diet. *(Courtesy of Peter Beyer, University of Freiburg, Germany)*

Advancing Food Quality and Processing Genetic engineering is also being used to improve the appeal and quality of food. The first genetically modified whole food available on the market was the Flavr Savr tomato, introduced in 1994. In this case, rather than adding a gene, an existing gene for an enzyme that controls ripening was inactivated to slow the ripening process. This prolonged the tomato's shelf life and made it easier to harvest and transport.

Biotechnology is also used in food processing. For example, the enzyme preparation rennet, which is used in cheese production, used to be extracted from calf stomachs, but it is now also produced by genetically modified bacteria (Figure 20.16). About 60% of the hard cheese made in the United States is made with genetically engineered enzymes.[11] Other enzymes, such as those used in the production of high-fructose corn syrup and the enzyme lactase, which is used to reduce the lactose content of milk, are also produced by genetically modified microorganisms. Many food color and flavor additives are also produced in the laboratory. For example, vanilla can be produced by plant cells grown in culture.

Improving Food Safety Biotechnology can improve food safety by engineering foods in which naturally occurring allergens and antinutritional compounds have been reduced or eliminated. For example, people who are allergic to peanuts may someday enjoy peanut butter sandwiches made with peanuts that have been genetically modified to eliminate the proteins or portions of the proteins to which they are allergic.

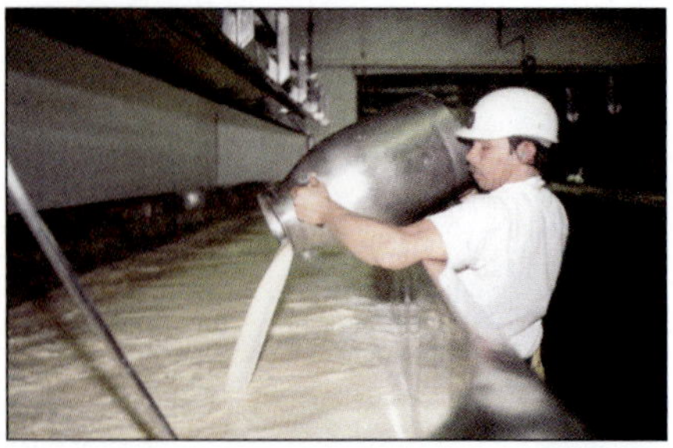

FIGURE 20.16 During cheese production, an enzyme preparation known as rennet is added to clot the milk. Much of the hard cheese produced in the United States today relies on rennet produced by genetically modified bacteria. *(© Inga Spence/Visuals Unlimited)*

Web Menu: For more information on human gene therapy, go to the Institute for Human Gene Therapy at health.upenn.edu/ihgt/.

Improving Animal Production Genetic engineering is being used to improve the prevention, diagnosis, and treatment of animal disease as well as to enhance growth efficiency and fertility in food animals. The first FDA-approved application of biotechnology in animal production was recombinant bovine somatotropin (bST) in dairy cows.[16] To produce recombinant bST, scientists isolated the gene from cow cells and then inserted it into bacterial cells. The bST, which is produced in large amounts by the bacterial cells, was then isolated, purified, and injected into dairy cows to increase milk production. Genetic engineering has also been used to increase growth rate in a species of Atlantic salmon. These fish grow to market weight in about 18 months, compared to 24 to 30 months for unmodified fish.[17]

Combating Human Disease Biotechnology has impacted human health and the treatment of disease in many ways. Cells from other organisms can be used to produce large amounts of human medicines. In 1978, bacteria were engineered to produce human insulin. Before this, diabetics relied on insulin extracted from pigs or cows. Other engineered proteins used to treat human disease include tissue plasminogen activator to dissolve blood clots in heart attack victims; growth factors to stimulate cell replication in bone marrow transplants; hepatitis B vaccine; and interferon to attack viruses and stimulate the immune system.

Critical Thinking

Organic versus Biotechnology

Padma is from India but has come to the United States for her college education. She has seen famine in her country and wants to learn more about biotechnology because she believes genetically modified foods can increase food production and help eliminate hunger and malnutrition in her country. Allen, her classmate, disagrees. He believes genetically modified foods have the potential to cause environmental damage. He promotes organic agricultural methods because he believes these foods are safer and that preserving the environment is the key to eliminating hunger.

Can organic farming help alleviate hunger?

A switch to organic farming would initially produce less food because more crops would be lost to insect pests and disease, but organic methods are more sustainable and ecologically sound. These methods help preserve the environment so food production can be sustained for future generations.

How can genetically modified crops help alleviate hunger and malnutrition?

Answer:

Padma argues that many genetically modified crops offer similar benefits to those produced organically. For example, the biological pesticide Bt can be used in organic farming. Some crops developed by genetic modification produce Bt on their own, so it does not need to be sprayed on the fields. Allen argues that harmful fertilizers and pesticides are still used when growing genetically modified crops, particularly those that have been modified in ways that do not target insect resistance.

Do you think that genetically modified crops raised using organic techniques should be considered organic? Why or why not?

Answer:

Regulation of Genetically Engineered Food Products

Although the federal government does not scrutinize every step of the development of new plant varieties, it is involved in overseeing the process. The government sets guidelines to help researchers address safety and environmental issues at all stages of the process, from the early development of genetically engineered plants through field-testing and, eventually, commercialization. Companies that develop new plant varieties must provide data to support the safety and wholesomeness of the product. Crops created by both traditional breeding and biotechnology methods must be field-tested for several seasons to make sure only desirable changes have been made. Plants are examined to ensure that they look right, grow right, and produce food that is safe and tastes right. Analytical tests must be performed to determine if the levels of nutrients in the new variety are different and if the food is safe to eat.[10] The FDA, the USDA, and the EPA are all involved in the oversight of plant biotechnology.

Food and Drug Administration The FDA has jurisdiction over the safety of foods in the marketplace and therefore regulates the safety and labeling of all foods and animal feeds derived from crops, including genetically modified crops. The FDA policy is that the safety of a food product should be determined based on the characteristics of the food or food product, not the method used to produce it. Foods developed using biotechnology are therefore evaluated to determine their equivalence to foods produced by traditional plant breeding. Emphasis is placed on whether the food creates a new or increased allergenic risk, has an increased level of a naturally occurring toxin, contains a substance not previously present in the food supply, or is nutritionally different from the traditional plant. Currently, premarket approval is required only when the new food contains substances not commonly found in foods or contains a substance that does not have a history of safe use in foods. However, the FDA has proposed a rule regarding plant-derived bioengineered foods that, if approved, would mandate that developers of such foods notify the FDA 120 days prior to the date at which they intend to market the food. The new rule would also require that specific information be submitted to help the FDA determine whether the foods pose any potential safety, labeling, or adulteration issues.[18]

U.S. Department of Agriculture The USDA regulates agricultural products and research concerning the development of new plant varieties. The Animal and Plant Health Inspection Service (APHIS) of the USDA helps to ensure that the cultivation of a new plant variety poses no risk to agricultural production or to the environment. For example, if there is a high probability that a new plant variety will crossbreed with a weed and that the transfer of the new trait could allow the weed plant to survive better, APHIS may not allow further development of this plant. If a plant has been studied and tested and does not pose environmental risks, field-testing is allowed. APHIS continues to oversee the testing until it is determined that the plant is safe.

Environmental Protection Agency The EPA regulates any pesticides that may be present in foods and sets tolerance levels for these pesticides. This includes genetically modified plants that are able to protect themselves from insects or disease. The EPA assesses the safety of the protein that confers the insect or disease resistance for human consumption, for other organisms, and for the environment.

For more information on the development and regulation of bioengineered foods, go to www.fda.gov/cvm/biotechnology/bioengineered.html or to the National Genetic Resources Program at www.ars-grin.gov/.

Safety of Genetically Modified Foods

In 1994, there were no genetically modified crops grown commercially anywhere in the world, but by 1998, over 70 million acres were cultivated in the United States, Australia, Argentina, Canada, and Mexico. In 1999, about half the American soybean crop and a quarter of the corn crop planted were genetically modified varieties (Figure 20.17).[10] There is some concern that the rapid advancement of these techniques has created the potential for both health problems and environmental damage.

Panels of scientists that have evaluated these concerns have concluded that the risks posed by agricultural products produced by modern biotechnology are the same as those for products produced by traditional plant breeding. And, thus far, experience has backed their conclusions. In the two decades since the emergence of agricultural biotechnology, genetically engineered food products have not been shown to cause harm to humans or to the environment.[11] And, there is good evidence that foods on the market are safe to eat after genetic modification.[19]

Despite this, others believe that conclusions regarding the environmental and the health impact of these relatively new products are premature and that the impact of this booming technology has not yet become apparent. They believe that lack of sufficient regulation over the science and the foods produced is creating risks. This issue was brought to the public's attention in 2000 when genetically modified corn that had not been approved for human consumption was used to make taco shells. The product had to be recalled from grocery shelves.[20] The taco shells caused no health problems but served to highlight the fact that it is difficult to identify the presence of genetically modified ingredients and to segregate crops at all aspects of food production.

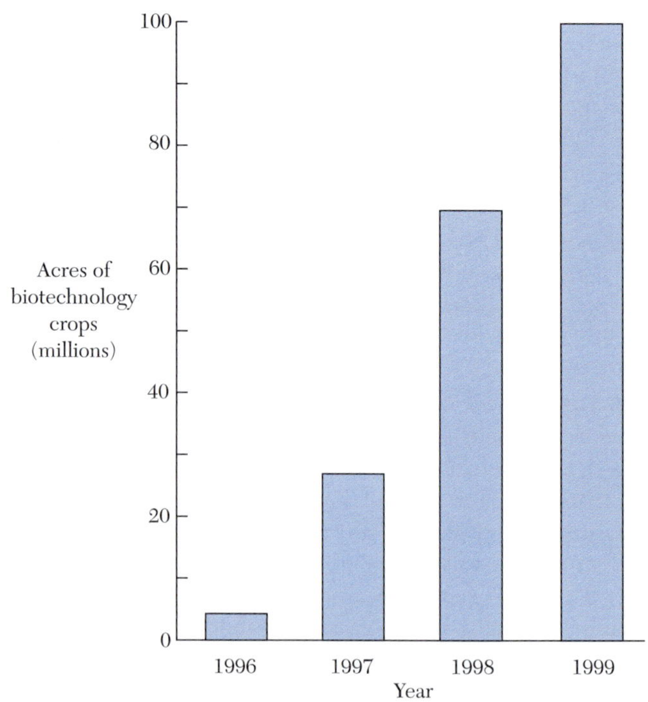

FIGURE 20.17 The use of genetically modified seeds has increased dramatically since 1996, when only 4.3 million acres of biotechnology crops were grown worldwide. *(Food and Ag Biotech. 1999 Acreage Data on Biotechnology Crops at* http://www.bio.org/food&ag/1999Acreage.html).

Opposition to genetically engineered foods is greater in Europe than in the United States. In 1998, U.S. farmers lost $200 million in corn sales to the European Union because the corn contained genetically modified varieties not approved for use in the European Union.

Consumer Safety Safety concerns related to bioengineered foods include the possibility that an allergen or toxin may have inadvertently been introduced into a previously safe food, or that the nutrient content of a food has been negatively affected. When these issues are a possibility, the food must be labeled to alert consumers. Another potential health concern is that the antibiotic resistance genes used in biotechnology may promote the development of antibiotic-resistant strains of bacteria.

Allergens and Toxins Genes code for proteins, so when a new gene is introduced into a food product, a new protein is made. If this new protein is an allergen, allergic individuals will now react to a food that was previously safe for them. Proper testing for the transfer of allergens is important in maintaining a safe food supply. For example, as was mentioned earlier, allergy testing successfully prevented soybeans containing a gene from a Brazil nut from entering the market (Figure 20.18).[1] However, despite mandatory testing programs, individuals with food allergies cannot assume that new foods are safe.

Similar policy is in place for toxins. When a product is created using either a donor or recipient organism that is known to produce a toxin, the manufacturer must verify that the resulting product does not have high levels of the toxin. Toxins are also an issue when plants are produced by traditional breeding. For example, toxic varieties of celery and potatoes have resulted from traditional breeding methods.

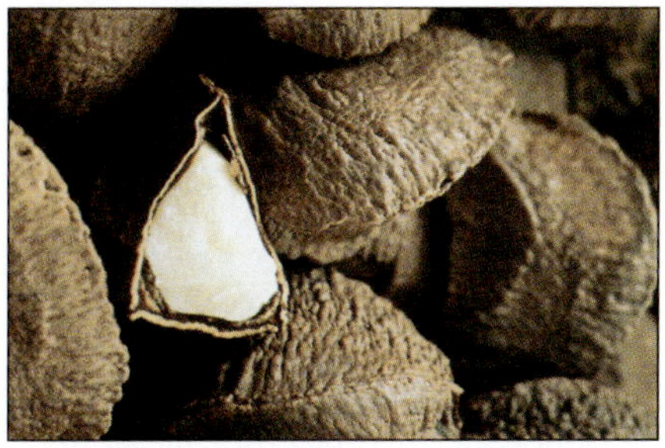

FIGURE 20.18 DNA from Brazil nuts, such as those shown here, was introduced into soybeans to enhance their protein content. Unfortunately, the resulting soy contained an allergen that could cause reactions in people allergic to nuts. *(© Steve Taylor/Stone)*

Labeling of Genetically Modified Foods Foods containing ingredients derived from plant biotechnology are not required to carry special labels unless they pose a potential risk. The introduction of an allergen or toxin is considered a potential risk. For example, if DNA from fish or peanuts—foods that commonly cause allergic reactions—was introduced into tomatoes or corn, these foods would have to be labeled. However, if the manufacturer can prove the food does not cause allergies, the label would not need to warn consumers. Another potential risk would be a significant change in nutrient content. For example, tomatoes are an excellent source of vitamin C. If a tomato were developed that had no vitamin C, it would have to be labeled to disclose this information. Foods and ingredients created by genetic engineering cannot be labeled as organic (see Chapter 19).[21] (See *Making Decisions*: "Labeling for Genetically Modified Foods")

Antibiotic Resistance There is a concern that the use of genetic engineering will spread antibiotic resistance traits to bacteria in the environment or the gut. If pathogenic bacteria were to acquire this trait, it would make some of the antibiotics used to treat disease ineffective. The reason for this concern is that genetic engineering techniques use antibiotic resistance genes as marker genes. By inserting a marker gene along with the gene they want to transfer, scientists are able to check to see that the gene transfer was successful. Antibiotic resistant genes are used for this purpose because it is easy to verify that the transfer has occurred by exposing the bacteria to antibiotics—those that survive the antibiotic contain the transferred genes. Current techniques are unlikely to cause problems because the marker genes used are already widespread in the normal bacteria that inhabit the gut and in harmless environmental bacteria. In addition, markers are not used if they confer resistance to clinically important antibiotics.[10] Newer techniques are under development that will remove the antibiotic resistance markers before the plants leave the laboratory.[22]

Web Menu For more information on antibiotic resistance, go to the National Antimicrobial Resistance Monitoring System at www.fda.gov/cvm/index/narms/narms_pg.html.

Making Decisions

Labeling for Genetically Modified Foods

Should foods containing ingredients made by genetic modification be specially labeled? The FDA currently requires special labels only on foods containing genetically modified ingredients that pose a potential risk to consumers. But, some people feel that all foods containing genetically modified ingredients should be labeled as such.

Proponents of mandatory labeling argue that many consumers want to know if a food contains a genetically modified ingredient regardless of whether a potential risk has been identified. They feel access to this information is a consumer right and that the reasons for knowing whether a food is genetically modified may be ethical or philosophical and unrelated to the quality or safety of the food. Others favor labeling because they believe it would help ensure that the regulatory measures set up to protect consumer and environmental safety are working. In the event of a food-related incident, such as an allergic reaction, labeling would help to track its source in the food supply. Opponents of mandatory labeling believe that labeling all genetically modified foods would be misleading to the consumer. Even foods that are not different in quality, nutrient composition, and safety would be viewed as somehow different from the traditional food. Ethical, religious, and economic issues are all involved in deciding which foods should be labeled.

Ethical and Religious Issues Can a tomato that contains some DNA from a fish be included in a vegan diet? Is corn that contains DNA from a pig appropriate for Jews and Muslims to eat? The FDA currently believes that the answer to these questions is yes, since plants and animals already share some of the same DNA segments.[a] Jewish organizations agree with this and have taken the position that a single gene or even several genes transferred from an animal or shellfish source do not embody the essence of the being and creates no automatic conflict with a kosher diet. Despite this, some have suggested that foods developed with the use of animal- or shellfish-derived genes be specially labeled for kosher and vegetarian dietary requirements.[b]

Economic Issues Labeling will increase costs at many levels. There are hundreds, if not thousands, of food products that contain genetically modified ingredients and would therefore need to be labeled. For example, products such as cake mixes and margarine contain ingredients from corn and soybeans and other commodity crops that have been improved through biotechnology. Even the cheese on a pizza could be subject to labeling under a mandatory system. In order to label genetically modified foods as such, DNA-modified plants would need to be segregated during planting and harvesting and products containing ingredients from these plants would require different manufacturing, transport, and storage facilities. Despite this, the need to sell to markets such as the European Union that do not want genetically modified crops may force U.S. farmers to keep genetically modified crops segregated and labeled.

The Role of the FDA The FDA is responsible for the labeling of all foods. Historically, when considering the safety and labeling of foods, the FDA has focused on the characteristics of a food, not on how it is produced. Virtually all plants have been genetically modified through traditional plant breeding, and the FDA does not require declarations regarding these modifications. Under this precedent, labeling decisions are based on whether there are differences between the new food and the traditional food. Labeling of foods containing genetically modified ingredients is therefore only required if the nutritional composition of the food has been altered; if it contains potentially harmful allergens, toxins, pesticides, or herbicides; if it contains ingredients that are new to the food supply; or if it has been changed significantly enough that its traditional name no longer applies. If the consumer's right to know leads to mandatory labeling of genetically modified foods, it would represent a shift in regulatory precedent that might ultimately impact the labeling of other types of foods.

An Appropriate Label Designing an appropriate label is a complex issue. Some companies are voluntarily labeling foods as "Grown from genetically modified seed." The FDA feels that these simple labels will imply to some people that the product is inherently better than other products, while other people will feel this means that the food is more dangerous than others. However, a more detailed label that describes the way that a particular product was modified would be too lengthy and would not be understood by many consumers. Regardless of whether labeling of all food products containing genetically modified ingredients becomes mandatory, guidance about labeling is important to assure that the label provides the information consumers need without being misleading.

References

[a] Kendall, P. Food biotechnology: boon or threat? J. Nutr. Ed. 29:112–115, 1997.
[b] Center for Consumer Research. Biotechnology Questions and Answers. Available online at **http://ccr.ucdavis.edu/biot/index.html.** Accessed 29 Oct 2000.

Environmental Concerns One of the arguments against the use of these foods is that they will harm the environment by reducing diversity, promoting the evolution of pesticide-resistant insects and creating "superweeds" that will overgrow our agricultural and forest lands.

Diversity If every farmer begins to use only genetically modified rice, then the varieties of rice that carry other traits will die off and those traits will be lost. (This process also occurs when plants produced by traditional breeding are used to the exclusion of others.) Farmers prefer the new resistant, high-yielding varieties and stop planting other varieties, causing them to eventually become extinct. This is a concern because the ability of populations of organisms to adapt to new conditions, diseases, or other hazards depends on the presence of many different species that provide a diversity of genes. To preserve diversity and ensure a large supply of traits for use in future breeding, molecular biology techniques are being applied to establish gene banks and seed banks and to identify and characterize the genes in many species. The USDA maintains the National Plant Germplasm System, which contains seeds for over 400,000 varieties of plants that are no longer in use or were never grown commercially.[23] These precautions are designed to help prevent genes from being lost, but they will not prevent our agricultural land from being dominated by only a few varieties of crops.

Superweeds and Superbugs Another environmental concern that has been raised with regard to genetically modified crops is that they will promote the development of superweeds and superbugs. A superweed might arise if a plant that has been modified to grow faster or to better survive begins growing in areas beyond the farmer's field. Most experts do not feel this is a major concern because domesticated crops depend on a managed agricultural environment and carry traits that make them unable to compete in the wild.[11]

It has also been suggested that the genes inserted to produce hardy, high-yield, fast-growing crops can be transferred to wild relatives by natural cross-breeding. This could result in fast-growing superweeds. Although a possibility, this scenario is unlikely for a number of reasons. First, the probability that a weed growing near a genetically modified plant is closely enough related to crossbreed is small. Even if it does occur, the chances that the new plant will survive and have inherited traits that enhance its survival is even smaller. As a further safeguard to prevent environmental risks, most developers avoid adding traits that could increase the competitiveness or other undesirable properties of weedy relatives.

There is also concern that crops engineered to produce pesticides will promote the evolution of pesticide-resistant insects. Although this is an important concern, the risk of it occurring is no greater for such crops than it is for pesticides that are sprayed on crops. An illustration of this problem involves insects that are resistant to the Bt toxin. As more and more of the insect's food supply is made up of plants that produce this pesticide, only insects that carry genes making them resistant to Bt can survive and reproduce. This increases the number of Bt-resistant insects and therefore reduces the effectiveness of Bt as a method of pest control. It has been reported that 1 in 350 tobacco budworms, a major cotton pest, carry a gene for resistance to the Bt toxin.[24] To address this problem, strategies are being developed to prevent the number of Bt-resistant insects from increasing. Farmers who grow pesticide-resistant crops are required to grow nonmodified plants in adjacent fields. This provides a food supply for—and encourages the continued existence of—nonresistant insect pests, thereby reducing the likelihood that the number of pesticide-resistant insects will increase.[11]

Summary

1. Technology has been used for centuries to improve the quantity and quality of the food supply. Some old techniques are still used today, and new techniques have been developed.
2. Traditional methods of food preservation involve changing the temperature, pH, atmosphere, and water availability in foods.
3. Both heat and cold can be used to improve the safety of food. High temperatures used in cooking, canning, heat pasteurization, and sterilization kill microorganisms. Cold temperatures used in refrigeration and freezing slow or prevent microbial growth.
4. Because most bacteria grow best at a neutral pH, raising or lowering pH can help prevent bacterial growth. During

fermentation, bacteria produce acids, which inhibit the growth of harmful bacteria.
5. Water activity is a measure of the amount of water available in a food. Reducing water activity by drying or by adding salt, sugar, or other solutes prevents spoilage because bacteria need water to survive.
6. Reducing exposure to oxygen can prevent the growth of aerobic bacteria. Oxygen availability is reduced by canning and by newer techniques such as modified atmosphere packaging. Some bacteria are anaerobic and so can grow in a low-oxygen environment.
7. Irradiation preserves food by exposing it to X rays or high-energy electrons, which kill microorganisms, destroy insects, and slow the germination and ripening of fruits and vegetables. Irradiation has little effect on the nutritive value of food, and irradiated foods are carefully regulated.
8. New varieties of plants and animals and new food products can be produced by traditional breeding methods or genetic engineering. Genetic engineering alters the DNA of plants or animals to produce new varieties with desired traits, such as disease resistance, increased nutrient content, or delayed spoilage.
9. Genetic engineering has been used to improve crop yields by producing plants that are resistant to insects and herbicides and better able to withstand adverse environmental conditions. Genetic engineering is also used to improve the nutritional composition, flavor, and storage properties of plant products, and to combat human and animal disease.
10. Careful monitoring and regulation of genetic engineering and the products produced by this technology help to ensure its safety. Despite existing regulation, there is concern that genetic engineering poses risks both to human health and to the environment. Health concerns include the possibility that an allergen or toxin may be introduced into a food, or that the nutrient content of a food has been negatively affected. The possibility of antibiotic resistance being introduced into pathogenic bacteria is also an issue. Environmental concerns include the possibility that this technology may contribute to a reduction in biological diversity, the evolution of pesticide-resistant insects, and the creation of superweeds.

Review Questions

1. List some ways in which food processing reduces foodborne illnesses.
2. Define "water activity" and give an example of how it is used in food preservation.
3. Identify some methods of food packaging that preserve food by reducing exposure to oxygen.
4. Explain how irradiation is used to preserve food. Is it safe?
5. Describe how food irradiation is regulated in the United States.
6. Describe how biotechnology can be used to improve the food supply.
7. Compare and contrast the use of traditional breeding and modern biotechnology to develop superior products.
8. How does genetic engineering introduce new traits into plants or animals?
9. List some ways in which genetic engineering is being used to enhance the food supply.
10. List some potential risks associated with genetic modification.

Applying Critical Thinking Skills

Personal nutrition:

1. Assume you live in a cold climate with a limited growing season. Describe how your diet would change if you lived without the following technologies:
   a. Refrigeration.
   b. Canning.
   c. Pesticides.
   d. Refrigerated trucks to transport foods.
   e. Packaged convenience food.
   f. Irradiation.
2. Using one day of the food intake record you kept in Chapter 2, list the food preservation methods used for each component of your diet.
   a. What are the benefits of each?
   b. List any risks associated with each.

General nutrition issues:

1. A new plant variety has just been developed. This plant provides iron in a readily absorbable form. It is being introduced as a staple of the diet in a developing country.
   a. What are the potential benefits of this product?
   b. What are the potential risks?
2. Plan a debate around these questions:
   a. Is irradiated food safe to eat?
   b. Does irradiated food create an environmental hazard?
   c. Are genetically engineered foods safe for human consumption?
   d. Are genetically engineered plants safe for the environment?

References

1. Nordlee, J. A., Taylor, S. L., Townsend, J. A., et al. Identification of a Brazil-nut allergen in transgenic soybeans. N. Engl. J. Med. 334:688–692, 1996.
2. Gould, G. W. Methods of preservation and extension of shelf life. Int. J. Food Microbiol. 33:51–64, 1996.
3. Birds Eye Co. A Man Named Birdseye: A Company History. Available online at **http://www.birdseye.com/about.html**. Accessed 1 Nov 2000.
4. Marth, E. H. Scientific Status Summary: extended-shelf-life refrigerated foods: microbiological quality and safety. Food Technol. 52:57–62, 1998.
5. U.S. General Accounting Office. Food Irradiation: Available Research Indicates That Benefits Outweigh Risks. Washington D.C., August, 2000. Available online at **http://www.foodsafety.gov/~fsg/irradiat.html**. Accessed 6 March, 2001.
6. American Dietetic Association. Position paper of the American Dietetic Association: food irradiation. J. Am. Diet. Assoc. 100:246–252, 2000.
7. Henkel, J. Irradiation: a safe measure for safer food. FDA Consumer 32:12–17, May/June 1998.
8. Diehl, J. F. *Safety of Irradiated Foods.* New York: Marcel Dekker, 1995.
9. Cook, J. R. Testimony before the U.S. House of Representatives Subcommittee on Basic Research hearing on "Plant Genome Research: From the Lab to the Field to the Market." October 5, 1999, Serial No. 106-60. Government Printing Office, Washington, D.C., 1999.
10. Thompson, L. Are bioengineered foods safe? FDA Consumer 18–23, Jan./Feb. 2000.
11. Smith, N. Seeds of opportunity: an assessment of the benefits, safety and oversight of plant genomics and agricultural biotechnology. U.S. House of Representatives report, 13 Apr 2000. Available online at **http://www.house.gov/science/documents.htm.** Accessed 25 Oct 2000.
12. McHughen, A. *Biotechnology and Food*, 2nd ed. New York: American Council on Science and Health, 2000.
13. Goto, F., Yoshihara, T., Shigemoto, N., et al. Iron fortification of rice seed by the soybean ferritin gene. Nat. Biotechnol. 17:282–286, 1999.
14. Ye, X., Al-Babili, S., Kloti, A., et al. Engineering the provitamin A (beta-carotene) biosynthetic pathway into (carotenoid-free) rice endosperm. Science 303–305, 2000.
15. Shintani, D., and DellaPenna, D. Elevating the vitamin E content of plants through metabolic engineering. Science 282:2098–2100, 1998.
16. American Dietetic Association. Position of the American Dietetic Association: biotechnology and the future of food. J. Am. Diet. Assoc. 95:1429–1432, 1995.
17. Lewis, C. Kind of fish story: the coming of biotech animals. FDA Consumer 35:15–20, Jan./Feb. 2001.
18. U.S. Department of Health and Human Services. FDA to strengthen premarket review of bioengineered foods. HHS News, May 3, 2000. Available online at **http://www.fda.gov/bbs/topics/NEWS/NEW00726.html.** Accessed 27 Oct 2000.
19. National Academy of Sciences, National Research Council. *Genetically Modified Pest-Protected Plants: Science and Regulation.* Washington, D.C.: National Academy Press, 2000.
20. FDA Recalls and Field Corrections of Foods Class I Enforcement Report. November 1, 2000. Available online at **http://www.fda.gov/bbs/topics/enforce/enf00666.htm#Star.** Accessed 15 Dec 2000.
21. U.S. Department of Agriculture, Agricultural Marketing Service, National Organic Program. Final Rule. Available online at **http://www.ams.usda.gov/nop/nop2000/nop/finalrulepages/finalrulemap.htm.** Accessed 1 March 2001.
22. Iamtham, S., and Day, A. Removal of antibiotic resistance genes from transgenic tobacco plastids. Nat. Biotechnol. 18:1172–1176, 2000.
23. National Plant Germplasm System. Available online at **http://www.ars-grin.gov/npgs/.** Accessed 6 Mar 2001.
24. Prakash, C. S. Boom and bust of insect resistant *Bt* Cotton? ISB NewsReport, July 1997. Available online at **http://www.biotech-info.net/boom.html.** Accessed 6 Mar 2001.

Appendices

Appendix A

Nutrient Composition of Foods

Key: Qty = quantity; Meas = measurement; Wgt = weight; Wtr = water; Cals = kcalories; Prot = protein; Carb = carbohydrate; Fib = fiber; SatF = saturated fat; MonoF = monounsaturated fat; PolyF = polyunsaturated fat; Choles = cholesterol; Calc = calcium; Phos = phosphorus; Sod = sodium; Pot = potassium; Zn = zinc; Magn = magnesium; VitA = vitamin A; VitE = vitamin E; VitC = vitamin C; Thia = thiamin; Ribo = riboflavin; Nia = niacin; B6 = vitamin B6; Fola = folate; B12 = vitamin B12.

Food Item	Qty	Meas	Wgt (g)	Wtr (g)	Cals	Prot (g)	Carb (g)	Fib (g)	Fat (g)	SatF (g)
Ac'cent flavor enhancer	0.25	tsp	1	—	0	0	0	0	0	0
Acorns, dried	1	oz.	28	1	144	2	15	1.2	9	1.2
Allspice, ground	0.25	tsp	0	0	1	0	0	0.1	0	0
Almond butter, honey+cinnamon	2	Tbs	31	1	188	5	8	1.2	16	1.6
Almond butter, plain, salted	2	Tbs	31	0	198	5	7	1.2	18	1.8
Almond butter, plain, unsalted	2	Tbs	32	0	203	5	7	1.2	19	1.8
Almond chicken	0.5	cup	121	93	137	10	9	1.9	7	1
Almond meal, partially defatted	1	oz.	28	2	116	11	8	1	5	0.5
Almond paste, packed	2	Tbs	28	4	131	3	14	1.4	8	0.8
Almond, dried, unblanched, whole	0.25	cup	36	2	209	7	7	3.9	18	1.8
Almond, dry roasted, unsalted, whole	0.25	cup	34	1	203	6	8	4.7	18	1.7
Almonds, blanched, slices	0.25	cup	26	1	154	5	5	1.8	14	1.3
Almonds, blanched, whole	0.25	cup	36	2	212	7	7	2.4	19	1.8
Almonds, blanched, whole	0.25	cup	36	2	222	8	7	4.8	18	—
Almonds, dried, unblanched, chopped	0.25	cup	32	1	191	6	7	3.5	17	1.6
Almonds, dried, unblanched, slivered	0.25	cup	34	1	199	7	7	3.7	18	1.7
Almonds, dry roasted, salted	0.25	cup	34	1	203	6	8	4.7	18	1.7
Almonds, dry roasted, whole	0.25	cup	34	1	206	7	7	3.7	18	1.5
Almonds, natural, whole	0.25	cup	36	2	213	7	7	4.4	18	1.3
Almonds, oil roasted, blanched	0.25	cup	36	1	218	7	6	4	20	1.9
Almonds, oil roasted, salted	0.25	cup	39	1	243	8	6	4.4	23	2.2
Almonds, oil roasted, unsalted	0.25	cup	39	1	243	8	6	4.4	23	2.2
Almonds, oil roasted, whole	0.25	cup	39	1	244	9	5	3.7	23	1.7
Almonds, whole, toasted	1	oz.	28	1	167	6	6	3.2	14	1.4
Amaranth leaves, cooked, drained	0.5	cup	66	60	14	1	3	1.2	0	0
Amaranth leaves, raw, chopped	0.5	cup	14	13	3	0	1	0.2	0	0
Amaranth, grain	0.5	cup	98	10	365	14	64	14.8	6	1.6
Amaranth, raw leaf	1	each	14	13	3	0	1	0.2	0	0
Anise seed	1	tsp	2	0	8	0	1	0.3	0	0
Annatto seed	1	oz.	28	3	102	4	19	10.2	1	—
Apple brown betty	0.75	cup	155	96	264	4	46	3.8	8	4.2
Apple butter	1	Tbs	17	10	30	0	7	0.3	0	0
Apple crisp, recipe	1	cup	282	173	460	5	91	4.8	10	2.1
Apple dumpling	1	each	190	62	670	7	84	2.9	35	8.6
Apple juice, canned/bottled	1	cup	248	218	117	0	29	0.2	0	0

This table of food composition has been prepared for Harcourt, Inc. and is copyrighted by ESHA Research in Salem, Oregon, developer and publisher of The Food Processor® and Genesis™ nutrition and labeling software systems. The table includes nutrient data for over 3900 foods, including brand-name items, ethnic foods, vegetarian products, nonfat and low-sodium alternatives, baby foods and formulas, and a large selection of common food items. The foods are presented alphabetically with corresponding units of measure. Over 1000 sources of scientific information are researched to provide the most accurate, reliable data available. Government sources of information are the base for all the data: the USDA Handbook series and its current supplemental data, as well as current data from both published and unpublished provisional data. Even with all the government data available, there are still missing values for some nutrients. Dashes in the table appear where there are no data available. Considerable effort has been made to report the most accurate data available and to eliminate missing values. Please be advised that the folate values in this table include the amount added in fortification for all non–brand-name items. Values for brand-name items may or may not include added folic acid. The authors welcome any suggestions or comments for future editions.

MonoF	PolyF	Choles	Calc	Phos	Sod	Pot	Zn	Iron	Magn	VitA	VitE	VitC	Thia	Ribo	Nia	B6	Fola	B12
(g)	(g)	(mg)	(mg)	(mg)	(mg)	(mg)	(mg)	(mg)	(mg)	(μg RE)	(mg α-TE)	(mg)	(mg)	(mg)	(mg)	(mg)	(μg)	(μg)
0	0	0	0	—	160	—	—	0	—	0	—	0	—	—	—	—	—	0
5.6	1.7	0	15	29	0	201	0.2	0.3	23	0	—	0	0.04	0.04	0.7	0.2	33	0
0	0	0	3	1	0	5	0	0	1	0	0	0	0	0	0	0	0	0
10.6	3.4	0	84	162	3	234	0.9	1.1	94	0	5.63	0	0.04	0.19	0.9	0.02	20	0
12	3.9	0	84	163	141	237	1	1.2	95	0	6.34	0	0.04	0.19	0.9	0.02	20	0
12.3	4	0	86	167	4	243	1	1.2	97	0	6.5	0	0.04	0.2	0.9	0.02	21	0
2.6	2.9	18	40	119	307	275	0.8	1	30	38	1.32	5	0.04	0.1	4.3	0.21	16	0.12
3.4	1.1	0	120	259	2	397	0.8	2.4	82	0	3.8	0	0.09	0.48	1.8	0.03	16	0
5.1	1.7	0	49	74	3	90	0.4	0.5	37	0	5.79	0	0.02	0.12	0.4	0.01	21	0
12	3.9	0	94	185	4	260	1	1.3	105	0	8.52	0	0.08	0.28	1.2	0.04	21	0
11.6	3.7	0	97	189	4	266	1.7	1.3	105	0	1.91	0	0.04	0.21	1	0.03	22	0
9	2.9	0	65	140	3	197	0.8	1	75	0	5.33	0	0.04	0.18	0.8	0.03	10	0
12.4	4	0	90	193	4	272	1.2	1.3	104	0	7.36	0	0.06	0.24	1.2	0.04	14	0
—	—	0	94	192	0	221	1.2	1.4	109	—	7.5	—	0.05	0.23	1.1	0.04	14	0
11	3.6	0	86	169	4	238	0.9	1.2	96	0	7.8	0	0.07	0.25	1.1	0.04	19	0
11.4	3.7	0	90	176	4	247	1	1.2	100	0	8.1	0	0.07	0.26	1.1	0.04	20	0
11.6	3.7	0	97	189	269	266	1.7	1.3	105	0	1.91	0	0.04	0.21	1	0.03	22	0
11.5	3.2	0	111	—	1	243	—	—	—	—	7.62	—	0.02	0.49	0.8	—	15	0
11.2	4.1	0	—	—	—	—	—	—	—	—	8.09	—	0.07	0.32	1.1	0.04	16	0
13	4.2	0	69	205	4	246	0.5	1.9	103	0	1.95	0	0.03	0.1	1.4	0.03	22	0
14.7	4.8	0	92	215	306	268	1.9	1.5	119	0	2.18	0	0.05	0.39	1.4	0.03	25	0
14.7	4.8	0	92	215	4	268	1.9	1.5	119	0	2.18	0	0.05	0.39	1.4	0.03	25	0
13.1	5.4	0	120	196	0	232	1.2	1.5	101	—	8.6	—	0.04	0.43	1.4	—	12	0
9.4	3	0	80	156	3	219	1.4	1.4	86	0	4.54	0	0.04	0.17	0.8	0.02	18	0
0	0.1	0	138	48	14	423	0.6	1.5	36	183	0.33	27	0.01	0.09	0.4	0.12	38	0
0	0	0	30	7	3	87	0.1	0.3	8	42	0.11	6	0	0.02	0.1	0.03	12	0
1.4	2.8	0	149	444	20	357	3.1	7.4	259	0	1	4	0.08	0.2	1.3	0.22	48	0
0	0	0	30	7	3	86	0.1	0.3	8	41	0.11	6	0	0.02	0.1	0.03	12	0
0.2	0.1	0	14	10	0	32	0.1	0.8	4	1	0.02	0	0.01	0.01	0.1	0.01	0	0
—	—	—	51	—	4	—	—	9.2	—	2	—	1	—	—	—	—	—	0
2.3	0.9	17	70	49	295	147	0.4	1.9	16	61	0.42	0	0.22	0.13	1.9	0.07	7	0.02
0	0	0	2	2	1	16	0	0.1	1	2	0	0	0	0	0	0.01	0	0
4.3	3.3	0	79	70	513	274	0.5	2.1	20	87	—	6	0.24	0.2	2.2	0.12	14	0
15.2	9.2	0	14	75	607	129	0.5	3.1	16	10	3.2	2	0.39	0.3	3.5	0.05	11	0
0	0.1	0	17	17	7	295	0.1	0.9	7	0	0.02	2	0.05	0.04	0.2	0.07	0	0

A

Food Item	Qty	Meas	Wgt (g)	Wtr (g)	Cals	Prot (g)	Carb (g)	Fib (g)	Fat (g)	SatF (g)
Apple juice, prepared from frozen	1	cup	239	210	112	0	28	0.2	0	0
Apple rings, dried	10	each	64	20	156	1	42	5.6	0	0
Apple slices, canned, sweetened	0.5	cup	102	84	68	0	17	1.7	0	0.1
Apple slices, frozen, heated	0.5	cup	103	90	48	0	12	2	0	0.1
Apple slices, peeled, cooked	0.5	cup	85	72	48	0	12	2.4	0	0.1
Apple strudel	1	each	71	31	195	2	29	1.6	8	1.4
Apple turnover	1	each	82	27	289	3	36	1.2	15	3.7
Apple, baked, unsweetened	1	each	161	133	102	0	26	3.8	1	0.1
Apple, dried, cooked w/o sugar	0.5	cup	128	108	73	0	20	2.6	0	0
Apple, dried, cooked w/sugar	0.5	cup	140	110	116	0	29	2.7	0	0
Apple, no peel	1	each	128	108	73	0	19	2.4	0	0.1
Apple, peeled slices	0.5	cup	55	46	31	0	8	1	0	0
Apple, w/peel	1	each	138	116	81	0	21	3.7	0	0.1
Apple, w/peel, slices	0.5	cup	55	46	32	0	8	1.5	0	0
Applesauce, canned, sweetened	0.5	cup	128	101	97	0	25	1.5	0	0
Applesauce, unsweetened	0.5	cup	122	108	52	0	14	1.5	0	0
Apricot halves w/skin, canned in water	3	each	84	78	23	1	5	1.3	0	0
Apricot halves, dried, cooked	0.5	cup	125	94	106	2	27	4	0	0
Apricot halves, dried, sulfured	10	each	35	11	83	1	22	3.2	0	0
Apricot nectar, canned	1	cup	251	213	141	1	36	1.5	0	0
Apricot nectar, canned, vitamin C added	1	cup	251	213	141	1	36	1.5	0	0
Apricot, pitted, fresh	3	each	106	92	51	1	12	2.5	0	0
Apricot, w/skin, canned in heavy syrup	0.5	cup	129	100	107	1	28	2.1	0	0
Apricot, w/skin, canned in light syrup	0.5	cup	126	104	80	1	21	2	0	0
Apricot, w/skin, canned w/juice	0.5	cup	124	107	60	1	15	2	0	0
Apricots, frozen, sweetened	0.5	cup	121	89	119	1	30	2.7	0	0
Apricots, halves, fresh	0.5	cup	78	67	37	1	9	1.9	0	0
Apricots, peeled, canned in water	2	each	90	84	20	1	5	1	0	0
Arby's Bac'n cheddar sandwich, deluxe	1	each	231	136	512	21	39	0.3	32	8.7
Arby's Philly beef'n swiss sandwich	1	each	197	105	467	24	38	—	25	9.6
Arby's Q sandwich	1	each	190	104	389	18	48	—	15	5.4
Arby's chicken sandwich, grilled, deluxe	1	each	230	143	430	24	42	—	20	3.5
Arby's roast beef sandwich, Junior	1	each	89	42	233	12	23	0.5	11	3.8
Arby's roast beef sandwich, regular	1	each	155	72	383	22	35	1.1	18	6.9
Arby's sandwich, light roast beef, deluxe	1	each	182	118	294	18	33	—	10	3.4
Arby's sandwich, light roast chicken, deluxe	1	each	195	129	276	24	33	—	7	1.7
Arby's sauce	0.5	oz.	14	10	15	0	3	—	0	0
Arby's sub sandwich, Italian	1	each	297	174	671	34	47	—	39	12.8
Arby's sub sandwich, roast beef	1	each	305	185	623	38	47	—	32	11.5
Arby's sub sandwich, tuna	1	each	284	118	663	74	50	—	37	8.2
Arby's sub sandwich, turkey	1	each	277	173	486	33	46	—	19	5.3
Arby's, Cheddar fries	5	oz.	142	64	399	6	46	—	22	9
Arby's, Steak'n cheddar sandwich	1	each	194	96	508	25	43	—	26	7.7
Arby's, curly fries	3.5	oz.	99	31	337	4	43	—	18	7.4
Arby's, roast chicken club sandwich	1	each	238	142	503	30	37	—	27	6.9
Artichoke heart, marinated	6	oz.	170	138	168	4	13	7.5	14	2
Artichoke heart, raw	0.5	cup	84	73	37	2	9	5	0	0
Artichoke heart, raw	0.5	cup	84	73	37	2	9	5	0	0
Artichoke, Jerusalem, raw, freshly harvested	0.5	cup	75	58	57	2	13	1.2	0	0
Artichoke, frozen, cooked	9	oz.	240	208	108	7	22	11	1	0.3
Artichoke, globe, cooked	1	each	120	101	60	4	13	6.5	0	0
Arugula leaf, raw	5	each	10	9	2	0	0	0.2	0	0
Arugula, chopped, raw	0.5	cup	10	9	2	0	0	0.2	0	0
Asparagus spears, canned, drained	4	each	80	75	15	2	2	1.3	1	0.1
Asparagus spears, canned, not drained, low sodium	4	each	80	75	12	1	2	0.8	0	0
Asparagus spears, cooked, unsalted	4	each	60	55	14	2	3	1	0	0
Asparagus spears, frozen, cooked	4	each	60	55	17	2	3	1	0	0.1
Asparagus, canned w/liquid, low sodium	0.5	cup	122	115	18	2	3	1.2	0	0.1
Asparagus, frozen, uncooked spears	4	each	58	53	14	2	2	1.1	0	0
Asparagus, raw spears	4	each	58	54	13	1	3	1.2	0	0
Aunt Anne's pretzel, original, soft	1	each	138	—	390	12	84	3	1	0
Aunt Anne's pretzel, whole wheat, soft	1	each	140	—	390	13	82	8	2	0
Avocado cubes	0.5	cup	75	56	121	1	6	3.8	12	1.8
Avocado slices	1	piece	10	7	16	0	1	0.5	2	0.2
Avocado, California	1	each	173	126	306	4	12	8.5	30	4.5

MonoF	PolyF	Choles	Calc	Phos	Sod	Pot	Zn	Iron	Magn	VitA	VitE	VitC	Thia	Ribo	Nia	B6	Fola	B12
(g)	(g)	(mg)	(mg)	(mg)	(mg)	(mg)	(mg)	(mg)	(mg)	(μg RE)	(mg α-TE)	(mg)	(mg)	(mg)	(mg)	(mg)	(μg)	(μg)
0	0.1	0	14	17	17	301	0.1	0.6	12	0	0.02	1	0.01	0.04	0.1	0.08	1	0
0	0.1	0	9	24	56	288	0.1	0.9	10	0	0.35	2	0	0.1	0.6	0.08	0	0
0	0.1	0	4	5	3	69	0	0.2	2	5	0.01	0	0.01	0.01	0.1	0.04	0	0
0	0.1	0	5	8	3	78	0.1	0.2	3	2	0.21	0	0.01	0.01	0	0.03	1	0
0	0.1	0	4	7	1	79	0	0.1	3	3	0.01	0	0.01	0.01	0.1	0.04	1	0
2.3	3.8	4	11	23	191	106	0.1	0.3	6	6	2.19	1	0.03	0.02	0.2	0.03	10	0.16
6.6	4	0	6	32	262	56	0.2	1.3	7	4	1.38	1	0.17	0.13	1.5	0.02	5	0
0	0.2	0	12	12	0	179	0.1	0.3	9	7	1.02	8	0.02	0.02	0.1	0.08	3	0
0	0	0	4	12	26	134	0.1	0.4	5	3	0	1	0.01	0.02	0.2	0.06	0	0
0	0	0	4	11	27	137	0.1	0.4	4	3	0.34	1	0.01	0.02	0.2	0.07	0	0
0	0.1	0	5	9	0	145	0.1	0.1	4	5	0.1	5	0.02	0.01	0.1	0.06	1	0
0	0	0	2	4	0	62	0	0	2	2	0.04	2	0.01	0.01	0	0.02	0	0
0	0.1	0	10	10	0	159	0.1	0.2	7	7	0.44	8	0.02	0.02	0.1	0.07	4	0
0	0.1	0	4	4	0	63	0	0.1	3	3	0.18	3	0.01	0.01	0	0.03	2	0
0	0.1	0	5	9	4	78	0.1	0.4	4	1	0.01	2	0.02	0.04	0.2	0.03	1	0
0	0	0	4	9	2	92	0	0.1	4	4	0.01	1	0.02	0.03	0.2	0.03	1	0
0.1	0	0	7	11	3	161	0.1	0.3	6	108	0.75	3	0.02	0.02	0.3	0.04	1	0
0.1	0	0	20	51	4	611	0.3	2.1	21	295	0.62	2	0.01	0.04	1.2	0.14	0	0
0.1	0	0	16	41	4	482	0.3	1.6	16	253	0.52	1	0	0.05	1	0.06	4	0
0.1	0	0	18	23	8	286	0.2	1	13	331	0.2	2	0.02	0.04	0.7	0.06	3	0
0.1	0	0	18	23	8	286	0.2	1	13	331	0.23	137	0.02	0.04	0.7	0.06	3	0
0.2	0.1	0	15	20	1	314	0.3	0.6	8	277	0.94	11	0.03	0.04	0.6	0.06	9	0
0	0	0	12	16	5	181	0.1	0.4	9	159	1.15	4	0.03	0.03	0.5	0.07	2	0
0	0	0	14	16	5	175	0.1	0.5	10	167	1.13	3	0.02	0.02	0.4	0.07	2	0
0	0	0	15	25	5	205	0.1	0.4	12	210	1.1	6	0.02	0.02	0.4	0.07	2	0
0.1	0	0	12	23	5	277	0.1	1.1	11	203	1.08	11	0.02	0.05	1	0.07	2	0
0.1	0.1	0	11	15	1	229	0.2	0.4	6	202	0.69	8	0.02	0.03	0.5	0.04	7	0
0	0	0	7	14	10	139	0.1	0.5	8	163	0.8	2	0.02	0.02	0.4	0.05	2	0
12.7	10.1	38	110	—	1094	491	3	4.3	—	40	—	11	0.34	0.46	9.6	—	—	—
10.6	5.1	53	290	—	1144	409	3.8	4.1	—	—	—	19	0.28	0.46	8.8	—	—	—
6.3	3.5	29	70	—	1268	456	—	9.2	—	—	—	—	0.27	0.39	9.2	—	—	—
5.1	4.4	44	70	—	901	659	—	2.5	—	80	—	8	0.32	0.29	13.6	—	—	—
4.8	2.3	22	40	60	519	201	1.5	2.7	8	—	—	—	0.18	0.26	6.6	0.1	7	—
7.9	3.4	43	60	120	936	422	3.8	4.9	16	0	—	1	0.28	0.48	11	0.2	14	—
4.6	2	42	130	—	826	392	—	4.5	—	40	—	8	0.27	0.49	8.4	—	—	—
2.9	2.5	33	130	—	326	392	—	2.9	—	40	—	7	0.44	0.75	9.4	—	—	—
0.1	0.1	0	—	—	113	28	—	0.4	—	—	—	—	—	—	—	—	—	—
15.7	8.5	69	410	—	2062	565	—	4.3	—	100	—	11	0.92	0.49	8.2	—	—	—
13	6.8	73	410	—	1847	708	—	7.7	—	100	—	9	0.56	0.71	10.1	—	—	—
11.8	17	43	410	—	1847	708	—	7.7	—	100	—	9	0.56	0.71	14.2	—	—	—
6	7	51	400	—	2033	500	—	4.7	—	20	—	—	13.2	0.54	18.8	—	—	—
10	1.7	9	80	—	443	742	0.9	1.4	—	—	—	—	0.06	0.14	2	—	—	0
12	6.8	52	150	—	1166	321	3	6.1	—	—	—	1	0.42	0.63	9.8	—	—	—
7.6	1.5	0	20	—	167	724	0.6	1.4	—	0	—	—	0.06	0.07	2	—	—	0
9.8	10.4	46	180	—	1143	534	2.2	2.9	—	—	—	8	0.51	0.71	10.6	—	—	—
3	7.7	0	39	102	899	439	0.5	1.6	48	28	1.87	52	0.06	0.17	1.4	0.15	149	0
0	0.1	0	33	50	55	221	0.3	1.1	33	12	0.17	6	0.05	0.04	0.5	0.07	37	0
0	0.1	0	33	50	55	221	0.3	1.1	33	12	0.17	6	0.05	0.04	0.5	0.07	37	0
0	0	0	10	58	3	322	0.1	2.6	13	2	0.14	3	0.15	0.04	1	0.06	10	0
0	0.5	0	50	146	127	634	0.9	1.3	74	38	0.46	12	0.15	0.38	2.2	0.21	286	0
0	0.1	0	54	103	114	425	0.6	1.6	72	22	0.23	12	0.08	0.08	1.2	0.13	61	0
0	0	0	16	5	3	37	0	0.1	5	24	0.04	2	0	0.01	0	0.01	10	0
0	0	0	16	5	3	37	0	0.1	5	24	0.04	2	0	0.01	0	0.01	10	0
0	0.2	0	13	34	230	138	0.3	1.5	8	42	0.34	15	0.05	0.08	0.8	0.09	76	0
0	0.1	0	12	30	227	138	0.4	0.5	7	42	1.72	13	0.04	0.07	0.7	0.08	68	0
0	0.1	0	12	32	7	96	0.3	0.4	6	32	0.23	6	0.07	0.08	0.6	0.07	88	0
0	0.1	0	14	33	2	131	0.3	0.4	8	49	0.75	15	0.04	0.06	0.6	0.01	81	0
0	0.1	0	18	46	32	210	0.6	0.7	11	65	0.15	20	0.07	0.11	1	0.12	104	0
0	0.1	0	14	37	5	147	0.3	0.4	8	55	1.25	18	0.07	0.08	0.7	0.06	111	0
0	0.1	0	12	32	1	158	0.3	0.5	10	34	1.16	8	0.08	0.07	0.7	0.08	74	0
—	—	0	40	—	1100	—	—	2.7	—	0	—	—	—	—	—	—	—	—
—	—	0	40	—	1290	—	—	2.7	—	0	—	—	—	—	—	—	—	—
7.2	1.5	0	8	31	8	449	0.3	0.8	29	46	1.01	6	0.08	0.09	1.4	0.21	46	0
1	0.2	0	1	4	1	60	0	0.1	4	6	0.13	1	0.01	0.01	0.2	0.03	6	0
19.4	3.5	0	19	73	21	1096	0.7	2	71	106	2.32	14	0.19	0.21	3.3	0.48	113	0

Food Item	Qty	Meas	Wgt (g)	Wtr (g)	Cals	Prot (g)	Carb (g)	Fib (g)	Fat (g)	SatF (g)
Avocado, California, mashed	0.5	cup	115	84	204	2	8	5.6	20	3
Avocado, Florida	1	each	304	242	340	5	27	16.1	27	5.4
Avocado, Florida, mashed	0.5	cup	115	92	129	2	10	6.1	10	2
Avocado, average	1	each	201	149	324	4	15	10.1	31	4.9
Baby Food, bananas, strained, Heinz	1	Tbs	16	12	16	0	4	0.3	0	0
Baby Food, beef dinner supreme, stage 2, Beech-nut	1	each	128	106	147	2	9	1.1	10	—
Baby Food, beef stew, toddler	1	Tbs	14	12	7	1	1	0.2	0	0.1
Baby Food, carrots, stage 1, Beech-nut	1	oz.	28	26	12	0	2	1	0	0
Baby Food, cereal, mixed, w/formula	1	Tbs	18	14	22	1	3	—	1	—
Baby Food, cereal, rice w/fruit, Gerber	1	Tbs	14	12	11	0	3	0.1	0	—
Baby Food, chicken w/broth, stage 1, jar, Beech-nut	1	each	71	59	70	8	0	0	3	—
Baby Food, chicken-rice dinner, stage 2, Beech-nut	4	oz.	113	100	80	1	9	1	3	—
Baby Food, peaches, strained, Heinz	1	Tbs	16	13	12	0	3	0.4	0	0
Baby Food, pudding, cherry vanilla, Gerber	1	Tbs	14	12	10	0	2	0	0	—
Baby Food, spaghetti w/meat sauce, toddler	1	Tbs	14	12	11	1	2	—	0	—
Baby Food, sweet potatoes, stage 3, jar, Beech-nut	1	each	170	148	110	1	25	1	0	0
Baby Food, tropical fruit medley, Gerber	1	Tbs	14	12	9	0	2	0	0	—
Baby Food, turkey sticks, Gerber	1	each	10	8	13	1	0	0	1	0.3
Baby Formulat, similac, liquid, 27cal/oz, Ross Labs	0.46	cup	114	95	100	3	10	—	5	—
Bacon, Canadian style, grilled	2	piece	47	29	87	11	1	0	4	1.3
Bacon, cooked, regular	3	piece	19	2	109	6	0	0	9	3.3
Bagel chips	2	piece	28	1	119	2	21	2.2	3	0.5
Bagel, 100% whole wheat	1	each	55	16	145	6	31	5.4	1	0.1
Bagel, cinnamon raisin	1	each	71	23	195	7	39	1.6	1	0.2
Bagel, cinnamon raisin, toasted	1	each	66	18	194	7	39	1.6	1	0.2
Bagel, egg	1	each	71	23	197	8	38	1.6	1	0.3
Bagel, egg, toasted	1	each	66	18	197	8	38	1.6	1	0.3
Bagel, oat bran	1	each	71	23	181	8	38	2.6	1	0.1
Bagel, oat bran, toasted	1	each	66	18	181	8	38	2.5	1	0.1
Bagel, plain	1	each	68	22	187	7	36	1.6	1	0.2
Bagel, plain, toasted	1	each	66	18	195	7	38	1.6	1	0.2
Baking chips, butterscotch	0.5	cup	85	1	458	2	57	0	25	20.5
Baking chips, peanut butter	0.5	cup	85	5	422	16	38	7.1	25	11.1
Baking chips, white chocolate	0.5	cup	85	1	458	5	50	0	27	16.5
Baking chocolate, bar, semi-sweet, Nestle	1	oz.	28	0	142	2	18	4	8	5.1
Baking chocolate, bar, unsweetened, Nestle	1	oz.	28	0	162	4	9	6.1	14	4
Baking chocolate, unsweetened, liquid, pkt	1	each	28	0	134	3	10	5.1	14	7.2
Baking chocolate, unsweetened, premelted, ChocoBake	1	oz.	28	1	162	0	10	6.1	16	10.2
Baking mix, reduced fat, Bisquick	1	cup	120	—	450	9	84	1.5	8	1.5
Baking powder, double acting, Calumet	1	tsp	5	0	2	0	1	0	0	0
Baking powder, double acting, Rumford	1	tsp	5	0	2	0	1	0	0	0
Baking powder, low sodium	1	tsp	4	0	4	0	2	0.1	0	0
Baking soda/sodium bicarbonate	1	tsp	5	0	0	0	0	0	0	0
Baklava	1	piece	78	20	333	5	29	1.6	23	9.3
Balsam pear, leaftips, cooked	0.5	cup	29	26	10	1	2	0.6	0	0
Balsam pear, pods, cooked	0.5	cup	62	58	12	1	3	1.2	0	0
Bamboo shoot, sliced, canned	0.5	cup	66	62	12	1	2	0.9	0	0.1
Bamboo shoot, sliced, raw	0.5	cup	76	69	20	2	4	1.7	0	0.1
Bamboo shoots, cooked slices	0.5	cup	60	58	7	1	1	0.6	0	0
Bamboo shoots, cooked, whole	1	each	144	138	17	2	3	1.4	0	0.1
Banana	1	each	114	85	105	1	27	2.7	1	0.2
Banana chips, fried	0.5	cup	46	2	239	1	27	3.5	16	13.3
Banana nectar	1	cup	250	202	177	1	46	1.4	0	0.2
Banana slices	0.5	cup	75	56	69	1	18	1.8	0	0.1
Banana split w/whipped cream	1	each	425	221	1076	15	120	1.2	66	37.9
Banana, chocolate-covered, w/nuts	1	each	145	74	336	7	43	4.6	19	7
Banana, dehydrated	0.5	cup	50	2	173	2	44	3.8	1	0.3
Banana, ripe, fried	1	each	91	54	184	1	24	1.6	11	2.2
Barley, pearled, cooked	0.5	cup	78	54	97	2	22	3	0	0.1
Barley, pearled, dry	0.5	cup	100	10	352	10	78	15.6	1	0.2
Barley, whole, cooked	0.5	cup	100	65	135	4	30	6.8	1	0.2
Barley, whole, dry	0.5	cup	92	9	326	12	68	15.9	2	0.4
Basil, dried	0.25	tsp	0	0	1	0	0	0.2	0	0
Basil, fresh leaves	5	each	2	2	1	0	0	0.1	0	0
Basil, fresh, chopped	1	Tbs	3	2	1	0	0	0.1	0	0

MonoF	PolyF	Choles	Calc	Phos	Sod	Pot	Zn	Iron	Magn	VitA	VitE	VitC	Thia	Ribo	Nia	B6	Fola	B12
(g)	(g)	(mg)	(mg)	(mg)	(mg)	(mg)	(mg)	(mg)	(mg)	(μg RE)	(mg α-TE)	(mg)	(mg)	(mg)	(mg)	(mg)	(μg)	(μg)
12.9	2.4	0	13	48	14	729	0.5	1.4	47	70	1.54	9	0.12	0.14	2.2	0.32	75	0
14.8	4.5	0	33	119	15	1483	1.3	1.6	103	185	2.37	24	0.33	0.37	5.8	0.85	162	0
5.6	1.7	0	13	45	6	561	0.5	0.6	39	70	0.9	9	0.12	0.14	2.2	0.32	61	0
19.3	3.9	0	22	82	20	1203	0.8	2	78	123	2.69	16	0.22	0.24	3.9	0.56	124	0
—	—	—	1	3	0	52	0	0.1	—	2	—	6	0	0.02	0.1	0.04	—	—
—	—	—	27	—	51	192	—	0.3	—	813	—	0	0.01	0.06	1	—	—	—
0.1	0	2	1	6	49	20	0.1	0.1	2	36	0.03	0	0	0.01	0.2	0.01	1	0.07
0	0	—	6	—	25	40	—	0	—	300	—	0	0	0	0.1	—	—	—
—	—	—	7	—	3	—	—	0.9	—	7	—	1	0.02	0.02	0.3	0.04	—	—
—	—	—	2	3	1	7	0.1	0.4	1	0	—	1	0.02	0.02	0.3	0.02	—	—
—	—	—	12	—	55	120	—	0.6	—	0	—	0	0.02	0.08	1.2	—	—	—
—	—	—	36	—	70	115	—	0.6	—	1260	—	0	0.02	0.03	0.6	—	—	—
—	—	—	1	1	0	34	0	0.1	—	16	—	10	0	0.01	0.2	0	—	—
—	—	—	1	1	1	6	—	0	0	0	—	0	0	0	0	0	—	—
—	—	—	3	6	51	23	0.1	0.1	2	12	—	1	0.01	0.01	0.2	0.01	5	0.03
0	0	—	12	—	15	360	—	0.3	—	855	—	0	0.03	0.04	0.5	—	—	—
—	—	—	1	0	1	6	—	0	1	2	—	2	0	0	0	0.01	—	—
—	—	9	10	13	43	12	0.2	0.1	1	0	—	0	0	0.02	0.2	0.01	—	—
—	—	—	90	70	34	132	0.8	0.2	7	90	2.01	9	0.1	0.15	1	0.06	15	0.25
1.9	0.4	27	5	139	727	183	0.8	0.4	10	0	0.12	0	0.39	0.09	3.2	0.21	2	0.37
4.5	1.1	16	2	64	303	92	0.6	0.3	5	0	0.1	0	0.13	0.05	1.4	0.05	1	0.33
0.8	1.4	0	4	58	168	67	0.4	0.6	16	0	0.19	0	0.05	0.05	0.6	0.08	23	0
0.1	0.3	0	16	159	270	190	1.3	1.8	59	0	0.49	0	0.17	0.14	2.8	0.18	40	0
0.1	0.5	0	14	71	229	105	0.8	2.7	20	6	0.11	0	0.27	0.2	2.2	0.04	64	0
0.1	0.5	0	13	55	228	108	0.5	2.7	15	5	0.12	0	0.22	0.18	2	0.04	51	0
0.3	0.5	17	9	60	359	48	0.5	2.8	18	23	0.1	0	0.38	0.17	2.4	0.06	62	0.11
0.3	0.5	17	9	59	358	48	0.5	2.8	18	21	0.07	0	0.3	0.15	2.2	0.06	11	0.11
0.2	0.3	0	9	78	360	82	0.6	2.2	22	0	0.1	0	0.24	0.24	2.1	0.03	58	0
0.2	0.3	0	9	117	360	145	1.5	2.2	41	0	0.17	0	0.19	0.22	1.9	0.13	23	0
0.1	0.5	0	50	65	363	69	0.6	2.4	20	0	0.03	0	0.37	0.21	3.1	0.04	60	0
0.1	0.5	0	53	68	379	72	0.6	2.5	20	0	0.02	0	0.31	0.2	2.9	0.03	50	0
1.9	0.4	0	29	27	76	159	0.1	0.1	4	0	1.91	0	0.07	0	0.1	0.01	1	0.08
8.2	4.5	0	94	264	213	429	1.7	1.4	94	2	2.55	0	0.04	0.17	7	0.19	82	0.05
7.7	0.9	18	169	150	76	243	0.6	0.2	10	3	1.91	0	0.05	0.24	0.6	0.05	14	0.52
—	—	0	0	—	0	109	—	0.7	—	0	—	0	0.02	0	0.2	—	—	—
5.2	0.7	0	0	—	0	239	—	0	—	0	—	0	0.03	0.04	0.4	—	—	—
2.6	3	0	15	96	3	331	1	1.2	75	0	1.71	0	0.01	0.08	0.6	0.02	5	0
—	—	0	0	—	0	—	—	1.5	—	0	—	0	0.04	0.04	0.4	—	—	—
—	—	0	120	—	1380	90	—	4.3	—	—	—	—	0.45	0.31	4.8	—	—	—
0	0	0	270	101	488	1	0	0.5	1	0	0	0	0	0	0	0	0	0
0	0	0	339	456	363	0	0	0.5	2	0	0	0	0	0	0	0	0	0
0	0	0	186	295	4	434	0	0.4	1	0	0	0	0	0	0	0	0	0
0	0	0	0	0	1258	0	0	0	0	0	0	0	0	0	0	0	0	0
8.5	3.8	36	34	88	291	139	0.5	1.7	34	124	1.99	1	0.17	0.13	1.3	0.05	9	0.02
0	0	0	12	22	4	175	0.1	0.3	27	50	0.14	16	0.04	0.08	0.3	0.22	25	0
0	0	0	6	22	4	198	0.5	0.2	10	7	0.43	20	0.03	0.03	0.2	0.02	32	0
0	0.1	0	5	16	5	52	0.4	0.2	3	1	0.25	1	0.02	0.02	0.1	0.09	2	0
0	0.1	0	10	44	3	402	0.8	0.4	2	2	0.76	3	0.11	0.05	0.5	0.18	5	0
0	0.1	0	7	12	2	320	0.3	0.1	2	0	0.4	0	0.01	0.03	0.2	0.06	1	0
0	0.1	0	17	29	6	768	0.7	0.3	4	0	0.96	0	0.03	0.07	0.4	0.14	3	0
0	0.1	0	7	23	1	451	0.2	0.4	33	9	0.31	10	0.05	0.11	0.6	0.66	22	0
0.9	0.3	0	8	26	3	247	0.3	0.6	35	4	2.48	3	0.04	0.01	0.3	0.12	6	0
0	0.1	0	8	18	5	347	0.2	0.3	27	7	0.24	8	0.04	0.09	0.5	0.5	17	0
0	0.1	0	4	15	1	297	0.1	0.2	22	6	0.2	7	0.03	0.08	0.4	0.43	14	0
18.8	5	209	468	477	354	779	2.7	1.5	89	545	0.49	2	0.15	0.9	0.5	0.17	19	1.41
7.5	3.2	0	28	153	7	596	1.8	1.4	93	8	1.92	9	0.1	0.19	3.3	0.63	42	0
0.1	0.2	0	11	37	2	746	0.3	0.6	54	16	0	4	0.09	0.12	1.4	0.22	7	0
4.8	3.4	0	10	23	120	366	0.2	0.3	30	142	1.89	6	0.04	0.1	0.5	0.53	10	0.01
0	0.2	0	9	42	2	73	0.6	1	17	1	0.04	0	0.06	0.05	1.6	0.09	13	0
0.1	0.6	0	29	221	9	280	2.1	2.5	79	2	0.13	0	0.19	0.11	4.6	0.26	23	0
0.1	0.6	0	13	115	1	115	0.8	1	22	0	0.6	0	0.08	0.03	1.4	0.09	8	0
0.3	1	0	30	243	11	416	2.6	3.3	122	2	0.55	0	0.59	0.26	4.2	0.29	18	0
0	0	0	8	2	0	13	0	0.2	2	4	0.01	0	0	0	0	0	1	0
0	0	0	4	2	0	12	0	0.1	2	10	—	0	0	0	0	0	2	0
0	0	0	4	2	0	12	0	0.1	2	10	—	0	0	0	0	0	2	0

Food Item	Qty	Meas	Wgt (g)	Wtr (g)	Cals	Prot (g)	Carb (g)	Fib (g)	Fat (g)	SatF (g)
Bay leaf, crumbled	1	tsp	1	0	2	0	0	0.2	0	0
Bean cake, Japanese style	1	each	32	7	130	2	16	0.9	7	1
Bean paste, sweetened	1	oz.	28	13	60	2	14	1.5	0	0
Bean sprouts, mung, canned, drained	0.5	cup	62	60	8	1	1	0.5	0	0
Bean sprouts, mung, cooked, drained	0.5	cup	1	1	0	0	0	0	0	0
Bean sprouts, mung, raw	0.5	cup	52	47	16	2	3	0.9	0	0
Bean sprouts, mung, stir fried	0.5	cup	62	52	31	3	7	1.2	0	0
Bean, Italian green, canned, drained, low sodium	0.5	cup	120	112	24	1	5	2.3	0	0
Bean, winged/goabean, dry, cooked	0.5	cup	86	58	126	9	13	2.1	5	0.7
Beans, Adzuki, canned, sweetened	0.5	cup	145	59	344	6	80	4.2	0	0
Beans, Adzuki, cooked	0.5	cup	115	76	147	9	28	1	0	0
Beans, B & M baked, fat free	0.5	cup	130	—	160	8	31	7	1	0
Beans, baked, canned, vegetarian	0.5	cup	127	92	118	6	26	6.4	1	0.1
Beans, baked, canned, w/pork	0.5	cup	126	90	134	7	25	6.9	2	0.8
Beans, baked, home prepared	0.5	cup	126	82	190	7	27	6.9	6	2.5
Beans, baked, low sodium	0.5	cup	126	92	118	6	26	7	1	0.2
Beans, black turtle soup, canned w/liquid	0.5	cup	120	91	109	7	20	8.3	0	0.1
Beans, black turtle soup, cooked	0.5	cup	92	60	120	8	22	4.9	0	0.1
Beans, black, dry, cooked, no added salt	0.5	cup	86	56	114	8	20	7.5	0	0.1
Beans, broadbean/fava dry, cooked	0.5	cup	85	61	94	6	17	4.6	0	0.1
Beans, broadbean/fava, canned w/liquid	0.5	cup	128	103	91	7	16	4.7	0	0
Beans, cranberry, cooked	0.5	cup	88	57	120	8	22	8.8	0	0.1
Beans, french, cooked	0.5	cup	86	57	111	6	21	8.1	1	0.1
Beans, garbanzo/chickpeas, canned w/liquid	0.5	cup	120	84	143	6	27	5.3	1	0.1
Beans, Garbanzo/chickpeas, cooked from dry	0.5	cup	82	49	134	7	22	6.2	2	0.2
Beans Garbanzo/Chickpeas, dry	0.25	cup	50	6	182	10	30	8.7	3	0.3
Beans, great northern, dry, cooked	0.5	cup	88	61	104	7	19	6.2	0	0.1
Beans, green, Italian, canned, drained	0.5	cup	68	63	14	1	3	1.3	0	0
Beans, green, Italian, canned, not drained	0.5	cup	120	114	18	1	4	1.8	0	0
Beans, green, Italian, cooked	0.5	cup	62	56	22	1	5	2	0	0
Beans, green, Italian, frozen, cooked, drained	0.5	cup	68	62	19	1	4	2	0	0
Beans, green, Italian, raw	0.5	cup	55	50	17	1	4	1.9	0	0
Beans, green, canned, drained, low sodium	0.5	cup	68	63	14	1	3	1.3	0	0
Beans, green, canned, not drained, low sodium	0.5	cup	120	114	18	1	4	1.8	0	0
Beans, green, seasoned, canned	0.5	cup	114	108	18	1	4	1.7	0	0.1
Beans, green, snap/string, canned, drained	0.5	cup	68	63	14	1	3	1.3	0	0
Beans, green, snap/string, frozen, cooked, drained	0.5	cup	68	62	19	1	4	2	0	0
Beans, green, string, pickled	0.5	cup	68	61	19	1	4	1.1	0	0
Beans, green/snap/string, raw	0.5	cup	55	50	17	1	4	1.9	0	0
Beans, green/snap/string, raw, cooked	0.5	cup	62	56	22	1	5	2	0	0
Beans, hyacinth, dry, cooked	0.5	cup	97	67	113	8	20	3.5	1	0.1
Beans, Italian green, canned, not drained, low sodium	0.5	cup	120	114	18	1	4	1.8	0	0
Beans, kidney, California red, cooked	0.5	cup	88	59	109	8	20	8.2	0	0
Beans, kidney, all, canned w/liquid	0.5	cup	128	100	104	7	19	4.5	0	0.1
Beans, kidney, red, canned w/liquid, low sodium	0.5	cup	128	99	109	7	20	8.2	0	0.1
Beans, kidney, red, canned, drained	0.5	cup	128	88	151	9	28	11.4	1	—
Beans, kidney, red, cooked	0.5	cup	88	59	112	8	20	6.5	0	0.1
Beans, kidney, royal red, cooked	0.5	cup	88	59	108	8	19	8.2	0	0
Beans, lima, baby, canned, w/liquid, low sodium	0.5	cup	87	71	62	4	12	3.1	0	0.1
Beans, lima, baby, dry	0.25	cup	48	6	159	10	30	9.8	0	0.1
Beans, lima, baby, dry, cooked	0.5	cup	91	61	115	7	21	7	0	0.1
Beans, lima, baby, frozen, cooked	0.5	cup	90	65	94	6	18	5.4	0	0.1
Beans, lima, canned, drained	0.5	cup	85	57	82	5	16	3.7	0	0.1
Beans, lima, fordhook, frozen, cooked	0.5	cup	85	62	85	5	16	4.9	0	0.1
Beans, lima, immature, canned w/liquid	0.5	cup	124	101	88	5	16	4.5	0	0.1
Beans, lima, immature, raw, cooked	0.5	cup	85	57	105	6	20	4.5	0	0.1
Beans, lima, large, canned, not drained	0.5	cup	120	93	95	6	18	5.8	0	0
Beans, lima, large, dry, cooked	0.5	cup	94	66	108	7	20	6.6	0	0.1
Beans, mung, cooked, unsalted	0.5	cup	101	73	106	7	19	7.7	0	0.1
Beans, mungo, cooked	0.5	cup	90	65	94	7	16	5.8	0	0
Beans, Navy, dry, cooked	0.5	cup	91	58	129	8	24	5.8	1	0.1
Beans, pink, cooked	0.5	cup	84	51	125	8	23	4.4	0	0.1
Beans, pinto, canned w/liquid	0.5	cup	120	93	103	6	18	5.5	1	0.2
Beans, pinto, dry, cooked	0.5	cup	86	55	117	7	22	7.4	0	0.1
Beans, red kidney, dry	0.25	cup	46	5	155	10	28	7	0	0.1

A

MonoF	PolyF	Choles	Calc	Phos	Sod	Pot	Zn	Iron	Magn	VitA	VitE	VitC	Thia	Ribo	Nia	B6	Fola	B12
(g)	(g)	(mg)	(mg)	(mg)	(mg)	(mg)	(mg)	(mg)	(mg)	(μg RE)	(mg α-TE)	(mg)	(mg)	(mg)	(mg)	(mg)	(μg)	(μg)
0	0	0	5	1	0	3	0	0.3	1	4	0.01	0	0	0	0	0.01	1	0
2.9	2.6	0	3	21	55	58	0.2	0.7	6	0	1.14	0	0.07	0.05	0.5	0.02	9	0
0	0	0	4	23	30	105	0.2	0.5	9	0	0.04	0	0.03	0.01	0.1	0.03	17	0
0	0	0	9	20	88	17	0.2	0.3	6	1	0.01	0	0.02	0.04	0.1	0.02	6	0
0	0	0	0	0	0	1	0	0	0	0	0	0	0	0	0	0	0	0
0	0	0	7	28	3	78	0.2	0.5	11	1	0	7	0.04	0.06	0.4	0.05	32	0
0	0	0	8	49	6	136	0.6	1.2	20	2	0.01	10	0.09	0.11	0.7	0.08	43	0
0	0.1	0	31	23	2	131	0.3	1.1	16	42	0.17	6	0.02	0.07	0.2	0.04	38	0
1.8	1.3	0	122	132	11	241	1.2	3.7	46	0	0.09	0	0.25	0.11	0.7	0.04	9	0
0	0	0	32	107	316	173	2.3	1.6	45	1	0.04	0	0.15	0.08	0.9	0.12	155	0
0	0	0	32	193	9	612	2	2.3	60	1	0.12	0	0.13	0.07	0.8	0.11	139	0
0	0.5	0	60	—	220	—	—	3.6	—	0	—	0	—	—	—	—	—	—
0	0.2	0	64	132	504	376	1.8	0.4	41	22	0.67	4	0.19	0.08	0.5	0.17	30	0
0.8	0.3	9	67	136	522	389	1.8	2.1	43	23	0.49	3	0.07	0.05	0.6	0.08	46	0
2.7	0.9	6	77	137	532	451	0.9	2.5	54	0	0.66	1	0.17	0.06	0.5	0.11	61	0
0.1	0.2	0	63	132	1	374	1.8	0.4	40	22	0.67	4	0.19	0.08	0.5	0.16	30	0
0	0.2	0	42	130	461	370	0.6	2.3	42	0	0.31	3	0.17	0.14	0.7	0.07	73	0
0	0.1	0	51	140	3	398	0.7	2.6	45	1	0.28	0	0.21	0.05	0.5	0.07	79	0
0	0.2	0	23	120	1	305	1	1.8	60	1	0.07	0	0.21	0.05	0.4	0.06	128	0
0.1	0.1	0	31	106	4	228	0.9	1.3	37	2	0.08	0	0.08	0.08	0.6	0.06	88	0
0.1	0.1	0	33	101	580	310	0.8	1.3	41	1	0.1	2	0.03	0.06	1.2	0.06	42	0
0	0.2	0	44	119	1	341	1	1.8	44	0	0.09	0	0.18	0.06	0.5	0.07	182	0
0	0.4	0	54	88	5	318	0.6	0.9	48	0	0.1	1	0.11	0.05	0.5	0.09	64	0
0.3	0.6	0	38	108	359	206	1.3	1.6	35	2	0.18	5	0.04	0.04	0.2	0.57	80	0
0.5	1	0	40	138	6	239	1.2	2.4	39	2	0.29	1	0.1	0.05	0.4	0.11	141	0
0.7	1.4	0	52	183	12	438	1.7	3.1	58	4	0.41	2	0.24	0.11	0.8	0.27	279	0
0	0.2	0	60	146	2	346	0.8	1.9	44	0	0.27	1	0.14	0.05	0.6	0.1	90	0
0	0	0	18	13	177	74	0.2	0.6	9	24	0.1	3	0.01	0.04	0.1	0.02	22	0
0	0.1	0	29	23	311	110	0.2	1.1	16	38	0.14	4	0.03	0.06	0.2	0.04	22	0
0	0.1	0	29	24	2	187	0.2	0.8	16	42	0.09	6	0.05	0.06	0.4	0.04	21	0
0	0.1	0	33	21	6	85	0.3	0.6	16	27	0.1	3	0.02	0.06	0.3	0.04	16	0
0	0	0	20	21	3	115	0.1	0.6	14	37	0.23	9	0.05	0.06	0.4	0.04	20	0
0	0	0	18	13	1	74	0.2	0.6	9	24	0.1	3	0.01	0.04	0.1	0.02	22	0
0	0.1	0	29	23	17	110	0.2	1.1	16	38	0.17	4	0.03	0.06	0.2	0.04	22	0
0	0.1	0	25	18	425	106	0.2	0.5	15	60	0.14	4	0.03	0.06	0.3	0.05	20	0
0	0	0	18	13	177	74	0.2	0.6	9	24	0.1	3	0.01	0.04	0.1	0.02	22	0
0	0.1	0	33	21	6	85	0.3	0.6	16	27	0.1	3	0.02	0.06	0.3	0.04	16	0
0	0	0	22	23	148	127	0.1	0.6	16	38	0.24	8	0.04	0.06	0.4	0.04	18	0
0	0	0	20	21	3	115	0.1	0.6	14	37	0.23	9	0.05	0.06	0.4	0.04	20	0
0	0.1	0	29	24	2	187	0.2	0.8	16	42	0.09	6	0.05	0.06	0.4	0.04	21	0
0.1	0.3	0	39	116	7	327	2.8	4.4	80	0	0.1	0	0.26	0.04	0.4	0.04	4	0
0	0.1	0	29	23	17	110	0.2	1.1	16	38	0.17	4	0.03	0.06	0.2	0.04	22	0
0	0	0	58	121	4	369	0.8	2.6	42	0	0.18	1	0.11	0.06	0.5	0.09	65	0
0	0.2	0	35	134	444	329	0.7	1.6	40	0	0.26	2	0.14	0.09	0.6	0.09	63	0
0	0.2	0	31	120	436	329	0.7	1.6	36	0	0.06	1	0.13	0.11	0.6	0.03	65	0
—	—	0	—	166	—	—	1	—	50	0	—	—	0.19	0.16	0.8	0.04	90	0
0	0.2	0	25	125	2	355	0.9	2.6	40	0	0.07	1	0.14	0.05	0.5	0.11	114	0
0	0.1	0	39	125	4	333	0.8	2.4	37	0	0.07	1	0.08	0.06	0.5	0.09	65	0
0	0.1	0	24	62	3	248	0.6	1.4	30	13	0.25	8	0.02	0.04	0.5	0.05	14	0
0	0.2	0	38	176	6	666	1.2	2.9	89	0	0.19	0	0.27	0.1	0.8	0.16	190	0
0	0.2	0	26	116	3	365	0.9	2.2	48	0	0.16	0	0.15	0.05	0.6	0.07	137	0
0	0.1	0	25	101	26	370	0.5	1.8	50	15	0.58	5	0.06	0.05	0.7	0.1	14	0
0	0.2	0	24	60	201	189	0.8	1.5	35	16	0.26	5	0.03	0.04	0.4	0.02	20	0
0	0.1	0	19	54	45	347	0.4	1.2	29	16	0.25	11	0.06	0.05	0.9	0.1	18	0
0	0.2	0	35	88	312	353	0.8	2	42	19	0.36	9	0.04	0.05	0.7	0.08	20	0
0	0.1	0	27	111	14	485	0.7	2.1	63	32	0.12	9	0.12	0.08	0.9	0.16	22	0
0	0.1	0	25	89	405	265	0.8	2.2	47	0	0.12	0	0.07	0.04	0.3	0.11	61	0
0	0.2	0	16	104	2	478	0.9	2.2	40	0	0.17	0	0.15	0.05	0.4	0.15	78	0
0.1	0.1	0	27	100	2	269	0.8	1.4	48	2	0.52	1	0.17	0.06	0.6	0.07	161	0
0	0.3	0	48	140	6	208	0.7	1.6	57	3	0.14	1	0.14	0.07	1.4	0.05	85	0
0	0.2	0	64	143	1	335	1	2.3	54	0	0.36	1	0.18	0.06	0.5	0.15	127	0
0	0.2	0	44	139	2	427	0.8	1.9	55	0	0.33	0	0.22	0.05	0.5	0.15	141	0
0.2	0.3	0	52	110	353	292	0.8	1.8	32	3	1.13	1	0.12	0.08	0.4	0.09	72	0
0.1	0.2	0	41	137	2	400	0.9	2.2	47	0	0.8	2	0.16	0.08	0.3	0.13	147	0
0	0.3	0	38	187	6	625	1.3	3.1	64	0	0.1	2	0.28	0.1	1	0.18	181	0

Food Item	Qty	Meas	Wgt (g)	Wtr (g)	Cals	Prot (g)	Carb (g)	Fib (g)	Fat (g)	SatF (g)
Beans, red kidney, dry, cooked	0.5	cup	88	59	112	8	20	5.7	0	0.1
Beans, red mexican, dry, cooked	0.5	cup	112	78	126	8	24	9	0	0.1
Beans, refried/frijoles, canned	1	cup	253	192	238	14	39	13.4	3	1.2
Beans, small white, dry, cooked	0.5	cup	90	57	127	8	23	9.3	1	0.1
Beans, white, canned w/liquid	0.5	cup	131	92	153	10	29	6.3	0	0.1
Beans, white, dry, cooked, unsalted	0.5	cup	90	57	125	9	23	5.7	0	0.1
Beans, winged/goabean, dry, mature	0.5	cup	91	8	372	27	38	6.2	15	2.1
Beans, yardlong, dry, cooked	0.5	cup	86	59	101	7	18	3.2	0	0.1
Beans, yardlong, dry, mature	0.5	cup	84	7	290	20	52	9.2	1	0.3
Beans, yellow snap, canned, low sodium	0.5	cup	68	63	14	1	3	0.9	0	0
Beans, yellow wax, canned, drained	0.5	cup	68	63	14	1	3	0.9	0	0
Beans, yellow wax, cooked, drained	0.5	cup	62	56	22	1	5	2.1	0	0
Beans, yellow wax, frozen, cooked, drained	0.5	cup	68	62	19	1	4	2	0	0
Beans, yellow, dry, cooked	0.5	cup	88	55	127	8	22	9.2	1	0.2
Beans, yokan adzuki, confection, slices	3	piece	43	15	112	1	26	0.9	0	0
Beechnuts, dried	1	oz.	28	2	163	2	10	1	14	1.6
Beef & noodles, w/tomato sauce, Hamburger Helper	0.5	cup	124	93	140	15	10	1.4	4	1.4
Beef (roast) hash	0.5	cup	95	65	158	11	10	1.1	8	2.5
Beef cube steak, fried, lean	4	oz.	113	63	261	38	0	0	11	3.8
Beef jerky	1	each	20	5	81	7	2	0.4	5	2.2
Beef pot pie, Banquet	1	each	198	134	330	9	38	3	15	7
Beef pot pie, Swanson	1	each	198	120	415	11	41	2	23	9
Beef round steak, fried, lean	4	oz.	113	63	261	38	0	0	11	3.8
Beef sirloin steak, fried, lean	4	oz.	113	63	261	38	0	0	11	3.8
Beef stroganoff	0.5	cup	128	91	202	13	8	0.7	13	5.3
Beef, London Broil, broiled, lean	1	piece	21	13	44	6	0	0	2	0.9
Beef, London Broil, broiled, lean	3	oz.	85	52	176	23	0	0	9	3.7
Beef, bacon, Sizzlean	2	piece	22	6	99	7	0	0	8	3.2
Beef, bottom round, pot roast, braised, lean	3	oz.	85	49	178	27	0	0	7	2.4
Beef, bottom round, pot roast, braised, lean	4	oz.	113	65	237	36	0	0	9	3.1
Beef, brisket, corned, cooked, lean	1	piece	42	25	105	8	0	0	8	2.7
Beef, brisket, corned, cooked, lean	3	oz.	85	51	213	16	0	0	16	5.4
Beef, chuck, arm pot roast, braised, lean	3	oz.	85	49	184	28	0	0	7	2.6
Beef, chuck, arm pot roast, braised, lean	4	oz.	113	66	245	37	0	0	9	3.4
Beef, corned, canned	4	oz.	113	65	284	31	0	0	17	7
Beef, cube steak, bread/flour fried, lean	4	oz.	113	54	313	30	12	0.7	15	4.5
Beef, dried, cured	0.75	piece	28	16	47	8	0	0	1	0.5
Beef, filet mignon steak, broiled, lean	4	oz.	113	68	239	32	0	0	11	4.2
Beef, ground, baked, well done, extra lean	4	oz.	113	60	311	34	0	0	18	7.1
Beef, ground, broiled, well done, extra lean	4	oz.	113	61	301	32	0	0	18	7
Beef, ground, broiled, well done, lean	1	each	88	47	246	25	0	0	16	6.1
Beef, ground, broiled, well done, lean	4	oz.	113	60	318	32	0	0	20	7.9
Beef, ground, broiled, well done, regular	4	oz.	113	59	331	31	0	0	22	8.7
Beef, ground, extra lean, broiled, well done	1	each	96	52	254	28	0	0	15	6
Beef, ground, fried, well done, lean	4	oz.	113	61	314	31	0	0	20	7.9
Beef, ground, fried, well, extra lean	4	oz.	113	61	298	32	0	0	18	7.1
Beef, ground, patty, baked, well done, lean	1	each	88	45	257	26	0	0	16	6.3
Beef, heart, simmered	4	oz.	113	73	198	33	0	0	6	1.9
Beef, liver, fried	3	oz.	85	47	184	23	7	0	7	2.3
Beef, lunchmeat, thin sliced	1	oz.	28	16	50	8	2	0	1	0.5
Beef, meat stick, smoked	1	each	20	4	109	4	1	—	10	4.1
Beef, meatloaf	1	piece	108	67	230	18	7	0.4	14	5
Beef, porterhouse steak, choice, broiled, lean	1	each	170	102	366	44	0	0	20	6.9
Beef, rib eye steak, broiled, lean	4	oz.	113	67	255	32	0	0	13	5.4
Beef, rib steak, broiled, lean	4	oz.	113	66	251	32	0	0	13	5.1
Beef, rib, whole, roasted, lean	1	piece	42	24	102	12	0	0	6	2.4
Beef, rib, whole, roasted, lean	3	oz.	85	49	207	23	0	0	12	4.8
Beef, rib, whole, roasted, lean & fat	3	oz.	85	39	320	19	0	0	26	10.7
Beef, rib, whole, roasted, lean & fat	4	oz.	113	52	426	25	0	0	35	14.3
Beef, roast, rump, braised, lean	3	oz.	85	50	167	27	0	0	6	2
Beef, roast, rump, braised, lean	4	oz.	113	66	222	36	0	0	8	2.6
Beef, roast, rump, braised, lean & fat	3	oz.	85	45	220	25	0	0	13	4.8
Beef, roast, rump, braised, lean & fat	4	oz.	113	61	294	33	0	0	17	6.5
Beef, round steak, fried, lean & fat	4	oz.	113	57	327	35	0	0	20	7.5
Beef, round tip, sirloin roast, roasted, lean	4	oz.	113	74	210	32	0	0	8	2.7

A

MonoF	PolyF	Choles	Calc	Phos	Sod	Pot	Zn	Iron	Magn	VitA	VitE	VitC	Thia	Ribo	Nia	B6	Fola	B12
(g)	(g)	(mg)	(mg)	(mg)	(mg)	(mg)	(mg)	(mg)	(mg)	(μg RE)	(mg α-TE)	(mg)	(mg)	(mg)	(mg)	(mg)	(μg)	(μg)
0	0.2	0	25	126	2	357	0.9	2.6	40	0	0.19	1	0.14	0.05	0.5	0.11	115	0
0.1	0.2	0	42	139	240	369	0.9	1.9	48	0	0.08	2	0.13	0.07	0.4	0.12	94	0
1.4	0.4	20	89	218	756	676	3	4.2	84	0	0	15	0.07	0.04	0.8	0.36	28	0
0	0.2	0	65	151	2	414	1	2.5	61	0	0.36	0	0.21	0.05	0.2	0.11	123	0
0	0.2	0	96	119	7	595	1.5	3.9	67	0	0.24	0	0.13	0.05	0.1	0.1	86	0
0	0.1	0	81	102	5	505	1.2	3.3	57	0	0.2	0	0.11	0.04	0.1	0.08	73	0
5.5	3.9	0	400	410	35	889	4.1	12.2	163	0	0.26	0	0.94	0.41	2.8	0.16	41	0
0	0.2	0	36	155	4	269	0.9	2.3	84	2	0.24	0	0.18	0.06	0.5	0.08	125	0
0.1	0.5	0	115	467	14	966	2.9	7.2	282	4	0.24	1	0.74	0.2	1.8	0.31	549	0
0	0	0	18	13	1	74	0.2	0.6	9	7	0.2	3	0.01	0.04	0.1	0.02	22	0
0	0	0	18	13	169	74	0.2	0.6	9	7	0.2	3	0.01	0.04	0.1	0.02	22	0
0	0.1	0	29	24	2	187	0.2	0.8	16	5	0.18	6	0.05	0.06	0.4	0.04	21	0
0	0.1	0	33	21	6	85	0.3	0.6	16	7	0.1	3	0.02	0.06	0.3	0.04	16	0
0.1	0.4	0	55	161	4	286	0.9	2.2	65	0	0.44	2	0.16	0.09	0.6	0.11	71	0
0	0	0	12	17	36	19	0	0.5	8	0	0.02	0	0	0	0	0	4	0
6.2	5.7	0	0	0	11	288	0.1	0.7	0	0	—	4	0.09	0.1	0.2	0.19	32	0
1.7	0.3	47	13	144	343	390	2.4	2.1	28	50	0.8	6	0.13	0.16	2.9	0.32	10	1.39
2.9	1.7	29	10	103	427	294	2.5	1.2	18	0	0.62	4	0.08	0.1	1.9	0.25	8	0.91
4.6	1	110	9	317	345	555	6.1	3.9	38	0	0.16	0	0.14	0.34	5.6	0.63	13	4
2.2	0.2	10	4	81	438	118	1.6	1.1	10	0	0.1	0	0.03	0.03	0.3	0.04	26	0.2
—	—	25	20	—	1000	—	—	1.1	—	150	—	0	—	—	—	—	—	—
—	—	25	20	—	740	—	—	1.8	—	150	—	0	—	—	—	—	—	—
4.6	1	110	9	317	345	555	6.1	3.9	38	0	0.16	0	0.14	0.34	5.6	0.63	13	4
4.6	1	110	9	317	345	555	6.1	3.9	38	0	0.16	0	0.14	0.34	5.6	0.63	13	4
3.7	3.3	42	46	153	610	276	2.4	1.8	20	49	0.78	1	0.09	0.19	2.2	0.14	10	1.29
0.9	0.1	14	1	50	17	87	1	0.5	5	0	0.04	0	0.02	0.04	1.1	0.07	2	0.68
3.5	0.3	57	6	201	71	352	4.1	2.2	20	0	0.14	0	0.09	0.16	4.3	0.29	7	2.76
3.7	0.3	26	2	52	496	91	1.4	0.7	6	0	0.05	0	0.02	0.06	1.4	0.07	2	0.76
3	0.3	82	4	231	43	262	4.7	2.9	21	0	0.12	0	0.06	0.22	3.5	0.31	9	2.1
4.1	0.4	109	6	308	58	349	6.2	3.9	28	0	0.16	0	0.08	0.3	4.6	0.41	12	2.8
3.9	0.3	41	3	52	476	61	1.9	0.8	5	0	0.07	0	0.01	0.07	1.3	0.1	3	0.68
7.8	0.6	83	7	106	964	123	3.9	1.6	10	0	0.14	0	0.02	0.14	2.6	0.2	5	1.39
3	0.3	86	8	228	56	246	7.4	3.2	20	0	0.12	0	0.07	0.25	3.2	0.28	9	2.89
3.9	0.4	115	10	304	75	328	9.8	4.3	27	0	0.16	0	0.09	0.33	4.2	0.37	12	3.86
6.8	0.7	98	14	126	1140	154	4	2.4	16	0	0.17	0	0.02	0.17	2.8	0.15	10	1.84
5.5	3.7	86	36	260	386	438	5.7	4	35	3	0.55	0	0.17	0.34	4.4	0.44	14	3.23
0.5	0.1	12	2	49	986	126	1.5	1.3	9	0	0.04	0	0.02	0.06	1.6	0.1	3	0.76
4.3	0.4	95	8	270	71	475	6.3	4.1	34	0	0.16	0	0.15	0.34	4.4	0.5	8	2.91
7.9	0.7	121	10	184	73	330	7.9	3.4	25	0	0.2	0	0.06	0.35	6.1	0.33	12	2.11
7.8	0.7	112	10	215	93	418	7.3	3.1	28	0	0.2	0	0.08	0.36	6.6	0.36	12	2.9
6.8	0.6	89	11	160	78	307	5.5	2.2	21	0	0.18	0	0.05	0.21	5.2	0.26	10	2.39
8.8	0.7	115	14	206	101	396	7	2.8	27	0	0.23	0	0.07	0.27	6.8	0.34	12	3.08
9.7	0.8	115	14	217	105	371	6.6	3.1	25	0	0.26	0	0.04	0.24	7.3	0.34	11	3.72
6.6	0.6	95	9	182	79	354	6.2	2.7	24	0	0.17	0	0.07	0.31	5.6	0.31	11	2.46
8.8	0.7	108	12	205	99	386	6.7	2.8	26	0	0.22	0	0.07	0.27	6.2	0.36	11	2.93
7.9	0.7	105	9	210	92	408	7.1	3.1	27	0	0.2	0	0.08	0.34	6.2	0.35	11	2.63
7.1	0.6	87	11	144	62	252	5.7	2.3	18	0	0.18	0	0.06	0.21	4.8	0.23	11	1.99
1.4	1.6	219	7	284	71	264	3.6	8.5	28	0	0.82	2	0.16	1.75	4.6	0.24	2	16.2
1.4	1.4	410	9	392	90	309	4.6	5.3	20	9119	0.54	20	0.18	3.52	12.2	1.22	187	95.2
0.5	0.1	12	3	48	409	122	1.1	0.8	5	0	0.05	0	0.02	0.05	1.5	0.1	3	0.73
4.1	0.9	26	14	36	293	51	0.5	0.7	4	34	0.06	1	0.03	0.09	0.9	0.04	0	0.2
6	0.7	90	43	161	409	293	3.6	2	22	17	0.17	1	0.08	0.28	4	0.14	12	1.64
8.9	0.6	117	12	359	117	624	9	5.3	46	0	0.24	0	0.19	0.42	7.9	0.68	14	3.86
5.6	0.4	91	15	236	78	447	7.9	2.9	31	0	0.18	0	0.11	0:25	5.4	0.45	9	3.76
5.4	0.4	91	15	236	78	447	7.9	2.9	31	0	0.16	0	0.11	0.25	5.4	0.45	9	3.76
2.5	0.2	34	4	90	30	157	2.9	1.2	10	0	0.06	0	0.03	0.09	1.8	0.11	3	1.22
5	0.4	68	8	182	61	318	5.9	2.4	21	0	0.12	0	0.07	0.18	3.5	0.23	7	2.47
11.4	0.9	72	9	146	54	252	4.4	2	16	0	0.2	0	0.06	0.14	2.9	0.2	6	2.14
15.2	1.3	96	12	195	71	336	5.9	2.6	22	0	0.27	0	0.08	0.19	3.8	0.26	8	2.86
2.5	0.2	82	4	231	43	262	4.7	2.9	21	0	0.08	0	0.06	0.22	3.5	0.31	9	2.1
3.4	0.3	109	6	308	58	349	6.2	3.9	28	0	0.1	0	0.08	0.3	4.6	0.41	12	2.8
5.6	0.5	82	5	210	42	241	4.2	2.7	20	0	0.09	0	0.06	0.2	3.2	0.28	8	2.01
7.4	0.6	109	7	280	57	321	5.6	3.6	26	0	0.12	0	0.08	0.27	4.2	0.37	11	2.68
8.4	1.2	110	10	287	340	500	5.5	3.6	34	0	0.2	0	0.13	0.31	5.1	0.57	12	3.71
3.1	0.3	92	6	274	74	438	8	3.3	31	0	0.16	0	0.11	0.31	4.2	0.45	9	3.28

Food Item	Qty	Meas	Wgt (g)	Wtr (g)	Cals	Prot (g)	Carb (g)	Fib (g)	Fat (g)	SatF (g)
Beef, round, bottom, braised, lean	1	piece	42	24	92	13	0	0	4	1.3
Beef, round, bottom, braised, lean	3	oz.	85	48	187	27	0	0	8	2.7
Beef, round, broiled, lean & fat	4	oz.	113	62	311	29	0	0	21	9.2
Beef, round, pot roasted, lean & fat	1	piece	42	22	116	12	0	0	7	2.7
Beef, round, pot roasted, lean & fat	3	oz.	85	44	234	24	0	0	14	5.4
Beef, sandwich steak, Steak Ums	1	each	41	24	105	10	0	0	7	2.6
Beef, short ribs, choice, braised, lean	2	each	102	51	301	31	0	0	18	7.9
Beef, shortrib, braised, lean & fat	4	oz.	113	40	534	24	0	0	48	20.2
Beef, sirloin steak, broiled, lean	1	each	156	96	315	47	0	0	12	4.8
Beef, sirloin steak, broiled, lean	3	oz.	85	52	172	26	0	0	7	2.6
Beef, sirloin strip steak, broiled, lean	4	oz.	113	68	235	32	0	0	11	4.1
Beef, stew meat, cooked, lean & fat	4	oz.	113	57	345	32	0	0	23	9.2
Beef, stew meat, cooked, lean only	0.5	cup	70	39	164	22	0	0	8	3
Beef, t-bone steak, broiled, lean	1	each	184	113	377	49	0	0	19	6.6
Beef, t-bone steak, broiled, lean	3	oz.	85	52	174	23	0	0	9	3.1
Beef, t-bone steak, broiled, lean & fat	1	each	219	114	677	51	0	0	51	19.9
Beef, t-bone steak, broiled, lean & fat	3	oz.	85	44	263	20	0	0	20	7.7
Beef, tenderloin steak, broiled, lean	4	oz.	113	68	239	32	0	0	11	4.2
Beef, top round steak, broiled, lean	4	oz.	113	70	204	36	0	0	6	1.9
Beef, top sirloin steak, broiled, lean	4	oz.	113	70	221	34	0	0	8	3.2
Beef, tripe, pickled	1	oz.	28	25	18	3	0	0	0	0.1
Beefalo, roasted	4	oz.	113	70	213	35	0	0	7	3
Beer, Lowenbrau Special	1	cup	237	—	105	1	10	—	0	0
Beer, Lowenbrau dark, 12 fl oz	1	each	356	—	158	1	14	—	0	0
Beer, Milwaukee's Best Ice	1	cup	237	—	90	1	5	—	0	0
Beer, Red Dog	1	cup	237	—	98	0	9	—	0	0
Beer, lager, bottled 355ml can	1	each	357	336	107	1	6	0.7	—	—
Beer, light	1	cup	236	225	66	0	3	0	0	0
Beer, non-alcoholic, Sharp's	1	cup	237	—	39	0	8	—	0	0
Beer, regular, alcoholic	1	cup	237	219	97	1	9	0.5	0	0
Beerwurst/beer salami	1	piece	23	12	76	3	0	0	7	3
Beet greens, cooked, no added salt	0.5	cup	72	64	19	2	4	2.1	0	0
Beets & onions, pickled	0.5	cup	84	72	42	1	10	1.2	0	0
Beets, canned, drained	0.5	cup	85	77	26	1	6	1.4	0	0
Beets, canned, w/liquid, low sodium	0.5	cup	123	113	34	1	8	1.5	0	0
Beets, canned, w/liquid, regular	0.5	cup	123	113	34	1	8	1.5	0	0
Beets, cooked, no added salt	0.5	cup	85	74	37	1	8	1.7	0	0
Beets, pickled slices	0.5	cup	114	93	74	1	19	2.3	0	0
Beets, raw slices	0.5	cup	68	60	29	1	6	1.9	0	0
Beets, raw, whole	1	each	82	71	35	1	8	2.3	0	0
Beets, w/Harvard sauce	0.5	cup	123	91	135	1	25	1.5	4	0.8
Beets, whole, cooked, no added salt	2	each	100	87	44	2	10	2	0	0
Beets, whole, pickled	1	each	50	41	32	0	8	1	0	0
Berry turnover	1	each	78	25	277	3	36	1.4	14	3.4
Biscuit dough, higher fat, chilled	1	oz.	28	10	90	2	12	0.4	4	1
Biscuit dough, higher fat, chilled, baked	1	each	27	8	93	2	13	0.4	4	1
Biscuit dough, lower fat, chilled, baked	1	each	21	6	63	2	12	0.4	1	0.3
Biscuit mix, dry, prepared	1	each	28	8	95	2	14	0.5	3	0.8
Biscuit, cheese	1	each	30	8	115	3	12	0.4	6	2.2
Biscuit, homemade	1	each	28	8	101	2	13	0.4	5	1.2
Biscuit, mixed grain, chilled, baked	1	each	41	11	125	3	23	1.1	3	0.7
Biscuit, plain, fast food	1	each	74	20	276	4	34	1.4	13	8.7
Biscuit, plain/buttermilk, baked	1	each	35	9	127	2	17	0.5	6	0.9
Biscuit, whole wheat	1	each	63	17	201	6	29	4.8	8	2.2
Bison, roasted	4	oz.	113	75	162	32	0	0	3	1
Blackberries, fresh	0.5	cup	72	62	37	1	9	3.8	0	0
Blackberries, frozen, unsweetened	0.5	cup	76	62	48	1	12	3.8	0	0
Blackberry, canned w/heavy syrup	0.5	cup	128	96	118	2	30	4.4	0	0
Blackeyed cowpeas, frozen, cooked	0.5	cup	85	56	112	7	20	5.4	1	0.1
Blackeyed peas, cooked from raw, drained	0.5	cup	82	62	80	3	17	4.1	0	0.1
Blintz, fruit-filled	1	each	70	44	124	4	17	0.4	5	1.4
Blueberries, canned w/heavy syrup	0.5	cup	128	98	113	1	28	1.9	0	0
Blueberries, fresh	0.5	cup	72	61	41	0	10	2	0	0
Blueberries, frozen, sweetened, pkg	0.5	cup	115	89	93	0	25	2.4	0	0
Blueberries, frozen, unsweetened	0.5	cup	78	67	40	0	9	2.1	0	0

MonoF (g)	PolyF (g)	Choles (mg)	Calc (mg)	Phos (mg)	Sod (mg)	Pot (mg)	Zn (mg)	Iron (mg)	Magn (mg)	VitA (μg RE)	VitE (mg α-TE)	VitC (mg)	Thia (mg)	Ribo (mg)	Nia (mg)	B6 (mg)	Fola (μg)	B12 (μg)
1.7	0.2	40	2	114	21	129	2.3	1.4	10	0	0.08	0	0.03	0.11	1.7	0.15	5	1.04
3.5	0.3	82	4	231	43	262	4.7	2.9	21	0	0.15	0	0.06	0.22	3.5	0.31	9	2.1
10.5	0.9	95	8	239	68	415	4.7	2.7	27	0	0.29	0	0.1	0.23	4.2	0.5	10	3.12
3.1	0.3	40	3	103	21	118	2.1	1.3	9	0	0.08	0	0.03	0.1	1.6	0.14	4	0.99
6.2	0.5	82	5	208	42	240	4.2	2.6	19	0	0.16	0	0.06	0.2	3.2	0.28	8	2
3	0.2	33	3	66	29	128	2.2	1	9	0	0.07	0	0.02	0.11	1.9	0.11	4	0.82
8.1	0.6	95	11	240	59	319	8	3.4	22	0	0.14	0	0.07	0.21	3.3	0.29	7	3.53
21.4	1.7	107	14	184	57	254	5.5	2.6	17	0	0.33	0	0.06	0.17	2.8	0.25	6	2.97
5.3	0.5	139	17	381	103	629	10.2	5.2	50	0	0.22	0	0.2	0.45	6.7	0.7	16	4.45
2.9	0.3	76	9	207	56	343	5.5	2.9	27	0	0.12	0	0.11	0.25	3.6	0.38	8	2.42
4.3	0.4	86	9	247	77	449	5.9	2.8	31	0	0.16	0	0.1	0.23	6.1	0.48	9	2.27
10.1	0.8	113	12	248	333	285	8.5	3.5	23	0	0.2	0	0.08	0.27	3.3	0.32	8	2.78
3.4	0.3	71	7	172	208	193	6.1	2.5	16	0	0.1	0	0.06	0.19	2.2	0.21	5	1.83
8.3	0.6	109	11	396	131	696	9.8	5.8	52	0	0.26	0	0.2	0.46	8.5	0.72	15	4.18
3.8	0.3	50	5	183	60	321	4.5	2.7	24	0	0.12	0	0.09	0.21	3.9	0.33	7	1.93
22.3	1.8	147	18	403	140	703	9.8	5.9	50	0	0.46	0	0.2	0.46	8.6	0.72	15	4.66
8.7	0.7	57	7	156	54	273	3.8	2.3	20	0	0.18	0	0.08	0.18	3.4	0.28	6	1.81
4.3	0.4	95	8	270	71	475	6.3	4.1	34	0	0.16	0	0.15	0.34	4.4	0.5	8	2.91
2.2	0.2	95	7	279	69	501	6.3	3.3	35	0	0.16	0	0.14	0.31	6.8	0.64	14	2.81
3.5	0.3	101	12	277	75	457	7.4	3.8	36	0	0.16	0	0.15	0.33	4.8	0.51	11	3.23
0.1	0	19	36	24	13	5	0.5	0.5	2	0	0.03	0	0	0.04	0.5	0	0	0.26
3	0.2	66	27	284	93	521	7.3	3.5	0	0	0.2	10	0.03	0.12	5.6	0.45	20	2.89
0	0	0	—	—	5	—	—	—	—	—	—	—	—	—	—	—	—	0
0	0	0	—	—	7	—	—	—	—	—	—	—	—	—	—	—	—	0
0	0	0	—	—	3	—	—	—	—	—	—	—	—	—	—	—	—	0
0	0	0	—	—	3	—	—	—	—	—	—	—	—	—	—	—	—	0
—	—	0	14	—	14	121	0	—	—	—	—	0	—	0.07	—	0.07	14	0.5
0	0	0	12	28	7	42	0.1	0.1	12	0	0	0	0.02	0.07	0.9	0.08	10	0.02
0	0	0	—	—	2	—	—	—	—	—	—	—	—	—	—	—	—	0
0	0	0	12	28	12	59	0	0.1	14	0	0	0	0.01	0.06	1.1	0.12	14	0.05
3.2	0.3	14	2	22	236	40	0.6	0.3	3	0	0.04	0	0.02	0.03	0.8	0.04	1	0.45
0	0	0	82	30	174	654	0.4	1.4	49	367	0.22	18	0.08	0.21	0.4	0.1	10	0
0	0	0	8	21	209	211	0.2	0.5	27	1	0.22	3	0.02	0.01	0.2	0.02	27	0
0	0	0	13	14	165	126	0.2	1.6	14	1	0.26	3	0.01	0.03	0.1	0.05	26	0
0	0	0	16	20	26	175	0.3	0.8	20	4	0.37	3	0.01	0.05	0.2	0.07	36	0
0	0	0	16	20	310	162	0.3	0.8	20	4	0.35	3	0.01	0.05	0.2	0.07	36	0
0	0.1	0	14	32	66	259	0.3	0.7	20	3	0.26	3	0.02	0.03	0.3	0.06	68	0
0	0	0	12	19	301	169	0.3	0.5	17	1	0.15	3	0.01	0.06	0.3	0.06	30	0
0	0	0	11	27	53	221	0.2	0.5	16	3	0.2	3	0.02	0.03	0.2	0.05	74	0
0	0	0	13	33	64	265	0.3	0.7	19	3	0.24	4	0.02	0.03	0.3	0.06	89	0
1.7	1.2	0	12	30	287	288	0.2	0.7	36	53	0.87	5	0.03	0.02	0.2	0.03	45	0
0	0.1	0	16	38	77	305	0.4	0.8	23	4	0.3	4	0.03	0.04	0.3	0.07	80	0
0	0	0	6	8	132	74	0.1	0.2	8	0	0.06	1	0	0.02	0.1	0.02	13	0
6.1	3.7	0	6	32	230	54	0.2	1.3	8	2	1.51	3	0.18	0.13	1.5	0.02	6	0
2.1	0.5	0	5	100	314	41	0.1	0.7	4	0	0.51	0	0.11	0.06	0.9	0.01	16	0
2.2	0.5	0	5	104	325	42	0.1	0.7	4	0	0.49	0	0.09	0.06	0.8	0.01	12	0
0.6	0.2	0	4	98	305	39	0.1	0.6	4	0	0.14	0	0.09	0.05	0.7	0.01	14	0
1.2	1.2	1	52	133	271	53	0.2	0.6	7	7	0.11	0	0.1	0.1	0.9	0.02	2	0.06
2.4	1.2	6	80	70	197	42	0.3	0.7	6	17	0.43	0	0.1	0.1	0.8	0.01	3	0.04
2	1.2	1	67	47	165	34	0.2	0.8	5	7	0.37	0	0.1	0.09	0.8	0.01	17	0.02
1.4	0.4	0	8	158	319	217	0.3	1.3	14	0	0.57	0	0.15	0.09	1.5	0.02	4	0
3.4	0.5	5	90	260	584	87	0.3	1.6	9	24	0.44	0	0.27	0.18	1.6	0.03	6	0.1
2.4	2.2	0	17	151	368	78	0.2	1.2	6	0	1.03	0	0.15	0.1	1.2	0.02	21	0.05
3	1.9	4	120	177	468	200	1.2	1.5	56	9	0.98	0	0.14	0.12	2.2	0.13	13	0.06
1.1	0.3	93	9	237	65	409	4.2	3.9	30	0	0.16	0	0.11	0.31	4.2	0.45	9	3.24
0	0.2	0	23	15	0	141	0.2	0.4	14	12	0.51	15	0.02	0.03	0.3	0.04	24	0
0	0.2	0	22	23	1	106	0.2	0.6	17	8	0.54	2	0.02	0.04	0.9	0.05	26	0
0	0.1	0	27	18	4	127	0.2	0.8	22	28	0.91	4	0.04	0.05	0.4	0.05	34	0
0.1	0.2	0	20	104	4	319	1.2	1.8	42	7	0.33	2	0.22	0.05	0.6	0.08	120	0
0	0.1	0	106	42	3	345	0.8	0.9	43	65	0.18	2	0.08	0.12	1.2	0.05	105	0
1.8	1	50	33	56	151	75	0.3	0.8	6	78	0.69	1	0.05	0.13	0.3	0.04	8	0.2
0.1	0.2	0	6	13	4	51	0.1	0.4	5	8	1.28	1	0.04	0.07	0.1	0.05	2	0
0	0.1	0	4	7	4	64	0.1	0.1	4	7	0.72	9	0.04	0.04	0.3	0.03	5	0
0	0.1	0	7	8	1	69	0.1	0.4	2	5	0.82	1	0.02	0.06	0.3	0.07	8	0
0.1	0.2	0	6	9	1	42	0.1	0.1	4	6	0.78	2	0.02	0.03	0.4	0.05	5	0

A

Food Item	Qty	Meas	Wgt (g)	Wtr (g)	Cals	Prot (g)	Carb (g)	Fib (g)	Fat (g)	SatF (g)
Bologna, beef	1	piece	23	13	72	3	0	0	7	2.8
Bologna, beef & pork	1	piece	28	15	90	3	1	0	8	3
Bologna, cured pork	1	piece	23	14	57	4	0	0	5	1.6
Bologna, turkey	1	piece	28	18	56	4	0	0	4	1.4
Boysenberries, canned w/heavy syrup	0.5	cup	128	98	113	1	28	3.3	0	0
Boysenberries, fresh	0.5	cup	72	62	37	1	9	3.8	0	0
Boysenberries, frozen, unsweetened	0.5	cup	66	57	33	1	8	2.6	0	0
Bratwurst, cooked link	1	each	85	48	256	12	2	0	22	7.9
Bread crumbs, dry, grated, plain	0.25	cup	25	2	99	3	18	0.6	1	0.3
Bread crumbs, seasoned, dry, grated	0.25	cup	30	2	110	4	21	1.3	1	0.2
Bread crumbs, soft	0.25	cup	11	4	30	1	6	0.2	1	0.2
Bread stick, w/o salt coating, plain	10	each	100	6	412	12	68	3	10	1.4
Bread stick, w/salt coating	1	each	35	2	134	4	26	0.8	1	0.2
Bread stuffing, homemade	1	cup	203	132	341	8	45	4	15	3
Bread stuffing, mix, prepared	1	cup	140	91	249	4	30	4.1	12	2.4
Bread, 7-grain, Pepperidge Farm	1	piece	38	15	100	3	18	2	2	0
Bread, Armenian	1	piece	20	7	55	2	10	0.6	1	0.1
Bread, Armenian, toasted	1	piece	18	5	55	2	10	0.6	1	0.1
Bread, Boston brown, canned	1	piece	45	21	88	2	20	2.1	1	0.1
Bread, Cuban-Spanish-Portuguese	1	piece	20	6	58	2	11	0.5	1	0.1
Bread, Cuban-Spanish-Portuguese, toasted	1	piece	18	3	61	2	12	0.6	1	0.1
Bread, French	1	piece	35	12	96	3	18	1	1	0.2
Bread, Hollywood, dark	1	piece	18	7	39	2	8	1.4	0	0.1
Bread, Hollywood, dark, toasted	1	piece	16	6	39	2	8	—	0	0.1
Bread, Hollywood, light	1	piece	18	7	41	2	8	0.9	0	0
Bread, Hollywood, light, toasted	1	piece	16	6	40	2	8	—	0	0
Bread, Indian fry, 5 inch diameter	1	piece	90	24	296	6	48	1.6	9	2.1
Bread, Italian	1	piece	30	11	81	3	15	0.8	1	0.3
Bread, Italian, toasted	1	piece	27	8	80	3	15	0.8	1	0.3
Bread, Spanish coffee	1	each	85	21	292	7	49	1.6	7	1.1
Bread, banana, homemade, w/margarine	1	piece	50	15	163	2	27	0.6	5	1.1
Bread, banana, recipe, w/vegetable shortening	1	piece	60	17	203	3	33	0.8	7	1.8
Bread, barley	1	piece	26	10	69	2	13	1.2	1	0.3
Bread, batter	1	piece	33	12	93	3	15	0.6	2	0.7
Bread, buckwheat	1	piece	27	10	71	2	13	1	1	0.3
Bread, buckwheat, toasted	1	piece	25	7	73	2	14	1	1	0.3
Bread, cheese	1	piece	26	10	71	2	12	0.6	1	0.5
Bread, cheese, toasted	1	piece	24	7	71	2	12	0.6	1	0.5
Bread, corn & molasses	1	piece	32	12	86	2	15	0.6	2	0.6
Bread, corn & molasses, toasted	1	piece	29	9	87	2	15	0.6	2	0.6
Bread, cracked wheat	1	piece	25	9	65	2	12	1.4	1	0.2
Bread, cracked wheat, toasted	1	piece	21	6	59	2	11	1.3	1	0.2
Bread, crumpet biscuit	1	each	45	24	80	3	17	0.8	0	0.1
Bread, crumpet biscuit, toasted	1	each	41	19	82	3	18	0.8	0	0.1
Bread, dark pumpernickel, Pepperidge Farm	1	piece	32	12	80	3	15	1	1	0.5
Bread, date nut	1	piece	56	12	217	3	30	0.8	10	2.2
Bread, egg/challah	1	piece	23	8	66	2	11	0.5	1	0.4
Bread, egg/challah, toasted	1	piece	21	6	66	2	11	0.5	1	0.3
Bread, fruit, w/o nuts	1	piece	41	10	150	2	23	0.5	6	1.5
Bread, hoecake, 1/8 pone	1	piece	61	29	136	3	25	3.6	3	0.7
Bread, milk & honey	1	piece	28	10	74	2	15	0.6	1	0.2
Bread, milk & honey, toasted	1	piece	29	9	84	2	17	0.6	1	0.2
Bread, mixed grain	1	piece	25	9	62	2	12	1.6	1	0.2
Bread, mixed grain, toasted	1	piece	23	7	63	3	12	1.5	1	0.2
Bread, multigrain, low calorie, high fiber	1	piece	23	10	46	2	10	2.8	1	0
Bread, multigrain, low calorie, high fiber, toasted	1	piece	21	8	47	2	10	2.8	1	0
Bread, oat bran	1	piece	30	13	71	3	12	1.4	1	0.2
Bread, oat bran, low calorie	1	piece	28	13	56	2	12	3.4	1	0.1
Bread, oat bran, low calorie, toasted	1	piece	25	9	60	2	12	3.6	1	0.1
Bread, oat bran, toasted	1	piece	27	10	70	3	12	1.3	1	0.2
Bread, oatmeal	1	piece	25	9	67	2	12	1	1	0.2
Bread, oatmeal, low calorie	1	piece	23	10	48	2	10	—	1	0.1
Bread, oatmeal, low calorie, toasted	1	piece	19	6	48	2	10	—	1	0.1
Bread, oatmeal, toasted	1	piece	23	7	67	2	12	1	1	0.2
Bread, onion cheese	1	piece	26	10	71	2	12	0.6	1	0.5

MonoF (g)	PolyF (g)	Choles (mg)	Calc (mg)	Phos (mg)	Sod (mg)	Pot (mg)	Zn (mg)	Iron (mg)	Magn (mg)	VitA (μg RE)	VitE (mg α-TE)	VitC (mg)	Thia (mg)	Ribo (mg)	Nia (mg)	B6 (mg)	Fola (μg)	B12 (μg)
3.2	0.3	13	3	20	226	36	0.5	0.4	3	0	0.04	0	0.01	0.02	0.6	0.04	1	0.33
3.8	0.7	16	3	26	289	51	0.6	0.4	3	0	0.06	0	0.05	0.04	0.7	0.05	1	0.38
2.2	0.5	14	3	32	272	65	0.5	0.2	3	0	0.06	0	0.12	0.04	0.9	0.06	1	0.21
1.4	1.2	28	24	37	249	56	0.5	0.4	4	0	0.15	0	0.02	0.05	1	0.06	2	0.08
0	0.1	0	23	13	4	115	0.2	0.6	14	5	0.91	8	0.03	0.04	0.3	0.05	44	0
0	0.2	0	23	15	0	141	0.2	0.4	14	12	0.51	15	0.02	0.03	0.3	0.04	24	0
0	0.1	0	18	18	1	92	0.1	0.6	11	5	0.3	2	0.04	0.02	0.5	0.04	42	0
10.4	2.3	51	37	127	473	180	2	1.1	13	0	0.21	1	0.43	0.16	2.7	0.18	2	0.81
0.6	0.3	0	57	37	216	55	0.3	1.5	12	0	0.14	0	0.19	0.11	1.7	0.02	27	0
0.3	0.2	0	30	40	795	81	0.3	1	11	1	0.04	0	0.05	0.05	0.8	0.04	33	0.01
0.2	0.1	0	9	11	57	12	0.1	0.3	2	0	0.02	0	0.04	0.03	0.4	0	4	0
3.6	3.6	0	22	121	657	124	0.9	4.3	32	0	1.48	0	0.59	0.55	5.3	0.07	122	0
0.4	0.3	1	10	35	586	32	0.2	1.5	7	0	0.04	0	0.23	0.18	2.2	0.01	4	0
6.5	4.3	0	130	100	936	266	0.6	3.3	30	140	2.44	3	0.34	0.29	3.2	0.11	34	0
5.3	3.6	0	45	59	760	104	0.4	1.5	17	113	1.96	0	0.19	0.15	2.1	0.06	141	0.01
0.5	0	0	0	—	180	—	—	0.7	—	0	—	0	0.12	0.07	1.2	—	—	—
0.1	0.3	0	16	15	117	15	0.2	0.6	5	0	0.05	0	0.08	0.05	0.7	0.01	5	0
0.1	0.3	0	16	15	116	15	0.2	0.6	5	0	0.04	0	0.06	0.05	0.7	0.01	4	0
0.1	0.3	0	32	50	284	143	0.2	0.9	28	5	0.25	0	0.01	0.05	0.5	0.04	5	0
0.2	0.2	0	9	17	116	18	0.1	0.6	4	0	0.02	0	0.08	0.05	0.7	0.01	6	0
0.2	0.2	0	9	18	121	19	0.1	0.6	4	0	0.01	0	0.07	0.05	0.7	0.01	6	0
0.4	0.2	0	26	37	213	40	0.3	0.9	9	0	0.1	0	0.18	0.12	1.7	0.02	33	0
0.1	0.2	0	139	29	92	36	0.3	0.6	12	0	0.02	0	0.08	0.07	0.7	0.02	5	0
0.1	0.2	0	137	29	91	36	0.3	0.6	12	0	0.02	0	0.06	0.06	0.6	0.02	4	0
0.1	0.2	0	130	15	124	34	0.2	0.6	7	0	0.04	0	0.08	0.06	0.7	0.01	4	0
0.1	0.1	0	128	14	123	34	0.2	0.6	7	0	0.03	0	0.06	0.05	0.7	0	3	0.01
3.6	2.3	0	210	141	626	67	0.4	3.2	14	0	0.7	0	0.39	0.27	3.3	0.02	67	0
0.2	0.4	0	23	31	175	33	0.3	0.9	8	0	0.11	0	0.14	0.09	1.3	0.01	28	0
0.2	0.4	0	23	31	173	33	0.3	0.9	8	0	0.05	0	0.11	0.08	1.2	0.01	6	0
4.8	0.8	32	12	81	12	82	0.5	2.6	14	15	1.08	0	0.34	0.31	3	0.05	34	0.06
2.2	1.6	22	10	29	151	67	0.2	0.7	7	60	0.9	1	0.09	0.1	0.7	0.08	16	0.05
3	1.8	26	11	34	119	79	0.2	0.8	8	14	0.84	1	0.1	0.12	0.9	0.09	7	0.05
0.3	0.3	1	10	31	96	39	0.3	0.7	8	2	0.06	0	0.09	0.08	1.1	0.02	9	0.01
0.9	0.5	14	20	41	127	50	0.2	0.9	7	9	0.25	0	0.12	0.13	1	0.03	13	0.05
0.4	0.3	1	11	38	100	57	0.3	0.8	18	2	0.12	0	0.1	0.08	1.2	0.04	10	0.01
0.4	0.3	1	11	40	103	59	0.3	0.8	19	2	0.12	0	0.1	0.08	1.2	0.04	11	0.01
0.4	0.3	2	38	32	144	30	0.2	0.7	7	4	0.02	0	0.12	0.09	1	0.01	9	0.01
0.4	0.3	1	38	32	145	30	0.2	0.7	6	4	0.02	0	0.1	0.09	1	0.01	7	0.01
0.7	0.4	2	27	35	261	100	0.2	0.9	16	6	0.17	0	0.11	0.11	1	0.05	11	0.03
0.7	0.4	2	27	35	263	101	0.2	0.9	16	6	0.17	0	0.11	0.11	1	0.06	11	0.03
0.5	0.2	0	11	38	135	44	0.3	0.7	13	0	0.15	0	0.09	0.06	0.9	0.08	15	0
0.4	0.2	0	10	35	123	40	0.3	0.6	12	0	0.13	0	0.07	0.05	0.8	0.06	6	0.01
0	0.2	0	50	72	324	37	0.2	0.4	7	0	0.02	0	0.08	0.01	0.4	0.02	4	0
0	0.2	0	51	74	332	38	0.2	0.5	7	0	0.02	0	0.08	0.01	0.4	0.02	4	0
0	0.5	0	20	—	230	—	—	1.1	—	0	—	0	0.12	0.07	1.2	—	—	—
3.8	3.5	28	47	54	140	100	0.3	1	15	14	0.88	1	0.12	0.12	0.9	0.12	9	0.05
0.5	0.3	12	21	24	113	26	0.2	0.7	4	5	0.14	0	0.1	0.1	1.1	0.02	24	0.02
0.6	0.2	12	21	25	113	26	0.2	0.7	4	5	0.18	0	0.08	0.09	1	0.01	19	0.02
2.5	1.5	22	34	32	109	62	0.2	0.7	7	11	0.61	1	0.08	0.09	0.7	0.08	5	0.04
1.2	1	0	69	94	245	94	0.6	1.1	41	0	0.27	0	0.1	0.06	1.1	0.09	6	0
0.1	0.2	1	10	29	53	35	0.2	0.9	5	2	0.08	0	0.12	0.1	1	0.02	13	0.01
0.1	0.3	1	12	33	60	40	0.2	1	6	2	0.1	0	0.11	0.12	1.2	0.03	13	0.01
0.4	0.2	0	23	44	122	51	0.3	0.9	13	0	0.16	0	0.1	0.09	1.1	0.08	20	0.02
0.4	0.2	0	23	44	122	51	0.3	0.9	13	0	0.15	0	0.08	0.08	1	0.08	16	0.02
0	0.1	2	18	57	117	40	0.5	0.6	20	0	0.04	0	0.1	0.07	0.9	0.03	14	0
0	0.1	2	18	58	118	40	0.5	0.6	20	0	0.04	0	0.08	0.07	0.9	0.03	12	0
0.5	0.5	0	20	42	122	44	0.3	0.9	10	0	0.19	0	0.15	0.1	1.4	0.02	24	0
0.2	0.5	0	16	39	98	29	0.3	0.9	15	0	0.13	0	0.1	0.06	1	0.03	18	0
0.2	0.5	0	17	36	105	30	0.3	0.9	14	0	0.13	0	0.08	0.05	1	0.02	14	0
0.5	0.5	0	19	31	121	33	0.3	0.9	9	0	0.12	0	0.12	0.09	1.3	0.01	19	0
0.4	0.4	0	16	32	150	36	0.3	0.7	9	0	0.15	0	0.1	0.06	0.8	0.02	16	0.01
0.2	0.3	0	26	23	89	28	0.2	0.5	6	0	0.09	0	0.08	0.06	0.7	0.01	13	0.02
0.2	0.3	0	26	27	88	35	0.2	0.5	6	0	0.08	0	0.06	0.06	0.6	0.01	5	0.03
0.4	0.4	0	17	32	150	35	0.3	0.7	9	0	0.09	0	0.08	0.05	0.7	0.02	12	0
0.4	0.3	2	38	32	144	30	0.2	0.7	7	4	0.02	0	0.12	0.09	1	0.01	9	0.01

A

Food Item	Qty	Meas	Wgt (g)	Wtr (g)	Cals	Prot (g)	Carb (g)	Fib (g)	Fat (g)	SatF (g)
Bread, onion cheese, toasted	1	piece	24	7	71	2	12	0.6	1	0.5
Bread, pita pocket, white	1	each	60	19	165	5	33	1.3	1	0.1
Bread, pita pocket, whole wheat	1	each	45	14	120	4	25	3.3	1	0.2
Bread, pita, 100% whole wheat, toasted	1	each	41	9	120	5	26	4.7	1	0.1
Bread, potato	1	piece	26	10	69	2	13	0.6	1	0.2
Bread, potato, toasted	1	piece	24	7	70	2	13	0.6	1	0.2
Bread, protein	1	piece	19	8	47	2	8	0.6	0	0.1
Bread, protein, toasted	1	piece	17	6	46	2	8	0.6	0	0.1
Bread, pumpernickel	1	piece	32	12	80	3	15	2.1	1	0.1
Bread, pumpernickel, toasted	1	piece	29	9	80	3	15	2.1	1	0.1
Bread, raisin	1	piece	25	8	68	2	13	1.1	1	0.3
Bread, raisin, toasted	1	piece	21	6	62	2	12	1	1	0.2
Bread, rice	1	piece	25	9	79	2	10	0.6	4	0.4
Bread, rice bran, low calorie	1	piece	27	11	66	2	12	1.3	1	0.2
Bread, rice bran, toasted, low calorie	1	piece	25	9	66	2	12	1.3	1	0.2
Bread, rice, toasted	1	piece	23	6	81	2	10	0.6	4	0.4
Bread, rye	1	piece	25	9	65	2	12	1.4	1	0.2
Bread, rye, light, toasted	1	piece	22	7	62	2	12	1.4	1	0.2
Bread, rye, low calorie	1	piece	23	11	47	2	9	2.8	1	0.1
Bread, rye, low calorie, toasted	1	piece	19	7	46	2	9	—	1	0.1
Bread, sourdough	1	piece	25	9	68	2	13	0.8	1	0.2
Bread, sourdough starter	1	Tbs	16	10	22	1	4	0.3	0	0
Bread, sourdough, toasted	1	piece	23	7	68	2	13	0.8	1	0.2
Bread, soy	1	piece	26	10	69	3	12	0.7	1	0.4
Bread, soy, toasted	1	piece	24	7	71	3	12	0.7	1	0.4
Bread, sprouted wheat	1	piece	26	10	68	2	12	1.4	1	0.2
Bread, sunflower meal	1	piece	27	10	75	3	12	0.5	1	0.5
Bread, sunflower meal, toasted	1	piece	25	7	76	3	12	0.5	1	0.5
Bread, sweet potato	1	piece	25	8	72	2	12	0.6	2	0.3
Bread, triticale	1	piece	25	9	63	2	12	1.6	1	0.2
Bread, triticale, toasted	1	piece	23	7	64	2	12	1.7	1	0.2
Bread, vienna	1	piece	25	9	68	2	13	0.8	1	0.2
Bread, wheat	1	piece	28	10	74	3	13	1.2	1	0.3
Bread, wheat berry	1	piece	26	10	68	2	12	1.1	1	0.2
Bread, wheat berry, toasted	1	piece	24	8	68	2	12	1.3	1	0.2
Bread, wheat bran	1	piece	36	14	89	3	17	1.4	1	0.3
Bread, wheat bran, toasted	1	piece	33	10	90	3	17	1.4	1	0.3
Bread, wheat, low calorie, thin sliced	1	piece	23	10	46	2	10	2.8	1	0.1
Bread, wheat, low calorie, thin sliced, toasted	1	piece	21	7	50	2	11	2.8	1	0.1
Bread, wheat, toasted	1	piece	25	8	70	2	13	1.3	1	0.2
Bread, white, composite, firm & soft, toasted	1	piece	23	7	67	2	12	0.6	1	0.2
Bread, white, compostite, firm & soft	1	piece	25	9	67	2	12	0.6	1	0.2
Bread, white, firm	1	piece	33	12	91	3	17	0.7	1	0.4
Bread, white, firm, toasted	1	piece	29	7	93	3	17	0.8	1	0.4
Bread, white, low calorie, thin sliced	1	piece	20	9	41	2	9	1.9	0	0.1
Bread, white, low calorie, thin sliced, toasted	1	piece	18	6	44	2	9	2	1	0.1
Bread, white, recipe, w/2% milk	1	piece	42	15	120	3	21	0.8	2	0.5
Bread, white, recipe, w/2% milk, toasted	1	piece	38	11	119	3	21	0.8	2	0.5
Bread, white, recipe, w/nonfat dry milk	1	piece	44	15	121	3	24	0.9	1	0.2
Bread, white, recipe, w/nonfat dry milk, toasted	1	piece	40	11	120	3	24	0.9	1	0.2
Bread, white, soft	0.25	cup	8	3	20	1	4	0.2	0	0.1
Bread, white, soft	1	piece	28	10	76	2	14	0.6	1	0.4
Bread, white, soft, toasted	1	piece	24	6	75	2	14	0.6	1	0.3
Bread, white, very low sodium	1	piece	26	10	69	2	13	0.6	1	0.2
Bread, white, very low sodium, toasted	1	piece	24	7	70	2	13	0.6	1	0.2
Bread, whole wheat	1	piece	35	13	86	3	16	2.4	1	0.3
Bread, whole wheat, recipe	1	piece	23	8	64	2	12	1.4	1	0.2
Bread, whole wheat, recipe, toasted	1	piece	42	11	128	4	24	2.8	2	0.4
Bread, whole wheat, toasted	1	piece	29	9	80	3	15	2.2	1	0.3
Breadfruit, raw	0.5	cup	110	78	113	1	30	5.4	0	0.1
Breath Savers, spearmint breath mints	1	each	2	—	10	0	0	0	0	0
Broccoflower, raw	0.5	cup	50	45	16	1	3	1.6	0	0
Broccoflower, steamed	0.5	cup	78	70	25	2	5	2.5	0	0
Broccoli floweret, raw	5	each	55	50	15	2	3	1.6	0	0
Broccoli pieces, cooked, no added salt	0.5	cup	78	71	22	2	4	2.3	0	0

MonoF	PolyF	Choles	Calc	Phos	Sod	Pot	Zn	Iron	Magn	VitA	VitE	VitC	Thia	Ribo	Nia	B6	Fola	B12
(g)	(g)	(mg)	(mg)	(mg)	(mg)	(mg)	(mg)	(mg)	(mg)	(μg RE)	(mg α-TE)	(mg)	(mg)	(mg)	(mg)	(mg)	(μg)	(μg)
0.4	0.3	1	38	32	145	30	0.2	0.7	6	4	0.02	0	0.1	0.09	1	0.01	7	0.01
0.1	0.3	0	52	58	322	72	0.5	1.6	16	0	0.02	0	0.36	0.2	2.8	0.02	57	0
0.2	0.5	0	7	81	239	76	0.7	1.4	31	0	0.41	0	0.15	0.04	1.3	0.12	22	0
0.1	0.3	0	13	133	173	161	1.1	1.5	50	0	0.43	0	0.14	0.12	2.3	0.15	34	0
0.3	0.3	0	30	27	143	30	0.2	0.8	6	0	0.01	0	0.12	0.09	1	0.01	9	0
0.3	0.3	0	31	27	145	31	0.2	0.8	7	0	0.01	0	0.1	0.09	1	0.01	8	0
0	0.2	0	24	35	104	61	0.3	0.8	12	0	0.07	0	0.07	0.08	0.8	0.01	20	0
0	0.2	0	23	32	102	59	0.2	0.8	10	0	0.01	0	0.05	0.07	0.7	0.01	13	0
0.3	0.4	0	22	57	215	67	0.5	0.9	17	0	0.14	0	0.1	0.1	1	0.04	26	0
0.3	0.4	0	22	57	214	66	0.5	0.9	17	0	0.17	0	0.08	0.09	0.9	0.04	20	0
0.6	0.2	0	16	27	98	57	0.2	0.7	6	0	0.13	0	0.08	0.1	0.9	0.02	22	0
0.5	0.2	0	15	25	89	52	0.2	0.7	6	0	0.17	0	0.06	0.08	0.7	0.01	16	0
0.6	2.7	0	3	52	69	93	0.3	0.3	14	0	1.32	0	0.05	0.04	0.9	0.08	19	0
0.4	0.5	0	19	48	119	58	0.4	1	22	0	0.22	0	0.18	0.08	1.8	0.07	18	0
0.4	0.5	0	19	44	120	53	0.3	1	19	0	0.2	0	0.14	0.07	1.7	0.05	14	0
0.6	2.8	0	3	53	71	96	0.3	0.3	15	0	1.36	0	0.05	0.05	0.9	0.08	20	0
0.3	0.2	0	18	31	165	42	0.3	0.7	10	0	0.09	0	0.11	0.08	1	0.02	22	0
0.3	0.2	0	18	30	160	40	0.3	0.7	9	0	0.13	0	0.08	0.07	0.8	0.02	16	0
0.2	0.2	0	18	18	93	22	0.2	0.7	5	0	0.06	0	0.08	0.06	0.6	0.02	11	0.01
0.2	0.2	0	17	19	92	22	0.2	0.7	4	0	0.03	0	0.07	0.05	0.5	0.01	4	0.02
0.3	0.2	0	19	26	152	28	0.2	0.6	7	0	0.07	0	0.13	0.08	1.2	0.01	24	0
0	0	0	8	18	3	26	0.1	0.3	2	4	0.02	0	0.06	0.07	0.5	0.01	16	0.02
0.3	0.2	0	19	26	152	28	0.2	0.6	7	0	0.06	0	0.1	0.07	1.1	0.01	19	0
0.4	0.3	1	23	44	74	110	0.2	0.9	14	3	0.07	0	0.1	0.08	0.9	0.03	12	0.02
0.4	0.3	1	24	46	76	112	0.2	0.9	14	3	0.07	0	0.1	0.09	1	0.03	13	0.02
0.3	0.4	0	23	33	138	35	0.4	0.7	13	0	0.28	0	0.09	0.06	0.8	0.02	7	0
0.5	0.4	1	17	40	61	34	0.3	0.8	13	3	0.12	0	0.15	0.09	1.2	0.03	10	0.02
0.5	0.4	1	17	40	62	34	0.3	0.8	13	3	0.12	0	0.16	0.1	1.2	0.03	10	0.02
0.6	0.4	14	5	28	228	40	0.2	0.8	5	50	0.3	1	0.09	0.1	0.9	0.03	14	0.03
0.2	0.4	0	22	47	136	52	0.4	0.7	17	0	0.06	0	0.07	0.04	0.7	0.02	12	0
0.2	0.4	0	22	47	137	53	0.4	0.7	17	0	0.07	0	0.06	0.04	0.7	0.02	10	0
0.3	0.2	0	19	26	152	28	0.2	0.6	7	0	0.07	0	0.13	0.08	1.2	0.01	24	0
0.5	0.3	0	30	43	151	57	0.3	0.9	13	0	0.15	0	0.12	0.08	1.2	0.03	22	0
0.4	0.2	0	27	39	138	52	0.3	0.9	12	0	0.14	0	0.11	0.07	1.1	0.02	20	0
0.4	0.2	0	27	39	138	52	0.3	0.9	12	0	0.14	0	0.09	0.07	1	0.02	16	0
0.6	0.2	0	27	67	175	82	0.5	1.1	29	0	0.17	0	0.14	0.1	1.6	0.06	25	0
0.6	0.2	0	27	67	176	82	0.5	1.1	29	0	0.24	0	0.12	0.09	1.4	0.06	7	0
0.1	0.2	0	18	24	118	28	0.3	0.7	9	0	0.03	0	0.1	0.07	0.9	0.03	16	0
0.1	0.2	0	20	23	128	31	0.2	0.7	7	0	0.04	0	0.08	0.07	0.9	0.03	5	0.02
0.5	0.2	0	28	41	144	54	0.3	0.9	12	0	0.15	0	0.09	0.07	1	0.02	16	0
0.4	0.2	0	27	24	136	30	0.2	0.8	6	0	0.07	0	0.1	0.08	0.9	0.01	19	0
0.4	0.2	0	27	24	135	30	0.2	0.8	6	0	0.1	0	0.12	0.08	1	0.02	24	0.01
0.5	0.2	1	32	34	163	40	0.2	0.9	7	0	0.25	0	0.13	0.08	1.1	0.01	12	0
0.5	0.2	1	32	34	163	40	0.2	0.9	7	0	0.26	0	0.11	0.08	1.1	0.01	12	0
0.2	0.1	0	19	24	91	15	0.3	0.6	5	0	0.03	0	0.08	0.06	0.7	0.01	19	0.06
0.2	0.1	0	20	29	97	16	0.3	0.7	6	0	0.04	0	0.07	0.06	0.7	0.01	5	0.05
0.5	1.2	1	24	48	151	61	0.3	1.2	8	9	0.36	0	0.17	0.16	1.5	0.02	38	0.03
0.5	1.2	1	24	48	150	61	0.3	1.2	8	8	0.46	0	0.14	0.14	1.4	0.02	12	0.03
0.2	0.6	0	14	42	148	49	0.3	1.4	7	5	0.17	0	0.19	0.16	1.6	0.02	37	0.01
0.2	0.6	0	14	42	148	49	0.3	1.4	8	5	0.16	0	0.15	0.14	1.5	0.01	8	0.01
0.1	0.1	0	6	7	38	8	0	0.2	2	0	0.01	0	0.03	0.02	0.2	0	3	0
0.5	0.2	1	24	28	143	30	0.2	0.8	6	0	0.05	0	0.11	0.07	0.9	0.01	10	0
0.3	0.2	1	24	27	142	30	0.2	0.8	6	0	0.05	0	0.09	0.07	0.9	0.01	10	0
0.4	0.2	0	28	24	7	31	0.2	0.8	6	0	0.1	0	0.12	0.09	1	0.02	25	0.01
0.4	0.2	0	29	25	7	31	0.2	0.8	6	0	0.08	0	0.1	0.08	0.9	0.02	23	0
0.6	0.4	0	25	80	184	88	0.7	1.2	30	0	0.3	0	0.12	0.07	1.3	0.06	18	0
0.3	0.7	0	8	43	80	72	0.3	0.7	19	0	0.31	0	0.07	0.05	0.9	0.05	14	0
0.5	1.4	0	15	86	160	145	0.7	1.4	37	0	0.67	0	0.11	0.1	1.6	0.08	24	0
0.5	0.3	0	24	75	172	82	0.6	1.1	28	0	0.34	0	0.09	0.06	1.1	0.05	10	0
0	0.1	0	19	33	2	539	0.1	0.6	28	4	1.23	32	0.12	0.03	1	0.11	15	0
0	0	0	—	—	0	0	—	—	—	—	—	—	—	—	—	—	—	—
0	0.1	0	16	32	12	161	0.2	0	10	4	0.15	37	0.04	0.05	0.4	0.1	28	0
0	0.1	0	25	50	18	251	0.4	0.5	16	5	0.23	49	0.06	0.07	0.6	0.14	38	0
0	0.1	0	26	36	15	179	0.2	0.5	14	165	0.91	51	0.04	0.06	0.4	0.09	39	0
0	0.1	0	36	46	20	228	0.3	0.7	19	108	1.32	58	0.04	0.09	0.4	0.11	39	0

Food Item	Qty	Meas	Wgt (g)	Wtr (g)	Cals	Prot (g)	Carb (g)	Fib (g)	Fat (g)	SatF (g)
Broccoli pieces, frozen, cooked, no added salt	0.5	cup	92	83	26	3	5	2.8	0	0
Broccoli pieces, raw	0.5	cup	44	40	12	1	2	1.3	0	0
Broccoli pieces, steamed	0.5	cup	62	56	17	2	3	1.9	0	0
Broccoli pieces, stir fried	0.5	cup	78	71	22	2	4	2.3	0	0
Broccoli spears, cooked, no added salt	1	each	180	163	50	5	9	5.2	1	0.1
Broccoli spears, frozen, cooked	1	piece	30	27	8	1	2	0.9	0	0
Broccoli spears, raw	1	each	151	137	42	4	8	4.5	1	0.1
Broccoli, Chinese, Gai Lan	4	oz.	113	104	34	3	5	—	0	—
Broccoli, batter-dipped, fried	0.5	cup	42	32	61	2	4	1	4	0.7
Broccoli, cooked w/cheese sauce	0.5	cup	114	92	110	6	6	2	7	3.5
Broccoli, stalk only, raw	0.5	cup	44	40	12	1	2	1.4	0	0
Broth, beef, fat free, Health Valley	4	oz.	113	111	14	2	1	0	0	0
Broth, chicken, dry, cube	1	each	5	0	10	1	1	0	0	0.1
Broth, chicken, dry, prepared	0.5	cup	122	118	11	1	1	0	1	0.1
Brownie, mix, low calorie, low sodium, prepared	1	each	22	3	84	1	16	0.8	2	1.1
Brownie, mix, w/nuts, prepared	1	each	33	4	140	1	20	0.9	7	1.4
Brownie, peanut butter fudge, Weight Watchers	1	each	35	8	110	2	21	3	2	0.5
Brownie, w/nuts	1	each	25	3	101	1	16	0.5	4	1.1
Brownie, w/walnuts, homemade	1	each	20	3	93	1	10	0.4	6	1.5
Brussels sprouts, cooked, drained	4	each	84	73	33	2	7	2.2	0	0.1
Brussels sprouts, cooked, drained, cup measure	0.5	cup	78	68	30	2	7	2	0	0.1
Brussels sprouts, frozen, cooked	0.5	cup	78	67	33	3	6	3.2	0	0.1
Brussels sprouts, raw	4	each	76	65	33	3	7	2.9	0	0
Brussels sprouts, raw, cup measure	0.5	cup	44	38	19	1	4	1.7	0	0
Buckwheat groats, roasted/cooked	0.5	cup	99	75	91	3	20	2.7	1	0.1
Buckwheat, w/outside skin	0.5	cup	85	8	292	11	61	8.5	3	0.6
Bulgur wheat, cooked	0.5	cup	91	71	76	3	17	4.1	0	0
Bun, hamburger	1	each	45	15	129	4	23	1.2	2	0.5
Bun, hamburger/hot dog, low calorie, extra fiber	1	each	43	20	84	4	18	2.7	1	0.1
Bun, hamburger/hot dog, mixed grain	1	each	43	16	113	4	19	1.6	3	0.4
Bun, hotdog/frankfurter	1	each	40	14	114	3	20	1.1	2	0.5
Burger King, BK broiler, chicken sandwich	1	each	248	146	550	30	41	2	29	6
Burger King, Whopper sandwich	1	each	270	157	640	27	45	3	39	11
Burger King, Whopper sandwich, w/cheese	1	each	294	167	730	33	46	3	46	16
Burger King, cheeseburger, double	1	each	213	104	609	42	28	1	36	17.2
Burger King, chicken sandwich	1	each	229	104	710	26	54	2	43	9
Burger King, fish fillet sandwich, Ocean Catch	1	each	255	130	700	26	56	3	41	6
Burger King, whopper Jr. w/cheese	1	each	180	96	468	23	30	2	28	10.2
Burger King, whopper junior sandwich	1	each	168	90	430	22	30	2	25	8.2
Burrito, apple, small	1	each	155	55	484	5	73	—	20	9.6
Burrito, bean & cheese	2	each	186	100	378	15	55	—	12	6.8
Burrito, black bean, Life Choice	1	each	374	269	410	12	86	13	2	0
Burrito, sausage, Great Starts	1	each	99	52	240	9	24	1	12	4
Butter replacement, dry (Butter Buds)	1	Tbs	5	0	19	0	4	0	0	0
Butter, lightly salted	1	Tbs	14	2	102	0	0	0	12	7.2
Butter, regular, salted	1	Tbs	14	2	100	0	0	0	11	7.1
Butter, regular, salted, pat	1	each	5	1	36	0	0	0	4	2.5
Butter, unsalted	1	Tbs	14	3	102	0	0	0	12	7.2
Butter, whipped	1	Tbs	9	2	68	0	0	0	8	4.8
Butter/vegetable oil blend, Blue Bonnet spread	1	Tbs	14	2	102	0	0	0	12	4
Butterbur (fuki), canned pieces	0.5	cup	62	61	2	0	0	—	0	—
Butterbur (fuki), raw	0.5	cup	47	44	7	0	2	0.6	0	—
Butterbur (fuki), stalks, cooked	3	each	45	44	4	0	1	0.6	0	—
Buttermilk, skim, cultured	1	cup	245	221	99	8	12	0	2	1.3
Butternuts, dried	1	oz.	28	1	174	7	3	1.3	16	0.4
Butterscotch morsels, Toll House	0.25	cup	42	0	243	0	30	0	12	12.3
Cabbage, Chinese, steamed	0.5	cup	85	81	11	1	2	0.8	0	0
Cabbage, Japanese, pickled	0.5	cup	75	69	16	1	3	2.3	0	0
Cabbage, bok choy, cooked, drained	0.5	cup	85	81	10	1	2	1.4	0	0
Cabbage, bok choy, shredded, raw	0.5	cup	35	33	5	1	1	0.4	0	0
Cabbage, head, cooked, no added salt, drained	1	each	1262	1181	278	13	56	29	5	0.7
Cabbage, head, raw	1	each	908	837	227	13	49	20.9	2	0.3
Cabbage, kim chee style	0.5	cup	75	69	16	1	3	0.9	0	0
Cabbage, mustard, salted	0.5	cup	64	59	13	1	3	2	0	0
Cabbage, pe tsai, chopped, raw	0.5	cup	38	36	6	0	1	1.2	0	0

MonoF	PolyF	Choles	Calc	Phos	Sod	Pot	Zn	Iron	Magn	VitA	VitE	VitC	Thia	Ribo	Nia	B6	Fola	B12
(g)	(g)	(mg)	(mg)	(mg)	(mg)	(mg)	(mg)	(mg)	(mg)	(µg RE)	(mg α-TE)	(mg)	(mg)	(mg)	(mg)	(mg)	(µg)	(µg)
0	0.1	0	47	51	22	166	0.3	0.6	18	174	1.52	37	0.05	0.08	0.4	0.12	52	0
0	0.1	0	21	29	12	143	0.2	0.4	11	68	0.73	41	0.03	0.05	0.3	0.07	31	0
0	0.1	0	30	41	17	201	0.2	0.5	16	91	0.3	49	0.04	0.07	0.4	0.09	37	0
0	0.1	0	37	51	21	253	0.3	0.7	20	108	0.37	62	0.05	0.09	0.5	0.12	44	0
0	0.3	0	83	106	47	526	0.7	1.5	43	250	3.04	134	0.1	0.2	1	0.26	90	0
0	0	0	15	16	7	54	0.1	0.2	6	57	0.31	12	0.02	0.02	0.1	0.04	9	0
0	0.3	0	72	100	41	491	0.6	1.3	38	233	2.51	141	0.1	0.18	1	0.24	107	0
—	—	—	—	—	—	—	—	—	—	186	—	32	—	—	—	—	—	0
1.1	2.4	8	34	35	31	121	0.2	0.5	10	51	1.05	27	0.04	0.07	0.4	0.06	22	0.03
2.4	1	15	148	128	365	269	0.7	0.8	24	176	0.76	57	0.06	0.17	0.5	0.13	41	0.18
0	0.1	0	21	29	12	143	0.2	0.4	11	18	0.73	41	0.03	0.05	0.3	0.07	31	0
0	0	0	0	—	76	93	—	0	—	0	—	2	—	—	0.5	—	—	—
0.1	0.1	1	9	9	1152	18	0	0.1	3	4	0.04	0	0.01	0.02	0.2	0	2	0.01
0.2	0.2	0	7	6	742	12	0	0	2	6	0.01	0	0	0.02	0.1	0	1	0.01
1	0.2	0	3	11	21	69	0	0.3	1	0	0.36	0	0.02	0.03	0.2	0	7	0
2	2.8	9	6	26	83	61	0.2	0.6	11	4	0.66	0	0.04	0.05	0.5	0.01	3	0.02
—	—	0	20	—	140	100	—	1.1	—	0	—	0	—	—	—	—	—	—
2.2	0.6	4	7	25	78	37	0.2	0.6	8	2	0.52	0	0.06	0.05	0.4	0.01	5	0.02
2.2	1.9	15	11	26	69	35	0.2	0.4	11	40	0.58	0	0.03	0.04	0.2	0.02	6	0.03
0	0.2	0	30	47	18	266	0.3	1	17	60	0.71	52	0.09	0.07	0.5	0.15	50	0
0	0.2	0	28	44	16	247	0.3	0.9	16	56	0.66	48	0.08	0.06	0.5	0.14	47	0
0	0.2	0	19	42	18	252	0.3	0.6	19	46	0.45	35	0.08	0.09	0.4	0.22	78	0
0	0.1	0	32	52	19	296	0.3	1.1	18	67	0.67	65	0.11	0.07	0.6	0.17	46	0
0	0.1	0	18	30	11	171	0.2	0.6	10	39	0.39	37	0.06	0.04	0.3	0.1	27	0
0.2	0.2	0	7	69	4	87	0.6	0.8	50	0	0.23	0	0.04	0.04	0.9	0.08	14	0
0.9	0.9	0	15	295	1	391	2	1.9	196	0	0.88	0	0.09	0.36	6	0.18	26	0
0	0.1	0	9	36	5	62	0.5	0.9	29	0	0.03	0	0.05	0.02	0.9	0.08	16	0
0.4	1.1	0	63	40	252	64	0.3	1.4	9	0	0.7	0	0.22	0.14	1.8	0.02	43	0.03
0.2	0.3	0	25	36	190	34	0.3	1.3	9	0	0.07	0	0.17	0.08	2.1	0.02	41	0.04
0.8	0.4	0	41	52	197	69	0.5	1.7	19	0	0.24	0	0.2	0.13	1.9	0.04	41	0
0.3	1	0	56	35	224	56	0.2	1.3	8	0	0.62	0	0.19	0.12	1.6	0.02	38	0.02
—	—	80	60	—	480	—	—	5.4	—	60	—	6	—	—	—	—	—	—
—	—	90	80	—	870	—	—	4.5	—	100	—	9	0.33	0.41	7	0.35	—	—
—	—	115	250	—	1350	—	—	4.5	—	150	—	9	0.34	0.48	7	0.33	—	—
—	—	137	203	—	1075	—	—	4.6	—	81	—	0	—	—	—	—	—	—
—	—	60	100	—	1400	—	—	3.6	—	0	—	0	—	—	—	—	—	—
—	—	90	60	—	980	—	—	2.7	—	20	—	1	—	—	—	—	—	—
—	—	76	153	—	783	—	—	3.7	—	81	—	5	—	—	—	—	—	—
—	—	62	62	—	543	—	—	3.7	—	41	—	5	—	—	—	—	—	—
7.2	2.2	8	33	31	443	219	0.8	2.2	16	78	—	2	0.36	0.37	3.9	0.16	51	1.07
2.5	1.8	28	214	180	1166	497	1.6	2.3	80	238	—	2	0.22	0.71	3.6	0.24	74	0.89
—	—	0	150	—	570	—	—	3.6	—	20	—	9	—	—	—	—	—	—
—	—	90	60	—	500	—	—	1.4	—	20	—	1	—	—	—	—	—	—
0	0	0	1	0	60	0	0	0.1	0	0	0	0	0	0	0	0	0	0
3.5	0.4	31	3	3	106	4	0	0	0	107	0.22	0	0	0	0	0	0	0.02
3.4	0.4	31	3	3	116	4	0	0	0	106	0.22	0	0	0	0	0	0	0.02
1.2	0.2	11	1	1	41	1	0	0	0	38	0.08	0	0	0	0	0	0	0.01
3.3	0.4	31	3	3	2	4	0	0	0	107	0.22	0	0	0	0	0	0	0.02
2.2	0.3	21	2	2	78	2	0	0	0	71	0.15	0	0	0	0	0	0	0.01
4.7	2.3	12	4	3	127	5	0	0	0	113	1.08	0	0	0	0	0	0	0.01
—	—	0	21	2	2	7	0	0.4	1	0	—	7	0	0	0.1	0.02	2	0
—	—	0	48	6	3	308	0.1	0	7	2	—	15	0.01	0.01	0.1	0.04	5	0
—	—	0	27	3	2	159	0	0	4	1	—	9	0	0	0	0.02	2	0
0.6	0.1	9	284	219	257	370	1	0.1	27	20	0.15	2	0.08	0.38	0.1	0.08	12	0.54
3	12.1	0	15	126	0	119	0.9	1.1	67	3	0.99	1	0.11	0.04	0.3	0.16	19	0
0	0	0	0	—	46	79	—	0	—	0	—	0	0.03	0.04	0	—	—	—
0	0.1	0	89	31	55	213	0.2	0.7	16	8	0.1	3	0.03	0.06	0.4	0.15	47	0
0	0	0	36	32	208	640	0.2	0.4	9	14	0.09	1	0	0.03	0.1	0.08	32	0
0	0.1	0	79	25	29	315	0.1	0.9	9	218	0.1	22	0.03	0.05	0.4	0.14	34	0
0	0	0	37	13	23	88	0.1	0.3	7	105	0.04	16	0.01	0.02	0.2	0.07	23	0
0.4	2.5	0	391	189	101	1224	1.1	2.2	101	164	1.33	254	0.72	0.69	3.6	1.43	252	0
0.2	1.1	0	427	209	163	2233	1.6	5.4	136	118	0.95	292	0.45	0.36	2.7	0.87	390	0
0	0.1	0	73	30	498	188	0.2	0.6	14	213	0.12	40	0.04	0.05	0.4	0.17	44	0
0	0	0	43	17	459	157	0.2	0.4	10	62	0.01	0	0.03	0.06	0.5	0.19	46	0
0	0	0	29	11	3	90	0.1	0.1	5	46	0.05	10	0.02	0.02	0.2	0.09	30	0

Food Item	Qty	Meas	Wgt (g)	Wtr (g)	Cals	Prot (g)	Carb (g)	Fib (g)	Fat (g)	SatF (g)
Cabbage, pe tsai, cooked, drained	0.5	cup	60	57	8	1	1	1.6	0	0
Cabbage, raw, fresh harvest	0.5	cup	35	32	8	0	2	0.8	0	0
Cabbage, red, cooked, drained	0.5	cup	75	70	16	1	3	1.5	0	0
Cabbage, red, pickled	0.5	cup	75	45	110	0	29	0.6	0	0
Cabbage, red, raw	0.5	cup	35	32	9	0	2	0.7	0	0
Cabbage, red, sweet & sour	0.5	cup	75	45	110	0	29	0.6	0	0
Cabbage, savoy, cooked, drained	0.5	cup	72	67	17	1	4	2	0	0
Cabbage, savoy, raw	0.5	cup	35	32	9	1	2	1.1	0	0
Cabbage, shredded, cooked, no added salt, drained	0.5	cup	75	70	16	1	3	1.7	0	0
Cabbage, shredded, raw	0.5	cup	35	32	9	1	2	0.8	0	0
Cactus pad/nopales, cooked	1	each	29	25	12	0	3	1	0	0
Cactus/nopales, raw	0.5	cup	59	52	24	0	6	2.1	0	0.1
Cajun seasoning	0.25	tsp	1	0	2	0	0	0.1	0	—
Cake, German chocolate, mix, prepared, w/frosting	1	piece	111	30	404	4	55	1.5	21	5.3
Cake, angel food	1	piece	53	18	137	3	31	0.8	0	0.1
Cake, angel food, mix, prepared	1	piece	50	16	129	3	29	0.1	0	0
Cake, angel food, recipe	1	piece	53	17	142	4	32	0.2	0	0
Cake, apple spice crumb, fat free, Entenmann's	1	piece	50	—	130	2	30	2	0	0
Cake, applesauce w/nuts & icing	1	piece	108	21	399	3	70	1.5	13	3.2
Cake, applesauce, no icing	1	piece	87	19	313	3	52	1.7	11	2.9
Cake, apricot, no icing	1	piece	87	19	313	3	52	1.7	11	2.9
Cake, banana loaf, fat free, Entenmann's	1	piece	57	—	150	2	34	1	0	0
Cake, banana w/icing	1	piece	108	37	309	3	58	1.1	8	1.6
Cake, banana, no icing	1	piece	87	32	245	3	43	1.1	7	1.6
Cake, blackberry, no icing	1	piece	87	19	313	3	52	1.7	11	2.9
Cake, carrot w/cream cheese frosting, recipe	1	piece	112	23	488	5	53	1.3	30	5.5
Cake, carrot, mix, prepared, no frosting	1	piece	70	22	239	4	33	1.4	11	1.8
Cake, cherry fudge, w/chocolate frosting	1	piece	71	33	187	2	27	0.9	9	3.6
Cake, chocolate crunch, fat free, Entenmann's	1	piece	50	—	130	2	32	2	0	0
Cake, chocolate w/fluffy white icing	1	piece	91	30	262	4	48	1	8	1.8
Cake, chocolate, mix, low sodium, prepared	1	piece	38	9	116	1	23	0.6	3	1.4
Cake, chocolate, mix, prepared	1	piece	65	21	198	4	32	1.4	8	1.8
Cake, chocolate, mix, pudding type, prepared	1	piece	77	23	270	4	34	1.5	14	3
Cake, chocolate, recipe, no frosting	1	piece	95	23	340	5	51	1.5	14	5.2
Cake, chocolate, w/chocolate icing-commercial	1	piece	69	16	253	3	38	1.9	11	3.3
Cake, chocolate, w/cream cheese icing	1	piece	103	26	355	4	57	1	14	3.7
Cake, chocolate, w/vanilla icing	1	piece	103	26	358	4	58	1	14	3.6
Cake, coffee, cheese	1	piece	76	24	258	5	34	0.8	12	4.1
Cake, coffee, cheese, Entenmann's	1	piece	54	17	190	4	24	0	8	3.5
Cake, coffee, cinnamon, w/crumb topping	1	piece	63	14	263	4	29	1.3	15	3.6
Cake, coffee, cinnamon, w/crumb topping, recipe	1	piece	60	13	240	4	30	0.9	12	2.2
Cake, coffee, creme filled, w/chocolate frosting	1	piece	90	26	298	4	48	1.8	10	2.6
Cake, coffee, fruit	1	piece	50	16	156	3	26	1.2	5	1.2
Cake, coffee, mix, prepared	1	piece	72	22	229	4	38	0.9	7	1.3
Cake, date pudding	1	piece	42	14	131	2	19	0.9	6	3
Cake, fruit, recipe	1	piece	43	8	155	2	28	1.6	5	0.6
Cake, funnel, 6 inch diameter	1	each	90	37	285	7	29	0.9	15	3.9
Cake, gingerbread, mix, prepared	1	piece	63	21	195	3	32	0.7	6	1.6
Cake, gingerbread, recipe	1	piece	110	31	392	4	54	0.9	18	4.5
Cake, golden loaf, fat free, Entenmann's	1	piece	48	—	120	2	28	0.5	0	0
Cake, graham cracker	1	piece	45	13	156	3	22	0.4	7	1.7
Cake, ice cream roll, chocolate	1	piece	34	13	102	1	14	0.3	5	2.2
Cake, ice cream roll, chocolate	1	each	340	134	1015	14	136	3.5	50	22
Cake, lemon, w/icing, 2-layer	1	piece	109	23	388	3	70	0.5	11	2.6
Cake, marble w/chocolate icing	1	piece	111	28	404	3	59	0.9	19	4.4
Cake, marble, mix, pudding type, dry	1	oz.	28	1	118	1	22	0.8	3	0.7
Cake, mix, Angle Food, prepared	1	piece	53	5	192	5	43	0	0	0
Cake, mix, Devil's Food, prep w/oil & egg	1	piece	44	6	210	3	25	0	10	3
Cake, oatmeal w/icing	1	piece	110	21	410	3	70	1.5	14	3.4
Cake, pineapple upside-down cake, recipe	1	piece	115	37	367	4	58	0.9	14	3.4
Cake, plum pudding	1	piece	42	14	131	2	19	0.9	6	3
Cake, poppyseed, no icing	1	piece	90	21	354	7	43	1	18	6.5
Cake, pound w/butter	1	piece	29	7	113	2	14	0.1	6	3.4
Cake, pound, commercial, not w/butter	1	piece	30	7	117	2	16	0.3	5	1.4
Cake, pound, old fashion, w/butter	1	piece	53	11	229	3	25	0.4	13	7.6

MonoF	PolyF	Choles	Calc	Phos	Sod	Pot	Zn	Iron	Magn	VitA	VitE	VitC	Thia	Ribo	Nia	B6	Fola	B12
(g)	(g)	(mg)	(mg)	(mg)	(mg)	(mg)	(mg)	(mg)	(mg)	(μg RE)	(mg α-TE)	(mg)	(mg)	(mg)	(mg)	(mg)	(μg)	(μg)
0	0	0	19	23	5	134	0.1	0.2	6	58	0.07	9	0.03	0.03	0.3	0.1	32	0
0	0	0	16	8	6	86	0.1	0.2	5	5	0.04	18	0.02	0.01	0.1	0.03	20	0
0	0.1	0	28	22	6	105	0.1	0.3	8	2	0.09	26	0.03	0.02	0.2	0.1	9	0
0	0	0	36	16	14	153	0.1	0.6	13	1	0.03	9	0.01	0.01	0.1	0.06	4	0
0	0	0	18	15	4	72	0.1	0.2	5	1	0.04	20	0.02	0.01	0.1	0.07	7	0
0	0	0	36	16	14	153	0.1	0.6	13	1	0.03	9	0.01	0.01	0.1	0.06	4	0
0	0	0	22	24	17	133	0.2	0.3	17	64	0.08	12	0.04	0.02	0	0.11	34	0
0	0	0	12	15	10	80	0.1	0.1	10	35	0.04	11	0.02	0.01	0.1	0.07	28	0
0	0.1	0	23	11	6	73	0.1	0.1	6	10	0.08	15	0.04	0.04	0.2	0.08	15	0
0	0	0	16	8	6	86	0.1	0.2	5	5	0.04	11	0.02	0.01	0.1	0.03	15	0
0	0.1	0	15	7	68	57	0	0.1	24	1	0	3	0	0.02	0.1	0.02	1	0
0.1	0.1	0	33	14	3	130	0.1	0.2	50	3	0.01	8	0.01	0.04	0.3	0.04	4	0
—	—	—	—	—	119	7	—	—	—	—	—	—	—	—	—	—	—	0
8.7	5.5	53	53	173	369	151	0.5	1.2	19	23	1.18	0	0.11	0.14	1.1	0.02	4	0.1
0	0.2	0	74	17	397	49	0	0.3	6	0	0.05	0	0.05	0.26	0.5	0.02	19	0.03
0	0.1	0	42	116	255	68	0.1	0.1	4	0	0	0	0.05	0.1	0.1	0	15	0.02
0	0	0	3	13	96	116	0.1	0.4	5	0	0.01	0	0.05	0.17	0.4	0	2	0.05
0	0	0	0	—	140	65	—	0	—	20	—	0	—	—	—	—	—	—
5.7	3.6	21	20	45	293	137	0.2	1.3	10	49	1.5	1	0.12	0.12	1	0.05	5	0.05
4.9	2.9	22	17	46	285	145	0.2	1.4	11	10	1.15	1	0.14	0.13	1.1	0.06	6	0.04
4.9	2.9	22	17	46	285	145	0.2	1.4	11	10	1.15	1	0.14	0.13	1.1	0.06	6	0.04
0	0	0	20	—	190	140	—	0	—	0	—	0	—	—	—	—	—	—
3.2	2.3	31	28	48	292	198	0.3	1	17	105	1.36	4	0.13	0.18	1.1	0.25	12	0.08
3.1	2.2	29	26	46	257	186	0.3	1	16	100	1.3	3	0.12	0.16	1	0.24	12	0.07
4.9	2.9	22	17	46	285	145	0.2	1.4	11	10	1.15	1	0.14	0.13	1.1	0.06	6	0.04
7.3	15.2	60	28	80	276	125	0.5	1.4	20	430	4.73	1	0.15	0.18	1.1	0.08	13	0.11
3.4	5	51	77	123	249	84	0.2	0.9	5	173	2.94	2	0.09	0.12	0.8	0.06	8	0.81
3.1	1.7	30	34	75	160	118	0.2	0.8	14	72	0.85	10	0.02	0.14	0.5	0.04	7	0.15
0	0	0	0	—	170	200	—	1.1	—	0	—	0	—	—	—	—	—	—
3.1	2.3	35	71	133	411	173	0.5	2.1	22	16	—	0	0.06	0.11	0.8	0.02	8	0.07
1.2	0.2	0	11	102	130	82	0.3	0.8	14	0	0.11	0	0.05	0.06	0.5	0	2	0.01
3.1	2.3	35	70	132	370	153	0.4	2.1	22	16	1.14	0	0.06	0.1	0.6	0.02	7	0.06
4.7	5.9	53	64	146	402	161	0.5	1.4	19	24	1.37	0	0.08	0.13	0.9	0.03	8	0.32
5.7	2.6	55	57	101	299	133	0.7	1.5	30	38	1.51	0	0.13	0.2	1.1	0.04	26	0.15
6	1.3	29	30	84	230	138	0.5	1.5	24	17	1.17	0	0.02	0.09	0.4	0.03	12	0.1
6.5	3.2	35	71	133	460	167	0.4	2.2	22	60	—	0	0.06	0.1	0.6	0.02	7	0.06
6.4	3.2	35	71	147	404	168	0.4	2.1	22	102	—	0	0.06	0.1	0.6	0.02	7	0.06
5.4	1.2	65	45	77	258	220	0.4	0.5	11	66	1.19	0	0.08	0.1	0.5	0.04	30	0.26
—	—	30	40	—	160	55	—	0	—	20	—	0	—	—	—	—	—	—
8.2	2	20	34	68	221	78	0.5	1.2	14	21	2.15	0	0.13	0.14	1.1	0.02	38	0.11
4.6	4.6	36	67	83	233	143	0.5	1.3	24	99	1.5	0	0.11	0.12	0.7	0.06	9	0.09
5.1	1.3	62	34	68	291	70	0.4	0.5	14	33	1.62	0	0.07	0.07	0.8	0.04	37	0.18
2.8	0.7	4	22	59	193	45	0.3	1.2	8	10	0.43	0	0.02	0.1	1.3	0.02	24	0.01
2.8	2.3	35	98	155	303	81	0.3	1	13	29	1.2	0	0.12	0.13	1.1	0.04	49	0.1
1.9	0.3	16	40	35	56	196	0.2	0.8	23	8	0.26	0	0.04	0.06	0.4	0.08	3	0.05
2	2	12	28	34	62	133	0.3	0.8	15	6	1.08	2	0.07	0.05	0.5	0.04	4	0.02
4.5	5.9	66	115	128	236	153	0.6	1.8	18	46	1	0	0.24	0.32	1.9	0.05	14	0.24
3.6	0.8	22	44	106	289	152	0.3	2.1	10	10	0.86	0	0.12	0.12	1	0.02	6	0.04
7.8	4.6	35	78	59	360	483	0.4	3.2	77	15	2.64	0	0.21	0.18	1.9	0.21	36	0.07
0	0	0	0	—	160	75	—	0	—	20	—	0	—	—	—	—	—	—
3	1.8	34	44	52	176	78	0.3	0.7	8	80	1.12	0	0.04	0.14	0.6	0.02	5	0.09
1.8	0.7	16	43	38	69	57	0.2	0.5	9	22	0.25	0	0.04	0.07	0.3	0.01	2	0.08
18.4	7	156	431	380	688	569	2.4	4.7	90	215	2.47	1	0.4	0.71	3	0.14	23	0.79
5.2	2.7	33	70	136	248	55	0.2	0.9	6	79	2.09	1	0.1	0.12	0.8	0.02	6	0.07
7.4	6.2	53	43	172	311	143	0.4	1.4	18	99	—	0	0.07	0.12	0.7	0.03	7	0.1
1.4	1.1	0	22	78	147	35	0.1	0.5	5	0	0.51	0	0.05	0.04	0.4	0.01	10	0
0	0	0	24	—	320	56	—	0	—	0	—	0	0	0	0	—	—	—
3	3.5	25	20	—	270	170	—	1.1	—	0	—	0	0.09	0.1	0.4	—	—	—
6.1	3.8	20	20	56	257	135	0.3	1.8	14	57	1.56	1	0.15	0.11	1.1	0.05	5	0.05
6	3.8	25	138	94	367	129	0.4	1.7	15	75	1.54	1	0.18	0.18	1.4	0.04	30	0.09
1.9	0.3	16	40	35	56	196	0.2	0.8	23	8	0.26	0	0.04	0.06	0.4	0.08	3	0.05
4.6	5.3	79	107	122	251	138	0.7	1.7	20	94	1.03	1	0.25	0.29	1.7	0.05	16	0.18
1.7	0.3	64	10	40	115	34	0.1	0.4	3	45	0.19	0	0.04	0.07	0.4	0.01	12	0.07
3	0.7	17	19	40	120	32	0.1	0.5	4	10	0.72	0	0.04	0.08	0.4	0.01	11	0.04
3.9	0.7	92	13	44	153	37	0.3	0.9	5	134	0.4	0	0.1	0.14	0.8	0.02	8	0.13

Food Item	Qty	Meas	Wgt (g)	Wtr (g)	Cals	Prot (g)	Carb (g)	Fib (g)	Fat (g)	SatF (g)
Cake, pound, old fashion, w/margarine	1	piece	53	11	230	3	25	0.4	13	2.8
Cake, pound, recipe, w/margarine	1	piece	54	13	206	3	28	0.4	9	2
Cake, raisin loaf, fat free, Entenmann's	1	piece	53	—	140	2	33	1	0	0
Cake, rhubarb, no icing	1	piece	87	19	313	3	52	1.7	11	2.9
Cake, shortcake, biscuit type, recipe	1	each	65	18	225	4	32	0.8	9	2.5
Cake, snack, chocolate, creme filled, w/icing	1	each	28	6	107	1	17	0.2	4	0.8
Cake, snack, cream filled, Twinkie	1	each	42	8	153	1	27	0.2	5	1.1
Cake, spice, w/icing	1	piece	109	27	374	4	65	1	11	3.8
Cake, sponge, 1/12th	1	piece	65	19	188	4	40	0.4	2	0.5
Cake, sponge, chocolate, no icing	1	piece	66	20	195	5	36	1	4	1.4
Cake, sponge, fruit-cream filled, Twinkie	1	each	43	12	146	2	24	0.4	5	1.4
Cake, sponge, recipe	1	piece	63	18	187	5	36	0.4	3	0.8
Cake, white, mix, low sodium, prepared	1	piece	38	10	118	1	23	0.2	2	0.4
Cake, white, mix, prepared, pkg	1	each	739	228	2261	30	409	4.9	57	8.6
Cake, white, mix, pudding type, prepared	1	each	826	235	2915	30	427	3.7	122	23.1
Cake, white, no yolk, chocolate icing	1	piece	109	22	397	3	70	1.2	12	5.7
Cake, white, w/coconut frosting, recipe	1	piece	70	14	249	3	44	0.7	7	2.7
Cake, white, w/white frosting	1	piece	71	14	266	2	45	0.7	10	4.3
Cake, yellow, mix, prepared	1	piece	69	21	221	3	38	0.6	6	1.1
Cake, yellow, w/chocolate frosting, commercial	1	piece	69	15	262	3	38	1.2	12	3.2
Cake, yellow, w/vanilla frosting	1	piece	121	27	451	4	71	0.4	18	2.9
Candy, milk chocolate-covered peanuts	0.25	cup	42	1	221	6	21	2	14	6.2
Candy, 3 Musketeers bar	1	each	60	4	251	2	46	1	8	3.9
Candy, 3 Musketeers bar, snack size	1	each	18	1	75	1	14	0.3	2	1.2
Candy, 5th Avenue bar	1	each	56	1	276	5	37	1.2	12	4.4
Candy, Almond Joy bar	1	each	49	5	229	2	29	2.4	13	8.5
Candy, Alpine White bar, w/almonds	1	each	35	0	193	3	18	1.9	13	7
Candy, Baby Ruth bar	1	each	60	3	289	4	39	1.7	13	7.1
Candy, Bar None bar	1	each	42	2	219	3	22	1.4	14	9.2
Candy, Bit-o-Honey chews	6	piece	48	3	186	1	39	—	4	—
Candy, Butterfinger bar	1	each	61	1	293	8	40	1.5	11	6.3
Candy, Butterfinger bar, snack size	1	each	21	0	101	3	14	0.5	4	2.2
Candy, Caramello bar	1	each	45	3	213	3	28	0.7	10	6.3
Candy, Chunky bar, small	1	each	35	1	173	3	20	1.7	10	8.1
Candy, Crisped Rice bar, almond	1	each	28	2	130	2	18	1	6	1.1
Candy, Crisped Rice bar, chocolate chip	1	each	28	2	115	1	21	0.6	4	1.5
Candy, Demet's Turtles	10	piece	170	10	825	11	99	4.4	47	18.4
Candy, English toffee bar, Skor	1	each	39	1	217	2	22	0.6	13	8.5
Candy, Golden Almond Solitaires	1	each	85	2	484	10	40	3.7	32	12.9
Candy, Golden Almond bar	1	each	85	2	488	10	39	4.1	32	13.9
Candy, Golden III bar	1	each	91	3	471	6	51	5.2	30	—
Candy, Kit Kat bar	1	each	42	1	216	3	27	0.8	11	6.8
Candy, Krackel bar	1	each	41	1	218	3	25	0.9	12	7.4
Candy, M&M's, peanut, pieces	10	piece	20	0	103	2	12	0.7	5	2.1
Candy, M&M's, peanut, pkg	1	each	49	1	254	5	30	1.7	13	5.1
Candy, M&M's, plain, pieces	10	piece	7	0	34	0	5	0.2	1	0.9
Candy, M&M's, plain, pkg	1	each	48	1	236	2	34	1.2	10	6.3
Candy, Mars almond bar	1	each	50	2	234	4	31	1	12	3.6
Candy, Milky Way bar	1	each	61	4	258	3	44	1	10	4.8
Candy, Milky Way bar, snack size	1	each	18	1	76	1	13	0.3	3	1.4
Candy, Mounds bar	1	each	53	6	253	2	31	3.1	13	10.8
Candy, Mr. Goodbar bar	1	each	49	0	267	5	25	1.7	17	7.3
Candy, Nestle 100 Grand bar	1	each	42	2	198	2	30	0.6	8	4.8
Candy, Nestle Crunch bar	1	each	40	0	209	2	26	1	10	6.1
Candy, Nestle Crunch bar, snack size	1	each	10	0	52	1	7	0.3	3	1.5
Candy, Oh Henry! bar	1	each	57	3	246	6	37	2	10	3.8
Candy, Planter's peanut bar	1.5	oz.	43	1	222	7	20	1.4	14	1.8
Candy, Reese's Pieces	10	piece	8	0	39	1	5	0.2	2	1.4
Candy, Reese's peanut butter cups	2	each	45	1	243	5	25	1.4	14	5
Candy, Rolo chocolate-covered caramels	10	piece	55	11	225	3	29	0.4	11	6.7
Candy, Skittles, bite size	10	piece	11	0	45	0	10	0	0	0.1
Candy, Snickers bar, 2.2 oz	1	each	59	3	281	5	35	1.5	14	5.3
Candy, Special Dark Sweet bar	1	each	41	0	226	2	25	2	13	8.3
Candy, Starburst fruit chews	6	piece	59	4	232	0	50	0	5	0.7
Candy, Symphony bar	1	each	42	0	232	3	24	0.8	14	—

MonoF (g)	PolyF (g)	Choles (mg)	Calc (mg)	Phos (mg)	Sod (mg)	Pot (mg)	Zn (mg)	Iron (mg)	Magn (mg)	VitA (μg RE)	VitE (mg α-TE)	VitC (mg)	Thia (mg)	Ribo (mg)	Nia (mg)	B6 (mg)	Fola (μg)	B12 (μg)
5.6	3.9	60	13	44	169	39	0.3	0.9	5	147	1.96	0	0.1	0.14	0.8	0.02	8	0.13
3.8	2.6	41	39	52	172	49	0.3	0.9	6	104	1.35	0	0.11	0.14	0.9	0.02	6	0.1
0	0	0	20	—	150	120	—	0	—	20	—	0	—	—	—	—	—	—
4.9	2.9	22	17	46	285	145	0.2	1.4	11	10	1.15	1	0.14	0.13	1.1	0.06	6	0.04
4	2.4	2	133	93	329	69	0.3	1.6	10	12	1.3	0	0.2	0.18	1.7	0.02	6	0.05
1.6	1.5	5	21	26	121	35	0.1	1	12	1	0.96	0	0.06	0.08	0.7	0.01	8	0.02
1.7	1.4	7	19	78	153	36	0.1	0.5	3	2	0.85	0	0.06	0.06	0.5	0.01	12	0.05
5.1	1.4	48	77	201	271	150	0.4	1.6	15	40	2.2	0	0.13	0.18	1.1	0.04	9	0.11
0.6	0.3	66	46	89	159	64	0.3	1.8	7	30	0.18	0	0.16	0.18	1.2	0.03	25	0.16
1.5	0.5	141	22	89	115	98	0.6	1.6	20	63	0.7	1	0.09	0.21	0.7	0.05	14	0.26
2.2	0.8	23	46	92	132	34	0.1	0.6	4	11	0.92	0	0.06	0.08	0.6	0.01	5	0.05
1	0.4	107	26	63	144	89	0.4	1	6	48	0.32	0	0.1	0.19	0.8	0.04	25	0.23
1	0.9	0	8	87	83	50	0.1	0.6	3	0	0.39	0	0.07	0.07	0.6	0	2	0.01
23.8	21.4	0	1019	1780	3591	702	2.5	7.3	66	1	9.53	1	0.99	1.19	5.2	0.13	37	0.66
45.4	48.9	0	421	1470	3650	504	1.4	7.2	58	0	14.1	1	1.18	1.25	11.6	0.11	33	0.58
3.9	1.9	20	84	144	336	78	0.2	0.7	6	64	1.06	0	0.08	0.1	0.4	0.01	3	0.07
2.6	1.5	1	63	49	199	69	0.2	0.8	8	8	0.5	0	0.09	0.13	0.7	0.02	15	0.04
3.8	1	6	34	46	166	41	0.1	0.6	4	23	1.28	0	0.07	0.09	0.6	0.01	4	0.04
2.7	2.2	40	70	165	327	50	0.2	0.9	6	17	1.07	0	0.08	0.13	0.8	0.05	6	0.13
6.6	1.5	38	26	111	233	123	0.4	1.4	21	23	1.57	0	0.08	0.11	0.9	0.02	15	0.12
7.4	6.2	67	75	173	416	64	0.3	1.3	7	23	2.3	0	0.12	0.08	0.6	0.03	33	0.18
5.5	1.8	4	44	90	17	213	0.8	0.6	40	0	1.08	0	0.05	0.07	1.8	0.09	3	0.12
2.6	0.3	7	51	55	117	80	0.3	0.4	18	14	0.38	0	0.02	0.08	0.1	0.01	0	0.1
0.8	0.1	2	15	16	35	24	0.1	0.1	5	4	0.11	0	0.01	0.02	0	0	0	0.03
5.6	1.9	3	41	86	92	166	0.7	0.7	36	8	1.29	0	0.08	0.07	1.9	0.05	21	0.07
3.2	0.7	2	30	69	72	121	0.4	0.7	32	2	1.1	0	0.02	0.07	0.2	0.03	—	0.06
5	0.9	4	81	82	26	146	0.4	0.2	13	9	1.33	0	0.03	0.15	0.3	0.03	5	0.3
3.7	1.9	2	25	91	136	238	0.8	0.1	48	0	1.13	0	0.06	0.06	1.7	0.04	19	0.03
3.3	0.9	7	61	84	44	164	0.5	0.5	30	10	0.63	0	0.02	0.11	0.7	0.03	12	0.18
—	—	0	27	32	124	60	0.2	0.1	10	0	—	0	0	0.12	0	0.01	2	0
3.4	1.7	1	16	80	121	232	0.7	0.5	48	0	0.99	0	0.05	0.04	1.5	0.04	16	0.01
1.2	0.6	0	6	28	42	80	0.2	0.2	17	0	0.34	0	0.02	0.02	0.5	0.01	6	0
3.2	0.3	12	83	72	62	153	0.4	0.3	19	35	0.76	0	0.02	0.18	0.5	0.02	—	0.28
0.1	1.5	4	50	73	19	187	0.6	0.4	26	4	0.52	0	0.03	0.14	0.7	0.04	8	0.13
2.1	2.2	0	21	47	66	65	1.5	1.8	20	75	—	3	0.37	0.42	5	0.5	0	0
1.1	1	0	6	38	79	48	0.2	1.8	14	50	0.03	0	0.15	0.17	2	0.2	40	0
18.9	7.9	37	269	335	160	524	2.4	2.3	89	58	—	1	0.26	0.41	0.6	0.09	17	0.68
4.3	0.5	20	51	58	108	93	0.3	0.2	13	27	0.53	0	0.01	0.13	0	0.01	—	0.11
15	3.6	11	160	255	48	428	1.6	2	100	8	1.93	0	0.05	0.42	0.9	0.04	—	0.4
15	3.3	13	190	230	57	400	1.4	1.5	94	32	0.51	0	0.05	0.45	0.9	0.04	—	0.37
—	—	17	275	200	79	413	1	0.5	61	20	1.18	1	0.06	0.26	0.1	0.1	11	0.41
3.1	0.3	3	69	100	32	122	0.5	0.4	16	20	0.34	0	0.07	0.23	1.1	0.05	60	0.07
3.9	0.4	8	72	91	57	140	0.5	0.4	23	5	0.53	0	0.02	0.12	0.2	0.01	—	0.24
2.2	0.8	2	20	46	10	69	0.5	0.2	15	5	0.49	0	0.02	0.03	0.8	0.02	7	0.04
5.4	2.1	4	50	112	24	171	1.1	0.6	36	12	1.2	0	0.05	0.08	1.8	0.04	17	0.09
0.5	0	1	7	10	4	19	0.1	0.1	3	4	0.06	0	0	0.02	0	0	0	0.02
3.3	0.3	7	50	72	29	127	0.5	0.5	20	25	0.41	0	0.03	0.1	0.1	0.01	3	0.13
5.4	2	8	84	117	85	163	0.6	0.6	36	25	2.33	0	0.02	0.16	0.5	0.03	10	0.18
3.7	0.4	9	79	88	146	147	0.4	0.5	21	20	0.4	1	0.02	0.14	0.2	0.03	6	0.2
1.1	0.1	3	23	26	43	43	0.1	0.1	6	6	0.12	0	0.01	0.04	0.1	0.01	2	0.06
2.3	0.3	1	8	48	79	131	0.5	1.1	30	1	0.36	0	0.02	0.03	0.2	0.05	2	0
5.7	2.4	4	53	122	73	219	0.9	0.6	42	18	1.34	0	0.08	0.12	1.6	0.04	19	0.15
2.5	0.3	8	48	57	88	96	0.4	0.1	16	10	0.31	0	0.12	0.18	1.4	0.14	30	0.11
3.4	0.3	5	68	81	53	138	0.6	0.2	23	8	0.44	0	0.14	0.22	1.6	0.16	32	0.15
0.9	0.1	1	17	20	13	34	0.1	0	6	2	0.11	0	0.03	0.06	0.4	0.04	8	0.04
3.8	1.6	5	62	94	135	185	0.7	0.3	35	5	1.08	0	0.01	0.09	1.6	0.04	17	0.12
7.1	4.5	3	33	65	102	173	0.6	0.4	32	22	0.41	0	0.04	0.06	3.4	0.04	26	0.01
0.2	0.1	0	7	11	12	18	0.1	0.1	4	0	0.17	0	0.01	0.01	0.2	0.01	2	0.02
5.9	2.5	2	35	91	143	158	0.8	0.5	40	9	1.83	0	0.11	0.08	2.1	0.07	25	0.07
3.4	0.3	10	84	82	96	136	0.5	0.3	21	20	0.46	0	0.03	0.12	0.1	0.02	3	0.15
0.3	0	0	0	0	2	1	0	0	0	0	0.03	7	0	0	0	0	0	0
6.2	2.9	8	55	130	156	190	1.4	0.4	42	23	0.9	0	0.06	0.09	2.5	0.05	24	0.09
4.6	0.4	0	11	62	3	123	0.6	1	46	2	0.18	0	0.01	0.03	0.2	0.01	1	0
2.1	1.8	0	2	4	33	1	0	0.1	1	0	0.89	31	0	0	0	0	0	0
—	—	9	90	105	39	162	0.5	0.5	23	5	0.52	0	0.04	0.16	0.1	0.02	—	0.16

Food Item	Qty	Meas	Wgt (g)	Wtr (g)	Cals	Prot (g)	Carb (g)	Fib (g)	Fat (g)	SatF (g)
Candy, Twix Cookie bar, caramel	1	each	57	2	283	3	37	0.6	14	5
Candy, Twix Cookie bar, peanut butter	1	each	48	1	257	5	26	1.6	16	5.5
Candy, Whatchamacallit bar	1	each	48	5	214	4	29	1	9	4.5
Candy, Y&S Nibs, cherry	1	oz.	28	0	106	1	26	0	1	—
Candy, Y&S Twizzlers, strawberry	1	each	71	12	237	2	55	1	1	0.3
Candy, York Peppermint Patty	1	each	42	4	165	1	34	0.8	3	1.8
Candy, almonds, chocolate-coated	0.25	cup	41	1	234	5	16	3.5	18	3
Candy, butterscotch	5	piece	30	0	119	0	29	0	1	0.3
Candy, caramel, plain or chocolate	5	piece	40	3	153	2	31	0.5	3	2.6
Candy, carob bar	1	each	87	1	470	7	49	3.3	27	25.2
Candy, cherries, chocolate-covered	2	each	28	2	102	1	22	0.3	3	1.5
Candy, chewing gum	1	piece	4	0	14	0	4	0	0	0
Candy, chewing gum, uncoated, sugarless	1	piece	4	0	11	0	4	0	0	0
Candy, chocolate Kisses	6	piece	28	0	145	2	17	0.8	9	5.2
Candy, chocolate, sweet	1	each	41	0	207	2	24	2.3	14	8.2
Candy, chocolate-covered mint patty	1	each	11	1	40	0	9	0.2	1	0.6
Candy, divinity, no nuts	1	piece	20	2	70	0	18	0	0	0
Candy, fondant/candy corn	1	cup	200	14	716	0	186	0	0	0
Candy, fudge, brown sugar w/nuts, recipe	1	piece	14	1	55	0	11	0.1	1	0.2
Candy, fudge, chocolate marshmallow, recipe	1	piece	20	2	84	0	14	0	3	2
Candy, fudge, chocolate marshmallow, w/nuts, recipe	1	piece	22	2	96	1	15	0.4	4	2.1
Candy, fudge, chocolate w/nuts, recipe	1	piece	19	1	81	1	14	0.2	3	1.1
Candy, fudge, chocolate, recipe	1	piece	17	2	65	0	14	0.1	1	0.9
Candy, fudge, peanut butter, recipe	1	piece	16	2	59	1	12	0.1	1	0.2
Candy, fudge, vanilla, recipe	1	piece	16	2	59	0	13	0	1	0.5
Candy, fudge, vanilla, w/nuts, recipe	1	piece	15	1	62	0	11	0.1	2	0.6
Candy, gumdrops	10	piece	35	0	135	0	35	0	0	0
Candy, gummy bears	10	each	35	0	135	0	35	0	0	0
Candy, hard, all flavor	1	oz.	28	0	112	0	28	0	0	0
Candy, hard, dietetic	1	piece	3	0	11	0	3	0	0	0
Candy, jellybeans	10	piece	11	1	40	0	10	0	0	0
Candy, licorice	1	oz.	28	1	120	0	24	0	3	3.1
Candy, licorice, Good & Plenty	1.5	oz.	43	3	156	0	40	0	0	0.1
Candy, lollipop	1	each	6	0	24	0	6	0	0	0
Candy, malted milk balls, Whoppers	10	each	29	1	144	2	18	0.8	8	4.6
Candy, milk chocolate bar	1	each	44	1	226	3	26	1.5	14	8.1
Candy, milk chocolate bar w/almonds	1	each	41	1	216	4	22	2.5	14	7
Candy, milk chocolate w/peanuts	1	each	43	1	238	7	17	2.4	18	5.2
Candy, milk chocolate w/rice cereal	1	each	40	1	198	3	25	1.2	11	6.4
Candy, milk chocolate-covered peanuts, Goobers	10	piece	10	0	51	1	5	0.6	3	1.2
Candy, milk chocolate-covered raisins	0.25	cup	48	5	185	2	32	2	7	4.2
Candy, milk chocolate-covered raisins,Raisinets	1	each	45	3	185	2	32	2.3	7	3.3
Candy, peanut brittle, recipe	0.25	cup	37	1	166	3	26	0.7	7	1.8
Candy, peanut butter cup, dietetic	2	each	16	1	88	2	7	1.1	6	5.1
Candy, praline, recipe	1	piece	39	4	177	1	24	1	9	0.7
Candy, sesame crunch	20	piece	35	1	181	4	18	2.8	12	1.6
Candy, sugar-coated almonds, Jordan	7	each	28	1	129	2	20	1.3	5	0.4
Candy, taffy, recipe	1	piece	15	1	56	0	14	0	0	0.3
Candy, toffee, Almond Roca	1	piece	11	1	48	1	7	0.3	2	1.1
Candy, toffee, recipe	4	piece	48	1	260	1	31	0	16	9.8
Candy, tootsie roll, bite size	7	each	35	3	126	1	31	0.2	1	0.2
Candy, yogurt-covered peanuts	0.25	cup	42	2	193	4	16	1.8	13	2.5
Candy, yogurt-covered raisins	0.25	cup	48	4	190	2	34	1.5	6	3.6
Candy, truffle, recipe	1	piece	12	2	59	1	5	0.3	4	2.1
Cantaloupe Nectar	1	cup	250	210	151	1	38	0.8	0	0.2
Capers	1	tsp	5	4	0	0	0	0.2	0	—
Carambola, raw (starfruit)	1	each	127	115	42	1	10	3.4	0	0
Caraway seed	0.25	tsp	1	0	2	0	0	0.2	0	0
Cardamom, ground	0.25	tsp	0	0	1	0	0	0.1	0	0
Carissa, raw (natal plum)	1	each	20	17	12	0	3	—	0	—
Carob chips, unsweetened	0.25	cup	42	—	201	6	23	0	9	8.4
Carob flavor mix, prepared w/milk	1	cup	256	215	195	8	22	1	8	5.1
Carrot chips, dried	0.5	cup	37	1	136	3	27	7.3	1	0.1
Carrot juice, canned	1	cup	246	219	98	2	23	2	0	0.1
Carrot slices, cooked, no added salt, drained	0.5	cup	78	68	35	1	8	2.6	0	0

MonoF	PolyF	Choles	Calc	Phos	Sod	Pot	Zn	Iron	Magn	VitA	VitE	VitC	Thia	Ribo	Nia	B6	Fola	B12
(g)	(g)	(mg)	(mg)	(mg)	(mg)	(mg)	(mg)	(mg)	(mg)	(μg RE)	(mg α-TE)	(mg)	(mg)	(mg)	(mg)	(mg)	(μg)	(μg)
7.6	0.5	3	51	68	109	115	0.4	0.5	18	14	0.69	0	0.09	0.13	0.7	0.02	14	0.1
7.2	2	2	37	92	132	173	0.7	0.4	36	9	0.54	0	0.05	0.07	2	0.07	12	0.06
2.8	1.5	5	55	87	99	148	0.6	0.3	29	9	0.71	0	0.22	0.29	3.5	0.27	5	0.16
—	—	0	18	88	67	18	0	0.2	2	1	0.17	0	0.01	0.01	0	0	0	0
—	—	0	5	220	175	45	0.1	0.2	4	0	—	0	0.01	0.03	0.1	0.01	—	0
1	0.1	0	6	40	10	54	0.3	0.4	26	0	0.13	0	0.01	0.04	0.4	0	—	0.01
12	3.2	0	83	141	24	225	1	1.2	91	0	5.21	0	0.05	0.22	0.7	0.03	32	0
0.2	0	3	1	1	110	1	0	0	0	10	0.02	0	0	0	0	0	0	0
0.3	0.1	3	55	46	98	86	0.2	0.1	7	3	0.18	0	0	0.07	0.1	0.01	2	0
0.4	0.3	3	264	110	93	551	3.1	1.1	31	7	1.37	0	0.09	0.16	0.9	0.11	24	0.87
0.9	0.1	0	5	27	7	47	0.1	0.4	18	1	0.1	0	0.01	0.02	0.2	0	0	0
0	0	0	0	0	0	0	0	0	0	0	0	0	0	0	0	0	0	0
0	0	0	1	0	0	0	0	0	0	0	0	0	0	0	0	0	0	0
2.8	0.3	6	54	61	23	109	0.4	0.4	17	14	0.35	0	0.02	0.08	0.1	0.01	2	0.11
4.6	0.4	0	10	60	7	119	0.6	1.1	46	1	0.49	0	0.01	0.1	0.3	0.02	1	0
0.3	0	0	2	10	3	18	0	0.2	7	0	0.04	0	0	0.01	0.1	0	0	0
0	0	0	0	1	9	4	0	0	0	0	—	0	0	0.01	0	0	0	0
0	0	0	4	4	80	32	0.1	0.1	2	1	0	0	0	0.03	0	0	0	0
0.3	0.8	1	16	12	14	52	0.1	0.3	7	2	—	0	0.01	0.01	0	0.02	2	0
1	0.1	5	9	13	21	28	0.1	0.2	7	16	—	0	0	0.02	0	0	0	0.01
1.3	0.7	5	11	18	21	37	0.2	0.2	10	16	—	0	0.01	0.02	0	0.01	2	0.01
0.8	1	3	10	18	11	30	0.1	0.1	9	9	0.08	0	0.01	0.02	0	0.02	2	0.01
0.4	0.1	2	7	10	10	18	0.1	0.1	4	8	0.02	0	0	0.01	0	0	0	0.01
0.5	0.3	1	7	10	12	21	0.1	0	4	2	—	0	0	0.01	0.2	0.01	2	0.01
0.2	0	3	6	5	11	8	0	0	1	8	0.03	0	0	0.01	0	0	0	0.01
0.5	0.8	2	7	11	9	17	0.1	0.1	4	7	0.07	0	0.01	0.01	0	0.01	2	0.01
0	0	0	1	0	15	2	0	0.1	0	0	0	0	0	0	0	0	0	0
0	0	0	1	0	15	2	0	0.1	0	0	0	0	0	0	0	0	0	0
0	0	0	1	1	11	1	0	0.1	1	0	0	0	0	0	0	0	0	0
0	0	0	0	0	0	0	0	0	0	0	0	0	0	0	0	0	0	0
0	0	0	0	0	3	4	0	0.1	0	0	0	0	0	0	0	0	0	0
—	—	0	0	—	80	54	0.1	0	3	0	—	0	—	—	—	—	—	—
0.1	0	0	1	2	11	16	0	0.5	1	0	0	0	0	0	0	0	0	0
0	0	0	0	0	2	0	0	0	0	0	0	0	0	0	0	0	0	0
2.5	0.2	6	50	56	42	100	0.3	0.2	14	3	0.36	0	0.02	0.08	0.1	0.02	3	0.11
4.4	0.5	10	84	95	36	169	0.6	0.6	26	24	0.55	0	0.04	0.13	0.1	0.02	4	0.17
5.5	0.9	8	92	108	30	182	0.5	0.7	37	6	0.78	0	0.02	0.18	0.3	0.02	5	0.14
7.8	3.9	4	50	126	17	230	1	0.8	53	9	1.99	0	0.12	0.08	3.2	0.07	36	0.08
3.5	0.3	8	68	77	58	137	0.4	0.3	20	4	0.44	0	0.02	0.12	0.2	0.02	4	0.14
1.5	0.5	1	13	30	4	50	0.2	0.1	12	0	0.26	0	0.01	0.02	0.5	0.02	1	0.03
2.2	0.2	1	41	68	17	244	0.4	0.8	21	3	0.46	0	0.04	0.08	0.2	0.04	2	0.09
2.7	0.9	2	49	65	16	231	0.4	0.5	20	4	0.47	0	0.04	0.1	0.2	0.05	2	0.1
3.1	1.7	5	11	41	166	76	0.4	0.5	18	17	0.6	0	0.07	0.02	1.3	0.04	26	0
0.7	0.1	1	48	53	17	97	0.4	0.2	21	0	0.63	0	0.03	0.08	0.4	0.03	10	0.12
5.9	2.4	0	12	42	24	82	0.8	0.5	20	2	0.58	0	0.12	0.02	0.1	0.03	5	0
4.4	5.1	0	229	148	58	113	1.3	1.5	88	0	0.53	0	0.19	0.06	1.3	0.19	23	0
3.6	1.1	0	28	47	6	72	0.5	0.5	46	0	0.52	0	0.01	0.08	0.3	0.02	16	0
0.1	0	1	0	0	13	1	0	0	0	5	0.08	0	0	0	0	0	0	0
0.6	0.2	1	16	19	20	34	0.1	0.1	5	2	0.17	0	0.01	0.02	0.2	0.01	3	0.01
4.6	0.6	50	16	16	90	24	0.1	0	2	153	0.96	0	0	0.03	0	0	1	0.03
0.4	0.3	0	9	14	28	36	0.2	0.1	11	1	0.08	0	0.01	0.03	0	0.01	0	0.02
6.4	3.5	1	17	63	14	107	0.9	0.5	25	10	2.04	1	0.05	0.03	2.4	0.05	48	0.17
1.9	0.2	4	55	65	21	269	0.2	0.6	10	13	0.64	1	0.05	0.08	0.3	0.08	4	0.15
1.8	0.2	6	19	21	9	37	0.1	0.1	6	17	0.14	0	0.01	0.03	0	0	0	0.04
0	0	0	13	18	13	279	0.2	0.2	12	242	0.15	30	0.03	0.02	0.5	0.1	8	0
—	—	0	2	—	105	—	—	0.1	—	1	—	0	—	—	—	—	—	0
0	0.2	0	5	20	3	207	0.1	0.3	11	62	0.47	27	0.04	0.03	0.5	0.13	18	0
0	0	0	4	3	0	8	0	0.1	1	0	0.01	0	0	0	0	0	0	0
0	0	0	2	1	0	5	0	0.1	1	0	—	0	0	0	0	—	—	0
—	—	0	2	1	1	52	—	0.3	3	1	—	8	0.01	0.01	0	—	—	0
—	—	4	269	—	187	—	—	0.4	—	5	—	2	—	—	—	—	—	—
2.4	0.3	33	292	228	133	369	0.9	0.7	33	77	0.1	2	0.1	0.39	0.3	0.12	12	0.87
0	0.3	0	81	125	111	921	0.6	1.5	45	3699	0.14	21	0.26	0.18	2.6	0.44	31	0
0	0.2	0	59	103	71	718	0.4	1.1	34	2693	0.02	21	0.23	0.14	1	0.53	9	0
0	0.1	0	24	23	52	177	0.2	0.5	10	1914	0.33	2	0.03	0.04	0.4	0.19	11	0

Food Item	Qty	Meas	Wgt (g)	Wtr (g)	Cals	Prot (g)	Carb (g)	Fib (g)	Fat (g)	SatF (g)
Carrot slices, steamed	0.5	cup	78	68	34	1	8	2.3	0	0
Carrot slices, stir fried	0.5	cup	78	68	34	1	8	2.3	0	0
Carrot, baby, raw (2.75inch)	1	each	10	9	4	0	1	0.2	0	0
Carrot, glazed	0.5	cup	80	56	117	1	17	2.1	6	1.1
Carrot, raw, grated	0.5	cup	55	48	24	1	6	1.6	0	0
Carrot, whole, raw	1	each	72	63	31	1	7	2.2	0	0
Carrots, canned, drained	0.5	cup	73	68	18	0	4	1.1	0	0
Carrots, canned, drained, low sodium	0.5	cup	73	68	18	0	4	1.1	0	0
Carrots, canned, not drained	0.5	cup	123	114	28	1	7	2.2	0	0
Carrots, frozen, cooked	0.5	cup	73	66	26	1	6	2.6	0	0
Carrots, julienne	0.5	cup	55	48	24	1	6	1.7	0	0
Carrots, whole, cooked, no added salt, drained	1	each	46	40	21	1	5	1.5	0	0
Cashew butter, salted	1	Tbs	16	0	94	3	4	0.3	8	1.6
Cashew butter, unsalted	2	Tbs	32	1	188	6	9	0.6	16	3.1
Cashew chicken	1	cup	162	91	409	27	11	2	29	4.8
Cashew, dry roasted, salted	0.25	cup	34	1	197	5	11	1	16	3.1
Cashews, dry roasted, unsalted	0.25	cup	34	1	197	5	11	1	16	3.1
Cashews, oil roasted, salted	0.25	cup	32	1	187	5	9	1.2	16	3.1
Cashews, oil roasted, unsalted	0.25	cup	32	1	187	5	9	1.2	16	3.1
Cassava (yuca blanca), pieces, cooked	0.5	cup	68	46	82	2	18	0.1	0	0.1
Cassava, raw	4	oz.	113	68	181	2	43	2	0	0.1
Catsup/ketchup	1	Tbs	15	10	16	0	4	0.2	0	0
Catsup/ketchup, low sodium	1	Tbs	15	10	16	0	4	0.2	0	0
Catsup/ketchup, packet	1	each	6	4	6	0	2	0.1	0	0
Cauliflower flowerets, cooked, drained	3	each	54	50	12	1	2	1.5	0	0
Cauliflower, cooked, drained, cup measure	0.5	cup	62	58	14	1	3	1.7	0	0
Cauliflower, flowerets, batter-dipped, fried	5	piece	130	89	250	6	13	2.1	20	4.8
Cauliflower, flowerets, pickled	3	each	81	71	34	1	8	1.5	0	0
Cauliflower, frozen, cooked, drained	0.5	cup	90	85	17	1	3	2.4	0	0
Cauliflower, raw flowerets	3	each	56	52	14	1	3	1.4	0	0
Cauliflower, raw, cup measure	0.5	cup	50	46	12	1	3	1.2	0	0
Cauliflower, w/cheese sauce	0.5	cup	81	67	73	3	5	0.9	5	2.2
Celeriac/celery root, cooked	0.5	cup	78	72	21	1	5	0.9	0	0
Celery pieces, cooked, no added salt	0.5	cup	75	71	14	1	3	1.2	0	0
Celery seed	0.25	tsp	0	0	2	0	0	0.1	0	0
Celery, chopped, raw	0.5	cup	60	57	10	0	2	1	0	0
Celery, chopped, steamed	0.5	cup	75	71	12	1	3	1.3	0	0
Celery, chopped, stir fried	0.5	cup	75	71	12	1	3	1.3	0	0
Celery, pickled	0.5	cup	75	71	11	0	3	1.1	0	0
Celery, raw, large outer stalk	1	each	40	38	6	0	1	0.7	0	0
Celery, stuffed w/cheese	1	piece	32	25	44	2	1	0.3	4	2.4
Cereal, 100% Bran	0.5	cup	33	1	89	4	24	9.8	2	0.3
Cereal, 100% Natural	0.5	cup	52	1	231	5	36	3.9	9	3.7
Cereal, 100% Natural w/apple cinnamon	0.5	cup	52	1	239	6	35	3.4	10	7.8
Cereal, 100% Natural w/raisins & dates	0.5	cup	55	2	248	6	36	3.6	10	6.8
Cereal, All Bran	0.5	cup	43	1	114	5	33	13.9	1	0.3
Cereal, Alpha Bits	1	cup	28	0	111	2	25	1.2	1	0.1
Cereal, Amaranth flakes	0.5	cup	19	1	67	2	13	1.8	2	0.5
Cereal, Apple Jacks	1	cup	28	1	109	1	25	0.5	0	0.1
Cereal, Bran Buds	0.5	cup	43	1	119	4	34	17.1	1	0.2
Cereal, Bran Chex	1	cup	49	1	156	5	39	7.9	1	0.2
Cereal, Bran Flakes, Kellogg's	1	cup	39	1	128	4	31	6.2	1	0.2
Cereal, Bran Flakes, Post	1	cup	47	1	152	5	37	9.2	1	0.1
Cereal, Bran'ola raisin, Post	1	cup	110	3	400	8	88	10	6	1
Cereal, C.W. Post w/raisins	1	cup	103	4	446	9	74	13.6	15	11
Cereal, C.W. Post, plain	1	cup	97	2	421	9	73	7.2	13	1.7
Cereal, Cap'n Crunch	1	cup	37	1	147	2	32	1.2	2	0.5
Cereal, Cap'n Crunch, peanut butter	1	cup	35	1	146	3	28	1	3	0.7
Cereal, Cap'n Crunchberries	1	cup	35	1	140	2	30	0.8	2	0.5
Cereal, Cheerios	1	cup	23	1	83	2	17	2	1	0.3
Cereal, Clusters	0.5	cup	28	1	111	4	20	2.9	3	0.4
Cereal, Cocoa Krispies	1	cup	36	1	140	2	32	0.5	1	0.7
Cereal, Cocoa Pebbles	1	cup	32	1	131	2	28	0.5	2	1.1
Cereal, Corn Bran	1	cup	36	1	120	2	30	6.4	1	0.3
Cereal, Corn Chex	1	cup	28	1	111	2	25	0.5	0	0

MonoF	PolyF	Choles	Calc	Phos	Sod	Pot	Zn	Iron	Magn	VitA	VitE	VitC	Thia	Ribo	Nia	B6	Fola	B12
(g)	(g)	(mg)	(mg)	(mg)	(mg)	(mg)	(mg)	(mg)	(mg)	(μg RE)	(mg α-TE)	(mg)	(mg)	(mg)	(mg)	(mg)	(μg)	(μg)
0	0.1	0	21	34	27	252	0.2	0.4	12	1977	0.33	5	0.07	0.04	0.7	0.11	10	0
0	0.1	0	21	34	27	252	0.2	0.4	12	1977	0.33	6	0.07	0.04	0.7	0.11	10	0
0	0	0	2	4	4	28	0	0.1	1	150	0.04	1	0	0	0.1	0.01	3	0
2.5	1.8	0	31	24	131	189	0.2	0.6	12	1717	1.16	2	0.02	0.04	0.3	0.17	9	0.01
0	0	0	15	24	19	178	0.1	0.3	8	1547	0.25	5	0.05	0.03	0.5	0.08	8	0
0	0.1	0	19	32	25	233	0.1	0.4	11	2025	0.33	7	0.07	0.04	0.7	0.11	10	0
0	0.1	0	18	18	177	131	0.2	0.5	6	1005	0.31	2	0.01	0.02	0.4	0.08	7	0
0	0.1	0	18	18	31	131	0.2	0.5	6	1005	0.31	2	0.01	0.02	0.4	0.08	7	0
0	0.1	0	38	25	295	213	0.4	0.6	11	1189	0.49	2	0.02	0.03	0.5	0.14	10	0
0	0	0	20	19	43	115	0.2	0.3	7	1292	0.31	2	0.02	0.03	0.3	0.09	8	0
0	0	0	15	24	19	178	0.1	0.3	8	1554	0.25	5	0.05	0.03	0.5	0.08	8	0
0	0	0	14	14	30	104	0.1	0.3	6	1129	0.19	1	0.02	0.03	0.2	0.11	6	0
4.7	1.3	0	7	73	98	87	0.8	0.8	41	0	0.25	0	0.05	0.03	0.3	0.04	11	0
9.3	2.7	0	14	146	5	175	1.6	1.6	83	0	0.5	0	0.1	0.06	0.5	0.08	22	0
13	9.1	60	47	249	988	415	1.4	1.9	60	93	3.65	9	0.14	0.14	12.5	0.56	40	0.24
9.4	2.7	0	15	168	219	194	1.9	2.1	89	0	0.2	0	0.07	0.07	0.5	0.09	24	0
9.4	2.7	0	15	168	5	194	1.9	2.1	89	0	0.2	0	0.07	0.07	0.5	0.09	24	0
9.2	2.6	0	13	138	203	172	1.5	1.3	83	0	0.51	0	0.14	0.06	0.6	0.08	22	0
9.2	2.6	0	13	138	6	172	1.5	1.3	83	0	0.51	0	0.14	0.06	0.6	0.08	22	0
0.1	0.1	0	60	43	165	473	0.2	2.4	43	1	0.13	22	0.12	0.06	0.9	0.19	10	0
0.1	0.1	0	18	31	16	307	0.4	0.3	24	2	0.22	23	0.1	0.05	1	0.1	31	0
0	0	0	3	6	182	74	0	0.1	3	16	0.22	2	0.01	0.01	0.2	0.03	2	0
0	0	0	3	6	3	72	0	0.1	3	15	0.22	2	0.01	0.01	0.2	0.03	2	0
0	0	0	1	2	71	29	0	0	1	6	0.09	1	0	0	0.1	0.01	1	0
0	0.1	0	9	17	8	77	0.1	0.2	5	1	0.02	24	0.02	0.03	0.2	0.09	24	0
0	0.1	0	10	20	9	88	0.1	0.2	6	1	0.02	28	0.03	0.03	0.3	0.11	27	0
5.2	9.1	30	167	173	239	332	0.6	0.9	19	45	3.43	47	0.1	0.16	0.7	0.19	40	0.17
0.1	0.1	0	20	28	129	192	0.1	0.4	10	30	0.08	35	0.04	0.03	0.3	0.12	24	0
0	0.1	0	15	22	16	125	0.1	0.4	8	2	0.04	28	0.03	0.05	0.3	0.08	37	0
0	0.1	0	12	25	17	170	0.2	0.2	8	1	0.02	26	0.03	0.04	0.3	0.12	32	0
0	0	0	11	22	15	152	0.1	0.2	8	1	0.02	23	0.03	0.03	0.3	0.11	28	0
1.7	0.8	10	88	73	258	183	0.4	0.2	10	41	0.29	21	0.04	0.1	0.3	0.1	22	0.17
0	0.1	0	20	51	47	134	0.2	0.3	9	0	0.16	3	0.02	0.03	0.3	0.08	3	0
0	0.1	0	32	19	68	213	0.1	0.3	9	10	0.27	5	0.03	0.04	0.2	0.06	16	0
0.1	0	0	9	3	1	7	0	0.2	2	0	0	0	0	0	0	0	0	0
0	0	0	24	15	52	172	0.1	0.2	7	8	0.22	4	0.03	0.03	0.2	0.05	17	0
0	0.1	0	30	19	65	216	0.1	0.3	8	10	0.27	4	0.1	0.03	0.2	0.06	18	0
0	0.1	0	30	19	65	215	0.1	0.3	8	9	0.27	4	0.1	0.03	0.2	0.06	17	0
0	0	0	26	15	183	177	0.1	0.3	8	8	0.24	3	0.02	0.03	0.2	0.05	12	0
0	0	0	16	10	35	115	0.1	0.2	4	5	0.14	3	0.02	0.02	0.1	0.04	11	0
1.1	0.1	12	45	50	110	75	0.2	0.2	4	46	0.16	2	0.01	0.04	0.1	0.02	7	0.06
0.3	0.9	0	23	401	229	326	2.9	4.1	156	0	0.77	31	0.79	0.89	10.5	1.06	23	3.14
3.7	1.1	1	50	161	14	228	1.2	1.6	55	1	0.59	0	0.18	0.08	0.9	0.09	13	0.06
0.9	0.7	0	78	175	26	257	1	1.4	36	3	0.36	1	0.17	0.29	0.9	0.05	8	0.15
1.9	0.9	0	80	174	24	269	1.1	1.6	62	3	0.38	0	0.15	0.32	1	0.08	23	0.07
0.3	0.8	0	152	422	87	490	5.4	6.4	185	323	0.79	22	0.56	0.6	7.2	0.73	129	2.15
0.2	0.2	0	8	51	180	55	1.5	2.7	17	376	0.02	0	0.37	0.43	5	0.51	100	1.51
0.4	0.9	0	3	63	7	67	0	0.3	5	2	1.61	0	0.01	0.02	0.5	0.01	2	0
0.1	0.2	0	3	28	127	30	3.5	4.2	8	213	0.05	14	0.37	0.4	4.7	0.48	100	0
0.2	0.6	0	29	238	286	386	9.2	6.4	119	323	0.68	22	0.56	0.6	7.2	0.73	129	0
0.3	0.7	0	29	173	345	216	6.5	14	69	11	0.56	26	0.64	0.26	8.6	0.88	173	2.6
0.2	0.5	0	19	202	304	236	5	10.9	81	488	7.22	20	0.51	0.58	6.7	0.66	138	1.95
0.1	0.4	0	21	296	431	251	2.5	13.4	102	622	0.54	0	0.61	0.7	8.3	0.85	166	2.49
—	—	0	0	200	440	440	3	9	80	751	—	0	0.75	0.85	10	1	200	3
1.7	1.4	0	50	232	161	261	1.6	16.4	74	1363	0.72	0	1.34	1.55	18.1	1.85	364	5.46
6	4.7	0	47	224	167	198	1.6	15.4	67	1284	0.68	0	1.26	1.46	17.1	1.75	342	5.14
0.4	0.3	0	7	39	286	47	5.1	6.2	13	5	0.18	0	0.51	0.58	6.8	0.68	137	0
1.1	0.7	0	4	67	264	80	4.9	5.8	24	5	0.19	0	0.49	0.55	6.5	0.65	130	0
0.4	0.3	0	9	40	256	49	5.4	6.1	13	6	0.25	0	0.5	0.57	6.7	0.67	135	0.01
0.5	0.2	0	42	86	215	67	2.8	6.1	25	284	0.16	11	0.28	0.32	3.8	0.38	76	0
1.4	1.4	0	51	106	135	137	0.4	4.5	27	373	0.97	16	0.39	0.48	6	0.52	100	0
0.1	0.1	0	5	34	244	70	1.7	2.1	13	261	0.17	17	0.43	0.5	5.8	0.58	108	0
0.4	0.1	0	5	25	180	53	1.7	2	13	424	0.04	0	0.42	0.48	5.6	0.58	113	1.7
0.3	0.4	0	27	48	338	75	5	10.1	19	5	0.19	0	0.1	0.56	6.7	0.67	134	0
0	0	0	3	11	310	23	0.1	8.1	4	14	0.07	15	0.37	0.07	5	0.51	100	1.5

Food Item	Qty	Meas	Wgt (g)	Wtr (g)	Cals	Prot (g)	Carb (g)	Fib (g)	Fat (g)	SatF (g)
Cereal, Corn Flakes, USDA	1	cup	25	1	91	2	22	0.7	0	0
Cereal, Corn Pops USDA	1	cup	28	1	108	1	26	0.4	0	0.1
Cereal, Cracklin' Oat Bran	0.5	cup	30	1	123	3	22	3.6	4	1.6
Cereal, Crispy Wheat `N Raisins	1	cup	43	3	150	3	35	2.7	1	0.1
Cereal, Farina, enriched, cooked	0.5	cup	116	102	58	2	12	1.6	0	0
Cereal, Froot Loops	1	cup	28	1	111	1	25	0.5	1	0.4
Cereal, Frosted Flakes	1	cup	38	1	146	1	34	0.8	0	0.1
Cereal, Fruit & Fibre, date-raisin-nut	0.5	cup	28	3	96	2	22	3.8	1	0.2
Cereal, Fruity Pebbles	1	cup	32	1	130	1	28	0.4	2	1.4
Cereal, Golden Grahams	1	cup	39	1	150	2	33	1.2	1	0.2
Cereal, Granola, Nature Valley	0.5	cup	56	2	255	6	37	3.6	10	1.3
Cereal, Granola, low fat	0.5	cup	47	1	182	5	38	3	3	0
Cereal, Grape Nuts	0.5	cup	54	2	195	7	45	5.4	0	0
Cereal, Grape Nuts Flakes	1	cup	39	1	144	4	32	3.9	1	0.6
Cereal, Heartwise, plain	1	cup	39	1	113	4	31	8.6	1	0.2
Cereal, Honey & Nut Corn Flakes	667	cup	28	1	115	2	24	0.5	1	0.3
Cereal, Honey Bran	1	cup	35	1	119	3	29	3.9	1	0.3
Cereal, Honey Buckwheat Crisp	1	cup	38	2	147	4	31	3.4	1	0.2
Cereal, Honey Bunches of Oats	1	cup	43	1	173	3	36	2.1	2	0.5
Cereal, Honey Comb	1	cup	22	0	86	1	20	0.6	0	0.2
Cereal, Honey Nut Cheerios	1	cup	33	1	126	3	27	1.7	1	0.3
Cereal, Honey Smacks	1	cup	38	1	144	2	33	1.3	1	0.4
Cereal, Just Right	1	cup	43	1	152	5	36	3	1	0.2
Cereal, King Vitaman	1	cup	21	0	81	2	18	0.8	1	0.2
Cereal, Kix	1	cup	19	0	72	1	16	0.5	0	0.1
Cereal, Life, plain/cinnamon	1	cup	44	2	167	4	35	2.8	2	0.3
Cereal, Lucky Charms	1	cup	32	1	124	2	27	1.3	1	0.2
Cereal, Maypo, cooked, no salt added	0.5	cup	120	99	85	3	16	2.9	1	0.2
Cereal, Most	1	cup	52	2	175	7	40	7.3	1	0.1
Cereal, Mueslix Five Grain Muesli	0.5	cup	41	2	139	4	32	3.7	2	0.3
Cereal, Multi-grain, cooked	0.5	cup	123	96	100	3	20	2	1	0.2
Cereal, Oat flakes, fortified	1	cup	48	1	180	8	36	1.4	1	0.2
Cereal, Oatmeal, instant, packet, prepared, plain	1	each	177	151	104	4	18	3	2	0.3
Cereal, Post Toasties	1	cup	24	1	93	2	21	0.8	0	0
Cereal, Product 19	1	cup	33	1	121	3	28	1.1	0	0
Cereal, Quisp	1	cup	30	1	121	2	26	0.8	2	0.5
Cereal, Raisin Bran, Kellogg's	1	cup	56	5	171	5	43	7.5	1	0
Cereal, Raisin Bran, Post	1	cup	56	5	172	5	42	7.9	1	0.2
Cereal, Raisin Nut Bran	1	cup	57	3	221	4	42	5.6	6	1
Cereal, Ralston, cooked	0.5	cup	126	109	67	3	14	3	0	0.1
Cereal, Rice Chex	1	cup	25	1	99	1	22	0.5	0	0
Cereal, Rice Krispies	1	cup	28	1	111	2	25	0.3	0	0
Cereal, Roman meal, cooked	0.5	cup	120	99	73	3	16	4.1	0	0.1
Cereal, Shredded Wheat, large biscuit	1	each	24	1	85	3	19	2.3	0	0.1
Cereal, Shredded Wheat, small	1	cup	43	2	152	5	34	4.2	1	0.1
Cereal, Special K	1	cup	28	1	105	6	20	0.9	0	0
Cereal, Super Golden Crisp	1	cup	33	0	123	2	30	0.5	0	0.1
Cereal, Team Rice	1	cup	42	2	164	3	36	0.5	1	0.1
Cereal, Total, wheat	1	cup	33	1	116	3	26	2.9	1	0.2
Cereal, Trix	1	cup	28	1	114	1	24	0.7	2	0.4
Cereal, Uncle Sam's High Fiber	0.5	cup	55	3	213	8	40	14.5	2	0.2
Cereal, Wheat Chex	1	cup	46	1	169	5	38	4.1	1	0.2
Cereal, Wheatena, cooked, unsalted	0.5	cup	122	104	68	2	14	3.3	1	0.1
Cereal, Wheaties	1	cup	29	1	106	3	23	2	1	0.2
Cereal, cream of rye, cooked	0.5	cup	126	111	54	1	12	2.2	0	0
Cereal, cream of wheat, cooked	0.5	cup	122	107	63	1	14	0.1	0	0
Cereal, cream of wheat, cooked	0.5	cup	122	106	66	2	14	0.6	0	0
Cereal, cream of wheat, mix'n eat, prep, plain	1	each	142	117	102	3	21	0.4	0	0
Cereal, farina, unenriched, cooked w/o salt	0.5	cup	116	102	58	2	12	1.6	0	0
Cereal, frosted mini wheats, biscuits	4	each	31	2	105	3	26	3.3	0	0.1
Cereal, frosted rice krispies	1	cup	19	0	71	1	17	0.2	0	0
Cereal, honey cluster flake crunch, fat free	1	cup	41	1	173	4	35	5.3	0	0
Cereal, malt-o-meal, plain, cooked	0.5	cup	120	105	61	2	13	0.5	0	0
Cereal, oat bran, cooked, Mother's brand	0.5	cup	121	109	31	2	8	2	1	0.2
Cereal, oatmeal, cooked	0.5	cup	117	100	72	3	13	2	1	0.2

MonoF	PolyF	Choles	Calc	Phos	Sod	Pot	Zn	Iron	Magn	VitA	VitE	VitC	Thia	Ribo	Nia	B6	Fola	B12
(g)	(g)	(mg)	(mg)	(mg)	(mg)	(mg)	(mg)	(mg)	(mg)	(μg RE)	(mg α-TE)	(mg)	(mg)	(mg)	(mg)	(mg)	(μg)	(μg)
0	0.1	0	1	10	266	23	0.2	7.8	3	188	0.03	12	0.32	0.35	4.2	0.42	88	0
0.1	0	0	2	6	113	21	1.4	1.7	2	213	0.03	14	0.37	0.4	4.7	0.48	100	0
1.8	0.4	0	14	102	107	139	0.9	1.1	42	138	0.2	9	0.23	0.26	3.1	0.31	83	0
0.1	0.1	0	54	110	223	180	0.8	3.5	33	293	0.45	0	0.29	0.33	3.9	0.39	78	0
0	0	0	2	14	0	15	0.1	0.6	2	0	0.02	0	0.09	0.06	0.6	0.01	27	0
0.2	0.3	0	3	20	133	30	3.5	4	8	200	0.1	13	0.37	0.4	4.7	0.48	85	0
0	0.1	0	1	10	244	25	0.2	5.5	3	274	0.05	18	0.45	0.53	6.1	0.6	113	0
0.6	0.5	0	15	110	134	167	1.5	5.1	40	361	0.66	0	0.38	0.43	5	0.5	100	1.5
0.1	0.1	0	4	19	178	24	1.7	2	9	424	0.03	0	0.42	0.48	5.6	0.58	113	1.7
0.4	0.2	0	19	47	357	69	4.9	5.8	12	293	0.29	20	0.49	0.55	6.5	0.65	130	0
6.7	1.9	0	42	164	92	188	1.1	1.8	54	0	3.98	0	0.18	0.06	0.6	0.08	8	0
—	—	0	—	121	91	144	5.7	2.7	36	227	7.61	—	0.57	0.64	7.6	0.76	152	2.27
0	0.1	0	5	137	379	182	1.2	15.6	36	722	0.14	0	0.71	0.82	9.6	0.98	192	2.89
0.1	0.2	0	16	116	220	136	0.8	11.2	43	516	0.1	0	0.51	0.58	6.9	0.7	138	2.07
0.3	0.4	0	30	154	168	265	2.1	6.2	55	310	0.02	0	0.52	0.58	7	0.69	137	1.95
0.6	0.4	0	3	19	191	31	0.2	2.3	3	116	0.07	8	0.2	0.23	2.6	0.26	57	0
0.1	0.3	0	16	132	202	151	0.9	5.6	46	463	0.81	19	0.46	0.52	6.2	0.63	24	1.86
0.3	0.6	0	53	107	359	141	0.7	10.8	43	908	8.94	36	0.9	1.02	12	1.87	11	3.6
1.4	0.3	0	8	66	272	77	0.7	6	24	838	0.3	0	0.55	0.74	8.3	1.04	196	3.67
0.1	0.1	0	4	22	124	25	1.2	2.1	7	291	0.09	0	0.29	0.33	3.9	0.4	78	1.17
0.5	0.2	0	22	113	285	94	4.1	5	32	248	0.34	16	0.41	0.47	5.5	0.55	110	0
0.1	0.3	0	4	56	71	59	0.5	2.5	22	315	0.19	21	0.53	0.6	7	0.72	140	0
0.2	0.4	0	11	94	288	98	22.8	27.3	29	341	45.6	0	2.27	2.58	30.3	3.03	607	9.1
0.3	0.2	0	3	54	176	58	2.6	5.9	18	212	1.42	8	0.26	0.3	3.5	0.35	71	1.06
0.1	0	0	27	26	166	26	2.4	5.1	6	236	0.05	9	0.24	0.27	3.2	0.32	63	0
0.6	0.8	0	134	187	240	109	5.5	12.3	43	2	0.22	0	0.55	0.62	7.4	0.73	147	0
0.4	0.2	0	35	81	217	58	4	4.8	21	240	0.14	16	0.4	0.45	5.3	0.53	107	0
0.4	0.4	0	62	124	5	106	0.7	4.2	25	352	0.84	14	0.36	0.36	4.7	0.48	5	1.44
0.2	0.3	0	79	361	276	340	2.8	33	103	2753	55	110	2.76	3.13	36.7	3.69	734	11
0.5	0.6	0	19	107	53	185	3.7	4.5	41	374	4.47	0	0.37	0.42	4.9	0.5	98	1.64
0.5	0.3	0	35	92	380	68	0.5	2.7	33	57	1.71	0	0.2	0.23	2.2	0.23	9	0
0.3	0.4	0	68	176	220	228	2.5	13.7	58	636	0.34	0	0.62	0.72	8.4	0.86	169	2.54
0.6	0.7	0	163	133	285	99	0.9	6.3	42	453	0.21	0	0.53	0.28	5.5	0.74	150	0
0	0	0	1	11	252	28	0.1	0.6	4	318	0.06	0	0.31	0.36	4.2	0.43	85	1.27
0.2	0.2	0	3	36	238	45	16.5	19.8	14	248	24.4	66	1.65	1.88	22	2.21	429	6.6
0.4	0.2	0	6	47	216	40	4.3	5.1	15	4	0.16	0	0.42	0.48	5.7	0.56	113	0
0.2	0.7	0	32	197	325	401	3.8	4.6	82	230	0.51	0	0.39	0.45	5.1	0.5	112	1.51
0.1	0.5	0	26	235	365	345	3	8.9	95	741	1.3	0	0.73	0.84	9.9	1.01	198	2.97
1.6	2.9	0	80	201	302	302	1.7	9	64	753	1.32	0	0.75	0.86	10.1	1	201	0
0.1	0.2	0	6	73	3	77	0.7	0.8	29	0	0.13	0	0.1	0.09	1	0.06	9	0.05
0	0	0	4	25	210	29	0.3	7.2	6	2	0.03	13	0.33	0.01	4.4	0.45	89	1.33
0	0	0	5	30	206	27	0.5	0.7	12	371	0.03	15	0.52	0.59	6.9	0.69	138	0.08
0.1	0.2	0	14	107	1	150	0.9	1.1	54	0	0.22	0	0.12	0.06	1.5	0.06	12	0
0.1	0.2	0	10	86	0	77	0.6	0.7	40	0	0.12	0	0.07	0.07	1.1	0.06	12	0
0.1	0.4	0	16	151	4	154	1.4	1.8	56	0	0.23	0	0.11	0.12	2.2	0.11	21	0
0	0.2	0	4	46	229	50	3.4	8	16	206	0.07	14	0.48	0.54	6.4	0.65	85	0
0.1	0.1	0	7	44	51	48	1.8	2.1	20	437	0.12	0	0.43	0.5	5.8	0.59	116	1.75
0.2	0.3	0	6	65	260	71	0.6	12	12	556	0.1	22	0.55	0.63	7.4	0.76	7	2.23
0.1	0.1	0	284	232	218	107	16.5	19.8	35	413	25.8	66	1.65	1.87	22.1	2.2	440	8.45
0.8	0.3	0	30	24	184	16	3.5	4.2	3	210	0.56	14	0.35	0.4	4.7	0.47	93	0
0.5	1.5	0	38	208	125	259	1.5	2	67	0	0.79	0	1.31	1.39	11.6	0.07	43	0
0.1	0.5	0	18	182	308	173	1.2	13.2	58	0	0.17	24	0.6	0.17	8.1	0.83	162	2.44
0.1	0.3	0	5	73	2	94	0.8	0.7	24	0	0.45	0	0.01	0.02	0.7	0.02	9	0
0.2	0.1	0	53	92	215	101	0.7	7.8	31	218	0.36	14	0.36	0.41	4.8	0.48	97	0
0	0.1	0	6	27	175	33	0.3	0.3	11	0	0.08	0	0.04	0.01	0.1	0.03	2	0
0	0	0	4	21	1	24	0.2	0.2	4	0	0.02	0	0	0	0.5	0.03	4	0
0	0.1	0	26	51	71	23	0.2	5.2	6	0	0.02	0	0.12	0	0.7	0.02	55	0
0	0.2	0	20	20	241	38	0.2	8.1	7	376	0.02	0	0.43	0.28	5	0.57	101	0
0	0	0	2	14	0	15	0.1	0	2	0	0.02	0	0.01	0.01	0.1	0.01	2	0
0.1	0.3	0	11	90	1	103	0.9	8.7	31	0	0.28	0	0.22	0.25	3	0.28	62	0.9
0	0.1	0	1	15	138	15	0.2	1.3	5	164	0.02	11	0.26	0.3	3.6	0.36	76	0
0	0	0	0	—	27	—	—	0.5	—	40	—	2	—	—	—	—	—	—
0	0	0	2	12	1	16	0.1	4.8	2	0	0.02	0	0.24	0.12	2.9	0.01	2	0
0.3	0.4	0	10	89	127	69	0.4	0.7	31	0	0.22	0	0.12	0.02	0.1	0.02	5	0
0.4	0.4	0	9	89	1	66	0.6	0.8	28	2	0.12	0	0.13	0.02	0.2	0.02	5	0

Food Item	Qty	Meas	Wgt (g)	Wtr (g)	Cals	Prot (g)	Carb (g)	Fib (g)	Fat (g)	SatF (g)
Cereal, oatmeal, instant packet, prepared, apple-ci	1	each	149	117	125	3	26	2.5	1	0.3
Cereal, oatmeal, instant packet, prepared, cinn-spi	1	each	161	118	177	5	35	2.6	2	0.4
Cereal, oatmeal, instant packet, prepared, maple	1	each	155	116	153	4	32	2.6	2	0.4
Cereal, oatmeal, instant, prepared, raisin-spice	1	each	158	119	161	4	32	2.2	2	0.3
Cereal, puffed rice, fortified	1	cup	14	1	54	1	12	0.2	0	0
Cereal, puffed wheat, fortified	1	cup	12	0	44	2	9	1.1	0	0
Cereal, rolled wheat, cooked	0.5	cup	120	100	74	2	16	1.9	0	0.1
Cerealm, Tasteeos	1	cup	24	1	94	3	19	2.5	1	0.2
Chayote fruit, raw	1	each	203	191	39	2	9	3.4	0	0.1
Chayote, cooked pieces	0.5	cup	80	75	19	0	4	2.2	0	0.1
Cheese food, American cold pack	1	oz.	28	12	94	6	2	0	7	4.4
Cheese food, swiss processed, slice	1	piece	21	9	68	5	1	0	5	3.3
Cheese product, nonfat (Kraft Free Singles)	1	piece	19	12	30	4	3	0	0	0
Cheese puffs (Cheetos)	1	cup	20	0	111	2	11	0.2	7	1.3
Cheese spread, American	1	Tbs	15	7	44	2	1	0	3	2
Cheese spread, American	2	Tbs	30	14	88	5	3	0	6	4.1
Cheese spread, Velveeta	1	oz.	28	13	80	5	3	0	6	4
Cheese spread, lowfat, low sodium (Velveeta)	1	Tbs	15	9	27	4	1	0	1	0.7
Cheese spread, lowfat, low sodium (Velveeta)	1	piece	34	21	61	9	1	0	2	1.5
Cheese, American food slice	1	piece	21	9	69	4	2	0	5	3.2
Cheese, American processed	1	piece	21	8	79	5	0	0	7	4.1
Cheese, American processed, lowfat	1	oz.	28	17	51	7	1	0	2	1.2
Cheese, Gjetost	1	piece	28	4	132	3	12	0	8	5.4
Cheese, Mexican, nonfat, Lifetime	1	oz.	28	18	40	8	1	0	0	0
Cheese, asiago, shredded	0.25	cup	27	10	102	8	1	0	7	4.8
Cheese, beer	1	oz.	28	12	105	7	1	0	8	5.3
Cheese, blue	1	oz.	28	12	100	6	1	0	8	5.3
Cheese, brick w/salami	1	oz.	28	12	102	6	1	0	8	5
Cheese, brick, shredded	0.25	cup	28	12	105	7	1	0	8	5.3
Cheese, brick, shredded	1	oz.	28	12	105	7	1	0	8	5.3
Cheese, brie, sliced	1	oz.	28	14	95	6	0	0	8	4.9
Cheese, camembert	0.25	cup	28	15	85	6	0	0	7	4.3
Cheese, camembert	1	oz.	28	15	85	6	0	0	7	4.3
Cheese, caraway	1	piece	28	11	107	7	1	0	8	5.3
Cheese, cheddar, low fat, Alpine Lace	1	oz.	28	14	81	9	1	0	5	3
Cheese, cheddar, low sodium	1	oz.	28	11	113	7	1	0	9	5.9
Cheese, cheddar, lowfat, low sodium	0.25	cup	28	18	49	7	1	0	2	1.2
Cheese, cheddar, nonfat, Lifetime	1	oz.	28	18	40	8	1	0	0	0
Cheese, cheddar, shredded	0.25	cup	28	10	114	7	0	0	9	6
Cheese, cheshire	1	oz.	28	11	110	7	1	0	9	5.5
Cheese, cheshire	1	piece	28	11	110	7	1	0	9	5.5
Cheese, colby, cubed	0.25	cup	33	13	130	8	1	0	11	6.7
Cheese, colby, cubed	1	oz.	28	11	112	7	1	0	9	5.7
Cheese, colby, low sodium	1	oz.	28	11	113	7	1	0	9	5.9
Cheese, colby, lowfat, low sodium	1	oz.	28	18	49	7	1	0	2	1.3
Cheese, colby, shredded	0.25	cup	28	11	111	7	1	0	9	5.7
Cheese, cottage, 1% lowfat	0.5	cup	113	93	82	14	3	0	1	0.7
Cheese, cottage, 2% lowfat	0.5	cup	113	18	810	1	0	0	92	57.2
Cheese, cottage, creamed w/fruit	0.5	cup	113	82	140	11	15	0	4	2.4
Cheese, cottage, creamed, large curd	0.5	cup	113	89	116	14	3	0	5	3.2
Cheese, cottage, lowfat, low sodium	0.5	cup	112	94	81	14	3	0	1	0.7
Cheese, cottage, nonfat (Knudsen)	0.5	cup	122	103	80	15	4	0	0	0
Cheese, cottage, small curd	0.5	cup	105	83	108	13	3	0	5	3
Cheese, cream	2	Tbs	29	16	101	2	1	0	10	6.4
Cheese, cream, lowfat	2	Tbs	30	19	69	3	2	0	5	3.3
Cheese, cream, nonfat (Philadelphia Free)	2	Tbs	33	26	30	5	2	0	0	0
Cheese, cream, nonfat (Philadelphia)	1	oz.	28	22	25	4	2	0	0	0
Cheese, cream, soft (Philadelphia)	2	Tbs	30	17	100	2	1	0	10	7
Cheese, edam	1	oz.	28	12	101	7	0	0	8	5
Cheese, feta, shredded	0.25	cup	62	34	162	9	3	0	13	9.2
Cheese, feta, shredded	1	oz.	28	16	75	4	1	0	6	4.2
Cheese, fontina	1	oz.	28	11	110	7	0	0	9	5.4
Cheese, goat, hard	1	oz.	28	8	128	9	1	0	10	7
Cheese, goat, soft	0.5	cup	62	37	165	11	1	0	13	9

MonoF	PolyF	Choles	Calc	Phos	Sod	Pot	Zn	Iron	Magn	VitA	VitE	VitC	Thia	Ribo	Nia	B6	Fola	B12
(g)	(g)	(mg)	(mg)	(mg)	(mg)	(mg)	(mg)	(mg)	(mg)	(μg RE)	(mg α-TE)	(mg)	(mg)	(mg)	(mg)	(mg)	(μg)	(μg)
0.5	0.6	0	104	113	121	106	0.7	3.9	30	305	0.12	0	0.3	0.35	4.1	0.41	94	0
0.6	0.7	0	172	145	280	105	1	6.6	52	473	0.35	0	0.56	0.34	5.6	0.77	153	0
0.6	0.7	0	105	132	234	112	0.9	3.9	39	302	0.16	0	0.3	0.34	4	0.4	81	0
0.6	0.6	0	166	133	226	150	0.7	6.6	36	441	0.16	0	0.51	0.36	5.5	0.75	150	0
0	0	0	1	16	1	16	0.2	0.4	4	0	0.01	0	0.06	0.01	0.9	0	1	0
0	0.1	0	3	40	1	44	0.4	0.6	16	0	0.08	0	0.05	0.03	1.4	0.02	4	0.05
0.1	0.2	0	8	83	0	85	0.6	0.7	26	0	0.24	0	0.08	0.06	1.1	0.09	13	0
0.2	0.2	0	11	96	183	71	0.7	6.9	26	318	0.17	13	0.31	0.36	4.2	0.43	85	1.27
0	0.1	0	34	36	4	254	1.5	0.7	24	12	0.24	16	0.05	0.06	1	0.15	189	0
0	0.2	0	10	23	1	138	0.2	0.2	10	4	0.1	6	0.02	0.03	0.3	0.09	14	0
2	0.2	18	141	113	274	103	0.9	0.2	8	57	0.19	0	0.01	0.13	0	0.04	2	0.36
1.4	0.1	17	152	110	326	60	0.7	0.1	6	51	0.14	0	0	0.08	0	0.01	1	0.48
0	0	2	150	714	290	55	—	0	—	86	0	0	—	0.07	—	—	—	—
4.1	1	1	12	22	210	33	0.1	0.5	4	7	1.02	0	0.05	0.07	0.6	0.03	24	0.03
0.9	0.1	8	84	107	202	36	0.4	0	4	28	0.11	0	0.01	0.06	0	0.02	1	0.06
1.9	0.2	17	171	217	410	74	0.8	0.1	9	58	0.22	0	0.02	0.13	0	0.04	2	0.12
—	—	20	150	250	420	80	0.6	0	8	86	—	0	—	0.14	—	—	—	0.24
0.3	0	5	103	124	1	27	0.5	0.1	4	10	0.08	0	0	0.06	0	0.01	1	0.12
0.7	0.1	12	233	281	2	61	1.1	0.1	8	22	0.17	0	0.01	0.13	0	0.03	3	0.26
1.5	0.2	13	121	96	250	59	0.6	0.2	6	46	0.15	0	0.01	0.09	0	0.03	2	0.24
1.9	0.2	20	129	156	300	34	0.6	0.1	5	61	0.1	0	0.01	0.07	0	0.02	2	0.15
0.6	0.1	10	194	234	405	51	0.9	0.1	7	18	0.14	0	0.01	0.11	0	0.02	3	0.22
2.2	0.3	27	114	126	170	400	0.3	0.1	20	78	0.17	0	0.09	0.39	0.2	0.08	1	0.69
0	0	5	405	—	223	—	—	—	—	87	—	—	—	—	—	—	—	—
2	0.3	25	259	163	70	30	1	0	10	68	0.14	0	0.01	0.1	0	0.02	2	0.45
2.4	0.2	27	191	128	159	39	0.7	0.1	7	86	0.14	0	0	0.1	0	0.02	6	0.36
2.2	0.2	21	150	110	395	73	0.8	0.1	6	65	0.18	0	0.01	0.11	0.3	0.05	10	0.35
2.4	0.3	26	172	118	173	40	0.7	0.2	7	77	0.13	0	0.01	0.1	0.1	0.02	5	0.42
2.4	0.2	27	190	127	158	38	0.7	0.1	7	85	0.14	0	0	0.1	0	0.02	6	0.36
2.4	0.2	27	190	127	158	38	0.7	0.1	7	85	0.14	0	0	0.1	0	0.02	6	0.36
2.3	0.2	28	52	53	178	43	0.7	0.1	6	52	0.19	0	0.02	0.15	0.1	0.07	18	0.47
2	0.2	20	110	98	238	53	0.7	0.1	6	71	0.18	0	0.01	0.14	0.2	0.06	18	0.37
2	0.2	20	110	98	239	53	0.7	0.1	6	71	0.19	0	0.01	0.14	0.2	0.06	18	0.37
2.4	0.2	26	191	139	196	26	0.8	0.2	6	82	0.14	0	0.01	0.13	0.1	0.02	5	0.08
—	—	15	253	—	96	—	—	0.4	—	87	—	1	—	—	—	—	—	—
2.6	0.3	28	199	137	6	32	0.9	0.2	8	82	0.1	0	0.01	0.11	0	0.02	5	0.24
0.6	0.1	6	199	137	6	32	0.9	0.2	8	18	0.05	0	0.01	0.01	0	0.02	5	0.23
0	0	5	405	—	223	—	—	—	—	87	—	—	—	—	—	—	—	—
2.6	0.3	30	204	145	175	28	0.9	0.2	8	78	0.1	0	0.01	0.11	0	0.02	5	0.23
2.5	0.2	29	183	132	199	27	0.8	0.1	6	70	0.18	0	0.01	0.08	0	0.02	5	0.24
2.5	0.2	29	183	132	199	27	0.8	0.1	6	70	0.18	0	0.01	0.08	0	0.02	5	0.24
3.1	0.3	31	226	151	199	42	1	0.3	9	91	0.12	0	0	0.12	0	0.03	6	0.27
2.6	0.3	27	194	130	171	36	0.9	0.2	7	78	0.1	0	0	0.11	0	0.02	5	0.23
2.6	0.3	28	199	137	6	32	0.9	0.2	8	82	0.1	0	0.01	0.11	0	0.02	5	0.24
0.6	0.1	6	199	137	6	32	0.9	0.2	8	18	0.05	0	0.01	0.01	0	0.02	5	0.24
2.6	0.3	27	194	129	171	36	0.9	0.2	7	78	0.1	0	0	0.11	0	0.02	5	0.23
0.3	0	5	69	151	459	97	0.4	0.2	6	12	0.12	0	0.02	0.19	0.1	0.08	14	0.72
27.1	3.4	247	27	26	933	29	0.1	0.2	2	852	1.79	0	0.01	0.04	0	0	3	0.14
1.1	0.1	13	54	119	458	76	0.3	0.1	5	41	0.1	0	0.02	0.15	0.1	0.06	11	0.56
1.5	0.2	17	68	149	458	95	0.4	0.2	6	54	0.14	0	0.02	0.18	0.1	0.08	14	0.7
0.3	0	4	69	151	15	97	0.4	0.2	6	12	0.12	0	0.02	0.18	0.1	0.08	14	0.71
0	0	10	60	150	370	75	—	0	—	57	—	0	0	0.17	—	0.03	—	0.6
1.4	0.1	16	63	139	425	88	0.4	0.1	6	50	0.13	0	0.02	0.17	0.1	0.07	13	0.65
2.8	0.4	32	23	30	86	34	0.2	0.3	2	111	0.27	0	0	0.06	0	0.01	4	0.12
1.7	0.2	17	34	44	89	50	0.2	0.5	2	66	0.14	0	0.01	0.08	0	0.02	5	0.18
0	0	2	100	150	160	65	0.3	0	0	143	—	0	—	0.34	—	—	—	0.12
0	0	3	81	101	137	51	0.3	0	0	145	—	0	—	0.07	—	—	—	0.12
—	—	30	20	20	100	40	0	0	0	86	—	0	—	0.03	—	—	—	0
2.3	0.2	25	207	152	274	53	1.1	0.1	8	72	0.21	0	0.01	0.11	0	0.02	5	0.44
2.8	0.4	55	303	207	686	38	1.8	0.4	12	79	0.02	0	0.1	0.52	0.6	0.26	20	1.04
1.3	0.2	25	140	96	316	18	0.8	0.2	5	36	0.01	0	0.04	0.24	0.3	0.12	9	0.48
2.5	0.5	33	156	98	227	18	1	0.1	4	82	0.1	0	0.01	0.06	0	0.02	2	0.48
2.3	0.2	30	254	207	98	14	0.5	0.5	15	135	0.22	0	0.04	0.34	0.7	0.02	1	0.03
3	0.3	28	86	157	226	16	0.6	1.2	10	174	0.28	0	0.04	0.23	0.3	0.15	7	0.12

Food Item	Qty	Meas	Wgt (g)	Wtr (g)	Cals	Prot (g)	Carb (g)	Fib (g)	Fat (g)	SatF (g)
Cheese, goat, soft	1	oz.	28	17	76	5	0	0	6	4.1
Cheese, gouda	1	oz.	28	12	101	7	1	0	8	5
Cheese, gruyere	1	oz.	28	9	117	8	0	0	9	5.4
Cheese, havarti	1	oz.	28	12	105	7	1	0	8	5.3
Cheese, imitation mozzarella, shredded	0.25	cup	28	17	51	4	3	0	2	1.3
Cheese, light neufchatel (Kraft Philadelphia)	1	oz.	28	18	71	3	1	0	6	4
Cheese, limburger	1	oz.	28	14	93	6	0	0	8	4.7
Cheese, monterey jack, cubed	0.25	cup	33	14	123	8	0	0	10	6.3
Cheese, monterey jack, nonfat, Lifetime	1	oz.	28	18	40	8	1	0	0	0
Cheese, monterey jack, shredded	0.25	cup	28	12	105	7	0	0	9	5.4
Cheese, mozzarella nuggets, Banquet	8	piece	35	15	110	5	8	1	6	2.5
Cheese, mozzarella sting/stick	1	each	28	15	72	7	1	0	5	2.9
Cheese, mozzarella, low sodium	1	oz.	28	14	79	8	1	0	5	3.1
Cheese, mozzarella, low sodium string/stick	1	each	28	14	79	8	1	0	5	3.1
Cheese, mozzarella, lowfat, shredded	0.25	cup	28	14	79	8	1	0	5	3.1
Cheese, mozzarella, nonfat, Lifetime	1	oz.	28	18	40	8	1	0	0	0
Cheese, mozzarella, part skim, low moisture	0.25	cup	28	14	79	8	1	0	5	3.1
Cheese, mozzarella, part skim, shredded	0.25	cup	28	15	72	7	1	0	4	2.8
Cheese, mozzarella, whole milk, low moisture	0.25	cup	28	14	90	6	1	0	7	4.4
Cheese, mozzarella, whole milk, shredded	0.25	cup	28	15	79	5	1	0	6	3.7
Cheese, muenster	0.25	cup	28	12	104	7	0	0	8	5.4
Cheese, muenster, low sodium	1	oz.	28	12	104	7	0	0	9	5.4
Cheese, neufchatel	1	oz.	28	18	74	3	1	0	7	4.2
Cheese, parmesan, grated	1	Tbs	6	1	28	3	0	0	2	1.2
Cheese, parmesan, hard, cubed	1	each	10	3	40	4	0	0	3	1.7
Cheese, parmesan, low sodium, grated	0.25	cup	25	6	114	10	1	0	8	4.9
Cheese, parmesan, shredded	2	oz.	57	14	235	22	2	0	16	9.9
Cheese, pimento processed	1	oz.	28	11	106	6	0	0	9	5.6
Cheese, port du salut	1	oz.	28	13	100	7	0	0	8	4.7
Cheese, provolone	0.25	cup	33	14	116	8	1	0	9	5.6
Cheese, ricotta, part skim	1	oz.	28	21	39	3	1	0	2	1.4
Cheese, ricotta, whole milk	0.33	cup	82	59	143	9	2	0	11	6.8
Cheese, romano, grated	0.33	cup	33	10	128	10	1	0	9	5.6
Cheese, roquefort, crumbled	0.25	cup	34	13	125	7	1	0	10	6.5
Cheese, roquefort, cubed	1	each	17	7	64	4	0	0	5	3.3
Cheese, roquefort, cubed	1	oz.	28	11	105	6	1	0	9	5.5
Cheese, sharp cheddar, nonfat, Lifetime	1	oz.	28	18	40	8	1	0	0	0
Cheese, swiss	1	oz.	28	10	107	8	1	0	8	5
Cheese, swiss, low fat, Alpine Lace	1	oz.	28	12	91	8	1	0	6	4
Cheese, swiss, low sodium	1	oz.	28	11	107	8	1	0	8	5
Cheese, swiss, nonfat, Lifetime	1	oz.	28	18	40	8	1	0	0	0
Cheese, swiss, shredded	0.25	cup	27	10	102	8	1	0	7	4.8
Cheese, tilsit, whole milk	1	oz.	28	12	96	7	1	0	7	4.8
Cheese, white, fat free, Apine Lace	1	oz.	28	18	25	5	1	0	0	0
Cheese, yogurt	1	oz.	28	21	22	2	3	0	0	0
Cherimoya, raw	1	each	547	402	514	7	131	13.1	2	—
Cherries, ground, raw	0.5	cup	70	60	37	1	8	1.9	0	—
Cherries, maraschino	0.5	cup	80	56	93	0	24	—	0	0
Cherries, sour, canned in extra heavy syrup	0.5	cup	130	91	149	1	38	1	0	0
Cherries, sour, canned in water	0.5	cup	122	110	44	1	11	1.3	0	0
Cherries, sour, frozen, unsweetened	0.5	cup	78	68	36	1	9	1.2	0	0.1
Cherries, sour, red, fresh, pitted	0.5	cup	78	67	39	1	9	1.2	0	0.1
Cherries, sweet, canned in heavy syrup	0.5	cup	128	100	107	1	27	1.9	0	0
Cherries, sweet, canned in juice	0.5	cup	125	106	68	1	17	1.9	0	0
Cherries, sweet, fresh	10	each	68	55	49	1	11	1.6	1	0.1
Cherries, sweet, fresh, cup measure	0.5	cup	72	59	52	1	12	1.7	1	0.2
Cherries, sweet, frozen, sweetened	0.5	cup	130	98	115	1	29	2.7	0	0
Cherry crisp	1	cup	246	97	710	5	112	2.3	28	6.2
Cherry crisp, piece, 3x3 in	1	piece	138	106	146	2	24	1.3	5	0.9
Cherry turnover	1	each	78	32	238	3	31	0.9	12	2.9
Chervil, dried	0.25	tsp	0	0	0	0	0	0	0	0
Chestnuts, Chinese, cooked	1	oz.	28	18	43	1	10	0.3	0	0
Chestnuts, Chinese, dried	1	oz.	28	3	103	2	23	0.6	1	0.1
Chestnuts, Chinese, raw	1	oz.	28	12	64	1	14	0.4	0	0
Chestnuts, Chinese, roasted	1	oz.	28	11	68	1	15	0.4	0	0

MonoF	PolyF	Choles	Calc	Phos	Sod	Pot	Zn	Iron	Magn	VitA	VitE	VitC	Thia	Ribo	Nia	B6	Fola	B12
(g)	(g)	(mg)	(mg)	(mg)	(mg)	(mg)	(mg)	(mg)	(mg)	(μg RE)	(mg α-TE)	(mg)	(mg)	(mg)	(mg)	(mg)	(μg)	(μg)
1.4	0.1	13	40	73	104	7	0.3	0.5	5	80	0.13	0	0.02	0.11	0.1	0.07	3	0.05
2.2	0.2	32	198	155	232	34	1.1	0.1	8	49	0.1	0	0.01	0.1	0	0.02	6	0.44
2.8	0.5	31	287	172	95	23	1.1	0	10	85	0.1	0	0.02	0.08	0	0.02	3	0.45
2.4	0.2	27	191	128	159	39	0.7	0.1	7	86	0.14	0	0	0.1	0	0.02	6	0.36
0.6	0.1	5	161	206	324	65	0.7	0	8	23	0.05	0	0.01	0.11	0.1	0.04	1	0.13
—	—	20	20	40	122	30	0	0	0	58	—	0	—	0.03	—	—	—	0
2.4	0.1	26	141	111	227	36	0.6	0	6	90	0.18	0	0.02	0.14	0	0.02	16	0.3
2.9	0.3	29	246	147	177	27	1	0.2	9	84	0.11	0	0	0.13	0	0.03	6	0.27
0	0	5	405	—	223	—	—	—	—	87	—	—	—	—	—	—	—	—
2.5	0.3	25	211	125	151	23	0.8	0.2	8	72	0.1	0	0	0.11	0	0.02	5	0.23
—	—	10	100	290	200	60	—	0.4	—	0	—	0	0.06	0.1	0.2	—	—	—
1.3	0.1	16	183	131	132	24	0.8	0.1	7	50	0.12	0	0	0.09	0	0.02	2	0.23
1.4	0.1	15	207	149	5	27	0.9	0.1	7	54	0.13	0	0.01	0.1	0	0.02	3	0.26
1.4	0.1	15	207	149	5	27	0.9	0.1	7	54	0.13	0	0.01	0.1	0	0.02	3	0.26
1.4	0.1	15	207	148	149	27	0.9	0.1	7	54	0.13	0	0.01	0.1	0	0.02	3	0.26
0	0	5	405	—	223	—	—	—	—	87	—	—	—	—	—	—	—	—
1.4	0.1	15	207	148	149	27	0.9	0.1	7	54	0.13	0	0.01	0.1	0	0.02	3	0.26
1.3	0.1	16	182	131	132	24	0.8	0.1	7	50	0.12	0	0	0.09	0	0.02	2	0.23
2	0.2	25	162	116	117	21	0.7	0.1	6	77	0.19	0	0	0.08	0	0.02	2	0.2
1.9	0.2	22	146	105	105	19	0.6	0.1	5	68	0.1	0	0	0.07	0	0.02	2	0.18
2.5	0.2	27	203	132	177	38	0.8	0.1	8	89	0.13	0	0	0.09	0	0.02	3	0.42
2.5	0.2	27	203	133	5	38	0.8	0.1	8	90	0.13	0	0	0.09	0	0.02	3	0.42
1.9	0.2	22	21	39	113	32	0.1	0.1	2	85	0.27	0	0	0.06	0	0.01	3	0.08
0.5	0	5	86	50	116	7	0.2	0.1	3	11	0.05	0	0	0.02	0	0.01	0	0.09
0.8	0.1	7	122	72	165	10	0.3	0.1	4	15	0.08	0	0	0.03	0	0.01	1	0.12
2.2	0.2	20	344	202	16	27	0.8	0.2	13	43	0.2	0	0.01	0.1	0.1	0.02	2	0.35
5	0.4	41	710	417	962	55	1.8	0.5	29	98	0.48	0	0.02	0.2	0.2	0.06	5	0.79
2.5	0.3	27	174	211	405	46	0.8	0.1	6	91	0.13	1	0.01	0.1	0	0.02	2	0.2
2.6	0.2	35	184	102	151	39	0.7	0.1	7	105	0.14	0	0	0.07	0	0.02	5	0.42
2.4	0.3	23	249	164	289	46	1.1	0.2	9	87	0.12	0	0.01	0.11	0.1	0.02	3	0.48
0.7	0.1	9	77	52	35	35	0.4	0.1	4	32	0.06	0	0.01	0.05	0	0.01	4	0.08
3	0.3	42	170	130	69	86	1	0.3	9	110	0.29	0	0.01	0.16	0.1	0.04	10	0.28
2.6	0.2	34	351	251	396	28	0.9	0.3	14	46	0.24	0	0.01	0.12	0	0.03	2	0.37
2.9	0.4	30	223	132	611	31	0.7	0.2	10	101	0.26	0	0.01	0.2	0.2	0.04	16	0.22
1.5	0.2	16	115	68	313	16	0.4	0.1	5	52	0.13	0	0.01	0.1	0.1	0.02	8	0.11
2.4	0.4	26	188	111	513	26	0.6	0.2	8	85	0.22	0	0.01	0.17	0.2	0.04	14	0.18
0	0	5	405	—	223	—	—	—	—	87	—	—	—	—	—	—	—	—
2.1	0.3	26	272	172	74	32	1.1	0	10	72	0.14	0	0.01	0.1	0	0.02	2	0.48
—	—	20	253	—	35	—	—	0.4	—	87	—	1	—	—	—	—	—	—
2.1	0.3	26	272	172	4	32	1.1	0	10	72	0.14	0	0.01	0.1	0	0.02	2	0.48
0	0	5	405	—	223	—	—	—	—	87	—	—	—	—	—	—	—	—
2	0.3	25	259	163	70	30	1	0	10	68	0.14	0	0.01	0.1	0	0.02	2	0.45
2	0.2	29	198	142	213	18	1	0.1	4	82	0.2	0	0.02	0.1	0.1	0.02	6	0.6
0	0	5	150	—	420	—	—	0.4	—	57	—	1	—	—	—	—	—	—
0	0	1	56	44	22	72	0.3	0	5	1	0	0	0.01	0.06	0	0.01	3	0.17
—	—	0	126	219	16	—	—	2.7	—	5	—	49	0.55	0.6	7.1	—	—	0
—	—	0	6	28	1	191	—	0.7	—	50	0.31	8	0.08	0.03	2	—	—	0
0	0	0	12	10	1	101	—	0.2	—	0	0.1	0	0	0	0	—	—	0
0	0	0	13	12	9	119	0.1	1.6	7	91	0.16	2	0.02	0.05	0.2	0.06	10	0
0	0	0	13	12	9	120	0.1	1.7	7	92	0.16	3	0.02	0.05	0.2	0.05	10	0
0.1	0.1	0	10	12	1	96	0.1	0.4	7	67	0.1	1	0.03	0.03	0.1	0.05	3	0
0.1	0.1	0	12	12	2	134	0.1	0.2	7	99	0.1	8	0.02	0.03	0.3	0.03	6	0
0.1	0.1	0	12	23	4	186	0.1	0.4	12	19	0.08	5	0.03	0.05	0.5	0.04	5	0
0	0	0	18	28	4	164	0.1	0.7	15	16	0.12	3	0.02	0.03	0.5	0.04	5	0
0.2	0.2	0	10	13	0	152	0	0.3	7	14	0.09	5	0.03	0.04	0.3	0.02	3	0
0.2	0.2	0	11	14	0	162	0	0.3	8	15	0.09	5	0.04	0.04	0.3	0.03	3	0
0	0.1	0	16	21	1	258	0.1	0.5	13	25	0.17	1	0.04	0.06	0.2	0.05	5	0
13.2	7.3	0	157	284	592	223	0.3	3.7	20	305	5.26	3	0.27	0.27	2.2	0.09	16	0.02
2.5	1.8	0	26	23	74	154	0.2	2.1	11	150	0.93	3	0.06	0.08	0.6	0.06	11	0.01
5.1	3.1	0	8	28	212	58	0.2	1.6	7	27	1.09	1	0.14	0.11	1.2	0.02	6	0
0	0	0	2	1	0	8	0	0.1	0	1	0	0	0	0	0	0	0	0
0.1	0.1	0	3	19	1	87	0.2	0.3	16	4	0.11	7	0.03	0.04	0.2	0.08	13	0
0.3	0.1	0	8	44	1	206	0.4	0.6	39	9	0.26	17	0.07	0.08	0.4	0.19	31	0
0.2	0.1	0	5	27	1	127	0.2	0.4	24	6	0.17	10	0.04	0.05	0.2	0.12	19	0
0.2	0.1	0	5	29	1	135	0.3	0.4	26	0	0.17	11	0.04	0.03	0.4	0.12	20	0

Food Item	Qty	Meas	Wgt (g)	Wtr (g)	Cals	Prot (g)	Carb (g)	Fib (g)	Fat (g)	SatF (g)
Chestnuts, European, cooked	1	oz.	28	19	37	1	8	1.4	0	0.1
Chestnuts, European, raw, peeled	1	oz.	28	15	56	0	12	2.2	0	0.1
Chestnuts, European, roasted, cup measure	0.25	cup	36	14	88	1	19	1.8	1	0.1
Chestnuts, European, roasted, whole	17	each	143	58	350	5	76	7.3	3	0.6
Chewing gum, Care Free sugarless	1	piece	2	—	5	0	2	—	0	0
Chex party mix	1	oz.	28	1	120	3	18	1.6	5	1.5
Chia seeds, dried	1	oz.	28	2	134	5	14	7.2	7	3
Chicken & dumplings, Chicken Helper	0.5	cup	122	87	187	13	10	0.3	10	2.9
Chicken & noodles, recipe	1	cup	240	171	367	22	26	1.8	18	5.9
Chicken hearts, simmered	1	each	3	2	6	1	0	0	0	0.1
Chicken nuggets, fast food serving	1	each	102	52	276	17	15	0	16	3.5
Chicken parmigiana	1	piece	182	120	317	28	15	1.4	16	5.4
Chicken patty, breaded, cooked	1	each	75	37	213	12	11	0.3	13	4.1
Chicken pot pie, Banquet	1	each	198	133	350	10	36	3	18	7
Chicken salad, w/celery	0.5	cup	78	41	268	11	1	0.2	25	3.1
Chicken teriyaki, breast	1	each	128	85	176	26	7	0.2	4	0.9
Chicken teriyaki, drumstick	1	each	68	45	93	14	4	0.1	2	0.5
Chicken, back, skinless, fried	0.5	each	58	28	167	17	3	0	9	2.4
Chicken, back, skinless, roasted	0.5	each	40	24	96	11	0	0	5	1.4
Chicken, back, w/skin, flour fried	1	each	72	32	238	20	5	0.1	15	4
Chicken, back, w/skin, roasted	1	each	53	28	159	14	0	0	11	3.1
Chicken, boned, w/broth, can	1	each	142	98	234	31	0	0	11	3.1
Chicken, breast meat, skinless, stewed	1	each	95	65	143	28	0	0	3	0.8
Chicken, breast w/skin, roasted	1	each	98	61	193	29	0	0	8	2.2
Chicken, breast, skinless, fried	1	each	86	52	161	29	0	0	4	1.1
Chicken, breast, skinless, roasted	1	each	86	56	142	27	0	0	3	0.9
Chicken, breast, w/skin, flour fried	1	each	98	56	218	31	2	0.1	9	2.4
Chicken, breast, w/skin, stewed	1	each	110	73	202	30	0	0	8	2.3
Chicken, canned in water, Swanson	0.5	cup	124	94	131	24	2	0	2	1.1
Chicken, canned, diced, dark meat	0.5	cup	102	70	169	22	0	0	8	2.3
Chicken, canned, diced, light & dark meat	0.5	cup	102	70	169	22	0	0	8	2.3
Chicken, canned, diced, light meat	0.5	cup	102	70	169	22	0	0	8	2.3
Chicken, dark meat, skinless, fried	4	oz.	113	63	271	33	3	0	13	3.5
Chicken, dark meat, skinless, roasted	4	oz.	113	72	232	31	0	0	11	3
Chicken, drumstick, batter fried	1	each	72	38	193	16	6	0.2	11	3
Chicken, drumstick, flour fried	1	each	49	28	120	13	1	0	7	1.8
Chicken, drumstick, roasted	1	each	52	33	112	14	0	0	6	1.6
Chicken, drumstick, skinless, fried	1	each	42	26	82	12	0	0	3	0.9
Chicken, drumstick, skinless, roasted	1	each	44	29	76	12	0	0	2	0.7
Chicken, fried, dark meat, 2 piece serving	1	each	148	72	431	30	16	0.9	27	7
Chicken, fried, white meat, 2 piece serving	1	each	163	74	494	36	20	1.1	30	7.8
Chicken, gizzard, simmered	1	each	22	15	34	6	0	0	1	0.2
Chicken, light meat, skinless, fried	4	oz.	113	68	218	37	0	0	6	1.7
Chicken, light meat, skinless, roasted	4	oz.	113	74	196	35	0	0	5	1.4
Chicken, liver pate, canned	0.5	cup	104	68	209	14	7	0.2	14	4.2
Chicken, liver, simmered	7	each	140	96	220	34	1	0	8	2.6
Chicken, meat, all types, skinless, fried	4	oz.	113	65	248	35	2	0.1	10	2.8
Chicken, meat, all types, skinless, roasted	4	oz.	113	72	215	33	0	0	8	2.3
Chicken, meat, all types, skinless, stewed	0.5	cup	70	47	124	19	0	0	5	1.3
Chicken, roaster, skinless, roasted	4	oz.	113	76	189	28	0	0	8	2
Chicken, skinless, stewed	0.5	cup	70	40	166	21	0	0	8	2.2
Chicken, stewer w/giblets, cooked	1	each	593	322	1636	157	0	0	107	29.1
Chicken, thigh, skinless, fried	1	each	52	31	113	15	1	0	5	1.4
Chicken, thigh, skinless, roasted	1	each	52	33	109	14	0	0	6	1.6
Chicken, thigh, w/skin, flour fried	1	each	62	34	162	17	2	0.1	9	2.5
Chicken, thigh, w/skin, roasted	1	each	62	37	153	16	0	0	10	2.7
Chicken, whole, roasted	1	each	598	356	1429	163	0	0	81	22.7
Chicken, whole, stewed	1	each	668	427	1462	165	0	0	84	23.4
Chicken, wing, flour fried	1	each	32	16	103	8	1	0	7	1.9
Chicken, wing, skinless, fried	1	each	20	12	42	6	0	0	2	0.5
Chicken, wing, skinless, roasted	1	each	21	13	43	6	0	0	2	0.5
Chicken, wing, w/skin, roasted	3	each	102	56	296	27	0	0	20	5.6
Chicken, wings, buffalo type/spicy	1	piece	16	8	49	4	0	0	3	0.9
Chile, banana, cooked	4	oz.	113	101	17	1	4	1.8	0	—
Chile, banana, raw	0.5	cup	75	68	10	1	3	1	0	—

MonoF (g)	PolyF (g)	Choles (mg)	Calc (mg)	Phos (mg)	Sod (mg)	Pot (mg)	Zn (mg)	Iron (mg)	Magn (mg)	VitA (µg RE)	VitE (mg α-TE)	VitC (mg)	Thia (mg)	Ribo (mg)	Nia (mg)	B6 (mg)	Fola (µg)	B12 (µg)
0.1	0.2	0	13	28	8	203	0.1	0.5	15	1	0.2	8	0.04	0.03	0.2	0.07	11	0
0.1	0.1	0	5	11	1	137	0.1	0.3	9	1	0.2	11	0.04	0	0.3	0.1	16	0
0.3	0.3	0	10	38	1	212	0.2	0.3	12	1	0.43	9	0.09	0.06	0.5	0.18	25	0
1.1	1.2	0	42	153	3	847	0.8	1.3	47	3	1.72	37	0.35	0.25	1.9	0.71	100	0
0	0	—	—	—	0	0	—	—	—	—	—	—	—	—	—	—	—	—
2.6	0.7	0	10	53	288	76	0.6	7	18	4	0.07	14	0.44	0.14	4.8	0.44	0	3.52
2.1	2.1	0	150	171	11	292	1.5	2.8	22	1	—	4	0.25	0.05	1.6	0.2	32	0
4	2.2	47	55	125	503	151	1	1.1	17	24	0.37	1	0.11	0.15	4.8	0.15	5	0.16
7.1	3.5	96	26	247	600	149	1.5	2.2	26	10	—	0	0.05	0.17	4.3	0.19	10	0.25
0.1	0.1	8	1	7	2	4	0.2	0.3	1	0	0.05	0	0	0.02	0.1	0.01	3	0.24
7.1	3.4	59	13	278	494	294	1	0.9	24	0	1.35	0	0.11	0.15	7.2	0.3	30	0.3
4.4	4.3	138	189	317	767	463	2.3	2.1	44	146	1.84	9	0.15	0.33	8.2	0.36	18	0.43
6.4	1.6	45	12	150	399	185	0.8	0.9	15	22	1.46	0	0.07	0.1	5	0.23	8	0.22
—	—	40	20	—	950	—	—	1.1	—	200	—	0	—	—	—	—	—	—
4.5	15.8	48	16	80	201	138	0.8	0.6	11	31	6.27	1	0.03	0.07	3.3	0.34	8	0.19
1	0.9	80	27	199	1866	309	1.9	1.8	36	16	0.35	3	0.08	0.2	8.7	0.46	13	0.28
0.6	0.5	43	14	105	991	164	1	0.9	19	8	0.18	2	0.04	0.1	4.6	0.24	7	0.15
3.3	2.1	54	15	102	57	146	1.6	1	14	17	0.34	0	0.06	0.15	4.4	0.2	5	0.18
1.9	1.2	36	10	66	38	95	1.1	0.6	9	11	0.11	0	0.03	0.09	2.8	0.14	3	0.12
5.9	3.5	64	17	120	65	163	1.8	1.2	17	27	0.6	0	0.08	0.17	5.3	0.22	11	0.2
4.4	2.4	47	11	82	46	111	1.2	0.8	11	52	0.14	0	0.03	0.1	3.6	0.14	3	0.14
4.5	2.5	88	20	158	714	196	2	2.2	17	48	0.3	3	0.02	0.18	9	0.5	6	0.41
1	0.6	73	12	157	60	178	0.9	0.8	23	6	0.25	0	0.04	0.11	8	0.31	3	0.22
3	1.6	82	14	210	70	240	1	1	26	26	0.26	0	0.06	0.12	12.4	0.55	4	0.31
1.5	0.9	78	14	212	68	237	0.9	1	27	6	0.36	0	0.07	0.11	12.7	0.55	3	0.32
1.1	0.7	73	13	196	64	220	0.9	0.9	25	5	0.23	0	0.06	0.1	11.8	0.52	3	0.29
3.4	1.9	87	16	228	74	254	1.1	1.2	29	15	0.56	0	0.08	0.13	13.4	0.57	6	0.33
3.2	1.7	82	14	172	68	196	1.1	1	24	26	0.29	0	0.04	0.13	8.6	0.32	3	0.23
—	—	54	0	—	500	—	—	0	—	0	—	0	—	—	—	—	—	—
3.2	1.8	64	14	114	516	141	1.4	1.6	12	35	0.22	2	0.02	0.13	6.5	0.36	4	0.3
3.2	1.8	64	14	114	516	141	1.4	1.6	12	35	0.22	2	0.02	0.13	6.5	0.36	4	0.3
3.2	1.8	64	14	114	516	141	1.4	1.6	12	35	0.22	2	0.02	0.13	6.5	0.36	4	0.3
4.9	3.1	109	20	212	110	287	3.3	1.7	28	27	0.66	0	0.1	0.28	8	0.42	10	0.37
4	2.6	105	17	203	105	272	3.2	1.5	26	25	0.3	0	0.08	0.26	7.4	0.41	9	0.36
4.6	2.7	62	12	106	194	134	1.7	1	14	19	0.88	0	0.08	0.16	3.7	0.19	13	0.2
2.7	1.6	44	6	86	44	112	1.4	0.7	11	12	0.41	0	0.04	0.11	3	0.17	5	0.16
2.2	1.3	47	6	91	47	119	1.5	0.7	12	16	0.14	0	0.04	0.11	3.1	0.18	4	0.17
1.2	0.8	40	5	78	40	105	1.4	0.6	10	8	0.21	0	0.03	0.1	2.6	0.16	4	0.15
0.8	0.6	41	5	81	42	108	1.4	0.6	11	8	0.12	0	0.03	0.1	2.7	0.17	4	0.15
10.9	6.3	166	36	240	755	445	3.2	1.6	37	67	1.33	0	0.13	0.43	7.2	0.33	25	0.83
12.2	6.8	148	60	306	975	566	1.6	1.5	38	59	1.52	0	0.15	0.29	12	0.57	29	0.67
0.2	0.2	43	2	34	15	39	1	0.9	4	12	0.26	0	0.01	0.05	0.9	0.03	12	0.43
2.2	1.4	102	18	262	92	298	1.4	1.3	33	10	0.34	0	0.08	0.14	15.2	0.71	5	0.41
1.8	1.1	96	17	245	87	280	1.4	1.2	31	10	0.3	0	0.07	0.13	14.1	0.68	5	0.39
5.5	2.6	407	10	182	401	99	2.2	9.6	14	226	1.02	10	0.05	1.46	7.8	0.27	334	8.4
1.9	1.3	883	20	437	71	196	6.1	11.9	29	6878	2.02	22	0.21	2.45	6.2	0.81	1078	27.2
3.8	2.4	107	19	232	103	291	2.5	1.5	31	20	0.52	0	0.1	0.22	11	0.54	8	0.39
3	1.9	101	17	221	98	276	2.4	1.4	28	18	0.3	0	0.08	0.2	10.4	0.53	7	0.37
1.7	1.1	58	10	105	49	126	1.4	0.8	15	10	0.19	0	0.03	0.11	4.3	0.18	4	0.15
2.8	1.7	85	14	218	85	260	1.7	1.4	24	14	0.47	0	0.07	0.17	8.9	0.46	6	0.33
2.8	2	58	9	143	55	141	1.4	1	15	23	0.21	0	0.08	0.19	4.5	0.22	4	0.18
40.5	23.8	605	77	1079	421	1049	12	10.9	119	1630	2.09	3	0.55	1.8	33.4	1.54	213	5.93
2	1.3	53	7	103	49	135	1.4	0.8	14	11	0.3	0	0.05	0.13	3.7	0.2	5	0.17
2.2	1.3	49	6	95	46	124	1.3	0.7	12	10	0.14	0	0.04	0.12	3.4	0.18	4	0.16
3.6	2.1	60	9	116	55	147	1.6	0.9	16	18	0.52	0	0.06	0.15	4.3	0.2	7	0.19
3.8	2.1	58	7	108	52	138	1.5	0.8	14	30	0.16	0	0.04	0.13	4	0.19	4	0.18
31.9	17.8	526	90	1088	490	1333	11.6	7.5	138	281	1.58	0	0.38	1	50.8	2.39	30	1.79
32.9	18.3	521	87	929	448	1108	11.8	7.8	127	281	1.77	0	0.31	0.99	37.3	1.47	33	1.34
2.8	1.6	26	5	48	25	57	0.6	0.4	6	12	0.18	0	0.02	0.04	2.1	0.13	2	0.09
0.6	0.4	17	3	33	18	42	0.4	0.2	4	4	0.06	0	0.01	0.03	1.4	0.12	1	0.07
0.5	0.4	18	3	35	19	44	0.4	0.2	4	4	0.06	0	0.01	0.03	1.5	0.12	1	0.07
7.8	4.2	86	15	154	84	188	1.9	1.3	19	48	0.27	0	0.04	0.13	6.8	0.43	3	0.3
1.4	0.8	13	2	24	30	29	0.3	0.2	3	9	0.12	0	0.01	0.02	1	0.07	0	0.04
—	—	0	23	—	5	255	0.5	0.5	19	10	—	136	0.06	0.04	0.7	—	—	0
—	—	0	16	—	3	188	0.3	0.3	14	8	—	113	0.04	0.03	0.5	—	—	0

Food Item	Qty	Meas	Wgt (g)	Wtr (g)	Cals	Prot (g)	Carb (g)	Fib (g)	Fat (g)	SatF (g)
Chiles rellenos	1	each	143	75	425	23	7	1	35	17
Chili & beans, canned	1	cups	255	193	286	15	30	11.2	14	6
Chili pepper, dried, Foran Spice	0.5	gram	0	0	2	0	0	0.1	0	—
Chili powder	1	Tbs	8	1	24	1	4	2.6	1	0.2
Chilies, green, canned, Santiago	1	each	62	58	13	0	3	0.7	0	0
Chilies, green, whole, Old El Paso	1	each	35	33	10	0	2	1	0	0
Chimichanga, beef	1	each	174	88	425	20	43	2	20	8.5
Chimichanga, beef & bean	1	each	118	68	249	11	26	3.1	12	3.4
Chives, freeze dried	0.25	cup	1	0	2	0	1	0.2	0	0
Chives, fresh	1	Tbs	3	3	1	0	0	0.1	0	0
Chocolate brownie, Weight Watchers	1	each	182	136	190	6	35	4	4	1
Chocolate chips, milk chocolate	0.25	cup	42	1	218	3	25	1.4	13	7.9
Chocolate chips, semi-sweet	0.25	cup	42	0	204	2	27	2.5	13	7.6
Chocolate drink (syrup w/whole milk)	1	cup	250	203	205	8	30	0.5	8	4.7
Chocolate drink, syrup w/lowfat milk	1	cup	250	206	181	8	30	0.6	4	2.8
Chocolate drink, syrup w/skim milk	1	cup	250	209	149	8	30	0.6	1	0.4
Chocolate fudge shake, Weight Watchers	1	cup	250	206	158	10	30	4.8	2	0
Chocolate morsels, milk chocolate, Toll House	0.25	cup	42	1	213	0	27	0	14	7.6
Chocolate morsels, semi-sweet, Toll House	0.25	cup	42	2	213	0	27	0.1	12	6
Chocolate morsels, semi-sweet, Toll House mini	0.25	cup	42	2	213	0	27	0.1	12	6
Chocolate, baking, unsweetened, grated	0.25	cup	33	0	172	3	9	5.1	18	10.8
Chocolate, baking, unsweetened, square	1	each	28	0	148	3	8	4.4	16	9.2
Chocolate, bittersweet, square	1	each	28	1	135	2	13	0.9	11	6.3
Chow mein entree, chicken, Chun King	1	each	369	292	370	16	45	4	14	5
Chow mein, chicken, canned	1	cup	250	222	95	6	18	2	1	0
Chow mein, pork, no noodles	0.5	cup	110	83	144	11	6	1.2	8	2.2
Chowder, Manhattan clam, chunky, RTS	0.5	cup	120	103	67	4	9	1.4	2	1.1
Chowder, Manhattan clam, chunky, RTS, can	1	each	539	464	302	16	42	6.5	8	4.7
Chowder, Manhattan clam, w/water	0.5	cup	122	112	39	1	6	0.7	1	0.2
Chowder, New England clam, w/milk	0.5	cup	124	106	82	5	8	0.7	3	1.5
Chowder, New England clam, w/water	0.5	cup	122	110	48	2	6	0.7	1	0.2
Chowder, fish/seafood	0.5	cup	122	100	98	12	6	0.3	3	1.5
Chutney	1	Tbs	17	10	26	0	7	0.4	0	0
Cinnamon	0.25	tsp	1	0	1	0	0	0.3	0	0
Citron, candied, chopped	2	Tbs	28	5	89	0	23	0.4	0	0
Citrus drink, concentrate, frozen, prepared	1	cup	252	221	116	1	29	0	0	0
Citrus fruit juice drink, frozen concentrate	0.5	cup	141	81	228	2	57	0.1	0	0
Citrus juice drink, Citrus Hill	1	cup	240	210	112	1	28	0.1	0	0
Clam nectar, canned	1	cup	240	234	5	1	0	0	0	0
Clam patty	1	each	120	33	429	24	40	1.2	18	4.4
Clam, baked/broiled, small	15	each	150	108	209	22	5	0	10	1.9
Cloves, ground	0.25	tsp	1	0	2	0	0	0.2	0	0
Cobbler, apple, piece, 3 x 3	1	piece	104	59	199	2	35	2.1	6	1.2
Cobbler, berry	1	cup	217	103	506	6	92	3.8	14	3.7
Cobbler, cherry	1	cup	217	120	430	5	78	2	12	3.1
Cobbler, cherry, piece, 3 x 3	1	piece	129	85	198	2	34	1.2	6	1.2
Cobbler, peach, piece, 3x3 in	1	piece	130	84	204	2	36	1.7	6	1.2
Cobbler, plum	1	cup	217	115	446	5	84	3	11	2.9
Cobbler, rhubarb	1	cup	217	93	548	5	102	2.9	15	3.6
Cocoa mix, prep w/water, sugar free	1	cup	250	231	62	5	11	0.5	0	0.3
Cocoa mix, w/water (fortified)	1	cup	279	237	159	3	32	1.1	4	2.4
Cocoa powder unsweetened, European	1	Tbs	5	0	21	1	3	1.6	0	0.3
Cocoa powder w/lowfat milk added	1	cup	250	205	186	8	30	1.2	5	3.1
Cocoa powder w/skim milk added	1	cup	250	208	152	8	30	1.2	1	0.6
Cocoa powder, dutch processed, unsweetened	1	Tbs	5	0	12	1	3	1.6	1	0.4
Cocoa powder, unsweetened	1	Tbs	5	0	12	1	3	1.8	1	0.4
Cocoa, baking type	1	oz.	28	1	85	6	16	11.3	3	0
Cocoa, dry, low fat	1	oz.	28	1	53	6	16	—	2	1.1
Cocoa, sugar free w/lowfat milk (Swiss Miss)	1	cup	250	218	136	9	14	1.5	6	3.3
Coconut cream, canned	0.5	cup	148	105	284	4	12	3.3	26	23.2
Coconut milk, raw	1	cup	240	162	552	6	13	5.3	57	50.6
Coconut water, raw	1	cup	240	228	46	2	9	2.6	0	0.4
Coconut, dried, sweetened, shredded	0.25	cup	23	3	116	1	11	1	8	7.3
Coconut, dried, toasted	1	oz.	28	0	168	2	13	1.8	13	11.8
Coconut, dried, unsweetened	0.25	cup	20	1	129	1	5	3.2	13	11.2

A

MonoF	PolyF	Choles	Calc	Phos	Sod	Pot	Zn	Iron	Magn	VitA	VitE	VitC	Thia	Ribo	Nia	B6	Fola	B12
(g)	(g)	(mg)	(mg)	(mg)	(mg)	(mg)	(mg)	(mg)	(mg)	(μg RE)	(mg α-TE)	(mg)	(mg)	(mg)	(mg)	(mg)	(μg)	(μg)
10.2	5.4	165	595	409	620	337	2.8	1.6	39	641	1.84	88	0.07	0.46	0.8	0.22	29	0.54
5.9	0.9	43	120	393	1331	931	5.1	8.8	115	87	1.87	4	0.12	0.27	0.9	0.34	58	0
—	—	0	0	2	0	10	—	0	—	26	—	0	0	0.01	0.1	—	—	0
0.3	0.6	0	21	23	76	144	0.2	1.1	13	262	0.08	5	0.03	0.06	0.6	0.14	8	0
0	0.1	0	39	9	122	77	—	0.8	—	35	—	23	0.01	0.01	0.3	0.3	—	0
0	0	0	0	—	230	—	—	—	—	20	—	9	—	—	—	—	—	0
8.1	1.1	9	63	124	910	586	5	4.5	63	16	—	5	0.49	0.64	5.8	0.28	84	1.51
4.9	2.3	24	46	132	242	386	1.8	2.6	34	40	1.73	9	0.2	0.17	2.8	0.18	55	0.69
0	0	0	6	4	1	24	0	0.2	5	55	0.02	5	0.01	0.01	0	0.02	1	0
0	0	0	3	2	0	9	0	0	1	13	0.01	2	0	0	0	0	3	0
2	1	5	80	—	160	230	—	1.1	—	0	—	0	0.06	0.03	0.2	0.03	—	—
4.2	0.5	9	81	92	35	164	0.6	0.6	26	23	0.53	0	0.03	0.13	0.1	0.02	3	0.17
4.2	0.4	0	14	56	5	155	0.7	1.3	49	1	0.51	0	0.02	0.04	0.2	0.02	1	0
2.2	0.3	30	263	245	138	403	1.1	0.8	50	68	0.2	2	0.08	0.37	0.3	0.09	12	0.78
1.3	0.2	16	268	249	140	410	1.1	0.8	52	124	0.16	2	0.09	0.38	0.3	0.1	12	0.79
0.2	0	4	272	262	144	434	1.1	0.8	46	133	0.1	2	0.08	0.32	0.3	0.09	13	0.82
2.2	0.2	5	396	278	175	443	4.3	5	110	277	5.53	16	0.43	0.48	5.5	0.55	110	1.65
—	—	9	0	—	0	123	—	0	—	0	—	0	0.03	0.08	0.1	—	—	—
—	—	0	0	67	0	136	—	0	—	0	—	0	0.03	—	0.2	—	—	—
4.4	0.5	0	0	67	0	136	—	0	—	0	—	0	0.03	—	0.2	—	—	—
6.1	0.6	0	24	138	5	275	1.3	2.1	102	3	0.41	0	0.03	0.06	0.4	0.03	2	0
5.2	0.5	0	21	118	4	236	1.1	1.8	88	3	0.35	0	0.02	0.05	0.3	0.03	2	0
4.2	0.2	0	16	80	1	174	1.1	1.4	28	3	0.35	0	0.01	0.05	0.3	0.01	3	0
—	—	45	40	200	2010	260	—	1.4	—	100	—	9	1.5	0.17	3	—	—	—
0.1	0.8	8	45	85	725	418	1.3	1.2	14	28	0.05	12	0.05	0.1	1	0.09	12	0.05
3.7	1.9	28	24	113	385	264	1.2	0.9	20	77	1.07	12	0.32	0.17	2.4	0.22	20	0.24
0.5	0.1	7	34	42	500	192	0.8	1.3	10	164	0.05	6	0.03	0.03	0.9	0.13	5	3.96
2.2	0.3	32	151	189	2247	862	3.8	5.9	43	738	0.22	28	0.13	0.14	4.2	0.59	21	17.8
0.2	0.6	1	13	21	289	94	0.5	0.8	6	49	0.37	2	0.02	0.02	0.4	0.05	5	2.03
1.1	0.5	11	93	78	496	150	0.4	0.7	11	20	0.07	2	0.03	0.12	0.5	0.06	5	5.12
0.6	0.5	2	22	27	458	73	0.4	0.7	4	0	0.04	1	0.01	0.02	0.5	0.04	2	4
1	0.3	30	73	146	251	351	0.5	0.3	24	22	0.19	4	0.08	0.13	1.4	0.18	8	0.61
0	0	0	5	7	38	65	0	0.2	4	8	0.1	3	0.01	0.01	0.1	0.02	2	0
0	0	0	7	0	0	3	0	0.2	0	0	0	0	0	0	0	0	0	0
0	0	0	24	7	82	34	—	0.2	—	0	—	0	0	0	0	0	—	0
0	0	0	23	25	8	282	0.1	2.8	15	10	0	68	0.04	0.03	0.5	0.06	5	0
0	0	0	35	51	4	554	0.2	5.6	28	21	0	134	0.07	0.05	0.9	0.12	10	0
0	0	0	316	20	4	196	0.1	0.2	17	1	0.07	80	0.06	0.03	0.3	0.06	5	0
0	0	7	31	274	516	358	0.2	0.7	26	22	2.4	2	0.02	0.05	0.4	0.02	5	12
7.5	4.8	117	191	336	567	496	2.4	21.2	24	168	2.57	12	0.37	0.56	4.6	0.11	29	56.7
4.1	3.3	60	84	299	622	556	2.4	24.5	16	253	3.16	22	0.13	0.3	2.9	0.1	27	82.4
0	0	0	4	1	1	6	0	0	1	0	0.01	0	0	0	0	0.01	1	0
2.8	2	1	22	30	288	106	0.2	0.8	6	76	1.11	0	0.1	0.09	0.7	0.04	3	0.04
5.8	3.6	4	141	105	347	189	0.5	2	19	18	2.35	12	0.29	0.28	2.4	0.06	12	0.06
5	3	3	118	86	354	195	0.4	3.4	18	106	1.29	2	0.21	0.23	1.8	0.08	12	0.05
2.8	2	1	28	34	294	133	0.2	1.8	9	135	1.01	2	0.1	0.11	0.8	0.05	9	0.04
2.8	1.9	1	24	40	291	159	0.2	0.9	10	105	1.16	3	0.09	0.09	1.2	0.03	6	0.04
4.9	2.7	3	107	85	258	291	0.4	1.5	20	42	1.74	10	0.24	0.3	2.2	0.12	8	0.05
6.2	4	3	184	89	408	356	0.4	1.9	24	83	1.84	6	0.24	0.23	2.1	0.04	11	0.05
0.2	0	2	118	175	225	528	0.7	1	42	0	0.08	0	0.05	0.27	0.2	0.06	3	0.38
1.3	0.1	0	139	148	276	541	0.4	2.4	31	201	0.11	8	0.2	0.23	2.7	0.05	0	0.56
0.2	0	0	8	45	3	273	0.4	2.2	30	0	0.02	0	0	0.01	0.2	0.01	—	0
1.5	0.2	17	287	245	158	476	1.2	0.8	52	131	0.24	2	0.1	0.41	0.3	0.1	13	0.84
0.3	0	4	291	258	162	502	1.2	0.7	46	140	0.18	2	0.09	0.35	0.3	0.1	13	0.87
0.2	0	0	6	39	1	135	0.3	0.8	26	0	0.02	0	0.01	0.02	0.1	0.01	2	0
0.2	0	0	7	40	1	82	0.4	0.7	27	0	0.02	0	0	0.01	0.1	0.01	2	0
0.9	0.1	0	0	—	0	493	—	2	—	0	—	0	0.05	0.07	0.7	—	—	—
0.9	0.2	0	43	213	2	431	—	3	—	0	—	0	0.03	0.13	0.7	—	—	—
1.6	0.3	18	303	268	160	495	1.3	0.8	56	140	0.22	2	0.1	0.44	0.3	0.12	14	0.9
1.1	0.3	0	1	33	74	149	0.9	0.8	25	0	1.08	3	0.03	0.06	0.1	0.04	21	0
2.4	0.6	0	38	240	36	631	1.6	3.9	89	0	1.75	7	0.06	0	1.8	0.08	39	0
0	0	0	58	48	252	600	0.2	0.7	60	0	0	6	0.07	0.14	0.2	0.08	6	0
0.4	0.1	0	3	25	61	78	0.4	0.4	12	0	0.31	0	0.01	0	0.1	0.06	2	0
0.6	0.1	0	8	60	10	157	0.6	1	26	0	0.28	0	0.02	0.03	0.2	0.09	3	0
0.5	0.1	0	5	40	7	106	0.4	0.6	18	0	0.26	0	0.01	0.02	0.1	0.06	2	0

A

Food Item	Qty	Meas	Wgt (g)	Wtr (g)	Cals	Prot (g)	Carb (g)	Fib (g)	Fat (g)	SatF (g)
Coconut, fresh piece, 2.5 x 2 inch	1	piece	45	21	159	2	7	4	15	13.4
Coconut, fresh, grated	0.25	cup	20	9	71	1	3	1.8	7	5.9
Coffee substitute, cereal grain, dry	1	Tbs	7	0	23	0	6	0.6	0	0
Coffee substitute, dry, prepared, Postum	1	cup	240	237	12	0	2	0	0	0
Coffee, brewed	1	cup	240	238	5	0	1	0	0	0
Coffee, brewed. decaffeinated	1	cup	240	238	5	0	1	0	0	0
Coffee, cappuccino, mix, prepared	1	cup	256	237	82	1	14	0	3	2.4
Coffee, chicory, instant, dry	1	Tbs	3	0	9	0	2	0	0	0
Coffee, chicory, instant, prepared	1	cup	239	236	10	0	2	0	0	0
Coffee, decaffeinated, instant, prepared	1	cup	239	236	5	0	1	0	0	0
Coffee, demi tasse	1	cup	240	238	5	0	1	0	0	0
Coffee, espresso	1	cup	240	238	5	0	1	0	0	0
Coffee, espresso, decaffeinated	1	cup	240	238	5	0	1	0	0	0
Coffee, french, mix, prepared	1	cup	252	237	76	1	9	0	5	3.9
Coffee, mocha, instant, dry	1	Tbs	9	0	38	0	6	0.1	1	1.2
Coffee, mocha, mix, prepared	1	cup	251	236	68	1	11	0.3	3	2.2
Coffee, prepared from instant	1	cup	240	238	5	0	1	0	0	0
Coffee, swiss mocha, mix, prepared	1	cup	251	235	67	1	11	0.2	2	2.2
Coffee, vending machine, creamer	1	each	180	174	27	0	3	0	2	1.5
Coffee, vending machine, sugared	1	each	180	172	28	0	7	0	0	0
Coffee, vending machine, sugared, creamed	1	each	180	168	51	0	9	0	2	1.4
Coleslaw salad	0.5	cup	60	44	89	1	8	1	7	1
Collard greens, cooked, no added salt	0.5	cup	64	59	17	1	3	1.8	0	0
Collard greens, frozen, cooked, no added salt	0.5	cup	85	75	31	3	6	2.4	0	0.1
Collard greens, raw	0.5	cup	18	16	5	0	1	0.6	0	0
Comfrey leaves	1	oz.	28	25	9	1	2	—	0	—
Consomme, beef, w/gelatin, prep w/water	0.5	cup	120	116	14	3	1	0	0	0
Cookie crust, chocolate, recipe, baked	1	each	219	12	1130	11	122	3.4	69	15
Cookie dough, chocolate chip, refrigerated	4	each	48	6	213	2	30	0.7	10	3.2
Cookie mix, oatmeal, dry	8	oz.	227	12	1047	15	153	6.4	44	10.8
Cookie mix, oatmeal, dry, prepared	2	each	32	2	148	2	21	1.2	6	1.6
Cookie, Fig bar	4	each	56	9	195	2	40	2.6	4	0.6
Cookie, Ladyfinger	2	each	22	4	80	2	13	0.2	2	0.7
Cookie, Nilla wafers	7	each	28	—	124	1	21	0.4	4	0.9
Cookie, almond	2	each	20	1	104	2	10	0.5	6	1
Cookie, animal, small box	1	each	67	3	299	4	50	—	9	3.5
Cookie, apple filled oatmeal, Archway	1	each	28	4	111	1	18	0.6	4	0.8
Cookie, applesauce, large	2	each	36	6	133	2	23	1.1	4	0.9
Cookie, apricot filled, Archway	1	each	28	4	112	1	18	0.4	4	1.5
Cookie, blueberry filled, Archway	1	each	28	—	110	1	19	0.5	4	1.5
Cookie, butter, commercially prepared	5	each	25	1	117	2	17	0.2	5	2.8
Cookie, butterscotch brownie	1	each	34	4	149	2	22	0.3	7	1.2
Cookie, carob	2	each	26	1	103	2	17	1.6	4	0.8
Cookie, chocolate brownie, fat free, Entenmann's	1	each	12	1	40	0	10	0.5	0	0
Cookie, chocolate brownie, fat-free, Entenmann's	2	each	24	2	80	1	20	1	0	0
Cookie, chocolate chip, Archway	3	each	27	—	130	1	17	0	7	2
Cookie, chocolate chip, commercial	1	each	10	0	45	1	7	0.4	2	0.4
Cookie, chocolate chip, dietetic	5	each	25	1	125	1	16	1.2	7	2.2
Cookie, chocolate chip, homemade, w/butter	2	each	32	2	156	2	19	0.8	9	4.5
Cookie, chocolate chip, homemade, w/margarine	2	each	20	1	98	1	12	0.6	6	1.6
Cookie, chocolate chip, mix, prepared	2	each	32	1	159	2	20	0.4	8	2.7
Cookie, chocolate chip, no sodium, w/fructose	4	each	28	1	126	1	21	0.4	5	1.2
Cookie, chocolate chip, refrigerated dough, baked	2	each	24	1	118	1	16	0.4	5	1.9
Cookie, chocolate chip, rich	1	each	10	0	48	1	7	0.2	2	0.7
Cookie, chocolate chip, small box	1	each	55	3	233	3	36	—	12	5.3
Cookie, chocolate chip, soft	2	each	21	2	96	1	12	0.7	5	1.6
Cookie, chocolate sandwich, Snackwell's	1	oz.	28	1	116	1	22	0.7	3	0.7
Cookie, chocolate sandwich, creme-filled	2	each	20	0	94	1	14	0.6	4	0.7
Cookie, chocolate sandwich, low sodium, w/fructose	3	each	30	1	138	1	20	1.2	7	1.2
Cookie, chocolate sandwich, w/chocolate icing	2	each	34	1	164	1	22	1.8	9	2.5
Cookie, chocolate sandwich, w/extra creme	2	each	26	0	130	1	18	0.5	7	1
Cookie, chocolate wafer	4	each	24	1	104	2	17	0.8	3	1
Cookie, cinnamon honey, fat free, Archway	3	each	30	3	106	1	25	0.4	0	0.1
Cookie, coconut macaroon, Archway	1	each	23	2	111	1	13	0.5	6	5.7
Cookie, coconut macaroon, recipe	1	each	24	3	97	1	17	0.4	3	2.7

MonoF (g)	PolyF (g)	Choles (mg)	Calc (mg)	Phos (mg)	Sod (mg)	Pot (mg)	Zn (mg)	Iron (mg)	Magn (mg)	VitA (μg RE)	VitE (mg α-TE)	VitC (mg)	Thia (mg)	Ribo (mg)	Nia (mg)	B6 (mg)	Fola (μg)	B12 (μg)
0.6	0.2	0	6	51	9	160	0.5	1.1	14	0	0.33	1	0.03	0.01	0.2	0.02	12	0
0.3	0.1	0	3	23	4	71	0.2	0.5	6	0	0.15	1	0.01	0	0.1	0.01	5	0
0	0.1	0	4	40	5	127	0	0.3	17	0	0.07	0	0.04	0.01	1.2	0.06	2	0
0	0	0	7	17	10	58	0.1	0.1	10	0	0	0	0.02	0	0.5	0.03	1	0
0	0	0	5	2	5	130	0	0.1	12	0	0	0	0	0	0.5	0	0	0
0	0	0	5	2	5	130	0	0.1	12	0	0	0	0	0	0.5	0	0	0
0.2	0.1	0	10	36	138	159	0.1	0.2	13	0	0.1	0	0.02	0.01	0.4	0	0	0
0	0	0	3	7	7	92	0	0.1	6	0	0	0	0	0.01	0.6	0	0	0
0	0	0	7	7	14	81	0.1	0.1	7	0	0	0	0	0.01	0.5	0	0	0
0	0	0	7	7	7	84	0.1	0.1	10	0	0	0	0	0.03	0.7	0	0	0
0	0	0	5	2	5	130	0	0.1	12	0	0	0	0	0	0.5	0	0	0
0	0	0	5	2	5	130	0	0.1	12	0	0	0	0	0	0.5	0	0	0
0	0	0	5	2	5	130	0	0.1	12	0	0	0	0	0	0.5	0	0	0
0.3	0.1	0	10	55	40	181	0	0	3	0	0	0	0	0	0.9	0	0	0
0.1	0	0	3	22	23	89	0.1	0.2	6	0	0	0	0	0	0.2	0	0	0
0.1	0	0	10	38	48	158	0.2	0.3	12	0	0.02	0	0	0	0.3	0	0	0
0	0	0	7	7	7	86	0.1	0.1	10	0	0	0	0	0	0.7	0	0	0
0.1	0	0	10	38	48	158	0.2	0.3	13	0	0	0	0	0	0.3	0	0	0
0	0	0	6	22	14	72	0.1	0.1	5	1	0.01	0	0	0.01	0.3	0	0	0
0	0	0	5	3	6	35	0.1	0.1	5	0	0	0	0	0	0.3	0	0	0
0	0	0	6	21	13	70	0.1	0.1	5	1	0.01	0	0	0.01	0.3	0	0	0
1.5	3.9	3	20	22	162	107	0.1	0.4	5	30	2.4	5	0.02	0.02	0	0.07	23	0.11
0	0.1	0	76	17	6	166	0.3	0.3	11	200	0.56	12	0.03	0.07	0.4	0.08	60	0
0	0.2	0	179	23	42	213	0.2	1	26	508	0.42	22	0.04	0.1	0.5	0.1	65	0
0	0	0	26	2	4	30	0	0	2	69	0.41	6	0.01	0.02	0.1	0.03	30	0
—	—	—	90	15	—	—	—	0.9	—	275	—	7	0.03	0.06	0.4	—	—	0
0	0	0	5	16	318	77	0.2	0.3	0	0	0.01	0	0.01	0.01	0.4	0.01	1	0
32.9	17.2	4	68	234	1502	374	1.8	6.7	90	488	—	0	0.34	0.46	4.8	0	0	0.04
5	1	12	12	33	100	86	0.2	1.1	12	8	1.11	0	0.09	0.09	1	0.02	27	0.04
24	6.3	0	57	370	1072	415	1.8	5	109	5	5.9	0	0.32	0.32	3	0.1	113	0
3.4	0.9	13	9	56	150	60	0.3	0.7	15	7	0.9	0	0.09	0.05	0.4	0.02	4	0.03
1.7	1.6	0	36	35	196	116	0.2	1.6	15	2	0.7	0	0.09	0.12	1	0.04	15	0.05
0.9	0.3	80	10	38	32	25	0.3	0.8	3	37	0.28	1	0.06	0.09	0.5	0.03	17	0.16
1.3	0	2	18	—	89	27	—	1	—	—	—	—	—	—	—	—	—	—
3.2	1.8	9	15	34	49	42	0.2	0.5	14	57	1.7	0	0.05	0.07	0.5	0.01	4	0.02
3.8	1	11	11	64	273	56	0.3	1.5	11	8	0.32	1	0.25	0.24	2.5	0.02	81	0.05
1.4	0.3	2	8	—	116	51	—	0.9	—	1	—	0	0.07	0.04	0.5	—	15	—
1.9	1.4	9	22	44	109	76	0.2	0.7	11	55	0.74	0	0.07	0.05	0.4	0.03	3	0.02
1.2	0.2	8	6	—	9	35	—	0.6	—	3	—	0	0.07	0.06	0.5	—	—	—
—	—	5	0	—	115	—	—	0.7	—	0	—	0	—	—	—	—	—	—
1.4	0.2	29	7	26	88	28	0.1	0.6	3	42	0.13	0	0.09	0.08	0.8	0.01	10	0.09
2.6	2.3	18	24	26	96	80	0.2	0.7	10	76	0.96	0	0.05	0.06	0.4	0.02	4	0.04
2	1.4	16	70	59	80	140	0.4	0.6	17	7	0.7	0	0.04	0.09	0.5	0.05	6	0.08
0	0	0	0	—	45	62	—	0.4	—	0	—	0	—	—	—	—	—	—
0	0	0	0	—	90	125	—	0.7	—	0	—	0	—	—	—	—	—	—
—	—	10	0	—	70	—	—	0.7	—	0	—	0	—	—	—	—	—	—
0.6	0.5	0	2	8	38	12	0.1	0.3	3	0	0.18	0	0.03	0.03	0.3	0.03	7	0
2.2	1.9	3	8	14	3	21	0.2	0.3	6	2	0.64	0	0.04	0.04	0.3	0.02	2	0.03
2.6	1.4	22	12	32	109	71	0.3	0.8	18	47	0.29	0	0.06	0.06	0.4	0.03	11	0.03
2.1	1.7	6	8	20	72	45	0.2	0.5	11	33	0.57	0	0.04	0.04	0.3	0.02	7	0.02
4.2	0.9	13	15	30	94	68	0.2	0.7	12	6	0.83	0	0.05	0.07	0.6	0.01	3	0.03
1.9	1.4	0	13	30	3	56	0.1	1	6	0	0.69	0	0.1	0.05	0.8	0	13	0
2.7	0.6	6	7	18	56	48	0.1	0.6	6	4	0.49	0	0.04	0.05	0.5	0	2	0.02
1.2	0.2	0	2	11	32	14	0.1	0.3	3	0	0.26	0	0.02	0.03	0.3	0.01	4	0
5	1	12	20	52	188	82	0.3	1.5	16	15	0.37	1	0.09	0.19	1.4	0.03	33	0.1
2.7	0.7	0	3	10	68	20	0.1	0.5	7	0	0.61	0	0.02	0.04	0.3	0.03	8	0
0.8	0.2	0	16	58	217	45	0.2	0.8	13	0	—	0	0.04	0.05	0.6	0.01	—	0
1.7	1.4	0	5	20	121	35	0.2	0.8	9	0	0.69	0	0.02	0.04	0.4	0	9	0.01
2.8	2.4	0	29	60	73	88	0.2	1.4	8	0	1.13	0	0.16	0.09	1.2	0.01	19	0.01
5	1	0	12	31	111	82	0.2	1.1	13	0	1.13	0	0.03	0.07	0.5	0.02	6	0.02
2.8	2.4	0	6	24	128	32	0.2	0.7	9	0	1.17	0	0.02	0.04	0.4	0.01	11	0
1.2	1	0	7	32	139	50	0.3	1	13	1	0.38	0	0.05	0.06	0.7	0.01	12	0.02
0.1	0.1	0	6	—	123	20	—	0.8	—	0	—	0	0.1	0.06	0.8	—	24	—
0.4	0.1	0	4	—	40	6	—	0.4	—	0	—	0	0.01	0.01	0.1	—	1	—
0.1	0	0	2	10	59	37	0.2	0.2	5	0	0.07	0	0	0.03	0	0.02	1	0.01

Food Item	Qty	Meas	Wgt (g)	Wtr (g)	Cals	Prot (g)	Carb (g)	Fib (g)	Fat (g)	SatF (g)
Cookie, date filled oatmeal, Archway	1	each	28	4	111	1	19	0.8	3	0.8
Cookie, devil's food, Snackwell's	1	oz.	28	5	97	1	22	0.4	0	0
Cookie, double fudge, fat free, Snackwell's	1	oz.	28	4	94	1	21	0.5	0	0.2
Cookie, fortune	4	each	32	3	121	1	27	0.5	1	0.2
Cookie, fruit bar, no fat, Archway	1	each	28	—	90	2	21	0	0	0
Cookie, fudge cake type	1	each	21	2	73	1	16	0.6	1	0.2
Cookie, fudge, fat free, Snackwell's	2	each	32	5	106	2	24	0.6	0	0.2
Cookie, gingerbread, iced, Archway	3	each	32	1	149	1	23	0.4	6	1.8
Cookie, gingersnap	4	each	28	1	116	2	22	0.6	3	0.7
Cookie, graham cracker, chocolate-coated	2	each	28	1	136	2	19	0.9	6	3.8
Cookie, granola	2	each	26	1	119	2	17	1.1	4	3.7
Cookie, lemon bar	2	each	32	4	139	2	20	0.3	6	1.2
Cookie, marshmallow, chocolate-coated	2	each	26	3	109	1	18	0.5	4	1.2
Cookie, molasses	2	each	30	2	129	2	22	0.3	4	1
Cookie, molasses, old fashioned, Archway	1	each	28	3	113	1	20	0.3	3	0.8
Cookie, oatmeal	2	each	36	2	162	2	25	1	7	1.6
Cookie, oatmeal chocolate chip, fat free, Entenmann	1	each	12	—	40	0	10	0.5	0	0
Cookie, oatmeal raisin, Archway	1	each	28	—	110	2	19	0.5	4	1
Cookie, oatmeal raisin, fat free, Entenmann's	1	each	24	4	80	1	18	0.5	0	0
Cookie, oatmeal raisin, no fat, Archway	1	each	28	4	96	1	22	0.9	0	0.1
Cookie, oatmeal raisin, recipe	2	each	26	2	113	2	18	0.8	4	0.8
Cookie, oatmeal raisin, w/fructose, no sodium	4	each	28	2	126	1	20	0.8	5	0.8
Cookie, oatmeal w/raisins, dietetic	3	each	33	3	144	2	21	0.8	6	1.5
Cookie, oatmeal, Archway	1	each	27	3	115	2	18	0.8	4	0.9
Cookie, oatmeal, chilled dough, baked	2	each	24	1	113	1	16	0.7	5	1.3
Cookie, oatmeal, recipe	2	each	30	2	134	2	20	0.9	5	1.1
Cookie, oatmeal, soft	2	each	30	3	123	2	20	0.8	4	1.1
Cookie, oreo sandwich	2	each	28	—	138	2	20	0.9	6	1.3
Cookie, peanut butter sandwich	2	each	28	1	134	2	18	0.5	6	1.4
Cookie, peanut butter sandwich, low sodium, w/fructose	3	each	30	1	161	3	15	0.5	10	1.5
Cookie, peanut butter, Archway	1	each	28	2	134	3	16	0.8	7	1.5
Cookie, peanut butter, chilled dough, baked	2	each	24	1	121	2	14	0.3	7	1.5
Cookie, peanut butter, homemade	2	each	24	1	114	2	14	0.5	6	1.1
Cookie, peanut butter, soft type	2	each	30	3	137	2	17	0.5	7	1.8
Cookie, pecan sandies	2	each	30	1	149	2	20	0.5	7	1.8
Cookie, pecan shortbread	2	each	28	1	152	1	16	0.5	9	2.3
Cookie, raisin oatmeal, Archway	3	each	28	—	130	2	19	1	6	1.5
Cookie, raisin, soft type	2	each	30	4	120	1	20	0.4	4	1
Cookie, raspberry filled, Archway	1	each	28	4	113	1	18	0.4	4	1.5
Cookie, raspberry oatmeal, no fat, Archway	1	each	28	3	98	1	22	0.9	0	0.1
Cookie, sandwich-type, dietetic	3	each	33	4	151	2	18	0.3	8	2
Cookie, shortbread, commercial, plain	4	each	32	1	161	2	21	0.6	8	2
Cookie, shortbread, homemade, w/butter	2	each	28	1	155	2	16	0.4	9	5.8
Cookie, shortbread, homemade, w/margarine	3	each	33	1	180	2	19	0.5	11	2.1
Cookie, snickerdoodle	1	each	20	4	81	1	12	0.4	3	2.1
Cookie, sugar	2	each	30	1	143	2	20	0.2	6	1.6
Cookie, sugar wafer, cream-filled w/fructose, no sodium	7	each	28	1	141	1	18	0.5	7	1.1
Cookie, sugar wafer, creme-filled	8	each	28	0	143	1	20	0.2	7	1
Cookie, sugar, Archway	1	each	28	—	120	2	20	0	4	1
Cookie, sugar, homemade, w/butter	2	each	28	2	132	2	17	0.4	7	4
Cookie, sugar, homemade, w/margarine	2	each	28	2	132	2	17	0.3	7	1.3
Cookie, sugar, no sodium, w/fructose	4	each	28	2	121	1	22	0.2	4	0.5
Cookie, sugar, refrigerated dough, baked	2	each	24	1	116	1	16	0.2	6	1.4
Cookie, sugar, soft, Archway	1	each	28	3	115	1	19	0.3	4	0.9
Cookie, sugar/plain, dietetic	5	each	30	3	139	1	18	0.1	7	1.4
Cookie, vanilla sandwich	3	each	30	1	145	1	22	0.4	6	0.9
Cookie, vanilla sandwich, Snackwell's	1	oz.	28	1	119	1	23	0.6	3	0.6
Cookie, vanilla wafer, Archway	5	each	30	—	130	2	22	0	4	1
Cookie, vanilla wafer, made w/egg	7	each	28	1	123	1	21	0.5	4	1.1
Cookie, vanilla wafer, no egg	4	each	24	1	114	1	17	0.5	5	1.2
Cookie, whole wheat fruit & nut	2	each	28	4	121	2	16	1.3	6	1
Cooking wine, red, Fleischmann's	1	Tbs	15	13	10	0	0	0	0	0
Cooking wine, white, Fleischmann's	1	Tbs	15	13	10	0	0	0	0	0
Coriander leaf, dried	0.25	tsp	0	0	0	0	0	0	0	0
Coriander seed	0.25	tsp	0	0	1	0	0	0.2	0	0

MonoF (g)	PolyF (g)	Choles (mg)	Calc (mg)	Phos (mg)	Sod (mg)	Pot (mg)	Zn (mg)	Iron (mg)	Magn (mg)	VitA (μg RE)	VitE (mg α-TE)	VitC (mg)	Thia (mg)	Ribo (mg)	Nia (mg)	B6 (mg)	Fola (μg)	B12 (μg)
1.3	0.3	4	10	—	110	59	—	0.6	—	1	—	0	0.07	0.05	0.5	—	—	—
0.2	0	0	9	22	48	30	0.1	0.4	6	0	—	0	0.03	0.04	0.4	0.01	—	0.02
0.1	0.1	0	5	20	125	47	0.1	0.5	9	0	0	0	0.03	0.03	0.5	0.01	—	0
0.4	0.1	1	4	11	88	13	0.1	0.5	2	0	0.11	0	0.06	0.04	0.6	0	18	0
0	0	0	0	—	95	—	—	0.4	—	0	0.01	0	—	—	—	—	—	—
0.4	0.1	0	7	17	40	29	0.1	0.5	7	0	0.12	0	0.05	0.04	0.3	0.01	9	0.02
0.1	0.1	0	6	22	141	53	0.2	0.6	10	0	0	0	0.03	0.04	0.5	0.01	—	0
1.9	0.7	0	7	—	114	22	—	0.1	—	0	—	0	0.06	0.09	0.8	—	22	—
1.5	0.4	0	22	23	183	97	0.2	1.8	14	0	0.36	0	0.06	0.08	0.9	0.03	20	0
2.2	0.3	0	16	38	82	58	0.3	1	16	0	0.32	0	0.04	0.06	0.6	0.02	5	0
0.3	0.1	0	18	93	86	94	0.4	0.8	26	0	0.03	0	0.16	0.06	0.5	0.09	21	0
2.6	1.8	25	12	22	78	22	0.1	0.5	3	83	1	1	0.06	0.07	0.4	0.01	4	0.05
2.4	0.5	0	12	25	44	47	0.2	0.7	9	0	0.56	0	0.02	0.05	0.2	0.02	5	0.04
2.1	0.5	0	22	28	138	104	0.1	1.9	16	0	0.51	0	0.11	0.08	0.9	0.03	22	0
1.2	0.2	9	10	—	148	32	—	1.3	—	3	—	0	0.08	0.07	0.7	—	—	—
3.6	0.9	0	13	50	138	51	0.3	0.9	12	1	0.91	0	0.1	0.08	0.8	0.02	16	0
0	0	0	0	—	55	40	—	0.2	—	0	—	0	—	—	—	—	—	—
—	—	2	0	—	115	—	—	1.1	—	0	—	0	—	—	—	—	—	—
0	0	0	0	—	120	60	—	0	—	0	—	0	—	—	—	—	—	—
0.1	0.2	0	10	—	149	79	—	0.9	—	0	—	0	0.07	0.04	0.5	—	13	—
1.8	1.3	9	26	42	140	62	0.2	0.7	11	43	0.65	0	0.06	0.04	0.3	0.02	8	0.02
2.1	1.9	0	15	34	3	49	0.1	1.1	5	0	0.9	0	0.13	0.06	0.9	0.01	15	0
2.6	1.6	1	7	46	1	55	0.3	0.7	9	0	0.82	0	0.08	0.03	0.3	0.01	4	0.04
1.5	0.4	3	8	—	94	50	—	0.6	—	1	—	0	0.08	0.05	0.5	—	—	—
2.8	0.7	6	8	28	78	39	0.2	0.6	8	3	0.72	0	0.05	0.04	0.4	0.01	2	0.01
2.3	1.7	11	32	50	179	55	0.3	0.8	13	55	0.81	0	0.08	0.05	0.4	0.02	10	0.03
2.4	0.7	2	27	63	105	40	0.1	0.8	9	2	0.6	0	0.06	0.07	0.5	0.03	10	0
2.6	0.4	0	—	—	189	52	—	0.6	—	—	—	—	—	—	—	—	—	—
3.1	1.1	0	15	53	103	54	0.3	0.7	14	0	0.91	0	0.09	0.07	1	0.04	12	0.06
4.6	3.6	0	13	46	124	88	0.3	0.8	15	0	1.72	0	0.1	0.04	1.6	0.02	16	0
2.9	1.2	10	10	—	113	59	—	0.8	—	3	—	0	0.07	0.06	1.2	—	—	—
3.5	1.2	7	27	63	105	81	0.2	0.4	10	3	0.96	0	0.04	0.04	1	0.02	2	0.01
2.6	1.7	7	9	28	124	55	0.2	0.5	9	37	0.91	0	0.05	0.05	0.8	0.02	13	0.02
4.1	1	0	4	26	101	32	0.2	0.3	10	0	1.17	0	0.07	0.05	0.6	0.01	20	0
3.9	0.9	10	21	47	18	20	0.1	0.9	5	7	0.89	0	0.14	0.08	0.9	0.01	3	0.02
5.2	1.2	9	8	24	79	20	0.2	0.7	5	0	1.06	0	0.08	0.06	0.7	0.01	18	0
—	—	10	0	—	55	—	—	0.7	—	0	—	0	—	—	—	—	—	—
2.3	0.5	1	14	25	101	42	0.1	0.7	6	0	0.58	0	0.06	0.06	0.6	0.02	13	0.01
1.2	0.2	8	7	—	94	35	—	0.6	—	2	—	0	0.09	0.06	0.5	—	—	—
0.2	0.2	0	11	—	150	80	—	0.9	—	0	—	0	0.08	0.04	0.5	—	13	—
3.6	2.2	0	12	21	4	32	0.2	0.4	10	0	1.32	0	0.05	0.05	0.4	0.01	2	0
4.3	1	6	11	35	146	32	0.2	0.9	5	4	1.03	0	0.11	0.1	1.1	0.03	19	0.03
2.7	0.4	25	5	20	132	20	0.1	0.7	4	87	0.23	0	0.1	0.07	0.8	0.01	3	0.01
4.8	3.5	0	7	23	169	25	0.1	0.9	4	114	1.65	0	0.12	0.08	1	0.01	4	0.01
1	0.2	9	8	10	74	24	0.1	0.5	2	32	0.1	0	0.05	0.04	0.4	0.01	2	0.02
3.5	0.8	15	6	24	107	19	0.1	0.6	4	8	0.85	0	0.07	0.06	0.8	0.02	14	0.06
3	2.7	0	15	10	3	17	0.1	0.4	2	0	1.13	0	0.05	0.03	0.4	0	12	0
2.9	2.6	0	5	16	41	16	0.1	0.5	3	0	1.23	0	0.03	0.06	0.7	0	12	0
—	—	2	0	—	190	—	—	0.7	—	0	—	0	—	—	—	—	—	—
1.9	0.3	24	20	25	129	20	0.1	0.7	3	62	0.2	0	0.08	0.07	0.7	0.01	3	0.02
2.9	2	7	20	25	137	22	0.1	0.7	3	70	1.02	0	0.08	0.07	0.7	0.01	15	0.02
1.5	1.3	0	7	20	1	29	0.1	1.1	3	0	0.62	0	0.14	0.06	1	0	16	0
3.1	0.7	8	22	45	112	39	0.1	0.4	2	3	0.77	0	0.04	0.03	0.6	0.01	13	0.02
1.3	0.2	6	9	—	189	23	—	0.6	—	2	—	0	0.09	0.06	0.7	—	—	—
3.1	2.2	18	2	11	0	12	0.1	0.4	4	0	0.96	0	0.06	0.03	0.4	0.01	3	0.03
2.5	2.3	0	8	22	105	27	0.1	0.7	4	0	1.08	0	0.08	0.07	0.8	0	18	0
0.8	0.2	0	19	40	104	31	0.2	0.7	5	0	—	0	0.05	0.07	0.7	0.01	—	0.02
—	—	5	0	—	130	—	—	1.1	—	0	—	0	—	—	—	—	—	—
1.8	1.1	14	13	29	87	27	0.1	0.7	4	2	0.36	0	0.08	0.09	0.9	0.02	14	0.04
2.7	0.6	0	6	15	73	26	0.1	0.5	3	0	0.34	0	0.09	0.05	0.7	0.01	10	0.01
2.2	2.7	15	18	49	59	111	0.4	0.7	20	50	0.81	0	0.05	0.04	0.5	0.06	6	0.03
0	0	—	1	2	90	12	—	0.1	—	0	—	0	0.08	0.08	0.1	—	—	0
0	0	—	1	2	90	13	—	0.1	—	0	—	0	0.08	0.08	0.1	—	—	0
0	0	0	2	1	0	7	0	0.1	1	1	0	1	0	0	0	0	0	0
0.1	0	0	3	2	0	5	0	0.1	1	0	—	0	0	0	0	—	0	0

Food Item	Qty	Meas	Wgt (g)	Wtr (g)	Cals	Prot (g)	Carb (g)	Fib (g)	Fat (g)	SatF (g)
Coriander/cilantro, fresh	0.25	cup	4	4	1	0	0	0.1	0	0
Corn bran, crude	0.25	cup	19	1	43	2	16	16.2	0	0
Corn chips, BBQ flavor	10	piece	18	0	94	1	10	0.9	6	0.8
Corn chips/Fritos	1	cup	26	0	140	2	15	1.3	9	1.2
Corn chips/Fritos, grab bag	1	each	85	1	458	6	48	4.2	28	3.9
Corn cones, nacho flavor, Bugles	1	oz.	28	1	152	2	16	0.3	9	7.6
Corn cones, plain, Bugles	1	oz.	28	1	145	2	18	0.3	8	6.5
Corn flour patties, fried	1	each	10	4	23	0	5	0.7	0	0.1
Corn grits, instant, w/imitation bacon bits, prepared	0.5	cup	105	86	70	2	16	1	0	0
Corn grits, white, enriched, cooked	0.5	cup	121	103	73	2	16	0.2	0	0
Corn grits, white, packet, prepared	1	each	137	113	89	2	21	1.2	0	0
Corn grits, white, unenriched, cooked	0.5	cup	121	103	73	2	16	0.2	0	0
Corn grits, yellow, enriched, cooked	0.5	cup	121	103	73	2	16	0.2	0	0
Corn grits, yellow, enriched, dry	0.5	cup	78	8	289	7	62	1.2	1	0.1
Corn grits, yellow, unenriched, cooked	0.5	cup	121	103	73	2	16	0.2	0	0
Corn on cob, small, frozen, cooked	1	each	77	56	72	2	17	2.2	1	0.1
Corn w/sweet peppers, canned, w/liquid	0.5	cup	114	88	85	3	21	2.3	1	0.1
Corn, canned, not drained	0.5	cup	128	104	82	2	20	2.2	1	0.1
Corn, creamed, canned	0.5	cup	128	101	92	2	23	1.5	1	0.1
Corn, sweet, yellow, canned, drained	0.5	cup	82	63	66	2	15	1.6	1	0.1
Corn, white, canned, drained, salted	0.5	cup	82	63	66	2	15	1.6	1	0.1
Corn, white, canned, w/liquid, salted	0.5	cup	128	104	82	2	20	2.2	1	0.1
Corn, white, canned, w/liquid, unsalted	0.5	cup	128	104	82	2	20	0.9	1	0.1
Corn, white, cream style, canned, drained, salted	0.5	cup	128	101	92	2	23	1.5	1	0.1
Corn, white, cream style, canned, w/salt	0.5	cup	128	101	92	2	23	1.5	1	0.1
Corn, white, creamed, canned w/liquid, salted	0.5	cup	128	101	92	2	23	1.5	1	0.1
Corn, white, fresh, cooked	0.5	cup	82	57	89	3	21	2.2	1	0.2
Corn, white, kernel, frozen, cooked	0.5	cup	82	63	66	2	16	2	0	0.1
Corn, yellow, canned, not drained, low sodium	0.5	cup	128	104	82	2	20	2.2	1	0.1
Corn, yellow, creamed, low sodium	0.5	cup	128	101	92	2	23	1.5	1	0.1
Corn, yellow, fresh, cooked	0.5	cup	82	57	89	3	21	2.3	1	0.2
Corn, yellow, frozen, cooked, no added salt	0.5	cup	82	63	66	2	16	2	0	0.1
Corn, yellow, on cob, cooked ear	1	each	77	54	83	3	19	2.2	1	0.2
Cornbread mix, dry, 8.5 oz pkg	1	each	241	19	1007	17	167	15.7	29	7.4
Cornbread mix, dry, prepared	1	piece	60	19	188	4	29	1.4	6	1.6
Cornbread, dry, recipe, w/2% milk, 1/6th	1	piece	60	24	160	4	26	1.7	4	0.9
Cornbread, dry, recipe, w/whole milk, 1/9th	1	piece	65	25	176	4	28	2.3	5	1.2
Cornbread, jalapeno, piece	1	piece	65	31	161	4	23	1.9	6	2.1
Corndog (hotdog w/coating)	1	each	175	82	460	17	56	—	19	5.2
Corndog, chicken	1	each	113	59	272	13	26	—	13	—
Corned beef hash, canned	0.5	cup	110	74	199	10	12	0.6	12	6
Cornish game hen, whole, roasted (20 oz hen)	1	each	306	181	727	83	0	0	41	11.5
Cornish game hen, whole, skinless, roasted	1	each	249	158	470	72	0	0	18	5
Cornmeal mush, fried slice	1	piece	51	32	84	2	15	0.8	2	0.4
Cornmeal mush, made w/milk	0.5	cup	120	80	180	7	25	1.2	6	3.3
Cornmeal, white, degermed, enriched	1	cup	138	16	505	12	107	10.2	2	0.3
Cornmeal, white, whole grain	1	cup	122	13	442	10	94	8.9	4	0.6
Cornmeal, yellow, degermed, enriched	0.5	cup	69	8	253	6	54	5.1	1	0.2
Cornmeal, yellow, enriched, baked value	1	cup	138	16	505	12	107	10.2	2	0.3
Cornmeal, yellow, self rising, degermed	1	cup	138	14	490	12	103	9.8	2	0.3
Cornmeal, yellow, whole grain	0.5	cup	61	6	221	5	47	4.4	2	0.3
Cornnuts, BBQ flavor	10	piece	18	0	78	2	13	1.5	3	0.5
Cornnuts, plain	10	piece	18	0	79	2	13	1.2	3	0.5
Cornstarch	1	tsp	3	0	10	0	2	0	0	0
Couscous, cooked	0.5	cup	90	65	100	3	21	1.2	0	0
Cowpea, catjang, dry, cooked	0.5	cup	86	60	101	7	18	3.1	1	0.2
Crab cake, blue crab	1	each	60	43	93	12	0	0	5	0.9
Crab imperial	0.5	cup	130	94	196	20	4	0.2	10	2.5
Crab salad	0.5	cup	104	76	142	14	6	0.3	7	1
Crab thermidor	0.5	cup	122	75	306	15	5	0.1	25	14.8
Crab, deviled	0.5	cup	88	54	171	11	12	0.7	9	1.8
Crabapple, raw, slices	0.5	cup	55	43	42	0	11	0.6	0	0
Cracker bread, Armenian/Ak Mak	4	piece	24	1	94	3	20	0.7	0	0
Cracker meal	1	cup	115	9	440	11	93	2.9	2	0.3
Cracker, Better Cheddar, low sodium	4	each	5	0	25	1	3	0	1	0.4

MonoF	PolyF	Choles	Calc	Phos	Sod	Pot	Zn	Iron	Magn	VitA	VitE	VitC	Thia	Ribo	Nia	B6	Fola	B12
(g)	(g)	(mg)	(mg)	(mg)	(mg)	(mg)	(mg)	(mg)	(mg)	(μg RE)	(mg α-TE)	(mg)	(mg)	(mg)	(mg)	(mg)	(μg)	(μg)
0	0	0	4	1	1	22	0	0.1	1	11	0.1	0	0	0	0	0	0	0
0	0.1	0	8	14	1	8	0.3	0.5	12	1	0.44	0	0	0.02	0.5	0.03	1	0
1.7	2.9	0	24	37	137	42	0.2	0.3	14	11	0.24	0	0.01	0.04	0.3	0.04	7	0
2.5	4.3	0	33	48	164	37	0.3	0.3	20	2	0.35	0	0.01	0.04	0.3	0.06	5	0
8.2	14	0	108	157	536	121	1.1	1.1	65	8	1.16	0	0.02	0.12	1	0.21	17	0
0.6	0.2	1	10	22	270	35	0.1	0.4	7	11	0.6	0	0.06	0.03	0.4	0.03	1	0
0.5	0.2	0	1	12	290	23	0.1	0.7	3	9	0.54	0	0.09	0.07	0.4	0.01	1	0
0.1	0.2	0	8	12	40	16	0.1	0.4	6	0	0.06	0	0.06	0.04	0.5	0.02	1	0
0.1	0.1	0	9	28	247	50	0.2	6	7	0	0.02	0	0.12	0.06	1	0.05	34	0
0.1	0.1	0	0	14	0	27	0.1	0.8	5	0	0.06	0	0.12	0.07	1	0.03	38	0
0	0.1	0	8	29	289	38	0.2	8.2	11	0	0.03	0	0.15	0.08	1.4	0.06	47	0
0.1	0.1	0	0	14	0	27	0.1	0.2	5	0	0.06	0	0.02	0.01	0.2	0.03	1	0
0.1	0.1	0	0	14	0	27	0.1	0.8	5	7	0.06	0	0.12	0.07	1	0.03	38	0
0.2	0.4	0	2	57	1	107	0.3	3	21	34	0.2	0	0.5	0.3	3.9	0.12	146	0
0.1	0.1	0	0	14	0	27	0.1	0.2	5	7	0.06	0	0.02	0.01	0.2	0.03	1	0
0.2	0.3	0	2	58	3	193	0.5	0.5	22	16	0.07	4	0.13	0.05	1.2	0.17	24	0
0.2	0.3	0	6	70	394	174	0.4	0.9	28	26	1.25	10	0.02	0.09	1.1	0.11	38	0
0.2	0.3	0	5	65	273	210	0.5	0.5	20	19	0.15	7	0.03	0.08	1.2	0.05	49	0
0.2	0.3	0	4	65	365	172	0.7	0.5	22	13	0.12	6	0.03	0.07	1.2	0.08	57	0
0.2	0.4	0	4	53	175	160	0.3	0.7	16	13	0.12	7	0.03	0.06	1	0.04	40	0
0.2	0.4	0	4	53	265	160	0.3	0.7	16	0	0.07	7	0.03	0.06	1	0.04	40	0
0.2	0.3	0	5	65	273	210	0.5	0.5	20	0	0.09	7	0.03	0.08	1.2	0.05	49	0
0.2	0.3	0	5	65	15	210	0.5	0.5	20	0	0.09	7	0.03	0.08	1.2	0.05	49	0
0.2	0.3	0	4	65	4	172	0.7	0.5	22	0	0.12	6	0.03	0.07	1.2	0.08	57	0
0.2	0.3	0	4	65	365	172	0.7	0.5	22	0	0.12	6	0.03	0.07	1.2	0.08	57	0
0.2	0.3	0	4	65	365	172	0.7	0.5	22	0	0.12	6	0.03	0.07	1.2	0.08	57	0
0.3	0.5	0	2	84	14	204	0.4	0.5	26	0	0.07	5	0.18	0.06	1.3	0.05	38	0
0.1	0.2	0	3	47	4	121	0.3	0.3	16	0	0.07	3	0.07	0.06	1.1	0.11	25	0
0.2	0.3	0	5	65	15	210	0.5	0.5	20	19	0.15	7	0.03	0.08	1.2	0.05	49	0
0.2	0.3	0	4	65	4	172	0.7	0.5	22	13	0.12	6	0.03	0.07	1.2	0.08	57	0
0.3	0.5	0	2	84	14	204	0.4	0.5	26	18	0.07	5	0.18	0.06	1.3	0.05	38	0
0.1	0.2	0	3	47	4	121	0.3	0.3	16	18	0.07	3	0.07	0.06	1.1	0.11	25	0
0.3	0.5	0	2	79	13	192	0.4	0.5	25	17	0.07	5	0.17	0.06	1.2	0.05	36	0
16.2	4	5	137	1178	2677	272	1.4	6	58	29	3.98	0	1.03	0.66	8	0.31	253	0.22
3.1	0.7	37	44	226	467	77	0.4	1.1	12	26	0.72	0	0.15	0.16	1.2	0.06	7	0.1
1.1	1.9	24	149	101	395	88	0.4	1.5	15	32	0.54	0	0.18	0.18	1.4	0.07	38	0.09
1.3	2.1	28	161	109	428	95	0.4	1.6	16	28	0.65	0	0.19	0.19	1.5	0.07	12	0.1
2.1	1	40	61	188	369	94	0.4	0.8	15	39	0.95	0	0.09	0.15	0.7	0.06	7	0.17
9.1	3.5	79	102	166	973	263	1.3	6.2	18	37	0.7	0	0.28	0.7	4.2	0.09	103	0.44
—	—	65	—	—	670	—	—	—	—	—	—	—	—	—	—	—	—	—
5.5	0.4	36	14	74	594	220	1.6	2.2	18	0	0.24	0	0.01	0.1	2.3	0.22	10	0.67
16.2	9	268	46	554	957	678	5.9	3.8	70	143	0.8	0	0.19	0.51	25.8	1.22	15	0.91
6.6	4.2	220	38	483	788	602	5.2	3	62	40	0.66	0	0.17	0.44	22.7	1.16	15	0.82
0.8	0.5	0	2	20	265	23	0.3	0.8	11	7	0.31	0	0.06	0.05	0.6	0.04	3	0
1.6	0.4	21	187	165	262	273	0.8	1	30	57	0.23	1	0.18	0.34	1.2	0.11	14	0.44
0.6	1	0	7	116	4	224	1	5.7	55	0	0.46	0	0.99	0.56	6.9	0.36	258	0
1.2	2	0	7	294	43	350	2.2	4.2	155	0	0.4	0	0.47	0.24	4.4	0.37	31	0
0.3	0.5	0	3	58	2	112	0.5	2.8	28	28	0.23	0	0.49	0.28	3.5	0.18	129	0
0.6	1	0	7	116	4	224	1	5.7	55	57	0.5	0	0.79	0.5	6.2	0.32	181	0
0.6	1	0	483	860	1860	235	1.4	6.5	68	57	0.28	0	0.94	0.53	6.3	0.54	258	0
0.6	1	0	4	147	21	175	1.1	2.1	78	29	0.41	0	0.24	0.12	2.2	0.18	16	0
1.3	0.6	0	3	51	176	52	0.3	0.3	20	6	0.18	0	0.06	0.03	0.3	0.03	0	0
1.3	0.6	0	2	50	99	50	0.3	0.3	20	0	0.18	0	0.01	0.02	0.3	0.04	0	0
0	0	0	0	0	0	0	0	0	0	0	0	0	0	0	0	0	0	0
0	0.1	0	7	20	4	52	0.2	0.3	7	0	0.01	0	0.06	0.02	0.9	0.05	13	0
0.1	0.3	0	22	122	16	323	1.6	2.6	83	1	0.32	0	0.14	0.04	0.6	0.08	122	0
1.7	1.4	90	63	128	198	194	2.4	0.6	20	49	0.9	2	0.05	0.05	1.7	0.1	32	3.56
4	2.8	162	125	229	336	345	3.8	1.2	34	125	2.23	7	0.13	0.19	2.8	0.19	49	6.27
1.8	3.6	72	79	147	513	266	2.9	0.7	24	18	1.43	3	0.08	0.05	2.3	0.14	40	4.93
7.3	1.3	212	124	193	446	266	2	1.2	27	263	1.49	1	0.07	0.2	1.5	0.11	22	2.48
3.5	2.6	81	70	126	576	255	2	1.1	23	121	1.91	6	0.11	0.12	2	0.12	31	3.17
0	0	0	10	8	1	107	—	0.2	4	2	0.32	4	0.02	0.01	0.1	—	—	0
0	0.1	0	4	28	120	27	0.2	1.2	6	0	0.1	0	0.16	0.11	1.4	0.01	5	0
0.2	0.8	0	26	120	32	132	0.8	5.3	28	0	0.06	0	0.8	0.54	6.6	0.04	132	0
0.5	0.1	2	18	16	24	6	0	0.2	1	2	0.03	0	0.02	0.02	0.2	0.01	1	0.02

Food Item	Qty	Meas	Wgt (g)	Wtr (g)	Cals	Prot (g)	Carb (g)	Fib (g)	Fat (g)	SatF (g)
Cracker, Cuban	4	each	20	1	80	2	15	0.4	1	0.3
Cracker, Finn Ry Krisp, thin	3	each	6	0	21	1	5	0.5	0	0
Cracker, Matzoh, egg	1	each	28	2	111	3	22	0.8	1	0.2
Cracker, Matzoh, egg & onion	1	each	28	2	111	3	22	1.4	1	0.3
Cracker, Matzoh, plain	1	each	28	1	112	3	24	0.9	0	0.1
Cracker, Matzoh, whole wheat	1	each	28	1	100	4	22	3.4	0	0.1
Cracker, Melba Toast, unsalted	4	piece	20	1	78	2	15	1.3	1	0.1
Cracker, Melba Toast, wheat	2	piece	10	1	37	1	8	0.7	0	0
Cracker, Melba toast, plain	1	piece	5	0	20	1	4	0.3	0	0
Cracker, Norwegian flatbread	4	each	23	1	85	2	19	3.8	0	0
Cracker, Premium, unsalted tops	4	each	12	—	50	2	8	0	1	0
Cracker, Saltine, unsalted top	4	each	20	1	87	2	14	0.6	2	0.6
Cracker, Saltine, whole wheat	4	each	12	0	52	1	8	0.8	2	0.4
Cracker, Wasa rye crispbread	2	piece	17	1	58	2	13	1.5	0	0
Cracker, Wheatsworth	6	each	18	1	86	1	12	1	4	1.6
Cracker, buttery, Ritz	10	each	30	1	151	2	18	0.5	8	1.1
Cracker, cheese w/peanut butter filling	4	each	30	1	145	4	17	0.8	7	1.6
Cracker, crispbread, Wasa extra crisp	4	each	24	1	95	3	18	1.7	2	0.4
Cracker, crispbread, wheat	4	each	24	1	94	3	20	0.7	0	0
Cracker, crispbread, white/rye, fat added	4	each	24	1	95	3	18	1.7	2	0.4
Cracker, graham, crumbs	0.25	cup	30	1	127	2	23	0.8	3	0.5
Cracker, graham, crust, baked	1	piece	54	2	268	2	35	0.8	14	2.8
Cracker, graham, plain/honey	2	each	14	1	59	1	11	0.4	1	0.2
Cracker, milk, New England Biscuit	2	each	22	1	100	2	15	0.4	3	0.7
Cracker, oat bran-oat thins	3	each	6	0	26	1	4	0.3	1	0.1
Cracker, rusk toast	2	each	20	1	81	3	14	0.4	1	0.3
Cracker, rye crispbread	3	each	30	2	110	2	25	5	0	0
Cracker, rye crispbread, low sodium	2	piece	14	1	48	2	11	2.3	0	0
Cracker, rye, Melba Toast	2	each	10	0	39	1	8	0.8	0	0
Cracker, rye, cheese filled	4	each	28	1	135	3	17	1	6	1.7
Cracker, rye, seasoned, triple	1	each	22	1	84	2	16	4.6	2	0.3
Cracker, sesame seed	8	each	24	1	120	2	15	0.4	6	0.9
Cracker, snack type, cheese-filled	4	each	28	1	134	3	17	0.5	6	1.7
Cracker, snack type, peanut butter-filled	4	each	28	1	137	3	16	0.8	7	1.6
Cracker, wheat	15	each	30	1	142	3	20	1.4	6	1.6
Cracker, wheat thin type, low sodium	10	each	20	1	92	2	14	0.4	4	1.1
Cracker, wheat'n bran, Triscuits	4	each	16	1	64	1	11	1.7	2	0.4
Cracker, wheat, 100% stoned wheat	4	each	16	1	64	1	11	1.7	2	0.4
Cracker, wheat, cheese-filled	4	each	28	1	139	3	16	0.9	7	1.2
Cracker, wheat, peanut butter-filled	4	each	28	1	139	4	15	1.2	7	1.3
Cracker, wheat, thin type	10	each	20	1	95	1	13	1.1	4	1.8
Cracker, whole wheat, Triscuit	2	each	9	0	40	1	6	0.9	2	0.3
Crackers, Cracked Pepper, Snackwell's	1	oz.	28	0	113	3	24	0.9	1	0.2
Crackers, Fire, chilis and cheese, fat free, Health Valley	6	each	15	1	50	2	11	2	0	0
Crackers, Pizza, zesty cheese, fat free, Health Valley	6	each	15	1	50	2	11	2	0	0
Crackers, buttery snack type (Club/Waverly)	7	each	28	1	141	2	17	0.4	7	1.1
Crackers, cheese, Cheez-its	10	each	10	0	50	1	6	0.2	3	0.9
Crackers, cheese, reduced fat, Snackwell's	1	oz.	28	1	119	3	22	0.9	2	0.6
Crackers, classic golden, reduced fat, Snackwell's	1	oz.	28	0	117	2	23	0.7	2	0.4
Crackers, cracked pepper, Snackwell's	1	each	15	0	60	2	12	0.5	0	0.1
Crackers, oyster	1	each	1	0	4	0	1	0	0	0
Crackers, oyster, crushed	0.25	cup	18	1	76	2	12	0.5	2	0.5
Crackers, saltine	4	each	12	0	52	1	9	0.4	1	0.4
Crackers, wheat, fat free, Snackwell's	1	oz.	28	0	113	3	23	1.2	1	0.2
Crackers, whole grain rye, Ry Krisp	2	each	14	1	47	1	11	3.2	0	0
Cranberries, fresh	0.5	cup	48	41	23	0	6	2	0	0
Cranberries, fresh, cooked, sauce	0.5	cup	138	84	209	0	54	1.4	0	0
Cranberry juice cocktail	1	cup	253	216	144	0	36	0.3	0	0
Cranberry juice cocktail, frozen, prepared	1	cup	249	214	137	0	35	0.2	0	0
Cranberry juice, low calorie, bottled	1	cup	237	226	45	0	11	0	0	0
Cranberry sauce, sweetened, canned	0.5	cup	138	84	209	0	54	1.4	0	0
Cranberry-apple drink, w/vitamin C, bottled	1	cup	253	209	170	0	43	0.3	0	0
Cranberry-apple juice drink, low calorie	1	cup	240	228	46	0	11	0.2	0	0
Cranberry-apricot juice drink, low calorie	1	cup	240	228	46	0	11	0.2	0	0
Cranberry-blackberry juice drink, low calorie	1	cup	240	228	46	0	11	0.2	0	0

MonoF	PolyF	Choles	Calc	Phos	Sod	Pot	Zn	Iron	Magn	VitA	VitE	VitC	Thia	Ribo	Nia	B6	Fola	B12
(g)	(g)	(mg)	(mg)	(mg)	(mg)	(mg)	(mg)	(mg)	(mg)	(μg RE)	(mg α-TE)	(mg)	(mg)	(mg)	(mg)	(mg)	(μg)	(μg)
0.7	0.2	0	15	18	52	52	0.1	0.3	9	0	0.22	0	0.02	0.01	0.2	0.02	3	0
0	0	0	3	23	53	36	0.2	0.2	7	0	0.11	0	0.02	0.02	0.1	0.02	3	0
0.2	0.1	24	11	42	6	42	0.2	0.8	7	4	0.28	0	0.22	0.18	1.4	0.02	33	0.05
0.3	0.3	13	10	25	81	24	0.2	1.2	9	2	0.17	0	0.16	0.12	1.4	0.03	45	0.06
0	0.2	0	4	25	1	32	0.2	0.9	7	0	0.02	0	0.11	0.08	1.1	0.03	33	0
0.1	0.2	0	7	86	1	90	0.7	1.3	38	0	0.38	0	0.1	0.08	1.5	0.04	14	0
0.2	0.3	0	19	39	4	40	0.4	0.7	12	0	0.01	0	0.08	0.06	0.8	0.02	25	0
0.1	0.1	0	4	16	84	15	0.2	0.4	6	0	0.04	0	0.04	0.03	0.5	0.01	13	0
0	0.1	0	5	10	42	10	0.1	0.2	3	0	0	0	0.02	0.01	0.2	0	6	0
0	0.1	0	7	62	61	74	0.6	0.6	18	0	0.31	0	0.06	0.03	0.2	0.05	11	0
0	0	0	—	—	100	10	—	0.7	—	—	0.2	—	—	—	—	—	—	—
1.3	0.3	0	24	21	127	145	0.2	1.1	5	0	0.31	0	0.11	0.09	1	0.01	25	0
0.9	0.2	0	3	23	124	26	0.2	0.5	8	0	0.28	0	0.06	0.04	0.6	0.02	3	0
0	0.1	0	9	66	150	102	0.5	0.7	20	0	0.32	0	0.05	0.04	0.2	0.05	8	0
1.8	0.4	4	6	32	157	36	0.3	0.6	11	1	0.05	0	0.09	0.06	0.8	0.02	3	0.08
3.2	2.9	0	36	68	254	40	0.2	1.1	8	0	1.36	0	0.12	0.1	1.2	0.02	23	0
3.5	1.4	2	24	97	298	74	0.3	0.9	17	10	1.12	0	0.12	0.1	2	0.45	26	0
0.8	0.3	0	20	45	153	68	0.3	0.8	11	0	0.34	0	0.1	0.08	0.8	0.03	4	0.03
0	0.1	0	4	28	120	27	0.2	1.2	6	0	0.1	0	0.16	0.11	1.4	0.01	5	0
0.8	0.3	0	20	45	153	68	0.3	0.8	11	0	0.34	0	0.1	0.08	0.8	0.03	4	0.03
1.2	1.2	0	7	31	182	40	0.2	1.1	9	0	0.61	0	0.07	0.09	1.2	0.02	18	0
6.2	3.8	0	11	35	309	48	0.3	1.2	10	109	2.21	0	0.06	0.1	1.2	0.02	13	0.01
0.6	0.5	0	3	15	85	19	0.1	0.5	4	0	0.29	0	0.03	0.04	0.6	0.01	8	0
1.9	0.5	2	38	67	130	25	0.1	0.8	5	2	0.6	0	0.12	0.09	1	0.01	18	0.02
0.3	0.3	0	5	17	36	12	0.1	0.2	4	0	0.14	0	0.03	0.02	0.2	0	1	0
0.6	0.5	16	5	31	51	49	0.2	0.5	7	2	0.1	0	0.08	0.08	0.9	0.01	17	0.04
0	0.2	0	9	81	79	96	0.7	0.7	23	0	0.4	0	0.07	0.04	0.3	0.06	14	0
0	0.1	0	7	54	33	84	0.4	0.5	17	0	0.26	0	0.04	0.04	0.2	0.04	6	0
0.1	0.1	0	8	18	90	19	0.1	0.4	4	0	0.06	0	0.05	0.03	0.5	0.01	8	0
3.4	0.8	3	62	95	292	96	0.2	0.7	10	11	0.56	0	0.17	0.14	1	0.02	23	0.03
0.7	0.8	0	10	68	195	100	0.6	0.7	23	0	0.44	0	0.07	0.05	0.5	0.04	3	0
2.5	2.3	0	29	55	203	32	0.2	0.9	6	0	1.08	0	0.1	0.08	1	0.01	18	0
3.2	0.7	1	72	114	392	120	0.2	0.7	10	5	0.14	0	0.12	0.19	1.1	0.01	24	0.03
3.5	1.2	0	27	68	264	62	0.3	0.9	15	0	1.04	0	0.12	0.09	1.6	0.03	24	0
3.4	0.8	0	15	66	239	55	0.5	1.3	19	0	0.97	0	0.15	0.1	1.5	0.04	13	0
1.3	0.9	0	6	38	50	43	0.2	0.8	10	3	0.12	0	0.1	0.07	0.9	0.03	5	0
1.2	0.3	0	4	32	86	22	0.2	0.5	11	0	0.59	0	0.08	0.05	0.7	0.02	4	0.15
1.2	0.3	0	4	30	88	19	0.2	0.5	10	0	0.59	0	0.08	0.05	0.7	0.02	4	0.16
2.9	2.6	2	57	107	256	86	0.2	0.7	15	3	0.17	0	0.1	0.12	0.9	0.07	18	0.03
3.3	2.5	0	48	97	226	83	0.2	0.7	11	0	0.17	0	0.11	0.08	1.6	0.04	20	0
2	0.5	4	6	36	174	40	0.3	0.7	13	1	0.05	0	0.1	0.07	0.8	0.03	4	0.08
0.5	0.6	0	4	27	59	27	0.2	0.3	9	0	0.1	0	0.02	0.01	0.4	0.02	4	0
0.1	0.3	0	49	96	280	36	0.3	1.4	7	0	—	0	0.1	0.12	1.5	0.02	—	—
0	0	0	0	—	80	—	—	0	—	20	—	1	—	—	—	—	—	—
0	0	0	0	—	140	—	—	0	—	20	—	1	—	—	—	—	—	—
3	2.7	0	34	64	237	37	0.2	1	8	0	1.27	0	0.11	0.1	1.1	0.02	22	0
1.2	0.2	1	15	22	100	14	0.1	0.5	4	3	0.26	0	0.06	0.04	0.5	0.06	8	0.05
0.6	0.2	2	18	45	320	43	0.3	1.4	8	12	—	0	0.11	0.16	1.8	0.03	—	0.01
0.6	0.2	0	56	104	292	31	0.2	1.2	6	0	—	0	0.18	0.12	1.4	0.02	—	0.01
0	0.1	0	26	51	148	19	0.1	0.7	4	0	—	0	0.05	0.06	0.8	0.01	—	—
0.1	0	0	1	1	13	1	0	0.1	0	0	0.02	0	0.01	0	0.1	0	1	0
1.1	0.3	0	21	18	228	22	0.1	0.9	5	0	0.27	0	0.1	0.08	0.9	0.01	22	0
0.8	0.2	0	14	13	156	15	0.1	0.6	3	0	0.19	0	0.07	0.06	0.6	0	15	0
0.2	0.3	0	52	116	320	81	0.4	1.1	13	0	—	0	0.08	0.14	1.4	0.03	—	0.04
0	0.1	0	6	47	111	69	0.4	0.8	17	0	0.2	0	0.06	0.04	0.2	0.04	2	0
0	0	0	3	4	0	34	0.1	0.1	2	2	0.05	6	0.01	0.01	0	0.03	1	0
0	0.1	0	6	8	40	36	0.1	0.3	4	3	0.14	3	0.02	0.03	0.1	0.02	1	0
0	0.1	0	8	5	5	46	0.2	0.4	5	1	0	90	0.02	0.02	0.1	0.05	1	0
0	0	0	12	2	7	35	0.1	0.2	5	2	0.02	25	0.02	0.02	0	0.04	0	0
0	0	0	21	2	7	52	0	0.1	5	1	0	76	0.02	0.02	0.1	0.04	0	0
0	0.1	0	6	8	40	36	0.1	0.3	4	3	0.14	3	0.02	0.03	0.1	0.02	1	0
0	0	0	18	8	5	68	0.1	0.2	5	1	0	81	0.01	0.05	0.2	0.05	1	0
0	0	0	17	7	5	65	0.1	0.1	5	1	0	77	0	0.05	0.1	0.05	0	0
0	0	0	17	7	5	65	0.1	0.1	5	1	0	77	0	0.05	0.1	0.05	0	0
0	0	0	17	7	5	65	0.1	0.1	5	1	0	77	0	0.05	0.1	0.05	0	0

Food Item	Qty	Meas	Wgt (g)	Wtr (g)	Cals	Prot (g)	Carb (g)	Fib (g)	Fat (g)	SatF (g)
Cranberry-grape juice drink, low calorie	1	cup	240	228	46	0	11	0.2	0	0
Cranberry-raspberry juice drink, low calorie	1	cup	240	228	46	0	11	0.2	0	0
Cream of tartar	0.25	tsp	1	0	2	0	1	0	0	0
Cream of tartar	0.25	tsp	1	0	1	0	0	0	0	0
Cream puff shell, recipe	1	each	66	27	239	6	15	0.5	17	3.7
Cream puff, custard-filled	1	each	110	59	284	7	25	0.4	17	4
Cream, coffee/table	1	Tbs	15	11	29	0	1	0	3	1.8
Cream, half & half	2	Tbs	30	24	39	1	1	0	3	2.2
Cream, medium, 25% fat	1	Tbs	15	10	36	0	1	0	4	2.3
Cream, sour, cultured	2	Tbs	29	20	62	1	1	0	6	3.7
Cream, sour, imitation, IMO	2	Tbs	29	20	60	1	2	0	6	5.1
Cream, sour, low cal, half & half	2	Tbs	30	24	40	1	1	0	4	2.2
Cream, whipped, pressurized	2	Tbs	8	5	19	0	1	0	2	1
Cream, whipping, heavy	2	Tbs	30	17	103	1	1	0	11	6.8
Cream, whipping, heavy	2	Tbs	15	9	51	0	0	0	6	3.4
Cream, whipping, light	1	Tbs	30	19	87	1	1	0	9	5.8
Cream, whipping, light	2	Tbs	15	9	44	0	0	0	5	2.9
Creamer, non-dairy, Cremora	1	tsp	2	—	10	0	1	—	0	0.5
Creamer, non-dairy, Mocha Mix	1	Tbs	14	11	19	0	1	0	2	0.3
Creamer, non-dairy, powdered coffee whitener	1	tsp	2	0	11	0	1	0	1	0.6
Crepe suzette w/sauce	1	each	66	36	161	4	16	0.3	9	4.2
Crepe, chocolate-filled	1	each	78	53	119	4	15	0.6	5	2
Crepe, fruit-filled	1	each	78	49	131	4	21	0.9	4	1.2
Cress, garden, cooked, drained	0.5	cup	68	62	16	1	3	0.5	0	0
Cress, garden, raw	0.5	cup	25	22	8	1	1	0.3	0	0
Cress, garden, raw sprigs	20	each	20	18	6	1	1	0.2	0	0
Croissant, apple	1	each	57	26	145	4	21	1.4	5	2.8
Croissant, butter	1	each	57	13	231	5	26	1.5	12	6.7
Croissant, cheese	1	each	57	12	236	5	27	1.5	12	6
Croissant, chocolate	1	each	56	12	233	5	23	1.6	14	8.2
Croissant, egg & cheese	1	each	127	58	368	13	24	—	25	14.1
Croutons, dry	0.25	cup	8	0	30	1	6	0.4	0	0.1
Croutons, seasoned	3	Tbs	7	0	33	1	4	0.4	1	0.4
Cucumber salad, cucumber & vinegar	0.5	cup	80	72	24	0	6	0.6	0	0
Cucumber, kim chee	0.5	cup	75	68	16	1	4	1.1	0	0
Cucumber, w/peel, raw slices	0.5	cup	52	50	7	0	1	0.4	0	0
Cucumber, w/peel, raw, whole	1	each	301	289	39	2	8	2.4	0	0.1
Cumin seed	0.25	tsp	0	0	2	0	0	0.1	0	0
Cupcake, chocolate w/chocolate icing-commercial	1	each	42	10	154	2	23	1.2	7	2
Currants, black, fresh	0.5	cup	56	46	35	1	9	4.1	0	0
Currants, dried (Zante)	0.5	cup	72	14	204	3	53	4.9	0	0
Currants, red/white, fresh	0.5	cup	56	47	31	1	8	2.4	0	0
Curry powder	0.25	tsp	1	0	2	0	0	0.2	0	0
Custard apple, raw	4	oz.	113	81	115	2	29	4.2	1	0.1
Custard, egg, baked, recipe	0.5	cup	141	111	148	7	15	0	7	3.3
Custard, egg, mix, w/2% milk	0.5	cup	133	99	149	6	24	0	4	1.9
Custard, egg, prepared mix w/whole milk	0.5	cup	133	97	162	5	23	0	5	3
Dairy Queen blizzard, heath, regular size	1	each	404	236	820	14	119	1	33	20
Dairy Queen breeze, heath, frozen yogurt	1	each	379	229	666	14	115	0.9	17	10.3
Dairy Queen shake, chocolate	1	each	397	273	567	12	96	0	15	9.6
Dairy Queen, Buster bar	1	each	149	67	450	10	41	2	28	12
Dairy Queen, Dilly Bar	1	each	85	47	210	3	21	0	13	7
Dairy Queen, Mr. Misty, regular size	1	each	330	267	250	0	63	0	0	0
Dairy Queen, banana split	1	each	369	249	510	8	96	3	12	8
Dairy Queen, blizzard, strawberry	1	each	383	259	570	12	95	1	16	11
Dairy Queen, breeze, strawberry frozen yogurt	1	each	354	246	425	12	92	0.9	1	0.9
Dairy Queen, cheeseburger, single	1	each	156	86	349	20	30	2	17	8.2
Dairy Queen, choc dipped vanilla cone, regular	1	each	156	92	340	6	42	0.7	17	8.7
Dairy Queen, chocolate cone, regular	1	each	142	90	240	6	37	0	7	5.3
Dairy Queen, hamburger, single	1	each	142	80	298	18	30	2.1	12	5.1
Dairy Queen, hot fudge brownie delight	1	each	305	160	710	11	102	0.6	29	14
Dairy Queen, hotdog	1	each	99	57	240	9	19	1	14	5
Dairy Queen, hotdog, w/cheese	1	each	113	62	290	12	20	1	18	8
Dairy Queen, malt, vanilla, regular size	1	each	418	285	610	13	106	0.3	14	8
Dairy Queen, peanut buster parfait	1	each	305	156	730	16	99	2	31	17

MonoF	PolyF	Choles	Calc	Phos	Sod	Pot	Zn	Iron	Magn	VitA	VitE	VitC	Thia	Ribo	Nia	B6	Fola	B12
(g)	(g)	(mg)	(mg)	(mg)	(mg)	(mg)	(mg)	(mg)	(mg)	(μg RE)	(mg α-TE)	(mg)	(mg)	(mg)	(mg)	(mg)	(μg)	(μg)
0	0	0	17	7	5	65	0.1	0.1	5	1	0	77	0	0.05	0.1	0.05	0	0
0	0	0	17	7	5	65	0.1	0.1	5	1	0	77	0	0.05	0.1	0.05	0	0
0	0	0	0	0	0	137	0	0	0	0	0	0	0	0	0	0	0	0
0	0	0	0	0	58	30	—	0	—	0	—	0	0	0	0	—	—	—
7.3	4.9	129	24	78	368	64	0.5	1.3	8	203	2.54	0	0.14	0.24	1	0.05	32	0.26
7.2	4.6	147	73	120	375	127	0.7	1.3	13	219	2.43	0	0.13	0.31	0.9	0.07	31	0.4
0.8	0.1	10	14	12	6	18	0	0	1	27	0.02	0	0	0.02	0	0	0	0.03
1	0.1	11	32	29	12	39	0.2	0	3	32	0.03	0	0.01	0.04	0	0.01	1	0.1
1.1	0.1	13	14	10	6	17	0	0	1	35	0.09	0	0	0.02	0	0	0	0.03
1.7	0.2	13	33	24	15	41	0.1	0	3	56	0.16	0	0.01	0.04	0	0	3	0.09
0.2	0	0	1	13	29	46	0.3	0.1	2	0	0.04	0	0	0	0	0	0	0
1	0.1	12	31	28	12	39	0.2	0	3	34	0.1	0	0.01	0.04	0	0	3	0.09
0.5	0.1	6	8	7	10	11	0	0	1	16	0.04	0	0	0	0	0	0	0.02
3.2	0.4	41	19	19	11	22	0.1	0	2	125	0.19	0	0.01	0.03	0	0.01	1	0.05
1.6	0.2	20	10	9	6	11	0	0	1	63	0.09	0	0	0.02	0	0	1	0.03
2.7	0.3	33	21	18	10	29	0.1	0	2	88	0.18	0	0.01	0.04	0	0.01	1	0.06
1.4	0.1	17	10	9	5	14	0	0	1	44	0.09	0	0	0.02	0	0	1	0.03
—	—	—	—	—	5	15	—	—	—	—	—	—	—	—	—	—	—	—
0	0.7	0	1	8	7	20	—	—	0	—	—	—	—	—	—	—	—	—
0	0	0	0	8	4	16	0	0	0	0	0	0	0	0	0	0	0	0
3.2	1.2	84	45	68	163	84	0.4	0.8	8	76	0.72	3	0.08	0.17	0.6	0.04	11	0.22
1.7	0.7	58	81	89	148	126	0.5	0.7	12	58	0.52	0	0.07	0.2	0.4	0.04	8	0.27
1.5	0.8	63	38	59	124	90	0.3	0.7	8	59	0.92	4	0.08	0.16	0.6	0.04	9	0.19
0.1	0.1	0	41	32	5	238	0.1	0.5	18	520	0.47	16	0.04	0.11	0.5	0.11	25	0
0.1	0.1	0	20	19	4	152	0.1	0.3	10	233	0.18	17	0.02	0.06	0.2	0.06	20	0
0	0	0	16	15	3	121	0	0.3	8	186	0.14	14	0.02	0.05	0.2	0.05	16	0
1.4	0.4	18	17	33	156	51	0.6	0.6	7	56	0.11	0	0.13	0.09	0.9	0.02	32	0.11
3.2	0.6	38	21	60	424	67	0.4	1.2	9	106	0.25	0	0.22	0.14	1.2	0.03	35	0.09
3.7	1.4	32	30	74	316	75	0.5	1.2	14	112	0.59	0	0.3	0.18	1.2	0.04	42	0.18
4.2	0.7	56	31	82	257	113	0.6	1.7	28	105	0.42	0	0.19	0.21	2	0.05	19	0.1
7.5	1.4	216	244	348	551	174	1.8	2.2	22	255	—	0	0.19	0.38	1.5	0.1	47	0.78
0.2	0.1	0	6	9	52	9	0.1	0.3	2	0	0.02	0	0.05	0.02	0.4	0	10	0
0.4	0.2	0	7	10	87	13	0.1	0.2	3	1	0.15	0	0.04	0.03	0.3	0.01	6	0.01
0	0	0	10	13	175	105	0.1	0.3	10	2	0.05	3	0.02	0.01	0.2	0.04	8	0
0	0	0	7	10	766	88	0.4	3.6	6	25	0.12	3	0.02	0.02	0.3	0.08	17	0
0	0	0	7	10	1	75	0.1	0.1	6	11	0.04	3	0.01	0.01	0.1	0.02	7	0
0	0.2	0	42	60	6	433	0.6	0.8	33	63	0.24	16	0.07	0.07	0.7	0.13	39	0
0.1	0	0	5	2	1	9	0	0.3	2	1	0	0	0	0	0	0	0	0
3.7	0.8	18	18	51	140	84	0.3	0.9	14	10	0.71	0	0.01	0.06	0.2	0.02	7	0.06
0	0.1	0	31	33	1	180	0.2	0.9	13	13	0.06	101	0.03	0.03	0.2	0.04	2	0
0	0.1	0	62	90	6	642	0.5	2.4	30	5	0.07	3	0.12	0.1	1.2	0.21	7	0
0	0	0	18	25	1	154	0.1	0.6	7	7	0.06	23	0.02	0.03	0.1	0.04	4	0
0	0	0	2	2	0	8	0	0.2	1	1	0	0	0	0	0	0	1	0
0.2	0.1	0	34	24	5	433	0.5	0.8	20	3	—	22	0.09	0.11	0.6	0.25	—	0
2.1	0.5	123	158	159	109	216	0.7	0.4	20	85	0.34	1	0.05	0.32	0.1	0.07	14	0.44
1.2	0.3	74	197	176	200	287	0.7	0.3	27	74	0.27	1	0.07	0.29	0.2	0.08	11	0.61
1.7	0.3	81	194	174	198	283	0.7	0.3	25	44	0.13	1	0.07	0.29	0.2	0.08	11	0.6
—	—	60	450	450	580	730	—	1.8	—	300	—	1	0.15	0.76	—	—	—	—
—	—	19	422	449	544	539	—	2.5	—	19	—	2	0.12	0.76	—	—	—	—
—	—	52	442	400	309	600	—	2	—	295	—	2	0.12	0.59	0.8	—	—	—
—	—	15	150	250	280	400	—	1.1	—	80	—	0	0.09	0.17	3	0.08	—	—
3	3	10	100	80	75	170	—	0.4	—	60	—	0	0.03	0.14	—	0.06	—	—
0	0	0	0	—	10	—	—	0	—	0	—	2	0	0	—	0	—	—
—	—	30	250	40	180	860	—	1.8	—	200	—	15	0.15	0.26	0.4	0.2	—	—
—	—	50	450	350	260	700	—	1.8	—	300	—	9	0.15	0.68	—	—	—	—
0	0	9	416	349	250	490	—	2.5	—	0	—	8	0.12	0.68	—	—	—	—
—	—	56	154	249	872	270	—	3.7	—	62	—	4	0.3	0.34	4	—	—	—
—	—	20	200	150	133	290	—	1.2	—	100	—	2	0.06	0.26	0.1	0.09	—	—
—	—	20	167	200	120	350	—	1.2	—	133	—	1	0.06	0.26	—	—	—	—
6.2	1	46	62	149	648	259	—	2.8	—	41	—	4	0.3	0.25	4	—	—	—
12	2	35	300	600	340	510	—	5.4	—	80	—	1	0.15	0.68	0.3	0.18	—	—
—	—	25	60	60	730	170	—	1.8	—	20	—	4	0.22	0.14	2	—	—	—
8	2	40	150	150	950	180	—	1.8	—	60	—	4	0.22	0.17	2	—	—	—
2	2	45	400	350	230	570	—	1.4	—	80	—	0	0.12	0.6	0.8	0.19	—	—
—	—	35	300	450	400	660	—	1.8	—	150	—	1	0.15	0.51	3	0.22	—	—

Food Item	Qty	Meas	Wgt (g)	Wtr (g)	Cals	Prot (g)	Carb (g)	Fib (g)	Fat (g)	SatF (g)
Dairy Queen, quarter pound super hotdog	1	each	198	98	590	20	41	—	38	16
Dairy Queen, sundae, chocolate, regular	1	each	177	110	301	6	54	0	7	4.4
Dairy Queen, sundae, nutty double fudge	1	each	276	—	570	10	85	—	22	10
Dairy Queen, ultimate burger, double bacon-cheese	1	each	276	159	687	41	30	2	44	19.5
Dandelion greens, cooked, drained	0.5	cup	52	47	17	1	3	1.5	0	0.1
Danish pastry, cheese	1	each	91	31	353	6	29	—	25	5.1
Danish pastry, cinnamon	1	each	88	18	349	5	47	0.3	17	3.5
Danish pastry, cinnamon	1	each	88	18	349	5	47	0.3	17	3.5
Danish pastry, fruit filled	1	each	94	27	335	5	45	—	16	3.3
Dates, chopped	0.5	cup	89	20	245	2	65	6.7	0	0.2
Dates, whole	10	each	83	19	228	2	61	6.2	0	0.2
Deer/venison steak, fried	1	each	85	52	146	28	0	0	3	1.2
Deer/venison, roasted	4	oz.	113	74	179	34	0	0	4	1.4
Dessert topping, low cal, mix, prepared	1	Tbs	5	4	3	0	1	0	0	0.3
Dessert topping, low cal, mix, prepared	2	Tbs	10	8	5	0	1	0	1	0.6
Dessert topping, mix w/whole milk (Dream Whip)	1	Tbs	5	3	9	0	1	0	1	0.5
Dessert topping, mix w/whole milk (Dream Whip)	2	Tbs	10	7	19	0	2	0	1	1.1
Dessert topping, non-dairy, frozen (Cool Whip)	1	Tbs	5	2	15	0	1	0	1	1
Dessert topping, non-dairy, frozen (Cool Whip)	2	Tbs	9	5	30	0	2	0	2	2
Dessert topping, non-dairy, pressurized	1	Tbs	4	3	12	0	1	0	1	0.8
Dessert topping, non-dairy, pressurized	2	Tbs	9	5	23	0	1	0	2	1.6
Dill seed	1	tsp	2	0	7	0	1	0.5	0	0
Dill weed, dried	0.25	tsp	0	0	1	0	0	0	0	0
Dill weed, fresh sprig	0.25	cup	2	2	1	0	0	0	0	0
Dip, Jalapeno pepper bean	1	Tbs	33	22	46	2	6	2.2	2	0.2
Dip, caramel, Marie's	2	cup	35	5	150	0	24	1	5	4
Dip, sour cream, buttermilk/onion	2	Tbs	30	20	67	1	2	0.2	6	3.7
Dip, sour cream, low calorie	2	Tbs	30	22	44	1	2	0.2	3	2.1
Distilled spirits, 100 proof	1	oz.	28	16	84	0	0	0	0	0
Distilled spirits, 80 proof, all	1	oz.	28	19	66	0	0	0	0	0
Distilled spirits, 86 proof, all	1	oz.	28	18	71	0	0	0	0	0
Distilled spirits, 90 proof, all	1	oz.	28	18	75	0	0	0	0	0
Distilled spirits, 94 proof	1	oz.	28	17	78	0	0	0	0	0
Dock/sorrel greens, cooked	0.5	cup	50	47	10	1	1	1.3	0	—
Domino's pizza, pepperoni, deep dish	2	piece	218	94	622	26	63	3.3	29	11.3
Domino's pizza, pepperoni, hand tossed	2	piece	159	72	406	18	50	2.6	15	6.5
Domino's pizza, pepperoni, thin crust	1	piece	59	26	169	7	15	0.8	9	3.5
Domino's pizza, sausage mushroom, deep dish	2	piece	236	111	618	26	66	3.8	28	10.8
Domino's pizza, vegetarian, hand tossed	2	piece	176	95	360	15	52	3	10	4.6
Domino's pizza, veggie, deep dish	2	piece	236	117	576	24	65	3.8	25	9.2
Domino's pizza, veggie, thin crust	1	piece	68	37	146	6	16	1	6	2.4
Doo Dads, original flavor	0.5	cup	28	1	129	3	18	1.9	5	1
Doughnut, Eclair, chocolate, custard-filled	1	each	94	49	246	6	23	0.6	15	3.9
Doughnut, French cruller, glazed	1	each	41	7	169	1	24	0.5	8	1.9
Doughnut, Mexican crueller	1	each	26	6	116	1	12	0.2	7	1.4
Doughnut, cake, chocolate w/choc icing	1	each	42	7	175	2	24	0.9	8	2.2
Doughnut, cake, chocolate-iced	1	each	43	6	204	2	21	0.9	13	3.5
Doughnut, cake, plain	1	each	50	10	211	2	25	0.8	12	1.8
Doughnut, cake, sugared/glazed	1	each	45	9	192	2	23	0.7	10	2.7
Doughnut, custard filled, Bismarck	1	each	70	20	261	3	34	1	13	5.9
Doughnut, eggless, carob-coated, raised	1	each	78	21	285	5	32	5.4	18	2.6
Doughnut, fritter, apple	1	each	24	9	87	1	8	0.3	6	1.6
Doughnut, oriental, Okinawan	1	each	18	3	75	1	10	0.2	4	0.9
Doughnut, wheat, sugared/glazed	1	each	45	13	162	3	19	1	9	1.4
Doughnut, yeast, chocolate, w/choc icing	1	each	71	20	273	4	30	2.5	16	7.5
Doughnut, yeast, creme-filled	1	each	85	32	307	5	26	0.7	21	4.6
Doughnut, yeast, glazed	1	each	60	15	242	4	27	0.7	14	3.5
Doughnut, yeast, jelly-filled	1	each	65	23	221	4	25	0.6	12	3.2
Drink mix, citrus, Crystal Light	1	cup	238	237	5	0	0	0	0	0
Duck meat, skinless, roasted	4	oz.	113	73	228	27	0	0	13	4.7
Duck, domestic, w/skin, roasted	4	oz.	113	59	382	22	0	0	32	11
Dumpling, apple	1	each	151	78	357	2	53	2.5	16	3.6
Dumpling, plain, medium	1	each	32	22	42	1	7	0.2	1	0.4
Egg Beaters, Fleischmann's	0.5	cup	122	—	60	12	2	0	0	0
Egg Delight, frozen, prepared	0.5	cup	70	51	92	9	5	0	4	0.7

MonoF (g)	PolyF (g)	Choles (mg)	Calc (mg)	Phos (mg)	Sod (mg)	Pot (mg)	Zn (mg)	Iron (mg)	Magn (mg)	VitA (μg RE)	VitE (mg α-TE)	VitC (mg)	Thia (mg)	Ribo (mg)	Nia (mg)	B6 (mg)	Fola (μg)	B12 (μg)
16	4	60	100	150	1360	340	—	2.7	—	—	—	—	0.45	0.34	5	—	—	—
—	—	22	184	150	154	289	—	1.1	—	110	—	0	0.06	0.26	0.3	0.14	—	—
9	3	35	300	300	170	450	—	3.6	—	60	—	—	0.12	0.6	—	—	—	—
—	—	139	616	399	1241	479	—	2.8	—	41	—	4	0.44	0.5	7.9	—	—	—
0	0.1	0	74	22	23	122	0.1	0.9	13	614	1.31	9	0.07	0.09	0.3	0.08	7	0
15.6	2.4	20	70	80	319	116	0.6	1.8	16	43	—	3	0.26	0.21	2.6	0.06	55	0.23
10.6	1.6	27	37	74	326	96	0.5	1.8	14	5	0.79	3	0.26	0.19	2.2	0.05	55	0.22
10.6	1.6	27	37	74	326	96	0.5	1.8	14	5	0.79	3	0.26	0.19	2.2	0.05	55	0.22
10.1	1.6	19	22	69	333	110	0.5	1.4	14	24	0.85	2	0.29	0.21	1.8	0.06	31	0.24
0.1	0	0	28	36	3	580	0.3	1	31	4	0.09	0	0.08	0.09	2	0.17	11	0
0.1	0	0	27	33	2	541	0.2	1	29	4	0.08	0	0.08	0.08	1.8	0.16	10	0
0.9	0.6	102	6	206	331	305	2.5	4.1	24	0	0.24	0	0.14	0.55	5.7	0.22	5	5.3
1	0.7	127	8	256	61	380	3.1	5.1	27	0	0.28	0	0.2	0.68	7.6	0.43	5	3.61
0	0	0	0	2	5	1	0	0	0	0	0	0	0	0	0	0	0	0
0	0	0	0	3	11	3	0	0	0	0	0	0	0	0	0	0	0	0
0	0	0	5	4	3	8	0	0	0	2	0.01	0	0	0.01	0	0	0	0.01
0.1	0	1	9	9	7	15	0	0	1	5	0.01	0	0	0.01	0	0	0	0.03
0.1	0	0	0	0	1	1	0	0	0	4	0.01	0	0	0	0	0	0	0
0.2	0	0	1	1	2	2	0	0	0	8	0.02	0	0	0	0	0	0	0
0.1	0	0	0	1	3	1	0	0	0	2	0.01	0	0	0	0	0	0	0
0.2	0	0	0	2	5	2	0	0	0	4	0.02	0	0	0	0	0	0	0
0.2	0	0	33	6	0	26	0.1	0.4	6	0	0.02	0	0.01	0.01	0.1	0.01	0	0
0	0	0	5	1	1	9	0	0.1	1	2	—	0	0	0	0	0	—	0
0	0	0	5	1	1	16	0	0.1	1	17	—	2	0	0.01	0	0	3	0
0.4	1	0	11	34	382	96	0.2	0.5	12	18	0.38	4	0.03	0.02	0.1	0.03	23	0
—	—	5	20	—	75	—	—	0	—	0	—	0	—	—	—	—	—	—
1.8	0.2	13	36	32	228	56	0.1	0.1	5	55	0.18	0	0.02	0.06	0.1	0.01	3	0.08
1	0.1	11	32	34	212	51	0.2	0.1	4	31	0.11	0	0.02	0.06	0.1	0.01	3	0.08
0	0	0	0	1	0	1	0	0	0	0	0	0	0	0	0	0	0	0
0	0	0	0	1	0	1	0	0	0	0	0	0	0	0	0	0	0	0
0	0	0	0	1	0	1	0	0	0	0	0	0	0	0	0	0	0	0
0	0	0	0	1	0	1	0	0	0	0	0	0	0	0	0	0	0	0
0	0	0	0	1	0	1	0	0	0	0	0	0	0	0	0	0	0	0
—	—	0	19	26	2	161	0.1	1	44	174	0.5	13	0.02	0.04	0.2	0.05	4	0
—	—	44	456	—	1382	—	—	5	—	155	—	3	—	—	—	—	—	—
—	—	32	282	—	1179	—	—	4.3	—	94	—	3	—	—	—	—	—	—
—	—	16	162	—	484	—	—	0.7	—	44	—	1	—	—	—	—	—	—
—	—	43	460	—	1355	—	—	5.2	—	158	—	4	—	—	—	—	—	—
—	—	19	286	—	1028	—	—	4.4	—	99	—	13	—	—	—	—	—	—
—	—	32	460	—	1232	—	—	5.2	—	160	—	13	—	—	—	—	—	—
—	—	10	164	—	408	—	—	0.7	—	47	—	6	—	—	—	—	—	—
3.2	0.9	0	21	84	360	78	0.6	0.7	17	12	0.04	0	0.1	0.07	1.5	0.06	11	0
6.1	3.7	119	59	101	317	110	0.6	1.1	14	180	1.97	0	0.11	0.25	0.8	0.06	26	0.32
4.3	0.9	5	11	50	141	32	0.1	1	5	1	1.02	0	0.07	0.09	0.9	0.01	14	0.02
3	2.6	2	2	8	37	8	0.1	0.3	2	6	1.11	0	0.04	0.03	0.4	0	1	0
4.8	1	24	90	68	143	44	0.2	1	14	5	1.13	0	0.02	0.03	0.2	0.01	16	0.04
7.5	1.6	26	15	87	184	84	0.3	1.1	17	5	1.79	0	0.06	0.04	0.6	0.02	12	0.1
4.6	3.9	18	22	135	273	64	0.3	1	10	8	1.92	0	0.11	0.12	0.9	0.03	24	0.14
5.7	1.3	14	27	53	181	46	0.2	0.5	8	1	0.45	0	0.1	0.09	0.7	0.01	21	0.11
5.3	0.9	20	27	43	125	50	0.6	1	13	4	1.91	0	0.11	0.12	0.9	0.04	13	0.17
6.4	7.4	0	77	146	74	218	1.1	1.6	56	0	2.74	0	0.14	0.13	2.3	0.16	30	0
2.4	1.4	21	13	22	10	34	0.1	0.3	3	12	0.55	0	0.04	0.06	0.3	0.02	3	0.06
1.5	0.9	13	19	19	49	15	0.1	0.4	2	7	0.34	0	0.04	0.05	0.4	0.01	2	0.03
3.6	3.2	9	22	47	160	67	0.3	0.5	10	7	1.62	0	0.1	0.11	0.8	0.04	9	0.08
6.5	1.2	22	31	74	129	110	0.9	1.6	35	10	2.17	0	0.12	0.14	1	0.04	15	0.18
10.3	2.6	20	21	65	263	68	0.7	1.6	17	16	2.35	0	0.29	0.13	1.9	0.06	54	0.12
7.7	1.7	4	26	56	205	65	0.5	1.2	13	2	1.84	0	0.22	0.13	1.7	0.03	26	0.05
6.6	1.6	17	16	55	190	51	0.5	1.1	13	10	1.6	0	0.2	0.09	1.4	0.06	40	0.14
0	0	0	0	—	0	45	—	0	—	0	—	6	—	—	—	—	—	0
4.2	1.6	101	14	230	74	286	3	3.1	23	26	0.79	0	0.3	0.53	5.8	0.28	11	0.45
14.6	4.1	95	12	177	67	231	2.1	3.1	18	71	0.79	0	0.2	0.3	5.5	0.2	7	0.34
8.2	3.4	0	50	38	302	212	0.2	1.3	16	94	3.24	5	0.1	0.07	0.8	0.07	6	0.01
0.4	0.2	1	33	22	105	21	0.1	0.4	3	2	0.1	0	0.06	0.05	0.5	0.01	2	0.02
0	0	0	80	—	200	170	—	2.2	—	80	0.59	—	—	—	—	—	—	—
1.6	1.2	46	12	21	113	103	0.1	0.2	7	172	0.59	0	0.01	0.21	0.1	0.01	12	0.12

A

Food Item	Qty	Meas	Wgt (g)	Wtr (g)	Cals	Prot (g)	Carb (g)	Fib (g)	Fat (g)	SatF (g)
Egg foo yung patty	1	each	86	67	113	6	3	0.6	8	1.9
Egg omelet, ham & cheese, 1 egg	1	each	78	55	142	10	1	0	11	3.9
Egg omelet, mushroom, 1 egg	1	each	69	54	91	6	1	0.1	7	2.6
Egg omelet, onion, peppper, tomato, mushroom, 3 egg	1	each	145	122	125	5	7	1.6	9	2
Egg omelet, plain, 1 large egg	1	each	59	45	90	6	1	0	7	1.9
Egg omelet, sausage & mushroom, 1 egg	1	each	95	68	172	11	1	0.2	13	4.9
Egg omelet, spanish, 1 egg	1	each	145	122	125	5	7	1.6	9	2
Egg omelet, spinach, 1 egg	1	each	84	68	95	7	2	0.7	7	2.2
Egg roll, chicken, Chun King	6	piece	106	62	210	6	30	3	7	1.5
Egg roll, shrimp, Chun King	6	piece	106	65	190	5	29	3	6	1
Egg salad	0.5	cup	92	52	293	8	1	0	28	5.3
Egg substitute, frozen	0.25	cup	60	44	96	7	2	0	7	1.2
Egg substitute, liquid	0.25	cup	63	52	53	8	0	0	2	0.4
Egg substitute, liquid, prepared	0.5	cup	105	84	100	14	1	0	4	0.8
Egg substitute, powder	1	oz.	28	1	126	16	6	0	4	1.1
Egg substitute, w/cholesterol, frozen, prepared	0.5	cup	70	51	92	9	5	0	4	0.7
Egg white, cooked	1	each	33	29	17	4	0	0	0	0
Egg white, fresh or frozen, raw	2	each	67	59	33	7	1	0	0	0
Egg white, fresh or frozen, raw, large	1	each	33	29	17	4	0	0	0	0
Egg yolk, cooked	1	each	17	8	59	3	0	0	5	1.6
Egg yolk, fresh, raw, large	1	each	17	8	59	3	0	0	5	1.6
Egg yolk, frozen, raw, salted	0.5	cup	122	62	333	17	2	0	28	8.5
Egg, Second Nature, prepared	0.5	cup	105	84	100	14	1	0	4	0.8
Egg, creamed	1	each	145	107	230	11	8	0.2	17	5.2
Egg, deviled	2	each	62	43	125	7	1	0	10	2.5
Egg, hard cooked, extra large	1	each	58	43	90	7	1	0	6	1.9
Egg, hard cooked/boiled, chopped, large	1	cup	136	101	211	17	2	0	14	4.4
Egg, hard cooked/boiled, large	1	each	50	37	78	6	1	0	5	1.6
Egg, hard cooked/boiled, medium	1	each	44	33	68	6	0	0	5	1.4
Egg, poached, extra large	1	each	57	43	85	7	1	0	6	1.8
Egg, poached, large	1	each	50	38	74	6	1	0	5	1.6
Egg, poached, medium size	1	each	44	33	66	5	1	0	4	1.4
Egg, scrambled, dry, prepared	0.5	cup	107	73	238	10	1	0	21	5.1
Egg, scrambled, frozen, prepared, no cholesterol	0.5	cup	76	53	139	10	3	0	10	1.7
Egg, scrambled, w/cheese, no chol, frozen, prepared	0.5	cup	76	62	64	10	2	0	2	1
Egg, scrambled, w/milk & margarine, large	1	each	61	45	101	7	1	0	7	2.2
Egg, substitute, dry, prepared	0.5	cup	94	64	181	11	4	0	13	2.8
Egg, substitute, frozen, prepared	0.5	cup	76	53	139	10	3	0	10	1.7
Egg, whole, dried	0.5	cup	42	1	252	20	2	0	17	5.4
Egg, whole, fresh or frozen, raw	1	each	50	38	74	6	1	0	5	1.6
Egg, whole, fresh or frozen, raw, jumbo	1	each	65	49	97	8	1	0	6	2
Egg, whole, fresh or frozen, raw, medium	1	each	44	33	66	6	1	0	4	1.4
Egg, whole, fresh or frozen, raw, small	1	each	37	28	55	5	0	0	4	1.2
Egg, whole, fresh or frozen, raw, extra large	1	each	58	44	86	7	1	0	6	1.8
Egg, whole, fried in margarine, large	1	each	46	32	92	6	1	0	7	1.9
Eggnog, made w/2% lowfat milk	1	cup	254	215	189	12	17	0	8	3.8
Eggnog, w/whole milk, commercial	1	cup	254	189	343	10	34	0	19	11.3
Eggplant slices, batter-dipped, fried	1	piece	50	37	75	1	6	1.2	5	1.3
Eggplant slices, cooked, drained, no added salt	1	piece	54	50	15	0	4	1.4	0	0
Eggplant, pieces, steamed	0.5	cup	48	44	12	0	3	1.2	0	0
Eggplant, pieces, stir fried, no oil	0.5	cup	48	44	12	0	3	1.2	0	0
Eggplant, raw, cubes	0.5	cup	41	38	11	0	2	1	0	0
Eggplant, whole, cooked, drained, no added salt	1	each	538	494	151	4	36	13.5	1	0.2
Eggs, scrambled, plain	2	each	100	75	155	13	1	0	11	3.3
Elderberries, cooked or canned	0.5	cup	128	87	152	1	39	6.6	0	0
Elderberries, raw	0.5	cup	72	58	53	0	13	5.1	0	0
Elk, roasted	4	oz.	113	75	166	34	0	0	2	0.8
Emu, thigh, raw	4	oz.	113	—	105	23	—	—	2	—
Enchilada suiza, chicken, Stouffer's Lean Cuisine	1	each	255	187	290	12	48	5	5	2
Enchilada suiza, chicken, Weight Watchers	1	each	255	203	250	15	28	4	8	3
Enchilada, cheese	1	each	163	103	319	10	28	—	19	10.6
Enchilada, cheese, Stouffer's Entrees	1	each	276	197	370	12	48	5	14	5
Enchilada, chicken	1	each	120	81	192	13	16	1.9	9	3.5
Enchirito, beef-bean-cheese	1	each	193	121	344	18	34	5.5	16	8
English muffin, cheese	1	each	63	28	148	6	25	1.5	2	1

MonoF (g)	PolyF (g)	Choles (mg)	Calc (mg)	Phos (mg)	Sod (mg)	Pot (mg)	Zn (mg)	Iron (mg)	Magn (mg)	VitA (μg RE)	VitE (mg α-TE)	VitC (mg)	Thia (mg)	Ribo (mg)	Nia (mg)	B6 (mg)	Fola (μg)	B12 (μg)
3.4	2.1	184	31	93	310	118	0.7	1	12	86	1.57	5	0.04	0.26	0.4	0.09	30	0.37
4.1	1.6	231	70	163	368	98	1	0.8	9	138	1.69	0	0.08	0.29	0.4	0.1	19	0.54
2.6	1.3	204	25	97	158	99	0.6	0.8	6	109	1.53	0	0.04	0.28	0.5	0.07	19	0.41
3.6	2.3	126	28	118	251	325	0.7	1.2	15	147	1.88	14	0.09	0.34	1.9	0.15	28	0.26
2.7	1.3	207	25	87	159	60	0.5	0.7	5	110	0.76	0	0.03	0.24	0	0.06	17	0.41
5.6	2.2	254	35	140	454	145	1.1	1.1	10	128	1.82	0	0.17	0.32	1	0.14	21	0.79
3.6	2.3	126	28	118	251	325	0.7	1.2	15	147	1.88	14	0.09	0.34	1.9	0.15	28	0.26
3	1.4	201	44	101	201	152	0.7	1.2	16	198	1.69	16	0.04	0.27	0.2	0.11	38	0.4
—	—	10	20	90	260	120	—	0.4	—	3	—	1	0.1	0.06	0.7	—	—	—
—	—	10	20	50	360	80	—	0.4	—	20	—	4	0.09	0.03	0.4	—	—	—
8.7	12.1	287	37	117	333	90	0.7	0.9	7	130	4.44	0	0.04	0.33	0	0.23	31	0.79
1.5	3.7	1	44	43	119	128	0.6	1.2	9	81	1.27	0	0.07	0.23	0.1	0.08	10	0.2
0.6	1	1	33	76	111	207	0.8	1.3	5	136	0.3	0	0.07	0.19	0.1	0	9	0.19
1.1	1.9	1	63	144	211	394	1.6	2.5	10	258	0.58	0	0.11	0.34	0.1	0	13	0.3
1.5	0.5	162	92	136	227	211	0.5	0.9	18	105	0.46	0	0.06	0.5	0.2	0.04	35	1
1.6	1.2	46	12	21	113	103	0.1	0.2	7	172	0.59	0	0.01	0.21	0.1	0.01	12	0.12
0	0	0	2	4	106	48	0	0	4	0	0	0	0	0.14	0	0	1	0.06
0	0	0	4	9	110	96	0	0	7	0	0	0	0	0.3	0.1	0	2	0.13
0	0	0	2	4	55	48	0	0	4	0	0	0	0	0.15	0	0	1	0.07
1.9	0.7	212	23	81	33	16	0.5	0.6	1	97	0.49	0	0.02	0.1	0	0.06	18	0.44
1.9	0.7	213	23	81	7	16	0.5	0.6	1	97	0.52	0	0.03	0.11	0	0.06	24	0.52
10.8	3.8	1160	139	524	4592	142	3.4	4.6	12	434	2.74	0	0.16	0.52	0	0.32	130	3.06
1.1	1.9	1	63	144	211	394	1.6	2.5	10	258	0.58	0	0.11	0.34	0.1	0	13	0.3
6.7	3.4	281	125	185	484	193	1	0.9	16	216	2.33	1	0.08	0.46	0.3	0.11	33	0.98
3.5	3	242	29	98	187	73	0.6	0.7	6	99	1.72	0	0.04	0.29	0	0.1	26	0.65
2.4	0.8	246	29	100	72	73	0.6	0.7	6	97	0.61	0	0.04	0.3	0	0.07	26	0.64
5.6	1.9	577	68	234	169	171	1.4	1.6	14	228	1.43	0	0.09	0.7	0.1	0.16	60	1.51
2	0.7	212	25	86	62	63	0.5	0.6	5	84	0.52	0	0.03	0.26	0	0.06	22	0.56
1.8	0.6	187	22	76	55	55	0.5	0.5	4	74	0.46	0	0.03	0.23	0	0.05	19	0.49
2.2	0.8	241	28	101	160	68	0.6	0.8	6	108	0.6	0	0.03	0.24	0	0.07	20	0.46
1.9	0.7	212	24	88	140	60	0.6	0.7	5	95	0.52	0	0.02	0.22	0	0.06	18	0.4
1.7	0.6	186	22	78	123	53	0.5	0.6	4	84	0.46	0	0.02	0.19	0	0.05	15	0.35
9.3	5.1	411	52	149	468	111	1.2	1.7	11	291	3.13	0	0.06	0.24	0.1	0.08	30	1.83
2.1	5.4	2	63	62	173	185	0.9	1.7	13	117	1.84	0	0.09	0.32	0.1	0.11	11	0.25
0.4	0	4	66	87	271	135	0.3	0.1	12	14	0.04	0	0.01	0.37	0.1	0.01	2	0.15
2.9	1.3	215	43	104	171	84	0.6	0.7	7	119	0.8	0	0.03	0.27	0	0.07	18	0.47
6.1	3.9	108	67	93	281	146	0.4	0.6	13	216	2.04	0	0.04	0.32	0.1	0.03	18	0.58
2.1	5.4	2	63	62	173	185	0.9	1.7	13	117	1.84	0	0.09	0.32	0.1	0.11	11	0.25
6.5	2.5	729	98	353	222	210	2.2	2.9	18	115	1.86	0	0.08	0.66	0.1	0.16	73	1.68
1.9	0.7	213	24	89	63	60	0.6	0.7	5	96	0.52	0	0.03	0.25	0	0.07	24	0.5
2.5	0.9	276	32	116	82	79	0.7	0.9	6	124	0.68	0	0.04	0.33	0	0.09	31	0.65
1.7	0.6	187	22	78	55	53	0.5	0.6	4	84	0.46	0	0.03	0.22	0	0.06	21	0.44
1.4	0.5	157	18	66	47	45	0.4	0.5	4	71	0.39	0	0.02	0.19	0	0.05	17	0.37
2.2	0.8	247	28	103	73	70	0.6	0.8	6	111	0.61	0	0.04	0.3	0	0.08	27	0.58
2.8	1.3	211	25	89	162	61	0.5	0.7	5	114	0.75	0	0.03	0.24	0	0.07	18	0.42
2.7	0.7	194	269	269	155	367	1.3	0.7	32	197	1.01	2	0.11	0.55	0.2	0.15	30	1.17
5.7	0.9	149	330	277	138	419	1.2	0.5	47	203	0.58	4	0.09	0.48	0.3	0.13	2	1.14
2.3	1.5	9	27	26	31	107	0.1	0.5	6	5	0.45	1	0.06	0.04	0.5	0.04	7	0.06
0	0	0	3	12	2	134	0.1	0.2	7	3	0.02	1	0.04	0.01	0.3	0.05	8	0
0	0	0	3	11	1	104	0.1	0.1	5	3	0.01	1	0.04	0.01	0.3	0.04	9	0
0	0	0	3	11	1	104	0.1	0.1	5	3	0.01	1	0.04	0.01	0.3	0.04	9	0
0	0	0	3	9	1	89	0.1	0.1	6	3	0.01	1	0.02	0.01	0.2	0.03	8	0
0.1	0.5	0	32	118	16	1334	0.8	1.9	70	32	0.16	7	0.41	0.11	3.2	0.46	78	0
4.1	1.4	424	50	172	124	126	1	1.2	10	168	1.05	0	0.07	0.51	0.1	0.12	44	1.11
0.1	0.2	0	34	37	6	236	0.1	1.5	5	42	0.94	24	0.05	0.06	0.4	0.19	3	0
0.1	0.2	0	28	28	4	203	0.1	1.2	4	44	0.72	26	0.05	0.04	0.4	0.17	4	0
0.5	0.5	83	6	204	69	372	3.6	4.1	27	0	0.03	0	0.25	0.91	6.6	0.28	5	7.37
—	—	56	—	—	—	—	—	5.7	—	—	—	—	—	—	—	—	—	—
1.5	1.5	25	150	—	530	360	—	0.7	—	60	—	4	—	—	—	—	—	—
—	—	25	300	—	570	470	—	1.4	—	40	—	1	0.15	0.26	4	—	—	—
6.3	0.8	44	324	134	784	240	2.5	1.3	50	186	1.47	1	0.08	0.42	1.9	0.39	65	0.75
—	—	25	200	—	890	310	—	1.4	—	200	—	12	—	—	—	—	—	—
2.5	2	36	159	212	307	199	1.3	1	34	108	0.73	16	0.08	0.13	3.1	0.25	15	0.2
6.5	0.3	50	218	224	1250	560	2.8	2.4	71	133	1.54	5	0.17	0.7	3	0.21	60	1.62
0.7	0.5	3	118	78	184	80	0.6	1.8	14	10	0.1	0	0.26	0.27	3	0.1	55	0.02

Food Item	Qty	Meas	Wgt (g)	Wtr (g)	Cals	Prot (g)	Carb (g)	Fib (g)	Fat (g)	SatF (g)
English muffin, cheese, toasted	1	each	56	21	151	6	26	1.5	2	1
English muffin, mixed grain	1	each	61	24	143	6	28	1.7	1	0.1
English muffin, mixed grain, toasted	1	each	61	21	156	6	31	1.8	1	0.2
English muffin, plain	1	each	57	24	134	4	26	1.5	1	0.1
English muffin, raisin cinnamon	1	each	57	22	139	4	28	1.6	2	0.2
English muffin, raisin cinnamon, toasted	1	each	52	17	137	4	28	1.6	2	0.2
English muffin, sourdough	1	each	56	24	132	4	26	1.5	1	0.1
English muffin, sourdough, toasted	1	each	50	19	128	4	25	1.4	1	0.1
English muffin, toasted	1	each	50	19	128	4	25	1.4	1	0.1
English muffin, w/butter, fast food	1	each	63	20	189	5	30	1.9	6	2.4
English muffin, wheat	1	each	57	24	127	5	26	2.6	1	0.2
English muffin, wheat, toasted	1	each	52	19	126	5	25	2.6	1	0.2
English muffin, whole wheat	1	each	50	23	102	4	20	3.4	1	0.6
English muffin, whole wheat, toasted	1	each	50	20	111	5	22	3.6	1	0.2
Escarole/curly endive, raw, chopped	0.5	cup	25	24	4	0	1	0.8	0	0
Escargot, snail, steamed	2	each	10	6	18	3	0	0	0	0.1
Fajita, w/beef	1	each	223	140	409	17	46	3.8	18	5.1
Falafel, fava bean patty	1	piece	17	6	57	2	5	0.9	3	0.4
Fat replacer, plum puree	0.5	cup	124	25	391	2	95	7.2	0	0
Fat, beef/tallow, drippings	1	Tbs	13	0	116	0	0	0	13	6.4
Fat, chicken	1	Tbs	13	0	115	0	0	0	13	3.8
Feijoa fruit, raw	1	each	50	43	24	1	5	2.1	0	0.1
Fennel seed	0.25	tsp	0	0	2	0	0	0.2	0	0
Fenugreek seed	0.25	tsp	1	0	3	0	1	0.2	0	0
Fig, canned in heavy syrup	3	each	85	65	75	0	20	1.9	0	0
Figs, canned in water	3	each	80	68	42	0	11	1.8	0	0
Figs, dried	10	each	187	53	477	6	122	22.8	2	0.4
Figs, dried DFA	10	each	187	52	527	6	124	22.8	1	0
Figs, dried, cooked, unsweetened	0.5	cup	130	90	140	2	36	6.6	1	0.1
Figs, fresh	1	each	50	40	37	0	10	1.6	0	0
Filbert/hazelnut, dried, ground	0.25	cup	19	1	119	2	3	1.1	12	0.9
Filbert/hazelnut, dried, unblanched, chopped	0.25	cup	29	2	182	4	4	1.8	18	1.3
Filbert/hazelnut, dried, unblanched, whole	0.25	cup	34	2	213	4	5	2.1	21	1.6
Filberts/hazelnuts, dry roasted, unsalted	1	oz.	28	1	188	3	5	2	19	1.4
Filberts/hazelnuts, dry roasted, w/salt	1	oz.	28	1	188	3	5	2.2	19	1.4
Filberts/hazelnuts, oil roasted, salted	1	oz.	28	0	187	4	5	1.8	18	1.3
Filberts/hazelnuts, oil roasted, unsalted	1	oz.	28	0	187	4	5	1.8	18	1.3
Fish ball, cod	1	each	63	39	125	9	8	0.7	7	1.7
Fish cake, cod	1	each	120	74	239	16	15	1.4	13	3.3
Fish cake, fried	1	each	69	41	150	14	5	0.3	8	2
Fish cake, fried, frozen, heated	1	each	85	45	230	8	15	0.8	15	6
Fish dinner, lemon pepper, Healthy Choice	1	each	303	236	320	14	50	5	7	2
Fish patty, heated from frozen	1	each	57	26	155	9	14	0	7	1.8
Fish stick/portion, heated, from frozen	2	each	57	26	155	9	14	0	7	1.8
Fish, Abalone, canned	4	oz.	113	91	91	18	3	0	6	0.3
Fish, Anchovies, canned in oil, drained	10	each	40	20	84	12	0	0	4	0.9
Fish, Gefiltefish, sweet, commercial	1	piece	42	34	35	4	3	0	1	0.2
Fish, Kamaboko (Japanese fish cake)	1	piece	16	11	18	2	2	0	0	0
Fish, King Crab leg, baked/broiled	1	each	119	87	164	23	0	0	8	1.4
Fish, Lingcod, baked/broiled fillet	0.5	each	151	114	165	34	0	0	2	0.4
Fish, Queen crab, baked/broiled	0.5	cup	59	44	68	14	0	0	1	0.1
Fish, Snow Crab leg, baked/broiled	1	each	10	7	14	2	0	0	1	0.1
Fish, Spiny lobster, steamed	1	each	229	153	327	60	7	0	4	0.7
Fish, abalone, floured, fried	4	oz.	113	68	214	22	13	0	8	1.9
Fish, abalone, fried	4	oz.	113	68	214	22	13	0	8	1.9
Fish, abalone, mixed species, raw	4	oz.	113	85	119	19	7	0	1	0.2
Fish, abalone, steamed/poached	4	oz.	113	56	238	39	14	0	2	0.3
Fish, anchovies, cooked	10	each	40	20	84	12	0	0	4	0.9
Fish, butterfish, baked/broiled fillet	1	each	25	17	47	6	0	0	3	0.8
Fish, butterfish, baked/broiled fillet	3	oz.	85	57	159	19	0	0	9	2.6
Fish, calamari, dried	1	oz.	28	6	95	16	3	0	1	0.4
Fish, carp, baked/broiled fillet	1	each	170	118	275	39	0	0	12	2.4
Fish, carp, baked/broiled fillet	3	oz.	85	59	138	20	0	0	6	1.2
Fish, catfish, breaded fried fillet	1	each	87	51	199	16	7	0.7	12	2.9
Fish, catfish, breaded fried fillet	3	oz.	85	50	195	15	7	0.6	11	2.8

MonoF (g)	PolyF (g)	Choles (mg)	Calc (mg)	Phos (mg)	Sod (mg)	Pot (mg)	Zn (mg)	Iron (mg)	Magn (mg)	VitA (μg RE)	VitE (mg α-TE)	VitC (mg)	Thia (mg)	Ribo (mg)	Nia (mg)	B6 (mg)	Fola (μg)	B12 (μg)
0.7	0.5	3	121	79	188	82	0.6	1.9	15	9	0.1	0	0.21	0.28	3	0.1	48	0.02
0.5	0.3	0	120	49	254	95	0.8	1.8	25	0	0.17	0	0.26	0.19	2.2	0.02	49	0
0.5	0.4	0	130	99	276	103	0.6	2	29	1	0.76	0	0.23	0.19	2.1	0.06	41	0
0.2	0.5	0	99	76	264	75	0.4	1.4	12	0	0.1	0	0.25	0.16	2.2	0.02	46	0.02
0.3	0.8	0	84	39	255	119	0.6	1.4	9	0	0.23	0	0.22	0.17	2	0.04	46	0
0.3	0.8	0	83	44	253	118	0.6	1.4	9	0	0.1	0	0.17	0.15	1.8	0.04	36	0
0.2	0.5	0	97	74	260	73	0.4	1.4	12	0	0.1	0	0.25	0.16	2.2	0.02	45	0.02
0.2	0.5	0	94	72	252	72	0.4	1.4	11	0	0.09	0	0.19	0.14	1.9	0.02	37	0.02
0.2	0.5	0	94	72	252	72	0.4	1.4	11	0	0.09	0	0.19	0.14	1.9	0.02	37	0.02
1.5	1.4	13	103	85	386	69	0.4	1.6	13	33	0.13	1	0.25	0.32	2.6	0.04	57	0.02
0.2	0.5	0	101	61	218	106	0.6	1.6	21	0	0.28	0	0.25	0.17	1.9	0.05	31	0
0.2	0.5	0	100	65	216	105	0.6	1.6	22	0	0.18	0	0.2	0.15	1.7	0.05	24	0
0.4	0	0	133	141	319	105	0.8	1.2	36	0	0.35	0	0.15	0.07	1.7	0.08	21	0
0.3	0.5	0	144	154	346	114	0.9	1.3	38	0	0.38	0	0.13	0.07	1.7	0.08	18	0
0	0	0	13	7	6	78	0.2	0.2	4	51	0.11	2	0.02	0.02	0.1	0	36	0
0.1	0.1	10	2	38	12	54	0.2	0.6	42	5	1	0	0	0.02	0.2	0.02	1	0.06
7.6	3.9	26	76	200	850	427	2.4	3.7	38	52	2.08	29	0.46	0.3	4.7	0.32	25	1.18
1.7	0.7	0	9	33	50	100	0.3	0.6	14	0	0.19	0	0.02	0.03	0.2	0.02	16	0
—	—	—	16	—	45	443	—	1	—	27	—	4	—	—	—	—	—	—
5.4	0.5	14	0	0	0	0	0	0	0	0	0.35	0	0	0	0	0	0	0
5.7	2.7	11	0	0	0	0	0	0	0	0	0.35	0	0	0	0	0	0	0
0	0.2	0	8	10	2	78	0	0	4	0	—	10	0	0.02	0.1	0.02	19	0
0	0	0	6	2	0	8	0	0.1	2	0	—	0	0	0	0	—	—	0
—	—	0	2	3	1	7	0	0.3	2	0	—	0	0	0	0	—	1	0
0	0	0	23	8	1	84	0.1	0.2	8	3	0.76	1	0.02	0.03	0.4	0.06	2	0
0	0	0	22	8	1	82	0.1	0.2	8	3	0.71	1	0.02	0.03	0.4	0.06	2	0
0.5	1	0	269	127	21	1331	1	4.2	110	24	0	2	0.13	0.16	1.3	0.42	14	0
—	—	0	249	134	23	1138	1	5.7	115	2	—	1	0.14	0.17	1.4	0.63	33	0
0.1	0.3	0	79	38	6	390	0.3	1.2	32	21	0	6	0.01	0.14	0.8	0.17	1	0
0	0.1	0	18	7	0	116	0.1	0.2	8	7	0.44	1	0.03	0.02	0.2	0.06	3	0
9.2	1.1	0	35	58	1	83	0.4	0.6	53	1	4.48	0	0.09	0.02	0.2	0.12	14	0
14.1	1.7	0	54	90	1	128	0.7	0.9	82	2	6.87	0	0.14	0.03	0.3	0.18	21	0
16.6	2	0	64	105	1	150	0.8	1.1	96	2	8.07	0	0.17	0.04	0.4	0.21	24	0
14.7	1.8	0	55	92	1	131	0.7	1	84	2	6.78	0	0.06	0.06	0.8	0.18	21	0
14.7	1.8	0	55	92	221	131	0.7	1	84	0	7.09	0	0.06	0.06	0.8	0.18	21	0
14.1	1.7	0	56	92	223	132	0.7	1	84	2	7.09	0	0.06	0.06	0.8	0.18	21	0
14.1	1.7	0	56	92	1	132	0.7	1	84	2	6.78	0	0.06	0.06	0.8	0.18	21	0
2.8	1.7	35	18	108	175	274	0.3	0.4	20	13	0.64	2	0.07	0.07	1.3	0.16	7	0.33
5.3	3.2	66	34	206	333	522	0.7	0.8	38	25	1.21	5	0.13	0.13	2.5	0.31	13	0.63
3.2	2	47	24	139	267	255	0.4	0.6	24	13	1.89	1	0.07	0.09	2.2	0.13	8	0.94
3.4	3.4	22	9	142	150	296	0.3	0.3	15	17	0.51	0	0.03	0.06	1.4	0.04	10	0.85
—	—	30	20	—	480	—	—	1.1	—	100	—	30	—	—	—	—	—	—
2.9	1.8	64	11	103	332	149	0.4	0.4	14	18	0.78	0	0.07	0.1	1.2	0.03	10	1.03
2.9	1.8	64	11	103	332	149	0.4	0.4	14	18	0.78	0	0.07	0.1	1.2	0.03	10	1.03
2.6	3.6	91	16	145	794	318	1	2.6	57	2	5.67	1	0.14	0.08	2	0.17	2	0.79
1.5	1	34	93	101	1467	218	1	1.8	28	8	2	0	0.03	0.14	8	0.08	5	0.35
0.3	0.1	13	10	31	220	38	0.3	1	4	11	0.06	0	0.03	0.02	0.4	0.03	1	0.35
0	0.1	8	7	24	135	39	0.1	0.1	7	1	0.02	0	0	0.02	0.4	0.03	0	0.33
2.8	2.5	111	118	231	642	364	4.7	1	37	78	2.01	4	0.11	0.06	3.7	0.2	57	8.13
0.7	0.6	101	27	390	115	846	0.9	0.6	50	26	0.44	0	0.05	0.21	3.5	0.52	15	6.27
0.2	0.3	42	20	76	408	118	2.1	1.7	37	31	0.67	4	0.06	0.14	1.7	0.1	25	6.14
0.2	0.2	9	10	19	54	31	0.4	0.1	3	7	0.17	0	0.01	0	0.3	0.02	5	0.68
0.8	1.7	206	144	524	520	476	16.6	3.2	117	14	4.58	5	0.02	0.13	11.2	0.4	2	9.25
3.1	1.9	107	42	246	670	322	1.1	4.3	64	2	6.8	2	0.25	0.15	2.2	0.17	16	0.78
3.1	1.9	107	42	246	670	322	1.1	4.3	64	2	6.8	2	0.25	0.15	2.2	0.17	16	0.78
0.1	0.1	96	35	215	341	284	0.9	3.6	54	2	4.54	2	0.22	0.11	1.7	0.17	6	0.83
0.2	0.2	193	67	302	580	397	1.9	6.5	92	4	9.07	3	0.39	0.17	2.6	0.29	9	0.99
1.5	1	34	93	101	1467	218	1	1.8	28	8	2	0	0.03	0.14	8	0.08	5	0.35
0.9	0.8	21	7	77	28	120	0.2	0.2	8	8	0.15	0	0.04	0.05	1.4	0.09	4	0.46
3.1	2.7	71	24	262	97	409	0.8	0.5	27	28	0.52	0	0.12	0.16	4.9	0.29	14	1.56
0.1	0.5	240	33	228	165	253	1.6	0.7	34	9	1.24	4	0.02	0.42	2.2	0.06	5	1.27
5.1	3.1	143	88	903	107	726	3.2	2.7	65	15	1.82	3	0.24	0.12	3.6	0.37	29	2.5
2.5	1.6	71	44	451	54	363	1.6	1.4	32	8	0.91	1	0.12	0.06	1.8	0.19	15	1.25
4.9	2.9	70	38	188	244	296	0.7	1.2	24	7	1.11	0	0.06	0.12	2	0.16	26	1.65
4.8	2.8	69	37	184	238	289	0.7	1.2	23	7	1.09	0	0.06	0.11	1.9	0.16	26	1.62

A

Food Item	Qty	Meas	Wgt (g)	Wtr (g)	Cals	Prot (g)	Carb (g)	Fib (g)	Fat (g)	SatF (g)
Fish, catfish, steamed/poached	4	oz.	113	78	191	22	0	0	11	2.5
Fish, caviar, black/red, granular	2	Tbs	32	15	81	8	1	0	6	1.3
Fish, clam, breaded, fried	0.5	cup	75	46	152	11	8	0.1	8	2
Fish, clam, breaded, fried, small	0.5	cup	75	46	152	11	8	0.1	8	2
Fish, clam, smoked, canned in oil	10	each	100	69	175	14	3	0	12	2.7
Fish, clams, canned, drained	4	oz.	113	72	168	29	6	0	2	0.2
Fish, clams, minced, w/liquid, small can	1	each	183	146	145	25	5	0	2	0.2
Fish, clams, steamed, large	8	each	150	95	222	38	8	0	3	0.3
Fish, clams, steamed, small	20	each	90	57	133	23	5	0	2	0.2
Fish, cod, Pacific, baked/broiled fillet	1	each	90	68	94	21	0	0	1	0.1
Fish, cod, Pacific, baked/broiled fillet	3	oz.	85	65	89	20	0	0	1	0.1
Fish, cod, batter fried pieces	3	piece	48	32	83	8	3	0.1	4	0.9
Fish, cod, steamed/poached	4	oz.	113	87	116	25	0	0	1	0.2
Fish, crab leg, Alaskan King, steamed	1	each	134	104	130	26	0	0	2	0.2
Fish, crab, baked/broiled	0.5	cup	59	43	81	11	0	0	4	0.7
Fish, crab, blue, canned meat	4	oz.	113	86	112	23	0	0	1	0.3
Fish, crab, blue, steamed	1	cup	118	91	120	24	0	0	2	0.3
Fish, crab, blue, steamed, whole	1	each	48	37	49	10	0	0	1	0.1
Fish, crab, dungeness, steamed	4	oz.	113	83	125	25	1	0	1	0.2
Fish, crab, dungeness, whole, steamed	1	each	127	93	140	28	1	0	2	0.2
Fish, crab, imitation	4	oz.	113	84	116	14	12	0	1	0.3
Fish, crab, soft shell, floured/breaded, fried	1	each	65	26	217	13	11	0.5	13	3.2
Fish, crayfish/Crawdads, steamed	4	oz.	113	90	93	19	0	0	1	0.2
Fish, crayfish/crawdads wild, raw	8	each	27	22	21	4	0	0	0	0
Fish, cuttlefish, steamed	4	oz.	113	69	179	37	2	0	2	0.3
Fish, eel, baked/broiled fillet	1	each	159	94	375	38	0	0	24	4.8
Fish, eel, steamed/poached	4	oz.	113	68	261	26	0	0	16	3.3
Fish, grouper, baked/broiled fillet	1	each	202	148	238	50	0	0	3	0.6
Fish, grouper, baked/broiled fillet	3	oz.	85	62	100	21	0	0	1	0.3
Fish, haddock patty	1	each	120	74	239	16	15	1.4	13	3.3
Fish, haddock, baked/broiled fillet	1	each	150	111	168	36	0	0	1	0.3
Fish, haddock, baked/broiled fillet	3	oz.	85	63	95	21	0	0	1	0.1
Fish, haddock, breaded, fried fillet	1	each	81	45	189	16	10	0.6	9	2.3
Fish, haddock, breaded, fried fillet	3	oz.	85	47	199	16	11	0.6	10	2.4
Fish, haddock, steamed/poached	3	oz.	85	64	92	20	0	0	1	0.1
Fish, haddock, steamed/poached	4	oz.	113	85	123	27	0	0	1	0.2
Fish, halibut, Pacific, steamed	4	oz.	113	81	159	30	0	0	3	0.5
Fish, herring, Atlantic, baked/broiled fillet	1	each	143	92	290	33	0	0	17	3.8
Fish, herring, Atlantic, baked/broiled fillet	3	oz.	85	55	173	20	0	0	10	2.2
Fish, herring, Atlantic, pickled	6	piece	90	50	236	13	9	0	16	2.1
Fish, herring, Pacific, baked/broiled fillet	1	each	144	91	360	30	0	0	26	6
Fish, jellyfish, pickled	0.5	cup	29	20	10	2	0	0	0	0.1
Fish, lobster pieces, baked/broiled	0.5	cup	72	54	84	14	1	0	2	1.2
Fish, lobster tail, baked/broiled	1	each	125	92	145	25	2	0	4	2
Fish, lobster, battered, fried	1	each	111	67	235	21	9	0.2	12	3
Fish, lobster, battered, fried	3	oz.	85	51	180	16	7	0.2	9	2.3
Fish, lobster, northern, raw	1	each	150	115	135	28	1	0	1	0.3
Fish, lobster, northern, raw	3	oz.	85	65	76	16	0	0	1	0.2
Fish, lobster, northern, steamed	4	oz.	113	86	111	23	1	0	1	0.1
Fish, lobster, w/butter sauce	0.5	cup	94	59	224	15	1	0	18	10.9
Fish, mackerel patty	1	each	120	65	298	19	16	1.5	18	4.8
Fish, mackerel, Atlantic, baked/broiled fillet	1	each	88	47	231	21	0	0	16	3.7
Fish, mackerel, Atlantic, baked/broiled fillet	3	oz.	85	45	223	20	0	0	15	3.6
Fish, mackerel, Jack, canned, drained	1	cup	190	131	296	44	0	0	12	3.5
Fish, mackerel, king, baked/broiled fillet	0.5	piece	154	106	206	40	0	0	4	0.7
Fish, moochim, Korean (dried fish & soy sauce)	0.5	cup	40	9	133	15	4	0.2	6	0.9
Fish, mullet, baked/broiled fillet	1	each	93	66	140	23	0	0	5	1.3
Fish, mullet, baked/broiled fillet	3	oz.	85	60	128	21	0	0	4	1.2
Fish, mussels, blue, raw	4	oz.	113	91	98	14	4	0	3	0.5
Fish, mussels, blue, steamed	4	oz.	113	69	195	27	8	0	5	1
Fish, mussels, smoked, canned, in oil, drained	0.5	cup	75	46	146	16	3	0	8	—
Fish, mussels, w/tomato-based sauce	0.5	cup	120	87	134	15	12	1.8	3	0.6
Fish, octopus, cooked	4	oz.	113	69	186	34	5	0	2	0.5
Fish, octopus, dried	0.5	cup	26	5	90	15	3	0	1	0.3
Fish, octopus, dried, cooked	0.5	cup	53	30	97	16	3	0	1	0.4

MonoF (g)	PolyF (g)	Choles (mg)	Calc (mg)	Phos (mg)	Sod (mg)	Pot (mg)	Zn (mg)	Iron (mg)	Magn (mg)	VitA (μg RE)	VitE (mg α-TE)	VitC (mg)	Thia (mg)	Ribo (mg)	Nia (mg)	B6 (mg)	Fola (μg)	B12 (μg)
5.1	2.2	67	13	258	68	360	1	0.7	29	17	1.7	1	0.41	0.1	2.8	0.21	11	2.98
1.5	2.4	188	88	114	480	58	0.3	3.8	96	179	2.24	0	0.06	0.2	0	0.1	16	6.4
3.4	2.2	46	47	141	273	245	1.1	10.4	10	68	1.88	8	0.08	0.18	1.6	0.04	27	30.2
3.4	2.2	46	47	141	273	245	1.1	10.4	10	68	1.88	8	0.08	0.18	1.6	0.04	27	30.2
4.8	3.1	38	52	188	321	349	1.5	15.6	10	100	1.97	14	0.08	0.24	2	0.07	18	55
0.2	0.6	76	104	383	127	712	3.1	31.8	20	194	1.13	25	0.17	0.48	3.8	0.12	33	112
0.2	0.5	65	101	328	293	609	2.8	27.1	28	166	1.46	3	0.01	0.41	3.3	0.08	4	98.8
0.3	0.8	101	138	507	168	942	4.1	42	27	257	2.94	33	0.22	0.64	5	0.16	43	148
0.2	0.5	60	83	304	101	565	2.5	25.2	16	154	1.76	20	0.14	0.38	3	0.1	26	89
0.1	0.3	42	8	201	82	465	0.5	0.3	28	9	0.31	3	0.02	0.05	2.2	0.42	7	0.94
0.1	0.3	40	8	190	77	439	0.4	0.3	26	8	0.29	3	0.02	0.04	2.1	0.39	7	0.88
1.5	1.1	27	18	98	52	188	0.3	0.4	15	7	0.39	0	0.05	0.06	1.1	0.1	4	0.41
0.1	0.3	61	23	259	69	498	0.6	0.5	41	14	0.32	1	0.09	0.08	2.5	0.28	8	1.09
0.2	0.7	71	79	375	1436	351	10.2	1	84	12	1.21	10	0.07	0.07	1.8	0.24	68	15.4
1.4	1.2	55	59	115	319	180	2.3	0.5	18	38	0.99	2	0.06	0.03	1.8	0.1	28	4.03
0.2	0.5	101	115	295	378	424	4.6	1	44	2	1.13	3	0.09	0.1	1.6	0.17	48	0.52
0.3	0.8	118	123	243	329	382	5	1.1	39	2	1.18	4	0.12	0.06	3.9	0.21	60	8.61
0.1	0.3	48	50	99	134	156	2	0.4	16	1	0.48	2	0.05	0.02	1.6	0.09	24	3.5
0.2	0.5	86	67	198	429	463	6.2	0.5	66	35	1.28	4	0.06	0.23	4.1	0.2	48	11.8
0.3	0.5	96	75	222	480	518	7	0.5	74	39	1.44	5	0.07	0.26	4.6	0.22	53	13.2
0.2	0.8	23	15	320	954	102	0.4	0.4	49	23	0.11	0	0.04	0.03	0.2	0.03	2	1.81
5.4	3.4	80	71	141	336	203	2.4	1.2	23	14	1.63	1	0.13	0.12	2.4	0.1	28	3.34
0.3	0.4	151	68	306	107	336	2	0.9	37	17	1.7	1	0.06	0.1	2.6	0.09	50	2.44
0	0.1	31	7	69	16	82	0.4	0.2	7	4	0.77	0	0.02	0.01	0.6	0.03	10	0.54
0.2	0.3	254	204	658	844	722	3.9	12.2	68	230	5.1	10	0.02	1.96	2.5	0.31	27	6.12
14.7	1.9	256	41	440	103	555	3.3	1	41	1806	8.11	3	0.29	0.08	7.1	0.12	28	4.6
10.2	1.3	179	28	276	65	328	2.3	0.7	26	1256	5.67	2	0.17	0.05	4.2	0.08	17	3.61
0.5	0.8	95	42	289	107	960	1	2.3	75	101	1.26	0	0.16	0.01	0.8	0.71	21	1.4
0.2	0.3	40	18	122	45	404	0.4	1	32	42	0.53	0	0.07	0	0.3	0.3	9	0.59
5.3	3.2	66	34	206	333	522	0.7	0.8	38	25	1.21	5	0.13	0.13	2.5	0.31	13	0.63
0.2	0.5	111	63	362	131	599	0.7	2	75	28	0.73	0	0.06	0.07	7	0.52	20	2.09
0.1	0.3	63	36	205	74	339	0.4	1.2	42	16	0.42	0	0.03	0.04	3.9	0.29	11	1.18
3.8	2.4	68	45	163	375	247	0.4	1.4	33	24	1.12	0	0.06	0.1	3.2	0.2	14	0.81
4	2.5	72	48	171	393	259	0.4	1.4	35	25	1.17	0	0.06	0.11	3.4	0.21	15	0.85
0.1	0.3	61	35	180	65	281	0.4	1.1	37	14	0.41	0	0.03	0.04	3.4	0.26	10	1.09
0.2	0.3	81	47	240	87	375	0.5	1.5	50	19	0.55	0	0.04	0.05	4.6	0.34	13	1.45
1.1	1.1	46	68	323	78	653	0.6	1.2	121	61	1.24	0	0.08	0.1	8.1	0.45	16	1.55
6.8	3.9	110	106	433	164	599	1.8	2	59	44	1.92	1	0.16	0.43	5.9	0.5	16	18.7
4.1	2.3	66	63	258	98	356	1.1	1.2	35	26	1.14	1	0.1	0.25	3.5	0.3	10	11.1
10.7	1.5	12	69	80	783	62	0.5	1.1	7	232	0.9	0	0.03	0.12	3	0.15	2	3.84
12.7	4.5	143	153	420	137	780	1	2.1	59	50	1.87	0	0.1	0.37	4.1	0.75	9	13.9
0.1	0.2	1	1	6	2809	1	0.1	0.7	1	1	0.01	0	0	0	0.1	0	0	0.01
0.6	0.1	55	43	130	451	247	2	0.3	24	35	0.73	0	0	0.05	0.7	0.05	8	2.18
1.1	0.2	95	75	224	777	425	3.5	0.5	42	60	1.27	0	0.01	0.08	1.3	0.09	14	3.75
5.2	3.4	88	83	203	426	363	2.9	0.9	37	30	1.91	0	0.06	0.12	1.5	0.08	12	2.64
4	2.6	68	64	155	326	278	2.2	0.7	28	23	1.46	0	0.05	0.1	1.1	0.06	9	2.02
0.4	0.2	143	72	216	444	413	4.5	0.4	40	32	2.21	0	0.01	0.07	2.2	0.1	14	1.39
0.2	0.1	81	41	122	252	234	2.6	0.3	23	18	1.25	0	0	0.04	1.2	0.05	8	0.79
0.2	0.1	82	69	210	431	399	3.3	0.4	40	30	1.13	0	0.01	0.08	1.2	0.09	13	3.53
5.1	0.7	99	49	139	453	261	2.1	0.3	26	180	1.06	0	0.01	0.06	0.8	0.06	9	2.29
7.3	4.5	91	193	265	478	349	1	2	40	97	2.18	5	0.12	0.24	5.4	0.3	12	3.76
6.2	3.8	66	13	245	73	353	0.8	1.4	85	48	1.63	0	0.14	0.36	6	0.4	1	16.7
6	3.7	64	13	236	71	341	0.8	1.3	82	46	1.57	0	0.14	0.35	5.8	0.39	1	16.2
4.2	3.1	150	458	572	720	369	1.9	3.9	70	247	2.66	2	0.08	0.4	11.7	0.4	10	13.2
1.5	0.9	105	62	490	313	859	1.1	3.5	63	388	2.66	2	0.18	0.89	16.2	0.78	14	27.7
2.3	2.5	34	54	230	2015	349	0.5	1	38	9	0.37	1	0.08	0.07	2	0.22	8	2.22
1.3	0.9	59	29	227	66	426	0.8	1.3	31	39	1.13	1	0.09	0.09	5.9	0.46	9	0.23
1.2	0.8	54	26	207	60	389	0.7	1.2	28	36	1.04	1	0.08	0.08	5.4	0.42	8	0.21
0.6	0.7	32	30	223	324	363	1.8	4.5	39	54	0.84	9	0.18	0.24	1.8	0.06	48	13.6
1.2	1.4	64	37	323	418	304	3	7.6	42	103	1.64	15	0.34	0.48	3.4	0.11	86	27.2
—	—	69	51	—	341	104	2.8	7	74	90	—	0	—	0.36	1.7	—	—	—
0.6	0.7	34	37	193	745	457	2	4.5	44	72	1.91	12	0.21	0.26	2.2	0.1	52	13
0.4	0.5	109	120	316	522	714	3.8	10.8	68	92	1.36	9	0.06	0.09	4.3	0.74	27	40.8
0.1	0.5	227	31	215	156	240	1.5	0.7	32	9	1.17	4	0.02	0.4	2.1	0.05	5	1.2
0.1	0.6	246	34	233	169	259	1.6	0.7	35	9	1.26	4	0.02	0.43	2.3	0.06	5	1.3

Food Item	Qty	Meas	Wgt (g)	Wtr (g)	Cals	Prot (g)	Carb (g)	Fib (g)	Fat (g)	SatF (g)
Fish, octopus, raw	4	oz.	113	91	93	17	2	0	1	0.3
Fish, octopus, smoked	4	oz.	113	75	158	29	4	0	2	0.4
Fish, orange roughy baked/broiled	0.5	cup	66	46	59	12	0	0	1	0
Fish, oyster, Eastern, breaded, fried	6	each	88	57	173	8	10	0.1	11	2.8
Fish, oyster, Eastern, breaded, fried, cup measure	1	cup	131	85	258	12	15	0.2	16	4.2
Fish, oyster, Pacific, raw	1	each	50	41	40	5	2	0	1	0.3
Fish, oyster, baked/broiled	4	oz.	113	94	82	9	5	0	2	0.6
Fish, oyster, eastern, canned, w/liquid	0.5	cup	124	106	86	9	5	0	3	0.8
Fish, oyster, eastern, raw	4	oz.	113	97	77	8	4	0	3	0.9
Fish, oyster, eastern, steamed	6	each	42	30	58	6	3	0	2	0.6
Fish, oysters, Pacific, steamed/boiled	4	oz.	113	73	185	21	11	0	5	1.2
Fish, perch, mixed, baked/broiled fillet	1	each	46	34	54	12	0	0	1	0.1
Fish, perch, mixed, baked/broiled fillet	3	oz.	85	62	100	21	0	0	1	0.2
Fish, pollock, walleye, baked/broiled	1	each	60	44	68	14	0	0	1	0.1
Fish, pollock, walleye, baked/broiled	3	oz.	85	63	96	20	0	0	1	0.2
Fish, salmon cake/patty	1	each	120	71	261	16	14	1.3	16	4.1
Fish, salmon croquette	1	each	63	37	137	9	7	0.7	8	2.2
Fish, salmon loaf	1	each	105	63	210	16	9	0.4	12	3.1
Fish, salmon loaf	3	oz.	85	51	170	13	7	0.3	9	2.5
Fish, salmon, Atlantic, baked/broiled fillet	0.5	each	154	92	280	39	0	0	12	1.9
Fish, salmon, Atlantic, baked/broiled fillet	3	oz.	85	51	155	22	0	0	7	1.1
Fish, salmon, chinook, baked/broiled	4	oz.	113	74	262	29	0	0	15	3.6
Fish, salmon, chinook, smoked/lox	4	oz.	113	82	133	21	0	0	5	1
Fish, salmon, chinook, smoked/lox	4	oz.	113	82	133	21	0	0	5	1
Fish, salmon, chum, baked/broiled	4	oz.	113	78	175	29	0	0	5	1.2
Fish, salmon, chum, canned, drained	0.5	cup	75	53	106	16	0	0	4	1.1
Fish, salmon, coho, steamed/poached fillet	3	oz.	85	56	156	23	0	0	6	1.4
Fish, salmon, coho, steamed/poached fillet	4	oz.	113	74	209	31	0	0	9	1.8
Fish, salmon, pink, baked/broiled	4	oz.	113	79	169	29	0	0	5	0.8
Fish, salmon, pink, w/bone, #1 can, drained	1	cup	150	103	209	30	0	0	9	2.3
Fish, salmon, sockeye, baked/broiled fillet	1	each	155	96	335	42	0	0	17	3
Fish, salmon, sockeye, canned, drained	0.5	cup	75	52	115	15	0	0	5	1.2
Fish, sardine, Atlantic, canned in oil, drained	4	each	48	29	100	12	0	0	6	0.7
Fish, sardines in soy oil	1	each	84	—	150	18	1	0	8	4
Fish, sardines, Pacific, canned in tomato sauce	2	each	76	52	135	12	0	0	9	2.4
Fish, sardines, canned, w/mustard	4	oz.	113	73	222	21	2	0	14	4.4
Fish, sardines, skinless, water pack	4	each	84	50	182	21	0	0	10	2.3
Fish, scallop, battered, fried	10	each	80	44	184	14	11	0.4	9	2.2
Fish, scallop, raw, small	5	each	30	24	26	5	1	0	0	0
Fish, scallops, baked/broiled	4	each	100	70	133	21	3	0	4	0.7
Fish, scallops, breaded, fried, large	2	each	31	18	67	6	3	0	3	0.8
Fish, scallops, imitation, from surimi	4	oz.	113	84	112	14	12	0	0	0.1
Fish, scallops, steamed	4	oz.	113	86	121	18	3	0	4	0.6
Fish, sea bass, baked/broiled fillet	1	each	101	73	125	24	0	0	3	0.7
Fish, sea bass, baked/broiled fillet	3	oz.	85	61	105	20	0	0	2	0.6
Fish, sea bass, striped, baked/broiled	4	oz.	113	83	141	26	0	0	3	0.7
Fish, shark, baked/broiled w/marg, lemon juice, salt	4	oz.	113	74	203	28	0	0	9	1.9
Fish, shark, batter fried	4	oz.	113	68	259	21	7	0	16	3.6
Fish, shrimp cocktail	0.5	cup	115	89	98	13	10	2.1	1	0.3
Fish, shrimp w/butter sauce	0.5	cup	68	47	110	15	1	0	5	2.6
Fish, shrimp, baked/broiled, medium size	2	each	10	7	16	2	0	0	1	0.1
Fish, shrimp, batter fried	12	each	90	48	218	19	10	0.3	11	1.9
Fish, shrimp, canned, drained	10	each	32	23	38	7	0	0	1	0.1
Fish, shrimp, canned, drained, cup	1	cup	128	93	154	30	1	0	3	0.5
Fish, shrimp, dried	1	cup	38	12	115	22	1	0	2	0.4
Fish, shrimp, dried, whole	60	each	30	9	91	18	1	0	1	0.3
Fish, shrimp, imitation, made from surimi	4	oz.	113	85	115	14	10	0	2	0.3
Fish, shrimp, large/prawns, breaded, fried	5	each	85	45	206	18	10	0.3	10	1.8
Fish, shrimp, large/prawns, steamed	10	each	55	42	54	12	0	0	1	0.2
Fish, shrimp, popcorn, baked/broiled	15	each	15	10	23	4	0	0	1	0.1
Fish, shrimp, raw (1 large=7 gram)	4	each	28	21	30	6	0	0	0	0.1
Fish, shrimp, small, breaded, fried	12	each	72	38	174	15	8	0.3	9	1.5
Fish, shrimp, small, steamed	10	each	40	31	40	8	0	0	0	0.1
Fish, shrimp, sweet & sour	0.5	cup	88	42	240	9	21	0.4	14	2.1
Fish, smelt, rainbow, baked/broiled	4	oz.	113	83	141	26	0	0	4	0.7

MonoF (g)	PolyF (g)	Choles (mg)	Calc (mg)	Phos (mg)	Sod (mg)	Pot (mg)	Zn (mg)	Iron (mg)	Magn (mg)	VitA (μg RE)	VitE (mg α-TE)	VitC (mg)	Thia (mg)	Ribo (mg)	Nia (mg)	B6 (mg)	Fola (μg)	B12 (μg)
0.2	0.3	54	60	211	261	397	1.9	6	34	51	1.36	6	0.03	0.04	2.4	0.41	18	22.7
0.3	0.5	93	102	359	444	676	3.2	10.2	58	78	2.32	8	0.06	0.08	4.1	0.66	29	36.7
0.4	0	17	25	169	54	254	0.6	0.2	25	16	0.42	0	0.08	0.12	2.4	0.23	5	1.52
4.1	2.9	71	55	140	367	215	76.6	6.1	51	79	2.01	3	0.13	0.18	1.4	0.06	27	13.7
6.2	4.3	106	81	208	546	320	114	9.1	76	118	2.99	5	0.2	0.26	2.2	0.08	41	20.4
0.2	0.4	25	4	80	53	83	8.2	2.5	11	40	0.42	4	0.03	0.12	1	0.02	5	7.94
0.3	0.9	56	51	154	277	191	83.5	4.9	52	0	0.96	5	0.1	0.09	1.9	0.11	20	31.5
0.3	0.9	68	56	172	139	284	113	8.3	67	112	1.05	6	0.19	0.21	1.5	0.12	11	23.7
0.4	1.1	60	51	153	239	177	103	7.6	53	34	0.96	4	0.11	0.11	1.6	0.07	11	22.1
0.3	0.8	44	38	85	177	118	76.4	5	40	23	0.67	3	0.08	0.08	1	0.05	6	14.7
0.8	2	113	18	276	240	342	37.6	10.4	50	166	2.01	14	0.14	0.5	4.1	0.1	17	32.7
0.1	0.2	53	47	118	36	158	0.7	0.5	18	5	0.7	1	0.04	0.06	0.9	0.06	3	1.01
0.2	0.4	98	87	218	67	292	1.2	1	32	8	1.28	1	0.07	0.1	1.6	0.12	5	1.87
0.1	0.3	58	4	289	70	232	0.4	0.2	44	14	0.12	0	0.04	0.05	1	0.04	2	2.52
0.1	0.4	82	5	410	99	329	0.5	0.2	62	20	0.17	0	0.06	0.06	1.4	0.06	3	3.57
6.4	4	56	180	275	657	385	0.9	0.9	32	27	2.11	4	0.09	0.18	5.4	0.37	20	2.19
3.4	2.1	30	95	144	345	202	0.5	0.5	17	14	1.11	2	0.05	0.1	2.9	0.2	10	1.15
4.3	3.2	122	188	276	791	289	1	1.3	30	120	2.01	2	0.09	0.3	4.5	0.22	22	2.35
3.5	2.6	99	153	223	640	234	0.8	1	25	97	1.63	2	0.07	0.24	3.7	0.18	18	1.9
4.2	5	109	23	394	86	967	1.3	1.6	57	20	1.94	0	0.42	0.75	15.6	1.45	45	4.7
2.3	2.8	60	13	218	48	534	0.7	0.9	32	11	1.07	0	0.23	0.41	8.6	0.8	25	2.59
6.5	3	96	32	421	68	573	0.6	1	138	169	1.94	5	0.05	0.18	11.3	0.52	40	3.25
2.3	1.1	26	12	186	889	198	0.4	1	20	30	1.53	0	0.03	0.12	5.4	0.32	2	3.7
2.3	1.1	26	12	186	2268	198	0.4	1	20	30	1.53	0	0.03	0.12	5.4	0.32	2	3.7
2.2	1.3	108	16	412	73	624	0.7	0.8	32	39	1.94	0	0.1	0.25	9.7	0.52	6	3.92
1.4	1.1	29	187	266	365	225	0.8	0.5	22	14	1.2	0	0.02	0.12	5.2	0.28	15	3.3
2.3	2.1	48	39	253	45	387	0.4	0.6	30	27	0.69	1	0.1	0.14	6.6	0.47	8	3.81
3.1	2.9	65	52	338	60	516	0.6	0.8	40	36	0.92	1	0.13	0.18	8.8	0.63	10	5.08
1.4	2	76	19	335	98	469	0.8	1.1	37	46	1.43	0	0.22	0.08	9.7	0.26	6	3.92
2.7	3.1	82	320	494	831	489	1.4	1.3	51	26	2.03	0	0.04	0.28	9.8	0.45	23	6.6
8.2	3.7	135	11	428	102	581	0.8	0.9	48	98	1.95	0	0.33	0.26	10.3	0.34	8	8.99
2.4	1.4	33	179	245	404	283	0.8	0.8	22	40	1.2	0	0.01	0.14	4.1	0.22	7	0.22
1.9	2.5	68	183	235	242	191	0.6	1.4	19	32	0.14	0	0.04	0.11	2.5	0.08	6	4.29
—	—	100	250	—	310	—	—	1.4	—	0	—	0	—	—	—	—	—	—
4.2	1.8	46	182	278	315	259	1.1	1.8	26	53	2.81	1	0.03	0.18	3.2	0.09	18	6.84
4.8	3.2	125	344	401	862	295	0.6	5.9	11	10	1.13	0	0.03	0.23	6.1	0.14	18	7.94
4.3	2.4	69	71	273	771	375	1.1	1.3	39	33	0.84	1	0.11	0.27	3.7	0.35	12	15.7
3.7	2.3	65	29	182	374	248	0.8	0.9	43	29	1.55	2	0.07	0.14	1.3	0.11	15	0.98
0	0.1	10	7	66	48	97	0.3	0.1	17	4	0.3	1	0	0.02	0.3	0.04	5	0.46
1.4	1.3	40	30	265	511	390	1.2	0.4	68	56	1.69	3	0.01	0.06	1.3	0.17	18	1.75
1.4	0.9	19	13	73	144	103	0.3	0.3	18	7	0.59	1	0.01	0.03	0.5	0.04	12	0.41
0.1	0.2	25	9	320	902	117	0.4	0.4	49	23	0.12	0	0.01	0.02	0.4	0.03	2	1.81
1.3	1.2	36	28	180	465	318	1	0.3	61	52	1.53	3	0.01	0.07	1.1	0.16	13	1.51
0.5	1	54	13	250	88	331	0.5	0.4	54	65	0.64	0	0.13	0.15	1.9	0.46	6	0.3
0.5	0.8	45	11	211	74	279	0.4	0.3	45	54	0.54	0	0.11	0.13	1.6	0.39	5	0.26
1	1.2	117	22	288	100	372	0.6	1.2	58	35	0.69	0	0.13	0.04	2.9	0.39	11	5
3.5	3	68	47	279	455	219	0.6	1.1	65	124	1.86	2	0.05	0.08	3.9	0.48	4	1.48
6.7	4.2	67	57	220	138	176	0.5	1.3	49	61	1.19	0	0.08	0.11	3.2	0.34	17	1.37
0.2	0.4	87	43	138	496	277	0.7	1.7	27	36	2.32	12	0.05	0.05	1.9	0.12	27	0.56
1.3	0.6	120	38	149	146	134	0.8	1.7	26	47	1.66	1	0.02	0.02	1.8	0.07	1	0.72
0.2	0.2	18	6	25	50	22	0.1	0.3	4	10	0.39	0	0	0	0.3	0.01	0	0.13
3.4	4.6	159	60	196	310	203	1.2	1.1	36	50	1.35	1	0.12	0.12	2.8	0.09	7	1.68
0.1	0.2	55	19	75	54	67	0.4	0.9	13	6	0.3	1	0.01	0.01	0.9	0.04	1	0.36
0.4	1	221	76	298	216	269	1.6	3.5	52	23	1.19	3	0.04	0.05	3.5	0.14	2	1.43
0.3	0.7	166	57	224	163	202	1.2	2.6	39	17	2.41	2	0.03	0.04	2.6	0.11	2	1.08
0.2	0.6	131	45	177	128	159	1	2.1	31	14	1.9	2	0.02	0.03	2.1	0.08	1	0.85
0.2	0.9	41	22	320	799	101	0.4	0.7	49	23	0.12	0	0.03	0.04	0.2	0.03	2	1.81
3.2	4.3	150	57	185	292	191	1.2	1.1	34	48	1.28	1	0.11	0.12	2.6	0.08	7	1.59
0.1	0.2	107	22	75	123	100	0.9	1.7	19	36	0.28	1	0.02	0.02	1.4	0.07	2	0.82
0.2	0.3	28	10	37	75	34	0.2	0.4	7	14	0.59	0	0	0	0.4	0.02	1	0.2
0.1	0.2	43	15	57	41	52	0.3	0.7	10	15	0.23	1	0.01	0.01	0.7	0.03	1	0.32
2.7	3.7	127	48	157	248	162	1	0.9	29	40	1.08	1	0.09	0.1	2.2	0.07	6	1.35
0.1	0.2	78	16	55	90	73	0.6	1.2	14	26	0.2	1	0.01	0.01	1	0.05	1	0.6
3.3	8.2	60	29	98	409	183	0.6	1.5	23	25	2.07	5	0.03	0.04	1.4	0.1	3	0.39
0.9	1.3	102	87	335	87	422	2.4	1.3	43	19	0.71	0	0.01	0.17	2	0.19	5	4.5

Food Item	Qty	Meas	Wgt (g)	Wtr (g)	Cals	Prot (g)	Carb (g)	Fib (g)	Fat (g)	SatF (g)
Fish, snapper, baked/broiled fillet	4	oz.	113	80	145	30	0	0	2	0.4
Fish, sole/flounder, baked/broiled fillet	1	each	127	93	149	31	0	0	2	0.5
Fish, sole/flounder, baked/broiled fillet	3	oz.	85	62	100	21	0	0	1	0.3
Fish, sole/flounder, batter fried pieces	4	piece	64	42	121	13	5	0.1	5	1
Fish, sole/flounder, breaded, fried fillet	1	each	81	48	176	16	6	0.4	9	2.3
Fish, sole/flounder, breaded, fried fillet	3	oz.	85	50	185	17	7	0.4	10	2.4
Fish, sole/flounder, steamed/poached	4	oz.	113	84	129	27	0	0	2	0.4
Fish, squid, canned	0.5	cup	94	70	99	17	3	0	1	0.4
Fish, squid, flour fried	0.5	cup	75	48	131	13	6	0	6	1.4
Fish, squid, pickled	4	oz.	113	85	104	17	5	0	2	0.4
Fish, squid/calamari, baked/broiled	4	oz.	113	80	156	21	4	0	5	1.2
Fish, steelhead, baked/broiled fillet	3	oz.	85	61	113	18	0	0	4	1.1
Fish, steelhead, baked/broiled fillet	4	oz.	113	82	151	24	0	0	5	1.5
Fish, sturgeon, baked/broiled	4	oz.	113	79	153	24	0	0	6	1.3
Fish, sturgeon, smoked	4	oz.	113	71	196	35	0	0	5	1.2
Fish, surimi (processed pollock)	4	oz.	113	86	112	17	8	0	1	0.2
Fish, swordfish, broiled/baked	1	piece	106	73	164	27	0	0	5	1.5
Fish, swordfish, broiled/baked	3	oz.	85	58	132	22	0	0	4	1.2
Fish, swordfish, steamed/poached	4	oz.	113	78	174	28	0	0	6	1.6
Fish, trout, floured/breaded, fried	1	each	125	63	334	29	12	0.7	18	4
Fish, trout, mixed, baked/broiled	4	oz.	113	72	215	30	0	0	10	1.7
Fish, trout, rainbow, baked/broiled fillet	1	each	62	44	93	14	0	0	4	1
Fish, trout, rainbow, baked/broiled fillet	3	oz.	85	60	128	20	0	0	5	1.4
Fish, tuna cake/patty	1	each	120	64	300	22	14	1.3	17	4.2
Fish, tuna, bluefin, baked/broiled	4	oz.	113	67	209	34	0	0	7	1.8
Fish, tuna, light, canned in oil, drained	1	cup	146	87	289	42	0	0	12	2.2
Fish, tuna, skipjack, baked/broiled	4	oz.	113	71	150	32	0	0	1	0.5
Fish, tuna, smoked pieces	4	piece	64	38	140	15	0	0	8	2.2
Fish, tuna, yellowfin, baked/broiled	4	oz.	113	71	158	34	0	0	1	0.3
Fish, whelk, steamed	4	oz.	113	36	312	54	18	0	1	0.1
Fish, whiting, baked/broiled	4	oz.	113	85	132	27	0	0	2	0.5
Flan caramel custard mix w/2% milk	0.5	cup	133	100	136	4	26	0.1	2	1.5
Flan caramel custard mix w/whole milk	0.5	cup	133	99	150	4	25	0.1	4	2.5
Flauta, beef	1	each	113	55	360	16	13	1.7	27	4.9
Flauta, chicken	1	each	113	59	343	14	13	1.7	27	4.3
Flour, Soy, lowfat	1	cup	88	2	325	45	30	9	6	0.9
Flour, arrowroot	1	cup	128	15	457	0	113	4.4	0	0
Flour, bread, white, Pillsbury	1	cup	113	16	396	14	81	2.7	1	0.3
Flour, brown rice	1	cup	158	19	574	11	121	7.3	4	0.9
Flour, buckwheat, whole groat	1	cup	98	11	328	12	69	9.8	3	0.7
Flour, carob	1	cup	103	4	229	5	92	41	1	0.1
Flour, chickpea	1	cup	85	8	313	17	51	3.1	6	—
Flour, corn, white, whole grain	1	cup	117	13	422	8	90	11.2	5	0.6
Flour, corn, yellow	1	cup	114	10	416	11	87	15.3	4	0.6
Flour, corn, yellow, whole grain	1	cup	117	13	422	8	90	15.7	5	0.6
Flour, corn/masa harina, enriched	1	cup	114	10	416	11	87	10.9	4	0.6
Flour, gluten	1	cup	140	12	529	58	66	1.2	3	0
Flour, masa harina, enriched, baked value	1	cup	114	10	416	11	87	10.9	4	0.6
Flour, potato	1	cup	179	12	639	12	149	10.6	1	0.2
Flour, rye, dark	1	cup	128	14	415	18	88	28.9	3	0.4
Flour, rye, light	1	cup	102	9	374	9	82	14.9	1	0.1
Flour, rye, light, baked value	1	cup	102	9	374	9	82	14.9	1	0.1
Flour, rye, medium	1	cup	102	10	361	10	79	14.9	2	0.2
Flour, rye, medium, baked value	1	cup	102	10	361	10	79	14.9	2	0.2
Flour, rye-wheat, bohemian style, Pillsbury	1	cup	113	16	395	13	82	6.5	2	0.3
Flour, semolina, enriched	1	cup	167	21	601	21	122	6.5	2	0.3
Flour, sesame, high fat	1	oz.	28	0	149	9	8	1.8	10	1.5
Flour, sesame, lowfat	1	oz.	28	2	94	14	10	1.4	0	0.1
Flour, sesame, partially defatted	1	oz.	28	2	108	11	10	1.7	3	0.5
Flour, shake and blend, Pillsbury	1	cup	216	30	756	23	158	5.8	3	1.1
Flour, soy, whole fat	1	cup	85	4	369	32	27	8.2	18	2.5
Flour, sunflower seed, partially defatted	1	cup	80	6	261	38	29	4.2	1	0.1
Flour, triticale, whole grain	1	cup	130	13	439	17	95	19	2	0.4
Flour, white rice	1	cup	158	19	578	9	127	3.8	2	0.6
Flour, white, all purpose, enriched	1	cup	125	15	455	13	95	3.4	1	0.2

A

MonoF	PolyF	Choles	Calc	Phos	Sod	Pot	Zn	Iron	Magn	VitA	VitE	VitC	Thia	Ribo	Nia	B6	Fola	B12
(g)	(g)	(mg)	(mg)	(mg)	(mg)	(mg)	(mg)	(mg)	(mg)	(μg RE)	(mg α-TE)	(mg)	(mg)	(mg)	(mg)	(mg)	(μg)	(μg)
0.4	0.7	53	45	228	65	592	0.5	0.3	42	40	0.71	2	0.06	0	0.4	0.52	7	3.97
0.3	0.8	86	23	367	133	437	0.8	0.4	74	14	2.4	0	0.1	0.14	2.8	0.3	12	3.19
0.2	0.5	58	15	246	89	292	0.5	0.3	49	9	1.61	0	0.07	0.1	1.8	0.2	8	2.13
2	1.8	31	44	145	105	277	0.3	0.8	50	66	1.04	0	0.07	0.08	3.7	0.18	9	0.7
3.8	2.4	56	28	163	314	300	0.5	0.7	28	15	2.22	1	0.08	0.1	2.6	0.15	10	1.1
4	2.5	58	30	171	329	315	0.5	0.7	29	16	2.33	1	0.09	0.11	2.8	0.16	10	1.16
0.3	0.5	68	26	235	103	435	0.6	0.5	40	11	2.68	2	0.1	0.1	3.5	0.24	9	1.83
0.1	0.6	250	35	190	292	211	1.6	0.7	32	9	1.29	4	0.02	0.35	1.9	0.04	4	1.05
2.1	1.6	195	29	188	230	209	1.3	0.8	28	8	1.39	3	0.04	0.34	2	0.04	10	0.92
0.1	0.6	254	37	229	1585	273	1.7	0.7	36	10	1.31	4	0.02	0.45	2.2	0.05	5	1.35
1.7	1.8	318	45	303	420	338	2.1	0.9	45	58	2.19	6	0.02	0.45	2.8	0.07	6	1.69
1	0.8	90	19	273	63	371	0.5	0.3	34	30	0.21	0	0.06	0.18	2.5	0.39	5	2.94
1.3	1	120	25	364	84	496	0.7	0.4	45	40	0.28	0	0.08	0.24	3.3	0.52	7	3.92
2.8	1	87	19	307	78	413	0.6	1	51	274	0.85	0	0.09	0.1	11.5	0.26	20	2.84
2.7	0.5	91	19	319	838	430	0.6	1	53	318	0.57	0	0.1	0.1	12.6	0.31	23	3.29
0.2	0.5	34	10	320	162	127	0.4	0.3	49	23	0.28	0	0.02	0.02	0.2	0.03	2	1.81
2.1	1.2	53	6	357	122	391	1.6	1.1	36	44	0.67	1	0.05	0.12	12.5	0.4	2	2.14
1.7	1	42	5	286	98	314	1.2	0.9	29	35	0.54	1	0.04	0.1	10	0.32	2	1.72
2.2	1.3	56	6	340	116	351	1.6	1.2	35	44	0.72	1	0.04	0.12	11.8	0.38	2	2.14
7.4	5.5	106	80	341	530	484	1	2.6	34	34	1.24	1	0.41	0.48	6.2	0.24	23	8.74
4.7	2.2	84	62	356	76	525	1	2.2	32	22	0.3	1	0.48	0.48	6.5	0.26	17	8.49
1.1	1.1	43	53	167	35	278	0.3	0.2	19	9	0.31	1	0.09	0.06	3.6	0.22	12	3.91
1.5	1.6	59	73	229	48	381	0.4	0.3	26	13	0.43	2	0.13	0.08	4.9	0.29	16	5.36
7.2	4.9	43	28	252	421	325	0.9	1.4	33	30	1.87	4	0.1	0.15	9.2	0.21	11	1.38
2.3	2.1	56	11	370	57	366	0.9	1.5	73	857	1.43	0	0.32	0.35	11.9	0.6	2	12.4
4.3	4.2	26	19	454	517	302	1.3	2	45	34	1.75	0	0.06	0.18	18.1	0.16	8	3.21
0.3	0.5	68	42	323	53	592	1.2	1.8	50	20	1.43	1	0.04	0.14	21.3	1.11	11	2.48
3.3	2.2	61	42	163	179	192	0.4	0.9	19	30	0.96	0	0.01	0.18	2.1	0.32	6	4.48
0.2	0.4	66	24	278	53	645	0.8	1.1	73	23	0.71	1	0.57	0.06	13.5	1.18	2	0.68
0.1	0.1	147	128	320	467	787	3.7	11.5	195	56	0.3	8	0.06	0.24	2.3	0.74	13	20.5
0.5	0.7	95	70	323	150	492	0.6	0.5	31	39	0.34	0	0.08	0.07	1.9	0.2	17	2.95
0.7	0.1	9	153	116	66	194	0.5	0.1	17	62	0.07	1	0.04	0.2	0.1	0.05	5	0.36
1.2	0.2	16	150	114	65	192	0.5	0.1	16	35	0.13	1	0.04	0.2	0.1	0.05	5	0.35
11.6	9.1	45	50	199	187	292	4.2	2.2	29	15	4	14	0.07	0.15	2.1	0.25	10	1.45
11.1	9.6	37	52	146	189	243	1.2	1	28	22	4.06	14	0.05	0.1	3.2	0.22	8	0.09
1.3	3.3	0	165	522	16	2261	1	5.3	202	4	0.17	0	0.33	0.25	1.9	0.46	361	0
0	0.1	0	51	6	3	14	0.1	0.4	4	0	—	0	0	0	0	0.01	9	0
—	—	0	23	—	1	—	—	5	—	0	—	0	0.68	0.45	6	—	175	—
1.6	1.6	0	17	532	13	457	3.9	3.1	177	0	1.14	0	0.7	0.13	10	1.16	25	0
0.9	0.9	0	40	330	11	565	3.1	4	246	0	1.01	0	0.41	0.19	6	0.57	53	0
0.2	0.2	0	358	81	36	852	0.9	3	56	1	0.65	0	0.06	0.48	2	0.38	30	0
—	—	—	85	296	—	—	—	6	92	—	—	—	0.1	0.28	0.6	—	—	0
1.2	2.1	0	8	318	6	369	2	2.8	109	0	0.29	0	0.29	0.09	2.2	0.43	29	0
1.1	2	0	161	254	6	340	2	8.2	125	54	0.95	0	1.63	0.86	11.2	0.42	213	0
1.2	2.1	0	8	318	6	369	2	2.8	109	55	0.29	0	0.29	0.09	2.2	0.43	29	0
1.1	2	0	161	254	6	340	2	8.2	125	0	0.28	0	1.63	0.86	11.2	0.42	213	0
0	0	0	56	196	3	84	—	0.6	—	0	—	0	0.04	0.04	0.7	—	30	0
1.1	2	0	161	254	6	340	2	8.2	125	0	0.95	0	1.63	0.77	10.1	0.38	149	0
0	0.3	0	116	301	98	1791	1	2.5	116	0	0.45	7	0.41	0.09	6.3	1.38	45	0
0.4	1.5	0	72	809	1	934	7.2	8.3	317	0	3.3	0	0.4	0.32	5.5	0.57	77	0
0.2	0.6	0	21	198	2	238	1.8	1.8	71	0	0.57	0	0.34	0.09	0.8	0.24	22	0
0.2	0.6	0	21	198	2	238	1.8	1.8	71	0	0.57	0	0.27	0.08	0.7	0.22	16	0
0.2	0.8	0	24	211	3	347	2	2.2	76	0	1.36	0	0.29	0.12	1.8	0.27	19	0
0.2	0.8	0	24	211	3	347	2	2.2	76	0	0.81	0	0.24	0.1	1.6	0.25	14	0
—	—	0	22	—	0	—	—	5	—	0	—	0	0.68	0.45	6	—	—	—
0.2	0.7	0	28	227	2	311	1.8	7.3	78	0	0.1	0	1.35	0.95	10	0.17	257	0
4	4.6	0	45	229	12	120	3	4.3	102	2	0.44	0	0.76	0.08	3.8	0.04	9	0
0.2	0.2	0	42	215	11	113	2.8	4	96	2	0.02	0	0.71	0.08	3.5	0.04	8	0
1.2	1.4	0	42	230	12	120	3	4	103	2	0.16	0	0.72	0.08	3.6	0.04	8	0
—	—	0	43	—	2	—	—	9.5	—	0	—	0	1.3	0.86	11.4	—	—	—
3.9	10	0	175	420	11	2137	3.3	5.4	365	10	1.66	0	0.49	0.99	3.7	0.39	293	0
0.2	0.7	0	91	551	2	54	4	5.3	277	4	1.3	1	2.55	0.21	5.8	0.6	178	0
0.2	1	0	46	417	3	606	3.5	3.4	199	0	2.48	0	0.49	0.17	3.7	0.52	96	0
0.7	0.6	0	16	155	0	120	1.3	0.6	55	0	0.2	0	0.22	0.03	4.1	0.69	6	0
0.1	0.5	0	19	135	2	134	0.9	5.8	28	0	0.08	0	0.98	0.62	7.4	0.06	193	0

Food Item	Qty	Meas	Wgt (g)	Wtr (g)	Cals	Prot (g)	Carb (g)	Fib (g)	Fat (g)	SatF (g)
Flour, white, all purpose, enriched, baked value	1	cup	125	15	455	13	95	4.1	1	0.2
Flour, white, all purpose, enriched, unbleached	1	cup	125	15	455	13	95	3.4	1	0.2
Flour, white, all purpose, sifted	1	cup	115	14	419	12	88	3.1	1	0.2
Flour, white, cake, baked value	1	cup	109	14	395	9	85	1.8	1	0.1
Flour, white, cake, enriched, sifted	1	cup	96	12	348	8	75	1.6	1	0.1
Flour, white, cake, sifted, baked value	1	cup	96	12	348	8	75	1.6	1	0.1
Flour, white, self-rising, enriched	1	cup	125	13	443	12	93	3.4	1	0.2
Flour, whole wheat	1	cup	120	12	407	16	87	14.6	2	0.4
Flour, whole wheat, Pillsbury	1	cup	113	16	397	16	77	13.4	3	0.6
Flour, whole wheat, baked value	1	cup	120	12	407	16	87	14.6	2	0.4
Forza energy bar	1	each	70	12	231	10	45	4	1	—
French toast, homemade, w/2% milk	1	piece	65	36	149	5	16	0.6	7	1.8
French toast, recipe, w/whole milk	1	piece	65	35	151	5	16	0.5	7	2
Fritter, banana	1	each	34	13	116	2	11	0.4	7	2
Fritter, berry	1	each	34	15	111	2	10	0.6	7	1.9
Fritter, wheat, no syrup	1	each	22	8	99	2	4	0.1	9	2
Frog legs, steamed	2	each	100	74	106	24	0	0	0	0.1
Frosting, chocolate cream, recipe, w/margarine	2	Tbs	34	3	138	0	27	0.6	4	0.9
Frosting, chocolate supreme, Pillsbury	2	Tbs	35	7	139	0	21	0.2	6	1.7
Frosting, chocolate, creamy, ready to eat, can	1	each	462	78	1834	5	292	2.8	81	25.5
Frosting, chocolate, creamy, w/butter	2	Tbs	34	5	131	0	25	0.6	4	1.9
Frosting, chocolate, creamy, w/margarine	2	Tbs	34	5	132	0	25	0.6	4	0.6
Frosting, coconut nut, ready to eat, can	1	each	462	97	1903	7	244	6.5	111	32.5
Frosting, cream cheese flavor, ready to eat	1	each	462	70	1908	0	308	0	80	23.3
Frosting, creamy chocolate butter, recipe	2	Tbs	34	3	138	0	27	0.6	4	2.4
Frosting, french vanilla supreme, Pillsbury	2	Tbs	38	6	158	0	26	0	6	1.7
Frosting, lite, milk chocolate, Pillsbury	2	Tbs	58	11	209	1	41	1.6	5	1.4
Frosting, lite, vanilla, Pillsbury	2	Tbs	32	5	121	0	24	0.1	3	0.7
Frosting, seven minute, recipe	0.25	cup	80	14	254	1	64	0	0	0
Frosting, sour cream flavor, ready to eat, can	1	each	462	66	1903	0	312	0.5	80	23.1
Frosting, vanilla cream, recipe, w/butter	2	Tbs	40	7	137	0	31	0	2	1
Frosting, vanilla cream, recipe, w/margarine	2	Tbs	40	4	162	0	32	0	4	0.9
Frosting, vanilla, creamy, mix w/water & butter	2	Tbs	40	5	169	0	28	0	7	2.8
Frosting, white, fluffy, mix w/water, pkg	1	each	315	111	769	5	197	0	0	0
Frosting/Icing, chocolate, ready to spread	1	oz.	28	5	120	0	18	0	5	2
Frosting/glaze, recipe	0.25	cup	80	14	287	0	59	0	6	1.4
Frosting/icing, creamy vanilla, canned	2	Tbs	31	4	131	0	22	0	5	1.5
Frosting/icing, creamy, mix, prepared	2	Tbs	40	5	169	0	28	0	7	1.3
Frozen dessert bar, Treat, Weight Watchers	1	each	81	58	88	2	19	0	1	0.2
Frozen dessert, Weight Watchers	0.5	cup	66	47	73	3	14	0	1	0.3
Frozen yogurt cone, chocolate	1	each	78	44	157	4	22	1.1	7	3.9
Frozen yogurt cone, not chocolate	1	each	78	47	143	3	22	0.5	5	2.6
Frozen yogurt, Cherry Garcia, Ben & Jerry's	0.5	cup	106	—	170	4	31	0	3	2
Frozen yogurt, chocolate	0.5	cup	96	67	110	5	21	1.5	2	1.2
Frozen yogurt, chocolate-coated	1	each	41	21	109	1	12	0.1	7	5.4
Frozen yogurt, nonfat, chocolate	0.5	cup	96	67	104	5	21	1.5	1	0.5
Frozen yogurt, nonfat, fruit	0.5	cup	96	72	95	5	19	0	0	0.1
Frozen yogurt, soft serve, chocolate	0.5	cup	72	46	115	3	18	1.6	4	2.6
Frozen yogurt, soft serve, vanilla	0.5	cup	72	47	114	3	17	0	4	2.5
Frozen yogurt, vanilla	0.5	cup	96	71	102	4	18	0	1	0.8
Frozen yogurt, vanilla/fruit	0.5	cup	96	71	102	4	18	0	1	0.8
Fruit cocktail in light syrup	0.5	cup	126	106	72	1	19	1.3	0	0
Fruit cocktail, canned in heavy syrup	0.5	cup	128	103	93	0	24	1.3	0	0
Fruit cocktail, juice pack	0.5	cup	124	108	57	1	15	1.2	0	0
Fruit cocktail, water pack	0.5	cup	122	111	39	1	10	1.2	0	0
Fruit drink, Crystal Light, prepared	1	cup	240	239	3	0	0	0	0	0
Fruit drink, low cal (Wylers/Koolaid)	1	cup	240	228	43	0	11	0	0	0
Fruit drink, low calorie, dry mix (Crystal Light)	1	Tbs	12	1	27	1	12	0	0	0
Fruit drink, low calorie, powder, prepared	1	cup	240	228	43	0	11	0	0	0
Fruit drink, powder, prepared (Koolade)	1	cup	240	217	89	0	23	0	0	0
Fruit drink, punch flavor (Hi-C)	1	cup	240	228	43	0	11	0	0	0
Fruit juice bar, frozen	1	each	77	60	63	1	16	0	0	0
Fruit juice bar, w/cream, frozen	1	each	65	43	86	1	19	0.1	1	0.8
Fruit leather/roll ups, small	1	each	14	2	49	0	12	0.5	0	0.1
Fruit punch drink, canned	1	cup	253	223	119	0	30	0.3	0	0

MonoF	PolyF	Choles	Calc	Phos	Sod	Pot	Zn	Iron	Magn	VitA	VitE	VitC	Thia	Ribo	Nia	B6	Fola	B12
(g)	(g)	(mg)	(mg)	(mg)	(mg)	(mg)	(mg)	(mg)	(mg)	(μg RE)	(mg α-TE)	(mg)	(mg)	(mg)	(mg)	(mg)	(μg)	(μg)
0.1	0.5	0	19	135	2	134	0.9	5.8	28	0	0.46	0	0.78	0.56	6.6	0.05	135	0
0.1	0.5	0	19	135	2	134	0.9	5.8	28	0	0.46	0	0.98	0.62	7.4	0.06	193	0
0.1	0.5	0	17	124	2	123	0.8	5.3	25	0	0.07	0	0.9	0.57	6.8	0.05	177	0
0.1	0.4	0	15	93	2	114	0.7	8	17	0	0.08	0	0.78	0.42	6.7	0.03	118	0
0.1	0.4	0	13	82	2	101	0.6	7	15	0	0.06	0	0.86	0.41	6.5	0.03	148	0
0.1	0.4	0	13	82	2	101	0.6	7	15	0	0.06	0	0.86	0.41	6.5	0.03	148	0
0.1	0.5	0	423	744	1587	155	0.8	5.8	24	0	0.08	0	0.84	0.52	7.3	0.06	193	0
0.3	0.9	0	41	415	6	486	3.5	4.7	166	0	1.48	0	0.54	0.26	7.6	0.41	53	0
—	—	0	45	—	1	—	—	5.6	—	0	—	0	0.57	0.11	5.8	—	—	—
0.3	0.9	0	41	415	6	486	3.5	4.7	166	0	0.5	0	0.43	0.23	6.9	0.37	37	0
—	—	0	300	350	65	220	5.2	6.3	160	—	20	60	1.5	1.7	20	2	400	6
2.9	1.7	75	65	76	311	87	0.4	1.1	11	86	0.72	0	0.13	0.21	1.1	0.05	28	0.2
3	1.7	76	64	76	311	86	0.4	1.1	11	81	0.31	0	0.13	0.21	1.1	0.05	15	0.2
3.1	1.8	25	16	29	19	86	0.2	0.4	8	23	0.75	1	0.05	0.09	0.4	0.1	5	0.07
3.1	1.8	25	16	27	20	41	0.2	0.4	4	23	0.87	2	0.05	0.08	0.4	0.02	4	0.08
3.8	2.4	36	6	21	56	17	0.1	0.3	2	67	1.11	0	0.03	0.06	0.3	0.01	4	0.08
0.1	0.2	72	26	160	84	372	1.4	2	29	20	1.45	0	0.19	0.34	1.6	0.16	16	0.52
1.7	1.1	0	6	16	70	32	0.1	0.3	9	38	0.69	0	0	0.01	0	0	1	0.01
—	—	0	4	—	78	—	—	0.6	—	0	—	0	—	—	—	—	—	—
41.7	9.8	0	37	365	845	906	1.3	6.6	97	915	10.9	0	0.06	0.08	0.6	0.02	0	0
0.9	0.1	8	4	17	52	49	0.2	0.3	10	21	0.69	0	0	0.01	0	0.02	0	0
1.4	1	0	4	17	56	50	0.2	0.3	10	23	0.69	0	0	0.01	0	0.02	0	0
56.4	15.8	0	60	291	901	859	1.9	2.5	88	0	5.27	1	0.16	0.09	1	0.25	28	0
41.7	10.9	0	14	14	1094	162	0	0.7	9	536	9.33	0	0	0.03	0.1	0	0	0
1.1	0.1	10	6	16	65	31	0.1	0.3	9	34	0.69	0	0	0.01	0	0	1	0.01
—	—	0	1	—	76	—	—	0	—	0	—	0	—	—	—	—	—	—
—	—	0	5	—	144	—	—	0.9	—	0	—	0	—	—	—	—	—	—
—	—	0	1	—	58	—	—	0	—	0	—	0	—	—	—	—	—	—
0	0	0	2	2	136	51	0	0.1	2	0	0	0	0	0.07	0	0	0	0.02
41.5	10.8	0	9	18	942	896	0	0.3	9	564	9.33	0	0.05	0.09	3.1	0.02	5	0.05
0.5	0.1	5	9	7	26	12	0	0	1	15	0.81	0	0	0.01	0	0	0	0.03
1.9	1.3	0	5	4	82	7	0	0	1	45	0.81	0	0	0.01	0	0	0	0.02
2.2	1.3	10	4	11	83	8	0	0.1	1	38	0.28	0	0.01	0.01	0.1	0	0	0
0	0	0	13	16	491	243	0.1	0.2	6	0	0	0	0	0.08	2.1	0	6	0.03
2	0	0	0	—	40	40	—	0	—	0	—	0	0	0	0	—	—	—
2.7	1.8	2	18	14	75	24	0.1	0	2	65	0.61	0	0.01	0.02	0	0.01	1	0.06
2.7	0.7	0	1	12	28	12	0	0	0	70	1.47	0	0	0	0	0	0	0
2.7	2.3	0	4	11	88	9	0	0.1	1	43	0.81	0	0.01	0.01	0.1	0	0	0
0.1	0.4	1	82	66	47	111	0.3	0.1	10	38	0.07	1	0.03	0.11	0.1	0.03	3	0.24
0.2	0	3	111	88	61	156	0.3	0.1	10	5	0.01	0	0.03	0.13	0.1	0.03	1	0.44
2.5	0.5	1	115	119	70	193	0.5	0.6	29	42	0.34	1	0.05	0.17	0.3	0.08	6	0.2
1.8	0.4	1	118	107	74	167	0.4	0.4	17	44	0.3	1	0.04	0.17	0.3	0.08	6	0.21
—	—	10	150	—	70	—	—	0.4	—	40	—	1	—	—	—	—	—	—
0.6	0.1	5	150	150	56	311	1	0.8	38	13	0.05	1	0.04	0.19	0.2	0.04	10	0.44
0.8	0.2	1	46	43	28	74	0.2	0.1	6	18	0.05	0	0.01	0.07	0.1	0.03	2	0.09
0.3	0	1	163	160	62	327	1.1	0.9	39	2	0.02	1	0.04	0.21	0.2	0.05	11	0.48
0	0	2	167	132	64	214	0.8	0.1	16	2	0	1	0.04	0.2	0.1	0.04	10	0.51
1.3	0.2	4	106	100	71	188	0.4	0.9	19	31	0.1	0	0.03	0.15	0.2	0.05	8	0.21
1.1	0.2	1	103	93	63	152	0.3	0.2	10	41	0.04	1	0.03	0.16	0.2	0.06	4	0.21
0.4	0	5	153	121	59	197	0.8	0.1	15	13	0.04	1	0.04	0.18	0.1	0.04	9	0.47
0.4	0	5	153	121	59	197	0.8	0.1	15	13	0.04	1	0.04	0.18	0.1	0.04	9	0.47
0	0	0	8	14	8	112	0.1	0.4	6	26	0.36	2	0.02	0.02	0.5	0.06	3	0
0	0	0	8	14	8	112	0.1	0.4	6	26	0.37	2	0.02	0.02	0.5	0.06	3	0
0	0	0	10	17	5	118	0.1	0.3	9	38	0.25	3	0.02	0.02	0.5	0.06	3	0
0	0	0	6	14	5	115	0.1	0.3	9	31	0.36	3	0.02	0.01	0.4	0.06	3	0
0	0	0	38	15	7	45	0.1	0	2	0	0	6	0	0	0	0	0	0
0	0	0	17	5	50	50	0.3	0.6	5	2	0	78	0.02	0.05	0	0	5	0
0	0	0	342	156	1	465	0	0	0	0	0	62	0	0	0	0	0	0
0	0	0	17	5	50	50	0.3	0.6	5	2	0	78	0.02	0.05	0	0	5	0
0	0	0	38	48	34	2	0.1	0.1	2	0	0	28	0	0	0	0	0	0
0	0	0	17	5	50	50	0.3	0.6	5	2	0	78	0.02	0.05	0	0	5	0
0	0	0	4	5	3	41	0	0.1	3	2	0	7	0.01	0.01	0.1	0.02	5	0
0.4	0	5	29	5	20	64	0	0.1	2	8	0.03	8	0.01	0.06	0.1	0.03	3	0.05
0.2	0.1	0	4	4	9	41	0	0.1	3	2	0.04	1	0.01	0	0	0.04	1	0
0	0	0	20	3	56	63	0.3	0.5	5	4	0	75	0.06	0.06	0.1	0	3	0

Food Item	Qty	Meas	Wgt (g)	Wtr (g)	Cals	Prot (g)	Carb (g)	Fib (g)	Fat (g)	SatF (g)
Fruit punch drink, frozen concentrate, prepared	1	cup	247	218	114	0	29	0.2	0	0
Fruit punch juice drink, frozen, prepared	1	cup	248	217	124	0	30	0.2	0	0.1
Fruit punch, powder	1	Tbs	6	0	24	0	6	0	0	0
Fruit salad, canned in light syrup	0.5	cup	126	106	73	0	19	1.3	0	0
Fruit salad, includes citrus	0.5	cup	88	74	50	0	13	1.2	0	0.1
Fruit salad, no citrus	0.5	cup	88	73	51	1	13	1.5	0	0.1
Fruit salad, tropical, canned in heavy syrup	0.5	cup	128	99	111	1	29	1.7	0	0
Fruit spread, strawberry, low calorie, Kraft	1	Tbs	20	—	20	0	5	0	0	0
Garlic clove, fresh	1	each	3	2	4	0	1	0.1	0	0
Garlic clove, fresh, chopped	0.25	cup	34	20	51	2	11	0.7	0	0
Garlic powder	0.25	tsp	1	0	2	0	1	0.1	0	0
Garlic, dehydrated	0.25	tsp	1	0	2	0	1	0.1	0	—
Gatorade	1	cup	241	93	60	0	15	0	0	0
Gelatin dessert/Jello, prepared	0.5	cup	135	114	80	2	19	0	0	0
Gelatin dessert/Jello, sugar-free	0.5	cup	117	115	8	1	1	0	0	0
Gelatin, dry mix, sweetened, pkg	1	each	85	1	324	7	77	0	0	0
Gelatin, dry, unsweetened, envelope	1	each	7	1	24	6	0	0	0	0
Gelatin/Jello dessert w/fruit (Jello)	0.5	cup	106	86	73	1	18	0.6	0	0.1
Gelatin/Jello frozen fruit bar	1	each	44	36	31	1	7	0	0	—
Gherkin in sweetened brine	1	each	19	14	19	0	5	0.4	0	0
Ginger root, raw slices	1	piece	2	2	2	0	0	0	0	0
Ginger root, raw, chopped	0.25	cup	24	20	17	0	4	0.5	0	0
Ginger, ground	0.25	tsp	0	0	2	0	0	0.1	0	0
Gnocchi, cheese	0.5	cup	35	24	62	3	3	0.1	4	1.6
Gnocchi, potato	0.5	cup	94	68	136	2	17	0.9	7	4.2
Goat meat, cooked	4	oz.	113	66	237	37	0	0	9	3.7
Goat ribs, cooked	1	each	46	31	66	12	0	0	1	0.4
Goose, liver pate, smoked, canned	0.5	cup	104	38	480	12	5	0	46	15.1
Goose, roasted	4	oz.	113	59	346	29	0	0	25	7.8
Goose, skinless, roasted	4	oz.	113	65	270	33	0	0	14	5.2
Gooseberries canned in light syrup	0.5	cup	126	101	92	1	24	3	0	0
Gooseberries, cooked	0.5	cup	126	101	92	1	24	3	0	0
Gooseberries, fresh	0.5	cup	75	66	33	1	8	3.2	0	0
Graham cracker crust, chilled, not baked	1	oz.	28	2	137	1	18	0.4	7	1.4
Granola bar, New Trail, raisin-coconut, soft	1	each	40	2	182	4	27	1.2	7	4.6
Granola bar, hard, almond	1	each	24	1	117	2	15	1.1	6	3
Granola bar, hard, chocolate chip	1	each	24	1	103	2	17	1	4	2.7
Granola bar, hard, peanut butter	1	each	24	1	114	2	15	0.7	6	0.8
Granola bar, hard, plain	1	each	28	1	134	3	18	1.5	6	0.7
Granola bar, high fiber, yogurt coating, Fi-Bar	1	each	28	3	96	3	19	2.2	3	1
Granola bar, soft, choc chip w/granola & marshmallow	1	each	28	2	121	2	20	1.1	4	2.6
Granola bar, soft, chocolate chocolate chip	1	each	35	1	165	2	23	1.2	9	5
Granola bar, soft, chocolate peanut butter	1	each	37	1	187	4	20	1	11	6.2
Granola bar, soft, chocolate raisin	1	each	42	3	190	3	28	1.8	8	4.1
Granola bar, soft, nut & raisin	1	each	28	2	129	2	18	1.6	6	2.7
Granola bar, soft, peanut butter	1	each	24	2	101	2	15	1	4	0.9
Granola bar, soft, peanut butter chocolate chip	1	each	28	2	122	3	18	1.2	6	1.6
Granola bar, soft, uncoated, chocolate	1	each	42	2	179	3	29	2	7	4.3
Granola bar, soft, uncoated, plain	1	each	28	2	126	2	19	1.3	5	2
Granola clusters, Nature Valley	1	each	34	1	140	2	24	1.4	5	1.9
Grape drink, canned	1	cup	251	222	113	0	29	0	0	0
Grape drink, low calorie	1	cup	240	228	43	0	11	0	0	0
Grape juice drink, canned	1	cup	250	218	125	0	32	0.2	0	0
Grape juice, bottle/canned, unsweetened	1	cup	253	213	154	1	38	0.3	0	0.1
Grape juice, frozen conc w/vit C, prepared	1	cup	250	217	128	0	32	0.2	0	0.1
Grape leaves, raw	1	oz.	28	22	19	1	4	—	0	—
Grape, American type/slip skin, no seeds	0.5	cup	46	37	31	0	8	0.5	0	0.1
Grape, Thompson seedless, cup measure	0.5	cup	80	64	57	1	14	0.8	0	0.2
Grape, Tokay/Red Flame, seedless, cup measure	0.5	cup	80	64	57	1	14	0.8	0	0.2
Grape, adherent skin type	0.5	cup	80	64	57	1	14	0.8	0	0.2
Grapefruit juice, canned, unsweetened	1	cup	247	223	94	1	22	0.2	0	0
Grapefruit juice, fresh	1	cup	247	222	96	1	23	0.2	0	0
Grapefruit juice, frozen concentrate, prepared	1	cup	247	221	101	1	24	0.2	0	0
Grapefruit sections canned in juice	0.5	cup	124	112	46	1	12	0.5	0	0
Grapefruit sections, canned in light syrup	0.5	cup	127	106	76	1	20	0.5	0	0

MonoF (g)	PolyF (g)	Choles (mg)	Calc (mg)	Phos (mg)	Sod (mg)	Pot (mg)	Zn (mg)	Iron (mg)	Magn (mg)	VitA (μg RE)	VitE (mg α-TE)	VitC (mg)	Thia (mg)	Ribo (mg)	Nia (mg)	B6 (mg)	Fola (μg)	B12 (μg)
0	0	0	10	2	10	32	0.1	0.2	5	2	0	108	0.02	0.03	0.1	0.02	2	0
0.1	0.1	0	17	0	12	191	0.5	0.6	10	2	0	14	0	0.16	0.1	0.03	0	0
0	0	0	9	13	8	0	0	0	0	0	0	8	0	0	0	0	0	0
0	0	0	9	11	8	103	0.1	0.4	6	54	0.82	3	0.02	0.02	0.5	0.04	3	0
0	0.1	0	8	9	0	154	0.1	0.2	9	7	0.39	14	0.03	0.03	0.2	0.12	7	0
0	0.1	0	7	10	0	164	0.1	0.2	10	17	0.39	7	0.04	0.04	0.4	0.1	7	0
0	0	0	17	9	3	168	0.1	0.7	17	17	0.64	22	0.07	0.06	0.7	0.15	12	0
0	0	0	0	—	20	25	—	0	—	0	—	0	—	—	—	—	—	—
0	0	0	5	5	1	12	0	0.1	1	0	0	1	0.01	0	0	0.04	0	0
0	0.1	0	62	52	6	136	0.4	0.6	8	0	0	11	0.07	0.04	0.2	0.42	1	0
0	0	0	1	3	0	8	0	0	0	0	0	0	0	0	0	0.02	0	0
—	—	—	1	0	0	10	0	0	1	0	—	0	0	0	—	—	—	0
0	0	0	0	22	96	26	.05	.12	2	0	0	0	.01	0	0	0	0	0
0	0	0	3	30	57	1	0	0	1	0	0	0	0	0	0	0	0	0
0	0	0	2	32	56	0	0	0	1	0	0	0	0	0	0	0	0	0
0	0	0	3	121	216	6	0	0.1	2	0	0	0	0	0.02	0	0.01	3	0
0	0	0	4	3	14	1	0	0.1	2	0	0	0	0	0.02	0	0	2	0
0	0.1	0	5	22	30	110	0.1	0.1	7	3	0.11	4	0.03	0.03	0.2	0.13	4	0
—	—	0	1	0	20	1	0	0	0	0	—	0	0	0	0	0	0	0
0	0	0	4	—	99	2	—	0.1	—	1	—	0	0	0	—	0.01	3	0
0	0	0	0	1	0	10	0	0	1	0	0.01	0	0	0	0	0	0	0
0	0	0	4	6	3	100	0.1	0.1	10	0	0.06	1	0.01	0.01	0.2	0.04	3	0
0	0	0	1	1	0	6	0	0.1	1	0	0	0	0	0	0	0	0	0
1.6	0.8	24	68	52	92	25	0.3	0.3	4	52	0.47	0	0.02	0.06	0.2	0.01	4	0.1
1.9	0.3	18	22	39	71	121	0.2	0.7	10	65	0.2	2	0.11	0.09	1.1	0.08	5	0.05
3.3	0.5	192	42	271	368	320	4.9	1.5	30	0	0.44	0	0.07	0.41	11.3	0.29	18	1.83
0.6	0.1	34	8	92	40	186	2.4	1.7	0	0	0.02	0	0.04	0.28	1.8	0	2	0.55
26.6	0.9	156	73	208	725	144	1	5.7	14	1040	1.79	2	0.09	0.31	2.6	0.06	62	9.78
11.7	2.9	103	15	306	79	373	3	3.2	25	24	1.97	0	0.09	0.37	4.7	0.42	2	0.46
4.9	1.8	109	16	350	86	440	3.6	3.2	28	14	1.76	0	0.1	0.44	4.6	0.53	14	0.56
0	0.1	0	20	9	3	97	0.1	0.4	8	18	0.47	13	0.02	0.07	0.2	0.02	4	0
0	0.1	0	20	9	3	97	0.1	0.4	8	18	0.47	13	0.02	0.07	0.2	0.02	4	0
0	0.2	0	19	20	1	149	0.1	0.2	8	22	0.28	21	0.03	0.02	0.2	0.06	4	0
3.2	1.9	0	6	18	159	24	0.1	0.6	5	56	1.15	0	0.03	0.05	0.6	0.01	10	0.01
1	1	0	24	111	111	130	0.6	1.3	40	0	0.28	0	0.11	0.04	0.7	0.14	32	0
1.8	0.9	0	8	54	60	64	0.4	0.6	19	1	0.42	0	0.07	0.02	0.1	0.01	3	0
0.6	0.3	0	18	48	81	59	0.5	0.7	17	1	0.21	0	0.04	0.02	0.1	0.01	3	0
1.6	2.9	0	10	33	67	69	0.3	0.6	13	0	0.31	0	0.05	0.02	0.5	0.02	4	0
1.2	3.4	0	17	79	84	95	0.6	0.8	28	4	0.38	0	0.08	0.03	0.4	0.02	7	0
1	0.7	0	15	107	6	107	0.6	0.7	36	0	0.56	0	0.12	0.05	0.8	0.04	8	0.01
0.8	0.7	0	25	57	90	78	0.4	0.7	20	1	0.26	0	0.04	0.04	0.3	0.01	6	0
2.8	0.6	2	36	70	71	111	0.5	0.8	23	2	0.35	0	0.03	0.09	0.3	0.04	9	0.2
2.4	0.7	4	40	83	71	124	0.5	0.5	25	13	0.48	0	0.04	0.08	1.2	0.04	9	0
1.2	1.4	0	43	94	120	154	0.6	1	31	0	0.47	0	0.1	0.07	0.5	0.04	9	0.08
1.2	1.6	0	24	68	72	111	0.5	0.6	26	1	0.31	0	0.05	0.05	0.7	0.03	9	0.07
1.6	1	0	22	59	96	69	0.4	0.5	20	0	0.29	0	0.05	0.04	0.7	0.02	8	0.05
2.4	1.3	0	23	74	93	107	0.5	0.6	25	1	0.37	0	0.03	0.03	0.9	0.03	9	0.13
1.5	0.8	0	40	98	116	145	0.6	1.1	33	2	0.42	0	0.1	0.06	0.4	0.04	9	0.07
1.1	1.5	0	30	65	79	92	0.4	0.7	21	0	0.35	0	0.08	0.05	0.1	0.03	7	0.11
1.1	1.6	0	15	55	48	77	0.5	0.6	16	2	0.58	0	0.08	0.05	0.3	0.05	10	0.01
0	0	0	8	3	15	12	0.3	0.4	5	0	0	86	0.01	0.01	0.1	0.02	1	0
0	0	0	17	5	50	50	0.3	0.6	5	2	0	78	0.02	0.05	0	0	5	0
0	0	0	8	10	2	88	0.1	0.2	10	0	0	40	0.02	0.02	0.2	0.05	2	0
0	0.1	0	23	28	8	334	0.1	0.6	25	3	0	0	0.07	0.09	0.7	0.16	7	0
0	0.1	0	10	10	5	52	0.1	0.2	10	2	0.12	60	0.04	0.06	0.3	0.1	3	0
—	—	0	203	11	6	72	—	2	—	765	—	3	0.06	0.02	0.3	—	—	0
0	0	0	6	5	1	88	0	0.1	2	5	0.16	2	0.04	0.03	0.1	0.05	2	0
0	0.1	0	9	10	2	148	0	0.2	5	6	0.56	9	0.07	0.05	0.2	0.09	3	0
0	0.1	0	9	10	2	148	0	0.2	5	6	0.56	9	0.07	0.05	0.2	0.09	3	0
0	0.1	0	9	10	2	148	0	0.2	5	6	0.56	9	0.07	0.05	0.2	0.09	3	0
0	0.1	0	17	27	2	378	0.2	0.5	25	2	0.12	72	0.1	0.05	0.6	0.05	26	0
0	0.1	0	22	37	2	400	0.1	0.5	30	2	0.12	94	0.1	0.05	0.5	0.11	25	0
0	0.1	0	20	35	2	336	0.1	0.3	27	2	0.12	83	0.1	0.05	0.5	0.11	9	0
0	0	0	19	15	9	210	0.1	0.3	14	0	0.31	42	0.04	0.02	0.3	0.02	11	0
0	0	0	18	13	3	164	0.1	0.5	13	0	0.32	27	0.05	0.02	0.3	0.02	11	0

Food Item	Qty	Meas	Wgt (g)	Wtr (g)	Cals	Prot (g)	Carb (g)	Fib (g)	Fat (g)	SatF (g)
Grapefruit sections, fresh	1	piece	15	14	5	0	1	0.2	0	0
Grapefruit sections, fresh, cup measure	0.5	cup	115	105	37	1	9	1.3	0	0
Grapefruit, pink/red	0.5	each	123	112	37	1	9	1.7	0	0
Grapefruit, pink/red	0.5	each	123	110	46	1	12	1.6	0	0
Grapefruit, white	0.5	each	118	107	39	1	10	1.3	0	0
Grapefruit, white, California	0.5	each	118	106	44	1	11	1.5	0	0
Grapes, Concord	0.5	cup	46	37	31	0	8	0.5	0	0.1
Grapes, Thompson seedless, canned in heavy syrup	0.5	cup	128	102	93	1	25	0.5	0	0
Gravy, au jus, canned	0.25	cup	60	56	10	1	1	0	0	0.1
Gravy, au jus, dry w/water	0.25	cup	62	59	8	0	1	0	0	0.2
Gravy, beef, canned	0.25	cup	58	51	31	2	3	0.2	1	0.7
Gravy, beef, recipe	0.25	cup	34	29	22	1	2	0.1	1	0.4
Gravy, brown, from dry, w/water	0.25	cup	64	59	19	1	3	0.1	0	0.2
Gravy, chicken giblet, recipe	0.25	cup	32	28	24	2	2	0.1	1	0.3
Gravy, chicken, canned	0.25	cup	60	51	47	1	3	0.2	3	0.8
Gravy, chicken, dry mix w/water	0.25	cup	65	59	21	1	4	0.1	0	0.1
Gravy, mushroom, canned	0.25	cup	60	53	30	1	3	0.2	2	0.2
Gravy, mushroom, dry mix w/water	0.25	cup	64	59	17	1	3	0.3	0	0.1
Gravy, swiss steak	0.25	cup	58	51	31	2	3	0.2	1	0.7
Gravy, turkey, canned	0.25	cup	60	53	30	2	3	0.2	1	0.4
Gravy, turkey, dry, w/water	0.25	cup	65	59	22	1	4	0.3	0	0.1
Green pepper, stuffed	1	each	172	128	229	11	20	1.8	12	5
Grits, Soy HS	0.5	cup	78	7	218	41	23	—	1	—
Guava juice drink, vitamin C added	1	cup	253	218	132	0	34	2	0	0.1
Guava nectar	1	cup	250	211	149	0	38	2	0	0.1
Guava sauce, cooked	0.5	cup	119	107	43	0	11	4.3	0	0
Guava turnover	1	each	78	33	240	3	29	2.6	13	3.2
Guava, raw	1	each	90	78	46	1	11	4.9	1	0.2
Guava, strawberry, raw	1	each	6	5	4	0	1	0.4	0	0
Ham hocks, diced meat, cooked	0.5	cup	70	33	229	20	0	0	16	5.9
Ham patty, cured, grilled	1	each	70	36	238	9	1	0	22	7.7
Ham salad spread	0.5	cup	120	75	259	10	13	0	19	6.1
Ham, canned, unheated, extra lean (7% fat)	0.5	cup	70	50	101	13	0	0	5	1.7
Ham, smoked, sliced, 95% fat free	1	oz.	28	—	31	5	0	—	1	0.3
Ham, whole, roasted, lean	4	oz.	28	19	44	7	0	0	2	0.5
Ham, whole, roasted, lean & fat	4	oz.	113	66	276	24	0	0	19	6.8
Hamburger macaroni & cheese, Hamburger Helper	0.5	cup	122	85	178	17	8	0.7	8	4
Hardee's Big Country Breakfast, bacon	1	each	217	66	740	25	81	—	43	13
Hardee's Biscuit 'n gravy	1	each	221	126	510	10	55	—	28	9
Hardee's ham'n cheese sandwich, hot	1	each	201	101	530	18	49	—	30	9
Hardee's mushroom & swiss hamburger	1	each	203	107	520	30	37	—	27	13
Hardee's roast beef sandwich, regular	1	each	124	68	270	15	28	—	11	5
Hardee's sundae, Cool Twist, hot fudge	1	each	156	91	290	7	51	—	6	3
Hardee's, Frisco hamburger	1	each	242	—	760	36	43	—	50	18
Hardee's, ice cream cone, Cool Twist, vanilla/choc	1	each	118	77	180	4	34	—	2	0.7
Hardee's, shake, peach	1	each	345	—	390	10	77	—	4	3
Healthy Choice Meal, Beef Broccoli Bejing	1	each	340	261	300	21	45	5	4	1.5
Healthy Choice Meal, Beef Burrito Ranchero, mild	1	each	306	240	300	13	45	7	7	2.5
Healthy Choice Meal, Beef Macaroni Casserole	1	each	241	191	210	14	34	5	2	0.5
Healthy Choice Meal, Beef Tips Francais	1	each	262	196	280	20	40	4	5	1.5
Healthy Choice Meal, Beef/Peppers Cantonese	1	each	326	264	270	22	32	5	6	2.5
Healthy Choice Meal, Cacciatore Chicken	1	each	354	292	270	22	36	5	4	1
Healthy Choice Meal, Cheddar Broccoli Potatoes	1	each	298	226	330	13	53	6	7	3
Healthy Choice Meal, Cheese Ravioli Parmigiana	1	each	255	195	260	11	44	6	5	2.5
Healthy Choice Meal, Chicken & Vegetable Marsala	1	each	326	270	240	20	32	3	4	2
Healthy Choice Meal, Chicken Broccoli Alfredo	1	each	326	259	300	25	34	2	7	3
Healthy Choice Meal, Chicken Cantonese	1	each	305	242	280	22	34	2	6	3
Healthy Choice Meal, Chicken Con Queso Burrito	1	each	299	218	350	14	60	6	6	2.5
Healthy Choice Meal, Chicken Enchilada Suprema	1	each	320	253	300	13	46	4	7	3
Healthy Choice Meal, Chicken Enchiladas Suiza	1	tsp	284	217	280	14	43	5	6	3
Healthy Choice Meal, Chicken Fettuccini Alfredo	1	each	241	183	260	22	35	3	4	2
Healthy Choice Meal, Chicken Francesca Classic	1	each	354	270	330	23	46	4	6	2.5
Healthy Choice Meal, Country Herb Chicken	1	each	344	293	310	18	44	3	6	2.5
Healthy Choice Meal, Country Inn Roast Turkey	1	each	284	224	250	20	28	4	6	2
Healthy Choice Meal, Country Roast Turkey with Mush	1	each	241	189	230	19	26	2	5	1.5

MonoF	PolyF	Choles	Calc	Phos	Sod	Pot	Zn	Iron	Magn	VitA	VitE	VitC	Thia	Ribo	Nia	B6	Fola	B12
(g)	(g)	(mg)	(mg)	(mg)	(mg)	(mg)	(mg)	(mg)	(mg)	(µg RE)	(mg α-TE)	(mg)	(mg)	(mg)	(mg)	(mg)	(µg)	(µg)
0	0	0	2	1	0	21	0	0	1	2	0.04	5	0	0	0	0.01	2	0
0	0	0	14	9	0	160	0.1	0.1	9	14	0.29	40	0.04	0.02	0.3	0.05	12	0
0	0	0	14	11	0	159	0.1	0.1	10	32	0.31	47	0.04	0.02	0.2	0.05	15	0
0	0	0	14	15	1	181	0.1	0.1	11	32	0.31	47	0.04	0.02	0.2	0.05	15	0
0	0	0	14	9	0	175	0.1	0.1	11	1	0.3	39	0.04	0.02	0.3	0.05	12	0
0	0	0	14	14	0	169	0.1	0.1	11	1	0.3	39	0.04	0.02	0.3	0.05	14	0
0	0	0	6	5	1	88	0	0.1	2	5	0.16	2	0.04	0.03	0.1	0.05	2	0
0	0	0	13	22	6	132	0.1	1.2	8	8	0.9	1	0.04	0.03	0.2	0.08	3	0
0	0	0	2	18	30	48	0.6	0.4	1	0	0	1	0.01	0.04	0.5	0.01	1	0.06
0.1	0	1	6	0	241	0	0	0	2	0	0	0	0	0	0	0	0	0
0.6	0	2	4	18	326	47	0.6	0.4	1	0	0.04	0	0.02	0.02	0.4	0.01	1	0.06
0.6	0.2	1	4	10	192	32	0.3	0.2	1	19	0.04	0	0.01	0.01	0.2	0	1	0.03
0.2	0	1	17	11	269	14	0.1	0.1	3	0	0.01	0	0.01	0.02	0.2	0	0	0
0.5	0.3	14	4	16	171	38	0.4	0.4	1	82	0.08	0	0.01	0.05	0.4	0.01	12	0.58
1.5	0.9	1	12	17	343	65	0.5	0.3	1	66	0.09	0	0.01	0.03	0.3	0.01	1	0.06
0.2	0.1	1	10	12	283	16	0.1	0.1	3	0	0.01	1	0.01	0.04	0.2	0.01	1	0.04
0.7	0.6	0	4	9	339	63	0.4	0.4	1	0	0.05	0	0.02	0.04	0.4	0.01	7	0
0.1	0	0	12	11	350	14	0.1	0.1	2	0	0.01	0	0.01	0.02	0.2	0.01	1	0.04
0.6	0	2	4	18	326	47	0.6	0.4	1	0	0.04	0	0.02	0.02	0.4	0.01	1	0.06
0.5	0.3	1	2	17	343	65	0.5	0.4	1	0	0.04	0	0.01	0.05	0.8	0.01	1	0.06
0.2	0.1	1	12	12	374	16	0.1	0.1	3	0	0.01	0	0.01	0.03	0.3	0.01	1	0.06
4.9	0.5	34	16	85	201	233	2.3	1.8	20	44	0.75	55	0.15	0.1	2.7	0.3	17	0.67
—	—	0	250	569	8	1926	4.1	7.8	244	0	0	0	0.47	0.24	2	0.39	0	0
0	0.1	0	11	10	7	105	0.1	0.1	6	29	0.41	85	0.02	0.02	0.4	0.05	5	0
0	0.1	0	11	10	7	93	0.1	0.2	5	22	0.4	46	0.02	0.02	0.4	0.05	3	0
0	0.1	0	8	13	5	268	0.2	0.2	8	33	0	174	0.03	0.02	0.5	0.11	6	0
5.6	3.5	0	14	34	105	124	0.2	1.1	9	36	1.59	49	0.15	0.12	1.5	0.06	7	0
0	0.2	0	18	22	3	256	0.2	0.3	9	71	1.01	166	0.04	0.04	1.1	0.13	13	0
0	0	0	1	2	2	18	0	0	1	1	0.03	2	0	0	0	0	0	0
7.2	1.6	76	13	147	223	257	2.9	1.1	13	2	0.18	0	0.38	0.21	3.6	0.24	3	0.45
10.2	2.3	50	6	70	739	170	1.3	1.1	7	0	0.18	0	0.24	0.13	2.3	0.11	2	0.49
8.6	3.2	44	10	144	1094	180	1.3	0.7	12	0	2.09	0	0.52	0.14	2.5	0.18	1	0.91
2.5	0.5	27	4	145	893	234	1.3	0.6	11	0	0.18	0	0.62	0.16	3.2	0.32	4	0.56
0.6	0.3	14	—	—	357	—	—	—	—	—	—	—	—	—	—	—	—	—
0.7	0.2	16	2	64	376	90	0.7	0.3	6	0	0.07	0	0.19	0.07	1.4	0.13	1	0.2
8.9	2	70	8	243	1346	324	2.6	1	22	0	0.3	0	0.68	0.25	5.1	0.43	3	0.73
2.9	0.4	54	86	181	952	223	2.8	1.9	20	34	0.14	0	0.1	0.17	2.4	0.21	8	1.3
22	8	305	166	—	1800	530	—	5	—	—	—	—	—	—	—	—	—	—
14	5	15	150	—	1500	210	—	2	—	—	—	—	—	—	—	—	—	—
—	—	65	288	—	—	300	—	3	—	—	—	—	—	—	—	—	—	—
12	2	45	294	—	890	370	—	5	—	—	—	—	—	—	—	—	—	—
4	2	25	105	—	780	260	—	4	—	—	—	—	—	—	—	—	—	—
1.6	0.2	20	152	—	310	173	—	0.4	—	—	—	—	—	—	—	—	—	—
—	—	70	—	—	1280	—	—	—	—	—	—	—	—	—	—	—	—	—
1.3	0	10	123	—	120	180	—	2	—	—	—	—	—	—	—	—	—	—
—	—	25	—	—	290	—	—	—	—	—	—	—	—	—	—	—	—	—
—	—	25	40	—	420	—	—	2.7	—	200	—	12	—	—	—	—	—	—
—	—	15	20	—	480	—	—	1.1	—	40	—	5	—	—	—	—	—	—
—	—	15	40	—	450	—	—	2.7	—	100	—	54	—	—	—	—	—	—
—	—	30	20	—	520	—	—	1.8	—	0	—	0	—	—	—	—	—	—
—	—	55	40	—	480	—	—	1.8	—	100	—	21	—	—	—	—	—	—
—	—	35	40	—	550	—	—	1.8	—	40	—	6	—	—	—	—	—	—
—	—	25	200	—	550	—	—	1.1	—	60	—	27	—	—	—	—	—	—
—	—	30	150	—	290	—	—	1.8	—	60	—	0	—	—	—	—	—	—
—	—	30	40	—	440	—	—	0.7	—	100	—	4	—	—	—	—	—	—
—	—	50	100	—	530	—	—	1.8	—	20	—	2	—	—	—	—	—	—
—	—	50	40	—	480	—	—	1.8	—	600	—	6	—	—	—	—	—	—
—	—	35	40	—	590	—	—	1.8	—	300	—	15	—	—	—	—	—	—
—	—	40	100	—	560	—	—	0.7	—	150	—	18	—	—	—	—	—	—
—	—	40	150	—	440	—	—	1.1	—	60	—	6	—	—	—	—	—	—
—	—	40	100	—	410	—	—	1.4	—	0	—	0	—	—	—	—	—	—
—	—	30	100	—	600	—	—	1.8	—	20	—	15	—	—	—	—	—	—
—	—	45	40	—	540	—	—	0.7	—	250	—	0	—	—	—	—	—	—
—	—	40	40	—	530	—	—	1.8	—	100	—	0	—	—	—	—	—	—
—	—	45	0	—	440	—	—	0.7	—	150	—	0	—	—	—	—	—	—

Food Item	Qty	Meas	Wgt (g)	Wtr (g)	Cals	Prot (g)	Carb (g)	Fib (g)	Fat (g)	SatF (g)
Healthy Choice Meal, Fiesta Chicken Fajitas	1	each	198	136	260	21	36	5	4	1
Healthy Choice Meal, Garden Potato Casserole	1	each	262	216	210	11	30	6	5	1.5
Healthy Choice Meal, Ginger Chicken Hunan	1	each	357	271	380	24	59	5	5	1
Healthy Choice Meal, Honey Mustard Chicken	1	each	269	205	270	21	38	2	4	1.5
Healthy Choice Meal, Imperial Chicken	1	each	255	201	240	17	31	3	5	1.5
Healthy Choice Meal, Macaroni and Cheese	1	each	255	189	320	15	50	4	7	2.5
Healthy Choice Meal, Mandarin Chicken	1	each	284	216	280	20	44	4	2	0
Healthy Choice Meal, Mesquite Beef Barbeque	1	each	312	239	320	21	38	5	9	3
Healthy Choice Meal, Mesquite Chicken Barbeque	1	each	298	221	310	18	48	6	5	2
Healthy Choice Meal, Pasta Shells Marinara	1	each	340	252	380	25	55	5	6	3.5
Healthy Choice Meal, Salisbury Steak Classics	1	each	312	255	310	16	40	4	9	3
Healthy Choice Meal, Sesame Chicken Shanghai	1	each	340	268	300	24	40	6	5	1
Healthy Choice Meal, Shrimp & Vegetable Maria	1	each	354	290	290	15	46	5	5	2
Healthy Choice Meal, Shrimp Marinara	1	each	298	243	250	10	44	5	4	2
Healthy Choice Meal, Smokey Chicken Barbeque	1	each	361	273	290	25	57	7	5	3
Healthy Choice Meal, Three Cheese Manicotti	1	each	312	245	300	15	40	5	9	3
Healthy Choice Meal, Traditional Beef Tips	1	each	319	261	280	20	32	4	8	3
Healthy Choice Meal, Vegetable Pasta Italiano	1	each	284	230	250	9	48	6	3	1.5
Healthy Choice Meal, Yankee Pot Roast	1	each	312	249	290	19	38	4	7	3
Healthy Choice Meal, Zucchini Lasagna	1	each	383	318	280	13	47	5	4	2.5
Hi-C, punch	1	cup	240	207	125	0	33	0	0	0
Hickory nuts, dried	1	oz.	28	1	186	4	5	1.8	18	2
Hominy, cooked	0.5	cup	82	62	73	2	17	4.7	1	0.1
Hominy, white, canned	0.5	cup	80	66	58	1	11	2	1	0.1
Hominy, yellow, canned	0.5	cup	80	66	58	1	11	2	1	0.1
Honey	1	Tbs	21	4	64	0	18	0	0	0
Horseradish, prepared	1	tsp	5	4	2	0	1	0.2	0	0
Hot cocoa, homemade, w/whole milk	1	cup	250	203	193	10	30	2	6	3.6
Hot dog, beef, fat free, Oscar Mayer	1	piece	50	39	39	7	3	0	0	0.1
Hot dog, turkey	1	oz.	28	18	64	4	0	0	5	1.7
Hotdog, w/chili	1	each	114	54	296	14	31	—	14	4.9
Hotdog/frankfurter, beef & pork, 8 per pkg	1	each	57	31	182	6	1	0	17	6.2
Hotdog/frankfurter, beef, 8 per pkg	1	each	57	31	180	7	1	0	16	6.9
Hotdog/frankfurter, turkey	1	each	45	28	102	6	1	0	8	2.6
Hummus/hummous	0.5	cup	123	80	210	6	25	6.3	10	1.6
Hungry Man dinner, Mexican	1	each	567	420	690	26	87	13	27	9
Hush puppies, recipe	1	each	22	6	74	2	10	0.6	3	0.5
Ice Cream sundae, hot fudge	1	each	158	94	284	6	48	0	9	5
Ice Cream sundae, strawberry	1	each	153	93	268	6	45	0	8	3.7
Ice cream bar, Creamsicle	1	each	66	44	92	2	18	0	2	1.2
Ice cream bar, Drumstick	1	each	60	29	157	3	18	0.7	9	4.3
Ice cream bar, Fudgesicle	1	each	73	49	90	4	19	0.1	0	0.1
Ice cream bar, Heath	1	each	68	33	206	2	17	0.2	15	11.6
Ice cream bar, Nutty Buddy	1	each	78	37	215	4	23	1.3	13	5.5
Ice cream bar, chocolate coated w/nuts	1	each	54	23	171	2	17	0.3	11	6.4
Ice cream cone, cake/wafer type	1	each	4	0	17	0	3	0.1	0	0
Ice cream cone, chocolate	1	each	78	42	171	3	25	0.6	7	4.4
Ice cream cone, sugar/rolled type	1	each	10	0	40	1	8	0.2	0	0.1
Ice cream cone, vanilla	1	each	78	44	167	3	22	0.1	8	4.9
Ice cream cone, vanilla, choc dipped	1	each	78	41	185	3	24	0.4	9	5.6
Ice cream cookie sandwich, Chipwich	1	each	59	28	144	3	22	0.6	6	3.2
Ice cream pie, cookie crust, fudge topping	1	each	1836	723	5579	70	723	11	297	141
Ice cream sandwich	1	each	59	28	144	3	22	0.6	6	3.2
Ice cream sandwich, mini Oreo	1	each	29	14	71	1	11	0.3	3	1.6
Ice cream, Choc Chip Cookie Dough, Ben & Jerry's	0.5	cup	106	—	270	4	30	0	17	9
Ice cream, Chunky Monkey, Ben & Jerry's	0.5	cup	106	—	280	4	29	1	19	10
Ice cream, brandied cherry, HaagenDaz	0.5	cup	106	—	250	4	24	—	15	0.5
Ice cream, chocolate Dove bar	1	each	101	38	339	3	36	2.1	23	13.8
Ice cream, chocolate chip, low fat, Healthy Choice	0.5	cup	71	44	120	3	21	0.5	2	1
Ice cream, chocolate, Breyers	0.5	cup	70	38	160	3	20	0.5	8	5
Ice cream, chocolate, regular	0.5	cup	66	37	143	3	19	0.8	7	4.5
Ice cream, cookie & cream, Healthy Choice	0.5	cup	71	44	120	3	21	0.5	2	1.5
Ice cream, deep choc pnut butter, HaagenDaz	0.5	cup	106	—	330	7	25	—	19	—
Ice cream, imitation, chocolate, Mellorine	0.5	cup	66	40	134	3	16	0.5	7	6
Ice cream, imitation, strawberry, Mellorine	0.5	cup	66	41	132	2	16	0	7	5.9

MonoF (g)	PolyF (g)	Choles (mg)	Calc (mg)	Phos (mg)	Sod (mg)	Pot (mg)	Zn (mg)	Iron (mg)	Magn (mg)	VitA (μg RE)	VitE (mg α-TE)	VitC (mg)	Thia (mg)	Ribo (mg)	Nia (mg)	B6 (mg)	Fola (μg)	B12 (μg)
—	—	30	20	—	410	—	—	1.8	—	150	—	36	—	—	—	—	—	—
—	—	10	100	—	520	—	—	0.7	—	250	—	21	—	—	—	—	—	—
—	—	30	60	—	430	—	—	2.7	—	100	—	0	—	—	—	—	—	—
—	—	40	20	—	520	—	—	0.4	—	200	—	0	—	—	—	—	—	—
—	—	50	20	—	470	—	—	1.4	—	150	—	6	—	—	—	—	—	—
—	—	25	250	—	580	—	—	1.4	—	0	—	0	—	—	—	—	—	—
—	—	35	20	—	520	—	—	0.7	—	150	—	15	—	—	—	—	—	—
—	—	55	40	—	490	—	—	1.1	—	250	—	0	—	—	—	—	—	—
—	—	55	40	—	480	—	—	1.4	—	350	—	9	—	—	—	—	—	—
—	—	25	400	—	390	—	—	1.8	—	100	—	0	—	—	—	—	—	—
—	—	45	20	—	550	—	—	1.8	—	200	—	0	—	—	—	—	—	—
—	—	40	40	—	550	—	—	1.8	—	150	—	5	—	—	—	—	—	—
—	—	40	40	—	540	—	—	2.7	—	20	—	12	—	—	—	—	—	—
—	—	55	60	—	260	—	—	1.8	—	60	—	1	—	—	—	—	—	—
—	—	50	40	—	450	—	—	1.8	—	450	—	6	—	—	—	—	—	—
—	—	35	250	—	550	—	—	0.2	—	150	—	0	—	—	—	—	—	—
—	—	50	20	—	480	—	—	1.8	—	600	—	42	—	—	—	—	—	—
—	—	10	60	—	480	—	—	2.7	—	100	—	2	—	—	—	—	—	—
—	—	55	40	—	460	—	—	1.8	—	450	—	6	—	—	—	—	—	—
—	—	10	200	—	310	—	—	1.8	—	250	—	0	—	—	—	—	—	—
0	0	—	—	—	29	—	—	—	—	0	—	96	—	—	—	—	—	0
9.2	6.2	0	17	95	0	124	1.2	0.6	49	4	1.48	1	0.25	0.04	0.3	0.05	11	0
0.2	0.5	0	8	35	146	8	0.9	0.8	14	0	0.04	0	0	0	0	0.01	1	0
0.2	0.3	0	8	28	168	7	0.8	0.5	13	0	0.04	0	0	0	0	0	1	0
0.2	0.3	0	8	28	168	7	0.8	0.5	13	9	0.08	0	0	0	0	0	1	0
0	0	0	1	1	1	11	0	0.1	0	0	0	0	0	0.01	0	0	0	0
0	0	0	3	2	16	12	0	0	1	0	0	1	0	0	0	0	3	0
1.7	0.2	20	315	293	128	500	1.5	1.2	70	138	0.26	2	0.1	0.44	0.4	0.12	15	0.92
0.1	0.1	15	10	64	484	234	1.2	1	10	0	—	0	—	—	—	—	—	—
1.6	1.4	30	30	38	404	51	0.9	0.5	4	0	0.18	0	0.01	0.05	1.2	0.06	2	0.08
6.6	1.2	51	19	192	480	166	0.8	3.3	10	6	—	3	0.22	0.4	3.7	0.05	73	0.3
7.8	1.6	28	6	49	638	95	1	0.7	6	0	0.14	0	0.11	0.07	1.5	0.07	2	0.74
7.8	0.8	35	11	50	585	95	1.2	0.8	2	0	0.11	0	0.03	0.06	1.4	0.07	2	0.88
2.5	2.2	48	48	60	642	81	1.4	0.8	6	0	0.28	0	0.02	0.08	1.9	0.1	4	0.13
4.4	3.9	0	62	138	300	214	1.4	1.9	36	2	1.23	10	0.11	0.06	0.5	0.49	73	0
—	—	35	300	—	2170	—	—	3.6	—	300	—	36	—	—	—	—	—	—
0.7	1.6	10	61	42	147	32	0.1	0.7	5	9	0.52	0	0.08	0.07	0.6	0.02	16	0.04
2.3	0.8	20	207	228	182	395	0.9	0.6	33	57	0.66	2	0.06	0.3	1.1	0.13	9	0.65
2.7	1	21	161	155	92	271	0.7	0.3	24	58	0.78	2	0.06	0.28	0.9	0.08	18	0.64
0.6	0.1	7	62	48	42	102	0.4	0.1	7	22	0	1	0.02	0.1	0.1	0.02	4	0.24
3	1	21	72	86	48	151	0.7	0.4	21	55	0.4	0	0.04	0.14	0.9	0.04	7	0.18
0.1	0	1	129	99	55	173	0.3	0.1	14	2	0.01	0	0.03	0.18	0.1	0.05	1	0.62
2.3	0.4	24	70	62	43	126	0.4	0.2	11	63	0.07	0	0.02	0.13	0.1	0.03	3	0.21
5.4	1.3	26	104	123	60	206	0.9	0.6	40	69	0.53	0	0.05	0.25	0.6	0.04	9	0.23
2.6	0.8	1	136	62	50	129	0.3	0.4	16	25	0.36	0	0.02	0.1	0.5	0.12	6	0.2
0.1	0.1	0	1	4	6	4	0	0.1	1	0	0.07	0	0.01	0.01	0.2	0	4	0
2	0.3	18	96	89	51	176	0.4	0.4	17	62	0.22	0	0.04	0.14	0.3	0.03	4	0.27
0.1	0.1	0	4	10	32	14	0.1	0.4	3	0	0.05	0	0.05	0.04	0.5	0	8	0
2.3	0.4	32	102	88	72	158	0.5	0.2	11	84	0.03	0	0.04	0.2	0.3	0.04	4	0.28
2.8	0.4	29	95	89	66	169	0.6	0.4	18	77	0.1	0	0.04	0.19	0.3	0.04	4	0.26
1.7	0.4	20	60	64	36	122	0.4	0.3	13	53	0.09	0	0.03	0.12	0.2	0.03	5	0.18
94.1	45.4	505	1733	2076	2765	3607	11.6	13.5	441	1377	8.17	7	0.75	4.33	8.9	0.75	94	4.98
1.7	0.4	20	60	64	36	122	0.4	0.3	13	53	0.09	0	0.03	0.12	0.2	0.03	5	0.18
0.8	0.2	10	30	31	18	60	0.2	0.1	6	26	0.05	0	0.02	0.06	0.1	0.01	2	0.09
—	—	80	100	—	95	—	—	1.1	—	150	—	1	—	—	—	—	—	—
—	—	70	100	—	50	—	—	1.1	—	100	—	1	—	—	—	—	—	—
7.5	7	100	107	107	80	170	—	—	—	160	—	—	0.16	0.18	—	—	—	—
7.1	0.7	38	74	139	56	260	1.1	1.1	63	95	0.72	0	0.03	0.21	0.3	0.04	2	0.23
1	0	2	100	141	50	240	—	0	—	40	—	0	—	—	—	—	—	—
2	0	20	48	32	30	150	—	—	—	40	0.21	—	—	0.1	—	—	—	0.04
2.1	0.3	22	72	71	50	164	0.4	0.6	19	78	0.22	0	0.03	0.13	0.1	0.04	11	0.19
0.5	0	2	100	141	90	254	—	—	—	60	—	2	0.03	0.15	—	—	—	—
—	—	—	107	213	90	300	—	1.2	—	21	—	—	0.1	0.14	2.1	—	—	—
0.5	0.1	0	90	81	48	179	0.8	0.3	17	0	0.06	0	0.03	0.15	0.1	0.04	2	0.38
0.4	0.1	0	90	71	48	144	0.7	0.1	10	0	0.05	0	0.03	0.15	0.1	0.04	1	0.39

Food Item	Qty	Meas	Wgt (g)	Wtr (g)	Cals	Prot (g)	Carb (g)	Fib (g)	Fat (g)	SatF (g)
Ice cream, imitation, vanilla, Mellorine	0.5	cup	66	41	132	2	16	0	7	5.9
Ice cream, orange sorbet & vanilla, HaagenDaz	0.5	cup	106	62	199	3	30	—	8	4
Ice cream, praline & cream, Healthy Choice	0.5	cup	71	40	130	3	25	0.5	2	0.5
Ice cream, rocky road, low fat, Healthy Choice	0.5	cup	71	37	140	3	28	2	2	1
Ice cream, soft serve, chocolate	0.5	cup	173	100	355	6	48	1.4	17	10.4
Ice cream, soft serve, french vanilla	0.5	cup	86	51	185	4	19	0	11	6.4
Ice cream, strawberry	0.5	cup	66	40	127	2	18	0.2	6	3.4
Ice cream, strawberry, Breyers	0.5	cup	70	45	130	2	16	0.1	6	4
Ice cream, triple choc chunk, Healthy Choice	0.5	cup	71	44	110	3	21	1	2	1
Ice cream, vanilla	0.5	cup	66	40	133	2	16	0	7	4.5
Ice cream, vanilla, Breyers	0.5	cup	70	43	150	3	15	0.1	8	5
Ice cream, vanilla, Healthy Choice	0.5	cup	71	47	100	3	18	1	2	0.5
Ice cream, vanilla, rich, 16% fat	0.5	cup	74	42	178	3	17	0	12	7.4
Ice milk, chocolate	0.5	cup	66	43	94	3	17	0.3	2	1.3
Ice milk, chocolate, Breyer's Light	0.5	cup	68	41	122	3	19	0.3	4	2.6
Ice milk, premium, strawberry, Breyer's Light	0.5	cup	68	41	122	3	19	0	4	2.5
Ice milk, vanilla, Breyer's Light	0.5	cup	68	41	122	3	19	0	4	2.5
Ice milk, vanilla, hard	0.5	cup	66	45	92	3	15	0	3	1.7
Ice milk, vanilla, soft, 3% fat	0.5	cup	88	61	111	4	19	0	2	1.4
Ice slushy	1	cup	193	129	151	1	63	0	0	0
Ices, fruit flavor, sugar-free	1	each	51	48	12	0	3	0	0	0
Ices, lime	1	cup	192	128	246	1	63	0	0	0
Injera (Ethiopian bread), 12 inch loaf	1	piece	21	13	29	1	6	0.2	0	0.1
Instant breakfast, vanilla, Carnation	1	cup	281	—	975	56	167	0	0	0
Instant breakfast, w/1% milk	1	cup	281	222	233	15	36	0.2	3	2
Instant breakfast, w/2% milk	1	cup	281	220	252	16	36	0.2	5	3.3
Instant breakfast, w/nonfat milk	1	cup	282	225	216	16	36	0.2	1	0.7
Instant breakfast, w/whole milk	1	cup	281	217	280	15	36	0.2	9	5.4
Jack in the Box, BreakfastJack sandwich	1	each	121	59	300	18	30	0	12	4.8
Jack in the Box, Jumbo Jack	1	each	229	126	560	26	41	0	32	10
Jack in the Box, Jumbo Jack w/cheese	1	each	242	133	610	29	41	0	36	12
Jack in the Box, bacon cheeseburger	1	each	242	119	710	35	41	0	45	15
Jack in the Box, chicken caesar pita sandwich	1	each	237	139	520	27	44	4	26	6
Jack in the Box, chicken sandwich	1	each	160	83	400	20	38	0	18	4
Jack in the Box, cinnamon churritos, serving	1	each	75	16	330	3	34	3	21	5
Jack in the Box, fajita, chicken pita	1	each	189	127	290	24	29	3	8	3
Jack in the Box, fried steak sandwich	1	each	153	70	450	14	42	0	25	7
Jack in the Box, hamburger, sourdough, grilled	1	each	223	107	670	32	39	0	43	16
Jack in the Box, monterey roast beef sandwich	1	each	238	135	540	30	40	3	30	9
Jack in the Box, sourdough breakfast sandwich	1	each	147	73	380	21	31	0	20	7
Jack in the Box, ultimate breakfast sandwich	1	each	242	128	620	36	39	—	35	11
Jackfruit, raw	4	oz.	113	83	107	2	27	1.8	0	0.1
Jam, cherry/strawberry	1	Tbs	20	6	54	0	14	—	0	0
Jam, not cherry/strawberry	1	Tbs	20	6	54	0	14	0.2	0	0
Jam/marmalade, artificially sweetened	1	Tbs	20	9	2	0	11	0.5	0	0
Jam/preserves, 1 pkt	1	Tbs	20	7	48	0	13	0.2	0	0
Jam/preserves/marmalade, reduced sugar	1	Tbs	20	10	36	0	9	0.6	0	0
Java plum/jambolan, fresh	3	each	9	7	5	0	1	0.1	0	—
Jelly	1	Tbs	18	5	49	0	13	0.2	0	0
Jelly, dietetic	1	Tbs	19	8	6	0	11	0.2	0	0
Jelly, packet	1	each	14	4	38	0	10	0.1	0	0
Jelly, reduced sugar, all flavors	1	Tbs	19	10	34	0	9	0.2	0	0
Jicama, raw	0.5	cup	60	54	23	1	5	2.9	0	0
Jicama/Yambean tuber, sliced, cooked	0.5	cup	50	45	19	0	4	2.4	0	0
Jicama/Yambean tuber, sliced, raw	0.5	cup	60	54	23	0	5	2.9	0	0
Juice drink, cranberry apricot, w/vitamin C	1	cup	253	209	170	0	43	0.3	0	0
Juice drink, cranberry blueberry, w/vitamin C	1	cup	253	209	170	0	43	0.3	0	0
Juice drink, cranberry grape, w/vitamin C	1	cup	253	209	170	0	43	0.3	0	0
Juice drink, cranberry raspberry, w/vitamin C	1	cup	253	209	170	0	43	0.3	0	0
Juice drink, orange, CapriSun Natural	1	cup	176	—	83	0	22	0	0	0
Juice, acerola, fresh	1	cup	242	228	56	1	12	0.7	1	0.2
Juice, apple, frozen w/vit C, prepared	1	cup	239	210	112	0	28	0.2	0	0
Juice, apple, w/vit C, canned/bottled	1	cup	248	218	117	0	29	0.2	0	0
Juice, apple-cherry	1	cup	250	219	117	1	29	0.8	0	0.1
Juice, apple-grape	1	cup	244	211	128	1	32	0.2	0	0.1

MonoF (g)	PolyF (g)	Choles (mg)	Calc (mg)	Phos (mg)	Sod (mg)	Pot (mg)	Zn (mg)	Iron (mg)	Magn (mg)	VitA (µg RE)	VitE (mg α-TE)	VitC (mg)	Thia (mg)	Ribo (mg)	Nia (mg)	B6 (mg)	Fola (µg)	B12 (µg)
0.4	0.1	0	90	71	48	144	0.7	0.1	10	0	0.05	0	0.03	0.15	0.1	0.04	1	0.39
—	—	60	64	64	30	114	—	0	—	85	—	6	0.03	0.11	0.8	—	—	—
0.1	1.4	2	100	141	70	226	—	0	—	40	—	0	0.03	0.15	—	—	—	—
0.5	0	2	100	9	60	168	—	0	—	40	—	0	0.03	0.15	—	—	—	—
4.9	0.6	43	206	184	89	384	1	0.7	37	147	0.46	1	0.07	0.27	0.2	0.06	9	0.64
3	0.4	78	113	100	52	152	0.4	0.2	10	132	0.32	1	0.04	0.16	0.1	0.04	8	0.43
1.6	0.2	19	79	66	40	124	0.2	0.1	9	52	0.13	5	0.03	0.17	0.1	0.03	8	0.2
2	0	20	64	48	40	125	—	—	—	40	0.14	—	0.03	0.14	—	—	—	0.08
—	—	2	100	—	60	—	—	0.4	—	8	—	0	—	—	—	—	—	—
2.1	0.3	29	84	69	53	131	0.5	0.1	9	77	0	0	0.03	0.16	0.1	0.03	3	0.26
2	0.3	25	80	80	50	140	—	0.1	—	60	0.21	—	0.03	0.15	—	—	—	0.12
1.5	0	5	100	141	50	254	—	—	—	60	—	2	0.05	0.22	—	—	—	—
3.4	0.4	45	87	70	41	118	0.3	0	8	136	0	1	0.03	0.12	0.1	0.03	4	0.27
0.6	0.1	6	94	78	41	155	0.4	0.2	13	18	0.06	0	0.03	0.12	0.1	0.03	4	0.3
1.2	0.2	12	105	87	46	172	0.4	0.2	14	37	0.12	1	0.04	0.13	0.1	0.03	4	0.33
0.8	0.2	16	109	80	63	162	0.3	0.1	11	27	0.08	0	0.05	0.2	0.1	0.05	2	0.51
0.8	0.2	16	109	80	63	162	0.3	0.1	11	27	0.08	0	0.05	0.2	0.1	0.05	2	0.51
0.8	0.1	9	92	72	56	139	0.3	0.1	10	31	0	1	0.04	0.18	0.1	0.04	4	0.44
0.7	0.1	11	138	106	62	194	0.5	0.1	12	26	0	1	0.05	0.17	0.1	0.04	5	0.44
0	0	0	4	2	42	6	0	0.3	2	0	0	2	0	0	0	0	0	0
—	—	0	1	0	3	13	0	0.1	1	0	0	0	0	0	0.1	0	0	0
0	0	0	4	2	42	6	0	0.3	2	0	0	2	0	0	0	0	0	0
0	0.1	0	12	24	42	12	0.1	6.2	2	0	0	0	0.02	0.02	0.3	0.01	6	0
0	0	36	4869	1390	1253	3478	41.9	62.7	1112	7311	70	376	4.19	1.88	69.7	5.56	1390	8.35
0.9	0.1	14	406	393	266	731	4.1	4.9	118	698	5.36	31	0.41	0.48	5.5	0.53	118	1.53
1.5	0.2	23	401	390	264	726	4.1	4.9	118	693	5.41	31	0.41	0.48	5.5	0.53	118	1.52
0.3	0	9	407	406	268	755	4.1	4.8	112	703	5.3	31	0.4	0.42	5.5	0.52	118	1.56
2.5	0.3	38	396	385	262	719	4.1	4.9	117	630	5.51	31	0.41	0.47	5.5	0.52	118	1.5
4.8	2.4	185	200	—	890	220	—	2.7	—	80	—	9	0.47	0.41	3	—	—	—
13	8	65	100	—	700	450	—	4.5	—	40	—	6	0.36	0.29	1.8	—	—	—
15	9	80	200	—	780	460	—	5.4	—	60	—	6	0.36	0.44	1.6	—	—	—
15.7	8.7	110	250	—	1240	540	—	5.4	—	80	—	9	0.24	0.48	8.8	0.39	—	—
—	—	55	250	—	1050	490	—	2.7	—	80	—	2	—	—	—	—	—	—
—	—	45	150	—	1290	180	—	1.8	—	40	—	0	—	—	—	—	—	—
—	—	20	20	—	200	170	—	5.4	—	0	—	0	—	—	—	—	—	—
3.6	1.4	35	250	—	700	430	—	2.7	—	100	—	6	0.75	0.17	6	—	—	—
—	—	35	60	—	890	270	—	2.7	—	20	—	5	—	—	—	—	—	—
17.8	7.9	110	200	—	1140	510	—	4.5	—	150	—	6	0.65	0.48	8	0.33	—	—
—	—	75	300	—	1270	500	—	3.6	—	80	—	5	—	—	—	—	—	—
—	—	235	250	—	1120	260	—	3.6	—	150	—	9	—	—	—	—	—	—
—	—	455	250	—	1800	450	—	4.5	—	150	—	9	—	—	—	—	—	—
0	0.1	0	39	41	3	344	0.5	0.7	42	34	0.17	8	0.03	0.12	0.5	0.12	16	0
—	—	0	4	2	2	18	—	0.2	—	0	—	3	0	0.01	0	—	—	—
0	0	0	4	2	2	18	0	0.2	1	0	0.02	0	0	0.01	0	0	2	0
0	0	0	2	2	0	14	0	0.1	1	0	0.01	0	0	0	0	0	2	0
0	0	0	4	2	8	15	0	0.1	1	0	0	2	0	0	0	0	7	0
0	0.1	0	1	1	5	12	0	0.2	1	0	0.03	8	0	0.02	0.1	0.03	2	0
—	—	0	2	2	1	7	0	0	1	0	—	1	0	0	0	0	—	0
0	0	0	1	1	6	12	0	0	1	0	0	0	0	0	0	0	0	0
0	0	0	1	1	0	12	0	0	1	0	0.02	0	0	0	0	0.01	0	0
0	0	0	1	1	5	9	0	0	1	0	0	0	0	0	0	0	0	0
0	0	0	1	1	0	13	0	0	1	0	0	0	0	0	0	0.01	0	0
0	0	0	7	11	2	90	0.1	0.4	7	1	2.74	12	0.01	0.02	0.1	0.02	7	0
0	0	0	6	8	2	68	0.1	0.3	6	1	0.23	7	0.01	0.01	0.1	0.02	4	0
0	0	0	7	11	2	90	0.1	0.4	7	1	0.27	12	0.01	0.02	0.1	0.02	7	0
0	0	0	18	8	5	68	0.1	0.2	5	1	0	81	0.01	0.05	0.2	0.05	1	0
0	0	0	18	8	5	68	0.1	0.2	5	1	0	81	0.01	0.05	0.2	0.05	1	0
0	0	0	18	8	5	68	0.1	0.2	5	1	0	81	0.01	0.05	0.2	0.05	1	0
0	0	0	18	8	5	68	0.1	0.2	5	1	0	81	0.01	0.05	0.2	0.05	1	0
0	0	0	0	—	21	92	—	0	—	0	—	0	—	—	—	—	—	0
0.2	0.2	0	24	22	7	235	0.2	1.2	29	123	0.1	3872	0.05	0.14	1	0.01	34	0
0	0.1	0	14	17	17	301	0.1	0.6	12	0	0.02	60	0.01	0.04	0.1	0.08	1	0
0	0.1	0	17	17	7	295	0.1	0.9	7	0	0.02	103	0.05	0.04	0.2	0.07	0	0
0.1	0.2	0	21	24	6	308	0.1	0.9	12	13	0.12	3	0.05	0.06	0.5	0.08	4	0
0	0.1	0	19	21	7	303	0.1	0.8	14	1	0.02	1	0.06	0.06	0.4	0.11	3	0

Food Item	Qty	Meas	Wgt (g)	Wtr (g)	Cals	Prot (g)	Carb (g)	Fib (g)	Fat (g)	SatF (g)
Juice, apple-raspberry	1	cup	239	212	108	0	26	0.2	0	0
Juice, beef broth & tomato, canned	0.5	cup	122	110	45	1	10	0.1	0	0
Juice, clam and tomato	1	cup	241	210	115	1	26	0.5	0	0.1
Juice, grapefruit, canned, sweetened	0.5	cup	125	109	58	1	14	0.1	0	0
Juice, orange, chilled	1	cup	249	220	110	2	25	0.5	1	0.1
Juice, orange, fresh	1	cup	248	219	112	2	26	0.5	0	0.1
Juice, orange, frozen concentrate, prepared	1	cup	249	219	112	2	27	0.5	0	0
Juice, orange, unsweetened, canned	1	cup	249	222	105	1	24	0.5	0	0
Juice, orange, unsweetened, frozen concentrate	0.5	cup	106	62	169	3	41	0.9	0	0
Juice, passion fruit, purple, fresh	0.5	cup	124	106	63	0	17	0.2	0	0
Juice, passion fruit, yellow	0.5	cup	124	104	74	1	18	0.2	0	0
Juice, pineapple, canned, unsweetened	1	cup	250	214	140	1	34	0.5	0	0
Juice, pineapple, frozen concentrate, prepared	1	cup	250	216	130	1	32	0.5	0	0
Juice, pineapple, sweetened	1	cup	252	211	158	1	39	0.2	0	0
Juice, prune, bottled	1	cup	256	208	182	2	45	2.6	0	0
Juice, strawberry	1	cup	237	217	71	1	17	0.2	1	0
Juice, tangerine, canned, sweetened	0.5	cup	124	108	62	1	15	0.2	0	0
Juice, tangerine, fresh, unsweetened	1	cup	247	220	106	1	25	0.5	0	0.1
Juice, tangerine, frozen, sweetened, prepared	1	cup	241	212	111	1	27	0.5	0	0
Juice, tangerine, frozen, unswt, prepared	1	cup	247	220	106	1	25	0.5	0	0.1
Juice, watermelon, fresh	1	cup	238	218	76	1	17	1.2	1	0.1
Jujube fruit, raw	4	oz.	113	88	90	1	23	1.4	0	—
Jute/potherb, cooked	0.5	cup	43	38	16	2	3	0.9	0	0
KFC chicken leg, original	1	each	57	30	152	14	3	0.2	8	2.2
KFC, Chicken Little sandwich	1	each	47	16	169	6	14	0.4	10	2
KFC, Chicken breast, side, original	1	each	90	42	266	20	10	0.2	16	4.5
KFC, Chicken sandwich, Colonel's	1	each	166	76	482	21	39	—	27	6
KFC, Red beans & rice	1	each	111	84	113	4	18	3	3	1
KFC, chicken breast, center, original	1	each	115	60	290	28	10	0.1	16	4.2
KFC, chicken breast, crispy	1	each	135	65	378	30	16	0.1	22	5.5
KFC, chicken leg, crispy	1	each	69	34	202	14	6	0.1	13	3.4
KFC, chicken, dark quarter, no skin, rotisserie gold	1	each	117	77	217	27	0	0	12	3.5
KFC, chicken, hot wings pieces (6)	1	each	119	45	415	24	16	—	29	—
KFC, chicken, white quarter, no skin, rotisserie gold	1	each	117	73	199	37	0	0	6	1.7
KFC, chicken, wing, whole, Hot and Spicy	1	each	61	23	220	14	5	—	16	4
Kale, fresh, chopped	0.5	cup	34	28	17	1	3	0.7	0	0
Kale, fresh, cooked, drained, no added salt	0.5	cup	65	59	18	1	4	1.3	0	0
Kale, frozen, cooked, drained, no added salt	0.5	cup	65	59	20	2	3	1.3	0	0
Kiwi fruit, freshly harvested	1	each	76	63	46	1	11	2.6	0	0
Kiwi fruit, raw slices	10	piece	70	58	43	1	10	2.4	0	0
Kiwi fruit, raw, stored	1	each	76	63	46	1	11	2.6	0	0
Kohlrabi slices, raw	0.5	cup	70	64	19	1	4	2.5	0	0
Kohlrabi, cooked, drained, no added salt	0.5	cup	82	74	24	1	6	0.9	0	0
Kool-aid, mix, unsweetened, grape, prepared	1	cup	246	221	100	0	25	0	0	0
Kudos nutty fudge snack bar	1	each	37	1	200	3	20	—	12	—
Kumquat, raw	1	each	19	16	12	0	3	1.2	0	0
LJS, chicken plank, 2 piece	1	each	112	62	240	16	22	—	12	3.2
LJS, clam dinner	1	each	361	168	990	24	114	—	52	10.9
LJS, fish & fryes, batter fried, 2 piece	1	each	261	142	610	27	52	—	37	7.9
LJS, fish & more, 2 piece w/fries & slaw	1	each	407	233	890	31	92	—	48	10.1
LJS, fish sandwich, batter dipped	1	each	159	86	340	18	40	—	13	3.1
LJS, fish shrimp chicken dinner	1	each	513	—	1160	45	113	—	65	14.2
LJS, fish w/lemon dinner, 3 piece	1	each	493	352	610	39	86	—	13	2.2
LJS, fish, batter fried, svg	1	each	88	52	180	12	12	—	11	2.7
LJS, fish, light portion dinner	1	each	334	257	330	24	46	—	5	0.9
LJS, fish-shrimp-clams dinner	1	each	512	—	1240	44	123	—	70	15.2
LJS, herb chicken a la carte	1	each	100	74	120	22	—	—	4	1.2
LJS, malt vinegar, serving	1	each	8	—	1	0	0	0	—	—
LJS, seafood gumbo w/cod	1	each	198	175	120	9	4	—	8	2.1
Lamb curry	0.5	cup	118	93	141	14	1	0.3	9	2.2
Lamb kabob meat, broiled, lean	4	oz.	113	72	211	32	0	0	8	3
Lamb stew meat, braised, lean	4	oz.	113	64	253	38	0	0	10	3.6
Lamb, arm chop, broiled, lean	1	each	74	46	148	20	0	0	7	2.5
Lamb, arm chop, broiled, lean	3	oz.	85	53	170	24	0	0	8	2.9
Lamb, chop, loin, broiled, lean	1	each	46	28	99	14	0	0	4	1.6

MonoF	PolyF	Choles	Calc	Phos	Sod	Pot	Zn	Iron	Magn	VitA	VitE	VitC	Thia	Ribo	Nia	B6	Fola	B12
(g)	(g)	(mg)	(mg)	(mg)	(mg)	(mg)	(mg)	(mg)	(mg)	(μg RE)	(mg α-TE)	(mg)	(mg)	(mg)	(mg)	(mg)	(μg)	(μg)
0	0.2	0	19	19	6	309	0.1	1.1	16	7	0.09	6	0.05	0.05	0.3	0.08	5	0
0	0	0	13	16	160	117	0	0.7	4	16	0.49	1	0	0.04	0.2	0.03	5	0.06
0	0	0	29	188	871	217	2.6	1.4	53	53	1.2	10	0.1	0.07	0.5	0.2	38	73.6
0	0	0	10	14	2	203	0.1	0.4	12	0	0.06	34	0.05	0.03	0.4	0.02	13	0
0.1	0.2	0	25	27	2	473	0.1	0.4	27	20	0.47	82	0.28	0.05	0.7	0.13	45	0
0.1	0.1	0	27	42	2	496	0.1	0.5	27	50	0.22	124	0.22	0.07	1	0.1	75	0
0	0	0	22	40	2	473	0.1	0.2	25	20	0.47	97	0.2	0.04	0.5	0.11	109	0
0.1	0.1	0	20	35	5	436	0.2	1.1	27	45	0.22	86	0.15	0.07	0.8	0.22	45	0
0	0	0	34	61	3	718	0.2	0.4	36	30	0.34	147	0.3	0.07	0.8	0.17	165	0
0	0	0	5	16	7	343	0.1	0.3	21	89	0.06	37	0	0.16	1.8	0.06	9	0
0	0.1	0	5	31	7	343	0.1	0.4	21	298	0.06	22	0	0.12	2.8	0.07	10	0
0	0.1	0	42	20	2	335	0.3	0.6	32	1	0.05	27	0.14	0.06	0.6	0.24	58	0
0	0	0	28	20	2	340	0.3	0.8	22	2	0.02	30	0.18	0.05	0.5	0.18	26	0
0	0.1	0	42	20	3	331	0.3	0.6	32	1	0.05	26	0.14	0.06	0.6	0.24	57	0
0.1	0	0	31	64	10	707	0.5	3	36	1	0.03	10	0.04	0.18	2	0.56	1	0
0.1	0.4	0	33	45	2	393	0.3	0.9	24	5	0.33	67	0.05	0.14	0.5	0.12	21	0
0	0	0	22	17	1	222	0	0.2	10	52	0.11	27	0.08	0.02	0.1	0.04	6	0
0.1	0.1	0	44	35	2	440	0.1	0.5	20	104	0.22	77	0.15	0.05	0.2	0.1	11	0
0	0	0	19	19	2	272	0.1	0.2	19	137	0.1	58	0.12	0.05	0.2	0.1	11	0
0.1	0.1	0	44	35	2	440	0.1	0.5	20	104	0.22	77	0.15	0.05	0.2	0.1	11	0
0.3	0.3	0	19	21	5	276	0.2	0.4	26	88	0.36	23	0.19	0.05	0.5	0.34	5	0
—	—	0	24	26	3	284	0.1	0.5	11	5	—	78	0.02	0.04	1	0.09	—	0
0	0	0	91	31	5	237	0.3	1.4	27	223	0.3	14	0.04	0.08	0.4	0.24	45	0
4.1	1.3	75	21	—	269	—	—	1.1	—	15	—	—	0.05	0.12	3.2	—	—	—
4.7	3.4	18	23	—	331	—	—	1.7	—	5	—	—	0.16	0.12	2.2	—	—	—
9.4	2.4	85	74	—	655	—	—	1.3	—	16	—	—	0.06	0.14	7.5	—	—	—
—	—	47	50	—	1060	—	—	1.3	—	15	—	6	—	—	—	—	—	—
—	—	4	10	—	312	—	—	0.7	—	—	—	—	—	—	—	—	—	—
8.7	2.2	103	34	—	680	—	—	0.8	—	17	—	—	0.1	0.19	12.8	—	—	—
12.4	2.4	86	38	—	847	—	—	0.9	—	17	—	—	0.13	0.15	15	—	—	—
7.7	1.7	69	21	—	329	—	—	0.4	—	32	—	—	0.06	0.13	3.9	—	—	—
—	—	128	10	—	772	—	—	0.2	—	15	—	1	—	—	—	—	—	—
—	—	132	35	—	1084	—	—	2.9	—	13	—	5	—	—	—	—	—	—
—	—	97	10	—	667	—	—	0.2	—	15	—	1	—	—	—	—	—	—
—	—	65	20	—	440	—	—	0.7	—	30	—	—	—	—	—	—	—	—
0	0.1	0	45	19	14	150	0.1	0.6	11	298	0.27	40	0.04	0.04	0.3	0.09	10	0
0	0.1	0	47	18	15	148	0.2	0.6	12	481	0.55	27	0.03	0.05	0.3	0.09	9	0
0	0.2	0	90	18	10	209	0.1	0.6	12	413	0.12	16	0.03	0.07	0.4	0.06	9	0
0	0.2	0	20	30	4	252	0.1	0.3	23	14	0.85	74	0.02	0.04	0.4	0.07	29	0
0	0.2	0	18	28	4	232	0.1	0.3	21	13	0.78	52	0.01	0.04	0.4	0.04	7	0
0	0.2	0	20	30	4	252	0.1	0.3	23	14	0.85	57	0.02	0.04	0.4	0.04	8	0
0	0	0	17	32	14	245	0	0.3	13	3	0.34	43	0.04	0.01	0.3	0.1	11	0
0	0	0	21	37	17	281	0.3	0.3	16	3	1.38	45	0.03	0.02	0.3	0.13	10	0
0	0	0	0	—	15	0	—	0	—	0	—	6	—	—	—	—	—	0
—	—	—	40	—	55	—	—	0.4	—	—	—	—	—	0.1	—	—	—	—
0	0	0	8	4	1	37	0	0.1	2	6	0.05	7	0.02	0.02	0.1	0.01	3	0
8.4	0.2	30	—	—	790	320	0.6	1.1	—	—	—	—	0.15	0.26	7	—	—	—
31.3	9.9	75	200	—	1830	910	3	4.5	—	40	—	12	0.75	0.42	12	—	—	—
23.5	5.3	60	40	—	1480	900	1.2	1.8	—	—	—	9	0.38	0.34	8	—	—	—
28.5	9.5	75	200	—	1790	1230	2.2	3.6	—	40	—	9	0.52	0.51	12	—	—	—
8.9	1	30	80	—	890	370	1.5	3.6	—	—	—	1	0.38	0.34	6	—	—	—
40.3	9.6	135	200	—	2590	1450	3.8	4.5	—	40	—	9	0.75	0.68	16	—	—	—
3.9	5.3	125	200	—	1420	990	2.2	5.4	—	700	—	6	0.75	0.6	24	—	—	—
8.1	0.2	30	—	—	490	260	0.3	0.4	—	—	—	—	0.15	0.17	3	—	—	—
1.6	1.2	75	80	—	640	440	0.9	1.8	—	1000	—	18	0.3	0.26	14	—	—	—
44.2	9.9	140	200	—	2630	1390	3.8	5.4	—	40	—	9	0.9	0.68	16	—	—	—
1.7	1.1	60	—	—	570	270	0.6	0.7	—	—	—	—	0.09	0.26	—	—	—	—
—	—	—	—	—	15	10	—	—	—	—	—	—	—	—	—	—	—	—
3.2	2.6	25	100	—	740	310	1.5	1.8	—	200	—	—	0.15	0.17	3	—	—	—
2.9	2.8	44	15	137	237	235	3.2	1.3	18	0	1	1	0.04	0.14	3.9	0.09	13	1.41
3.4	0.8	102	15	254	86	380	6.5	2.6	35	0	0.23	0	0.12	0.34	7.5	0.16	26	3.44
4	0.9	122	17	232	79	295	7.5	3.2	32	0	0.23	0	0.08	0.27	6.8	0.14	24	3.1
2.7	0.6	68	13	162	61	252	4.2	1.7	22	0	0.15	0	0.07	0.22	5	0.1	17	2.22
3.1	0.7	78	14	186	70	289	4.9	2	26	0	0.17	0	0.08	0.25	5.8	0.12	20	2.55
2	0.3	44	9	104	39	173	1.9	0.9	13	0	0.07	0	0.05	0.13	3.2	0.07	11	1.16

Food Item	Qty	Meas	Wgt (g)	Wtr (g)	Cals	Prot (g)	Carb (g)	Fib (g)	Fat (g)	SatF (g)
Lamb, chop, loin, broiled, lean	3	oz.	85	52	184	26	0	0	8	3
Lamb, chop, loin, broiled, lean & fat	1	each	64	33	202	16	0	0	15	6.3
Lamb, chop, loin, broiled, lean & fat	3	oz.	85	44	269	21	0	0	20	8.4
Lamb, ground, broiled	4	oz.	113	62	321	28	0	0	22	9.2
Lamb, leg, roasted, lean	3	oz.	85	54	162	24	0	0	7	2.4
Lamb, leg, sirloin, roasted, lean	4	oz.	113	71	231	32	0	0	10	3.7
Lamb, leg, sirloin, roasted, lean & fat	4	oz.	113	61	331	28	0	0	24	9.9
Lamb, rib, roast, cooked, lean	4	oz.	113	68	263	30	0	0	15	5.4
Lamb, rib, roast, cooked, lean & fat	4	oz.	113	54	407	24	0	0	34	14.5
Lamb, shoulder, roasted, lean	4	oz.	113	72	231	28	0	0	12	4.6
Lamb, shoulder, roasted, lean & fat	4	oz.	113	64	313	26	0	0	23	9.6
Lambsquarter, raw, chopped	0.5	cup	28	24	12	1	2	1.1	0	0
Lambsquarters, cooked, drained	0.5	cup	90	80	29	3	4	1.9	1	0
Lard, pork fat	1	Tbs	13	0	116	0	0	0	13	5.1
Lasagna, w/meat, recipe	1	piece	245	165	382	22	39	3.3	15	7.8
Lasagna, zucchini, Healthy Choice	1	each	397	330	290	14	49	5.2	4	2.6
Leek, whole, drained	1	each	124	113	38	1	9	1.2	0	0
Leek, whole, raw	1	each	124	103	76	2	18	2.2	0	0
Leeks, chopped, cooked, drained	0.5	cup	52	47	16	0	4	0.5	0	0
Leeks, chopped, raw	0.5	cup	52	43	32	1	7	0.9	0	0
Lemon grass, leaves	1	oz.	28	20	19	0	4	—	0	—
Lemon juice, bottled	1	cup	244	226	51	1	16	1	1	0.1
Lemon juice, fresh	1	cup	244	221	61	1	21	1	0	0
Lemon juice, frozen, unsweetened	1	cup	244	225	54	1	16	1	1	0.1
Lemon peel, candied	1.5	oz.	43	7	134	0	34	—	0	0
Lemon peel, fresh	1	Tbs	6	5	3	0	1	0.6	0	0
Lemon pepper	0.25	tsp	1	0	2	0	0	0	0	—
Lemon turnover	1	each	78	33	238	3	29	0.6	12	3.1
Lemon, fresh, peeled	1	each	58	52	17	1	5	1.6	0	0
Lemonade drink, powder	1	Tbs	15	0	56	0	14	0	0	0
Lemonade flavor drink, dry, prepared	1	cup	266	237	112	0	29	0	0	0
Lemonade, low calorie	1	cup	240	228	43	0	11	0.2	0	0
Lemonade, low calorie, dry, prepared (Country Time)	1	cup	238	236	5	0	1	0	0	0
Lemonade, pink, frozen, prepared	1	cup	248	221	99	0	26	0	0	0
Lemonade, powder	1	Tbs	14	0	51	0	14	0	0	0
Lemonade, powder, prepared, Country Time	1	cup	264	237	103	0	27	0	0	0
Lemonade, white, frozen, prepared	1	cup	248	221	99	0	26	0.2	0	0
Lentil loaf	1	piece	47	30	82	4	9	3.1	3	0.4
Lentil sprouts, raw	0.5	cup	38	26	41	3	9	1.6	0	0
Lentil, sprouted, stir fried	4	oz.	113	78	115	10	24	4.4	1	0.1
Lentils, dry	0.25	cup	48	5	162	14	27	14.6	0	0.1
Lentils, dry, cooked	0.5	cup	99	69	115	9	20	7.8	0	0.1
Lettuce, butterhead, chopped	0.5	cup	28	27	4	0	1	0.3	0	0
Lettuce, butterhead, leaves	2	piece	15	14	2	0	0	0.2	0	0
Lettuce, butterhead, whole head	1	each	163	156	21	2	4	1.6	0	0
Lettuce, iceberg/crisphead leaves	1	piece	20	19	2	0	0	0.3	0	0
Lettuce, iceberg/crisphead, chopped	0.5	cup	28	27	3	0	1	0.4	0	0
Lettuce, iceberg/crisphead, whole head	1	each	539	517	65	5	11	7.6	1	0.1
Lettuce, looseleaf, chopped	0.5	cup	28	26	5	0	1	0.5	0	0
Lettuce, looseleaf, leaves	1	piece	10	9	2	0	0	0.2	0	0
Lettuce, romaine, chopped	0.5	cup	28	27	4	0	1	0.5	0	0
Lettuce, romaine, inner leaf	1	piece	10	9	1	0	0	0.2	0	0
Lime juice, bottled	1	cup	246	228	52	1	16	1	1	0.1
Lime juice, fresh	1	cup	246	222	66	1	22	1	0	0
Lime, fresh, peeled	0.5	each	67	59	20	0	7	1.9	0	0
Limeade, concentrate, frozen	0.5	cup	145	73	272	0	72	0.6	0	0
Limeade, from frozen	1	cup	247	220	101	0	27	0.2	0	0
Liqueur, coffee, 53 proof	1	oz.	28	9	95	0	13	0	0	0
Liqueur, coffee, 63 proof	1	oz.	28	12	87	0	9	0	0	0
Liqueur, de menthe, 72 proof	1	oz.	28	8	105	0	12	0	0	0
Liqueur, kahlua, 1 shot	1	each	30	9	106	0	13	0	0	0
Liver, chopped, w/egg & onion	0.5	cup	104	66	230	13	3	0.4	18	5.5
Liverwurst	1	oz.	28	15	92	4	1	0	8	3
Liverwurst	1	piece	18	9	59	3	0	0	5	1.9

MonoF	PolyF	Choles	Calc	Phos	Sod	Pot	Zn	Iron	Magn	VitA	VitE	VitC	Thia	Ribo	Nia	B6	Fola	B12
(g)	(g)	(mg)	(mg)	(mg)	(mg)	(mg)	(mg)	(mg)	(mg)	(µg RE)	(mg α-TE)	(mg)	(mg)	(mg)	(mg)	(mg)	(µg)	(µg)
3.6	0.5	81	16	192	71	320	3.5	1.7	24	0	0.14	0	0.09	0.24	5.8	0.14	20	2.14
6.2	1.1	64	13	125	49	209	2.2	1.2	15	0	0.08	0	0.06	0.16	4.5	0.08	12	1.58
8.2	1.4	85	17	167	66	278	3	1.5	20	0	0.11	0	0.08	0.21	6	0.11	15	2.1
9.4	1.6	110	25	228	92	384	5.3	2	27	0	0.28	0	0.11	0.28	7.6	0.16	22	2.96
2.9	0.4	76	7	175	58	287	4.2	1.8	22	0	0.15	0	0.09	0.25	5.4	0.14	20	2.24
4.6	0.7	104	9	230	80	378	5.5	2.5	28	0	0.19	0	0.14	0.35	7.1	0.19	24	2.93
9.9	1.7	110	12	208	77	341	4.7	2.3	25	0	0.15	0	0.12	0.32	7.5	0.16	19	2.87
6.6	1	100	24	221	92	357	5.1	2	26	0	0.17	0	0.1	0.26	7	0.17	25	2.45
14.2	2.5	110	25	188	83	307	4	1.8	23	0	0.11	0	0.1	0.24	7.6	0.12	17	2.53
4.9	1.1	99	22	227	77	301	6.8	2.4	28	0	0.2	0	0.1	0.3	6.5	0.17	28	3.06
9.3	1.8	104	23	209	75	285	5.9	2.2	26	0	0.16	0	0.1	0.27	7	0.15	24	2.99
0	0.1	0	86	20	12	127	0.1	0.3	10	325	0.43	22	0.04	0.12	0.3	0.08	8	0
0.1	0.3	0	232	40	26	259	0.3	0.6	21	873	1.21	33	0.09	0.23	0.8	0.16	12	0
5.4	1.8	12	0	0	0	0	0	0	0	0	0.15	0	0	0	0	0	0	0
5	0.9	56	258	289	745	461	3.2	3.2	50	158	1.15	16	0.23	0.33	4	0.21	19	0.78
—	—	10	207	—	321	—	—	1.9	—	259	—	0	—	—	—	—	—	—
0	0.1	0	37	21	12	108	0.1	1.4	17	6	0.76	5	0.03	0.02	0.2	0.14	30	0
0	0.2	0	73	43	25	223	0.1	2.6	35	12	1.14	15	0.07	0.04	0.5	0.29	80	0
0	0.1	0	16	9	5	45	0	0.6	7	3	0.32	2	0.01	0.01	0.1	0.06	13	0
0	0.1	0	31	18	10	94	0.1	1.1	15	5	0.48	6	0.03	0.02	0.2	0.12	33	0
—	—	—	46	12	—	—	—	1.5	—	1143	—	7	0.01	0.03	0.1	—	—	0
0	0.2	0	27	22	51	249	0.1	0.3	20	5	0.22	60	0.1	0.02	0.5	0.1	25	0
0	0	0	17	15	2	303	0.1	0.1	15	5	0.22	112	0.07	0.02	0.2	0.12	32	0
0	0.2	0	20	20	2	217	0.1	0.3	20	2	0.22	77	0.14	0.03	0.3	0.15	23	0
—	—	0	0	0	0	0	—	0	—	0	—	0	0	0	0	—	—	0
0	0	0	8	1	0	10	0	0	1	0	0.01	8	0	0	0	0.01	1	0
—	—	—	—	—	98	3	—	—	—	—	—	—	—	—	—	—	—	0
5.4	3.2	47	10	41	228	31	0.3	1.1	5	32	1.16	1	0.13	0.12	1.1	0.02	8	0.09
0	0.1	0	15	9	1	80	0	0.3	5	2	0.14	31	0.02	0.01	0.1	0.05	6	0
0	0	0	12	1	6	0	0	0	0	0	0	17	0	0	0	0	0	0
0	0	0	29	3	19	3	0.1	0.1	3	0	0	34	0	0	0	0	0	0
0	0	0	7	2	7	38	0.1	0.4	5	2	0	16	0.02	0.02	0	0	7	0
0	0	0	50	24	7	0	0.1	0.1	2	0	0	6	0	0	0	0	0	0
0	0	0	7	5	7	37	0.1	0.4	5	0	0	10	0.02	0.05	0	0.02	5	0
0	0	0	33	17	3	16	0	0.1	0	0	0	4	0	0	0	0	2	0
0	0	0	71	34	13	34	0.1	0.2	3	0	0	8	0	0	0	0.01	3	0
0	0	0	7	5	7	37	0.1	0.4	5	5	0	10	0.02	0.05	0	0.02	5	0
0.7	2.1	0	15	88	40	155	0.6	1.4	26	0	2.01	1	0.13	0.04	0.6	0.09	62	0
0	0.1	0	10	67	4	124	0.6	1.2	14	2	0.04	6	0.09	0.05	0.4	0.07	38	0
0.1	0.2	0	16	174	11	322	1.8	3.5	40	5	0.1	14	0.25	0.1	1.4	0.19	76	0
0.1	0.2	0	24	218	5	434	1.7	4.3	51	2	0.16	3	0.23	0.12	1.3	0.26	208	0
0.1	0.2	0	19	178	2	365	1.3	3.3	36	1	0.11	1	0.17	0.07	1	0.18	179	0
0	0	0	9	6	1	72	0	0.1	4	27	0.12	2	0.02	0.02	0.1	0.01	20	0
0	0	0	5	3	1	39	0	0	2	15	0.07	1	0.01	0.01	0	0.01	11	0
0	0.2	0	52	38	8	419	0.3	0.5	21	158	0.72	13	0.1	0.1	0.5	0.08	119	0
0	0	0	4	4	2	32	0	0.1	2	7	0.06	1	0.01	0.01	0	0.01	11	0
0	0	0	5	6	3	44	0.1	0.1	3	9	0.08	1	0.01	0.01	0.1	0.01	16	0
0	0.5	0	102	108	48	852	1.2	2.7	48	178	1.51	21	0.25	0.16	1	0.22	302	0
0	0	0	19	7	3	74	0.1	0.4	3	53	0.12	5	0.01	0.02	0.1	0.02	14	0
0	0	0	7	2	1	26	0	0.1	1	19	0.04	2	0	0.01	0	0.01	5	0
0	0	0	10	13	2	81	0.1	0.3	2	73	0.12	7	0.03	0.03	0.1	0.01	38	0
0	0	0	4	4	1	29	0	0.1	1	26	0.04	2	0.01	0.01	0	0	14	0
0.1	0.2	0	30	25	39	185	0.1	0.6	17	5	0.17	16	0.08	0.01	0.4	0.07	19	0
0	0.1	0	22	17	2	268	0.1	0.1	15	2	0.22	72	0.05	0.02	0.2	0.11	20	0
0	0	0	22	12	1	68	0.1	0.4	4	1	0.16	20	0.02	0.01	0.1	0.03	5	0
0	0	0	7	9	0	86	0.1	0.1	6	0	0	17	0.02	0.02	0.1	0	6	0
0	0	0	7	2	5	32	0	0.1	2	0	0	7	0	0	0.1	0	2	0
0	0	0	0	2	2	9	0	0	1	0	0	0	0	0	0	0	0	0
0	0	0	0	2	2	9	0	0	1	0	0	0	0	0	0	0	0	0
0	0	0	0	0	1	0	0	0	0	0	0	0	0	0	0	0	0	0
0	0	0	0	1	2	4	0	0	0	0	0	0	0	0	0	0	0	0
7.4	3.5	367	21	178	1078	125	2.2	4.1	14	2230	1.38	9	0.09	0.88	2	0.31	358	8.89
3.8	0.7	45	7	65	244	48	0.7	1.8	3	2353	0.08	0	0.08	0.29	1.2	0.05	9	3.83
2.4	0.5	28	5	41	155	31	0.4	1.2	2	1494	0.05	0	0.05	0.18	0.8	0.03	5	2.43

Food Item	Qty	Meas	Wgt (g)	Wtr (g)	Cals	Prot (g)	Carb (g)	Fib (g)	Fat (g)	SatF (g)
Lobster newburg	0.5	cup	122	75	306	15	6	0.1	25	14.8
Loganberries, canned w/heavy syrup	0.5	cup	128	98	113	1	28	3.3	0	0
Loganberries, fresh	0.5	cup	75	64	39	1	10	4	0	0
Loganberries, frozen	0.5	cup	74	62	40	1	10	3.6	0	0
Longan, raw	1	each	3	3	2	0	0	0	0	—
Loquat, raw	1	each	10	9	5	0	1	0.2	0	0
Lotus root, cooked	10	each	89	72	59	1	14	2.8	0	0
Lotus root, slices, raw	10	each	81	64	60	2	14	4	0	0
Lunchables, bologna & American, regular	1	each	128	—	450	18	19	0	34	15
Lunchables, ham & cheddar, regular	1	each	128	—	340	21	19	0	20	11
Lunchmeat, Spam, canned	1	piece	28	14	95	4	1	0.1	9	—
Lunchmeat, chicken/turkey sandwich spread	1	Tbs	13	9	26	2	1	0	2	0.4
Lunchmeat, chopped ham, slices	2	piece	42	27	96	7	0	0	7	2.4
Lunchmeat, pickle & pimento loaf	2	piece	57	32	149	7	3	0	12	4.5
Lychee, raw	1	each	10	8	6	0	2	0.1	0	0
Lychees, canned, sweetened	3.5	oz.	100	76	91	1	23	0.3	0	0.1
Macadamia nut, dried	0.25	cup	34	1	235	3	5	3.1	25	3.7
Macadamia nuts, oil roasted, salted	0.25	cup	34	1	241	2	4	3.1	26	3.8
Macadamia nuts, oil roasted, unsalted	11	each	28	0	204	2	4	2.6	22	3.3
Macaroni & cheese, canned	0.5	cup	120	96	114	5	13	0.7	5	2.1
Macaroni & cheese, recipe, w/margarine	0.5	cup	100	58	215	8	20	0.6	11	4.4
Mace, ground	0.25	tsp	0	0	2	0	0	0.1	0	0
Mamey apple, raw	1	each	846	729	431	4	106	25.4	4	1.2
Mango nectar	1	cup	250	210	147	1	38	2	0	0.1
Mango, fresh slices	0.5	cup	82	67	54	0	14	1.5	0	0.1
Mango, fresh, whole	1	each	207	169	135	1	35	3.7	1	0.1
Margarine, Blue Bonnet, stick	1	Tbs	14	2	102	0	0	0	11	2.4
Margarine, Fleischmann's corn oil, tub type	1	Tbs	14	2	102	0	0	0	11	2
Margarine, Parkay Squeeze	1	Tbs	14	2	102	0	0	0	11	1.9
Margarine, Parkay, soft, tub	1	Tbs	14	2	102	0	0	0	11	1.9
Margarine, Saffola, stick	1	Tbs	14	2	102	0	0	0	11	1.9
Margarine, Saffola, tub	1	Tbs	14	2	102	0	0	0	11	1.5
Margarine, hard, pat	1	each	3	0	22	0	0	0	2	0.4
Margarine, hard, stick	1	Tbs	14	2	102	0	0	0	11	1.9
Margarine, hard, unsalted	1	Tbs	14	3	101	0	0	0	11	2.1
Margarine, liquid	1	Tbs	14	2	102	0	0	0	11	1.9
Margarine, soft, tub	1	Tbs	14	2	102	0	0	0	11	1.9
Margarine, spread, Blue Bonnet, tub	1	Tbs	14	8	49	0	0	0	6	0.9
Margarine, spread, Fleischmann's light, tub	1	Tbs	14	8	49	0	0	0	6	0.9
Margarine, spread, Shedd's Spread, tub	1	Tbs	14	8	60	0	0	0	6	0.8
Margarine, spread, Touch of Butter, stick	1	Tbs	14	4	90	0	0	0	10	2
Margarine, spread, Weight Watcher's XLight, tub	1	Tbs	14	8	49	0	0	0	6	1.1
Margarine, unsalted, Saffola	1	Tbs	14	3	101	0	0	0	11	2
Marjoram, dried	0.25	tsp	0	0	0	0	0	0.1	0	0
Marmalade, orange	1	Tbs	20	7	49	0	13	0	0	0
Marmalade, orange, packet	1	each	14	5	34	0	9	0	0	0
Marshmallow	4	each	28	5	90	1	23	0	0	0
Marshmallow creme, Kraft	1	oz.	28	5	93	0	23	0	0	0
Marshmallow, miniature, not packed	0.5	cup	23	4	73	0	19	0	0	0
Mayonnaise, fat free (Kraft Free)	1	Tbs	16	14	10	0	2	0	0	0
Mayonnaise, imitation	1	Tbs	15	9	35	0	2	0	3	0.5
Mayonnaise, low calorie	1	Tbs	16	10	36	0	2	0	3	0.5
Mayonnaise, low calorie, low sodium	1	Tbs	14	9	32	0	2	0	3	0.5
Mayonnaise, soybean, w/salt	1	Tbs	14	2	99	0	0	0	11	1.6
McDonald's Egg McMuffin	1	each	137	78	289	17	27	1.5	13	0.7
McDonald's Fillet-O-Fish sandwich	1	each	145	71	364	14	41	1.5	16	3.7
McDonald's McDonaldland cookies	1	each	56	2	258	4	41	1	9	1.7
McDonald's McLean Deluxe, w/cheese	1	each	228	143	397	26	38	2.2	16	6.8
McDonald's McLean deluxe	1	each	214	137	345	24	37	2.2	12	4.4
McDonald's Sausage McMuffin	1	each	112	48	361	13	26	1.5	23	8.3
McDonald's cheeseburger	1	each	122	56	319	15	36	1.9	13	5.6
McDonald's frozen yogurt cone, vanilla	1	each	90	61	118	4	24	0.4	1	0.5
McDonald's frozen yogurt shake, small, choc	1	each	295	—	348	13	62	0.9	6	3.5
McDonald's frozen yogurt shake, small, strawberry	1	each	294	—	343	12	63	0.3	5	3.4
McDonald's frozen yogurt shake, small, vanilla	1	each	293	—	308	12	54	0.3	5	3.3

A

MonoF (g)	PolyF (g)	Choles (mg)	Calc (mg)	Phos (mg)	Sod (mg)	Pot (mg)	Zn (mg)	Iron (mg)	Magn (mg)	VitA (μg RE)	VitE (mg α-TE)	VitC (mg)	Thia (mg)	Ribo (mg)	Nia (mg)	B6 (mg)	Fola (μg)	B12 (μg)
7.3	1.1	184	120	199	323	304	2	0.6	28	261	1	0	0.05	0.21	0.8	0.08	16	2.01
0	0.1	0	23	13	4	115	0.2	0.6	14	5	0.91	8	0.03	0.04	0.3	0.05	44	0
0	0.2	0	24	16	0	146	0.2	0.4	15	12	0.53	16	0.02	0.03	0.3	0.04	25	0
0	0.1	0	19	19	1	107	0.2	0.5	15	3	1.62	11	0.04	0.02	0.6	0.05	19	0
—	—	0	0	1	0	9	0	0	0	0	—	3	0	0	0	—	—	0
0	0	0	2	3	0	26	0	0	1	15	0.09	0	0	0	0	0.01	1	0
0	0	0	23	69	40	323	0.3	0.8	20	0	0.01	24	0.11	0.01	0.3	0.19	7	0
0	0	0	36	81	32	450	0.3	0.9	19	0	0.01	36	0.13	0.18	0.3	0.21	10	0
—	—	85	300	—	1620	—	—	2.7	—	60	—	0	—	—	—	—	—	—
—	—	75	250	—	1830	—	—	1.8	—	60	—	—	—	—	—	—	—	—
—	—	16	2	—	445	54	0.7	0.4	3	5	—	—	0.03	0.05	0.9	—	—	—
0.4	0.8	4	1	4	49	24	0.1	0.1	1	5	0.29	0	0	0.01	0.2	0.01	1	0.05
3.4	0.9	21	3	65	576	134	0.8	0.3	7	0	0.11	0	0.26	0.09	1.6	0.15	0	0.39
5.5	1.5	21	54	80	792	194	0.8	0.6	10	4	0.14	0	0.17	0.14	1.2	0.11	3	0.67
0	0	0	0	3	0	16	0	0	1	0	0.07	7	0	0.01	0.1	0.01	1	0
0	0.1	0	4	20	1	100	0.1	0.2	7	0	0.45	32	0.01	0.04	0.4	0.06	5	0
19.5	0.4	0	24	46	2	123	0.6	0.8	39	0	0.14	0	0.12	0.04	0.7	0.07	5	0
20.2	0.4	0	15	67	87	110	0.4	0.6	39	0	0.14	0	0.07	0.04	0.7	0.07	5	0
17.1	0.4	0	13	57	2	93	0.3	0.5	33	0	0.12	0	0.06	0.03	0.6	0.06	5	0
1.5	0.7	12	100	91	365	70	0.6	0.5	16	37	0.07	0	0.06	0.12	0.5	0.01	4	0.1
4.4	1.8	21	181	161	543	120	0.6	0.9	18	117	0.06	0	0.1	0.2	0.9	0.02	5	0.15
0	0	0	1	0	0	2	0	0.1	1	0	0.01	0	0	0	0	0	0	0
1.7	0.7	0	93	93	127	398	0.8	5.9	135	195	4.99	118	0.17	0.34	3.4	0.85	118	0
0.1	0.1	0	12	11	6	141	0.1	0.2	10	292	1.12	19	0.05	0.06	0.5	0.12	7	0
0.1	0	0	8	9	2	129	0	0.1	7	321	0.92	23	0.05	0.05	0.5	0.11	12	0
0.2	0.1	0	21	23	4	323	0.1	0.3	19	805	2.32	57	0.12	0.12	1.2	0.28	29	0
5.6	3	0	4	3	134	6	0	0	0	113	1.48	0	0	0	0	0	0	0.01
4.5	4.4	0	4	3	153	5	0	0	0	113	2.13	0	0	0	0	0	0	0.01
4	5.1	0	9	7	111	13	0	0	1	113	0.74	0	0	0.01	0	0	0	0.03
5.2	3.8	0	4	3	153	5	0	0	0	113	1.85	0	0	0	0	0	0	0.01
3.3	5.8	0	4	3	134	6	0	0	0	113	2.7	0	0	0	0	0	0	0.01
4.4	5	0	4	3	153	5	0	0	0	113	2.41	0	0	0	0	0	0	0.01
1.1	0.8	0	1	1	28	1	0	0	0	24	0.49	0	0	0	0	0	0	0
5.3	3.7	0	4	3	134	6	—	0	0	113	1.82	0	0	0	0	0	0	0.01
5.2	3.6	0	2	2	0	4	0	0	0	113	1.82	0	0	0	0	0	0	0.01
4	5.1	0	9	7	111	13	0	0	1	113	0.74	0	0	0.01	0	0	0	0.03
5.2	3.8	0	4	3	153	5	0	0	0	113	1.85	0	0	0	0	0	0	0.01
2.4	2	0	3	2	136	4	0	0	0	113	1.21	0	0	0	0	0	0	0.01
2.1	2.3	0	3	2	136	4	0	0	0	113	1.56	0	0	0	0	0	0	0.01
2.4	2.4	0	3	2	110	4	0	0	0	144	0.48	0	0	0	0	0	0	0.01
—	—	0	0	—	110	0	—	0	—	122	—	0	—	—	—	—	—	—
2.2	2	0	3	2	136	4	0	0	0	154	0.33	0	0	0	0	0	0	0.01
3	4.6	—	0	—	0	—	—	0	—	52	—	0	—	—	—	—	—	—
0	0	0	3	0	0	2	0	0.1	0	1	0	0	0	0	0	0	0	0
0	0	0	8	1	11	7	0	0	0	1	0	1	0	0	0	0	7	0
0	0	0	5	1	8	5	0	0	0	1	0	1	0	0	0	0	5	0
0	0	0	1	2	13	1	0	0.1	1	0	0	0	0	0	0	0	0	0
0	0	0	0	—	23	0	—	0	—	0	0	0	—	—	—	—	—	—
0	0	0	1	2	11	1	0	0.1	0	0	0	0	0	0	0	0	0	0
0	0	0	0	—	105	5	—	0	—	0	—	0	—	—	—	—	—	—
0.7	1.6	4	0	0	75	2	0	0	0	0	0.96	0	0	0	0	0	0	0
0.7	1.6	4	0	0	78	2	0	0	0	0	1	0	0	0	0	0	0	0
0.6	1.4	3	0	0	15	1	0	0	0	1	0.53	0	0	0	0	0	0	0.01
3.1	5.7	8	2	4	78	5	0	0.1	0	12	1.63	0	0	0	0	0.08	1	0.04
4.5	1.6	234	151	270	730	199	1.6	2.4	24	100	0.85	2	0.49	0.45	3.3	0.15	33	0.67
3.8	5.6	37	124	183	708	266	0.7	1.8	32	21	1.52	0	0.32	0.23	2.6	0.07	30	0.58
6.3	0.8	0	10	70	267	62	0.4	1.7	11	0	0.99	0	0.24	0.16	2	0.03	—	—
4.6	1.3	72	139	291	1045	558	5.3	4.3	43	115	0.85	8	0.42	0.39	7.2	0.3	47	2.05
3.6	1.2	59	131	226	809	537	4.9	4.3	40	74	0.63	8	0.42	0.34	7.2	0.29	44	1.9
8.2	2.8	46	132	157	751	191	1.5	2.1	22	48	0.66	0	0.56	0.27	3.8	0.14	16	0.5
3.8	1.1	42	134	178	768	282	2.6	2.7	27	64	0.46	2	0.33	0.31	3.8	0.15	24	1.2
0.2	0	3	132	101	84	175	—	0.2	—	4	—	1	0	0.02	0.2	—	—	—
0.1	0.7	24	371	354	241	542	—	1	—	46	—	3	0.12	0.51	0.4	0.1	—	—
0.1	0.6	24	366	329	170	542	—	0.3	—	46	—	3	0.12	0.51	0.4	0.11	—	—
0.1	0.6	24	360	327	194	534	—	0.3	—	45	—	3	0.12	0.51	0.3	—	—	—

A

Food Item	Qty	Meas	Wgt (g)	Wtr (g)	Cals	Prot (g)	Carb (g)	Fib (g)	Fat (g)	SatF (g)
McDonald's hashed browns	1	each	53	29	130	1	14	1.4	8	1.4
McDonald's turnover, apple	1	each	85	40	225	2	32	1.2	11	2.6
McDonald's, Big Mac sandwich	1	each	216	115	510	25	46	3.3	26	9.3
McDonald's, Chicken McNuggets	4	piece	73	37	198	12	10	0	12	2.5
McDonald's, Fajita, chicken	1	each	82	42	190	11	20	1	8	2
McDonald's, McChicken sandwich	1	each	189	98	492	17	42	1.7	29	5.5
McDonald's, Quarter-Pounder	1	each	171	89	415	23	36	1.7	20	7.8
McDonald's, Quarter-Pounder, w/cheese	1	each	199	100	520	28	37	1.7	29	12.6
McDonald's, biscuit w/spread	1	each	76	24	260	4	32	1.1	13	3.8
McDonald's, burrito, breakfast	1	each	105	52	290	12	21	1	17	5
McDonald's, chicken salad, chunky	1	each	296	259	164	23	8	3.2	5	1.3
McDonald's, chicken sandwich, McGrilled	1	each	188	126	254	24	33	2	3	0.7
McDonald's, chicken, drumstick, hot & spicy	1	each	63	29	180	14	6	—	12	3
McDonald's, danish pastry, apple	1	each	105	—	360	5	51	1.5	17	5.2
McDonald's, danish pastry, cinnamon raisin	1	each	105	20	435	5	56	1.4	22	7.4
McDonald's, danish pastry, raspberry	1	each	105	24	396	5	58	1.4	16	5.2
McDonald's, french fries, regular order	1	each	97	37	320	4	36	1.7	17	3.5
McDonald's, hamburger	1	each	108	54	266	12	36	1.9	9	3.2
McDonald's, scrambled eggs, serving	1	each	102	75	170	13	1	0	12	3.6
Meatless hot dog, Tofu Pups, Lightlife	1	each	42	3	60	8	28	0	2	1
Meatless patty, Garden Burger	2.5	oz.	71	41	130	8	18	5	3	1
Meatless patty, Garden Burger, Veggie Medley	2.5	oz.	71	41	130	8	18	5	3	1
Meatless patty, Garden Burger, vegan	2.5	oz.	71	36	140	11	23	4	0	0
Melon balls, mixed, frozen	0.5	cup	86	78	28	1	7	0.6	0	0.1
Melon, cantaloupe, cubes	0.5	cup	80	72	28	1	7	0.6	0	0.1
Melon, cantaloupe, cubes	0.5	each	267	240	94	2	22	2.1	1	0.2
Melon, casaba/crenshaw	1	each	1640	1508	426	15	102	13.1	2	0.4
Melon, casaba/crenshaw cubes	0.5	cup	85	78	22	1	5	0.7	0	0
Melon, honeydew, 1/10th melon=piece	1	piece	129	116	45	1	12	0.8	0	0
Melon, honeydew, cubes	0.5	cup	85	76	30	0	8	0.5	0	0
Milk drink, malted, chocolate (Ovaltine)	1	cup	265	215	225	9	29	0.3	9	5.5
Milk drink, malted, chocolate, unfortified	1	cup	265	215	228	9	30	0.3	9	5.5
Milk drink, malted, natural (Ovaltine)	1	cup	265	215	231	10	28	0	9	5.4
Milk, 1% fat, low lactose	1	cup	246	222	103	9	12	0	3	1.6
Milk, 1% fat, low lactose	1	cup	247	222	103	9	12	0	3	1.6
Milk, 1% lowfat	1	cup	244	220	102	8	12	0	3	1.6
Milk, 1% lowfat, protein fortified	1	cup	246	218	119	10	14	0	3	1.8
Milk, 2% lowfat	1	cup	244	218	121	8	12	0	5	2.9
Milk, 2% lowfat, protein+vitamin A fortified	1	cup	246	216	137	10	14	0	5	3
Milk, Goat	1	cup	244	212	168	9	11	0	10	6.5
Milk, chocolate, 1% lowfat	1	cup	250	211	158	8	26	1.2	2	1.5
Milk, chocolate, 2% lowfat	1	cup	250	209	179	8	26	1.2	5	3.1
Milk, chocolate, nonfat	1	cup	250	211	144	9	27	1.5	1	0.7
Milk, chocolate, syrup w/milk	1	cup	263	220	197	8	24	0.3	8	5.2
Milk, chocolate, whole fat	1	cup	250	206	209	8	26	2	8	5.2
Milk, condensed, sweetened, canned	3	Tbs	57	16	184	5	31	0	5	3.2
Milk, dry, nonfat, instant, w/vitamin A added	1	Tbs	4	0	15	1	2	0	0	0
Milk, evaporated, 2% fat	2	Tbs	32	25	29	2	4	0	1	0.4
Milk, evaporated, skim, canned	0.5	cup	128	101	99	10	14	0	0	0.2
Milk, human breast, mature	1	cup	246	215	171	3	17	0	11	4.9
Milk, imitation, (Vitamite)	1	cup	244	220	112	4	13	0	5	1
Milk, imitation, fluid, soy based	1	cup	244	215	150	4	15	0	8	1.9
Milk, malted, natural, powder, unfortified	1	cup	265	5	1097	30	201	1.6	21	11.1
Milk, nonfat skim	1	cup	245	222	86	8	12	0	0	0.3
Milk, nonfat, dry, reconstituted,	1	cup	245	223	82	8	12	0	0	0.1
Milk, nonfat, low lactose	1	cup	245	222	86	9	12	0	0	0.3
Milk, rice, Arroz con leche	1	cup	245	219	100	0	25	0.2	0	0
Milk, skim, protein fortified	1	cup	245	219	100	10	14	0	1	0.4
Milk, strawberry mix w/milk (Nestle's Quik)	1	cup	250	202	220	8	31	0	8	4.8
Milk, whole, 3.3% fat	1	cup	244	215	150	8	11	0	8	5.1
Milk, whole, extra rich, 3.7% fat	1	cup	244	214	157	8	11	0	9	5.6
Milk, whole, fluid, low sodium	1	cup	244	215	149	8	11	0	8	5.2
Milkshake, chocolate	1	cup	226	162	288	8	46	1.8	8	5.2
Milkshake, strawberry	1	cup	226	168	256	8	43	0.9	6	3.9
Milkshake, vanilla	1	cup	226	169	251	8	40	0.9	7	4.2

A

MonoF	PolyF	Choles	Calc	Phos	Sod	Pot	Zn	Iron	Magn	VitA	VitE	VitC	Thia	Ribo	Nia	B6	Fola	B12
(g)	(g)	(mg)	(mg)	(mg)	(mg)	(mg)	(mg)	(mg)	(mg)	(μg RE)	(mg α-TE)	(mg)	(mg)	(mg)	(mg)	(mg)	(μg)	(μg)
2.3	1.9	0	7	51	332	213	0.2	0.3	11	0	0.58	3	0.08	0.02	0.9	0.08	8	0
4.6	2.8	0	6	24	179	67	0.2	1	6	10	1.62	1	0.13	0.09	1	0.03	20	0
7.5	4.1	76	202	267	931	455	4.8	4.3	46	66	1.01	3	0.49	0.44	6.1	0.25	49	2.25
3.7	2.4	42	9	199	353	210	0.7	0.6	17	0	0.96	0	0.08	0.11	5.2	0.21	—	0.21
—	—	35	80	—	310	—	—	0.7	—	20	—	6	—	—	—	—	—	—
8.5	10.2	52	129	223	799	320	1.1	2.5	33	29	6.17	1	0.91	0.24	7.8	0.39	37	0.05
6.7	1.3	70	127	207	692	405	4.7	4.3	34	33	0.36	3	0.39	0.32	6.8	0.24	27	2.58
8.7	1.6	97	143	—	1160	—	—	4.5	—	115	0.81	3	0.39	0.43	6.8	0.26	33	2.89
3.7	0.8	0	68	353	836	105	0.3	1.8	9	2	0.81	0	0.29	0.23	2.2	0.03	5	—
—	—	135	100	—	580	—	—	1.4	—	100	—	6	—	—	—	—	—	—
1.6	1	76	54	277	318	673	1.5	1.6	44	1973	1.28	30	0.51	0.21	8.5	0.52	83	0.28
0.5	1.1	47	117	327	506	433	0.9	2.4	42	46	0.3	5	0.43	0.28	12.1	0.55	38	0.16
—	—	55	—	—	320	—	—	—	—	15	—	6	—	—	—	—	—	—
—	—	42	78	0	291	113	—	1	—	100	—	1	0.3	0.17	2	—	—	—
—	—	51	92	0	280	112	—	1.6	—	100	—	1	0.3	0.26	3	—	—	—
—	—	44	86	0	296	94	—	1	—	101	—	1	0.3	0.17	2	—	—	—
12	1.5	0	14	—	150	—	—	0.7	—	0	—	12	0.23	0	3	—	—	0
2.8	0.9	28	126	113	533	261	2.3	2.7	24	23	0.23	2	0.33	0.26	3.8	0.14	21	1.05
5.3	1.7	424	50	172	143	126	1.1	1.2	10	168	0.92	0	0.07	0.51	0.1	0.12	44	1.11
—	—	0	20	—	140	—	—	1.8	—	0	—	2	—	—	—	—	—	—
1.5	0.5	11	84	132	290	193	0.9	0	30	10	0.2	0	0.11	0.15	1.1	0.08	10	0.11
1.5	0.5	11	84	132	290	193	0.9	0	30	10	0.2	1	0.11	0.15	1.1	0.08	10	0.11
0	0	0	20	—	250	—	—	1.1	—	0	—	0	—	—	—	—	—	—
0	0.1	0	9	10	27	242	0.1	0.3	12	153	0.13	5	0.14	0.02	0.6	0.09	22	0
0	0.1	0	9	14	7	247	0.1	0.2	9	258	0.12	34	0.03	0.02	0.5	0.09	14	0
0	0.3	0	29	45	24	825	0.4	0.6	29	860	0.4	113	0.1	0.06	1.5	0.31	45	0
0	0.6	0	82	115	197	3444	2.6	6.6	131	49	2.46	262	0.98	0.33	6.6	1.97	279	0
0	0	0	4	6	10	179	0.1	0.3	7	3	0.13	14	0.05	0.02	0.3	0.1	14	0
0	0	0	8	13	13	350	0.1	0.1	9	5	0.19	32	0.1	0.02	0.8	0.08	8	0
0	0	0	5	8	8	230	0.1	0.1	6	3	0.13	21	0.06	0.02	0.5	0.05	5	0
2.6	0.4	34	384	313	244	620	1.2	3.8	53	901	0.32	34	0.73	1.26	10.9	1.02	32	0.88
2.6	0.4	34	305	265	172	498	1.1	0.6	48	80	0.26	3	0.13	0.44	0.6	0.14	16	0.93
2.5	0.4	34	371	307	204	572	1.1	3.6	48	742	0.32	29	0.71	1.14	10.4	0.87	22	1.03
0.8	0.1	10	303	237	124	384	1	0.1	34	145	0.1	2	0.1	0.41	0.2	0.11	12	0.9
0.8	0.1	10	550	237	125	385	1	0.1	34	146	0.1	2	0.1	0.41	0.2	0.11	13	0.91
0.7	0.1	10	300	235	123	381	1	0.1	34	144	0.1	2	0.1	0.41	0.2	0.1	12	0.9
0.8	0.1	10	349	273	143	443	1.1	0.1	39	145	0.1	3	0.11	0.47	0.2	0.12	14	1.05
1.4	0.2	18	298	232	122	376	1	0.1	33	139	0.17	2	0.1	0.4	0.2	0.1	12	0.89
1.4	0.2	19	352	276	145	448	1.1	0.1	40	140	0.17	3	0.11	0.48	0.2	0.12	15	1.05
2.7	0.4	28	327	271	122	498	0.7	0.1	34	137	0.22	3	0.12	0.34	0.7	0.11	1	0.16
0.8	0.1	7	288	258	152	425	1	0.6	33	148	0.06	2	0.1	0.42	0.3	0.1	12	0.86
1.5	0.2	17	285	255	151	423	1	0.6	33	143	0.13	2	0.09	0.41	0.3	0.1	12	0.85
0.4	0	4	292	265	121	486	1.2	0.7	46	142	0.11	2	0.09	0.34	0.3	0.1	14	0.88
2.4	0.3	34	292	229	147	460	0.9	2.7	32	321	0.21	2	0.1	0.55	6.5	0.1	12	0.87
2.5	0.3	30	280	253	149	418	1	0.6	32	72	0.23	2	0.09	0.4	0.3	0.1	12	0.84
1.4	0.2	20	163	145	73	213	0.5	0.1	15	46	0.12	1	0.05	0.24	0.1	0.03	6	0.26
0	0	1	52	42	23	72	0.2	0	5	30	0	0	0.02	0.07	0	0.02	2	0.17
0.2	0	3	90	60	36	103	0.3	0.1	8	41	0.02	0	0.01	0.1	0.1	0.02	3	0.07
0.1	0	5	370	249	147	423	1.2	0.4	34	149	0.01	2	0.06	0.39	0.2	0.07	11	0.3
4.1	1.2	34	79	34	42	126	0.4	0.1	8	157	2.21	12	0.03	0.09	0.4	0.03	13	0.11
2.7	0.9	0	200	244	134	366	0.2	0.2	2	149	0	0	0	0	0.2	0	0	0
4.9	1.2	0	79	181	191	278	2.9	1	16	0	2.56	0	0.03	0.22	0	0	0	0
5.4	3.2	53	790	949	1306	2008	2.6	1.9	246	233	1.06	8	1.34	2.44	13.9	1.09	122	2.07
0.1	0	4	301	247	126	407	1	0.1	28	149	0.1	2	0.09	0.34	0.2	0.1	13	0.93
0.1	0	4	284	224	131	388	1.1	0.1	29	162	0	1	0.09	0.4	0.2	0.08	11	0.91
0.1	0	4	302	247	126	406	1	0.1	28	149	0.1	2	0.09	0.34	0.2	0.1	13	0.93
0	0	0	12	5	7	6	0.1	0.3	4	0	0	0	0.02	0.01	0.1	0.01	0	0
0.2	0	5	350	274	144	446	1.1	0.1	39	149	0.1	3	0.11	0.48	0.2	0.12	15	1.05
2.2	0.3	30	275	215	120	348	0.9	0.2	30	70	0.25	2	0.09	0.4	0.2	0.1	12	0.82
2.4	0.3	33	290	228	120	371	0.9	0.1	33	76	0.24	2	0.09	0.4	0.2	0.1	12	0.87
2.6	0.3	35	290	227	119	368	0.9	0.1	33	83	0.24	4	0.09	0.39	0.2	0.1	12	0.87
2.4	0.3	33	246	209	6	617	0.9	0.1	12	78	0.24	2	0.05	0.26	0.1	0.08	12	0.88
2.4	0.3	29	256	231	220	453	0.9	0.7	38	52	0.15	1	0.13	0.56	0.4	0.11	8	0.77
1.8	0.3	25	256	226	188	412	0.8	0.2	29	66	0.29	2	0.1	0.44	0.4	0.1	7	0.7
2	0.3	25	276	231	186	394	0.8	0.2	27	72	0.13	2	0.1	0.41	0.4	0.12	7	0.82

Food Item	Qty	Meas	Wgt (g)	Wtr (g)	Cals	Prot (g)	Carb (g)	Fib (g)	Fat (g)	SatF (g)
Millet, cooked	0.5	cup	120	86	143	4	28	1.6	1	0.2
Miso (soybean)	1	Tbs	17	7	36	2	5	0.9	1	0.2
Miso sauce	0.25	cup	62	36	96	3	18	1.5	2	0.2
Mixed fruit canned in heavy syrup	0.5	cup	128	103	92	0	24	1.3	0	0
Mixed fruit, dried	0.5	cup	68	21	165	2	44	5.3	0	0
Mixed fruit, frozen-sweetened-thawed	0.5	cup	125	92	123	2	30	2.4	0	0
Mixed nuts, no peanuts, oil roasted, salted	0.25	cup	36	1	221	6	8	2	20	3.3
Mixed nuts, no peanuts, oil roasted, unsalted	0.25	cup	36	1	221	6	8	2	20	3.3
Mixed nuts, w/peanuts, dry roasted, salted	0.25	cup	34	1	203	6	9	3.1	18	2.4
Mixed nuts, w/peanuts, dry roasted, unsalted	0.25	cup	34	1	203	6	9	3.1	18	2.4
Mixed nuts, w/peanuts, oil roasted, salted	0.25	cup	36	1	219	6	8	3.2	20	3.1
Mixed nuts, w/peanuts, oil roasted, unsalted	0.5	cup	71	1	438	12	15	7	40	6.2
Mixed vegetables, Chinese, LaChoy	4	oz.	113	108	14	1	3	1.7	0	0
Mixed vegetables, canned, drained	0.5	cup	82	71	38	2	8	2.4	0	0
Mixed vegetables, canned, low sodium	0.5	cup	91	82	33	1	6	2.8	0	0
Mixed vegetables, canned, w/liquid	0.5	cup	122	110	44	2	9	4.7	0	0.1
Mixed vegetables, dried-Salad Crunchies	1	Tbs	6	0	22	1	3	0.8	1	0.1
Mixed vegetables, frozen	4	oz.	113	93	73	4	15	4.5	1	0.1
Mixed vegetables, frozen, cooked	0.5	cup	91	76	54	3	12	4	0	0
Mocha mix, vanilla	1	Tbs	8	5	17	0	2	—	1	0.2
Mock chicken leg, cooked	4	oz.	113	66	262	23	6	0.2	16	4.9
Molasses, blackstrap cane	1	Tbs	20	6	48	0	12	0	0	0
Molasses, light cane	1	Tbs	20	5	54	0	14	0	0	0
Moo goo gai pan	0.5	cup	108	84	140	8	6	1.4	10	2.4
Mothbean, cooked, no salt	0.5	cup	88	61	103	7	18	3.3	0	0.1
Moussaka, lamb & eggplant	1	cup	250	205	237	16	13	3.6	13	4.6
Mousse, chocolate, recipe	0.5	cup	202	125	446	9	33	1.2	33	18.5
Muffin, blueberry, Weight Watchers	1	each	71	14	250	4	46	4	5	1
Muffin, blueberry, commercial	1	each	57	22	158	3	27	1.5	4	0.8
Muffin, blueberry, mix, prepared	1	each	45	16	135	2	22	0.5	4	0.7
Muffin, blueberry, recipe, w/2% milk	1	each	57	22	162	4	23	1.1	6	1.2
Muffin, blueberry, recipe, w/whole milk	1	each	45	18	131	3	18	0.8	5	1.1
Muffin, buckwheat	1	each	47	16	144	4	20	1.4	6	1.7
Muffin, carrot w/raisins & nuts	1	each	58	20	177	4	26	1	7	1.1
Muffin, cheese	1	each	58	21	184	5	23	0.7	8	3
Muffin, chocolate chip	1	each	58	18	190	4	27	1	8	2.8
Muffin, cornmeal, commercial	1	each	57	19	174	3	29	1.9	5	0.8
Muffin, cornmeal, mix, prepared	1	each	45	14	144	3	22	1.1	5	1.3
Muffin, cornmeal, recipe w/2% milk	1	each	57	19	180	4	25	1.9	7	1.3
Muffin, cornmeal, recipe, w/whole milk	1	each	45	15	144	3	20	1.5	6	1.2
Muffin, cranberry nut	1	each	58	22	164	4	25	0.8	5	1.5
Muffin, egg-bacon-cheese, Great Starts	1	each	116	59	290	14	25	2	15	6
Muffin, oat bran	1	each	57	20	154	4	28	2.6	4	0.6
Muffin, oatmeal	1	each	47	22	112	3	17	0.7	3	1
Muffin, plain, recipe, w/2% milk	1	each	57	22	169	4	24	1.5	6	1.2
Muffin, plain, recipe, w/whole milk	1	each	45	17	135	3	19	1.2	5	1.2
Muffin, pumpkin, w/raisins	1	each	58	16	181	3	34	1.1	4	0.8
Muffin, toaster type, blueberry	1	each	33	10	103	2	18	0.6	3	0.5
Muffin, toaster type, blueberry, toasted	1	each	31	8	103	2	18	0.6	3	0.5
Muffin, toaster type, corn	1	each	33	8	114	2	19	0.5	4	0.6
Muffin, toaster type, cornmeal, toasted	1	each	31	6	114	2	19	0.5	4	0.6
Muffin, toaster type, wheat bran-raisin	1	each	36	11	106	2	19	2.8	3	0.5
Muffin, toaster type, wheat bran-raisin, toasted	1	each	34	9	106	2	19	2.8	3	0.5
Muffin, wheat bran, mix, prepared	1	each	45	16	124	3	21	1.9	4	1.1
Muffin, wheat bran, recipe, w/2% milk	1	each	57	20	161	4	24	2.2	7	1.3
Muffin, wheat bran, recipe, w/whole milk	1	each	45	16	130	3	19	3.2	6	1.2
Muffin, whole wheat	1	each	47	16	142	4	20	2.5	6	1.7
Muffin, zucchini	1	each	58	17	210	3	26	0.8	10	1.7
Mulberries, raw	0.5	cup	70	61	30	1	7	1.2	0	0
Mushroom pieces, cooked, drained	0.5	cup	78	71	21	2	4	1.7	0	0
Mushroom pieces, raw	0.5	cup	35	32	9	1	2	0.4	0	0
Mushroom pieces, steamed	0.5	cup	78	72	20	2	4	0.9	0	0
Mushroom pieces, stir fried, no oil	0.5	cup	78	72	20	2	4	0.9	0	0
Mushroom, batter-dipped, fried	5	each	70	46	148	2	8	0.7	12	2.1
Mushroom, chanterelle, dried	0.5	cup	72	9	246	13	38	14.2	5	0.5

A

MonoF (g)	PolyF (g)	Choles (mg)	Calc (mg)	Phos (mg)	Sod (mg)	Pot (mg)	Zn (mg)	Iron (mg)	Magn (mg)	VitA (μg RE)	VitE (mg α-TE)	VitC (mg)	Thia (mg)	Ribo (mg)	Nia (mg)	B6 (mg)	Fola (μg)	B12 (μg)
0.2	0.6	0	4	120	2	74	1.1	0.8	53	0	0.22	0	0.13	0.1	1.6	0.13	23	0
0.2	0.6	0	11	26	629	28	0.6	0.5	7	2	0	0	0.02	0.04	0.1	0.04	6	0
0.4	0.9	0	19	43	1003	52	0.9	0.8	13	2	0	0	0.03	0.07	0.2	0.06	9	0
0	0.1	0	1	13	5	107	0.1	0.5	6	24	0.51	88	0.02	0.05	0.8	0.05	4	0
0.2	0.1	0	26	52	12	541	0.3	1.8	26	166	0.43	3	0.03	0.11	1.3	0.11	3	0
0	0.1	0	9	15	4	164	0.1	0.4	8	40	0.75	94	0.02	0.04	0.5	0.03	10	0
11.9	4.1	0	38	162	252	196	1.7	0.9	90	1	2.16	0	0.18	0.18	0.7	0.06	20	0
11.9	4.1	0	38	162	4	196	1.7	0.9	90	1	2.16	0	0.18	0.18	0.7	0.06	20	0
10.8	3.7	0	24	149	229	204	1.3	1.3	77	0	2.06	0	0.07	0.07	1.6	0.1	17	0
10.8	3.7	0	24	149	4	204	1.3	1.3	77	0	2.06	0	0.07	0.07	1.6	0.1	17	0
11.3	4.7	0	38	165	231	206	1.8	1.1	83	1	2.13	0	0.18	0.08	1.8	0.08	30	0
22.5	9.4	0	77	329	8	413	3.6	2.3	167	1	4.26	0	0.35	0.16	3.6	0.17	59	0
—	—	0	14	—	59	—	—	0.2	—	1	—	8	—	—	—	—	—	0
0	0.1	0	22	34	121	237	0.3	0.9	13	949	0.49	4	0.04	0.04	0.5	0.06	19	0
0	0.1	0	19	34	24	126	0.5	0.6	14	462	0.19	3	0.03	0.04	0.4	0.07	16	0
0	0.1	0	26	45	274	169	0.6	0.8	18	622	0.55	5	0.04	0.05	0.6	0.09	22	0
0.1	0.4	0	17	23	28	106	0.2	0.8	10	194	0.47	13	0.05	0.03	0.4	0.06	13	0.01
0	0.3	0	28	67	53	240	0.5	1.1	27	576	0.34	12	0.14	0.1	1.4	0.11	33	0
0	0.1	0	23	46	32	154	0.4	0.7	20	389	0.33	3	0.06	0.11	0.8	0.07	17	0
0.3	0.4	0	3	5	10	12	—	0.1	0	0	—	0	0	0	0	—	—	—
6.5	2.6	98	24	211	648	320	3.8	1.3	24	4	0.78	0	0.31	0.34	5.6	0.31	11	1.25
0	0	0	176	8	11	511	0.2	3.6	44	0	0	0	0.01	0.01	0.2	0.14	0	0
0	0	0	42	6	8	300	0.1	1	50	0	0	0	0.01	0	0.2	0.14	0	0
3.2	3.7	19	65	98	163	238	0.8	0.8	16	101	1.03	17	0.07	0.16	2.2	0.16	22	0.18
0	0.2	0	3	132	9	268	0.5	2.8	92	1	0.09	1	0.11	0.02	0.6	0.08	126	0
5.4	1.9	97	68	179	432	557	2.6	1.8	40	105	0.81	6	0.15	0.31	4.1	0.23	45	1.41
10.3	1.7	299	202	259	87	297	1.4	1.3	44	323	0.98	1	0.08	0.41	0.3	0.13	32	0.93
3	1	45	480	—	384	92	—	0.1	—	540	—	0	—	—	—	—	—	—
1.1	1.4	17	32	112	255	70	0.3	0.9	9	5	0.6	1	0.08	0.07	0.6	0.01	26	0.33
1.6	1.4	21	11	85	197	35	0.2	0.5	5	10	0.63	0	0.07	0.14	1	0.03	5	0.04
1.5	3.1	21	108	83	251	70	0.3	1.3	9	22	0.97	1	0.16	0.16	1.3	0.02	27	0.08
1.2	2.4	18	85	65	198	55	0.2	1	7	13	0.81	1	0.12	0.13	1	0.02	5	0.06
2.4	1.3	21	88	85	284	106	0.5	1	31	14	0.6	0	0.1	0.12	1.1	0.07	8	0.07
1.6	3.6	18	82	69	251	112	0.3	1.2	10	263	0.61	1	0.15	0.15	1.2	0.04	7	0.08
3	1.4	30	111	115	274	80	0.5	1.3	11	35	0.6	0	0.16	0.2	1.3	0.03	8	0.11
3	1.4	24	74	75	186	92	0.4	1.4	16	17	0.65	0	0.17	0.18	1.4	0.03	7	0.09
1.2	1.8	15	42	162	297	39	0.3	1.6	18	20	1.05	0	0.16	0.19	1.2	0.05	35	0.05
2.4	0.6	28	34	173	358	59	0.3	0.9	9	20	0.68	0	0.11	0.12	0.9	0.05	5	0.07
1.7	3.5	24	148	101	333	83	0.3	1.5	13	29	1.03	0	0.17	0.18	1.4	0.05	35	0.09
1.4	2.8	20	116	79	263	65	0.3	1.2	10	18	0.86	0	0.14	0.14	1.1	0.04	8	0.07
2	1.1	39	81	72	326	71	0.3	1.2	9	23	0.61	0	0.16	0.18	1.3	0.03	8	0.11
—	—	95	150	—	750	—	—	1.8	—	0	—	0	—	—	—	—	—	—
1	2.4	0	36	214	224	289	1	2.4	90	0	0.75	0	0.15	0.05	0.2	0.09	30	0.01
1.2	0.7	18	69	62	161	58	0.3	0.9	10	13	0.32	0	0.13	0.13	0.9	0.02	6	0.07
1.6	3.3	22	114	87	266	69	0.3	1.4	10	23	1.03	0	0.16	0.17	1.3	0.02	29	0.09
1.3	2.6	19	90	68	210	54	0.3	1.1	7	13	0.81	0	0.13	0.14	1	0.02	5	0.07
1	2.1	26	31	40	154	87	0.2	1.1	9	331	0.59	1	0.1	0.11	0.8	0.03	6	0.05
0.7	1.8	2	4	20	158	27	0.1	0.2	4	22	0.57	0	0.08	0.1	0.7	0.01	18	0.01
0.7	1.7	2	4	60	158	27	0.1	0.2	5	20	0.24	0	0.06	0.09	0.6	0.01	15	0
0.9	2.1	4	6	50	142	30	0.1	0.5	5	7	0.53	0	0.1	0.12	0.8	0.02	19	0.01
0.9	1.9	2	6	80	142	30	0.1	0.5	4	6	0.5	0	0.08	0.11	0.7	0.01	3	0.01
0.7	1.7	6	13	71	178	60	0.2	1	11	18	0.62	0	0.09	0.11	0.9	0.04	12	0.01
0.8	1.7	3	13	97	179	60	0.2	1	7	16	0.42	0	0.07	0.1	0.8	0.02	7	0.01
2.1	0.6	31	14	150	210	66	0.5	1.1	26	14	0.68	0	0.09	0.11	1.3	0.08	7	0.06
1.7	3.6	19	107	162	335	181	1.6	2.4	44	143	1.31	4	0.19	0.25	2.3	0.18	30	0.08
1.4	2.8	16	84	128	265	143	1.2	1.9	35	108	1.04	4	0.15	0.2	1.8	0.14	23	0.06
2.3	1.4	21	89	110	283	119	0.7	0.9	31	14	0.7	0	0.08	0.09	1.2	0.07	9	0.07
2.6	5.7	37	41	44	169	69	0.3	1.2	8	22	0.84	1	0.12	0.12	0.9	0.03	9	0.07
0	0.1	0	27	27	7	136	0.1	1.3	13	2	0.32	26	0.02	0.07	0.4	0.04	4	0
0	0.1	0	5	68	2	278	0.7	1.4	9	0	0.09	3	0.06	0.23	3.5	0.07	14	0
0	0.1	0	2	36	1	130	0.3	0.4	4	0	0.04	1	0.04	0.16	1.4	0.03	7	0
0	0.1	0	4	81	3	289	0.6	1	8	0	0.09	2	0.07	0.34	3.1	0.07	14	0
0	0.1	0	4	81	3	289	0.6	1	8	0	0.09	2	0.07	0.33	3.1	0.07	13	0
3	6.4	14	54	103	121	180	0.4	0.8	8	10	0.92	1	0.07	0.22	1.6	0.05	8	0.06
2.3	2	1	34	—	23	—	—	8.2	—	2	—	1	—	—	—	—	—	0

Food Item	Qty	Meas	Wgt (g)	Wtr (g)	Cals	Prot (g)	Carb (g)	Fib (g)	Fat (g)	SatF (g)
Mushroom, enoki, raw	1	each	3	3	1	0	0	0.1	0	0
Mushroom, oyster, dried	0.5	cup	72	5	262	20	39	7.5	3	0.3
Mushroom, patty straw, dried	0.5	cup	72	9	228	17	35	5.2	2	0.4
Mushroom, raw, sliced	0.5	cup	34	31	8	1	2	0.4	0	0
Mushroom, shiitake, cooked pieces	0.5	cup	72	60	40	1	10	1.5	0	0
Mushroom, shiitake, cooked, whole	4	each	72	60	40	1	10	1.5	0	0
Mushroom, shiitake, dried	4	each	15	1	44	1	11	1.7	0	0
Mushroom, shiitake, dried	0.5	cup	72	9	241	19	37	9.1	2	0.3
Mushroom, whole, pickled	1	each	12	11	3	0	1	0.1	0	0
Mushrooms, canned, drained	0.5	cup	78	71	19	1	4	1.9	0	0
Mushrooms, canned, drained	10	each	120	109	29	2	6	2.9	0	0
Mushrooms, whole, cooked, drained	10	each	120	109	32	3	6	2.6	1	0.1
Mushrooms, whole, raw	5	each	90	83	22	2	4	1.1	0	0
Mustard greens, cooked, drained, no added salt	0.5	cup	70	66	10	2	1	1.4	0	0
Mustard greens, frozen, cooked, drained	0.5	cup	75	70	14	2	2	2.1	0	0
Mustard greens, raw	0.5	cup	28	25	7	1	1	0.9	0	0
Mustard seed, yellow	1	tsp	4	0	18	1	1	0.5	1	0.1
Mustard, Chinese Gai Choy	1	tsp	5	5	1	0	0	—	0	—
Mustard, brown, prepared	1	tsp	5	4	5	0	0	0.1	0	0
Mustard, yellow, prepared	1	tsp	5	4	4	0	0	0.1	0	0
Nacho chips, w/cinnamon & sugar	7	piece	109	1	592	7	63	3.3	36	18.2
Nachos, w/cheese	7	piece	113	46	346	9	36	—	19	7.8
Nectarine, fresh	1	each	136	117	67	1	16	2.2	1	0.1
Noodle roni, prepared	0.5	cup	82	55	123	4	20	1.8	3	0.6
Noodles, Japanese soba, buckwheat, cooked	0.5	cup	57	42	56	3	12	0.6	0	0
Noodles, Japanese somen, wheat, cooked	0.5	cup	88	60	115	4	24	1.4	0	0
Noodles, Ramen, cooked	5	cup	114	93	78	3	15	1.4	1	0.2
Noodles, buckwheat, dry, cooked	0.5	cup	70	50	81	2	17	0.1	0	—
Noodles, chow mein, dry	0.25	cup	11	0	59	1	6	0.4	3	0.5
Noodles, egg, enriched, cooked	0.5	cup	80	55	106	4	20	0.9	1	0.2
Noodles, mug-o-lunch, prepared	1	each	198	132	295	9	48	4.2	7	1.5
Noodles, rice, cooked	0.5	cup	80	65	62	0	15	0.1	0	0
Noodles, rice, freshly made	0.5	cup	70	36	142	2	32	0.4	0	—
Nutmeg, ground	0.25	tsp	1	0	3	0	0	0.1	0	0.2
Oat bran, cooked	1	Tbs	14	12	5	0	2	0.4	0	0
Oat bran, dry	2	Tbs	12	1	29	2	8	1.8	1	0.2
Oats, rolled, baked value	1	cup	80	7	307	13	54	8.5	5	0.9
Oats, rolled, dry	0.25	cup	20	2	78	3	14	2.2	1	0.2
Oats, whole grain	0.5	cup	78	6	303	13	52	8.3	5	1
Oil, almond	1	Tbs	14	0	120	0	0	0	14	1.1
Oil, apricot kernel	1	Tbs	14	0	120	0	0	0	14	0.9
Oil, butter	1	Tbs	13	0	112	0	0	0	13	7.9
Oil, canola	1	Tbs	14	0	120	0	0	0	14	1
Oil, cocoa butter	1	Tbs	14	0	120	0	0	0	14	8.1
Oil, coconut	1	Tbs	14	0	117	0	0	0	14	11.8
Oil, cod liver	1	Tbs	14	0	123	0	0	0	14	3.1
Oil, corn	1	Tbs	14	0	120	0	0	0	14	1.7
Oil, cottonseed	1	Tbs	14	0	120	0	0	0	14	3.5
Oil, grapeseed	1	Tbs	14	0	120	0	0	0	14	1.3
Oil, herring	1	Tbs	14	0	123	0	0	0	14	2.9
Oil, menhaden, not fully hydrogenated	1	Tbs	14	0	123	0	0	0	14	4.1
Oil, olive	1	Tbs	14	0	119	0	0	0	14	1.8
Oil, palm	1	Tbs	14	0	120	0	0	0	14	6.7
Oil, palm kernel	1	Tbs	14	0	117	0	0	0	14	11.1
Oil, peanut	1	Tbs	14	0	119	0	0	0	14	2.3
Oil, safflower	1	Tbs	14	0	120	0	0	0	14	1.2
Oil, salmon	1	Tbs	14	0	123	0	0	0	14	2.7
Oil, sardine	1	Tbs	14	0	123	0	0	0	14	4.1
Oil, sesame	1	Tbs	14	0	120	0	0	0	14	1.9
Oil, soybean & cottonseed	1	Tbs	14	0	120	0	0	0	14	2.4
Oil, soybean (Crisco/Wesson)	1	Tbs	14	0	120	0	0	0	14	2
Oil, sunflower (Wesson Sunlite)	1	Tbs	14	0	120	0	0	0	14	1.4
Oil, walnut	1	Tbs	14	0	120	0	0	0	14	1.2
Oil, wheat germ	1	Tbs	14	0	120	0	0	0	14	2.6
Okra pods, frozen, cooked, drained	0.5	cup	92	84	26	2	5	2.6	0	0.1

MonoF (g)	PolyF (g)	Choles (mg)	Calc (mg)	Phos (mg)	Sod (mg)	Pot (mg)	Zn (mg)	Iron (mg)	Magn (mg)	VitA (μg RE)	VitE (mg α-TE)	VitC (mg)	Thia (mg)	Ribo (mg)	Nia (mg)	B6 (mg)	Fola (μg)	B12 (μg)
0	0	0	0	3	0	11	0	0	0	0	0	0	0	0	0.1	0	1	0
0.7	1.9	1	7	—	70	—	—	6.8	—	1	—	5	—	—	—	—	—	0
0.1	1.6	1	29	—	65	—	—	45.9	—	1	—	1	—	—	—	—	—	0
0	0.1	0	2	35	1	126	0.2	0.4	3	0	0.04	1	0.04	0.15	1.4	0.03	7	0
0	0	0	2	21	3	85	1	0.3	10	0	0.09	0	0.03	0.12	1.1	0.12	15	0
0	0	0	2	21	3	84	1	0.3	10	0	0.09	0	0.03	0.12	1.1	0.11	15	0
0	0	0	2	44	2	230	1.2	0.3	20	0	0.02	1	0.04	0.19	2.1	0.14	24	0
0.1	1.5	1	28	—	61	—	—	11.5	—	1	—	1	—	—	—	—	—	0
0	0	0	1	10	24	36	0.1	0.1	1	0	0.01	0	0.01	0.04	0.4	0.01	1	0
0	0.1	0	9	52	332	101	0.6	0.6	12	0	0.09	0	0.07	0.02	1.2	0.05	10	0
0	0.1	0	13	79	510	155	0.9	0.9	18	0	0.14	0	0.1	0.02	1.9	0.07	15	0
0	0.2	0	7	104	2	427	1	2.1	14	0	0.14	5	0.09	0.36	5.4	0.11	22	0
0	0.2	0	4	94	4	333	0.7	1.1	9	0	0.11	3	0.09	0.4	3.7	0.09	19	0
0.1	0	0	52	29	11	141	0.1	0.5	10	212	1.41	18	0.03	0.04	0.3	0.07	51	0
0.1	0	0	76	18	19	104	0.2	0.8	10	335	1.31	10	0.03	0.04	0.2	0.08	52	0
0	0	0	29	12	7	99	0.1	0.4	9	148	0.56	20	0.02	0.03	0.2	0.05	52	0
0.7	0.2	0	19	31	0	25	0.2	0.4	11	0	0.09	0	0.02	0.01	0.3	0.01	3	0
—	—	—	—	—	—	—	—	—	—	—	—	—	—	—	—	—	—	0
0	0.2	0	6	7	65	6	—	0.1	—	0	—	0	0	0	0	—	—	—
0.2	0	0	4	4	65	7	0	0.1	2	0	0.09	0	0	0	0	0	0	0
11.9	4.1	39	85	33	439	78	0.6	2.9	20	11	—	8	0.18	0.45	3.9	0.17	8	1.72
8	2.2	18	272	276	816	172	1.8	1.3	55	92	—	1	0.19	0.37	1.5	0.2	10	0.82
0.2	0.3	0	7	22	0	288	0.1	0.2	11	101	1.21	7	0.02	0.06	1.4	0.03	5	0
1.2	0.9	26	10	56	163	23	0.5	1.3	15	30	0.34	0	0.15	0.07	1.2	0.03	6	0.07
0	0	0	2	14	34	20	0.1	0.3	5	0	—	0	0.05	0.02	0.3	0.02	4	0
0	0.1	0	7	24	142	26	0.2	0.5	2	0	0.01	0	0.02	0.03	0.1	0.01	2	0
0.2	0.2	19	10	41	675	25	0.4	0.9	12	102	0.04	0	0.11	0.05	0.9	0.03	5	0.05
—	—	—	7	56	—	—	—	0.7	—	—	—	0	0.04	0.02	0.3	—	—	—
0.9	2	0	2	18	49	14	0.2	0.5	6	1	0.02	0	0.06	0.05	0.7	0.01	10	0
0.3	0.3	26	10	55	6	22	0.5	1.3	15	5	0.04	0	0.15	0.07	1.2	0.03	51	0.07
2.8	2.2	63	25	133	391	56	1.2	3	37	72	0.82	0	0.36	0.16	2.8	0.07	14	0.18
0	0	0	5	5	3	1	0.1	0.3	1	0	0.02	0	0.02	0	0	0.01	0	0
—	—	—	7	26	—	—	—	1.7	—	—	—	0	0.03	0.01	0.9	—	—	—
0	0	0	1	1	0	2	0	0	1	0	0.02	0	0	0	0	0	0	0
0	0	0	1	16	0	13	0.1	0.1	5	0	0.03	0	0.02	0	0	0	1	0
0.3	0.3	0	7	86	0	66	0.4	0.6	28	0	0.2	0	0.14	0.03	0.1	0.02	6	0
1.6	1.8	0	42	379	3	280	2.5	3.4	118	8	0.91	0	0.47	0.1	0.6	0.09	18	0
0.4	0.5	0	10	96	1	71	0.6	0.9	30	2	0.14	0	0.15	0.03	0.2	0.02	6	0
1.7	2	0	42	408	2	335	3.1	3.7	138	0	0.55	0	0.6	0.11	0.8	0.09	44	0
9.5	2.4	0	0	0	0	0	0	0	0	0	5.36	0	0	0	0	0	0	0
8.2	4	0	0	0	0	0	0	0	0	0	1.18	0	0	0	0	0	0	0
3.7	0.5	33	0	0	0	1	0	0	0	118	0.36	0	0	0	0	0	0	0
8	4	0	0	0	0	0	0	0	0	0	2.86	0	0	0	0	0	0	0
4.5	0.4	0	0	0	0	0	0	0	0	0	0.24	0	0	0	0	0	0	0
0.8	0.2	0	0	0	0	0	0	0	0	0	0.04	0	0	0	0	0	0	0
6.4	3.1	78	0	0	0	0	0	0	0	4080	2.99	0	0	0	0	0	0	0
3.3	8	0	0	0	0	0	0	0	0	0	2.88	0	0	0	0	0	0	0
2.4	7.1	0	0	0	0	0	0	0	0	0	5.22	0	0	0	0	0	0	0
2.2	9.5	0	0	0	0	0	0	0	0	0	4.36	0	0	0	0	0	0	0
7.7	2.1	104	0	0	0	0	0	0	0	0	1.25	0	0	0	0	0	0	0
3.6	4.6	71	0	0	0	0	0	0	0	0	1.77	0	0	0	0	0	0	0
10	1.1	0	0	0	0	0	0	0.1	0	0	1.67	0	0	0	0	0	0	0
5	1.3	0	0	0	0	0	0	0	0	0	2.97	0	0	0	0	0	0	0
1.6	0.2	0	0	0	0	0	0	0	0	0	0.52	0	0	0	0	0	0	0
6.2	4.3	0	0	0	0	0	0	0	0	0	1.74	0	0	0	0	0	0	0
1.6	10.2	0	0	0	0	0	0	0	0	0	5.87	0	0	0	0	0	0	0
3.9	5.5	66	0	0	0	0	0	0	0	0	2.6	0	0	0	0	0	0	0
4.6	4.3	97	0	0	0	0	0	0	0	0	1.63	0	0	0	0	0	0	0
5.4	5.7	0	0	0	0	0	0	0	0	0	0.56	0	0	0	0	0	0	0
4	6.6	0	0	0	0	0	0	0	0	0	3.84	0	0	0	0	0	0	0
3.2	7.9	0	0	0	0	0	0	0	0	0	2.48	0	0	0	0	0	0	0
2.7	9	0	0	0	0	0	0	0	0	0	6.9	0	0	0	0	0	0	0
3.1	8.6	0	0	0	0	0	0	0	0	0	0.44	0	0	0	0	0	0	0
2	8.4	0	0	0	0	0	0	0	0	0	26.1	0	0	0	0	0	0	0
0	0.1	0	88	42	3	215	0.6	0.6	47	47	0.64	11	0.09	0.11	0.7	0.04	134	0

Food Item	Qty	Meas	Wgt (g)	Wtr (g)	Cals	Prot (g)	Carb (g)	Fib (g)	Fat (g)	SatF (g)
Okra, Chinese/luffa, cooked	0.5	cup	89	80	28	2	6	2.8	0	0
Okra, batter-dipped, fried	0.5	cup	46	32	88	1	6	1	7	1.1
Okra, fresh pods, cooked, drained	8	each	85	76	27	2	6	2.1	0	0
Okra, fresh slices, cooked, drained	0.5	cup	80	72	26	2	6	2	0	0
Olive, green, no pits	10	each	39	30	45	1	1	0.4	5	0.5
Olive, green, stuffed	5	each	20	16	21	0	0	0.2	2	0.2
Olive, ripe, jumbo/super colossal	1	each	15	13	12	0	1	0.4	1	0.1
Olive, ripe, large, no pits	10	each	45	36	52	0	3	1.4	5	0.6
Olive, ripe, large, no pits, slices	0.5	cup	68	54	78	1	4	2.2	7	1
Olives, Calamata	1	oz.	28	16	80	0	3	0.2	7	0.9
Onion flakes, dehydrated	0.25	cup	14	1	49	1	12	1.3	0	0
Onion powder	0.25	tsp	1	0	2	0	0	0	0	0
Onion rings, breaded, fried, serving	8.5	piece	83	31	276	4	31	—	16	7
Onion rings, breaded, fried, svg	1	each	83	31	276	4	31	—	16	7
Onion rings, heated from frozen	2	each	20	6	81	1	8	0.3	5	1.7
Onion slices, cooked	2	piece	24	21	11	0	2	0.3	0	0
Onion slices, raw	1	piece	14	13	5	0	1	0.3	0	0
Onion, canned w/liquid	1	each	63	59	12	1	3	0.8	0	0
Onion, chopped, frozen, cooked	0.5	cup	105	97	29	1	7	1.9	0	0
Onion, chopped, steamed	0.5	cup	105	94	40	1	9	1.9	0	0
Onion, chopped, stir fried	0.5	cup	105	94	40	1	9	1.9	0	0
Onion, creamed	0.5	cup	114	94	100	3	11	1.3	5	1.7
Onion, medium size, cooked	1	each	94	83	41	1	10	1.3	0	0
Onion, pearl, cooked, whole	3	each	45	39	20	1	5	0.7	0	0
Onion, raw, chopped	0.5	cup	80	72	30	1	7	1.4	0	0
Onion, raw, red, chopped	0.5	cup	80	72	30	1	7	1.4	0	0
Onion, raw, whole, medium size	1	each	110	99	42	1	9	2	0	0
Onion, red, raw	0.5	cup	80	72	30	1	7	1.4	0	0
Onion, red, slices	2	piece	28	25	11	0	2	0.5	0	0
Onion, red, whole	1	each	110	99	42	1	9	2	0	0
Onion, spring/green, chopped	0.5	cup	50	45	16	1	4	1.3	0	0
Onion, spring/green, top only	0.5	cup	50	46	17	1	3	1.2	0	0.1
Onion, spring/green, white part	0.5	cup	50	46	25	0	5	1.2	0	0
Onion, welsh, raw	0.5	cup	80	72	27	2	5	1.1	0	0.1
Onion, whole, frozen, cooked	1	each	63	58	18	0	4	0.9	0	0
Onions, cooked, drained	0.5	cup	105	92	46	1	11	1.5	0	0
Orange & apricot juice drink, canned	1	cup	250	217	128	1	32	0.2	0	0
Orange Julius	1	cup	215	183	133	0	33	0.2	0	0.1
Orange breakfast drink, frozen, prepared	1	cup	248	216	122	0	30	0.2	0	0.1
Orange breakfast drink, powder	1	Tbs	12	0	44	0	11	0	0	0
Orange breakfast drink, prepared w/water	1	cup	248	218	114	0	29	0	0	0
Orange drink, Sunny Delight	1	cup	249	216	127	0	32	0.2	0	0
Orange drink, carbonated	1	cup	248	217	119	0	30	0	0	0
Orange drink, frozen, prepared	1	cup	248	218	112	0	28	0	0	0
Orange drink/Sunny Delight	1	cup	248	216	126	0	32	0.2	0	0
Orange peel, candied	1.5	oz.	43	7	134	0	34	—	0	0
Orange peel, fresh, grated	1	Tbs	6	4	6	0	2	0.6	0	0
Orange sections, fresh, cup measure	0.5	cup	90	78	42	1	11	2.2	0	0
Orange, California Navel	1	each	140	122	64	1	16	3.4	0	0
Orange, California Valencia	1	each	121	104	59	1	14	3	0	0
Orange, Florida	1	each	151	132	70	1	17	3.6	0	0
Orange, fresh	1	each	131	114	62	1	16	3.1	0	0
Orange, mandarin, canned	0.5	cup	126	113	47	1	12	0.9	0	0
Orange-grapefruit juice, canned	0.5	cup	124	109	53	1	13	0.1	0	0
Oregano, Mexican	0.25	tsp	0	0	1	0	0	0.1	0	—
Oregano, fresh	0.25	cup	18	15	12	0	2	—	0	—
Oregano, ground	0.25	tsp	0	0	1	0	0	0.2	0	0
Oriental snack mix	1	oz.	28	1	156	5	15	3.7	7	1.1
Oysters Rockefeller	0.5	cup	112	84	131	8	11	1.8	6	2.4
Palm heart, cooked slices	0.5	cup	73	51	75	2	19	1.1	0	0.1
Pancake mix, buckwheat, prepared	1	each	27	14	56	2	8	0.6	2	0.5
Pancake, Chinese	1	each	28	14	58	1	13	0.2	0	0
Pancake, French/crepe	1	each	102	57	239	9	22	0.6	12	4
Pancake, Indian	1	each	29	16	52	2	10	0.7	0	0.2
Pancake, blueberry, recipe	2	each	76	40	169	5	22	0.9	7	1.5

MonoF	PolyF	Choles	Calc	Phos	Sod	Pot	Zn	Iron	Magn	VitA	VitE	VitC	Thia	Ribo	Nia	B6	Fola	B12
(g)	(g)	(mg)	(mg)	(mg)	(mg)	(mg)	(mg)	(mg)	(mg)	(μg RE)	(mg α-TE)	(mg)	(mg)	(mg)	(mg)	(mg)	(μg)	(μg)
0	0	0	56	50	210	285	0.5	0.4	50	51	0.61	14	0.12	0.05	0.8	0.17	40	0
1.7	3.6	8	52	53	68	107	0.2	0.4	18	21	1.54	5	0.07	0.05	0.4	0.06	19	0.04
0	0	0	54	48	4	274	0.5	0.4	48	49	0.59	14	0.11	0.05	0.7	0.16	39	0
0	0	0	50	45	4	258	0.4	0.4	46	46	0.55	13	0.11	0.04	0.7	0.15	37	0
3.8	0.3	0	24	7	936	22	0	0.6	9	12	1.17	0	0	0	0	0.01	0	0
1.6	0.2	0	11	3	413	16	0	0.3	4	12	0.54	3	0	0	0	0.01	1	0
0.8	0.1	0	14	0	136	1	0	0.5	1	5	0.46	0	0	0	0	0	0	0
3.6	0.4	0	40	1	392	4	0.1	1.5	2	18	1.35	0	0	0	0	0	0	0
5.3	0.6	0	59	2	589	5	0.1	2.2	3	27	2.03	1	0	0	0	0.01	0	0
5.7	0.9	0	10	—	462	—	—	0.2	—	2	—	0	—	—	—	—	—	—
0	0	0	36	42	3	227	0.3	0.2	13	0	0.19	10	0.07	0.01	0.1	0.22	23	0
0	0	0	2	2	0	5	0	0	1	0	0	0	0	0	0	0.01	1	0
6.6	0.7	14	73	86	430	129	0.3	0.8	16	1	0.33	1	0.08	0.1	0.9	0.06	55	0.12
6.6	0.7	14	73	86	430	129	0.3	0.8	16	1	0.33	1	0.08	0.1	0.9	0.06	55	0.12
2.2	1	0	6	16	75	26	0.1	0.3	4	5	0.14	0	0.06	0.03	0.7	0.02	13	0
0	0	0	5	8	1	40	0	0.1	3	0	0.03	1	0.01	0.01	0	0.03	4	0
0	0	0	3	5	0	22	0	0	1	0	0.02	1	0.01	0	0	0.02	3	0
0	0	0	28	18	234	70	0.2	0.1	4	0	0.05	3	0.02	0	0	0.09	6	0
0	0	0	17	20	13	113	0.1	0.3	6	3	0.2	3	0.02	0.03	0.1	0.07	14	0
0	0.1	0	21	35	3	165	0.2	0.2	10	0	0.33	5	0.04	0.02	0.1	0.12	16	0
0	0.1	0	21	35	3	165	0.2	0.2	10	0	0.33	5	0.04	0.02	0.1	0.12	16	0
2.2	1.3	5	65	64	334	177	0.3	0.3	13	58	0.66	4	0.05	0.09	0.2	0.11	13	0.14
0	0.1	0	21	33	3	156	0.2	0.2	10	0	0.12	5	0.04	0.02	0.2	0.12	14	0
0	0	0	10	16	105	74	0.1	0.1	5	0	0.06	2	0.02	0.01	0.1	0.06	7	0
0	0	0	16	26	2	126	0.2	0.2	8	0	0.1	5	0.03	0.02	0.1	0.09	15	0
0	0	0	16	26	2	126	0.2	0.2	8	0	0.1	5	0.03	0.02	0.1	0.09	15	0
0	0.1	0	22	36	3	173	0.2	0.2	11	0	0.14	7	0.05	0.02	0.2	0.13	21	0
0	0	0	16	26	2	126	0.2	0.2	8	0	0.1	5	0.03	0.02	0.1	0.09	15	0
0	0	0	6	9	1	44	0.1	0.1	3	0	0.04	2	0.01	0.01	0	0.03	5	0
0	0.1	0	22	36	3	173	0.2	0.2	11	0	0.14	7	0.05	0.02	0.2	0.13	21	0
0	0	0	36	18	8	138	0.2	0.7	10	20	0.06	9	0.03	0.04	0.3	0.03	32	0
0	0.1	0	28	20	4	130	0.1	1.1	10	20	0.15	26	0.04	0.05	0.3	0	40	0
0	0	0	20	20	4	115	0.1	0.4	8	0	0.06	13	0.03	0.02	0.2	0.05	18	0
0	0.1	0	14	39	14	170	0.4	1	18	93	0.04	22	0.04	0.07	0.3	0.06	13	0
0	0	0	17	1	5	64	0.1	0.2	5	1	0.08	3	0.01	0.01	0.1	0.04	8	0
0	0.1	0	23	37	3	174	0.2	0.3	12	0	0.14	5	0.04	0.02	0.2	0.14	16	0
0.1	0.1	0	12	20	5	200	0.1	0.2	10	145	0	50	0.05	0.02	0.5	0.07	14	0
0	0	0	32	—	8	145	—	0.1	—	0	—	29	0.07	0.07	—	0.04	—	0
0.2	0.1	0	82	55	22	308	0.1	0.2	2	0	0.74	172	0.3	0.09	0	0	56	0
0	0	0	44	20	1	23	0	0	0	72	0.96	29	0	0.08	1	0.1	0	0
0	0	0	62	37	12	50	0.1	0.2	2	551	0	121	0	0.04	0	0	143	0
0	0	0	15	2	40	45	0.2	0.7	5	5	0	85	0.02	0.01	0.1	0.02	5	0
0	0	0	12	2	30	5	0.2	0.1	2	0	0	0	0	0	0	0	0	0
0	0	0	290	82	25	335	0.1	0.2	27	2	0.01	137	0.26	2.58	0.6	0.18	80	0
0	0	0	15	2	40	45	0.2	0.7	5	5	0	85	0.02	0.01	0.1	0.02	5	0
—	—	0	0	0	0	0	—	0	—	0	—	0	0	0	0	—	—	—
0	0	0	10	1	0	13	0	0	1	3	0.01	8	0.01	0	0.1	0.01	2	0
0	0	0	36	13	0	163	0.1	0.1	9	19	0.22	48	0.08	0.04	0.3	0.05	27	0
0	0	0	56	27	1	249	0.1	0.2	14	25	0.17	80	0.12	0.06	0.4	0.1	47	0
0.1	0.1	0	48	21	0	217	0.1	0.1	12	28	0.36	59	0.1	0.05	0.3	0.08	47	0
0.1	0.1	0	65	18	0	255	0.1	0.1	15	30	0.36	68	0.15	0.06	0.6	0.08	26	0
0	0	0	52	18	0	237	0.1	0.1	13	28	0.31	70	0.11	0.05	0.4	0.08	40	0
0	0	0	14	13	6	168	0.6	0.3	14	107	0.63	43	0.1	0.04	0.6	0.05	6	0
0	0	0	10	17	4	195	0.1	0.6	12	15	0.09	36	0.07	0.04	0.4	0.03	18	0
—	—	—	4	—	0	—	—	0.1	—	3	—	0	—	—	—	—	—	0
—	—	—	56	7	1	59	0.2	—	10	24	—	8	0.01	—	—	—	—	0
0	0	0	6	1	0	6	0	0.2	1	3	0.01	0	0	0	0	0	1	0
2.8	3	0	15	74	117	93	0.8	0.7	34	0	2.39	0	0.09	0.04	0.9	0.02	11	0
2.1	1	39	89	130	445	331	50.2	5.1	62	423	1.05	16	0.19	0.21	1.8	0.12	64	10.6
0	0	0	13	102	10	1318	2.7	1.2	7	5	0.36	5	0.03	0.12	0.6	0.53	15	0
0.5	0.8	18	69	110	144	63	0.3	0.5	15	18	0.56	0	0.05	0.07	0.4	0.04	5	0.09
0	0	0	5	18	1	18	0.2	0.1	4	0	0.02	0	0.01	0.01	0.3	0.03	1	0
4.9	2.4	163	93	145	274	159	0.8	1.6	17	88	1.43	0	0.17	0.37	1.3	0.08	19	0.48
0.1	0.1	1	29	40	59	84	0.3	0.2	10	2	0.06	0	0.04	0.04	0.3	0.04	9	0.08
1.8	3.2	43	157	115	313	105	0.4	1.3	12	39	0.76	2	0.15	0.21	1.2	0.04	27	0.15

Food Item	Qty	Meas	Wgt (g)	Wtr (g)	Cals	Prot (g)	Carb (g)	Fib (g)	Fat (g)	SatF (g)
Pancake, buttermilk, recipe	2	each	76	40	173	5	22	0.6	7	1.4
Pancake, cornmeal	1	each	21	12	43	1	7	0.3	1	0.3
Pancake, frozen, ready to eat, 6 inch	2	each	146	66	334	8	64	2.6	5	1.1
Pancake, mix, incomplete, prepared	2	each	76	40	166	6	22	1.4	6	1.6
Pancake, mix, prepared, low calorie	2	each	44	22	88	2	19	0.7	0	0.1
Pancake, plain, mix, prepared	1	each	27	14	52	1	10	0.4	1	0.1
Pancake, plain, recipe	1	each	27	14	61	2	8	0.4	3	0.6
Pancake, rye, 4 inch	1	each	21	7	63	1	9	0.6	2	0.6
Pancake, sourdough, 4 inch	1	each	21	11	46	1	7	0.3	1	0.3
Pancake, whole wheat, mix, prepared	1	each	52	28	108	4	15	1.5	3	0.9
Pancakes w/butter & syrup, Fast Food	3	each	232	101	582	9	105	2	14	2.5
Pannetone-Italian sweetbread	1	piece	27	8	86	2	15	0.7	2	1.2
Papaya nectar, canned	1	cup	250	213	143	0	36	1.5	0	0.1
Papaya, fresh slices	0.5	cup	70	62	27	0	7	1.3	0	0
Papaya, whole, fresh	1	each	304	270	119	2	30	5.5	0	0.1
Paprika	0.25	tsp	1	0	2	0	0	0.1	0	0
Parsley, dried	0.25	tsp	0	0	0	0	0	0	0	0
Parsley, freeze dried	0.25	tsp	0	0	0	0	0	0	0	0
Parsley, fresh sprigs	10	each	10	9	4	0	1	0.3	0	0
Parsley, fresh, chopped	0.5	cup	30	26	11	1	2	1	0	0
Parsnip, cooked from raw, drained	0.5	cup	78	61	63	1	15	3.1	0	0
Parsnip, sliced, raw	0.5	cup	66	53	50	1	12	3.3	0	0
Passion fruit, purple, fresh	1	each	18	13	18	0	4	1.9	0	0
Pasta, spaghetti, whole wheat, cooked	0.5	cup	70	47	87	4	19	3.2	0	0.1
Pasta/Noodle, spaghetti, spinach, cooked	0.5	cup	70	48	91	3	18	2.4	0	0.1
Pasta/Noodles, cellophane, cooked	0.5	cup	95	75	80	0	20	0.1	0	0
Pasta/Noodles, corn-based, cooked	0.5	cup	60	41	75	2	17	2.9	0	0.1
Pasta/Noodles, corn-based, spaghetti, cooked	0.5	cup	60	41	75	2	17	2.9	0	0.1
Pasta/Noodles, egg, fried	0.5	cup	84	63	129	2	10	0.4	10	1.7
Pasta/Noodles, egg, spinach, cooked	0.5	cup	80	55	106	4	19	1.8	1	0.3
Pasta/Noodles, fresh, cooked	2	oz.	57	39	74	3	14	1	1	0.1
Pasta/Noodles, homemade w/egg, cooked	0.5	cup	80	55	104	4	19	3.1	1	0.3
Pasta/Noodles, homemade, no egg, cooked	2	oz.	57	39	70	2	14	0.9	1	0.1
Pasta/Noodles, jumbo shells, enriched, cooked	2.5	oz.	70	46	99	3	20	0.9	0	0.1
Pasta/Noodles, lasagna cuts, cooked	0.5	cup	70	46	99	3	20	0.9	0	0.1
Pasta/Noodles, lasagna, enriched, cooked	2.5	oz.	70	46	99	3	20	0.9	0	0.1
Pasta/Noodles, linguini, cooked	0.5	cup	70	46	99	3	20	1.2	0	0.1
Pasta/Noodles, macaroni, corn-based, cooked	0.5	cup	60	41	75	2	17	2.9	0	0.1
Pasta/Noodles, macaroni, enriched, cooked	1	cup	140	92	197	7	40	1.8	1	0.1
Pasta/Noodles, macaroni, vegetable, cooked	0.5	cup	67	46	86	3	18	2.9	0	0
Pasta/Noodles, rotini, enriched, cooked	0.5	cup	70	46	99	3	20	0.9	0	0.1
Pasta/Noodles, small shells, enriched, cooked	0.5	cup	58	38	81	3	16	0.7	0	0.1
Pasta/Noodles, spaghetti, cooked	0.5	cup	70	46	99	3	20	1.2	0	0.1
Pasta/Noodles, spaghetti, cooked w/salt	0.5	cup	70	46	99	3	20	1.2	0	0.1
Pasta/Noodles, spinach, fresh, cooked	2	oz.	57	39	74	3	14	1.3	1	0.1
Pasta/Noodles, spirals, enriched, cooked	0.5	cup	67	44	94	3	19	0.9	0	0.1
Pasta/Noodles, vermicelli, cooked	0.5	cup	70	46	99	3	20	1.2	0	0.1
Pasta/Noodles, wagon wheels, enriched, cooked	0.5	cup	70	46	99	3	20	0.9	0	0.1
Pasta/Noodles, whole wheat, lasagna cuts, cooked	0.5	cup	70	47	87	4	19	2	0	0.1
Pasta/Noodles, whole wheat, lasagna, cooked	2.5	oz.	70	47	87	4	19	2	0	0.1
Pasta/Noodles, whole wheat, macaroni, cooked	0.5	cup	70	47	87	4	19	2	0	0.1
Pasta/Noodles, whole wheat, rotini, cooked	0.5	cup	70	47	87	4	19	2	0	0.1
Pasta/Noodles, whole wheat, shells, cooked	0.5	cup	70	47	87	4	19	2	0	0.1
Pasta/Noodles, whole wheat, spirals, cooked	0.5	cup	70	47	87	4	19	2	0	0.1
Pasta/Noodles, whole wheat, wagon wheels, cooked	0.5	cup	70	47	87	4	19	2	0	0.1
Pastrami, turkey	2	piece	57	40	80	10	1	0	4	1
Pastry cookie, apple, dietetic	1	each	24	3	115	1	12	0.2	7	3.5
Pastry, Chinese	1	oz.	28	13	67	1	13	0.1	1	0.2
Patty tart shell, frozen, baked	1	each	71	5	396	5	32	1.1	27	3.9
Patty tart shells, frozen	1	each	47	4	259	3	21	0.7	18	4.5
Pea pod (snow pea), stir fried	0.5	cup	82	73	35	2	6	2.2	0	0
Pea sprouts, cooked	4	oz.	113	84	134	8	25	4.9	1	0.1
Pea sprouts, raw	0.5	cup	60	37	77	5	17	2.4	0	0.1
Peach crisp, piece, 3x3 in	1	piece	139	104	155	2	27	2	5	0.9
Peach halves, cooked from dry	0.5	cup	129	101	99	2	25	3.5	0	0

MonoF	PolyF	Choles	Calc	Phos	Sod	Pot	Zn	Iron	Magn	VitA	VitE	VitC	Thia	Ribo	Nia	B6	Fola	B12
(g)	(g)	(mg)	(mg)	(mg)	(mg)	(mg)	(mg)	(mg)	(mg)	(μg RE)	(mg α-TE)	(mg)	(mg)	(mg)	(mg)	(mg)	(μg)	(μg)
1.8	3.4	44	119	106	397	110	0.5	1.3	11	23	1.06	0	0.16	0.22	1.2	0.03	29	0.14
0.5	0.4	9	25	19	42	21	0.1	0.4	4	19	0.21	0	0.05	0.05	0.4	0.02	3	0.03
1.8	1.4	13	90	543	743	107	1	5.1	20	42	0.58	0	0.55	0.68	5.8	0.12	73	0.26
1.6	2.2	54	163	238	384	151	0.6	1	17	55	0.65	0	0.15	0.24	0.9	0.08	8	0.26
0.1	0.2	0	26	150	115	170	0.3	0.8	12	4	0.04	0	0.07	0.05	0.7	0.01	2	0
0.2	0.2	3	34	90	170	47	0.1	0.4	5	2	0.23	0	0.06	0.06	0.5	0.02	2	0.05
0.7	1.2	16	59	43	119	36	0.2	0.5	4	15	0.26	0	0.05	0.08	0.4	0.01	10	0.06
0.9	0.6	8	22	24	54	96	0.2	0.5	15	4	0.26	0	0.04	0.05	0.3	0.04	2	0.03
0.4	0.6	8	3	16	46	17	0.1	0.5	3	4	0.12	0	0.06	0.06	0.5	0.02	8	0.02
0.9	1.2	32	130	194	297	145	0.5	1.6	24	33	0.44	0	0.1	0.28	1.2	0.06	11	0.15
4.9	6.1	11	113	525	780	298	0.6	2.1	28	125	1.25	0	0.25	0.27	2	0.09	0	0.28
0.6	0.2	19	16	39	96	53	0.2	0.8	6	22	0.13	0	0.1	0.12	1	0.05	24	0.05
0.1	0.1	0	25	0	12	78	0.4	0.8	8	28	0.05	8	0.02	0.01	0.4	0.02	5	0
0	0	0	17	4	2	180	0	0.1	7	20	0.78	43	0.02	0.02	0.2	0.01	27	0
0.1	0.1	0	73	15	9	781	0.2	0.3	30	85	3.4	188	0.08	0.1	1	0.06	116	0
0	0	0	1	2	0	14	0	0.1	1	35	0	0	0	0.01	0.1	0.01	1	0
0	0	0	2	0	0	4	0	0.1	0	3	0	0	0	0	0	0	0	0
0	0	0	0	0	0	2	0	0	0	2	0	0	0	0	0	0	0	0
0	0	0	14	6	6	55	0.1	0.6	5	52	0.18	13	0.01	0.01	0.1	0.01	15	0
0.1	0	0	41	17	17	166	0.3	1.9	15	156	0.54	40	0.03	0.03	0.4	0.03	46	0
0.1	0	0	29	54	8	286	0.2	0.5	23	0	0.78	10	0.06	0.04	0.6	0.07	45	0
0.1	0	0	24	47	7	249	0.4	0.4	19	0	0.66	11	0.06	0.03	0.5	0.06	44	0
0	0.1	0	2	12	5	63	0	0.3	5	13	0.2	5	0	0.02	0.3	0.02	3	0
0.1	0.1	0	10	62	2	31	0.6	0.7	21	0	0.04	0	0.08	0.03	0.5	0.06	4	0
0	0.2	0	21	76	10	41	0.8	0.7	43	10	0.01	0	0.07	0.07	1.1	0.07	8	0
0	0	0	7	7	4	2	0.1	0.5	1	0	0.03	0	0.03	0	0	0.01	0	0
0.1	0.2	0	1	45	0	18	0.4	0.1	21	4	0.2	0	0.03	0.01	0.3	0.04	4	0
0.1	0.2	0	1	45	0	18	0.4	0.1	21	4	0.2	0	0.03	0.01	0.3	0.04	4	0
2	2.8	4	5	—	71	24	0.3	0.3	—	2	—	0	0.01	0.01	—	0.01	1	0
0.4	0.3	26	15	46	10	30	0.5	0.9	19	11	0.04	0	0.2	0.1	1.2	0.09	51	0.11
0.1	0.2	19	3	36	3	14	0.3	0.6	10	3	0.08	0	0.12	0.08	0.6	0.02	36	0.08
0.4	0.4	33	8	42	66	17	0.4	0.9	11	14	0.17	0	0.14	0.14	1	0.03	34	0.08
0.1	0.3	0	3	23	42	11	0.2	0.6	8	0	0.08	0	0.1	0.08	0.8	0.02	24	0
0.1	0.2	0	5	38	1	22	0.4	1	13	0	0.02	0	0.14	0.07	1.2	0.02	49	0
0.1	0.2	0	5	38	1	22	0.4	1	13	0	0.02	0	0.14	0.07	1.2	0.02	49	0
0.1	0.2	0	5	38	1	22	0.4	1	13	0	0.02	0	0.14	0.07	1.2	0.02	49	0
0.1	0.2	0	5	38	1	22	0.4	1	13	0	0.04	0	0.14	0.07	1.2	0.02	49	0
0.1	0.2	0	1	45	0	18	0.4	0.1	21	4	0.2	0	0.03	0.01	0.3	0.04	4	0
0.1	0.4	0	10	76	1	43	0.7	2	25	0	0.04	0	0.29	0.14	2.3	0.05	98	0
0	0	0	7	34	4	21	0.3	0.3	13	3	0.03	0	0.08	0.04	0.7	0.02	44	0
0.1	0.2	0	5	38	1	22	0.4	1	13	0	0.02	0	0.14	0.07	1.2	0.02	49	0
0	0.2	0	4	31	1	18	0.3	0.8	10	0	0.02	0	0.12	0.06	1	0.02	40	0
0.1	0.2	0	5	38	1	22	0.4	1	13	0	0.04	0	0.14	0.07	1.2	0.02	49	0
0.1	0.2	0	5	38	70	22	0.4	1	13	0	0.19	0	0.14	0.07	1.2	0.02	49	0
0.2	0.1	19	10	32	3	21	0.4	0.6	14	8	0.12	0	0.1	0.08	0.6	0.06	36	0.08
0.1	0.2	0	5	36	1	21	0.4	0.9	12	0	0.02	0	0.14	0.07	1.1	0.02	47	0
0.1	0.2	0	5	38	1	22	0.4	1	13	0	0.04	0	0.14	0.07	1.2	0.02	49	0
0.1	0.2	0	5	38	1	22	0.4	1	13	0	0.02	0	0.14	0.07	1.2	0.02	49	0
0.1	0.1	0	10	62	2	31	0.6	0.7	21	0	0.07	0	0.08	0.03	0.5	0.06	4	0
0.1	0.1	0	10	62	2	31	0.6	0.7	21	0	0.07	0	0.08	0.03	0.5	0.06	4	0
0.1	0.1	0	10	62	2	31	0.6	0.7	21	0	0.07	0	0.08	0.03	0.5	0.06	4	0
0.1	0.1	0	10	62	2	31	0.6	0.7	21	0	0.07	0	0.08	0.03	0.5	0.06	4	0
0.1	0.1	0	10	62	2	31	0.6	0.7	21	0	0.07	0	0.08	0.03	0.5	0.06	4	0
0.1	0.1	0	10	62	2	31	0.6	0.7	21	0	0.07	0	0.08	0.03	0.5	0.06	4	0
0.1	0.1	0	10	62	2	31	0.6	0.7	21	0	0.07	0	0.08	0.03	0.5	0.06	4	0
1.2	0.9	31	5	114	596	148	1.2	0.9	8	0	0.12	0	0.03	0.14	2	0.15	3	0.14
2.6	0.6	0	2	12	0	22	0.1	0.3	7	0	1.54	0	0.04	0.02	0.3	0.01	2	0.02
0.4	0.8	0	8	16	3	28	0.2	0.5	6	0	0.25	0	0.05	0	0.4	0.02	1	0
6.3	15.8	0	7	43	180	44	0.4	1.8	11	0	1.69	0	0.23	0.18	2.7	0.01	33	0
10.2	2.3	0	5	28	117	29	0.2	1.2	8	0	2.4	0	0.19	0.13	2	0.01	44	0
0	0.1	0	36	44	3	165	0.2	1.7	20	11	0.32	42	0.11	0.06	0.5	0.12	28	0
0.1	0.3	0	30	27	3	304	0.9	1.9	46	12	0.01	7	0.24	0.32	1.2	0.14	41	0
0	0.2	0	22	99	12	229	0.6	1.4	34	10	0.01	6	0.14	0.09	1.8	0.16	86	0
2.5	1.8	0	20	31	70	189	0.2	0.9	12	108	1.13	5	0.06	0.05	1.1	0.03	6	0.01
0.1	0.2	0	12	49	3	413	0.2	1.7	17	26	0	5	0.01	0.03	2	0.05	0	0

Food Item	Qty	Meas	Wgt (g)	Wtr (g)	Cals	Prot (g)	Carb (g)	Fib (g)	Fat (g)	SatF (g)
Peach halves, dried	10	each	130	41	311	5	80	10.7	1	0.1
Peach nectar, canned	1	cup	249	213	134	1	35	1.5	0	0
Peach nectar, canned, sweetened	1	cup	249	213	134	1	35	1.5	0	0
Peach nectar, canned, vit C added	1	cup	249	213	134	1	35	1.5	0	0
Peach slices, frozen, sweetened	1	each	284	212	267	2	68	5.1	0	0
Peach turnover	1	each	78	28	261	3	33	1.3	13	3.3
Peach, fresh, whole (2.5in)	1	each	87	76	37	1	10	1.7	0	0
Peach, peeled slices, fresh	0.5	cup	85	74	37	1	9	1.7	0	0
Peaches, canned in heavy syrup	0.5	cup	128	102	95	1	26	1.7	0	0
Peaches, canned in juice	0.5	cup	124	109	55	1	14	1.6	0	0
Peaches, canned in light syrup	0.5	cup	126	106	68	1	18	1.6	0	0
Peanut butter, chunky, salted	2	Tbs	32	0	188	8	7	2.1	16	3.1
Peanut butter, chunky, unsalted	2	Tbs	32	0	188	8	7	2.1	16	3.1
Peanut butter, natural, salted	2	Tbs	32	0	187	8	7	2.1	16	2.2
Peanut butter, natural, unsalted	2	Tbs	32	0	187	8	7	2.1	16	2.2
Peanut butter, smooth, salted	2	Tbs	32	0	190	8	6	1.9	16	3.3
Peanut butter, smooth, unsalted	2	Tbs	32	0	190	8	6	1.9	16	3.3
Peanut, Spanish, raw	0.5	cup	36	2	208	10	6	3.5	18	2.8
Peanuts, Spanish, oil roasted, unsalted	0.25	cup	37	1	213	10	6	3.3	18	2.8
Peanuts, Valencia, oil roasted, unsalted	0.25	cup	36	1	212	10	6	3.2	18	2.8
Peanuts, Virginia, oil roasted, unsalted	0.25	cup	36	1	207	9	7	3.2	17	2.3
Peanuts, dry roasted, unsalted	0.25	cup	36	1	214	9	8	2.9	18	2.5
Peanuts, oil roasted, unsalted	0.25	cup	36	1	209	10	7	2.5	18	2.5
Pear halves canned in water	1	each	77	71	22	0	6	1.2	0	0
Pear halves, dried	10	each	175	47	459	3	122	13.1	1	0.1
Pear nectar, canned	1	cup	250	210	150	0	40	1.5	0	0
Pear nectar, canned, vit C added	1	cup	250	210	150	0	40	1.5	0	0
Pear, Asian, raw	1	each	122	108	51	1	13	4.4	0	0
Pear, candied	1.5	oz.	43	9	129	1	32	—	0	0
Pear, canned in heavy syrup	0.5	cup	128	103	94	0	24	2	0	0
Pear, fresh slices	0.5	cup	82	69	49	0	12	2	0	0
Pear, fresh, Bartlett	1	each	166	139	98	1	25	4	1	0
Pear, fresh, Bosc	1	each	139	116	82	1	21	3.3	1	0
Pear, fresh, D'Anjou	1	each	209	175	123	1	32	5	1	0
Pears, canned in juice	0.5	cup	124	107	62	0	16	2	0	0
Pears, canned in light syrup	0.5	cup	126	106	72	0	19	2	0	0
Peas & carrots, canned w/liquid, low sodium	0.5	cup	128	113	49	3	11	4.2	0	0.1
Peas & carrots, canned, not drained	0.5	cup	128	113	49	3	11	2.6	0	0.1
Peas & carrots, frozen, cooked	0.5	cup	80	69	38	2	8	2.5	0	0.1
Peas & carrots, frozen, unheated	0.5	cup	70	59	37	2	8	2.4	0	0.1
Peas & onions, canned w/liquid	0.5	cup	60	52	31	2	5	1.4	0	0
Peas, edible pod/snow pea, cooked	0.5	cup	80	71	34	3	6	2.2	0	0
Peas, blackeyed/cowpea, canned w/liquid	0.5	cup	120	96	92	6	16	4	1	0.2
Peas, blackeyed/cowpea, dry	0.5	cup	84	10	281	20	50	8.8	1	0.3
Peas, blackeyed/cowpea, dry, cooked	0.5	cup	86	60	99	7	18	5.6	0	0.1
Peas, edible pod/snow pea, frozen, cooked	0.5	cup	80	69	42	3	7	2.5	0	0.1
Peas, edible pod/snow pea, raw	0.5	cup	72	64	30	2	5	1.9	0	0
Peas, edible pods/snow peas, steamed	0.5	cup	82	73	35	2	6	2.2	0	0
Peas, green, canned, drained	0.5	cup	85	69	59	4	11	3.5	0	0.1
Peas, green, canned, low sodium	0.5	cup	85	69	59	4	11	3.5	0	0.1
Peas, green, canned, not drained	0.5	cup	124	107	66	4	12	4	0	0.1
Peas, green, canned, not drained, low sodium	0.5	cup	124	107	66	4	12	4	0	0.1
Peas, green, frozen, cooked	0.5	cup	80	64	62	4	11	4.4	0	0
Peas, green, frozen, unheated	0.5	cup	72	58	55	4	10	3.4	0	0
Peas, green, raw	0.5	cup	72	57	59	4	10	3.7	0	0.1
Peas, green, raw, cooked	0.5	cup	80	62	67	4	12	4.4	0	0
Peas, pigeon/red gram, cooked	0.5	cup	84	58	102	6	20	5.6	0	0.1
Peas, seasoned, canned, not drained	0.5	cup	114	99	57	4	10	2.3	0	0.1
Peas, split, dry	0.5	cup	98	11	336	24	60	25.1	1	0.2
Peas, split, dry, cooked	0.5	cup	98	68	116	8	21	8.1	0	0.1
Pecan halves, oil roasted, unsalted	15	each	28	1	194	2	5	1.9	20	1.6
Pecan, dry roasted, salted	0.25	cup	28	0	187	2	6	2.6	18	1.5
Pecans, dried halves	0.25	cup	27	1	180	2	5	2	18	1.5
Pecans, dried, chopped	0.25	cup	30	1	198	2	5	2.3	20	1.6
Pecans, dried, ground	0.25	cup	24	1	158	2	4	1.8	16	1.3

MonoF (g)	PolyF (g)	Choles (mg)	Calc (mg)	Phos (mg)	Sod (mg)	Pot (mg)	Zn (mg)	Iron (mg)	Magn (mg)	VitA (μg RE)	VitE (mg α-TE)	VitC (mg)	Thia (mg)	Ribo (mg)	Nia (mg)	B6 (mg)	Fola (μg)	B12 (μg)
0.4	0.5	0	36	155	9	1294	0.7	5.3	55	281	0	6	0	0.28	5.7	0.09	0	0
0	0	0	12	15	17	100	0.2	0.5	10	65	0.02	13	0.01	0.04	0.7	0.02	3	0
0	0	0	12	15	17	100	0.2	0.5	10	65	0.02	13	0.01	0.04	0.7	0.02	3	0
0	0	0	12	15	17	100	0.2	0.5	10	65	0.2	67	0.01	0.04	0.7	0.02	3	0
0.1	0.2	0	9	31	17	369	0.1	1	14	80	2.53	268	0.04	0.1	1.8	0.05	9	0
5.9	3.5	0	6	32	218	89	0.2	1.2	8	14	1.4	2	0.16	0.13	1.7	0.02	5	0
0	0	0	4	10	0	171	0.1	0.1	6	47	0.61	6	0.02	0.04	0.9	0.02	3	0
0	0	0	4	10	0	167	0.1	0.1	6	46	0.6	6	0.01	0.04	0.8	0.02	3	0
0	0.1	0	4	14	8	118	0.1	0.3	6	42	1.14	4	0.01	0.03	0.8	0.02	4	0
0	0	0	7	21	5	159	0.1	0.3	9	47	1.86	4	0.01	0.02	0.7	0.02	4	0
0	0	0	4	14	6	122	0.1	0.5	6	44	1.12	3	0.01	0.03	0.7	0.02	4	0
7.6	4.5	0	13	101	156	239	0.9	0.6	51	0	2.4	0	0.04	0.04	4.4	0.14	29	0
7.6	4.5	0	13	101	5	239	0.9	0.6	51	0	3.2	0	0.04	0.04	4.4	0.14	29	0
7.9	5	0	17	114	80	210	1.1	0.7	56	0	2.59	0	0.04	0.03	4.3	0.13	46	0
7.9	5	0	17	115	2	211	1.1	0.7	56	0	2.4	0	0.14	0.03	4.3	0.13	46	0
7.8	4.4	0	12	118	149	214	0.9	0.6	51	0	3.2	0	0.03	0.03	4.3	0.14	24	0
7.8	4.4	0	12	118	5	214	0.9	0.6	51	0	3.2	0	0.03	0.03	4.3	0.14	24	0
8.1	6.3	0	39	142	8	272	0.8	1.4	69	0	2.7	0	0.25	0.05	5.8	0.13	88	0
8.1	6.2	0	37	142	2	285	0.7	0.8	62	0	2.72	0	0.12	0.03	5.5	0.09	46	0
8.3	6.4	0	19	115	2	220	1.1	0.6	58	0	2.77	0	0.03	0.06	5.2	0.09	45	0
9	5.3	0	31	181	2	233	2.4	0.6	67	0	2.61	0	0.1	0.04	5.3	0.09	45	0
9	5.7	0	20	131	297	240	1.2	0.8	64	0	2.7	0	0.16	0.04	4.9	0.09	53	0
8.8	5.6	0	32	186	2	246	2.4	0.7	67	0	2.67	0	0.09	0.04	5.2	0.09	45	0
0	0	0	3	5	2	41	0.1	0.2	3	0	0.38	1	0.01	0.01	0	0.01	1	0
0.2	0.3	0	60	103	10	933	0.7	3.7	58	1	0	12	0.01	0.25	2.4	0.13	0	0
0	0	0	12	8	10	32	0.2	0.6	8	0	0.25	3	0	0.03	0.3	0.04	3	0
0	0	0	12	8	10	32	0.2	0.6	8	0	0.25	68	0	0.03	0.3	0.04	3	0
0.1	0.1	0	5	13	0	148	0	0	10	0	0.61	5	0.01	0.01	0.3	0.03	10	0
—	—	0	15	20	3	244	—	0.6	—	3	—	3	0	0.08	0.3	—	—	—
0	0	0	6	9	6	83	0.1	0.3	5	0	0.64	1	0.01	0.03	0.3	0.02	2	0
0.1	0.1	0	9	9	0	103	0.1	0.2	5	2	0.41	3	0.02	0.03	0.1	0.02	6	0
0.1	0.2	0	18	18	0	208	0.2	0.4	10	3	0.83	7	0.03	0.07	0.2	0.03	12	0
0.1	0.1	0	15	15	0	174	0.2	0.3	8	3	0.7	6	0.03	0.06	0.1	0.02	10	0
0.2	0.2	0	23	23	0	261	0.3	0.5	12	4	1.05	8	0.04	0.08	0.2	0.04	15	0
0	0	0	11	15	5	119	0.1	0.4	9	1	0.62	2	0.01	0.01	0.2	0.02	1	0
0	0	0	6	9	6	83	0.1	0.4	5	0	0.63	1	0.01	0.02	0.2	0.02	2	0
0	0.2	0	29	59	5	128	0.7	1	18	739	0.54	8	0.1	0.07	0.7	0.11	23	0
0	0.2	0	29	59	333	128	0.7	1	18	739	0.24	8	0.1	0.07	0.7	0.11	23	0
0	0.2	0	18	39	54	126	0.4	0.8	13	621	0.26	6	0.18	0.05	0.9	0.07	21	0
0	0.2	0	19	42	55	136	0.4	0.8	13	665	0.22	8	0.13	0.06	1	0.07	25	0
0	0.1	0	10	31	265	58	0.3	0.5	10	10	0.17	2	0.06	0.04	0.8	0.12	16	0
0	0.1	0	34	44	3	192	0.3	1.6	21	10	0.31	38	0.1	0.06	0.4	0.12	23	0
0.1	0.3	0	24	84	359	206	0.8	1.2	34	1	0.12	3	0.09	0.09	0.4	0.05	61	0
0.1	0.5	0	92	354	13	929	2.8	6.9	154	4	0.33	1	0.71	0.19	1.7	0.3	529	0
0	0.2	0	20	133	3	238	1.1	2.2	45	2	0.24	0	0.17	0.05	0.4	0.09	178	0
0	0.1	0	47	46	4	174	0.4	1.9	22	14	0.17	18	0.05	0.1	0.4	0.14	28	0
0	0.1	0	31	38	3	145	0.2	1.5	17	10	0.28	44	0.11	0.06	0.4	0.12	30	0
0	0.1	0	36	44	3	165	0.2	1.7	20	11	0.32	42	0.11	0.06	0.5	0.12	29	0
0	0.1	0	17	57	214	147	0.6	0.8	14	66	0.32	8	0.1	0.07	0.6	0.05	38	0
0	0.1	0	17	57	2	147	0.6	0.8	14	66	0.32	8	0.1	0.07	0.6	0.05	38	0
0	0.2	0	22	66	310	124	0.9	1.3	21	47	0.34	12	0.14	0.09	1	0.08	35	0
0	0.2	0	22	66	11	124	0.9	1.3	21	47	0.47	12	0.14	0.09	1	0.08	35	0
0	0.1	0	19	72	70	134	0.8	1.3	23	54	0.14	8	0.23	0.08	1.2	0.09	47	0
0	0.1	0	16	58	81	107	0.6	1.1	18	53	0.12	13	0.19	0.07	1.2	0.09	38	0
0	0.1	0	18	78	4	177	0.9	1.1	24	46	0.28	29	0.19	0.1	1.5	0.12	47	0
0	0.1	0	22	94	2	217	1	1.2	31	48	0.31	11	0.21	0.12	1.6	0.17	51	0
0	0.2	0	36	100	4	323	0.8	0.9	39	0	0.08	0	0.12	0.05	0.7	0.04	93	0
0	0.1	0	17	62	290	139	0.7	1.4	17	49	0.34	13	0.11	0.08	0.8	0.11	33	0
0.2	0.5	0	54	361	15	966	3	4.4	113	15	0.3	2	0.72	0.21	2.8	0.17	270	0
0.1	0.2	0	14	97	2	355	1	1.3	35	1	0.38	0	0.19	0.06	0.9	0.05	64	0
12.6	5	0	10	83	0	102	1.6	0.6	37	4	0.94	1	0.09	0.03	0.3	0.05	11	0
11.4	4.5	0	10	86	222	105	1.6	0.6	38	4	0.85	1	0.09	0.03	0.3	0.06	12	0
11.4	4.5	0	10	79	0	106	1.5	0.6	35	4	0.84	1	0.23	0.04	0.2	0.05	11	0
12.6	5	0	11	87	0	117	1.6	0.6	38	4	0.92	1	0.25	0.04	0.3	0.06	12	0
10	4	0	9	69	0	93	1.3	0.5	30	3	0.74	0	0.2	0.03	0.2	0.04	9	0

Food Item	Qty	Meas	Wgt (g)	Wtr (g)	Cals	Prot (g)	Carb (g)	Fib (g)	Fat (g)	SatF (g)
Pecans, dry roasted, unsalted	0.24	cup	28	0	187	2	6	2.6	18	1.5
Pecans, oil roasted, salted	0.25	cup	28	1	188	2	4	1.8	20	1.6
Pecans, oil roasted, unsalted	0.25	cup	28	1	188	2	4	1.8	20	1.6
Pepper, black	0.25	tsp	1	0	1	0	0	0.1	0	0
Pepper, cayenne/red	0.25	tsp	0	0	1	0	0	0.1	0	0
Pepper, hot green chili, canned, w/liquid, no seeds	0.5	cup	68	63	14	1	3	0.9	0	0
Pepper, hot green chili, raw, whole	1	each	45	40	18	1	4	0.7	0	0
Pepper, hot jalapeno, pickled	2	each	16	13	8	0	2	0.2	0	0
Pepper, hot red chili, canned, not drained	1	Tbs	8	8	2	0	0	0.1	0	0
Pepper, hot red chili, raw pod	1	each	45	40	18	1	4	0.7	0	0
Pepper, hot red chili, raw, chopped	1	Tbs	9	8	4	0	1	0.1	0	0
Pepper, hot red, dried pods	0.25	cup	2	0	5	0	1	—	0	0
Pepper, jalapeno, chopped, canned	1	Tbs	8	8	2	0	0	0.2	0	0
Pepper, jalapeno, raw	1	each	45	40	11	0	2	—	0	—
Pepper, lemon	0.25	tsp	0	0	1	0	0	0	0	0
Pepper, pickled	1	each	20	18	8	0	2	0.3	0	0
Pepper, serrano, raw	1	each	45	40	20	—	—	—	—	—
Pepper, sweet green bell, freeze dried	0.5	cup	3	0	10	1	2	0.7	0	0
Pepper, sweet green bell, frozen, cooked	0.5	cup	68	64	12	1	3	0.6	0	0
Pepper, sweet green, canned w/liquid	0.5	cup	70	64	13	1	3	0.8	0	0
Pepper, sweet green, chopped, cooked	0.5	cup	68	62	19	1	5	0.8	0	0
Pepper, sweet green, chopped, steamed	0.5	cup	68	63	18	1	4	1.2	0	0
Pepper, sweet green, chopped, stir fried	0.5	cup	68	63	18	1	4	1.2	0	0
Pepper, sweet green, raw, chopped	0.5	cup	50	46	14	0	3	0.9	0	0
Pepper, sweet green, raw, whole	1	each	74	68	20	1	5	1.3	0	0
Pepper, sweet green, whole, cooked	1	each	73	67	20	1	5	0.9	0	0
Pepper, sweet red bell, canned, w/liquid	0.5	cup	70	64	13	1	3	0.8	0	0
Pepper, sweet red bell, chopped, cooked	0.5	cup	68	62	19	1	5	0.8	0	0
Pepper, sweet red bell, freeze dried	0.5	cup	3	0	10	1	2	0.7	0	0
Pepper, sweet red bell, frozen, cooked	0.5	cup	68	64	12	1	3	1.1	0	0
Pepper, sweet red bell, steamed	0.5	cup	68	63	18	1	4	1.2	0	0
Pepper, sweet red bell, stir fried, no oil	0.5	cup	68	63	18	1	4	1.2	0	0
Pepper, sweet red, raw, chopped	0.5	cup	50	46	14	0	3	1	0	0
Pepper, sweet yellow, raw strips	10	piece	52	48	14	1	3	0.5	0	0
Pepper, sweet yellow, raw, large	1	each	186	171	50	2	12	1.7	0	0.1
Pepper, white	0.25	tsp	1	0	2	0	0	0.2	0	0
Pepperoncini, Greek	1	oz.	28	26	8	0	1	0.4	0	0
Pepperoncini, Italian	1	oz.	28	26	6	0	1	0.2	0	0
Peppers, hot green chili, raw, chopped	1	Tbs	9	8	4	0	1	0.1	0	0
Peppers, sweet cherry	1	oz.	28	24	16	1	2	0.5	0	0.1
Persimmon, Japanese, dried	1	each	34	8	93	0	25	4.9	0	0.1
Persimmon, Japanese, large, raw	1	each	168	135	118	1	31	6	0	0
Persimmon, native, fresh	1	each	25	16	32	0	8	0.4	0	—
Phyllo dough	1	each	19	6	57	1	10	0.4	1	0.3
Pickle, chow chow	1	Tbs	15	10	18	0	4	0.2	0	0
Pickle, cucumber, dill, low sodium, slices	4	each	30	28	3	0	1	0.4	0	0
Pickle, cucumber, dill, low sodium, spears	1	each	30	28	3	0	1	0.4	0	0
Pickle, cucumber, dill, low sodium, whole	1	each	65	61	7	0	1	0.8	0	0
Pickle, cucumber, fresh slices	4	piece	30	24	22	0	5	0.4	0	0
Pickle, dill	1	each	65	60	12	0	3	0.8	0	0
Pickle, dill, slices	10	piece	60	55	11	0	2	0.7	0	0
Pickle, dill, low sodium	1	each	65	60	12	0	3	0.8	0	0
Pickle, dill, low sodium, slices	10	piece	60	55	11	0	2	0.7	0	0
Pickle, mustard	0.25	cup	61	42	71	1	16	0.9	1	0
Pickle, sour	1	each	35	33	4	0	1	0.4	0	0
Pickle, sour cucumber, slices	10	piece	70	66	8	0	2	0.8	0	0
Pickle, sour, low sodium	1	each	35	33	4	0	1	0.4	0	0
Pickle, sour, low sodium, slices	10	piece	70	66	8	0	2	0.8	0	0
Pickle, sweet butter chips, low sodium	5	each	30	20	35	0	10	0.4	0	0
Pickle, sweet cucumber, low sodium, slices	5	each	30	20	35	0	10	0.4	0	0
Pickle, sweet relish	1	Tbs	15	10	21	0	5	0.3	0	0
Pickle, sweet, low sodium	1	each	35	23	41	0	11	0.4	0	0
Pickle, sweet, low sodium, slices	10	piece	60	39	70	0	19	0.7	0	0
Pickle, sweet, medium size	1	each	35	23	41	0	11	0.4	0	0
Pickles, Japanese, tsukemono	0.5	cup	68	62	14	1	3	1.8	0	0

MonoF (g)	PolyF (g)	Choles (mg)	Calc (mg)	Phos (mg)	Sod (mg)	Pot (mg)	Zn (mg)	Iron (mg)	Magn (mg)	VitA (μg RE)	VitE (mg α-TE)	VitC (mg)	Thia (mg)	Ribo (mg)	Nia (mg)	B6 (mg)	Fola (μg)	B12 (μg)
11.4	4.5	0	10	86	0	105	1.6	0.6	38	4	0.88	1	0.09	0.03	0.3	0.06	12	0
12.2	4.8	0	9	81	208	99	1.5	0.6	36	4	0.91	1	0.08	0.03	0.2	0.05	11	0
12.2	4.8	0	9	81	0	99	1.5	0.6	36	4	0.91	1	0.08	0.03	0.2	0.05	11	0
0	0	0	2	1	0	7	0	0.2	1	0	0	0	0	0	0	0	0	0
0	0	0	1	1	0	9	0	0	1	18	0.02	0	0	0	0	0.01	0	0
0	0	0	5	12	798	127	0.1	0.3	10	42	0.47	46	0.01	0.03	0.5	0.1	7	0
0	0	0	8	21	3	153	0.1	0.5	11	35	0.31	109	0.04	0.04	0.4	0.12	10	0
0	0	0	3	6	121	43	0	0.1	3	124	0.08	28	0.01	0.01	0.1	0.03	3	0
0	0	0	1	1	100	16	0	0	1	101	0.06	6	0	0	0.1	0.01	1	0
0	0	0	8	21	3	153	0.1	0.5	11	484	0.31	109	0.04	0.04	0.4	0.12	10	0
0	0	0	2	4	1	32	0	0.1	2	101	0.06	23	0.01	0.01	0.1	0.03	2	0
—	—	0	2	4	6	19	—	0.1	—	123	—	0	0	0.02	0.2	—	—	0
0	0	0	2	2	142	16	0	0.2	1	14	0.06	1	0	0	0	0.02	1	0
—	—	—	—	—	2	2	—	—	—	30	0.37	53	—	—	—	—	—	0
0	0	0	1	0	115	1	0	0	0	0	0	0	0	0	0	0	0	0
0	0	0	2	4	26	31	0	0.1	2	46	0.1	21	0.01	0	0.1	0.04	4	0
—	—	—	—	—	2	2	—	—	—	63	—	37	—	—	—	—	—	0
0	0.1	0	4	10	6	101	0.1	0.3	6	20	0.13	61	0.04	0.04	0.2	0.07	7	0
0	0.1	0	5	9	3	49	0	0.4	5	20	0.42	28	0.04	0.02	0.7	0.07	7	0
0	0.1	0	29	14	958	102	0.1	0.6	8	11	0.42	33	0.02	0.02	0.4	0.12	11	0
0	0.1	0	6	12	1	113	0.1	0.3	7	40	0.47	51	0.04	0.02	0.3	0.16	11	0
0	0.1	0	6	13	1	120	0.1	0.3	7	41	0.47	52	0.04	0.02	0.3	0.15	13	0
0	0.1	0	6	13	1	120	0.1	0.3	7	39	0.47	52	0.04	0.02	0.3	0.15	12	0
0	0.1	0	4	10	1	88	0.1	0.2	5	32	0.34	45	0.03	0.02	0.3	0.12	11	0
0	0.1	0	7	14	1	131	0.1	0.3	7	47	0.51	66	0.05	0.02	0.4	0.18	16	0
0	0.1	0	7	13	1	121	0.1	0.3	7	43	0.5	54	0.04	0.02	0.3	0.17	12	0
0	0.1	0	29	14	958	102	0.1	0.6	8	36	0.48	33	0.02	0.02	0.4	0.12	11	0
0	0.1	0	6	12	1	113	0.1	0.3	7	256	0.47	116	0.04	0.02	0.3	0.16	11	0
0	0.1	0	4	10	6	101	0.1	0.3	6	247	0.14	61	0.04	0.04	0.2	0.07	7	0
0	0.1	0	5	9	3	49	0	0.4	5	227	0.42	28	0.04	0.02	0.7	0.07	7	0
0	0.1	0	6	13	1	120	0.1	0.3	7	368	0.47	110	0.04	0.02	0.3	0.15	13	0
0	0.1	0	6	13	1	120	0.1	0.3	7	349	0.47	110	0.04	0.02	0.3	0.15	12	0
0	0.1	0	4	10	1	88	0.1	0.2	5	285	0.34	95	0.03	0.02	0.3	0.12	11	0
0	0.1	0	6	12	1	110	0.1	0.2	6	12	0.36	96	0.02	0.01	0.5	0.09	14	0
0	0.2	0	20	45	4	394	0.3	0.9	22	45	1.28	342	0.05	0.05	1.7	0.31	48	0
0	0	0	2	1	0	0	0	0.1	1	0	0.02	0	0	0	0	0	0	0
0	0.1	0	11	—	369	—	—	0.2	—	7	—	2	—	—	—	—	—	—
0	0.1	0	14	—	598	—	—	0.4	—	12	—	0	—	—	—	—	—	—
0	0	0	2	4	1	32	0	0.1	2	7	0.06	23	0.01	0.01	0.1	0.03	2	0
0	0.3	0	4	—	323	—	—	0.5	—	52	—	12	—	—	—	—	—	—
0	0.1	0	8	28	1	273	0.1	0.3	10	19	0.34	0	—	0.01	0.1	0.04	3	0
0.1	0.1	0	13	29	2	270	0.2	0.3	15	365	0.99	13	0.05	0.03	0.2	0.17	13	0
—	—	0	7	6	0	78	—	0.6	—	0	0.25	16	—	—	—	—	2	0
0.6	0.2	0	2	14	92	14	0.1	0.6	3	0	0.19	0	0.1	0.06	0.8	0.01	14	0
0.1	0	0	4	3	81	31	0	0.2	3	1	0.02	1	0	0	0	0	1	0
0	0	0	0	4	5	7	0	0.1	1	4	0.02	0	0	0	0	0	0	0
0	0	0	0	4	5	7	0	0.1	1	4	0.02	0	0	0	0	0	0	0
0	0.1	0	0	9	12	15	0	0.3	3	10	0.03	1	0	0.01	0	0.01	0	0
0	0	0	10	8	202	60	0	0.5	2	4	0.05	3	0	0.01	0	0	0	0
0	0	0	6	14	833	75	0.1	0.3	7	22	0.1	1	0.01	0.02	0	0.01	1	0
0	0	0	5	13	769	70	0.1	0.3	7	20	0.1	1	0.01	0.02	0	0.01	1	0
0	0	0	6	14	12	75	0.1	0.3	7	22	0.1	1	0.01	0.02	0	0.01	1	0
0	0	0	5	13	11	70	0.1	0.3	7	20	0.09	1	0.01	0.02	0	0.01	1	0
0.3	0.1	0	14	14	323	123	0.1	0.9	13	6	0.1	4	0	0.01	0	0.01	3	0
0	0	0	0	5	423	8	0	0.1	1	5	0.06	0	0	0	0	0	0	0
0	0.1	0	0	10	846	16	0	0.3	3	10	0.11	1	0	0.01	0	0.01	0	0
0	0	0	0	5	6	8	0	0.1	1	5	0.02	0	0	0	0	0	0	0
0	0.1	0	0	10	13	16	0	0.3	3	10	0.04	1	0	0.01	0	0.01	0	0
0	0	0	1	4	5	10	0	0.2	1	4	0.05	0	0	0.01	0.1	0	0	0
0	0	0	1	4	5	10	0	0.2	1	4	0.05	0	0	0.01	0.1	0	0	0
0	0	0	3	2	109	31	0	0.1	1	2	0.02	1	0	0	0	0	0	0
0	0	0	1	4	6	11	0	0.2	1	5	0.06	0	0	0.01	0.1	0	0	0
0	0.1	0	2	7	11	19	0	0.4	2	8	0.1	1	0	0.02	0.1	0.01	1	0
0	0	0	1	4	329	11	0	0.2	1	5	0.06	0	0	0.01	0.1	0	0	0
0	0.1	0	26	25	360	400	0.1	0.2	7	6	0.04	0	0.01	0.02	0.2	0.07	17	0

Food Item	Qty	Meas	Wgt (g)	Wtr (g)	Cals	Prot (g)	Carb (g)	Fib (g)	Fat (g)	SatF (g)
Pie crust, double, recipe, baked	1	each	320	31	1686	20	152	5.4	111	27.6
Pie crust, frozen, baked	1	piece	21	2	108	1	10	0.2	7	2.2
Pie crust, frozen, ready to bake	1	each	14	3	64	1	6	0.1	4	0.6
Pie crust, homemade, not baked, double	1	each	194	38	910	11	82	6.6	60	14.9
Pie crust, homemade, not baked, single	1	each	320	63	1500	18	135	10.9	99	24.5
Pie crust, mix, prepared, baked	1	each	180	19	902	12	91	3.2	55	13.9
Pie crust, single, recipe, baked	1	each	180	18	949	12	86	3	62	15.5
Pie filling, apple	1	cup	255	187	258	0	67	2.6	0	0.1
Pie filling, blueberry	1	cup	262	190	272	2	68	3.7	1	0.1
Pie filling, cherry	1	cup	264	184	304	1	77	1.6	1	0.1
Pie filling, cherry, low calorie	1	cup	264	208	211	2	51	1.6	2	0.4
Pie filling, lemon	1	cup	266	49	927	13	185	1.2	18	4.4
Pie filling, pumpkin, canned	0.5	cup	135	96	140	1	36	11.2	0	0.1
Pie, Boston cream, thaw'n serve, Mrs. Smith	1	piece	106	51	240	3	48	0.8	4	1.5
Pie, Plush Pippin, 9", apple	1	piece	126	—	350	2	41	2	21	4
Pie, Plush Pippin, 9", cherry	1	piece	120	—	340	3	45	1	22	4
Pie, Plush Pippin, chocolate creme	1	piece	124	—	280	4	36	1	14	4
Pie, Plush Pippin, lemon meringue	1	piece	119	—	250	2	41	0.5	9	2
Pie, Plush Pippin, pumpkin	1	piece	121	—	260	3	34	1	13	3
Pie, banana cream, mix, no bake, prepared	125	each	92	47	231	3	29	0.6	12	6.4
Pie, banana cream, mix, no bake, prepared	1	each	737	375	1849	25	233	4.6	95	50.9
Pie, blackberry, 1/5th pie, Banquet	1	piece	113	47	300	3	45	3	12	5
Pie, cheesecake	1	piece	92	42	295	5	24	0.4	21	9.1
Pie, cheesecake, chocolate	1	piece	128	37	501	8	48	1.9	32	15.5
Pie, cheesecake, no bake mix, prepared	1	piece	103	46	282	6	37	2	13	6.9
Pie, cheesecake, recipe	1	piece	128	52	457	9	32	0.5	33	18.4
Pie, cheesecake, triple chocolate, svg, Weight Watc	1	each	89	46	200	7	32	1	5	2.5
Pie, cheesecake, w/cherry topping, recipe	1	piece	142	70	408	7	38	0.6	26	14.5
Pie, cherry, fried, turnover	1	each	85	32	269	3	36	2.2	14	2.1
Pie, chocolate cream, individual	1	each	117	47	357	6	44	1.7	19	6.7
Pie, chocolate mousse, mix, no bake, prepared	125	each	95	47	247	3	28	—	15	7.8
Pie, chocolate mousse, mix, no bake, prepared	1	each	760	378	1976	27	225	—	117	62.3
Pie, coconut cream, mix, no bake, prepared	125	each	94	47	260	3	27	0.5	17	8.4
Pie, coconut cream, mix, no bake, prepared	1	each	754	375	2081	21	215	3.8	133	67.3
Pie, fried, apple, turnover	1	each	85	34	266	2	33	1.5	14	6.5
Pie, pecan, individual, Bama pie	1	each	85	14	366	4	45	1.4	20	3.4
Pimento/pimiento, canned	1	Tbs	12	11	3	0	1	0.2	0	0
Pimento/pimiento, canned slices	20	piece	20	19	5	0	1	0.4	0	0
Pine nut, pignola, dried	1	oz.	28	2	160	7	4	1.3	14	2.2
Pine nut, pinon, dried	1	oz.	28	2	178	3	5	3	17	2.7
Pineapple chunks, fresh	0.5	cup	78	67	38	0	10	0.9	0	0
Pineapple chunks, frozen, sweetened	0.5	cup	122	94	104	0	27	1.4	0	0
Pineapple grapefruit juice drink, canned	1	cup	250	220	118	0	29	0.2	0	0
Pineapple juice, canned, vit C, unsweetened	1	cup	250	214	140	1	34	0.5	0	0
Pineapple orange drink, canned	1	cup	250	217	125	3	30	0.2	0	0
Pineapple pieces in heavy syrup	0.5	cup	128	101	100	0	26	1	0	0
Pineapple rings in heavy syrup	1	each	58	46	45	0	12	0.5	0	0
Pineapple slices, fresh	1	piece	84	73	41	0	10	1	0	0
Pineapple, canned in juice	0.5	cup	125	104	75	1	20	1	0	0
Pineapple, canned in light syrup	0.5	cup	126	108	66	0	17	1	0	0
Pistachio nut, dried, meat	0.25	cup	32	1	185	7	8	3.5	16	2
Pistachio nut, dry roasted, salted	0.25	tsp	32	1	194	5	9	3.5	17	2.1
Pistachio nuts, dry roasted, unsalted	0.25	cup	32	1	194	5	9	3.5	17	2.1
Pitanga, raw	1	each	7	6	2	0	1	0.1	0	—
Pizza Hut, pizza, cheese, pan	2	piece	205	106	495	23	53	3.8	21	9.5
Pizza Hut, pizza, pepperoni, pan	2	piece	211	103	539	22	57	4.1	24	8.1
Pizza Hut, pizza, supreme, pan	2	piece	255	143	581	28	52	5.6	28	11.2
Pizza Hut, pizza, pepperoni, hand-tossed	2	piece	197	100	452	23	55	3.8	15	7.6
Pizza Hut, pizza, pepperoni, personal pan	1	each	256	128	639	27	69	5	28	10
Pizza Hut, pizza, supreme, personal pan	1	each	264	152	582	27	56	4.8	27	9.7
Pizza Hut, pizza, supreme, thin/crispy	2	piece	200	114	443	24	36	3.4	22	8.6
Pizza, deluxe, Tombstone	2	piece	250	131	597	28	54	3.7	30	13.1
Pizza, supreme, light, Tombstone	2	piece	276	—	540	50	60	4	18	7
Plantain chips	32	piece	35	1	180	1	20	2.7	12	10
Plantain slices, cooked	0.5	cup	77	52	89	1	24	1.8	0	0.1

MonoF (g)	PolyF (g)	Choles (mg)	Calc (mg)	Phos (mg)	Sod (mg)	Pot (mg)	Zn (mg)	Iron (mg)	Magn (mg)	VitA (μg RE)	VitE (mg α-TE)	VitC (mg)	Thia (mg)	Ribo (mg)	Nia (mg)	B6 (mg)	Fola (μg)	B12 (μg)
48.6	29.2	0	32	214	1734	214	1.4	9.2	45	0	17.7	0	1.25	0.89	10.6	0.08	214	0
3.3	0.8	0	4	12	136	23	0.1	0.5	4	0	1.07	0	0.06	0.08	0.5	0.02	8	0
1.7	1.5	0	3	7	81	14	0	0.3	2	0	0.74	0	0.04	0.05	0.3	0.01	10	0
26.2	15.8	0	18	116	935	114	0.8	5	23	0	4.93	0	0.68	0.48	5.7	0.04	122	0
43.2	26	0	29	192	1542	189	1.2	8.2	38	0	8.13	0	1.11	0.79	9.4	0.07	202	0
31.1	6.9	0	108	151	1312	112	0.7	3.9	27	0	9.94	0	0.55	0.34	4.3	0.1	22	0
27.4	16.4	0	18	121	976	121	0.8	5.2	25	0	9.94	0	0.7	0.5	6	0.04	121	0
0	0.1	0	10	18	112	115	0.1	0.7	5	3	0	3	0.03	0.03	0.1	0.04	0	0
0.1	0.3	0	13	26	68	97	0.2	1	10	16	2.45	3	0.08	0.13	0.3	0.08	5	0
0.2	0.2	0	29	40	24	277	0.1	0.6	18	55	0.58	10	0.07	0.04	0.4	0.1	11	0
1	0.7	0	24	21	24	201	0.2	0.6	13	53	0.58	4	0.03	0.08	0.4	0.08	11	0
7.3	4.2	349	58	177	216	198	1.1	2.2	16	284	3.31	28	0.18	0.53	1.2	0.15	38	0.67
0	0	0	50	61	281	186	0.4	1.4	22	1120	1.08	5	0.02	0.16	0.5	0.22	47	0
1.7	0.8	4	43	—	240	105	—	0.5	—	7	—	1	0.02	0.12	0.3	0.05	—	—
6	0.5	0	—	—	220	75	—	1.1	—	—	—	1	—	—	—	—	—	—
7	0.5	0	—	—	220	90	—	1.4	—	—	—	1	—	—	—	—	—	—
4	0	45	80	—	300	130	—	1.1	—	20	—	—	—	—	—	—	—	—
3	0	35	—	—	180	25	—	0.7	—	—	—	—	—	—	—	—	—	—
4	0	55	60	—	210	180	—	1.4	—	200	—	2	—	—	—	—	—	—
4.2	0.7	27	67	154	267	104	0.3	0.4	11	92	1.47	0	0.09	0.14	0.7	0.03	19	0.19
33.6	5.6	214	538	1230	2137	833	2.4	3.4	88	737	11.8	4	0.75	1.08	5.2	0.26	155	1.55
—	—	5	80	—	430	—	—	1.1	—	0	—	4	0.02	0.03	0.3	—	—	—
7.9	1.5	51	47	86	190	83	0.5	0.6	10	134	1.45	0	0.03	0.18	0.2	0.05	17	0.16
11	3.9	118	72	144	403	188	0.9	2.2	37	347	2.31	0	0.16	0.29	1.3	0.05	14	0.23
4.7	0.8	30	177	241	391	217	0.5	0.5	20	102	1.13	1	0.12	0.27	0.5	0.05	31	0.32
10.4	2.6	155	74	123	362	131	0.7	1.6	10	411	2.94	1	0.04	0.27	0.5	0.06	15	0.32
—	—	10	80	—	200	170	—	1.1	—	0	—	0	—	—	—	—	—	—
8.3	2.2	121	61	101	288	132	0.6	1.8	10	342	2.27	1	0.04	0.23	0.5	0.06	14	0.24
6.3	4.6	0	19	37	318	55	0.2	1	8	14	0.37	1	0.12	0.09	1.2	0.03	15	0.07
7.5	3.6	58	81	126	277	169	0.8	1.8	34	41	1.31	0	0.18	0.24	1.5	0.05	12	0.21
4.8	0.8	33	73	219	437	271	0.6	1	30	96	1.43	0	0.05	0.14	0.6	0.03	25	0.2
38.6	6.2	266	585	1755	3496	2166	4.6	8.2	243	768	11.4	4	0.39	1.12	4.5	0.22	198	1.6
6.2	1.2	22	68	159	310	133	0.4	0.4	16	94	1.41	1	0.03	0.1	0.1	0.04	14	0.2
49.4	9.2	173	543	1274	2480	1063	2.9	3	128	754	11.3	5	0.21	0.78	1	0.34	113	1.58
5.8	1.2	13	13	37	325	51	0.2	0.9	8	33	0.37	1	0.1	0.08	1	0.03	4	0.08
10.7	5.1	38	19	83	210	104	1	1.4	27	19	1.47	0	0.23	0.15	1.1	0.05	11	0.07
0	0	0	1	2	2	19	0	0.2	1	32	0.08	10	0	0.01	0.1	0.03	1	0
0	0	0	1	3	3	32	0	0.3	1	53	0.14	17	0	0.01	0.1	0.04	1	0
5.4	6	0	7	144	1	170	1.2	2.6	66	1	0.99	1	0.23	0.05	1	0.03	16	0
6.5	7.3	0	2	10	20	178	1.2	0.9	66	1	0.99	1	0.35	0.06	1.2	0.03	16	0
0	0.1	0	5	5	1	88	0.1	0.3	11	2	0.08	12	0.07	0.03	0.3	0.07	8	0
0	0	0	11	5	2	123	0.1	0.5	12	4	0.12	10	0.12	0.04	0.4	0.09	13	0
0	0.1	0	18	15	35	153	0.2	0.8	15	10	0	115	0.08	0.04	0.7	0.1	26	0
0	0.1	0	42	20	2	335	0.3	0.6	32	1	0.05	60	0.14	0.06	0.6	0.24	58	0
0	0	0	12	10	8	115	0.2	0.7	15	133	0	56	0.08	0.05	0.5	0.12	27	0
0	0.1	0	18	9	1	133	0.2	0.5	20	1	0.13	9	0.12	0.03	0.4	0.09	6	0
0	0	0	8	4	1	60	0.1	0.2	9	1	0.06	4	0.05	0.02	0.2	0.04	3	0
0	0.1	0	6	6	1	95	0.1	0.3	12	2	0.08	13	0.08	0.03	0.4	0.07	9	0
0	0	0	18	8	1	153	0.1	0.4	18	5	0.12	12	0.12	0.02	0.4	0.09	6	0
0	0	0	18	9	1	132	0.2	0.5	20	1	0.13	9	0.12	0.03	0.4	0.09	6	0
10.5	2.3	0	43	161	2	350	0.4	2.2	51	7	1.67	2	0.26	0.06	0.3	0.08	19	0
11.4	2.6	0	22	152	250	310	0.4	1	42	8	2.06	2	0.14	0.08	0.5	0.08	19	0
11.4	2.6	0	22	152	2	310	0.4	1	42	8	1.67	2	0.14	0.08	0.5	0.08	19	0
—	—	0	1	1	0	7	—	0	1	10	—	2	0	0	0	—	—	0
6.4	3.2	48	273	—	951	320	4.1	2.8	60	200	—	7	0.57	0.61	5.2	0.17	—	—
10.1	3.8	49	209	—	1156	405	4.2	3.2	56	193	—	8	0.63	0.49	5.4	0.16	0	—
11.2	3.9	56	219	—	1428	580	5.6	4.3	76	182	—	10	0.8	0.78	6	0.31	—	—
—	—	46	192	—	1307	578	5.7	3	80	177	—	12	0.68	0.53	7.2	—	—	—
11.8	4.5	55	251	—	1344	408	3.8	4	60	234	—	10	0.56	0.66	8.2	0.2	—	—
11.9	4.5	53	223	—	1419	487	3.8	4.2	60	194	—	11	0.59	0.66	8	0.32	—	—
—	—	54	205	—	1371	544	4.7	3.1	68	170	—	10	0.6	0.49	5.4	—	—	—
—	—	56	466	—	1194	—	—	2.7	—	187	—	17	—	—	—	—	—	—
—	—	40	800	—	1420	—	—	3.6	—	400	—	12	—	—	—	—	—	—
0.7	0.2	0	6	19	2	185	0.3	0.4	26	3	1.87	2	0.03	0.01	0.2	0.09	5	0
0	0	0	2	22	4	358	0.1	0.4	25	70	0.11	8	0.04	0.04	0.6	0.18	20	0

Food Item	Qty	Meas	Wgt (g)	Wtr (g)	Cals	Prot (g)	Carb (g)	Fib (g)	Fat (g)	SatF (g)
Plantain slices, raw	0.5	cup	74	48	90	1	24	1.7	0	0.1
Plantain, ripe, fried	0.5	cup	84	40	216	1	30	2.2	12	1.8
Plum slices, fresh	0.5	cup	82	70	45	1	11	1.2	1	0
Plum, fresh	1	each	66	56	36	1	9	1	0	0
Plum, purple, canned in light syrup	0.5	cup	126	105	79	0	20	1.3	0	0
Plums, canned in heavy syrup	0.5	cup	129	98	115	0	30	1.3	0	0
Plums, purple, canned in juice	0.5	cup	126	106	73	1	19	1.3	0	0
Pochito, frank w/chili in tortilla	1	each	122	72	268	9	22	3.3	16	5.9
Pokeberry shoots/poke greens, cooked	0.5	cup	78	72	16	2	2	1.2	0	0.1
Pokeberry shoots/poke greens, cooked, drained	0.5	cup	82	77	16	2	3	1.2	0	0.1
Pokeberry shoots/poke greens, raw	0.5	cup	80	73	18	2	3	1.4	0	0.1
Polenta, dry	1	piece	57	7	190	5	39	1.6	1	—
Pomegranate, raw (3.5-in. diameter)	1	each	154	125	105	1	26	0.9	0	0.1
Pop Tarts, raspberry frosted	1	each	52	6	210	2	37	1	6	1
Popcorn cake	1	each	10	0	38	1	8	0.3	0	0
Popcorn, air popped, plain	1	cup	8	0	31	1	6	1.2	0	0
Popcorn, caramel corn	1	cup	35	1	152	1	28	1.8	5	1.3
Popcorn, caramel-coated, w/peanuts, Cracker Jacks	1	oz.	28	1	113	2	23	1.1	2	0.3
Popcorn, cheese-flavored	1	cup	11	0	58	1	6	1.1	4	0.7
Popcorn, cooked in oil, salted	1	cup	11	0	55	1	6	1.1	3	0.5
Popcorn, microwave, lowfat, low sodium	1	cup	6	0	24	1	4	0.8	1	0.1
Popcorn, microwave, pop & serve bag	1	each	87	2	435	8	50	8.7	24	4.2
Popcorn, white, air-popped	1	cup	8	0	31	1	6	1.2	0	0
Popover mix, prepared, 2 x 2	1	each	33	18	67	3	10	0.3	1	0.4
Popover, homemade, w/2% milk	1	each	40	22	88	3	11	0.4	3	0.8
Popover, homemade, w/whole milk	1	each	54	29	122	5	15	0.4	5	1.4
Poppyseed	0.25	tsp	1	0	4	0	0	0.1	0	0
Popsicle/ice pop, double stick	1	each	128	102	92	0	24	0	0	0
Pork & beans, w/sweet sauce, canned	0.5	cup	126	89	140	7	27	6.6	2	0.7
Pork & beans, w/tomato sauce, canned	0.5	cup	126	92	124	7	24	6.1	1	0.5
Pork loin, top roast, prime, roasted, lean	1	piece	42	26	82	13	0	0	3	1.1
Pork skins/rinds, BBQ flavor	1	cup	32	1	172	18	1	—	10	3.7
Pork, blade chop, fried, lean & fat	1	each	89	44	304	19	0	0	25	9.1
Pork, chop, blade, fried, lean	1	each	62	37	149	15	0	0	9	3.2
Pork, chop, breaded, baked/broiled, lean	1	each	80	44	184	21	5	0.2	8	2.9
Pork, chop, center loin, fried, lean	1	each	67	38	155	22	0	0	7	2.4
Pork, chop, center loin, fried, lean & fat	1	each	89	47	247	27	0	0	15	5.4
Pork, chop, loin, broiled, lean	1	each	66	40	139	19	0	0	6	2.4
Pork, chop, loin, roasted, lean & fat	1	piece	42	24	104	11	0	0	6	2.3
Pork, chop, smoked/cured, cooked, lean	1	each	67	43	114	17	0	0	5	1.6
Pork, composite cuts, cooked, lean	4	oz.	113	68	240	33	0	0	11	3.9
Pork, loin, slice, roasted, lean	1	piece	42	26	88	12	0	0	4	1.5
Pork, loin, sparerib, braised, lean	4	oz.	113	67	265	30	0	0	15	5.6
Pork, rib, country style, roasted, lean	4	oz.	113	66	280	30	0	0	17	6
Pork, sausage link, cooked	1	each	13	6	48	3	0	0	4	1.4
Pork, sausage patty, cooked	1	each	27	12	100	5	0	0	8	2.9
Pork, shoulder, braised, lean	4	oz.	113	62	281	37	0	0	14	4.7
Pork, sirloin steak, broiled, lean	4	oz.	113	69	242	32	0	0	12	4.1
Pork, sparerib, braised, lean & fat	4	oz.	113	46	450	33	0	0	34	12.6
Pork, steak/cutlet, breaded, fried	4	oz.	113	56	325	26	10	0.6	20	6.2
Pork, tenderloin, roasted, lean & fat	4	oz.	113	74	196	32	0	0	7	2.4
Pork, tenderloin, tipless, roasted, lean	4	oz.	113	75	186	32	0	0	5	1.9
Potato chips	10	piece	20	0	107	1	11	0.9	7	2.2
Potato chips, BBQ flavor	20	piece	26	0	128	2	14	1.1	8	2.1
Potato chips, Pringles, can	1	each	198	3	1104	12	101	7.1	76	18.7
Potato chips, cheese flavor	1	cup	20	0	99	2	12	1	5	1.7
Potato chips, cheese, Pringles, can	1	each	191	4	1052	13	97	6.4	71	18.3
Potato chips, crushed	0.25	cup	14	0	75	1	7	0.6	5	1.5
Potato chips, grab bag	1	each	57	1	304	4	30	2.6	20	6.2
Potato chips, light	20	piece	40	0	188	3	27	2.3	8	1.7
Potato chips, light, Pringle, can	1	each	170	2	852	10	110	6.1	44	8.7
Potato chips, light, Pringle, can	1	oz.	28	0	142	2	18	1	7	1.4
Potato chips, no salt added	10	each	20	1	105	1	10	1	7	1.8
Potato chips, plain, unsalted	1	oz.	28	1	152	2	15	1.4	10	3.1
Potato chips, rippled	10	piece	30	1	161	2	16	1.4	10	3.3

MonoF (g)	PolyF (g)	Choles (mg)	Calc (mg)	Phos (mg)	Sod (mg)	Pot (mg)	Zn (mg)	Iron (mg)	Magn (mg)	VitA (μg RE)	VitE (mg α-TE)	VitC (mg)	Thia (mg)	Ribo (mg)	Nia (mg)	B6 (mg)	Fola (μg)	B12 (μg)
0	0.1	0	2	25	3	369	0.1	0.4	27	84	0.2	14	0.04	0.04	0.5	0.22	16	0
2.7	6.6	0	3	32	4	427	0.1	0.6	35	81	0.96	12	0.04	0.05	0.6	0.26	10	0
0.3	0.1	0	3	8	0	142	0.1	0.1	6	26	0.5	8	0.04	0.08	0.4	0.07	2	0
0.3	0.1	0	3	7	0	114	0.1	0.1	5	21	0.4	6	0.03	0.06	0.3	0.05	1	0
0.1	0	0	11	16	25	117	0.1	1.1	6	33	0.88	1	0.02	0.05	0.4	0.03	3	0
0.1	0	0	12	17	24	117	0.1	1.1	6	34	0.9	1	0.02	0.05	0.4	0.04	3	0
0	0	0	13	19	1	194	0.1	0.4	10	127	0.88	4	0.03	0.07	0.6	0.03	3	0
7.3	1.8	30	86	211	728	279	2	2.4	46	20	0.54	10	0.13	0.12	1.7	0.18	16	0.5
0	0.1	0	41	26	14	143	0.1	0.9	11	674	0.66	64	0.05	0.19	0.9	0.09	7	0
0	0.1	0	44	27	15	152	0.2	1	12	718	0.7	68	0.06	0.21	0.9	0.09	7	0
0	0.1	0	42	35	18	194	0.2	1.4	14	696	0.68	109	0.06	0.26	1	0.12	13	0
—	—	0	2	—	1	86	0.3	0.4	24	12	—	0	0.35	0.01	0.3	—	—	—
0.1	0.1	0	5	12	5	399	0.2	0.5	5	0	0.85	9	0.05	0.05	0.5	0.16	9	0
—	—	0	0	40	210	—	0.6	1.8	8	150	—	0	0.15	0.17	2	0.2	40	—
0.1	0.1	0	1	28	29	33	0.4	0.2	16	1	0.01	0	0.01	0.02	0.6	0.02	2	0
0.1	0.2	0	1	24	0	24	0.3	0.2	10	2	0.01	0	0.02	0.02	0.2	0.02	2	0
1	1.6	2	15	29	72	38	0.2	0.6	12	4	0.42	0	0.02	0.02	0.8	0.01	1	0
0.8	0.9	0	19	36	84	101	0.4	1.1	23	2	0.42	0	0.01	0.04	0.6	0.05	5	0
1.1	1.7	1	12	40	98	29	0.2	0.2	10	5	0.01	0	0.01	0.03	0.2	0.03	1	0.06
0.9	1.5	0	1	28	97	25	0.3	0.3	12	2	0.01	0	0.02	0.02	0.2	0.02	2	0
0.2	0.3	0	1	15	28	14	0.2	0.1	9	1	0.06	0	0.02	0.01	0.1	0.01	1	0
7.1	11.7	0	9	218	769	196	2.3	2.4	94	13	0.1	0	0.12	0.12	1.4	0.18	15	0
0.1	0.2	0	1	24	0	24	0.3	0.2	10	0	0.01	0	0.02	0.02	0.2	0.02	2	0
0.6	0.2	37	9	30	143	25	0.2	0.6	5	16	0.36	0	0.05	0.06	0.4	0.02	6	0.08
0.9	1	46	38	56	82	65	0.3	0.8	7	34	0.43	0	0.09	0.15	0.7	0.03	7	0.13
1.3	1.4	64	50	75	110	87	0.4	1	10	37	0.2	0	0.12	0.2	1	0.04	10	0.18
0	0.2	0	11	6	0	5	0.1	0.1	2	0	0.02	0	0.01	0	0	0	0	0
0	0	0	0	0	15	5	0	0	1	0	0	0	0	0	0	0	0	0
0.8	0.2	9	77	133	425	336	1.9	2.1	43	14	0.68	4	0.06	0.08	0.4	0.11	47	0
0.6	0.2	9	71	148	557	380	7.4	4.2	44	15	0.68	4	0.07	0.06	0.6	0.09	28	0
1.4	0.2	33	2	93	19	149	1	0.4	10	1	0.15	0	0.27	0.13	2.2	0.17	4	0.23
4.8	1.1	37	14	70	853	58	0.2	0.3	0	58	—	0	0.03	0.14	1.1	0.05	10	0.04
10.4	2.8	76	27	183	60	295	2.8	0.8	19	3	0.23	1	0.55	0.26	3.5	0.3	4	0.75
3.9	1.2	51	14	137	48	226	2.4	0.7	16	1	0.16	0	0.45	0.22	2.8	0.25	2	0.6
3.7	0.9	57	17	197	333	331	1.8	0.8	22	1	0.36	1	0.68	0.25	4	0.36	5	0.52
3	0.9	62	15	182	58	301	1.6	0.7	21	1	0.17	1	0.83	0.22	4	0.34	4	0.51
6.3	1.7	82	24	231	71	378	2.1	0.8	26	2	0.23	1	1.01	0.27	5	0.42	5	0.65
2.9	0.5	52	11	167	42	289	1.6	0.6	19	1	0.17	0	0.61	0.22	3.5	0.32	4	0.48
2.7	0.5	34	8	102	25	171	1	0.4	11	1	0.11	0	0.42	0.13	2.3	0.22	3	0.3
2.2	0.5	32	7	163	825	196	2	0.7	11	0	0.17	0	0.49	0.15	3.2	0.25	3	0.74
4.9	0.9	98	24	269	67	425	3.4	1.2	30	2	0.3	0	0.96	0.39	5.9	0.49	7	0.85
1.8	0.3	34	8	105	24	179	1.1	0.5	12	1	0.11	0	0.43	0.14	2.5	0.23	3	0.31
6.7	1.2	98	28	191	71	391	4.5	1.6	20	2	0.5	1	0.62	0.32	4.6	0.41	3	0.84
7.3	1.2	105	33	251	33	396	4.3	1.5	27	2	0.55	0	0.65	0.39	5.3	0.5	6	0.91
2	0.4	11	4	24	168	47	0.3	0.2	2	0	0.03	0	0.1	0.03	0.6	0.04	0	0.23
4.2	0.8	22	9	50	349	98	0.7	0.3	5	0	0.07	0	0.2	0.07	1.2	0.09	1	0.47
6.6	1.3	129	9	256	116	459	5.6	2.2	25	2	0.3	0	0.68	0.41	6.7	0.46	6	0.8
5	1	96	15	291	82	455	3.1	1.2	35	2	0.3	1	1.17	0.42	5.4	0.68	6	0.9
15.3	3.1	137	53	296	105	363	5.2	2.1	27	3	0.3	0	0.46	0.43	6.2	0.4	5	1.22
7.7	3.7	109	44	233	458	343	3.3	1.7	28	15	0.71	1	0.77	0.4	4.4	0.38	11	0.86
2.8	0.6	90	7	291	62	491	3	1.6	31	2	0.3	0	1.05	0.44	5.3	0.47	7	0.62
2.2	0.5	90	7	294	64	496	3	1.7	32	2	0.3	0	1.07	0.44	5.3	0.48	7	0.62
2	2.4	0	5	33	119	255	0.2	0.3	13	0	0.98	6	0.03	0.04	0.8	0.13	9	0
1.7	4.3	0	13	48	195	328	0.2	0.5	20	6	1.3	9	0.06	0.06	1.2	0.16	22	0
14.4	39.6	0	48	311	1298	1995	1.2	3	115	0	9.66	16	0.41	0.24	6.2	0.29	14	0
1.5	1.9	1	14	60	159	306	0.2	0.4	15	2	0.98	11	0.03	0.03	1	0.07	0	0
13.6	35.7	8	210	311	1442	728	1.2	3.1	101	0	9.32	16	0.34	0.23	5	1	34	0
1.4	1.7	0	3	23	83	179	0.2	0.2	9	0	0.68	4	0.02	0.03	0.5	0.09	6	0
5.6	6.9	0	14	94	337	723	0.6	0.9	38	0	2.77	18	0.1	0.11	2.2	0.37	26	0
1.9	4.4	0	8	77	197	698	0	0.5	36	0	1.16	10	0.08	0.11	2.8	0.27	11	0
10.1	23	0	58	262	728	1708	1	2.6	107	0	8.5	20	0.32	0.1	7.1	1.33	39	0
1.7	3.8	0	10	44	121	285	0.2	0.4	18	0	1.42	3	0.05	0.02	1.2	0.22	7	0
1.2	3.6	0	5	31	2	260	0.2	0.2	12	0	0.86	8	0.03	0	0.8	0.1	9	0
2.8	3.5	0	7	47	2	361	0.3	0.5	19	0	1.38	9	0.05	0.06	1.1	0.19	13	0
3	3.7	0	7	50	178	383	0.3	0.5	20	0	1.46	9	0.05	0.06	1.2	0.2	14	0

A

Food Item	Qty	Meas	Wgt (g)	Wtr (g)	Cals	Prot (g)	Carb (g)	Fib (g)	Fat (g)	SatF (g)
Potato chips, sour cream & onion	1	oz.	28	1	151	2	15	1.5	10	2.5
Potato chips, sour cream & onion, Pringles, can	1	each	191	4	1044	13	98	2.3	71	18.1
Potato pancake, large	1	each	76	36	207	5	22	1.5	12	2.3
Potato pieces, canned, drained	0.5	cup	90	76	54	1	12	2.1	0	0
Potato salad w/mayonnaise & eggs	0.5	cup	125	95	179	3	14	1.6	10	1.8
Potato salad, German	0.5	cup	88	68	79	2	15	1.4	2	0.6
Potato skin, cooked	1	each	34	26	26	1	6	1.1	0	0
Potato skin, microwave cooked	1	each	58	37	77	3	17	3.2	0	0
Potato skin, oven baked	1	each	58	27	115	2	27	4.6	0	0
Potato skins, chips, Tato Skins	10	piece	20	0	112	1	10	0.7	7	1.9
Potato, Tater Tots, frozen, oven heated	10	each	70	37	155	2	21	2.2	7	3.6
Potato, au gratin, prep from dry mix	0.5	cup	122	97	114	3	16	1.1	5	3.2
Potato, au gratin, recipe, w/margarine	0.5	cup	122	91	162	6	14	2.2	9	4.3
Potato, baked, flesh only, medium size	1	each	122	92	113	2	26	1.8	0	0
Potato, boiled in skin, peeled after, diced	0.5	cup	78	60	68	1	16	1.4	0	0
Potato, boiled, peeled after	1	each	136	105	118	3	27	2.4	0	0
Potato, canned, 1 in diam, drained	2	each	70	59	42	1	10	1.6	0	0
Potato, cottage fries, frozen, oven heated	10	each	50	26	109	2	17	1.6	4	2
Potato, flesh, raw, diced	0.5	cup	75	59	59	2	14	1.2	0	0
Potato, french fried, veg oil, reg svg	1	each	76	31	232	3	29	2.7	11	2
Potato, french fries, frozen, oven heated	10	piece	50	18	167	2	20	1.6	9	3
Potato, french fries, frozen, restaurant fried	10	each	50	19	158	2	20	1.6	8	1.9
Potato, french fries, fried in animal & veg oil	10	each	50	19	158	2	20	1.6	8	1.9
Potato, hash browns-fast food serving	1	each	65	39	137	2	15	—	8	3.9
Potato, hashed brown patty, frozen, fried	1	each	66	37	144	2	18	1.3	8	3
Potato, hashed brown w/butter sauce, frozen, cooked	0.5	cup	72	46	129	2	18	2.8	6	2.4
Potato, hashed browns, frozen, cooked	0.5	cup	78	44	170	2	22	1.6	9	3.5
Potato, mashed w/milk & margarine	0.5	cup	105	80	111	2	18	2.1	4	1.1
Potato, mashed w/whole milk	0.5	cup	105	82	81	2	18	2.1	1	0.4
Potato, mashed w/whole milk & butter	0.5	cup	105	80	111	2	18	2.1	4	2.9
Potato, mashed, flakes prep w/milk & butter	0.5	cup	105	80	119	2	16	2.4	6	3.6
Potato, mashed, flakes prep w/whole milk & margarine	0.5	cup	110	84	124	2	16	2.5	6	1.6
Potato, mashed, granules w/whole milk & butter	0.5	cup	105	81	113	2	15	2.3	5	3.2
Potato, microwaved w/skin, flesh only, medium size	1	each	92	68	92	2	21	1.5	0	0
Potato, o'brien, frozen, cooked	0.5	cup	97	60	198	2	21	1.6	13	3.2
Potato, o'brien, recipe	0.5	cup	97	77	79	2	15	1	1	0.8
Potato, peeled, boiled, diced	0.5	cup	78	60	67	1	16	1.4	0	0
Potato, peeled, boiled, whole	1	each	135	105	116	2	27	2.4	0	0
Potato, prepared mix, Twice Baked	0.5	cup	118	54	324	8	33	2.7	18	9
Potato, scalloped, prep from dry mix	0.5	cup	122	97	114	3	16	1.4	5	3.2
Potato, scalloped, recipe w/margarine	0.5	cup	122	99	105	4	13	2.3	5	1.7
Potato, small, whole, frozen, cooked	1	each	70	58	46	1	10	1	0	0
Potato, w/skin, medium size, baked	1	each	122	87	133	3	31	2.9	0	0
Potato, w/skin, medium size, microwaved	1	each	93	67	98	2	22	2.1	0	0
Potato, white, roasted	1	each	93	58	132	3	30	2.7	0	0
Potato, whole, canned w/liquid	0.5	cup	150	132	66	2	15	2.1	0	0
Potato, whole, raw, flesh only	1	each	112	88	88	2	20	1.8	0	0
Poultry seasoning	0.25	tsp	0	0	1	0	0	0	0	0
Power bar	1	each	65	—	230	10	45	3	2	—
Power bar, mocha	1	each	65	7	230	10	45	3	2	1
Power bar, apple cinnamon	1	each	65	7	230	10	45	3	2	0.5
Pretzel, hard twist, unenriched, unsalted	10	each	60	2	229	5	48	1.7	2	0.4
Pretzel, hard, twist	10	each	60	2	229	5	48	1.9	2	0.4
Pretzel, hard, whole wheat	1	oz.	28	1	103	3	23	2.2	1	0.2
Pretzel, soft	1	each	55	8	190	5	38	0.9	2	0.7
Pretzel, sticks	10	each	5	0	19	0	4	0.2	0	0
Pretzel, thick Dutch twist	1	each	16	1	61	1	13	0.5	1	0.1
Pretzel, yogurt-covered	6	each	25	1	115	2	17	0.2	5	3.6
Pretzels, cheddar, Combos snack	10	piece	30	1	139	3	20	—	5	—
Prickly pear fruit, raw	1	each	103	90	42	1	10	3.7	1	0.1
Prunes, canned in heavy syrup	0.5	cup	117	83	123	1	32	4.4	0	0
Prunes, dried	10	each	84	27	201	2	53	6	0	0
Prunes, dry, stewed, no sugar added	0.5	cup	106	74	113	1	30	7	0	0
Pudding pop, chocolate	1	each	47	30	72	2	12	0.2	2	2.1
Pudding pop, vanilla	1	each	47	30	75	2	13	0	2	2.1

MonoF	PolyF	Choles	Calc	Phos	Sod	Pot	Zn	Iron	Magn	VitA	VitE	VitC	Thia	Ribo	Nia	B6	Fola	B12
(g)	(g)	(mg)	(mg)	(mg)	(mg)	(mg)	(mg)	(mg)	(mg)	(μg RE)	(mg α-TE)	(mg)	(mg)	(mg)	(mg)	(mg)	(μg)	(μg)
1.7	4.9	2	20	50	177	377	0.3	0.5	21	6	1.38	11	0.05	0.06	1.1	0.19	18	0.28
13.6	35.9	6	122	323	1375	947	1.4	2.7	105	187	9.32	18	0.34	0.19	4.8	0.91	44	0
3.5	5	73	18	84	386	597	0.6	1.2	25	11	1.52	17	0.1	0.13	1.6	0.29	12	0.14
0	0.1	0	4	25	197	206	0.3	1.1	13	0	0.04	5	0.06	0.01	0.8	0.17	6	0
3.1	4.7	85	24	65	661	318	0.4	0.8	19	41	2.33	12	0.1	0.08	1.1	0.18	8	0
0.7	0.2	3	7	42	201	277	0.3	0.3	18	1	0.07	10	0.09	0.02	1.1	0.21	9	0.05
0	0	0	15	18	5	138	0.2	2.1	10	0	0.01	2	0.01	0.01	0.4	0.08	3	0
0	0	0	27	48	9	377	0.3	3.4	22	0	0.02	9	0.04	0.04	1.3	0.28	10	0
0	0	0	20	59	12	332	0.3	4.1	25	0	0.02	8	0.07	0.06	1.8	0.36	12	0
1.2	3.9	0	5	31	131	202	0.1	0.3	12	0	0.98	2	0.04	0.02	0.6	0.03	1	0
3	0.6	0	21	34	522	266	0.2	1.1	13	1	0.04	5	0.14	0.05	1.5	0.16	12	0
1.4	0.2	18	102	116	538	268	0.3	0.4	18	38	1.47	4	0.02	0.1	1.2	0.05	8	0
3.2	1.3	18	146	138	530	485	0.8	0.8	24	47	0.65	12	0.08	0.14	1.2	0.21	14	0
0	0.1	0	6	61	6	477	0.4	0.4	30	0	0.05	16	0.13	0.03	1.7	0.37	11	0
0	0	0	4	34	3	296	0.2	0.2	17	0	0.04	10	0.08	0.02	1.1	0.23	8	0
0	0.1	0	7	60	5	515	0.4	0.4	30	0	0.07	18	0.14	0.03	2	0.41	14	0
0	0.1	0	4	20	153	160	0.2	0.9	10	0	0.04	4	0.05	0.01	0.6	0.13	4	0
1.7	0.3	0	5	32	22	240	0.2	0.7	11	0	0.1	5	0.06	0.02	1.2	0.12	8	0
0	0	0	5	34	4	407	0.3	0.6	16	0	0.04	15	0.07	0.03	1.1	0.2	10	0
5	2.8	0	11	98	150	524	0.4	0.6	30	0	0.93	9	0.06	0.03	2.2	0.27	29	0
5.6	0.7	0	6	48	307	270	0.2	0.8	12	0	0.25	3	0.04	0.02	1.3	0.11	11	0
4.7	0.7	0	10	46	108	366	0.2	0.4	17	0	0.25	5	0.09	0.01	1.6	0.12	14	0
4.7	0.7	6	10	46	108	366	0.2	0.4	17	0	0.25	5	0.09	0.01	1.6	0.12	14	0
3.5	0.4	8	6	62	262	241	0.2	0.4	14	3	0.11	5	0.07	0.01	1	0.15	7	0.01
3.4	0.9	0	10	48	22	288	0.2	1	11	0	0.12	4	0.07	0.01	1.6	0.08	4	0
2.3	1.3	17	24	28	73	237	0.2	0.7	11	12	0.1	3	0.04	0.02	1	0.19	10	0
4	1	0	12	56	26	340	0.2	1.2	13	0	0.15	5	0.09	0.02	1.9	0.1	5	0
1.9	1.3	2	27	48	310	303	0.3	0.3	19	21	0.32	6	0.09	0.04	1.1	0.24	8	0
0.2	0.1	2	27	50	318	314	0.3	0.3	19	6	0.05	7	0.09	0.04	1.2	0.24	9	0
1.2	0.2	13	27	48	310	303	0.3	0.3	19	21	0.32	6	0.09	0.04	1.1	0.24	8	0
1.7	0.3	15	52	59	349	245	0.2	0.2	19	22	0.73	10	0.12	0.05	0.7	0.01	8	0.08
2.5	1.7	4	54	62	365	256	0.2	0.2	20	23	0.77	11	0.12	0.06	0.7	0.01	8	0
1.5	0.2	15	37	63	270	151	0.3	0.2	20	20	0.03	6	0.08	0.08	0.8	0.01	8	0
0	0	0	5	100	6	378	0.3	0.4	23	0	0.04	14	0.12	0.02	1.5	0.29	11	0
5.6	3.4	0	19	90	42	459	0.5	0.9	33	18	0.18	10	0.05	0.13	1.4	0.37	12	0
0.3	0.1	4	35	48	210	258	0.3	0.5	18	55	0.12	16	0.07	0.05	1	0.21	8	0
0	0	0	6	31	4	256	0.2	0.2	16	0	0.04	6	0.08	0.02	1	0.21	7	0
0	0.1	0	11	54	7	443	0.4	0.4	27	0	0.07	10	0.13	0.03	1.8	0.36	12	0
6.5	1.3	155	83	153	936	515	0.7	0.8	34	155	1.38	25	0.34	0.26	2.2	0.32	23	0.36
1.5	0.2	14	44	69	418	249	0.3	0.5	17	26	0.18	4	0.02	0.07	1.3	0.05	12	0
1.6	0.9	7	70	77	410	463	0.5	0.7	23	23	0.4	13	0.08	0.11	1.3	0.22	14	0
0	0	0	5	18	14	201	0.2	0.6	8	0	0.04	7	0.07	0.02	0.9	0.14	6	0
0	0.1	0	12	70	10	510	0.4	1.7	33	0	0.06	16	0.13	0.04	2	0.42	13	0
0	0	0	10	98	7	416	0.3	1.2	25	0	0.05	14	0.11	0.03	1.6	0.32	11	0
0	0.1	0	12	77	10	905	0.6	1.3	35	0	0.1	26	0.12	0.06	2.4	0.41	19	0
0	0.1	0	58	33	326	308	0.6	1.1	21	0	0.06	11	0.05	0.03	1.3	0.21	7	0
0	0	0	8	52	7	608	0.4	0.9	24	0	0.07	22	0.1	0.04	1.7	0.29	14	0
0	0	0	3	1	0	2	0	0.1	1	1	0	0	0	0	0	0	0	0
—	—	0	300	350	110	150	5.2	5.4	140	—	—	60	1.5	1.7	20	2	400	6
1	0.5	0	300	350	90	145	5.2	6.3	140	0	20	60	1.5	1.7	20	2	400	6
1.5	0.5	0	300	350	90	110	5.2	6.3	140	0	20	60	1.5	1.7	20	2	400	6
0.8	0.7	0	22	68	173	88	0.5	1	21	0	0.13	0	0.11	0.06	1.2	0.07	50	0
0.8	0.7	0	22	68	1029	88	0.5	2.6	21	0	0.13	0	0.28	0.37	3.2	0.07	103	0
0.3	0.2	0	8	35	58	122	0.2	0.8	9	0	0.07	0	0.12	0.08	1.8	0.08	15	0
0.8	0.2	2	13	44	772	48	0.5	2.2	12	0	0.02	0	0.23	0.16	2.4	0.01	8	0
0.1	0.1	0	2	6	86	7	0	0.2	2	0	0.01	0	0.02	0.03	0.3	0.01	9	0
0.2	0.2	0	6	18	274	23	0.1	0.7	6	0	0.03	0	0.07	0.1	0.8	0.02	27	0
0.5	0.1	1	37	36	16	60	0.2	0.4	5	19	0.17	0	0.08	0.09	0.7	0.01	4	0.12
—	—	2	59	43	335	39	0.2	0.3	7	2	0.06	0	0.09	0.17	1	0.01	2	0.04
0.1	0.2	0	58	25	5	227	0.1	0.3	88	5	0.01	14	0.01	0.06	0.5	0.06	6	0
0.2	0	0	20	30	4	264	0.2	0.5	18	94	0.29	3	0.04	0.14	1	0.24	0	0
0.3	0.1	0	43	66	3	626	0.4	2.1	38	167	1.22	3	0.07	0.14	1.6	0.22	3	0
0.2	0.1	0	24	37	2	354	0.3	1.2	21	33	0	3	0.02	0.11	0.8	0.23	0	0
0	0	1	66	53	78	105	0.2	0.2	10	16	0.01	0	0.02	0.08	0.1	0.02	1	0.25
0	0	1	61	48	50	65	0.2	0	5	24	0.01	0	0.02	0.09	0	0.02	2	0.17

Food Item	Qty	Meas	Wgt (g)	Wtr (g)	Cals	Prot (g)	Carb (g)	Fib (g)	Fat (g)	SatF (g)
Pudding, banana, instant w/2% milk	0.5	cup	147	110	153	4	29	0	2	1.5
Pudding, banana, instant w/whole milk	0.5	cup	147	108	166	4	29	0	4	2.6
Pudding, banana, mix w/whole milk	0.5	cup	140	104	157	4	25	0	4	2.6
Pudding, banana, regular w/2% milk	0.5	cup	140	106	143	4	26	0	2	1.5
Pudding, bread, w/raisins	0.5	cup	126	79	212	7	31	1.3	7	2.9
Pudding, chocolate, instant w/2% milk	0.5	cup	147	110	150	5	28	0.6	3	1.6
Pudding, chocolate, instant w/whole milk	0.5	cup	147	108	163	5	28	1.5	5	2.7
Pudding, chocolate, recipe w/2% milk	0.5	cup	157	106	206	5	40	1.4	4	2
Pudding, chocolate, reg mix w/whole milk	0.5	cup	142	106	158	5	26	1.4	5	3
Pudding, chocolate, regular w/2% milk	0.5	cup	142	105	151	5	28	0.4	3	1.8
Pudding, chocolate, w/whole milk, recipe	0.5	cup	157	105	221	5	40	1.3	6	3.1
Pudding, coconut cream, instant w/2% milk	0.5	cup	147	109	157	4	28	0.1	3	2
Pudding, coconut cream, reg w/2% milk	0.5	cup	140	106	146	4	25	0.3	4	2.5
Pudding, coconut, instant w/whole milk	0.5	cup	147	108	172	4	28	0.1	5	3.1
Pudding, lemon, instant w/2% milk	0.5	cup	147	109	154	4	30	0	2	1.5
Pudding, lemon, instant w/whole milk	0.5	cup	147	108	169	4	30	0	4	2.6
Pudding, lemon, mix+sugar+egg yolk+water	0.5	cup	146	106	164	1	36	0	2	0.6
Pudding, low cal mix w/milk, D-Zerta	0.5	cup	130	110	88	4	12	0	2	1.5
Pudding, low calorie mix w/milk, D-Zerta	0.5	cup	125	108	60	5	11	1	0	0
Pudding, rice w/raisins, recipe	0.5	cup	152	101	217	5	40	0.8	4	2.6
Pudding, rice, mix w/2% milk	0.5	cup	144	105	161	5	30	0.1	2	1.4
Pudding, rice, mix w/whole milk, cooked	0.5	cup	144	104	176	5	30	0.1	4	2.5
Pudding, tapioca, mix w/2% milk	0.5	cup	141	105	147	4	28	0	2	1.5
Pudding, tapioca, reg mix w/whole milk	0.5	cup	141	104	161	4	28	0	4	2.5
Pudding, tapioca, w/whole milk, recipe	0.5	cup	82	60	103	4	14	0	4	1.8
Pudding, vanilla, fat free, snack size, Jell-o	1	each	113	87	100	2	23	0	0	0
Pudding, vanilla, instant w/2% milk	0.5	cup	142	106	148	4	28	0	2	1.4
Pudding, vanilla, instant w/whole milk	0.5	cup	142	104	162	4	28	0	4	2.5
Pudding, vanilla, reg mix w/2% milk	0.5	cup	140	106	141	4	26	0	2	1.5
Pudding, vanilla, reg mix w/whole milk	0.5	cup	140	104	155	4	26	0	4	2.6
Pudding, vanilla, w/whole milk, recipe	0.5	cup	123	94	130	4	20	0	4	2.5
Puff pastry, frozen	1	each	47	4	259	3	21	0.7	18	4.5
Puff pastry, frozen, baked	1	each	40	3	223	3	18	0.6	15	2.2
Pummelo, raw sections	0.5	cup	95	85	36	1	9	1	0	—
Pumpkin leaves, cooked	0.5	cup	35	32	7	1	1	0.9	0	0
Pumpkin leaves, raw	0.5	cup	20	19	4	1	0	0.2	0	0
Pumpkin pie spice	0.25	tsp	0	0	2	0	0	0.1	0	0
Pumpkin seed kernel, dry roasted, unsalted	0.25	cup	34	2	187	8	6	1.4	16	3
Pumpkin seed kernels, roasted, salted	0.25	cup	57	4	296	19	8	2.2	24	4.5
Pumpkin seed kernels, roasted, unsalted	0.25	cup	57	4	296	19	8	2.2	24	4.5
Pumpkin seeds, roasted, salted	0.25	cup	16	1	71	3	9	0.8	3	0.6
Pumpkin turnover	1	each	78	41	198	4	20	1.3	11	3.5
Pumpkin, canned, low sodium	0.5	cup	123	111	42	1	10	3.6	0	0.2
Pumpkin, fresh, cooked	0.5	cup	122	115	24	1	6	1.4	0	0
Quesadilla	1	each	54	16	199	6	21	1.2	10	3.6
Quiche Lorraine, 1/8th pie	1	piece	176	95	508	20	20	0.6	39	17.6
Rabbit, domestic, roasted	4	oz.	113	69	223	33	0	0	9	2.7
Radicchio leaf, raw	10	each	80	74	18	1	4	0.7	0	0
Radicchio, raw, shredded	0.5	cup	20	19	5	0	1	0.2	0	0
Radish, Daikon/Chinese, cooked slices	0.5	cup	74	70	12	0	3	1.2	0	0.1
Radish, red	10	each	45	43	9	0	2	0.7	0	0
Radish, red, slices	0.5	cup	58	55	12	0	2	0.9	0	0
Radish, white icicle, raw slices	0.5	cup	50	48	7	1	1	0.7	0	0
Radish, white icicle, raw, whole	3	each	51	49	7	1	1	0.7	0	0
Radishes, Chinese/Daikon, slices, raw	0.5	cup	44	42	8	0	2	0.7	0	0
Radishes, Daikon/Chinese, whole, raw	1	each	338	320	61	2	14	5.4	0	0.1
Raisin, seedless, packed	0.5	cup	82	13	248	3	65	3.3	0	0.1
Raisin, seedless, unpacked	0.5	cup	72	11	218	2	57	2.9	0	0.1
Raisins, golden seedless, packed	0.5	cup	82	12	249	3	66	3.3	0	0.1
Raspberries, canned in heavy syrup	0.5	cup	128	96	116	1	30	4.2	0	0
Raspberries, fresh	0.5	cup	62	53	30	1	7	4.2	0	0
Raspberries, frozen, sweetened	10	oz.	284	207	293	2	74	12.5	0	0
Ravioli, cheese-filled, w/tomato sauce, serving	1	each	250	178	336	14	38	2.2	14	6.3
Ravioli, meat filled	0.5	cup	125	85	194	10	18	1.3	9	3
Refried beans/frijoles, w/cheese	8	oz.	167	115	225	11	29	—	8	4.1

MonoF	PolyF	Choles	Calc	Phos	Sod	Pot	Zn	Iron	Magn	VitA	VitE	VitC	Thia	Ribo	Nia	B6	Fola	B12
(g)	(g)	(mg)	(mg)	(mg)	(mg)	(mg)	(mg)	(mg)	(mg)	(μg RE)	(mg α-TE)	(mg)	(mg)	(mg)	(mg)	(mg)	(μg)	(μg)
0.7	0.2	9	150	318	435	193	0.5	0.1	18	66	0.07	1	0.05	0.2	0.1	0.05	6	0.44
1.2	0.2	16	147	315	434	188	0.5	0.1	18	37	0.07	1	0.05	0.2	0.1	0.05	6	0.44
1.2	0.2	17	151	116	231	189	0.5	0.1	18	38	0.07	1	0.04	0.2	0.1	0.05	6	0.35
0.7	0.1	10	154	118	232	193	0.5	0.1	18	70	0.07	1	0.04	0.2	0.1	0.05	6	0.36
2.7	1.2	83	144	137	291	282	0.7	1.4	24	82	0.63	1	0.12	0.28	0.8	0.09	16	0.33
0.9	0.2	9	153	353	417	247	0.6	0.4	26	56	0.15	1	0.05	0.21	0.1	0.06	6	0.46
1.4	0.3	16	150	351	417	244	0.6	0.4	26	31	0.09	1	0.05	0.21	0.1	0.06	6	0.44
1.3	0.4	9	155	149	138	256	0.8	0.7	39	78	0.11	1	0.05	0.22	0.2	0.05	6	0.36
1.4	0.2	17	158	132	146	231	0.6	0.5	21	37	0.08	1	0.04	0.25	0.1	0.05	6	0.36
0.8	0.1	10	160	138	149	240	0.7	0.5	30	68	0.08	1	0.04	0.21	0.2	0.05	6	0.36
1.8	0.5	17	152	148	137	253	0.8	0.7	38	49	0.14	1	0.05	0.22	0.2	0.05	6	0.34
0.9	0.3	9	150	295	362	194	0.5	0.2	21	69	0.06	1	0.05	0.2	0.1	0.06	6	0.44
0.7	0.1	10	158	125	228	223	0.5	0.3	22	70	0.1	1	0.04	0.2	0.1	0.2	6	0.36
1.4	0.4	16	147	294	362	190	0.5	0.2	21	37	0.09	1	0.05	0.2	0.1	0.05	6	0.44
0.7	0.1	9	148	304	394	190	0.5	0.1	16	69	0.07	1	0.05	0.2	0.1	0.05	6	0.44
1.2	0.2	16	146	301	392	187	0.5	0.1	16	38	0.07	1	0.05	0.2	0.1	0.05	6	0.44
0.7	0.2	77	12	31	93	7	0.2	0.3	3	35	0.07	0	0.01	0.05	0	0.02	9	0.19
0.7	0.1	9	151	211	303	191	0.5	0.1	18	70	0.09	1	0.05	0.2	0.1	0.05	6	0.45
0	0	0	150	210	65	290	0.5	0.4	27	40	0.09	1	0.05	0.2	0.1	0.05	6	0.42
1.2	0.2	17	155	143	85	269	0.7	1	24	38	0.08	1	0.12	0.21	0.8	0.08	6	0.24
0.6	0.1	9	151	127	158	190	0.6	0.5	19	52	0.06	1	0.11	0.2	0.6	0.05	6	0.36
1.2	0.2	16	148	124	157	186	0.5	0.5	19	29	0.09	1	0.11	0.2	0.6	0.05	6	0.35
0.7	0.1	8	149	117	172	189	0.5	0.1	17	69	0.07	1	0.04	0.2	0.1	0.06	6	0.35
1.2	0.2	17	147	116	171	186	0.5	0.1	17	38	0.11	1	0.04	0.2	0.1	0.05	6	0.35
1.2	0.3	68	86	87	157	117	0.4	0.3	11	47	0.07	0	0.03	0.18	0.1	0.04	7	0.3
0	0	0	80	—	240	125	—	0	—	20	—	0	—	—	—	—	—	—
0.7	0.1	9	146	283	406	185	0.5	0.1	17	64	0.07	1	0.05	0.2	0.1	0.05	6	0.43
1.2	0.2	16	143	280	406	182	0.5	0.1	17	36	0.08	1	0.05	0.19	0.1	0.05	6	0.43
0.7	0.1	10	153	118	224	193	0.5	0.1	18	70	0.07	1	0.04	0.2	0.1	0.05	6	0.36
1.2	0.2	17	150	115	224	190	0.5	0.1	18	38	0.08	1	0.04	0.2	0.1	0.05	6	0.35
1.2	0.2	16	145	114	113	185	0.5	0.1	16	37	0.1	1	0.03	0.2	0.1	0.04	5	0.23
10.2	2.3	0	5	28	117	29	0.2	1.2	8	0	2.4	0	0.19	0.13	2	0.01	44	0
3.5	8.9	0	4	24	101	25	0.2	1	6	0	0.95	0	0.13	0.1	1.5	0.01	19	0
—	—	0	4	16	1	205	0.1	0.1	6	0	0.09	58	0.03	0.03	0.2	0.03	25	0
0	0	0	15	28	3	153	0.1	1.1	13	86	0.34	0	0.02	0.05	0.3	0.07	9	0
0	0	0	8	21	2	87	0	0.4	8	39	0.35	2	0.02	0.03	0.2	0.04	7	0
0	0	0	3	1	0	3	0	0.1	1	0	0	0	0	0	0	0	0	0
4.9	7.2	0	15	405	6	278	2.6	5.2	185	13	0.34	1	0.07	0.11	0.6	0.08	20	0
7.4	10.9	0	24	665	326	457	4.2	8.5	303	22	0.57	1	0.12	0.18	1	0.05	33	0
7.4	10.9	0	24	665	10	457	4.2	8.5	303	22	0.57	1	0.12	0.18	1	0.05	33	0
1	1.4	0	9	15	92	147	1.6	0.5	42	1	0.08	0	0	0.01	0	0.01	1	0
4.7	2.5	34	72	84	103	153	0.4	1.3	16	635	1.26	1	0.12	0.19	1	0.04	10	0.07
0	0	0	32	43	6	253	0.2	1.7	28	2713	1.3	5	0.03	0.07	0.5	0.07	15	0
0	0	0	18	37	1	282	0.3	0.7	11	132	1.3	6	0.04	0.1	0.5	0.05	10	0
3.6	2.3	14	123	112	255	66	0.7	1.3	13	55	1.16	3	0.15	0.14	1.2	0.03	5	0.06
13.8	4.9	205	201	271	549	271	1.7	1.9	27	243	1.91	3	0.23	0.44	4.7	0.2	17	0.99
2.5	1.8	93	22	298	53	434	2.6	2.6	24	0	0.96	0	0.1	0.24	9.6	0.53	12	9.41
0	0.1	0	15	32	18	242	0.5	0.5	10	2	1.81	6	0.01	0.02	0.2	0.05	48	0
0	0	0	4	8	4	60	0.1	0.1	3	1	0.45	2	0	0.01	0.1	0.01	12	0
0	0.1	0	12	18	10	209	0.1	0.1	7	0	0	11	0	0.02	0.1	0.03	13	0
0	0	0	9	8	11	104	0.1	0.1	4	0	0	10	0	0.02	0.1	0.03	12	0
0	0	0	12	10	14	135	0.2	0.2	5	1	0	13	0	0.03	0.2	0.04	16	0
0	0	0	14	14	8	140	0.1	0.4	4	0	0	14	0.02	0.01	0.2	0.04	7	0
0	0	0	14	14	8	143	0.1	0.4	5	0	0	15	0.02	0.01	0.2	0.04	7	0
0	0	0	12	10	9	100	0.1	0.2	7	0	0	10	0.01	0.01	0.1	0.02	12	0
0.1	0.2	0	91	78	71	767	0.5	1.4	54	0	0	74	0.07	0.07	0.7	0.16	95	0
0	0.1	0	40	80	10	620	0.2	1.7	27	1	0.58	3	0.13	0.07	0.7	0.2	3	0
0	0.1	0	36	70	9	544	0.2	1.5	24	1	0.51	2	0.11	0.06	0.6	0.18	2	0
0	0.1	0	44	95	10	615	0.3	1.5	29	3	0.58	3	0.01	0.16	0.9	0.27	3	0
0	0.1	0	14	12	4	120	0.2	0.5	15	4	0.58	11	0.03	0.04	0.6	0.05	13	0
0	0.2	0	14	7	0	94	0.3	0.4	11	8	0.28	15	0.02	0.06	0.6	0.04	16	0
0	0.3	0	43	48	3	324	0.5	1.8	37	17	1.28	47	0.05	0.13	0.7	0.1	74	0
4.8	2	160	166	214	1541	400	1.4	3.1	32	245	2.36	9	0.31	0.42	2.9	0.19	30	0.38
3.6	1	84	32	109	619	259	1.7	2	20	94	1.52	11	0.15	0.22	3	0.14	14	0.81
2.6	0.7	37	189	175	882	605	1.7	2.2	85	70	—	2	0.13	0.33	1.5	0.2	112	0.68

A

Food Item	Qty	Meas	Wgt (g)	Wtr (g)	Cals	Prot (g)	Carb (g)	Fib (g)	Fat (g)	SatF (g)
Relish, corn	1	Tbs	15	11	13	0	3	0.4	0	0
Relish, cranberry orange	0.5	cup	138	73	245	0	64	0	0	0
Relish, hotdog	1	Tbs	15	10	18	0	4	0.2	0	0
Relish, pickle, sweet	1	Tbs	15	10	21	0	5	0.3	0	0
Relish, sweet pickle, 2/3 Tbsp packet	1	each	10	6	14	0	3	0.2	0	0
Relish, vegetable	1	Tbs	9	8	4	0	1	0.1	0	0
Relish/preserves, tomato	1	Tbs	20	10	30	0	8	0.4	0	0
Rennin dessert mix w/2% milk, chocolate	0.5	cup	136	109	110	4	18	0.7	3	1.7
Rennin dessert mix w/2% milk, vanilla	0.5	cup	133	109	101	4	16	0	2	1.5
Rennin dessert mix w/whole milk, chocolate	0.5	cup	136	108	125	4	18	0.7	4	2.8
Rennin dessert mix w/whole milk, vanilla	0.5	cup	133	108	116	4	16	0	4	2.5
Rhubarb crisp	1	cup	246	130	513	3	96	4.2	16	3.1
Rhubarb, frozen, cooked w/sugar	0.5	cup	120	81	139	0	37	2.4	0	0
Rhubarb, raw, diced	0.5	cup	61	57	13	1	3	1.1	0	0
Rice bran, crude	0.25	cup	21	1	66	3	10	4.4	4	0.9
Rice cake, brown, buckwheat	2	each	18	1	68	2	14	0.7	1	0.1
Rice cake, brown, corn	2	each	18	1	69	2	15	0.5	1	0.1
Rice cake, brown, multi-grain	2	each	18	1	70	2	14	0.5	1	0.1
Rice cake, brown, plain	1	each	9	1	35	1	7	0.4	0	0.1
Rice cake, brown, rye	2	each	18	1	70	1	14	0.7	1	0.1
Rice cake, brown, sesame seed	2	each	18	1	71	1	15	1	1	0.1
Rice cake, puffed, w/o salt	2	each	18	1	70	1	15	0.8	1	0.1
Rice Krispie bar	1	each	28	3	109	1	21	0.1	3	0.5
Rice paste (mochi)	1	Tbs	17	7	40	1	9	0.3	0	0
Rice pilaf	0.5	cup	103	73	134	2	23	0.6	3	0.7
Rice polishings	1	Tbs	7	1	17	1	4	0.5	1	0.2
Rice w/cheddar/broccoli sauce, Lipton	0.5	cup	63	5	250	6	48	1	3	1
Rice, Spanish	0.5	cup	122	95	108	2	21	1.9	2	0.3
Rice, basmati, brown, premium, dry	0.25	cup	49	5	173	4	38	2.3	2	0.4
Rice, basmati, white, premium, dry	0.25	cup	51	6	183	4	41	0.3	1	0.2
Rice, brown, glutinous	0.5	cup	92	11	333	7	71	0.7	2	—
Rice, brown, long grain, cooked	0.5	cup	98	71	108	3	22	1.8	1	0.2
Rice, brown, long grain, cooked, cold	0.5	cup	72	53	80	2	17	1.3	1	0.1
Rice, brown, long grain, dry	0.25	cup	46	5	171	4	36	1.6	1	0.3
Rice, brown, med grain, cooked	0.5	cup	98	72	110	2	23	1.8	1	0.2
Rice, fried, meatless	0.5	cup	83	57	132	3	17	0.7	6	0.9
Rice, organic, basmati CA white, dry	0.25	cup	51	7	179	4	39	1.1	1	—
Rice, organic, basmati, CA brown, dry	0.25	cup	49	6	167	4	36	2.2	2	0.4
Rice, white, enriched, long grain, cooked, hot	0.5	cup	102	70	133	3	29	0.4	0	0.1
Rice, white, enriched, long grain, dry	0.25	cup	46	5	169	3	37	0.6	0	0.1
Rice, white, glutinous/sticky, cooked	0.5	cup	120	92	117	2	25	1.2	0	0
Rice, white, instant, long grain, cooked, cold	0.5	cup	65	50	64	1	14	0.4	0	0
Rice, white, instant, long grain, cooked, hot	0.5	cup	82	63	81	2	18	0.5	0	0
Rice, white, instant, long grain, dry	0.25	cup	24	2	90	2	20	0.4	0	0
Rice, white, long grain, cooked, cold	0.5	cup	72	50	94	2	20	0.3	0	0.1
Rice, white, long grain, parboiled, cooked, cold	0.5	cup	72	53	83	2	18	0.3	0	0.1
Rice, white, long grain, parboiled, cooked, hot	0.5	cup	88	63	100	2	22	0.4	0	0.1
Rice, white, long grain, parboiled, dry	0.25	cup	46	5	172	3	38	0.8	0	0.1
Rice, white, med grain, unenriched, cooked	0.5	cup	102	70	133	2	29	0.3	0	0.1
Rice, white, short grain, cooked	1	cup	205	140	267	5	59	2.1	0	0.1
Rice, wild, cooked	0.5	cup	82	61	83	3	18	1.5	0	0
Rockfish, Pacific, baked/broiled	1	each	149	109	180	36	0	0	3	0.7
Roll dough, cinnamon, frosted, refrigerated, baked	1	each	30	7	109	2	17	0.6	4	1
Roll dough, sweet, cinnamon, w/frosting, refrigerated	1	each	30	9	100	2	16	0.6	4	0.9
Roll, French	1	each	38	13	105	3	19	1.2	2	0.4
Roll, Mexican bolillo	1	each	117	46	295	10	58	2.2	2	0.4
Roll, Mexican sweet (pan dulce), crumb topping	1	each	79	17	291	5	48	1.1	9	2
Roll, butterhorn	1	each	55	17	174	5	27	0.7	5	1.3
Roll, cheese bread	1	each	41	13	124	4	21	0.7	3	1
Roll, cinnamon w/raisins & nuts, homemade	1	each	57	15	196	4	30	1.1	7	1.4
Roll, dinner	1	each	28	9	85	2	14	0.9	2	0.5
Roll, dinner, bran	1	each	28	10	76	3	14	1.2	2	0.2
Roll, dinner, bran, toasted	1	each	25	8	73	2	12	1.2	1	0.2
Roll, dinner, egg	1	each	35	11	107	3	18	1.3	2	0.6
Roll, dinner, homemade, w/2% milk	1	each	35	10	111	3	19	0.7	3	0.6

MonoF	PolyF	Choles	Calc	Phos	Sod	Pot	Zn	Iron	Magn	VitA	VitE	VitC	Thia	Ribo	Nia	B6	Fola	B12
(g)	(g)	(mg)	(mg)	(mg)	(mg)	(mg)	(mg)	(mg)	(mg)	(μg RE)	(mg α-TE)	(mg)	(mg)	(mg)	(mg)	(mg)	(μg)	(μg)
0	0	0	2	7	55	28	0	0.1	3	9	0.03	4	0.01	0.01	0.1	0.02	4	0
0	0.1	0	15	11	44	52	0.1	0.3	6	10	0.07	25	0.04	0.03	0.1	0.03	4	0
0.1	0	0	4	3	81	31	0	0.2	3	1	0.02	1	0	0	0	0	1	0
0	0	0	3	2	109	31	0	0.1	1	2	0.02	1	0	0	0	0	0	0
0	0	0	2	1	71	20	0	0.1	0	1	0.02	1	0	0	0	0	0	0
0	0	0	2	2	41	16	0	0	1	2	0.02	1	0	0	0	0	1	0
0	0	0	9	9	452	79	0	0.3	6	25	0.1	10	0.01	0.01	0.1	0.03	2	0
0.8	0.1	10	171	133	71	248	0.7	0.4	27	60	0.07	1	0.05	0.21	0.1	0.06	7	0.45
0.7	0.1	9	161	126	61	189	0.5	0.1	17	69	0.07	1	0.05	0.2	0.1	0.05	7	0.44
1.3	0.2	16	169	132	69	243	0.7	0.4	27	33	0.11	1	0.05	0.21	0.1	0.06	7	0.44
1.2	0.2	17	158	124	61	186	0.5	0.1	16	33	0.11	1	0.05	0.2	0.1	0.05	7	0.44
6.9	5	0	294	46	193	289	0.3	1.8	34	221	2.9	6	0.15	0.14	1.4	0.05	14	0.02
0	0	0	174	10	1	115	0.1	0.3	14	8	0.24	4	0.02	0.03	0.2	0.02	6	0
0	0.1	0	52	9	2	176	0.1	0.1	7	6	0.12	5	0.01	0.02	0.2	0.02	4	0
1.6	1.6	0	12	348	1	308	1.2	3.8	162	0	1.26	0	0.57	0.06	7.1	0.84	13	0
0.2	0.2	0	2	68	21	54	0.4	0.2	27	0	0.02	0	0.01	0.02	1.5	0.02	4	0
0.2	0.2	0	2	58	52	50	0.4	0.2	20	0	0	0	0.01	0.02	1.2	0.02	3	0
0.2	0.3	0	4	67	45	53	0.5	0.4	25	0	0	0	0.01	0.03	1.2	0.02	4	0
0.1	0.1	0	1	32	29	26	0.3	0.1	12	0	0.06	0	0	0.02	0.7	0.01	2	0
0.2	0.3	0	4	68	20	56	0.5	0.3	26	0	0	0	0.02	0.02	1.3	0.03	1	0
0.2	0.2	0	2	68	41	52	0.5	0.3	24	0	0.02	1	0.01	0.02	1.3	0.03	3	0
0.2	0.2	0	2	65	5	52	0.5	0.3	24	1	0.02	0	0.01	0.03	1.4	0.03	4	0
1.2	0.8	0	3	12	141	11	0.2	0.6	3	103	0.42	5	0.11	0.13	1.5	0.16	30	0
0	0	0	6	16	1	37	0.2	0.6	7	0	0.02	0	0.01	0	0.5	0.02	1	0
1.5	1.1	0	13	39	377	54	0.4	1.2	10	43	0.56	0	0.14	0.02	1.3	0.06	4	0
0.3	0.3	0	5	73	0	47	0.5	0.7	39	0	0.4	0	0.12	0.01	1.8	0.03	7	0
—	—	2	40	—	940	—	—	1.8	—	0	—	2	—	—	—	—	—	—
0.7	0.7	0	35	47	162	271	0.4	1.2	20	58	0.65	20	0.12	0.04	1.5	0.16	10	0
0.7	0.6	0	5	—	3	—	—	0.5	—	0	—	0	—	—	—	—	—	—
0.2	0.2	0	4	—	—	—	—	0.2	—	0	—	0	—	—	—	—	—	—
—	—	—	19	225	10	266	—	3.2	—	0	0.48	—	0.28	0.11	4.6	—	—	—
0.3	0.3	0	10	81	5	42	0.6	0.4	42	0	0.7	0	0.09	0.02	1.5	0.14	4	0
0.2	0.2	0	7	60	4	31	0.5	0.3	31	0	0.52	0	0.07	0.02	1.1	0.1	3	0
0.5	0.5	0	11	154	3	103	0.9	0.7	66	0	0.33	0	0.18	0.04	2.4	0.24	9	0
0.3	0.3	0	10	76	1	77	0.6	0.5	43	0	0.32	0	0.1	0.01	1.3	0.15	4	0
1.5	3.2	21	15	47	143	67	0.4	0.9	12	10	1.23	2	0.1	0.05	1.1	0.08	11	0.06
—	—	0	4	—	4	—	—	0.2	—	0	—	1	—	—	—	—	—	—
0.6	0.6	0	4	—	4	—	—	0.7	—	0	—	0	—	—	—	—	—	—
0.1	0.1	0	10	44	1	36	0.5	1.2	12	0	0.05	0	0.17	0.01	1.5	0.1	60	0
0.1	0.1	0	13	53	2	53	0.5	2	12	0	0.06	0	0.27	0.02	1.9	0.08	107	0
0.1	0.1	0	2	10	6	12	0.5	0.2	6	0	0.04	0	0.02	0.02	0.3	0.03	1	0
0	0	0	5	9	2	3	0.2	0.4	3	0	0.03	0	0.05	0.03	0.6	0.01	27	0
0	0	0	7	12	2	3	0.2	0.5	4	0	0.04	0	0.06	0.04	0.7	0.01	34	0
0	0	0	4	16	1	4	0.2	1	3	0	0.03	0	0.15	0.01	1.3	0.01	55	0
0.1	0.1	0	7	31	1	25	0.4	0.9	9	0	0.04	0	0.12	0.01	1.1	0.07	42	0
0.1	0.1	0	14	30	2	27	0.2	0.8	9	0	0.04	0	0.18	0.01	1	0.01	36	0
0.1	0.1	0	17	37	3	32	0.3	1	10	0	0.04	0	0.22	0.02	1.2	0.02	44	0
0.1	0.1	0	28	63	2	56	0.4	1.6	14	0	0.06	0	0.28	0.03	1.7	0.16	107	0
0.1	0.1	0	3	38	0	30	0.4	1.5	13	0	0.05	0	0.17	0.02	1.9	0.05	60	0
0.1	0.1	0	2	68	0	53	0.8	3	16	0	0.09	0	0.34	0.03	3	0.12	121	0
0	0.2	0	2	67	2	83	1.1	0.5	26	0	0.19	0	0.04	0.07	1.1	0.11	21	0
0.7	0.9	66	18	340	115	775	0.8	0.8	51	98	1.86	0	0.07	0.12	5.8	0.4	16	1.79
2.2	0.5	0	10	104	250	19	0.1	0.8	4	0	0.48	0	0.12	0.07	1.1	0.01	2	0.02
2	0.5	0	9	96	230	17	0.1	0.7	3	0	0.45	0	0.14	0.08	1.1	0.01	15	0.01
0.7	0.3	0	35	32	231	43	0.3	1	8	0	0.17	0	0.2	0.11	1.6	0.02	36	0
0.2	0.6	1	14	88	347	96	0.8	3.7	22	4	0.05	0	0.67	0.45	6.3	0.06	47	0
3.9	2.7	26	13	56	140	57	0.4	1.8	10	88	1.35	0	0.23	0.21	2	0.04	22	0.06
2.6	0.7	18	58	59	214	68	0.3	1.2	10	12	0.66	0	0.2	0.18	1.2	0.06	17	0
1.3	0.4	2	54	44	210	39	0.3	1.1	9	6	0.04	0	0.16	0.1	1.3	0.02	15	0.01
2.7	2.8	13	36	63	185	123	0.4	1.5	16	60	0.91	0	0.16	0.16	1.3	0.05	18	0.06
1	0.3	0	34	33	148	38	0.2	0.9	7	0	0.25	0	0.14	0.09	1.1	0.02	27	0.02
0.6	0.6	0	6	54	126	53	0.3	0.9	15	0	0.22	0	0.13	0.1	1.1	0.04	22	0
0.5	0.6	0	6	52	118	50	0.3	0.9	14	0	0.21	0	0.1	0.09	0.9	0.04	15	0
1	0.4	18	21	35	191	36	0.4	1.2	9	3	0.25	0	0.18	0.18	1.2	0.02	37	0.08
1	0.7	12	21	44	145	53	0.2	1	7	32	0.34	0	0.14	0.14	1.2	0.02	32	0.05

Food Item	Qty	Meas	Wgt (g)	Wtr (g)	Cals	Prot (g)	Carb (g)	Fib (g)	Fat (g)	SatF (g)
Roll, dinner, recipe, w/whole milk	1	each	35	10	112	3	19	1	3	0.8
Roll, dinner, wheat	1	each	28	10	77	2	13	1.1	2	0.4
Roll, dinner, whole wheat	1	each	35	12	93	3	18	2.6	2	0.3
Roll, garlic	1	each	35	11	104	3	18	0.7	2	0.5
Roll, hard, white, enriched	1	each	50	16	147	5	26	1.2	2	0.3
Roll, jelly filled	1	each	55	17	173	4	28	0.9	5	1.2
Roll, oatmeal, toasted	1	each	33	14	78	3	13	1.4	2	0.2
Roll, rye, light	1	each	28	9	81	3	15	1.4	1	0.2
Roll, sourdough	1	each	45	14	131	4	25	1.2	1	0.3
Roll, submarine/hoagie	1	each	135	41	392	12	75	3.6	4	0.9
Roll, sweet, cheese	1	each	66	19	238	5	29	0.8	12	4
Roll, sweet, cinnamon raisin, commercial	1	each	39	10	145	2	20	0.9	6	1.2
Rose apple, raw	4	oz.	113	105	28	1	6	1.5	0	—
Rosemary, dried	0.25	tsp	0	0	1	0	0	0.1	0	0
Rutabaga, cooked cubes	0.5	cup	85	76	33	1	7	1.5	0	0
Rutabaga, cooked, mashed	0.5	cup	120	107	47	2	10	2.2	0	0
Rutabaga, raw, cubes/pieces	0.5	cup	70	63	25	1	6	1.8	0	0
Rye, whole grain	0.5	cup	79	9	265	12	55	11.5	2	0.2
Saffron	0.25	tsp	0	0	1	0	0	0	0	0
Saffron safflower, flowers	1	oz.	28	4	68	5	—	—	1	—
Sage, fresh	0.25	cup	8	5	10	0	1	—	0	—
Sage, ground	0.25	tsp	0	0	1	0	0	0.1	0	0
Salad dressing, Blue Cheese, low calorie	2	Tbs	31	24	30	2	1	0	2	0.3
Salad dressing, Catalina, fat free, Kraft	2	Tbs	35	4	124	5	24	1.6	1	0.5
Salad dressing, Dijon Vinaigrette Lite	2	Tbs	30	25	32	0	1	0	3	0.4
Salad dressing, Italian, fat free, Kraft	2	Tbs	35	32	11	0	2	0	0	0
Salad dressing, Italian, fat free, Lipton	2	Tbs	30	28	15	0	2	0	0	0
Salad dressing, Seven Seas Viva	2	Tbs	30	12	140	0	3	0	14	2.1
Salad dressing, bacon & tomato, low calorie	2	Tbs	32	24	65	1	1	0.1	7	1.1
Salad dressing, blue cheese	2	Tbs	31	10	154	1	2	0	16	3
Salad dressing, buttermilk, light	2	Tbs	29	21	58	1	2	—	5	—
Salad dressing, caesar's	2	Tbs	23	8	107	3	1	0.1	10	1.9
Salad dressing, caesar, low calorie	2	Tbs	30	22	33	0	6	0	1	0.2
Salad dressing, cooked	2	Tbs	32	22	50	1	5	0	3	0.9
Salad dressing, creamy Italian	2	Tbs	29	11	143	0	2	0	16	2.3
Salad dressing, creamy bacon	2	Tbs	29	11	143	0	2	0	16	2.3
Salad dressing, creamy cucumber	2	Tbs	29	11	143	0	2	0	16	2.3
Salad dressing, creamy cucumber, low calorie	2	Tbs	30	22	48	0	2	0	4	0.6
Salad dressing, creamy, oil free, low calorie	2	Tbs	30	22	48	0	2	0	4	0.6
Salad dressing, french	2	Tbs	31	12	134	0	5	0	13	3
Salad dressing, french, fat free, Kraft	2	Tbs	35	23	40	0	12	0.5	0	0
Salad dressing, french, homemade	2	Tbs	28	7	177	0	1	0	20	3.5
Salad dressing, french, low calorie	2	Tbs	32	23	44	0	7	0	2	0.3
Salad dressing, honey dijon, fat free, Kraft	2	Tbs	35	23	50	0	11	1	0	0
Salad dressing, honey mustard	2	Tbs	31	11	101	0	14	0.2	6	0.8
Salad dressing, Italian	2	Tbs	29	11	137	0	3	0	14	2.1
Salad dressing, Italian, low calorie	2	Tbs	30	25	32	0	1	0	3	0.4
Salad dressing, light, cholesterol free	1	Tbs	15	9	48	0	2	0	4	1.1
Salad dressing, low calorie, Miracle Whip Light	1	Tbs	14	8	36	0	3	0	3	0.4
Salad dressing, mayonnaise type	1	Tbs	15	6	57	0	4	0	5	0.7
Salad dressing, oil free, low calorie	2	Tbs	30	26	7	0	2	0	0	0
Salad dressing, ranch	2	Tbs	30	16	109	1	1	0	11	1.7
Salad dressing, ranch, fat free, Kraft	2	Tbs	35	23	50	0	11	0.5	0	0
Salad dressing, roquefort, low calorie	2	Tbs	31	24	30	2	1	0	2	0.3
Salad dressing, russian	2	Tbs	31	11	151	0	3	0	16	2.2
Salad dressing, russian, low calorie	2	Tbs	33	21	46	0	9	0.1	1	0.2
Salad dressing, sesame seed	2	Tbs	31	12	136	1	3	0.3	14	1.9
Salad dressing, thousand island	2	Tbs	31	14	118	0	5	0	11	1.9
Salad dressing, thousand island, low calorie	2	Tbs	31	21	49	0	5	0.4	3	0.5
Salad dressing, vinaigrette	2	Tbs	29	11	137	0	3	0	14	2.1
Salad dressing, vinegar & oil	2	Tbs	32	15	144	0	1	0	16	2.9
Salad dressing, vinegar & sugar & water	2	Tbs	32	27	16	0	4	0	0	0
Salad dressing, yogurt	2	Tbs	31	26	22	1	2	0	1	0.6
Salad dressing/marinade, Korean	2	Tbs	30	27	10	0	2	0.2	0	0
Salad topping, Bac-O-Bits	2	Tbs	12	1	50	5	3	—	2	—

MonoF (g)	PolyF (g)	Choles (mg)	Calc (mg)	Phos (mg)	Sod (mg)	Pot (mg)	Zn (mg)	Iron (mg)	Magn (mg)	VitA (μg RE)	VitE (mg α-TE)	VitC (mg)	Thia (mg)	Ribo (mg)	Nia (mg)	B6 (mg)	Fola (μg)	B12 (μg)
1.1	0.7	13	21	44	145	53	0.2	1	7	28	0.35	0	0.14	0.14	1.2	0.02	15	0.05
0.9	0.3	0	50	30	96	33	0.3	1	10	0	0.27	0	0.12	0.08	1.2	0.02	14	0
0.4	0.8	0	37	78	167	95	0.7	0.8	30	0	0.48	0	0.09	0.05	1.3	0.07	11	0
1	0.3	0	35	30	176	34	0.3	1	7	0	0.03	0	0.14	0.08	1.2	0.02	13	0
0.6	0.9	0	48	50	272	54	0.5	1.6	14	0	0.16	0	0.24	0.17	2.1	0.02	48	0
2.4	0.7	17	56	58	199	92	0.3	1.2	10	11	0.64	0	0.2	0.17	1.2	0.07	16	0
0.5	0.5	0	28	38	136	40	0.3	1.4	11	0	0.23	0	0.15	0.1	1.6	0.02	31	0
0.4	0.2	0	9	45	253	51	0.3	0.8	15	0	0.1	0	0.11	0.08	1.1	0.02	24	0
0.4	0.5	0	40	38	261	40	0.3	1.3	9	0	0.03	0	0.18	0.11	1.5	0.02	14	0
1.3	1.4	0	122	115	783	122	0.9	3.8	27	0	0.1	0	0.54	0.33	4.5	0.05	40	0
6	1.3	50	78	65	236	90	0.4	0.5	12	51	1.25	0	0.1	0.09	0.5	0.05	28	0.2
1.9	2.9	26	28	30	149	43	0.2	0.6	7	25	1.68	1	0.13	0.1	0.9	0.04	20	0.06
—	—	0	33	9	0	139	0.1	0.1	6	39	—	25	0.02	0.03	0.9	—	—	0
0	0	0	4	0	0	3	0	0.1	1	1	—	0	0	—	0	—	—	0
0	0.1	0	41	48	17	277	0.3	0.5	20	48	0.13	16	0.07	0.04	0.6	0.09	13	0
0	0.1	0	58	67	24	391	0.4	0.6	28	67	0.18	23	0.1	0.05	0.9	0.12	18	0
0	0.1	0	33	41	14	236	0.2	0.4	16	41	0.21	18	0.06	0.03	0.5	0.07	15	0
0.2	0.9	0	26	295	5	209	3	2.1	96	0	1.48	0	0.25	0.2	3.4	0.23	47	0
0	0	0	0	0	0	3	0	0	0	0	0	0	0	0	0	0	0	0
—	—	—	175	73	—	—	—	5.7	—	5	—	6	0.04	0.11	2.4	—	—	0
—	—	—	48	3	0	31	0.1	—	13	17	—	—	0.01	—	—	—	—	0
0	0	0	3	0	0	2	0	0	1	1	0	0	0	0	0	0	0	0
0.9	0.8	0	27	25	367	2	0.1	0.2	2	1	0.28	0	0.01	0.03	0	0.01	1	0.07
0.5	0.3	0	162	188	48	78	2.8	3.4	75	0	10.8	32	0.81	0.92	10.8	1.08	215	3.23
0.6	1.8	2	1	2	236	4	0	0.1	0	0	0.45	0	0	0	0	0	0	0
0	0	0	0	—	327	45	—	0	—	0	—	0	—	—	—	—	—	—
0	0	0	0	—	280	—	—	0	—	0	—	0	—	—	—	—	—	—
3.4	8.4	0	3	2	236	4	0	0.1	0	7	3.12	0	0	0.01	0	0	1	0.05
1.8	3.6	1	1	8	351	35	0.1	0.1	2	9	1.3	3	0.01	0.01	0.2	0.03	0	0.03
3.8	8.5	5	25	23	335	11	0.1	0.1	0	20	2.85	1	0	0.03	0	0.01	2	0.08
—	—	—	—	—	167	35	—	—	—	—	—	—	—	—	—	—	—	—
7.2	1	24	43	37	396	40	0.2	0.4	5	13	1.38	1	0.01	0.05	1	0.02	3	0.11
0.6	0.5	1	7	6	323	9	0	0.1	1	1	0.12	0	0	0	0	0	1	0.01
1.2	0.7	18	27	28	235	39	0.1	0.2	3	39	0.61	0	0.02	0.05	0.1	0.01	3	0.11
3.8	8.7	1	4	3	347	8	0	0	1	6	3.15	0	0	0	0	0	0	0.01
3.8	8.7	1	4	3	347	8	0	0	1	6	3.15	0	0	0	0	0	0	0.01
3.8	8.7	1	4	3	347	8	0	0	1	6	3.15	0	0	0	0	0	0	0.01
1.8	1.6	0	2	2	307	11	0	0	1	2	0.57	0	0	0	0	0.01	4	0.02
1.8	1.6	0	2	2	307	11	0	0	1	2	0.57	0	0	0	0	0.01	4	0.02
2.5	6.8	0	3	4	428	25	0	0.1	0	41	2.63	0	0	0	0	0	1	0.04
0	0	0	0	—	300	40	—	0	—	150	—	0	—	—	—	—	—	—
5.8	9.4	0	2	1	184	7	0	0.1	0	43	3.36	0	0	0.01	0	0	0	0
0.5	1.1	0	4	5	256	26	0.1	0.1	0	42	0.39	0	0	0	0	0	0	0
0	0	0	0	—	330	50	—	0.4	—	0	—	0	—	—	—	—	—	—
1.4	3.2	0	6	5	181	20	0.1	0.2	3	0	0.44	0	0	0.01	0.1	0.01	1	0
3.3	8.2	0	3	1	231	4	0	0.1	0	7	3.06	0	0	0.01	0	0	1	0.05
0.6	1.8	2	1	2	236	4	0	0.1	0	0	0.45	0	0	0	0	0	0	0
1.1	2.1	0	0	0	102	0	0	0	0	2	0.64	0	0	0	0	0	0	0
0.7	1.4	4	2	4	99	1	0	0	0	9	0.6	0	0	0	0	0	1	0.03
1.3	2.6	4	2	4	104	1	0	0	0	12	0.59	0	0	0	0	0	1	0.03
0	0	0	2	2	512	15	0	0.1	3	0	0	0	0	0	0	0	0	0
4.8	4.2	12	30	25	131	40	0.1	0.1	3	22	1.19	0	0.01	0.04	0	0.01	2	0.08
0	0	0	0	—	310	50	—	0	—	0	—	0	—	—	—	—	—	—
0.9	0.8	0	27	25	367	2	0.1	0.2	2	1	0.28	0	0.01	0.03	0	0.01	1	0.07
3.6	9	6	6	11	266	48	0.1	0.2	0	63	3.12	2	0.02	0.02	0.2	0.01	3	0.09
0.3	0.8	2	6	12	283	51	0	0.2	0	5	0.25	2	0	0	0	0	1	0.04
3.6	7.7	0	6	11	306	48	0	0.2	0	63	1.53	0	0	0	0	0	0	0
2.6	6.2	8	3	5	219	35	0	0.2	1	30	0.36	0	0	0.01	0	0	2	0.06
0.7	1.9	5	3	5	306	35	0	0.2	0	29	0.36	0	0	0.01	0	0	2	0.06
3.3	8.2	0	3	1	231	4	0	0.1	0	7	3.06	0	0	0.01	0	0	1	0.05
4.7	7.7	0	0	0	0	2	0	0	0	0	2.82	0	0	0	0	0	0	0
0	0	0	1	1	331	9	0	0.1	2	0	0	0	0	0	0	0	0	0
0.3	0.2	3	31	24	118	45	0.1	0.1	4	7	0.04	1	0.01	0.04	0	0.01	2	0.09
0	0	0	8	8	77	31	0	0.2	4	41	0.03	9	0.01	0.01	0.2	0.03	3	0
—	—	0	26	—	205	328	—	0.8	—	—	—	—	1.03	0.04	0.2	—	—	—

Food Item	Qty	Meas	Wgt (g)	Wtr (g)	Cals	Prot (g)	Carb (g)	Fib (g)	Fat (g)	SatF (g)
Salad, carrot raisin	0.5	cup	88	50	202	1	21	2	14	2
Salad, chef style w/turkey+ham+cheese	1.5	cup	326	269	267	26	5	—	16	8.2
Salad, crab, w/imitation crab	0.5	cup	104	72	150	9	14	0.4	6	0.9
Salad, fruit, canned, juice pack	0.5	cup	124	107	62	1	16	1.2	0	0
Salad, mixed greens/lettuce	0.5	cup	28	26	5	0	1	0.5	0	0
Salad, spinach, no dressing	0.5	cup	37	27	44	2	5	0.8	2	0.5
Salad, taco	1.5	cup	198	143	279	13	24	—	15	6.8
Salad, three bean	0.5	cup	75	61	70	2	7	1.5	4	0.6
Salad, tossed green	0.5	cup	69	66	12	1	2	0.8	0	0
Salad, Waldorf	0.5	cup	68	40	204	2	6	1.2	20	2.1
Salami, beef, cooked	1	piece	23	13	60	3	1	0	5	2.1
Salami, dry, beef & pork	2	piece	20	7	84	5	1	0	7	2.4
Salami, turkey, cooked	2	piece	57	38	112	9	0	0	8	2.3
Salisbury steak, 4-compartment, Swanson	1	each	298	231	325	15	33	5.7	14	5.7
Salsa cruda (uncooked salsa)	2	Tbs	30	28	6	0	1	0.3	0	0
Salsify, cooked, drained	0.5	cup	68	55	46	2	10	2.1	0	0
Salt	0.25	tsp	1	0	0	0	0	0	0	0
Salt Free 17	0.25	tsp	2	0	5	0	1	0.2	0	—
Salt blend, light, Papa Dash	0.25	tsp	2	0	1	0	0	—	0	0
Salt substitute, Morton	0.25	tsp	1	0	0	0	0	—	0	0
Salt, Sea	1	Tbs	16	0	0	0	0	0	0	0
Salt, light, Morton	0.25	tsp	2	0	0	0	0	—	0	0
Salt, light, Morton Lite	0.25	tsp	1	—	—	—	—	—	—	—
Salt, seasoning, Morton	0.25	tsp	0	0	0	0	0	—	0	—
Sandwich, BLT, on firm white	1	each	145	75	366	12	35	2	19	4.9
Sandwich, avocado & cheese, on wheat	1	each	196	116	433	14	34	6.5	28	8.4
Sandwich, bologna	1	each	83	34	257	7	26	1.2	14	4.2
Sandwich, chicken frank on bun	1	each	85	38	235	9	24	0.8	11	3
Sandwich, chicken salad, on firm white	1	each	114	45	381	11	34	1.6	22	3.5
Sandwich, corned beef & swiss, on rye	1	each	147	73	396	26	20	0.1	24	8.9
Sandwich, egg salad, on firm white	1	each	121	50	394	10	34	1.5	24	4.2
Sandwich, fish w/tartar sauce & cheese	1	each	183	83	523	21	48	0.4	28	8.1
Sandwich, french dip au jus	1	each	193	118	359	26	34	1.7	12	4.8
Sandwich, grilled cheese, on firm white	1	each	127	46	426	19	34	1.5	24	13.1
Sandwich, grilled chicken, Weight Watchers	1	each	113	65	210	18	24	2	5	2
Sandwich, gyro	1	each	105	67	169	12	20	1.1	4	1.5
Sandwich, ham & swiss, on rye	1	each	145	79	328	22	21	0.1	18	6.3
Sandwich, ham salad, on wheat	1	each	126	60	343	10	34	3.3	19	4.4
Sandwich, ham, on wheat	1	each	123	68	259	17	22	2.7	11	2.2
Sandwich, hotdog, plain	1	each	98	53	242	10	18	—	14	5.1
Sandwich, pastrami	1	each	134	71	334	14	27	1.7	18	6.3
Sandwich, patty melt, on rye	1	each	177	81	546	36	21	2.9	36	12.9
Sandwich, peanut butter & jam, on soft white	1	each	101	26	351	12	47	3	15	3.1
Sandwich, reuben	1	each	181	91	496	23	31	4.1	31	10.6
Sandwich, roast beef, on wheat	1	each	123	57	314	23	25	2.6	13	2.5
Sandwich, submarine w/coldcuts	1	each	228	132	456	22	51	1.7	19	6.8
Sandwich, tuna salad, on firm white	1	each	126	57	342	14	38	1.8	14	2.3
Sandwich, turkey ham & cheese, on wheat	1	each	152	76	385	22	27	3.3	21	8
Sandwich, turkey ham, on rye	1	each	116	70	217	16	16	0.1	10	1.9
Sandwich, turkey, on whole wheat	1	each	136	72	294	21	26	3.5	12	1.8
Sapodilla, raw	1	each	170	133	141	1	34	9	2	0.3
Sapotes, raw	1	each	170	106	228	4	58	4.4	1	0.2
Sauce, Alfredo, Di Girono	0.5	cup	124	—	460	8	4	0	44	20
Sauce, Alfredo, low fat, Di Girono	0.5	cup	138	—	340	10	32	0	20	12
Sauce, Tabasco brand pepper	1	tsp	5	5	1	0	0	0	0	0
Sauce, alfredo, Progresso	0.5	cup	124	81	310	10	5	0	27	15
Sauce, armanino pesto	0.25	cup	58	30	195	4	4	0.9	18	3
Sauce, barbecue	2	Tbs	31	25	23	1	4	0.4	1	0.1
Sauce, bechamel	0.25	cup	72	61	71	1	3	0.2	6	3.7
Sauce, black bean	1	tsp	6	5	5	0	1	0.1	0	0
Sauce, bordelaise	0.25	cup	116	100	104	1	5	0.3	6	3.9
Sauce, cheese	0.25	cup	50	32	110	5	4	0.1	8	4.6
Sauce, cheese, dry mix w/milk	0.25	cup	70	54	77	4	6	0.2	4	2.3
Sauce, cheese, low fat	1	cup	243	177	338	23	16	0.3	20	8.2
Sauce, chili, hot green	1	tsp	5	5	1	0	0	—	0	0

MonoF (g)	PolyF (g)	Choles (mg)	Calc (mg)	Phos (mg)	Sod (mg)	Pot (mg)	Zn (mg)	Iron (mg)	Magn (mg)	VitA (μg RE)	VitE (mg α-TE)	VitC (mg)	Thia (mg)	Ribo (mg)	Nia (mg)	B6 (mg)	Fola (μg)	B12 (μg)
3.9	7.2	10	26	46	117	315	0.2	0.7	14	1444	5	5	0.08	0.05	0.6	0.22	9	0.05
5.2	1.4	140	235	401	743	401	3.1	2	49	137	—	16	0.39	0.39	6	0.42	101	0.85
1.6	3.4	37	37	110	892	211	0.3	0.4	33	22	0.86	1	0.03	0.1	1.5	0.14	7	1.41
0	0	0	14	17	6	144	0.2	0.3	10	74	0.74	4	0.01	0.02	0.4	0.03	3	0
0	0	0	15	9	7	87	0.1	0.4	7	75	0.18	4	0.02	0.03	0.1	0.02	32	0
0.7	0.4	30	26	37	78	138	0.3	0.8	17	120	0.5	5	0.06	0.13	0.7	0.05	38	0.08
5.2	1.8	44	192	143	762	416	2.7	2.3	52	77	—	4	0.1	0.36	2.5	0.22	83	0.63
1	2.4	0	18	32	257	112	0.3	0.7	13	11	0.98	2	0.04	0.05	0.2	0.02	26	0.01
0	0.1	0	10	16	7	134	0.1	0.3	7	139	0.26	7	0.04	0.03	0.3	0.04	24	0
3.7	13.5	10	21	42	118	135	0.3	0.4	20	20	4.34	3	0.05	0.02	0.2	0.18	14	0.04
2.2	0.2	15	2	26	270	52	0.5	0.5	3	0	0.04	0	0.02	0.04	0.7	0.04	0	0.7
3.4	0.6	16	2	28	372	76	0.6	0.3	3	0	0.06	0	0.12	0.06	1	0.1	0	0.38
2.6	2	47	11	60	572	139	1	0.9	9	0	0.32	0	0.04	0.1	2	0.14	2	0.12
—	—	29	76	—	879	—	—	2.6	—	955	—	6	—	—	—	—	—	—
0	0	0	3	6	117	48	0	0.1	3	44	0.08	11	0.01	0.01	0.1	0.02	4	0
0	0	0	32	38	11	191	0.2	0.4	12	0	0.13	3	0.04	0.12	0.3	0.15	10	0
0	0	0	0	0	535	0	0	0	0	0	0	0	0	0	0	0	0	0
—	—	—	—	—	1	18	—	—	—	—	—	—	—	—	—	—	—	0
0	0	0	—	—	694	0	—	—	—	0	0	0	0	0	0	0	0	0
0	0	—	8	6	0	694	—	—	—	—	—	—	—	—	—	—	—	0
0	0	0	6	0	6905	3	0	0	1	0	0	0	0	0	0	0	0	0
0	0	—	1	—	293	390	—	—	1	—	—	—	—	—	—	—	—	0
—	—	—	0	—	290	386	—	—	1	—	—	—	—	—	—	—	—	0
—	—	—	—	—	0	217	—	—	—	—	—	—	—	—	—	—	—	0
6.7	6.6	24	73	145	686	275	1.1	2.4	24	34	2.95	13	0.42	0.23	3.8	0.16	41	0.36
11.1	7.2	30	284	254	512	602	1.9	3	65	137	4.44	11	0.34	0.38	3.8	0.34	78	0.26
6.2	2.5	16	63	79	608	111	0.8	1.9	16	54	0.73	6	0.28	0.21	2.7	0.08	18	0.38
5	2.2	45	83	82	819	76	0.8	2	13	17	0.13	0	0.19	0.15	2.7	0.16	17	0.1
5.8	11.5	32	73	110	478	152	0.8	2.2	19	23	6.27	1	0.28	0.19	3.8	0.24	28	0.12
7	5.9	77	252	257	1311	212	3.4	2.9	26	77	2.44	1	0.18	0.31	2.6	0.16	18	1.63
6.5	11.5	152	84	129	545	128	0.8	2.3	17	73	4.74	0	0.28	0.32	2.2	0.19	40	0.42
8.9	9.4	68	185	311	939	353	1.2	3.5	37	97	1.83	3	0.46	0.42	4.2	0.11	92	1.08
5.2	0.9	58	66	212	608	355	5.3	3.7	31	0	0.15	0	0.3	0.31	5.4	0.24	26	2.11
7.4	2	56	412	488	1174	173	2.1	2.1	26	210	1.52	0	0.28	0.36	2.2	0.06	28	0.4
—	—	20	60	—	420	220	—	1.4	—	0	—	0	—	—	—	—	—	—
1.4	0.4	34	44	117	212	209	2.3	2.2	20	11	0.28	4	0.21	0.25	3.5	0.16	30	0.9
5	5.8	55	249	317	1548	333	2.5	2.2	28	76	2.43	15	0.7	0.35	3.9	0.34	15	1.13
6.6	7.2	28	66	160	901	207	1.3	2.3	32	8	3.55	4	0.5	0.23	3.6	0.2	25	0.48
3.5	4.7	36	56	218	1285	332	1.8	2.1	34	6	2.15	17	0.81	0.28	5.1	0.39	22	0.52
6.8	1.7	44	24	97	670	143	2	2.3	13	0	0.27	0	0.24	0.27	3.6	0.05	48	0.51
8.9	1.2	53	71	142	1341	242	2.7	2.6	24	3	0.21	4	0.29	0.27	4.8	0.13	21	0.99
11.4	8.2	110	215	319	682	380	6.9	4.1	35	119	3.4	0	0.24	0.45	6	0.34	24	2.36
6.7	3.9	2	60	141	293	245	1.1	2.2	56	0	0.12	0	0.27	0.17	5.3	0.13	40	0
9.9	7.6	89	319	321	1308	247	4.2	2.9	36	101	0.7	11	0.18	0.32	3.1	0.22	30	1.45
3.4	6.5	34	56	183	1267	382	3.2	3.4	34	9	2.91	10	0.24	0.25	5.4	0.33	27	1.76
8.2	2.3	36	189	287	1650	394	2.6	2.5	68	80	—	12	1	0.8	5.5	0.14	87	1.09
3.6	7.6	15	74	161	582	174	0.7	2.4	24	22	3	1	0.28	0.2	5.6	0.12	28	0.64
5.1	6.6	62	239	400	1350	345	3.1	3.6	43	88	3.11	0	0.26	0.39	4.2	0.26	29	0.35
2.2	5.4	42	40	166	917	264	2.3	3.1	19	6	2.16	0	0.17	0.26	3.3	0.22	13	0.21
2.8	6.8	35	47	289	1340	336	1.9	2.2	62	9	2.8	0	0.23	0.18	7.9	0.41	32	1.43
0.9	0	0	36	20	20	328	0.2	1.4	20	10	0.42	25	0	0.03	0.3	0.06	24	0
0.5	0	0	66	48	17	585	0.2	1.7	51	70	0.73	34	0.02	0.03	3.1	0.1	41	0
—	—	90	200	200	1100	150	—	0	0	160	—	0	0	0.2	0	—	—	—
—	—	60	300	200	1200	160	—	0	16	160	—	0	0	0.2	0	—	—	—
0	0	0	1	1	31	7	0	0.1	0	22	0.04	0	0	0	0	0.01	0	3.12
7	1	75	300	—	670	—	—	0	—	150	—	0	—	—	—	—	—	—
—	—	11	169	—	372	—	—	1.2	—	279	—	0	—	—	—	—	—	—
0.2	0.2	0	6	6	255	54	0.1	0.3	6	27	0.35	2	0.01	0.01	0.3	0.02	1	0
1.8	0.3	16	7	9	563	14	0	0.2	2	57	0.14	0	0.03	0.03	0.3	0	2	0.02
0.1	0.1	0	1	2	55	8	0	0	1	0	0.03	0	0	0	0	0	1	0
1.9	0.3	16	16	23	261	102	0.1	0.8	9	63	0.19	4	0.04	0.05	0.8	0.03	6	0.06
2.5	1.1	18	134	101	258	63	0.6	0.3	9	84	0.59	0	0.04	0.12	0.2	0.02	5	0.22
1.3	0.4	13	142	110	391	138	0.2	0.1	12	29	0.08	1	0.04	0.14	0.1	0.04	3	0.28
7.5	3.6	44	661	724	1549	397	2.9	1	40	231	2.18	2	0.14	0.56	0.6	0.12	16	1.08
—	—	0	0	1	1	29	—	0	—	3	—	3	0	0	0	—	—	—

Food Item	Qty	Meas	Wgt (g)	Wtr (g)	Cals	Prot (g)	Carb (g)	Fib (g)	Fat (g)	SatF (g)
Sauce, chili, tomato base	1	tsp	6	4	6	0	1	0.1	0	0
Sauce, chili, unsalted, bottled	0.25	cup	68	46	71	2	17	—	0	0
Sauce, curry	0.25	cup	58	51	37	1	2	0.1	3	0.5
Sauce, enchilada, green	0.5	cup	62	54	44	1	4	0.7	3	1.8
Sauce, enchilada, red	0.25	cup	62	50	83	1	3	0.6	8	4.1
Sauce, fish/bagoong	0.25	cup	68	44	71	14	0	0	1	0.2
Sauce, hoisin	2	Tbs	34	16	70	1	14	0	2	0
Sauce, hollandaise, dry mix w/water	2	Tbs	32	27	30	1	2	0.1	2	1.4
Sauce, horseradish	1	tsp	5	3	10	0	0	0	1	0.6
Sauce, horseradish, Kraft	1	tsp	5	5	0	0	0	0	0	0
Sauce, hot chili/red pepper	1	tsp	5	5	1	0	0	0	0	0
Sauce, lobster	0.25	cup	58	41	95	6	4	0.3	6	1.3
Sauce, marinara tomato	0.5	cup	125	103	85	2	13	—	4	0.6
Sauce, mole poblano	0.25	cup	66	47	109	2	9	2.8	7	2.2
Sauce, mole verde	0.25	cup	66	57	39	2	4	1.1	2	0.4
Sauce, Mornay	0.25	cup	86	57	183	6	6	0.2	15	7
Sauce, pesto	0.25	cup	58	12	311	10	4	0.9	29	7.3
Sauce, soy (wheat & soy)	1	Tbs	18	13	10	1	2	0.1	0	0
Sauce, soy, lite, LaChoy	1	Tbs	18	13	15	1	2	0	0	0
Sauce, soy, tamari	1	Tbs	14	10	9	2	1	0.1	0	0
Sauce, spaghetti w/meat, recipe	0.5	cup	124	94	144	8	11	2.1	8	2.3
Sauce, spaghetti w/meatballs, canned	0.5	cup	125	94	128	6	14	0.9	5	1.3
Sauce, spaghetti, Prego	0.5	cup	125	94	135	2	22	1.9	4	1.4
Sauce, spaghetti, canned	0.5	cup	124	94	136	2	20	4.2	6	0.8
Sauce, spaghetti, meat flavor, canned	0.5	cup	125	92	150	4	19	4	7	1.4
Sauce, spaghetti, w/mushrooms, canned	0.5	cup	123	103	108	2	13	1.2	3	0.4
Sauce, spaghetti/marinara	0.5	cup	125	102	94	2	13	2.5	5	0.7
Sauce, stroganoff w/milk & water	0.25	cup	62	48	57	2	7	0.1	2	1.4
Sauce, Szechuan	1	Tbs	16	13	12	0	2	0.2	0	0
Sauce, tartar	2	Tbs	28	10	149	0	1	0.1	16	3.1
Sauce, tartar, nonfat, Kraft	2	Tbs	30	—	23	0	5	0.5	0	0
Sauce, teriyaki	1	Tbs	18	12	15	1	3	0	0	0
Sauce, teriyaki, dry w/water	1	Tbs	18	15	8	0	2	—	0	0
Sauce, tomato, canned, no added salt	0.5	cup	122	109	37	2	9	1.7	0	0
Sauce, white clam	0.25	cup	60	34	149	11	2	0	11	1.4
Sauce, white, dry mix, prep w/milk	0.25	cup	66	54	60	3	5	0.1	3	1.6
Sauce, white, recipe	0.25	cup	62	48	89	2	5	0.1	7	2
Sauce, Worcestershire	1	tsp	6	4	4	0	1	0	0	0
Sauerkraut, canned, low sodium	0.5	cup	71	66	14	1	3	1.8	0	0
Sauerkraut, canned, w/liquid	0.5	cup	118	109	22	1	5	3	0	0
Sausage, Polish, pork	1	oz.	28	15	93	4	0	0	8	2.9
Sausage, braunschweiger	2	piece	57	27	205	8	2	0	18	6.2
Sausage, chorizo, link	1	each	60	19	273	14	1	0	23	8.6
Sausage, kielbasa	1	piece	26	14	81	3	1	0	7	2.6
Sausage, pepperoni, pork/beef	4	piece	22	6	109	5	1	0	10	3.5
Sausage, pork, Chinese	4	oz.	113	44	403	24	7	0	33	—
Sausage, pork, Italian link, cooked	1	each	67	34	216	13	1	0	17	6.1
Sausage, summer, thuringer, beef & pork	1	piece	23	12	77	4	0	0	7	2.8
Sausage, turkey, breakfast type	1	piece	28	17	65	6	0	0	5	1.6
Sausage, turkey, smoked	1	oz.	28	19	55	4	0	0	4	1.3
Savory, ground	0.25	tsp	0	0	1	0	0	0.2	0	0
Scone	1	each	42	12	150	4	18	0.6	7	2.1
Scone, apple kiwi, fat free, Health Valley	1	each	60	35	80	7	15	7	0	0
Scone, whole wheat	1	each	42	11	145	5	18	2.8	7	2.1
Seafood salad	0.5	cup	104	76	166	12	2	0.4	12	1.6
Seafood souffle	0.5	cup	80	57	129	9	4	0.1	8	2.4
Seaweed, Irishmoss, raw	0.5	cup	40	32	20	1	5	0.5	0	0
Seaweed, agar, dried	0.5	cup	8	1	23	0	6	0.6	0	0
Seaweed, agar, raw	0.5	cup	40	36	10	0	3	0.2	0	0
Seaweed, kelp, raw	0.5	cup	40	33	17	1	4	0.5	0	0.1
Seaweed, laver, raw	0.5	cup	40	34	14	2	2	0.1	0	0
Seaweed, spirulina, dried	0.5	cup	8	0	22	4	2	0.3	1	0.2
Seeds, lupin, cooked, no salt	0.5	cup	83	59	99	13	8	2.3	2	0.3
Sego diet drink	1	cup	256	—	180	9	27	0	4	0.1
Sego lite diet drink	1	cup	256	—	120	9	16	0	2	0.4

MonoF (g)	PolyF (g)	Choles (mg)	Calc (mg)	Phos (mg)	Sod (mg)	Pot (mg)	Zn (mg)	Iron (mg)	Magn (mg)	VitA (μg RE)	VitE (mg α-TE)	VitC (mg)	Thia (mg)	Ribo (mg)	Nia (mg)	B6 (mg)	Fola (μg)	B12 (μg)
0	0	0	1	3	76	21	0	0	1	8	0.02	1	0	0	0.1	0.01	0	0
—	—	0	14	36	14	253	—	0.5	—	96	—	11	0.06	0.05	1.1	—	—	—
1.3	0.9	0	4	19	196	52	0.1	0.3	2	31	0.41	0	0.01	0.03	0.8	0.01	1	0.06
0.9	0.3	10	20	30	92	146	0.2	0.4	11	138	0.26	27	0.03	0.04	0.7	0.05	4	0.03
2.4	0.8	22	16	22	84	98	0.1	0.3	8	195	0.43	5	0.02	0.05	0.3	0.06	6	0.03
0.2	0.3	42	126	157	5440	442	1.4	2.2	7	29	2.63	0	0.02	0.15	4	0.09	12	5.24
—	—	0	0	—	500	—	—	0	—	0	—	0	—	—	—	—	—	—
0.7	0.1	6	16	16	196	16	0.1	0.1	1	28	0.08	0	0.01	0.02	0	0.06	3	0.1
0.3	0	2	5	4	14	7	0	0	1	9	0.03	0	0	0.01	0	0	0	0.01
0	0	0	0	—	47	9	—	0	—	0	—	1	—	—	—	—	—	—
0	0	0	0	1	1	29	0	0	1	50	0.04	2	0	0	0	0.01	1	0
1.8	2.5	42	11	67	484	114	0.6	0.5	8	12	0.43	1	0.1	0.1	1.2	0.09	13	0.2
2.1	1.2	0	22	44	786	530	0.3	1	30	120	2	16	0.06	0.07	2	0.31	17	0
3.2	1.9	1	16	54	89	216	0.3	1.2	21	254	0.96	0	0.02	0	1.1	0.17	19	0.03
0.6	0.8	0	11	67	235	191	0.4	0.9	25	41	0.22	12	0.03	0.04	1.3	0.06	9	0.04
5	2.6	79	158	127	402	108	0.6	0.4	12	163	1.14	1	0.06	0.16	0.3	0.05	10	0.39
18.1	2.1	18	417	207	422	206	1	2.4	33	86	2.9	5	0.02	0.1	0.4	0.09	16	0.32
0	0	0	3	20	1028	32	0.1	0.4	6	0	0	0	0.01	0.02	0.6	0.03	3	0
—	—	0	3	—	505	—	—	0.1	—	0	—	0	—	—	—	—	—	—
0	0	0	3	19	810	31	0.1	0.3	6	0	0	0	0.01	0.02	0.6	0.03	3	0
2.8	2.4	23	29	86	565	542	1.7	2	31	229	2.14	18	0.09	0.13	2.9	0.26	12	0.71
2.4	0.8	16	26	56	553	123	1.1	1.6	14	220	2	2	0.08	0.1	1.2	0.16	7	1.18
—	—	0	38	—	587	—	—	1.4	—	96	—	9	—	—	—	—	—	0
3	1.6	0	35	45	618	478	0.3	0.8	30	153	2.49	14	0.07	0.07	1.9	0.44	27	0
3.5	1.6	8	34	57	590	476	0.7	1	30	288	2.96	13	0.07	0.08	2.2	0.44	26	0.25
1.5	0.8	0	15	30	496	333	0.3	1	15	241	1.36	9	0.08	0.08	0.9	0.16	13	0
1.1	2.7	0	32	51	657	565	0.5	1.6	31	138	2.52	21	0.09	0.1	1.7	0.23	12	0
0.6	0.1	8	109	63	381	140	0.2	0.3	8	26	—	0	0.18	0.16	0.2	0.02	2	0.12
0.1	0.1	0	3	3	127	27	0	0.1	3	14	0.17	1	0	0	0.1	0.01	1	0
5.2	8.1	14	5	9	198	22	0	0.3	1	18	4.48	0	0	0.01	0	0.01	1	0
0	0	0	0	—	197	14	—	0	—	0	—	0	—	—	—	—	—	—
0	0	0	4	28	690	40	0	0.3	11	0	0	0	0	0.01	0.2	0.02	4	0
0	0	0	7	13	299	13	0	0.2	5	0	0	0	0	0	0.1	0.01	2	0
0	0.1	0	17	39	741	454	0.3	0.9	23	120	1.72	16	0.08	0.07	1.4	0.19	12	0
7.3	1.1	28	42	141	245	265	1.2	11.7	8	72	1.6	9	0.06	0.18	1.4	0.05	12	40.8
1.2	0.4	9	106	64	199	111	0.1	0.1	66	23	0.4	1	0.02	0.11	0.1	0.02	4	0.26
2.3	2.2	7	65	54	92	86	0.2	0.2	8	78	0.85	1	0.05	0.1	0.2	0.02	4	0.19
0	0	0	6	3	56	45	0	0.3	1	1	0	1	0	0.01	0	0	0	0
0	0	0	21	14	219	121	0.1	1	9	1	0.07	10	0.01	0.01	0.1	0.06	17	0
0	0.1	0	35	24	780	201	0.2	1.7	15	2	0.12	17	0.02	0.03	0.2	0.15	28	0
3.8	0.9	20	3	39	249	67	0.5	0.4	4	0	0.06	0	0.14	0.04	1	0.05	1	0.28
8.5	2.1	89	5	96	652	113	1.6	5.3	6	2405	0.2	0	0.14	0.87	4.8	0.19	25	11.5
11	2.1	53	5	90	741	239	2	1	11	0	0.13	0	0.38	0.18	3.1	0.32	1	1.2
3.4	0.8	17	11	38	280	70	0.5	0.4	4	0	0.06	0	0.06	0.06	0.7	0.05	1	0.42
4.6	1	17	2	26	449	76	0.6	0.3	4	0	0.05	0	0.07	0.06	1.1	0.06	1	0.55
—	—	—	27	245	998	—	—	3.4	—	0	—	0	0.52	0.31	5.3	—	—	—
8	2.2	52	16	114	618	204	1.6	1	12	0	0.17	1	0.42	0.16	2.8	0.22	3	0.87
3	0.3	17	3	26	286	62	0.6	0.6	3	0	0.05	0	0.04	0.08	1	0.06	0	1.27
1.8	1.2	23	5	52	191	76	1	0.5	6	0	0.14	0	0.03	0.08	1.4	0.08	1	0.5
1.6	1	19	5	37	219	59	0.7	0.4	5	0	0.14	0	0.02	0.06	1.2	0.06	1	0.56
—	—	0	8	1	0	4	0	0.1	1	2	—	0	0	—	0	—	—	0
2.5	1.4	51	62	61	246	50	0.3	1.2	7	85	0.9	0	0.14	0.16	1.2	0.03	8	0.1
0	0	0	20	—	160	—	—	0.1	—	200	—	12	—	—	—	—	—	—
2.5	1.5	50	55	153	174	189	0.8	1	32	84	1.07	0	0.09	0.11	1.3	0.08	11	0.1
8.3	1.2	64	45	137	274	249	1.6	1	27	27	2.29	7	0.04	0.05	1.2	0.09	16	0.89
3.3	2	112	65	116	303	136	0.8	0.8	14	117	1.49	1	0.05	0.19	1.3	0.08	13	0.53
0	0	0	29	63	27	25	0.8	3.6	58	5	0.35	1	0.01	0.19	0.2	0.03	73	0
0	0	0	47	4	8	84	0.4	1.6	58	0	0.38	0	0	0.02	0	0.02	44	0
0	0	0	22	2	4	90	0.2	0.7	27	0	0.35	0	0	0.01	0	0.01	34	0
0	0	0	67	17	93	36	0.5	1.1	48	5	0.35	1	0.02	0.06	0.2	0	72	0
0	0	0	28	23	19	142	0.4	0.7	1	208	0.4	16	0.04	0.18	0.6	0.06	58	0
0.1	0.2	0	9	9	79	102	0.2	2.1	15	4	0.38	1	0.18	0.28	1	0.03	7	0
1	0.6	0	42	106	3	203	1.2	1	45	1	0.08	1	0.11	0.04	0.4	0.01	49	0
1.7	1.5	3	200	200	289	481	3	3.6	80	300	—	12	0.3	0.34	4	0.4	80	1.2
0.4	0.9	3	200	200	289	481	3	3.6	80	300	—	12	0.3	0.34	4	0.4	80	1.2

Food Item	Qty	Meas	Wgt (g)	Wtr (g)	Cals	Prot (g)	Carb (g)	Fib (g)	Fat (g)	SatF (g)
Sesame butter, tahini, f/roasted/toasted kernels	1	Tbs	15	0	89	3	3	1.4	8	1.1
Sesame meal, partially defatted	1	oz.	28	1	161	5	7	1.1	14	1.9
Sesame seed kernels, dried	0.25	cup	38	2	221	10	4	4.4	21	2.9
Sesame seed, whole, dried	0.25	cup	36	2	206	6	8	4.2	18	2.5
Shallot, freeze dried, chopped	0.25	cup	4	0	12	0	3	0.2	0	0
Shallot, raw, chopped	1	Tbs	10	8	7	0	2	0.1	0	0
Shasta Soda, cherry cola, diet	1	cup	240	239	0	0	0	0	0	0
Shasta Soda, cream soda, diet	1	cup	240	239	0	0	0	0	0	0
Shasta Soda, ginger ale, diet	1	cup	240	239	0	0	0	0	0	0
Sherbet, orange	0.5	cup	96	64	132	1	29	0	2	1.1
Sherry, medium	1	cup	240	206	336	1	19	0	0	0
Shortening, vegetable (Crisco/Fluffo)	1	Tbs	13	0	113	0	0	0	13	3.2
Shrimp jambalaya	0.5	cup	122	88	153	14	13	0.9	5	0.9
Shrimp marinara dinner, Healthy Choice	1	each	298	243	250	10	44	5	4	2
Shrimp patty burger	1	each	120	72	248	18	15	1.3	13	3.4
Shrimp salad	0.5	cup	91	65	141	13	3	0.4	8	1.3
Shrimp w/lobster sauce	0.25	cup	46	32	72	9	2	0.1	3	0.6
Shrimp, curried	0.5	cup	118	88	157	14	7	0.2	8	2.5
Soda, 7-Up, Gold	1	cup	240	215	104	0	25	—	0	0
Soda, 7-Up, Gold, diet	1	cup	240	239	3	0	1	—	0	0
Soda, 7-Up, diet	1	cup	240	240	2	0	0	0	0	0
Soda, 7-Up, regular	1	cup	240	233	28	0	7	0	0	0
Soda, Coca Cola, can/bottle	1	cup	240	215	100	0	26	0	0	0
Soda, Coca Cola, classic, can/bottle	1	cup	240	218	94	0	26	0	0	0
Soda, Coca Cola, diet, can/bottle	1	cup	240	240	1	0	0	0	0	0
Soda, Dr. Pepper type	1	cup	245	219	101	0	26	0	0	0.2
Soda, Dr. Pepper type, decaf, sugar free, 12 oz can	1	each	355	354	4	0	0	0	0	0
Soda, Pepsi, diet	1	cup	240	239	0	0	0	0	0	0
Soda, Pepsi, regular	1	cup	240	212	100	0	27	0	0	0
Soda, Slice, apple, diet	1	cup	237	233	0	0	0	0	0	0
Soda, Slice, mandarin orange, diet	1	cup	237	233	0	0	0	0	0	0
Soda, Slice, mandarin orange, diet	1	cup	240	236	0	0	0	0	0	0
Soda, Sprite, can/bottle	1	cup	240	213	93	0	25	0	0	0
Soda, Sprite, diet, can/bottle	1	cup	240	240	3	0	0	0	0	0
Soda, Tab, can/bottle	1	cup	240	239	1	0	0	0	0	0
Soda, cherry cola, Slice	1	cup	248	217	119	0	30	0	0	0
Soda, club	1	cup	237	236	0	0	0	0	0	0
Soda, cola, caffeine-free, can/bottle	1	cup	240	212	107	0	27	0	0	0
Soda, cola, diet, w/aspartame+saccharin	1	cup	237	236	2	0	0	0	0	0
Soda, cola-type, regular	1	cup	247	221	101	0	26	0	0	0
Soda, cola/coke, diet, caffeine-free	1	cup	240	239	0	0	0	0	0	0
Soda, cola/coke, diet, w/aspartame, can/bottle	1	cup	237	236	2	0	0	0	0	0
Soda, cola/pepper type, diet, w/saccharin	1	cup	237	236	0	0	0	0	0	0
Soda, cream	1	cup	247	214	126	0	33	0	0	0
Soda, cream, sugar-free, 12 fl oz can	1	each	355	354	0	0	0	0	0	0
Soda, diet, lemon lime, Slice	1	cup	240	234	0	0	1	0	0	0
Soda, ginger ale	1	cup	244	223	83	0	21	0	0	0
Soda, ginger ale, sugar-free, 12 fl oz can	1	each	355	354	0	0	0	0	0	0
Soda, grape, carbonated	1	cup	248	220	107	0	28	0	0	0
Soda, lemon lime	1	cup	245	220	98	0	26	0	0	0
Soda, Mountain Dew	1	cup	240	—	113	0	31	0	0	0
Soda, orange, Minute Maid, can/bottle	1	cup	240	209	113	0	31	0	0	0
Soda, Pepsi, diet, caffeine free	1	cup	240	239	0	0	0	0	0	0
Soda, root beer	1	cup	247	220	101	0	26	0	0	0
Sorbet, fruit, citrus flavor	0.5	cup	100	76	92	0	23	0.1	0	0
Sorbet, fruit, non-citrus flavor	0.5	cup	100	82	70	1	17	0	0	0
Souffle, cheese	0.5	cup	56	40	98	6	3	0	7	2.8
Souffle, spinach	0.5	cup	68	50	109	5	1	1.4	9	3.6
Soup, Home Cookin', hearty lentil, RTS	0.5	cup	122	105	65	4	12	2.5	0	0.2
Soup, Pasta Fagioli, fat free, Health Valley	0.5	cup	120	107	40	3	8	2	0	0
Soup, Scotch broth, w/water	0.5	cup	120	111	40	2	5	0.6	1	0.6
Soup, bean & ham, RTS, can	1	each	546	429	519	28	61	25.1	19	7.5
Soup, bean & ham, chunky, RTS	0.5	cup	122	96	115	6	14	5.6	4	1.7
Soup, bean and 'frank', w/water	0.5	cup	125	104	94	5	11	2.9	3	1.1
Soup, bean and 'frank', w/water	1	cup	150	125	113	6	13	3.4	4	1.3

MonoF	PolyF	Choles	Calc	Phos	Sod	Pot	Zn	Iron	Magn	VitA	VitE	VitC	Thia	Ribo	Nia	B6	Fola	B12
(g)	(g)	(mg)	(mg)	(mg)	(mg)	(mg)	(mg)	(mg)	(mg)	(μg RE)	(mg α-TE)	(mg)	(mg)	(mg)	(mg)	(mg)	(μg)	(μg)
3	3.5	0	64	110	17	62	0.7	1.3	14	1	0.34	0	0.18	0.07	0.8	0.02	15	0
5.1	6	0	43	219	11	115	2.9	4.1	98	2	0.64	0	0.73	0.08	3.6	0.04	8	0
7.8	9	0	49	291	15	153	3.9	2.9	130	3	0.85	0	0.27	0.03	1.8	0.06	36	0
6.8	7.8	0	351	226	4	168	2.8	5.3	126	0	0.82	0	0.28	0.09	1.6	0.28	35	0
0	0	0	7	11	2	59	0.1	0.2	4	202	0.01	1	0.01	0	0	0.06	4	0
0	0	0	4	6	1	33	0	0.1	2	12	0.01	1	0.01	0	0	0.04	3	0
0	0	0	—	49	37	0	—	—	—	—	—	—	—	—	—	—	—	0
0	0	0	—	0	37	0	—	—	—	—	—	—	—	—	—	—	—	0
0	0	0	—	—	37	0	—	—	—	—	—	—	—	—	—	—	—	0
0.5	0.1	6	52	38	44	92	0.5	0.1	8	13	0.08	3	0.02	0.08	0.1	0.02	5	0.18
0	0	0	19	16	18	200	0.2	0.6	19	0	0	0	0.02	0.06	0.3	0.02	0	0
5.7	3.3	0	0	0	0	0	0	0	0	0	1.06	0	0	0	0	0	0	0
1.8	1.6	93	51	158	327	227	0.9	2.7	31	82	2.12	9	0.09	0.05	2.3	0.12	5	0.6
—	—	55	60	—	260	—	—	1.8	—	60	—	1	—	—	—	—	—	—
5.4	3.5	143	58	197	299	328	1.1	2.3	39	29	2.7	5	0.1	0.1	2.7	0.22	9	0.78
2.2	4.2	103	43	140	195	183	0.8	1.7	26	21	2.56	3	0.02	0.03	1.6	0.14	8	0.65
0.8	1.3	64	21	91	248	105	0.6	0.9	15	10	0.86	1	0.05	0.05	1.2	0.07	6	0.39
2.9	2	91	113	181	316	218	0.9	1.5	30	94	2.04	2	0.06	0.15	1.6	0.08	6	0.67
0	0	—	—	45	47	—	—	—	—	0	—	—	—	—	—	—	—	0
0	0	—	—	45	47	—	—	—	—	0	—	—	—	—	—	—	—	0
0	0	0	5	—	7	18	—	0.1	—	0	—	0	0	0	—	0	—	0
0	0	0	1	—	2	5	—	0	—	0	0	0	0	0	—	0	—	0
0	0	0	7	35	5	2	0	0.1	2	0	0	0	0	0	0	0	0	0
0	0	0	9	40	9	0	0	0.1	3	0	0	0	0	0	0	0	0	0
0	0	0	10	18	4	12	0.2	0.1	2	0	0	0	0.02	0.05	0	0	0	0
0	0	0	7	27	24	2	0.1	0.1	0	0	0	0	0	0	0	0	0	0
0	0	0	14	32	21	0	0.3	0.1	4	0	0	0	0.02	0.08	0	0	0	0
0	0	0	0	27	23	5	—	0	—	0	—	0	—	—	—	—	—	0
0	0	0	0	35	23	—	—	0	—	0	—	0	—	—	—	—	—	0
0	0	0	0	0	33	—	—	0	—	0	—	0	—	—	—	—	—	0
0	0	0	0	0	33	—	—	0	—	0	—	0	—	—	—	—	—	0
0	0	0	0	0	33	—	—	0	—	0	—	0	—	—	—	—	—	0
0	0	0	5	0	22	0	0.1	0.2	2	0	0	0	0	0	0	0	0	0
0	0	0	10	0	0	67	0.1	0.1	—	0	0	0	0	0	0	0	0	0
0	0	0	8	30	4	12	—	0.1	—	0	0	0	0	0	—	0	0	0
0	0	0	12	2	30	5	0.2	0.1	2	0	0	0	0	0	0	0	0	0
0	0	0	12	0	50	5	0.2	0	2	0	0	0	0	0	0	0	0	0
0	0	0	—	33	30	0	—	—	—	—	—	—	—	—	—	—	—	0
0	0	0	9	21	21	0	0.2	0.1	2	0	0	0	0.01	0.05	0	0	0	0
0	0	0	7	30	10	2	0	0.1	2	0	0	0	0	0	0	0	0	0
0	0	0	—	33	37	36	—	—	—	—	—	—	—	—	—	—	—	0
0	0	0	9	21	14	0	0.2	0.1	2	0	0	0	0.01	0.05	0	0	0	0
0	0	0	9	26	38	5	0.1	0.1	2	0	0	0	0	0	0	0	0	0
0	0	0	12	0	30	2	0.2	0.1	2	0	0	0	0	0	0	0	0	0
0	0	0	14	39	57	7	0.2	0.1	4	0	0	0	0	0	0	0	0	0
0	0	0	0	0	23	—	—	0	—	0	—	0	—	—	—	—	—	0
0	0	0	7	0	17	2	0.1	0.4	2	0	0	0	0	0	0	0	0	0
0	0	0	14	39	57	7	0.2	0.1	4	0	0	0	0	0	0	0	0	0
0	0	0	7	0	37	2	0.2	0.2	2	0	0	0	0	0	0	0	0	0
0	0	0	5	0	27	2	0.1	0.2	2	0	0	0	0	0	0	0	0	0
0	0	—	0	0	47	—	—	0	—	0	—	0	—	—	—	—	—	0
0	0	0	5	0	0	13	0.1	0.2	2	0	0	0	0	0	0	0	0	0
0	0	—	0	27	23	—	—	0	—	0	—	0	—	—	—	—	—	0
0	0	0	12	0	32	2	0.2	0.1	2	0	0	0	0	0	0	0	0	0
0	0	0	9	13	8	100	0	0.5	8	27	0.05	26	0.01	0.03	0.2	0.02	22	0
0	0	0	2	0	46	2	0	0	1	0	0	0	0	0	0	0	0	0
2.4	1.4	97	105	100	149	73	0.5	0.4	8	84	0.64	0	0.04	0.18	0.1	0.04	12	0.39
3.4	1.5	92	115	116	381	101	0.6	0.7	19	337	0.61	2	0.05	0.15	0.2	0.06	40	0.68
0	0	0	20	—	430	—	—	1.8	—	200	—	0	—	—	—	—	—	—
0	0	0	20	—	125	—	—	0.1	—	200	—	8	—	—	—	—	—	—
0.4	0.3	2	7	28	506	80	0.8	0.4	2	108	0.04	0	0.01	0.02	0.6	0.04	5	0.13
8.6	2.1	49	175	322	2184	956	2.4	7.3	104	890	0.27	10	0.33	0.33	3.8	0.27	66	0.16
1.9	0.5	11	39	72	486	213	0.5	1.6	23	198	0.06	2	0.07	0.07	0.9	0.06	15	0.04
1.4	0.8	6	44	82	546	239	0.6	1.2	24	44	—	0	0.06	0.03	0.5	0.07	15	0.04
1.6	1	8	52	99	656	287	0.7	1.4	28	52	—	1	0.07	0.04	0.6	0.08	18	0.04

A

Food Item	Qty	Meas	Wgt (g)	Wtr (g)	Cals	Prot (g)	Carb (g)	Fib (g)	Fat (g)	SatF (g)
Soup, bean w/bacon, dry, w/water	0.5	cup	132	119	53	3	8	4.5	1	0.5
Soup, bean with bacon, prep w/water	0.5	cup	126	107	86	4	11	4.3	3	0.8
Soup, beef and mushroom, w/water	0.5	cup	122	113	37	3	3	0.1	2	0.7
Soup, beef broth/bouillon, condensed, prepared	0.5	cup	120	117	8	1	0	0	0	0.1
Soup, beef broth/bouillon, ready to serve can	1	cup	236	230	16	3	0	0	1	0.3
Soup, beef broth/bouillon, ready to serve can	1	each	397	387	28	5	0	0	1	0.4
Soup, beef noodle, dry, w/water	0.5	cup	126	120	20	1	3	0.4	0	0.1
Soup, beef noodle, prep w/water	0.5	cup	122	112	42	2	4	0.4	2	0.6
Soup, beef stroganoff, chunky style	0.5	cup	120	96	118	6	11	0.7	6	2.5
Soup, beef, chunky, RTS	0.5	cup	120	100	85	6	10	0.7	3	1.3
Soup, beef, chunky, RTS	1	cup	240	200	170	12	20	1.4	5	2.5
Soup, beef, chunky, RTS, can	1	each	539	449	383	26	44	3.2	12	5.7
Soup, bisque, tomato, prepared, w/milk	0.5	cup	126	102	99	3	15	0.3	3	1.6
Soup, bisque, tomato, w/water	0.5	cup	124	108	62	1	12	0.2	1	0.3
Soup, black bean, w/water	0.5	cup	124	108	58	3	10	2.2	1	0.2
Soup, bouillabaisse	0.5	cup	114	88	121	17	2	0.3	4	1
Soup, broth, chicken, dry cube, prepared	0.5	cup	122	118	6	0	1	0	0	0
Soup, broth/bouillon, beef, canned, low sodium	0.5	cup	120	115	19	2	0	0	1	0.2
Soup, broth/bouillon, beef, condensed	1	each	298	286	36	7	2	0	0	0
Soup, broth/bouillon, beef, dry cube, prepared	0.5	cup	120	118	4	0	0	0	0	0
Soup, broth/bouillon, beef, dry, w/water	0.5	cup	122	118	10	1	1	0	0	0.2
Soup, broth/bouillon, chicken, condensed, prepared	0.5	cup	122	117	20	2	0	0	1	0.2
Soup, cauliflower, dry, w/water	0.5	cup	128	119	35	1	5	0.1	1	0.1
Soup, cheese, condensed	1	cup	257	198	311	11	21	2.1	21	13.3
Soup, cheese, condensed, can	1	each	312	241	378	13	26	2.5	25	16.2
Soup, cheese, prepared w/milk	0.5	cup	126	103	115	5	8	0.5	7	4.6
Soup, cheese, prepared w/water	0.5	cup	124	109	78	3	5	0.5	5	3.3
Soup, chicken & vegetable chunky, RTS	1	each	539	450	372	28	42	0.5	11	3.2
Soup, chicken & vegetable, chunky, RTS	1	cup	240	200	166	12	19	0.2	5	1.4
Soup, chicken and dumpling, prep w/water	0.5	cup	120	111	48	3	3	0.2	3	0.7
Soup, chicken gumbo, prep w/water	0.5	cup	122	114	28	1	4	1	1	0.2
Soup, chicken mushroom, w/water	0.5	cup	122	110	66	2	5	0.1	5	1.2
Soup, chicken noodle & meatballs, RTS	0.5	cup	124	112	50	4	4	0.3	2	0.5
Soup, chicken noodle, chunky, RTS	0.5	cup	120	101	88	6	9	1.9	3	0.7
Soup, chicken noodle, chunky, RTS	1	cup	240	202	175	13	17	3.8	6	1.4
Soup, chicken noodle, chunky, RTS, can	1	each	539	453	393	29	38	8.6	14	3.1
Soup, chicken noodle, dry, prep w/water	0.5	cup	126	119	26	1	4	0.4	1	0.1
Soup, chicken noodle, prep w/water	0.5	cup	120	111	37	2	5	0.4	1	0.3
Soup, chicken rice, chunky, RTS	0.5	cup	120	104	64	6	6	0.5	2	0.5
Soup, chicken rice, chunky, RTS, can	1	each	539	468	286	28	29	2.2	7	2.2
Soup, chicken rice, dry, w/water	0.5	cup	126	119	30	1	5	0.4	1	0.2
Soup, chicken rice, w/water	0.5	cup	120	113	30	2	4	0.4	1	0.2
Soup, chicken vegetable, dry, prep w/water	0.5	cup	126	119	25	1	4	0.3	0	0.1
Soup, chicken vegetable, prep w/water	0.5	cup	120	112	37	2	4	0.5	1	0.4
Soup, chicken, chunky, ready to serve	0.5	cup	126	106	89	6	9	0.8	3	1
Soup, chicken, chunky, ready to serve	1	cup	251	211	178	13	17	1.5	7	2
Soup, chicken, chunky, ready to serve, can	1	each	305	257	217	15	21	1.8	8	2.4
Soup, chili beef, w/water	0.5	cup	125	106	85	3	11	4.8	3	1.7
Soup, consomme, w/gelatin, prepared mix	0.5	cup	124	118	9	1	1	0	0	0
Soup, crab bisque	0.5	cup	124	100	127	10	6	0.2	7	2.3
Soup, crab, RTS	0.5	cup	122	112	38	3	5	0.4	1	0.2
Soup, crab, RTS	1	cup	244	223	76	5	10	0.7	2	0.4
Soup, crab, RTS, can	1	each	369	338	114	8	16	1.1	2	0.6
Soup, cream of asparagus, condensed	1	cup	251	211	173	5	21	1	8	2.1
Soup, cream of asparagus, condensed, can	1	each	305	257	210	6	26	1.2	10	2.5
Soup, cream of asparagus, dry, w/water	0.5	cup	126	118	29	1	4	0.2	1	0
Soup, cream of asparagus, w/milk	0.5	cup	124	107	81	3	8	0.4	4	1.7
Soup, cream of asparagus, w/water	0.5	cup	122	112	43	1	5	0.2	2	0.5
Soup, cream of bacon, prepared w/water	0.5	cup	122	111	59	2	5	0.1	4	1
Soup, cream of broccoli	0.5	cup	118	96	117	4	8	0.9	8	3
Soup, cream of celery, condensed	1	cup	251	213	181	3	18	1.5	11	2.8
Soup, cream of celery, condensed, can	1	each	305	259	220	4	21	1.8	14	3.4
Soup, cream of celery, dry, w/water	0.5	cup	127	119	32	1	5	0.2	1	0.1
Soup, cream of celery, w/milk	0.5	cup	124	107	82	3	7	0.4	5	2
Soup, cream of celery, w/water	0.5	cup	122	113	45	1	4	0.4	3	0.7

MonoF (g)	PolyF (g)	Choles (mg)	Calc (mg)	Phos (mg)	Sod (mg)	Pot (mg)	Zn (mg)	Iron (mg)	Magn (mg)	VitA (μg RE)	VitE (mg α-TE)	VitC (mg)	Thia (mg)	Ribo (mg)	Nia (mg)	B6 (mg)	Fola (μg)	B12 (μg)
0.5	0.1	1	28	45	464	163	0.3	0.7	15	3	0.13	1	0.03	0.13	0.2	0.01	4	0.01
1.1	0.9	1	40	66	476	201	0.5	1	23	44	0.04	1	0.04	0.02	0.3	0.02	16	0.02
0.6	0.1	4	2	17	471	77	0.7	0.4	5	0	—	2	0.02	0.03	0.5	0.02	5	0.1
0.1	0	0	7	16	391	65	0	0.2	2	0	0	0	0	0.02	0.9	0.01	2	0.08
0.2	0	0	14	31	769	127	0	0.4	5	0	0	0	0	0.05	1.8	0.02	5	0.16
0.4	0	0	24	52	1294	214	0	0.7	8	0	0	0	0.01	0.08	3.1	0.04	8	0.28
0.2	0.1	1	3	20	521	40	0	0.2	5	1	0.01	0	0.06	0.03	0.3	0.02	8	0
0.6	0.2	2	7	23	476	50	0.8	0.5	2	32	0	0	0.03	0.03	0.5	0.02	10	0.1
2.1	1.2	25	24	60	522	168	1.3	1.1	2	98	0.76	0	0.05	0.11	0.1	0.07	7	0.31
1.1	0.1	7	16	60	433	168	1.3	1.2	2	131	0.08	3	0.03	0.08	1.4	0.07	7	0.31
2.1	0.2	14	31	120	866	336	2.6	2.3	5	262	0.17	7	0.06	0.15	2.7	0.13	13	0.62
4.8	0.5	32	70	270	1945	755	5.9	5.2	11	588	0.38	16	0.13	0.34	6.1	0.3	30	1.4
0.9	0.6	11	93	87	555	302	0.3	0.4	13	55	0.5	4	0.06	0.13	0.6	0.07	11	0.21
0.3	0.6	2	20	30	524	209	0.3	0.4	5	36	0.37	3	0.03	0.04	0.6	0.04	7	0
0.3	0.2	0	22	53	599	137	0.7	1.1	21	25	0.04	0	0.04	0.03	0.3	0.05	12	0.01
2	0.7	45	41	170	208	366	0.9	2	37	44	1.15	6	0.12	0.09	2.5	0.19	14	5.21
0.1	0	0	6	6	396	12	0	0.1	1	2	0.02	0	0.01	0.01	0.1	0	1	0.01
0.3	0.1	0	5	36	36	103	0.1	0.3	1	0	0.02	0	0	0.04	1.6	0.01	2	0.12
0	0	12	0	39	2162	161	0	0.9	6	0	0	0	0	0.05	2.3	0.02	6	0.22
0	0	0	1	6	578	10	0	0.1	1	0	0	0	0	0.01	0.1	0	1	0
0.1	0	0	5	12	681	18	0	0	4	1	0.01	0	0	0.01	0.2	0	0	0
0.3	0.1	0	5	37	388	105	0.1	0.3	1	0	0.02	0	0	0.04	1.7	0.01	2	0.12
0.4	0.3	0	5	26	421	52	0.1	0.3	1	0	—	1	0.04	0.04	0.3	0.01	1	0.09
5.9	0.6	59	285	272	1919	308	1.3	1.5	8	218	0.41	0	0.03	0.27	0.8	0.05	8	0
7.2	0.7	72	346	331	2330	374	1.6	1.8	9	265	0.5	0	0.04	0.33	1	0.06	9	0
2	0.2	24	144	126	510	171	0.3	0.4	10	74	0.13	1	0.03	0.17	0.3	0.04	5	0.21
1.5	0.1	15	70	68	479	77	0.3	0.4	2	54	—	0	0.01	0.07	0.2	0.01	2	0
4.8	2.3	38	59	237	2398	825	4.8	3.3	22	1347	0.16	12	0.09	0.37	7.4	0.22	27	0.54
2.2	1	17	26	106	1068	367	2.2	1.5	10	600	0.07	6	0.04	0.17	3.3	0.1	12	0.24
1.3	0.7	17	7	30	430	58	0.2	0.3	2	26	0.07	0	0.01	0.04	0.9	0.02	1	0.08
0.3	0.2	2	12	12	477	38	0.2	0.5	2	7	0.02	2	0.01	0.02	0.3	0.03	2	0.01
2	1.2	5	15	13	471	77	0.5	0.4	5	56	0.61	0	0.01	0.06	0.8	0.02	0	0.02
0.8	0.4	5	15	42	520	77	0.2	0.9	5	117	—	4	0.06	0.06	1.2	0.02	11	0.12
1.3	0.8	10	12	36	425	54	0.5	0.7	5	61	0.4	0	0.04	0.08	2.2	0.02	19	0.16
2.7	1.5	19	24	72	850	108	1	1.4	10	122	0.79	0	0.07	0.17	4.3	0.05	38	0.31
6	3.4	43	54	162	1908	243	2.2	3.2	22	275	1.78	0	0.16	0.38	9.7	0.11	86	0.7
0.3	0.2	1	16	16	641	15	0.1	0.3	4	3	0.01	0	0.04	0.03	0.4	0	9	0
0.6	0.3	4	8	18	553	28	0.2	0.4	2	36	0.04	0	0.03	0.03	0.7	0.01	11	0.07
0.7	0.3	6	17	36	444	54	0.5	0.9	5	293	0.04	2	0.01	0.05	2	0.02	2	0.16
3.2	1.5	27	76	162	1994	243	2.2	4.2	22	1315	0.19	9	0.05	0.22	9.2	0.11	9	0.7
0.3	0.2	1	4	5	491	5	0.1	0	0	0	0.02	0	0	0	0.2	0.01	0	0.04
0.5	0.2	4	8	11	407	51	0.1	0.4	0	32	0.03	0	0.01	0.01	0.6	0.01	0	0.07
0.2	0.1	1	8	16	404	34	0.1	0.3	11	1	—	1	0.04	0.02	0.3	0.04	1	0.05
0.6	0.3	5	8	20	472	77	0.2	0.4	4	133	0.04	0	0.02	0.03	0.6	0.02	2	0.06
1.5	0.7	15	13	56	444	88	0.5	0.9	4	65	0.09	1	0.04	0.09	2.2	0.02	2	0.13
3	1.4	30	25	113	889	176	1	1.7	8	131	0.18	1	0.08	0.17	4.4	0.05	5	0.25
3.6	1.7	37	30	137	1079	214	1.2	2.1	9	159	0.21	2	0.1	0.21	5.4	0.06	5	0.3
1.4	0.1	6	21	74	518	263	0.7	1.1	15	75	0.09	2	0.03	0.04	0.5	0.08	9	0.16
0	0	0	4	20	1649	29	0	0.1	4	0	0	0	0	0.01	0.3	0.01	2	0.06
2.5	1.5	46	125	149	290	242	1.9	0.5	23	74	1.06	2	0.08	0.15	1.5	0.1	23	2.9
0.3	0.2	5	33	44	617	163	0.7	0.6	7	26	0.12	0	0.1	0.04	0.7	0.06	7	0.1
0.7	0.4	10	66	88	1234	327	1.5	1.2	15	51	0.24	0	0.2	0.07	1.3	0.12	15	0.2
1	0.6	15	100	133	1867	494	2.2	1.8	22	78	0.37	0	0.3	0.11	2	0.18	22	0.3
1.9	3.7	10	58	78	1962	346	1.8	1.6	8	90	1.26	6	0.11	0.16	1.6	0.02	48	0.1
2.3	4.4	12	70	95	2385	421	2.1	2	9	110	1.53	7	0.13	0.19	1.9	0.03	58	0.12
0.4	0.3	0	11	15	400	66	0.3	0.3	1	14	—	0	0.02	0.02	0.3	0	4	0.01
1	1.1	11	87	77	521	180	0.5	0.4	10	42	0.42	2	0.05	0.14	0.4	0.03	15	0.25
0.5	0.9	2	15	20	490	87	0.4	0.4	2	22	0.33	1	0.03	0.04	0.4	0.01	11	0.02
1.6	0.7	5	17	18	493	44	0.3	0.3	1	28	0.1	0	0.02	0.03	0.4	0.01	1	0.05
3	1.7	12	123	104	394	214	0.4	0.3	18	104	0.74	22	0.05	0.19	0.3	0.08	19	0.31
2.6	5	28	80	75	1900	246	0.3	1.3	13	60	0.38	1	0.06	0.1	0.7	0.02	5	0.1
3.1	6.1	34	98	92	2308	299	0.4	1.5	15	73	0.46	1	0.07	0.12	0.8	0.03	6	0.12
0.4	0.3	0	18	16	419	55	0.1	0.3	3	14	0.13	0	0.01	0.02	0.2	0	1	0.02
1.2	1.3	16	93	76	505	155	0.1	0.3	11	34	0.48	1	0.04	0.12	0.2	0.03	4	0.25
0.6	1.3	7	20	18	475	61	0.1	0.3	4	16	0.45	0	0.02	0.02	0.2	0.01	1	0.12

Food Item	Qty	Meas	Wgt (g)	Wtr (g)	Cals	Prot (g)	Carb (g)	Fib (g)	Fat (g)	SatF (g)
Soup, cream of chicken, condensed, can	1	each	305	249	284	8	22	0.6	18	5.1
Soup, cream of chicken, dry, prep w/water	0.5	cup	130	119	54	1	7	0.1	3	1.7
Soup, cream of chicken, w/milk	0.5	cup	124	105	96	4	7	0.1	6	2.3
Soup, cream of chicken, w/water	0.5	cup	122	111	59	2	5	0.1	4	1
Soup, cream of mushroom, condensed	1	cup	251	204	259	4	19	0.8	19	5.2
Soup, cream of mushroom, condensed, can	1	each	305	248	314	5	23	0.9	23	6.2
Soup, cream of mushroom, low sodium, RTS	1	each	298	262	200	3	18	3	14	4
Soup, cream of mushroom, w/milk	0.5	cup	124	105	102	3	8	0.2	7	2.6
Soup, cream of mushroom, w/water	0.5	cup	122	110	65	1	5	0.2	4	1.2
Soup, cream of mushroom, w/water	0.5	cup	122	110	65	1	5	0.2	5	1.2
Soup, cream of onion, condensed, can	1	each	305	247	268	7	32	1.2	13	3.6
Soup, cream of onion, w/milk	0.5	cup	124	105	93	3	9	0.4	5	2
Soup, cream of onion, w/water	0.5	cup	122	110	54	1	6	0.5	3	0.7
Soup, cream of potato, w/milk	0.5	cup	124	108	74	3	9	0.2	3	1.9
Soup, cream of potato, w/water	0.5	cup	122	113	37	1	6	0.2	1	0.6
Soup, cream of salmon	0.5	cup	124	96	129	14	3	0.1	6	1.7
Soup, cream of shrimp, w/milk	0.5	cup	124	107	82	3	7	0.1	5	2.9
Soup, cream of shrimp, w/water	0.5	cup	122	112	45	1	4	0.1	3	1.6
Soup, cream of vegetable, dry, prep w/water	0.5	cup	130	119	53	1	6	0.3	3	0.7
Soup, egg drop	0.5	cup	122	114	36	4	1	0	2	0.6
Soup, escarole, RTS	0.5	cup	124	120	14	1	1	—	1	0.3
Soup, escarole, RTS, can	1	each	553	536	61	3	4	—	4	1.2
Soup, gazpacho, RTS	0.5	cup	122	114	23	4	2	0.2	0	0
Soup, gazpacho, RTS, can	1	each	369	346	70	11	7	0.7	0	0
Soup, green pea, canned, w/milk	0.5	cup	127	99	119	6	16	1.4	4	2
Soup, green pea, w/water	0.5	cup	125	104	82	4	13	1.4	1	0.7
Soup, hot & sour/hot & spicy	0.5	cup	122	107	66	6	3	0.2	3	1
Soup, leek, dry, w/water	0.5	cup	127	118	36	1	6	1.5	1	0.5
Soup, lentil & ham, RTS	0.5	cup	124	106	69	5	10	1	1	0.6
Soup, lentil & ham, RTS, can	1	each	567	486	318	21	46	4.3	6	2.6
Soup, lobster bisque	0.5	cup	124	98	136	10	6	0.1	8	2.9
Soup, lobster gumbo	0.5	cup	122	102	89	5	10	2	4	0.7
Soup, minestrone, Real Italian, Health Valley	4	oz.	113	99	38	4	10	5.2	0	0
Soup, minestrone, chunky, RTS	0.5	cup	120	104	64	3	10	2.9	1	0.7
Soup, minestrone, chunky, RTS, can	1	each	539	467	286	12	47	12.9	6	3.3
Soup, minestrone, dry, prepared	0.5	cup	127	116	39	2	6	0.7	1	0.4
Soup, minestrone, w/water	0.5	cup	120	110	41	2	6	0.5	1	0.3
Soup, mushroom & beef stock, w/water	0.5	cup	122	112	43	2	5	0.4	2	0.8
Soup, mushroom barley, w/water	0.5	cup	122	113	37	1	6	0.4	1	0.2
Soup, mushroom, dry, prep w/water	0.5	cup	126	116	48	1	6	0.4	2	0.4
Soup, onion, canned, condensed, can	1	each	298	257	137	9	20	2.1	4	0.6
Soup, onion, dry packet	1	each	7	0	21	1	4	0.7	0	0.1
Soup, onion, dry, prep w/water	0.5	cup	123	118	14	1	3	0.5	0	0.1
Soup, onion, w/water	0.5	cup	120	112	29	2	4	0.5	1	0.1
Soup, oxtail, dry, w/water	0.5	cup	126	118	35	1	4	0.3	1	0.6
Soup, pea, prepared w/water, low sodium	0.5	cup	125	104	82	4	13	0.4	2	0.7
Soup, pepper pot, prep w/water	0.5	cup	120	109	52	3	5	0.2	2	1
Soup, pork rice and vegetable	0.5	cup	122	109	61	6	4	0.5	2	0.7
Soup, split pea & ham, chunky, RTS	0.5	cup	120	97	92	6	13	2	2	0.8
Soup, split pea & ham, chunky, RTS, can	1	each	539	437	415	25	60	9.2	9	3.6
Soup, split pea and carrot, Health Valley	4	oz.	113	101	52	4	8	1.9	0	0
Soup, split pea and ham, w/water	0.5	cup	126	103	95	5	14	1.1	2	0.9
Soup, split pea, low sodium, RTS	1	each	305	250	240	12	38	5	4	3
Soup, split pea, prep w/watery	0.5	cup	128	111	62	4	11	1.4	1	0.2
Soup, stock pot, w/water	0.5	cup	124	112	50	2	6	0.2	2	0.4
Soup, sweet and sour	0.5	cup	122	110	37	2	8	0.9	0	0.1
Soup, tomato beef noodle, w/water	0.5	cup	122	106	70	2	11	0.7	2	0.8
Soup, tomato rice, w/water	0.5	cup	124	109	59	1	11	0.7	1	0.3
Soup, tomato vegetable, dry, prep w/water	0.5	cup	126	118	28	1	5	0.3	0	0.2
Soup, tomato, dry, prep w/water	0.5	cup	132	119	52	1	10	0.3	1	0.5
Soup, tomato, low sodium, RTS	0.5	cup	122	105	70	2	12	0.8	2	1
Soup, tomato, w/milk	0.5	cup	124	105	81	3	11	1.4	3	1.4
Soup, tomato, w/water	0.5	cup	122	110	43	1	8	0.2	1	0.2
Soup, turkey noodle, w/water	0.5	cup	122	113	34	2	4	0.4	1	0.3
Soup, turkey vegetable, w/water	0.5	cup	120	112	36	2	4	0.2	2	0.4

MonoF	PolyF	Choles	Calc	Phos	Sod	Pot	Zn	Iron	Magn	VitA	VitE	VitC	Thia	Ribo	Nia	B6	Fola	B12
(g)	(g)	(mg)	(mg)	(mg)	(mg)	(mg)	(mg)	(mg)	(mg)	(μg RE)	(mg α-TE)	(mg)	(mg)	(mg)	(mg)	(mg)	(μg)	(μg)
8	3.6	24	82	92	2397	214	1.5	1.5	6	137	0.4	0	0.07	0.15	2	0.04	4	0.21
0.6	0.2	1	38	48	592	107	0.8	0.1	3	61	0.07	0	0.05	0.1	1.3	0.03	3	0.13
2.2	0.8	14	90	76	523	136	0.3	0.3	9	47	0.12	1	0.04	0.13	0.5	0.03	4	0.27
1.6	0.7	5	17	18	493	44	0.3	0.3	1	28	0.1	0	0.02	0.03	0.4	0.01	1	0.05
3.6	8.9	3	65	85	1736	168	1.2	1	10	0	2.61	2	0.06	0.17	1.6	0.02	8	0.25
4.4	10.8	3	79	104	2110	204	1.4	1.3	12	0	3.17	3	0.07	0.2	2	0.03	9	0.3
—	—	20	60	—	65	—	—	1.1	—	0	—	0	—	—	—	—	—	—
1.5	2.3	10	89	78	459	135	0.3	0.3	10	19	0.67	1	0.04	0.14	0.5	0.03	5	0.25
0.9	2.1	1	23	24	440	50	0.3	0.3	2	0	0.62	0	0.02	0.04	0.4	0.01	2	0.02
0.9	0.9	1	23	24	24	50	0.3	0.3	2	0	0.62	0	0.02	0.05	0.4	0.01	2	0.02
5.1	3.5	37	82	92	2318	299	0.4	1.5	15	73	2.07	3	0.12	0.18	1.2	0.06	17	0.12
1.6	0.8	16	89	77	502	155	0.3	0.3	11	35	0.04	1	0.05	0.14	0.3	0.04	11	0.25
1	0.7	7	17	18	464	60	0.1	0.3	2	15	0.37	1	0.03	0.04	0.3	0.01	3	0.02
0.9	0.3	11	83	81	531	161	0.3	0.3	9	34	0.05	1	0.04	0.12	0.3	0.04	5	0.25
0.3	0.2	2	10	23	500	68	0.3	0.2	1	15	0.01	0	0.02	0.02	0.3	0.02	1	0.02
2.2	1.8	37	144	225	767	262	0.8	0.8	22	30	0.89	0	0.03	0.14	4.8	0.2	11	2.77
1.3	0.2	17	82	73	518	124	0.4	0.3	11	27	0.43	1	0.03	0.11	0.3	0.22	5	0.52
0.7	0.1	9	9	16	488	29	0.4	0.3	5	7	0.42	0	0.01	0.01	0.2	0.02	2	0.29
1.3	0.7	0	16	27	585	48	0.1	0.3	5	1	0.62	2	0.61	0.05	0.3	0.01	4	0.06
0.8	0.3	52	10	54	364	110	0.2	0.4	2	20	0.26	0	0.01	0.09	1.5	0.03	8	0.25
0.4	0.2	1	16	40	1931	133	1.1	0.4	2	109	—	2	0.04	0.02	1.2	0.11	17	0.25
1.8	0.8	6	72	177	8615	592	5	1.7	11	487	—	10	0.17	0.11	5.1	0.5	77	1.11
0	0	0	12	18	370	112	0.1	0.5	4	131	0.23	4	0.02	0.01	0.5	0.07	5	0
0	0.1	0	37	55	1118	339	0.4	1.5	11	395	0.7	11	0.07	0.04	1.4	0.22	15	0
1.1	0.3	9	86	119	485	188	0.9	1	28	29	0.09	1	0.08	0.13	0.7	0.05	4	0.22
0.5	0.2	0	14	62	459	95	0.9	1	20	10	0.05	1	0.05	0.03	0.6	0.03	1	0
1.2	0.5	11	15	80	781	176	0.6	0.9	14	1	0.06	0	0.1	0.11	2.3	0.07	6	0.17
0.4	0	1	15	15	483	44	0.1	0.3	5	0	0.08	1	0.02	0.01	0.1	0.01	4	0.01
0.6	0.2	4	21	92	660	179	0.4	1.3	11	17	0.12	2	0.09	0.06	0.7	0.11	25	0.15
3	0.7	17	96	420	3016	816	1.7	6.1	51	79	0.57	10	0.4	0.26	3.1	0.51	113	0.68
2.9	1.6	36	135	153	429	269	1.3	0.3	25	97	1.14	1	0.05	0.18	0.5	0.07	9	1.29
1.5	1.2	12	54	64	335	305	0.8	0.9	27	103	1.11	14	0.1	0.06	1.1	0.1	34	0.51
0	0	0	19	—	99	—	—	1.7	—	945	—	2	—	—	—	—	—	—
0.5	0.1	2	30	55	432	306	0.7	0.9	7	217	0.36	2	0.03	0.06	0.6	0.12	26	0
2	0.6	11	135	248	1940	1374	3.2	4	32	976	1.62	11	0.12	0.26	2.6	0.54	119	0
0.4	0.1	1	19	30	513	170	0.4	0.5	4	15	0.02	1	0.04	0.02	0.5	0.05	18	0
0.3	0.6	1	17	28	455	157	0.4	0.5	4	117	0.04	1	0.03	0.02	0.5	0.05	18	0
0.7	0.4	4	5	18	484	79	0.7	0.4	5	62	0.28	0	0.02	0.05	0.6	0.02	5	0
0.5	0.4	0	6	30	445	46	0.2	0.3	5	10	0.18	0	0.01	0.04	0.4	0.08	2	0
1.1	0.8	0	33	38	510	100	0	0.3	3	0	0.32	1	0.14	0.06	0.2	0.01	3	0.13
1.8	1.6	0	66	27	2562	167	1.5	1.6	6	0	0.68	3	0.08	0.06	1.5	0.12	37	0
0.2	0	0	10	23	636	47	0	0.1	5	0	0.08	0	0.02	0.04	0.4	0.01	1	0
0.2	0	0	6	15	424	32	0	0.1	2	0	0.05	0	0.01	0.03	0.2	0	1	0
0.4	0.3	0	13	6	527	34	0.3	0.3	1	0	0.14	1	0.02	0.01	0.3	0.02	8	0
0.5	0.1	1	5	30	605	42	0	0.1	5	2	0.04	0	0.01	0.01	0.4	0.01	3	0.13
0.5	0.2	0	14	62	12	95	0.8	1	20	10	0.05	1	0.05	0.04	0.6	0.02	1	0
1	0.2	5	12	20	486	76	0.6	0.4	2	43	0.04	1	0.03	0.02	0.6	0.03	5	0.08
1	0.2	19	9	48	301	110	1	0.5	8	247	0.11	1	0.12	0.07	1.2	0.11	4	0.12
0.8	0.3	4	17	89	482	152	1.6	1.1	19	244	0.07	3	0.06	0.05	1.3	0.11	2	0.12
3.7	1.3	16	76	399	2166	685	7	4.8	86	1094	0.32	16	0.26	0.21	5.7	0.48	10	0.54
0	0	0	19	—	109	208	—	2.6	—	945	—	4	0.05	0.08	2.7	0.21	—	—
0.9	0.3	4	11	106	503	200	0.7	1.1	24	23	0.08	1	0.07	0.04	0.7	0.03	1	0.13
—	—	5	40	—	50	—	—	1.8	—	250	—	0	—	—	—	—	—	—
0.3	0.1	1	10	62	574	112	0.3	0.5	22	3	0.06	0	0.1	0.07	0.6	0.02	20	0.13
0.5	0.9	2	11	27	526	119	0.6	0.4	2	200	—	1	0.02	0.03	0.6	0.04	5	0
0.1	0.1	2	14	24	661	139	0.2	0.3	9	15	0.26	9	0.04	0.03	0.5	0.06	9	0.02
0.9	0.3	2	9	28	459	110	0.4	0.6	4	27	0.39	0	0.04	0.04	0.9	0.04	10	0.1
0.3	0.7	1	11	17	408	165	0.3	0.4	2	38	0.4	7	0.03	0.02	0.5	0.04	7	0
0.2	0	0	4	15	573	52	0.1	0.3	10	10	0.4	3	0.03	0.02	0.4	0.02	5	0
0.5	0.1	0	26	33	472	147	0.1	0.2	7	41	0.42	2	0.03	0.02	0.4	0.05	3	0.04
—	—	4	16	—	25	—	—	0.6	—	51	—	15	—	—	—	—	—	—
0.8	0.6	9	79	74	372	224	0.1	0.9	11	55	1.3	34	0.07	0.12	0.8	0.08	10	0.22
0.2	0.5	0	6	17	348	132	0.1	0.9	4	34	1.24	33	0.04	0.03	0.7	0.06	7	0
0.4	0.2	2	6	24	407	38	0.3	0.5	2	15	0.03	0	0.04	0.03	0.7	0.02	10	0.07
0.7	0.3	1	8	20	453	88	0.3	0.4	2	122	0.07	0	0.01	0.02	0.5	0.02	2	0.08

Food Item	Qty	Meas	Wgt (g)	Wtr (g)	Cals	Prot (g)	Carb (g)	Fib (g)	Fat (g)	SatF (g)
Soup, turkey, chunky, RTS	0.5	cup	118	102	67	5	7	0.5	2	0.6
Soup, turkey, chunky, RTS, can	1	each	532	460	303	23	32	2.3	10	2.8
Soup, turtle and vegetable	0.5	cup	122	110	59	6	2	0.3	2	0.4
Soup, vegetable & beef broth, w/water	0.5	cup	120	110	41	1	7	0.2	1	0.2
Soup, vegetable beef, dry, prep w/water	0.5	cup	126	119	27	1	4	0.3	1	0.3
Soup, vegetable beef, w/water	0.5	cup	122	112	39	3	5	0.2	1	0.4
Soup, vegetable chicken, low sodium, w/water	0.5	cup	120	100	83	6	10	0.5	2	0.7
Soup, vegetable, canned, low sodium	0.5	cup	120	110	41	1	6	0.4	1	0.2
Soup, vegetable, chunky, RTS	0.5	cup	120	105	61	2	10	0.6	2	0.3
Soup, vegetable, chunky, RTS, can	1	each	539	472	275	8	43	2.7	8	1.2
Soup, vegetable, from dry mix, low sodium	0.5	cup	126	118	28	1	5	0.3	0	0.2
Soup, vegetable, vegetarian, w/water	0.5	cup	120	111	36	1	6	0.2	1	0.1
Soup, vichyssoise	0.5	cup	124	108	74	3	9	0.2	3	1.9
Soup, won ton	0.5	cup	120	101	94	7	8	0.5	3	1.1
Sour cream, nonfat	2	Tbs	28	21	31	2	5	0	0	0
Soursop, raw pulp	1	each	225	183	149	2	38	7.4	1	0.1
Soy drink, So Good Lite	1	cup	260	229	114	9	17	2.1	2	0.3
Soy drink, So Good	1	cup	255	222	158	8	13	2	8	0.8
Soy flour, defatted, stirred	1	cup	88	6	290	41	34	15.4	1	0.1
Soy milk	1	cup	240	224	79	7	4	3.1	5	0.5
Soy milk, fat-free, Soy Moo, Health Valley	1	cup	54	48	25	1	5	0.2	0	0
Soybean sprouts, raw	0.5	cup	35	24	43	5	3	0.4	2	0.3
Soybean sprouts, steamed	0.5	cup	47	37	38	4	3	0.4	2	0.3
Soybean, fermented/Natto	0.5	cup	88	48	186	16	13	4.7	10	1.4
Soybeans, dry, cooked	0.5	cup	86	54	149	14	9	5.2	8	1.1
Soybeans, dry, roasted	0.5	cup	86	1	387	34	28	7	19	2.7
Soybeans, green, cooked	0.5	cup	90	62	127	11	10	3.8	6	0.7
Spaghetti, w/meatballs, canned	1	cup	250	195	258	12	28	5.8	10	2.2
Spaghetti, w/sauce & cheese, canned	1	cup	250	200	190	6	38	2.5	2	0
Spaghetti, w/white clam sauce	0.5	cup	124	78	228	13	21	1.1	10	1.3
Spearmint leaves	1	oz.	28	3	94	7	14	8.5	1	—
Spinach, canned w/liquid	0.5	cup	117	109	22	2	3	1.9	0	0.1
Spinach, canned w/liquid, low sodium	0.5	cup	117	109	22	2	3	2.6	0	0.1
Spinach, canned, drained, no added salt	0.5	cup	107	98	25	3	4	2.6	1	0.1
Spinach, cooked, drained, no added salt	0.5	cup	90	82	21	3	3	2.2	0	0
Spinach, frozen, cooked, drained, no added salt	0.5	cup	95	86	27	3	5	2.8	0	0
Spinach, frozen, unprepared	0.5	cup	78	71	19	2	3	2.3	0	0
Spinach, raw, chopped	0.5	cup	28	26	6	1	1	0.8	0	0
Spinach, steamed	0.5	cup	14	13	3	0	0	0.4	0	0
Spinach, stir fried	0.5	cup	90	82	20	3	3	2.4	0	0
Sport drink, orange, All Sport	1	cup	240	—	47	0	13	0	0	0
Sports bar, Tiger	1	each	65	11	230	11	40	4	2	—
Spread, Touch of Butter, tub	1	Tbs	14	5	77	0	0	0	9	2
Spring roll w/meat	1	each	64	42	114	5	9	0.7	6	1.5
Squash, acorn, baked cubes	0.5	cup	102	85	57	1	15	4.5	0	0
Squash, acorn, baked, mashed	0.5	cup	122	102	69	1	18	5.4	0	0
Squash, acorn, boiled, mashed	0.5	cup	122	110	42	1	11	3.2	0	0
Squash, butternut, baked cubes	0.5	cup	102	90	41	1	11	2.9	0	0
Squash, butternut, baked, mashed	0.5	cup	122	108	49	1	13	3.4	0	0
Squash, butternut, frozen, cooked	0.5	cup	120	105	47	1	12	3.4	0	0
Squash, crookneck, canned slices, drained	0.5	cup	108	104	14	1	3	1.5	0	0
Squash, crookneck, cooked	0.5	cup	90	84	18	1	4	1.3	0	0.1
Squash, hubbard, baked	0.5	cup	120	102	60	3	13	3.2	1	0.2
Squash, scallop, cooked, mashed	0.5	cup	120	114	19	1	4	2.3	0	0
Squash, scallop, slices, cooked	0.5	cup	90	86	14	1	3	1.7	0	0
Squash, spaghetti, cooked	0.5	cup	78	72	21	1	5	1.1	0	0
Squash, summer, cooked slices	0.5	cup	90	84	18	1	4	1.3	0	0.1
Squash, summer, raw slices	0.5	cup	65	61	13	1	3	1.2	0	0
Squash, winter, baked cubes	0.5	cup	102	91	40	1	9	2.9	1	0.1
Squash, winter, cooked w/salt, no sugar, no fat	0.5	cup	120	106	46	1	10	3.3	1	0.2
Squash, zucchini slices, steamed	0.5	cup	90	86	13	1	3	1.1	0	0
Squash, zucchini w/peel, frozen, cooked	0.5	cup	112	106	19	1	4	1.4	0	0
Squash, zucchini, baby, raw	1	each	16	15	3	0	0	0.2	0	0
Squash, zucchini, canned, Italian style	0.5	cup	114	103	33	1	8	2.3	0	0
Squash, zucchini, cooked	0.5	cup	90	85	14	1	4	1.3	0	0

A

MonoF (g)	PolyF (g)	Choles (mg)	Calc (mg)	Phos (mg)	Sod (mg)	Pot (mg)	Zn (mg)	Iron (mg)	Magn (mg)	VitA (μg RE)	VitE (mg α-TE)	VitC (mg)	Thia (mg)	Ribo (mg)	Nia (mg)	B6 (mg)	Fola (μg)	B12 (μg)
0.9	0.5	5	25	52	461	181	1.1	1	12	358	0.06	3	0.02	0.05	1.8	0.15	6	1.06
4	2.4	21	112	234	2080	814	4.8	4.3	53	1611	0.27	14	0.08	0.24	8.1	0.69	25	4.79
0.6	0.9	30	34	59	236	140	0.3	0.6	9	21	0.33	3	0.04	0.08	0.8	0.05	9	0.28
0.3	0.4	1	8	19	405	96	0.4	0.5	4	105	0.16	1	0.02	0.02	0.5	0.03	5	0
0.2	0	0	6	18	501	38	0.1	0.4	11	11	0.02	1	0.02	0.02	0.2	0.03	4	0.13
0.4	0.1	2	9	21	395	87	0.8	0.6	2	95	0.16	1	0.02	0.02	0.5	0.04	5	0.16
1.1	0.5	8	13	53	42	184	1.1	0.7	5	301	0.06	3	0.02	0.08	1.6	0.05	6	0.12
0.5	0.5	0	19	11	21	133	1.1	0.6	3	198	0.27	2	0.02	0.02	0.4	0.06	6	0
0.8	0.7	0	28	36	505	198	1.6	0.8	4	294	0.3	3	0.04	0.03	0.6	0.1	8	0
3.6	3.1	0	124	162	2269	889	7	3.7	16	1320	1.35	14	0.16	0.15	2.7	0.43	37	0
0.1	0	0	4	15	25	52	0.1	0.3	10	10	0.4	3	0.02	0.02	0.4	0.02	5	0
0.4	0.4	0	11	17	411	105	0.2	0.5	4	151	0.4	1	0.03	0.02	0.5	0.03	5	0
0.9	0.3	11	83	81	531	161	0.3	0.3	9	34	0.05	1	0.04	0.12	0.3	0.04	5	0.25
1.5	0.5	27	16	77	380	157	0.6	0.9	10	48	0.26	2	0.21	0.14	2.3	0.1	10	0.2
0	0	0	36	36	22	62	—	0	—	43	—	0	0	0.06	—	—	—	0.11
0.2	0.2	0	32	61	32	626	0.2	1.4	47	0	0.9	46	0.16	0.11	2	0.13	32	0
0.5	1	0	257	—	94	322	0.5	2.1	—	101	—	5	0.16	0.49	—	0.16	26	0.78
2	4.6	0	252	—	92	316	0.5	2	—	100	—	5	0.15	0.48	—	0.15	26	0.76
0.2	0.5	0	212	593	18	2097	2.2	8.1	255	4	0.17	0	0.61	0.22	2.3	0.5	268	0
0.8	2	0	10	118	29	338	0.6	1.4	46	7	0.02	0	0.39	0.17	0.4	0.1	4	0
0	0	0	90	—	14	4	—	0.3	—	0	—	0	0.02	0.02	0.7	—	—	0
0.5	1.3	0	24	57	5	169	0.4	0.7	25	0	0	5	0.12	0.04	0.4	0.06	60	0
0.5	1.2	0	28	64	5	167	0.5	0.6	28	0	0	4	0.1	0.02	0.5	0.05	38	0
2.1	5.4	0	190	152	6	638	2.6	7.5	101	0	0.01	11	0.14	0.17	0	0.11	7	0
1.7	4.4	0	88	211	1	443	1	4.4	74	1	1.68	1	0.13	0.24	0.3	0.2	46	0
4.1	10.5	0	120	558	2	1173	4.1	3.4	196	2	3.96	4	0.37	0.65	0.9	0.19	176	0
1.1	2.7	0	131	142	13	485	0.8	2.2	54	14	0.01	15	0.23	0.14	1.1	0.05	100	0
3.9	3.9	22	52	113	1220	245	2.4	3.2	20	100	1.5	5	0.15	0.18	2.2	0.12	5	0.82
0.4	0.5	8	40	88	955	303	1.1	2.8	21	120	2.13	10	0.35	0.28	4.5	0.13	6	0
6.6	1.1	24	42	162	218	256	1.4	11.3	20	64	1.46	8	0.19	0.22	2.4	0.07	16	36.2
—	—	—	471	—	99	—	—	54.4	—	184	—	0	—	—	—	—	—	0
0	0.2	0	97	37	373	269	0.5	1.8	66	752	1.25	16	0.02	0.12	0.3	0.09	68	0
0	0.2	0	97	37	88	269	0.5	1.8	66	752	1.13	16	0.02	0.12	0.3	0.09	68	0
0	0.2	0	136	47	29	370	0.5	2.5	81	939	1.39	15	0.02	0.15	0.4	0.11	105	0
0	0.1	0	122	50	63	419	0.7	3.2	78	737	0.86	9	0.09	0.21	0.4	0.22	131	0
0	0.1	0	139	46	82	283	0.7	1.4	66	739	0.91	12	0.06	0.16	0.4	0.14	103	0
0	0.1	0	87	32	58	252	0.3	1.6	45	605	0.74	19	0.07	0.12	0.3	0.11	94	0
0	0	0	28	14	22	156	0.1	0.8	22	188	0.53	8	0.02	0.05	0.2	0.06	54	0
0	0	0	13	6	11	73	0.1	0.4	11	89	0.26	2	0.01	0.02	0.1	0.02	18	0
0	0.1	0	89	44	71	502	0.5	2.4	71	545	1.7	22	0.06	0.16	0.6	0.17	149	0
0	0	—	0	23	37	37	—	0	—	0	—	0	—	—	—	—	—	0
—	—	—	350	400	100	280	—	4.5	140	50	20	60	1.5	1.7	20	2	400	6
4.4	1.9	1	3	2	140	4	0	0	0	152	0.43	0	0	0	0	0	0	0.01
2.7	1.6	37	13	58	304	124	0.5	0.8	10	14	0.78	2	0.16	0.13	1.3	0.1	9	0.12
0	0.1	0	45	46	4	448	0.2	1	44	44	0.12	11	0.17	0.01	0.9	0.2	19	0
0	0.1	0	54	55	5	535	0.2	1.1	53	53	0.15	13	0.2	0.02	1.1	0.24	23	0
0	0	0	32	33	4	322	0.1	0.7	32	32	0.15	8	0.12	0.01	0.6	0.14	14	0
0	0	0	42	28	4	291	0.1	0.6	30	718	0.17	16	0.07	0.02	1	0.13	20	0
0	0	0	50	33	5	348	0.2	0.7	36	858	0.21	18	0.09	0.02	1.2	0.15	24	0
0	0	0	23	17	2	160	0.1	0.7	11	401	0.16	4	0.06	0.05	0.6	0.08	20	0
0	0	0	13	23	5	104	0.3	0.8	14	13	0.13	3	0.02	0.03	0.5	0.04	11	0
0	0.1	0	24	35	1	173	0.4	0.3	22	26	0.11	5	0.04	0.04	0.5	0.08	18	0
0.1	0.3	0	20	28	10	430	0.2	0.6	26	725	0.14	11	0.09	0.06	0.7	0.21	19	0
0	0.1	0	18	34	1	168	0.3	0.4	23	11	0.14	13	0.06	0.03	0.6	0.1	25	0
0	0.1	0	14	25	1	126	0.2	0.3	17	8	0.11	10	0.05	0.02	0.4	0.08	19	0
0	0.1	0	16	11	14	91	0.2	0.3	9	9	0.09	3	0.03	0.02	0.6	0.08	6	0
0	0.1	0	24	35	1	173	0.4	0.3	22	26	0.11	5	0.04	0.04	0.5	0.06	18	0
0	0.1	0	13	23	1	127	0.2	0.3	15	13	0.08	10	0.04	0.02	0.4	0.07	17	0
0	0.3	0	14	20	1	448	0.3	0.3	8	365	0.12	10	0.09	0.02	0.7	0.07	29	0
0.1	0.3	0	17	24	279	521	0.3	0.4	10	425	0.14	12	0.1	0.03	0.8	0.09	33	0
0	0.1	0	14	29	3	223	0.2	0.4	20	29	0.11	7	0.06	0.03	0.3	0.07	17	0
0	0.1	0	19	28	2	216	0.2	0.5	14	48	0.34	4	0.05	0.04	0.4	0.05	9	0
0	0	0	3	15	0	73	0.1	0.1	5	8	0.04	5	0.01	0.01	0.1	0.02	3	0
0	0.1	0	19	33	424	311	0.3	0.8	16	61	0.11	3	0.05	0.04	0.6	0.17	34	0
0	0	0	12	36	3	228	0.2	0.3	20	22	0.11	4	0.04	0.04	0.4	0.07	15	0

Food Item	Qty	Meas	Wgt (g)	Wtr (g)	Cals	Prot (g)	Carb (g)	Fib (g)	Fat (g)	SatF (g)
Squash, zucchini, raw	0.5	cup	65	62	9	1	2	0.8	0	0
Squash, zucchini, stir fried, no oil	0.5	cup	90	86	13	1	3	1.1	0	0
Stew, beef & vegetable, canned	1	cup	245	202	194	14	17	2.4	8	2.4
Stew, Brunswick	1	cup	250	208	174	16	21	3.2	4	1
Stew, lamb, tomato base sauce	0.5	cup	126	96	136	9	14	2.9	5	2.2
Stew, oyster, prep w/milk	1	cup	245	218	135	6	10	0	8	5
Stew, oyster, prep w/water	0.5	cup	120	114	29	1	2	0	2	1.2
Stew, seafood, tomato base sauce	0.5	cup	126	104	84	10	8	1.2	1	0.4
Stew, veal, tomato base sauce	0.5	cup	126	105	95	8	8	1.3	3	1.4
Stew, venison, tomato base sauce	0.5	cup	126	105	81	9	9	1.5	1	0.3
Strawberries, cooked, unsweetened	0.5	cup	121	114	24	0	6	2.1	0	0
Strawberries, fresh	0.5	cup	83	76	25	1	6	1.9	0	0
Strawberries, fresh slices	1	each	32	29	10	0	2	0.7	0	0
Strawberries, frozen, unsweetened	0.5	cup	74	67	26	0	7	1.6	0	0
Strawberries, sliced, frozen, sweetened, thawed	0.5	cup	128	93	122	1	33	2.4	0	0
Strawberry Julius	1	cup	215	183	170	0	41	0.4	0	0.1
Strudel, berry	1	piece	64	28	159	2	29	1.4	4	0.8
Strudel, cheese	1	piece	64	24	195	6	24	0.4	8	3.9
Strudel, cherry	1	piece	64	25	179	3	29	1.1	6	0.9
Strudel, peach	1	piece	64	36	123	2	23	1.2	3	0.6
Stuffing mix, cornbread, prepared	0.5	cup	100	65	179	3	22	2.9	9	1.8
Subway, Club sandwich on a 6-in. white roll	1	each	246	179	297	21	40	3	5	1
Subway, Cold Cut Trio salad	1	each	330	294	191	13	11	1	11	3
Subway, Spicy Italian sandwich on a 6-in. white roll	1	each	232	148	467	20	38	3	24	9
Subway, Veggie Delite sandwich on a 6-in. white roll	1	each	175	124	222	9	38	3	3	0
Subway, chicken taco salad	1	each	370	322	250	18	15	2	14	5
Subway, meatball sandwich on a 6-in. white roll	1	each	260	181	404	18	44	3	16	6
Subway, pizza salad	1	each	335	288	277	12	13	2	20	8
Subway, seafood & crab salad w/light mayonnaise	1	each	331	298	161	13	11	2	8	1
Subway, tuna salad w/light mayonnaise	1	each	331	294	205	12	11	1	13	2
Subway, tuna sandwich w/light mayonnaise	1	each	178	119	279	11	38	2	9	2
Succotash, cooked from fresh	0.5	cup	96	66	110	5	23	4.3	1	0.1
Succotash, frozen, cooked	0.5	cup	85	63	79	4	17	3.5	1	0.1
Succotash, whole corn & lima beans, canned	0.5	cup	128	105	80	3	18	3.3	1	0.1
Sugar apple (sweetsop), raw	1	each	155	113	146	3	37	6.8	0	0.1
Sugar cane juice	8	oz.	227	198	79	0	21	—	0	—
Sugar, brown, Sugar Twin	1	tsp	0	0	1	0	0	0	0	0
Sugar, brown, packed	1	tsp	3	0	11	0	3	0	0	0
Sugar, maple, piece	1	each	28	2	100	0	26	0	0	0
Sugar, raw	1	tsp	4	0	15	0	4	0	0	0
Sugar, white, granulated	1	tsp	4	0	16	0	4	0	0	0
Sugar, white, powdered, sifted	0.25	cup	25	0	97	0	25	0	0	0
Sugar, white, powdered, unsifted	0.25	cup	30	0	117	0	30	0	0	0
Sukiyaki	0.5	cup	81	63	88	10	3	0.6	4	1.5
Sunflower seed butter, salted	1	Tbs	16	0	93	3	4	2	8	0.8
Sunflower seed butter, unsalted	2	Tbs	32	0	185	6	9	2	15	1.6
Sunflower seed kernels, dry	0.25	cup	36	2	205	8	7	3.8	18	1.9
Sunflower seed kernels, oil roasted, unsalted	0.25	cup	34	1	208	7	5	2.3	19	2
Sunflower seed, dry roasted	0.25	cup	32	0	186	6	8	3.6	16	1.7
Sunflower seed, oil roasted, salted	0.25	cup	34	1	208	7	5	2.3	19	2
Sunflower seeds, dry roasted, salted	0.25	cup	32	0	186	6	8	2.9	16	1.7
Supplement, Osmolite, prepared, Ross Labs	1	cup	253	199	250	9	36	—	8	—
Supplement, shake, vanilla, prepared, MenuMagic	1	cup	260	172	400	12	63	0	12	2
Sushi, w/egg, rolled in seaweed	0.5	cup	83	62	102	5	12	0.2	4	1
Sushi, w/vegetables & fish	0.5	cup	83	53	119	4	24	0.7	0	0.1
Sushi, w/vegetables, rolled in seaweed	0.5	cup	83	59	97	2	22	0.5	0	0.1
Swamp cabbage, chopped, cooked	0.5	cup	49	46	10	1	2	0.9	0	0
Sweet & sour chicken breast	1	each	131	103	117	8	15	0.8	3	0.6
Sweet potato leaves, raw	0.5	cup	18	15	6	1	1	0.4	0	0
Sweet potato leaves, steamed	0.5	cup	32	28	11	1	2	0.6	0	0
Sweet potato, baked, then peeled	1	each	114	83	117	2	28	3.4	0	0
Sweet potato, baked, then peeled	0.5	cup	100	73	103	2	24	3	0	0
Sweet potato, candied	1	piece	52	35	71	0	14	1.2	2	0.7
Sweet potato, candied, cup measure	0.5	cup	98	66	134	1	27	2.4	3	1.3
Sweet potato, canned, w/syrup	0.5	cup	114	88	101	1	24	2.8	0	0

MonoF	PolyF	Choles	Calc	Phos	Sod	Pot	Zn	Iron	Magn	VitA	VitE	VitC	Thia	Ribo	Nia	B6	Fola	B12
(g)	(g)	(mg)	(mg)	(mg)	(mg)	(mg)	(mg)	(mg)	(mg)	(μg RE)	(mg α-TE)	(mg)	(mg)	(mg)	(mg)	(mg)	(μg)	(μg)
0	0	0	10	21	2	161	0.1	0.3	14	22	0.08	6	0.05	0.02	0.3	0.06	14	0
0	0.1	0	14	29	3	223	0.2	0.4	20	28	0.11	7	0.06	0.03	0.3	0.07	16	0
3.1	0.4	34	29	110	1006	426	4.2	2.2	39	262	0.34	7	0.07	0.12	2.4	0.2	31	1.59
1.3	1	34	37	168	451	538	1.4	1.7	46	51	0.57	18	0.12	0.16	5.8	0.37	44	0.18
1.9	0.4	26	18	100	512	361	1.6	1.1	27	157	0.54	7	0.12	0.14	2.7	0.2	17	0.74
2.1	0.3	32	167	162	1041	235	10.3	1	20	44	0.49	4	0.07	0.23	0.3	0.06	10	2.62
0.5	0.1	7	11	24	490	24	5.2	0.5	2	4	0.12	2	0.01	0.02	0.1	0.01	1	1.1
0.5	0.3	48	40	111	493	405	0.9	4.7	22	266	1.27	16	0.09	0.1	1.7	0.17	17	12.2
1.3	0.3	28	18	96	303	273	1	0.7	18	307	0.25	6	0.07	0.12	3.5	0.2	13	0.28
0.2	0.2	29	16	104	339	383	1	1.8	22	267	0.43	13	0.11	0.2	2.8	0.2	15	1.61
0	0.2	0	12	15	2	135	0.1	0.3	9	2	0.11	44	0.02	0.05	0.2	0.05	14	0
0	0.2	0	12	16	1	138	0.1	0.3	8	2	0.12	47	0.02	0.06	0.2	0.05	15	0
0	0.1	0	4	6	0	53	0	0.1	3	1	0.04	18	0.01	0.02	0.1	0.02	6	0
0	0	0	12	10	1	110	0.1	0.6	8	3	0.2	31	0.02	0.03	0.3	0.02	12	0
0	0.1	0	14	17	4	125	0.1	0.8	9	3	0.18	53	0.02	0.06	0.5	0.04	19	0
0.1	0.1	0	27	—	8	82	—	0.1	—	0	—	6	0.01	0.06	—	0.01	—	0
1.7	1.2	11	15	26	103	55	0.2	0.8	6	53	1.04	5	0.09	0.09	0.8	0.02	6	0.03
2.8	1.1	42	90	87	116	64	0.6	0.8	8	95	0.69	0	0.08	0.16	0.7	0.03	8	0.12
2	2.9	9	19	40	88	100	0.3	0.8	15	79	0.7	3	0.09	0.08	0.8	0.05	8	0.02
1.2	0.9	8	12	22	75	102	0.2	0.6	7	59	0.82	3	0.06	0.07	1	0.02	4	0.02
3.9	2.7	0	26	34	455	62	0.2	0.9	13	85	1.39	1	0.12	0.09	1.2	0.04	97	0.01
—	—	26	29	—	1341	—	—	4	—	120	—	15	—	—	—	—	—	—
—	—	64	46	—	1127	—	—	2	—	282	—	33	—	—	—	—	—	—
—	—	57	40	—	1592	—	—	4	—	169	—	15	—	—	—	—	—	—
—	—	0	25	—	582	—	—	3	—	120	—	15	—	—	—	—	—	—
—	—	52	115	—	990	—	—	3	—	361	—	35	—	—	—	—	—	—
—	—	33	32	—	1035	—	—	4	—	142	—	16	—	—	—	—	—	—
—	—	50	100	—	1336	—	—	2	—	390	—	33	—	—	—	—	—	—
—	—	32	25	—	599	—	—	2	—	284	—	32	—	—	—	—	—	—
—	—	32	29	—	654	—	—	2	—	298	—	32	—	—	—	—	—	—
—	—	16	26	—	583	—	—	3	—	126	—	14	—	—	—	—	—	—
0.1	0.4	0	16	112	16	394	0.6	1.5	51	28	0.32	8	0.16	0.09	1.3	0.11	32	0
0.1	0.4	0	13	60	38	225	0.4	0.8	20	20	0.31	5	0.06	0.06	1.1	0.08	28	0
0.1	0.3	0	14	70	282	208	0.6	0.7	24	19	0.26	6	0.04	0.07	0.8	0.06	40	0
0.2	0.1	0	37	50	14	383	0.2	0.9	33	2	0.92	56	0.17	0.18	1.4	0.31	22	0
—	—	—	30	20	—	—	—	0.2	—	—	—	—	0.02	0.02	0.2	—	—	—
0	0	0	4	0	2	0	0	0	0	0	0	0	0	0	0	0	0	0
0	0	0	3	1	1	10	0	0.1	1	0	0	0	0	0	0	0	0	0
0	0	0	26	1	3	78	1.7	0.5	5	1	0	0	0	0	0	0	0	0
0	0	0	3	1	2	14	0	0.1	1	0	0	0	0	0	0	0	0	0
0	0	0	0	0	0	0	0	0	0	0	0	0	0	0	0	0	0	0
0	0	0	0	0	0	0	0	0	0	0	0	0	0	0	0	0	0	0
0	0	0	0	1	0	1	0	0	0	0	0	0	0	0	0	0	0	0
1.6	0.4	77	31	105	381	234	1.8	1.7	24	132	0.55	2	0.06	0.21	1.6	0.18	31	0.78
1.5	5	0	20	118	83	12	0.8	0.8	59	1	7.68	0	0.05	0.04	0.9	0.13	38	0
2.9	10.1	0	39	236	1	23	1.7	1.5	118	2	15.4	1	0.1	0.09	1.7	0.26	76	0
3.4	11.8	0	42	254	1	248	1.8	2.4	127	2	18.1	1	0.82	0.09	1.6	0.28	82	0
3.7	12.8	0	19	384	1	163	1.8	2.3	43	2	17	0	0.11	0.1	1.4	0.27	79	0
3	10.5	0	22	370	1	272	1.7	1.2	41	0	16.1	0	0.03	0.08	2.2	0.26	76	0
3.7	12.8	0	19	384	204	163	1.8	2.3	43	2	13.5	0	0.11	0.1	1.4	0.27	79	0
3	10.5	0	22	370	250	272	1.7	1.2	41	0	16.1	0	0.03	0.08	2.2	0.26	76	0
—	—	—	125	125	150	240	2.8	2.2	50	125	3.78	38	0.38	0.43	5	0.5	100	1.5
—	—	5	400	267	267	467	4	4.8	160	267	5.33	16	0.4	0.45	5.3	0.53	107	1.6
1.6	0.9	98	22	72	274	70	0.6	0.9	12	66	0.8	1	0.07	0.14	0.8	0.07	14	0.21
0.1	0.1	6	13	55	172	108	0.4	1.2	14	86	0.3	2	0.14	0.04	1.5	0.08	8	0.17
0.1	0.1	0	12	34	76	56	0.4	0.8	11	33	0.07	1	0.11	0.02	1	0.07	5	0
0	0	0	26	21	60	139	0.1	0.6	15	255	0.01	8	0.02	0.04	0.2	0.04	17	0
0.8	1.5	23	16	75	732	187	0.7	0.8	21	20	0.39	12	0.06	0.08	3.1	0.18	6	0.08
0	0	0	6	16	2	91	0.1	0.2	11	18	0.17	2	0.03	0.06	0.2	0.03	14	0
0	0	0	8	19	4	153	0.1	0.2	20	29	0.31	0	0.04	0.08	0.3	0.05	16	0
0	0.1	0	32	63	11	397	0.3	0.5	23	2487	0.32	28	0.08	0.14	0.7	0.28	26	0
0	0	0	28	55	10	348	0.3	0.4	20	2182	0.28	25	0.07	0.13	0.6	0.24	23	0
0.3	0.1	4	14	14	36	98	0.1	0.6	6	218	1.98	3	0.01	0.02	0.2	0.02	6	0
0.6	0.1	8	26	26	69	185	0.1	1.1	11	411	3.72	7	0.02	0.04	0.4	0.04	11	0
0	0.1	0	17	31	50	211	0.2	0.9	15	652	0.26	12	0.03	0.05	0.5	0.06	7	0

Food Item	Qty	Meas	Wgt (g)	Wtr (g)	Cals	Prot (g)	Carb (g)	Fib (g)	Fat (g)	SatF (g)
Sweet potato, canned, w/syrup, drained	0.5	cup	98	71	106	1	25	2.9	0	0.1
Sweet potato, flakes prep w/water	0.5	cup	128	96	121	1	29	—	0	0
Sweet potato, peeled, boiled, mashed	0.5	cup	100	73	105	2	24	1.8	0	0.1
Sweet potato, peeled, boiled, medium size	1	each	156	114	164	3	38	2.8	0	0.1
Sweetener, NutraSweet, low calorie	5	gram	5	0	19	5	0	0	0	0
Sweetener, saccharin, tablet	1	each	0	0	0	0	0	0	0	0
Sweetener, sugar substitute, saccharin-based, liqui	1	tsp	5	5	0	0	0	0	0	0
Swiss chard, chopped, raw	0.5	cup	18	17	3	0	1	0.3	0	0
Swiss chard, cooked, no added salt	0.5	cup	88	81	18	2	4	1.8	0	0
Swiss chard, raw leaf	1	each	48	44	9	1	2	0.8	0	0
Syrup, chocolate, thin	2	Tbs	38	14	82	1	22	0.7	0	0.2
Syrup, chocolate, thin	2	Tbs	38	11	92	1	25	0.7	0	0.3
Syrup, corn, dark	1	Tbs	20	5	58	0	16	0	0	0
Syrup, corn, light	2	Tbs	41	9	116	0	31	0	0	0
Syrup, maple	2	Tbs	40	13	105	0	27	0	0	0
Syrup, pancake	2	Tbs	39	9	113	0	30	0	0	0
Syrup, pancake, Pillsbury Lite	2	Tbs	39	25	55	0	14	0.5	0	0
Syrup, pancake, Pillsbury regular	2	Tbs	39	14	103	0	26	0.1	0	0
Syrup, pancake, buttery, Mrs. Butterworth's	2	Tbs	39	9	117	0	29	0	1	0.4
Syrup, pancake, buttery, low cal, Butterworth's	2	Tbs	36	20	58	0	15	0	0	0
Syrup, pancake, reduced-calorie	2	Tbs	36	20	59	0	16	0	0	0
Syrup, pancake, w/2% maple	2	Tbs	39	12	104	0	27	0	0	0
Tabbouleh/tabbuli	0.5	cup	80	62	93	2	8	2.3	7	0.9
Taco Bell, Pintos & cheese	1	each	128	87	203	10	19	10.7	10	4.3
Taco Bell, burrito, big beef supreme	1	each	298	192	520	24	54	11	23	10
Taco Bell, burrito, chicken	1	each	171	99	345	17	41	—	13	5
Taco Bell, burrito, seven layer	1	each	234	143	438	13	55	10.7	19	5.8
Taco Bell, cinnamon twist	1	each	35	2	175	1	24	0	8	0
Taco Bell, mexican pizza	1	each	223	119	578	21	43	8.1	36	10.1
Taco Bell, nachos, bellgrande, svg	1	each	287	148	708	19	77	15.6	36	10.1
Taco Bell, nachos, supreme, serving	1	each	145	81	330	10	33	6.6	18	5.9
Taco Bell, taco	1	each	78	46	180	9	12	3	10	4
Taco Bell, taco, soft, chicken	1	each	128	81	212	15	22	2.1	7	2.6
Taco Bell, taco, soft, steak	1	each	100	63	180	12	16	1.6	8	2
Taco Bell, taco, soft, supreme	1	each	124	79	227	10	20	2.6	12	6.1
Taco Bell, taco, supreme	1	each	106	68	206	9	13	2.8	13	6.6
Taco Time, Mexi-fries, svg	1	each	130	75	330	3	31	1	20	7
Taco Time, burrito, bean, crispy	1	each	149	82	354	11	34	4	21	4
Taco Time, burrito, beef, crispy	1	each	149	65	466	22	32	1	28	10
Taco Time, burrito, combo, soft	1	each	255	153	520	27	48	4	25	10
Taco Time, chicken fajita salad	1	each	297	198	541	28	39	2	31	7
Taco Time, taco, natural super	1	each	283	173	575	28	49	4	31	13
Taco shell, Ortega	2	each	30	0	140	2	20	2	7	1
Taco shell, baked	2	each	26	2	122	2	16	2	6	0.8
Taco, chicken	1	each	78	44	174	16	9	1.2	8	3.2
Tahini (sesame butter)	1	Tbs	15	0	91	3	3	1.4	8	1.2
Tamale, w/meat	1	each	70	36	183	7	16	2.9	10	3.7
Tamales, Old El Paso	1	each	69	49	110	2	10	1.7	6	2.3
Tamarind, raw	5	each	10	3	24	0	6	0.5	0	0
Tangelo, fresh	1	each	95	82	45	1	11	2.3	0	0
Tangerine, canned in light syrup	0.5	cup	126	105	77	1	20	0.9	0	0
Tangerine, fresh	1	each	84	74	37	1	9	1.9	0	0
Taro chips	10	each	23	0	115	1	16	1.7	6	1.5
Taro shoots, cooked slices	0.5	cup	70	67	10	1	2	0.4	0	0
Taro slices, cooked	0.5	cup	66	42	94	0	23	3.4	0	0
Taro, raw slices	0.5	cup	52	37	58	1	14	2.1	0	0
Taro, tahitian, cooked slices	0.5	cup	68	59	30	3	5	0.7	0	0.1
Tarragon, ground	0.25	tsp	0	0	1	0	0	0	0	0
Tart, lemon meringue	1	each	117	53	329	4	43	0.6	16	4
Tea, brewed	1	cup	240	239	2	0	1	0	0	0
Tea, camomile	1	cup	240	239	2	0	0	0	0	0
Tea, decaf, low calorie, frozen, prepared	1	cup	245	243	7	0	2	0	0	0
Tea, from instant, sweetened, w/lemon	1	cup	262	239	89	0	22	0	0	0
Tea, from instant, unsweetened	1	cup	237	236	2	0	0	0	0	0
Tea, herbal, brewed	1	cup	237	237	2	0	0	0	0	0

MonoF	PolyF	Choles	Calc	Phos	Sod	Pot	Zn	Iron	Magn	VitA	VitE	VitC	Thia	Ribo	Nia	B6	Fola	B12
(g)	(g)	(mg)	(mg)	(mg)	(mg)	(mg)	(mg)	(mg)	(mg)	(µg RE)	(mg α-TE)	(mg)	(mg)	(mg)	(mg)	(mg)	(µg)	(µg)
0	0.1	0	17	24	38	189	0.2	0.9	12	702	0.27	11	0.02	0.04	0.3	0.06	8	0
0	0.1	0	19	26	57	179	—	0.8	—	1530	—	14	0.03	0.04	0.4	—	—	0
0	0.1	0	21	27	13	184	0.3	0.6	10	1705	0.28	17	0.05	0.14	0.6	0.24	11	0
0	0.2	0	33	42	20	287	0.4	0.9	16	2659	0.44	27	0.08	0.22	1	0.38	17	0
0	0	0	0	0	2	0	—	0.1	—	0	—	0	0	0	0	—	—	0
0	0	0	0	0	0	1	0	0	0	0	0	0	0	0	0	0	0	0
0	0	0	0	0	1	5	0	0	0	0	0	0	0	0	0	0	0	0
0	0	0	9	8	38	68	0.1	0.3	15	59	0.34	5	0.01	0.02	0.1	0.02	2	0
0	0	0	51	29	157	480	0.3	2	75	275	1.65	16	0.03	0.08	0.3	0.07	8	0
0	0	0	24	22	102	182	0.2	0.9	39	158	0.91	14	0.02	0.04	0.2	0.05	7	0
0.1	0	0	5	48	36	84	0.3	0.8	24	1	0.01	0	0	0.02	0.1	0	2	0
0.2	0	0	5	48	57	180	0.3	5.1	24	488	0.01	0	0	0.31	12.6	0.01	2	0
0	0	0	4	2	32	9	0	0.1	2	0	0	0	0	0	0	0	0	0
0	0	0	1	1	50	2	0	0	1	0	0	0	0	0	0	0	0	0
0	0	0	27	1	4	82	1.7	0.5	6	0	0	0	0	0	0	0	0	0
0	0	0	0	4	33	1	0	0	1	0	0	0	0	0	0	0	0	0
0	0	0	2	—	104	—	—	0	—	0	—	0	—	—	—	—	—	—
0	0	0	1	—	45	—	—	0.2	—	0	—	0	—	—	—	—	—	—
0.2	0	2	1	4	39	1	0	0	1	6	0.01	0	0	0	0	0	0	0
0	0	0	3	2	74	12	0	0.6	2	0	0	0	0.02	0.01	0	0	0	0
0	0	0	0	16	72	1	0	0	0	0	0	0	0	0	0	0	0	0
0	0	0	2	4	24	2	0.1	0	1	0	0	0	0	0.01	0	0	0	0
4.7	0.6	0	27	37	321	168	0.3	1.2	23	83	1.08	26	0.04	0.03	0.7	0.06	29	0
—	—	16	160	—	693	384	2.2	1.9	110	267	—	0	0.05	0.15	0.4	0.21	68	0
—	—	55	150	—	1520	—	—	2.7	—	600	—	5	—	—	—	—	—	—
—	—	57	140	—	854	—	—	2.5	—	440	—	1	—	—	—	—	—	—
—	—	21	165	—	1058	—	—	3	—	248	—	5	—	—	—	—	—	—
—	—	0	0	—	238	28	—	0.4	—	50	—	0	0.1	0.04	0.7	0.04	—	—
—	—	46	253	—	1054	408	5.4	3.6	80	405	—	5	0.32	0.34	3	1.12	60	—
—	—	32	184	—	1205	674	—	3.3	—	138	—	3	0.1	0.34	2.2	—	—	—
—	—	22	110	—	593	—	—	2	—	73	—	3	—	—	—	—	—	—
—	—	25	80	—	330	159	—	1.1	—	100	—	0	0.05	0.14	1.2	0.12	—	—
—	—	37	85	—	571	—	—	0.8	—	64	—	1	—	—	—	—	—	—
—	—	20	62	—	797	—	—	1.1	—	31	—	0	—	—	—	—	—	—
—	—	31	87	—	515	—	—	1.6	—	131	—	3	—	—	—	—	—	—
—	—	33	94	—	328	—	—	1	—	141	—	0	—	—	—	—	—	—
9	4	—	13	46	360	315	—	1	—	0	—	4	0.06	0.01	1	—	—	0
11	6	11	143	216	302	347	2	4	—	12	—	—	0.33	0.2	2	0.35	13	—
12	6	52	180	253	571	463	4	4	—	28	—	2	0.24	0.37	5	0.33	68	—
14	1	54	271	392	826	713	5	7	—	90	—	5	0.45	0.44	5	0.6	70	—
10	11	73	177	267	490	442	2	3	—	127	—	20	0.26	0.36	9	0.44	66	—
17	1	66	300	414	763	749	5	7	—	107	—	5	0.46	0.48	5	0.58	74	—
3	1	0	60	—	200	70	—	0.7	—	20	—	—	—	—	—	—	—	—
2.3	2.2	0	42	64	95	46	0.4	0.6	27	0	0.95	0	0.06	0.01	0.4	0.08	27	0
3.2	1.4	46	95	154	106	167	1.3	1	28	39	0.85	1	0.08	0.13	4.2	0.25	16	0.2
3.2	3.7	0	21	119	0	69	1.6	1	53	1	0.34	0	0.24	0.02	0.8	0.02	15	0
4.3	1.4	24	32	80	229	154	1.1	1.9	29	18	0.43	4	0.24	0.18	2.9	0.12	5	0.18
2.7	0.5	10	13	—	197	—	—	0.6	—	—	—	—	—	—	—	—	—	—
0	0	0	7	11	3	63	0	0.3	9	0	0.07	0	0.04	0.02	0.2	0.01	1	0
0	0	0	38	13	0	172	0.1	0.1	10	20	0.23	50	0.08	0.04	0.3	0.06	29	0
0	0	0	9	13	8	98	0.3	0.5	10	106	0.43	25	0.07	0.06	0.6	0.05	6	0
0	0	0	12	8	1	132	0.2	0.1	10	77	0.2	26	0.09	0.02	0.1	0.06	17	0
1	3	0	14	30	79	174	0.1	0.3	19	0	1.13	1	0.04	0.01	0.1	0.1	5	0
0	0	0	10	18	1	241	0.4	0.3	6	4	0.7	13	0.03	0.04	0.6	0.08	2	0
0	0	0	12	50	10	319	0.2	0.5	20	0	0.29	3	0.07	0.02	0.3	0.22	13	0
0	0	0	22	44	6	307	0.1	0.3	17	0	1.24	2	0.05	0.01	0.3	0.15	12	0
0	0.2	0	102	46	37	427	0.1	1.1	35	121	1.85	26	0.03	0.14	0.3	0.08	5	0
0	0	0	5	1	0	12	0	0.1	1	2	0.01	0	0	0	0	0	1	0
6.8	3.9	74	14	56	272	54	0.4	1.3	8	34	1.56	3	0.15	0.19	1.2	0.04	11	0.14
0	0	0	0	2	7	89	0	0	7	0	0	0	0	0.03	0	0	12	0
0	0	0	5	0	2	22	0.1	0.2	2	5	0.19	0	0.02	0.01	0	0	1	0
0	0	0	0	2	7	90	0	0	7	0	0	0	0	0.03	0	0	13	0
0	0	0	5	3	8	50	0.1	0.1	5	0	0	0	0	0.05	0.1	0	10	0
0	0	0	5	2	7	47	0.1	0	5	0	0	0	0	0	0.1	0	1	0
0	0	0	5	0	2	21	0.1	0.2	2	0	0	0	0.02	0.01	0	0	1	0

Food Item	Qty	Meas	Wgt (g)	Wtr (g)	Cals	Prot (g)	Carb (g)	Fib (g)	Fat (g)	SatF (g)
Tea, instant, w/lemon, diet, dry, prepared	1	cup	238	236	5	0	1	0	0	0
Tea, instant, w/lemon, prepared	1	cup	238	237	5	0	1	0	0	0
Tea, presweetened, w/low calorie sweetener	1	cup	245	243	5	0	1	0	0	0
Tempeh	0.5	cup	83	46	165	16	14	4.5	6	0.9
Thyme, fresh	0.25	cup	17	12	16	1	3	—	0	—
Thyme, ground	0.25	tsp	0	0	1	0	0	0.1	0	0
Toaster pastry, Pop Tarts, brown sugar cinnamon	1	each	50	5	220	3	32	1	9	1
Toaster pastry, fruit filled, Pop Tart	1	each	52	6	204	2	37	1.1	5	0.8
Tofu (soybean curd, reg)	0.5	cup	124	108	76	8	2	0.2	5	0.7
Tofu yogurt	1	cup	262	203	254	9	43	0.5	5	0.7
Tofu, fried, w/Nigari	1	oz.	28	14	77	5	3	1.1	6	0.8
Tofu, fried, w/Nigari	1	piece	13	7	35	2	1	0.5	3	0.4
Tofu, okara, w/Nigari	0.5	cup	61	50	47	2	8	2.5	1	0.1
Tofu, raw, firm, prepared, w/Nigari	0.5	cup	126	105	97	10	4	0.5	6	0.8
Tofu, salted, fermented (fuyu), w/Nigari, block	1	each	11	8	13	1	1	0	1	0.1
Tomatillo, raw, chopped	0.5	cup	66	60	21	1	4	1.2	1	0.1
Tomatillo, raw, whole	1	each	34	31	11	0	2	0.6	0	0
Tomato juice, canned, low sodium	1	cup	244	229	42	2	10	2	0	0
Tomato juice, canned, w/salt	1	cup	244	229	42	2	10	1	0	0
Tomato paste, canned	0.25	cup	66	48	54	2	13	2.7	0	0.1
Tomato paste, canned, no added salt	0.5	cup	66	48	54	2	13	2.7	0	0.1
Tomato puree, canned, low sodium	0.5	cup	125	109	50	2	12	2.5	0	0
Tomato puree, canned, w/salt	0.5	cup	125	109	50	2	12	2.5	0	0
Tomato sauce w/mushrooms, canned	0.5	cup	122	108	43	2	10	1.8	0	0
Tomato slices, raw	2	piece	40	38	8	0	2	0.4	0	0
Tomato wedge w/tomato juice, canned	0.5	cup	130	120	34	1	8	1.3	0	0
Tomato, Italian/plum, raw, whole	1	each	62	58	13	1	3	0.7	0	0
Tomato, Roma, raw	1	each	62	58	13	1	3	0.7	0	0
Tomato, cherry	10	each	170	159	36	1	8	1.9	1	0.1
Tomato, fresh, stewed w/bread crumbs	0.5	cup	50	41	40	1	7	0.9	1	0.3
Tomato, green, fried	1	each	144	104	237	4	16	2	18	4.7
Tomato, green, raw slices	1	piece	44	41	11	1	2	0.5	0	0
Tomato, green, raw, chopped	0.5	cup	90	84	22	1	5	1	0	0
Tomato, green, raw, whole	1	each	123	114	30	1	6	1.4	0	0
Tomato, raw, chopped	0.5	cup	90	84	19	1	4	1	0	0
Tomato, raw, wedge	1	piece	31	29	7	0	1	0.3	0	0
Tomato, raw, whole, medium size	1	each	123	115	26	1	6	1.4	0	0.1
Tomato, red, fried	1	each	101	74	164	3	11	1.2	13	3.3
Tomato, ripe (June-Oct)	1	each	123	115	26	1	6	1.4	0	0.1
Tomato, ripe (Nov-May)	1	each	123	115	26	1	6	1.4	0	0.1
Tomato, stewed, canned, low sodium	0.5	cup	128	116	36	1	9	1.3	0	0
Tomato, sun dried pieces	10	piece	20	3	52	3	11	2.5	1	0.1
Tomato, sun dried, oil pack, drained	10	each	30	16	64	2	7	1.7	4	0.6
Tomato, yellow, sun dried	0.5	cup	27	6	79	3	15	3.2	1	0.2
Tomatoes w/green chilies, canned	0.5	cup	120	114	18	1	4	1.2	0	0
Tomatoes, canned, no salt added	0.5	cup	120	112	23	1	5	1.2	0	0
Tomatoes, raw, diced, cooked	0.5	cup	120	111	32	1	7	1.2	0	0.1
Tomatoes, sun dried, whole	0.5	cup	27	4	70	4	15	3.3	1	0.1
Topping, Marshmallow creme	2	Tbs	38	8	122	0	30	0	0	0
Topping, butterscotch	2	Tbs	41	13	103	1	27	0.4	0	0
Topping, caramel	2	Tbs	41	13	103	1	27	0.4	0	0
Topping, chocolate hot fudge	2	Tbs	42	9	149	2	27	1.2	4	1.7
Topping, nuts in syrup	2	Tbs	41	8	167	2	22	0.7	9	0.8
Topping, pineapple	2	Tbs	42	14	108	0	28	0.4	0	0
Topping, strawberry	2	Tbs	42	14	108	0	28	0.4	0	0
Tortellini, spinach	0.5	cup	61	37	116	6	13	0.5	4	1.6
Tortilla chips, Doritos	20	piece	36	1	180	3	23	2.3	9	1.8
Tortilla chips, Doritos, grab bag	1	each	64	1	319	4	40	4.1	17	3.2
Tortilla chips, baked, low fat, Tostitos	1	oz.	28	—	111	3	24	2	1	0
Tortilla chips, baked, low fat, unsalted, Tostitos	1	oz.	28	—	111	3	24	2	1	0
Tortilla chips, nacho flavor (Doritos)	1	cup	26	0	129	2	16	1.4	7	1.3
Tortilla chips, nacho flavor (Doritos), grab bag	1	each	64	1	317	5	40	3.4	16	3.1
Tortilla chips, nacho flavor, light	10	each	16	0	71	1	12	0.8	2	0.5
Tortilla chips, ranch flavor, Doritos	10	piece	18	0	88	1	12	0.7	4	0.8
Tortilla chips, taco flavor, Doritos	1	oz.	28	0	136	2	18	1.5	7	1.3

MonoF	PolyF	Choles	Calc	Phos	Sod	Pot	Zn	Iron	Magn	VitA	VitE	VitC	Thia	Ribo	Nia	B6	Fola	B12
(g)	(g)	(mg)	(mg)	(mg)	(mg)	(mg)	(mg)	(mg)	(mg)	(μg RE)	(mg α-TE)	(mg)	(mg)	(mg)	(mg)	(mg)	(μg)	(μg)
0	0	0	5	2	24	40	0.1	0.1	5	0	0	0	0	0.01	0.1	0	5	0
0	0	0	5	2	14	50	0.1	0	5	0	0	0	0	0.02	0.1	0	1	0
0	0	0	5	2	24	42	0.1	0.1	5	0	0	0	0	0.01	0.1	0	5	0
1.4	3.6	0	77	171	5	305	1.5	1.9	58	57	0.02	0	0.11	0.09	3.8	0.25	43	0.83
—	—	—	108	12	3	46	0.4	—	13	22	—	—	0.03	—	—	—	—	0
0	0	0	7	1	0	3	0	0.4	1	1	0.01	0	0	0	0	0	1	0
—	—	0	0	40	210	—	0.6	1.8	—	150	—	0	0.15	0.17	2	0.2	40	—
2.2	2	0	14	58	218	58	0.3	1.8	9	150	1.19	0	0.15	0.19	2	0.2	34	0
1	2.6	0	138	114	10	149	0.8	1.4	34	1	0.01	0	0.06	0.05	0.7	0.06	55	0
1.1	2.7	0	309	100	92	123	0.8	2.8	105	8	0.81	7	0.16	0.05	0.6	0.05	16	0
1.3	3.2	0	105	81	5	41	0.6	1.4	17	0	0.01	0	0.05	0.01	0	0.03	8	0
0.6	1.5	0	48	37	2	19	0.3	0.6	8	0	0	0	0.02	0.01	0	0.01	3	0
0.2	0.5	0	49	37	5	130	0.3	0.8	16	0	0	0	0.01	0.01	0.1	0.07	16	0
1.2	3.2	0	204	185	10	222	1.3	1.8	58	1	0.02	0	0.12	0.13	0	0.08	42	0
0.2	0.5	0	5	8	316	8	0.2	0.2	6	2	0	0	0.02	0.01	0	0.01	3	0
0.1	0.3	0	5	26	1	177	0.1	0.4	13	7	0.25	8	0.03	0.02	1.2	0.04	5	0
0.1	0.1	0	2	13	0	91	0.1	0.2	7	4	0.13	4	0.02	0.01	0.6	0.02	2	0
0	0.1	0	22	46	24	537	0.3	1.4	27	137	2.22	45	0.12	0.08	1.6	0.27	49	0
0	0.1	0	22	46	881	537	0.3	1.4	27	137	2.22	45	0.12	0.08	1.6	0.27	49	0
0.1	0.1	0	23	52	517	614	0.5	1.3	33	160	2.82	28	0.1	0.12	2.1	0.25	15	0
0.1	0.1	0	23	52	58	614	0.5	1.3	33	160	2.82	28	0.1	0.12	2.1	0.25	15	0
0	0.1	0	21	50	42	533	0.3	1.6	30	160	3.15	13	0.09	0.07	2.2	0.19	14	0
0	0.1	0	21	50	499	533	0.3	1.6	30	160	3.15	13	0.09	0.07	2.2	0.19	14	0
0	0.1	0	16	39	554	466	0.3	1.1	23	116	1.72	15	0.09	0.13	1.6	0.16	12	0
0	0.1	0	2	10	4	89	0	0.2	4	25	0.15	8	0.02	0.02	0.3	0.03	6	0
0	0.1	0	34	30	283	328	0.2	0.6	14	76	0.5	19	0.07	0.04	0.9	0.15	13	0
0	0.1	0	3	15	6	138	0.1	0.3	7	38	0.24	12	0.04	0.03	0.4	0.05	9	0
0	0.1	0	3	15	6	138	0.1	0.3	7	38	0.24	12	0.04	0.03	0.4	0.05	9	0
0.1	0.2	0	8	41	15	377	0.2	0.8	19	105	0.65	32	0.1	0.08	1.1	0.14	26	0
0.5	0.4	0	13	19	230	125	0.1	0.5	8	34	0.64	9	0.06	0.04	0.6	0.04	6	0
7.7	4.5	32	85	84	242	269	0.3	1.3	17	81	1.93	24	0.15	0.16	1.2	0.1	12	0.11
0	0	0	6	12	6	90	0	0.2	4	28	0.17	10	0.03	0.02	0.2	0.04	4	0
0	0.1	0	12	25	12	184	0.1	0.5	9	58	0.34	21	0.05	0.04	0.4	0.07	8	0
0	0.1	0	16	34	16	251	0.1	0.6	12	79	0.47	29	0.07	0.05	0.6	0.1	11	0
0	0.1	0	4	22	8	200	0.1	0.4	10	56	0.34	17	0.05	0.04	0.6	0.07	14	0
0	0	0	2	7	3	69	0	0.1	3	19	0.12	6	0.02	0.02	0.2	0.02	5	0
0.1	0.2	0	6	30	11	273	0.1	0.6	14	76	0.47	24	0.07	0.06	0.8	0.1	18	0
5.4	3.2	23	54	56	167	202	0.2	0.8	12	58	1.35	14	0.1	0.12	0.9	0.07	12	0.08
0.1	0.2	0	6	30	11	273	0.1	0.6	14	76	0.47	32	0.07	0.06	0.8	0.1	18	0
0.1	0.2	0	6	30	11	273	0.1	0.6	14	76	0.47	12	0.07	0.06	0.8	0.1	18	0
0	0.1	0	42	26	282	303	0.2	0.9	15	69	0.48	14	0.06	0.04	0.9	0.02	7	0
0.1	0.2	0	22	71	419	685	0.4	1.8	39	17	0	8	0.11	0.1	1.8	0.07	14	0
2.6	0.6	0	14	42	80	470	0.2	0.8	24	39	0.16	31	0.06	0.12	1.1	0.1	7	0
0.4	0	0	32	—	23	—	—	2.3	—	49	—	5	—	—	—	—	—	0
0	0	0	24	17	483	129	0.2	0.3	13	47	0.46	7	0.04	0.02	0.8	0.12	11	0
0	0.1	0	36	23	178	265	0.2	0.7	14	72	0.38	17	0.05	0.04	0.9	0.11	9	0
0.1	0.2	0	7	37	13	335	0.1	0.7	17	89	0.46	27	0.08	0.07	0.9	0.11	16	0
0.1	0.3	0	30	96	566	925	0.5	2.4	52	24	0	11	0.14	0.13	2.4	0.09	18	0
0	0	0	1	3	19	2	0	0.1	1	0	0	0	0	0	0	0	0	0
0	0	0	22	19	143	34	0.1	0.1	3	11	0	0	0	0.04	0	0.01	1	0.04
0	0	0	22	19	143	34	0.1	0.1	3	11	0	0	0	0.04	0	0.01	1	0.04
1.6	0.1	1	34	57	147	154	0.3	0.6	22	2	1.24	0	0.02	0.09	0.1	0.03	2	0.09
2	5.6	0	16	46	17	86	0.4	0.4	26	2	0.36	0	0.07	0.05	0.2	0.08	9	0
0	0	0	9	3	27	135	0.2	0.2	1	1	0	25	0.01	0	0	0.01	1	0
0	0	0	10	6	9	31	0.2	0.4	2	1	0.06	11	0	0.01	0.1	0.01	1	0
1.6	0.7	79	72	84	126	69	0.5	1.2	12	95	0.66	1	0.12	0.19	0.9	0.05	17	0.24
5.6	1.3	0	55	74	190	71	0.6	0.5	32	7	0.49	0	0.03	0.07	0.5	0.1	4	0
9.9	2.3	0	98	131	336	125	1	1	56	13	0.87	0	0.05	0.12	0.8	0.18	6	0
—	—	0	—	—	142	—	—	—	—	—	—	—	—	—	—	—	—	—
—	—	0	—	—	0	—	—	—	—	—	—	—	—	—	—	—	—	—
3.9	0.9	1	38	63	184	56	0.3	0.4	21	11	0.35	0	0.03	0.05	0.4	0.07	4	0.01
9.6	2.2	2	94	155	451	138	0.8	0.9	52	26	0.87	1	0.08	0.12	0.9	0.18	9	0.03
1.4	0.3	0	25	51	160	44	—	0.3	16	7	0.13	0	0.04	0.04	0.1	0.04	4	0
2.5	0.6	0	25	43	110	44	0.2	0.3	16	5	0.24	0	0.02	0.04	0.3	0.04	3	0
4.1	1	1	44	68	224	62	0.4	0.6	25	26	0.39	0	0.07	0.06	0.6	0.08	6	0

Food Item	Qty	Meas	Wgt (g)	Wtr (g)	Cals	Prot (g)	Carb (g)	Fib (g)	Fat (g)	SatF (g)
Tortilla, corn, 6 inch	1	each	30	13	67	2	14	1.6	1	0.1
Tortilla, corn, thin	1	each	17	8	38	1	8	0.9	0	0.1
Tortilla, corn/taco shell	1	each	14	1	62	1	9	1.1	3	0.4
Tortilla, flour, 10.5 inch	1	each	57	15	185	5	32	1.9	4	1
Tortilla, flour, 8 inch	1	each	35	9	115	3	20	1.2	3	0.6
Tortilla, whole wheat	1	each	35	11	73	3	20	1.9	0	0.1
Tostada, bean & chicken	1	each	157	106	250	20	18	3.4	11	5.4
Tostada, beef & cheese	1	each	163	101	315	19	23	—	16	10.4
Tostada, w/guacamole	2	each	261	189	360	12	32	—	23	9.9
Trail mix, regular	0.5	cup	75	7	347	10	34	3.8	22	4.2
Trail mix, regular, unsalted	0.5	cup	75	7	347	10	34	3.8	22	4.2
Trail mix, regular, w/chocolate chips, salted	0.5	cup	73	5	353	10	33	4	23	4.4
Trail mix, regular, w/chocolate chips, unsalted	0.5	cup	73	5	353	10	33	4	23	4.4
Trail mix, tropical	0.5	cup	70	6	285	4	46	4.5	12	5.9
Tuna noodle casserole, recipe	1	cup	202	151	237	17	25	1.4	7	1.9
Tuna salad	0.5	cup	102	65	192	16	10	0	9	1.6
Tuna, bass, freshwater, baked/broiled fillet	1	each	62	43	90	15	0	0	3	0.6
Tuna, light, canned in water, drained	1	cup	154	115	179	39	0	0	1	0.4
Turkey breast, roasted, Healthy Favorites	1	oz.	28	—	22	4	1	0	0	0
Turkey patty, breaded, fried	1	each	64	32	181	9	10	0.3	12	3
Turkey patty, breaded, fried	3	oz.	85	42	241	12	13	0.4	15	4
Turkey pot pie, Banquet	1	each	198	129	370	10	38	3	20	8
Turkey roll, light & dark meat	2	piece	57	40	84	10	1	0	4	1.2
Turkey roll, light meat	2	piece	57	41	83	11	0	0	4	1.2
Turkey, canned in water, Swanson	0.5	cup	124	78	180	32	8	2	4	1
Turkey, dark & light meat, skinless, roasted	4	oz.	113	74	193	33	0	0	6	1.9
Turkey, dark meat, roasted	4	oz.	113	68	251	31	0	0	13	4
Turkey, dark meat, skinless, roasted	4	oz.	113	72	212	32	0	0	8	2.7
Turkey, fryer, breast meat, roasted	1	each	612	419	826	184	0	0	5	1.5
Turkey, fryer, breast meat, roasted	3	oz.	85	58	115	26	0	0	1	0.2
Turkey, ground, cooked patty	1	each	82	49	194	23	0	0	11	2.8
Turkey, hickory smoked, fat free, Louis Rich	1	piece	28	22	23	4	1	0	0	0.1
Turkey, light meat, roasted	4	oz.	113	71	223	32	0	0	9	2.6
Turkey, roast, seasoned, frozen, roasted	4	oz.	113	77	176	24	3	0	7	2.2
Turkey, roasted	4	oz.	113	70	236	32	0	0	11	3.2
Turkey, tom, breast, roasted	4	oz.	113	72	214	32	0	0	8	2.4
Turkey, tom, leg, roasted	4	oz.	113	69	234	32	0	0	11	3.4
Turkey, tom, roasted	4	oz.	113	70	229	32	0	0	10	3
Turkey, tom, skinless, roasted	4	oz.	113	74	191	33	0	0	5	1.8
Turkey, w/gravy, frozen, heated	1	cup	240	204	161	14	11	0	6	2
Turkey, white meat, skinless, roasted	4	oz.	113	78	159	34	0	0	1	0.4
Turmeric, ground	0.25	tsp	1	0	2	0	0	0.1	0	0
Turnip greens, frozen, cooked	0.5	cup	82	74	25	3	4	2.8	0	0.1
Turnip greens, raw, chopped	0.5	cup	28	25	7	0	2	0.9	0	0
Turnip greens, raw, cooked	0.5	cup	72	67	14	1	3	2.5	0	0
Turnip, raw cubes	0.5	cup	65	60	18	1	4	1.2	0	0
Turnip, raw cubes, cooked, no added salt	0.5	cup	78	73	16	1	4	1.6	0	0
Turtle meat, cooked	4	oz.	113	80	152	27	0	0	4	0.9
Vanilla cookie crust, recipe, baked	1	each	173	12	936	6	89	2.4	64	13.1
Vanilla cookie crust, recipe, chilled	1	piece	29	2	156	1	15	0	11	2.2
Vanilla extract, Single Fold	1	tsp	5	3	9	0	0	0	0	0
Vanillan (no alcohol)	1	tsp	5	0	22	—	5	—	—	—
Veal patty, breaded, cooked	1	each	79	42	209	16	6	0.4	13	4.4
Veal patty, breaded, cooked	3	oz.	85	45	225	18	7	0.4	14	4.8
Veal scallopini	1	piece	96	55	257	18	1	0.2	19	5.6
Veal, ground, broiled	4	oz.	113	76	195	28	0	0	9	3.4
Veal, leg, pan fried, lean	1	each	85	52	156	28	0	0	4	1.1
Veal, leg, pan fried, lean	3	oz.	85	52	156	28	0	0	4	1.1
Veal, leg, roasted, lean	4	oz.	113	76	170	32	0	0	4	1.4
Veal, leg, roasted, lean & fat	4	oz.	113	75	181	31	0	0	5	2.1
Veal, loin chop, braised, lean	1	each	69	39	156	23	0	0	6	1.8
Veal, loin, cutlet/chop, braised, lean & fat	1	each	80	42	227	24	0	0	14	5.4
Veal, rib, roasted, lean	4	oz.	113	73	201	29	0	0	8	2.4
Veal, rib, roasted, lean & fat	4	oz.	113	68	259	27	0	0	16	6.1
Veal, shoulder, whole, braised, lean	4	oz.	113	67	226	38	0	0	7	1.9

A

MonoF	PolyF	Choles	Calc	Phos	Sod	Pot	Zn	Iron	Magn	VitA	VitE	VitC	Thia	Ribo	Nia	B6	Fola	B12
(g)	(g)	(mg)	(mg)	(mg)	(mg)	(mg)	(mg)	(mg)	(mg)	(μg RE)	(mg α-TE)	(mg)	(mg)	(mg)	(mg)	(mg)	(μg)	(μg)
0.2	0.3	0	52	94	48	46	0.3	0.4	20	0	0.05	0	0.03	0.02	0.4	0.07	34	0
0.1	0.2	0	30	54	28	27	0.2	0.2	11	0	0.03	0	0.02	0.01	0.3	0.04	20	0
1.5	0.6	0	34	31	24	33	0.2	0.4	14	6	0.57	0	0.04	0.02	0.2	0.04	4	0
2.1	0.6	0	71	70	272	74	0.4	1.9	15	0	0.52	0	0.3	0.17	2	0.03	70	0
1.3	0.4	0	44	44	169	46	0.3	1.2	9	0	0.32	0	0.19	0.1	1.3	0.02	44	0
0.1	0.2	0	10	82	171	82	0.5	0.7	26	0	0.43	0	0.1	0.02	0.9	0.07	8	0
4	1.6	54	169	239	436	367	2.3	1.8	48	87	1.88	4	0.11	0.2	4.6	0.32	54	0.26
3.3	1	41	217	179	897	572	3.7	2.9	64	96	—	3	0.1	0.55	3.2	0.23	75	1.17
8.5	3	39	423	232	799	650	4.1	1.6	73	217	—	4	0.13	0.57	2	0.26	115	0.99
9.4	7.2	0	58	259	172	514	2.4	2.3	119	2	2.66	1	0.35	0.15	3.5	0.22	53	0
9.4	7.2	0	58	259	8	514	2.4	2.3	119	2	2.66	1	0.35	0.15	3.5	0.22	53	0
9.9	8.2	3	80	283	88	473	2.3	2.5	118	4	7.81	1	0.3	0.16	3.2	0.19	48	0
9.9	8.2	3	80	283	20	473	2.3	2.5	118	4	7.81	1	0.3	0.16	3.2	0.19	48	0
1.7	3.6	0	40	130	7	496	0.8	1.8	67	4	1.55	5	0.32	0.08	1	0.23	29	0
1.5	3.2	41	34	155	772	182	1.2	2.3	30	13	1.18	1	0.18	0.15	7.8	0.2	10	1.52
3	4.2	13	17	182	412	182	0.6	1	20	28	0.97	2	0.03	0.07	6.9	0.08	8	1.23
1.1	0.8	54	64	159	56	283	0.5	1.2	24	22	0.46	1	0.05	0.06	0.9	0.09	10	1.43
0.2	0.5	46	17	251	521	365	1.2	2.4	42	26	0.82	0	0.05	0.11	20.5	0.54	6	4.6
0	0	8	—	—	333	—	—	0.4	—	—	—	—	—	—	—	—	—	—
4.8	3	40	9	173	512	176	0.9	1.4	10	7	1.53	0	0.06	0.12	1.5	0.13	18	0.14
6.4	4	53	12	230	680	234	1.2	1.9	13	9	2.03	0	0.08	0.16	2	0.17	24	0.19
—	—	45	40	—	850	—	—	1.1	—	150	—	0	—	—	—	—	—	—
1.3	1	31	18	95	332	153	1.1	0.8	10	0	0.19	0	0.05	0.16	2.7	0.15	3	0.13
1.4	1	24	23	104	277	142	0.9	0.7	9	0	0.08	0	0.05	0.13	4	0.18	2	0.14
—	—	70	0	—	440	—	—	0	—	0	—	0	—	—	—	—	—	—
1.2	1.6	86	28	242	79	338	3.5	2	30	0	0.37	0	0.07	0.21	6.2	0.52	8	0.42
4.1	3.5	101	37	222	86	311	4.7	2.6	26	0	0.69	0	0.07	0.27	4	0.36	10	0.41
1.9	2.4	96	36	231	90	329	5.1	2.6	27	0	0.73	0	0.07	0.28	4.1	0.41	10	0.42
0.8	1.2	508	73	1370	318	1787	10.6	9.4	177	0	0.55	0	0.26	0.8	45.8	3.43	37	2.39
0.1	0.2	71	10	190	44	248	1.5	1.3	25	0	0.08	0	0.04	0.11	6.4	0.48	5	0.33
4	2.7	84	21	162	88	222	2.4	1.6	20	0	0.28	0	0.04	0.14	4	0.32	6	0.27
0.1	0	10	3	70	304	62	0.3	0.3	8	0	—	0	—	—	—	—	—	—
3.2	2.3	86	24	236	71	323	2.3	1.6	30	0	0.15	0	0.06	0.15	7.1	0.53	7	0.4
1.4	1.9	60	6	277	771	338	2.9	1.8	25	0	0.43	0	0.05	0.18	7.1	0.31	6	1.72
3.6	2.8	93	30	230	77	318	3.4	2	28	0	0.38	0	0.06	0.2	5.8	0.46	8	0.4
2.8	2	85	24	238	76	328	2.4	1.6	31	0	0.2	0	0.07	0.15	6.9	0.56	7	0.41
3.2	3	102	40	227	91	319	4.9	2.6	26	0	0.92	0	0.07	0.29	3.9	0.39	10	0.42
3.4	2.6	93	31	230	82	320	3.4	2	28	0	0.47	0	0.07	0.21	5.6	0.48	8	0.41
1.1	1.5	87	28	243	84	341	3.6	2	30	0	0.48	0	0.08	0.21	6	0.53	9	0.43
2.3	1.1	43	34	194	1329	146	1.7	2.2	19	31	0.84	0	0.06	0.3	4.3	0.24	10	0.58
0.2	0.4	98	17	245	64	314	2.4	1.8	32	0	0.12	0	0.05	0.15	7.9	0.65	7	0.44
0	0	0	1	2	0	14	0	0.2	1	0	0	0	0	0	0	0.01	0	0
0	0.1	0	125	28	12	184	0.3	1.6	21	654	2.39	18	0.04	0.06	0.4	0.06	32	0
0	0	0	52	12	11	81	0.1	0.3	9	209	0.8	16	0.02	0.03	0.2	0.07	53	0
0	0.1	0	99	21	21	146	0.1	0.6	16	396	1.24	20	0.03	0.05	0.3	0.13	85	0
0	0	0	20	18	44	124	0.2	0.2	7	0	0.02	14	0.03	0.02	0.3	0.06	9	0
0	0	0	17	15	39	105	0.2	0.2	6	0	0.02	9	0.02	0.02	0.2	0.05	7	0
1.6	1.3	68	163	247	454	316	1.4	1.9	28	83	1.23	0	0.15	0.21	1.4	0.15	18	1.23
27.7	18.9	69	74	137	910	140	0.4	2.9	19	503	9	0	0.33	0.4	3.7	0.09	12	0.16
4.6	3.1	11	12	23	151	23	0.1	0.5	3	84	1.48	0	0.06	0.07	0.6	0.02	14	0.03
0	0	0	0	0	0	0	0	0	0	0	0	0	0	0	0	0	0	0
—	—	—	0	0	0	0	—	0	0	—	—	—	—	—	—	—	—	0
5.1	1.9	80	25	152	309	221	1.9	0.9	19	8	0.74	0	0.06	0.22	5.7	0.28	12	0.73
5.5	2	86	27	164	333	237	2.1	1	20	9	0.8	0	0.06	0.23	6.1	0.3	13	0.79
8.3	4.2	62	45	170	381	228	1.9	0.7	19	165	2.2	0	0.05	0.19	3.6	0.22	10	0.95
3.2	0.6	117	19	246	94	382	4.4	1.1	27	0	0.17	0	0.08	0.31	9.1	0.44	12	1.44
1.4	0.3	91	6	247	66	376	2.9	0.7	27	0	0.36	0	0.06	0.32	10.7	0.43	14	1.28
1.4	0.3	91	6	247	66	376	2.9	0.7	27	0	0.36	0	0.06	0.32	10.7	0.43	14	1.28
1.4	0.3	117	7	268	77	446	3.5	1	32	0	0.62	0	0.07	0.37	11.5	0.35	18	1.34
2	0.4	117	7	265	77	441	3.4	1	32	0	0.56	0	0.07	0.36	11.3	0.35	18	1.33
2.3	0.6	86	22	164	58	205	2.8	0.8	19	0	0.29	0	0.04	0.24	7	0.19	10	0.91
5.4	0.9	94	22	176	64	224	2.9	0.9	19	0	0.32	0	0.03	0.24	7.2	0.21	11	0.97
3	0.8	130	14	235	110	353	5.1	1.1	27	0	0.41	0	0.07	0.33	8.5	0.31	16	1.79
6.2	1.1	125	12	223	104	335	4.6	1.1	25	0	0.4	0	0.06	0.31	7.9	0.28	15	1.66
2.5	0.6	147	42	295	110	362	7.9	1.6	32	0	0.51	0	0.07	0.4	7.6	0.3	18	2.2

A

Food Item	Qty	Meas	Wgt (g)	Wtr (g)	Cals	Prot (g)	Carb (g)	Fib (g)	Fat (g)	SatF (g)
Veal, sirloin, braised, lean	4	oz.	113	66	231	39	0	0	7	2.1
Veal, sirloin, roasted, lean	4	oz.	113	74	191	30	0	0	7	2.7
Veal, sirloin, roasted, lean & fat	4	oz.	113	71	229	28	0	0	12	5.1
Vegetable juice cocktail (V8), low sodium	1	cup	242	226	46	2	11	1.9	0	0
Vegetable tempura	0.5	cup	32	22	50	1	4	0.4	3	0.6
Vegetables, Japanese stir fry, Bird's Eye	0.5	cup	58	53	18	1	4	1.1	0	0
Vegetables, pickled, giardiniera	0.5	cup	82	74	22	1	5	1.7	0	0
Vegetarian, Garden dog, hotdog	1	each	57	30	120	19	4	1	2	—
Vegetarian, Garden veggie	1	each	96	56	176	11	24	6.8	4	1.3
Vegetarian, Garden(R) burger, meat only	2.5	oz.	71	41	130	8	18	5	3	1
Vegetarian, Garden(R) sausage patty, meat only	1	each	35	21	65	4	9	2	2	1
Vegetarian, Garden(R) steak, meat only, large	1	each	142	115	369	23	51	14.2	8	2.8
Vegetarian, Garden(R) taco/Veg Mexi 1	0.25	oz.	35	9	107	6	18	4.8	1	0.6
Vegetarian, bacon bits	4	each	57	5	253	18	16	5.8	15	2.3
Vegetarian, bacon strips	3	each	24	12	74	3	2	0.6	7	1.1
Vegetarian, breakfast links	1	each	25	13	64	5	2	0.7	5	0.7
Vegetarian, breakfast sausage patty	1	each	38	19	97	7	4	1.1	7	1.1
Vegetarian, chicken, breaded, fried	1	oz.	28	20	48	3	1	1.2	3	0.5
Vegetarian, chicken, breaded, fried	1	piece	57	40	97	6	3	2.5	7	1
Vegetarian, chili	0.5	cup	107	69	141	19	15	3.9	2	0.3
Vegetarian, fish sticks	2	each	57	26	165	13	5	3.5	10	1.6
Vegetarian, frankfurter	1	each	51	30	102	10	4	2.4	5	0.8
Vegetarian, luncheon slice	1	piece	67	31	188	17	6	3.4	11	1.7
Vegetarian, meat loaf/patties	1	each	71	41	142	15	6	3.3	6	1
Vegetarian, meatballs	7	each	70	41	140	15	6	3.2	6	1
Vegetarian, scallops, breaded, fried	0.5	cup	85	36	257	20	8	5.4	16	2.5
Vegetarian, soyburger	1	each	71	41	142	15	6	3.3	6	1
Vegetarian, soyburger	1	oz.	28	16	57	6	2	1.3	3	0.4
Vegetarian, soyburger, w/cheese, serving	1	each	135	67	316	21	30	4.1	13	4.2
Vegetarian, soyburger, w/cheese, serving	1	oz.	28	14	66	4	6	0.9	3	0.9
Vermouth, dry	0.5	cup	120	92	144	0	7	0	0	0
Vinegar, balsamic	1	Tbs	15	13	10	0	2	0	0	—
Vinegar, cider	1	Tbs	15	14	2	0	1	0	0	0
Vinegar, palm	1	oz.	28	28	2	0	1	—	—	—
Vinegar, rice, natural, Nakano	1	Tbs	15	14	0	0	0	0	0	0
Waffle, Special K, Eggo	1	each	30	11	72	3	15	0	0	0
Waffle, blueberry, 7 inch round	1	each	75	32	186	6	30	1.3	5	1.8
Waffle, blueberry, 9 inch square	1	each	200	85	496	15	81	3.4	13	4.8
Waffle, buttermilk, Eggo	1	each	39	16	110	2	15	0	4	0.8
Waffle, buttermilk, recipe	1	each	75	32	217	6	25	1.1	10	1.9
Waffle, cornmeal, 7 inch round	1	each	75	31	209	6	28	1.3	8	2
Waffle, cornmeal, 9 inch square	1	each	200	83	557	17	75	3.4	21	5.2
Waffle, cornmeal, frozen, 4 inch	1	each	38	16	106	3	14	0.6	4	1
Waffle, frozen toasted	1	each	35	15	92	2	14	0.8	3	0.5
Waffle, mix prepared w/water	1	each	75	32	218	5	26	1	10	1.7
Waffle, mixed grain, frozen, 4 inch	1	each	38	12	116	3	17	2.1	5	1.2
Waffle, oat bran, Common Sense	1	each	39	18	100	3	14	1.5	4	0.8
Waffle, oat bran, Eggo	1	each	38	16	107	3	15	2.1	4	0.6
Waffle, plain, recipe	1	each	75	32	218	6	25	1.1	11	2.2
Waffle, whole grain, 4 inch round	1	each	39	17	107	4	13	1	5	1.6
Waffle, whole grain, frozen	1	each	39	17	107	4	13	1	5	1.6
Walnut, English/Persian, dried, chopped	0.25	cup	30	1	193	4	5	1.4	19	1.7
Walnut, English/Persian, dried, cup measure	0.25	cup	25	1	161	4	5	1.2	16	1.4
Walnut, black, dried, ground	0.25	cup	20	1	121	5	2	1	11	0.7
Walnuts, black, dried	0.25	cup	31	1	190	8	4	1.6	18	1.1
Water	1	cup	237	237	0	0	0	0	0	0
Water, Perrier, 6.5 fl oz bottle	1	each	192	192	0	0	0	0	0	0
Water, bottled, Poland Springs	1	cup	237	237	0	0	0	0	0	0
Water, sparkling mineral, sweet, bottled	1	each	488	445	166	0	43	0	0	0
Water, tonic, sugar-free, 12 fl oz can	1	each	355	354	0	0	0	0	0	0
Water, tonic/quinine/carbonated	1	cup	244	222	83	0	22	0	0	0
Water chestnut, Chinese, raw slices	0.5	cup	62	46	60	1	15	1.9	0	0
Water chestnut, Chinese, slices, canned w/liquid	0.5	cup	70	60	35	1	9	1.8	0	0
Water chestnut, Chinese, whole, canned w/liquid	4	each	28	24	14	0	4	0.7	0	0
Watercress, fresh	0.5	cup	17	16	2	0	0	0.3	0	0

MonoF (g)	PolyF (g)	Choles (mg)	Calc (mg)	Phos (mg)	Sod (mg)	Pot (mg)	Zn (mg)	Iron (mg)	Magn (mg)	VitA (μg RE)	VitE (mg α-TE)	VitC (mg)	Thia (mg)	Ribo (mg)	Nia (mg)	B6 (mg)	Fola (μg)	B12 (μg)
2.6	0.7	128	22	294	92	384	5.4	1.4	33	0	0.5	0	0.07	0.43	8	0.43	18	1.8
2.6	0.5	118	16	262	96	414	4	1	31	0	0.52	0	0.07	0.42	10.6	0.39	18	1.69
4.6	0.8	116	15	253	94	398	3.8	1	30	0	0.48	0	0.07	0.4	10.1	0.36	17	1.61
0	0.1	0	27	41	653	467	0.5	1	27	283	0.77	67	0.1	0.07	1.8	0.34	51	0
0.9	1.3	20	8	22	10	56	0.1	0.4	4	73	0.32	1	0.04	0.06	0.4	0.02	7	0.04
—	—	0	16	21	219	96	—	0.4	8	37	—	16	0.03	0.06	0.5	0.05	18	0
0	0.1	0	18	23	562	186	0.1	0.3	10	624	0.23	26	0.04	0.03	0.4	0.11	14	0
—	—	0	20	—	310	500	—	1.4	—	0	—	4	—	—	—	—	—	—
2	0.7	15	114	179	394	262	1.2	0	41	14	0.27	1	0.14	0.2	1.5	0.11	14	0.15
1.5	0.5	11	84	132	289	193	0.9	0	30	10	0.2	0	0.11	0.15	1.1	0.08	10	0.11
0.4	0.1	5	40	68	150	71	0.4	0.2	14	12	0.1	0	0.05	0.07	0.5	0.04	5	0.06
4.2	1.2	31	239	375	822	548	2.5	0	86	28	0.61	0	0.3	0.42	3	0.21	29	0.31
0.4	0.2	0	118	—	80	152	—	0.4	—	18	—	1	—	—	—	—	—	0
3.6	7.7	0	58	124	1008	83	1.1	0.4	54	0	3.93	1	0.34	0.04	0.9	0.05	72	0.68
1.7	3.7	0	6	17	352	41	0.1	0.6	5	2	1.66	0	1.06	0.12	1.8	0.12	10	0
1.1	2.3	0	16	56	222	58	0.4	0.9	9	16	0.52	0	0.58	0.1	2.8	0.21	6	0
1.7	3.5	0	24	86	337	88	0.6	1.4	14	24	0.8	0	0.89	0.15	4.3	0.32	10	0
1.5	1.3	0	7	70	113	85	0.2	0.5	3	0	0.55	0	0.2	0.14	1.3	0.14	16	0.6
2.9	2.5	0	13	140	228	171	0.4	1	7	0	1.11	0	0.4	0.27	2.7	0.28	32	1.2
0.6	0.9	0	53	216	526	362	1.3	4.2	36	78	1.24	16	0.12	0.07	1.2	0.15	82	0
2.5	5.4	0	54	257	279	342	0.8	1.1	13	0	2.25	0	0.63	0.51	6.8	0.86	58	2.39
1.2	2.7	0	17	175	219	76	0.6	0.9	9	0	0.98	0	0.56	0.61	8.2	0.5	40	1.22
2.6	5.6	0	28	296	576	188	1.1	1.5	15	0	2.01	0	0.64	0.37	7.4	0.74	67	1.74
1.5	3.3	0	21	244	391	128	1.3	1.5	13	0	1.23	0	0.64	0.43	7.1	0.85	55	1.7
1.5	3.3	0	20	241	385	126	1.3	1.5	13	0	1.21	0	0.63	0.42	7	0.84	55	1.68
3.8	8.3	0	84	398	434	531	1.2	1.8	20	0	3.5	0	0.97	0.8	10.6	1.33	90	3.72
1.5	3.3	0	21	244	391	128	1.3	1.5	13	0	1.23	0	0.64	0.43	7.1	0.85	55	1.7
0.6	1.3	0	8	98	156	51	0.5	0.6	5	0	0.49	0	0.26	0.17	2.8	0.34	22	0.68
4	3.7	13	146	372	931	211	2	2.7	26	45	1.43	1	0.77	0.55	8.1	0.86	70	1.71
0.8	0.8	3	31	78	196	44	0.4	0.6	6	9	0.3	0	0.16	0.12	1.7	0.18	15	0.36
0	0	0	8	8	20	48	0	0.4	6	0	0	0	0.02	0.02	0	0.01	0	0
—	—	0	5	—	4	12	—	0.1	—	0	—	0	—	—	—	—	—	—
0	0	0	1	1	0	15	0	0.1	3	0	0	0	0	0	0	0	0	0
—	—	—	3	2	—	—	—	0.9	—	—	—	—	0	0	0.1	—	—	—
0	0	0	—	—	1	—	—	—	—	—	—	—	—	—	—	—	—	—
0	0	0	21	—	129	16	—	1.9	—	155	—	0	0.16	0.18	2.1	0.21	41	0.62
1.6	0.9	34	219	262	523	154	0.5	1.2	16	29	0.89	2	0.15	0.23	1	0.06	7	0.2
4.2	2.4	90	584	699	1394	411	1.4	3.2	43	78	2.38	6	0.39	0.6	2.6	0.16	20	0.54
—	—	12	20	—	240	32	—	1.8	—	150	—	0	0.15	0.17	2	0.2	40	0.6
2.5	5.1	50	137	124	451	128	0.6	1.6	14	26	1.5	0	0.2	0.27	1.6	0.04	11	0.16
2.2	3	75	110	108	312	124	0.6	1.6	17	50	1.41	0	0.21	0.27	1.6	0.08	16	0.27
5.7	8.1	199	294	289	832	330	1.5	4.3	45	133	3.77	1	0.55	0.71	4.2	0.22	43	0.73
1.1	1.5	38	56	55	158	63	0.3	0.8	9	25	0.72	0	0.1	0.14	0.8	0.04	8	0.14
1.1	1	8	81	147	275	45	0.2	1.6	8	127	0.29	0	0.14	0.17	1.6	0.31	16	0.88
2.7	5.2	38	93	252	458	134	0.4	1.2	15	20	1.5	0	0.16	0.19	1.2	0.08	9	0.2
1.2	2	28	83	104	146	123	0.9	1.4	25	60	0.93	3	0.14	0.19	1.4	0.11	23	0.12
2.2	0.5	0	20	—	175	18	—	1.8	—	150	—	0	0.15	0.17	2	0.2	40	0.6
1.1	2	0	8	131	214	189	0.7	0.7	38	57	0.57	0	0.06	0.06	0.8	0.03	15	0.23
2.6	5.1	52	191	143	383	119	0.5	1.7	14	49	1.73	0	0.2	0.26	1.6	0.04	34	0.19
1.9	1	39	84	83	150	91	0.4	0.7	16	25	0.53	0	0.08	0.13	0.7	0.04	7	0.15
1.9	1	39	84	83	150	91	0.4	0.7	16	25	0.53	0	0.08	0.13	0.7	0.04	7	0.15
4.3	11.7	0	28	95	3	151	0.8	0.7	51	4	0.79	1	0.12	0.04	0.3	0.17	20	0
3.6	9.8	0	24	79	2	126	0.7	0.6	42	3	0.66	1	0.1	0.04	0.3	0.14	16	0
2.5	7.5	0	12	93	0	105	0.7	0.6	40	6	0.52	1	0.04	0.02	0.1	0.11	13	0
4	11.7	0	18	145	0	164	1.1	1	63	9	0.82	1	0.07	0.03	0.2	0.17	20	0
0	0	0	5	0	7	0	0.1	0	2	0	0	0	0	0	0	0	0	0
0	0	0	27	0	2	0	0	0	0	0	0	0	0	0	0	0	0	0
0	0	0	2	0	2	0	0	0	2	0	0	0	0	0	0	0	0	0
0	0	0	5	0	20	0	0.5	0	0	0	0	0	0	0	0	0	0	0
0	0	0	14	39	57	7	0.2	0.1	4	0	0	0	0	0	0	0	0	0
0	0	0	2	0	10	0	0.2	0	0	0	0	0	0	0	0	0	0	0
0	0	0	7	39	9	362	0.3	0	14	0	0.74	2	0.09	0.12	0.6	0.2	10	0
0	0	0	3	13	6	83	0.3	0.6	4	0	0.35	1	0.01	0.02	0.3	0.11	4	0
0	0	0	1	5	2	34	0.1	0.2	1	0	0.14	0	0	0.01	0.1	0.04	2	0
0	0	0	20	10	7	56	0	0	4	80	0.17	7	0.02	0.02	0	0.02	2	0

Food Item	Qty	Meas	Wgt (g)	Wtr (g)	Cals	Prot (g)	Carb (g)	Fib (g)	Fat (g)	SatF (g)
Watercress, fresh sprigs	10	each	25	24	3	1	0	0.4	0	0
Watermelon, fresh pieces	0.5	cup	80	73	26	0	6	0.4	0	0
Waxgourd, cooked cubes	0.5	cup	87	84	11	0	3	0.9	0	0
Waxgourd, raw, cubes	0.5	cup	66	63	9	0	2	1.9	0	0
Weiner wraps, franks in dough	1	each	85	39	278	7	15	0.4	21	6.8
Wendy's, Frosty dairy dessert, medium	1	each	324	219	478	12	79	0	12	7.6
Wendy's, Jr cheeseburger, deluxe	1	each	179	104	358	18	36	3	17	6
Wendy's, bacon cheeseburger, w/bun	1	each	170	94	389	20	35	2	20	7.2
Wendy's, chicken sandwich, grilled	1	each	177	109	290	25	33	1.9	7	1.4
Wendy's, hamburger, big classic, w/cheese	1	each	287	170	590	35	47	3	30	12.2
Wendy's, hamburger, single, deluxe	1	each	219	136	420	25	37	3	20	7
Wendy's, junior hamburger	1	each	117	56	268	15	34	2	10	3.5
Wheat berries, whole, cooked	0.5	cup	75	65	42	2	10	1.7	0	0
Wheat bran, baked value	0.5	cup	18	2	39	3	12	7.7	1	0.1
Wheat bran, crude	0.25	cup	15	1	32	2	10	6.4	1	0.1
Wheat germ, crude, raw	2	Tbs	12	1	45	3	6	1.6	1	0.2
Wheat germ, defatted, Viobin	0.5	oz.	15	1	45	4	9	3	0	0
Wheat germ, toasted	2	Tbs	14	1	54	4	7	1.8	2	0.3
Wheat germ, w/brown sugar/honey	1	cup	113	4	420	30	66	11.5	9	1.5
Wheat grain, cracked, dry	4	oz.	113	12	384	16	82	13.1	2	0.4
Wheat sprouts	0.5	cup	54	26	107	4	23	0.6	1	0.1
Whiskey sour mix, packet	1	each	17	0	64	0	16	0	0	0
Whiskey sour, canned	2	Tbs	31	24	37	0	4	0	0	0
Wine, dessert, dry	1	cup	236	189	297	0	10	0	0	0
Wine, dessert, sweet	0.5	cup	118	86	181	0	14	0	0	0
Wine, nonalcoholic	1	cup	232	228	14	1	3	0	0	0
Wine, nonalcoholic, light	1	cup	251	246	15	1	3	0	0	0
Wine, red	1	cup	236	209	170	0	4	0	0	0
Wine, rice	4	oz.	113	89	152	1	6	0	0	0
Wine, rose'	1	cup	236	210	168	0	3	0	0	0
Wine, sangria	4	oz.	113	94	93	0	13	0	0	0
Wine, sherry, dry	0.5	cup	117	104	82	0	2	0	0	0
Wine, sweet vermouth	0.5	cup	120	87	184	0	14	0	0	0
Wine, white, dry	1	cup	238	213	158	0	1	0	0	0
Wine, white, medium	1	cup	236	211	160	0	2	0	0	0
Winged bean/goabean leaves, raw	0.5	cup	50	38	37	3	7	1.2	1	0.1
Winged bean/goabean tuber, raw	0.5	cup	50	29	74	6	14	2.8	0	0.1
Wonton, fried, meat filled	3	piece	57	25	183	8	12	0.6	11	2.2
Wonton/eggroll wrapper	3	each	24	7	70	2	14	0.4	0	0.1
Yam, Hawaii Mountain, steamed	0.5	cup	72	56	60	1	14	2.2	0	0
Yam, orange, canned in syrup	0.5	cup	114	88	101	1	24	2.8	0	0
Yam, white, cooked	0.5	cup	68	48	79	1	19	2.6	0	0
Yams, orange, baked, then peeled, mashed	0.5	cup	100	73	103	2	24	3	0	0
Yams, orange, canned, mashed	0.5	cup	128	95	129	3	30	2.2	0	0.1
Yams, orange, peeled, boiled, mashed	0.5	cup	100	73	105	2	24	1.8	0	0.1
Yeast, baker's, compressed cake	1	each	17	12	18	1	3	1.4	0	0
Yeast, baker's, dry active	1	Tbs	8	1	22	3	3	1.6	0	0
Yeast, brewer's	1	Tbs	8	0	23	3	3	2.5	0	0
Yogurt chips	1	oz.	28	1	146	3	16	0.5	8	2.1
Yogurt, custard fruit, lowfat	1	cup	245	183	250	11	47	0	3	1.7
Yogurt, frozen, banana-strawberry, HaagenDaz	0.5	cup	98	—	170	6	27	—	4	2
Yogurt, frozen, peach, HaagenDaz	0.5	cup	98	—	170	6	26	—	4	2
Yogurt, fruit, lowfat	1	cup	245	183	250	11	47	0	3	1.7
Yogurt, fruit, nonfat, low cal sweetener	1	cup	241	208	122	12	19	1.3	0	0.2
Yogurt, lowfat, fruit & nuts	1	cup	245	178	290	11	47	0.5	7	2
Yogurt, lowfat, maple	1	cup	245	194	209	12	34	0	3	2
Yogurt, lowfat, vanilla/lemon	1	cup	245	194	209	12	34	0	3	2
Yogurt, mixed berry, nonfat, Knudsen	6	oz.	170	—	170	8	33	0	0	0
Yogurt, nonfat, lemon	1	cup	245	187	223	12	43	0	0	0.3
Yogurt, nonfat, lemon	1	cup	245	187	223	12	43	0	0	0.3
Yogurt, nonfat, vanilla	1	each	227	173	207	12	40	0	0	0.2
Yogurt, peach, nonfat, Knudsen	6	oz.	170	—	170	8	33	0	0	0
Yogurt, plain, lowfat	1	cup	245	208	155	13	17	0	4	2.4
Yogurt, plain, nonfat	1	cup	245	209	137	14	19	0	0	0.3
Yogurt, plain, whole milk	1	cup	245	215	150	8	11	0	8	5.2

MonoF (g)	PolyF (g)	Choles (mg)	Calc (mg)	Phos (mg)	Sod (mg)	Pot (mg)	Zn (mg)	Iron (mg)	Magn (mg)	VitA (μg RE)	VitE (mg α-TE)	VitC (mg)	Thia (mg)	Ribo (mg)	Nia (mg)	B6 (mg)	Fola (μg)	B12 (μg)
0	0	0	30	15	10	82	0	0	5	118	0.25	11	0.02	0.03	0	0.03	2	0
0.1	0.1	0	6	7	2	93	0.1	0.1	9	30	0.12	8	0.06	0.02	0.2	0.12	2	0
0	0.1	0	16	15	93	4	0.5	0.3	9	0	0.34	9	0.03	0	0.3	0.03	3	0
0	0.1	0	12	12	73	4	0.4	0.3	7	0	0.26	9	0.03	0.07	0.3	0.02	3	0
9.6	3.4	22	137	103	818	131	1	1.2	10	14	0.82	10	0.19	0.16	2	0.06	5	0.59
—	—	54	446	356	260	776	1.4	1.6	65	217	—	0	0.15	0.67	0.5	0.17	25	1.2
—	—	50	179	—	885	—	—	3.4	—	99	—	6	—	—	—	—	—	—
10.5	1.4	61	174	342	870	384	6	3.5	39	82	—	6	0.31	0.32	6.6	0.27	29	2.04
—	—	61	94	—	740	—	—	2.5	—	38	—	6	—	—	—	—	—	—
—	—	102	254	—	1485	588	—	5.5	—	153	—	15	0.46	1.55	6.1	—	—	—
—	—	70	130	—	920	468	—	4.7	—	60	—	6	0.43	0.33	5.8	—	—	—
—	—	30	109	—	605	—	—	3	—	20	—	1	—	—	—	—	—	—
0	0.1	0	4	39	0	50	0.4	0.4	17	0	0.15	0	0.06	0.02	0.8	0.04	6	0
0.1	0.4	0	13	182	0	213	1.3	1.9	110	0	0.47	0	0.08	0.09	2.2	0.21	10	0
0.1	0.3	0	11	152	0	177	1.1	1.6	92	0	0.35	0	0.08	0.09	2	0.2	12	0
0.2	0.8	0	5	105	2	112	1.5	0.8	30	0	2.25	0	0.24	0.06	0.9	0.16	35	0
0	0.1	0	10	179	1	174	2.1	1.5	52	250	0.01	—	0.15	0.08	1.2	0.22	63	0.08
0.2	0.9	0	6	162	1	134	2.4	1.3	45	0	2.56	1	0.24	0.12	0.8	0.14	50	0
1.2	5.5	0	56	1142	12	1089	15.7	9.1	307	11	24.9	0	1.51	0.78	5.3	0.56	376	0
0.3	0.9	0	39	392	6	459	3.3	4.4	156	0	0.48	0	0.51	0.24	7.2	0.39	50	0
0.1	0.3	0	15	108	9	91	0.9	1.2	44	0	0.03	1	0.12	0.08	1.7	0.14	20	0
0	0	0	45	2	46	3	0	0.1	3	1	0	0	0	0	0	0	0	0
0	0	0	0	2	14	3	0	0	0	0	0	0	0	0	0	0	0	0
0	0	0	19	21	21	217	0.2	0.6	21	0	0	0	0.04	0.04	0.5	0	1	0
0	0	0	9	11	11	109	0.1	0.3	11	0	0	0	0.02	0.02	0.3	0	0	0
0	0	0	21	35	16	204	0.2	0.9	23	0	0	0	0	0.02	0.2	0.05	2	0
0	0	0	23	38	18	221	0.2	1	25	0	0	0	0	0.02	0.3	0.05	3	0
0	0	0	19	33	12	264	0.2	1	31	0	0	0	0.01	0.07	0.2	0.08	5	0.02
0	0	0	6	7	2	28	0	0.1	7	0	0	0	0	0	0	0	0	0
0	0	0	19	35	12	234	0.1	0.9	24	0	0	0	0.01	0.04	0.2	0.06	3	0.02
0	0	0	5	6	8	40	0.1	0.1	4	1	0.01	4	0.01	0.01	0	0.01	2	0
0	0	0	9	16	9	104	0.1	0.5	12	0	0	0	0	0.02	0.1	0.03	1	0.01
0	0	0	10	11	11	110	0.1	0.3	11	0	0	0	0.02	0.02	0.3	0	0	0
0	0	0	22	14	10	146	0.2	0.8	22	0	0	0	0	0.01	0.2	0.05	0	0
0	0	0	21	33	12	189	0.2	0.8	24	0	0	0	0.01	0.01	0.2	0.03	0	0
0.1	0.1	0	112	32	4	88	0.6	2	4	405	—	22	0.42	0.3	1.7	0.12	8	0
0.1	0.1	0	15	22	18	293	0.7	1	12	0	—	0	0.19	0.08	0.8	0.04	10	0
4.9	3.6	39	17	72	250	114	0.7	1.2	13	65	1.71	1	0.24	0.17	1.8	0.1	10	0.17
0	0.1	2	11	19	137	20	0.2	0.8	5	1	0.02	0	0.12	0.09	1.3	0.01	21	0
0	0	0	6	29	9	359	0.2	0.3	7	0	—	0	0.06	0.01	0.1	0.15	9	0
0	0.1	0	17	31	50	211	0.2	0.9	15	652	0.26	12	0.03	0.05	0.5	0.06	7	0
0	0	0	10	33	5	456	0.1	0.4	12	0	0.11	8	0.06	0.02	0.4	0.16	11	0
0	0	0	28	55	10	348	0.3	0.4	20	2182	0.28	25	0.07	0.13	0.6	0.24	23	0
0	0.1	0	38	67	96	269	0.3	1.7	31	1936	0.35	7	0.04	0.12	1.2	0.3	14	0
0	0.1	0	21	27	13	184	0.3	0.6	10	1705	0.28	17	0.05	0.14	0.6	0.24	11	0
0.2	0	0	3	57	5	102	1.7	0.6	7	0	0.01	0	0.32	0.19	2.1	0.07	133	0
0.2	0	0	5	97	4	150	0.5	1.2	7	0	0.01	0	0.18	0.41	3	0.12	176	0
0	0	0	17	140	10	151	0.6	1.4	18	0	—	0	1.25	0.34	3	0.4	313	0
3.5	2.1	1	37	47	13	63	0.3	0.9	7	3	0.69	0	0.12	0.12	1	0.02	5	0.08
0.7	0.1	10	372	292	143	478	1.8	0.2	36	27	0.07	2	0.09	0.44	0.2	0.1	23	1.14
2	0	60	146	195	50	170	—	0.4	—	—	—	4	—	0.17	—	—	—	—
2	0	40	146	146	45	160	—	0.4	—	—	—	—	—	0.17	—	—	—	—
0.7	0.1	10	372	292	143	478	1.8	0.2	36	27	0.07	2	0.09	0.44	0.2	0.1	23	1.14
0.1	0	3	369	291	139	550	1.8	0.6	41	6	0.17	26	0.1	0.45	0.5	0.11	32	1.11
3.7	1.3	10	364	305	139	490	2.2	0.3	44	27	0.29	2	0.15	0.43	0.3	0.11	25	1.11
0.8	0.1	12	419	331	161	537	2	0.2	40	32	0.08	2	0.1	0.49	0.3	0.11	26	1.29
0.8	0.1	12	419	331	161	537	2	0.2	40	32	0.08	2	0.1	0.49	0.3	0.11	26	1.29
0	0	5	250	200	105	370	—	0	—	0	—	0	0.03	0.26	—	—	—	0.9
0.1	0	4	436	343	168	559	2.1	0.2	42	4	0.01	2	0.1	0.52	0.3	0.12	27	1.34
0.1	0	4	436	343	168	559	2.1	0.2	42	4	0.01	2	0.1	0.52	0.3	0.12	27	1.34
0.1	0	4	404	318	155	518	2	0.2	39	4	0.01	2	0.1	0.48	0.3	0.11	25	1.24
0	0	5	250	200	105	370	—	—	—	0	—	0	0.03	0.26	—	—	—	0.9
1	0.1	15	448	353	172	573	2.2	0.2	43	39	0.1	2	0.11	0.52	0.3	0.12	27	1.38
0.1	0	4	488	385	187	625	2.4	0.2	47	5	0.01	2	0.12	0.57	0.3	0.13	30	1.5
2.2	0.2	31	296	233	114	380	1.4	0.1	28	74	0.22	1	0.07	0.35	0.2	0.08	18	0.91

A

Food Item	Qty	Meas	Wgt (g)	Wtr (g)	Cals	Prot (g)	Carb (g)	Fib (g)	Fat (g)	SatF (g)
Yogurt, red raspberry, nonfat, Knudsen	6	oz.	170	—	160	8	31	0	0	0
Yogurt, strawberry, nonfat, Knudsen	6	oz.	170	—	160	8	32	0	0	0

MonoF (g)	PolyF (g)	Choles (mg)	Calc (mg)	Phos (mg)	Sod (mg)	Pot (mg)	Zn (mg)	Iron (mg)	Magn (mg)	VitA (μg RE)	VitE (mg α-TE)	VitC (mg)	Thia (mg)	Ribo (mg)	Nia (mg)	B6 (mg)	Fola (μg)	B12 (μg)
0	0	5	250	200	105	360	—	0	—	0	—	0	0.03	0.26	—	—	—	0.9
0	0	5	250	200	105	380	—	0	—	0	—	0	0.03	0.26	—	—	—	0.9

A

Appendix B

Standards for Body Size

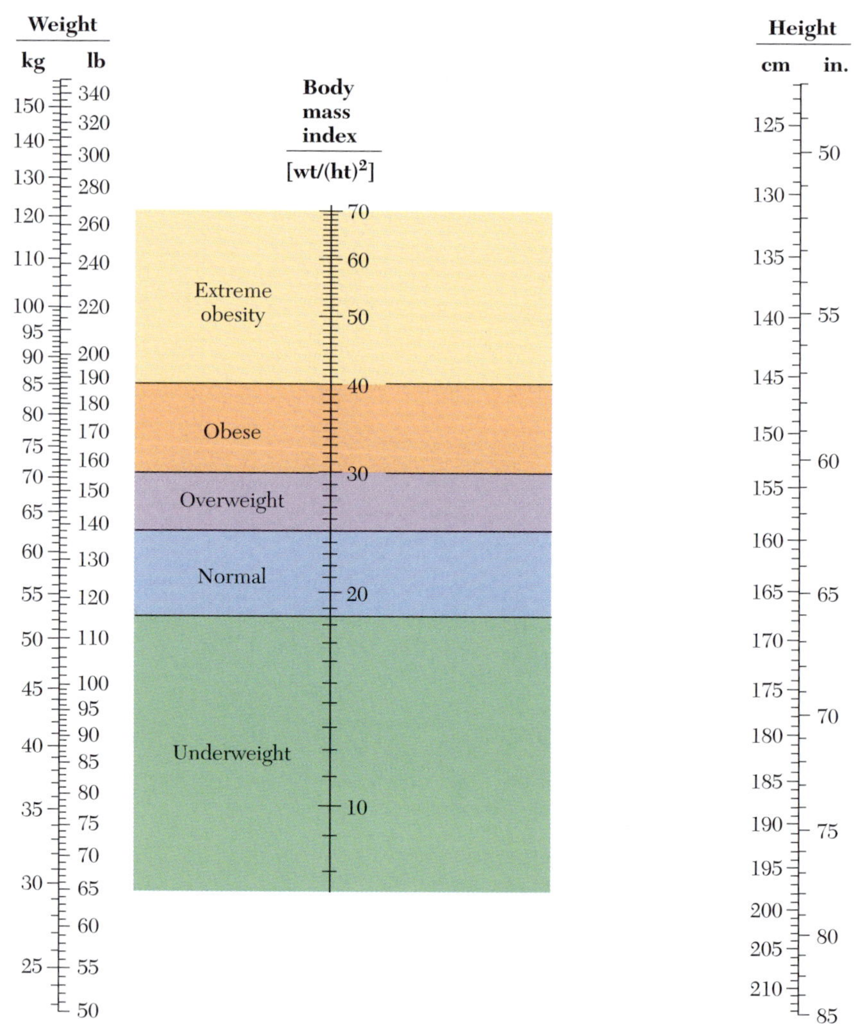

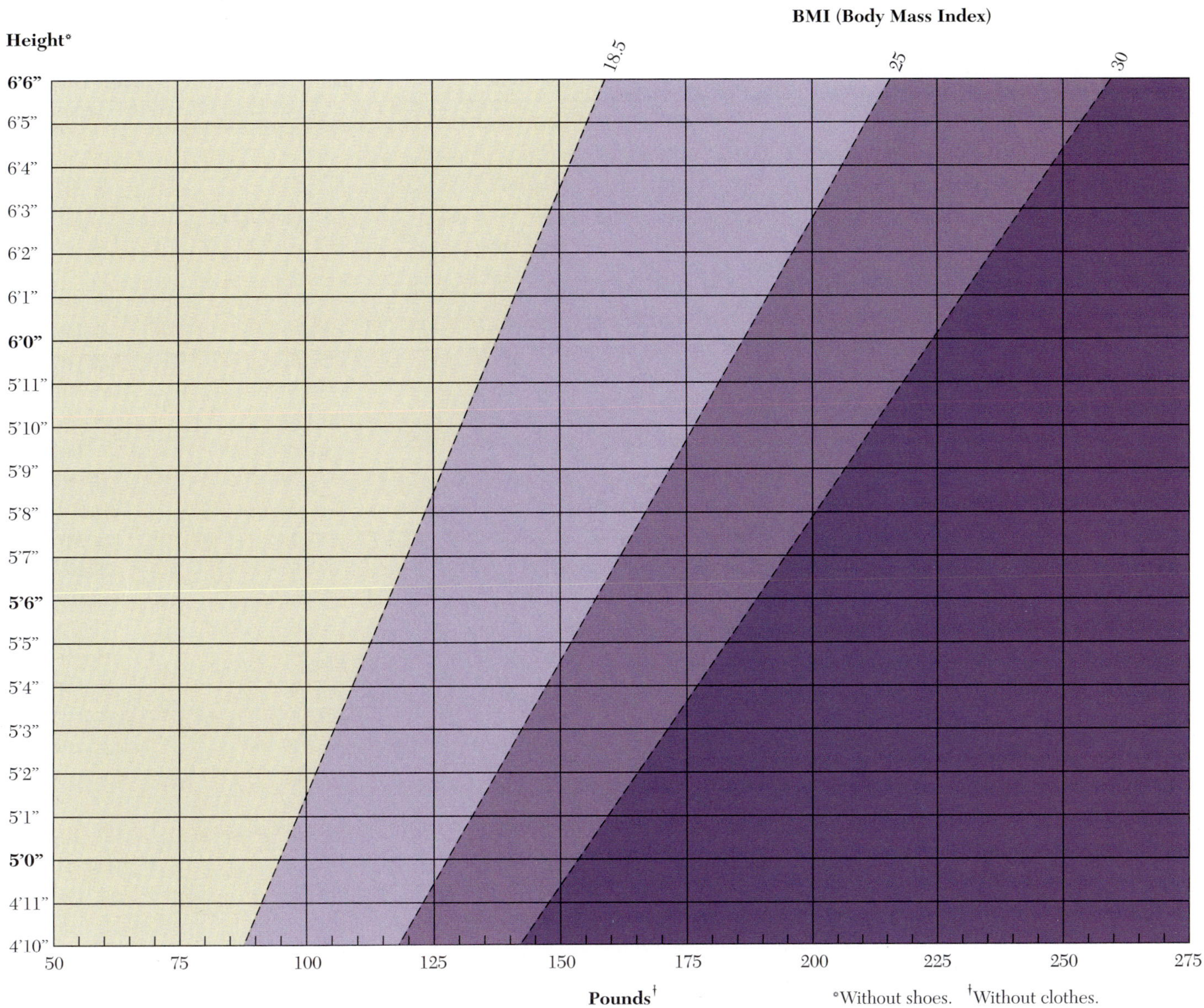

°Without shoes. †Without clothes.

Healthy Weight BMI from 18.5 up to 25 refers to healthy weight.

Overweight BMI from 25 up to 30 refers to overweight.

Obese BMI 30 or higher refers to obesity. Obese persons are also overweight.

BMI measures weight in relation to height. The BMI ranges shown above are for adults. They are not exact ranges of healthy and unhealthy weights. However, they show that health risk increases at higher levels of overweight and obesity. Even within the healthy BMI range, weight gains can carry health risks for adults.

Directions: Find your weight on the bottom of the graph. Go straight up from that point until you come to the line that matches your height. Then look to find your weight group.

Source: Report of the Dietary Guidelines Advisory Committee on the Dietary Guidelines for Americans, 2000, page 3.

B

1983 Metropolitan Life Insurance Co. Height and Weight Tables

Height	Small Frame	Medium Frame	Large Frame
	←	lb	→
Men*			
5′2″	128–134	131–141	138–150
5′3″	130–136	133–143	140–153
5′4″	132–138	135–145	142–156
5′5″	134–140	137–148	144–160
5′6″	136–142	139–151	146–164
5′7″	138–145	142–154	149–168
5′8″	140–148	145–157	152–172
5′9″	142–151	148–160	155–176
5′10″	144–154	151–163	158–180
5′11″	146–157	154–166	161–184
6′0″	149–160	157–170	164–188
6′1″	152–164	160–174	168–192
6′2″	155–168	164–178	172–197
6′3″	158–172	167–182	176–202
6′4″	162–176	171–187	181–207
Women†			
4′10″	102–111	109–121	118–131
4′11″	103–113	111–123	120–134
5′0″	104–115	113–126	122–137
5′1″	106–118	115–129	125–140
5′2″	108–121	118–132	128–143
5′3″	111–124	121–135	131–147
5′4″	114–127	124–138	134–151
5′5″	117–130	127–141	137–155
5′6″	120–133	130–144	140–159
5′7″	123–136	133–147	143–163
5′8″	126–139	136–150	146–167
5′9″	129–142	139–153	149–170
5′10″	132–145	142–156	152–173
5′11″	135–148	145–159	155–176
6′0″	138–151	148–162	158–179

*Weights at ages 25 to 59 based on lowest mortality. Weight in pounds according to frame (in indoor clothing weighing 5 lb, shoes with 1-in. heels).

†Weights at ages 25 to 59 based on lowest mortality. Weight in pounds according to frame (in indoor clothing weighing 3 lb, shoes with 1-in. heels).

Courtesy of Metropolitan Life Insurance Company.

Weight-for-Height Tables for Adults—Gerontology Research Center Recommendations

Height (ft and in)	Age-Specific Weight Range in Pounds for Men and Women*				
	20–29 yr	30–39 yr	40–49 yr	50–59 yr	60–69 yr
4′10″	84–111	92–119	99–127	107–135	115–142
4′11″	87–115	95–123	103–131	111–139	119–147
5′0″	90–119	98–127	106–135	114–143	123–152
5′1″	93–123	101–131	110–140	118–148	127–157
5′2″	96–127	105–136	113–144	122–153	131–163
5′3″	99–131	108–140	117–149	126–158	135–168
5′4″	102–135	112–145	121–154	130–163	140–173
5′5″	106–140	115–149	125–159	134–168	144–179
5′6″	109–144	119–154	129–164	138–174	148–184
5′7″	112–148	122–159	133–169	143–179	153–190
5′8″	116–153	126–163	137–174	147–184	158–196
5′9″	119–157	130–168	141–179	151–190	162–201
5′10″	122–162	134–173	145–184	156–195	167–207
5′11″	126–167	137–178	149–190	160–201	172–213
6′0″	129–171	141–183	153–195	165–207	177–219
6′1″	133–176	145–188	157–200	169–213	182–225
6′2″	137–181	149–194	162–206	174–219	187–232
6′3″	141–186	153–199	166–212	179–225	192–238
6′4″	144–191	157–205	171–218	184–231	197–244

*Values in this table are for height without shoes and weight without clothes.

Estimation of Frame Size Using Elbow Breadth*

MEN Height in 1-Inch Heels	Elbow Breadth	WOMEN Height in 1-Inch Heels	Elbow Breadth
5′2″ to 5′3″	2½ to 2⅞″	4′10″ to 4′11″	2¼ to 2½″
5′4″ to 5′7″	2⅝ to 2⅞″	5′0″ to 5′3″	2¼ to 2½″
5′8″ to 5′11″	2¾ to 3″	5′4″ to 5′7″	2⅜ to 2⅝″
6′0″ to 6′3″	2¾ to 3⅛″	5′8″ to 5′11″	2⅜ to 2⅝″
6′4″ and over	2⅞ to 3¼″	6′0″ and over	2½ to 2¾″

*If your measurement is within the range indicated, you have a medium frame. Measurements smaller than those listed indicate a small frame, and those larger indicate a large frame. Elbow breadth is measured as the distance between the bony protrusions of the elbow. For this measurement the right arm is raised to the horizontal, and the elbow flexed to 90 degrees, with the back of the hand facing the measurer.

Source: Metropolitan Life Insurance Company.

Growth Charts for Ages Birth to 20 Years

Infants (birth to 24 months) must be measured for length, and the sex-appropriate length-for-age or weight-for-length charts for infants from birth to 36 months must be used to plot the measurements. At age 24 months and older, if children stand unassisted and follow directions, stature should be measured and plotted on the stature-for-age chart for older children (2 to 20 years).

BMI-for-age charts are recommended to assess weight in relation to stature for older children (2 to 20 years). The weight-for-stature charts are available as an alternative to accommodate children ages 2–5 years who are not evaluated beyond the preschool years. However, all health-care providers should consider using the BMI-for-age charts to be consistent with current recommendations.

A complete set of growth charts is available on the Internet at www.cdc.gov/growthcharts. There are three sets, each with a different set of percentiles. Each set includes the following charts for girls and boys:

Weight-for-age percentiles: birth to 36 months
Length-for-age percentiles: birth to 36 months
Weight-for-length percentiles: birth to 36 months
Head circumference-for-age percentiles: birth to 36 months
Weight-for-age percentiles: 2 to 20 years
Stature-for-age percentiles: 2 to 20 years
Weight-for-stature percentiles
Body mass index–for-age percentiles: 2 to 20 years

Birth to 36 months: Boys
Length-for-age and Weight-for-age percentiles

NAME ______________________

RECORD # ____________

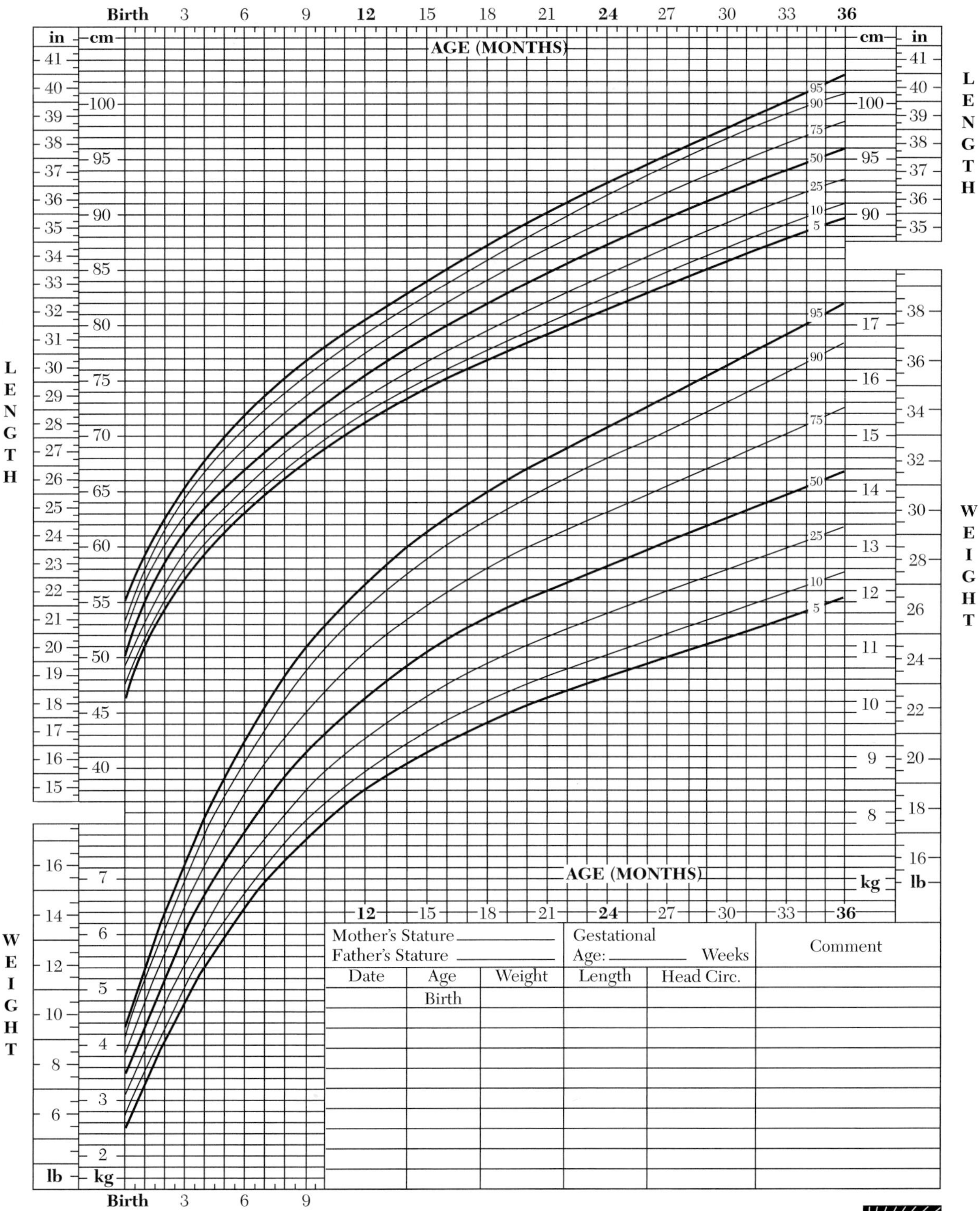

Revised November 28, 2000.
SOURCE: Developed by the National Center for Health Statistics in collaboration with the National Center for Chronic Disease Prevention and Health Promotion (2000).
http://www.cdc.gov/growthcharts

B

Birth to 36 months: Girls
Length-for-age and Weight-for-age percentiles

NAME ______________________

RECORD # ______________

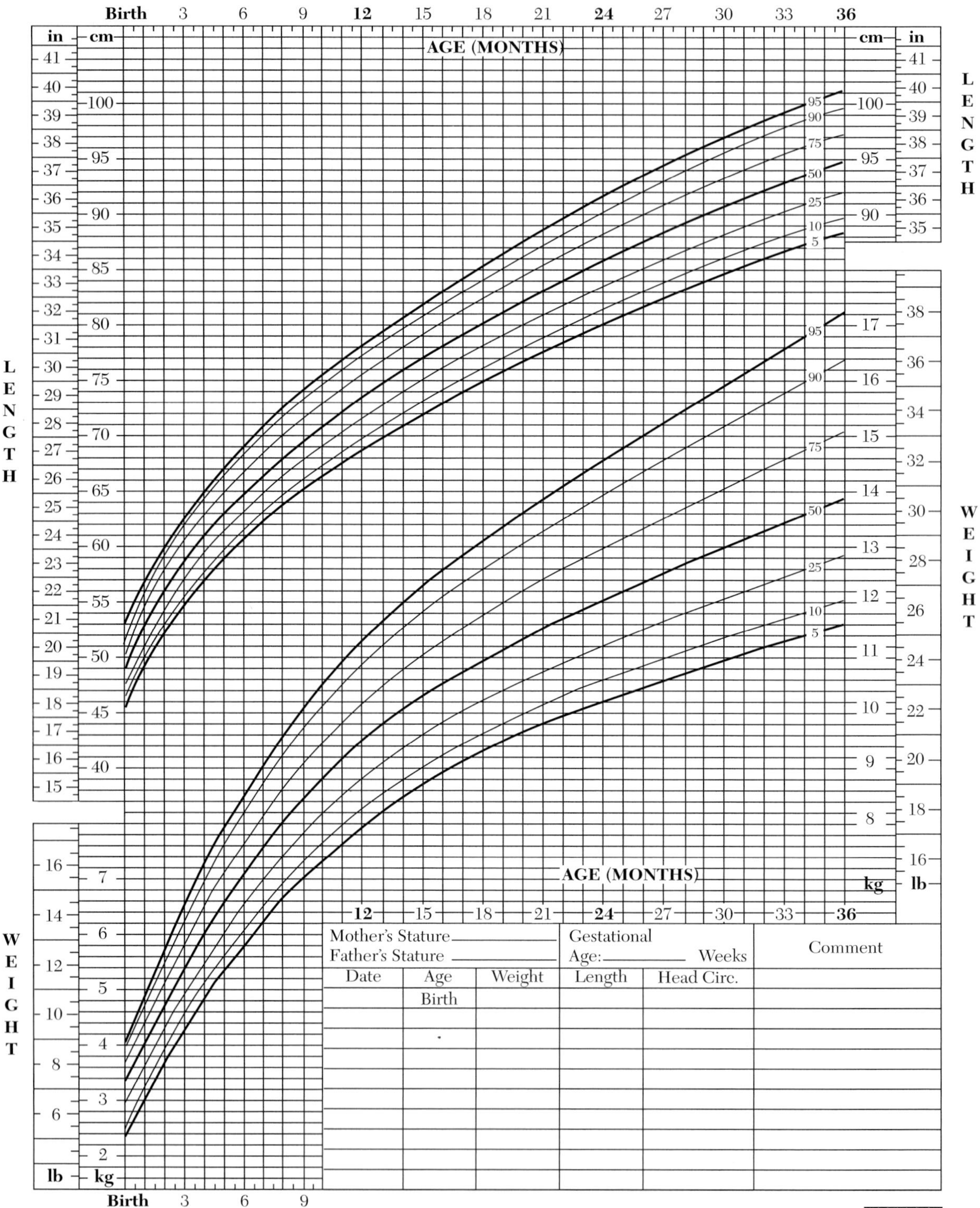

Date	Age	Weight	Length	Head Circ.	Comment
	Birth				

Mother's Stature ______

Father's Stature ______

Gestational Age: ______ Weeks

Revised November 28, 2000.

SOURCE: Developed by the National Center for Health Statistics in collaboration with the National Center for Chronic Disease Prevention and Health Promotion (2000).
http://www.cdc.gov/growthcharts

B

2 to 20 years: Boys
Body mass index-for-age percentiles

NAME ______________________

RECORD # ______________

Date	Age	Weight	Stature	BMI°	Comments

°To Calculate BMI: Weight (kg) ÷ Stature (cm) ÷ Stature (cm) × 10,000
or Weight (lb) ÷ Stature (in) ÷ Stature (in) × 703

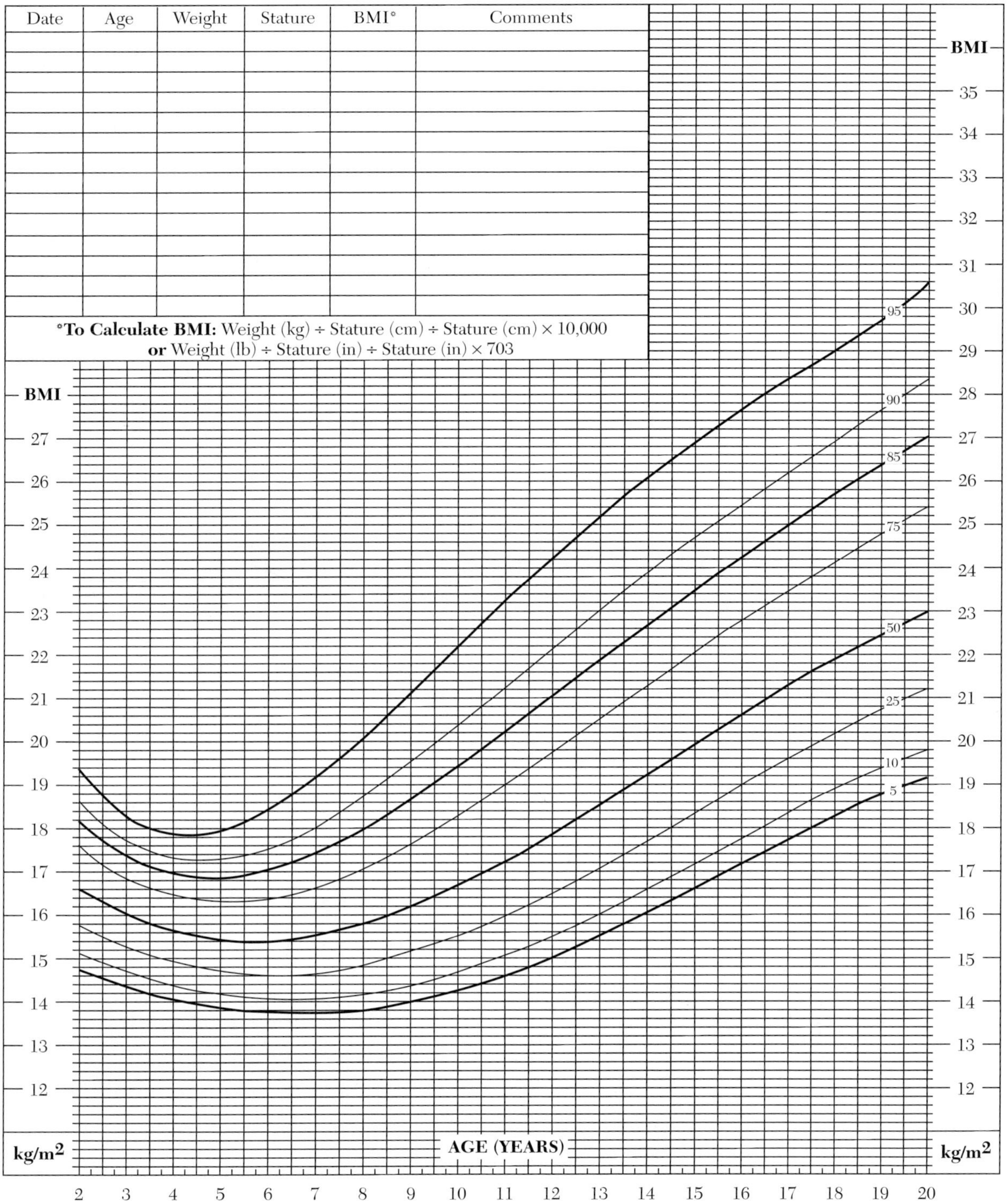

SOURCE: Developed by the National Center for Health Statistics in collaboration with the National Center for Chronic Disease Prevention and Health Promotion (2000).
http://www.cdc.gov/growthcharts

B

2 to 20 years: Girls
Body mass index-for-age percentiles

NAME ______________________

RECORD # ______________

Date	Age	Weight	Stature	BMI*	Comments

***To Calculate BMI:** Weight (kg) ÷ Stature (cm) ÷ Stature (cm) × 10,000
or Weight (lb) ÷ Stature (in) ÷ Stature (in) × 703

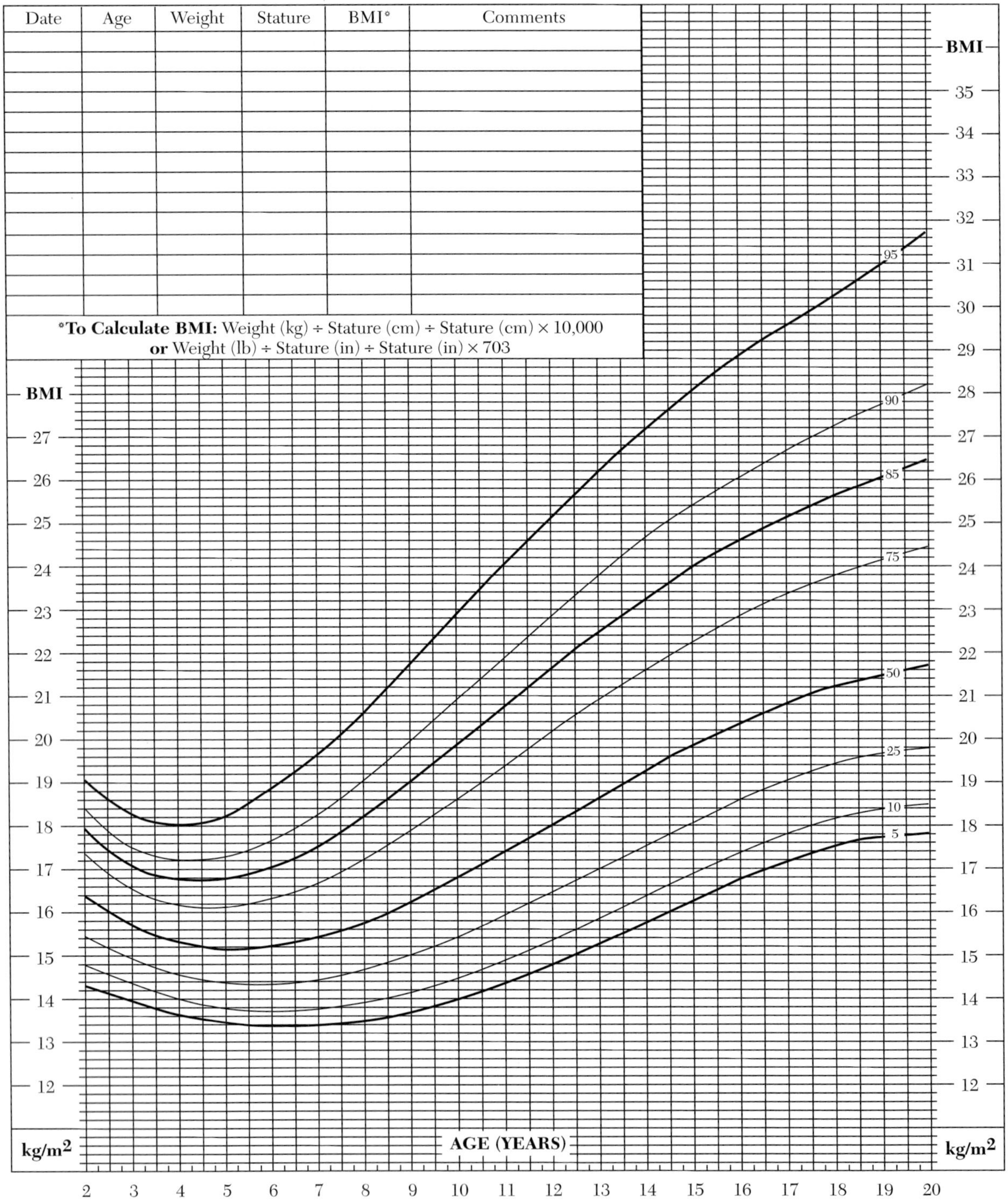

SOURCE: Developed by the National Center for Health Statistics in collaboration with the National Center for Chronic Disease Prevention and Health Promotion (2000).
http://www.cdc.gov/growthcharts

CDC

Appendix C

Normal Blood Values of Nutritional Relevance

C

Red blood cells	
Men	4.6–6.2 million/mm^3
Women	4.2–5.2 million/mm^3
White blood cells	5,000–10,000/mm^3
Hematocrit	
Men	40–45 ml/100 ml
Women	36–47 ml/100 ml
Children	35–49 ml/100 ml
Hemoglobin	
Men	14–18 g/100 ml
Women	12–15 g/100 ml
Children	11.2–16.5 g/100 ml
Ferritin	
Men	20–300 ng/ml
Women	20–120 ng/ml
Calcium	9–11 mg/100 ml
Iodine	3.8–8 μg/100 ml
Iron	
Men	75–175 μg/100 ml
Women	65–165 μg/100 ml
Zinc	0.75–1.4 μg/ml
Magnesium	1.8–3.0 mg/100 ml
Potassium	3.5–5.0 mEq/liter
Sodium	136–145 mEq/liter
Chloride	100–108 mEq/liter
Vitamin A	20–80 μg/100 ml
Vitamin B_{12}	200–800 pg/100 ml
Vitamin C	0.6–2.0 mg/100 ml
Carotene	48–200 μg/liter
Folate	2–20 ng/ml
pH	7.35–7.45
Total protein	6.6–8.0 g/100 ml
Albumen	3.0–4.0 g/100 ml
Cholesterol	$<$200 mg/100 ml
LDL cholesterol	$<$160 mg/100 ml
HDL cholesterol	$>$35 mg/100 ml
Triglycerides	$<$150 mg/100 ml
Glucose	60–100 mg/100 ml blood, 70–120 mg/100 ml serum

Blood Pressure Levels

Blood pressure is measured in millimeters of mercury (mm Hg). The classifications in the following table are for persons who are not taking antihypertensive drugs and are not acutely ill. When systolic and diastolic pressures fall into different categories, the physician will select the higher category to classify the person's blood pressure status. Diagnosis of high blood pressure is based on the average of two or more readings taken at each of two or more visits after an initial screening.

Classification of Blood Pressure for Adults Age 18 Years and Older, With Recommended Follow-Up

Category	Systolic (mm Hg)		Diastolic (mm Hg)	Recommended Follow-Up
Optimal*	<120	and	<80	Recheck in 2 years
Normal	<130	and	<85	Recheck in 2 years
High normal	130–139	or	85–89	Recheck in 1 year
Hypertension				
STAGE 1 (Mild)	140–159	or	90–99	Confirm within 2 months
STAGE 2 (Moderate)	160–179	or	100–109	Evaluate within 1 month
STAGE 3 (Severe)	≥180	or	≥110	Evaluate immediately or within 1 week, depending on clinical situation

*Unusually low readings should be evaluated for clinical significance.

Source: Sixth Report of the Joint National Committee on Detection, Evaluation, and Treatment of High Blood Pressure, NIH, 1997.

Appendix D

Sources of Information on Nutrition

Many publications are available at little or no cost from the government. For individual publications or catalogs, contact:

Superintendent of Documents
U.S. Government Printing Office
Washington, DC 20402
www.access.gpo.gov/su_docs/

National Technical Information Service
5285 Port Royal Road
Springfield, VA 22162

National Research Council
National Academy of Sciences
2102 Constitution Ave. N.W.
Washington, DC 20418
www.nas.edu/

Consumer Information Service
Department 609K
Pueblo, CO 81009
www.pueblo.gsa.gov/

Food Safety and Inspection Administration
U.S. Department of Agriculture
Washington, DC 20250
www.usda.gov/fsis/

National Council on Aging
1828 L Street NW
Washington, DC 20036
www.ncoa.org/

Alliance for Food & Fiber
Food Safety Hotline
(800) 266-0200
www.foodsafetyalliance.org/

Center for Food Safety and Applied Nutrition
Food and Drug Administration
200 C Street SW
Washington, DC 20204
(800) 332-4010
www.cfsan.fda.gov/

National Lead Information Center
(800) 424-5323
www.epa.gov/opptintr/lead/nlic.htm

Food and Agriculture Organization
North American Regional Office
1325 C St. S.W.
Washington, DC 20025
www.fao.org/

Food and Drug Administration
5600 Fishers Lane
Rockville, MD 20852
www.fda.gov/

The Food and Nutrition Information Center
National Agriculture Library
Room 304
10301 Baltimore Blvd.
Beltsville, MD 20705
www.nal.usda.gov/fnic/

National Center for Health Statistics
6265 Belcrest Road
Hyattsville, MD 20782
www.nchs.gov/

National Cancer Institute
Office of Cancer Communications
Building 31, Room 10A18
Bethesda, MD 20205
www.nih.nci.gov/

National Center for Complementary and Alternative Medicine
National Institutes of Health
Bethesda, MD 20205
nccam.nih.gov/

Seafood Safety Hotline
(800) 332-4010; (202) 205-4314

U.S. EPA Safe Drinking Water Hotline
(800) 426-4791

Office of Dietary Supplements
National Institutes of Health
Bethesda, MD 20205
www.odp.od.nih.gov/ods/

Agriculture Research Service
U.S. Department of Agriculture
3700 East West Hwy.
Hyattsville, MD 20782
www.usda.ars.gov/

National Institute on Aging
Information Office
Building 31, Room 5C35
Bethesda, MD 20205
www.nih.gov/nia/

National Heart, Lung, and Blood Institute
Information Office
Building 31, Room 4A21
Bethesda, MD 20205
www.nhlbi.nih.gov/

Health and Welfare Canada
Canadian Government Publishing Center
Minister of Supply and Services
Ottawa, Ontario K1A 0S9
www.hc-sc.gc.ca

National Weight Central Information Network
National Institutes of Health
Bethesda, MD 20205
www.niddk.nih.gov/WIN

World Health Org.
Geneva, Switzerland
www.who.int/

Many private organizations also publish reputable food and nutrition information. Some of these include:

American Dietetic Association
216 W. Jackson Blvd., Suite 800
Chicago, IL 60606-6995
www.eatright.org/

National Dairy Council
6300 North River Road
Rosemont, IL 60018-4233
www.nationaldairycouncil.org/

American Heart Association
7320 Grenville Ave.
Dallas, TX 75231
www.americanheart.org/

American Anorexia and Bulemia Assoc., Inc.
165 W. 46th St., Suite 1108
New York, NY 10036
www.aabainc.org

American College of Sports Medicine
401 W. Michigan Street
Indianapolis, IN 46202-3233
(317) 637-9200; fax: (317) 634-7817
www.acsm.org/

American Council on Exercise
5820 Oberlin Drive, Suite 102
San Diego, CA 92121
(800) 529-8227
www.acefitness.org/

American Diabetes Association
Diabetes Information Service Center
1660 Duke St.
Alexandria, VA 22314
www.diabetes.org/

American Cancer Society
90 Park Ave.
New York, NY 10016
www.cancer.org/

Canadian Dietetic Association
480 University Ave., Suite 601
Toronto, Ontario M5G 1V2 Canada
www.dietitians.ca/

American Academy of Pediatrics
141 Northwest Point Boulevard
Elk Grove Village, IL 60007-1098
(847) 434-4000; fax: (847) 434-8000
www.aap.org/

ILSI Human Nutrition Institute
1126 Sixteenth Street NW
Washington, DC 20036
(202) 659-0524; fax (202)659-3617
www.ilsi.org/hni.html

Institute of Food Technologists
221 N. LaSalle Street, Suite 300
Chicago, IL 60601-1291
(312) 782-8424; fax: (312) 782-8348
www.ift.org/

Appendix E

Canadian Recommendations and Guidelines

Recommended Nutrient Intakes (RNI): Summary of Examples of Recommended Nutrient Intake Based on Energy Expressed As Daily Rates*

Age	Sex	Energy (kcal)	Thiamin (mg)	Riboflavin (mg)	Niacin (NE‡)	N-3 PUFA† (g)	n-6 PUFA (g)
Months							
0–4	Both	600	0.3	0.3	4	0.5	3
5–12	Both	900	0.4	0.5	7	0.5	3
Years							
1	Both	1100	0.5	0.6	8	0.6	4
2–3	Both	1300	0.6	0.7	9	0.7	4
4–6	Both	1800	0.7	0.9	13	1.0	6
7–9	M	2200	0.9	1.1	16	1.2	7
	F	1900	0.8	1.0	14	1.0	6
10–12	M	2500	1.0	1.3	18	1.4	8
	F	2200	0.9	1.1	16	1.2	7
13–15	M	2800	1.1	1.4	20	1.5	9
	F	2200	0.9	1.1	16	1.2	7
16–18	M	3200	1.3	1.6	23	1.8	11
	F	2100	0.8	1.1	15	1.2	7
19–24	M	3000	1.2	1.5	22	1.6	10
	F	2100	0.8	1.1	15	1.2	7
25–49	M	2700	1.1	1.4	19	1.5	9
	F	1900	0.8§	1.0§	14§	1.1§	7§
50–74	M	2300	0.9	1.2	16	1.3	8
	F	1800	0.8§	1.0§	14§	1.1§	7§
75+	M	2000	0.8	1.0	14	1.1	7
	F‖	1700	0.8§	1.0§	14§	1.1§	7§
Pregnancy (additional)							
1st trimester		100	0.1	0.1	1	0.05	0.3
2nd trimester		300	0.1	0.3	2	0.16	0.9
3rd trimester		300	0.1	0.3	2	0.16	0.9
Lactation (additional)		450	0.2	0.4	3	0.25	1.5

* Recommendations for many of these nutrients have been replaced by Dietary Reference Intake Values.

† PUFA: polyunsaturated fatty acids.

‡ Niacin equivalents.

§ Level below which intake should not fall.

‖ Assumes moderate (more than average) physical activity.

Source: Reprinted from Health and Welfare Canada, *Nutrition Recommendations: The Report of the Scientific Review Committee* (Ottawa: Supply and Services Canada, 1990). Copyright, Health and Welfare Canada, with corrections.

Recommended Nutrient Intakes (RNI): Summary Examples of Recommended Nutrient Intake Based on Age and Body Weight Expressed As Daily Rates*

Age	Sex	Weight (kg)	Protein (g)	Vit. A (RE†)	Vit. D (μg)	Vit. E (mg)	Vit. C (mg)	Folate (μg)	Vit. B_{12} (μg)	Calcium (mg)	Phosphorus (mg)	Magnesium (mg)	Iron (mg)	Iodine (μg)	Zinc (mg)
Months															
0–4	Both	6.0	12[‡]	400	10	3	20	25	0.3	250[§]	150	20	0.3[‖]	30	2[‖]
5–12	Both	9.0	12	400	10	3	20	40	0.4	400	200	32	7	40	3
Years															
1	Both	11	13	400	10	3	20	40	0.5	500	300	40	6	55	4
2–3	Both	14	16	400	5	4	20	50	0.6	550	350	50	6	65	4
4–6	Both	18	19	500	5	5	25	70	0.8	600	400	65	8	85	5
7–9	M	25	26	700	2.5	7	25	90	1.0	700	500	100	8	110	7
	F	25	26	700	2.5	6	25	90	1.0	700	500	100	8	95	7
10–12	M	34	34	800	2.5	8	25	120	1.0	900	700	130	8	125	9
	F	36	36	800	2.5	7	25	130	1.0	1100	800	135	8	110	9
13–15	M	50	49	900	2.5	9	30[#]	175	1.0	1100	900	185	10	160	12
	F	48	46	800	2.5	7	30[#]	170	1.0	1000	850	180	13	160	9
16–18	M	62	58	1000	2.5	10	40[#]	220	1.0	900	1000	230	10	160	12
	F	53	47	800	2.5	7	30[#]	190	1.0	700	850	200	12	160	9
19–24	M	71	61	1000	2.5	10	40[#]	220	1.0	800	1000	240	9	160	12
	F	58	50	800	2.5	7	30[#]	180	1.0	700	850	200	13	160	9
25–49	M	74	64	1000	2.5	9	40[#]	230	1.0	800	1000	250	9	160	12
	F	59	51	800	2.5	6	30[#]	185	1.0	700	850	200	13	160	9
50–74	M	73	63	1000	5	7	40[#]	230	1.0	800	1000	250	9	160	12
	F	63	54	800	5	6	30[#]	195	1.0	800	850	210	8	160	9
75+	M	69	59	1000	5	6	40[#]	215	1.0	800	1000	230	9	160	12
	F	64	55	800	5	5	30[#]	200	1.0	800	850	210	8	160	9
Pregnancy (additional)															
1st trimester			5	0	2.5	2	0	200	0.2	500	200	15	0	25	6
2nd trimester			20	0	2.5	2	10	200	0.2	500	200	45	5	25	6
3rd trimester			24	0	2.5	2	10	200	0.2	500	200	45	10	25	6
Lactation (additional)			20	400	2.5	3	25	100	0.2	500	200	65	0	50	6

*Recommendations for many of these nutrients have been replaced by Dietary Reference Intake Values.

†Retinol equivalents.

‡Protein is assumed to be from breast milk and must be adjusted for infant formula.

§Infant formula with high phosphorus should contain 375 mg calcium.

‖Breast milk is assumed to be the source of the mineral.

#Smokers should increase vitamin C by 50%.

Source: Reprinted from Health and Welfare Canada, *Nutrition Recommendations: The Report of the Scientific Review Committee* (Ottawa: Supply and Services Canada, 1990). Copyright, Health and Welfare Canada, with corrections.

Nutrition Recommendations for Canadians

- The Canadian diet should provide energy consistent with the maintenance of *body weight* within the recommended range.
- The Canadian diet should include *essential nutrients* in amounts recommended.
- The Canadian diet should include no more than 30% of energy as *fat* (33 grams/1000 kcalories or 39 grams/5000 kilojoules) and no more than 10% as saturated fat (11 grams/1000 kcalories or 13 grams/5000 kilojoules).
- The Canadian diet should provide 55% of energy as *carbohydrate* (138 grams/1000 kcalories or 165 grams/5000 kilojoules) from a variety of sources.
- The *sodium* content of the Canadian diet should be reduced.
- The Canadian diet should include no more than 5% of total energy as *alcohol*, or two drinks daily, whichever is less.
- The Canadian diet should contain no more *caffeine* than the equivalent of four regular cups of coffee per day.
- Community water supplies containing less than 1 milligram per liter should be *fluoridated* to that level.

Note: Italics added to highlight areas of concern.

Source: Health and Welfare Canada, *Nutrition Recommendations: The Report of the Scientific Review Committee* (Ottawa: Canadian Government Publishing Centre, 1990).

Canada's Guidelines for Healthy Eating

1. Enjoy a VARIETY of foods.
2. Emphasize cereals, breads, other grain products, vegetables, and fruit.
3. Choose lower-fat dairy products, leaner meats, and foods prepared with little or no fat.
4. Achieve and maintain a healthy body weight by enjoying regular physical activity and healthy eating.
5. Limit salt, alcohol, and caffeine.

Source: Minister of Supply and Services, Canada, 1992. Cat. No. 1139-252/1992E.

CANADA'S

Food Guide

TO HEALTHY EATING

Enjoy a variety of foods from each group every day.

Choose lower-fat foods more often.

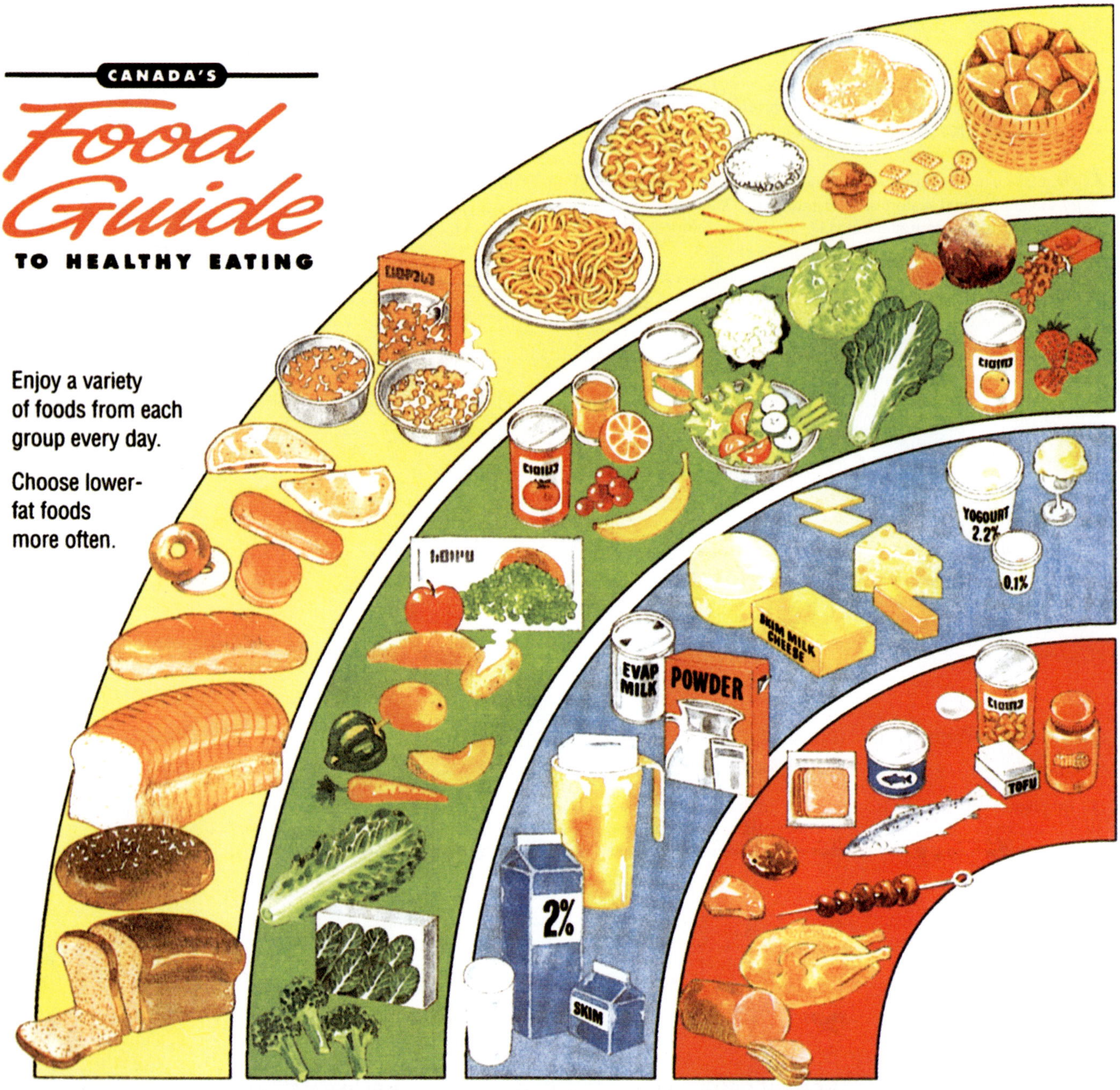

Grain Products
Choose whole grain and enriched products more often.

Vegetables & Fruit
Choose dark green and orange vegetables and orange fruit more often.

Milk Products
Choose lower-fat milk products more often.

Meat & Alternatives
Choose leaner meats, poultry and fish, as well as dried peas, beans and lentils more often.

CANADA'S

Food Guide

TO HEALTHY EATING

FOR PEOPLE FOUR YEARS AND OVER

Different People Need Different Amounts of Food

The amount of food you need every day from the 4 food groups and other foods depends on your age, body size, activity level, whether you are male or female and if you are pregnant or breast-feeding. That's why the Food Guide gives a lower and higher number of servings for each food group. For example, young children can choose the lower number of servings, while male teenagers can go to the higher number. Most other people can choose servings somewhere in between.

Grain Products
5–12
SERVINGS PER DAY

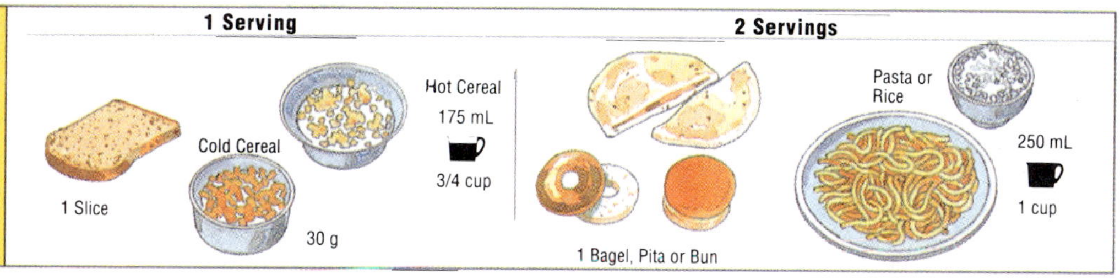

Vegetables & Fruit
5–10
SERVINGS PER DAY

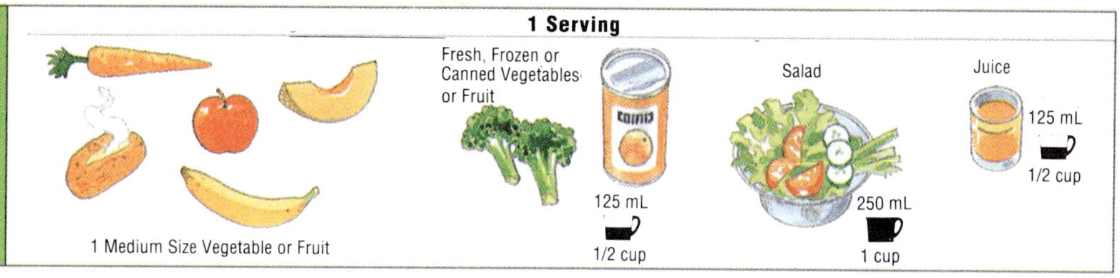
1 Serving
1 Medium Size Vegetable or Fruit
Fresh, Frozen or Canned Vegetables or Fruit
125 mL
1/2 cup
Salad
250 mL
1 cup
Juice
125 mL
1/2 cup

Milk Products
SERVINGS PER DAY
Children 4–9 years: 2–3
Youth 10–16 years: 3–4
Adults: 2–4
Pregnant & Breast-feeding Women: 3–4

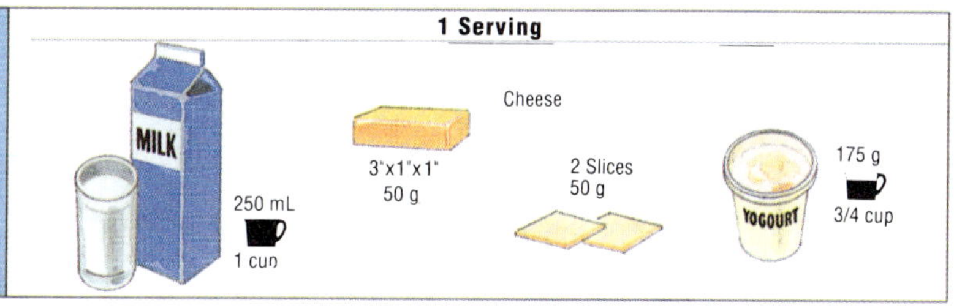

Meat & Alternatives
2–3
SERVINGS PER DAY

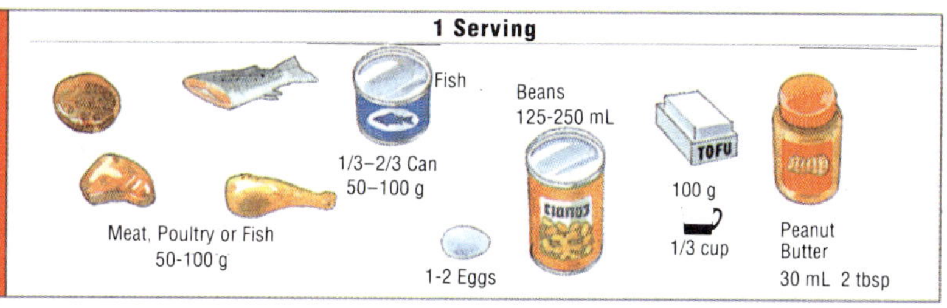

Other Foods

Taste and enjoyment can also come from other foods and beverages that are not part of the 4 food groups. Some of these foods are higher in fat or Calories, so use these foods in moderation.

Key Nutrients in Canada's Food Guide to Healthy Eating

Each food group is essential. That's because it provides its own set of nutrients.

Grain Products +	Vegetables & Fruits +	Milk Products +	Meat & Alternatives =	The Food Guide
protein		protein	protein	protein
		fat	fat	fat
carbohydrate	carbohydrate			carbohydrate
fibre	fibre			fibre
thiamin	thiamin		thiamin	thiamin
riboflavin		riboflavin	riboflavin	riboflavin
niacin			niacin	niacin
folacin	folacin		folacin	folacin
		vitamin B_{12}	vitamin B_{12}	vitamin B_{12}
	vitamin C			vitamin C
	vitamin A	vitamin A		vitamin A
		vitamin D		vitamin D
		calcium		calcium
iron	iron		iron	iron
zinc		zinc	zinc	zinc
magnesium	magnesium	magnesium	magnesium	magnesium

E

Guide to Food Labelling and Advertising, Canadian Food Inspection Agency

What Is Nutrition Labelling?

- It is a **standardized presentation** of the nutrient content of a food.
- It is designed to provide useful information that is **not misleading or deceptive.**
- It is **voluntary,** but if applied should comply with the Guidelines on Nutrition Labelling* and with the *Food and Drug Regulations*, which regulate the format, nutrient content information, nomenclature, units of measurement, per-serving basis, and declaration of serving size.
- It consists of the **heading,** a statement of the **serving size,** the **"core list"** (energy, protein, fat, and carbohydrate), plus optional nutrient declarations given equal prominence, in a standardized order.

**Guidelines on Nutrition Labelling*, Guideline No. 2 (Ottawa: Health Canada, Health Protection Branch, May 2, 1996).

Nomenclature, Order of Listing, and Units

1. **Heading**
2. **Serving size:** metric units as sold (household measure should be declared in brackets).
3. **Energy** (expressed in both Calories and kilojoules), **protein, fat** and **carbohydrate** constitute the "core list" and must be included when the nutrition labelling format is used. All must be expressed in grams.
4. If one of these **fat components,** excluding linoleic acid, is listed, all four (in addition to fat) must be listed. Linoleic acid may be listed provided the four fat components and fat are also listed.
5. Declaration of one **carbohydrate** component does not require the declaration of any others. All sugar alcohols must be declared by name when used.
6. If either **sodium or potassium** is listed, both must be listed. Both must be expressed in milligrams.
7. **Vitamins and mineral nutrients** must be stated as % of Recommended Daily Intake. If less than 5% of Recommended Daily Intake, they may be listed provided no claims relate to them. Only the names shown may be used in nutrition labelling.

Source: Online at http://www.cfia-acia.agr.ca/english/ppc/label/5-0-0.html.

Nutrition Information/Information Nutritionnelle

per × g or mL per serving (× cups, item, etc.)
par portion de × g ou mL (× tasses, unités, etc.)

Energy/Énergie	× Cal × kJ
Protein/Protéines	× g
Fat/Matières grasses	× g
polyunsaturates/polyinsaturés	× g
linoleic acid/acide linoléique	× g
monounsaturates/monoinsaturés	× g
saturates/saturés	× g
cholesterol/cholestérol	× mg
Carbohydrate/Glucides	× g
sugars/sucres	× g
sugar alcohols (named)	× g
polydextrose	× g
starch/amidon	× g
dietary fibre/fibres alimentaires	× g
Sucralose	× mg
Aspartame	× mg
Acesulfame-potassium/acésulfame-potassium	× mg
Sodium	× mg
Potassium	× mg

Percentage of Recommended Daily Intake
Pourcentage de l'Apport Quotidien Recommandé

Vitamin A/Vitamine A	× %
Vitamin D/Vitamine D	× %
Vitamin E/Vitamine E	× %
Vitamin C/Vitamine C	× %
Thiamine or/ou Vitamin B_1/Vitamine B_1	× %
Riboflavin/Riboflavine or/ou Vitamin B_2/Vitamine B_2	× %
Niacin/Niacine	× %
Vitamin B_6/Vitamine B_6	× %
Folacin/Folacine	× %
Vitamin B_{12}/Vitamine B_{12}	× %
Pantothenic Acid or Pantothenate/ Acide Pantothénique ou Pantothénate	× %
Calcium	× %
Phosphorus/Phosphore	× %
Magnesium/Magnésium	× %
Iron/Fer	× %
Zinc	× %
Iodine/Iode	× %

THE CANADIAN DIABETES ASSOCIATION FOOD CHOICE SYSTEM

The Canadian Diabetes Association (CDA) Food Choice System is a method of meal planning that is based on *Canada's Food Guide to Healthy Eating*. Foods are divided into choices according to carbohydrate, fat, and protein content. An energy value is given for each choice group and foods are interchangeable within a group. Most foods are eaten in measured amounts. The following examples of foods included in each list were selected from the Good Health Eating Guide Resource, copyright 1994, with permission of the Canadian Diabetes Association.

Canadian Food Choice System: Starch Foods

1 Starch Choice = 15 g carbohydrate (starch), 2 g protein, 290 kJ (68 kcal)

Food	Measure	Mass (weight)
Hamburger buns	½	30 g
Tortilla, flour	1-9 inch circle	30 g
White (French and Italian) bread	1 slice	25 g
Whole-wheat, cracked-wheat, rye, white enriched bread	1 slice	30 g
Ready-to-eat unsweetened cereals	125 mL (½ c)	20 g
Rice, cooked, brown and white (short and long grain)	75 mL (⅓ c)	60 g
Spaghetti, cooked	125 mL (½ c)	70 g
Beans and peas, dried, cooked	125 mL (½ c)	98 g
Corn, canned, whole kernel	125 mL (½ c)	85 g

Canadian Food Choice System: Fruits and Vegetables

1 Fruits and Vegetables Choice = 10 g carbohydrate, 1 g protein, 190 kJ (44 kcal)

Food	Measure	Mass (weight)
Fruits (fresh, frozen, without sugar, canned in water)		
Apples, raw (with or without skin)	½ medium	75 g
Bananas, with peel	½ small	75 g
Grapefruit, raw, with rind	½ small	185 g
Grapes, raw, slip skin	125 mL (½ c)	75 g
Oranges, raw, with rind	1 small	130 g
Watermelon, raw, with rind	1 wedge	310 g
Apricot, grape, guava, mango, prune juice	50 mL (½ c)	55 g
Peas, fresh or frozen	125 mL (½ c)	80 g
Tomatoes, canned	250 mL (1 c)	240 g

Canadian Food Choice System: Sugars

1 Sugar Choice = 10 g carbohydrate (sugar), 167 kJ (40 kcal)

Food	Measure	Mass (weight)
Regular soft drinks	125 mL (½ c)	
Sweet drink mixes	75 mL (⅓ c)	
Popsicle	1 stick (½ popsicle)	
Regular jam, jelly, marmalade	15 mL (1 Tbsp)	
Sugar, white, brown, icing, maple	10 mL (2 tsp)	10 g

Canadian Food Choice System: Protein Foods

1 Protein Choice = 7 g protein, 3 g fat, 230 kJ (55 kcal)

Food	Measure	Mass (weight)
Cottage cheese, 2% milkfat or less	50 mL (¼ c)	55 g
Canned, drained (e.g., mackerel, salmon, tuna packed in water)	50 mL (¼ c)	30 g
Cod tongues, cheeks	75 mL (⅓ c)	50 g
Fillet or steak (e.g., Boston blue, cod, flounder, haddock, halibut, mackerel, orange roughy, perch, pickerel, pike, salmon, shad, snapper, sole, swordfish, trout, tuna, whitefish)	1 piece	30 g
Meat and Poultry (e.g., beef, chicken, goat, ham, lamb, pork, turkey, veal, wild game)		
Chop	½ chop, with bone	40 g
Minced or ground, lean or extra-lean	30 mL (2 Tbsp)	30 g
Steak, lean	1 piece	30 g
Eggs, in shell, raw or cooked	1 medium	50 g

E

Canadian Food Choice System: Milk Foods

Milk Choice = 6 g carbohydrate, 4 g protein, 170–319 kJ (40–76 kcal)

Food	Measure	Mass (weight)
Milk	125 mL (½ c)	125 g
Plain yogurt	125 mL (½ c)	125 g

Canadian Food Choice System: Fats and Oils

1 Fat Choice = 5 g fat, 190 kJ (45 kcal)

Food	Measure	Mass (weight)
Avocado	⅛	30 g
Bacon, side, crisp	1 slice	5 g
Butter	5 mL (1 tsp)	5 g
Cream, half and half (cereal), 10%	30 mL (2 Tbsp)	30 g
Nuts, shelled:		
Almonds	8	5 g
Cashews	5	10 g
Peanuts	10	10 g
Oil, cooking and salad	5 mL (1 tsp)	5 g
Olives, green	10	45 g
Salad dressing: blue cheese, French, Italian,	10 mL (2 tsp)	10 g
mayonnaise	5 mL (1 tsp)	5 g
Thousand Island		

Canadian Food Choice System: Extras

Extras have no more than 2.5 g carbohydrate, 60 kJ (14 kcal)

Vegetables 125 mL (½ c)
Asparagus
Broccoli
Lettuce
Tomato wedges
Free Foods (may be used without measuring)
Artificial sweetener, such as cyclamate or aspartame
Bouillon or clear broth
Coffee, clear
Herbal teas, unsweetened
Lemon juice or lemon wedges

Canadian Food Choice System: Combined Food Choices

Food	Exchanges per Serving	Measures	Mass (weight)
Brownie	1 sugar + 1 fat	1	20 g
Potato chips	1 starch + 2 fats	15 chips	30 g
Egg roll	1 starch + ½ protein + 1 fat	1	75 g
Lasagna, regular cheese	1 starch + 1 fruits & vegetables + 3 proteins + 2 fats	3″ × 4″ piece	
Dried peas	2 starches + 2 protein	250 mL (1 c)	210 g
Pizza, cheese	1 starch + 1 protein + 1 fat	1 slice (⅛ of 12″)	50 g
Pork stir-fry	½–1 fruits & vegetables + 3 proteins	200 mL (¾ c)	
Stew	2 starches + 2 fruit & vegetables + 3 proteins + ½ fat	200 mL (¾ c)	
Sundae	4 sugars + 3 fats	125 mL (½ c)	

Appendix F

World Health Organization Nutrient Intake Recommendations

Recommended Intakes of Nutrients—WHO—1974

Age	Body Weight (kg)	Energy* (kcal)	Energy* (mJ)	Protein*,† (gm)	Vitamin A‡,§ (μg)	Vitamin D‖,# (μg)
Children						
<1	7.3	820	3.4	14	300	10.00
1–3	13.4	1360	5.7	16	250	10.0
4–6	20.2	1830	7.6	20	300	10.0
7–9	28.1	2190	9.2	25	400	2.5
Male adolescents						
10–12	36.9	2600	10.9	30	575	2.5
13–15	51.3	2900	12.1	37	725	2.5
16–19	62.9	3070	12.8	38	750	2.5
Female adolescents						
10–12	38.0	2350	9.8	29	575	2.5
13–15	49.9	2490	10.4	31	725	2.5
16–19	54.4	2310	9.7	30	750	2.5
Adult man (moderately active)	65.0	3000	12.6	37	750	2.5
Adult woman (moderately active)	55.0	2200	9.2	29	750	2.5
Pregnancy (latter half)		+350	+1.5	38	750	10.0
Lactation (first 6 months)		+550	+2.3	46	1200	10.0

* Energy and Protein Requirements. Report of a Joint FAO/WHO Expert Group, FAO, Rome, 1972. † As egg or milk protein. ‡ Requirements of vitamin A, thiamin, riboflavin and niacin. Report of a Joint FAO/WHO Expert Group, FAO, Rome, 1965. § As retinol. ‖ Requirements of ascorbic acid, vitamin D, vitamin B_{12}, folate, and iron. Report of a Joint Applied FAO/WHO Expert Group, FAO, Rome, 1970. # As cholecalciferol. ** Calcium requirements. Report of a FAO/WHO Expert Group, FAO, Rome, 1961. †† On each line the lower value applies when over 25% of calories in the diet come from animal foods, and the higher value when animal foods represent less than 10% of calories. ‡‡ For women whose iron intake throughout life has been at the level recommended in this table, the daily intake of iron during pregnancy and lactation should be the same as

Thiamin‡ (mg)	Riboflavin‡ (mg)	Niacin‡ (mg)	Folic Acid‖ (μg)	Vitamin B_{12}‖ (μg)	Ascorbic Acid‖ (mg)	Calcium** (gm)	Iron‖,†† (mg)
0.3	0.5	5.4	60	0.3	20	0.5–0.6	5–10
0.5	0.8	9.0	100	0.9	20	0.4–0.5	5–10
0.7	1.1	12.1	100	1.5	20	0.4–0.5	5–10
0.9	1.3	14.5	100	1.5	20	0.4–0.5	5–10
1.0	1.6	17.2	100	2.0	20	0.6–0.7	5–10
1.2	1.7	19.1	200	2.0	30	0.6–0.7	9–18
1.2	1.8	20.3	200	2.0	30	0.5–0.6	5–9
0.9	1.4	15.5	100	2.0	20	0.6–0.7	5–10
1.0	1.5	16.4	200	2.0	30	0.6–0.7	12–24
0.9	1.4	15.2	200	2.0	30	0.5–0.6	14–28
1.2	1.8	19.8	200	2.0	30	0.4–0.5	5–9
0.9	1.3	14.5	200	2.0	30	0.4–0.5	14–28
+0.1	+0.2	+2.3	400	3.0	50	1.0–1.2	(9)
+0.2	+0.4	+3.7	300	2.5	50	1.0–1.2	(9)

that recommended for nonpregnant, nonlactating women of childbearing age. For women whose iron status is not satisfactory at the beginning of pregnancy, the requirement is increased, and in the extreme situation of women with no iron stores, the requirement can probably not be met without supplementation.

Source: Passmore, Nicol, and Rao. *Handbook on Human Nutritional Requirements*. Geneva, WHO Monogr. Ser. No. 61, 1974, Table 1.

Addendum: Dietary allowances, official or unofficial, for many European countries, as of 1976 or earlier, appear in the Proceedings of the Second European Nutrition Conference, Munich, 1976. (Nutr. Metab. 21:210, 1977.)

F

The Population Nutrient Goals from WHO

	Limits for Population Average Intakes	
	Lower Limit	Upper Limit
Total fat	15% of energy	30% of energy*
Saturated fatty acids	0% energy	10% of energy
Polyunsaturated fatty acids	3% of energy	7% of energy
Dietary cholesterol	0 mg/day	300 mg/day
Total carbohydrate	55% of energy	75% of energy
Complex carbohydrates[†]	50% of energy	75% of energy
Dietary fibre[‡]		
As nonstarch polysaccharides (NSP)	16 g/day	24 g/day
As total dietary fibre	27 g/day	40 g/day
Free sugars[§]	0% of energy	10% of energy
Protein	10% of energy	15% of energy[‖]
Salt	—[‖]	6 g/day

Total energy
Energy intake needs to be sufficient to allow for normal childhood growth, for the needs of pregnancy and lactation, and for work and desirable physical activities, and to maintain appropriate body reserves of energy in children and adults. Adult populations on average should have a body mass index (BMI) of 20–22. (BMI = body mass in kg/[height in metres]^2).

The lower limit defines the minimum intake needed to prevent deficiency diseases, while the upper limit expressed the maximum intake compatible with the prevention of chronic diseases.

*An interim goal for nations with high fat intakes; further benefits would be expected by reducing fat intake towards 15% of total energy.

[†]A daily minimum intake of 400 g of vegetables and fruits, including at least 30 g of pulses, nuts, and seeds, should contribute to this component.

[‡]Dietary fibre includes the nonstarch polysaccharides (NSP), the goals for which are based on NSP obtained from mixed food sources. Since the definition and measurement of dietary fibre remain uncertain, the goals for total dietary fibre have been estimated from the NSP values.

[§]These sugars include monosaccharides, disaccharides, and other short-chain sugars extracted from carbohydrates by refining. These refined, or purified, sugars do not include the natural sugars consumed when eating fruits and vegetables or drinking milk.

[‖] Not defined.

Source: Diet, nutrition and the prevention of chronic diseases. A report of the WHO Study Group on Diet, Nutrition and Prevention of Noncommunicable Diseases. Nutr. Rev. 49:291–301, 1991.

F

Appendix G

Nutrition Goals and Guidelines

Nutrition and Your Health:
DIETARY GUIDELINES FOR AMERICANS

AIM FOR FITNESS...

- ▲ Aim for a healthy weight.
- ▲ Be physically active each day.

BUILD A HEALTHY BASE...

- ■ Let the Pyramid guide your food choices.
- ■ Choose a variety of grains daily, especially whole grains.
- ■ Choose a variety of fruits and vegetables daily.
- ■ Keep food safe to eat.

CHOOSE SENSIBLY...

- ● Choose a diet that is low in saturated fat and cholesterol and moderate in total fat.
- ● Choose beverages and foods to moderate your intake of sugars.
- ● Choose and prepare foods with less salt.
- ● If you drink alcoholic beverages, do so in moderation.

...for good health

Dietary Guidelines: Population Goals

1. Achieve an overall healthy eating pattern:
   - Choose an overall balanced diet with foods from all major food groups, emphasizing fruits, vegetables, and grains.
   - Consume a variety of fruits, vegetables, and grain products.
   - Include at least five daily servings of fruits and vegetables.
   - Include at least six daily servings of grain products, including whole grains.
   - Include fat-free and low-fat dairy products, fish, legumes, poultry, and lean meats.
   - Eat at least two servings of fish per week.
2. Achieve a healthy body weight.
   - Avoid excess intake of calories.
   - Maintain a level of physical activity that achieves fitness and balances energy expenditure with caloric intake; for weight reduction, expenditure should exceed intake.
   - Limit foods that are high in calories and/or low in nutritional quality, including those with a high amount of added sugar.
3. Achieve a desirable cholesterol level.
   - Limit foods with a high content of saturated fat and cholesterol. Substitute with grains and unsaturated fat from vegetables, fish, legumes, and nuts.
   - Limit cholesterol to 300 milligrams (mg) a day for the general population, and 200 mg a day for those with heart disease or its risk factors.
   - Limit *trans* fatty acids. *Trans* fatty acids are found in foods containing partially hydrogenated vegetable oils, such as packaged cookies, crackers, and other baked goods; commercially prepared fried foods; and some margarines.
4. Achieve a desirable blood pressure level.
   - Limit salt intake to less than 6 grams (2400 mg sodium) per day, slightly more than one teaspoon a day.
   - If you drink, limit alcohol consumption to no more than one drink per day for women and two drinks per day for men.

Dietary Guidelines for Americans, 1980 to 2000

1980	1985	1990	1995	2000	
7 Guidelines	***7 Guidelines***	***7 Guidelines***	***7 Guidelines***	***10 Guidelines, clustered into 3 groups***	
Eat a variety of foods.	Eat a variety of foods.	Eat a variety of foods.	Eat a variety of foods.		
Maintain ideal weight.	Maintain desirable weight.	Maintain healthy weight.	Balance the food you eat with physical activity—maintain or improve your weight.	Aim for a healthy weight.	**Aim for Fitness**
				Be physically active each day.	**Aim for Fitness**
Avoid too much fat, saturated fat, and cholesterol.	Avoid too much fat, saturated fat, and cholesterol.	Choose a diet low in fat, saturated fat, and cholesterol.		Let the Pyramid guide your food choices.	**Build a Healthy Base**
Eat foods with adequate starch and fiber.	Eat foods with adequate starch and fiber.	Choose a diet with plenty of vegetables, fruits, and grain products.	Choose a diet with plenty of grain products, vegetables, and fruits.	Choose a variety of grains daily, especially whole grains.	**Build a Healthy Base**
				Choose a variety of fruits and vegetables daily.	**Build a Healthy Base**
				Keep food safe to eat.	**Build a Healthy Base**
			Choose a diet low in fat, saturated fat, and cholesterol.	Choose a diet that is low in saturated fat and cholesterol and moderate in total fat.	**Choose Sensibly**
Avoid too much sugar.	Avoid too much sugar.	Use sugars only in moderation.	Choose a diet moderate in sugars.	Choose beverages and foods to moderate your intake of sugars.	**Choose Sensibly**
Avoid too much sodium.	Avoid too much sodium.	Use salt and sodium only in moderation.	Choose a diet moderate in salt and sodium.	Choose and prepare foods with less salt.	**Choose Sensibly**
If you drink alcohol, do so in moderation.	If you drink alcoholic beverages, do so in moderation.	If you drink alcoholic beverages, do so in moderation.	If you drink alcoholic beverages, do so in moderation.	If you drink alcoholic beverages, do so in moderation.	**Choose Sensibly**

Shading indicates how the order in which the guidelines are presented has changed over time

Source: Center for Nutrition Policy and Promotion, USDA, May 30, 2000.

G

Healthy People 2010

Goals

1. Increase quality and years of healthy life.
2. Eliminate health disparities.

Leading Health Indicators

1. *Physical activity*
2. *Overweight and obesity*
3. *Tobacco use*
4. *Substance abuse*
5. *Responsible sexual behavior*
6. *Mental health*
7. *Injury and violence*
8. *Environmental quality*
9. *Immunization*
10. *Access to health care*

Focus Areas

Access to quality health services
Arthritis, osteoporosis, and chronic back conditions
Cancer
Chronic kidney disease
Diabetes
Disability and secondary conditions
Educational and community-based programs
Environmental health
Family planning
Food safety
Health communication
Heart disease and stroke
HIV
Immunization and infectious diseases
Injury and violence prevention
Maternal, infant, and child health
Medical product safety
Mental health and mental disorders
Nutrition and overweight
Occupational safety and health
Oral health
Physical activity and fitness
Public health infrastructure
Respiratory diseases
Sexually transmitted diseases
Substance abuse
Tobacco use
Vision and hearing

Source: Healthy People 2010. Available online at **http://www.health.gov/healthypeople.**

American Heart Association Eating Plan for Healthy Americans*

Total kcalories should be adjusted to achieve and maintain a healthy body weight.

Saturated fatty acid intake should be 7 to 10% of total kcalories.

Polyunsaturated fatty acid intake should be up to 10% of total kcalories.

Monounsaturated fatty acids should make up the rest of the total fat intake, about 10 to 15% of total kcalories.

Total fat intake should be no more than 30% of total kcalories.

Cholesterol intake should be less than 300 milligrams per day.

Sodium intake should be less than 2400 milligrams per day, which is about 1 teaspoon of sodium chloride (salt).

Carbohydrate intake should make up 55 to 60% or more of kcalories, with emphasis on increasing sources of complex carbohydrates.

* Recommendations available online at http://americanheart.org/Heart_and_Stroke_A_Z_Guide/dietg.html.

National Cholesterol Education Program Step I and Step II Diets*

Nutrient	Recommended Intake As Percent of Total Kcalories: Step I	Step II
Total Fat	30% or less	30% or less
Saturated fatty acids	8–10%	Less than 7%
Polyunsaturated fatty acids	Up to 10%	Up to 10%
Monounsaturated fatty acids	Up to 15%	Up to 15%
Sodium	limit to 2400 mg	limit to 2400 mg
Carbohydrate	55% or more	55% or more
Protein	Approximately 15%	Approximately 15%
Cholesterol	Less than 300 mg/day	Less than 200 mg/day
Total kcalories	To achieve and maintain desired weight	To achieve and maintain desired weight

*Source: National Heart, Lung, and Blood Institute available online at http://www.nhlbisupport.com/cgi-bin/chd1/step2intro.cgi.

American Institute for Cancer Research Diet & Health Guidelines for Cancer Prevention

1. Choose a diet rich in a variety of plant-based foods.
2. Eat plenty of vegetables and fruits.
3. Maintain a healthy weight and be physically active.
4. Drink alcohol in moderation, if at all.
5. Select foods low in fat and salt.
6. Prepare and store foods safely.

   And, always remember. . .

   Do not smoke or use tobacco in any form.

Source: American Institute of Cancer Research. Available online at http://www.aicr.org/reduce.htm.

American Cancer Society*

Choose most foods you eat from plant sources.

Limit your intake of high-fat foods, particularly from animal sources.

Be physically active: Achieve and maintain a healthy weight.

Limit consumption of alcoholic beverages, if you drink at all.

*Available online at http://www.cancer.org/statistics/cff98/nutrition.html.

National Cancer Institute Dietary Guidelines*

Reduce fat intake to 30% of kcalories or less.

Increase fiber to 20–30 grams/day, with an upper limit of 35 grams.

Include a variety of fruits and vegetables in the daily diet.

Avoid obesity.

Consume alcoholic beverages in moderation, if at all.

Minimize consumption of salt-cured, salt-pickled, and smoked foods.

* Available online at http://rex.nci.nih.gov/NCI_Pub_Interface/ActionGd_Web/guidelns.html.

Dietary Approaches to Stop Hypertension: DASH Diet

When making changes, start small.

Center your meal around carbohydrates such as pasta, rice, beans, or vegetables.

Treat meat as one part of the whole meal instead of as the focus.

Use fruit and low-fat low-energy foods such as sugar-free gelatin for desserts and snacks.

A 2000-kcalorie diet should include
- 7–8 servings of grains and grain products
- 4–5 servings of vegetables
- 4–5 servings of fruit
- 2–3 servings of low-fat and nonfat dairy foods
- 2 or fewer servings of meat, poultry, and fish
- one-half serving of nuts, seeds, or legumes

Source: Dietary Approaches to Stop Hypertension. Online at http://dash.bwh.harvard.edu.

Food Guide Pyramid
A Guide to Daily Food Choices

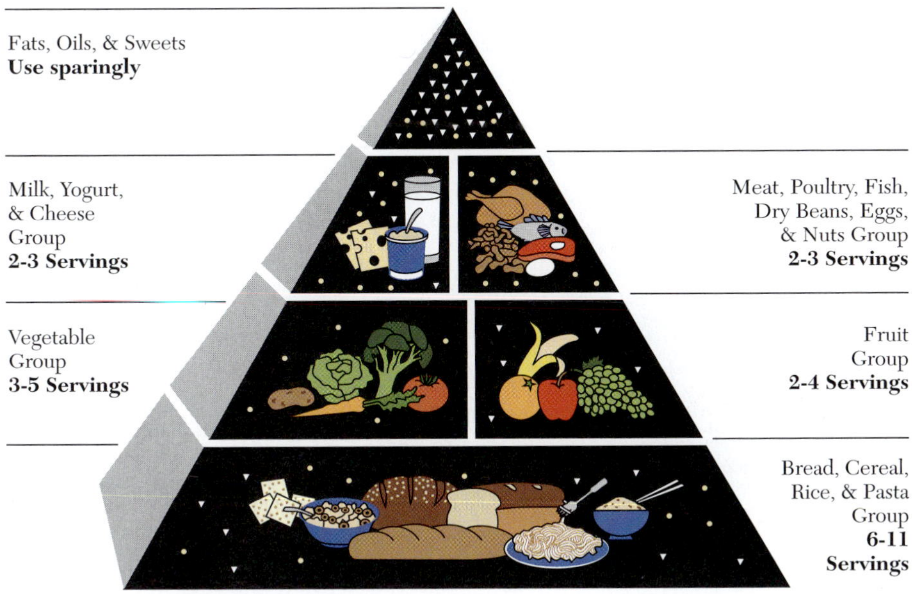

Key
• Fat (naturally occurring and added) ▼ Sugars (added)
These symbols show fats, oils, and added sugars in foods.

Number of Food Guide Pyramid Servings for Three Daily Energy Levels*

	1600 kcalories (sedentary women and some older adults)	2200 kcalories (children, teenage girls, active women, and many sedentary men)	2800 kcalories (teenage boys, many active men, and some very active women)
Bread, Cereal, Rice, & Pasta Group	6	9	11
Vegetable Group	3	4	5
Fruit Group	2	3	4
Milk, Yogurt, & Cheese Group	2–3†	2–3†	2–3†
Meat, Poultry, Fish, Dry Beans, Eggs, & Nuts Group	2 (5 oz total)	2 (6 oz total)	3 (7 oz total)

*Assumes that food choices are mostly low-fat and low kcalorie.

†Women who are pregnant or breastfeeding, teenagers, and young adults to age 24 need three servings.

U.S. Department of Agriculture. The Food Guide Pyramid. Home and Garden Bulletin 252, 1992, revised 1996.

A Modifed Food Guide Pyramid for Vegetarians

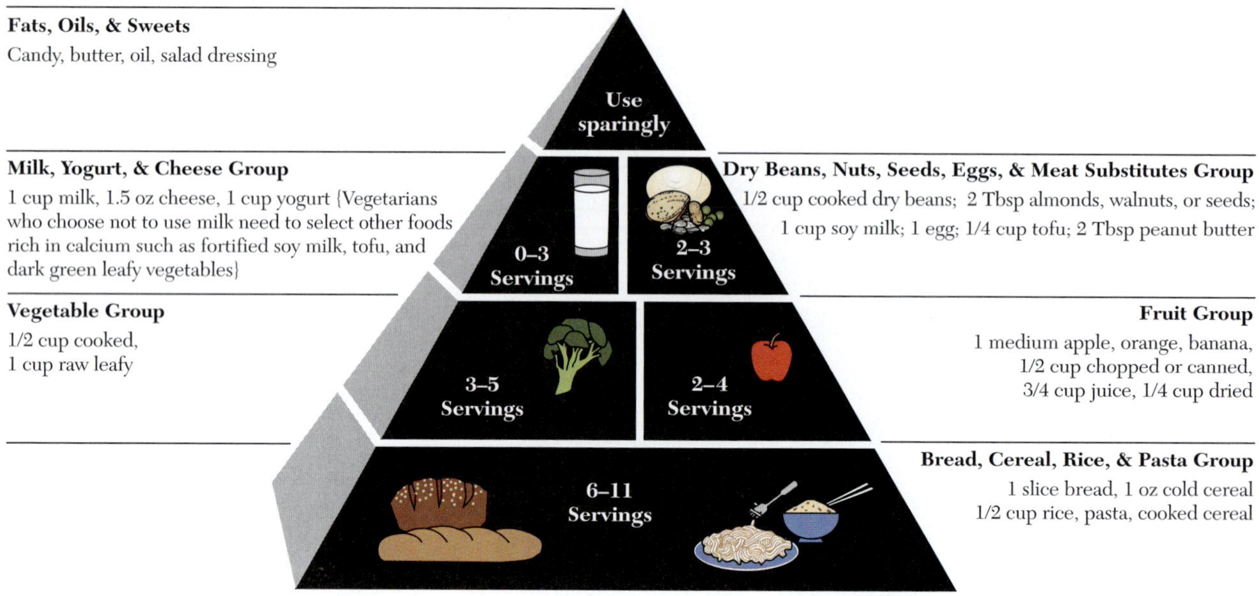

FOOD Guide PYRAMID

for Young Children

A Daily Guide for 2- to 6-Year-Olds

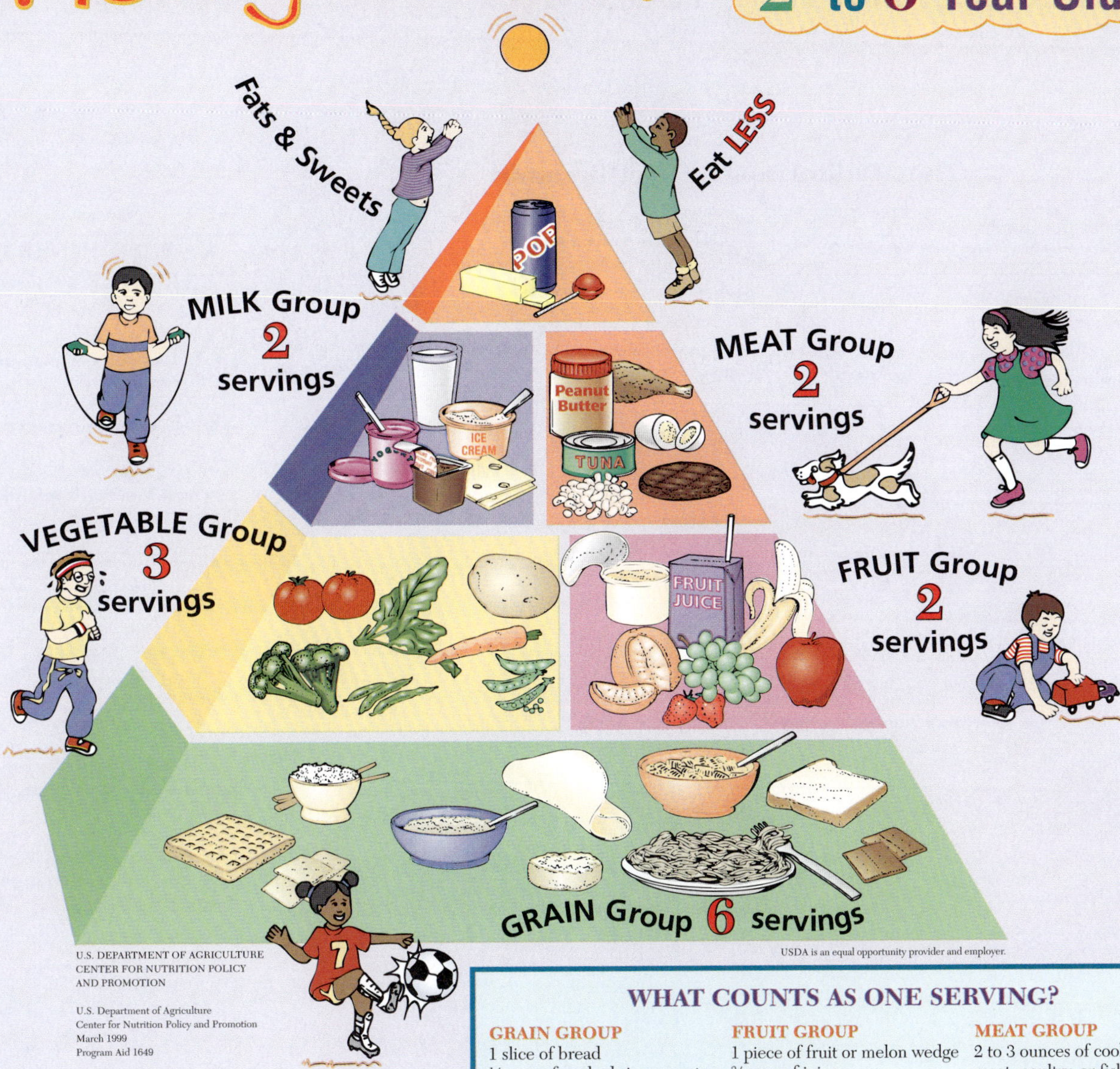

Fats & Sweets
Eat LESS
POP
MILK Group 2 servings
ICE CREAM
MEAT Group 2 servings
Peanut Butter
TUNA
VEGETABLE Group 3 servings
FRUIT JUICE
FRUIT Group 2 servings
GRAIN Group 6 servings
7

U.S. DEPARTMENT OF AGRICULTURE
CENTER FOR NUTRITION POLICY
AND PROMOTION

U.S. Department of Agriculture
Center for Nutrition Policy and Promotion
March 1999
Program Aid 1649

USDA is an equal opportunity provider and employer.

WHAT COUNTS AS ONE SERVING?

GRAIN GROUP
1 slice of bread
1/2 cup of cooked rice or pasta
1/2 cup of cooked cereal
1 ounce of ready-to-eat cereal

VEGETABLE GROUP
1/2 cup of chopped raw or cooked vegetables
1 cup of raw leafy vegetables

FRUIT GROUP
1 piece of fruit or melon wedge
3/4 cup of juice
1/2 cup of canned fruit
1/4 cup of dried fruit

MILK GROUP
1 cup of milk or yogurt
2 ounces of cheese

MEAT GROUP
2 to 3 ounces of cooked lean meat, poultry, or fish.

1/2 cup of cooked dry beans, or 1 egg counts as 1 ounce of lean meat. 2 tablespoons of peanut butter count as 1 ounce of meat.

FATS AND SWEETS
Limit calories from these.

Four- to 6-year-olds can eat these serving sizes. Offer 2- to 3-year-olds less, except for milk. Two- to 6-year-old children need a total of 2 servings from the milk group each day.

FOOD IS FUN and learning about food is fun, too. Eating foods from the Food Guide Pyramid and being physically active will help you grow healthy and strong.

EAT a variety of FOODS AND ENJOY!

G

Appendix H

Ethnic Diet Planning Tools

The Mediterranean Diet Pyramid

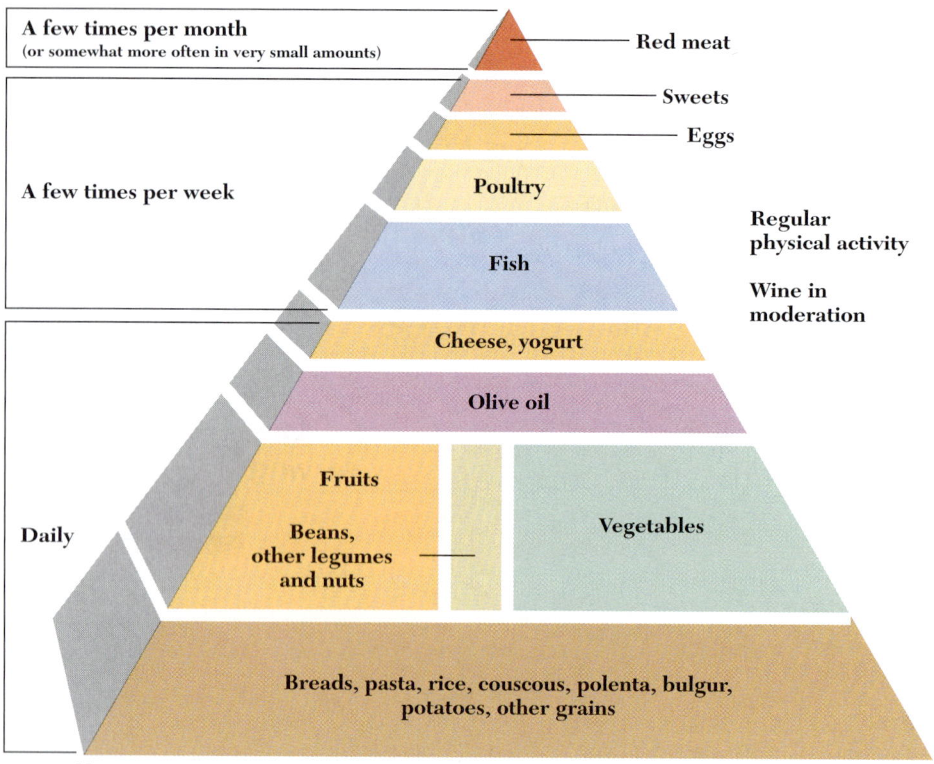

HEALTH HINTS FROM THE MEDITERRANEAN DIET PYRAMID

- Eat most food from plant sources, including fruits, vegetables, potatoes, breads, beans, nuts, and seeds.
- Use seasonally fresh, locally grown food with a minimum of processing.
- Let olive oil be your principal fat, replacing other fats, oils, butter, and margarine.
- Eat red meat only a few times per month and favor the lean cuts.
- If you drink wine, enjoy only 1 or 2 glasses a day, preferably with meals.
- Engage in regular exercise to promote a healthy weight, fitness, and well-being.

Asian Diet Pyramid

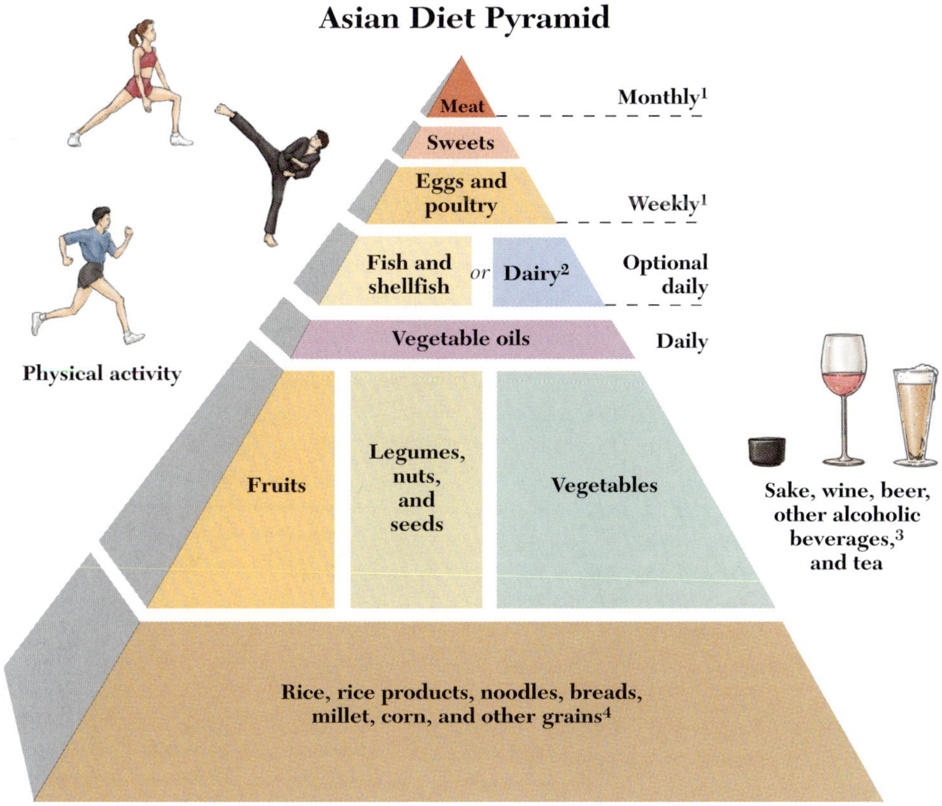

[1]Or more often in very small amounts.
[2]Dairy foods are generally not part of the healthy, traditional diets of Asia, with the notable exception of India. In light of current nutrition research, if dairy foods are consumed on a daily basis, they should be used in low to moderate amounts, and preferably be low in fat.
[3]Wine, beer, and other alcoholic beverages should be consumed in moderation and primarily with meals, and avoided whenever consumption would put an individual or others at risk.
[4]Minimally refined whenever possible.

Mexican-American Foods and the Food Guide Pyramid

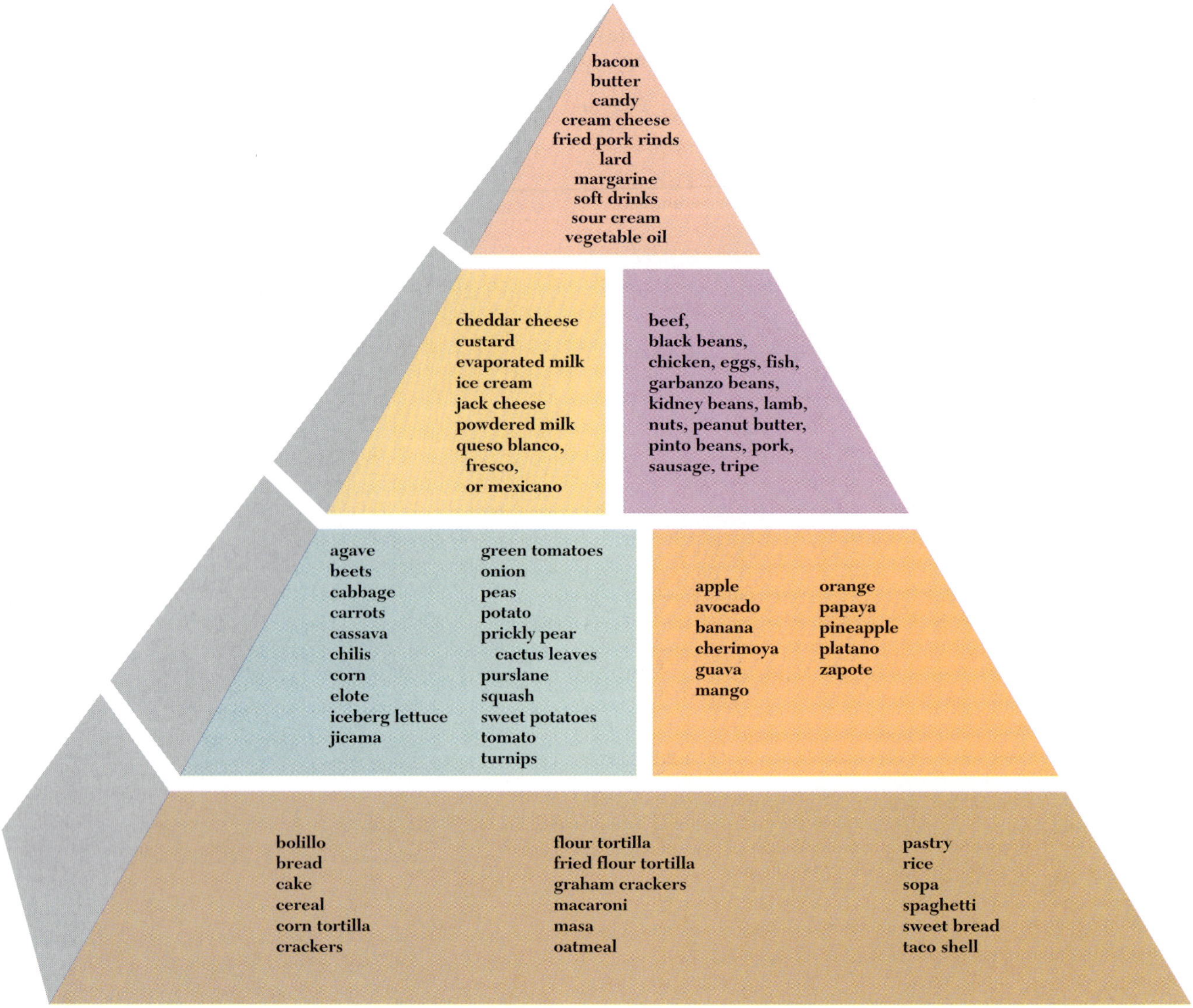

Sources: Algert, Susan J., and Teri Hall Ellison, Contributors. *Ethnic and Regional Food Practices—A Series: Mexican American Food Practices, Customs, and Holidays*; Diabetes Care and Education Practice Group of the American Dietetic Association, 1989; *Comidas Hispana en Dietas Diabetica (Spanish Foods in Diabetic Diets)*. Visiting Nurse Association of Milwaukee, 1975.

African-American Foods and the Food Guide Pyramid

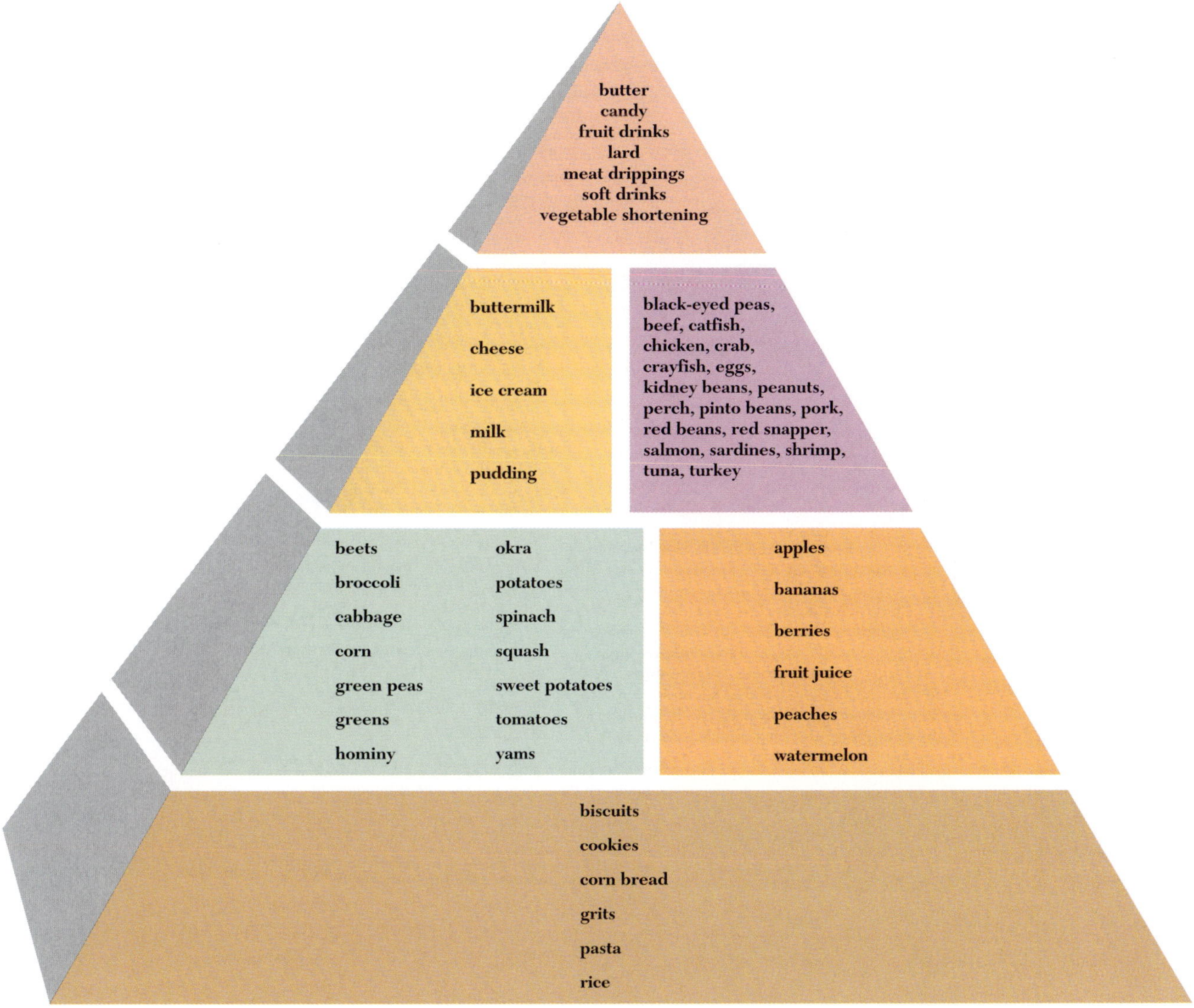

Source: Kittler, Pamela Goyan, and Kathryn Sucher. *Food and Culture in America* (New York: Van Nostrand Reinhold, 1989).

Chinese-American Foods and the Food Guide Pyramid

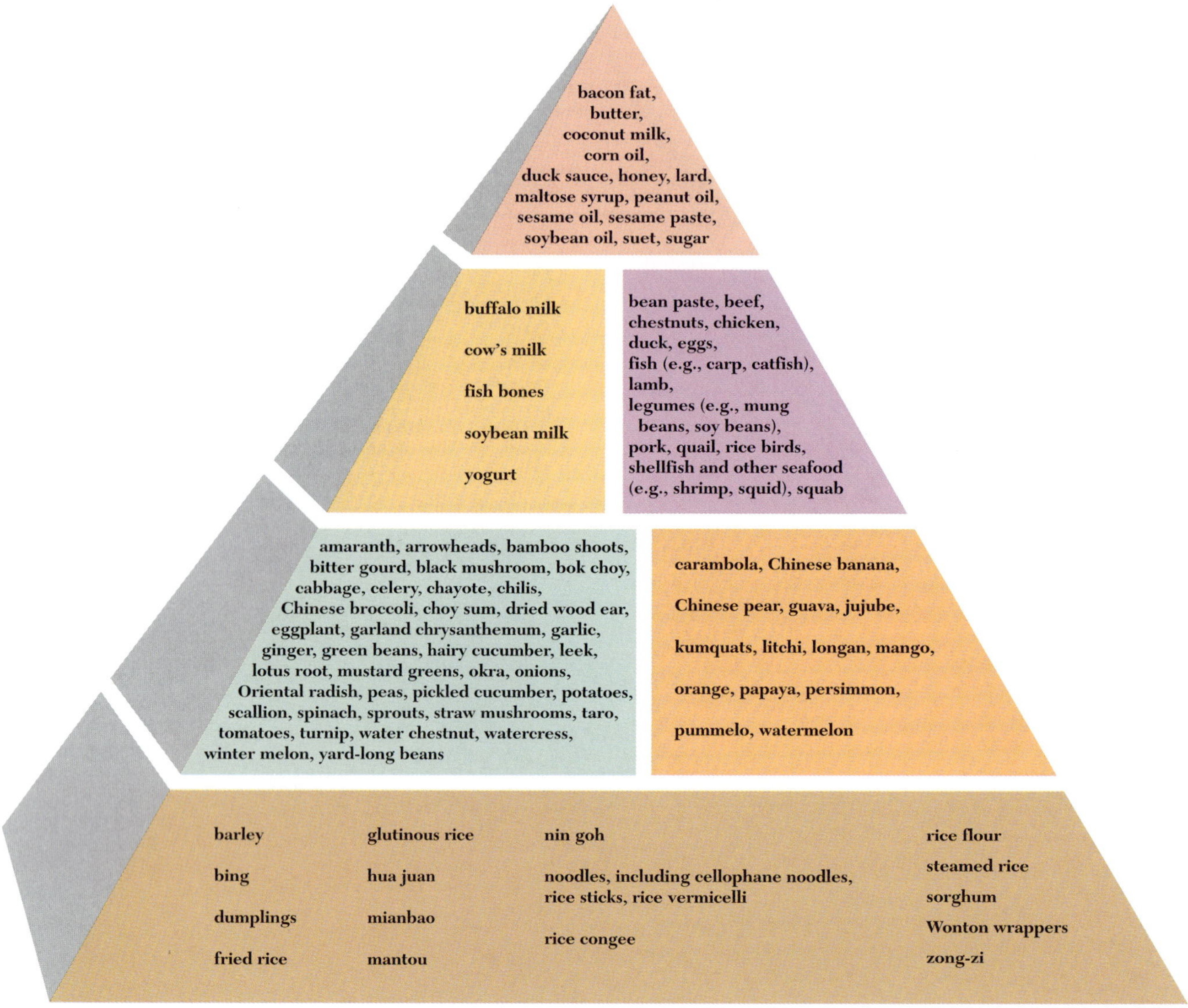

Sources: Kee Maggie Ma. *Ethnic and Regional Food Practices—A Series: Chinese American Food Practices, Customs and Holidays*. Diabetes Care and Education Practice Group of the American Dietetic Association, 1990; Kittler, Pamela Goyan, and Kathryn Sucher. *Food and Culture in America* (New York; Van Nostrand Reinhold, 1989).

Indian Foods and the Food Guide Pyramid

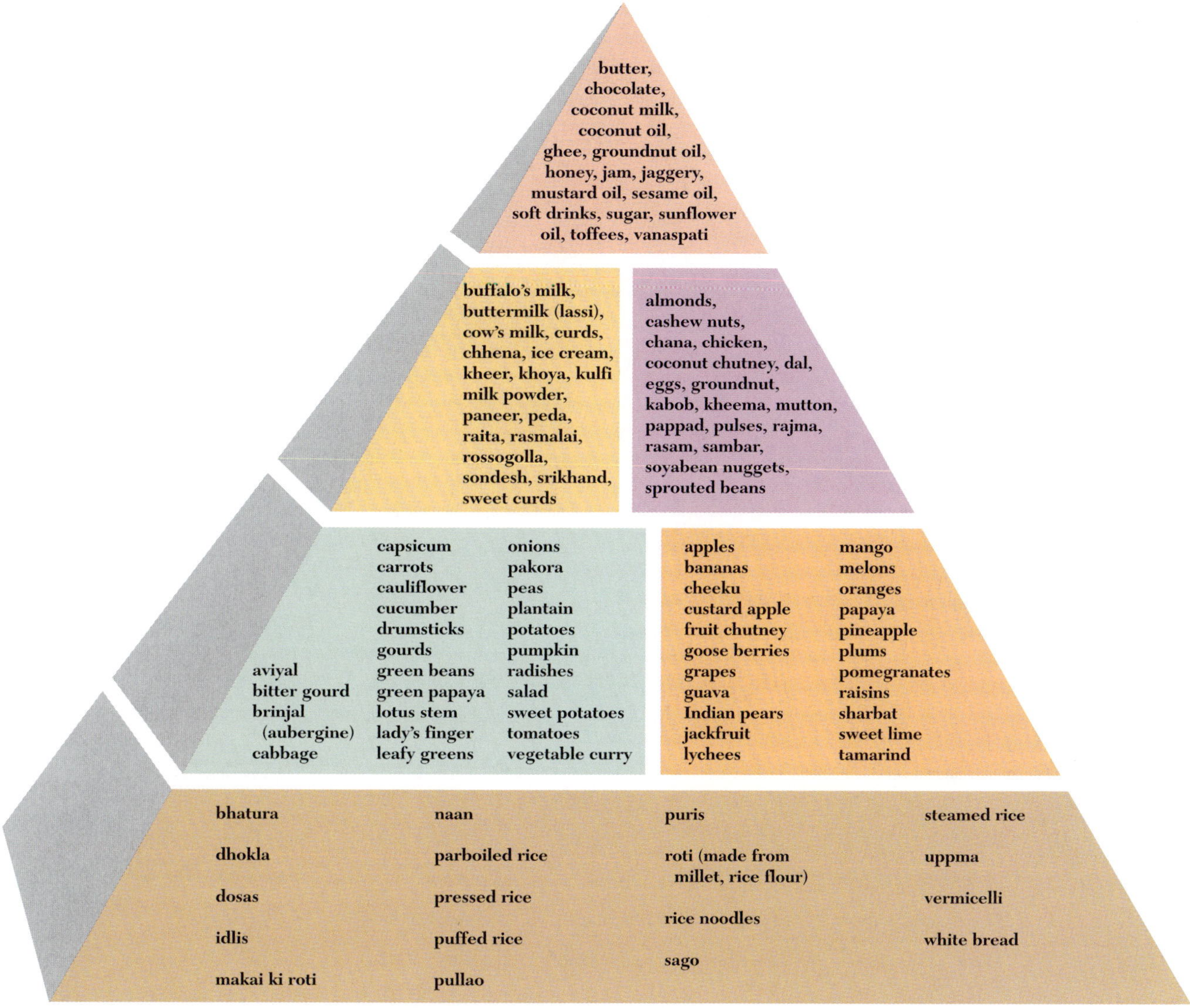

Sources: Barer-Stein, Thelma. *You Eat What You Are—A Study of Ethnic Food Traditions* (Toronto: McClelland and Stewart, Ltd., 1979); Dalal, *Tarla Dalal's New Indian Vegatarian Cooking* (Bombay: India Book Distributors, 1986); Kittler, Pamela Goyan, and Kathryn Sucher. *Food and Culture in America* (New York: Van Nostrand Reinhold, 1989); Madhur, Jaffrey. *A Taste of India* (London: Pan Books, Ltd., 1985); Sahni, Julie. *Classic Indian Cooking* (New York: William Morrow and Company, Inc. 1980); Santha, Rama Rau. *The Cooking of India* (New York: Time-Life Books [Foods of the World], 1969). Pyramid prepared by Uma Srinath.

Jewish Foods and the Food Guide Pyramid

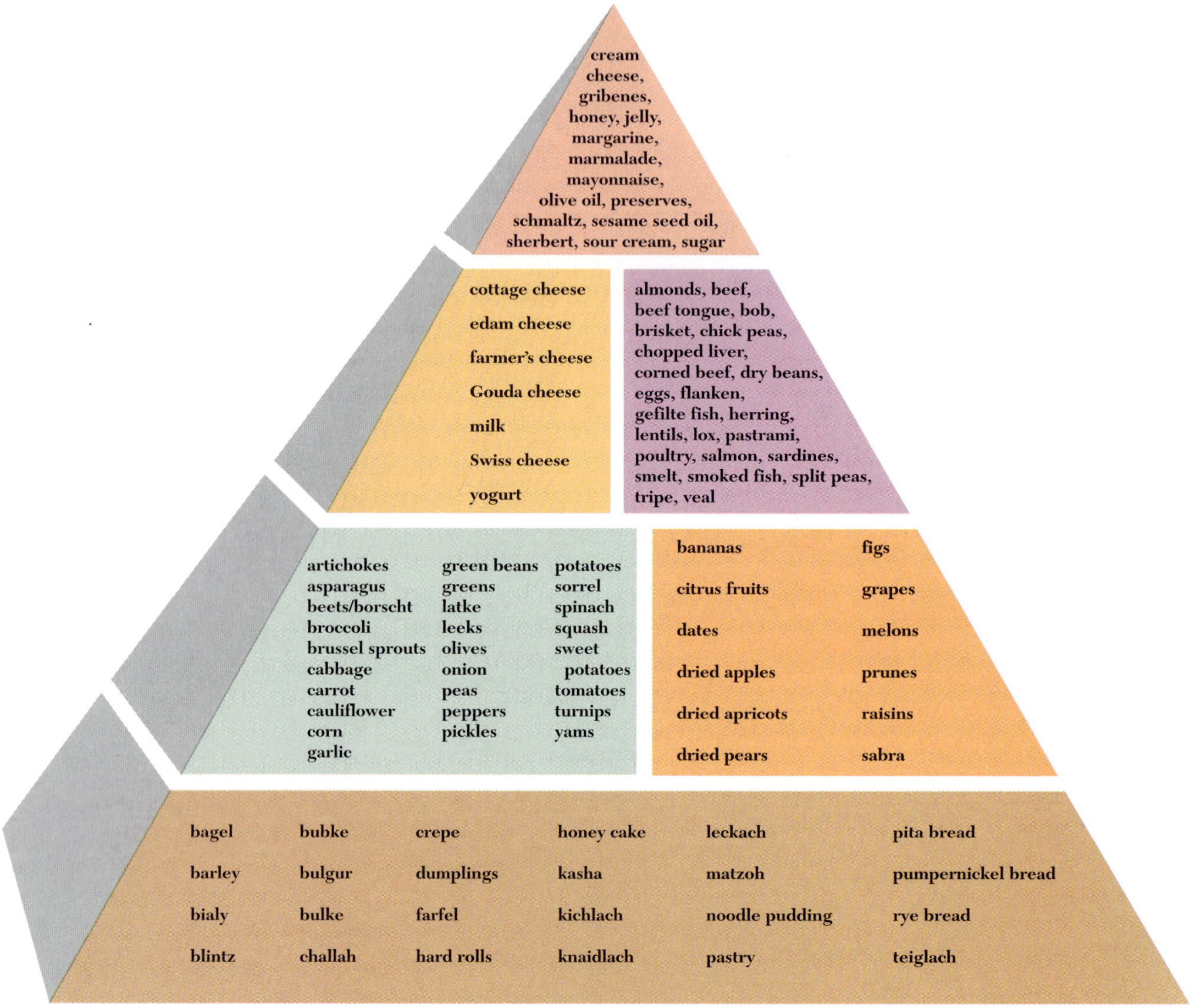

Sources: Higgins, Catherine, and Hope S. Warshaw, contributors. *Ethnic and Regional Food Practices—A Series: Jewish Food Practices, Customs, and Holidays.* Diabetes Care and Education Practice Group of the American Dietetic Association, 1989; Barer-Stein, Thelma. *You Eat What You Are—A Study of Ethnic Food Traditions* (Toronto: McClelland and Stewart Ltd., 1979).

Navajo Foods and the Food Guide Pyramid

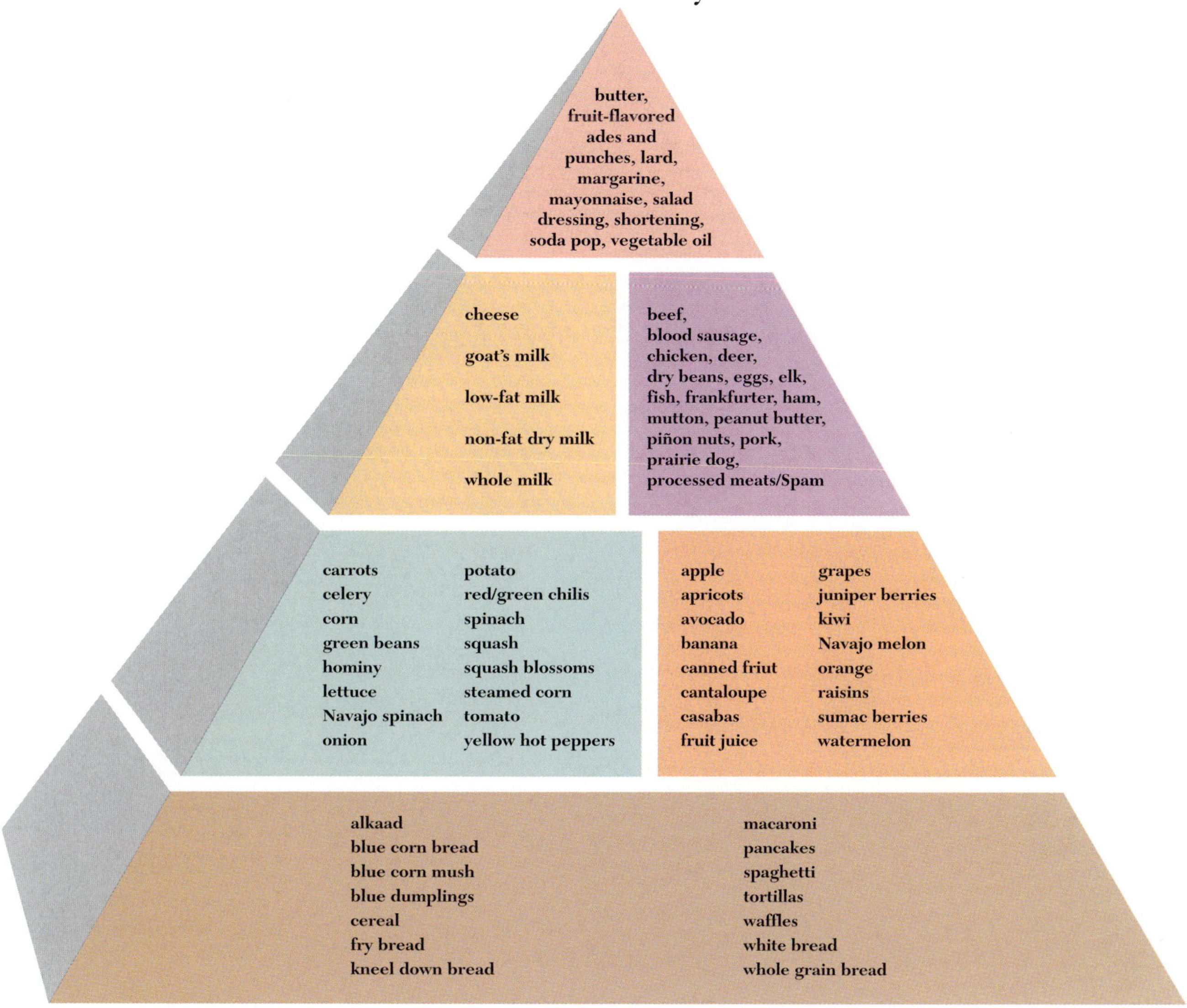

Sources: Pelican, Suzanne, and Karen Bachman-Carter. *Ethnic and Regional Food Practices—A Series: Navajo Food Practices, Customs, and Holidays.* Diabetes Care and Education Practice Group of the American Dietetic Association, 1991; Navajo Health and Nutrition Survey (unpublished). Navajo Area Indian Health Service.

Puerto Rican Foods and the Food Guide Pyramid*

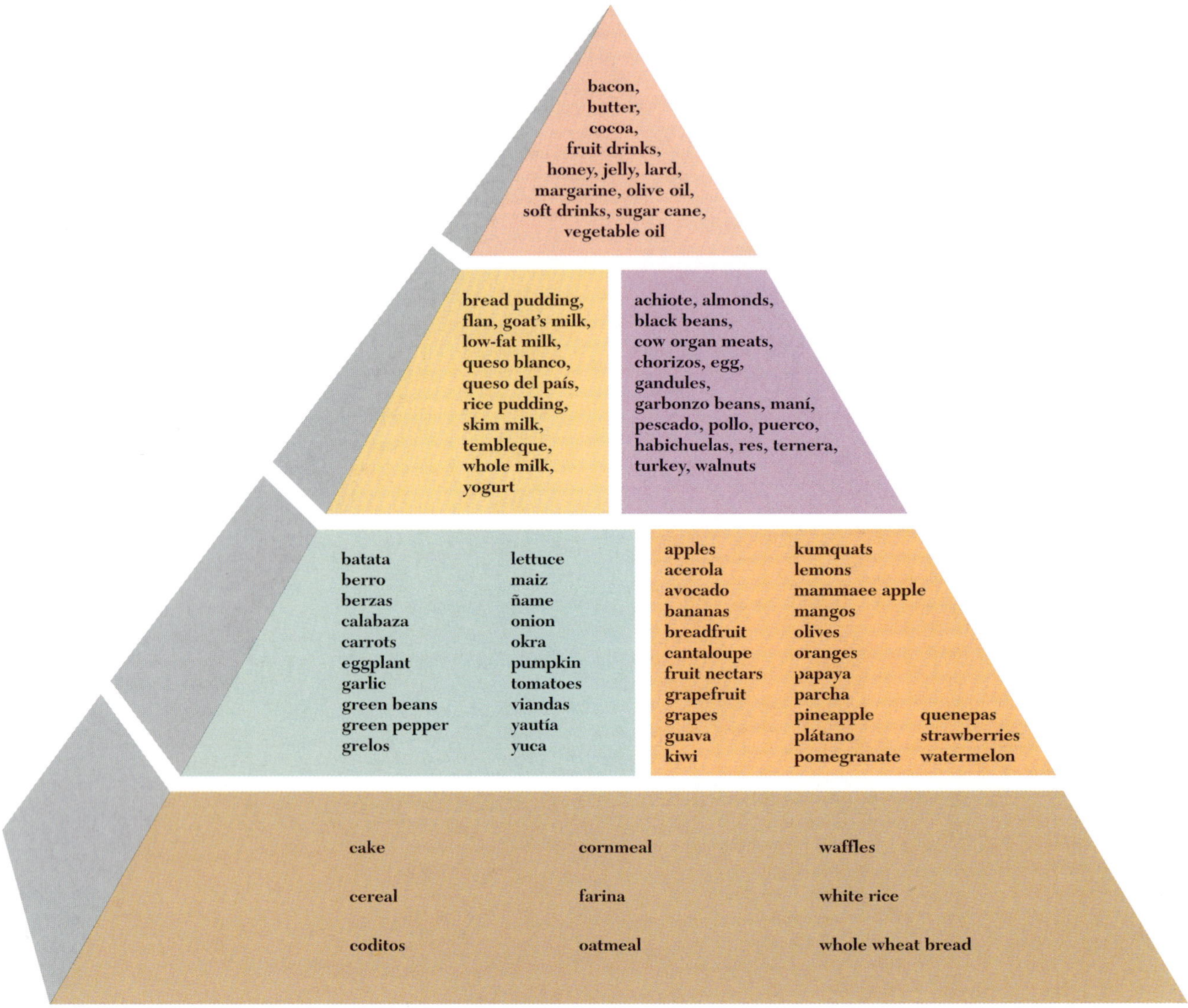

* May be used with Cuban and Dominican populations.

Sources: Dooley, Eliza B.K. *Puerto Rican Cookbook* (Virginia: Dietz, 1948); Internet: http://www.cu-online.com/~maggy/pr.html; Internet: http://pubweb.acns.nwu.edu/%7Ecotto/pr.html; Rivera, Jeanie. Personal interview, 1 April 1996; Ruíz, Leondro. Personal interview, 26 May 1996; "Buen Provecho..." *Bienvenidos* 1994; Vasquez, Susana. Personal Interview, 10 April 1996.

Vietnamese-American Foods and the Food Guide Pyramid

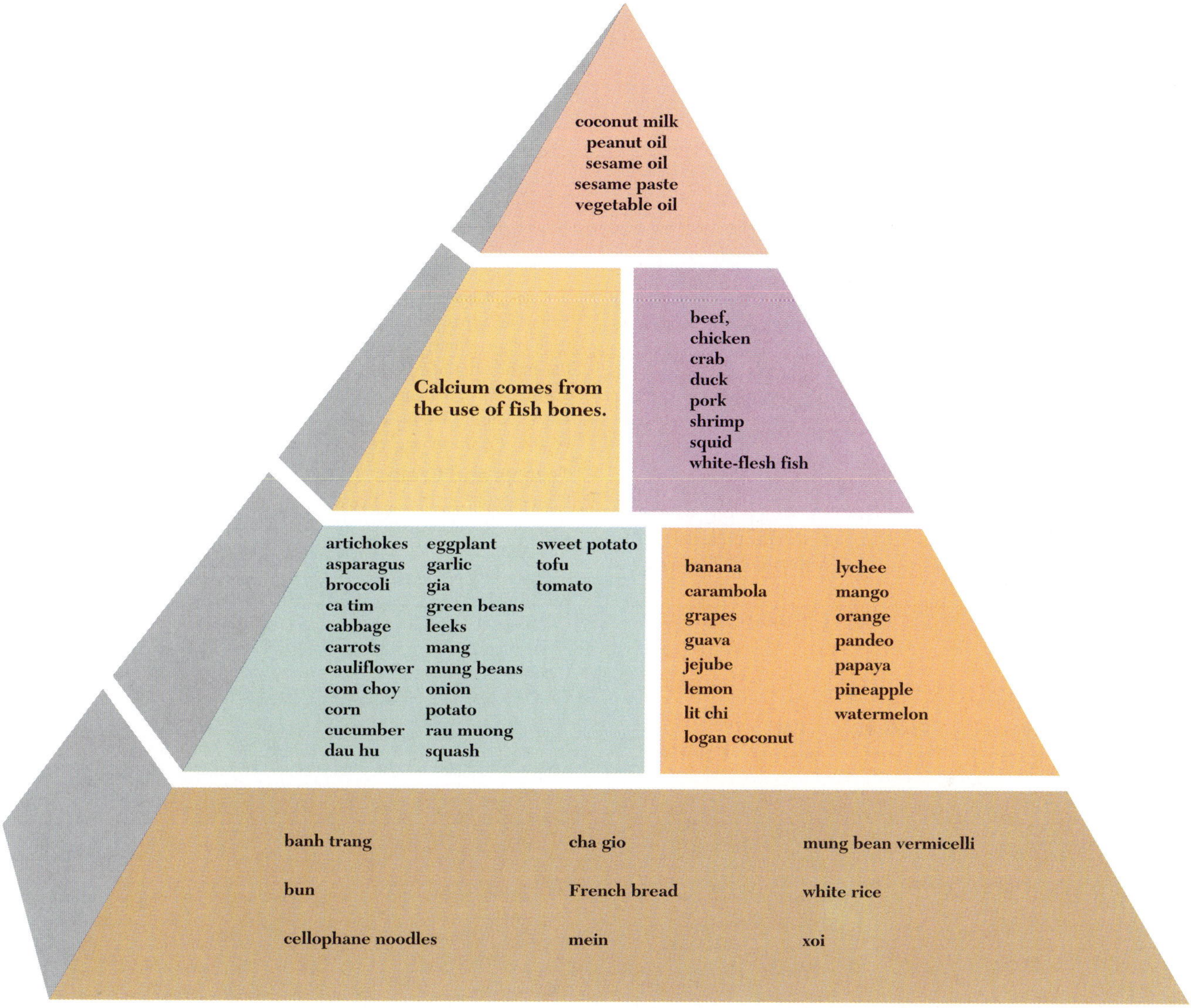

Sources: Passimore, Jackie. *Asia, the Beautiful Cookbook* (San Francisco: Collins Publishers, 1990); Routhier, Nicole. *The Foods of Vietnam* (New York: Stewart, Taborr and Chang, 1989); Solomon, Charmaine. *Complete Asian Cookbook* (New York: McGraw-Hill Book Co., 1982); Le, Laura, personal interview, April 1996; Le, Tuan, personal interview, April 1996; Waiter at The Pho Express Restaurant. personal interview, April 1996.

Appendix I

Exchange Lists

The exchange lists provide you with a lot of food choices (foods from the basic food groups, foods with added sugars, free foods, combination foods, and fast foods). This gives you variety in your meals. Several foods, such as dried beans and peas, bacon, and peanut butter, are on two lists. This gives you flexibility in putting your meals together. Whenever you choose new foods or vary your meal plan, monitor your blood glucose to see how these different foods affect your blood glucose level.

Foods are listed with their serving sizes, which are usually measured after cooking. When you begin, you should measure the size of each serving. This may help you learn to "eyeball" correct serving sizes.

The following chart shows the amount of nutrients in one serving from each list.

Groups/Lists	Carbohydrate (grams)	Protein (grams)	Fat (grams)	Calories
Carbohydrate Group				
Starch	15	3	1 or less	80
Fruit	15	—	—	60
Milk				
Skim	12	8	0–3	90
Low-fat	12	8	5	120
Whole	12	8	8	150
Other carbohydrates	15	Varies	Varies	Varies
Vegetables	5	2	—	25
Meat and Meat Substitute Group				
Very lean	—	7	0–1	35
Lean	—	7	3	55
Medium-fat	—	7	5	75
High-fat	—	7	8	100
Fat Group	—	—	5	45

Starch List

One starch exchange equals 15 grams carbohydrate, 3 grams protein, 0–1 grams fat, and 80 calories.

Bread

Bagel .... ½ (1 oz)
Bread, reduced-calorie .... 2 slices (1½ oz)
Bread, white, whole-wheat, pumpernickel, rye .... 1 slice (1 oz)
Bread sticks, crisp, 4 in. long × ½ in. .... 2 (⅔ oz)
English muffin .... ½
Hot dog or hamburger bun .... ½ (1 oz)
Pita, 6 in. across .... ½
Roll, plain, small .... 1 (1 oz)
Raisin bread, unfrosted .... 1 slice (1 oz)
Tortilla, corn, 6 in. across 1
Tortilla, flour, 7–8 in. across 1
Waffle, 4½ in. square, reduced-fat 1

Cereals and Grains

Bran cereals .... ½ cup
Bulgur .... ½ cup
Cereals .... ½ cup
Cereals, unsweetened, ready-to-eat .... ¾ cup
Cornmeal (dry) .... 3 Tbsp
Couscous .... ⅓ cup
Flour (dry) .... 3 Tbsp
Granola, low-fat .... ¼ cup
Grape-Nuts .... ¼ cup
Grits .... ½ cup
Kasha .... ½ cup
Millet .... ¼ cup
Muesli .... ¼ cup
Oats .... ½ cup
Pasta .... ½ cup
Puffed cereal .... 1½ cups
Rice, white or brown .... ⅓ cup
Rice milk .... ½ cup
Shredded Wheat .... ½ cup
Sugar-frosted cereal .... ½ cup
Wheat germ .... 3 Tbsp

Dried Beans, Peas, and Lentils

(Count as 1 starch exchange, plus 1 very lean meat exchange.)

Beans and peas (garbanzo, pinto, kidney, white, split, black-eyed) .... ½ cup
Lima beans .... ⅔ cup
Lentils .... ½ cup
Miso .... 3 Tbsp

= 400 mg or more of sodium per serving.

Starchy Vegetables

Baked beans .... ⅓ cup
Corn .... ½ cup
Corn on cob, medium .... 1 (5 oz)
Mixed vegetables with corn, peas, or pasta .... 1 cup
Peas, green .... ½ cup
Plantain .... ½ cup
Potato, baked or boiled .... 1 small (3 oz)
Potato, mashed .... ½ cup
Squash, winter (acorn, butternut) .... 1 cup
Yam, sweet potato, plain .... ½ cup

Crackers and Snacks

Animal crackers 8
Graham crackers, 2½ in. square 3
Matzoh .... ¾ oz

(continued)

Food	Serving
Melba toast	4 slices
Oyster crackers	24
Popcorn (popped, no fat added or low-fat microwave)	3 cups
Pretzels	¾ oz
Rice cakes, 4 in. across	2
Saltine-type crackers	6
Snack chips, fat-free (tortilla, potato)	15–20 (¾ oz)
Whole-wheat crackers, no fat added	2–5 (¾ oz)

Starchy Foods Prepared with Fat
(Count as 1 starch exchange, plus 1 fat exchange.)

Food	Serving
Biscuit, 2½ in. across	1
Chow mein noodles	½ cup
Corn bread, 2-in. cube	1 (2 oz)
Crackers, round butter type	6
Croutons	1 cup
French-fried potatoes	16–25 (3 oz)
Granola	¼ cup
Muffin, small	1 (1½ oz)
Pancake, 4 in. across	2
Popcorn, microwave	3 cups
Sandwich crackers, cheese or peanut butter filling	3
Stuffing, bread (prepared)	⅓ cup
Taco shell, 6 in. across	2
Waffle, 4½ in. square	1
Whole-wheat crackers, fat added	4–6 (1 oz)

Fruit List

One fruit exchange equals 15 grams carbohydrate and 60 calories. The weight includes skin, core, seeds, and rind.

Fruit

Food	Serving
Apple, unpeeled, small	1 (4 oz)
Applesauce, unsweetened	½ cup
Apples, dried	4 rings
Apricots, fresh	4 whole (5½ oz)
Apricots, dried	8 halves
Apricots, canned	½ cup
Banana, small	1 (4 oz)
Blackberries	¾ cup
Blueberries	¾ cup
Cantaloupe, small	⅓ melon (11 oz) or 1 cup cubes
Cherries, sweet, fresh	12 (3 oz)
Cherries, sweet, canned	½ cup
Dates	3
Figs, fresh	1½ large or 2 medium (3½ oz)
Figs, dried	1½
Fruit cocktail	½ cup
Grapefruit, large	½ (11 oz)
Grapefruit sections, canned	¾ cup
Grapes, small	17 (3 oz)
Honeydew melon	1 slice (10 oz) or 1 cup cubes
Kiwi	1 (3½ oz)
Mandarin oranges, canned	¾ cup
Mango, small	½ fruit (5½ oz) or ½ cup
Nectarine, small	1 (5 oz)
Orange, small	1 (6½ oz)
Papaya	½ fruit (8 oz) or 1 cup cubes
Peach, medium, fresh	1 (6 oz)
Peaches, canned	½ cup
Pear, large, fresh	½ (4 oz)
Pears, canned	½ cup
Pineapple, fresh	¼ cup
Pineapple, canned	½ cup
Plums, small	2 (5 oz)
Plums, canned	½ cup
Prunes, dried	3
Raisins	2 Tbsp
Raspberries	1 cup
Strawberries	1¼ cup whole berries
Tangerines, small	2 (8 oz)
Watermelon	1 slice (13½ oz) or 1¼ cup cubes

Fruit Juice

Food	Serving
Apple juice/cider	½ cup
Cranberry juice cocktail	⅓ cup
Cranberry juice cocktail, reduced-calorie	1 cup
Fruit juice blends, 100% juice	⅓ cup
Grape juice	⅓ cup
Grapefruit juice	½ cup
Orange juice	½ cup
Pineapple juice	½ cup
Prune juice	⅓ cup

Milk List

One milk exchange equals 12 grams carbohydrate and 8 grams protein.

Skim and Very Low-Fat Milk
(0–3 grams fat and 90 calories per serving)

Food	Serving
Skim milk	1 cup
½% milk	1 cup
1% milk	1 cup
Nonfat or low-fat buttermilk	1 cup
Evaporated skim milk	½ cup
Nonfat dry milk	⅓ cup dry
Plain nonfat yogurt	¾ cup
Nonfat or low-fat fruit-flavored yogurt sweetened with aspartame or with a non-nutritive sweetener	1 cup

Low-Fat
(5 grams fat and 120 calories per serving)

Food	Serving
2% milk	1 cup
Plain low-fat yogurt	¾ cup
Sweet acidophilus milk	1 cup

Whole Milk
(8 grams fat and 150 calories per serving)

Food	Serving
Whole milk	1 cup
Evaporated whole milk	½ cup
Goat's milk	1 cup
Kefir	1 cup

Other Carbohydrates List

One exchange equals 15 grams carbohydrate, or 1 starch, or 1 fruit, or 1 milk.

Food	Serving Size	Exchanges per Serving
Angel food cake, unfrosted	1/12 cake	2 carbohydrates
Brownie, small, unfrosted	2 in. square	1 carbohydrate, 1 fat
Cake, unfrosted	2 in. square	1 carbohydrate, 1 fat
Cake, frosted	2 in. square	2 carbohydrates, 1 fat
Cookie, fat-free	2 small	1 carbohydrate
Cookie or sandwich cookie with creme filling	2 small	1 carbohydrate, 1 fat
Cupcake, frosted	1 small	2 carbohydrates, 1 fat
Cranberry sauce, jellied	1/4 cup	2 carbohydrates
Doughnut, plain cake	1 medium (1½ oz)	1½ carbohydrates, 2 fats
Doughnut, glazed	3¾ in. across (2 oz)	2 carbohydrates, 2 fats
Fruit juice bars, frozen, 100% juice	1 bar (3 oz)	1 carbohydrate
Fruit snacks, chewy (pureed fruit concentrate)	1 roll (¾ oz)	1 carbohydrate
Fruit spread, 100% fruit	1 Tbsp	1 carbohydrate
Gelatin, regular	½ cup	1 carbohydrate
Gingersnaps	3	1 carbohydrate
Granola bar	1 bar	1 carbohydrate, 1 fat
Granola bar, fat-free	1 bar	2 carbohydrates
Hummus	1/3 cup	1 carbohydrate, 1 fat
Ice cream	½ cup	1 carbohydrate, 2 fats
Ice cream, light	½ cup	1 carbohydrate, 1 fat
Ice cream, fat-free, no sugar added	½ cup	1 carbohydrate
Jam or jelly, regular	1 Tbsp	1 carbohydrate
Milk, chocolate, whole	1 cup	2 carbohydrates, 1 fat
Pie, fruit, 2 crusts	1/6 pie	3 carbohydrates, 2 fats
Pie, pumpkin or custard	1/8 pie	1 carbohydrate, 2 fats
Potato chips	12–18 (1 oz)	1 carbohydrate, 2 fats
Pudding, regular (made with low-fat milk)	½ cup	2 carbohydrates
Pudding, sugar-free (made with low-fat milk)	½ cup	1 carbohydrate
Salad dressing, fat-free	¼ cup	1 carbohydrate
Sherbet, sorbet	½ cup	2 carbohydrates
Spaghetti or pasta sauce, canned	½ cup	1 carbohydrate, 1 fat
Sweet roll or Danish	1 (2½ oz)	2½ carbohydrates, 2 fats
Syrup, light	2 Tbsp	1 carbohydrate
Syrup, regular	1 Tbsp	1 carbohydrate
Syrup, regular	¼ cup	4 carbohydrates
Tortilla chips	6–12 (1 oz)	1 carbohydrate, 2 fats
Yogurt, frozen, low-fat, fat-free	1/3 cup	1 carbohydrate, 0–1 fat
Yogurt, frozen, fat-free, no sugar added	½ cup	1 carbohydrate
Yogurt, low-fat with fruit	1 cup	3 carbohydrates, 0–1 fat
Vanilla wafers	5	1 carbohydrate, 1 fat

= 400 mg or more of sodium per serving.

Vegetable List

Vegetables that contain small amounts of carbohydrates and calories are on this list. Vegetables contain important nutrients. Try to eat at least two or three vegetable choices each day. In general, one vegetable exchange is:

½ cup of cooked vegetable or vegetable juice, or
1 cup of raw vegetables

If you eat one to two vegetable choices at a meal or snack, you do not have to count the calories or carbohydrates because they contain small amounts of these nutrients.

One vegetable exchange equals 5 grams carbohydrate, 2 grams protein, 0 grams fat, and 25 calories.

Artichoke
Artichoke hearts
Asparagus
Beans (green, wax, Italian)
Bean sprouts
Beets
Broccoli
Brussels sprouts
Cabbage
Carrots
Cauliflower
Celery
Cucumber
Eggplant
Green onions or scallions
Greens(collard, kale, mustard, turnip)
Kohlrabi
Leeks
Mixed vegetables (without corn, peas, or pasta)
Mushrooms
Okra
Onions
Pea pods
Peppers (all varieties)
Radishes
Salad greens (endive, escarole, lettuce, romaine, spinach)
Sauerkraut
Spinach
Summer squash
Tomato
Tomatoes, canned
Tomato sauce
Tomato/vegetable juice
Turnips
Water chestnuts
Watercress
Zucchini

= 400 mg or more sodium per exchange.

Very Lean Meat and Substitutes List

One exchange equals 0 grams carbohydrate, 7 grams protein, 0–1 grams fat, and 35 calories.

One very lean meat exchange is equal to any one of the following items.

Poultry: Chicken or turkey (white meat, no skin), Cornish hen (no skin) .... 1 oz
Fish: Fresh or frozen cod, flounder, haddock, halibut, trout; tuna, fresh or canned in water .... 1 oz
Shellfish: Clams, crab, lobster, scallops, shrimp, imitation shellfish .... 1 oz
Game: Duck or pheasant (no skin), venison, buffalo, ostrich .... 1 oz
Cheese with 1 gram or less fat per ounce:
Nonfat or low-fat cottage cheese .... ¼ cup
Fat-free cheese .... 1 oz
Other: Processed sandwich meats with 1 gram or less fat per ounce, such as deli thin, shaved meats, chipped beef, turkey ham .... 1 oz
Egg whites 2
Egg substitutes, plain .... ¼ cup
Hot dogs with 1 gram or less fat per ounce .... 1 oz
Kidney (high in cholesterol) .... 1 oz
Sausage with 1 gram or less fat per ounce .... 1 oz

Count as one very lean meat and one starch exchange.

Dried beans, peas, lentils (cooked) .... ½ cup

= 400 mg or more sodium per exchange.

Lean Meat and Substitutes List

One exchange equals 0 grams carbohydrate, 7 grams protein, 3 grams fat, and 55 calories.

One lean meat exchange is equal to any one of the following items.

Beef: USDA Select or Choice grades of lean beef trimmed of fat, such as round, sirloin, and flank steak; tenderloin; roast (rib, chuck, rump); steak (T-bone, porterhouse, cubed), ground round .... 1 oz
Pork: Lean pork, such as fresh ham; canned, cured, or boiled ham; Canadian bacon; tenderloin, center loin chop .... 1 oz
Lamb: Roast, chop, leg .... 1 oz
Veal: Lean chop, roast .... 1 oz
Poultry: Chicken, turkey (dark meat, no skin), chicken white meat (with skin), domestic duck or goose (well-drained of fat, no skin) .... 1 oz
Fish:
Herring (uncreamed or smoked) .... 1 oz
Oysters .... 6 medium
Salmon (fresh or canned), catfish .... 1 oz
Sardines (canned) .... 2 medium
Tuna (canned in oil, drained) .... 1 oz
Game: Goose (no skin), rabbit .... 1 oz
Cheese:
4.5%-fat cottage cheese .... ¼ cup
Grated Parmesan .... 2 Tbsp
Cheeses with 3 grams or less fat per ounce .... 1 oz
Other:
Hot dogs with 3 grams or less fat per ounce .... 1½ oz
Processed sandwich meat with 3 grams or less fat per ounce, such as turkey pastrami or kielbasa .... 1 oz
Liver, heart (high in cholesterol) .... 1 oz

= 400 mg or more sodium per exchange.

Medium-Fat Meat and Substitutes List

One exchange equals 0 grams carbohydrate, 7 grams protein, 5 grams fat, and 75 calories.

One medium-fat meat exchange is equal to any one of the following items.

Beef: Most beef products fall into this category (ground beef, meatloaf, corned beef, short ribs, Prime grades of meat trimmed of fat, such as prime rib) .... 1 oz
Pork: Top loin, chop, Boston butt, cutlet .... 1 oz
Lamb: Rib roast, ground .... 1 oz
Veal: Cutlet (ground or cubed, unbreaded) .... 1 oz
Poultry: Chicken dark meat (with skin), ground turkey or ground chicken, fried chicken (with skin) .... 1 oz
Fish: Any fried fish product .... 1 oz
Cheese: With 5 grams or less fat per ounce
Feta .... 1 oz
Mozzarella .... 1 oz
Ricotta .... ¼ cup (2 oz)
Other:
Egg (high in cholesterol, limit to 3 per week) 1
Sausage with 5 grams or less fat per ounce .... 1 oz
Soy milk .... 1 cup
Tempeh .... ¼ cup
Tofu .... 4 oz or ½ cup

High-Fat Meat and Substitutes List

One exchange equals 0 grams carbohydrate, 7 grams protein, 8 grams fat, and 100 calories.

Remember, these items are high in saturated fat, cholesterol, and calories and may raise blood cholesterol levels if eaten on a regular basis. One high-fat meat exchange is equal to any one of the following items.

Pork: Spareribs, ground pork, pork sausage .... 1 oz
Cheese: All regular cheeses, such as American, cheddar, Monterey Jack, Swiss .... 1 oz
Other: Processed sandwich meats with 8 grams or less fat per ounce, such as bologna, pimento loaf, salami .... 1 oz
Sausage, such as bratwurst, Italian, knockwurst, Polish, smoked .... 1 oz
Hot dog (turkey or chicken) 1 (10/lb)
Bacon .... 2 slices (20 slices/lb)

Count as one high-fat meat plus one fat exchange.

Hot dog (beef, pork, or combination) 1 (10/lb)
Peanut butter (contains unsaturated fat) .... 2 Tbsp

= 400 mg or more sodium per exchange.

Fats List

One fat exchange equals 5 grams fat and 45 calories.

Monounsaturated Fats

Avocado, medium .... ⅛ (1 oz)
Oil (canola, olive, peanut) .... 1 tsp

(continued)

Food	Serving
Olives: ripe (black)	8 large
Green, stuffed	10 large
Nuts	
Almonds, cashews	6 nuts
Mixed (50% peanuts)	6 nuts
Peanuts	10 nuts
Pecans	4 halves
Peanut butter, smooth or crunchy	2 tsp
Sesame seeds	1 Tbsp
Tahini paste	2 tsp

= 400 mg or more sodium per exchange.

One fat exchange equals 5 grams fat and 45 calories.

Polyunsaturated Fats

Food	Serving
Margarine: stick, tub, or squeeze	1 tsp
Lower-fat (30 to 50% vegetable oil)	1 Tbsp
Mayonnaise: regular	1 tsp
Reduced-fat	1 Tbsp
Nuts, walnuts, English	4 halves
Oil (corn, safflower, soybean)	1 tsp
Salad dressing: regular	1 Tbsp
Reduced-fat	2 Tbsp
Miracle Whip Salad Dressing: regular	2 tsp
Reduced-fat	1 Tbsp
Seeds: pumpkin, sunflower	1 Tbsp

= 400 mg or more sodium per exchange.

One fat exchange equals 5 grams fat and 45 calories.

Saturated Fats*

Food	Serving
Bacon, cooked	1 slice (20 slices/lb)
Bacon, grease	1 tsp
Butter: stick	1 tsp
Whipped	2 tsp
Reduced-fat	1 Tbsp
Chitterlings, boiled	2 Tbsp (½ oz)
Coconut, sweetened, shredded	2 Tbsp
Cream, half and half	2 Tbsp
Cream cheese: regular	1 Tbsp (½ oz)
Reduced-fat	2 Tbsp (1 oz)
Fatback or salt pork†	
Shortening or lard	1 tsp
Sour cream: regular	2 Tbsp
Reduced-fat	3 Tbsp

*Saturated fats can raise blood cholesterol levels.

†Use a piece 1 in. × 1 in. × ¼ in. if you plan to eat the fatback cooked with vegetables. Use a piece 2 in. × 1 in. × ½ in. when eating only the vegetables with the fatback removed.

Free Foods List

A *free food* is any food or drink that contains less than 20 calories or less than 5 grams of carbohydrate per serving. Foods with a serving size listed should be limited to three servings per day. Be sure to spread them out throughout the day. If you eat all three servings at one time, it could affect your blood glucose level. Foods listed without a serving size can be eaten as often as you like.

Fat-Free or Reduced-Fat Foods

Food	Serving
Cream cheese, fat-free	1 Tbsp
Creamers, nondairy, liquid	1 Tbsp
Creamers, nondairy, powdered	2 tsp
Mayonnaise, fat-free	1 Tbsp
Mayonnaise, reduced-fat	1 tsp
Margarine, fat-free	4 Tbsp
Margarine, reduced-fat	1 tsp
Miracle Whip, nonfat	1 Tbsp
Miracle Whip, reduced-fat	1 tsp
Nonstick cooking spray	
Salad dressing, fat-free	1 Tbsp
Salad dressing, fat-free, Italian	2 Tbsp
Salsa	¼ cup
Sour cream, fat-free, reduced-fat	1Tbsp
Whipped topping, regular or light	2 Tbsp

Sugar-Free or Low-Sugar Foods

Food	Serving
Candy, hard, sugar-free	1 candy
Gelatin dessert, sugar-free	
Gelatin, unflavored	
Gum, sugar-free	
Jam or jelly, low-sugar or light	2 tsp
Sugar substitutes*	
Syrup, sugar-free	2 Tbsp

*Sugar substitutes, alternatives, or replacements that are approved by the Food and Drug Administration (FDA) are safe to use. Common brand names include: Equal (aspartame), Sprinkle Sweet (saccharin), Sweet One (acesulfame K), Sweet-10 (saccharin), Sugar Twin (saccharin), Sweet 'n Low (saccharin).

Drinks

Food	Serving
Bouillon, broth, consommé	
Bouillon or broth, low-sodium	
Carbonated or mineral water	
Cocoa powder, unsweetened	1 Tbsp
Coffee	
Club soda	
Diet soft drinks, sugar-free	
Drink mixes, sugar-free	
Tea	
Tonic water, sugar-free	

Condiments

Food	Serving
Catsup	1 Tbsp
Horseradish	
Lemon juice	
Lime juice	
Mustard	
Pickles, dill	1½ large
Soy sauce, regular or light	
Taco sauce	1 Tbsp
Vinegar	

Seasonings

Be careful with seasonings that contain sodium or are salts, such as garlic or celery salt, and lemon pepper.

Flavoring extracts
Garlic
Herbs, fresh or dried
Pimento
Spices
Tabasco or hot pepper sauce
Wine, used in cooking
Worcestershire sauce

= 400 mg or more of sodium per choice.

Combination Food List

Many of the foods we eat are mixed together in various combinations. These combination foods do not fit into any one exchange list. Often it is hard to tell what is in a casserole dish or prepared food item. This is a list of exchanges for some typical combination foods. This list will help you fit these foods into your meal plan. Ask your dietitian for information about any other combination foods you would like to eat.

Food	Serving Size	Exchanges per Serving
Entrees		
Tuna noodle casserole, lasagna, spaghetti with meatballs, chili with beans, macaroni and cheese	1 cup (8 oz)	2 carbohydrates, 2 medium-fat meats
Chow mein (without noodles or rice)	2 cups (16 oz)	1 carbohydrate, 2 lean meats
Pizza, cheese, thin crust	¼ of 10 in. (5 oz)	2 carbohydrates, 2 medium-fat meats, 1 fat
Pizza, meat topping, thin crust	¼ of 10 in. (5 oz)	2 carbohydrates, 2 medium-fat meats, 2 fats
Pot pie	1 (7 oz)	2 carbohydrates, 1 medium-fat meat, 4 fats
Frozen entrees		
Salisbury steak with gravy, mashed potato	1 (11 oz)	2 carbohydrates, 3 medium-fat meats, 3–4 fats
Turkey with gravy, mashed potato, dressing	1 (11 oz)	2 carbohydrates, 3 lean meats
Entree with less than 300 calories	1 (8 oz)	2 carbohydrates, 3 lean meats
Soups		
Bean	1 cup	1 carbohydrate, 1 very lean meat
Cream (made with water)	1 cup (8 oz)	1 carbohydrate, 1 fat
Split pea (made with water)	½ cup (4 oz)	1 carbohydrate
Tomato (made with water)	1 cup (8 oz)	1 carbohydrate
Vegetable beef, chicken noodle, or other broth-type	1 cup (8 oz)	1 carbohydrate

= 400 mg or more sodium per exchange.

Fast Foods List*

Food	Serving Size	Exchanges per Serving
Burritos with beef	2	4 carbohydrates, 2 medium-fat meats, 2 fats
Chicken nuggets	6	1 carbohydrate, 2 medium-fat meats, 1 fat
Chicken breast and wing, breaded and fried	1 each	1 carbohydrate, 4 medium-fat meats, 2 fats
Fish sandwich/tartar sauce	1	3 carbohydrates, 1 medium-fat meat, 3 fats
French fries, thin	20–25	2 carbohydrates, 2 fats
Hamburger, regular	1	2 carbohydrates, 2 medium-fat meats
Hamburger, large	1	2 carbohydrates, 3 medium-fat meats, 1 fat
Hot dog with bun	1	1 carbohydrate, 1 high-fat meat, 1 fat
Individual pan pizza	1	5 carbohydrates, 3 medium-fat meats, 3 fats
Soft-serve cone	1 medium	2 carbohydrates, 1 fat
Submarine sandwich	1 sub (6 in.)	3 carbohydrates, 1 vegetable, 2 medium-fat meats, 1 fat
Taco, hard shell	1 (6 oz)	2 carbohydrates, 2 medium-fat meats, 2 fats
Taco, soft shell	1 (3 oz)	1 carbohydrate, 1 medium-fat meat, 1 fat

= 400 mg or more of sodium per serving.

*Ask at your fast-food restaurant for nutrition information about your favorite fast foods.

Appendix J

Food Labeling Information

Sample Label for a Granola Bar

Nutrition Facts
Serving Size 1 bar (24g)
Servings Per Container 12

Amount Per Serving	
Calories 120	Calories from Fat 45
	% Daily Value*
Total Fat 5g	**8%**
Saturated Fat 1g	**5%**
Cholesterol 0mg	**0%**
Sodium 65mg	**3%**
Total Carbohydrate 17g	**6%**
Dietary Fiber 1g	**4%**
Sugars 6g	
Protein 2g	
Vitamin A 0% •	Vitamin C 0%
Calcium 0% •	Iron 4%

* Percent Daily Values are based on a 2,000 calorie diet. Your daily values may be higher or lower depending on your calorie needs:

	Calories:	2,000	2,500
Total Fat	Less than	65g	80g
Sat Fat	Less than	20g	25g
Cholesterol	Less than	300mg	300mg
Sodium	Less than	2,400mg	2,400mg
Total Carbohydrate		300g	375g
Dietary Fiber		25g	30g

Calories per gram:
Fat 9 • Carbohydrate 4 • Protein 4

Ingredients: Rolled oats, sugar, sunflower oil, brown sugar syrup, honey, salt, soy lecithin

Daily Reference Values

Food Component	Daily Reference Value (2000 kcal)
Total fat	Less than 65 g (30% of energy)
Saturated fat	Less than 20 g (10% of energy)
Cholesterol	Less than 300 mg
Total carbohydrate	300 g (60% of energy)
Dietary fiber	25 g (11.5 g/1000 kcal)
Sodium	Less than 2400 mg
Potassium	3500 mg
Protein	50 g (10% of energy)

Recommended Dietary Intakes (RDIs)*

Vitamins and Minerals	Units of Measurement	Adults and Children Age 4 Years or More	Infants	Children Under 4 Years of Age	Pregnant or Lactating Women
Vitamin A	International Units†	5000	1500	2500	8000
Vitamin D	International Units†	400	400	400	400
Vitamin E	International Units†	30	5	10	30
Vitamin C	Milligrams	60	35	40	60
Folic acid	Micrograms	400	0.1	0.2	0.8
Thiamin	Milligrams	1.5	0.5	0.7	1.7
Riboflavin	Milligrams	1.7	0.6	0.8	2.0
Niacin	Milligrams	20	8	9	20
Vitamin B_6	Milligrams	2.0	0.4	0.7	2.5
Vitamin B_{12}	Micrograms	6.0	2	3	8
Biotin	Micrograms	300	0.05	0.15	0.30
Pantothenic acid	Milligrams	10	3	5	10
Calcium	Milligrams	1000	0.6	0.8	1.3
Phosphorus	Milligrams	1000	0.5	0.8	1.3
Iodine	Micrograms	150	45	70	150
Iron	Milligrams	18	15	10	18
Magnesium	Milligrams	400	70	200	450
Copper	Milligrams	20	0.6	1.0	2.0
Zinc	Milligrams	15	5	8	15
Vitamin K	Micrograms	80	—‡	—‡	—‡
Chromium	Micrograms	120	—	—	—
Selenium	Micrograms	70	—	—	—
Molybdenum	Micrograms	75	—	—	—
Manganese	Milligrams	2	—	—	—
Chloride	Milligrams	3400	—	—	—

* Based on National Academy of Sciences' 1968 Recommended Dietary Allowances.

†The RDIs for fat-soluble vitamins are expressed in International Units (IU). The current RDAs use a newer system of measurement.

‡ No values yet established for vitamin K, chromium, selenium, molybdenum, manganese, or chloride for this population.

Nutrient Content Descriptors Commonly Used on Food Labels

Free	Means that a product contains no amount of, or a trivial amount of, fat, saturated fat, cholesterol, sodium, sugars, or kcalories. For example, "sugar free" and "fat free" both mean less than 0.5 g per serving. Synonyms for "free" include "without," "no," and "zero."
Low	Used for foods that can be eaten frequently without exceeding the Daily Value for fat, saturated fat, cholesterol, sodium, or kcalories. Specific definitions have been established for each of these nutrients. For example, "low-fat" means that the food contains 3 g or less per serving, and "low cholesterol" means that the food contains less than 20 mg of cholesterol per serving. Synonyms for "low" include "little," "few," and "low source of."
Lean and extra lean	Used to describe the fat content of meat, poultry, seafood, and game meats. "Lean" means that the food contains less than 10 g fat, less than 4.5 g saturated fat, and less than 95 mg of cholesterol per serving and per 100 g. "Extra lean" means that the food contains less than 5 g fat, less than 2 g saturated fat, and less than 95 mg of cholesterol per serving and per 100 g.
High	Can be used if a food contains 20% or more of the Daily Value for a particular nutrient. Synonyms for "high" include "rich in" and "excellent source of."
Good source	Means that a food contains 10 to 19% of the Daily Value for a particular nutrient per serving.
Reduced	Means that a nutritionally altered product contains 25% less of a nutrient or of energy than the regular or reference product.
Less	Means that a food, whether altered or not, contains 25% less of a nutrient or of energy than the reference food. For example, pretzels may claim to have "less fat" than potato chips. "Fewer" may be used as a synonym for "less."
Light	May be used in different ways. First, it can be used on a nutritionally altered product that contains one-third fewer kcalories or half the fat of a reference food. Second, it can be used when the sodium content of a low-calorie, low-fat food has been reduced by 50%. The term "light" can be used to describe properties such as texture and color as long as the label explains the intent—for example, "light and fluffy."
More	Means that a serving of food, whether altered or not, contains a nutrient that is at least 10% of the Daily Value more than the reference food. This definition also applies to foods using the terms "fortified," "enriched," or "added."
Healthy	May be used to describe foods that are low in fat and saturated fat and contain no more than 360 mg of sodium and no more than 60 mg of cholesterol per serving and provide at least 10% of the Daily Value for vitamins A or C, or iron, calcium, protein, or fiber.
Fresh	May be used on foods that are raw and have never been frozen or heated and contain no preservatives.

Source: Federal Register 58. Washington, D.C.: U.S. Government Printing Office, Superintendent of Documents, Jan. 6, 1993.

FDA-Approved Health Claims*

Calcium and osteoporosis	Adequate calcium intake throughout life helps maintain bone health and reduce the risk of osteoporosis.
Sodium and hypertension (high blood pressure)	Diets low in sodium may reduce the risk of high blood pressure in some people.
Dietary fat and cancer	Diets low in fat may reduce the risk of some types of cancer.
Saturated fat and cholesterol and risk of coronary heart disease	Diets low in saturated fat and cholesterol help reduce blood cholesterol and, thus, the risk of heart disease.
Fiber-containing grain products, fruits, and vegetables, and cancer risk	Diets low in fat and rich in fiber-containing grain products, fruits, and vegetables may reduce the risk of some types of cancer.
Fruits, vegetables, and grain products that contain fiber, particularly soluble fiber, and risk of coronary heart disease	Diets low in saturated fat and cholesterol and rich in fruits, vegetables, and grain products that contain fiber, particularly soluble fiber, may reduce the risk of coronary heart disease.
Fruits and vegetables and cancer	Diets low in fat and rich in fruits and vegetables may reduce the risk of some types of cancer.
Folic acid and neural tube birth defects	Adequate folic acid intake by the mother reduces the risk of birth defects of the brain or spinal cord in her baby.
Soluble fiber from certain foods and risk of coronary heart disease.	Diets low in fat, saturated fat, and cholesterol that include soluble fiber from whole oats or psyllium seed husk may reduce the risk of heart disease.
Dietary sugar alcohol and dental caries (cavities)	Sugar-free foods that are sweetened with sugar alcohols do not promote tooth decay and may reduce the risk of dental caries.
Soy protein and risk of coronary heart disease	Soy protein included in a diet that is low in saturated fat and cholesterol may reduce the risk of coronary heart disease by lowering blood cholesterol levels.
Plant sterol/stanol esters and risk of coronary heart disease	Plant sterols and plant stanols included in a diet that is low in saturated fat and cholesterol may reduce the risk of coronary heart disease by lowering blood cholesterol levels.

*A food carrying a health claim must be a naturally good source (10% or more of the Daily Value) for one of six nutrients (vitamin A, vitamin C, protein, calcium, iron, or fiber) and must not contain more than 20% of the Daily Value for fat, saturated fat, cholesterol, or sodium. These claims have been approved for use on food labels. The FDA continues to evaluate new claims, many of which are in various stages of approval.

Sample Label for a Dietary Supplement

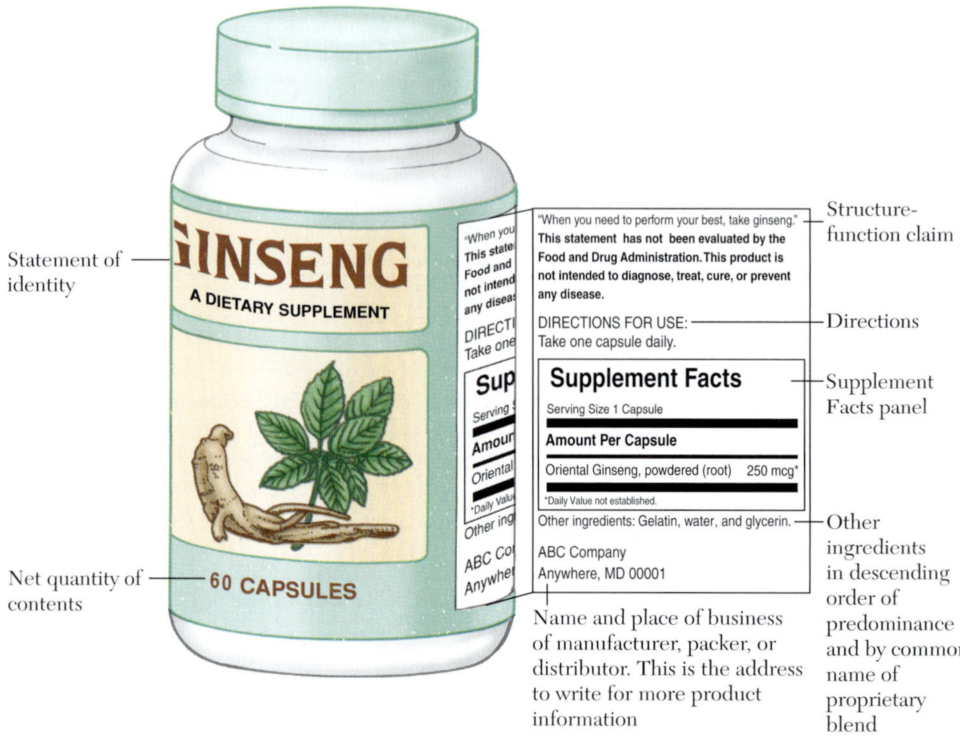

Appendix K

Energy Expenditure for Various Activities

Type of Activity	Kcalories per Hour (by Body Weight) 100 lb	120 lb	150 lb	180 lb	200 lb
Aerobics (heavy)	363	435	544	653	726
Aerobics (medium)	227	272	340	408	454
Aerobics (light)	136	163	204	245	272
Archery	159	190	238	286	317
Backpacking	408	490	612	735	816
Badminton (doubles)	181	218	272	327	363
Badminton (singles)	231	278	347	416	463
Basketball (nonvigorous)	431	517	646	776	862
Basketball (vigorous)	499	599	748	898	998
Bicycling (6 mph)	159	190	238	286	317
Bicycling (10 mph)	249	299	374	449	499
Bicycling (11 mph)	295	354	442	531	590
Bicycling (12 mph)	340	408	510	612	680
Bicycling (13 mph)	385	463	578	694	771
Billiards	91	109	136	163	181
Bowling	177	212	265	318	354
Boxing—competition	603	724	905	1086	1206
Boxing—sparring	376	452	565	678	753
Calisthenics (heavy)	363	435	544	653	726
Calisthenics (light)	181	218	272	327	363
Canoeing (2.5 mph)	150	180	224	269	299
Canoeing (5 mph)	340	408	510	612	680
Carpentry	227	272	340	408	454
Climbing (mountain)	454	544	680	816	907
Disco dancing	272	327	408	490	544
Ditch digging (hand)	263	316	395	473	526
Fencing	340	408	510	612	680
Fishing (bank/boat)	159	190	238	286	317
Fishing (in waders)	249	299	374	449	499
Football (touch)	340	408	510	612	680
Gardening	145	174	218	261	290
Golf (carry clubs)	227	272	340	408	454
Golf (pull cart)	163	196	245	294	327
Golf (ride in cart)	113	136	170	204	227
Handball (vigorous)	454	544	680	816	907
Hiking (X-country)	249	299	374	449	499

(continued)

K

Type of Activity	Kcalories per Hour (by Body Weight) 100 lb	120 lb	150 lb	180 lb	200 lb
Hiking (mountain)	340	408	510	612	680
Horseback trotting	231	278	347	416	463
Housework	181	218	272	327	363
Hunting (carry load)	272	327	408	490	544
Ice hockey (vigorous)	454	544	680	816	907
Ice skating (10 mph)	263	316	395	473	526
Jazzercize (heavy)	363	435	544	653	726
Jazzercise (medium)	227	272	340	408	454
Jazzercise (light)	136	163	204	245	272
Jogging (9 min/mile)	499	599	748	898	998
Jogging (10 min/mile)	454	544	680	816	907
Jogging (12 min/mile)	385	463	578	694	771
Jogging (13 min/mile)	317	381	476	571	635
Jogging (14 min/mile)	272	327	408	490	544
Jogging (15 min/mile)	227	272	340	408	454
Jogging (17 min/mile)	181	218	272	327	363
Lawn mowing (hand)	295	354	442	531	590
Lawn mowing (power)	163	196	245	294	327
Musical instrument playing	113	136	170	204	227
Racquetball (social)	385	463	578	694	771
Racquetball (vigorous)	454	544	680	816	907
Roller skating	231	278	347	416	463
Rowboating (2.5 mph)	200	239	299	359	399
Rowing (11 mph)	590	707	884	1061	1179
Running (5 min/mile)	816	980	1224	1469	1633
Running (6 min/mile)	703	844	1054	1265	1406
Running (7 min/mile)	612	735	918	1102	1224
Running (8 min/mile)	544	653	816	980	1088
Sailing	159	190	238	286	317
Shuffleboard/skeet	136	163	204	245	272
Skiing (X-country)	454	544	680	816	907
Skiing (downhill)	363	435	544	653	726
Square dancing	272	327	407	490	544
Swimming (competitive)	680	816	1020	1224	1361
Swimming (fast)	426	512	639	767	853
Swimming (slow)	349	419	524	629	698
Table tennis	236	283	354	424	472
Tennis (doubles)	227	272	340	408	454
Tennis (singles)	295	354	442	531	590
Tennis (vigorous)	385	463	578	694	771
Volleyball	231	278	347	416	463
Walking (20 min/mile)	159	190	238	286	317
Walking (26 min/mile)	136	163	204	245	272
Water skiing	317	381	476	571	635
Weight lifting (heavy)	408	490	612	735	816
Weight lifting (light)	181	218	272	327	363
Wood chopping (sawing)	295	354	442	531	590

Data reprinted with permission from N-Squared Computing, First Databank Division of the Hearst Corporation.

Appendix L

Amino Acid Structures

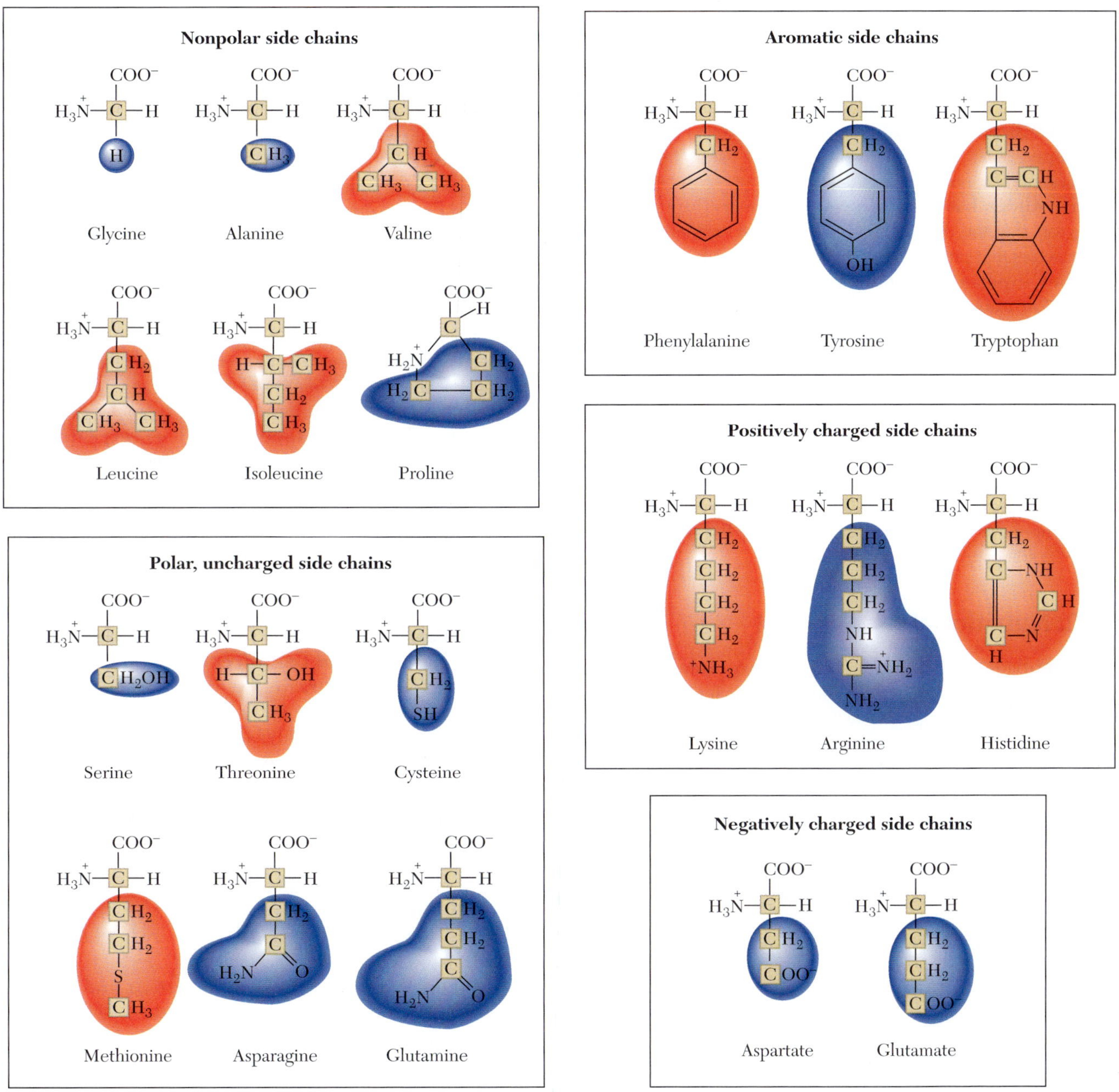

Essential amino acids side chain
Nonessential amino acids side chain

Source: Lehninger. *Principles of Biochemistry,* 2nd ed Worth Publishers

L

Appendix M

Answers to Critical Thinking Exercises

Chapter 1: The Scientific Method

What other possible reasons could explain a difference in cancer incidence between these two populations? The cancer could be caused by an infectious agent such as a bacterium or virus that is not found in Japan.

Which hypothesis has been disproved? The first hypothesis, which suggests that the difference in colon cancer incidence is due to genetic factors that protect the Japanese, has been disproved.

What other experiments could you propose to obtain more information about the causes of colon cancer in the United States? A group of Americans living in Japan could be evaluated for their incidence of colon cancer. A group of Americans could be asked to consume a traditional Japanese diet for a specific time period to see if it affects colon cancer incidence. Differences in the amounts of specific dietary components, such as fiber or antioxidant vitamins, between the American and Japanese diet could be evaluated for their effect on cancer incidence.

Propose a theory based on the evidence presented here. Some component of the American diet contributes to the development of colon cancer.

Chapter 2: Nutritional Assessment

What stage of nutrient deficiency is Angelica experiencing? Angelica's deficiency has progressed to the stage at which she is experiencing the outward symptoms of iron deficiency—fatigue and decreased work capacity. At this stage, she also has decreased iron stores and altered biochemical and physiological functions.

Should she be concerned about the nutrients she is consuming in excess of her goal? Look up the UL for vitamin A to determine if her intake is likely to pose a risk. Her protein intake exceeds the RDA, but this amount has not been shown to be toxic. The UL for vitamin C is 2000 mg and for vitamin A is 3000 μg of retinol. Although her intake exceeds the RDA for both these vitamins, it is far below the level that is likely to pose a risk of adverse effects. In addition, some of the vitamin A in her diet is likely to have come from carotenoids, which are not toxic.

M

Chapter 3: Gastrointestinal Problems Can Affect Nutritional Status

What effect would this have on nutrition? An individual who is taking medication that reduces the amount of saliva produced could have difficulty tasting and swallowing food. The lack of saliva may also result in dental problems, such as caries, because saliva serves to cleanse the mouth and inhibit microbial growth.

How will this affect the digestion and absorption of nutrients in the carrot? Partially chewed food consists of larger pieces. In the case of the carrot, these pieces contain indigestible fiber. Since enzymes can digest only the nutrients they come in contact with—those on the surface of the particles that have been freed of the fiber—many of the nutrients in the carrot will remain trapped and pass out in the feces.

Which person's stomach will empty faster? Why? The stomach of the man who had only cereal with skim milk and black coffee would empty more quickly because this meal is lower in fat than the scrambled eggs with sausage, biscuits with butter, and whole milk. Fat slows gastric emptying.

How will this affect the amount and types of food that can be consumed at any one time? Stomach stapling reduces the size of the stomach and therefore reduces the amount of food that can be consumed at a sitting. Foods must be soft or well-chewed.

What effect would this have on the digestion and absorption of protein? Without pancreatic enzymes, protein digestion will be significantly reduced. Some digestion will occur however, due to pepsin in the stomach and some protein-digesting enzymes in the brush border of the small intestine.

If the pancreas was not able to secrete bicarbonate into the duodenum, how would this affect digestion and absorption? Bicarbonate ions neutralize the acidic chyme so that enzymes that function in a more neutral pH can act on the chyme. Without bicarbonate, foods would not be completely digested and the nutrients could not be absorbed. The acid entering the duodenum could also damage the mucosal surface.

What type of foods should be avoided and why? An individual with gallstones may benefit from a low-fat diet because fat in the duodenum stimulates contraction of the gallbladder, causing pain.

How will this affect absorption? Her absorption of nutrients would be reduced; healthy villi are necessary for the efficient absorption of nutrients.

How might this affect nutrient digestion and absorption? Most digestion and absorption occurs in the small intestine. Her ability to digest food and absorb nutrients (including water) will be reduced; special feedings may be necessary to meet nutrient needs.

How would this affect fluid needs? Although most water absorption occurs in the small intestine, the large intestine is also responsible for some water absorption. Therefore, fecal water losses will increase, increasing her fluid needs.

How might this affect the feces? The amount of intestinal gas? Assuming sufficient fluids are consumed, the volume of the feces will increase and transit time will decrease. The increase in fiber will increase the amount of material available for microbial breakdown in the colon, causing an increase in intestinal gas production.

Chapter 4: Meeting Carbohydrate Recommendations

How does her new diet compare to the recommendations of the Food Guide Pyramid? Her diet provides about seven breads, four vegetables, three fruits, three meats, three milks, and few fats/sweets—therefore, it meets recommendations.

Chapter 5: Heart Disease Risk

What risk factors does she have for developing cardiovascular disease? She is at risk because her father had heart disease before age 55, she is moderately stressed, she has a sedentary lifestyle, and her total and LDL cholesterol levels are high and HDL cholesterol is low.

How does her diet compare to the serving recommendations of the Food Guide Pyramid? She consumes four breads (six are recommended); one vegetable (three are recommended); two fruits (two are recommended); one milk (two are recommended) and two meats (two are recommended). She also consumes about five servings of sweets and fat (limited recommendation).

Do her choices follow the selection tips of the Food Guide Pyramid? No; many of her choices are high in energy and fat—such as fish sticks, tater tots, potato chips, and cookies.

How does Selma's diet compare to the recommendations for fat intake—30% of energy as fat, 10% as saturated fat, and less than 300 mg of cholesterol per day? She consumes more than the recommended amount of fat ($102 \times 9/2210 = 41.5\%$), saturated fat ($30 \times 9/2210 = 15.1\%$), and *trans* fat ($8.7 \times 9/2210 = 3.5\%$ [goal is 2.6%]). Her cholesterol intake is within the recommendation of less than 300 mg per day.

What other dietary factors contribute to her risk of heart disease (see Table 5.2)? Her fiber intake is lower than the recommended 10 to 13 grams per 1000 kcals (or 26 to 28 grams). Soluble fiber helps lower cholesterol and reduce the risk of heart disease. Her diet is also low in grains, fruits, and vegetables, which are good sources of fiber, antioxidant nutrients, and phytochemicals, all of which can help protect against heart disease.

If Selma were to replace all of the added fat in her diet with olive oil, would she reduce her risk of cardiovascular disease to the level found in Mediterranean countries? No; changing one component of the diet does not provide the benefits of an entire dietary pattern and lifestyle.

Chapter 6: What Does Nitrogen Balance Tell Us?

What is his nitrogen balance? His output is equal to his intake, so he is in balance.

What is her nitrogen balance? Her intake exceeds her output by 2.4 grams per day. She is in positive balance.

Does her nitrogen balance make sense metabolically? Yes; she is pregnant so she is retaining more of the nitrogen that she consumes in order to build maternal and fetal tissues.

Chapter 6: Choosing a Vegetarian Diet

How much protein would her diet provide if she decided to eliminate dairy products? 47.7 grams.

Does her diet meet the Food Guide Pyramid recommendations for vegetarians? She meets the recommendations for all groups except for vegetables—she needs three to five servings, but she consumes only two.

Chapter 7: Balancing Energy: Genetics and Lifestyle

What is her BMI? Is it in the healthy range? Her BMI is 26.5, which is in the overweight range.

Is she in energy balance? No. she consumes 2650 kcalories per day and expends 2424 kcalories:

Her RMR is 1525 kcalories per day, or 63.5 kcal/hour (1525kcal/24 hour).

Her RMR + activity is equal to:

$$\begin{aligned} \text{8 hrs sleep} &= 8\text{ hrs} \times 1 \times 63.5 = 508\text{ kcal} \\ \text{14 hrs very light activity} &= 14\text{ hrs} \times 1.5 \times 63.5 = 1333.5\text{ kcal} \\ \text{2 hrs light activity} &= 2\text{ hrs} \times 2.5 \times 63.5 = 317.5\text{ kcal} \\ \text{RMR + activity} &= 2159\text{ kcal} \end{aligned}$$

Add the thermic effect of food (intake × 10% = 265):

$$\text{Total energy expenditure} = \text{RMR} + \text{activity} + \text{TEF} = 2424$$

Thus, energy balance = energy intake − energy expenditure, so 2650 − 2424 = an excess of about 226 kcalories per day.

If she replaces one hour of her very light activity with one hour of moderate activity, how much additional energy will this burn?

$63.5 \times 1.5 = 95.31$ kcal, and $63.5 \times 5 = 317.5$ kcal (difference = 222.2 kcal)

Chapter 8: Will This Weight-Loss Plan Work?

Does this program include an exercise component? No.

Does the program promote changes in eating habits and lifestyle that will encourage achieving and maintaining a healthy weight? No.

Chapter 9: Figuring Out Fortified Folate

Would you recommend Marcia take a folic acid supplement? Why or why not? If she cannot consistently consume the 400 μg of folic acid, she should take a supplement.

Chapter 10: Evaluating Vitamin Supplements

Will any of these prevent Miguel from getting sick or help boost his energy level? All of these nutrients are needed in adequate amounts to meet needs, but excess amounts will not prevent illness or boost energy.

Would you suggest that Miguel stop taking any of these supplements? Why or why not? He should stop taking all of them. The brain booster and B 50 contain potentially toxic amounts of some nutrients, and the others, while not harmful, are probably not beneficial.

Chapter 11: DASH: A Diet For Health

How does his modified diet compare to the recommendations of the Food Guide Pyramid? It meets or exceeds serving recommendations for all groups.

How could this diet be changed to reduce the energy content while still including eight servings of fruits and vegetables and three dairy servings per day? The juice and dried fruit could be replaced with fresh fruit, which has less energy per serving. She could use nonfat dairy products. And, she could reduce her added fats.

Chapter 12: Meeting Calcium Needs

Which of Laura's answers on the questionnaire suggest that she has an increased risk for osteoporosis? She is a female who drank little milk as an adolescent and still often consumes fewer than the recommended number of dairy servings. She smokes, gets little exercise, and she has a family history of the disease.

How does her intake compare to the recommendations for calcium intake? Her calcium intake is below recommendations.

How can she increase her calcium without increasing her energy intake? At lunch she could replace a slice of bologna with a slice of cheese on her sandwich. For a snack, she could have yogurt or a glass of milk, or replace the chips with an ounce of cheese. For dinner, she could have leafy green vegetables.

Do you think she should take a calcium supplement? Why or why not? Yes; she is approaching menopause and does not meet calcium or exercise recommendations.

Chapter 13: Increasing Iron Intake

Why would switching from iron to stainless steel cookware affect iron status? Iron leaches from the cookware into the food.

What other dietary factors could contribute to Odelia's poor iron status?

1. Her total iron intake is marginal at 12 mg per day, compared with the RDA for a young female vegetarian of 33 mg per day.
2. The iron in her diet comes from plant sources. This might contribute to iron deficiency because iron from plants is nonheme iron, which is poorly absorbed.
3. The diet is low in vitamin C–rich foods. This might contribute to iron deficiency because vitamin C enhances iron absorption.
4. The tannins in the tea she has at every meal reduce iron absorption.

M

What modifications could Odelia make to increase the iron content of her dinner? She could cook the meal in an iron pot. She could add tomatoes or lime juice to the meal; the acid would increase the amount of iron leached from the cookware into the food. She could have orange juice instead of apple juice with dinner, which would also enhance iron absorption from foods in that meal. She could add beans (a good vegetarian source of iron) to the rice. Tea, which contains tannins that inhibit iron absorption, could be consumed later in the evening.

Does Odelia's diet meet the recommendations of the Food Guide Pyramid for vegetarians? She needs to add a serving of dairy products and of legumes or nuts to her diet to meet the recommendations. Also, the only fruit she consumes is apples and apple juice; she should add more variety from this group.

Are there other nutrient deficiencies for which she may be at risk? Because she consumes dairy products, she is unlikely to be at risk for calcium, vitamin D, or vitamin B_{12} deficiency, but the lack of meat in her diet puts her at risk of zinc deficiency.

Chapter 14: A Sensible Exercise Strategy

If Fred's food intake does not change, how long will it take for him to lose five pounds? Each pound requires a deficit of 3500 kcal (for 5 pounds, 5×3500 kcal $= 17{,}500$ kcal). He is expending an additional 521 kcal/week, so it will take $17{,}500/521 = 33.6$ weeks or 8 to 9 months, to lose 5 pounds. If he also decreases his food intake, he can lose the weight more quickly.

Chapter 14: Can Supplements Safely Increase Speed?

What would you recommend Diana do? If Diana participates in a sport that requires short, rapid bursts of speed, bicarbonate may improve her performance. However, if she experiences the side effects of nausea and diarrhea, her performance will suffer. Diana should try the supplement during her practice schedule and evaluate her performance and any side effects before using it for a track meet.

Chapter 15: Nutrient Needs for a Successful Pregnancy

Does her diet meet the Food Guide Pyramid recommendations for a pregnant woman? If not, what food groups does she need to increase or decrease? No. She should increase her milk intake from 1.5 to three servings, her grain intake from six to eight servings, and her fruit intake from two to three servings.

Alice was about 10 pounds overweight when she started her pregnancy. How does this affect her energy and nutrient needs during pregnancy? Alice should still gain weight during her pregnancy in order to provide the nutrients her baby needs for healthy development. If she makes nutrient-dense food choices during her pregnancy, she will not gain excessive weight. She can diet to reduce her weight once the baby is born and weaned.

What substitutions would you suggest to increase her iron intake? With these substitutions, will Alice's diet meet the iron needs of pregnancy without supplements? Alice could increase her iron intake by consuming an iron-fortified cereal at breakfast and red meat at dinner. The RDA for iron during pregnancy is 27 mg—this is difficult to meet without supplements.

Chapter 15: Nourishing a New Baby

What options does she have? She can express her breast milk and have Grandma feed it to Henry in a bottle, or she could have Grandma feed him infant formula and she can breast-feed when she is available.

How often should infants be fed? What problems could be caused by feeding a formula that is too concentrated? Henry should be fed on demand every few hours. Feeding him concentrated formula without diluting it according to directions could cause dehydration because it does not provide enough fluid.

Chapter 16: Meeting But Not Exceeding Needs

Suggest some different meal and snack choices Sage could eat away from home to increase her iron without increasing her energy. Sage could stick with her original breakfast and lunch, which provide more iron than her current diet, and she could have a plain hamburger instead of the breaded chicken at dinner. For snacks, she could have dried fruit instead of the chocolate bar.

Chapter 17: Meeting the Needs of the Elderly

How does her diet compare to the serving recommendations of the Food Guide Pyramid for people over 70? Her meat intake does not meet recommendations and she consumes no vegetables.

Suggest some food choices that would increase Pauline's fiber intake. She could snack on fruit during the day and make a stew with vegetables and legumes for dinner.

Would you suggest nutrient supplements for Pauline? If so, which ones? Pauline would probably benefit from a multivitamin/multimineral supplement and a calcium supplement.

Chapter 18: How Can One Person Make a Difference?

What impact will the following changes have on the environment?

Instead of buying nonrecyclable juice boxes for her lunch, she brings juice in a Thermos: This reduces the amount of nonrecyclable waste.

She decides to begin composting the leftover vegetable scraps and other plant matter from her kitchen: This reduces the amount of trash that must be stored in landfills.

She can recycle the composted food waste by using it in her garden: This nutrient-rich material will reduce the need for fertilizers.

When she can afford it, she chooses organically grown produce: Organic produce is grown without the use of synthetic chemical pesticides or fertilizers.

She selects locally grown foods when possible: Locally grown foods are not shipped, so they do not require the pesticides and fungicides that are added to preserve foods during shipping.

What other changes could Sandra make to decrease her impact on the environment? She could buy foods in larger containers, thereby reducing the amount of packaging she has to discard. She could buy reusable containers to transport her lunch to school rather than using plastic or paper bags. She could start a recycling effort at school.

Chapter 19: Comparing the Risks with the Benefits

What other things can he do to minimize the risks associated with his typical diet while including foods that are beneficial? To decrease the risks associated with eating fish, he can try a wider variety of fresh and saltwater fish to avoid an excess of any one type. Because the risks of eating raw fish are greater, he can limit sushi to a rare treat purchased only from a restaurant that he knows buys the fish fresh daily. The pesticide risks from consuming produce are small compared with the benefits of a diet high in fruits and vegetables. To reduce the amounts of pesticides ingested, fruits and vegetables can be washed thoroughly or consumed without the skins. He can also reduce pesticide consumption by purchasing organic produce, but he must consider that it is more expensive. He can also buy locally grown produce and keep up his summer vegetable garden.

What safe food choices could he include? He could bring peanut butter and jelly sandwiches or other foods that do not require refrigeration.

Chapter 20: Organic versus Biotechnology

How can genetically modified crops help alleviate hunger and malnutrition? By increasing crop yields, decreasing crop losses, and improving the nutrient content of foods that are available.

Do you think that genetically modified crops raised using organic techniques should be considered organic? Why or why not? Such crops cannot be used in organic foods under current regulation. Thus, students will have their own opinion of the regulation itself.

Appendix N

Calculations and Conversions

Equations for Predicting Resting Metabolic Rate from Body Weight*

Sex and Age Range (years)	Equation to Derive RMR in kcal/day
Males	
0–3	$(60.9 \times wt^{\dagger}) - 54$
3–10	$(22.7 \times wt) + 495$
10–18	$(17.5 \times wt) + 651$
18–30	$(15.3 \times wt) + 679$
30–60	$(11.6 \times wt) + 879$
>60	$(13.5 \times wt) + 487$
Females	
0–3	$(61.0 \times wt) - 51$
3–10	$(22.5 \times wt) + 499$
10–18	$(12.2 \times wt) + 746$
18–30	$(14.7 \times wt) + 496$
30–60	$(8.7 \times wt) + 829$
>60	$(10.5 \times wt) + 596$

* From WHO (1985). These equations were derived from BMR data.
† Weight of person in kilograms.

Source: From National Research Council, *Recommended Dietary Allowances*, 10th ed. (Washington, D.C.: National Academy of Sciences, 1989).

Weights and Measures

Measure	Abbreviations	Equivalent
1 gram	g	1000 milligrams
1 milligram	mg	1000 micrograms
1 microgram	μg	1/1,000,000 of a gram
1 nanogram	ng	1/1,000,000,000 of a gram
1 picogram	pg	1/1,000,000,000,000 of a gram
1 kilogram	kg	1000 grams 2.2 lb
1 pound	lb	454 grams 16 ounces
1 teaspoon	tsp	approximately 5 grams
1 tablespoon	Tbsp	3 teaspoons
1 ounce	oz	28.4 grams
1 cup	c	8 ounces 16 tablespoon
1 pint	pt	2 cups 16 ounces
1 quart	qt	2 pints 32 ounces
1 gallon	gal	128 ounces 4 quarts
1 liter	l	10.6 quarts 1000 milliliters
1 milliliter	ml	1000 microliters
1 deciliter	dl	100 milliliters
1 kcalorie	kcal	1000 calories 4.18 kilojoules
1 kilojoule	kJ	1000 joules 0.24 kcalories

Calculating Dietary Folate Equivalents (DFEs) in Fortified Foods

The amount of folate in foods fortified with folic acid is equal to the folate naturally present in the food plus the amount of folic acid added. The % Daily Value on food labels is calculated assuming that all of the folate is the naturally occurring form, which is less well absorbed than the folic acid form. Therefore, in order to correctly account for the amount of folate that is available to the body from fortified foods, the % Daily Value must be corrected. This calculation assumes that all of the folate in fortified foods is from added folic acid.

- Determine the amount of folic acid in the fortified food.
- Multiply the μg folic acid by 1.7, because folic acid added in fortification provides 1.7 times more available folate than folate naturally present in foods.
- Example:

The Daily Value for folate is 400 μg.

A serving of breakfast cereal provides 50% of the Daily Value for folate; thus:

400 μg × 50% = 200 μg folic acid

200 μg folic acid × 1.7 = 340 μg DFE

Converting Vitamin A Units into μg Vitamin A

Form and source	Amount equal to 1μg vitamin A
Preformed vitamin A in food or supplements	1 μg = 1μg vitamin A
	1 RAE = 1 μg vitamin A
	1 μg RE = 1 μg vitamin A
	3.3 IU = 1 μg vitamin A
β-carotene in food*	12 μg = 1 μg vitamin A
	1 RAE = 1 μg vitamin A
	2 μg RE = 1 μg vitamin A
	20 IU = 1 μg vitamin A
α-carotene or β-cryptoxanthin in food	24 μg = 1 μg vitamin A
	1 RAE = 1 μg vitamin A
	2 μg RE = 1 μg vitamin A
	40 IU = 1 μg vitamin A

*Beta-carotene in supplements may be better absorbed than β-carotene in food and so provides more vitamin A activity. It is estimated that 2 μg of β-carotene dissolved in oil provides 1 μg of vitamin A activity.

Converting Vitamin E Values into mg α-Tocopherol

To estimate the α-tocopherol intake from foods:

- If values are given as mg α-TEs:

$$\text{mg } \alpha\text{-TE} \times 0.8^{*} = \text{mg } \alpha\text{-tocopherol}$$

- If values are given as IUs:

  First, determine if the source of the α-tocopherol is natural or synthetic.

  - For natural α-tocopherol:

$$\text{IU of natural } \alpha\text{-tocopherol} \times 0.67 = \text{mg } \alpha\text{-tocopherol}$$

  - For synthetic α-tocopherol (dl-α-tocopherol):

$$\text{IU of synthetic } \alpha\text{-tocopherol} \times 0.45 = \text{mg } \alpha\text{-tocopherol}$$

*Based on dietary data from the NHANES III study, approximately 80% of the α-tocopherol equivalents from food are from α-tocopherol and can thus contribute to the body's requirement for vitamin E.

Glossary

Absorption The process of taking substances from the gastrointestinal tract into the interior of the body.

Accidental contaminant Substance not regulated by the FDA that unexpectedly enters the food supply.

Accutane A drug that is used orally to treat severe acne. It is a derivative of vitamin A.

Acesulfame K (acesulfame potassium) An artificial sweetener that contains no energy and is 200 times as sweet as sugar.

Acetaldehyde A toxic intermediate compound (CH_3CHO) produced in the body during the metabolism of alcohol.

Acetylcholine A neurotransmitter that functions in the brain and other parts of the nervous system.

Acetyl-CoA A common intermediate consisting of a 2-carbon compound attached to a molecule of CoA that is produced from the metabolism of carbohydrate, fat, and protein.

Acid A substance that releases hydrogen ions (H^+) in solution.

Active transport The transport of substances across a cell membrane with the aid of a carrier molecule and the expenditure of energy. This may occur against a concentration gradient.

Acute Effects that develop rapidly.

Adaptive thermogenesis Adjustments in energy expenditure induced by factors such as changes in ambient temperature and food intake.

Adenosylocobalamin A coenzyme form of vitamin B_{12} that is active in metabolism.

Adequate Intake (AI) A DRI reference value that is used as a goal for intake that should be used when no RDA can be determined. These values are an approximation of the average nutrient intake that appears to sustain a desired indicator of health.

ADI (Acceptable Daily Intake) The amount of a sweetener that can be safely consumed daily over a lifetime without adverse effects.

Adipocyte Fat-storing cell.

Adipose tissue Tissue found under the skin and around body organs that is composed of fat-storing cells.

Adolescent growth spurt An 18- to 24-month period of peak growth velocity that begins at about ages 10 to 13 in girls and 12 to 15 in boys.

Adrenaline A hormone secreted by the adrenal gland in response to stress that causes changes, such as an increase in heart rate, in preparation for "fight or flight"; also called epinephrine.

Aerobic exercise Exercise such as jogging, swimming, or cycling that increases heart rate and requires oxygen in metabolism. This type of exercise improves cardiovascular fitness.

Aerobic metabolism Metabolism in the presence of oxygen. In aerobic metabolism, glycolysis, the citric acid cycle, and the electron transport chain break down carbohydrates, fatty acids, and amino acids to carbon dioxide and water and produce ATP.

Aflatoxin An extremely potent carcinogen that is produced by a mold that grows on peanuts, corn, and grains.

Agar A polysaccharide extract of seaweed that is used in foods as an emulsifier, stabilizer, and gel.

Age-related bone loss The bone loss that occurs in both cortical and trabecular bone of men and women as they advance in age.

Aging A process that occurs over a lifetime that is associated with and responsible for an ever-increasing susceptibility to disease and death.

AIDS (acquired immune deficiency syndrome) The syndrome resulting from HIV infection that causes the immune system to fail, leading to frequent recurrent infections that ultimately result in death.

Alcohol An energy-containing molecule that contains 7 kcalories per gram and is made by the fermentation of carbohydrates from plant products; the type of alcohol that is consumed in the diet is called ethanol.

Alcohol dehydrogenase An enzyme in the stomach and liver that converts ethanol to acetaldehyde.

Alcohol-related birth defects *See* Fetal alcohol effects.

Alcoholic hepatitis Inflammation of the liver caused by alcohol consumption.

Aldosterone A hormone secreted by the adrenal glands that increases sodium reabsorption and therefore enhances water retention by the kidney.

Alginate A polysaccharide extract of brown algae used in the processing of food—primarily dairy products.

Alimentary canal *See* Gastrointestinal tract.

Allergen A foreign substance, usually a protein, that stimulates an immune response.

Allergy An adverse reaction involving the immune system that results from exposure to a specific allergen.

Alpha-carotene A carotenoid, some of which can be converted into vitamin A, that is found in leafy green vegetables, carrots, and squash.

Alpha-linolenic acid An 18-carbon omega-3 polyunsaturated fatty acid known to be essential in humans.

Alpha-tocopherol (α-tocopherol) The only form of tocopherol (vitamin E) active in humans.

Alzheimer's disease A disease that results in the relentless and irreversible loss of mental function.

Amenorrhea Delayed onset of menstruation or the absence of three or more consecutive menstrual cycles.

Amino acid pool All of the amino acids in the body tissues and fluids that are available for protein synthesis.

Amino acids The building blocks of proteins. Each contains a carbon atom bound to a hydrogen atom, an amino group, an acid group, and a side chain.

Amniotic fluid The liquid in the amniotic sac that surrounds and protects the embryo and fetus during development.

Amniotic sac A membrane surrounding the embryo or fetus that contains the amniotic fluid.

Amylopectin A plant starch that is composed of long branched chains of glucose molecules.

Amylose A plant starch that is composed of long unbranched chains of glucose molecules.

Anabolic Refers to energy-requiring processes in which simpler molecules are combined to form more complex substances.

Anabolic reaction Energy-requiring reaction in which simpler molecules are combined to form more complex substances.

Anabolic steroid One of a group of synthetic fat-soluble hormones that mimics testosterone; used by some athletes to increase muscle strength and mass.

Anaerobic metabolism or **anaerobic glycolysis** Metabolism in the absence of oxygen. In glycolysis, two molecules of ATP are produced from each molecule of glucose. Glucose is metabolized in this way when the blood cannot deliver oxygen to the tissues quickly enough.

Androstenedione A compound (known as Andro) that can be converted into testosterone and estrogen inside the body. It is a dietary supplement used by athletes to increase muscle mass and strength.

Anecdotal Information based on a story of personal experience.

Anemia A condition in which there is a reduced number of red blood cells or a reduced amount of hemoglobin, which then reduces the oxygen-carrying capacity of the blood.

Angiotensin II A compound that causes blood vessel walls to constrict and stimulates the release of the hormone aldosterone.

Anisakis disease A disease caused by infection of the gastrointestinal tract with the Anisakis roundworm that contaminates raw fish.

Anorexia nervosa An eating disorder characterized by self-starvation, a distorted body image, and low body weight.

Antacid A drug used to neutralize acidity in the gastrointestinal tract.

Anthropometric measurements External measurements of the body, such as height, weight, limb circumference, and skinfold thickness.

Antibiotic A substance that inhibits the growth of or destroys microorganisms; used to treat or prevent microbial infection.

Antibiotic resistance A trait acquired by some bacteria that allows them to survive in the presence of antibiotics.

Antibody Protein molecule produced by the immune system that specifically binds antigen.

Anticaking agent A substance added to dry food products to prevent clumping.

Anticarcinogen A compound that can counteract the effect of cancer-causing substances.

Anticoagulant A substance that delays or prevents blood coagulation.

Antidiuretic hormone (ADH) A hormone secreted by the pituitary gland that increases the amount of water reabsorbed by the kidney and therefore retained in the body.

Antioxidant A substance that is able to neutralize reactive molecules and hence reduce the amount of oxidative damage.

Antithiamin factor One of a group of substances in food that destroys the vitamin thiamin. Some are enzymes and are destroyed by cooking; others are not inactivated by cooking.

Anus The lower opening of the digestive tract through which the feces leave the body.

Apolipoprotein B A protein embedded in the outer shell of low-density lipoprotein (LDL) particles that binds to LDL receptor proteins on body cells.

Appetite The desire to consume specific foods that is independent of hunger.

Arachidonic acid A 20-carbon omega-6 polyunsaturated fatty acid that can be synthesized from linoleic acid.

Arginine A nonessential amino acid found in protein.

Ariboflavinosis The condition resulting from a deficiency of riboflavin.

Arteriole A small artery that carries blood to capillaries.

Artery A blood vessel that carries blood away from the heart.

Arthritis A disease characterized by inflammation of the joints, pain, and sometimes change in joint structure.

Artificial sweetener A chemically manufactured sweetener that differs from simple sugars in chemical structure and often provides little or no energy when ingested.

Ascorbate or **ascorbic acid** Chemical terms for vitamin C.

Aseptic processing A method that places sterilized food in a sterilized package.

Asparagine A nonessential amino acid found in protein.

Aspartame An artificial sweetener that is 200 times as sweet as sugar and is composed of the amino acids phenylalanine and aspartic acid.

Aspartic acid A nonessential amino acid found in protein.

Asthma A respiratory disorder characterized by wheezing and difficulty in breathing.

Atherosclerosis A type of cardiovascular disease that involves the buildup of fatty material in the artery walls.

Atkins diet A popular weight-loss diet that severely restricts that amount of carbohydrate consumed.

Atom The smallest unit of an element that still retains the properties of that element.

ATP (adenosine triphosphate) The high-energy molecule used by the body to perform energy-requiring activities.

Atrophic gastritis An inflammation of the stomach lining that causes a reduction in stomach acid and allows bacterial overgrowth.

Atrophy A reduction in the size of a body structure that may occur from disuse.

Attention deficit hyperactive disorder (ADHD) A condition that is characterized by a short attention span and a high level of activity, excitability, and distractibility.

Autoimmune disease A disease that results from immune reactions that destroy normal body cells.

Avidin A protein found in raw egg whites that binds biotin, preventing its absorption.

Bacillus thuringiensis A bacterium that produces a protein that is toxic to certain insects but safe for humans and other animals.

Bacteria (singular, **bacterium**) Small single-celled organisms that have no nucleus or other membrane-bound organelles. They are found throughout the environment. Most are harmless or beneficial, but a few types can cause disease in humans.

Balance study A study that compares the total amount of a nutrient that enters the body with the total amount that leaves the body.

Basal metabolic rate (BMR) The minimum amount of energy that an awake, fasted, resting body needs to maintain itself. BMR measurements are performed in a warm room in the morning before the subject rises, and at least 12 hours after the last food intake and activity.

Base A substance that accepts hydrogen ions in solution.

Bee pollen A mixture of pollen, bee saliva, and plant nectar that collects on the legs of bees; sold as an ergogenic aid.

Behavior modification A process used to gradually and permanently change habitual behaviors.

Benzocaine A local anesthetic used in some weight-loss products.

Beriberi A thiamin deficiency disease that is characterized by muscle weakness, loss of appetite, and nerve degeneration.

Beta-carotene (β-carotene) A carotenoid pigment found in many yellow and red-orange fruits and vegetables that acts as an antioxidant and has more provitamin A activity than other carotenoids.

Beta-cryptoxanthin A carotenoid found in corn, green peppers, and lemons that can provide some vitamin A activity.

Bile A substance made in the liver and stored in the gallbladder. It is released into the small intestine to aid in fat digestion and absorption.

Bile acids Emulsifiers present in bile that are synthesized by the liver from cholesterol.

Binge A session involving the consumption of a large amount of food in a discrete period of time associated with feeling that eating is out of control.

Binge drinker Someone who consumes five or more drinks in a row on a single occasion.

Binge eating or **bingeing** The rapid consumption of a large amount of food in a discrete period of time; associated with feeling that eating is out of control.

Binge-eating disorder An eating disorder characterized by recurrent episodes of binge-eating in the absence of purging behavior.

Bioavailability A measure of how well a nutrient can be absorbed and used by the body.

Biochemistry The chemistry of living things.

Bioelectric impedance analysis A technique for estimating body composition that measures body water by directing electric current through the body and calculating resistance to flow.

Biological value A measure of protein quality determined by comparing the amount of nitrogen retained in the body with the amount absorbed from the diet.

Biotechnology A set of techniques used to manipulate DNA for the purpose of changing the characteristics of an organism or creating a new product; also called genetic engineering.

Blood cholesterol level A term generally used to describe the concentration of cholesterol in the blood, plasma, or serum.

Blood pressure The amount of force exerted by the blood against the artery walls.

Body mass index (BMI) An index of weight in relation to height that is used to compare body size with a standard; it is equal to body weight (in kilograms) divided by height squared (in meters squared).

Bolus A ball of chewed food mixed with saliva.

Bomb calorimeter An instrument used to determine the energy content of food. It measures the heat energy released when a food is combusted.

Bone remodeling The process whereby bone is continuously broken down and reformed to allow for growth and maintenance.

Botulism A severe form of foodborne intoxication that results from consumption of a food containing the botulism toxin produced by the bacterium *Clostridium botulinum.*

Bovine somatotropin (bST) A hormone naturally produced by cows that stimulates the production of milk. A synthetic version of this hormone is now being produced by genetic engineering.

Bran The protective outer layers of whole grains. It is a concentrated source of dietary fiber.

Brewer's yeast The type of yeast used in brewing beer; a good source of B vitamins and often used as a nutritional supplement.

Brown adipose tissue A type of fat tissue that has a greater number of mitochondria than the more common white adipose tissue. It can waste energy by producing heat and is believed to be responsible for some of the change in energy expenditure in adaptive thermogenesis in rodents.

Brush border The microvilli surface of the intestinal mucosa that contains some digestive enzymes.

Buffer A substance that reacts with an acid or base by picking up or releasing hydrogen ions to prevent changes in pH.

Bulimia nervosa An eating disorder characterized by the consumption of large amounts of food at one time (bingeing), followed by purging behavior such as vomiting and the use of laxatives to eliminate food energy from the body.

Caffeine A bitter white substance found in coffee, tea, chocolate, and other foods; a stimulant and a diuretic.

Calcitonin A hormone produced by the thyroid gland that stimulates bone mineralization and inhibits bone breakdown, thus lowering blood calcium levels.

Calorie The amount of heat required to raise the temperature of 1 g of water 1 degree Celsius; equal to 4.18 joules. A term used to express the amount of energy in foods. (see kilocalorie)

Calorimetry A technique for measuring energy expenditure.

Campylobacter jejuni A bacterium common in raw milk and undercooked meat that causes foodborne illness.

Cancer A disease characterized by cells that grow and divide without restraint and have the ability to grow in different locations in the body.

Capillaries Small, thin-walled blood vessels where the exchange of gases and nutrients between blood and cells occurs.

Caprenin An artificial fat made from a triglyceride containing poorly absorbed fatty acids; provides 5 kcal per gram.

Carbohydrate A compound containing carbon, hydrogen, and oxygen in the same proportions as in water; includes sugars, starches, and most fibers.

Carbohydrate loading *See* Glycogen supercompensation.

Carbon dioxide A waste product produced by cellular respiration that is eliminated from the body by the lungs.

Carboxypeptidase A protein-digesting enzyme produced in inactive form in the pancreas, released in pancreatic juice, and activated in the small intestine, where it aids digestion.

Carcinogen An agent that can cause cancer.

Cardiorespiratory system The circulatory and respiratory systems, which together deliver oxygen and nutrients to cells.

Cardiovascular Refers to the heart and blood vessels.

Cardiovascular disease Any disease affecting the heart and blood vessels.

Caries or **dental caries** Cavities, or decay of the tooth enamel caused by acid produced when bacteria growing on the teeth metabolize carbohydrate.

Carnitine A molecule synthesized in the body that is needed to transport fatty acids and some amino acids into the mitrochondria for metabolism. Supplements of carnitine are marketed to athletes as performance enhancers.

Carotenoid Natural pigment synthesized by plants and many microorganisms. Gives yellow and red-orange fruits and vegetables their color.

Carpal tunnel syndrome Numbness, tingling, weakness, and pain in the hand caused by pressure on the nerves.

Carrageenan A seaweed polysaccharide extracted from Irish moss algae and used as a thickener, mainly in dairy products.

Case-control study A type of epidemiological study that compares individuals with a particular condition to those without the condition and then explores other variables that are different between the groups that might correlate with the presence of the condition being studied.

Casein The predominant protein in cow's milk.

Cash crop A crop grown to be sold for monetary return rather than to be used for food locally.

Cassava A starchy root that is the staple of the diet in many parts of Africa.

Catabolic Refers to the processes by which substances are broken down into simpler molecules, releasing energy.

Catabolic reaction Energy-releasing reaction in which substances are broken down into simpler molecules.

Catalase An iron-containing enzyme that destroys peroxides.

Cataracts A disease of the eye that results in cloudy spots on the lens (and sometimes the cornea) that obscure vision.

Cell The basic structural and functional unit of plant and animal life.

Cell differentiation Structural and functional changes that cause cells to mature into specialized cells.

Cell membrane The barrier that surrounds the cell contents.

Cellular respiration The reactions that break down carbohydrates, fats, and proteins in the presence of oxygen to produce carbon dioxide, water, and energy in the form of ATP.

Cellulite Subcutaneous fat that has a lumpy appearance because strands of connective tissue connect it to underlying structures.

Cellulose An insoluble fiber that is the most prevalent structural material of plant cell walls.

Cephalic phase The phase of gastric secretion that is stimulated by the thought, sight, smell, and taste of food. It is characterized by an increase in the secretion of gastric juice.

Certified food color A food color that has been tested and certified for safety, quality, consistency, and strength of color.

Ceruloplasmin A copper-containing protein that converts iron to the ferric form, which can bind to iron storage and iron transport proteins.

Cesarean section The surgical removal of the fetus from the uterus.

Chemical bond A force that holds atoms together.

Chemical or **amino acid score** A measure of protein quality determined by comparing the amount of the limiting amino acid in a food with that in a reference protein.

Chief cell Cell in the gastric mucosa that produces pepsinogen.

Chinese restaurant syndrome *See* MSG symptom complex.

Choice grade A USDA-regulated grade of beef with a modest amount of marbled fat.

Cholecalciferol The chemical name for vitamin D_3. It can be formed in the skin of animals by the action of sunlight on a form of cholesterol called 7-dehydrocholesterol.

Cholecystokinin (CCK) A hormone released by the duodenum that signals the pancreas to secrete digestive enzymes and causes the gallbladder to contract and release bile into the duodenum.

Cholesterol A lipid made only by animal cells that consists of multiple chemical rings.

Cholic acid A bile acid.

Choline A compound needed for the synthesis of the phospholipid phosphatidylcholine and the neurotransmitter acetylcholine. It is important for a number of biochemical reactions, and there is evidence that it is essential in the diet during certain stages of life.

Chromium picolinate A well-absorbed form of chromium sold as a dietary supplement that is advertised to promote fat loss and increase lean body tissue.

Chronic Effects that develop slowly over a long period.

Chylomicron A lipoprotein that transports lipids from the mucosal cells of the intestine and delivers triglycerides to other body cells.

Chyme A mixture of partially digested food and stomach secretions.

Chymotrypsin A protein-digesting enzyme produced in an inactive form in the pancreas and activated in the small intestine, where it aids digestion.

Circulatory system The organ system, consisting of the heart, blood, and blood vessels, which transports material to and from cells.

Cirrhosis Chronic liver disease characterized by the loss of functioning liver cells and the accumulation of fibrous connective tissue.

Citric acid cycle Also known as the Krebs cycle or the tricarboxylic acid cycle, this is the stage of cellular respiration in which two carbons of acetyl-CoA are oxidized, producing two molecules of carbon dioxide.

Clone A copy that is identical to the original.

Clostridium botulinum A bacterium that produces a deadly toxin and grows in a low-acid, low-oxygen environment, such as inside certain canned goods.

Clostridium perfringens A bacterium found in meat and poultry that can cause foodborne illness.

Coagulation The process of blood clotting.

Cobalamin The chemical term for vitamin B_{12}.

Coenzyme A small nonprotein organic molecule that acts as a carrier of electrons or atoms in metabolic reactions and is necessary for the proper functioning of many enzymes.

Cofactor An inorganic ion or coenzyme required for enzyme activity.

Colic Inconsolable crying that is believed to be due either to pain from gas buildup in the gastrointestinal tract or to immaturity of the central nervous system.

Collagen The major protein in connective tissue.

Colon The largest portion of the large intestine.

Colostrum The first milk, which is secreted in late pregnancy and up to a week after birth. It is rich in protein and immune factors.

Commodity food Food purchased and stored by the government to eliminate excess in the marketplace.

Complete protein A protein that provides essential amino acids in the proportions needed to support cellular protein synthesis.

Complex carbohydrate Carbohydrate composed of sugar molecules linked together in straight or branching chains. Includes oligosaccharides, starches, and fibers.

Compression of morbidity The postponement of the onset of chronic disease so that disability occupies a smaller and smaller proportion of the life span.

Concentration gradient A condition that exists when the amount of a dissolved substance is greater in one area than it is in another.

Conception The union of sperm and egg (ovum) that results in pregnancy.

Condensation reaction A type of chemical reaction in which two molecules are joined to form a larger molecule and water is released.

Conditionally essential amino acid An amino acid that is essential in the diet only under certain conditions or at certain times of life; also called semiessential amino acid.

Connective tissue One of the four human tissue types; includes cartilage, bone, tendons, blood, and adipose tissue.

Constipation Infrequent or difficult defecation.

Continuing Survey of Food Intakes by Individuals (CSFII) A survey conducted by the U.S. Department of Agriculture that collects data on the food intake of individuals within households for the purpose of monitoring the nutritional health of the population.

Control group A group of participants in an experiment that are identical to the experimental group except that no experimental treatment is used. A control group is used as a basis of comparison.

Cornea The clear, transparent fibrous outer coat of the eye.

Coronary heart disease A disease of the heart and the blood vessels that supply blood to the heart.

Correlation Two or more factors occurring together.

Cortical or **compact bone** Dense bone that makes up the sturdy outer surface layer of bones.

Covalent bond A type of chemical bond formed when two atoms share a pair of electrons.

Creatine A compound that can be converted into creatine-phosphate, which replenishes muscle ATP during short bursts of activity. Creatine is a dietary supplement used by athletes to increase muscle mass and delay fatigue during short, intense exercise.

Creatine phosphate A high-energy compound found in muscle that can be broken down to make ATP.

Cretinism A condition resulting from poor maternal iodine intake during pregnancy that causes stunted growth and poor mental development in offspring.

Criterion of adequacy A measure or outcome that can be examined to determine the biological effect of a particular level of nutrient intake; established for each nutrient and gender and life-stage group when developing Dietary Reference Intakes.

Critical control point Possible point in the food production, manufacturing, and transportation processes where contamination could occur or be prevented or eliminated.

Critical period A time in growth and development when an organism is more susceptible to harm from poor nutrition or other environmental factors.

Crossbreeding Breeding animals with desirable characteristics to obtain offspring that have acquired these desirable traits.

Cross-contamination The transfer of contaminants from one food to another.

Cross-sectional data Information obtained by a single broad sampling of many different individuals in a population.

Crude fiber Fiber that remains after a food has been treated in the laboratory with acid and base. It consists primarily of cellulose and lignin.

Cyclamate An artificial sweetener that was common in the United States in the 1960s; banned after it was found to cause cancer in laboratory animals.

Cycle of malnutrition A cycle in which malnutrition is perpetuated by an inability to meet nutrient needs at all life stages.

Cysteine A conditionally essential sulfur-containing amino acid; when methionine is available in sufficient quantities, cysteine is not essential in the diet.

Cystic acne A chronic inflammatory disease of the skin in which cysts and nodules are common and scarring may occur.

Cytoplasm The cellular material outside the nucleus that is contained by the cell membrane.

Daily Reference Value (DRV) Reference value established for protein and for seven nutrients for which no RDA has been established. The values are based on dietary recommendations for reducing the risk of chronic disease

Daily Value Nutrient reference value used on food labels to help consumers see how a food fits into their overall diets.

DASH diet A dietary pattern that is plentiful in fruits and vegetables as well as low-fat dairy products, whole grains, and lean meat, fish, and poultry, making it high in potassium, magnesium, calcium, and fiber and low in saturated fat and cholesterol.

Deamination The removal of the amino group from an amino acid.

Dehydration A decrease of 1% or more of body fluids that results when the output of water exceeds water input due to either low water intake or excessive loss.

Delaney Clause A clause added to the 1958 Food Additives Amendment of U.S. Pure Food and Drug Act that prohibits the intentional addition to foods of any compound that has been shown to induce cancer in animals or humans at any dose.

Dementia A deterioration of mental state resulting in impaired memory, thinking, and/or judgment.

Denaturation The alteration of a protein's three-dimensional structure.

Dental caries *See* Caries.

Deoxyribonucleic acid *See* DNA.

Deoxyribose The 5-carbon sugar that is part of DNA.

Depletion-repletion study A study that feeds a diet devoid of a nutrient until signs of deficiency appear, and then adds the nutrient back to the diet to a level at which symptoms disappear.

Dermatitis An inflammation of the skin.

DHA *See* docosahexaenoic acid.

DHEA (dehydroepiandosterone) A precursor of the sex hormones testosterone, estrogen, and progesterone; sold as a dietary supplement to slow aging and to increase muscle mass.

Diabetes mellitus A group of metabolic diseases characterized by high blood glucose levels resulting from defects in insulin secretion, insulin action, or both.

Diacylglycerol or **diglyceride** A molecule of glycerol with two fatty acids attached.

Diaphragm A muscular wall separating the abdomen from the thoracic cavity containing the heart and lungs.

Diarrhea An intestinal disorder characterized by frequent or watery stools.

Dicumarol An anticoagulant isolated from moldy clover.

Diet history Information about dietary habits and patterns. It may include a 24-hour recall, a food record, or a food frequency questionnaire to provide information about current intake patterns.

Dietary antioxidant A substance in food that significantly decreases the adverse effects of reactive species, such as reactive oxygen and nitrogen species, on normal physiological function in humans.

Dietary fiber *See* Fiber.

Dietary folate equivalent (DFE) The unit used to express the amount of folate present in food. One DFE is equivalent to 1 μg of folate naturally occurring in food, 0.6 μg of synthetic folic acid from fortified food or supplements consumed with food, or 0.5 μg of synthetic folic acid consumed on an empty stomach.

Dietary Guidelines for Americans A set of diet and lifestyle recommendations designed to encourage active lives and promote healthy, safe food choices for the purpose of improving health and reducing the incidence of nutrition-related chronic disease.

Dietary Reference Intakes (DRIs) A set of four reference values for the intake of nutrients and food components that can be used for planning and assessing the diets of healthy people in the United States and Canada.

Dietary supplement Any product intended for ingestion as a supplement to the diet. These are classified as food and are regulated by the FDA.

Diet-induced thermogenesis *See* Thermic effect of food (TEF).

Diffusion The movement of molecules from an area of higher concentration to an area of lower concentration without the expenditure of energy.

Digestion The process of breaking food into components small enough to be absorbed into the body.

Digestive system The organ system responsible for the ingestion, digestion, and absorption of food and the elimination of food residues; includes the gastrointestinal tract as well as a number of accessory organs.

Digestive tract *See* Gastrointestinal tract.

Diglyceride *See* Diacylglycerol.

Dioxins A group of environmental contaminants that are produced naturally and as industrial by-products. Repeated ingestion causes them to accumulate in biological tissues over time, damages a number of body systems, and contributes to the development of cancer. The term "dioxin" is often used to refer to the most well-known and well-studied of these compounds.

Dipeptide Two amino acids linked by a peptide bond.

Direct calorimetry A method of determining energy use that measures the amount of heat produced.

Direct food additive A substance intentionally added to food; regulated by the FDA.

Disaccharide A sugar formed by linking two monosaccharides.

Dissociate To separate two charged ions.

Diuretic A substance that promotes water loss from the body by increasing the flow of urine.

Diverticula Sacs or pouches that protrude from the wall of the large intestine.

Diverticulitis A condition in which diverticula in the large intestine become inflamed.

Diverticulosis A condition in which diverticula (or sacs) form in the wall of the large intestine.

DNA (deoxyribonucleic acid) Genetic material found in the cell nucleus that codes for the synthesis of proteins.

DNA ligase An enzyme use in recombinant DNA technology to paste two pieces of DNA together.

Docosahexaenoic acid (DHA) A 22-carbon omega-3 polyunsaturated fatty acid found in fish that may be needed in the diet of newborns. It can be synthesized from alpha-linolenic acid.

Dolomite A calcium supplement composed of ground-up limestone.

Double-blind study An experiment in which neither the study participants nor the researchers know who is in the control or experimental groups.

Doubly-labeled water method An indirect calorimetry technique for measuring energy expenditure that is based on measuring the distribution of isotopes of hydrogen and oxygen in body fluids after consumption of a defined amount of isotopically labeled water.

Down syndrome A disorder caused by extra genetic material that results in distinctive facial characteristics, mental retardation, and other health problems.

Duodenum The upper segment of the small intestine that connects to the stomach.

Eating disorder A psychological disorder affecting eating behavior and the regulation of food intake or energy balance.

Eclampsia The most severe form of pregnancy-induced hypertension involving elevated blood pressure, protein in the urine, and in some cases convulsions and coma during pregnancy or shortly after delivery.

Edema Swelling due to an abnormal accumulation of fluids in the spaces between cells or in body cavities.

Eicosanoid or **prostaglandin** One of a group of hormone-like regulatory molecules that can be synthesized from omega-3 and omega-6 fatty acids.

Eicosapentaenoic acid (EPA) A 20-carbon omega-3 polyunsaturated fatty acid found in fish that can be synthesized from alpha-linolenic acid but may be essential in humans under some conditions.

Electrolyte Substance that separates in water to form positively and negatively charged ions and is able to conduct an electric current. In nutrition, this term refers to sodium, potassium, and chloride.

Electron High-energy particle carrying a negative charge that orbits the nucleus of an atom.

Electron transport chain The final stage of cellular respiration in which electrons are passed down a chain of molecules to oxygen to form water and produce ATP.

Element A substance that cannot be broken down into products with different properties.

Elimination diet An eating plan that eliminates one or more foods suspected of causing an adverse food reaction.

Embryo The developing human from the beginning of the third week to eight weeks after fertilization. All organ systems are formed during this time.

Empty kcalories A term that refers to foods that contribute energy but few other nutrients.

Emulsifier A substance with both water-soluble and fat-soluble portions that can break fat into tiny droplets and suspend it in a watery fluid.

Endocrine system Organ system composed of cells, tissues, and organs that secrete hormones to help control body functions.

Endoplasmic reticulum A cellular organelle involved in the synthesis of proteins and lipids and composed of a system of membranous tubules, channels, and sacs in the cytoplasm; rough endoplasmic reticulum has ribosomes on its outside surface.

Endorphin A peptide released by the brain during exercise that acts as a natural euphoric and reduces the perception of pain under certain stressful conditions; may be the cause of the euphoria known as runner's high.

Endosperm The largest portion of a kernel of grain. It is primarily starch and serves as a food supply for the sprouting seed.

Endurance The length of time one can perform a task.

Energy The capacity to do work.

Energy balance A state in which body weight remains stable because the amount of energy consumed in the diet equals the amount expended.

Enrichment The addition of nutrients to a food to restore those lost in processing to a level equal to or higher than that originally present.

Enteral or **tube feeding** Provision of nutrients to the gastrointestinal tract through a tube when oral intake is inadequate. The tube may enter the GI tract through the nose or be surgically placed so it enters through the abdominal wall.

Environmental Protection Agency (EPA) U.S. government agency responsible for determining acceptable levels of environmental contaminants in the food supply and for establishing water quality standards.

Enzyme A protein molecule that accelerates the rate of a specific chemical reaction without being changed itself.

EPA *See* Eicosapentaenoic acid or Environmental Protection Agency.

Epidemiology The study of the interrelationships between health and disease and other factors in the environment or lifestyle of different populations.

Epiglottis Elastic cartilage at the back of the throat that covers the opening of the larynx during swallowing.

Epinephrine The primary hormone produced by the adrenal medulla that stimulates functions such as heart rate and respiratory rate that are important in the body's handling of stress, injury, emotional excitement, and strenuous physical activity. Also called adrenaline.

Epithelial tissue One of the four human tissue types; includes the cells that cover external body surfaces and line internal cavities and tubes.

Ergogenic aid Anything designed to increase the ability to work or improve performance.

Ergot A toxin produced by a mold that grows on grains, particularly rye.

Erythropoeitin A hormone produced by the kidney that stimulates the synthesis of red blood cells. Genetically engineered erythropoeitin is an illegal ergogenic aid used by some athletes.

Esophagus A portion of the gastrointestinal tract that extends from the pharynx to the stomach.

Essential or **indispensable amino acid** An amino acid that cannot be synthesized by the human body in sufficient amounts to meet needs and therefore must be included in the diet.

Essential fatty acid A fatty acid that must be consumed in the diet because it cannot be made by the body or cannot be made in sufficient quantities to meet needs.

Essential fatty acid deficiency A condition characterized by dry scaly skin and poor growth that results when the diet does not supply sufficient amounts of the essential fatty acids.

Essential hypertension High blood pressure that has no obvious external cause.

Essential nutrient Nutrient that must be provided in the diet because the body either cannot make it or cannot make it in sufficient quantities to satisfy its needs.

Estimated Average Requirement (EAR) A DRI reference value that meets the estimated nutrient need (as defined by a specific indicator of adequacy) of 50% of individuals in a gender and life-stage group.

Estimated Safe and Adequate Daily Dietary Intake (ESADDI) A recommendation used prior to the development of the DRIs and established when data were sufficient to estimate a range of requirements but insufficient to develop a 1989 RDA.

Estrogen A steroid hormone secreted by the ovaries and by the placenta that is involved in the maintenance of pregnancy and the maintenance and development of female sex organs and secondary sex characteristics.

Exchange Lists A food group system that groups foods according to energy and macronutrient content. It is used extensively in planning diabetic and weight loss diets.

Excretory system Organ system involved in the elimination of metabolic waste products; includes the lungs, skin, and kidneys.

Experimental control A factor included in an experimental design that limits the number of variables, allowing an investigator to examine the effect of only the parameters of interest.

Experimental group A group of participants in an experiment who are subjected to an experimental treatment.

Extracellular fluid The fluid located outside cells. It includes fluid found in the blood, lymph, gastrointestinal tract, spinal column, eyes, and joints and that found between cells and tissues

Extreme or **morbid obesity** A condition in which body weight is 100 pounds (45.5 kg) above healthy body weight or body mass index is greater than 40.

Facilitated diffusion The movement of substances across a cell membrane from an area of higher concentration to an area of lower concentration with the aid of a carrier molecule. No energy is required.

Fad bulimia A type of bulimia that is more a trend than a psychological disorder; binge episodes are typically less dramatic and emotional than those of a true bulimic and are common among teenagers and young adults who are concerned about a few extra pounds of body weight.

Failure to thrive The inability of a child's growth to keep up with normal growth curves.

Fallopian tube (oviduct) Narrow duct leading from the ovary to the uterus.

Famine A widespread lack of access to food due to a disaster that causes a collapse in the food production and marketing systems.

Fasting hypoglycemia Low blood sugar that is not related to food intake; often caused by an insulin-secreting tumor.

Fat A lipid that is solid at room temperature; commonly used to refer to all lipids or specifically to triglycerides.

Fat-free mass Body mass composed of all tissue except adipose tissue.

Fatigue The inability to continue an activity at an optimal level.

Fat-soluble vitamin A vitamin that does not dissolve in water; includes vitamins A, D, E, and K.

Fatty acid An organic molecule made up of a chain of carbons linked to hydrogens with an acid group at one end.

Fatty liver The accumulation of fat in the liver.

Fatty streak A cholesterol deposit in the artery wall.

FDA *See* Food and Drug Administration.

Feces Body waste, including unabsorbed food residue, bacteria, mucus, and dead cells, which is excreted from the gastrointestinal tract through the anus.

Female athlete triad The combination of disordered eating, amenorrhea, and osteoporosis that occurs in some female athletes, particularly those involved in sports in which low body weight and appearance are important.

Fermentation A process in which microorganisms metabolize components of a food and therefore change the composition, taste, and storage properties of the food.

Ferritin The major iron storage protein.

Fertilization The union of sperm and egg (ovum).

Fetal alcohol effects (FAE) Also called alcohol-related birth defects (ARBD). A spectrum of abnormalities including learning and developmental disabilities and behavioral abnormalities in a child due to maternal alcohol consumption during pregnancy.

Fetal alcohol syndrome (FAS) A characteristic group of severe physical and mental abnormalities in an infant resulting from alcohol consumed by the mother during pregnancy.

Fetus The developing human from the ninth week after conception to birth. Growth and refinement of structures occur during this time.

Fiber Nonstarch polysaccharides in plant foods that are not broken down by human digestive enzymes.

Fitness The ability to perform routine physical activity without undue fatigue.

Flatulence Excessive gas in the stomach and intestines.

Flavin adenine dinucleotide (FAD) An active coenzyme form of riboflavin. The structure of this molecule allows it to pick up and donate hydrogens and electrons in chemical reactions.

Flavin mononucleotide (FMN) An active coenzyme form of riboflavin. The structure of this molecule allows it to pick up and donate hydrogens and electrons in chemical reactions.

Flexibility Range of motion.

Fluorohydroxyapatite A fluoride-containing mineral deposit in the tooth enamel that is resistant to acid.

Fluorosis Mottling of the tooth enamel caused by chronic overconsumption of the mineral fluoride.

Foam cell A cholesterol-filled white blood cell.

Folate A general term for the many forms of this B vitamin. The majority of folate found naturally in foods includes a string of glutamate molecules called a polyglutamate tail.

Folic acid A form of folate that is present in the diet in fortified foods and dietary supplements. Its structure contains only one glutamate molecule.

Food additive Substance that can reasonably be expected to become a component of a food during processing. The foods that may contain additives and the amounts that may be present are regulated by the FDA.

Food allergy An adverse reaction involving the immune system that results from the exposure, generally through consumption, to a specific food.

Food and Drug Administration (FDA) U.S. government agency responsible for the safety and wholesomeness of all food except red meat, poultry, and eggs; also sets standards and enforces regulations for food labeling and for food and color additives.

Food challenge The reintroduction of foods into the diet one at a time while the person is carefully observed in a medical setting for the recurrence of symptoms.

Food Code A set of recommendations published by the FDA for the handling and service of food sold in restaurants and other establishments that serve food.

Food diary A method of assessing nutrient intake that involves an individual keeping a written record of all food and drink consumed during a defined period.

Food disappearance survey A method that estimates the food use of a population by monitoring the amount of food that leaves the marketplace.

Food frequency questionnaire A method of assessing nutrient intake that gathers information about how often certain categories of food are consumed.

Food Guide Pyramid A guide for diet planning that is based on five major food groups. Following the Pyramid's serving and selection recommendations helps individuals select diets that meet nutrient requirements and the recommendations for health promotion and disease prevention.

Food insecurity The inability to obtain sufficient food for any reason.

Food intolerance An adverse reaction to a food that does not involve the immune system.

Food jag A temporary food fixation during which a child will eat only certain foods.

Food processing Any alteration of food from the way it is found in nature.

Food security A condition in which all people at all times have physical and economic access to sufficient, safe, and nutritious foods to meet their dietary needs and food preferences for an active, healthy life.

Food self-sufficiency The ability of an area to produce enough food to feed its population.

Food shortage Insufficient food to feed a population.

Foodborne illness An illness caused by consumption of food containing a contaminant such as a toxin or disease-causing microorganism.

Foodborne infection Illness produced by the ingestion of food containing microorganisms that can multiply inside the body and produce injurious effects.

Foodborne intoxication Illness caused by consuming a food containing a toxin.

Fortification A term used generally to describe the addition of nutrients to foods, such as the addition of vitamin D to milk.

Frame size An estimation of the proportion of body weight that is attributed to bone.

Free radical A type of highly reactive molecule that contains an atom with an unpaired electron. Many of these cause damage to biological molecules.

Freeze-drying A process in which substances are frozen and then exposed to a vacuum so the water is removed by sublimation (a change from solid ice to gaseous water vapor).

Fructose A monosaccharide found in fruits and honey that is composed of six carbon atoms arranged in a ring structure; commonly called fruit sugar.

Functional food A food that provides a health benefit beyond that provided by the traditional nutrients it contains.

Fungus An organism that obtains nutrients by secreting enzymes that digest food outside its body. The breakdown products are then absorbed into its cells. Fungi are important for the decomposition of organic material.

Galactose A monosaccharide composed of six carbon atoms arranged in a ring structure; when combined with glucose, it forms the disaccharide lactose.

Gallbladder An organ of the digestive system that stores bile, which is produced by the liver.

Gallstone A clump of solid material, typically made mostly of cholesterol, that forms in the gallbladder and can block a bile duct, causing pain.

Gastric gland A collection of cells in the stomach including mucus-producing cells, parietal cells, chief cells, and hormone-producing cells, which produce gastric juice.

Gastric juice A substance produced by the gastric glands of the stomach that contains mucus, pepsinogen, intrinsic factor, and hydrochloric acid.

Gastric phase The phase of gastric secretion triggered by the entry of food into the stomach. It is characterized by an increase in the secretion of gastric juice.

Gastric pits Deep depressions in the lining of the stomach that lead to the gastric glands that produce gastric juice.

Gastrin A hormone secreted by the stomach mucosa that stimulates the secretion of gastric juice.

Gastroesophageal sphincter A muscular valve, also known as the cardiac or lower esophageal sphincter, that is located at the upper end of the stomach. It allows food to enter the stomach from the esophagus and prevents the acidic stomach contents from leaking up into the esophagus.

Gastrointestinal tract A hollow tube consisting of the mouth, pharynx, esophagus, stomach, small intestine, large intestine, rectum, and anus in which digestion and absorption of nutrients occur; also called the alimentary canal and digestive tract.

Gel A jelly-like suspension of a liquid in a solid system that is semisolid in consistency.

Gelatin A protein derived from collagen that is deficient in the amino acid tryptophan.

Gene expression The events of protein synthesis in which the information coded in a gene is used to synthesize a protein.

Gene A length of DNA that contains the instructions for making a protein.

Generally recognized as safe (GRAS) A group of chemical additives defined by the FDA as generally recognized as safe based on their long-standing presence in the food supply without obvious harmful effects.

Genetic engineering *See* Biotechnology.

Germ The embryo or sprouting portion of a kernel of grain. It contains vegetable oil, vitamins, and minerals.

Gestation The time between conception and birth, which lasts about nine months (or about 40 weeks) in humans.

Gestational diabetes A consistently elevated blood glucose level that begins or is first recognized during pregnancy.

Gestational hypertension A mild form of pregnancy-induced hypertension involving an elevation in blood pressure that occurs after the 20th week of pregnancy.

Ginseng An herb used in traditional Chinese medicine; claims are made that it improves athletic performance and increases sexual potency.

Glomerulus A part of the nephron that consists of a cluster of capillaries where blood is filtered.

Glucagon A hormone secreted by the pancreas that stimulates the breakdown of liver glycogen and the synthesis of glucose via gluconeogenesis to increase blood sugar.

Gluconeogenesis The synthesis of glucose from simple noncarbohydrate molecules. Amino acids from protein are the primary source of carbons for glucose synthesis.

Glucose A monosaccharide that is the primary form of carbohydrate used to produce energy in the body. It is the sugar referred to as blood sugar.

Glutamic acid A nonessential amino acid that is found in protein and in monosodium glutamate (MSG).

Glutathione peroxidase A selenium-containing enzyme that protects cells from oxidative damage by neutralizing peroxides.

Glycemic index A ranking of the effect that the consumption of a single carbohydrate-containing food has on blood glucose relative to the same amount of a reference carbohydrate such as white bread or glucose.

Glycemic response The rate, magnitude, and duration of the rise in blood glucose that occurs after a meal or a food is consumed.

Glyceride The most common type of lipid; consists of one, two, or three fatty acids attached to a molecule of glycerol.

Glycerol A 3-carbon molecule that forms the backbone of triglycerides and phosphoglycerides; also used as a humectant in food.

Glycogen A carbohydrate made of many glucose molecules linked together in a highly branched structure. It is the storage form of carbohydrate in animals.

Glycogen supercompensation or **carbohydrate loading** A regimen of diet and exercise training designed to maximize muscle glycogen stores before an athletic event.

Glycolysis A metabolic pathway in the cytoplasm of the cell that splits glucose into two 3-carbon pyruvate molecules. The energy released from one molecule of glucose is used to make two ATP molecules.

Goblet cells Cells that produce mucus.

Goiter An enlargement of the thyroid gland that is caused by a deficiency of iodine.

Goitrogen A substance that interferes with thyroid hormone production or utilization.

Golden rice A genetically engineered variety of rice that synthesizes β-carotene, giving the rice kernel a golden color.

GRAS *See* Generally recognized as safe.

Growth hormone A hormone secreted by the pituitary gland that stimulates growth.

Guar gum A branched polysaccharide from guar plants used as an additive to increase the viscosity of food.

Gum A plant polysaccharide and its derivatives that can dissolve in water and swell to form viscous solutions.

Gum arabic A branched polysaccharide from acacia trees; it is colorless, odorless, and tasteless, and is used as an additive to increase the viscosity of food.

Gum karaya A branched polysaccharide from trees; used as an additive to increase the viscosity of food.

Gum tragacanth A branched polysaccharide from thorny shrubs that grow in the semidesert of the Near East; used as an additive to thicken foods and to stabilize emulsions.

Hazard Analysis Critical Control Point (HACCP) A management system in which food safety is addressed through the analysis and control of biological, chemical, and physical hazards from raw material production, procurement, and handling to manufacturing, distribution, and consumption of the finished product.

Health claim A statement made about the relationship between a nutrient or food and a disease or health condition.

Healthy People A set of national health promotion and disease prevention objectives for the U.S. population.

Heart attack A condition in which an artery supplying blood to the heart becomes blocked, cutting off blood flow and hence oxygen and nutrients to a segment of the heart muscle, resulting in tissue death.

Heartburn A burning sensation in the chest caused when acidic stomach contents leak into the esophagus through the gastroesophageal sphincter.

Heat cramp A muscle cramp caused by an imbalance of sodium and potassium as a result of excessive exercise without adequate fluid and electrolyte replacement.

Heat disorders or **thermal distress** Conditions including dehydration, heat cramps, heat exhaustion, and heat stroke, that can occur due to an unfavorable combination of exercise, hydration status, and climatic conditions.

Heat exhaustion Low blood pressure, rapid pulse, fainting, and sweating caused when dehydration decreases blood volume so much that blood can no longer both cool the body and provide oxygen to the muscles.

Heat stroke Elevated body temperature as a result of fluid loss and the failure of the temperature regulatory center of the brain.

Heavy drinker Someone who consumes five or more drinks on the same occasion on at least five different days.

Heimlich maneuver A procedure used to dislodge an object blocking an air passage; involves the application of sharp, firm pressure to the abdomen just below the rib cage.

Heme iron A readily absorbed form of iron found in animal products. This form of iron is present in proteins as a chemical complex in which the iron is associated with four nitrogen atoms.

Hemicellulose An insoluble fiber that is a structural component of plant cell walls.

Hemochromatosis An inherited condition that results in increased iron absorption and leads to iron deposits throughout the body and tissue damage.

Hemoglobin An iron-containing protein in red blood cells that binds and transports oxygen through the bloodstream to cells.

Hemolytic anemia A condition in which there is an insufficient number of red blood cells because many have burst open.

Hemorrhoids Swollen veins in the anal or rectal area.

Hemosiderin An insoluble iron-protein compound formed in the liver when the iron storage capacity of ferritin is exceeded.

Hepatic portal circulation The system of blood vessels that collects nutrient-laden blood from the digestive organs and delivers it to the liver.

Hepatic portal vein The vein that transports blood from the gastrointestinal tract to the liver.

Hepatitis Inflammation of the liver.

Herb The leaves, flowers, stems, roots, seeds, or any other part of a nonwoody seed-bearing plant that dies down to the ground after flowering.

Herbicide An agent that kills weeds.

Heterocyclic amine (HA) A mutagenic substance produced when there is incomplete combustion of amino acids during the cooking of meats—for example, when meat is charred.

High-density lipoprotein (HDL) A type of lipoprotein that picks up cholesterol from cells and transports it to the liver so that it can be eliminated from the body. A low level of HDL increases the risk of cardiovascular disease.

High-fructose corn syrup A sweetener made from corn syrup that is composed of approximately half fructose and half glucose.

Histamine A substance produced by cells of the immune system as part of a nonspecific response that leads to inflammation.

HIV (human immunodeficiency virus) A virus that infects cells of the immune system and eventually leads to AIDS.

Homeostasis A physiological state in which a stable internal body environment is maintained.

Homocysteine A sulfur-containing amino acid that is produced from the metabolism of methionine. Elevated blood levels increase the risk of cardiovascular disease.

Hormone A chemical messenger that is produced in one location, is released into the blood, and elicits responses at other locations in the body.

Hormone replacement therapy The administration of female sex hormones to postmenopausal women to alleviate the symptoms of menopause.

Hormone-sensitive lipase An enzyme present in adipose cells that responds to chemical signals by breaking down triglycerides into fatty acids and glycerol for release into the bloodstream.

Humectant A substance added to foods to retain moisture.

Hunger Internal signals that stimulate one to acquire and consume food.

Hybridization The process of cross-fertilizing two related plants with the goal of producing an offspring that has the desirable characteristics of both parent plants.

Hydrochloric acid An acid secreted by the gastric glands of the stomach to aid in digestion.

Hydrogen peroxide A reactive oxygen-containing compound that can form free radicals and cause oxidative damage. It can be eliminated by the selenium-containing enzyme glutathione peroxidase.

Hydrogenation The process whereby hydrogens are added to the carbon-carbon double bonds of unsaturated fatty acids, making them more saturated.

Hydrolysis A type of reaction in which a large molecule is broken into two smaller molecules by the addition of water.

Hydrolyzed protein *See* Protein hydrolysate.

Hydroxyapatite A compound composed of calcium and phosphorus that is deposited in the protein matrix of bone to give it strength and rigidity.

Hydroxyl A chemical group consisting of a hydrogen atom and an oxygen atom (OH).

Hyperactivity Overactive, excitable, distractible behavior that is characteristic of attention deficit hyperactive disorder.

Hypercarotenemia A condition caused by an accumulation of carotenoids in the adipose tissue, causing the skin to appear yellow-orange.

Hypertension Blood pressure that is consistently elevated to 140/90 mm of mercury or greater.

Hypertrophy The increase in the size or bulk of an organ that may occur due to an increase in usage.

Hypoglycemia A low blood glucose level, usually below 40 to 50 mg of glucose per 100 ml of blood.

Hypothalamus The region of the brain that monitors and regulates conditions and activities in the body, including food intake and energy expenditure.

Hypothermia A condition in which body temperature drops below normal. Hypothermia depresses the central nervous system, resulting in the inability to shiver, sleepiness, and eventually coma.

Hypothesis An educated guess made to explain an observation or to answer a question.

Ileocecal value A fold of mucous membrane that separates the ileum of the small intestine from the large intestine.

Ileum The 11-foot segment of the small intestine that connects the jejunum with the large intestine.

Immunization An injection of a killed or inactivated organism into the body to stimulate the immune system to develop antibodies against the active disease-causing organism.

Impaired glucose tolerance A fasting blood glucose between 110 and 126 mg per 100 ml; a level that is higher than normal but not high enough to be classified as diabetes.

Implantation The process that begins about a week after fertilization in humans by which the developing ball of cells embeds in the uterine lining.

Inbreeding Breeding between closely related animals. It can intensify desirable traits but may also intensify undesirable traits.

Incomplete protein A protein that is deficient in one or more of the amino acids required for protein synthesis in humans.

Indirect calorimetry A method of estimating energy use that compares the amount of oxygen consumed with the carbon dioxide expired.

Indirect food additive A substance that is expected to unintentionally enter foods during manufacturing or from packaging; regulated by the FDA.

Infant botulism A form of botulism that occurs in infants less than a year old because they consume spores of *Clostridium botulinum* that then germinate in the gastrointestinal tract and produce toxin.

Infant mortality rate The number of deaths during the first year of life per 1000 live births.

Inorganic molecule A molecule that does not contain carbon atoms in its structure.

Inositol A compound that is often included in B-vitamin supplements and functions as part of a phospholipid in the human brain but is not a dietary essential; also called myo-inositol.

Insensible losses Fluid losses that are not perceived by the senses, such as evaporation of water through the skin and lungs.

Insoluble fiber Fiber that, for the most part, does not dissolve in water. It includes cellulose, hemicelluloses, and lignin.

Insulin A hormone made in the pancreas that allows the uptake of glucose by body cells and has other metabolic effects such as stimulating the synthesis of glycogen in liver and muscle.

Insulin-dependent diabetes *See* Type 1 diabetes.

Integrated pest management Agricultural production that combines chemical and nonchemical methods of pest control and emphasizes the use of natural toxins and more effective pesticide application.

Intermediate-density lipoprotein (IDL) A lipoprotein produced by the removal of triglycerides from VLDLs, most of which are then transformed to LDLs.

International unit (IU) A unit of measure used to express recommended intake levels of some vitamins.

Interstitial fluid The portion of the extracellular fluid located in the spaces between cells.

Interstitial space The fluid-filled spaces between cells.

Intervention study or **clinical trial** A study of a population in which there is an experimental manipulation of some members of the population; observations and measurements are made to determine the effects of this manipulation.

Intestinal crypt A tubular intestinal gland located between the villi that secretes intestinal juice.

Intestinal microflora Microorganisms that inhabit the large intestine.

Intestinal phase The phase of gastric secretion that is begun by the entry of food into the small intestine. It is characterized by a decrease in stomach motility and a decrease in the secretion of gastric juice.

Intracellular fluid The fluid located inside cells.

Intrinsic factor A protein produced by the parietal cells in the stomach lining that function in the absorption of vitamin B_{12}.

Iodine deficiency disorders A spectrum of conditions that can occur at any stage of life due to inadequate dietary iodine.

Ion An atom or group of atoms that carries a negative or a positive electrical charge.

Iron deficiency anemia A condition that occurs when the oxygen-carrying capacity of the blood is decreased because there is insufficient iron to make hemoglobin. It is diagnosed in adults when hemoglobin concentration is less than 11 g per 100 ml of blood.

Irradiation A process in which foods are exposed to radiation to kill contaminating organisms and retard ripening and spoilage.

Isoleucine An essential amino acid found in protein.

Isomer A molecule with the same molecular formula as another but a different arrangement of molecular groups.

Isotope An alternative form of an element that has a different atomic mass, which may or may not be radioactive.

Jejunum The 8-foot-long section of the small intestine lying between the duodenum and ileum.

Juvenile-onset diabetes *See* Type 1 diabetes.

Keratin A hard protein that makes up hair and nails.

Keratomalacia Advanced xerophthalmia, characterized by a softening of the cornea that leads to blindness.

Keshan disease A type of heart disease that occurs in areas of China where the soil is very low in selenium content.

Ketone or **ketone body** A type of molecule formed in the liver when there is not sufficient carbohydrate to completely metabolize the acetyl-CoA produced from fat breakdown.

Ketosis High levels of ketones in the blood.

Kilocalorie (kcalorie or **kcal)** A unit of heat that is used to express the amount of energy provided by foods. It is the amount of heat required to raise the temperature of 1 kilogram of water 1 degree Celsius (1 kcalorie = 4.18 kjoules).

Kilojoule (kjoule or **kJ)** A measure of work that can be used to express energy intake and energy output. It is the amount of work required to move an object weighing 1 kilogram a distance of 1 meter under the force of gravity (4.18 kjoules = 1 kcalorie).

Kwashiorkor A form of protein-energy malnutrition in which only protein is deficient. It is most common in young children who are unable to meet their high protein needs with the available diet.

Lactase An enzyme located in the brush border of the small intestine that breaks the disaccharide lactose into glucose and galactose.

Lactation The production and secretion of milk by the mammary gland.

Lacteal A lymph vessel in the villus of the small intestine that can transport large particles such as the products of fat digestion.

Lactic acid An end product of anaerobic metabolism and an additive used in food to maintain acidity or form curds.

Lactitol The sugar alcohol formed from lactose.

Lacto-ovo vegetarian One who eats no animal flesh but eats eggs and dairy products such as milk and cheese.

Lactose A disaccharide that is formed by linking galactose and glucose. It is commonly known as milk sugar.

Lactose intolerance The inability to digest lactose because levels of the enzyme lactase are low or absent. It causes symptoms such as intestinal gas and bloating after dairy products are consumed.

Lacto-vegetarian One who eats no animal flesh or eggs but eats dairy products.

Large-for-gestational-age An infant weighing greater than 4 kg (8.8 lb) at birth.

Large intestine The portion of the gastrointestinal tract that includes the colon and rectum; some water and vitamins are absorbed and bacteria act on food residues here.

Laxative A substance that eases the excretion of feces.

LDL receptor *See* Low-density lipoprotein receptor.

Lean body mass Body mass attributed to nonfat body components such as bone, muscle, and internal organs. It is also called fat-free mass.

Leavening agent A substance added to food that causes the production of gas during processing, resulting in an increase in food volume.

Lecithin A phosphoglyceride composed of a glycerol backbone, two fatty acids, a phosphate group, and a molecule of choline; often used as an emulsifier in foods.

Legume The starchy seed or pod of a plant that produces a pod (leguminous plant). Examples of legumes include peas, beans, and peanuts.

Leptin A protein hormone produced by adipocytes that signals information about the amount of body fat.

Leptin receptor Protein that binds the hormone leptin. In response to this binding, it triggers events that cause changes in food intake and energy expenditure.

Let-down A hormonal reflex triggered by an infant's suckling that causes milk to be released from the milk glands and to flow through the duct system to the nipple.

Leucine An essential amino acid found in protein.

Leukocyte White blood cell.

Life expectancy The average length of life for a population of individuals.

Life span The maximum age to which a member of a species can live.

Life-stage group A grouping of individuals that have similar nutrient needs based on their stage of growth and development and whether they are pregnant or lactating.

Lignin An insoluble fiber responsible for the hard, woody nature of plant stems.

Limiting amino acid The essential amino acid that is available in the lowest concentration in relation to the body's needs.

Linoleic acid An omega-6 essential fatty acid with 18 carbons and 2 double bonds.

Lipase Fat-digesting enzyme.

Lipid One of a group of organic molecules, most of which do not dissolve in water, that provide energy and insulation and serve as precursors in the synthesis of certain hormones; include fatty acids, glycerides, phospholipids, and sterols.

Lipid bilayer Two layers of phosphoglyceride molecules oriented so that the fat-soluble fatty acid tails are sandwiched between the water-soluble phosphate-containing heads.

Lipoic acid A coenzyme needed in the reaction that forms acetyl-CoA; not a dietary essential.

Lipoprotein A particle containing a core of triglycerides and cholesterol surrounded by a shell of proteins, phospholipids, and cholesterol. Transports lipids in blood and lymph.

Lipoprotein lipase An enzyme that breaks down triglycerides into free fatty acids and glycerol; attached to the outside of the cells that line the blood vessels.

Liposuction A procedure that suctions out adipose tissue from under the skin; used to decrease the size of local fat deposits such as those on the abdomen or hips.

Locust bean gum A branched polysaccharide that is produced from the endosperm of the seed of the carob plant; used as an additive to increase viscosity in cheese products and sausages.

Long-chain fatty acid A fatty acid with more than 12 carbons; usually remains solid at room temperature.

Longevity The duration of an individual's life.

Longitudinal data Information obtained by repeatedly sampling the same individuals in a population over time.

Low birth weight A birth weight less than 2.5 kg (5.5 lb).

Low-density lipoprotein (LDL) A lipoprotein that transports cholesterol to cells. Elevated LDL cholesterol increases the risk of cardiovascular disease.

Low-density lipoprotein receptor A protein on the surface of cells that binds to LDL particles and allows them to be taken into the cells, making their contents available for use by the cell.

Lumen The inside cavity of a tube, such as the gastrointestinal tract.

Lutein A carotenoid found in corn and green peppers that provides some protection against macular degeneration.

Lycopene A carotenoid that gives the red color to tomatoes. It cannot be converted to vitamin A.

Lymphatic system The system of vessels, organs, and tissues that drains excess fluid from the spaces between cells, picks up fat-soluble substances absorbed from the digestive tract, and provides immune function.

Lymphocyte A type of white blood cell that is part of the specific branch of the immune system.

Lymph vessel or **lacteal** A tubular component of the lymphatic system that carries fluid away from body tissues. Lymph vessels in the intestine are known as lacteals and can transport large particles such as the products of fat digestion.

Lysosome A cellular organelle containing degradative enzymes.

Lysozyme An enzyme in saliva, tears, and sweat that is capable of destroying certain types of bacteria.

Macrocyte Larger-than-normal mature red blood cell that has a shortened life span.

Macronutrient Nutrient needed by the body in large amounts. Includes water and the energy-yielding nutrients carbohydrates, lipids, and proteins.

Macular degeneration A progressive degeneration of the central portion of the retina, causing gradual loss of central vision.

Major mineral A mineral needed in the diet in an amount greater than 100 mg per day or present in the body in an amount greater than 0.01% of body weight.

Malnutrition Poor nutritional status resulting from a dietary intake either above or below that which is optimal.

Maltase An enzyme found in the brush border of the small intestine that breaks maltose into two molecules of glucose.

Maltose A dissacharide made of two glucose molecules linked together.

Mannitol The sugar alcohol formed from the sugar mannose.

Marasmus A form of protein-energy malnutrition in which a deficiency of energy in the diet causes severe body wasting.

Maturity-onset diabetes *See* Type 2 diabetes.

Maximal oxygen consumption or **VO_2 max** The maximum amount of oxygen that can be consumed by the tissues during exercise.

Maximum heart rate The maximum number of beats per minute that the heart can attain. It declines with age and can be estimated by subtracting age in years from 220.

Mediterranean diet A dietary pattern that is associated with a low risk of heart disease. It is rich in whole grains, fruits, vegetables, and olive oil, and includes a glass of wine at meals.

Medium-chain fatty acid A fatty acid that contains 8 to 12 carbons.

Megaloblast Large immature red blood cell formed when developing red blood cells are unable to divide normally.

Megaloblastic or **macrocytic anemia** A condition in which there are abnormally large immature and mature red blood cells and a reduction in the total number of red blood cells.

Melatonin A hormone involved in regulating the body's cycles of sleep and wakefulness. Levels decline with age. Supplements claim to boost antioxidant defenses, improve immune function, and slow aging.

Menaquinones Originally called vitamin K_2; the forms of vitamin K synthesized by bacteria and found in animals.

Menarche The onset of menstruation, which occurs normally between the ages of 10 and 15.

Menopause Physiological changes that mark the end of a woman's menstrual cycles and capacity to bear children.

Menstruation The cyclic discharge of the uterine lining in the absence of pregnancy that occurs about every four weeks during the reproductive years of female humans.

Messenger RNA (mRNA) A class of RNA molecules that carries the genetic message from DNA in the nucleus to ribosomes in the cytoplasm of the cell so proteins can be synthesized.

Metabolism The sum of all the chemical reactions that take place in a living organism.

Metallothionein A protein that binds zinc and copper in intestinal cells and limits their absorption into the blood.

Methionine An essential sulfur-containing amino acid found in protein.

Methyl group A chemical group consisting of a carbon atom bound to three hydrogen atoms.

Methylcobalamin A coenzyme form of vitamin B_{12} that is active in metabolism.

Micelle Small particle—consisting of a core of fatty acids, monoglycerides, and other fat-soluble substances surrounded by bile acids—that aids the absorption of lipids in the small intestine.

Microbe An organism too small to be seen without a microscope; also called a microorganism.

Microflora *See* Intestinal microflora.

Micronutrient Nutrient needed by the body in small amounts. Includes vitamins and minerals.

Microorganism An organism such as a bacterium, too small to be seen without a microscope.

Microvilli Minute brushlike projections on the mucosal cell membrane that contain digestive enzymes and increase the absorptive surface area in the small intestine.

Mineral In nutrition, an element needed by the body in small amounts for structure and to regulate chemical reactions and body processes.

Miscarriage or **spontaneous abortion** Interruption of pregnancy prior to the seventh month.

Mitochondrion (mitochondria) The cellular organelle that is responsible for generating energy in the form of ATP via aerobic metabolism; the citric acid cycle and electron transport chain are located here.

Modified atmosphere packaging (MAP) A type of food packaging in which the gases inside the package are changed to control or retard chemical, physical, and microbiological changes.

Modified starch or **modified food starch** Starch that has been treated to enhance its ability to thicken or form a gel.

Mold Multicellular fungus that forms a filamentous branching growth.

Molecular biology The study of cellular function at the molecular level.

Molecule Unit of two or more atoms of the same or different elements bonded together.

Monoacylglycerol or **monoglyceride** A molecule of glycerol with one fatty acid attached.

Monosaccharide A single sugar molecule, such as glucose.

Monosodium glutamate (MSG) An additive used as a flavor enhancer, commonly found in Chinese food; made up of the amino acid glutamate bound to sodium.

Monounsaturated fatty acid A fatty acid containing one carbon-carbon double bond.

Morbid obesity *See* Extreme obesity.

Morbidity The incidence or state of disease or disability.

Morning sickness Nausea and vomiting that affects many women during the first few months of pregnancy and that in some women can continue throughout the pregnancy.

mRNA (messenger RNA) *See* Messenger RNA.

MSG symptom complex Symptoms of headache, flushing, tingling, burning sensations, and chest pain reported by some individuals after consuming monosodium glutamate (MSG); commonly referred to as Chinese restaurant syndrome.

Mucosa The layer of tissue lining the gastrointestinal tract and other body cavities.

Mucus A thick, viscous fluid secreted by glands in the gastrointestinal tract and other parts of the body. It acts to lubricate, moisten, and protect cells from harsh environments.

Mutagen A substance that causes changes in the molecular structure of DNA.

Mutation Change in DNA caused by chemical or physical agents.

Myelin A soft, white fatty substance that covers nerve fibers and aids in nerve transmission.

Myocardial infarction Heart attack.

Myoglobin An iron-containing protein in the cytoplasm of muscle cells. By binding oxygen, it helps increase the rate that oxygen diffuses from the blood into the muscle cells.

Myo-inositol *See* Inositol.

National Health and Nutrition Examination Survey (NHANES) An ongoing set of surveys designed to monitor the overall nutritional status of the U.S. population; combines food consumption information with medical histories, physical examinations, and laboratory measurements.

National Organic Program A U.S. Department of Agriculture program that provides information about certification, guidelines, and other aspects of organic food production.

Nephron Structural and functional unit of the kidney consisting of the glomerulus and renal tubules.

Nervous system A system of nerve cells organized in message sending, message receiving, and information processing pathways.

Net protein utilization A measure of protein quality determined by comparing the amount of nitrogen retained in the body with the amount eaten in the diet.

Neural tube A portion of the embryo that develops into the brain and spinal cord.

Neural tube closure A developmental event in which neural tissue forms a groove and the sides fold together to form a tube; is completed about 28 days after fertilization.

Neural tube defect A defect in the formation of the neural tube that occurs early in development and results in defects of the brain and spinal cord such as anencephaly and spina bifida.

Neurotransmitter A chemical substance produced by a nerve cell that can stimulate or inhibit another cell.

Niacin equivalent (NE) A unit used to express the amount of niacin present in food, including that which can be made from its precursor, tryptophan. One NE is equal to 1 mg of niacin or 60 mg of tryptophan.

Nicotinamide A form of niacin.

Nicotinamide adenine dinucleotide (NAD) An active coenzyme form of niacin that is able to pick up and donate hydrogens and electrons. It is important in the transfer of electrons to oxygen in cellular respiration.

Nicotinamide adenine dinucleotide phosphate (NADP) An active coenzyme form of niacin that is able to pick up and donate hydrogens and electrons. It is important in many synthetic reactions.

Nicotinic acid A form of niacin.

Nitrogen balance A state in which the amount of nitrogen consumed in the diet is equal to the nitrogen excreted by the body, indicating that the amount of body protein is constant and there is no net protein synthesis or degradation.

Nitrosamines Carcinogenic compounds produced by reactions between nitrites and amino acids.

Nonessential or **dispensable amino acid** An amino acid that can be synthesized by the human body in sufficient amounts to meet needs.

Nonheme iron Iron that is not associated with proteins or that is present in proteins that do not contain heme groups. This form of iron is less well absorbed than heme iron and is found in both animal and plant foods.

Noninsulin-dependent diabetes *See* Type 2 diabetes.

Nonrenewable resource A resource, such as fossil fuel, that is present in the Earth in limited amounts and, once depleted, cannot be replaced in a reasonable amount of time.

Nucleus The central core of an atom, consisting of positively charged protons and electrically neutral neutrons. In cells, it is an organelle containing DNA.

Nursing bottle syndrome Extreme tooth decay in the upper teeth resulting from putting a child to bed with a bottle containing milk or other sweetened liquid.

Nutrient density A measure of the nutrients provided by a food relative to the energy it contains.

Nutrient Chemical substance in foods that provides energy, forms body structures, and/or regulates body processes.

Nutrification The process of adding one or more nutrients to commonly consumed foods with the goal of adding to the nutrient intake of a group of people.

Nutrition A science that studies the interactions that occur between living organisms and food.

Nutritional assessment The process of determining the nutritional status of individuals or groups for the purpose of identifying nutritional needs and planning personal health-care or community programs to meet these needs.

Nutritional status State of health as it is influenced by the intake and utilization of nutrients.

Nutrition support claim Claim often included on the label of a dietary supplement that describes the relationship between a nutrient and a deficiency disease that could result if the nutrient were lacking in the diet.

Nutrition transition The shift in dietary pattern that occurs in developing countries as incomes increase—from a diet high in complex carbohydrates and fiber to a more varied diet higher in fats, saturated fat, and sugar.

Obesity A condition characterized by excess body fat. It is defined as a body mass index of 30 kg/m^2 or greater or a body weight that is 20% or more above the healthy body-weight standard.

Obesity gene A gene that codes for proteins involved in the regulation of body fat. When it is abnormal, the result is abnormal amounts of body fat.

Objective measurements Information that can be quantified and repeated by careful scientific methodology.

Oil A lipid that is liquid at room temperature.

Oleic acid A monounsaturated fatty acid with 18 carbons.

Olestra (sucrose polyester) An artificial fat made of sucrose with fatty acids linked to it that cannot be digested or absorbed. It has been approved by the FDA for use in certain snack foods.

Oligosaccharide Short-chain carbohydrate containing 3 to 10 sugar units.

Omega-3 (ω-3) fatty acid A fatty acid containing a carbon-carbon double bond between the third and fourth carbons from the omega end; includes alpha-linolenic acid found in vegetable oils and eicosapentaenoic acid (EPA) and docosahexaenoic acid (DHA) found in fish oils.

Omega-6 (ω-6) fatty acid A fatty acid containing a carbon-carbon double bond between the sixth and seventh carbons from the omega end; includes linoleic and arachidonic acids.

Opsin A protein in the retina of the eye involved in the visual cycle.

Organ A discrete structure composed of more than one tissue type that act together to perform a specialized function.

Organelle Cellular organ that carries out specific metabolic functions.

Organic food A food produced according to the production and handling standards established by the National Organic Program of the USDA. Foods produced using synthetic pesticides and fertilizers, sewage sludge, genetically modified ingredients, and irradiation do not meet the definition of organic.

Organic molecule Molecule containing carbon atoms in its structure.

Osmosis The passive movement of water across a semipermeable membrane in a direction that will equalize the concentration of dissolved solutes on both sides.

Osteoarthritis The form of arthritis common in the elderly that is characterized by a wearing down of the joint surfaces and pain when the joint is moved.

Osteoblast A type of cell responsible for the deposition of bone.

Osteoclast A type of large cell responsible for bone breakdown.

Osteomalacia A vitamin D–deficiency disease in adults characterized by a loss of minerals from the bone matrix. It causes weak bones and increases the likelihood of bone fractures.

Osteoporosis A bone disorder characterized by a reduction in bone mass, an increase in bone fragility, and an increased risk of fractures.

Outbreeding Breeding unrelated animals to reduce undesirable traits, increase variability, and introduce new traits into the offspring.

Overnutrition Poor nutritional status resulting from a dietary intake in excess of that needed to maintain health.

Overtraining syndrome A collection of emotional, behavioral, and physical symptoms that occur when over training persists for weeks to months.

Overweight A body mass index of 25 to 29.9 kg/m^2 or a body weight 10 to 19% above the healthy body weight standard.

Oviduct *See* Fallopian tube.

Ovum The female reproductive cell.

Oxalate An organic acid found in spinach, rhubarb, and other leafy green vegetables that can bind certain minerals and decrease their absorption.

Oxaloacetate A 4-carbon compound derived from carbohydrate that combines with acetyl-CoA in the first step of the citric acid cycle.

Oxidation The loss of electrons.

Oxidative damage Damage caused by highly reactive oxygen molecules that steal electrons from other compounds, causing changes in structure and function.

Oxidative stress A condition that occurs when there are more reactive oxygen molecules than can be neutralized by available antioxidant defenses. It occurs either because excessive amounts of reactive oxygen molecules are generated or because antioxidant defenses are deficient.

Oxidize To breakdown a molecule in the presence of oxygen to yield energy.

Oxidized LDL cholesterol A modified cholesterol formed when the cholesterol in LDL particles is oxidized by reactive oxygen molecules. It is key in the development of atherosclerosis because it is taken up by scavenger receptors on white blood cells.

Oxytocin A hormone produced by the posterior pituitary gland that acts on the breast to cause the movement of milk into the secretory ducts that lead to the nipple and on the uterus to cause uterine contractions.

Palmitic acid A saturated fatty acid containing 16 carbons.

Pancreas An organ that secretes digestive enzymes and bicarbonate ions into the small intestine during digestion. It also secretes the hormones insulin and glucagon into the blood.

Pancreatic amylase A starch-digesting enzyme found in pancreatic juice.

Pancreatic juice A secretion of the pancreas containing bicarbonate to neutralize acid and enzymes for the digestion of carbohydrates, fats, and proteins.

Papain A protein-digesting enzyme found in papaya.

Para-aminobenzoic acid (PABA) A chemical that is part of the folic acid molecule but that alone has no vitamin activity and cannot be used by the body to synthesize folic acid; effective at blocking ultraviolet (UV) light and thus is used in topical sunscreens.

Parasite An organism that lives at the expense of another without contributing to the survival of the host.

Parathyroid hormone (PTH) A hormone secreted by the parathyroid gland that acts to increase blood calcium levels.

Parietal cell Large cell in the stomach lining that produces and secretes intrinsic factor and hydrochloric acid.

Partially hydrogenated vegetable oil Vegetable oil that has been modified by hydrogenation to decrease the number of unsaturated bonds, therefore raising the melting point and improving the storage characteristics.

Pasteurization The process of treating food products to kill disease-causing organisms. Traditional pasteurization relies on heating to kill the microorganisms, but irradiation, referred to as cold pasteurization, can also be used.

Pathogen An organism capable of causing disease.

Peak bone mass The maximum bone density attained at any time in life, usually occurring in young adulthood.

Pectin A soluble fiber found in plant cell walls that forms a gel when mixed with acid and sugar.

Peer review Review of the design and validity of a research experiment by experts in the field of study who did not participate in the research.

Pellagra A niacin deficiency disease that is characterized by dermatitis, dementia, diarrhea, and, ultimately, death.

Pepsin A protein-digesting enzyme produced by the stomach. It is secreted in the gastric juice in an inactive form (pepsinogen) and activated by acid in the stomach.

Pepsinogen An inactive protein-digesting enzyme produced by gastric glands and activated to pepsin by acid in the stomach.

Peptic ulcer An open sore in the lining of the stomach, esophagus, or small intestine.

Peptidase A peptide-digesting enzyme.

Peptide Two or more amino acids joined by peptide bonds.

Peptide bond The chemical linkage formed between the amino group of one amino acid and the acid group of another by a condensation reaction in which water is eliminated.

Periodontal disease A degeneration of the area surrounding the teeth, specifically the gum and supporting bone.

Peristalsis Coordinated muscular contractions that move food through the gastrointestinal tract.

Pernicious anemia An anemia resulting from an autoimmune disorder in which parietal cells are destroyed, decreasing the production of intrinsic factor. This reduces the absorption of vitamin B_{12}, gradually resulting in deficiency.

Peroxide A reactive chemical that can form free radicals and cause cellular damage.

Pesticide A substance used to prevent or decrease damage to plants from insects and microorganisms.

pH A measure of the level of acidity or alkalinity of a solution compared to neutrality.

Pharynx A funnel-shaped opening that connects the nasal passages and mouth to the respiratory passages and esophagus. It is a common passageway for food and air and is responsible for swallowing.

Phenylalanine An essential amino acid found in protein that cannot be metabolized by individuals with phenylketonuria (PKU).

Phenylketone The product of phenylalanine breakdown produced when phenylalanine cannot be converted to tyrosine; when blood levels get too high, brain damage results.

Phenylketonuria (PKU) An inherited disease in which the body cannot metabolize the amino acid phenylalanine. If the disease is untreated, toxic by-products accumulate in the blood and cause mental retardation.

Phosphoglyceride A phospholipid composed of a glycerol backbone with two fatty acids and a phosphate group attached; mixes well with both watery and oily substances and is an important component of cell membranes.

Phospholipid A lipid containing a phosphate group.

Photosynthesis The metabolic process by which plants trap energy from the sun and use it to make sugars from carbon dioxide and water.

Phylloquinone Originally called vitamin K_1. The form of vitamin K found in plants.

Phytic acid or **phytate** An inorganic phosphorus storage compound found in seeds and grains that can bind minerals and decrease their absorption.

Phytochemical A substance found in plant foods (*phyto-* means plant) that is not an essential nutrient but may have health-promoting properties.

Phytoestrogen An estrogen-like molecule produced by plants.

Phytosterol A compound produced by plants that has a structure similar to that of cholesterol.

Pica An abnormal craving for and ingestion of unusual food and nonfood substances such as clay, laundry starch, and paint chips.

PKU *See* Phenylketonuria.

Placebo A fake medicine or supplement that is indistinguishable in appearance from the real thing. It is used to disguise the control and experimental groups in an experiment.

Placenta An organ produced from both maternal and embryonic tissues. It secretes hormones, transfers nutrients and oxygen from the mother's blood to the fetus, and removes fetal wastes.

Plaque The cholesterol-rich material that is deposited in the blood vessels of individuals with atherosclerosis. It consists of cholesterol, smooth muscle cells, fibrous tissue, and, eventually, calcium.

Plasma The liquid portion of the blood that remains when the blood cells are removed.

Plasmid A loop of bacterial DNA that is independent of the bacterial chromosome.

Platelet A cell fragment found in blood that is involved in blood clotting.

Polar A term used to describe a molecule that has a positive charge at one end and a negative charge at the other.

Polychlorinated biphenyls (PCBs) A group of carcinogenic industrial compounds that have found their way into the environment and, subsequently, the food supply. Repeated exposure causes them to accumulate in biological tissues over time.

Polycyclic aromatic hydrocarbons (PAHs) A class of mutagenic substances produced during cooking when there is incomplete combustion of organic materials—such as when fat drips on a grill.

Polypeptide A chain of three or more amino acids joined together by peptide bonds.

Polysaccharide Complex carbohydrate containing many sugar units linked together.

Polyunsaturated fatty acid A fatty acid that contains two or more double bonds between carbons in the carbon chain.

Postmenopausal bone loss The accelerated bone loss that occurs in women for about five years after estrogen production decreases.

Prebiotic An indigestible food product that stimulates the growth of a particular type of gut bacteria.

Precursor Inactive form of a substance that can be converted into the active form.

Preeclampsia A form of pregnancy-induced hypertension that is characterized by an increase in body weight, elevated blood pressure, protein in the urine, and edema.

Pregnancy-induced hypertension A spectrum of conditions involving elevated blood pressure that usually occurs after 20 weeks of gestation. It may be accompanied by protein in the urine, edema, and, rarely, convulsions and coma.

Premature or **preterm infant** An infant born before 37 weeks of gestation.

Premenstrual syndrome (PMS) A syndrome of mood swings, food cravings, bloating, tension and depression, headaches, acne, and anxiety, among other symptoms, that results from the hormonal changes during the days prior to menstruation.

Preservative A compound that prevents spoilage and extends the shelf life of a product by retarding chemical, physical, or microbiological changes.

Preterm infant *See* Premature infant.

Prime grade A USDA-regulated grade of beef with the largest amount of marbled fat.

Probiotic Foods or supplements that contain live microorganisms that survive passage through the upper GI tract and live temporarily in the gut.

Progesterone A female sex hormone needed for the development and function of the uterus and mammary glands.

Programmed cell death The death of cells at specific predictable times.
Prolactin A hormone released by the anterior pituitary that acts on the milk-producing glands in the breast to stimulate and sustain milk production.
Pro-oxidant A substance that promotes oxidative damage.
Prostaglandin *See* Eicosinoid.
Protein An organic molecule made up of one or more intertwining chains of amino acids.
Protein or **nitrogen balance** *See* Nitrogen balance.
Protein complementation A method of combining proteins from different sources so that they collectively provide the proportions of amino acids required to meet needs.
Protein digestibilty–corrected amino acid score A measure of protein quality that is calculated by adjusting the amino acid score with a correction factor for digestibility.
Protein efficiency ratio A measure of protein quality determined by comparing the weight gain of a laboratory animal fed a test protein with the weight gain of an animal fed a reference protein.
Protein-energy malnutrition (PEM) A condition characterized by wasting and an increased susceptibility to infection that results from the long-term consumption of insufficient energy and protein to meet needs.
Protein hydrolysate or **hydrolyzed protein** A mixture of amino acids or amino acids and polypeptides that results when a protein is completely or partially broken down by treatment with acid or enzymes.
Protein quality A measure of how efficiently a protein in the diet can be used to synthesize body proteins.
Protein-sparing modified fast A very-low-kcalorie diet with a high proportion of protein designed to maximize the loss of fat and minimize the loss of protein from the body.
Protein turnover The continuous synthesis and breakdown of body proteins.
Prothrombin A blood protein required for blood clotting.
Provitamin or **vitamin precursor** A compound that can be converted into the active form of a vitamin in the body.
Psyllium A plant product high in soluble fiber that is used in over-the-counter bulk-forming laxatives.
Puberty A period in life characterized by rapid growth and physical changes that ends in the attainment of sexual maturity.
Purging Behaviors such as self-induced vomiting and misuse of laxatives and diuretics used to rid the body of food energy.
Pyloric sphincter A muscular valve located at the lower end of the stomach that regulates the rate at which food leaves the stomach and enters the duodenum.
Pyridoxal phosphate The major active coenzyme form of vitamin B_6 that functions in more than 100 enzymatic reactions, most of which involve amino acid metabolism.
Pyridoxamine A form of vitamin B_6.
Pyridoxine One of a number of forms of vitamin B_6.
Pyruvate A 3-carbon molecule produced when glucose is broken down by glycolysis.

Raffinose An oligosaccharide found in beans and other legumes that cannot be digested by human enzymes in the stomach and small intestine.
Reactive hypoglycemia Low blood sugar that occurs an hour or so after the consumption of high-carbohydrate foods; results from an overproduction of insulin.
Recombinant DNA DNA that is produced by joining DNA from different sources to create a unique combination of genes.
Recommended Dietary Allowance (RDA) A DRI reference value that indicates a level of intake sufficient to meet the nutrient need of almost all healthy people in a specific life-stage and gender group.
Recommended Nutrient Intake (RNI) Recommended intake of nutrients established for Canadians by the Canadian government (Health Canada).
Rectum The portion of the large intestine that connects the colon and anus.
Reference Daily Intake (RDI) Reference value established for vitamins and minerals based on the highest amount of each nutrient recommended for any adult age group by the 1968 RDAs.
Refined Refers to the process whereby the coarse parts of foods are removed, leaving behind a product of more uniform composition.
Renewable resource A resource that can be restored and replaced by natural processes and can therefore be used forever.
Renin An enzyme produced by the kidney that aids in the conversion of angiotensin to its active form, angiotensin II.
Rennet A preparation of the enzyme rennin that is extracted from calf stomachs or made through genetic engineering and is used to form milk curd in the production of cheese.
Rennin An enzyme produced by the stomachs of infants and young children (and other animals) that acts on the milk protein casein to convert it to a curdy substance.
Reserve capacity The amount of functional capacity that an organ has above and beyond what is needed to sustain life.
Respiratory system Organ system that includes the lungs and air passageways involved in the exchange of oxygen from the environment with carbon dioxide waste from cells by way of the bloodstream.
Resting energy expenditure (REE) *See* Resting metabolic rate (RMR).
Resting heart rate The number of times that the heart beats per minute while a person is at rest.
Resting metabolic rate (RMR) or **resting energy expenditure (REE)** An estimate of basal metabolic rate that is determined by measuring energy utilization after 5 to 6 hours without food or exercise.
Restriction enzyme Bacterial enzyme used in genetic engineering that has the ability to cut DNA in a specific location.
Retin-A A drug that is a vitamin A derivative used topically to treat acne.
Retinal The aldehyde form of vitamin A, which is needed for the visual cycle.
Retinoic acid The acid form of vitamin A, which is needed for cell differentiation, growth, and reproduction.
Retinoid Preformed vitamin A; includes retinol, retinal, and retinoic acid.
Retinol The alcohol form of vitamin A, which can be interconverted with retinal.
Retinol activity equivalent (RAE) The amount of retinol, β-carotene, α-carotene, or β-cryptoxanthin that must be consumed to equal the vitamin A activity of 1 μg of retinol. One μg of retinol, 12 μg of β-carotene, or 24 μg α-carotene or β-cryptoxanthin is equal to 1 RAE.
Retinol-binding protein A protein that is needed to transport vitamin A from the liver to tissues in need.

Rhodopsin A light-sensitive compound found in the retina of the eye that is composed of the protein opsin loosely bound to retinal.

Ribonucleic acid *See* RNA.

Ribose The 5-carbon sugar that is part of RNA.

Ribosome The cell organelle where protein synthesis occurs.

Rickets A vitamin D deficiency disease in children that is characterized by poor bone development due to inadequate calcium deposition.

Risk-benefit analysis The process of weighing the risk associated with a substance against the benefits it provides; if the risk is small and the benefits great, small amounts of this substance may be acceptable.

Risk factor A characteristic or circumstance that is associated with the occurrence of a particular disease. Risk factors include variables such as genetic background, dietary and lifestyle habits, and environmental conditions.

RNA (ribonucleic acid) A single-stranded nucleic acid. It carries information in DNA from the nucleus to the cytoplasm, is a structural component of ribosomes, and delivers amino acids for protein synthesis.

Royal jelly The substance that is produced by worker bees to feed the queen; marketed as an ergogenic aid.

Saccharin An artificial sweetener used in diet products that contains no energy and is about 300 times sweeter than sugar.

Saliva A watery fluid produced and secreted into the mouth by the salivary glands. It contains lubricants, enzymes, and other substances.

Salivary amylase An enzyme secreted by the salivary glands that breaks down starch into smaller units.

Salivary gland One of the internal structures that secrete saliva; located at the sides of and below the face and in front of the ears.

Salmonella A bacterium that commonly causes foodborne illness.

Satiety The feeling of fullness and satisfaction caused by food consumption that eliminates the desire to eat.

Saturated fatty acid A fatty acid in which the carbon atoms are bound to as many hydrogens as possible and which therefore contains no carbon-carbon double bonds.

Scavenger receptor A protein on white blood cells that binds to oxidized LDL cholesterol, allowing it to enter the cell.

Scientific method The general approach of science that is used to explain observations about the world around us.

Scurvy A vitamin C deficiency disease.

Seasonal affective disorder A disorder characterized by depression and carbohydrate cravings during the fall and winter months.

Secondary lactase deficiency Lactase deficiency that occurs as a result of disease and may resolve after the disease has ended.

Secretin A hormone released by the duodenum that signals the pancreas to secrete bicarbonate ions and stimulates the liver to secrete bile into the gallbladder.

Segmentation Rhythmic local constrictions of the intestine that mix food with digestive juices and speed absorption by repeatedly moving different parts of the food mass over the intestinal wall.

Select grade A USDA-regulated grade of beef with a medium amount of marbled fat.

Selective breeding Technique to selectively control mating in plants and animals to produce organisms that better serve human needs.

Selectively permeable Describes a membrane or barrier that will allow some substances to pass freely but will restrict the passage of others.

Selenoprotein A protein that contains selenium as a structural component of its amino acids. Selenium is most often found as selenocysteine, which contains an atom of selenium in place of the sulfur atom of cysteine.

Semiessential amino acid *See* Conditionally essential amino acid.

Semivegetarian One who avoids only certain types of meat, fish, or poultry.

Serotonin A neurotransmitter that functions in the sleep center of the brain.

Set point theory A theory that suggests that body fat or body weight resists change despite changes in energy intake or output.

Short-chain fatty acid A fatty acid that contains four to seven carbons.

Sickle cell anemia An inherited disease in which hemoglobin structure is altered. Red blood cells containing the altered hemoglobin are sickle-shaped; rupture easily, causing anemia; and block small blood vessels, causing inflammation and pain.

Simple carbohydrates Carbohydrates known as sugars that include monosaccharides and disaccharides.

Simple diffusion The movement of substances from an area of higher concentration to an area of lower concentration. No energy is required.

Simple sugar *See* Simple carbohydrate.

Simplesse An artificial fat made from egg and milk proteins that contains about 1.3 kcalories per gram.

Single-blind study An experiment in which either the study participants or the researchers (but not both) are unaware of who is in a control or an experimental group.

Skinfold thickness A measurement of subcutaneous fat used to estimate total body fat.

Small-for-gestational-age An infant born at term weighing less than 2.5 kg (5.5 lb).

Small intestine A tube-shaped organ of the digestive tract where digestion of ingested food is completed and most of the absorption occurs.

Smooth muscle Involuntary muscles that cause constriction of the gastrointestinal tract, blood vessels, and glands.

Sodium bicarbonate A compound that is part of an important buffer system in pancreatic juice and in the bloodstream.

Sodium caseinate A form of the milk protein casein that is frequently used as a food additive.

Sodium-potassium ATPase An energy-requiring protein pump in the cell membrane that pumps sodium out of the cell and potassium into the cell.

Solanine A toxic substance naturally occurring in potatoes; inhibits the action of neurotransmitters.

Soluble fiber Fiber that either dissolves when placed in water or absorbs water. It includes pectins, gums, and some hemicelluloses.

Solutes Dissolved substances.

Solution A solvent containing a dissolved substance.

Solvent A fluid in which one or more substances dissolve.

Sorbitol A sugar alcohol formed from the sugar sorbose; used as a sweetener or humectant in food.

Sperm The male reproductive cell.

Sphincter A muscular valve that helps control the flow of materials in the gastrointestinal tract.

Spina bifida A neural tube defect in which part of the spinal cord is exposed through a gap in the backbone, causing varying degrees of disability.

Spontaneous abortion *See* Miscarriage.

Spore A dormant stage of some bacteria that is resistant to heat but can germinate and produce a new organism when environmental conditions are favorable.

Sports anemia A temporary decrease in hemoglobin concentration that occurs as part of a beneficial adaptation to aerobic exercise, in which expanded plasma volume dilutes red blood cells.

Stabilizer A substance added to food to stabilize its consistency.

Standards of identity Regulations that define the allowable ingredients, composition, and other characteristics of foods.

Staphylococcus A bacterium, commonly found in the nasal passages, that can contaminate food and cause foodborne illness.

Starch A carbohydrate made of many glucose molecules linked in straight or branching chains. The bonds that hold the glucose molecules together can be broken by the human digestive enzymes.

Starchyose An oligosaccharide found in beans and other legumes that cannot be digested by human enzymes in the stomach and small intestine.

Starvation The condition that occurs when insufficient food is ingested to maintain health.

Statistics The science of collecting and analyzing numerical information. It can be used to determine if an event is due to chance or to the effect of an experimental treatment.

Stearic acid An 18-carbon saturated fatty acid that, unlike other saturated fats, does not raise blood cholesterol levels.

Sterilization A process that kills all the living organisms in the treated material.

Steroid hormone A hormone that is made from cholesterol; includes the male and female sex hormones.

Sterol A lipid compound that contains atoms arranged in a multiple ring structure with a variety of side chains attached.

Stomach A muscular pouchlike organ of the digestive tract that mixes food and secretes gastric juice into the lumen and the hormone gastrin into the blood.

Stroke A blood clot or bleeding in the brain that causes brain tissue death.

Stroke volume The volume of blood pumped by each beat of the heart.

Stunting A decrease in linear growth rate, the frequency of which is an indicator of the nutritional well-being in populations of children.

Subcutaneous fat Adipose tissue located under the skin that is not associated with a great increase in the risk of chronic diseases.

Subscapular The region just below the shoulder blade that is a common location for measuring skinfold thickness.

Subsistence crop A crop grown as food for the local population.

Substrate cycling When opposing biochemical reactions occur together so that energy is expended but the concentration of molecules is not changed.

Sucralose An artificial sweetener that is about 600 times sweeter than sucrose; trichlorogalactosucrose. It is heat stable, and so can be used in baked products.

Sucrase An enzyme in the brush border of the small intestine that breaks sucrose into glucose and fructose.

Sucrose A disaccharide that is formed by linking fructose and glucose. It is commonly known as table sugar or white sugar.

Sudden infant death syndrome (SIDS or **crib death)** The unexplained death of infants, usually during sleep.

Sugar alcohol A sweetener that is structurally related to sugars but provides less energy than monosaccharides and disaccharides because it is not as well absorbed.

Sulfite A sulfur-containing compound used as a preservative to prevent oxidation in dried fruits and vegetables and to prevent bacterial growth in wine.

Sulforaphane A phytochemical found in broccoli and other cruciferous vegetables that boosts the activity of enzyme systems that detoxify carcinogens.

Superoxide dismutase (SOD) An enzyme that protects the cell from oxidative damage by neutralizing superoxide free radicals. One form of the enzyme requires zinc and copper for activity and another form requires manganese.

Superoxide radical A type of reactive oxygen molecule that can form free radicals leading to oxidative damage. They can be neutralized by the enzyme superoxide dismutase.

Sustainable Refers to methods of using resources that prevent overuse of natural systems and allow the environment to be maintained indefinitely without a decline.

Sustainable agriculture Methods of producing food that leave the environment able to restore itself and continue to produce food for future generations.

Tannin A substance found in tea and some grains that can bind certain minerals and decrease their absorption.

Taurine An amino acid found only in animal foods that is not used in protein synthesis but is necessary for nerve function and vision and the synthesis of bile acids; made in the adult human in sufficient quantities but may be essential in premature infants.

Teratogen A chemical, biological, or physical agent that causes birth defects.

Testosterone A steroid hormone secreted by the testes that is involved in the maintenance and development of male sex organs and secondary sex characteristics.

Texturizer A substance added to food to change its texture.

Theory An explanation based on scientific study and reasoning.

Thermal distress *See* heat disorders.

Thermic effect of food (TEF) or **diet induced thermogenesis** The energy required for the digestion of food and the absorption, metabolism, and storage of nutrients. It is equal to approximately 10% of daily energy intake.

Thiamin pyrophosphate The active coenzyme form of thiamin. It is the predominate form found inside cells where it aids reactions in which a carbon-containing group is lost as CO_2.

Threshold effect A reaction that occurs at a certain level of ingestion and increases as the dose increases.

Thyroid gland A gland located in the neck that produces thyroid hormones and calcitonin.

Thyroid hormones Hormones produced by the thyroid gland that regulates metabolic rate.

Thyroid-stimulating hormone A hormone that stimulates the synthesis and secretion of thyroid hormones from the thyroid gland.

Tissue A group of similar cells specialized to perform a specific function.

Tocopherol The chemical name for vitamin E.

Tolerable Upper Intake Level (UL) A DRI reference value that is the maximum daily intake by an individual that is unlikely to pose risks of adverse health effects to almost all individuals in the specified life-stage and gender group.

Tolerance The maximum amount of pesticide residue that may legally remain in food; set by the EPA.

Total parenteral nutrition (TPN) A method of providing complete nutrition by infusing nutrients into a large central vein.

Toxic The capacity to produce injury at some level of intake.

Toxin A substance with the ability to cause harm at some level of exposure; also called toxicant.

Trabecular or **spongy bone** The type of bone that forms an inner spongy lattice that lines the bone marrow cavity and supports the cortical shell.

Trace element or **trace mineral** A mineral required in the diet in an amount less than 100 mg per day or present in the body in an amount less than 0.01% of body weight.

Transamination The process by which an amino group from one amino acid is transferred to a carbon compound to form a new amino acid.

Transcription The process of copying the information in DNA to a molecule of mRNA.

***Trans* fatty acid** An unsaturated fatty acid in which the hydrogen atoms are on opposite sides of the double bond.

Transfer RNA A class of RNA molecule that interprets the mRNA code by delivering specific amino acids to the ribosome and by pairing with the mRNA code for those amino acids.

Transferrin An iron transport protein in the blood.

Transferrin receptor Protein found in cell membranes that binds to the iron-transferrin complex and allows it to be taken up by cells.

Transit time The time between the ingestion of food and the elimination of the solid waste from that food.

Translation The process of translating the mRNA code into the amino acid sequence of a protein.

Treatment group *See* Experimental group.

Triacylglycerol or **triglyceride** The major form of lipid in food and the major storage form of lipid in the body. It consists of three fatty acids attached to a glycerol molecule.

Triceps Region at the back of the upper arm that is a common site for measuring skin-fold thickness.

Trichinosis The disease caused by infection with the roundworm *Trichinella spiralis* after eating undercooked contaminated pork or game meats; the juvenile form of this roundworm migrates to the muscles and causes flulike symptoms and muscle pain and weakness.

Triglyceride *See* Triacylglycerol.

Trimester A term used to describe each three-month period, or one-third of a pregnancy.

Tripeptide Three amino acids linked together by peptide bonds.

Tropical oil A term used in the popular press to refer to the saturated oils—coconut, palm, and palm kernel oil—that are derived from plants grown in tropical regions.

Trypsin A protein-digesting enzyme that is secreted from the pancreas in inactive form and activated in the small intestine.

Tube feeding *See* Enteral feeding.

Tuber The starchy underground storage organ of plants.

Tumor A growth of tissue that forms an abnormal mass that serves no physiological function.

Tumor initiator A substance that causes mutations and therefore may predispose a cell to becoming cancerous.

Tumor promoter A substance that stimulates a mutated cell to begin dividing.

Twenty-four-hour recall A method of assessing dietary intake in which a trained interviewer asks an individual to report what they have eaten during the previous day.

Type 1 diabetes A form of diabetes that is caused by the autoimmune destruction of insulin-producing cells in the pancreas, usually leading to absolute insulin deficiency; previously known as insulin-dependent diabetes mellitus or juvenile-onset diabetes.

Type 2 diabetes A form of diabetes that is characterized by insulin resistance and usually relative (rather than absolute) insulin deficiency; previously know as non-insulin-dependent diabetes mellitus or adult-onset diabetes.

Tyrosine A conditionally essential amino acid; when phenylalanine is available in sufficient quantities, tyrosine is not essential in the diet.

U. S. Department of Agriculture (USDA) U.S. government agency responsible for monitoring the safety and wholesomeness of meat, poultry, and eggs.

U. S. Recommended Daily Allowance (U.S. RDA) A set of standard reference values for nutrients designed to be used on food labels; generally equal to the highest nutrient recommendation in any age or sex category from the published 1968 RDAs. Replaced by the RDI.

Ubiquinone A compound that transports electrons in the electron transport chain but that is not essential in the diet; also called coenzyme Q.

UL *See* Tolerable Upper Intake Level (UL).

Ulcer An open sore.

Undernutrition Any condition resulting from an energy or nutrient intake below that which meets nutritional needs.

Underwater weighing A technique that uses the difference between body weight underwater and body weight on land to estimate body composition.

Underweight A body mass index of less than 18.5 kg/m^2, or a body weight 10% or more below the desirable body weight standard.

Unsaturated fatty acid A fatty acid that contains one or more carbon-carbon double bonds.

Urea A nitrogen-containing waste product from the breakdown of proteins that is excreted in the urine.

Urine A fluid produced by the kidneys consisting of metabolic wastes, excess water, and dissolved substances.

USRDA *See* U.S. Recommended Daily Allowance.

Uterus A female organ for containing and nourishing the embryo and fetus from the time of implantation to the time of birth.

Variable A factor or condition that is monitored or changed in an experimental setting.

Vegan diet A pattern of food intake that eliminates all animal products.

Vegetarian diet A pattern of food intake that eliminates some or all animal products.

Vegetarianism A pattern of food intake the eliminates some or all animal products.

Vein Vessel that carries blood toward the heart.

Venule A small vein that drains blood from capillaries and passes it to larger veins for return to the heart.

Very low birth weight A birth weight less than 1.5 kg (3.3 lb).

Very-low-density lipoprotein (VLDL) A lipoprotein assembled by the liver that carries lipid from the liver and delivers triglycerides to body cells.

Very-low-kcalorie diet A weight-loss diet that provides fewer than 800 kcalories per day.

Villi (villus) Finger-like protrusions of the lining of the small intestine that participate in the digestion and absorption of foodstuffs.

Virus Minute particle not visible under an ordinary microscope that depends on cells for its metabolic and reproductive needs.

Visceral fat Adipose tissue deposited in the abdominal cavity around the internal organs. High levels are associated with an increased risk of heart disease, high blood pressure, stroke, diabetes, and breast cancer.

Vitamin An organic compound needed in the diet in small amounts to promote and regulate the chemical reactions and processes needed for growth, reproduction, and the maintenance of health.

Warfarin An anticoagulant drug that acts by inhibiting the action of vitamin K. It is a derivative of dicumarol; also used as rat poison.

Water A molecule composed of two hydrogen atoms and one oxygen atom; essential nutrient needed by the human body in large amounts.

Water activity A measure of the amount of available water in food.

Water-soluble vitamins Vitamins that dissolve in water. These include the B vitamins and vitamin C.

Wear and tear hypothesis A hypothesis that proposes that the changes that occur with age result from the accumulation of cellular damage over time.

Weight cycling or **yo-yo dieting** The cycle of repeatedly losing and regaining weight.

Wernicke-Korsakoff syndrome A condition involving loss of specific functions in the brain and in nerves throughout the body, due to malnutrition, specifically thiamin deficiency. It develops gradually and is most common in alcoholics.

Wheat germ oil An oil pressed from the germ of wheat; sold as an ergogenic aid.

Whole-wheat flour A flour that contains all components of the wheat kernel: the bran, the germ, and the endosperm.

Xanthan gum A plant extract used as a stabilizer in processed foods.

Xerophthalmia A spectrum of eye conditions resulting from vitamin A deficiency that may lead to blindness. An early symptom is night blindness, and as deficiency continues, a lack of mucus leaves the eye dry and vulnerable to cracking and infection.

Xylitol The sugar alcohol formed from the sugar xylose; used in sugarless gum.

Yo-yo diet syndrome *See* Weight cycling.

Zeaxanthin A carotenoid found in corn and green peppers that provides some protection against macular degeneration.

Zoochemicals Substances found in animal foods (*zoo-* means animal) that are not essential nutrients but may have health-promoting properties.

Zygote The cell produced by the union of sperm and ovum during fertilization.

Index

Note: Boldface numbers indicate the page where the term is defined. The letter "t" after a page number indicates a table.

G

J

K

L

O

P

Q

R

W

X

Y

Z

Dietary Reference Intakes (DRIs): Tolerable Upper Intake Levels (UL[a]): Vitamins

Life Stage Group	Vitamin A (μg/d)[b]	Vitamin D (μd/d)	Vitamin E (mg/d)[c,d]	Vitamin K	Vitamin C (mg/d)	Thiamin	Ribo-flavin	Niacin (mg/d)[d]	Vitamin B_6 (mg/d)	Folate (μg/d)[d]	Vitamin B_{12}	Pantothenic Acid	Biotin	Choline (g/d)	Carote-noids[e]
Infants															
0–6 mo	600	25	ND[f]	ND	ND	ND	ND	ND	ND	ND	ND	ND	ND	ND	ND
7–12 mo	600	25	ND	ND	ND	ND	ND	ND	ND	ND	ND	ND	ND	ND	ND
Children															
1–3 y	600	50	200	ND	400	ND	ND	10	30	300	ND	ND	ND	1.0	ND
4–8 y	900	50	300	ND	650	ND	ND	15	40	400	ND	ND	ND	1.0	ND
Males, Females															
9–13 y	1,700	50	600	ND	1,200	ND	ND	20	60	600	ND	ND	ND	2.0	ND
14–18 y	2,800	50	800	ND	1,800	ND	ND	30	80	800	ND	ND	ND	3.0	ND
19–70 y	3,000	50	1,000	ND	2,000	ND	ND	35	100	1,000	ND	ND	ND	3.5	ND
> 70 y	3,000	50	1,000	ND	2,000	ND	ND	35	100	1,000	ND	ND	ND	3.5	ND
Pregnancy															
≤ 18 y	2,800	50	800	ND	1,800	ND	ND	30	80	800	ND	ND	ND	3.0	ND
19–50 y	3,000	50	1,000	ND	2,000	ND	ND	35	100	1,000	ND	ND	ND	3.5	ND
Lactation															
≤ 18 y	2,800	50	800	ND	1,800	ND	ND	30	80	800	ND	ND	ND	3.0	ND
19–50 y	3,000	50	1,000	ND	2,000	ND	ND	35	100	1,000	ND	ND	ND	3.5	ND

[a]UL=The maximum level of daily nutrient intake that is likely to pose no risk of adverse effects. Unless otherwise specified, the UL represents total intake from food, water, and supplements. Due to lack of suitable data, ULs could not be established for vitamin K, thiamin, riboflavin, vitamin B_{12}, pantothenic acid, biotin, or carotenoids. In the absence of ULs, extra caution may be warranted in consuming levels above recommended intakes.

[b]As preformed vitamin A only.

[c]As α-tocopherol; applies to any form of supplemental α-tocopherol.

[d]The ULs for vitamin E, niacin, and folate apply to synthetic forms obtained from supplements, fortified foods, or a combination of the two.

[e]β-Carotene supplements are advised only to serve as a provitamin A source for individuals at risk of vitamin A deficiency.

[f]ND=Not determinable due to lack of data of adverse effects in this age group and concern with regard to lack of ability to handle excess amounts. Source of intake should be from food only to prevent high levels of intake.

Source: Trumbo, P., Schlicker, S., and Poos, M. *Dietary Reference Intakes: vitamin A, vitamin K, arsenic, boron, chromium, copper, iodine, manganese, molybdenum, nickel, silicon, vanadium, and zinc.* J. Am. Diet. Assoc. 101:294–301, 2001.

Dietary Reference Intakes (DRIs): Tolerable Upper Intake Levels (UL[a]): Minerals

Life Stage Group	Arsenic[b]	Boron (mg/d)	Calcium (g/d)	Chromium	Copper (μg/d)	Fluoride (mg/d)	Iodine (μg/d)	Iron (mg/d)	Magnesium (mg/d)[c]	Manganese (mg/d)	Molybdenum (μg/d)	Nickel (mg/d)	Phosphorus (g/d)	Selenium (μg/d)	Silicon[d]	Vanadium (mg/d)[e]	Zinc (mg/d)
Infants																	
0–6 mo	ND[f]	ND	ND	ND	ND	0.7	ND	40	ND	ND	ND	ND	ND	45	ND	ND	4
7–12 mo	ND	ND	ND	ND	ND	0.9	ND	40	ND	ND	ND	ND	ND	60	ND	ND	5
Children																	
1–3 y	ND	3	2.5	ND	1,000	1.3	200	40	65	2	300	0.2	3	90	ND	ND	7
4–8 y	ND	6	2.5	ND	3,000	2.2	300	40	110	3	600	0.3	3	150	ND	ND	12
Males, Females																	
9–13 y	ND	11	2.5	ND	5,000	10	600	40	350	6	1,100	0.6	4	280	ND	ND	23
14–18 y	ND	17	2.5	ND	8,000	10	900	45	350	9	1,700	1.0	4	400	ND	ND	34
19–70 y	ND	20	2.5	ND	10,000	10	1,100	45	350	11	2,000	1.0	4	400	ND	1.8	40
> 70 y	ND	20	2.5	ND	10,000	10	1,100	45	350	11	2,000	1.0	3	400	ND	1.8	40
Pregnancy																	
≤ 18 y	ND	17	2.5	ND	8,000	10	900	45	350	9	1,700	1.0	3.5	400	ND	ND	34
19–50 y	ND	20	2.5	ND	10,000	10	1,100	45	350	11	2,000	1.0	3.5	400	ND	ND	40
Lactation																	
≤ 18 y	ND	17	2.5	ND	8,000	10	900	45	350	9	1,700	1.0	4	400	ND	ND	34
19–50 y	ND	20	2.5	ND	10,000	10	1,100	45	350	11	2,000	1.0	4	400	ND	ND	40

[a]UL=The maximum level of daily nutrient intake that is likely to pose no risk of adverse effects. Unless otherwise specified, the UL represents total intake from food, water, and supplements. Due to lack of suitable data, ULs could not be established for arsenic, chromium, and silicon. In the absence of ULs, extra caution may be warranted in consuming levels above recommended intakes.

[b]Although the UL was not determined for arsenic, there is no justification for adding arsenic to food or supplements.

[c]The ULs for magnesium represent intake from a pharmacological agent only and do not include intake from food and water.

[d]Although silicon has not been shown to cause adverse effects in humans, there is no justification for adding silicon to supplements.

[e]Although vanadium in food has not been shown to cause adverse effects in humans, there is no justification for adding vanadium to food and vanadium supplements should be used with caution. The UL is based on adverse effects in laboratory animals and these data could be used to set a UL for adults but not children and adolescents.

[f]ND=Not determinable due to lack of data of adverse effects in this age group and concern with regard to lack of ability to handle excess amounts. Source of intake should be from food only to prevent high levels of intake.

Source: Trumbo, P., Schlicker, S., and Poos, M. *Dietary Reference Intakes: vitamin A, vitamin K, arsenic, boron, chromium, copper, iodine, manganese, molybdenum, nickel, silicon, vanadium, and zinc.* J. Am. Diet. Assoc. 101:294–301, 2001.